Essential Herbs & Natural Supplements

Essential Herbs & Natural Supplements

Lesley Braun

PhD, BPharm, DipAppSciNat

Associate Professor of Integrative Medicine (Hon) National Institute of Complementary Medicine, University of Western Sydney, NSW
Senior Research Fellow (Hon), Monash/Alfred Psychiatric Research Centre, Melbourne, VIC, Australia

Marc Cohen

MBBS(Hons), PhD, BMedSc(Hons), FAMAC, FICAE

Professor of Health Sciences, School of Health Sciences, RMIT University, Melbourne, VIC, Australia

ELSEVIER

ELSEVIER

Elsevier Australia. ACN 001 002 357
(a division of Reed International Books Australia Pty Ltd)
Tower 1, 475 Victoria Avenue, Chatswood, NSW 2067

Notice

This publication has been carefully reviewed and checked to ensure that the content is as accurate and current as possible at time of publication. We would recommend, however, that the reader verify any procedures, treatments, drug dosages or legal content described in this book. Neither the author, the contributors, nor the publisher assume any liability for injury and/or damage to persons or property arising from any error in or omission from this publication.

National Library of Australia Cataloguing-in-Publication Data

Braun, Lesley, author.

Essential herbs and natural supplements / Lesley Braun, Marc Cohen.

9780729542685 (paperback)

Herbs—Therapeutic use—Textbooks.
Dietary supplements—Textbooks.
Alternative medicine—Textbooks.

Cohen, Marc, author.

Senior Content Strategist: Larissa Norrie
Content Development Specialist: Lauren Santos
Senior Project Manager: Rochelle Deighton
Proofread by Tim Learner
Design by Tania Gomes
Cover image: iStockphoto/desy_sevdanova
Typeset by Toppan Best-set Premedia Limited
Printed in China by 1010 Printing International Limited

CONTENTS

ABOUT THE AUTHORS

Lesley Braun, PhD, BPharm, DipAppSciNat

Associate Professor of Integrative Medicine (Hon) National Institute of Complementary Medicine, University of Western Sydney, NSW, Senior Research Fellow (Hon), Monash/Alfred Psychiatric Research Centre, Melbourne, VIC, Australia

Dr Lesley Braun is a registered pharmacist and naturopath. She holds a PhD from RMIT University, Melbourne, in which she investigated the integration of complementary medicine into hospitals in Victoria. Dr Braun is an Adjunct Associate Professor of Integrative Medicine at the National Institute of Complementary Medicine (NICM) at the University of Western Sydney. NICM provides leadership and support for strategically directed research into complementary medicine and translation of evidence into clinical practice and relevant policy to benefit the health of all Australians.

Dr Braun serves on the Australian Therapeutic Goods Advisory Council, which oversees the implementation of TGA reforms and provides general strategic guidance to the TGA, advice on relationships and communication with stakeholders. She is also on the executive for the Complementary and Integrative Therapies interest group of the Clinical Oncology Society of Australia and is an advisory board member to the Australasian Integrative Medicine Association. As of 2014, she is also Director of Blackmore's Institute, the academic and professional arm of Blackmores, which entails engaging with a broad range of academics, government and industry bodies and overseeing a comprehensive academic and research program.

Since 1996 Lesley has authored numerous chapters for books and more than 100 articles, and since 2000 has written regular columns for the *Australian Journal of Pharmacy* and *Journal of Complementary Medicine*. She lectures to medical students at Monash University and to chiropractic students at RMIT University, and is regularly invited to present at national and international conferences about evidence-based complementary medicine, drug interactions, complementary medicine safety and her own clinical research.

Her role as the main author of *Herbs and Natural Supplements: an evidence-based guide* represents a continuation of a life-long goal to integrate evidence-based complementary medicine into standard practice and improve patient outcomes safely and effectively.

Marc Cohen, MBBS(Hons), PhD, BMedSc(Hons), FAMAC, FICAE

Professor of Health Sciences, School of Health Sciences, RMIT University, Melbourne, VIC, Australia

Professor Marc Cohen is one of Australia's pioneers of integrative and holistic medicine who has made significant impacts on education, research, clinical practice and policy. He is a medical doctor and Professor of Health Sciences at RMIT University, where he leads postgraduate wellness programs and supervises research into wellness and holistic health, including research on yoga, meditation, nutrition, herbal medicine, acupuncture, lifestyle and the health impact of pesticides, organic food and detoxification. Professor Cohen sits on the board of a number of national and international associations, including the Australasian Integrative Medicine Association, the Global Spa and Wellness Summit and the Australasian Spa and Wellness Association, as well as serving on the editorial boards of several international peer-reviewed journals. Professor Cohen has published more than 80 peer-reviewed journal articles and co-edited *Understanding the Global Spa Industry*, along with more than 10 other books on holistic approaches to health. He is a frequent speaker at many national and international conferences where he delivers inspiring, informative and uplifting presentations. His impact on the field has been recognised by four consecutive RMIT Media Star Awards, as well as the inaugural Award for Leadership and Collaboration from the National Institute of Complementary Medicine.

CONTRIBUTORS

Ayesha Amos, GCertEvidCompMed, GCertHigherEd, AdvDipAppSci(Nat)
Program Manager Naturopathy, Southern School of Natural Therapies, Victoria, Australia
Monographs contributed: Black Cohosh; Valerian

Surinder K. Baines, APD, PhD, BSc(Hons), GDip(Diet), GDip(Nutr)
Associate Professor of Nutrition and Dietetics, Faculty of Health and Medicine, University of Newcastle, NSW, Australia
Monographs contributed: L-Glutamine; L-Lysine

Liesl Blott, BPharm, PGDip(MM), BHSc(WHerbalMed), AdvDip(Nat)
School of Pharmacy, Curtin University, Perth, Australia
Monographs contributed: Andrographis; Calcium; Iodine; Iron; New Zealand green-lipped mussel

Helene de la Follye de Jeux, BNatr
Monographs contributed: Alpha lipoic acid; Chromium

Elizabeth Hammer, BHSc(CompMed/Nurs), AdvDipWHM, CertIVWTA(TAE)
Western Herbalist/ RN, Vice President National Herbalists Association of Australia, Tasmania, Australia
Monographs contributed: Garlic

Jason Hawrelak, PhD, BNat(Hons), DipN
Senior Lecturer, Course Coordinator, Graduate Certificate in Evidence-based Complementary Medicine, School of Medicine, University of Tasmania, Australia
Adjunct Lecturer, Master of Science in Human Nutrition and Functional Medicine program, University of Western States, Oregon, USA, Naturopathic practitioner, Goulds Naturopathica, Tasmania, Australia
Monographs contributed: Prebiotics; Probiotics

Leah Hechtman, PhD(candidate), MSciMed(RHHG), BHSc(Nat), DipN
Director and Clinician, The Natural Health and Fertility Centre
PhD Candidate — University of Sydney, Department of Obstetrics, Gynaecology and Neonatology, Faculty of Medicine, President, National Herbalists Association of Australia, NSW, Australia
Chapter updated: Chapter 5 Herbs and natural supplements in pregnancy
Monograph contributed: Vitamin C

Rebecca Hughes, BNatr
Naturopathic practitioner at ReMed and The Well Room, Victoria, Member of National Herbalists Association of Australia, Victoria, Australia
Monographs contributed: Astragalus; Siberian ginseng

Kate Levett, BEd(Hons), AdvDipAppSci(Acup), GradCertJapAcup, MPH(Merit), PhD
University of Notre Dame, School of Medicine, NSW, Australia
Monographs: Vitamin D

Amelia June McFarland, MPharm(Hons), BPharmSci
Registered Pharmacist, Clinical Tutor, School of Pharmacy, Griffith University, Queensland, Australia
Monographs contributed: Folate; Lutein; Selenium; Vitamin B_{12}

Teresa Mitchell-Paterson, AdvDipNatr, BHSc(CompMed), MHSc(HumNutr), DipCompMedSci
Senior Lecturer, Bachelor of Health Science Naturopathy, Nutrition and Western Herbal Medicine, Australasian College of Natural Therapies, Sydney, NSW, Australia
Integrative Natural Therapies Practitioner, Sydney Integrative Medicine, Sydney, Australia
Health and Medical Panellist, The Memorial Winston Churchill Trust Fund, Nutritional Advisor Bowel Cancer Australia
Monographs contributed: Magnesium; Vitamin E

Miranda Myles, MAppSc(Acu), BHSc(Nat), BA(Psych), CertNatFert, CertClinIntern, CertEsotAcu, CertIVTrain
Educator and Contract Lecturer at Southern School Natural Therapies and Endeavour College of Natural Health
Guest Lecturer at RMIT, Bundoora and La Trobe University, Bendigo, Victoria, Australia
Monographs contributed: Vitamin B_1; Vitamin B_2; Vitamin B_5; Vitamin B_6

Ses Salmond, PhD, BA, DipN, DipBotMed, DipHom, DipNutr
Herbalist/Naturopath, Leichhardt Women's Community Health Centre, Sydney Local Health District and Liverpool Women's Health Centre, South Western Local Health District, Private Practitioner, NSW, Australia
Monographs contributed: St Mary's thistle

Ondine Spitzer, MSocH, BHSci, BA, DipAppSciNat
Monographs contributed: Passionflower

Quilla Watt, BNat(Hons)
Monographs contributed: Schisandra; Slippery elm

Tanya Wells, BSc(Hons), BHSci(Nat), GCertHealthProfEd
Integrative Medicine Naturopath, Lecturer Synergy Health — Consulting, Seminars and Training — Drug–Herb/Nutrient Interaction Seminars for Medical and Nursing Practitioners, Victoria, Australia
Monographs contributed: Devil's claw; Ginger; SAMe

REVIEWERS

Robyn Carruthers, PGDip(HSc), BEd, DipTeach, BHSci(CompMed), AdvDipNat, AdvDipHerbMed
Deputy Director, Clinical and Research South Pacific College of Natural Medicine

Sandy Davidson, MPH, DipNat, AdvDipNat, DipNutr
Associate Program Leader — Nutritional Medicine, Endeavour College of Natural Health

Lauren Frail, Critical Care RN
Nurse Educator, Melbourne IVF, East Melbourne, Victoria, Australia

Chandrika Gibson, DipNat, MWell
Naturopathic practitioner, yoga therapist and project officer at Cancer Council WA, Australia
Former lecturer and clinical supervisor at Endeavour College of Natural Health and Paramount College of Natural Medicine, Perth, WA, Australia

Mara Goodridge, BHSc(Nat), ND, AdvDipAppSci(Nut), AdvDipHom, AdvDipWHM
Lecturer, Australasian College of Natural Therapies (ACNT), Think Education, NSW, Australia

Myfanwy Graham, MPharm
Associate Lecturer, School of Biomedical Sciences and Pharmacy, Faculty of Health and Medicine, University of Newcastle, NSW, Australia

Margot Jensen, AdvDipNat, BHSc(CompMed), BA/LLB
Population Health Coordinator, Canberra Institute of Technology, ACT, Australia

Elizabeth MacGregor, MEd(HighEd), BHSc(Nat)
Naturopathic Practitioner, Senior Lecturer of Naturopathic Medicine, Endeavour College, Perth, WA, Australia

Amanda Richardson, AdvDipNat, AdvDipWHM
Lecturer, Australasian College of Natural Therapies, Pyrmont, NSW, Australia

Kylie Seaton, BHSc(Nat), BA(Jour), PGDipComm, AdvDipNat, AdvDipHomeop, AdvDipWHM, DipNutr/Cert Iridology, Primary modules NutrEnvMed (ACNEM), IntegHeal(Kines), CertIV(TAE)
Owner, Kylie Seaton Naturopath Homeopath

Caroline van der Mey, BHSc(CompMed), PGDip(Phyto), AdvDipNat, DipHomeop
Private practitioner, Naturopathy, WA, Australia

Karen Wallace, BHSc(Nat), BBus (HAdm)
Naturopathic Practitioner, Lecturer, Endeavour College of Natural Health, Perth, WA, Australia

PREFACE

Welcome to the first edition of *Essential Herbs and Natural Supplements*.

Due to an increase in the evidence base over recent years we now have far more information available in the peer-reviewed literature about key active components in herbal medicines, pharmacological activity in vivo and clinical trials. In particular, the complexity of herbal medicines has become more evident as nearly all have multiple mechanisms of action and we have well and truly moved beyond using solely traditional evidence to guide their use. Overall reporting in herbal medicine studies is improving and where possible, we state the extract used, dose and administration form to help guide you in your practice.

Probably the biggest growth area has been in nutritional science and research. In this edition, the fish oil, vitamin D and probiotic monographs in particular have expanded significantly. They are among the most popular supplements bought in retail stores today. Fish oils are being intensively investigated for health conditions beyond cardiovascular disease, and there is work being done in mental health, neurological diseases, neonates and children and even cancer. Vitamin D is also being investigated for conditions unrelated to the musculoskeletal system, and population studies are indicating low vitamin D status is rife. Probiotics has been another areas to explode with new information about potential effects beyond the gastrointestinal tract. The effect of the microbiome on multiple diseases is only starting to be understood and the role of pre- and probiotics in influencing it is slowly being uncovered. In contrast, there have been relatively fewer studies published on vitamins E and C than in the past.

Our team of contributors have systematically searched the main medical databases, using primary literature where possible, to capture, collate and synthesise the best and most relevant information for busy clinicians. We used Medline, Science Direct and the Cochrane database as a starting point to identify articles published since our last edition. This means having access to over 24 million peer-reviewed articles. Despite our best efforts, no doubt we will have missed something. This is due to the intense research activity underway and almost weekly publication of new information making it extremely difficult to keep up.

In this book, we report on positive, negative and inconclusive results and try to put forward theories as to why results are inconsistent. Most adults in Western countries are using over-the-counter herbal and nutritional supplements, and informed advice from their healthcare practitioner is important and expected. I hope that this book will help expand your practice by unlocking the potential of natural medicines and safely guide your patients or clients to use them appropriately.

CHAPTER 1

INTRODUCTION TO HERBAL MEDICINE

Herbal medicine, also known as phytomedicine, can be broadly defined as both the science and the art of using botanical medicines to prevent and treat illness, and the study and investigation of these medicines. The term 'phytotherapy' is used to describe the therapeutic application of herbal medicines and was first coined by the French physician Henri Leclerc (1870–1955), who published numerous essays on the use of medicinal plants (Weiss 1988).

Phytotherapy can be considered one of the oldest forms of medicine. Since the dawn of time, plants have been used by people of all races, religions and cultures to sustain life and alter the course of disease. Over this time, the medicinal use of plants has evolved along two parallel paths, with the comparatively recent evolution of modern medicine. One path involves the accumulation of empirical knowledge over centuries. Gathered through careful observation of nature and disease, and from cumulative experiences of informed trial and error, the empirical knowledge base for herbal medicines is large and diverse. For example, the *Rig veda*, a text from India, and the Egyptian papyri *Antiquarium* both date from 3000 BC and contain extensive lists of medicinal plants used to treat illness (Berman et al 1999). In South America, the use of herbal medicine has also been documented, such as in the *Badianus* manuscript, a text written by the Aztecs (Walcott 1940). Their use of herbs, such as datura and passionflower, has been adopted in modern European and American pharmacopoeias. Native Americans were particularly knowledgeable about the botanical medicines in their environment. It has been estimated that more than 200 medicines used by one or more Indian nations have been incorporated into the US Pharmacopoeia or National Formulary (Vogel 1970).

Two of the most prominent historical figures in European herbal medicine were Dioscorides and Galen, who were physicians in ancient Greece.

Dioscorides was a Greek army surgeon in the service of the Roman emperor Nero (54–68 AD). He is best known for his *De materia medica*, which describes more than 600 herbs and their uses. Today this work is considered to be the first book ever written about medical botany as an applied science. Galen (131–201 AD) not only wrote several dozen books on pharmacy, but also developed an elaborate system of herbal polypharmacy in which herbal combinations were devised to produce more specific results. The modern term 'galenicals' is still used to describe herbal simples.

Alongside the 'empirical knowledge' approach a second path developed, which involved a more theoretical and formalised method of diagnosis and treatment. The resulting 'healthcare' systems were complex and often used herbal medicines as an important part of a more comprehensive approach to treatment that also included dietary control, lifestyle changes and spiritual practice. This approach reached its peak in the East with traditional Chinese medicine and Ayurvedic medicine in India.

Although contemporary clinical practice of herbal medicine still relies heavily on traditional wisdom, this knowledge is now being re-examined with the aid of modern analytical methods and scientific methodology. The use of science to establish an evidence base in modern healthcare is changing the way herbalism is being practised and who is using herbs. An emphasis on phytochemistry and an assessment of risk are inherent features of contemporary research into herbs. While these are important gains in knowledge about the actions and uses of herbs, there is an accompanying shift in the practice of herbal medicine, with less emphasis on the importance of traditional and empirical knowledge, which in time may lead to a loss of the paradigm of holistic and individualised care (Evans 2008). Whether this improves patient outcomes remains to be seen.

HERBS, DRUGS AND PHYTOCHEMICALS

Most pharmaceutical medicines contain a single, highly purified, often artificially produced substance that has a well-known (and occasionally specifically designed) chemical structure that can be patented and owned by the company that developed it. The dosage of these chemicals can also be precisely calculated down to the microgram and can usually be characterised by a very clear pharmacokinetic profile. Additionally, pharmaceutical drugs tend to have a generally agreed upon mechanism of action and series of indications that guide their use within the Western medical model.

As most of these drugs do not exist in nature, they must go through extensive testing to ensure efficacy and safety. New drugs are assessed in test-tube and animal studies for their potential to cause cancer, fetal malformations and other toxic effects, and are ultimately tested on humans to further define the safety profile, pharmacokinetics and drug effectiveness in a targeted disease (Wierenga & Eaton 2003). This process is very costly and requires the application of highly specialised knowledge and infrastructure, as well as many years of concentrated effort. It is estimated that the development of a new drug requires the investment of approximately US$800 million, but it is also extremely lucrative (Di Masi & Grabowski 2003).

PHARMACOGNOSY

In 2001 and 2002, approximately one-quarter of the best-selling drugs worldwide were natural products or derived from natural products. Research on natural products further accounted for approximately 48% of the new chemical entities reported from 1981 to 2002.

Modern drug discovery from medicinal plants has evolved to become a sophisticated process that includes numerous fields of enquiry and various methods of analysis. Typically, the process begins with a botanist, ethnobotanist, ethnopharmacologist or plant ecologist collecting and identifying plants based on the biological activity suggested by their traditional use. Additionally, plants are randomly selected for inclusion in screening programs based on molecular targets identified through the human genome project (Balunas & Kinghorn 2005).

Pharmacognosy is the term used to refer to the study of botanical supplements and herbal remedies, as well as to the search for single-compound drugs from plants. Increasingly, pharmaceutical medicines and preclinical research into herbal medicines are focused on identifying suitable chemical entities that may form the basis for novel treatments (Balunas & Kinghorn 2005).

CHEMICAL COMPLEXITY

In contrast to pharmaceutical drugs, which are based on single molecules that may or may not be derived from natural substances, herbal medicines are chemically complex and may contain many hundreds or even thousands of different 'phytochemicals', including various macro- and micro-nutrients such as fats, carbohydrates and proteins, enzymes, vitamins and minerals. A group of important secondary metabolites are also present, which are generally chemicals used to defend against herbivores, pathogens, insect attack and microbial decomposition, or which are produced in response to injury or infection, or used for signalling and growth regulation. It is these compounds, such as tannins, isoflavones, saponins, flavonoids, glycosides, coumarins, bitters, phyto-oestrogens etc, that are often responsible for the therapeutic properties of herbal medicines (Mills & Bone 2001).

As the secondary metabolites largely dictate a herb's pharmacological nature, a knowledge of herbal chemistry is essential to understand a herb's use and provide valuable insight into its clinical effects. It is sometimes tempting to take the modern reductionist approach and predict the pharmacological activity of a herbal medicine from an understanding of the effects of one key constituent or chemical group; however, this is unlikely to be entirely accurate. In practice, the overall pharmacological activity and safety of each herb is the result of the interaction of numerous constituents, some of which have demonstrated pharmacological effects, rather than the effect of a single active ingredient.

An example of this is the herb *Paullinia cupana*, commonly known as guarana. As there are limited clinical studies on guarana, it is often reported that the herb owes its pharmacological activity to one key constituent, caffeine, which may be present in concentrations as high as 10%. Studies referring to the isolate caffeine provide some clues about the effects of guarana, but are not entirely accurate, as other important constituents are also present in the remaining 90%. This has been borne out recently in clinical studies of low-caffeine-containing guarana preparations, which still demonstrated significant effects on cognitive function.

Because of the range of phytochemicals present in plants, herbal medicines often include many different active substances with different pharmacokinetics that work at different sites with different mechanisms of action. Herbal medicines therefore potentially have multiple pharmacological actions and many different clinical indications. Furthermore, in addition to the active ingredients, herbs may also contain substances that act to inhibit or promote the active properties, and/or potential unwanted side effects of the active agents. Thus, although specific components may not be active themselves, they may influence the activity of other components by altering their solubility, absorption, distribution or half-life.

For instance, berberine is a constituent of herbs such as goldenseal and barberry and exhibits numerous activities in vitro; however, in vivo, it has poor bioavailability (Pan et al 2002). Berberine has been shown to upregulate the expression and function of the drug transporter P-glycoprotein (P-gp) (Lin et al 1999), thereby reducing the absorption of P-gp substrates. Studies with the P-gp inhibitor cyclosporin have shown that it increases berberine absorption six-fold, as it counteracts the inducing effect of berberine (Pan et al 2002). P-gp inhibitors are also found in nature, such as the virtually ubiquitous quercetin, and when they are present in the same herb competing effects on P-gp expression and function will occur.

The herb St John's wort provides yet another example. The extraction method used in Germany in the product's commercial manufacture was modified in the late 1990s, resulting in higher concentrations of hyperforin than previously obtained (Madabushi et al 2006). Since then, numerous reports and studies have identified pharmacokinetic drug interactions with St John's wort, based on its ability to induce cytochromes and P-gp. It is now well established that hyperforin is the key constituent responsible for these unwanted effects, and St John's wort preparations manufactured with this newer extraction method, such as LI 160, can put people at risk of interactions. Meanwhile, studies with low-hyperforin preparations, such as Ze117, have found that it fails to induce the same interactions

(Madabushi et al 2006). Unfortunately, this distinction between St John's wort preparations is not well known, and many references and texts fail to mention this important point.

As these examples and many others in this book demonstrate, each herb is chemically complex and produces a pharmacological effect based on the total sum of actions produced by a myriad of constituents that may be acting in synergy. This complexity complicates the ability to test herbal medicines as they are most commonly used (that is, in their more natural states) and in combination with other herbal medicines.

SYNERGISTIC INTERACTIONS

The concept of synergistic interactions is another fundamental difference between herbs and drugs and explains how a single herb may have a number of seemingly unrelated mechanisms of actions and be indicated for a variety of conditions. Intra-herbal interactions between active and apparently non-active constituents also mean that tests performed with single, isolated constituents will not accurately represent the actions and safety of the entire herbal medicine. As such, these tests provide limited information. By and large, it is suspected that it is the intra-herbal interactions that give herbs a broad therapeutic range and very good tolerability.

St John's wort, popularised as a useful treatment for depression, is also an excellent example of intra-herbal interaction. It contains many different constituents, such as hypericin and pseudohypericin, flavonoids such as quercetin and rutin, vitamins C and A, phenolics such as hyperforin, sterols and an essential oil. Although many of the herb's pharmacological activities appear to be attributable to hypericin and hyperforin, it is now known that the flavonoid content also contributes to its antidepressant activity. In other words, the antidepressant effects identified for isolated hypericin or hyperforin are greater when the whole herb is used.

In practice, synergistic interactions are used in another important way — herbal polypharmacy. This is the combining of different herbal medicines within the same treatment for a more specific outcome, and is similar to the method Galen described centuries ago. In Chinese medicine the concept of synergistic interactions has reached a great level of sophistication, with Chinese formulas containing as many as 20 different herbs. In that system, the herb possessing the primary action of the formula is considered the 'emperor herb', while 'minister herbs' support the primary action and 'assistant herbs' modify the formula according to the needs of the individual. Finally 'messenger herbs' are used to aid absorption or reduce side effects of the formula. The practice is also common in Ayurvedic medicine and, in fact, in all traditional systems of herbal practice. Although it may be common in conventional medicine to give certain drugs specifically to reduce the side effects of other drugs, such as the administration of antiemetics and laxatives together with opiates, generally the giving of multiple drugs in combination is discouraged. In contrast, in herbal medicine this practice is often considered essential to provide both safety and the best effects.

KEY CONSTITUENT GROUPS

To better understand a herb's mechanisms of action, pharmacokinetics, pharmacodynamics, interactions and side effects, a basic knowledge of the key constituent groups is helpful. Here is a brief outline of the main constituent groups found in popular herbal medicines.

FLAVONOIDS

Flavonoids are plant pigments that are largely responsible for the colour of flowers, fruits and berries. There are many different types of flavonoids, including flavones, flavonols, isoflavones and flavins. They are generally anti-inflammatory, antioxidant and anti-allergic, and may decrease capillary fragility. Herbs that are well known for their flavonoid content are ginkgo (*Ginkgo biloba*), St Mary's thistle (*Silybum marianum*) and calendula (*Calendula officinale*).

Flavanols may be further oxidised to yield anthrocyanins. These bluish/purplish compounds contribute to the colour of blueberries and red grapes. They are greatly revered for their antioxidant and anti-inflammatory properties.

TANNINS

Tannins are astringent and often taste bitter. They can be divided into two groups, hydrolysable tannins and non-hydrolysable tannins (sometimes called condensed tannins or proanthocyanidins). Tannins have the ability to stabilise proteins and were used historically to tan or preserve animal hides. In herbal medicine, tannins are valued for their ability to dry and tone tissue. Some plants with appreciable levels of tannins include witch hazel (*Hamamelis virginiana*), oak bark (*Quercus robor*) and lady's mantle (*Alchemilla vulgaris*).

COUMARINS

Coumarins have a limited distribution in plants and may be either naturally present or synthesised by the plant in response to a bacteria or fungus (Heinrich et al 2004). They are a heterogeneous group, and thus different compounds have various effects on the body. For example, some coumarins demonstrate antispasmodic activity (for example, scopeletin from *Viburnum* spp), others anticoagulant activity (for example dicoumarol from sweet clover), and others anti-oedema effects (for example, coumarins from clivers and red clover).

ALKALOIDS

Alkaloids are so named for their alkaline properties. This group of phytochemicals has contributed much to modern medicine, and more than

10,000 have been isolated (Evans 2002). Consequently, they are perhaps the best-known constituent group. There are many different types of alkaloids with many different therapeutic properties; however, they commonly contain nitrogen, usually in a heterocyclic ring. Below is a brief outline of the main subgroups:

- **Pyridine, piperidine & pyrrolizidine alkaloids.** Nicotine (*Nicotiana tabacum*) is perhaps the best-known example of the pyridine class. The very poisonous piperidine alkaloid coniine is isolated from hemlock (*Conium maculatum*) and the pyrrolizidine alkaloid senecionine is the reason comfrey (*Symphytum officinale*) was withdrawn from sale in Australia due to concerns over hepatotoxicity.
- **Phenylalkylamine alkaloids.** This group of alkaloids differ in that nitrogen is not part of the heterocyclic ring. The most commonly known example is ephedrine, a central nervous system stimulant, bronchodilator and vasoconstrictive agent from *Ephedra sinica*.
- **Quinoline alkaloids.** The antimalarial quinine from *Cinchona* spp belongs in this category. Quinine was used in the synthetic production of many antimalarial drugs against *Plasmodium falciparum*. Interestingly, *Plasmodium* has become resistant to the synthesised medications such as chloroquinine, but not to naturally occurring quinine (Heinrich et al 2004).
- **Isoquinoline alkaloids.** Opium, from *Papaver somniferum*, contains over 30 alkaloids, including morphine, codeine, thebaine, papaverine and noscapine. Morphine is well known for its pain-relieving effects. Other examples are the protoberberines, consisting of berberine, berbamine and hydrastine. Golden seal (*Hydrastis canadensis*) contains berberine and hydrastine; barberry (*Berberis vulgaris*) contains berberine and berbamine; and oregon mountain grape (*Mahonia aquifolium*) contains all three. They are strongly antibacterial.
- **Indole alkaloids.** Examples include reserpine from *Rauwolfia serpentina*, which in the past has been used for hypertension; however, its use has largely been discontinued due to toxic side effects. The anticancer agents vincristine and vinblastine, from *Cantharanthus roseus*, are other notable examples.
- **Tropane alkaloids.** Hyoscyamine, from *Atropa belladonna*, is an anticholinergic agent. It has also been used to dilate the pupil of the eye for optical examinations.
- **Xanthine alkaloids.** These are the most widely known and used alkaloids, and include caffeine from tea (*Camellia sinensis*), coffee (*Coffea arabica*) and chocolate (*Theobroma cacao*), which is known to be beneficial to health in small amounts and detrimental in large amounts. Cocoa also contains theobromine and tea contains theophylline and theobromine, both of which are purine alkaloids.

TERPENES

Terpenes are widespread in the plant kingdom. There are many different types:

- **Monoterpene hydrocarbons.** Monoterpenes have a 10-carbon structure. They are major constituents of volatile oils and often have antimicrobial properties. Examples include limonene (lemon, caraway, peppermint and thyme) and alpha-pinene (rosemary, lemon, fennel and eucalyptus).
- **Sesquiterpene hydrocarbons.** Sesquiterpenes have a 15-carbon structure. They are also major constituents of volatile oils and are broadly antimicrobial and insecticidal. Subclasses include alcohols (linalool from lavender, menthol from peppermint), phenols (linalool from lavender), phenols (thymol from thyme, carvacrol from oregano), aldehydes (citronella from citronella), ketones (menthone from peppermint, thujone from wormwood), ethers (anethole from fennel) and esters (methyl salicylate from wintergreen).
- **Diterpene hydrocarbons.** Diterpenes have on average a 20-carbon structure and so are much denser molecules, with higher boiling points, than other hydrocarbons. They are often associated with volatile oils (oleoresins), gums (gum-resins) or with both (oleo-gum-resins) (Evans 2002). Examples include guaiacum resin obtained from *Guaiacum officinale* and gum-resins from frankincense (*Boswellia serrata*).

GLYCOSIDES

Glycosides are composed of two parts: the glycone (sugar molecule) and the aglycone (non-sugar molecule). The aglycone may be a terpene, a flavonoid or potentially any other natural compound (Heinrich et al 2004). Below are the most common classes:

- **Triterpene glycosides.** These may also be called saponins. They are a diverse group and exert many different effects on the human body. Depending on their structure, they may be anti-inflammatory (aescin from horse chestnut) or expectorant (senegin from snakeroot), or may demonstrate steroidal effects (glycyrrhetic acid from licorice, diosgenin from wild yam).
- **Glucosinolates.** Also called mustard oil glycosides, these important compounds are found in the Brassicaceae family of vegetables, such as broccoli, mustard and horseradish. They are topically mildly irritant and have digestive, circulatory and anticancer properties when ingested.
- **Cardiac glycosides.** These glycosides have a specific action on heart muscle. They are steroidal in structure and are related to steroidal saponins and phytosterols. A number of herbs contain cardioactive glycosides, including lily of the valley (*Convallaria majus*) and foxglove (*Digitalis* spp). Digoxin and digitoxin are naturally occurring compounds in digitalis, and digoxin is commonly used in drug form for heart failure.

- **Anthraquinone glycosides.** These compounds have osmotic and stimulant effects in the lower bowel and therefore have laxative properties. Examples of herbs that contain these compounds include cascara (*Rhamnus purshiana*), senna (*Cassia senna*), aloe (*Aloe vera*) and rhubarb root (*Rheum palmatum*).

CLINICAL NOTE — GERMAN COMMISSION E

The German Commission E is a German government regulatory agency composed of scientists, pharmacists, toxicologists, physicians and herbalists. It has produced a series of monographs based on the available scientific evidence, as well as evidence from traditional use, case studies and the experience of modern herbalists. These monographs are considered to provide authoritative information on herbs, as well as approved indications, contraindications, side effects, interactions, doses, and so on.

CHEMOTHERAPEUTICS VERSUS HERBALISM

In practice, drugs and herbs are prescribed quite differently. Drug prescription is often based on the results obtained from clinical trials that measure the effects in populations and use averages to predict outcomes. Investigation and usage is based on the Western medical model and is replicated in almost identical ways by each practitioner who uses this system. By contrast, the same herb may be understood and prescribed in distinctly different ways by different practitioners, depending on the prescribing system being used, with an emphasis on individual prescribing. For example, in Chinese medicine, a herb such as andrographis (*Andrographis paniculata*) is used to clear 'heat' from the blood, because it is considered to be a 'cold' herb, whereas in Western herbalism, it is used to boost immune function and treat the common cold. Further, traditional herbal practice entails combining a number of herbs into a prescription that is tailored to the individual. This customised approach to herbal prescribing is guided by the underpinning paradigm of herbal practice — holism and vitalism. This philosophical basis is lost when herbs are viewed as vehicles for one or two active components or with the increasing cultural emphasis on self-prescribing.

Not only are herbs described and prescribed differently by different medical systems, the properties of herbal medicines are often defined using unique terms not found in drug pharmacology. These properties have traditionally been classified into herbal actions. Thus herbs that relax the gastrointestinal tract and reduce flatulence may be described as carminatives, or those that stimulate bile flow as cholagogues. These actions may be due to particular chemical constituent groups found within the herb or some other property of the herb. Throughout this book, terms specific to herbal medicine and not generally used in drug pharmacology are explained in *Clinical notes*.

In contrast to pharmaceutical medicine, the evidence available to support herbal medicines originally comes from traditional sources, and scientific investigation has only recently been added. Over the past two to three decades there has been an exponential increase in the amount of scientific research being conducted on herbal medicines, chiefly in Europe and Asia, where there are fewer political, economic and regulatory reasons for rejecting traditional medicines. For some herbs there is now sufficient clinical trial evidence to enable meta-analyses to be performed. For many of the popular herbs available over the counter, clinical trial evidence is now being published that can be used to further clarify and determine their place in practice. For others, research may still be in its infancy, with only in vitro testing or testing in experimental models having been conducted so far. Although a general lack of resources, infrastructure, government funding and financial incentive for companies to invest in non-patentable medicines has slowed down investigation, great public popularity continues to fuel further study. Despite the limitations of randomised controlled trials in evaluating complex interventions characterised by traditional herbal practice (Evans 2008), data collections such as the German Commission E monographs are widely cited as gold-standard references, because they use a combination of traditional and scientific evidence to interpret data and make recommendations.

PRODUCT VARIATION AND STANDARDISATION

The chemical complexity of herbal medicines is compounded by the variation that occurs in their production, which starts with the quality of the original plant material. This may be influenced by the identification methods used (and any misidentification or contamination), genetic variability in the original cultivar and the growing conditions, including the soil type, geographical location, aspect, altitude and climate. Other factors further modify a herb's purity and quality, such as growing techniques (for example, wild harvesting, or organic or conventional farming methods), the timing and method of harvesting, drying, processing and storage, as well as the extraction techniques and solvents used. There are therefore numerous factors that determine the compositional profile of a given herbal extract, and attempts to ensure batch-to-batch consistency are confounded by the inherent chemical complexity of the herb and the natural variations that occur.

As a consequence, clinical research is never simply done on a herb itself. Rather, research must be done on a particular herbal preparation at a specific dose, and the evidence for the efficacy of herbal preparations must be related back to the preparation used in the research. The results of clinical trials are therefore only relevant to the specific herbal preparation that has been tested, at the specific dosage, dose form and route of administration used in the actual trial and cannot necessarily be used to support the use of other extracts or doses of the same herb. The challenge for manufacturers and clinicians, then, is to reproduce a particular preparation, administer it in the proven doses and achieve the expected result. More commonly in practice, herbs are used in variable ways, with different preparations, at a range of doses, and in combination with other herbs or treatments. It is thus hard to guarantee outcomes, either beneficial or adverse, based solely on controlled clinical trials.

STANDARDISATION

Efforts to ensure batch-to-batch reproducibility of herbal medicines have generated a great deal of controversy, particularly involving the term 'standardisation' or the production of so-called standardised extracts. The lack of an agreed definition and the variety of meanings attributed to these terms make them confusing to both consumers and health professionals. Yet they are still used as the basis for product labelling and promotion, where they are used by suppliers for marketing purposes to imply quality, safety or efficacy.

A commonly used (and some may say abused) definition of the term 'standardised' in relation to herbal extracts relies on measuring a specified concentration of an identified constituent or class of constituents known as 'markers'. Markers are usually stable components of a herb that can easily be identified, analysed and measured, but they may or may not be pharmacologically active. An example of this is seen with *Ginkgo biloba*, which is standardised to contain 24% flavonoid glycosides and 6% terpenoids in commercial herbal products, although the active constituents are largely unknown. Sophisticated laboratory techniques are now used to perform this analysis and measurement. Methods include chromatographic techniques, such as thin layer chromatography and high-performance liquid chromatography, both of which provide a visual characterisation of the presence of different chemical constituents, including 'marker' substances in the herb. The graphs produced from chromatographic testing are referred to as 'fingerprints' and are commonly used to determine the identity of herbal material and the integrity of the extraction process, as well as to measure quantities of individual constituents.

LIMITATIONS

Although it is generally accepted that herbal standardisation is a useful procedure, it does raise many problems and concerns. First, standardisation to non-active constituents does not necessarily reflect potency. Second, the more perplexing issue of identifying the exact active constituents in a herb is still the subject of much debate for many herbs. Lastly, individual chemical isolates do not fit the accepted definition of a herb, so if the concentration of an isolate is significantly altered for standardisation purposes, the final product may not be truly representative of the original herbal medicine and may even be considered to be 'adulterated' if marker substances are added. Furthermore, despite recent attempts to standardise herbal extracts, there are still no official standards, and herbal products can vary widely with regard to their quality and clinical effectiveness (American Herbal Products Association 2003).

Although conventional pharmaceutical thinking is based on milligrams of an active substance, such an approach is not appropriate for herbal medicines, which have many biologically active, often unmeasurable constituents. Because there can be hundreds of constituents in a complex herbal extract, standardisation is not possible by merely ensuring that one or two marker constituents are present in the same quantities from batch to batch. The therapeutic actions of herbal medicines rely on the complex combination and interactions of chemicals in the extract rather than on single constituents, and two total extracts can have very different profiles, despite there being a consistent level of one or two marker substances.

The biological activity of any compound, even a marker compound with demonstrated bioactivity, depends on the composition of the rest of the extract. Other components of the extract, even those with no direct physiological effect, may influence the uptake, distribution, metabolism and excretion of other components. Furthermore, this background matrix may affect the solubility, stability and bioavailability of any given compound (Eisner 2001). Thus the presence of chemical markers alone cannot be used to translate clinical evidence from one extract to another.

True standardisation requires more elegant procedures. The American Herbal Products Association has the following definition: 'Standardization refers to the body of information and controls that ensure product consistency from one batch to the next. This is achieved through minimising the inherent variation of natural product composition through quality assurance practices applied to agricultural and manufacturing processes' (American Herbal Products Association 2003). This definition accords more closely with the approach taken in Europe, where process control is an integral component of standardising herbal medicines. The methodology involves proceeding with the aim of standardising all the inputs and processes involved in making a particular extract, in order to ensure batch-to-batch consistency — from the genetic identity of the seed or plant, through to the agricultural processes employed and climatic factors (temperature, rainfall, sunlight), and finishing with drying, processing, extraction, solvent (or solvents), concentration, manufacture, storage, formulation and packaging of the finished product.

In addition to standardising the amount of certain chemical constituents in a herbal preparation, it is also necessary to have a means of standardising doses. Not only can different batches of the same herb have quite different potencies, there are many different formulations. Commercially available herbal preparations include fresh and dried herbs, teas, tinctures, fluid extracts, tablets, capsules and powders, as well as essential oils. When translating doses between different formulations, the amount of dried herb used to produce a set amount of the particular product is often used to give an indication of dosage strength. However, this may not give an accurate indication of potency; for example, fresh grapes, sultanas, grape juice, wine and sherry may all contain the same equivalent dry weight of grapes, but yield very different products with different biological properties.

Because of the lack of formalised standards and the need to prove 'phytoequivalence' for scientific rigour, it is increasingly common for clinical trials to specify the exact dose and extract used and for this information to be used as a basis for government regulation and for marketing purposes. When standardised extracts have been used in clinical trials, this information is included in each monograph.

HERBAL SAFETY

As with all medicines, a risk–benefit profile should be considered before using any herbal medicine. The vast majority of herbal medicines are generally considered to be safe, whether commercially or domestically produced. Most have a wide therapeutic index and only a few have toxic potential. However, adverse reactions may arise from a number of factors and may or may not be predictable. These include inappropriate usage (for example, dose, indication, time frame, administration route) and idiosyncratic reactions such as allergic responses and anaphylaxis.

In addition to adverse reactions arising from the properties of the herb itself, it is also possible for adverse events to arise from contamination or adulteration of herbal products. Contamination occurs when additional substances are inadvertently included in a herbal product. Contaminants can include toxic substances such as heavy metals, pesticide residues and microorganisms, as well as plant material from species other than the intended species, arising from either misidentification or poor quality control. Adulteration, on the other hand, is the intentional inclusion of foreign substances in herbal products, such as pharmaceutical steroids, NSAIDs or synthetic hormones, and may have very serious consequences. The standard of manufacture of commercial herbal products in Australia is generally very high.

REPRESENTING WESTERN HERBALISTS IN AUSTRALIA

In Australia, the knowledge and practice of contemporary herbal medicine has been preserved and nurtured mainly by Western herbalists. In fact, the National Herbalists Association of Australia (NHAA) has represented medical herbalists since 1920. Today, many industry insiders consider NHAA to be the industry standard setter for education in medical herbalism. Clinicians are encouraged to check whether herbal practitioners to whom they refer have undergone accredited courses. Further information can be found by contacting the association or accessing the website www.nhaa.org.au.

INTERACTIONS WITH PHARMACEUTICAL DRUGS

One safety issue that has become more recognised over the past decade is the potential for herbs to interact with pharmaceutical drugs. Evidence has emerged to suggest that some herb–drug interactions may be detrimental and have the potential to cause dangerous outcomes, whereas others may be beneficial when an interaction is manipulated to produce positive results (see Chapters 3 and 4).

The popularity of herbal medicine, and the increasing desire among patients for self-treatment and less use of pharmaceutical drugs, have meant that many medical doctors and pharmacists are now dealing with patients who regularly take these types of medicines. As neither doctors nor pharmacists receive comprehensive herbal training as part of their standard education, a potentially detrimental situation can arise in regard to not only patient safety but also negligence. Practical questions, such as whether a herb works in a particular scenario, or is dangerous in another, or compares favourably to a pharmaceutical drug, or can reasonably be expected to have an effect within a certain time frame, are important facts to know. It is hoped that resources such as this text will enable all health practitioners to ensure the safe and rational use of herbal medicines.

REFERENCES

American Herbal Products Association, Botanical Extracts Committee. Standardization of botanical products: White paper. Silver Spring, MD: American Herbal Products Association, 2003.

Balunas MJ, Kinghorn AD. Drug discovery from medicinal plants. Life Sci 78 (2005): 431–441.

Berman B et al. Essentials of complementary and alternative medicine. Philadelphia: Lippincott Williams & Wilkins, 1999.

Di Masi JH, Grabowski HG. The price of innovation: new estimates of drug development costs. J Health Econ 22 (2003): 151–185.

Eisner S (ed.). Guidance for manufacture and sale of bulk botanical extracts, Silver Spring, MD: Botanical Extracts Committee, American Herbal Products Association, 2001.

Evans WC. Trease and Evans pharmacognosy, 15th edn, Edinburgh: WB Saunders, 2002.

Evans S. Changing the knowledge base in Western herbal medicine. Soc Sci Med 67 (2008): 2098–2106.

Heinrich M et al. Fundamentals of pharmacognosy and phytotherapy. Philadelphia: Churchill Livingstone, 2004.

Lin HL et al. Up-regulation of multidrug resistance transporter expression by berberine in human and murine hepatoma cells. Cancer 85.9 (1999): 1937–1942.

Madabushi R et al. Hyperforin in St. John's wort drug interactions. Eur J Clin Pharmacol 62.3 (2006): 225–233.

Mills S, Bone K. Principles and practice of phytotherapy. London: Churchill Livingstone, 2001.

Pan GY et al. The involvement of P-glycoprotein in berberine absorption. Pharmacol Toxicol 91.4 (2002): 193–197.

Vogel V. American Indian medicine. Normal, OK: University of Oklahoma Press, 1970.

Walcott EE, transl. The Badianus Manuscript: An Aztec Herbal of 1552. Baltimore: Johns Hopkins Press, 1940.

Weiss R. Herbal medicine. Beaconsfield, UK: Beaconsfield Publishers, 1988.

Wierenga D, Eaton RC. Phases of product development. Canberra: Office of Research and Development, Australian Pharmaceutical Manufacturers Association, 2003.

CHAPTER 2

INTRODUCTION TO CLINICAL NUTRITION

Nutrition may be defined as the science of food, its nutrients and substances, and their association with the body in relation to health and disease. In every stage of life nutrition is important and influences clinical practice in many branches of healthcare. Clinical nutrition is the use of this information in the diagnosis, treatment and prevention of disease that may be caused by deficiency, excess or imbalance of nutrients, and in the maintenance of good health.

CONSEQUENCES OF POOR NUTRITION

Nutrition plays a vital role in the health of both individuals and society, with poor nutrition and inadequate intake having a devastating effect. Overall, it has been estimated that more than 60% of all deaths in Australia result from nutrition-related disorders, such as cardiovascular disease, diabetes and cancer (Sydney-Smith 2000).

MORTALITY RISK: CARDIOVASCULAR DISEASE AND CANCER

Atherosclerotic cardiovascular disease is the most common cause of death in most Western countries (Anderson 2003). In Australia, it is the leading cause of death, accounting for 34% of all deaths in 2006. Cardiovascular disease kills one Australian nearly every 10 minutes according to the Australian Heart Foundation website. It is well known that dietary factors such as carbohydrate and fat intake affect several important physiological parameters, along with risk factors, such as hypertension, lipid levels, diabetes and antioxidant status. With the exception of tobacco consumption, diet is probably the most important factor in the aetiology of human cancers, responsible for around one-third of all cases (Ferguson 2002).

Diet-related cancers have often been considered to relate to exogenous carcinogens; however, it is increasingly apparent that many carcinogens may be endogenously generated, and that diet plays an important role in modifying this process (Ferguson 1999).

Overeating and poorly balanced meals have also led to significant increases in metabolic syndrome (syndrome X) and obesity, which are now major health concerns. A 2003 review stated that the World Health Organization (WHO) estimates there are 1 billion people around the world who are now overweight or obese, and that 20–25% of the adult population in the USA have metabolic syndrome (Keller & Lemberg 2003).

Although overweight and obesity in adulthood is associated with decreased longevity, and the link with cardiovascular disease is well known, a recent series of meta-analyses revealed statistically significant associations for overweight with the incidence of type II diabetes, all cancers (except oesophageal [female], pancreatic and prostate), asthma, gall-bladder disease, osteoarthritis and chronic back pain (Guh et al 2009). It has further been established that obesity is associated with increased death rates from cancer (Peeters et al 2003). A large prospective study of more than 900,000 people found that a BMI above 40 was associated with a higher combined death rate from all cancers of 52% for obese men and 62% for obese women, compared with people of normal weight (Calle et al 2003). The adverse effects of obesity on health are not limited to adults. Overweight children and adolescents are now being diagnosed with impaired glucose tolerance and type 2 diabetes, and show early signs of insulin resistance syndrome and cardiovascular risk (Goran et al 2003).

A large body of research exists that attempts to isolate the influence of individual food groups and nutrients on morbidity and mortality. Research with macronutrients has found that the consumption of diets rich in plant-derived foods, wholegrains and fish reduces the risk of morbidity and mortality. However, numerous surveys have identified inadequate intakes of these foods in many Australian subpopulations (Barzi et al 2003, He et al 2002, Mozaffarian et al 2003, Rissanen et al 2003, Slavin 2003). The relative roles of micronutrients, phytochemicals and non-nutrients are still under debate.

FOOD UNDER THE MICROSCOPE

More than 25,000 different bioactive components are thought to occur in the foods consumed by human beings (Milner 2008). These components represent a veritable cocktail of chemicals that includes macronutrients (such as carbohydrates, protein, fat, water and fibre) and micronutrients (such as vitamins and minerals as well as phytochemicals), many of which are health-promoting, plant-based compounds (Table 2.1). Additives, such as preservatives, colourings and flavourings, together with contaminants introduced through farming or processing techniques, may also be present.

TABLE 2.1 THE CHEMICAL COMPLEXITY OF FOOD	
NUTRIENTS	
Micronutrients	Vitamins: A, B complex, C, D, E, K, coenzyme Q10 Minerals: iron, iodine, fluoride, zinc, chromium, selenium, manganese, molybdenum and copper Others?
Macronutrients	Carbohydrates: simple and complex Proteins: amino acids Lipids: saturated, monounsaturated and polyunsaturated fatty acids Fibre: soluble and insoluble Water Minerals: sodium, potassium, calcium, magnesium, phosphorus Others?
Phytochemicals	Bioflavonoids, carotenoids, isoflavones, glutathione, lipoic acid, caffeic acid, ferulic acid, lignans, allyl sulfides, indoles
NON-NUTRIENTS	
Food additives: natural or synthetic	Colourings: restore colours lost during processing or alter natural colour Flavourings: alter natural flavours Preservatives: prolong shelf-life by reducing bacterial, mould and yeast growth Thickeners: modify texture and consistency of food Humectants: control moisture levels and keep food moist (mainly used in baked foods) Food acids: used to standardise acid levels between different food batches Antioxidants: used to preserve foods mainly containing fats and oils
Contaminants	Natural contaminants Industrial pollutants Processing contaminants Others?

Source: Wahlqvist et al 1997, Wardlaw et al 1997.

Nutrients can be divided into two main subgroups — essential and non-essential. Essential nutrients are those that cannot be synthesised by the human body in sufficient quantities to meet average requirements, such as vitamin C, and therefore must be taken in through the diet. Non-essential nutrients can be synthesised in the body from other compounds, although they may also be ingested in foods.

MACRONUTRIENTS

Macronutrients supply energy and essential nutrients, making up the bulk of food. Carbohydrates, lipids, proteins, water and some minerals comprise this group and are all necessary to sustain life. Some macronutrients are produced in supplement form and are used as therapeutic agents. As a result, a number of these are reviewed in this book.

Carbohydrates

Simple carbohydrates, also known as sugars, are termed 'monosaccharides' because they are the single sugar units that form the basis of all sugar structures. Glucose is a monosaccharide and the primary source of energy for most human cells. Most glucose is not ingested through the diet, but rather synthesised from sucrose (common sugar) in the liver (Wardlaw et al 1997). More complex forms of carbohydrates, such as starches and fibres, are composed of many units of smaller carbohydrates found in grains, vegetables and fruit and are termed 'polysaccharides'. Overall, carbohydrates are important as a fuel. They are considered protein-sparing as they prevent the breakdown of proteins in the muscles, heart and liver into amino acids and ultimately glucose to produce fuel.

Lipids

The term 'lipid' is a generic one used to describe a number of chemicals that share two main characteristics: they are insoluble in water and contain fatty acids. When they are solid at room temperature they are called fats, whereas those that are liquid are called oils. Fatty acids are the simplest form of lipids, and more than 40 different types occur in nature (Wahlqvist et al 1997). Of all the various classes of lipids, only precursors of the omega-3 and omega-6 fatty acids are considered essential, meaning they are necessary in the diet to maintain health. The amount of dietary fat ingested and the ratios between saturated, monounsaturated and polyunsaturated fatty acids are important influences on overall health and disease.

Protein

Protein is formed by linking individual amino acids together, with the order of the amino acid sequence determining the protein's ultimate form and function. Proteins are crucial to the regulation and maintenance of many vital body processes, such as blood clotting and fluid balance, cell repair and hormone and enzyme production.

Amino acids can be divided into two broad groups: essential or non-essential. There are nine essential amino acids that must be ingested through the diet to maintain health. Protein foods that contain all nine essential amino acids are also referred to as complete protein sources (e.g. animal protein). By contrast, almost all plant foods are incomplete protein sources, with the possible exception of spirulina and soy. During times of growth, tissue repair or pronounced catabolism, such as after surgery, the body requires additional protein for efficient new tissue growth to occur. There is also emerging evidence that supplementation with individual amino acids produces a variety of pharmacological effects that can be manipulated to provide therapeutic benefits. Several of these amino acids are reviewed in the monograph section.

Minerals

Some minerals fall into the category of macronutrients because they are required in gram amounts every day, although they do not directly produce energy. These include sodium, potassium, calcium, phosphorus and magnesium.

MICRONUTRIENTS

Micronutrients do not in themselves provide energy or fuel for the body, but they may be involved in the chemical processes required to produce energy from macronutrients.

Vitamins and trace minerals fall into this category and are required to sustain life, typically through their roles as enzymatic co-factors in diverse biochemical processes. Many micronutrients are available in supplement preparations and are reviewed in this book.

Vitamins

Vitamins are organic substances (i.e. they contain a carbon atom) essential for normal growth and functioning of the body. They have been divided into two broad groups: vitamin C and the eight members of the B complex (B_1, B_2, B_3, B_5, B_6, B_{12}, biotin and folic acid) are defined as water-soluble vitamins, whereas vitamins A, D, E and K are fat-soluble. Levels in the body need to be replenished on a regular basis, as only vitamins A, E and B_{12} are stored to any significant extent. Just as a vitamin deficiency causes adverse outcomes, high doses of these supplements can also do so if used inappropriately.

Essential trace minerals

These are minerals required by the body, usually in milligram or microgram amounts. They include iron, iodine, fluoride, zinc, chromium, selenium, manganese, molybdenum and copper. All trace minerals have the potential to be toxic when consumed in high doses.

Phytochemicals

Phytochemicals are components in plant foods that appear to provide significant health benefits, yet are not essential. Considerable research has been undertaken in the past few decades to understand the role they play in maintaining health and preventing certain diseases, such as cancer, but there is still much to learn. Some of the better known phytochemicals include isoflavones (e.g. genistein), bioflavonoids (e.g. procyanidins), carotenoids (e.g. lycopene), glutathione and alpha-lipoic acid. Many of the phytochemicals found in food are also found in medicinal herbs and may partly explain their therapeutic qualities.

FOOD LABELS

According to Nutrition Australia, by law all packaged foods must carry labels that state the following information:

- name of food
- name and business address of manufacturer

- country of origin
- ingredients, listed by weight from greatest to smallest (including added water)
- percentage of the key ingredient or component present in the food product
- warnings about the presence of major allergens in the food, such as nuts, seafood, eggs, gluten and soy
- a nutrition information panel, unless the food is not packaged or the package is too small (e.g. tea bags)
- an expiry date.

For further information about labelling, see Food Standards Australia New Zealand (FSANZ) website.

Currently, more than 35 genetically modified (GM) foods have been approved for sale in Australia and New Zealand (FSANZ 2014), including foods derived from soy, sugar beet, corn, cottonseed oil, canola and potatoes. As from December 2001, labels must also state whether a food contains a GM-derived component or protein introduced through genetic modification.

Additives are listed as either numbers, known as additive codes, or by name. Up-to-date lists of the food additives found in Australian and New Zealand food products can be located on the FSANZ website.

NUTRITIONAL DEFICIENCIES

Malnutrition and other deficiency states, such as kwashiorkor (protein deficiency), scurvy or rickets, are major causes of morbidity and mortality in both developing and developed countries under conditions of deprivation. Malnutrition can occur as a result of alcoholism, medication use, fussy eating, anorexia, small bowel obstruction and numerous other medical conditions.

More specific or individual nutritional deficiencies can be classified as either a 'primary deficiency' or a 'secondary deficiency', according to their aetiology.

PRIMARY DEFICIENCY

Primary deficiency is defined as a state arising from inadequate dietary intake. Although considered to be rare in developed countries, inadequate intake and primary deficiency states are not uncommon, as evidenced by numerous dietary surveys both here and overseas.

Inadequate dietary intake

The Australian National Nutrition Survey (NNS), conducted in 1995, found that approximately 30% of 2–7-year-old children ate no fruit or vegetables. Among 8–11-year-olds, 44% of boys and 38% of girls ate no fruit on the previous day and approximately one in four older children consumed no vegetables. Additionally, neither age group consumed the minimum number of serves of dairy products (Cashel 2000). Later results from the Australian Institute of Health and Welfare in 1998 reported that approximately one in two Australian children under 12 were not eating fruit or fruit products, and more than one in five consumed no vegetables in a typical day.

The dietary intakes of adults are also far from ideal. The 1995 NNS also found that approximately 44% of adult males and 34% of females did not consume fruit in the 24 hours preceding the survey, and 20% of males and 17% of females did not consume vegetables (Giskes et al 2002).

Interestingly, dietary intakes were influenced by income level, with lower-income adults consuming a smaller variety of fruits and vegetables than their higher-income counterparts. Additional research has consistently identified other groups at risk of poor dietary habits, such as the elderly, institutionalised individuals and the indigenous population.

Surveys of individual vitamin and mineral intakes also identify a number of at-risk subpopulations. Calcium intakes for 1045 randomly selected Australian women (20–92 years), as estimated by questionnaire, showed that 76% of women aged 20–54 years, 87% of older women and 82% of lactating women had intakes below the recommended dietary intake (Pasco et al 2000). Of these, 14% had less than the minimum requirement of 300 mg/day and would, therefore, be in negative calcium balance and at risk of bone loss. The 1997 New Zealand National Nutrition Survey found that 20% of all New Zealanders and one in four women had calcium intakes below the UK estimated average requirements, and 15–20% of women aged 15–18 years were considered to have frank deficiency (Horwath et al 2001).

Surveys in Australia and New Zealand report that many adolescent girls have insufficient dietary intakes of iron and zinc to meet their high physiological requirements for growing body tissues, expanding red cell mass and onset of menarche (Gibson et al 2002).

More recent surveys do not show the situation improving. The 2007 Children's Survey, which assessed vegetable and fruit intakes against the recommendations for children aged 2–16 (1–3 serves fruit; 2–4 serves of vegetables) found a total of 22% of boys and girls aged 4–8 years met the recommended serves of vegetables, but this decreased to 11% of boys and 1% of girls aged 14–16 years (CSIRO & University of South Australia 2008).

About 9 in 10 children aged 2–13 years met the recommendation for fruit serves compared with only 1 in 4 boys aged 14–16 (25%) and about 1 in 5 girls (19%). This decreased substantially when fruit juice was excluded from the analysis, with only 2% of boys and 1% of girls aged 14–16 years meeting the recommendation

According to a 2012 government publication, 'Australia's Food and Nutrition', more than 9 in 10 (91%) people aged 16 years and over do not consume sufficient serves of vegetables, and about 50% do not consume sufficient serves of fruit (Australian Institute of Health and

Welfare 2012). When measures of sufficient serves of fruit and vegetables are combined, only 6% of people consume enough fruit and vegetables on a regular basis.

Evidence of deficiency in Australia and New Zealand

It is a common perception that although dietary intakes are not ideal, vitamin and mineral deficiencies are not a major health concern; however, research has shown that several subpopulations, such as children, pregnant and lactating women, older adults, institutionalised individuals, indigenous peoples and vegetarians, are at real risk.

For example, although severe iodine deficiency is rare in Australia and New Zealand, the Australian Population Health Development Principal Committee reports a high incidence of mild to moderate iodine deficiency in primary school aged children in Australia and New Zealand (APHDPC 2007).

This is of great concern because mild iodine deficiency during childhood and pregnancy has the potential to impair neurological development. One survey of Sydney schoolchildren, healthy adult volunteers, pregnant women and patients with diabetes found that all four groups had urinary iodine excretion values below those set by the WHO for iodine repletion (Li et al 2001). Another survey of 225 children in Tasmania identified evidence of mild iodine deficiency in 25% of boys and 21% of girls (Guttikonda et al 2002). A research group at Monash Medical Centre in Melbourne screened 802 pregnant women and found that 48.4% of Caucasian women had urinary iodine concentrations below 50 micrograms/L compared to 38.4% of Vietnamese women and 40.8% of Indian/Sri Lankan women (Hamrosi et al 2005). These figures are disturbing when one considers that normal levels are over 100 micrograms/L, mild deficiency is diagnosed at 51–100 micrograms/L and moderate to severe deficiency at < 50 micrograms/L (Gunton et al 1999). A study conducted at a Sydney hospital involving 81 women attending a 'high-risk' clinic found moderate to severe iodine deficiency in 19.8% of volunteers and mild iodine deficiency in another 29.6% (Gunton et al 1999).

In Australia and New Zealand, the prevalence of vitamin D deficiency varies, but it is now acknowledged to be much higher than previously thought (Nowson & Margerison 2002). The groups at greatest risk are dark-skinned and veiled women (particularly in pregnancy), their infants and older persons living in residential care. The study by Nowson and Margerison found marginal deficiency in 23% of women, and another frank deficiency in 80% of dark-skinned women in Australia. A study conducted in a large aged-care facility in Auckland identified frank vitamin D deficiency in 49% of elderly participants in midwinter and in 33% in midsummer (Ley et al 1999). Even in studies of 'healthy' adults, vitamin D insufficiency has been found to affect more than 40% of residents in Queensland (Kimlin et al 2007, van der Mei et al 2007) and over 65% of Tasmanians (van der Mei et al 2007).

Barriers to good nutrition

Clearly, living in a developed country is not a guarantee of healthy nutrition. Western first-world countries have a wide range of good-quality foods available at affordable prices, yet healthy eating is not commonplace. There are four key levels of influence on dietary behaviours:

1. individual factors
2. interpersonal factors
3. organisational factors
4. environmental factors.

At each level, barriers to healthy eating behaviours exist. Table 2.2 lists some of the more common barriers. Successful nutritional interventions that aim to modify individuals' eating patterns should help people develop new routines and simple internalised rules that they can use to navigate sensibly through the multitude of food choices and personal influences.

Nutritional intervention is a central component of disease prevention and management. Health professionals play a pivotal role in undertaking nutritional interventions with patients because of their knowledge, access to information and credibility as patient educators.

SECONDARY DEFICIENCY

Secondary deficiency may develop when there is reduced nutrient absorption, or increased metabolism or excretion of any given nutrient.

TABLE 2.2 INFLUENCES OVER FOOD CHOICES
• Nutritional knowledge • Religious beliefs and practices • Family beliefs and practices • Cultural beliefs and practices • Ethnicity • Education • Occupation • Peer and social influences • Advertising • Emotional factors: e.g. indulging in 'comfort' foods • Medication: dietary alterations may be necessary; side effects may alter appetite • Food: flavour, texture, appearance, odour • Income: food choices based on affordability • Childhood experiences • Dental health: e.g. ill-fitting dentures, sensitive teeth • Availability and convenience: e.g. convenience of fast food • Muscle weakness or joint pain: problems with shopping and cooking • Problems chewing and swallowing • Gastrointestinal problems: e.g. nausea, diarrhoea • Following a specific diet: e.g. fad diets • Psychosocial problems: loneliness, depression, confusion, isolation

Of these, malabsorption states are the most common and associated with many diseases such as those characterised by chronic diarrhoea (e.g. Crohn's disease), alterations to gastrointestinal tract architecture (e.g. coeliac disease) and liver cirrhosis. In these cases, malabsorption may be specific to certain nutrients and fats or may be more generalised.

The effects of pharmaceutical medicines on nutritional status must not be forgotten. A significant number of drugs affect appetite, nutrient absorption and synthesis, transport and storage, metabolism and excretion. In fact, some of the side effects of medicines may not be related to the medicine directly, but rather to the nutritional deficiencies that develop with their use over time. These will not always produce clinically significant adverse effects, but when combined with a poor diet, or when several medicines affecting the same nutrients are taken, the risk of deficiency is heightened.

Medicines that can reduce intake of nutrients include those that induce nausea, dyspepsia or decrease appetite, such as non-steroidal anti-inflammatory drugs (NSAIDs), and opioid drugs such as codeine and morphine. Medicines with the potential to reduce nutrient absorption include those that reduce gastric motility (e.g. opioid drugs), greatly increase gastric motility (e.g. metoclopramide), compromise digestive enzyme output and function (e.g. proton pump inhibitors) and bind nutrients, preventing their traversal across gastrointestinal membranes, such as anion exchange resins (e.g. cholestyramine). Certain medicines can also increase nutrient excretion, such as thiazide diuretics, which increase potassium excretion. Others can reduce vitamin biosynthesis, such as statins, which reduce the production of coenzyme Q10.

In each of these cases, either increased nutritional intakes may be required to offset possible depletions, or medicines should not be administered with meals or supplements to reduce the likelihood of more direct interactions.

RDA AND RDI REFERENCE VALUES FOR AUSTRALIA AND NEW ZEALAND

The concept of recommended daily allowances (RDAs) originated in the United States in the 1940s as a basis for setting the poverty threshold and food-stamp allocations for the military and civilian populations during times of war and/or economic depression (Russell 2007). At this time, the first RDAs were determined by observing a healthy population's usual dietary intakes and extrapolating RDAs from this information. Over subsequent decades, scientific research into health and nutrition became more sophisticated, rendering the original concept of RDAs incomplete and in need of modification. The main findings to emerge were as follows:

- Many additional nutrients found in food are important for health, so a longer list of nutrients with recommended levels will be required.
- Nutrient intake recommendations need to be related to a specific use, as requirements will vary for different subpopulations.

- Nutritional intake recommendations need to take into account longer-term disease prevention, not just deficiency prevention.
- Clearer endpoints will be required by which to set adequacy levels.
- Risk assessment of nutrients will be necessary.

In the mid-1990s a new framework was developed to address these issues. It aimed to establish new nutrient intake recommendations to meet a variety of uses and to base nutrient requirements on the reduction of chronic disease risk, with a clear rationale for the endpoints chosen. The new guidelines still contain RDAs, but have been expanded to include three new intake recommendations: estimated average requirements (EARs), adequate daily intake (ADI) and upper level (UL) of intake.

Revisions to the nutrient intake framework occurred all around the world and in 2006 the National Health and Medical Research Council (NHMRC) of Australia published its adjusted nutritional guidelines for the adequate intake of vitamins and minerals (NHMRC 2006). These guidelines were far more comprehensive than previous versions and incorporated some of the initiatives developed in the United States.

The NHMRC guidelines are intended for healthy people and specify requirements based on both gender and age, while assuming average body weights of 76 kg for the adult male and 61 kg for the adult female.

Four key dietary reference value terms are defined here:

1. Estimated average requirement (EAR). A daily nutrient level estimated to meet the needs of 50% of the healthy population in a particular life cycle and gender.
2. Recommended daily intake (RDI). A daily nutrient intake estimated to meet the needs of up to 98% of healthy people in a particular life cycle and gender. This remains the most common benchmark of individual nutrient adequacy.
3. Adequate daily intake (ADI). When RDI cannot be determined, this is based on observed or experimentally derived estimates of daily nutrient intake to meet the needs of healthy individuals.
4. Upper level (UL) of intake. An estimate of the highest level of regular intake that carries no appreciable risk of adverse health effects to almost all people in the general population. It is meant to apply to all groups of the general population, including sensitive individuals, throughout the life stages.

In some instances, the 2006 RDI values for specific nutrients represented a substantial increase (e.g. iron and folate), whereas others increased only marginally (e.g. calcium) or decreased (e.g. zinc requirements for adult females).

RDI and nutritional deficiencies

Although the RDIs provide a guide to preventing nutrient deficiency signs and symptoms in a 'healthy' population, they are only general recommendations and do not take into account each individual's requirements or specific circumstances. As a result, seemingly adequate food intake can provide false security, owing to a number of factors that influence the nutritional content of food and the way important nutrients are absorbed, utilised and excreted.

Unfavourable cooking and storage conditions can significantly reduce the nutritional content of food before it is consumed, no longer providing the expected vitamins and minerals. Many vitamins and minerals are sensitive to changes in temperature, light and oxygen. Up to 50% of vitamins A, D and E and 100% of vitamin C and folate can be lost during cooking (Wahlqvist et al 1997).

Issues relating to various farming techniques have often been cited as affecting the nutritional content of food and are readily reflected in the variability of resulting mineral composition. A good illustration of this is selenium, which, like most other minerals, enters the food chain through incorporation into plants from the soil. Plants grown in soils with low selenium levels are likely to contain smaller quantities than those grown in selenium-rich soils. Acid soils and complexation with metals, such as iron or aluminium, also reduce plant selenium content.

Beyond the actual quantities of nutrients provided by our food, reduced bioavailability of nutrients can occur as a result of interactions between food constituents. Phytates found in dietary fibre and tannins found in tea (and several herbal medicines) are able to bind to iron, zinc and other minerals, impairing the body's ability to absorb them. Therefore, adequate intake of mineral-rich food does not necessarily prevent deficiency. In addition to this, there are other potential contributors to secondary nutrient deficiencies, such as impaired absorption, compromised or accelerated utilisation and increased excretion of individual nutrients as well as genetic variables.

Serious deficiencies of reference values

Setting nutrient reference values is a complex task, which produces only approximate values. Robert Russell from the Human Nutrition Research Centre on Aging at Tufts University has outlined eight different obstacles that prevent accurate determination of reference values (Russell 2007):

1. Few long-term studies are available, so information is extrapolated from short-term studies (e.g. 1–2 weeks).
2. Little good-quality information is available about individual variability in response to the indicators in question.
3. Most research fails to consider the interaction between nutrients (which may be important for good health).
4. Many databases used when determining reference values provided information from studies that evaluated only dietary intakes and ignored supplemental intakes.
5. Most studies fail to consider the variation in nutrient bioavailability that is influenced by the food matrixes in which the nutrient presents.

6. Little good-quality information is available about children, adolescents and the elderly from which to establish reference values with any degree of certainty.
7. Little good-quality dose-response information is available (i.e. responses to multiple levels of the same nutrient in the same individual).
8. The cause and effect of a nutrient on a specific outcome is sometimes still speculative, as multiple factors may affect an outcome, not simply a single nutrient.

The obstacles outlined here clearly indicate that the scientific basis for many of the reference values is weak. They also indicate that for many nutrients and food components the RDI and UL levels are only approximations that are loosely relevant to the general healthy population, and even less relevant to the individual with comorbidities or special needs. Substantial research would be required to create a set of reference values with greater accuracy and relevance, but even then some values, such as ULs, may never be entirely accurate, as ethical considerations would prevent such research from ever being conducted.

OPTIMAL NUTRITION: A STATE BEYOND RDI

Dietary reference values are based on the concept of nutrient requirement. When considering these, it is important to keep in mind how we define or identify 'adequacy'. Historically, one measure of adequacy has been the dose of nutrient required to prevent the clinical manifestations of the corresponding deficiency. This method has yielded RDI reference values, which prevent overt deficiency presentations in most healthy people but do not guarantee the prevention of a less well-defined suboptimal intake which may over time contribute to other pathology.

There is considerable evidence that some nutrients may have health benefits at intake levels greater than the RDI. Higher intake levels appear to play a role in the prevention of many degenerative diseases such as cancer, cardiovascular disease, macular degeneration and cataract, cognitive decline and Alzheimer's dementia, as well as of developmental conditions such as neural tube defect. The NHMRC guidelines for the adequate intake of vitamins and minerals acknowledge this fact and state that 'there is some evidence that a range of nutrients could have benefits in chronic disease aetiology at levels above the RDI or AI' (NHMRC 2006).This has given rise to a new concept, 'suboptimal nutrition'.

The phrase 'suboptimal nutrition' was first coined by Fairfield and Fletcher in their 2002 systematic review evaluating the evidence indicating that certain nutrients had long-term disease prevention properties (Fairfield et al 2002, Fletcher et al 2002). They defined suboptimal nutrition as a state in which nutritional intake is sufficient to prevent the classical symptoms and signs of deficiency, yet insufficient to significantly reduce the risk of developmental or degenerative diseases. As such, avoiding a state of suboptimal nutrition requires adequate dietary intakes of all key food groups with an emphasis on health-promoting foods, and possibly the use of additional nutritional supplements. Furthermore, the balance between micronutrients or macronutrients is important, such as the ratio of omega-3 to omega-6 fatty acids and of high to low glycaemic carbohydrates.

As a reflection of these new developments, the term 'suggested dietary target' has been adopted by the NHMRC to describe the 'daily average intake from food and beverages for certain nutrients that may help in prevention of chronic disease'. It is a move that recognises food components offer more than just deficiency prevention; however, the general recommendations still relate only to the general healthy population.

Theoretically, it can be imagined that there is a level of intake that could be considered to provide optimal nutrition that is above the RDI yet below the UL levels. Figure 2.1 illustrates a theoretical description of beneficial health effects of a nutrient as a function of level of intake. The solid line in the figure represents risk of inadequacy in preventing nutritional deficiency and the broken line represents the risk of inadequacy in achieving a health benefit, that is, disease risk reduction (Renwick et al 2004). As intake falls below the RDI, the risk of adverse effects due to inadequate intake increases, and as intake increases beyond an optimal level, there is an increased risk of adverse effects due to toxicity. Naturally, however, such an optimal intake may be highly individualistic, based on the previous discussion of confounding factors.

REDEFINING AN ESSENTIAL NUTRIENT

Clearly the line between essential and non-essential nutrients has blurred as a result of modern scientific inquiry and experimentation (Yates 2005). In the first half of the 20th century, nutrients were termed 'essential' when their removal from the diet caused severe organ dysfunction or death.

FIGURE 2.1 A theoretical description of beneficial health effects of a nutrient as a function of level of intake (Renwick et al 2004)

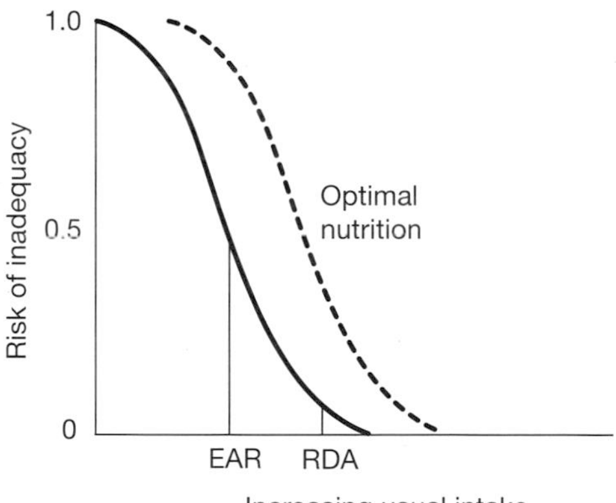

Since then, modern scientific techniques have enabled us to detect finer gradations of inadequacy well before organic pathology, such as a decline in health status or ability to function optimally, sets in. They have also allowed us to glimpse the potential of nutrients and certain food compounds to prevent genomic mutations, alter metabolic processes and ultimately prevent disease, possibly even extending longevity concomitantly. If we broaden the aim of nutrition beyond prevention of deficiency to include the promotion of wellness and optimal health, many additional nutrients and food components are also likely to be able to be termed 'essential'.

NUTRITIONAL GENOMICS

Nutritional genomics is a field that has emerged alongside the Human Genome Project. It has a unique focus on disease prevention and healthy ageing through the manipulation of gene–diet interactions. Several key scientific domains in nutritional genomics focus on specific areas of this interaction.

Nutrigenomics, also known as nutritional epigenetics, refers to the effect of nutrients and other food components on gene expression and gene regulation, i.e. diet–gene regulation. In contrast, nutrigenetics refers to the genetic makeup of an individual that affects their response to various dietary nutrients and can reveal why different people respond differently to the same nutrient. When understood together, these two emerging fields can help us understand how diet and nutrition affect human health and eventually lead to individualised dietary recommendations to reduce the risk of disease, possibly improve recovery and promote wellness (Gaboon 2011). In other words, from a clinical perspective, nutritional genomics may help clinicians bridge the gap from overarching public health messages aimed at the broader community to more individualised dietary guidance.

Another concept in nutritional genomics is systems biology, or nutritional engineering. This involves the identification, classification and characterisation of human genetic variants or polymorphisms (mutations) that modify individual responses to nutrients (Fig 2.2) and its application in the manipulation of biological pathways to produce health benefits.

From a public health and research perspective, it is possible that nutritional genomics could play an important role in the conduct and interpretation of clinical trials and epidemiological studies that investigate the associations between diet and/or nutritional supplementation and disease. This knowledge can be used to distinguish between responders and non-responders, and to determine which populations are most likely to benefit from nutritional intervention and which may be at increased risk of harm.

It has further been suggested that there is a need to establish genome-informed nutrient and food-based dietary guidelines for disease prevention and healthy ageing, and better targeted public health nutrition interventions

FIGURE 2.2 Nutrient genome interactions (from Stover and Caudill 2008)

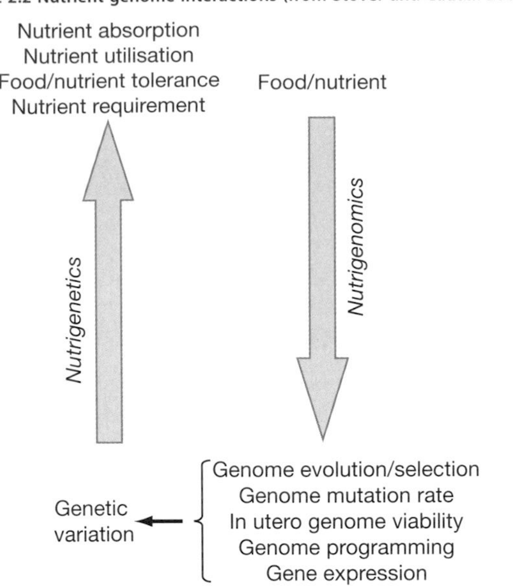

(including micronutrient fortification and supplementation) that maximise benefit and minimise adverse outcomes in genetically diverse human populations (Stover & Caudill 2008).

Whilst a better understanding of an individual's family history and genetic makeup may help inform practice in future, complex disorders, such as cancer, CVD and diabetes, are caused by genetic and environmental factors, and genetic mutations are only partially predictive of risk (Camp & Trujillo 2014). Our understanding of this complicated interplay between genetic variations, diet, lifestyle, environmental and even psychological influences is still far from clear.

The development of nutrigenomics holds great promise for individualised medicine and tailoring nutritional interventions for the individual; however, the science is still developing. The knowledge gained from nutritional genomics requires an evidence-based approach to validate that personalised recommendations result in health benefits to individuals and do not cause harm (Camp & Trujillo 2014). In addition, as with all emerging areas, ethical, legal and social issues need to be addressed, particularly with respect to how the public may access nutrigenetic tests and associated nutritional and lifestyle advice. There are five key areas identified by international experts in the context of both basic nutrigenomics research and its clinical and commercial uses:

1. health claims benefits arising from nutrigenomics
2. managing nutrigenomic information

3. delivery methods of nutrigenomics services
4. nutrigenomics products
5. equitable accessibility to nutrigenomics (Gaboon 2011).

NUTRITIONAL DEFICIENCY, GENOME DAMAGE AND CLINICAL PRACTICE

There is overwhelming evidence that several micronutrients (vitamins and minerals) are required as co-factors for enzymes or as part of the structure of proteins (metalloenzymes) involved in DNA synthesis and repair, prevention of oxidative damage to DNA as well as maintenance methylation of DNA. The main point is that genome damage caused by moderate micronutrient deficiency is of the same order of magnitude as the genome damage levels caused by exposure to significant doses of environmental genotoxins, such as chemical carcinogens, ultraviolet radiation and ionising radiation (Fenech 2008). For example, deficiency of vitamins B_{12}, folic acid, B_6, C, E or iron or zinc appears to damage DNA in the same way as radiation, by causing single- and double-strand breaks, oxidative lesions or both. Half of the population may be deficient in at least one of these micronutrients (Ames 2004). If moderate deficiency in just one micronutrient can cause significant DNA damage, it is possible that multiple moderate deficiencies may have additive or synergistic effects on genome stability.

Current research indicates the amount of micronutrients that appear to be protective against genome damage varies greatly between foods, and careful choice is needed to design dietary patterns optimised for genome health maintenance. Because dietary choices vary between individuals, several interventional options are required, and nutritional supplements may be necessary to fill in gaps not met by food intake, or to elevate intake levels beyond dietary intake to influence key metabolic pathways.

As the field of nutritional genomics matures, healthcare practitioners will have the opportunity to make genetically individualised dietary recommendations aimed at improving human health and preventing disease (Milner 2008). It is possible to envisage preventive medicine being practised in 'genome health clinics', where clinicians would diagnose and nutritionally prevent the most fundamental initiating cause of developmental and degenerative disease — genome damage itself (Fenech 2008).

NUTRITIONAL SUPPLEMENTATION

Nutritional supplements have traditionally been recommended only in cases of established deficiency; however, scientific evidence is accumulating to suggest they may be an important extension of healthy eating and necessary to achieve a level of health and disease prevention beyond what is possible through diet alone. As a consequence, many conservative medical bodies are being forced to reassess their long-established views.

SAFETY ISSUES

Nutritional supplements can be viewed as medicines that have both subtherapeutic and toxic doses, as well as the potential to induce adverse reactions and interactions.

Adverse reactions and interactions

The same subpopulations that have been identified to be at greater risk of adverse reactions to pharmaceutical medicines may be used for the safety assessment of nutritional supplements. These groups are the elderly, atopic patients, people with compromised liver or kidney function, anxiety or depression or serious illness, and those already taking many medicines. In clinical practice, the risk-versus-benefit decision of recommending a supplement or not is always considered and should be discussed with patients. In many cases, the risk of experiencing a minor adverse reaction that is short-lived and not serious may be an acceptable risk, whereas the risk of a more serious adverse reaction is not.

Toxicity

If a toxic dose is defined as one that is capable of causing death or a serious adverse reaction, then only a few nutrients are of special concern. In everyday practice, vitamins A, D and B_6 require special attention, as do the minerals iron, zinc, copper and selenium. Obviously, effects are dose-related and, in some cases, the doses are so large that they cannot practically be achieved in real life (see Appendix 6).

Natural versus synthetic

It is often asked whether natural and synthetic vitamins differ, and whether one is superior to and safer than the other. At this stage, very little research has been conducted to compare natural and synthetic forms, but some investigation into vitamin E has been undertaken.

The biological activity of vitamin E is based on the 'fetal resorption–gestation' method in rats. Using this test, the minimum amount of vitamin E required to sustain fetal growth in pregnant rats is determined. In the case of D-alpha tocopherol (RRR-alpha), which is considered to be the natural form, the highest activity is observed and therefore valued at 100%, whereas the biological activity of other vitamin E isomers has been estimated to be as low as 21% (Acuff et al 1998). Studies in humans have indicated that natural vitamin E has roughly twice the bioavailability of synthetic vitamin E; however, whether this also means that it has greater efficacy has yet to be clarified (Burton et al 1998).

It has also been speculated that the natural beta-carotene used in supplements, which is derived from algae and contains a mixture of carotenoids, may be safer and possibly more effective than synthetic beta-carotene.

RATIONAL USE OF SUPPLEMENTS

Nutritional supplements can never take the place of a balanced diet or provide all the health benefits of a whole food, but they can provide nutritional assistance and therapeutic effects in three different ways:

1. Supplementation to correct a gross deficiency. A patient presenting with clinical signs and symptoms of a nutritional deficiency will require nutritional counselling and possibly supplementation to quickly redress the situation (e.g. vitamin C supplementation and dietary education for patients with scurvy).
2. Supplementation to address a sub-clinical deficiency. A patient may not be presenting with overt clinical signs or symptoms of deficiency, but may benefit from an increased intake of certain nutrients or food components to prevent disease or reduce the incidence of other adverse outcomes (e.g. maternal folic acid supplementation and gestational health and development).
3. Supplementation to address symptoms not associated with nutrient deficiency. A patient presents with symptoms or disease unrelated to nutritional deficiency, but evidence indicates that nutritional supplementation can provide health benefits. This describes the use of nutritional supplements in pharmacological doses to achieve a specific health-related purpose, much like a therapeutic drug (e.g. high-dose riboflavin supplementation for migraine prophylaxis or coenzyme Q10 supplementation in hypertension). Many more examples are found in the monograph section of this book.

Table 2.3 provides a general guide for healthcare professionals when considering nutritional aspects of their patients' situation and nutritional supplementation.

TABLE 2.3 THE RATIONAL USE OF NUTRITIONAL SUPPLEMENTS
• Be informed and seek out unbiased information — do not rely on label claims, product information manuals or other commercial sources of information alone.
• Know the common nutrient deficiency signs and symptoms.
• Know the RDIs and where relevant suggested dietary targets.
• Know the benefits and risks of nutrients at levels beyond RDI and upper-limit levels (ULs) that increase the risk of adverse effects.
• Be able to detect inadequate dietary intakes or refer to a healthcare professional who can do so.
• Ensure that all healthcare professionals involved in a patient's care remain informed of nutritional supplement use.
• Take care with children, the elderly and pregnant or lactating women.
• Take care when high-risk medicines are being taken.
• Take care with HIV, cancer and other serious illnesses.
• Know the manufacturer or supplier details.
• Store medicines appropriately.

REFERENCES

Acuff RV et al. Transport of deuterium-labeled tocopherols during pregnancy. Am J Clin Nutr 67.3 (1998): 459–464.

Ames BN. A role for supplements in optimizing health: the metabolic tune-up. Arch Biochem Biophys 423.1 (2004): 227–234.

Anderson JW. Whole grains protect against atherosclerotic cardiovascular disease. Proc Nutr Soc 62.1 (2003): 135–142.

Australian Institute of Health and Welfare 2012. Australia's food & nutrition 2012. Cat. no. PHE 163. Canberra: AIHW.

Australian Population Health Development Principal Committee (APHDPC). The prevalence and severity of iodine deficiency in Australia. (2007). Available at: www.foodstandards.gov.au (accessed 24/01/2013).

Barzi F et al. Mediterranean diet and all-causes mortality after myocardial infarction: results from the GISSI-Prevenzione trial. Eur J Clin Nutr 57.4 (2003): 604–611.

Burton GW et al. Human plasma and tissue alpha-tocopherol concentrations in response to supplementation with deuterated natural and synthetic vitamin E. Am J Clin Nutr 67.4 (1998): 669–684.

Calle EE et al. Overweight, obesity, and mortality from cancer in a prospectively studied cohort of U.S. adults. N Engl J Med 348.17 (2003): 1625–1638.

Camp KM, Trujillo E. Position of the Academy of Nutrition and Dietetics: Nutritional Genomics. J Acad Nutrit Dietetics 114.2 (2014): 299–312.

Cashel K. What are Australian children eating? Med J Aust 173 (Suppl) (2000): S4–S5.

CSIRO, University of South Australia 2008. 2007 Australian national children's nutrition and physical activity survey — main findings. Canberra: Commonwealth of Australia.

Fairfield KM et al. Vitamins for chronic disease prevention in adults: scientific review. JAMA 287.23 (2002): 3116–3126.

Fenech M. Genome health nutrigenomics and nutrigenetics — diagnosis and nutritional treatment of genome damage on an individual basis. Food and Chemical Toxicology 46.4 (2008): 1365–1370.

Ferguson LR. Natural and man-made mutagens and carcinogens in the human diet. Mutat Res 443.1–2 (1999): 1–110.

Ferguson LR. Natural and human-made mutagens and carcinogens in the human diet. Toxicology 181.2 (2002): 79–82.

Fletcher RH, et al. Vitamins for chronic disease prevention in adults: clinical applications. JAMA 287.23 (2002): 3127–3129.

FSANZ (Food Standards Australia New Zealand). Food Standards Code; Standard 1.5.2 Available at: http://www.foodstandards.gov.au/code/Pages/default.aspx 20/7/2014.

FSANZ (Food Standards Australia New Zealand). Labelling. Available at: http://www.foodstandards.gov.au/consumer/labelling/Pages/default.aspx 20/7/2014.

Gaboon NEA. Nutritional genomics and personalized diet. Egyptian J Med Hum Genetics 12.1 (2011): 1–7.

Gibson RS et al. Risk of suboptimal iron and zinc nutriture among adolescent girls in Australia and New Zealand: causes, consequences, and solutions. Asia Pac J Clin Nutr 11 (Suppl 3) (2002): S543–S552.

Giskes K et al. Socio-economic differences in fruit and vegetable consumption among Australian adolescents and adults. Public Health Nutr 5.5 (2002): 663–669.

Goran MI et al. Obesity and risk of type 2 diabetes and cardiovascular disease in children and adolescents. J Clin Endocrinol Metab 88.4 (2003): 1417–1427.

Guh D et al. The incidence of co-morbidities related to obesity and overweight: A systematic review and meta-analysis. BMC Public Health 9.88 (2009): 1–20.

Gunton JE et al. Iodine deficiency in ambulatory participants at a Sydney teaching hospital: is Australia truly iodine replete? Med J Aust 171.9 (1999): 467–470.

Guttikonda K et al. Recurrent iodine deficiency in Tasmania, Australia: a salutary lesson in sustainable iodine prophylaxis and its monitoring. J Clin Endocrinol Metab 87.6 (2002): 2809–2815.

Hamrosi MA et al. Iodine status in pregnant women living in Melbourne differs by ethnic group. Asia Pac J Clin Nutr 14.1 (2005): 27–31.

He K et al. Fish consumption and risk of stroke in men. JAMA 288.24 (2002): 3130–3136.

Horwath C et al. Attaining optimal bone status: lessons from the 1997 National Nutrition Survey. NZ Med J 114.1128 (2001): 138–141.

Keller KB, Lemberg L. Obesity and the metabolic syndrome. Am J Crit Care 12.2 (2003): 167–170.

Kimlin M et al. Does a high UV environment ensure adequate vitamin D status? J Photochem Photobiol B 89.2–3 (2007): 139–147.

Ley SJ et al. Attention is needed to the high prevalence of vitamin D deficiency in our older population. NZ Med J 112.1101 (1999): 471–472.

Li M et al. Re-emergence of iodine deficiency in Australia. Asia Pac J Clin Nutr 10.3 (2001): 200–203.

Milner JA. Nutrition and cancer: essential elements for a road map. Cancer Letters 269.2 (2008): 189–198.

Mozaffarian D et al. Cardiac benefits of fish consumption may depend on the type of fish meal consumed: the Cardiovascular Health Study. Circulation 107.10 (2003): 1372–1377.

NHMRC (National Health and Medical Research Council). Nutrient reference values for Australia and New Zealand, 2006. Available online: http://www.nhmrc.gov.au/PUBLICATIONS/synopses/n35syn.htm 21-07-09.

Nowson CA, Margerison C. Vitamin D intake and vitamin D status of Australians. Med J Aust 177.3 (2002): 149–152.

Pasco JA et al. Calcium intakes among Australian women: Geelong Osteoporosis Study. Aust NZ J Med 30.1 (2000): 21–27.

Peeters A et al. Obesity in adulthood and its consequences for life expectancy: a life-table analysis. Ann Intern Med 138.1 (2003): 24–32.

Renwick AG et al. Risk-benefit analysis of micronutrients. Food Chem Toxicol 42.12 (2004): 1903–1922.

Rissanen TH et al. Low intake of fruits, berries and vegetables is associated with excess mortality in men: the Kuopio Ischaemic Heart Disease Risk Factor (KIHD) Study. J Nutr 133.1 (2003): 199–204.
Russell R. Setting dietary intake levels: problems and pitfalls. in: Bock G, Goode J (eds). Dietary supplements and health, 1st edn. Chichester: Wiley, 2007, pp 29–45.
Slavin J. Why whole grains are protective: biological mechanisms. Proc Nutr Soc 62.1 (2003): 129–134.
Stover PJ, Caudill MA. Genetic and epigenetic contributions to human nutrition and health: managing genome-diet interactions. J Am Diet Ass 108.9 (2008): 1480–1487.
Sydney-Smith M. Nutritional assessment in general practice. Curr Ther 41 (2000): 12–24.
van der Mei IA et al. The high prevalence of vitamin D insufficiency across Australian populations is only partly explained by season and latitude. Environ Health Perspect 115.8 (2007): 1132–1139.
Wahlqvist M et al. Food and nutrition. Sydney: Allen & Unwin, 1997.
Wardlaw G et al. Contemporary nutrition, 3rd edn. Dubuque: Brown and Benchmark, 1997.
Yates AA. Nutrient requirements, international perspectives. In: Benjamin C (ed). Encyclopedia of human nutrition. Oxford: Elsevier, 2005, pp 282–292.

CHAPTER 3

SAFETY OF COMPLEMENTARY MEDICINES

Complementary medicines (CMs) are widely used by the public as a non-pharmaceutical option that can be used to prevent, treat and manage disease (MacLennan et al 2002, Braun et al 2010b). They are used by people with a range of diseases and comorbidities such as low back pain, cancer, diabetes and cardiovascular disease (Broom et al 2012, Davis et al 2010, Grant et al 2012, Manya et al 2012). They are also used by people with no diagnosed disease but wanting to prevent disease, improve quality of life and general wellbeing, or for symptom relief. While MacLennan et al (2002) reported that people assumed if a medicine was 'natural' it must therefore be safe, times have changed and more people recognise that safety is relative and some CMs have the ability to cause drug interactions or even side effects (Braun 2007).

Finding information about CM safety is not straightforward for consumers as CM products are not accompanied by comprehensive consumer product information (CPI) in the same way that many pharmaceutical medicines are; many CMs are self-selected without professional advice, which means that much-needed information is not delivered with the product (Jamison 2003, MacLennan et al 2002).

Importantly, people who use CMs do not tend to use them as true alternatives to conventional treatment and it's not uncommon for care to be received from multiple healthcare providers over a similar time period. This situation is not necessarily dangerous and can produce significant benefits when well coordinated; however, if communication is poor, and complementary and conventional practitioners remain unaware of what the other has recommended, a potentially unsafe situation can arise. The prospect of interactions or adverse drug reactions leading to misdiagnosis, induction of withdrawal effects and misleading pathology test results are examples of unwanted outcomes when combined care is not coordinated.

In the real world, people are exposed to risk whenever they actively choose to undertake a treatment or choose to do without. Some risks are identifiable, while others are unknown. In practice, in order for patients to make an informed decision, these risks must be classified into those that are acceptable and those that are unacceptable, and then considered against the potential benefit, Over-the-counter (OTC) CMs that are produced under good manufacturing practice (GMP) conditions and meet government regulations offer a lower risk and potentially more cost-effective option than other treatments for some indications, and are generally considered safe when used appropriately under 'normal' circumstances; however,, they are not entirely devoid of risk.

A BRIEF HISTORY OF MEDICATION SAFETY

The potential for medical care to cause harm has been appreciated throughout history. In ancient times, knowledge of medicine, pharmacology and the healing arts developed through trial and error, with many adverse outcomes and deaths along the way. Although both practitioners and patients were aware that health could be compromised by the 'cures' used to alleviate disease, it was in ancient Greece that patient safety was formally acknowledged as the highest priority. The maxim *primum non nocere* (First, do no harm) is attributed by some historians to Galen (AD 131–201) and is still a basic tenet of modern medical practice (Ilan & Fowler 2005).

As societies developed over the centuries, so too did their systems of medicine and healing — particularly the Vedic system of medicine, which originated more than 3000 years ago in India, and Chinese medicine, which has an appreciation of the importance of dosage. Persian medicine had a major influence on the development of medicine in the Middle East and Europe, most notably with *The canon of medicine*, written by the Persian scientist Avicenna (AD 980–1037) in the 11th century. This major work documented 760 medicines, made comments about their use and effectiveness, and remained a standard medical text in western Europe for seven centuries. Avicenna recommended the testing of new medicines on animals and humans before general use, no doubt in recognition of their potential to have both beneficial and harmful effects.

In medieval Europe, there was a mixture of scientific and spiritual influences on the practice of medicine, so factors such as destiny, sin and astrology played a role in perceptions of health and disease. Two major trends appeared during this period, as the practice of medicine developed among both physicians of the upper classes and folk healers who lived in the villages. From the 14th to 17th centuries monasteries played a major role in the provision of medicine and developed great expertise in pharmacognosy. At the same time, the Christian church was instrumental in eliminating much of the practice of folk medicine through its witch hunts, which many believe retarded the development of medicine.

In the 16th century, Paracelsus (1493–1541) was one of the first physicians to believe that chemicals could cure and cause certain illnesses. He determined that specific chemicals were responsible for the toxicity of a plant or animal poison, and documented the body's responses to those chemicals. Paracelsus then concluded that the body's response was influenced by the dose received. He further discovered that a small dose of a substance may be harmless, or even beneficial, whereas a larger dose can be toxic. In essence, he started expounding the concept of a dose–response relationship. Paracelsus made an enormous contribution to medicine when he stated plainly, 'What is there that is not poison? All things are poison and nothing (is) without poison. Solely the dose determines that a thing is not a poison' (Watson 2005). As a result, he is sometimes referred to as the 'Father of Toxicology'.

In practice, this refers to the biological effect of chemicals that can be either beneficial or deleterious. Which of these effects occurs depends on the amount of active material present at the site of action (internal dose), and the concentration of the amount present relates to the amount of substance administered (external dose).

During the 18th and 19th centuries deliberate clinical testing of medicines began, and the study of dose–response relationships led to the safer use of medicines. From the 19th century onwards, developments in pharmacology, physiology and chemistry meant that drugs could be artificially synthesised and produced by large-scale manufacturing. During this time, animal- and plant-based medicines began to be replaced in clinical use by mass-produced pharmaceutical medicines which were being newly created in laboratories or synthesised from traditional medicines (e.g. morphine from *Papaver somniferum*).

Up to this point, Western herbalism had been intrinsically linked to the practice of medicine, and herbal products were an important source of treatment. Empirical knowledge accumulated and formed a body of evidence, now referred to as 'traditional evidence', a knowledge base built on the basic tenets of good clinical practice (i.e. careful observation of the patient, the environment and the diseases). This huge and diverse store of learning includes not only prescriptions for health, but also safety information. The traditional evidence base is still expanding and becoming more accessible as researchers investigate and document various healing practices worldwide. Although traditional evidence provides a valuable starting point, it has many limitations, especially with regard to issues of safety. Careful patient observation is likely to detect immediate or serious adverse effects, but is less likely to identify slow-onset responses or mild-to-moderate side effects that could be considered symptoms of a new disease. Additionally, many medicinal preparations contained multiple ingredients, making it difficult to identify which one might be responsible for inducing an adverse reaction.

More recently, the traditional evidence base has been joined by a scientific evidence base, which provides additional information about pharmacological actions, clinical effects and safety; however, much still remains unknown.

CLINICAL NOTE — HISTORY OF POISONS

The history of poisons dates back to the earliest times, when humans observed toxic effects in nature, most likely by chance. By 1500 BC, written records indicate that the poisons hemlock, opium and certain metals were used in warfare and in facilitating executions. Over time, poisons were used with greater sophistication; notable poisoning victims include Socrates, Cleopatra and Claudius. Today, the 'science of poisons' is known as toxicology. This field of learning investigates the chemical and physical properties of poisons and their physiological or behavioural effects on living organisms, and uses qualitative and quantitative methods for analysis and for the development of procedures to treat poisoning (Langman & Kapur 2006). The 20th century was marked by an advanced understanding of toxicology; DNA and various biochemicals that maintain cellular functions were discovered, so that today we are discovering the toxic effects on organs and cells at the molecular level.

This is particularly true regarding the safety of CMs in children and in women who are pregnant or lactating, and concerning drug interactions, which is a relatively new phenomenon. Just as Galen pronounced hundreds of years ago, 'First, do no harm' should remain the practitioner's guide.

WHAT IS SAFETY?

Safety is a complex issue that is determined by considering the interaction between 'likelihood' and 'consequence'. These two variables will differ for each medicine and individual. The likelihood can be graded from 'near impossible' to 'certainly likely', and the severity of consequence can be graded from 'negligible' to 'serious and life-threatening', with many outcomes lying somewhere between these extremes (Fig 3.1).

With regard to medication safety, avoidance of an adverse drug reaction (ADR) is paramount. Several factors are associated with an increased likelihood of developing an ADR, such as advanced age and polypharmacy, but most ADRs occur in people who are prescribed treatment within the limits of accepted clinical practice (Burgess et al 2005).

BENEFITS, RISK AND HARM

Many different sources of risk are associated with therapeutic products:

- **The product itself** — side effects and toxicity of ingredients, administration form, potential harm through excessive dosage and length of time used.

FIGURE 3.1 Interaction between the two variables of 'likelihood' and 'severity of consequence' with regard to medication safety

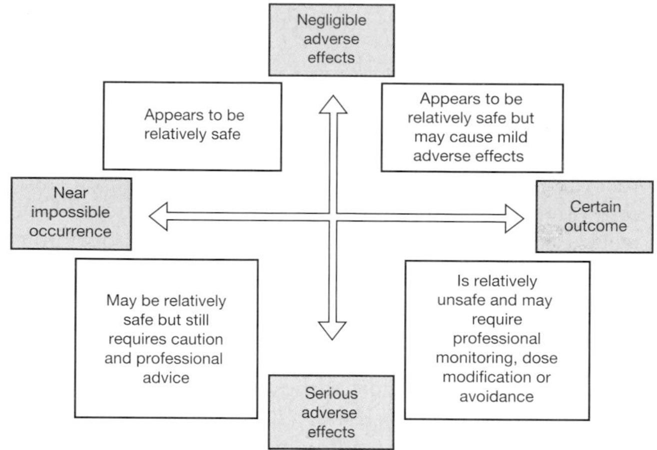

- **Manufacturing factors** — poor manufacturing process, which introduces contaminants, uses unsafe excipients or incorrect ingredients, incorrect labelling etc.
- **Prescribing faults** — incorrect product prescribed, based on insufficient information about it, the patient or the disease, or simply negligence.
- **Patient factors** — incorrect use of a product when information for appropriate use is poorly understood, or insufficient or inappropriate self-diagnosis and treatment.

Whenever a treatment is chosen, it is done so in the belief that its potential benefit will outweigh its potential to cause harm. Practice guidelines and traditions provide guidance when making risk–benefit evaluations and are based on common treatment decisions made many times before by many clinicians, together with the available evidence. Table 3.1 lists the potential risks associated with the use of complementary medicines. The safety information tends to come from a variety of sources, such as post-marketing surveillance and spontaneous reporting schemes, laboratory and animal studies, anecdotal reports, theoretical reasoning and, increasingly, formal studies.

The amount of safety literature published on pharmaceutical medicines is overwhelming. It has been estimated that 30% of the primary published literature about ADR appears in anecdotal reports and 35% as formal studies or randomised controlled trials (Aronson et al 2002). Regarding the safety of complementary medicines, traditional evidence and theoretical reasoning are heavily relied upon to provide guidance together with post-market surveillance studies and information from adverse event

TABLE 3.1 POTENTIAL RISKS ASSOCIATED WITH THE USE OF COMPLEMENTARY MEDICINES

TYPE OF HARM	CIRCUMSTANCES
Delay in diagnosis	When a patient has avoided or delayed seeking medical advice because they are self-treating with CMs. When a complementary medicine practitioner has not referred a patient to a medical practitioner for early diagnosis.
Adverse effects	Increased risk of adverse reactions with inappropriate use of CM products or when patients self-select CM products without professional advice. Increased risk if products used are not manufactured to pharmaceutical grade quality.
Drug interactions	Increased risk of drug interactions when patients: (a) self-select CM products without professional advice; (b) do not disclose use of CM products to their pharmacist or medical doctor; (c) do not disclose use of pharmaceutical drugs to their CM practitioner.
Financial cost	If an expensive medicine or therapy is not providing benefits and a patient continues to use it, this presents an unnecessary financial burden.
Lost opportunity to treat	Failure to undertake a different treatment with proven benefits, when the current treatment is ineffective but is being used to the exclusion of others.
False hope of a cure	When cure is unlikely, the use of any medicine or therapy that is associated with false hope may delay important considerations, such as attending to 'unfinished business'.

databases. Some clinical studies have looked at safety of the test intervention; however, this tends to be a secondary aim and often studies are not sufficiently powered to identify side effects. This poses a challenge for practitioners when making a rational decision about the relative risks of treatment and is one of the great difficulties of CM practice. For the public who are interested in using OTC products, it is just as difficult to find reliable and understandable information about their safety and efficacy.

ADVERSE DRUG REACTIONS (ADRs)

The World Health Organization (WHO) defines an ADR as a 'response to a medicine which is noxious and unintended that occurs at doses normally used in humans'. When two medicines interact in a way that produces an unwanted effect, this is also referred to as an ADR. Adverse reactions have been classified into different types depending on severity and likelihood or onset of reaction, and do not always result in serious outcomes; however, an ADR is considered serious when it is suspected of causing death, danger to life, admission to hospital, prolongation of hospital stay, absence from productive activity, increased investigational or treatment costs, or birth defects.

Adverse reactions can arise from either an intrinsic or an extrinsic effect. An intrinsic effect refers to the active ingredient itself, such as the herbal medicine present within a product, whereas an extrinsic effect relates to product characteristics resulting from poor manufacturing processes or quality control, such as contamination and adulteration. Intrinsic adverse effects can be categorised in a similar way to pharmaceutical medicines and are mainly type A or type B reactions.

Type A reactions

Type A reactions are the most common form and are typically dose-related, predictable from the known pharmacology of the medicine, associated with high morbidity but low mortality, and potentially avoidable (Routledge et al 2004). People most at risk of a type A reaction are frail, older patients who are also likely to be receiving a combination of medicines and those with altered hepatic or renal function. There is now mounting evidence to indicate that some type A adverse reactions are due to genetic polymorphisms, which affect an individual's drug clearance rate and therefore toxicological response. This may explain why certain individuals taking medicines in the recommended doses experience adverse reactions, whereas the majority of the population do not. Examples related to pharmaceutical medicine are bleeding with anticoagulants and hypoglycaemia with the use of insulin. An example for herbal medicine is licorice-associated hypertension, which is thought to be caused by increased renal sodium retention. The glycyrrhetinic acid in licorice inhibits renal 11-beta-hydroxysteroid dehydrogenase type 2 and, by that mechanism, increases the access of cortisol to the mineralocorticoid receptor that causes renal sodium retention and potassium loss. If continued for sufficient time, clinically significant changes in blood pressure and potassium status develop. This can be avoided by recommending that high-dose licorice herbal products not be used for longer than 2 weeks (Heilmann et al 1999). In recognition of this adverse effect, some manufacturers produce licorice products that do not contain glycyrrhetinic acid, so that they can be used more safely in the long term.

Table 3.2 gives some examples of known or suspected type A adverse reactions to herbs and natural supplements. For many herbal and natural medicines, there is insufficient reliable information about possible adverse reactions; where available, evidence from clinical trials, case reports and post-marketing surveillance systems are the main sources of information used in this book.

Type B reactions

Type B reactions are idiosyncratic and uncommon, difficult to predict and not dose related. They tend to have higher morbidity and mortality than type A reactions and are often immunologically mediated (Myers & Cheras 2004). Other factors contributing to type B reactions are receptor

TABLE 3.2 EXAMPLES OF KNOWN OR SUSPECTED TYPE A ADVERSE REACTIONS TO HERBS AND NATURAL SUPPLEMENTS

HERB OR NATURAL SUPPLEMENT	ADVERSE EFFECT/S
Andrographis paniculata	Vomiting, anorexia and gastrointestinal discomfort
Creatine	Nausea, vomiting, cramping, dehydration, fluid retention
Trigonella foenum (fenugreek)	Diarrhoea, flatulence
Fish oils	Gastrointestinal discomfort, diarrhoea
Allium sativum (garlic)	Breath and body odour, nausea, dyspepsia, flatulence, diarrhoea, increased bleeding
Zingiber officinale (ginger)	Gastric irritation, dyspepsia
Camellia sinensis (green or black tea)	CNS stimulation
Gymnema sylvestre	Hypoglycaemia
Paullinia cupana (guarana)	CNS stimulation
Selenium	Nausea, vomiting, irritability, fatigue, nail changes

or drug metabolism abnormalities and the unmasking of a biological deficiency (e.g. glucose-6-phosphate dehydrogenase deficiency) (Bryant et al 2003). They do not appear to relate to genetic polymorphisms.

An example of a type B reaction to a pharmaceutical drug is interstitial nephritis with the use of NSAIDs. With regard to CMs, *Asteraceae* dermatitis provides a good example of a type B hypersensitivity reaction — specifically, an allergic contact dermatitis caused by exposure to allergens from the *Asteraceae* family or the daisy group of plants and plant extracts. Some examples of common plants that belong to this family are arnica (*Arnica montana*), chamomile (*Chamomilla recucita*), marigold (*Calendula officinalis*), echinacea (*Echinacea* spp), tansy (*Tanacetum vulgare*), feverfew (*Tanacetum parthenium*) and yarrow (*Achillea millefolium*). The most important allergens in the *Asteraceae* family are the sesquiterpene lactones, which are present in the oleoresin fraction of the leaves, stems, flowers and possibly pollen (Gordon 1999). The condition is most frequently seen in middle-aged and elderly people; it typically starts in summer and disappears in the autumn or winter. The dermatitis manifests as eczema and can develop from exposure to airborne particles, direct topical application (such as cosmetics, perfumes, essential oils) or oral ingestion of allergenic components. The diagnosis of allergy can be difficult to establish, because there are few completely reliable laboratory tests and sometimes symptoms can mimic infectious disease symptoms. Table 3.3 gives examples of known or suspected type B adverse reactions.

TABLE 3.3 EXAMPLES OF KNOWN OR SUSPECTED TYPE B ADVERSE REACTIONS TO HERBS AND NATURAL SUPPLEMENTS

HERB OR NATURAL SUPPLEMENT	ADVERSE EFFECT/S
Andrographis paniculata	Urticaria
Aloe vera	Hypersensitivity and contact dermatitis
Chamomilla recutita	Asteraceae dermatitis
Echinacea spp	Asteraceae dermatitis and anaphylaxis
Tanacetum parthenium (feverfew)	Asteraceae dermatitis — lip swelling, mouth ulceration and soreness when the leaves are chewed
Zingiber officinale (ginger)	Contact dermatitis with topical use
Thymus vulgaris (thyme)	Contact dermatitis with topical use of the oil

Extrinsic factors

Extrinsic factors are also a consideration and of particular relevance when medicinal products are not manufactured according to the standards of good manufacturing practice, such as some produced in the USA and various Asian countries. Problems can result from a lack of standardisation, contamination, substitution of raw materials, adulteration or incorrect extraction, preparation or dosage information.

THE 'BOTANICAL ADULTERANTS PROGRAM'

Three leading nonprofit organisations — the American Botanical Council (ABC), the American Herbal Pharmacopoeia (AHP), and the University of Mississippi's National Center for Natural Products Research (NCNPR) initiated a large-scale program to educate members of the herbal and dietary supplement industry about ingredient and product adulteration. This arose because of concerns within the herbal and dietary supplement community about the suspected and confirmed practice of adulteration of numerous ingredients. This raises questions about the identity and quality of some popular herbal ingredients sold in dietary supplements in the United States and in other botanical products (e.g. medicines, cosmetics, etc.) in global markets.

It is understood that adulteration of herbal ingredients can be accidental or deliberate. The ABC-AHP-NCNPR Botanical Adulterants Program will focus on both accidental adulteration that occurs as a result of poor quality-control procedures, as well as the intentional adulteration of plant-based products for financial gain. This industry-funded program aspires to serve as a self-regulatory mechanism for industry to address adulteration problems through education rather than federal regulation.

For more information go to: http://abc.herbalgram.org/site/PageNavigator/About_Adulterants_Program.html

REGULATION AND PRODUCT INFORMATION

Numerous regulations are in place in Australia and New Zealand to protect people from potentially unsafe and dubious therapeutic products. Both countries have an international best-practice, risk-based regulatory system that encompasses both complementary and pharmaceutical medicines. Currently the Therapeutic Goods Administration (TGA) regulates the system in Australia, and aims to ensure the safety and quality of products and the truthful labelling of therapeutic goods. All products are entered onto the Australian Register of Therapeutic Goods (ARTG) and allocated an AUST L number if considered low risk (most CM products) or AUST R number if considered high risk, or low risk with a high-level claim (prescription drugs and many OTC pharmaceutical medicines). Products with either an Aust L or an Aust R number have been evaluated for safety and quality, whereas those with an AUST R number have also been evaluated for efficacy. Importantly, the TGA does not undertake the evaluation itself but relies on sponsors to provide the evidence.

The TGA also acts to ensure that all therapeutic products (complementary and pharmaceutical) are produced according to the code of Good Manufacturing Practice (GMP), and both licenses and audits manufacturers. Since the Pan Pharmaceuticals debacle in 2003, when more than 1000 CM products were recalled owing to quality control concerns, there have been calls for more frequent auditing of manufacturers in order to maintain closer control over product quality.

It appears that many people are unclear about the TGA's role in this regard and think it has a greater capacity to monitor product quality than actually occurs. According to a survey of more than 3000 people living in South Australia, approximately half assumed that CMs were independently tested by a government agency (MacLennan et al 2006).

It is important to note that the regulation of therapeutic goods varies greatly between countries and is influenced by ethnological, medical and historical factors. For instance, CM products are treated as foods by the Food and Drug Administration in the USA and not required to be manufactured to the same quality-control standards as pharmaceutical medicines (Brownie 2005).

While the regulation of CM products in Australia can always be improved, the current system employed by the TGA is providing an important safeguard for the public. This was clearly demonstrated in a national survey of over 1100 pharmacy customers attending 60 community pharmacies across Australia (Braun et al 2010a). Of the entire sample, 72% had taken a complementary medicine in the previous 12 months. Of these 7% (n = 55) thought they had experienced a side effect to a CM product at some time. Most (71%) described their reaction as mild, 22% as moderate and four people as severe. That works out at less than 0.5% of CM product users suspecting they had a serious reaction. As further details were not provided about the suspected reaction, causality could not be determined and the figures serve as a guide only.

RELIABLE INFORMATION SOURCES

When it comes to sources of information about herbal and natural medicines, Australian consumer reports consistently put family and friends as people's main sources of information about CM. This was first seen back in a 1999 Australian consumer report which found that 51% of people surveyed ask their friends or relatives for advice, with their mothers ranked as number one for healthcare advice (and it is open to debate as to where the mothers get their information from). In 2001, an Australian rural survey produced similar results, finding that 64.5% of people first ask family and friends for advice (Wilkinson & Simpson 2001). Interestingly, 78% of nursing, pharmacy or biomedical science students had used CAM in the previous 12 months, and 56% had visited a CAM practitioner. They, too, cited friends and family as their main sources of information (Wilkinson & Simpson 2001). More recent studies keep confirming that people seek advice from their family and friends and medical doctors and pharmacists are never ranked higher.

In recent years information technology has revolutionised the availability of health information for both practitioners and their patients. Besides relying on traditional sources of health information, such as healthcare providers, family and friends, people now have easy access to a variety of sources, particularly since the advent of the internet, email and text messaging.

Advertising plays a role in informing consumers about therapeutic products and is regulated by the government. Advertisements must comply with the Therapeutic Products Advertising Code and Therapeutic Product Act(s) and Rules, which state that advertising must be truthful, balanced and not misleading, and promote responsible use, and that the claims must be substantiated. The regulations relate to advertisements disseminated in all forms of media, including emails, websites and SMS messages. However, some information routes are exempt: bona fide news, editorial, public interest or entertainment programs are not restricted by the code, allowing for freedom of speech, but also allowing for sensationalism and inaccuracies.

In 2000, a study published in the *New England Journal of Medicine* found that media coverage of new drugs often exaggerates their benefits and downplays the associated risks (Moynihan et al 2000). The study analysed a sample of 207 stories released by 40 media outlets (36 newspapers, 4 television networks), which appeared between 1994 and 1998. Of the stories reviewed, 40% did not report benefits quantitatively and, of those that did, 83% used statistics to exaggerate the beneficial effect of the drug. Potential harm associated with use of the drug was not mentioned in 53% of stories, and 70% failed to mention costs. Based on the results of this study, it was concluded that news media stories about medicines may be inadequate or incomplete regarding benefits, risks and costs, and may fail to disclose financial ties between researchers and pharmaceutical companies.

It is clear that a number of factors influence the way journalists report health issues in the news media. One important factor relates to the information provided (or not provided) to the journalist by a medical journal, researcher or company in a press release. The following case about the safety of echinacea provides a local example. In 2002, an article entitled 'Adverse reactions associated with echinacea — the Australian experience' was published in a scientific journal. It described in detail five allergic reactions to different echinacea preparations, further stating that 51 adverse reaction reports involving echinacea had been reported to the Adverse Drug Reactions Advisory Committee (ADRAC) (Mullins & Heddle 2002). This was then reported in the news media as alarming and drew much debate about the safety of herbal medicines in general. Inspection of the original article reveals that the reports were collected over a 21-year period, an important fact that failed to be included in the original press release (Flinders Medical Centre 2006).

A study published in the *Journal of the American Medical Association* suggests that incomplete or inaccurate press releases may be more common than once thought (Woloshin & Schwartz 2002). The study assessed the quality of press releases from seven high-profile journals, which were selected for their professional influence and because they are frequently cited by the news media. It was identified that for 544 articles published in the journals over the study period, 127 press releases were issued. Of these press releases, only 23% reported study limitations, 65% quantified study results and only 22% reported the source of funding.

Ideally, journalists, program researchers and writers involved in the media need to be able to assess the scientific information provided to them, and then present it accurately to consumers in a way that is easy to understand, unambiguous and not misleading, so that they can make better personal health decisions. Inaccurate, incomplete and inconsistent information not only confuses consumers, it also confuses healthcare providers and makes it difficult for them to determine which resource is useful and reliable.

A 2008 study by the National Prescribing Service in Australia found that both general practitioners (GPs) and pharmacists seek or need information regarding complementary medicines, and are particularly interested in information about drug interactions, adverse effects, contraindications and evidence of effectiveness. GPs tend to refer to trade journals, MIMS, the internet in general, and peer-reviewed medical journals for information about CMs. Pharmacists' most common sources were the internet, MIMS and the Australian Pharmaceutical Products (APP) guide, colleagues and complementary medicine textbooks (Brown et al 2008). Interestingly, when asked which information sources were considered moderately or highly useful, CM textbooks came out on top for both groups of healthcare professionals. This implies that practitioners who only used standard drug information sources were not accessing the most useful resources available. Another consequence is the assumption by these practitioners that either little evidence exists (because little is available in standard pharmaceutical or medical texts or journals), or that there are no good resources.

Similarly, a study funded by the Department of Health and Ageing and the Pharmacy Guild that investigated the quality use of medicines in relation to complementary medicines found that pharmacists have trouble locating information they consider credible, and are keen for standardised information to be endorsed by a reputable organisation and made widely available.

MEDICAL DATABASES AND TEXTS: INCONSISTENCY

Unfortunately, some medical databases and textbooks that are widely used in the hospital system and universities are not always up to date; authors don't critically examine the evidence from primary sources and sometimes overstate the safety issues without considering the wider perspective. This makes it extremely difficult for a busy clinician to find accurate information in a timely manner.

An example presented here is the purported interaction between *Ginkgo biloba* and warfarin. Ginkgolides found in ginkgo leaf inhibit platelet aggregation according to in vitro and ex vivo studies. As a result, it has been assumed that the effect is clinically relevant, and ginkgo has been implicated as the causative factor in case reports where haemorrhage has been described in association with ginkgo use (Koch 2005). It has also led many writers and clinicians to assume that a pharmacodynamic interaction exists between ginkgo and drugs affecting haemostasis at the platelet level (Bone 2008). Evidence from multiple controlled studies published over the last 5 years casts doubt on the clinical significance of this theoretical interaction, indicating it is unsubstantiated (see monograph on *Ginkgo biloba* for further details). Major databases and textbooks on complementary medicines provide quite different information to readers about this issue, adding to the confusion (Table 3.4).

ADR INCIDENCE

Alarmingly, the rates of ADR-related hospital admissions are rising and account for considerable morbidity, mortality and costs. One Australian study found that one in ten patients who visited a GP had experienced a significant ADR within the previous 6 months, and almost 50% of these were assessed as moderate to severe by the GP (Miller et al 2006). An ADR is more likely to be experienced with increasing age, peaking at 65 years and older, and by females rather than males. Children aged between 1 and 4 years are three times more likely to have an ADR than children in other age groups. At this rate, ADRs rank as one of the most important

TABLE 3.4 EXAMPLES OF CURRENT DATABASES AND TEXTBOOKS REPORTING ON THE PURPORTED GINKGO–WARFARIN INTERACTION

RESOURCE	INTERACTION INFORMATION	COMMENTS
MIMS on CD	'Warfarin interacts with a wide range of complementary medicines, including vitamin and herbal preparations, e.g. Gingko biloba … have confirmed or potential interactions with warfarin.'	Accessed 10 July 2008 Ginkgo spelt incorrectly Insufficient information provided
eAMH (Australian Medicines Handbook)	No interaction information	Accessed 10 July 2008 Last updated Jan 2008
AltMedDex (Thomson Reuters 2008)	'Concomitant use of ginkgo and anticoagulants may increase the risk of bleeding complications. '*Adverse effect:* increased risk of bleeding '*Clinical management:* Avoid concomitant use of ginkgo and anticoagulants. '*Severity:* major '*Onset:* delayed '*Documentation:* fair '*Probable mechanism:* Ginkgolide B may inhibit platelet activating factor (PAF)-induced platelet aggregation'	Accessed 10 July 2008 Information does not reflect current evidence base.
The desktop guide to complementary and alternative medicine (Ernst et al 2006)	'Potentiation of anticoagulants is often mentioned, but a systematic review of the evidence refuted the notion.'	Published 2006 Succinct and evidence based
Herbs and natural supplements — an evidence based guide (Braun & Cohen 2007)	'Theoretically, ginkgo may increase bleeding risk when used together with warfarin; however, two randomised double-blind studies have found that *Ginkgo biloba* does not affect the pharmacokinetics or pharmacodynamics, INR or clinical effects of warfarin … and two clinical trials have not found evidence of significant effects on bleeding … Due to the potential seriousness of such an interaction, caution is still advised.'	Last updated 2006 Evidence based
The ABC clinical guide to herbs (Blumenthal 2003)	'Interaction with drugs inhibiting blood coagulation cannot be excluded.' Several case reports of bleeding reported, followed by RCTs showing no evidence of interaction with warfarin or aspirin.	Published 2003 Evidence based

causes of morbidity. Anticoagulants, NSAIDs and cardiovascular medicines feature prominently as preventable, high-impact problems in Australia and other countries (Pirmohamed et al 2004, Runciman et al 2003).

Although ADRs also occur with CMs, relatively few reports have been collected through spontaneous post-marketing surveillance systems. The most extensive database of ADRs to herbal medicines is held by the Uppsala Monitoring Centre, the coordinating centre for the WHO Programme for International Drug Monitoring (see www.who-umc.org). It receives data from national centres in 72 countries and, over the past 20 years, 11,716 case reports of suspected herbal ADR have been collected. The most commonly reported non-critical effects were (from higher to lower incidence): pruritus, urticaria, rash, erythematous rash, nausea, vomiting, diarrhoea, fever, abdominal pain and dyspnoea. The most common critical effects were: facial oedema, hepatitis, angio-oedema, thrombocytopenia, hypertension, chest pain, convulsions, purpurea, dermatitis and death.

In Australia, the ADRAC database holds reports of suspected ADRs. From 1 November 1972 to 19 April 2005, it has only 1112 reports related solely to CMs. This is reassuring, when one considers that in 2004 approximately 52% of the population were identified as users of at least one non-medically prescribed CM product in the previous 12 months (MacLennan et al 2006). The relatively small number of case reports can be interpreted as indicative of the comparative safety of CMs and the effectiveness of pre-market checks; however, the impact of under-reporting should not be dismissed.

Research on under-reporting of serious ADRs in the USA and Canada suggests that formal reporting rates may be as low as 1.5% of total ADRs (Miller et al 2006). In the specific case of CMs, CAM practitioners and retail staff may not report such events because:

- they are unaware of ADR schemes
- they are not qualified or trained to consider the possibility of ADRs
- they are not motivated to report any ADR that comes to their notice.

In addition, herbal medicine consumers may not be motivated to report ADRs to their doctor, as one British study suggests (Barnes et al 1998), or they may not consider the possibility that their symptoms may be related to the CM products they use.

CASE REPORTS AND POST-MARKETING SURVEILLANCE SYSTEMS

Given that current knowledge about CMs is incomplete and that controlled studies are often lacking for CAM, well-documented case reports can serve as a critical early warning system until further research is undertaken, whereas poorly documented case reports can be misleading. Unfortunately, reports of ADRs with herbal medicines often cause some controversy and contain incomplete data; for example, one systematic review, which assessed information from four electronic databases, located 108 cases of suspected medicine–herb interactions. Of these, 68.5% were classified as 'unable to be evaluated' and only 13% were described as 'well-documented' (Fugh-Berman & Ernst 2001). Table 3.5 lists the elements that should be included in a report of an adverse reaction.

Besides improving the quality of reporting, the ideal would be to chemically analyse the product to authenticate the ingredients and make sure that quality control issues are not involved. This is particularly important when the implicated product has not been manufactured under a strict GMP code.

Much of the information obtained from the current spontaneous post-marketing surveillance systems about CM safety is of limited value, as it does not provide an estimate of the incidence of adverse reactions. Without understanding the level of incidence, case reports can easily be interpreted as cause for alarm or alternatively dismissed as irrelevant. Additionally, authorities discourage reporting of less severe ADRs, so many mild-to-moderate side effects remain undetected and are a hidden source of patient morbidity.

Post-marketing surveillance systems aim to detect trends in ADR and become useful when a large number of reports relating to a specific medicine are received. When evidence gathers to suggest a significant problem, the TGA may issue an alert on its website, impose new conditions on the product's listing or registration, suspend or cancel listing or registration, impose new manufacturing conditions and, if considered sufficiently serious, issue a mandatory product recall. Alerts in recent years have included warnings about drug interactions with St John's wort (*Hypericum perforatum*), suspected hepatotoxicity with products containing kava kava and renal toxicity with Chinese herbal medicines containing the herb *Aristolochia*. The Advisory Committee on Complementary Medicines (ACCM) advises the TGA on matters regarding CMs and is made up of people considered expert in this area.

TABLE 3.5 IMPORTANT COMPONENTS OF AN ADVERSE REACTION REPORT
Patient demographics: male/female, age, social history if relevant
Suspected product details: formula as stated on label, batch number, expiry date and Aust L or Aust R number
Details of the person making the report
Manufacturer's details
Relevant medical history
Other medicines and treatments being used (including other complementary medicines)
Dose used, duration of use and administration form
Date and time of onset
Adverse effects: description of signs and symptoms
Outcome of event
Information regarding re-challenge, if applicable
Presence of confounding variables: e.g. additives

The two cases involving black cohosh and kava kava provide examples of how post-marketing surveillance systems can alert government agencies of a potential safety issue and the ensuing steps taken and research conducted to identify what the issue is and its prevalence.

Black cohosh

Rare, spontaneous hepatotoxicity has been reported in at least 42 case reports world-wide with treatment by *Cimicifuga racemosa rhizoma* (Levitsky et al 2005, Lynch et al 2006, Nisbet & O'Connor 2007, Teschke & Schwarzenboeck 2009, Whiting et al 2002). As a result, several safety reviews have been conducted to evaluate the available data and determine what risk exists with the use of this herb.

A 2008 safety review of black cohosh products was conducted by the Dietary Supplement Information Expert Committee of the US Pharmacopeia's Council of Experts. All the reports of liver damage were assigned possible causality, and none were probable or certain causality. The clinical pharmacokinetic and animal toxicological information did not reveal unfavourable information about black cohosh. The Expert Committee determined that in the United States black cohosh products should be labelled to include a cautionary statement, a change from their decision of 2002, which required no such statement (Mahady et al 2008).

Assessment of the 42 cases by European Medicines Agency (EMEA) has shown a possible or probable causality in only four out of 42 patients. A diagnostic algorithm has been applied in the four patients with suspected BC (Black cohosh) hepatotoxicity using several methods to allow objective assessment, scoring and scaling of the probability in each case. Due to incomplete data, the case of one patient was not assessable. For the remaining three patients, quantitative evaluation showed no causality for BC in any patient regarding the observed severe liver disease (Teschke & Schwarzenboeck 2009).

In Australia in February 2006, the TGA announced that based on the appraisal of case reports, a causal association between black cohosh and serious hepatitis exists; however, the incidence is very low considering its widespread use. As a result, products available in Australia containing black cohosh have to carry label warnings informing consumers of the risk. The conclusion made by the TGA is considered controversial by some experts because numerous confounding factors were present in many of the case reports, such as the use of multiple ingredient preparations, concurrent use of at least one pharmaceutical medicine and the presence of other medical conditions.

A 2008 study evaluated the effects of black cohosh extract on liver morphology and on levels of various hepatic function indices in an experimental model finding that at high doses, well above the recommended dosage, black cohosh appears quite safe (Mazzanti et al 2008).

More recently, Teschke (2010b) investigated data from 69 spontaneous or published case reports of suspected black cohosh-induced hepatotoxicity and found confounding variables such as uncertainty about the quality and authenticity of the black cohosh product, dose or insufficient adverse event description, missing or inadequate evaluation of a clear temporal association, the possible presence of other medications or comorbidities and lack of de-challenge or re-exposure. A clear causal relationship between black cohosh and hepatotoxicity was not found.

Even more recently, a 2011 meta-analysis investigated the potential hepatotoxicity of black cohosh (Remifemin) from published RCTs in perimenopausal and postmenopausal women. Liver function data (AST, ALT and γ-GT) from 1020 women was compared at baseline and after taking black cohosh (40–128 mg/day) for 3 to 6 months. No significant difference between the treatment and reference groups were found (Naser et al 2011).

Kava kava

Kava was well tolerated and considered as devoid of major side effects until 1998 when the first reports of kava hepatotoxicity appeared. Causality of hepatotoxicity for kava ± co-medicated drugs was evident after the use of predominantly ethanolic and acetonic kava extracts in Germany ($n = 7$), Switzerland ($n = 2$), United States ($n = 1$) and Australia ($n = 1$) as well as after aqueous extracts in New Caledonia ($n = 2$) (Teschke et al 2008a). Moreover, cases of tourists developing serious toxic liver disease after consumption of kava beverages in traditional Samoan kava ceremonies were reported (Christl et al 2009). For this reason, in 2002 the herb was withdrawn from various European countries (Sarris et al 2013), and the FDA issued a safety alert about kava and its liver problems (Teschke et al 2010a). In 2002 in Australia, the TGA posed a maximum limit of 125 mg kava lactones on kava tablets or capsules and a maximum of 3 g of dried rhizome per teabag with a maximum daily dose of 250 mg kava lactones allowed.

Various authors evaluated the reported cases. In an analysis of 36 cases of hepatotoxicity, the pattern of injury was both hepatocellular and cholestasis, the majority of patients were women, the culmative dose and latency were highly variable and liver transplant was necessary in eight of the cases (Stickel et al 2003). The WHO published a report in May 2007 entitled *Assessment of the risk of hepatotoxicity with kava products* (WHO 2007). It evaluated data from 93 case reports of which 8 were determined to have a close association between the use of kava kava and liver dysfunction; 53 cases were classified as having a possible relationship, but they could not be fully assessed due to insufficient data or other potential causes of liver damage; five cases had a positive rechallenge. Most of the other case reports could not be evaluated due to lack of information. It concluded that there is 'significant concern' for a cause and effect relationship between kava products and hepatotoxicity, especially for organic extracts. The report noted other risk factors such as heavy alcohol intake, preexisting liver disease, genetic polymorphisms of cytochrome P450 enzymes, excessive dosage and co-medication with other potentially hepatotoxic drugs and potentially interacting drugs.

Similarly, Teschke et al analysed 26 suspected cases of which causality was unassessable, unrelated or excluded for 16 cases owing to lack of temporal association and causes independent of kava or co-medicated drugs. Overall, the survey concluded that kava taken as recommended is associated with rare hepatotoxicity, whereas overdose, prolonged treatment and co-medication may carry an increased risk (Teschke et al 2008b, Teschke et al 2010a). However, several papers outlined pros and cons of the current methods of causality evaluation (Teschke et al 2011, Teschke & Wolff 2011).

The latest publications have accepted a causal relationship between the use of various kava extracts, including aqueous extracts, and liver injury, and have focused on an assessment of possible causes (Teschke et al 2009). Despite this, evidence is still lacking of in vivo hepatotoxicity in experimental animals under conditions similar to human kava use. Furthermore, in commercial Western kava extracts, pipermethystine was not detectable and flavokavain B was present as a natural compound in amounts much too low to cause experimental liver injury (Lechtenberg et al 2008).

More recent reports have postulated that mould hepatotoxins present in kava raw material may be the cause of hepatotoxicity (Teschke et al 2012, Teschke et al 2013). This could be the case given that aflatoxins have been detected in kava samples (Rowe & Ramzan 2012).

Strict guidelines for kava standardisation have now been suggested by several researchers. They include: (1) use of a noble kava cultivar such as Borogu, at least 5 years old at time of harvest, (2) use of peeled and dried rhizomes and roots, (3) aqueous extraction, (4) dosage recommendation of ≤ 250 mg kavalactones per day (for medicinal use), (5) systematic rigorous future research and (6) a Pan Pacific quality control system enforced by strict policing (Teschke et al 2011).

FACTORS THAT MAKE AN ADR MORE LIKELY

Although little investigation has been conducted into what factors influence the likelihood of ADRs with CMs, it can be assumed most factors that increase the risk of ADRs with pharmaceutical medicine will also apply to CMs. These factors can be grouped as patient-related or therapeutic.

Patient-related factors

- Older age. Declining liver and kidney function as a result of ageing can increase sensitivity to both therapeutic and adverse effects. During times of ill health, the elderly can experience a further loss of homeostatic reserve, once again increasing sensitivity to the effects of medicines and interactions (Atkinson et al 2001).
- Females appear to be more susceptible to ADRs.

- Concurrent disease, acute and/or severe.
- History of atopic disease.
- Confusion.
- Genetic factors: for example, variations in liver enzymes.
- Reduced renal or hepatic function. Altered metabolism or excretion of a medicine can increase the risk of toxicity.
- Self-medication. Prudent self-care can offer numerous benefits to the individual, society and the healthcare system if there is access to quality services, products and information. However, when people at higher risk of adverse effects self-medicate with OTC medicines, it can be potentially harmful. Additionally, interactions that do not produce a clinically obvious change, such as elevation in blood pressure, serum cholesterol or warfarin INR, can remain undetected and uncorrected unless professional advice is sought.
- Use of multiple healthcare practitioners. This is of concern when practitioners fail to communicate effectively with one another to ensure that interactions are avoided and identified.

Therapeutic factors

- Dose. Most ADRs are dose-related, with higher doses increasing risk.
- Route of administration (e.g. topical application) can cause delayed hypersensitivity.
- Prolonged and/or frequent therapy.
- Medicines not manufactured under a code of good manufacturing practice (GMP) have an increased risk of extrinsic effects.
- Use of concurrent high-risk medicines; for example, those with a narrow therapeutic index (NTI) such as warfarin, digoxin, lithium, cyclosporin, phenytoin, barbiturates, theophylline, many HIV medicines (e.g. saquinavir), antineoplastic agents (e.g. methotrexate) and anti-arrhythmic agents (e.g. quinidine). These medicines are particularly sensitive to pharmacokinetic alterations in which small changes to blood concentrations can cause a clinically significant change to drug activity. Depending on whether drug concentrations are reduced or increased, there is the potential to cause a loss of efficacy or induce toxic effects, respectively.
- Polypharmacy. This is of particular concern in the elderly, who may have chronic diseases and are known to use more medicines than any other age group, increasing the risk of interactions. Additionally, in many serious diseases such as cancer and HIV, multi-drug treatment is the standard of care.
- Use of medicines known to induce or inhibit cytochrome (CYP) enzymes, particularly CYP 3A4, which is responsible for the metabolism of many common pharmaceutical medicines.

STRATEGIES FOR PREVENTING AND LIMITING ADRs

Many countries are trying to cope with the growing problem of ADRs and their associated morbidity and mortality. Currently in Australia and New Zealand there are many structures and initiatives in place, such as regulatory agencies, the CMEC, 'quality use of medicines' organisations and information providers, safety and quality organisations and professional bodies; however, it is ultimately the practitioner and the patient who play the definitive roles.

Strategies for clinicians

- Encourage open and honest communication — between patient, carer and practitioner, and between fellow practitioners about treatments prescribed. One way of achieving this is for CM practitioners to label all dispensed herbal medicines with the botanical names of the herbs included in the product, together with suggested dosage, date of manufacture and practitioner's contact details.
- Take a careful medical and medicines history, including previous allergies and adverse effects.
- Consider non-medicinal treatments.
- Avoid polypharmacy and complicated treatment regimens.
- Become familiar with the potential safety issues associated with a medicine to avoid unnecessarily inducing an ADR or misdiagnosing one as a symptom of a new disease. An important adjunct to this is having access to reliable medical and CM information, and having a network of experts or informed colleagues to consult. Computer-generated prescriptions and decision-support systems are frequently advocated as possible solutions and can be useful if their information is accurate and updated frequently.
- Regularly review therapeutic goals and medicines being used. This provides an opportunity to promote patient compliance and ensure that the appropriate medicines are being taken safely.
- When problems do arise, practitioners need to be aware of their professional responsibility to report a suspected ADR to one of the following:
  - Adverse Drug Reactions Advisory Committee (Reporting is confidential, open to everyone and is now possible online at www.tga.gov.au.)
  - Relevant herbal and natural medicine associations such as the National Herbalists Association of Australia (www.nhaa.org.au)
  - Relevant manufacturer (Manufacturers keep their own records and are formally obliged to inform the TGA Prescriber, if applicable.)

Strategies for patients

Patients also play an important role in promoting a beneficial and harm-free outcome. They should ensure that they understand the benefits and potential risks associated with their treatment and be confident that they know how to take/use it appropriately. The Australian Commission on Safety and Quality in Health Care produced a patient information booklet entitled *10 tips for safer health care* (ACSQHC 2003) to encourage patients to become more active in their own healthcare while in hospital. Many of the steps outlined in the booklet are relevant to people taking CMs in the community or in hospital.

Below is a summary of recommendations for patients choosing to use or currently using CM, adapted from *10 tips for safer health care*.

- Choose a suitably experienced and qualified CM practitioner or ask for a referral from a trusted medical practitioner, pharmacist or other source.
- Become an active member of your own healthcare team. Help clinicians reach an accurate diagnosis, discuss appropriate management strategies, ensure treatment is administered and adhered to, identify side effects quickly and take appropriate action.
- Tell all healthcare practitioners about all the medicines being used (complementary and conventional). This includes telling doctors about complementary medicines and telling naturopaths and herbalists about pharmaceutical medicines.
- Make sure information given by the healthcare practitioner about the condition and the treatment options available is understood. In the case of lengthy explanations or recommendations, ask the practitioner to provide written information that can be taken home.
- Ask questions when you need more information because you are uncertain or the information provided is unclear.
- Be motivated to learn about the health condition being addressed, treatments being used and ways to improve wellbeing by referring to reliable information sources.

THE RATIONAL USE OF HERBAL AND NATURAL MEDICINES

Overall, when manufactured, prescribed and used appropriately, the safety of OTC CMs is high. Serious adverse effects and dangerous interactions are rare, particularly in comparison with the thousands of reports attributed to pharmaceutical medicines. Even so, the assessment of likely adverse reactions or interactions should remain integral to patient management.

Currently, there are few large-scale clinical studies confirming and clarifying the clinical significance of most suspected adverse reactions and interactions associated with CMs, and much remains unknown. It is important to recognise that the information presented in this book requires individual interpretation, because the clinical effects of any medicine or any potential interaction, no matter how well documented, will not occur consistently in each patient, each time or to the same degree of intensity.

Ultimately, the ideal in clinical practice is to combine knowledge about the medicine and the disease, experience of both, and information about the patient and the individual's circumstance in order to make wise treatment choices (Table 3.6). This requires the application of current knowledge, as well as good observational skills, open communication and clinical experience to reduce the risk of adverse reactions and maximise successful outcomes.

TABLE 3.6 FACTORS TO CONSIDER IN THE RATIONAL USE OF COMPLEMENTARY MEDICINES

FACTORS TO CONSIDER	RATIONALE
Products that are not produced under a code of GMP **should not be used.**	The quality of the product cannot be guaranteed.
Know the benefits, risks, potential adverse reactions and interactions and seek out reliable information. Additional training and/or access to accurate and updated information is important.	More than half the population use CMs and there is no sign of their popularity abating. Some CMs have proven benefits and offer cost-effective treatment options; however, safety issues also exist. Marketing/sales and company information is not sufficient, and education in the area of CM efficacy and safety may be limited.
Do not rely on label claims alone.	Although manufacturers must hold the evidence to support the claims made on a product label, often the label claims do not provide enough information to make an informed judgement.
Do not rely on label dose recommendations alone.	Some manufacturers state the lowest effective dose on the label to ensure that a patient's general requirements will be met; however, in practice, practitioners should prescribe a dose to meet the individual's needs, which may be higher than label doses, yet still be within safe limits.
Take care when high-risk medicines are involved.	In combination with drugs that have a narrow therapeutic index and many anticancer and HIV medicines, screen for interactions. In the case of herbal medicines, any product containing St John's wort (*Hypericum perforatum*) should be considered higher risk. Screen for interactions.
Take care with people considered to be at higher risk of adverse reactions or in 'at risk' circumstances.	Older age; reduced renal or liver function; acute or severe disease; polypharmacy; history of atopy and/or confusion; when drugs with a narrow therapeutic index are involved; during pregnancy or lactation; in children; before major surgery

(Continued)

TABLE 3.6 FACTORS TO CONSIDER IN THE RATIONAL USE OF COMPLEMENTARY MEDICINES *(continued)*

FACTORS TO CONSIDER	RATIONALE
Ensure that all health professionals involved in a patient's care are aware of CM use.	Effective communication will foster appropriate and safe use.
Do not assume all healthcare professionals have the knowledge to monitor safe use.	Few medical practitioners have had formal training in the safety issues of CM, and not all health practitioners have ready access to evidence-based safety data.
Know the manufacturer and supplier details.	If in doubt about a product, call the manufacturer or supplier for more information.
Know the prescriber's details (if relevant).	The original prescriber may have valuable information about the patient and the medicine, which may assist informed decision making.
Medicines should be stored appropriately.	Appropriate storage will depend on the patient's circumstance (e.g. at home, in hospital or in a hospice), level of vigilance and the type of medicine used.

REFERENCES

ACSQHC (Australian Commission on Safety and Quality in Health Care). 10 tips for safer health care. Commonwealth of Australia. 2003.

Aronson JK et al. Adverse drug reactions: keeping up to date. Fundam Clin Pharmacol 16 (2002): 49–56.

Atkinson AJ et al. Principles of clinical pharmacology. London: Academic Press, 2001.

Barnes J et al. Different standards for reporting ADRs to herbal remedies and conventional OTC medicines: face-to-face interviews with 515 users of herbal remedies. Br J Clin Pharmacol 45 (1998): 496–500.

Blumenthal M. ABC clinical guide to herbs. Austin: American Botanical Council, 2003.

Bone KM. Potential interaction of Ginkgo biloba leaf with antiplatelet or anticoagulant drugs: What is the evidence? Mol Nutr Food Res 52.7 (2008): 764–771.

Braun L. The integration of complementary medicine in Victorian hospitals — a focus on surgery and safety. Melbourne: RMIT, 2007.

Braun L, Cohen MM. Herbs and natural supplements: An evidence based guide, 2nd edn. Sydney: Elsevier, 2007.

Braun LA et al. Adverse reactions to complementary medicines: the Australian pharmacy experience. Int J Pharm Pract, 18.4 (2010a): 242–244.

Braun LA et al. Perceptions, use and attitudes of pharmacy customers on complementary medicines and pharmacy practice. BMC Complement Altern Med 10 (2010b): 38.

Broom AF et al. Use of complementary and alternative medicine by mid-age women with back pain: a national cross-sectional survey. BMC Complement Altern Med 12 (2012): 98.

Brown J et al. General practitioners and pharmacists. Complementary medicines information use and needs of health professionals. Sydney: National Prescribing Service, 2008.

Brownie S. The development of the US and Australian dietary supplement regulations: What are the implications for product quality? Complement Ther Med 13 (2005): 191–198.

Bryant B et al. Pharmacology for health professionals. Sydney: Elsevier, 2003.

Burgess CL et al. Adverse drug reactions in older Australians, 1981–2002. Med J Aust 182 (2005): 267–270.

Christl SU et al. Toxic hepatitis after consumption of traditional kava preparation. J Travel Med. Jan-Feb 16.1 (2009): 55–56.

Davis SR et al. Use of complementary and alternative therapy by women in the first 2 years after diagnosis and treatment of invasive breast cancer. Menopause 17.5 (2010): 1004–1009.

Ernst E et al. The desktop guide to complementary and alternative medicine, 2nd edn. London: Mosby, Elsevier, 2006.

Flinders Medical Centre, Government of South Australia. Media release 2006.

Fugh-Berman A, Ernst E. Herb–drug interactions: review and assessment of report reliability. Br J Clin Pharmacol 52 (2001): 587–595.

Gordon LA. Compositae dermatitis. Aust J Dermatol 40 (1999): 123–128.

Grant SJ et al. The use of complementary and alternative medicine by people with cardiovascular disease: a systematic review. BMC Public Health 12 (2012): 299.

Heilmann P et al. Administration of glycyrrhetinic acid: significant correlation between serum levels and the cortisol/cortisone-ratio in serum and urine. Exp Clin Endocrinol Diabetes 107 (1999): 370–378.

Ilan R, Fowler R. Brief history of patient safety culture and science. J Crit Care 20 (2005): 2–5.

Jamison JR. Herbal and nutrient supplementation practices of chiropractic patients: an Australian case study. J Manipulative Physiol Ther 26 (2003): 242.

Koch E. Inhibition of platelet activating factor (PAF)-induced aggregation of human thrombocytes by ginkgolides: considerations on possible bleeding complications after oral intake of Ginkgo biloba extracts. Phytomedicine 12.1–2 (2005): 10–16.

Langman LJ, Kapur BM. Toxicology: then and now. Clin Biochem 39.5 (2006): 498–510.

Lechtenberg M, et al. Is the alkaloid pipermethystine connected with the claimed liver toxicity of Kava products? Pharmazie. 63.1 (2008): 71–74.

Levitsky J et al. Fulminant liver failure associated with the use of black cohosh. Dig Dis Sci 50.3 (2005): 538–539.

Lynch CR et al. Fulminant hepatic failure associated with the use of black cohosh: a case report. Liver Transpl 12.6 (2006): 989–992.

MacLennan A et al. The escalating cost and prevalence of alternative medicine. Prev Med 35 (2002): 166–173.

MacLennan AH et al. The continuing use of complementary and alternative medicine in South Australia: costs and beliefs in 2004. Med J Aust 184 (2006): 27–31.

Mahady GB et al. United States Pharmacopeia review of the black cohosh case reports of hepatotoxicity. Menopause 15.4 Pt 1 (2008): 628–638.

Manya, K et al. The use of complementary and alternative medicine among people living with diabetes in Sydney. BMC Complement Altern Med 12 (2012): 2.

Mazzanti G et al. Effects of Cimicifuga racemosa extract on liver morphology and hepatic function indices. Phytomedicine 15.11 (2008): 1021–1024.

Miller GC et al. Adverse drug events in general practice patients in Australia. Med J Aust 184 (2006): 321–324.

Moynihan R et al. Coverage by the news media of the benefits and risks of medications. N Engl J Med 342 (2000): 1645–1650.

Mullins RJ, Heddle R. Adverse reactions associated with echinacea: the Australian experience. Ann Allergy Asthma Immunol 88 (2002): 42–51.

Myers SP, Cheras PA. The other side of the coin: Safety of complementary and alternative medicine. Med J Aust 181 (2004): 222–225.

Naser B et al. Suspected black cohosh hepatotoxicity: no evidence by meta-analysis of randomized controlled clinical trials for isopropanolic black cohosh extract. Menopause 18.4 (2011): 366–375.

Nisbet BC, O'Connor RE. Black cohosh-induced hepatitis. Del Med J 79.11 (2007): 441–444.

Pirmohamed M et al. Adverse drug reactions as cause of admission to hospital: prospective analysis of 18,820 patients. BMJ 329 (2004): 15–19.

Routledge PA et al. Adverse drug reactions in elderly patients. Br J Clin Pharmacol 57 (2004): 121–126.

Rowe A, Ramzan I. Are mould hepatotoxins responsible for kava hepatotoxicity? Phytother Res. 26.11 (2012):1768–1770.

Runciman WB et al. Adverse drug events and medication errors in Australia. Int J Qual Health Care 15 (Suppl 1) (2003): i49–i59.

Sarris J et al. Kava in the treatment of generalized anxiety disorder: a double-blind, randomized, placebo-controlled study. J Clin. Psychopharmacol. 33 (2013): 643–648.

Stickel F et al. Hepatitis induced by Kava (*Piper methysticum* rhizoma). J Hepatol. 39.1 (2003): 62–67.

Teschke R et al. Kava hepatotoxicity — a clinical review. Ann Hepatol. 9.3 (2010a): 251–265.

Teschke R. Black cohosh and suspected hepatotoxicity: inconsistencies, confounding variables, and prospective use of a diagnostic causality algorithm. A critical review. Menopause 17.2 (2010b): 426–440.

Teschke R, Schwarzenboeck A. Suspected hepatotoxicity by Cimicifugae racemosae rhizoma (black cohosh, root): critical analysis and structured causality assessment. Phytomedicine 16.1 (2009): 72–84.

Teschke R et al. Kava hepatotoxicity: regulatory data selection and causality assessment. Dig Liver Dis. 41.12 (2011): 891–901.

Teschke R et al. Contaminant hepatotoxins as culprits for kava hepatotoxicity — fact or fiction? Phytother Res. 27.3 (2013): 472–474.

Teschke R et al. Kava hepatotoxicity in traditional and modern use: the presumed Pacific kava paradox hypothesis revisited, Br J Clin Pharmacol. 73.2 (2012): 170–174.

Teschke R et al. Herbal hepatotoxicity by kava: update on pipermethystine, flavokavain B, and mould hepatotoxins as primarily assumed culprits. Dig Liver Dis. 43.9 (2011): 676–681.

Teschke R et al. Kava hepatotoxicity: comparison of aqueous, ethanolic, acetonic kava extracts and kava-herbs mixtures. J Ethnopharmacol. 123.3 (2009): 378–384.

Teschke R et al. Kava hepatotoxicity: a European view. NZ Med J 3.121 (2008a): 90–98.

Teschke R et al. Kava hepatotoxicity: a clinical survey and critical analysis of 26 suspected cases. Eur J Gastroenterol Hepatol 20.12 (2008b): 1182–1193.

Teschke R. Kava hepatotoxicity: pathogenetic aspects and prospective considerations. Liver Int. 30.9 (2010b):1270–1279.

Thomson Reuters publishers. Micromedex Health Care Series, AltMedDex 2008.

Watson KD. Toxicology, history of. In: Philip W (ed). Encyclopedia of toxicology. New York: Elsevier, 2005, pp 364–370.

Whiting PW et al. Black cohosh and other herbal remedies associated with acute hepatitis. Med J Aust 177 (2002): 440–443.

WHO. Assessment of the risk of hepatotoxicity with kava products. World Health Organization, May 2007.

Wilkinson JM, Simpson MD. Complementary therapy use by nursing, pharmacy and biomedical science students. Nurs Health Sci 3 (2001): 19–27.

Woloshin S, Schwartz LM. Press releases: translating research into news. JAMA 287 (2002): 2856–2858.

CHAPTER 4

INTERACTIONS WITH HERBAL AND NATURAL MEDICINES

A pharmacological interaction is said to occur when the response to one medicine varies from what is usually predicted because another substance has altered the response. Usually the term 'interaction' has a negative connotation when referring to medicines, because it can lead to drug toxicity or a loss of drug effect, and it may be difficult to predict. However, interactions can also benefit the patient by improving outcomes, reducing side effects or reducing costs. In order for health-care professionals to interpret interaction data and avoid or beneficially manipulate an interaction, or deal with an adverse effect due to an interaction, it is essential to have an understanding of the mechanisms involved.

Although thousands of drug interactions are studied each year, there has been far less scientific investigation into interactions with herbal and natural medicines. Research conducted with pharmaceutical medicines can provide some theoretical insights into the mechanisms of drug–herb interactions, but predicting clinical significance is difficult. Unlike conventional medicines, herbs and food-based supplements contain a complex mixture of bioactive chemicals, some of which may contribute to the overall therapeutic effect of the substances. The chemical composition is also variable and depends on factors such as the plant part used, seasonality, growing and harvesting conditions and extraction and manufacturing processes. Furthermore, some plant constituents have poor oral bioavailability, so in vitro screening for interactions will produce misleading results.

Evidence from controlled human studies has been steadily increasing in recent years; however, most information is still derived from in vitro and animal experiments. This approach is not without its limitations, as using evidence to predict what will happen in humans from studies not conducted in humans is bound to contain inaccuracies and therefore must be interpreted cautiously.

It must be mentioned that even when evidence from a controlled human study is available, predicting the likelihood and severity of a real-life interaction in a specific patient is still difficult and prone to error. Ultimately, the clinical importance of a herb–drug interaction depends on factors that relate to the medicines involved and the patients themselves. The chief medicinal factors will be dose, duration and frequency of use and administration route. Individual patient factors include age, gender, food intake, gastric and urinary pH, current state of health, preexisting disease and genetic polymorphism.

INTERACTION MECHANISMS

When one considers the great variation in physical properties and pharmacological effects of the numerous substances used as medicines, together with the variable nature of herbal medicines, it is apparent that a virtually endless number of interactions are possible. It is generally accepted, however, that there are two major interaction mechanisms, namely pharmacokinetic and pharmacodynamic interactions. A third minor category of physicochemical or pharmaceutical interactions also exists. Regardless of the mechanism involved, there can be three possible outcomes from an interaction:

1. increased therapeutic or adverse effects (additive or synergistic)
2. decreased therapeutic or adverse effects (additive or synergistic)
3. a unique response that does not occur when either agent is used alone.

PHARMACOKINETIC INTERACTIONS

Pharmacokinetics refers to the quantitative analysis of the absorption, distribution, metabolism and excretion of a medicine. Pharmacokinetic interactions occur when there is an alteration to any of these four processes, causing a change in the amount and persistence of available drug at receptor sites or target tissues. As a result, a change in the magnitude of effect or the duration of effect can occur without a change in the type of effect. Interactions of this type may have multiple mechanisms, making clinical predictions difficult. Additionally, there are many patient factors that influence the pharmacokinetics of a drug, such as age, liver and renal function, degree of physiological stress and the presence of other diseases such as hyperthyroidism.

Factors affecting absorption

Drug absorption is determined by the physicochemical properties of a drug, as well as by its formulation and route of administration. Because most herbal and nutritional medicines are administered orally, as tablets, capsules, teas and tinctures, this discussion will focus on interactions associated with these dose forms.

Most absorption of orally administered medicines occurs in the small intestine, which has a larger surface area than the stomach and greater membrane permeability. If a slow-release dosage form is taken and it continues to release the drug for more than 6 hours, then absorption will also occur in the large intestine. The absorption of oral dose forms is influenced by differences in pH along the gastrointestinal tract, surface area per luminal volume, blood perfusion, the presence of bile and mucus and the nature of epithelial membranes. Changes to gastrointestinal flora, transport systems, chelation and ion exchange also influence absorption.

Interactions at this level can alter the rate of absorption and/or extent of absorption of a medicine.

Changes in relative rate of absorption

Although a medicine may eventually be fully absorbed, a significantly slowed absorption rate may mean that it never reaches effective serum levels, or that an unwanted 'sustained release' effect causes prolonged activity or a delay in prompt relief. In some clinical situations, decreased rates of absorption are of no concern; however, in others it may be important. Generally, a decreased rate of absorption is less important for medicines that are given in multiple-dose regimens to achieve a steady state serum level than for those that are given as single doses or are required to produce a rapid effect (e.g. analgesics).

Changes in extent of absorption

Altering the extent of absorption may also have significant consequences. Increasing the amount of medicine absorbed may produce higher plasma levels and a higher risk of adverse reactions or toxicity. Alternatively, reducing the amount of medicine absorbed may result in reduced efficacy or therapeutic failure. This is of particular concern for medicines with a narrow therapeutic index, such as warfarin and digoxin.

Mucilaginous herbs

Although little research has been conducted to determine the effects of herbal medicines on the absorption of other medicines, one double-blind study found that guar gum slowed the absorption rate of digoxin, but did not alter the extent of absorption, whereas penicillin absorption was both slowed and reduced (Huupponen et al 1984). This brings into question the effects of other gums and highly mucilaginous herbal medicines, such as *Ulmus fulvus* (slippery elm), *Althea officinalis* (marshmallow) and *Plantago ovata* (psyllium). Poorly lipid soluble, the mucilaginous content forms an additional physical barrier to absorption, but whether this will have a clinically significant effect on rate and/or extent of absorption of other medicines is uncertain and remains to be tested.

Nutrients

More research has been conducted into the way nutrients interact and alter the absorption of pharmaceutical medicines than with herbal medicines. The interactions between iron and many minerals provide a useful example. Aluminium, calcium bicarbonate or magnesium trisilicate taken in antacid preparations are known to reduce the extent of iron absorption owing to an alteration in gastric pH. This type of interaction is easily avoided by separating the intake of iron by at least 2 hours from the last dose of antacid.

Intrinsic drug transporters

Until recently, when an orally administered medicine exhibited poor absorption, it was generally assumed that this was because of either physicochemical problems or significant first-pass hepatic metabolism. Recently, it has been recognised that for many medicines poor oral bioavailability could be related to the influence of transporter proteins (Benet & Cummins 2001). Transporter proteins are associated with the transfer of some medicines from the intestinal lumen, through the biological barrier of the intestinal mucosa, into the systemic circulation and back again. Transporters fall into two main categories: carriers and pumps. Carriers are involved in three types of transport processes: facilitated diffusion, co-transport and counter-transport. Pumps are distinguished from carriers by the linkage of transport to an external source of energy. Examples of transporters in the intestine are P-glycoprotein (P-gp), members of the multi-drug-resistance-associated protein family (breast-cancer resistance protein, organic cation and anion transporters) and members of the organic anion polypeptide family (Wagner et al 2001). Of these, P-gp is the most studied (see *Clinical note*).

Herbal and natural medicines affecting P-gp

The influence of herbal and natural medicines on P-gp expression has only recently been considered, so much is still unknown and speculative. To date, most research has centred on St John's wort, although clinical testing with other herbs has now gained momentum: every few months more studies investigating the likelihood and clinical significance of proposed interactions are published.

In 1999, clinical testing found that St John's wort significantly reduces serum levels of digoxin after 10 days' co-administration (Johne et al 1999). The suspected mechanism of interaction was chiefly liver enzyme induction; however, the magnitude of effect seen in this study, and in others, suggested that P-gp induction was involved (Hennessy et al 2002). More recently, several clinical tests have confirmed that St John's wort has significant P-gp induction effects. One study found up to a 4.2-fold increase in P-gp expression compared with a placebo after 16 days' administration.

CLINICAL NOTE — P-GLYCOPROTEIN: AN IMPORTANT DRUG TRANSPORTER

P-glycoprotein was first studied in the context of cancer research, where its overexpression in tumour cells is associated with multi-drug resistance (Jodoin et al 2002). In cancer cells, P-gp is one of the transporters responsible for actively expelling chemotherapeutic drugs from cells, thereby decreasing intracellular concentrations and thus drug efficacy. As a result, identification of those substances that reduce P-gp expression and can be administered safely with chemotherapeutic agents is being investigated.

P-gp is found on the surface of hepatocytes, and epithelial cells of the renal tubules, the intestine, placenta and capillaries in the brain (Lin 2003). It plays an important role in the processes of absorption, distribution, metabolism and excretion of medicines. P-gp has a counter-transport activity, meaning it can transport medicines from the blood back into the gastrointestinal tract, thereby reducing bioavailability.

In humans, P-gp demonstrates genetic polymorphism, which may partly account for the inter-individual variability seen in drug absorption. One study conducted in 25 volunteers supports this idea and found that a greater than eight-fold difference in expression of intestinal P-gp is possible (Lown et al 1997).

The expression of P-gp can be altered by a number of factors, such as everyday foods, herbs and pharmaceutical medicines. In the case of P-gp inhibition, there will be an increase in absorption, systemic exposure and tissue distribution of medicines that are P-gp substrates, whereas P-gp induction produces the opposite effect.

Interactions with substances that inhibit P-gp are of great interest, as they can potentially enhance the absorption of important medicines that are generally poorly absorbed, such as chemotherapeutic medicines. Alternatively, P-gp inhibition may theoretically increase the incidence of side effects or the toxicity of some medicines, producing unwanted effects.

Some important P-gp substrates are:

Berberine	Methotrexate
Colchicine	Morphine
Cortisol	Nifedipine
Cyclosporin	Progesterone
Digoxin	Protease inhibitors
Erythromycin	Taxol
Indinavir	Tamoxifen
Loperamide	*Vinca* alkaloids

Similar results were seen in another study in which 14 days' administration of St John's wort resulted in a 1.4-fold increased expression of duodenal P-gp (Durr et al 2000). Induction of P-gp is attributed to pregnane X receptor activation by the hyperforin constituent (Lin 2003). Low hyperforin products are therefore less likely to induce P-gp.

St John's wort is not the only natural substance found to influence P-gp. Other studies suggest that rosemary extract may have the opposite effect, inhibiting P-gp. Treating multi-drug-resistant mammary tumour cells with rosemary extract produced an increase in intracellular concentrations of doxorubicin and vinblastine (both P-gp substrates) (Plouzek et al 1999). The same effects were not seen in cells that lack P-gp expression, suggesting that rosemary extract inhibits P-gp activity. The isoflavone genistein has also been investigated, with some results suggesting inhibition of P-gp-mediated drug transport (Castro & Altenberg 1997). Other studies have found that different polyphenols, such as green tea polyphenols, resveratrol (a polyphenol from red wine), curcumin, caffeine, theanine and methoxyflavones from orange, may inhibit drug transport via P-gp (Jodoin et al 2002).

Grapefruit juice is well known to interact with a number of medicines, so it is not surprising that it has also been investigated for effects on P-gp. Currently, evidence is conflicting, as several studies have found that components in grapefruit juice inhibit P-gp (Eagling et al 1999, Ohnishi et al 2000, Soldner et al 1999, Spahn-Langguth & Langguth 2001), whereas a randomised, crossover clinical study found no significant effects (Becquemont et al 2001). A more recent in vitro study produced similar results with 5% normal concentration of grapefruit, orange and apple juices; however, inhibition of other transporter proteins was observed (Dresser et al 2002).

Research suggests that quercetin inhibits P-gp expression (Choi & Li 2005, Chung et al 2005, Kitagawa et al 2005, Wang et al 2004). Studies with experimental models have demonstrated that pretreatment with quercetin increases the bioavailability of the calcium-channel blocker, diltiazem (Choi & Li 2005), and of digoxin (Wang et al 2004). Intriguingly, one in vivo study found quercetin significantly decreased the oral bioavailability of cyclosporin, which is the opposite of what would be expected, suggesting that other mechanisms may also be involved (Hsiu et al 2002).

Although in vitro studies have also identified an inhibitory effect on P-gp for silymarin, the active constituent group in St Mary's thistle (Chung et al 2005, Zhang & Morris 2003), recent clinical testing found no significant effect in vivo (Gurley et al 2006). Additionally, the herb schisandra inhibits P-gp (Jin et al 2010). Table 4.1 lists herbal and natural medicines that have suspected or known effects on P-gp, together with the research that gives evidence for these effects.

Factors affecting metabolism

Metabolism can occur before and during absorption, thereby limiting the amount of drug reaching the systemic circulation. In the intestinal lumen,

TABLE 4.1 HERBAL AND NATURAL MEDICINES WITH SUSPECTED OR KNOWN EFFECTS ON P-GLYCOPROTEIN

HERBAL/ NATURAL MEDICINE	EFFECT	EVIDENCE
St John's wort	Induction	Clinical studies (Hennessy et al 2002, Johne et al 1999) In vivo and clinical study (Durr et al 2000) In vitro (Perloff et al 2001), also positive for hypericin Case report (Barone et al 2000)
Grapefruit juice	Inhibition	Clinical studies (Di Marco et al 2002, Edwards et al 1999) In vivo (Spahn-Langguth & Langguth 2001, Tian et al 2002) In vitro (Eagling et al 1999, Ohnishi et al 2000, Soldner et al 1999, Takanaga et al 1998)
Grapefruit juice	No effect	Clinical study (Becquemont et al 2001)
Orange and apple juice	Inhibition	Clinical study: Seville orange (Di Marco et al 2002) In vivo: orange (Tian et al 2002) In vitro (Ikegawa et al 2000, Takanaga et al 2000)
Rosemary extract	Inhibition	In vitro (Plouzek et al 1999)
Genistein and daidzein	Inhibition	In vitro (Evans 2000, Castro & Altenberg 1997)
Genistein and daidzein	Possible induction	In vitro (den Boer et al 1998)
Resveratrol	Inhibition	In vitro (Jodoin et al 2002)
Curcumin	Inhibition	In vitro (Anuchapreeda et al 2002, Romiti et al 1998)
Quercetin	Inhibition	In vitro and in vivo (Choi & Li 2005, Chung et al 2005, Kitagawa et al 2005, Scambia et al 1994, Wang et al 2004)
Green tea polyphenols, especially epigallocatechin gallate	Inhibition	In vitro (Jodoin et al 2002, Sadzuka et al 2000)
Piperine (a major component of black pepper)	Inhibition	In vivo (Bhardwaj et al 2002)
St Mary's thistle	Inhibition	In vitro tests (Chung et al 2005, Zhang & Morris 2003)
St Mary's thistle	No effect	Human study (Gurley et al 2006)

digestive enzymes and bowel flora are capable of causing a wide range of metabolic reactions. The intestinal mucosa is also capable of metabolising drugs, with new research suggesting it is a major metabolic organ for some medicines (Doherty & Charman 2002).

For many medicines, metabolism chiefly occurs in the liver in two apparent phases, known as phase I or functionalisation reactions and phase II or conjugation reactions. Phase I reactions include oxidation, hydroxylation, dealkylation and reduction. Examples of Phase I reactions include conversion of an active drug to an inactive, less active, more active or toxic metabolite, and conversion of an inactive prodrug to an active metabolite. Phase II reactions include glucuronidation, sulfation, acetylation and methylation glutathionation, glycination and other amino acid conjugations (taurine, glutamine, carnitine, arginine), and usually result in the formation of inactive compounds that are water-soluble and easily excreted (Blower et al 2005).

Although there are many enzymes responsible for phase I reactions, the most important enzyme group is the cytochrome P450 system (CYP), which comprises more than 50 enzymes and is responsible for the metabolism of many drugs, nutrients, endogenous substances and environmental toxins.

Cytochromes

Cytochrome P450 is a generic term for a super-family of enzymes (haem containing mono-oxygenases) that have existed throughout nature since the beginning of life more than 3.5 billion years ago (Pirmohamed & Park 2003). The P450s are found chiefly in the liver, but also to a lesser extent in the intestines, kidneys, skin and lungs. These enzymes are responsible for foreign compound metabolism, which evolved about 400–500 million years ago to enable animals to detoxify chemicals in plants. The cytochrome P450 (CYP) enzymes are the most powerful in vivo oxidising agents and are able to catalyse the oxidative biotransformation of a wide range of chemically and biologically unrelated exogenous and endogenous substrates. They are named by a root symbol CYP, followed by a number for family, a letter for subfamily, and another number for the specific gene. For example, CYP3A4 would refer to a specific enzyme from the cytochrome P450 system, family 3, subfamily A and gene 4. Three main CYP families (CYP1, 2, 3) are responsible for metabolism of therapeutic drugs. The different P450 isoforms vary in their abundance within the liver. Of these, the cytochromes CYP2C9, CYP2D6 and CYP3A4 are the most abundant in the human body (Pirmohamed & Park 2003).

The CYP2C sub-family accounts for 15–20% of the total P450 content of the liver, and metabolises approximately 20% of all drugs (Pirmohamed & Park 2003). The main member of this sub-family is CYP2C9, which is responsible for the metabolism of a number of compounds, including warfarin, phenytoin and various NSAIDs. Cytochrome 2D6 is responsible for

TABLE 4.2 SELECTED DRUGS THAT ACT AS SUBSTRATES FOR CYP ENZYMES	
CYP ENZYME	**DRUGS**
CYP1A2	amitriptyline, caffeine, melatonin, naproxen, paracetamol, tacrine, theophylline, verapamil, R-warfarin
CYP2B6	amitriptyline, diazepam, methadone, midazolam, tamoxifen, temazepam, testosterone
CYP2C9	amitriptyline, celecoxib, diclofenac, fluoxetine, ibuprofen, tamoxifen, S-warfarin
CYP2C19	amitriptyline, imipramine, indomethacin, omeprazole, progesterone, propranolol, R-warfarin
CYP2D6	amitriptyline, beta blockers, codeine, fluoxetine, flecainide, haloperidol, nicotine, ondansetron, paroxetine, sertraline, tamoxifen, tramadol
CYP3A4	alprazolam, caffeine, codeine, cyclosporin, erythromycin, HIV antivirals (e.g. indinavir), lovastatin, midazolam, oestradiol, ondansetron, progesterone, simvastatin, tamoxifen, taxol, testosterone

the metabolism of approximately 25% of therapeutically used drugs, although it accounts for only <5% of the total P450 content. The CYP3A sub-family accounts for 30% of the total P450 content and is responsible for metabolism of about 50% of therapeutic drugs. Table 4.2 provides examples of common drugs and the cytochromes chiefly responsible for their metabolism. For a more complete list that is frequently updated, see Flockhart 2007.

The expression and activity of many CYP isoenzymes vary enormously between individuals. Part of the inter-individual variability is environmentally determined by the concomitant intake of drugs and foodstuffs that cause induction and inhibition of the different P450 isoforms. P450 gene polymorphism may also influence expression and activity of CYP enzymes, as this can lead to:

- abolished activity of a CYP enzyme (e.g. CYP2C9, CYP2C19 and CYP2D6 can be genetically absent in some livers [USFDA 2014])
- reduced activity
- altered activity
- increased activity where there is gene duplication.

For example, one study identified that 30% of Ethiopians had multiple copies of the 2D6 gene (up to 13), resulting in ultra-rapid metabolism of CYP2D6 substrates (Aklillu et al 1996). As a result, standard doses of CYP2D6 substrates (e.g. beta-blockers, some opioids and tricyclic antidepressants) will not produce anticipated or adequate responses, and higher drug doses are necessary to produce therapeutic effects. It has also been estimated that 7% of Caucasians lack CYP2D6. These individuals will not experience the anticipated therapeutic effects of prodrugs that are CYP2D6 substrates, such as codeine, and will appear more sensitive to the side effects of CYP2D6 substrates (e.g. beta-blockers, some opioids and tricyclic antidepressants) (USFDA 2014).

Another example is the polymorphic distribution of CYP2C9, which is absent in 1% of Caucasians. More than 100 drugs in current use are known substrates of CYP2C9, corresponding to approximately 10–20% of commonly prescribed drugs. Of note, CYP2C9 is chiefly responsible for the metabolism of NSAIDs and COX-2-specific inhibitors (e.g. celecoxib).

Many other factors affect CYP activity, such as the ingestion of foreign compounds (e.g. environmental contaminants) or the ingestion of certain constituents found in food, beverages and medicines.

Because of overlapping substrates, many drug interactions involve both P-gp and CYP3A4.

Enzyme inhibition

Competitive CYP inhibition is dose-dependent and occurs when inhibitors compete with other substances for a particular enzyme. Non-competitive inhibition is also possible and occurs when a substance either destroys or binds irreversibly to a CYP enzyme. In both instances, serum levels of those drugs chiefly metabolised by the affected enzyme will become elevated and the inhibition process is rapid. This is of particular concern with medicines that have a narrow therapeutic index, as very small changes in dose or blood levels can produce significant changes in activity. In the case of enzyme inhibition, raised blood levels can lead to increased side effects and toxicity.

Although inhibition of a CYP enzyme is generally regarded as raising the serum levels of an active drug, this is not always the case. If the drug involved is a prodrug, then it is inactive in its administered form and must be converted to its active form, usually via metabolic processes. If metabolism is slowed, then the production of active metabolites will also be slowed. An example is codeine, which is primarily metabolised by CYP2D6 into its active analgesic metabolite morphine; therefore, CYP2D6 inhibition has the potential to slow or reduce its analgesic activity.

Inhibitors do not all have the same strength and can be classified as strong, moderate or weak, depending on their effect on drug clearance compared to normal values. For example, Flockhart describes a strong inhibitor as one that causes more than 80% decrease in clearance, a moderate inhibitor as one that causes a 50–80% decrease in drug clearance and a weak inhibitor as one that causes a 20–50% decrease in drug clearance (Flockhart 2007).

Enzyme inhibition is not always harmful and has been manipulated to raise serum drug levels without the need to increase the dose administered. The result has obvious cost advantages when extremely expensive drugs are involved and has been used in some hospitals for medicines such as cyclosporin.

To date, the most studied natural substance capable of significantly inhibiting CYP enzymes is grapefruit. The finding that grapefruit juice markedly increases the bioavailability of some orally administered medicines was based on an unexpected observation from an interaction study between the calcium-channel antagonist felodipine and ethanol. In the study, grapefruit juice was used to mask the taste of ethanol, but actually affected the results by reducing CYP3A4 by 62% and significantly raising felodipine levels (Bailey et al 1998). Since then, the constituents of grapefruit juice have been extensively studied and found to affect the transport and metabolism of many other medicines (Eagling et al 1999, Kane & Lipsky 2000).

Increasingly, research is being conducted to determine whether other commonly used herbal medicines have an affect on CYP activity in vivo. For example, one research group in the United States screened *Citrus aurantium*, *Echinacea purpurea*, milk thistle (*Silybum marianum*) and saw palmetto (*Serenoa repens*) extracts for effects on CYP1A2, CYP2D6, CYP2E1 and CYP3A4 activity in healthy subjects (Gurley et al 2004). Of the four herbs, only *E. purpurea* was found to have any effect on the CYP enzymes tested, with a minor influence on CYP1A2 and CYP3A4. Using the same method, extracts of the herbs goldenseal (*Hydrastis canadensis*), black cohosh (*Cimicifuga racemosa*), kava kava (*Piper methysticum*) and valerian (*Valeriana officinalis*) were tested for effects on CYP1A2, CYP2D6, CYP2E1 or CYP3A4/5 activity (Gurley et al 2005). Goldenseal strongly inhibited CYP2D6 and CYP3A4/5 activity in vivo, whereas kava kava inhibited CYP2E1, black cohosh weakly inhibited CYP2D6 and no effect was observed for valerian. In a separate study, testing *Panax ginseng* and *Ginkgo biloba*, no effect was observed on CYP activity; however, garlic oil inhibited CYP2E1 activity by 39% (Gurley et al 2002). More recently, a 2012 review considering which herbs are likely to induce clinically relevant drug interactions concluded that the herb schisandra is likely to inhibit CYP3A4 in humans, as is golden seal (Gurley et al 2012).

There are many other examples to be found in the individual monographs of this book.

Enzyme induction

Alternatively, many different medicines and everyday substances have been found to induce the CYP enzymes (e.g. broccoli, Brussels sprouts, chargrilled meat, high-protein diets, tobacco and alcohol). Research is now identifying a number of herbal medicines that cause CYP induction to various degrees; however, the most studied to date is St John's wort.

Clinical tests have confirmed that long-term administration of St John's wort has significant CYP inducer activity, particularly CYP3A4 (Durr et al 2000, Roby et al 2000, Ruschitzka et al 2000, Wang et al 2001). It appears that the hyperforin component is a potent ligand for the pregnane X receptor, which regulates expression of CYP3A4 mono-oxygenase. In this way, hyperforin increases the availability of CYP3A4, resulting in enzyme induction (Moore et al 2000).

Lack of in vitro–in vivo correlation

It is interesting to observe an apparent lack of in vitro–in vivo correlation with some studies of CYP. For example, in vitro investigations implicate milk thistle extract and/or silibinin as inhibitors of human CYP3A4, CYP2C9, CYP2D6 and CYP2E1; however, in vivo evidence for CYP-mediated interactions by milk thistle is less compelling (Gurley et al 2004). This may be owing to poor bioavailability of key constituents, large inter-individual differences in absorption of constituents, inter-product variability in the ratios of constituent, poor dissolution of dosage forms or other mechanisms.

Factors affecting excretion

The kidneys are the major organs of excretion, but it also occurs to a lesser extent via other routes such as saliva, sweat, faeces, breast milk and the lungs. If a medicine is chiefly eliminated by one pathway, then alterations to that particular pathway can theoretically have a significant influence on its excretion.

CLINICAL NOTE — PHARMACOGENETICS

Pharmacogenetics largely deals with genes encoding drug transporters, drug-metabolising enzymes and drug targets (Ingelman-Sundberg 2004). It is now well established that the polymorphism of metabolising enzymes, and in particular that of P450 cytochromes, has the greatest effect on inter-individual variability of drug response, as evidenced by many studies. These polymorphisms affect the response of individuals to drugs used in the treatment of depression, psychosis, cancer, cardiovascular disorders, ulcer and gastrointestinal disorders, pain and epilepsy, among others. The costs of genotyping are reducing and our knowledge about the benefits of predictive genotyping for more effective and safe drug therapy is increasing. This means that in future predictive genotyping for CYP enzymes will become routine, allowing individualised prescribing to produce better clinical outcomes with less risk of side effects.

With regard to urinary excretion, factors that alter renal function can interfere with the excretion of medicines and their metabolites. There are three main ways that renal function can be modified (Blower et al 2005):

- altered renal tubular reabsorption by substances that affect urinary pH
- changes in renal tubular secretion by agents that either compete for active secretion or that alter the activity of membrane transporter proteins
- changes in glomerular filtration induced by agents that alter cardiac output.

Alterations to urinary pH are easily achieved with regard to herbal and natural substances; for example, the half-life of an acidic medicine, such as a salicylate, can be increased with acidification of urine — for example, with high doses of ascorbic acid, because less is eliminated. Alternatively, the half-life of a weakly basic drug, such as amphetamine, may be decreased when urine is acidified. Alkalisation of urine produces the opposite effects and can occur with low-protein diets or the ingestion of substances such as potassium citrate.

PHARMACODYNAMIC INTERACTIONS

Pharmacodynamic interactions result when one substance alters the sensitivity or responsiveness of tissues to another. This type of interaction results in additive, synergistic or antagonistic drug effects and is of particular concern when medicines used simultaneously have overlapping toxicities.

In practice, clinicians frequently use additive or synergistic pharmacodynamic interactions to improve clinical outcomes. For example, medical doctors may prescribe a combination of antibiotics against difficult-to-eradicate microorganisms, or several antihypertensive drugs to one patient. Herbalists widely prescribe combinations of herbs with similar actions to strengthen clinical effects, and naturopaths may combine nutritional and herbal supplements in a similar way.

Pharmacodynamic interactions do not always produce wanted results, such as when several medicines with overlapping adverse effects or toxicities are used together, leading to more serious adverse effects. An example is the combined use of an opioid analgesic, which can induce drowsiness, and an antiemetic drug such as metoclopramide, which can also induce drowsiness. Other unwanted effects include potentiating drug activity to a clinically uncomfortable or dangerous level, or reducing activity and therefore the effectiveness of treatment.

Although pharmacodynamic interactions involving herbal and natural medicines and pharmaceutical medicines have not been thoroughly investigated, theoretical predictions are easy to produce. For example, case reports suggest that kava kava may have dopamine receptor antagonist activity and therefore theoretically can interact with dopamine agonists (e.g. L-dopa), opposing their effect (Meseguer et al 2002, Spillane et al 1997). Predicting real-life responses is difficult, because the evidence does not come from a controlled clinical study and individual factors such as dose, administration route and patient health further influence outcomes.

PHYSICOCHEMICAL INTERACTIONS

Physicochemical interactions occur when two substances come into contact and are either physically or chemically incompatible. This type of interaction can take place during the manufacture or administration of medicines and can affect both the rate and the extent of absorption of one or both medicines. Physicochemical interactions are a well-known concern among medical herbalists and naturopaths who prescribe and dispense their own herbal combinations.

Reduced absorption

Tannins

Herbs with significant tannin content have the potential to be involved in physicochemical interactions with other medicines, both outside and within the body, because they form precipitates with proteins, nitrogenous bases, polysaccharides and some alkaloids and glycosides (Mills 1991). Additionally, tannins will form complexes with metal ions such as iron, inhibiting their absorption (Glahn et al 2002). To avoid this interaction, herbal extracts containing tannins are traditionally not mixed with extracts containing alkaloids (Bone & Mills 2000).

In practice, herbal medicines containing tannins are used both internally and externally. When used internally, it is recommended that they be taken between meals or on an empty stomach to minimise precipitation of dietary proteins and digestive enzymes in the gut (Baxter et al 1997). Additionally, tannins can reduce the absorption of some minerals, so should not be taken at the same time. For example, the absorption of iron is significantly reduced in the presence of tannins, with one study finding amounts as small as 5 mg of tannic acid are able to inhibit iron absorption by 20% and higher levels of 100 mg by 88% (Brune et al 1989). Tannins are widely found in the plant kingdom, as shown in Table 4.3.

Chelation

Physicochemical interactions can also occur via a process of chelation, which is the chemical interaction of a metal ion and other substance that

TABLE 4.3 COMMON HERBS WITH SIGNIFICANT TANNIN CONTENT

COMMON NAME	BOTANICAL NAME
Agrimony	*Agrimony eupatorium*
Bearberry	*Arctostaphylus uva-ursi*
Bistort	*Polygonum bistorta*
Meadowsweet	*Filipendula ulmaria*
Raspberry	*Rubus idaeus*
Rhubarb	*Rheum* spp. root
Spinach	*Chenopodium* spp.
Tea	*Camellia sinensis*
Tormentil	*Potentilla tormentilla*

results in the formation of a molecular complex in which the metal is firmly bound and isolated. In other words, the metal ion irreversibly binds to a second molecule, leading to reduced activity or inactivation of that metal. A common example is the interaction between iron and various drugs, including tetracycline antibiotics.

A number of compounds found naturally in food have the potential to interact with medicines in this way. For example, oxalic acid found in spinach and rhubarb or phytic acid found in bran can form insoluble complexes with calcium, thereby reducing its absorption.

Increased absorption

Not all physicochemical interactions result in reduced absorption. It is widely accepted that interactions between plant components can enhance clinical effects by increasing the bioavailability of key pharmacologically active constituents.

The results of continuing investigation into the chemistry of St John's wort provide a good example. In vivo studies using hypericin and pseudohypericin found that the solubility of these two active constituents increases by approximately 60% in the presence of natural procyanidins (Butterweck et al 1998). Further research has isolated naturally occurring hyperoside, rutin and quercetin as some of the key components responsible for this interaction.

Although still largely speculative, the interaction between naturally occurring surfactant constituents, such as saponins, and poorly lipid soluble active constituents could feasibly result in increased absorption through a micellisation process. Besides improving oral bioavailability, the interaction could also improve dermal penetration.

Different forms of saponins are widely found in the plant kingdom and are used either internally or externally, depending on the particular herb (Table 4.4).

TABLE 4.4 COMMON HERBS CONTAINING SAPONINS

COMMON NAME	BOTANICAL NAME
Astragalus	*Astragalus membranaceus*
Bupleurum	*Bupleurum falcatum*
Horsechestnut	*Aesculus hippocastanum*
Japanese ginseng	*Panax japonicus*
Licorice	*Glycyrrhiza glabra*
Poke root	*Phytolacca decandra*
Soybean	*Glycine max*
Withania	*Withania somnifera*

SYNERGY HERBAL RESEARCH

In practice, herbalists use inter-herbal interactions to produce better outcomes. This practice is much the same as that of medical practitioners employing multi-target drug therapy in the treatment of cancer, hypertension and antibiotic resistance. Owing to the chemical complexity of herbal medicines, intra-herbal interactions are also being identified that largely explain the therapeutic superiority of many herbal drug extracts over single constituents isolated from the same herbal extracts. Synergistic effects can be produced if the constituents of an extract affect different targets or interact with one another in order to improve the solubility and thereby enhance the bioavailability of one or several substances of an extract. Synergy research in phytomedicine has established itself as a new activity in recent years and focuses on studying intra-herbal and inter-herbal interactions to better understand how therapeutic benefits can be harnessed.

INTERACTION SCREENING TOOLS

Information about interactions is derived from in vitro tests, studies with experimental animal models and, increasingly, clinical studies. Most studies of interactions conducted to date have focused on herbal constituents and their effects on cytochrome (CYP) enzymes and, increasingly, P-glycoprotein (P-gp), with few studies investigating effects on drug transport or phase II metabolism.

In vitro tests

Most studies conducted to investigate herb–drug interactions have used in vitro testing of herbal constituents in microsomal systems, supersomes, cytosols, expressed enzymes or cell-culture systems such as transfected cell lines, primary cultures of human hepatocytes and tumour-derived cells. While in vitro models provide a quick screening method for potential herb–drug interactions they do not always correlate with in vivo findings. One problem frequently encountered in the existing in vitro literature is the use of inappropriately high concentrations of single, isolated constituents obtained from commercial sources, and utilisation of these in experiments when only a small fraction of the compound may actually be bioavailable. Many natural products are generally subject to first-pass metabolism and to a much larger extent than conventional pharmaceutical agents, which are in most cases specifically developed to be substantially bioavailable or otherwise formulated as prodrugs. In addition, many are less bioavailable because of their hydrophilic nature or large molecular size (Markowitz et al 2008).

Animal studies

These studies may give important information on herb interactions. Probe substrates/inhibitors can be used to explore the effects of herbs on the activity of specific CYP enzyme in vivo, e.g. caffeine for CYP1A2, tolbutamide for CYP2C9, mephenytoin for CYP2C19, dextromethorphan or debrisoquine for CYP2D6, chlorzoxazone for CYP2E1 and midazolam or erythromycin for CYP3A4. In addition, a cocktail of probe drugs have been used to explore the activities of multiple CYPs in the same experiment. Ultimately, in vivo clinical studies are more reliable than in vitro tests as a means of determining the clinical importance of herb–drug interactions, although these studies can quickly be confounded by the documented variability found in specific constituents between individual botanical products as well as by the choice of probe substrates administered (Markowitz et al 2008).

Relying solely on in vitro or animal model experiments to predict clinically relevant herb–drug interactions is problematic and can provide inaccurate information. The herbs *Ginkgo biloba* and saw palmetto will be used here as examples to illustrate this point.

In vitro and/or tests with animal models have shown both cytochrome induction and inhibition for *Ginkgo biloba* (Chatterjee et al 2005, Chang et al 2006a, 2006b, Gaudineau et al 2004, He & Edeki 2004, Kubota et al 2004, Kuo et al 2004, Mohutsky et al 2006, Ohnishi et al 2003, Ryu & Chung 2003, Shinozuka et al 2002, Sugiyama et al 2004a, 2004b, von Moltke et al 2004, Zhao et al 2006). In contrast, four clinical studies have failed to identify a clinically significant effect on a variety of cytochromes. In one clinical study, Gurley et al (2002) demonstrated that *Ginkgo biloba* had no significant effect on CYP1A2, CYP2D6 or CYP3A4 activity. Markowitz et al (2003b) also conducted a human study and found no significant effects on CYP2D6 or CYP3A4 activity. Two further clinical studies found no significant effect for *Ginkgo biloba* on CYP2C9 activity (Greenblatt et al 2006, Mohutsky et al 2006). Overall, there have been at least 29 human studies investigating whether *Ginkgo biloba* alters the pharmacokinetics of multiple drugs (e.g. warfarin and digoxin) and affects various cytochromes. Of these, 23 studies found no observable effect, three a modest effect and three provided some evidence of CYP induction. However, when compared to FDA guidelines, these three studies do not suggest a clinically significant or important drug interaction potential (Gurley et al 2012).

Saw palmetto showed potent inhibition of CYP3A4, CYP2D6 and CYP2C9 in vitro (Yale & Glurich 2005); however, no significant effect was observed on CYP2D6 or CYP3A4 activity according to a clinical study by Markowitz et al (2003a). Gurley et al (2004) also found no significant effect for saw palmetto on CYP1A2, CYP2D6, CYP2E1 or CYP3A4 activity in healthy subjects.

To add to the complexity of the problem, in some instances researchers have conducted testing with individual herbal components or different forms of a herb and found different effects on CYPs. For example, using animal models Fukao et al (2004) demonstrated that diallyl sulphide (100 micromol/kg) increased cytochrome CYP2E1 activity slightly but significantly (1.6-fold versus control), whereas diallyl disulfide and diallyl trisulfide did not affect CYP2E1 activity or the hepatic total CYP level or CYP1A1/2 activity. The significance of these results in clinical practice is difficult to determine, as the overall effect on CYP activity will depend on the concentrations of these various constituents present in a garlic product. The example also highlights the general difficulty in extrapolating results for one herbal extract to another, as there may be a significant chemical variation between batches of the same herbal product and between different products of the same herb grown and produced by various manufacturers.

Clinical studies

These studies provide the most relevant information; however, they are costly to produce and are mostly conducted with young, healthy males, which may or may not accurately reflect the responses of other populations (e.g. women, the elderly).

Table 4.5 presents a summary of the strengths and limitations relevant to different types of research into interactions.

PUTTING THEORY INTO PRACTICE

It is clear that many patients will be taking herbal and natural medicines and pharmaceutical medicines at some stage of their lives. In some instances, use will overlap, so a patient will be taking several medicines at the same time. In order to promote the safe use of all medicines, the following section provides ideas for consideration and discussion, practical tools to aid in reducing the risk of interactions and in detection of adverse reactions and general recommendations.

INTERACTION MECHANISMS

Predicting the clinical importance of a herb–drug interaction is difficult and largely depends on factors that relate to the medicines administered and the individual patient. Having an understanding of the interaction mechanisms involved is also essential.

Medicine factors

Consider the types of medicines involved, administration route, dosage and duration of use. Drugs with a narrow therapeutic index are of most concern, as minor changes to serum levels can have clinically significant outcomes. Drugs that are administered intravenously will not always be subject to the same concerns as orally ingested drugs. In the case of herbal medicines, some preparations contain multiple CYP or transporter-modulating constituents, with some constituents causing induction and others inhibition. This means the overall outcome will depend on the amount of inducer/inhibitor constituents present, the CYPs or transporters affected and the relative strengths of inducers/inhibitors. Since herbal medicines naturally vary in constituent ratios owing to environmental and process factors, their effects on CYPs and transporters are more difficult to predict than for single-entity drugs.

TABLE 4.5 ADVANTAGES AND LIMITATIONS OF HERB–DRUG INTERACTION STUDIES		
STUDY TYPE	ADVANTAGES	LIMITATIONS
In vitro	Provides information about specific mechanisms under controlled conditions. Relatively simple to conduct compared with clinical studies. Inexpensive tests to conduct compared with clinical studies. Relatively quick to conduct.	Does not account for poor bioavailability of the test compound. May use one isolated constituent, whereas herbal extracts contain multiple constituents. Does not account for human genetic polymorphism. May use clinically irrelevant concentration. Metabolites of botanical extracts are poorly characterised for most extracts and may contribute to the net inhibitory or inductive effects observed, which will not be detected with in vitro testing.
In vivo using animal models	Can address some of the issues relating to bioavailability. Can produce quicker results than clinical studies. Can provide information when clinical studies are not able to be conducted.	Species variations make results difficult to interpret. Selection of appropriate dosage can be difficult and very large doses are often used. Does not account for human genetic polymorphism.
Clinical studies	Provide the most relevant information and are the most definitive.	Most studies conducted in healthy male subjects; however, most relevant results are obtained when conducted with the population that will be using the product. Inter-product variability in constituent ratios means tested product may not accurately represent effects of other products. Cannot differentiate between gut and liver effects (e.g. cytochromes). Does not provide information about mechanisms. Are costly and time consuming. May never be done for ethical reasons (e.g. safety studies in pregnancy).

Individual patient factors

The severity of the interaction is also influenced by factors such as age, gender, preexisting medical conditions and comorbidities, environmental influences and diet. Genetic polymorphism is increasingly becoming recognised as another significant factor that can alter a patient's risk of experiencing adverse drug reactions. The importance an interaction is given is also related to some extent to the setting in which it occurs. Risk can be minimised or managed when patients openly discuss their use of herbal and pharmaceutical medicines with all their healthcare providers and they are carefully supervised.

Problems and pitfalls interpreting the evidence

Firstly, understanding the basic mechanisms involved is essential, as is keeping in mind the type of evidence that might suggest the possibility of an interaction. It is important to note the general lack of correlation between in vitro and in vivo tests, and the inaccuracies of extrapolating data from animal models to predict clinical significance in humans. In many cases, interaction studies are absent, so clinicians must use their professional judgement to evaluate what is known about the medicines and the patient, and then the likelihood of a clinically relevant interaction.

A PREDICTIVE ALGORITHM

The METOPIA algorithm provides a framework for healthcare professionals when making rational decisions about the introduction of a second, potentially interacting medicine. In this chapter, it is assumed that a herbal medicine is involved. METOPIA stands for:

Medication and mechanisms

- What types of medicines are involved? High-risk medicines such as those with a narrow therapeutic index require closer monitoring.
- Is an interaction theoretically possible? This needs to be based on a fundamental understanding of the pharmacokinetic parameters and pharmacodynamic effects of the medicines involved.

Evidence available?

- Is there supportive evidence for an anticipated interaction?
- If so, what is the weight of that evidence (theoretical, in vitro, in vivo, case reports or clinical trials)?

If the information gathered so far suggests an interaction is possible, continue with the following steps.

Timing and dose — introducing which, when and for how long?

- When are the medicines being taken — at the same time or are doses separated by several hours? It is particularly important to determine the timing if a physicochemical interaction is anticipated.
- What is the duration of use? Interaction mechanisms may develop only over several days or weeks (such as CYP induction), or may occur more rapidly.

Outcomes possible

- What is the potential clinical outcome of an interaction — major, minor or neutral? In regard to herbal medicine, this is often speculative.

Practitioner considerations

- Is the practitioner in a position to monitor and manage an interaction should it become significant? In a hospital setting, an interaction is generally considered important if something must be done to relieve patient symptoms or if it will have a significant impact on critical therapy. Practitioners and nursing staff are in an ideal position to monitor for interactions and respond quickly should this be necessary. In a community setting, general practitioners, pharmacists, naturopaths and herbalists are better placed, and adequate patient self-monitoring becomes more important.

Individual considerations

- What are the patient's individual preferences and ability to self-monitor a potential interaction should it arise?

Action required

- Having established the criteria so far, five actions are possible:
  - *Avoid* — consider an alternative treatment that is unlikely to produce undesirable interaction effects.
  - *Avoid unless adequate medical monitoring is possible* — changing the dose and regimen may be required for safe combined use.
  - *Caution* — tell patients to be aware that a particular event is possible and to seek advice if they are concerned.
  - *Observe* — the practitioner is alert to the possibility of an interaction, even though it is unlikely to have clinical consequences and is likely to be a neutral interaction.
  - *Prescribe* — the outcome of the interaction is beneficial and can be used to improve clinical outcomes.

ASSESSING THE LIKELIHOOD OF AN ADVERSE DRUG–HERB INTERACTION

The likelihood that an adverse reaction is responsible for a patient's presenting signs and symptoms should always be considered. If suspicious, then it is essential to take appropriate steps to clarify the likelihood of an adverse reaction.

Patient evaluation

Factors to consider are:

- detailed description of the event — severity of symptoms, signs, onset, duration, frequency
- differential diagnoses (e.g. non-medicinal causes, such as exacerbation of condition, laboratory error or an interaction).

Causality and probability

Determining a cause-and-effect relationship between a medicine and an adverse reaction can be difficult. The degree of certainty that links a medicine to a specific reaction can be classified as definite, probable, possible, conditional or doubtful, and must be assessed in each individual case. Several algorithms exist to help clinicians determine the likelihood of an adverse reaction. Table 4.6 shows the Naranjo algorithm adapted for use as an interaction detection tool (Naranjo et al 1981). The adverse drug reaction possibility classification is based on the total score:

>8	highly probable
4–7	probable
1–3	possible
0	doubtful

TABLE 4.6 ASSESSING THE LIKELIHOOD THAT AN ADVERSE REACTION IS CAUSED BY AN INTERACTION

QUESTION	YES	NO	DON'T KNOW	SCORE
Do previous conclusive reports of this interaction exist?* It is suggested that several resources are examined to determine whether the report is a possible, probable or confirmed interaction.	+1	0	0	
Did the adverse event appear after the suspected medicine/herb/nutrient was co-administered?	+2	−1	0	
Did the adverse reaction improve after the suspected medicine/herb/nutrient was discontinued?	+1	0	0	
Did the adverse reaction reappear when the medicine/herb/nutrient was readministered?	+2	−1	0	
Are there alternative causes (other than the suspected medicine/s) that could produce this reaction?	−1	+2	0	
Was the medicine detected in the blood (or other fluids) at levels known to be toxic or subtherapeutic, when previous levels were within the normal range?	+1	0	0	
Was the reaction more severe when the dose of medicine/herb/nutrient was increased, or less severe when decreased?	+1	0	0	
Has the patient had a similar reaction to the same or similar medicine in any previous exposure, when concomitant complementary medicines were not used?	−2	+1	0	
Was the event confirmed by objective evidence?	+1	0	0	
TOTAL score				

*Although a rechallenge provides important evidence, this is not always appropriate.

NEXT STEPS IF INTERACTION IS LIKELY

Analysis of the medicine

If an interaction involving a herbal or natural medicine is highly likely, then it must be authenticated, botanically verified and analysed for the presence of contaminants. These essential steps will establish whether the interaction is due to an intrinsic property of the medicine itself, and therefore reproducible, or to extrinsic factors such as poor manufacturing processes.

Case reporting

All suspected adverse reactions should be reported to several authorities:

- The local government agency responsible for post-marketing surveillance and collecting adverse drug reaction case reports. In Australia this is the Adverse Drug Reactions Advisory Committee (ADRAC). (Reporting is confidential, open to everyone and is now possible online at www.tga.gov.au.)
- Relevant local herbal and natural medicine associations such as the National Herbalists Association of Australia (www.nhaa.org.au).
- Relevant product manufacturer. (Manufacturers keep their own records and are obligated to inform the TGA.)
- Prescriber, if applicable.

Chapter 3 provides further practical information about the safe use of CAM and risk factors for adverse events and interactions.

TWO MEDICINES REQUIRING SPECIAL ATTENTION

DIGOXIN

Digoxin is a drug indicated for the treatment of numerous cardiac ailments, such as atrial fibrillation and severe heart failure. It has a positive inotropic effect on both normal and failing hearts, although its primary benefit is mediated by neurohormonal modulation. It has a narrow therapeutic index and therefore minor changes in dose or serum levels can have clinically significant consequences. Digoxin is subject to pharmacokinetic and pharmacodynamic interactions with pharmaceutical, herbal and natural medicines, resulting in possible therapeutic failure or toxicity (Table 4.7).

Potassium changes

Potassium states are of special concern with digoxin because hypokalaemia lowers the threshold for drug toxicity. It is well known that pharmaceutical medicines such as thiazide diuretics and corticosteroids have the potential to induce a state of hypokalaemia. There are several herbal medicines that require attention such as *Glycyrrhiza glabra* (licorice), *Paullinia cupana*

TABLE 4.7 SUSPECTED OR KNOWN INTERACTIONS BETWEEN DIGOXIN AND HERBAL MEDICINES

INCREASED DIGOXIN EFFECTS POSSIBLE	DECREASED DIGOXIN EFFECTS POSSIBLE
Herbs that induce potassium loss with long-term use: • *Glycyrrhiza glabra* (licorice) • *Paullinia cupana* (guarana) • Anthraquinone-containing herbal laxatives (senna, cascara, aloes and buckthorn) Some herbal diuretics may also induce some degree of potassium loss; however, clinical significance is unknown.	Herbs currently known to induce P-gp and/or CYPs in a clinically significant manner: • *Hypericum perforatum* (St John's wort)
Herbs containing cardiac glycosides: • *Nerium oleander* (oleander) • *Adonis autumnalis* (false hellebore) • *Convallaria majalis* (lily of the valley)	Herbs containing > 50,000 ppm potassium: • *Avena sativa* (oats) • *Taraxacum officinale* (dandelion) • *Apium graveolens* (celery)
Pharmacodynamic interaction theoretically possible, although not seen in one clinical study: • *Crataegus oxyacantha* (hawthorn)	Foods containing >50,000 ppm potassium: • asparagus • beetroot • bok choy • cucumber • lettuce • rhubarb • spinach
Herbs and natural constituents known or suspected to inhibit P-gp or CYPs: • apple juice • curcumin • daidzein • genistein • grapefruit • green tea polyphenols • orange juice (seville oranges) • piperine • quercetin • resveratrol • rosemary extract	

(guarana) and anthraquinone laxatives (e.g. aloes, buckthorn, cascara and senna). As with potassium-depleting drugs, adequate potassium intake should be recommended and potassium levels monitored together with clinical signs and symptoms.

Alternatively, there are a number of herbal medicines and foods that contain significant amounts of potassium that could increase the threshold for drug efficacy. Some of the common herbs and foods containing greater than 50,000 ppm of potassium include asparagus, beetroot, bok choy, cucumber, lettuce, rhubarb, *Avena sativa* (oats), *Taraxacum officinale* (dandelion) and *Apium graveolens* (celery).

P-gp and changes to metabolism

Digoxin is a substrate for P-gp, therefore serum digoxin levels are altered when P-gp induction or inhibition occurs. It is known that drugs such as verapamil and quinidine, which affect P-gp, can significantly interact with digoxin and in recent years several herbal and natural medicines have also been identified with the potential to alter P-gp activity. Of these, the herb St John's wort has been investigated under controlled clinical conditions and found to decrease the digoxin area-under-the-curve by 25% after 10 days' treatment (Johne et al 1999). Monitoring of plasma digoxin concentration and clinical effects is required when patients commence or cease St John's wort while taking digoxin. As discussed earlier, several other herbs affect P-gp expression and concurrent use should be supervised.

Pharmacodynamic interactions

Pharmacodynamic interactions are theoretically possible when herbs containing naturally occurring cardiac glycoside constituents, such as oleander (*Nerium oleander*), false hellebore (*Adonis autumnalis*) and lily of the valley (*Convallaria majalis*), are ingested at the same time. Although not commonly prescribed for internal use, theoretically these plants may reinforce drug activity and induce symptoms of toxicity. Signs and symptoms of digoxin toxicity include anorexia, nausea, vomiting, diarrhoea, weakness, visual disturbances and ventricular tachycardia.

It has been speculated that the herb hawthorn (*Crataegus oxyacantha*) could potentiate the effects of cardiac glycosides, as both in vitro and in vivo studies indicate it has positive inotropic activity. Furthermore, the flavonoid components of hawthorn also affect P-gp function and cause interactions with drugs that are P-gp substrates, such as digoxin. In practice, however, results from a randomised crossover trial that evaluated co-administration of digoxin 0.25 mg with *Crataegus* special extract WS 1442 (hawthorn leaves with flowers) 450 mg twice daily for 21 days found no significant difference to any measured pharmacokinetic parameters (Tankanow et al 2003). Although this is reassuring, combined use should be supervised by a healthcare professional and drug requirements monitored.

In practice, the likelihood and significance of these interactions varies considerably, and the response required to ensure safe use of medicines can be multifaceted. For example, if Mr A has been taking St John's wort for several months and then digoxin is introduced, routine monitoring of digoxin levels enables appropriate doses to be determined and ensures the safe use of both medicines. However, it is essential to advise Mr A to inform his healthcare professional when use of St John's wort is going to be ceased or the dosage changed, as digoxin levels will require closer monitoring during the change. On the other hand, if Mrs B has been taking digoxin for some time and then St John's wort is to be introduced, additional monitoring is required for at least 3 weeks to determine whether a new effective digoxin dose is required. Once again, if there is to be an alteration to St John's wort use, Mrs B should be advised to see a health-care professional for monitoring during the transition.

Interference with therapeutic drug monitoring for digoxin

In 1996, a case was reported of a possible interaction between Siberian ginseng and digoxin (McRae 1996). More specifically, it involved an elderly man whose serum digoxin levels rose (but did not produce toxic symptoms) when he concurrently took a Siberian ginseng product, fell when the product was stopped and then rose again when use was resumed. Unfortunately, the report was inaccurate, as the product was later analysed and found to contain digitalis. Additionally, no case reports suggesting drug toxicity were published over the following years. Research published in 2010 suggests that eleutherosides found in the herb are chemically related to cardiac glycosides and may interfere with digoxin assays. Furthermore, several other herbal medicines have been identified with the ability to interfere with drug monitoring for digoxin, such as Dan Shen, Chan Su, *Uzara* root and Asian ginseng (Dasgupta 2003). According to Dasgupta, monitoring free digoxin eliminates the interference from Dan Shen and Chan Su, but is not useful in overcoming interference by Siberian or Asian ginseng. For these herbs, using the EMIT urine test or the Bayer, Randox, Roche or Beckman assays is appropriate.

WARFARIN

Warfarin is an important anticoagulant drug with a narrow therapeutic index. If blood levels become elevated, potentially serious consequences can arise if bleeding complications develop, whereas reduced blood levels can result in failure to protect the patient from thromboembolic events. Pharmacologically, the anticoagulant effect is dependent on its ability to interfere with hepatic synthesis of vitamin K-dependent clotting factors. As such, any significant changes to vitamin K ingestion can alter the drug's activity. Common foods with high vitamin K levels (>100 micrograms/100 g) are: beef (liver), broccoli, cabbage, cauliflower, egg yolk, kale, lettuce, spinach, canola oil (rapeseed) and soybean oil.

Pharmacodynamic interactions

Pharmacodynamic interactions can theoretically occur when other medicines with coagulant or anticoagulant activity are used concurrently. Medicines with antiplatelet activity, such as ginger and garlic, can theoretically increase the risk of bruising or bleeding when taken concurrently with warfarin. Other herbal medicines suspected to potentiate the pharmacological effects of warfarin include guarana and bilberry in very high doses. Alternatively, herbs containing naturally occurring coumarins exhibit weak anticoagulant activity, if any at all (unless converted to dicoumarol as a result of improper storage), so do not necessarily pose an additional bleeding risk.

The case of *Ginkgo biloba* is a curious one, as there is evidence that one of its components, ginkgolide B, is a potent platelet-activating factor antagonist (Smith et al 1996). However, multiple placebo-controlled studies have failed to detect a significant effect on platelet function or coagulation (see monograph for more details). One was an escalating dose study, which found that 120 mg, 240 mg or 480 mg given daily for 14 days did not alter platelet function or coagulation (Bal Dit et al 2003). Interaction studies have further found that the INR does not increase when patients are concurrently taking *Ginkgo biloba* with warfarin (Engelsen et al 2002, Jiang et al 2005). Owing to the serious nature of such potential interactions, a cautious approach is advised.

Pharmacokinetic interactions

Warfarin consists of a pair of enantiomers and is extensively metabolised by CYP1A2, 3A4 and 2C9. Metabolism of the more biologically active isomer, the S form, occurs chiefly by CYP2C9, whereas a minor metabolic pathway is CYP3A4. The less potent R isomer is chiefly metabolised by CYP1A2. Therefore, any alteration to the expression or activity of these specific enzymes can affect the drug's pharmacokinetics.

As is the case with nearly all herbal medicines, predicting the clinical significance of these theoretical interactions is difficult because most evidence currently comes from in vitro and in vivo tests and case reports.

THE RATIONAL USE OF HERBAL AND NATURAL MEDICINES

Since the first few human studies were conducted back in the late 1990s suggesting serious herb-drug interactions could occur, hundreds of further studies have been performed to test whether commonly used herbal medicines have the potential to interact with pharmaceutical drugs. At the time, the media touted the first studies as being the 'tip of the iceberg' and headlines of 'dangerous drug-herb cocktails' were commonplace.

Over the last 15 years, it has become apparent that the metaphorical iceberg has not emerged and there are, in fact, only a handful of commonly used herbal medicines with the potential to cause serious drug interactions. Medicines with a narrow therapeutic window are of greatest concern (such as warfarin), as are medications used in serious diseases and life-threatening situations such as anti-rejection, anticancer and anti-HIV medication.

As with all drug interactions, safety is greatly improved when patients openly discuss all the medications they are taking, clinicians are informed about the potential for interactions and appropriate steps are taken to avoid or minimise the interaction via separating doses, altering dosage regimens, ceasing some treatments or altering drug dosages. Often careful supervision is all that is required by an informed clinician and diligent patient.

TABLE 4.8 RATIONAL USE OF HERBAL AND NATURAL MEDICINES

- Be informed and seek out unbiased information — do not rely on label claims alone.
- Know the benefits, risks, potential adverse reactions and interactions — additional training and/or access to accurate and updated information is important.
- Do not assume all healthcare professionals have the knowledge to monitor safe use.
- Be aware that medical practitioners' and pharmacists' knowledge of herbal and natural medicines may be limited.
- Ensure that all healthcare professionals involved in a patient's care stay informed of herbal and natural medicine use.
- Take care with children, the elderly and pregnant or lactating women.
- Take care when high-risk medicines are being taken.
- Take care with HIV, cancer or other serious illnesses.
- Know the manufacturer or supplier details.
- Store medicines appropriately.

The two algorithms presented in this chapter provide a general guide to help in clinical practice and make sure the key factors are considered. As always, it is important to recognise that using this information in practice requires individual interpretation, because the clinical effects of any interaction, no matter how well documented, will not occur consistently in each patient, each time or to the same degree of intensity. Ultimately, it is the application of current knowledge, together with good observational skills, open communication and clinical experience that will reduce the risk of unwanted interactions and maximise successful outcomes. Table 4.8 lists key steps towards the rational use of herbal and natural medicines.

REFERENCES

Aklillu E et al. Frequent distribution of ultrarapid metabolizers of debrisoquine in an Ethiopian population carrying duplicated and multiduplicated functional CYP2D6 alleles. J Pharmacol Exp Ther 278.1 (1996): 441–446.

Anuchapreeda S et al. Modulation of P-glycoprotein expression and function by curcumin in multidrug-resistant human KB cells. Biochem Pharmacol 64.4 (2002): 573–582.

Bailey DG et al. Grapefruit juice–drug interactions. Br J Clin Pharmacol 46.2 (1998): 101–110.

Bal Dit SC et al. No alteration in platelet function or coagulation induced by EGb761 in a controlled study. Clin Lab Haematol 25.4 (2003): 251–253.

Barone GW et al. Drug interaction between St. John's wort and cyclosporine. Ann Pharmacother 34.9 (2000): 1013–1016.

Baxter NJ et al. Multiple interactions between polyphenols and a salivary proline-rich protein repeat result in complexation and precipitation. Biochemistry 36.18 (1997): 5566–5577.

Becquemont L et al. Effect of grapefruit juice on digoxin pharmacokinetics in humans. Clin Pharmacol Ther 70.4 (2001): 311–316.

Benet LZ, Cummins CL. The drug efflux–metabolism alliance: biochemical aspects. Adv Drug Deliv Rev 50 Suppl 1 (2001): S3–11.

Bhardwaj RK et al. Piperine, a major constituent of black pepper, inhibits human P-glycoprotein and CYP3A4. J Pharmacol Exp Ther 302.2 (2002): 645–650.

Blower P et al. Drug–drug interactions in oncology: why are they important and can they be minimized? Crit Rev Oncol Hematol 55.2 (2005): 117–142.

Bone K, Mills S. Principles and practice of phytotherapy. London: Elsevier, 2000.

Brune M et al. Iron absorption and phenolic compounds: importance of different phenolic structures. Eur J Clin Nutr 43.8 (1989): 547–557.

Butterweck V et al. Solubilized hypericin and pseudohypericin from Hypericum perforatum exert antidepressant activity in the forced swimming test. Planta Med 64.4 (1998): 291–294.

Castro AF, Altenberg GA. Inhibition of drug transport by genistein in multidrug-resistant cells expressing P-glycoprotein. Biochem Pharmacol 53.1 (1997): 89–93.

Chang TK et al. Distinct role of bilobalide and ginkgolide A in the modulation of rat CYP2B1 and CYP3A23 gene expression by Ginkgo biloba extract in cultured hepatocytes. Drug Metab Dispos 34.2 (2006a): 234–42.

Chang TK et al. Effect of Ginkgo biloba extract on procarcinogen-bioactivating human CYP1 enzymes: identification of isorhamnetin, kaempferol, and quercetin as potent inhibitors of CYP1B1. Toxicol Appl Pharmacol 213.1 (2006b): 18–26.

Chatterjee SS et al. Influence of the Ginkgo extract EGb 761 on rat liver cytochrome P450 and steroid metabolism and excretion in rats and man. J Pharm Pharmacol 57.5 (2005): 641–650.

Choi JS, Li X. Enhanced diltiazem bioavailability after oral administration of diltiazem with quercetin to rabbits. Int J Pharm 297.1–2 (2005): 1–8.

Chung SY et al. Inhibition of P-glycoprotein by natural products in human breast cancer cells. Arch Pharm Res 28.7 (2005): 823–828.

Dasgupta A. Review of abnormal laboratory test results and toxic effects due to use of herbal medicines. Am J Clin Pathol 120.1 (2003): 127–137.

Den Boer ML et al. The modulating effect of PSC 833, cyclosporin A, verapamil and genistein on in vitro cytotoxicity and intracellular content of daunorubicin in childhood acute lymphoblastic leukemia. Leukemia 12.6 (1998): 912–920.

Di Marco MP et al. The effect of grapefruit juice and Seville orange juice on the pharmacokinetics of dextromethorphan: the role of gut CYP3A and P-glycoprotein. Life Sci 71.10 (2002): 1149–1160.

Doherty MM, Charman WN. The mucosa of the small intestine: how clinically relevant as an organ of drug metabolism? Clin Pharmacokinet 41.4 (2002): 235–253.

Dresser GK et al. Fruit juices inhibit organic anion transporting polypeptide-mediated drug uptake to decrease the oral availability of fexofenadine. Clin Pharmacol Ther 71.1 (2002): 11–20.

Durr D et al. St John's Wort induces intestinal P-glycoprotein/MDR1 and intestinal and hepatic CYP3A4. Clin Pharmacol Ther 68.6 (2000): 598–604.

Eagling VA et al. Inhibition of the CYP3A4-mediated metabolism and P-glycoprotein-mediated transport of the HIV-1 protease inhibitor saquinavir by grapefruit juice components. Br J Clin Pharmacol 48.4 (1999): 543–552.

Edwards DJ et al. 6′,7′-Dihydroxybergamottin in grapefruit juice and Seville orange juice: effects on cyclosporine disposition, enterocyte CYP3A4, and P-glycoprotein. Clin Pharmacol Ther 65.3 (1999): 237–244.

Engelsen J et al. Effect of coenzyme Q10 and Ginkgo biloba on warfarin dosage in stable, long-term warfarin treated outpatients: A randomised, double blind, placebo-crossover trial. Thromb Haemost 87.6 (2002): 1075–1076.

Evans AM. Influence of dietary components on the gastrointestinal metabolism and transport of drugs. Ther Drug Monit 22.1 (2000): 131–136.

Flockhart DA. Drug interactions: cytochrome P450 drug interaction table. Indiana University School of Medicine (2007). Available: http://medicine.iupui.edu/flockhart/table.htm 23/7/2014.

Fukao T et al. The effects of allyl sulfides on the induction of phase II detoxification enzymes and liver injury by carbon tetrachloride. Food Chem Toxicol 42.5 (2004): 743–749.

Gaudineau C et al. Inhibition of human P450 enzymes by multiple constituents of the Ginkgo biloba extract. Biochem Biophys Res Commun 318.4 (2004): 1072–1078.

Glahn RP et al. Inhibition of iron uptake by phytic acid, tannic acid, and ZnCl2: studies using an in vitro digestion/Caco-2 cell model. J Agric Food Chem 50.2 (2002): 390–395.

Greenblatt DJ et al. Ginkgo biloba does not alter clearance of flurbiprofen, a cytochrome P450-2C9 substrate. J Clin Pharmacol 46.2 (2006): 214–221.

Gurley BJ et al. Cytochrome P450 phenotypic ratios for predicting herb–drug interactions in humans. Clin Pharmacol Ther 72.3 (2002): 276–287.

Gurley BJ et al. Effect of milk thistle (Silybum marianum) and black cohosh (Cimicifuga racemosa) supplementation on digoxin pharmacokinetics in humans. Drug Metab Dispos 34.1 (2006): 69–74.

Gurley BJ et al. In vivo assessment of botanical supplementation on human cytochrome P450 phenotypes: Citrus aurantium, Echinacea purpurea, milk thistle, and saw palmetto. Clin Pharmacol Ther 76.5 (2004): 428–440.

Gurley BJ et al. In vivo effects of goldenseal, kava kava, black cohosh, and valerian on human cytochrome P450 1A2, 2D6, 2E1, and 3A4/5 phenotypes. Clin Pharmacol Ther 77.5 (2005): 415–426.

Gurley BJ et al. Pharmacokinetic herb-drug interactions (part 2): drug interactions involving popular botanical dietary supplements and their clinical relevance. Planta Med, 78.13 (2012): 1490–1514.

He N, Edeki T. The inhibitory effects of herbal components on CYP2C9 and CYP3A4 catalytic activities in human liver microsomes. Am J Ther 11.3 (2004): 206–212.

Hennessy M et al. St John's wort increases expression of P-glycoprotein: implications for drug interactions. Br J Clin Pharmacol 53.1 (2002): 75–82.

Hsiu SL et al. Quercetin significantly decreased cyclosporin oral bioavailability in pigs and rats. Life Sci 72.3 (2002): 227–235.

Huupponen R et al. Effect of guar gum, a fibre preparation, on digoxin and penicillin absorption in man. Eur J Clin Pharmacol 26.2 (1984): 279–281.

Ikegawa T et al. Inhibition of P-glycoprotein by orange juice components, polymethoxyflavones in adriamycin-resistant human myelogenous leukemia (K562/ADM) cells. Cancer Lett 160.1 (2000): 21–28.

Ingelman-Sundberg M. Pharmacogenetics of cytochrome P450 and its applications in drug therapy: the past, present and future. Trends Pharmacol Sci 25.4 (2004): 193–200.

Jiang X et al. Effect of ginkgo and ginger on the pharmacokinetics and pharmacodynamics of warfarin in healthy subjects. Br J Clin Pharmacol 59.4 (2005): 425–432.

Jin et al. Enhancement of oral bioavailability of paclitaxel after oral administration of Schisandrol B in rats. Biopharmaceutics & Drug Disposition 31.4 (2010): 264–268.

Jodoin J et al. Inhibition of the multidrug resistance P-glycoprotein activity by green tea polyphenols. Biochim Biophys Acta 1542.1–3 (2002): 149–159.

Johne A et al. Pharmacokinetic interaction of digoxin with an herbal extract from St John's wort (Hypericum perforatum). Clin Pharmacol Ther 66.4 (1999): 338–345.

Kane GC, Lipsky JJ. Drug–grapefruit juice interactions. Mayo Clin Proc 75.9 (2000): 933–942.

Kitagawa S et al. Structure–activity relationships of the inhibitory effects of flavonoids on P-glycoprotein-mediated transport in KB-C2 cells. Biol Pharm Bull 28.12 (2005): 2274–2278.
Kubota Y et al. Pretreatment with Ginkgo biloba extract weakens the hypnosis action of phenobarbital and its plasma concentration in rats. J Pharm Pharmacol 56.3 (2004): 401–405.
Kuo I et al. Effect of Ginkgo biloba extract on rat hepatic microsomal CYP1A activity: role of ginkgolides, bilobalide, and flavonols. Can J Physiol Pharmacol 82.1 (2004): 57–64.
Lin JH. Drug–drug interaction mediated by inhibition and induction of P-glycoprotein. Adv Drug Deliv Rev 55.1 (2003): 53–81.
Lown KS et al. Role of intestinal P-glycoprotein (mdr1) in interpatient variation in the oral bioavailability of cyclosporine. Clin Pharmacol Ther 62.3 (1997): 248–260.
Markowitz JS et al. Multiple doses of saw palmetto (Serenoa repens) did not alter cytochrome P450 2D6 and 3A4 activity in normal volunteers. Clin Pharmacol Ther 74.6 (2003a): 536–542.
Markowitz JS et al. Multiple-dose administration of Ginkgo biloba did not affect cytochrome P-450 2D6 or 3A4 activity in normal volunteers. J Clin Psychopharmacol 23.6 (2003b): 576–581.
Markowitz JS et al. Predicting interactions between conventional medications and botanical products on the basis of in vitro investigations. Mol Nutr Food Res 52.7 (2008): 747–754.
McRae S. Elevated serum digoxin levels in a patient taking digoxin and Siberian ginseng. Can Med Assoc J 155.3 (1996): 293–295.
Meseguer E et al. Life-threatening parkinsonism induced by kava-kava. Mov Disord 17.1 (2002): 195–196.
Mills S. The essential book of herbal medicine. Arkana: Penguin Books, 1991.
Mohutsky MA et al. Ginkgo biloba: evaluation of CYP2C9 drug interactions in vitro and in vivo. Am J Ther 13.1 (2006a): 24–31.
Mohutsky MA et al. Ginkgo biloba: evaluation of CYP2C9 drug interactions in vitro and in vivo. Am J Ther 13.1 (2006b): 24–31.
Moore LB et al. St. John's wort induces hepatic drug metabolism through activation of the pregnane X receptor. Proc Natl Acad Sci USA 97.13 (2000): 7500–7502.
Naranjo CA et al. A method for estimating the probability of adverse drug reactions. Clin Pharmacol Ther 30.2 (1981): 239–245.
Ohnishi A et al. Effect of furanocoumarin derivatives in grapefruit juice on the uptake of vinblastine by Caco-2 cells and on the activity of cytochrome P450 3A4. Br J Pharmacol 130.6 (2000): 1369–1377.
Ohnishi N et al. Studies on interactions between functional foods or dietary supplements and medicines. I. Effects of Ginkgo biloba leaf extract on the pharmacokinetics of diltiazem in rats. Biol Pharm Bull 26.9 (2003): 1315–1320.
Perloff MD et al. Saint John's wort: an in vitro analysis of P-glycoprotein induction due to extended exposure. Br J Pharmacol 134.8 (2001): 1601–1608.
Pirmohamed M, Park BK. Cytochrome P450 enzyme polymorphisms and adverse drug reactions. Toxicology 192.1 (2003): 23–32.
Plouzek CA et al. Inhibition of P-glycoprotein activity and reversal of multidrug resistance in vitro by rosemary extract. Eur J Cancer 35.10 (1999): 1541–1545.
Roby CA et al. St John's Wort: effect on CYP3A4 activity. Clin Pharmacol Ther 67.5 (2000): 451–457.
Romiti N et al. Effects of curcumin on P-glycoprotein in primary cultures of rat hepatocytes. Life Sci 62.25 (1998): 2349–2358.
Ruschitzka F et al. Acute heart transplant rejection due to Saint John's wort. Lancet 355.9203 (2000): 548–549.
Ryu SD, Chung WG. Induction of the procarcinogen-activating CYP1A2 by a herbal dietary supplement in rats and humans. Food Chem Toxicol 41.6 (2003): 861–866.
Sadzuka Y et al. Efficacies of tea components on doxorubicin induced antitumor activity and reversal of multidrug resistance. Toxicol Lett 114.1–3 (2000): 155–162.
Scambia G et al. Quercetin potentiates the effect of adriamycin in a multidrug-resistant MCF-7 human breast-cancer cell line: P-glycoprotein as a possible target. Cancer Chemother Pharmacol 34.6 (1994): 459–464.
Shinozuka K et al. Feeding of Ginkgo biloba extract (GBE) enhances gene expression of hepatic cytochrome P-450 and attenuates the hypotensive effect of nicardipine in rats. Life Sci 70.23 (2002): 2783–2792.
Smith PF et al. The neuroprotective properties of the Ginkgo biloba leaf: a review of the possible relationship to platelet-activating factor (PAF). J Ethnopharmacol 50.3 (1996): 131–139.
Soldner A et al. Grapefruit juice activates P-glycoprotein-mediated drug transport. Pharm Res 16.4 (1999): 478–485.
Spahn-Langguth H, Langguth P. Grapefruit juice enhances intestinal absorption of the P-glycoprotein substrate talinolol. Eur J Pharm Sci 12.4 (2001): 361–367.
Spillane PK et al. Neurological manifestations of kava intoxication. Med J Aust 167.3 (1997): 172–173.
Sugiyama T et al. Ginkgo biloba extract modifies hypoglycemic action of tolbutamide via hepatic cytochrome P450 mediated mechanism in aged rats. Life Sci 75.9 (2004a): 1113–1122.
Sugiyama T et al. Induction and recovery of hepatic drug metabolizing enzymes in rats treated with Ginkgo biloba extract. Food Chem Toxicol 42.6 (2004b): 953–957.
Takanaga H et al. Inhibition of vinblastine efflux mediated by P-glycoprotein by grapefruit juice components in Caco-2 cells. Biol Pharm Bull 21.10 (1998): 1062–1066.
Takanaga H et al. Polymethoxylated flavones in orange juice are inhibitors of P-glycoprotein but not cytochrome P450 3A4. J Pharmacol Exp Ther 293.1 (2000): 230–236.
Tankanow R et al. Interaction study between digoxin and a preparation of hawthorn (Crataegus oxyacantha). J Clin Pharmacol 43.6 (2003): 637–642.
Tian R et al. Effects of grapefruit juice and orange juice on the intestinal efflux of P-glycoprotein substrates. Pharm Res 19.6 (2002): 802–809.
USFDA (United States Food and Drug Administration). [Cytochrome enzymes]. Available online: www.fda.gov/ 23/7/2014.

Von Moltke LL et al. Inhibition of human cytochromes P450 by components of Ginkgo biloba. J Pharm Pharmacol 56.8 (2004): 1039–1044

Wagner D et al. Intestinal drug efflux: formulation and food effects. Adv Drug Deliv Rev 50 (Suppl 1) (2001): S13–S31.

Wang YH et al. Lethal quercetin-digoxin interaction in pigs. Life Sci 74.10 (2004): 1191–1197.

Wang Z et al. The effects of St John's wort (Hypericum perforatum) on human cytochrome P450 activity. Clin Pharmacol Ther 70.4 (2001): 317–326.

Yale SH, Glurich I. Analysis of the inhibitory potential of Ginkgo biloba, Echinacea purpurea, and Serenoa repens on the metabolic activity of cytochrome P450 3A4, 2D6, and 2C9. J Altern Complement Med 11.3 (2005): 433–439.

Zhang S, Morris ME. Effect of the flavonoids biochanin A and silymarin on the P-glycoprotein-mediated transport of digoxin and vinblastine in human intestinal Caco-2 cells. Pharm Res 20.8 (2003): 1184–1191.

Zhao LZ et al. Induction of propranolol metabolism by Ginkgo biloba extract EGb 761 in rats. Curr Drug Metab 7.6 (2006): 577–587.

CHAPTER 5

HERBS AND NATURAL SUPPLEMENTS IN PREGNANCY

INTRODUCTION

Most women take over-the-counter (OTC) medicines at some point during their pregnancy. This may occur intentionally or inadvertently during the early stages of pregnancy. The advice on many product labels and package inserts is to 'consult your doctor' or 'consult your healthcare provider' before using a particular medicine, yet many healthcare providers are poorly equipped to weigh up the benefits of taking, or not taking, a particular medicine during pregnancy. The risk/benefit assessment is possibly even more complex when considering the safety and efficacy of complementary medicines (CMs).

Medical and complementary medicine practitioners, pharmacists and other healthcare providers face similar challenges when advising the pregnant patient about CMs. Despite their popularity, there is very little published evidence regarding the efficacy and safety of natural medicines during pregnancy and lactation. Modern and traditional texts may warn against use; however, little information is provided about the evidence used to come to such a recommendation. Information about the potential efficacy of CMs in pregnancy is also scarce.

This chapter aims to provide readers with an introduction to the fundamental concepts and concerns surrounding the use of CMs in pregnancy. Part 1 explores the use of herbs and natural supplements in pregnancy from a contemporary and traditional approach. Safety and evidence issues are discussed in Part 2. Central to this section is a discussion about the methods of establishing the safety of any medicine in pregnancy. Part 3 provides a guide as to how the information presented in this chapter may be used to shape clinical practice.

PART 1 — HERBS AND NATURAL SUPPLEMENTS USED IN PREGNANCY

It is commonly known that CM is widely used throughout the world. In many countries traditional medicine continues to form the basis of primary healthcare (WHO 2002). There is an increasing trend in developed countries, including Australia, for the use of traditional and complementary medicines (MacLennan et al 2002, Thomas et al 2001, Tindle et al 2005, Xue et al 2007). The literature indicates that women frequently use CM during pregnancy; however, usage estimates vary considerably due to variations in the definition of CM used, geographical location, socioeconomic and cultural influences. For example, surveys conducted in Europe, the United States and Canada indicate the prevalence of CM usage in pregnancy to range from 7.1 to 96% (Forster et al 2006). Australian statistics estimate that between 10% (Henry & Crowther 2000) and 91% (Forster et al 2007) of all pregnant women will use CM at some stage during their pregnancy. Specifically in regards to herbal medicines, although the majority of women discontinue taking herbal medicines once they are aware of their pregnancies, some others may commence taking them on the advice of their maternity care providers (Ranzini et al 2001).

Surveys of Australian women have identified that nutritional supplements are frequently taken before and throughout pregnancy. During the preconception period, the most common supplements used are folate (29–33%), multivitamins (11–12%) and other supplements including vitamin C, calcium and iron (12–15%). During pregnancy, folate use increases to 70–79% of women (particularly in the first trimester), multivitamins 27–35%, iron 38–52% and other supplements including calcium, vitamin B_6 (predominantly in the first trimester) and zinc. The herbal medicine most often used in pregnancy is raspberry leaf (particularly in the last trimester) (Forster et al 2007, Maats & Crowther 2002).

Despite the widespread use of CM, pregnant women do not always disclose their use of CMs to their healthcare providers. In one study only 1% of participants' medical records listed their CM use (Maats & Crowther 2002), while another study reported 75% of women had informed their primary care provider (Tsui et al 2001). This is problematic as it is a missed opportunity for women to receive informed advice about the effectiveness and safety of the medicines they have chosen to use and prevent unsafe outcomes. Unsupervised use potentially increases the risk of drug interactions with prescribed medicines and contributes to the under-reporting of side effects and adverse outcomes.

Some pregnant women are motivated to take CMs in lieu of conventional medicine as they regard them as safer treatments (Hollyer et al 2002). Sometimes self-prescribed use is justified, such as using nutritional supplements to meet increased nutritional requirements or to treat a pregnancy-related health issue (e.g. nausea or general pregnancy preparation) or to treat non-pregnancy specific problems (e.g. the common cold) (Henry & Crowther 2000, Maats & Crowther 2002, Nordeng & Havnen 2004).

Pregnant women appear to use a variety of information sources to aid their selection of CMs including healthcare practitioners (Forster et al 2007, Tsui et al 2001), friends, family members (Hollyer et al 2002, Maats & Crowther 2002, Nordeng & Havnen 2004, Tsui et al 2001) and media sources (e.g. magazines and internet) (Tsui et al 2001).

NUTRITIONAL MEDICINE

Pregnant women choose to use nutritional medicines as symptomatic treatment to improve their own health in general and to optimise the healthy development of the growing child and its safe delivery.

Most clinicians will be aware of the changes in nutritional requirements that occur in pregnancy and the need for women to increase their dietary intake of certain nutrients such as iron, calcium, folate and others. Nutritional supplements are sometimes used to help women achieve these higher intake levels and correct preexisting deficiencies. The National Health and Medical Research Council (NHMRC) nutritional guidelines for the adequate intake of vitamins and minerals (Australian Government 2006) provides guidelines for nutritional requirements during pregnancy; however, they are only estimates based on extrapolated data from other populations and models, and do not take into account the individual's specific needs. In practice, a detailed diet and lifestyle history is necessary and sometimes additional pathology testing to enable clinicians to make more appropriate individual recommendations.

Besides enabling women to meet their basic nutritional needs, nutritional supplements are also used in larger doses to act as pharmacological agents to ameliorate symptoms and address a specific health complaint. For example, calcium and magnesium supplements have been used to reduce the severity of leg cramps, pyridoxine to alleviate nausea and folate to reduce the incidence of neural tube defects. Appendix 5.1 (p. 116) lists common nutritional supplements and their use in pregnancy. Appendix 5.2 (p. 130) lists dosage recommendations for the nutrients.

Long-term impact of maternal nutrition

The 'developmental origins of disease' hypothesis suggests that the benefits of a nutritional intervention may extend much further than those more immediate outcomes. Environmental factors during development, such as maternal nutrition, have been shown to influence the expression of our phenotype. The most sensitive time for this influence has been shown in-utero. Fetal nutrition can alter the body's structure, function and metabolism, subsequently affecting the risk of developing diseases later in life (Barker 2004). Longitudinal studies from around the world have found low birth weight (in relation to gestational age) is associated with increased risk of coronary heart disease, stroke, hypertension and type 2 diabetes in adulthood (Barker 2007). Furthermore, maternal vitamin D status during pregnancy appears to influence the bone-mineral density of offspring, even in late childhood (Javaid et al 2006). Similarly, there is some evidence suggesting that calcium supplementation during pregnancy can reduce the offspring's blood pressure during their childhood (Hatton et al 2003).

HERBAL MEDICINE

Herbal medicines are used in pregnancy as pharmacological agents. They are used as foods, such as ginger, in extract form (liquid and solid dose forms) and also as teas. In many developing countries, herbal medicines have been used as the dominant form of medicine and continue to play a major role in healthcare, reproductive health and midwifery (WHO 2002).

A traditional approach

Although conception is a problem for some women nowadays, a more common problem throughout the ages was contraception. Ethnobotanical studies conducted in many parts of the world reveal that herbal medicines have been used widely to prevent conception and induce miscarriage for generations, and in some parts of the world, their use continues despite the availability of pharmaceutical contraceptive pills and devices. Besides this, herbal medicines have been used to enhance fertility, regulate menstruation, facilitate childbirth, help with expulsion of the placenta and promote lactation.

In many cultures, herbal healers have special reverence for herbs thought to have abortifacient or emmenagogue properties. These concepts are foreign in Western medicine and deserve some discussion.

Abortifacients

Plants have been used as a source of both contraceptives and early-term abortifacients since the times of ancient Egypt (Riddle 1991) and in some parts of the world this practice still occurs. The abortifacient effects of herbs are attributed to their inherent toxicity or ability to induce uterine contractions (Noumi & Tchakonang 2001). It is also suspected that abortifacient activity may be immune-mediated, hormonal or due to non-specific actions such as the ability to reduce uterine blood flow. Examples of western herbs with abortifacient potential due to suspected toxicity include: wormwood (*Artemisia absinthium*), pennyroyal (*Mentha pulegium*), poke root (*Phytolacca decandra*), pau d'arco (*Tabebuia avellanedae*), rue (*Ruta graveolens*) and tansy (*Tanacetum vulgare*) (Mills & Bone 2005).

Emmenagogues

The term 'emmenagogue' is used to describe a herb that will stimulate menstrual flow. These herbs have been traditionally indicated for delayed menstruation and developed a reputation as being contraindicated in pregnancy for fear they may induce miscarriage. Herbalists consider emmenagogues as exerting oxytocic-like effects which cause uterine contractions; however, this mechanism is unlikely to explain how they promote menses in a non-pregnant woman. Changes to lymph or blood flow and hormonal effects are more likely mechanisms. Examples of herbs found on many traditional lists thought to act as emmenagogues include aloe (*Aloe vera*), juniper (*Juniperus communis*), pennyroyal (*Mentha pulegium*), goldenseal (*Hydrastis canadensis*), black cohosh (*Cimicifuga racemosa*), blue cohosh (*Caulophyllum thalictroides*), dong quai (*Angelica polymorpha*), rue (*Ruta graveolens*), tansy (*Tanacetum vulgare*), and thuja (*Thuja occidentalis*). Some herbs considered as emmenagogues are also thought of as potential abortifacients if used in sufficient quantities (e.g. oxytocin agonists); however, not all abortifacients may act as emmenagogues, e.g. potentially toxic herbs with no hormonal or uterine effects.

Historical perspectives

The use of medicinal plants has occurred in Mexico since pre-Hispanic times. Nearly 10,000,000 indigenous people speaking nearly 85 different languages inhabit the region and many still depend upon plants for primary therapy from the diverse flora (almost 5000 medicinal plants) (Andrade-Cetto 2009). An ethnobotanical study of the medicinal plants from Tlanchinol, Hidalgo, Mexico identified several plants used as abortifacients: *Galium mexicanum* var *mexicanum, Ruta chalepensis, Zaluzania triloba* and *Tanacetum parthenium.* The herb *Cinnamomum verum* is generally considered useful to induce childbirth and *Pedilanthus tithymaloides* is used for ovarian pain.

The Criollo people of Argentina use a vast plant pharmacopoeia. To date, 189 species with 754 different medicinal applications have been recorded (Martinez 2008). The absence of a normal menstrual cycle and amenorrhoea are matters of concern among these people and are treated with emmenagogue plants, the most common being *Anemia tomentosa, Tripodanthus flagellaris, Lippia turbinata* and *Trixis divaricata.* Contraceptive herbs used in the region include: *Zea mays, Anemia tomentosa* and abortifacient herbs include: *Artemisia absinthium*; *Cheilantes buchtienii*; *Chenopodium aff. hircinum*; *Cuphea glutinosa*; *Ligaria cuneifolia*; *Lippia turbinata*; and *Pinus* spp. (Martinez 2008).

Rama midwives in eastern Nicaragua currently use a diverse group of plants in the practice of midwifery: 162 species from 125 genera and 62 families (Senes et al 2008). This extensive ethnopharmacopoeia is employed to treat the many health issues of pregnancy, parturition, postpartum care, neonatal care and primary healthcare of women and children. The 22 most popular midwifery species are medicinals that are widely used by practitioners other than midwives, not only in eastern Nicaragua, but elsewhere. Very few herbal species are used as contraceptives in this region, whereas abortifacients are well known and mostly made with bitter-tasting plants, probably due to alkaloids and other bitter-tasting compounds. The most widely used abortifacients are decoctions made from the leaves and seeds of soursap and the roots of guinea hen. Others are decoctions made with the leaves and/or flowers of barsley, broom weed, trompet, sorosi and wild rice and the root of ginja.

Interestingly, midwives in other parts of the world use many Rama midwifery species for the same purpose. For example, the two species sorosi and lime are both widely regarded as important in midwifery in many parts of the world. Sorosi is one of the most widely used medicinals in eastern Nicaragua and elsewhere where it is used as an abortifacient, with similar use in Africa, Australia, Brazil, India, Malaysia, Philippines and the West Indies (Senes et al 2008). Lime is a domesticated crop used by the Rama and other indigenous groups of eastern Nicaragua as an abortifacient and to accelerate labour. It is also used to induce abortion by tribal people in India, Honduran midwives and the Tikunas of north-western Amazonia.

Europe has a rich history of herbal medicine use, which continues to be popular today. Plants here were also used for reproductive health, to prevent conception and induce abortion, with women and midwives as the main keepers of herbal knowledge. Savin (*Juniperus sabina*) was one abortifacient herb of choice in Europe and pennyroyal, sage, thyme and rosemary were considered powerful emmenagogues (Belew 1999). Unlike some other parts of the world, information exchange down the generations was interrupted during the 18th and 19th centuries as there was a major shift in management of the birthing process (Schiebinger 2008). During this period, female practitioners with knowledge of herbal lore lost ground to obstetricians (men trained primarily as surgeons) and the use of plant-based treatments was gradually replaced with surgical procedures (Schiebinger 2008). As a result, much knowledge about European use of herbal medicines in fertility and reproduction was lost.

The North American Indians used herbal medicines extensively thoughout the reproductive life cycle and had many remedies for improving fertility, preventing miscarriage, treating symptoms during pregnancy and facilitating the birthing process. A large number of these treatments came to the knowledge of European settlers in North America through careful study, observation and subsequent clinical use. If repeated use indicated the treatments were effective, the herbs were recorded and prescribed by the Eclectic physicians who flourished from the mid-1800s to around 1920 in the United States (Belew 1999). Many of the herbal medicines used by the North American Indians and described by the Eclectic physicians are still in use today as part of the Western herbalists and traditional midwives cache of treatments.

The Eclectics considered black cohosh a 'remedy par excellence to stimulate normal functional activity of the uterus and ovaries' throughout the reproductive life cycle (Belew 1999). They reported that when used regularly at the end of pregnancy 'it will render labor easier and quicker, and give a better getting up'. Black haw was highly regarded by the Eclectic physicians, who used it both before and during pregnancy to prevent miscarriage, prepare for labour and relieve false labour pains and afterpains. The Eclectic physicians preferred to use cotton root (*Gossypium*) as an oxytocin agonist rather than the newly available sublingual oxytocin preparation because the herb was considered to have a more gentle action and produce more predictable results. Squaw vine (*Mitchella repens*) was well considered when enhanced fertility was called for. It was extensively used to promote menstruation and alleviate physical discomfort in the latter months of pregnancy, and was thought to be a good preparative to labour, rendering the birth of a child easier.

Contemporary use by Western herbalists

In Western herbal practice today, much knowledge about herbal safety and efficacy in pregnancy is drawn from North American and European traditions and traditional applications are largely used as a basis for prescriptions. Herbal medicines may be prescribed to regulate menstruation before conception, alleviate morning sickness and other symptoms related to pregnancy. A growing number of gynaecologists and obstetricians are working with herbalists to enhance patients' chances of conception and reduce miscarriage, sometimes in combination with IVF procedures.

Requests for abortifacient herbs in Western countries are virtually unheard of; however, some women still seek herbalists to provide '*partus* (birth) *preparatus* (prepare)' mixtures to prepare for childbirth and facilitate delivery. Traditionally the Eclectic physicians called these preparations 'mother's cordial'. They tend to be recommended in very low doses starting at 36 weeks gestation, increasing in dose each week until delivery. Herbs that have been used in *partus preparatus* preparations include: *Mitchella repens* (squaw vine), *Viburnum prunifolium* (black haw), *Rubus idaeus* (raspberry), *Chamaelirium luteum* (false unicorn), *Caulophyllum thalictroides* (blue cohosh) and *Cimicifuga racemosa* (black cohosh).

Today, Western herbalists are also asked for treatment to address pre- and postnatal depression, alleviate symptoms of dyspepsia, nausea and lower back pain and sometimes topical applications to reduce perineal discomfort and stretch marks associated with pregnancy. In addition, herbalists may be providing support for conditions unrelated to pregnancy, such as urinary tract or upper respiratory tract infections.

Unlike medical practitioners, Western herbalists are less concerned about teratogenicity than inducing miscarriage. To minimise the risk of harming the mother or fetus, several general guidelines are followed. Most importantly, traditional sources dictate that if known toxic herbs are avoided, then toxic side effects are unlikely to occur. In addition, other classes of herbs avoided during pregnancy include the following (Hess et al 2007):

- emmenagogues and abortifacients (discussed above)
- large quantities of herbs containing a high volatile oil content, especially during the first trimester. It is suspected that volatile oils contain constituents that could induce uterine contractions. Many kitchen spices contain

volatile oils, which are not believed to be a problem when used in dietary amounts but could pose problems when used in concentrated preparations, e.g. rosemary, peppermint, thyme, sage. This contraindication is likely to be derived from European tradition

- stimulant laxative herbs containing anthraquinones. These herbal medicines stimulate peristalsis and can induce loss of water and electrolytes, intestinal cramps, loose bowels and dependency with chronic use. It is believed these harsh irritant effects may exert a reflex stimulating effect on the uterus causing uterine contractions. Stimulant laxative herbs include buckthorn, cascara (*Rhamnus* species), rhubarb, castor, senna and aloe. Aloe gel is not a problem as it contains a part of the plant that does not contain significant levels of anthraquinones
- herbs with hormonal actions such as *Trifolium pratense* (red clover) and *Vitex agnus-castus* (chastetree) may adversely influence fetal development
- thujone-containing herbs, e.g. *Achillea millefolium* (yarrow), *Thuja occidentalis* (thuja) or *Artemisia absinthium* (wormwood) due to its inherent toxicity concerns

This approach is based on traditional evidence and theoretical concerns, usually without any scientific evidence to confirm lack of safety. As such, a herbalist's approach to these herbs may be overly cautious and not borne out if scientific testing takes place in the future. For example, senna is traditionally avoided during pregnancy as it is an anthraquinone-containing herb; however, it is widely recommended as a safe and effective short-term stimulant laxative for constipation by medical practitioners (Tytgat et al 2003). Some herbalists also recommend against the use of several aromatherapy oils during the first trimester; however, there is no scientific evidence to suggest external use of such oils poses any serious danger.

PART TWO — SAFETY IN PREGNANCY

All medicines have the potential to affect maternal health, cross the placenta and affect fetal development. The most serious risk associated with medicine use in pregnancy is the possibility of teratogenesis, which can manifest as a structural abnormality, dysfunctional growth in utero and/or long-term functional defects. Other risks include miscarriage and neonatal withdrawal.

Birth defects naturally occur in 2–4% of all newborns and in the vast majority of cases the cause is unknown. Medication use is not considered to be a major contributor to the incidence of birth defects as less than 1% of cases can be attributed to drug use (Webster & Freeman 2001). It is likely that the use of CMs in Western countries is a far less important factor.

CRITICAL PERIODS IN HUMAN DEVELOPMENT

The safe use of any medicine in pregnancy must take into account the safety of the treatment to be used, the seriousness of the patient's presenting problem and the timing of exposure.

In the first 2 weeks prior to implantation, an insult is thought to have an all or nothing effect. Assuming the embryo survives, the risk of structural malformations to the fetus is greatest 17–70 days post-conception, a critical stage of organ development (Freyer 2008). After this time, organs continue to mature, so later adverse effects tend to be functional rather than structural and major birth defects are unlikely. Functional defects are less obvious than structural ones and may only become obvious once the child is older. The central nervous system, eyes, teeth and external genitalia are the last to fully develop and continue to mature until the baby reaches full term.

If practitioner and patient agree that medicinal treatment is warranted, then minimising exposure during critical developmental times is essential. This means using the lowest effective dose of the least toxic substance for the shortest period of time.

TERATOGENESIS

Teratogens are agents that result in structural or functional defects in the development of fetal organs (Shehata & Nelson-Piercy 2000). Sources of exposure to these agents include: contaminated air, water, soil, food, beverages, household items and medicines (including CMs). Teratogens can cause a variety of effects, including embryo/fetal death, intrauterine growth restriction and increased risk of malformations and carcinogenesis (Shehata & Nelson-Piercy 2000). The exact mechanisms responsible for teratogenicity are unknown, but theories include damage to DNA, membranes, protein and mitochondria, enzyme inhibition and hormonal interference. Despite the potential for teratogens to have devastating consequences, only a relatively small number of fetuses exposed to these agents experience adverse effects (Freyer 2008). This relates to factors such as the dose and duration of exposure, genetic susceptibility of the fetus/embryo, timing of exposure, specific mode of action of the teratogen (Miller et al 2007) and nutritional and disease status of the mother–baby unit (Shehata & Nelson-Piercy 2000).

Data on herbal teratogens is limited and largely based on animal studies, which are not completely reliable. Blue cohosh is an example of a herb that has some evidence to suggest a potential teratogenic effect based on animal studies (Keeler 1976, Keeler et al 1976, Kennelly et al 1999). Other herbs that may increase the risk of fetal malformations (predominantly based on limited animal data) include aloe, andrographis, cat's claw, Jamaica dogwood, pau d'arco, pennyroyal, poke root, tribulus and white horehound (Mills & Bone 2005). There is very little evidence of teratogenic activity or adverse pregnancy outcomes from the use of nutritional supplements with the notable exception of high-dose vitamin A.

Interestingly, nutrient *deficiencies* such as vitamin A, folate, vitamin B_{12}, vitamin D, iodine and zinc have been found to have adverse effects including teratogenesis emphasising the important role these nutrients play in normal embryonic and fetal development.

Neonatal withdrawal

While the fetus is in utero, the placenta supplies it with nutrients and other substances, as well as drugs. When the baby is born, placental supply ceases, which can lead to neonatal withdrawal syndromes for certain drugs such as beta-blockers, SSRIs and other antidepressants, opiates and alcohol (Freyer 2008, Sanz et al 2005). It is not known whether the use of CMs during the final trimester can also induce withdrawal syndromes.

HOW IS SAFETY EVALUATED IN PREGNANCY?

One of the hardest challenges a clinician faces is advising a pregnant patient about the safety of a treatment. A key factor to consider is the strength of evidence indicating the treatment is safe or, as so often happens in pregnancy, the lack of evidence indicating it is unsafe. More specific factors are the dose of medicine to be used, precise timing of exposure and duration of exposure.

When evaluating the effectiveness of a treatment, prospective randomised trials and meta-analyses are widely considered the gold standards. When evaluating safety in pregnancy, there is a paucity of such trials because pregnant women tend to be excluded, so other methods of information-gathering are required. Epidemiological studies, tests with animal models, post-marketing surveillance systems, case reports and traditional use provide the main inputs into establishing safety; however, each method has limitations and should not stand alone without corroborating evidence from another source.

Epidemiological studies

Epidemiological studies are also known as population studies. Due to their large participant numbers, epidemiological studies can detect large and small size effects and sometimes rare outcomes, if the study population is sufficiently large and follow-up is sufficiently complete. As such, they may provide useful information regarding safety in pregnancy.

Considering that the incidence of fetal malformations is already small (2–4%) extremely large participant numbers would be required to detect a slight increase above what might normally be expected. For example, a study would require 35,000 women in order to establish with 95% confidence level that a medicine changes the naturally-occurring frequency of a congenital malformation by 1% (Lee et al 2000). Unfortunately, most epidemiological studies have inadequate statistical power to detect this outcome as they lack sufficient patient numbers. As such, no medicine (pharmaceutical or complementary) has proven safety based on reliable epidemiological data involving sufficient numbers of women.

Animal studies

Animal studies of reproductive toxicity are required for all new drugs before they are licensed; however, they are not required for CMs. While they can provide some assurance of safety, animal tests have limited usefulness as results do not always extrapolate accurately to humans. For example, the drug thalidomide did not cause birth defects in animal models; however, it had a potent effect in humans (Webster & Freeman 2001). Far more common is the problem of false positives, whereby medicines that produce defects in animals are later found to be relatively safe in humans (e.g. corticosteroids) (Lee et al 2000). It is likely that the excessive doses used in testing increase the risk of producing a false positive as there is greater embryonic and maternal exposure to the medicine than would be expected in clinical practice. This should be kept in mind when interpreting the results of drug or herbal medicine testing in animal models.

Post-marketing surveillance systems

In many cases, more meaningful safety data only become available once a medicine is in widespread use and women knowingly or inadvertently take it during pregnancy. Those medicines with high effect rates will be detected more quickly than less potent teratogens. For example, the teratogenic effect of isotretinoin was detected about one year after it came onto the market whereas the anti-epileptic drug valproic acid was available in Europe in the 1960s, yet it took approximately 20 years of use by millions of women before its teratogenic potential was identified (Webster & Freeman 2001).

Post-marketing surveillance systems are set up to detect unfavourable outcomes and highlight adverse events rather than establishing safety, an inherently more difficult endpoint.

Adverse event case reports

Adverse event case reports are an account of an individual's suspected response to a treatment. Case reports are notoriously unreliable, as they tend to lack sufficient detail to clearly establish causality and fully eliminate the influence of confounding factors. Individual case reports become more convincing when a series of similar reports are collected.

Several factors should be considered when interpreting a case report; firstly, was the exposure to the medicine at the appropriate critical stage in pregnancy (usually first trimester) and was the dose used clinically relevant and similar for all cases? Additionally, if a complementary medicine is implicated, has the medicine been tested for contaminants and adulteration to exclude extrinsic factors and did the treatment involve a single entity or combination therapy (the norm in complementary medicine)? Finally, the traditional body of evidence that accompanies herbal medicines may provide further insights when interpreting cases.

The following three cases are presented as examples of the literature. They involve the herbs dong quai, Korean ginseng and blue cohosh. The reports indicate a probable link between herbal use and adverse outcome; however, none of the products implicated was tested for herbal authenticity or the presence of contaminants or adulterants, an essential step towards drawing a definitive conclusion.

Examples of case reports:

A 32-year-old woman, 3 weeks postpartum, developed acute headache, weakness, light-headedness and vomiting with a blood pressure reading of 195/85 mmHg (Nambiar et al 1999). She reported using dong quai for postpartum weakness and had not been taking any other medicines. Her 3-week-old son's blood pressure was also raised at 115/69. Within 48 hours of stopping herbal treatment, blood pressure normalised for both the mother and the breastfed child.

In 1990, a case report published in *JAMA* described a 30-year-old mother who had taken *Panax ginseng* (650 mg twice a day) throughout pregnancy and during lactation of her 2-week-old baby (Koren et al 1990). The boy was noted to have signs of androgenisation, thick black pubic hair, hair over the entire forehead, swollen red nipples and enlarged testes. After 2 weeks, his pubic and forehead hair began to fall out and was scant by 7.5 weeks. Excessive androgen production was ruled out and the authors suspected the effects were producted by hormonal activity of the herbal product. Letters to the editor were subsequently exchanged suggesting the product contained Siberian ginseng and not *Panax ginseng* (Awang 1991). The story does not end here as Siberian ginseng has no significant androgenic activity in vivo which could account for the effects observed (Awang 1991, Waller et al 1992). It is now suspected that the herbal product was not substituted for Siberian ginseng but instead *Periploca sepium* (called Wu jia or silk vine), as American herb companies importing Siberian ginseng from China have been known to be supplied with two or three species of *Periploca* (Awang 1991).

A newborn infant presented with acute myocardial infarction associated with profound congestive heart failure and shock (Jones & Lawson 1998). The mother had been ingesting blue cohosh (*Caulophyllum thalictroides*) in the month prior to delivery to facilitate the birthing process. She had been instructed to take one tablet daily but elected to take three times the recommended dose in the 3 weeks prior to delivery. During this time she noticed an increase in uterine contractions and a decrease in fetal activity. The infant eventually recovered after being critically ill for several weeks. Attending doctors excluded other causes of myocardial infarction and indicated blue cohosh was responsible for the adverse event. On late follow-up at 2 years of age the child was doing well with good exercise tolerance and normal growth and development. However, cardiomegaly persisted, left ventricular function remained mildly reduced and he was still receiving digoxin therapy.

Clinical studies

While prospective clinical studies of herbal safety in pregnancy are problematic, retrospective studies are easier to conduct. Establishing cause–effect relationships beyond reasonable doubt are rare due to the myriad of confounding factors present; however, they may identify common or palpable problems that could be investigated in appropriate models.

Example: echinacea

A Canadian study involving 412 pregnant women investigated the safety of echinacea in pregnancy (Gallo et al 2000). These women had contacted a teratogen information service (Motherisk Program) between 1996 and 1998 with concerns about the safety of ingesting echinacea during pregnancy. Half the group had already taken the herb, whereas the others decided against use, so were enrolled as a control group. Of the 206 women in the echinacea group, 112 (54%) used the herb in the first trimester and 17 (8%) used it throughout their pregnancies. No significant differences were seen between the groups for rates of major and minor malformations or any pregnancy outcome including delivery method, maternal weight gain, gestational age, infant birth weight or fetal distress.

Long-term use

Long-term use of a medicine by large populations of women without apparent increase in adverse events is considered to contribute towards evidence of safety. For example, the Australian Drug Evaluation Committee (ADEC) has classified the drug metoclopramide as relatively low risk because the 'drug has already been taken by large numbers of pregnant women and women of child-bearing age without proven increase in fetal harm' (Bryant et al 2003).

The term 'long-term use' in relation to herbal medicine may actually refer to hundreds or even thousands of years of use, not just decades, as is the case with pharmaceutical medicines. In fact, many herbal medicines, such as ginger and garlic, have been used as both foods and medicines since antiquity. This has allowed a large body of longitudinal and retrospective evidence to accumulate which gives herbalists an extra dimension to consider.

Like all forms of evidence, traditional evidence has its limitations and must be interpreted carefully. It is likely that traditional healers would have found it easier to identify poisonous herbs and herbs that induce acute or obvious adverse effects than those which induce insidious, rare or delayed-onset adverse outcomes. There may also be significant differences in the way a herbal medicine is grown, prepared and used today compared with older times, thereby allowing larger doses to be taken and different herbal constituents to be absorbed (Tannis 2003).

WEIGHING UP THE EVIDENCE

For both pharmaceutical and complementary medicines, the evidence base is incomplete and insufficient to state with certainty that any medicine is safe in pregnancy. To build a case for safety, evidence from multiple sources must be considered to fill in as many gaps in knowledge as possible.

In regards to complementary medicines, any evidence supporting or contraindicating use during pregnancy must be based on the totality, quality and relevance of the evidence. In general, the greater the consistency of evidence from different sources, the stronger the evidence is overall.

In Australia, the Australian Drug Evaluation Committee (ADEC) has classified drugs on their potential to cause harm during pregnancy. Eight categories are listed and each describes the evidence used to indicate safety or lack of safety (see Table 5.1). They rely on evidence gathered from animal models and post-marketing surveillance systems and also consider the proven, suspected or expected potential of a drug to cause adverse outcomes (e.g. cytotoxic drugs).

Proposing a different system for complementary medicines

A similar grading system is required for CMs, which builds a case for safety or harm based on considering multiple forms of evidence. Ideally the new system should take into account the availability of a traditional body of evidence and the relative lack of data available from animal studies. It should also take into account the relative safety of OTC CMs in comparison to scheduled pharmaceutical drugs and whether the association between exposure and proposed adverse outcome is biologically plausible.

Table 5.2 (p. 107) is a safety matrix that synthesises different forms of evidence, including taking note of what is known and what remains unknown. Traditional and scientific evidence from various sources are compared and theoretical reasoning is considered. The matrix has been weighted so scientific evidence is given greater credence than traditional evidence; however, it must be acknowledged that, in many cases, scientific evidence to support safety will be unavailable.

USING THE SAFETY MATRIX

Clinicians are recommended to use information in the monographs of this text as a starting point for gathering information about evidence of safety in pregnancy. Supplementary information will be required from frequently updated databases and traditional monograph pharmacopeias. Five common herbs are reviewed here as examples of how the matrix may be used: echinacea, ginger, raspberry leaf, black cohosh and chaste tree.

Echinacea spp. (Echinacea)

Classification: Likely safe

- Traditional evidence: available? Y
  - Traditional evidence: cautions or contraindicates? NA
  - Traditional evidence: if cautions: biologically plausible? NA

TABLE 5.1 ADEC PREGNANCY CATEGORIES (AUSTRALIA)	
CATEGORY A	Drugs which have been taken by a large number of pregnant women and women of childbearing age without any proven increase in the frequency of malformations or other direct or indirect harmful effects on the fetus having been observed.
CATEGORY B1	Drugs which have been taken by only a limited number of pregnant women and women of childbearing age, without an increase in the frequency of malformation or other direct or indirect harmful effects on the human fetus having been observed. Studies in animals have not shown evidence of an increased occurrence of fetal damage.
CATEGORY B2	Drugs which have been taken by only a limited number of pregnant women and women of childbearing age, without an increase in the frequency of malformation or other direct or indirect harmful effects on the human fetus having been observed. Studies in animals are inadequate or may be lacking, but available data show no evidence of an increased occurrence of fetal damage.
CATEGORY B3	Drugs which have been taken by only a limited number of pregnant women and women of childbearing age, without an increase in the frequency of malformation or other direct or indirect harmful effects on the human fetus having been observed. Studies in animals have shown evidence of an increased occurrence of fetal damage, the significance of which is considered uncertain in humans.
CATEGORY C	Drugs which, owing to their pharmacological effects, have caused or may be suspected of causing harmful effects on the human fetus or neonate without causing malformations. These effects may be reversible. Accompanying texts should be consulted for further details.
CATEGORY D	Drugs which have caused, are suspected to have caused or may be expected to cause, an increased incidence of human fetal malformations or irreversible damage. These drugs may also have adverse pharmacological effects. Accompanying texts should be consulted for further details.
CATEGORY X	Drugs which have such a high risk of causing permanent damage to the fetus that they should not be used in pregnancy or when there is a possibility of pregnancy.

Note: For drugs in the B1, B2 and B3 categories, human data are lacking or inadequate and subcategorisation is therefore based on available animal data. The allocation of a B category does NOT imply greater safety than the C category. Drugs in category D are NOT absolutely contraindicated in pregnancy. Moreover, in some cases the D category has been assigned on the basis of suspicion.

Source: From Prescribing medicines in pregnancy database, 2016, Therapeutic Goods Administration, used by permission of the Australian Government. https://www.tga.gov.au/prescribing-medicines-pregnancy-database

TABLE 5.2 COMPLEMENTARY MEDICINE SAFETY MATRIX

→ TRADITIONAL EVIDENCE ↓ SCIENTIFIC EVIDENCE	WELL-DOCUMENTED TRADITIONAL EVIDENCE UNAVAILABLE	TRADITIONAL EVIDENCE DOES NOT CONTRAINDICATE AGAINST USE	TRADITIONAL EVIDENCE CAUTIONS OR CONTRAINDICATES USE DUE TO POSTULATED NON-SPECIFIC MECHANISMS THAT ARE NOT BIOLOGICALLY PLAUSIBLE	TRADITIONAL EVIDENCE CONTRAINDICATES USE BASED ON DESCRIPTIONS OF SPECIFIC ADVERSE EFFECTS OR IS USED AS AN ABORTIFACIENT
There are *no animal or human studies* available to support safety	Consider as unsafe because safety remains unknown	Likely to be safe but safety cannot be confirmed Scientific evidence unavailable to support or refute traditional safety claim	Likely to be safe but best used under professional guidance Scientific evidence unavailable to support or refute traditional contraindication	Unsafe Scientific evidence unavailable to support or refute traditional contraindication
Human and animal studies demonstrate there are *no known pharmacological activities* of the substance or its components relevant to therapeutic use in humans known to be associated with fetal damage, abortifacient activity or any other adverse reproductive effects	Safe	Safe Scientific evidence supports traditional safety claim	Likely to be safe but best used under professional guidance Scientific evidence does not support traditional contraindication	Likely to be safe but best used under professional guidance Scientific evidence does not support traditional contraindication
The toxicological or pharmacological profile of the substance indicates that there are *no known pharmacological actions* of the substance or its components relevant to therapeutic use in humans which could cause fetal damage, abortifacient activity or any other adverse reproductive effects	Safe	Safe Scientific evidence supports traditional safety claim	Likely to be safe but best used under professional guidance Scientific evidence does not support traditional contraindication	Likely to be safe but best used under professional guidance Scientific evidence does not support traditional contraindication
Human or animal studies *have shown* evidence of pharmacological activity for the substance or its components relevant to therapeutic use in humans which could cause fetal damage, abortifacient effects or any other adverse reproductive effects	Unsafe	Unsafe Scientific evidence refutes traditional safety claim	Unsafe Scientific evidence supports traditional contraindication	Unsafe Scientific evidence supports traditional contraindication

- Scientific evidence: available? Y
  - Scientific evidence: human or animal studies find NO known pharmacological effects of concern in pregnancy? Y
  - Scientific evidence: toxicological or pharmacological profile studies find NO known pharmacological effects of concern in pregnancy? NA
  - Scientific evidence: human and/or animal studies find evidence of pharmacological effects adverse to pregnancy, e.g. abortifacient? Y

One animal study highlighted concerns about use during the first trimester demonstrating the risk of spontaneous abortions, with pregnant mice fed *Echinacea purpurea* daily, increased as 50% of fetuses were lost by mid-pregnancy (Chow et al 2006). Human studies, however, indicate it is generally considered safe in pregnancy when used in recommended doses (Mills & Bone 2005). A recent study of a prospective cohort study found that oral consumption during the first trimester did not increase the risk of malformations and was recommended as safe for use during pregnancy (Perri et al 2006). Additional evidence from a prospective cohort study suggests it is safe during pregnancy with no increase in the risk for major malformations; however, large-scale controlled trials are unavailable (Gallo et al 2000). This particular study involved 206 women who used echinacea during their pregnancy (54% in the first trimester and 8% in all trimesters). Fifty-eight per cent of participants used capsules or tablets (doses ranging from 250 to 1000 mg/day) and 38% used tinctures (dose varied from 5 to 10 to a maximum of 30 drops per day). Most used the echinacea for only a short period of time compared with a control group matched by disease (upper respiratory tract ailments), maternal age, alcohol and cigarette use. There was no statistical differences between the groups for any of the end points analysed — major and minor malformations, miscarriages and neonatal complications.

Zingiber officinalis (Ginger)

Classification: Likely to be safe, but safety cannot be confirmed for high-dose supplements (concentrated extracts), safe for usual dietary intake

- Traditional evidence: available? Y
  - Traditional evidence: cautions or contraindicates? Y
  - Traditional evidence: if cautions: biologically plausible? N
- Scientific evidence: available? Y
  - Scientific evidence: human or animal studies find NO known pharmacological effects of concern in pregnancy? Y
  - Scientific evidence: toxicological or pharmacological profile studies find NO known pharmacological effects of concern in pregnancy? NA
  - Scientific evidence: human and/or animal studies find evidence of pharmacological effects adverse to pregnancy e.g. abortifacient? Y

Traditionally used as an anti-emetic, ginger has encouraging research to support its use during pregnancy for nausea and vomiting (Borrelli et al 2005) and no adverse effects have been reported in several studies examining ginger in treatment of nausea and vomiting in pregnancy. Ginger's anti-nausea and anti-emetic mechanism of action has not been fully elucidated, although several hypotheses have been proposed. It has been reported that symptoms of nausea and vomiting during pregnancy improve in a manner directly correlated to improvements in pregnancy-induced gastric dysrhythmias. Therefore, ginger's actions in pregnancy may be due to a direct effect of the medicine on the gastrointestinal tract (Chaiyakunapruk et al 2006, Matthews et al 2010).

A recent systematic review assessed 10 RCTs that investigated ginger in pregnancy. Five trials reported ginger to be more effective than placebo, four trials found ginger to be equally effective in the management of nausea and vomiting compared to vitamin B_6 and dimethhydrinate. Compared with dimenhydrinate, ginger caused fewer side effects and none of the studies raised any concerns about safety in pregnant women (Dante et al 2013). The Cochrane Collaboration reached the conclusion that the efficacy of ginger was equal to that of either vitamin B6 or dimenhydrinate (Matthews et al 2010).

Another systematic review of 4 double-blind RCTs (n = 449) and one prospective observational cohort study (n = 187) evaluated the effects of ginger on pregnancy outcomes. The preparation used in the trials was a ginger root powder or extract, taken 3–4 times daily (total dose ranging from 1.0–1.5 g) from 8 to 20 weeks' gestation. No dose was provided in the prospective study. No difference in the occurrence of spontaneous abortions, stillbirth, term delivery and caesarean deliveries, neonatal death, gestational age and congenital abnormalities were found between those women who took ginger compared to those taking vitamin B_6 or placebo, or the general population (Borrelli et al 2005).

Unfortunately, there is a lack of consensus regarding its safety during pregnancy. Soudamini et al (1995) suggest ginger contains possible mutagenic properties; however, this effect appears to be counteracted by zingerone, another constituent present in the whole rhizome (Nakamura & Yamamoto 1982). Traditionally, ginger has been contraindicated in labour due to the possibility of increased postpartum haemorrhage and in large doses it is traditionally thought to act as emmenagogue (Grieve 1971). German Commission E suggest that ginger is contraindicated in pregnancy, while more recent research suggests that doses up to 2 g/day of dried ginger root have been used safely. When considered in a comparison of recent research, the proposed notion of haemorrhage is unlikely. Teratogenicity studies in rats show that even at very large doses (ginger tea up to 50 g/L) it had no impact on maternal toxicity or fetal malformations; however, embryo losses were double compared to the controls. No evidence of maternal toxicity was found for a patented extract of ginger (EV.EXT 33) given in doses of up to 1000 mg/kg/body weight daily to pregnant rats during the period of organogenesis (Weidner & Sigwart 2001).

Rubus idaeus (raspberry leaf)

Classification: Likely to be safe, but safety cannot be confirmed (first trimester), likely to be safe (second and third trimester)

- Traditional evidence: available? Y
  - Traditional evidence: cautions or contraindicates? N
  - Traditional evidence: if cautions: biologically plausible? NA
- Scientific evidence: available? Y
  - Scientific evidence: human or animal studies find NO known pharmacological effects of concern in pregnancy? Y
  - Scientific evidence: toxicological or pharmacological profile studies find NO known pharmacological effects of concern in pregnancy? Y
  - Scientific evidence: human and/or animal studies find evidence of pharmacological effects adverse to pregnancy, e.g. abortifacient? Y

Raspberry leaves appear to have a dual effect on the uterus, acting as both a stimulant and a relaxant to the uterine musculature (Bamford et al 1970). The use of this herb in concentrated form is traditionally recommended only in the second and third trimesters due to its possible effects on the uterus. Traditional evidence and the select pharmacological studies highlight that this herbal medicine has an effect on uterine contractions (Bamford et al 1970). Unfortunately, there is limited research on both the efficacy and the safety of raspberry leaf. In one retrospective trial, raspberry leaf was associated with some shortening of labour and a decreased need for mechanical assistance (forceps or vacuum), although the difference was not statistically significant (Parsons et al 1999). In another study, raspberry did not shorten the first stage of labour. The only clinically significant findings were shortening of the second stage of labour (mean difference = 9.59 minutes) and lower rate of forceps deliveries between the treatment group and the control group (19.3% vs 30.4%) (Simpson et al 2001).

Two clinical studies evaluating the safety of raspberry leaf in pregnancy have reported no evidence of toxicity in either mother or child (Parsons et al 1999, Simpson et al 2001) although evidence from older animal studies is less clear (Burn & Withell 1941, Whitehouse 1941). In one systematic review, no adverse effects were described in the mothers (increase in blood pressure, increase in blood loss at birth, preterm or post-term labour), and no significant relationships were found between raspberry consumption and neonatal outcomes (Apgar score, birth weight) (Dante et al 2013).

Although raspberry leaf has been in traditional use for a very long time, the evidence regarding safety, efficacy and active constituents is weak. The chemical constituents responsible for the effect on uterus or other smooth muscle are not clearly determined. Some of the constituents, such as flavonoids, have repeatedly been shown to have a relaxing effect on smooth muscle (Mullen et al 2002); however, more research is required.

Cimicifuga racemosa (Black cohosh)

Classification: Unsafe (first and second trimester). Likely to be safe but cannot be confirmed (labour)

- Traditional evidence: available? Y
  - Traditional evidence: cautions or contraindicates? Y
  - Traditional evidence: if cautions: biologically plausible? Y
- Scientific evidence: available? Y
  - Scientific evidence: human or animal studies find NO known pharmacological effects of concern in pregnancy? N
  - Scientific evidence: toxicological or pharmacological profile studies find NO known pharmacological effects of concern in pregnancy? N
  - Scientific evidence: human and/or animal studies find evidence of pharmacological effects adverse to pregnancy, e.g. abortifacient? Y

Black cohosh was traditionally used by the Native Americans for a variety of ailments including arthritis, menopausal symptoms and respiratory symptoms, and was commonly used to induce labour. It was widely used by the Eclectics in traditional Western Herbal Medicine as a partum preparatory if taken in the last few weeks of pregnancy (Felter & Lloyd 1905, 1983). Black cohosh has a variety of actions such as selective oestrogen-receptor modulator activity, anti-inflammatory and dopaminergic effects. Traditionally it is avoided during early pregnancy, but could be used to assist birth under professional supervision.

Vitex agnus castus (Chaste tree)

Classification: Likely to be safe, but cannot be confirmed

- Traditional evidence: available? Y
  - Traditional evidence: cautions or contraindicates? N
  - Traditional evidence: if cautions — biologically plausible? NA
- Scientific evidence: available? Y
  - Scientific evidence: human or animal studies find NO known pharmacological effects of concern in pregnancy? Y
  - Scientific evidence: toxicological or pharmacological profile studies find NO known pharmacological effects of concern in pregnancy? Y
  - Scientific evidence: human and/or animal studies find evidence of pharmacological effects adverse to pregnancy, e.g. abortifacient? N

Chaste tree has been traditionally used for a variety of gynaecological conditions such as aiding the expulsion of the placenta after birth and promoting menstruation. In the first trimester it is sometimes used to promote conception and/or support the growth and development of the fetus. North American herbalists traditionally recommended vitex to improve fertility and after pregnancy as a galactagogue (Felter & Lloyd 1905, 1983). As it is most commonly used by women of childbearing age, it is likely that some women may consume it unknowingly when in the early stages of pregnancy (Dougoua et al 2008). Vitex is believed to act on dopamine receptors to decrease prolactin levels, (Mills & Bone 2005). According to in vitro studies, it may bind to alpha and beta oestrogen-receptors.

PART THREE — ADVISING PATIENTS IN CLINICAL PRACTICE

At some stage of practice most clinicians have to consider the question 'Is this treatment safe in pregnancy?' The answer to such a question is never straightforward, as establishing safety in pregnancy with any degree of certainty is difficult.

Over the years medical practitioners and pharmacists have generally held the view that all medicines should be avoided during pregnancy, where possible. This has referred to the use of pharmaceutical medicines and is wise counsel. With the increasing popularity and accessibility of CMs, many have extended this caution to include herbal medicines under the assumption that the same safety issues apply. Indeed, the safety issues are similar and prudence is still required.

Naturopaths and herbal medicine practitioners hold a more targeted view and recommend a small number of herbal and nutritional medicines during different stages of pregnancy, while being mindful of many others which are considered contraindicated for various reasons.

It is easy for clinicians to adopt the conservative view that all herbal medicines are to be avoided throughout pregnancy; however, this is not useful in practice, especially as women will continue to take them in the belief that they are safe. In fact, it could be argued that best practice means considering all treatment options for safety and efficacy in pregnancy, including herbs and natural supplements.

When medicinal treatments present unacceptable risks or are ineffective, CM as a treatment domain offers a broad range of non-medicinal treatment options which can be considered by clinicians. For example, lifestyle prescriptions, dietary manipulation, massage, acupuncture and aromatherapy provided by appropriately trained practitioners can address a range of symptoms during this sensitive time.

FACTORS TO CONSIDER IN PRACTICE

Individual prescribing

The decision to prescribe or withdraw a CM must be made on an individual case-by-case basis. The safe use of any medicine in pregnancy must take into account the safety of the treatment being considered, the seriousness of the patient's presenting problem, maternal age and gestational age of the fetus and timing of exposure. This includes a consideration of the dose to be used, dosing interval and timing in respect to other medicines and food. Additionally, the patient's presenting health and nutritional status, comorbidities, kidney and liver function and personal attitude to treatment are important factors.

If practitioner and patient agree that a medicine is to be used, steps should be taken to reduce harm, such as recommending the lowest effective dose for the shortest period possible. While special cautions exist for the first trimester, care must be taken at all stages of pregnancy as fetal growth and development continues.

Timing of the intervention

In practice, choosing the correct dose and administration form is essential and in pregnancy there is the additional consideration of correct timing, which is important for achieving a desired clinical result with a minimum of risk. For example, folate supplementation has been shown to prevent neural tube defects when administered in the preconception period and continued during the first trimester (Berry et al 1999, De-Reigil et al 2010). Similarly, antioxidant supplements appear to be ineffective in reducing preeclampsia when started later in pregnancy (Rumbold et al 2008); however, positive results in preeclampsia were reported in a study which commenced treatment in the first trimester with a broad spectrum antioxidant supplement (including vitamin A 1000 IU, vitamin C 200 mg, vitamin E 400 IU, folic acid 400 mcg, selenium 100 mcg, zinc 15 mg, copper 2 mg, N-acetyl cysteine 200 mg, iron 30 mg) (Rumiris et al 2006).

Informed consent

Evidence-based, patient-centred care means all clinicians are required to present risk/benefit information to their patient, who can then make an informed choice. This means an honest discussion between patient and practitioner about what is known and what remains unknown about the safety and efficacy of a treatment. Patients will no doubt vary in their interest and ability to comprehend and recall the necessary information, so written information and assurance that the woman understands the issues during the time of consultation is useful.

PRACTICE POINTS: GENERAL RULES FOR USING COMPLEMENTARY MEDICINES IN PREGNANCY

- Use CM within the Quality Use of Medicines (QUM) Framework.
- Consider the patient's presenting health status and comorbidities.
- Consider non-medicinal treatment options where appropriate, especially during the first trimester.
- Is such a treatment available and likely to be successful?

Risk–benefit analysis:
- If a CM is under consideration, what are the potential risks and benefits to the mother and fetus?
- What are the risks and benefits (for each) of not prescribing?

Timing of intervention:
- Avoid all medicinal agents where possible, especially in the first trimester.
- Carefully consider the timing of the intervention in regards to gestational age of the fetus: a fetus' susceptibility to toxic effects changes throughout gestation.
- Consider appropriate dose, dose frequency and duration of treatment.

Pharmacotherapy compared with complementary medicine:
- If the patient's condition is sufficiently severe that pharmacotherapy is being considered, clinicians should consider whether an appropriate CM treatment exists with a lower risk of harm.
- If clinician and patient decide a CM is to be used, the lowest possible dose should be used for the shortest period of time.
- CM is best prescribed by a qualified and appropriately trained health professional.

Counselling:
- Counsel pregnant women to avoid exposure to unnecessary medicines and chemicals.

Education and communication:
- If use of a CM is being considered, an open discussion about the potential benefits and potential risks must ensue, so patients can

make an informed decision. This includes providing information about what is known about the safety of the treatment and what remains unknown.

- Communication is essential among all health professionals involved in obstetric patient management and the patient.
- Encourage patients to disclose CM use to all their obstetric team of health professionals.
- Special caution should be considered by women due to have elective caesarean section or other surgery. Presurgery cautions and recommendations should be considered.

Additional rules relating to the specific use of herbal medicines in pregnancy

- Avoid all known toxic and poisonous plants at all times, e.g. aconite, pennyroyal, tansy.
- Avoid all thujone-containing herbal medicines, e.g. *Achillea millefolium* (yarrow), *Thuja occidentalis* (thuja) or *Artemisia absinthium* (wormwood).
- Avoid internal use of pure volatile oils from herbal medicines throughout pregnancy. Herbal teas and small concentrations of oils used as flavouring are the exception, e.g. peppermint oil or food quantities of essential oil containing herbal medicines.
- Avoid emmenagogue herbal medicines throughout pregnancy.
- Herbs used to assist delivery should only be used under close professional supervision in the final 6 weeks of pregnancy.

APPENDIX 5.1: NUTRIENTS DURING PREGNANCY

NUTRIENT	THERAPEUTIC FUNCTION/ JUSTIFICATION	DOSAGE RECOMMENDATIONS AND ISSUES
Vitamin A	Required for gene expression and cellular differentiation in organogenesis and embryonic development of the spinal cord and vertebrae, limbs, eyes and ears, and heart (Morriss-Kay & Sokolova 1996). Poor maternal status will result in risk of infant deficiency (Ortega et al 1997) associated with poor immune function and increased risk of infection morbidity and mortality in infants and children (Grubesic 2004, Huiming et al 2005). Maternal deficiency increases the risk of mortality (West et al 1999), premature rupture of membranes (Westney et al 1994), preterm delivery (Radhika et al 2002), reduced haemoglobin levels and anaemia (Bondevik et al 2000, Suharno et al 1993), night blindness (Livingstone et al 2003) and immune suppression (Cox et al 2006). A Cochrane review in 2011 (van den Broek et al 2010) pooled results of two large trials in Nepal and Ghana (95,000 women). These results indicated that there was no role for antenatal vitamin A supplementation to reduce maternal or perinatal mortality. However, the populations studied were probably different with regard to baseline vitamin A status and there were problems with follow-up. There is good evidence for antenatal vitamin A supplementation to reduce maternal anaemia for women who live in areas where vitamin A deficiency is common or who are HIV positive. There is also possibly some benefit to reduce maternal infection; however, these data sources are not high quality so further studies are required.	Excessive supplementation shown to be associated with adverse pregnancy outcomes particularly in the first trimester. No association with moderate intake (<10,000 IU) and fetal malformations (Botto et al 1996, Johansen et al 2008, Martinez-Frias & Salvador 1990, Mastroiacovo et al 1999, Mills et al 1997, Shaw et al 1997, Werler et al 1990). Supplement labels must carry the warning — when taken in excess of 3000 mcg retinol equivalents (10,000 IU), vitamin A may cause birth defects.

NUTRIENT	THERAPEUTIC FUNCTION/ JUSTIFICATION	DOSAGE RECOMMENDATIONS AND ISSUES
Vitamin B_6 (pyridoxine)	Beneficial in the treatment of nausea of pregnancy (Jamigorn & Phupong 2007, Jewell & Young 2003, Sripramote & Lekhyananda 2003). Poor vitamin B_6 status may decrease the possibility of conception (Ronnenberg et al 2007) and increase the risk of early pregnancy loss (Goddijn-Wessel et al 1996, Ronnenberg et al 2007, Wouters et al 1993). Unfortunately vitamin B_6 is insufficiently studied. A Cochrane review established that there were few trials reporting clinical outcomes and mostly had unclear trial methodology and inadequate follow-up. There was not enough evidence to detect clinical benefits of vitamin B_6 supplementation in pregnancy and/or labour, other than one trial suggesting protection against dental decay. It is recommended that future trials assessing this and other outcomes such as orofacial clefts, cardiovascular malformations, neurological development, preterm birth, preeclampsia and adverse events are required (Thaver et al 2006).	RDI during pregnancy is increased slightly to 1.9 mg, and upper recommended level is 50 mg with no evidence of teratogenicity. High dose supplementation (mean 132 mg/day) for 9 weeks during the first trimester appears to be safe with no associated increase in risk for major malformations (Shrim et al 2006). Doses used in studies for nausea are 30–75 mg/day.

(Continued)

NUTRIENT	THERAPEUTIC FUNCTION/ JUSTIFICATION	DOSAGE RECOMMENDATIONS AND ISSUES
Vitamin B_9 (folic acid)	Deficiency can lead to homocysteine accumulation, possibly associated with abnormalities of the placental vasculature and increased risk of miscarriage and preeclampsia (Dodds et al 2008, Napolitano et al 2008, Makedos et al 2007) and are associated with a two-fold increased risk of adult schizophrenia (Brown et al 2007). Intake of folic acid preconceptually and in the first 4–6 weeks of pregnancy reduces the risk of neural tube defects (NTD) by more than 50% (Berry et al 1999, Czeizel & Dudas 1992), and may also decrease risk of other congenital malformations including urinary tract and cardiovascular defects, limb deficiencies and hypertrophic pyloric stenosis (Czeizel 1998). The protective effects of higher folic acid intake was also demonstrated in a study from Chile, whereby fortification of flour with folic acid has led to a 55% reduction in NTD prevalence between 1999 and 2009. Individuals with polymorphisms in folate metabolism (methylenetetrahydrofolate reductase [MTHFR] gene) may be at greater risk of deficiency and subsequent adverse effects (Biselli et al 2008, Boyles et al 2008, Candito et al 2008, Coppede et al 2007, Steer et al 2008). In this instance, 5-methyl-tetrahydrofolate preparations are more advisable. A recent Cochrane review found a benefit for folic acid in improving mean birth weight (Lassi & Salam 2013).	Supplementation with folate has been linked with increased risk of multiple pregnancies (Czeizel 1998, Czeizel & Vargha 2004) although disputed by others (Li et al 2003). RDI in pregnancy is 600 mcg/day (200 mcg above non pregnancy state). Upper limit recommended in pregnancy is 1000 mcg due to the possibility of masking a vitamin B_{12} deficiency.

NUTRIENT	THERAPEUTIC FUNCTION/ JUSTIFICATION	DOSAGE RECOMMENDATIONS AND ISSUES
Vitamin B_{12} (cyanocobalamin)	Inadequate cobalamin status in pregnancy has been associated with several adverse outcomes such as preterm birth (Ronnenberg et al 2002), intrauterine growth-retardation (Muthayya et al 2006), increased risk for NTDs (Groenen et al 2004, Gaber et al 2007, Kirke et al 1993, Steen et al 1998, Suarez et al 2003, Wright 1995) and increased risk of miscarriage (Hubner et al 2008). It is also required for homocysteine metabolism, whereby increased levels have been associated with numerous conditions including preeclampsia (Napolitano et al 2008) and recurrent pregnancy loss (Hubner et al 2008). Inadequate maternal status may result in an infant with poor stores, and this may be further exacerbated by low stores in breast milk (Allen 1994).	The RDI is slightly increased to 2.6 mcg/day in pregnancy. There is no upper level of intake as there is no evidence of adverse effects. Deficiency (indicated by macrocytic changes) may be masked by high dose folic acid supplementation.
Vitamin C	Vitamin C deficiency has been suggested to play a role in several adverse pregnancy outcomes such as preeclampsia, intrauterine growth restriction and pre-labour rupture of fetal membranes (PROM). A Cochrane review reported no difference between women supplemented with vitamin C (alone or combined with other supplements) compared with placebo for the risk of stillbirth, miscarriage, birth weight, placental abruption or intrauterine growth restriction (Rumbold & Crowther 2005, Rumbold et al 2005). Required for healthy immune function and significantly reduces the risk of urinary tract infections during pregnancy (Ochoa-Brust et al 2007).	The recommended intake of vitamin C is slightly increased in pregnancy to 60 mg/ day. Early reports of high-dose maternal supplementation causing 'conditioned or rebound scurvy' in infants (Cochrane 1965, Rhead & Schrauzer 1971) have not been replicated in subsequent studies (Diplock et al 1998).

(Continued)

NUTRIENT	THERAPEUTIC FUNCTION/ JUSTIFICATION	DOSAGE RECOMMENDATIONS AND ISSUES
Vitamin D	Vitamin D supplementation in a single or continued dose during pregnancy increases serum vitamin D concentrations. A recent Cochrane review analysing results from three trials involving 463 women suggest that women who receive vitamin D supplements during pregnancy were less likely to have a low birth weight baby below 2500 grams compared to women receiving no treatment or a placebo (De-Regil et al 2012). High prevalence of vitamin D deficiency in pregnancy and lactation has been reported (Ainy et al 2006, Hollis & Wagner 2004, Judkins & Eagleton 2006, Sachan et al 2005, van der Meer et al 2006). Maternal status also affects the infant's vitamin D status (Hollis & Wagner 2004) and intrauterine growth of long bones (Morley et al 2006), poor infant skeletal growth and mineralisation (Zeghoud et al 1997). In severe maternal deficiency, there is an increased risk of rickets in the infant (Specker 1994). Glucose intolerance (Maghbooli et al 2008), bone health and risk of osteoporotic fracture risk later in life may also be influenced (Javaid et al 2006). It is important for normal brain development (Cui et al 2007, Eyles et al 2003) with fetal deficiency leading to alterations in brain structure and function (Almeras et al 2007, Feron et al 2005). Supplementation may protect against multiple sclerosis (Munger et al 2004, 2006) and reduce the risk of later preeclampsia in the infant (Hypponen et al 2007). Conversely, maternal concentrations of > 75 nmol/L of 25 (OH)-vitamin D in pregnancy may increase the risk of eczema in infants and asthma in children, but did not negatively influence the child's intelligence, psychological health or cardiovascular system (Gale et al 2008).	The amount of vitamin D required during pregnancy and lactation to avoid deficiency may be higher than the recommended amount (RDI 5.0 mcg) (Hollis 2005, 2007, Vieth et al 2001). The recommended upper limit is 80 mcg (Australian Government 2006). Vieth et al (2001), however, found no adverse effects even at doses of 100 mcg (4000 IU) per day. Toxicity is rare, but may occur with excessive supplementation (Koutkia et al 2001). Breast milk is a poor source of vitamin D, with infants requiring an exogenous source within a few months (Challa et al 2005, Daaboul et al 1997, Hatun et al 2005, Sills et al 1994).

NUTRIENT	THERAPEUTIC FUNCTION/ JUSTIFICATION	DOSAGE RECOMMENDATIONS AND ISSUES
Vitamin E	Antioxidant activity is valuable in protecting the embryo (in vitro) and fetus from damage due to oxidative stress (Cederberg et al 2001, Jishage et al 2001, Wang et al 2002). Although oxidative stress plays an important role in the pathogenesis of preeclampsia (Gupta et al 2005), there is little evidence for the role of vitamin E in its prevention (Polyzos et al 2007). Some evidence suggests it was beneficial in women with poor antioxidant status (Rumiris et al 2006). Low maternal levels contribute to increased risk of wheezing and asthma in childhood (Devereux et al 2006) and supplementation was useful in reducing pregnancy-related leg cramps (Shahraki 2006) and increasing birth weight for gestation (Scholl et al 2006, Valsecchi et al 1999).	The recommended intake for vitamin E (7 mg) is not increased for pregnancy. High dose supplementation of vitamin E (400–1200 IU) appears to be safe and does not increase risk for major malformations, preterm deliveries, miscarriages or stillbirths (Boskovic et al 2005). The recommended upper limit in pregnancy is 300 mg/day (Australian Government 2006).
Vitamin K	Poor maternal vitamin K levels can result in relative deficiency in newborn infants (Shearer 1992). Low intake combined with the reduced gastrointestinal bacterial synthesis puts infants at risk of Vitamin K deficiency bleeding (VKDB) due to the lack of activity of vitamin K-dependent clotting factors (II, VII, IX and X) (von Kries et al 1993). This is compounded in breastfed infants as breast milk contains lower levels compared to formula, although this may be increased with maternal supplementation during lactation (Greer et al 1997).	The recommended intake of vitamin K during pregnancy and lactation is the same as for a non-pregnant woman (60 mcg/day). To prevent infant health risks, prophylactic treatment of one intramuscular injection of 1 mg (0.1 mL) at birth, or 3 × 2 mg (0.2 mL) oral doses at birth, 3–5 days of age and at 4 weeks are recommended (Australian Government 2006).

(Continued)

NUTRIENT	THERAPEUTIC FUNCTION/ JUSTIFICATION	DOSAGE RECOMMENDATIONS AND ISSUES
Calcium	The newborn infant skeleton holds approximately 20–30 g calcium (Prentice 2003), 80% of which is acquired during the third trimester when the fetal skeleton is rapidly mineralising (Trotter & Hixon 1974). This increased demand for calcium during pregnancy is met by alterations to maternal calcium metabolism, particularly a two-fold increase in calcium absorption mediated by increases in 1,25-dihydroxyvitamin D and other mechanisms (Kovacs & Kronenberg 1997, Prentice 2003). A possible inverse relationship between calcium intake during pregnancy and risk of hypertension and preeclampsia has been suggested from epidemiological and clinical studies (Repke & Villar 1991, Villar & Belizan 2000, Villar et al 1983, 1987, 2003). Supplementation (1.0–2.0 g/day) is recommended to reduce the risk of preeclampsia, gestational hypertension (Hofmeyr et al 2006, 2007), and may also reduce the blood pressure of the offspring (Belizan et al 1997, Hatton et al 2003). Calcium supplementation during pregnancy has been shown to reduce maternal blood lead concentrations by an average of 11% by inhibiting the mobilisation of lead from bone and inhibiting intestinal absorption (Téllez-Rojo et al 2006). Supplementation (1200 mg) during lactation also reduces the risk of infant lead exposure by decreasing the concentration in breast milk by 5–10% (Ettinger et al 2006). A recent Cochrane review identified that calcium supplementation is associated with a significant protective benefit in the prevention of preeclampsia (Buppasiri et al 2011). Another Cochrane review determined that calcium supplementation halved the risk of preeclampsia, reduced the risk of preterm birth and reduced the occurrence of the composite outcome 'death or serious morbidity' (Hofmeyr et al 2010).	Although pregnancy is a time of high calcium requirement, there is no increase in the recommended daily intake for pregnancy (1000 mg). If supplementation is required, it appears to be safe to use (Hofmeyr et al 2006).

NUTRIENT	THERAPEUTIC FUNCTION/ JUSTIFICATION	DOSAGE RECOMMENDATIONS AND ISSUES
Chromium	Deficiency is believed to have an effect on glucose intolerance (Jovanovic-Peterson & Peterson 1996, Jovanovic & Peterson 1999). Chromium may protect against maternal insulin resistance and gestational diabetes (Morris & Samaniego 2000); however, studies are contradictory (Aharoni et al 1992, Gunton et al 2001, Woods et al 2008).	Recommended daily intake during pregnancy is slightly increased to 30 mcg/ day. Supplementation in gestational diabetes is likely to be safe (Jovanovic & Peterson 1999).
Iodine	Iodine deficiency occurs in both developing and developed countries (Becker et al 2006, Donnay et al 2013). Deficiency during pregnancy (defined as urinary iodine concentrations <150 mcg/L) has been found, even in areas considered to have generally adequate intake. In a study conducted in Rome where a salt iodination program has been introduced, only 4% of non-pregnant women were found to be iodine deficient (<100–199 mcg/L) compared to 92% of pregnant women, suggesting it may be necessary to monitor pregnant women even in regions where iodine deficiency is not common (Marchioni et al 2008). It enables the manufacture of maternal thyroid hormones, is protective against cretinism (Delange 2000) and development of fetal brain, protects against neurological damage (Perez-Lopez 2007), and is also supplied to the breastfed infant via breastmilk (Berbel et al 2007). Maternal hypothyroidism during early pregnancy is associated with other adverse outcomes including premature birth, preeclampsia, breech delivery and increased fetal mortality (Casey et al 2005, Haddow et al 1999, Pop 2004). It protects the mother from thyroid dysfunction which in turn protects the neonate's thyroid function and supports neurocognitive development in children (Ersino et al 2013). High-risk women (personal or family history of thyroid disorders or a personal history of other autoimmune diseases) have more than a six-fold increased risk of hypothyroidism during early pregnancy (Vaidya et al 2007).	Mild iodine deficiency (median UIE < 100 mcg/L) has been found in several areas in Australia including NSW and Victoria (Li et al 2006). To prevent iodine deficiency disorders, WHO, United Nations Children's Fund and International Council for the Control of Iodine Deficiency Disorders established that for a given population median urinary iodine concentrations (UIC) must be 150–249 mcg/L in clinically healthy pregnant women (Marchioni et al 2008). Iodine requirement increases during pregnancy and recommended intakes are 250–300 mcg/day (Delange 2007). To monitor iodine status, WHO suggest that a median urinary iodine concentration 250–500 mcg/day indicates adequate iodine intake in pregnancy (Zimmermann 2007).

(Continued)

NUTRIENT	THERAPEUTIC FUNCTION/ JUSTIFICATION	DOSAGE RECOMMENDATIONS AND ISSUES
Iron	Iron requirements increase significantly in pregnancy to support expansion of maternal red blood cell mass and fetal growth (Bothwell 2000). Accurate assessment of iron status during pregnancy is more challenging due to the physiological changes occurring at this time (Milman et al 1991). Haemodilution affects iron parameters, such as haemoglobin concentration, haematocrit, serum iron, ferritin and total-iron binding capacity. Serum ferritin is regarded as the most reliable indicator of iron stores (Byg et al 2000), while haemoglobin levels are used as an inexpensive marker to diagnose anaemia (Reveiz et al 2007). The evaluation of iron status and the future risk of anaemia developing during pregnancy may be more accurate when done early in pregnancy before the maternal plasma volume expands (Scholl 2005). Demands are partly met by a progressive increase in iron absorption as the pregnancy advances (Bothwell 2000); however, depending on initial iron reserves this may not be sufficient to prevent deficiency (Casanueva et al 2003). The risk of iron deficiency increases with parity (Looker et al 1997). Maternal iron stores at conception appear to be a strong predictor of the risk of anaemia in later pregnancy (Bothwell 2000, Casanueva et al 2003). WHO estimates indicate that iron deficiency anaemia affects 22% of women during pregnancy in industrialised countries and 52% in non-industrialised countries (WHO 1992).	The daily recommended intake of iron during pregnancy is increased to 27 mg/ day. Upper limit is 45 mg based on the risk for side effects and potential systemic toxicity. A daily supplement of 40 mg ferrous iron from 18 weeks of gestation appears adequate to prevent iron deficiency in 90% of women (Milman et al 2005). However, individual assessment of iron status in early pregnancy may be useful to tailor the appropriate prophylaxis to prevent iron deficiency and iron deficiency anaemia: Ferritin ≤ 30 mcg/L — 80–100 mg ferrous iron/day; ferritin 31–70 mcg/L — 40 mg ferrous iron/day; those with ferritin > 70 mcg/L do not require supplementation (Milman et al 2006).

NUTRIENT	THERAPEUTIC FUNCTION/ JUSTIFICATION	DOSAGE RECOMMENDATIONS AND ISSUES
	Supplementation raised haemoglobin levels by 7.5 g/dL and reduced the risk of iron deficiency and iron-deficiency anaemia at term (Casaneuva et al 2006, Pena-Rosas & Viteri 2006). Numerous studies have showed an association between adverse outcomes and iron deficiency anaemia, including increased risk of maternal mortality, infection, low birth weight and premature delivery. Fetal and infant iron deficiency may adversely impact on brain development, function and neurocognition (Grantham-McGregor & Ani 2001). Poor maternal iron status may contribute to reduced fetal stores (de Pee et al 2002, Emamghorashi & Heidari 2004, Preziosi et al 1997). However, in a recent cross-sectional study, pregnant women with iron deficiency or mild anaemia were not found to produce offspring with significantly altered iron levels (Paiva Ade et al 2007). Similarly, iron supplementation during the second half of pregnancy was not found to influence the iron status of the children at 6 months or 4 years of age (Zhou et al 2007). On a cautionary note, excessive iron supplementation resulting in high haemoglobin and increased iron stores may be associated with increased adverse pregnancy outcomes (Scholl 2005), including low birth weight and premature delivery (Casanueva & Viteri 2003). A recent Cochrane review involving more than 27,402 women concluded that prenatal supplementation with daily iron is effective in reducing the risk of low birth weight babies, and prevents maternal anaemia and iron deficiency in pregnancy (Peña-Rosas et al 2012).	High dose supplementation may reduce the absorption of zinc (Hambidge et al 1987, O'Brien et al 2000) and other divalent cations (copper, chromium, molybdenum, manganese, magnesium) (Rossander-Hulten et al 1991). Side effects of high dose supplementation typically include gastrointestinal disturbances — most commonly constipation and nausea (Melamed et al 2007).

(Continued)

NUTRIENT	THERAPEUTIC FUNCTION/ JUSTIFICATION	DOSAGE RECOMMENDATIONS AND ISSUES
Magnesium	Magnesium is involved as a cofactor in more than 300 enzyme pathways (Wacker & Parisi 1968) and acts as a neuromuscular relaxant. The infant will contain 750 mg at birth (Prentice 2003). Positive trials highlight benefits of magnesium supplementation for leg cramps (Dahle et al 1995) and possibly pre-ecclampsia although evidence is inconsistent for this last indication (Adam et al 2001, Ahmed 2004, Dawson et al 2000, Duley et al 2003a, 2003b, 2003c, Handwerker et al 1995, Kisters et al 2000, Makrides & Crowther 2001, Omu et al 2008, Sanders et al 1999, Seydoux et al 1992, Shamsuddin et al 2005).	The recommended daily intake for magnesium during pregnancy is increased slightly to 350 mg (19–30 years) and 360 mg (31–50 years). The upper level of intake from non-food sources is 350 mg/ day.
Zinc	Deficiency has been associated with adverse outcomes in pregnancy. Numerous animal models demonstrate an association between zinc deficiency and increased developmental abnormalities and fetal losses. Deficiency has also been associated with reduced interuterine growth, preterm delivery, labour and delivery complications, poor immunological development (Caulfield et al 1998) and congenital malformations (Hambidge et al 1977). A Cochrane review analysing results from studies assessed over 15,000 women and their babies concluded that zinc supplementation resulted in a small but significant reduction in preterm birth (Mori et al 2012). In humans acrodermatitis enteropathica, a genetic disease which produces severe zinc deficiency, has been found to increase fetal losses and malformations, most probably due to its key role in protein synthesis and cellular growth (King 2000).	Recommended daily intake during pregnancy is increased to 11 mg/day and recommended upper level of intake is the same as for adults at 40 mg/day. Vegans and vegetarians may need an additional 50%. The teratogenic effects of alcohol may be exacerbated by a concurrent zinc deficiency (Keppen et al 1985).

NUTRIENT	THERAPEUTIC FUNCTION/ JUSTIFICATION	DOSAGE RECOMMENDATIONS AND ISSUES
	The usefulness of zinc supplementation during pregnancy is unclear. Supplementation has been shown to reduce preterm birth (Mahomed et al 2007), assist the accumulation of lean tissue in the infant during the first year of growth (Iannotti et al 2008) and reduce the risk of delivering via caesarean section (Mahomed et al 2007). While women with preeclampsia have significantly lower zinc and SOD levels compared to healthy pregnant women (Ilhan et al 2002), zinc supplementation had no significant effect in pregnancy hypertension or preeclampsia (Mahomed et al 2007), and no significant differences were seen for several other maternal or infant outcomes including pre-labour rupture of membranes, antepartum haemorrhage, post-term birth, prolonged labour, retention of placenta, meconium in liquor, smell or taste dysfunction, maternal infections, gestational age at birth or birth weight (Mahomed et al 2007).	

(Continued)

NUTRIENT	THERAPEUTIC FUNCTION/ JUSTIFICATION	DOSAGE RECOMMENDATIONS AND ISSUES
Omega-3 (DHA/EPA)	High fetal demands for omega-3 fatty acids result in maternal stores progressively decreasing throughout pregnancy (Al et al 1995, Bonham et al 2008). Important for optimal fetal and infant neurodevelopment and may be associated with benefits for other pregnancy and infant health outcomes including growth and development of the fetal and infant brain (Horrocks & Yeo 1999, Rogers et al 2013), improvements to children's eye–hand coordination (Dunstan et al 2008) and higher infant cognitive function (Hibbeln et al 2007, Oken et al 2005). Lower maternal intake was associated with increased risk of infants with poorer outcomes for prosocial behaviour, fine motor, communication and social development scores (Hibbeln et al 2007), increase risk of infant asthma (Olsen et al 2008), increased risk of postnatal depression (Levant et al 2006, 2008) and increased depressive symptoms in postpartum women (Hibbeln 2002). However, more recent studies have found no association (Browne et al 2006, Freeman et al 2008, Rees et al 2008, Sontrop et al 2008) or mixed outcomes (Su et al 2008). Lower dietary intake of fish (Oken et al 2007) and biochemical markers of omega-3 fatty acid intake (Mehendale et al 2008, Qiu et al 2006, Velzing-Aarts et al 1999) have been reported in women who develop preeclampsia. However, intervention studies with fish oil supplementation generally have not found a protective effect. In a Cochrane review there was no significant difference in risk of gestational hypertension (five trials) or preeclampsia (four trials) in those taking the fish oil (133 mg/day to 3 g/day) compared with control groups (Makrides et al 2006).	Fish oil supplementation during pregnancy appears to be safe. Mild side effects such as belching and unpleasant taste are reported (Freeman & Sinha 2007, Makrides et al 2006). Recommendations for dietary intake of EPA/DHA (adequate intake) for pregnancy is 115 mg/day. Upper level of intake is recommended at 3 g for adults (no pregnancy specifications). Maternal dietary docosahexaenoic acid intake of at least 200 mg/day is associated with positive infant neurodevelopmental outcomes (Cetin & Koletzko 2008).

NUTRIENT	THERAPEUTIC FUNCTION/ JUSTIFICATION	DOSAGE RECOMMENDATIONS AND ISSUES
Probiotics	Prenatal and postnatal supplementation with probiotics may play a role in immune regulation and the prevention of allergies developing in the infant. Numerous positive studies in the prevention of allergies including eczema in the child have involved the following strains: *Lactobacillus reuteri* ATCC 55730 (Abrahamsson et al 2007) *Lactobacillus rhamnosus* strain GG (ATCC 53103) (Kalliomaki et al 2001, 2003, Rautava et al 2002) *Lactobacillus rhamnosus* GG (ATCC 53103); *L. rhamnosus* LC705 (DSM 7061); *Bifidobacterium breve* Bb99 (DSM 13692); and *Propionibacterium freudenreichii* ssp. *shermanii* JS (DSM 7076) (Kukkonen et al 2007) *Lactobacillus rhamnosus* strain GG and *Bifidobacterium lactis* Bb12 (Huurre et al 2008). Prophylactic enteral supplementation reduces the occurrence of necrotising enterocolitis and death in premature infants born less than 1500 g (Alfaleh & Bassler 2008), which may be due to normalisation of gut flora and stimulation of natural host defences (Hammerman & Kaplan 2006). Vaginal application reduces the risk of vaginal infections in pregnancy (Othman et al 2007).	Based on review of literature, prescription appears to be safe for internal and vaginal application.
Choline	Choline status in pregnancy influences the development of the memory centre (hippocampus) in the fetal brain, and may have a lifelong impact on memory (Zeisel 2004). It has been shown to improve cognitive function in the neonate and benefit extends into childhood (Boeke et al 2013).	The recommended daily intake is slightly increased at 440 mg/day, with an upper level of 3000 mg.

APPENDIX 5.2: NHMRC DOSAGE RECOMMENDATIONS FOR PREGNANCY

NUTRIENT	RDI (NHMRC)	NUTRIENT	RDI (NHMRC)
Vitamin A	2600 IU	PABA	No guidelines available
Vitamin B_1 (thiamine)	1.4 mg	Coenzyme Q10	No guidelines available
Vitamin B_2 (riboflavin)	1.4 mg	Alpha lipoic acid	No guidelines available
Vitamin B_3 (niacin)	18 mg	Calcium	1000–1300 mg
Vitamin B_5 (pantothenic acid)	5 mg	Chromium	30 mcg
Vitamin B_6 (pyridoxine)	1.9 mg	Copper	1.3 mg
Pyridoxal 5 phosphate (P5P)	No guidelines available	Iodine	220 mcg
Vitamin B_9 (folic acid)	600 mcg	Iron	27 mg
Folinic acid	No guidelines available	Magnesium	350 mg
L-5-MTHF	No guidelines available	Manganese	5 mg
Vitamin B_{12} (cyanocobalamin)	2.6 mcg	Potassium	2800 mg
Vitamin C	60 mg	Selenium	65 mcg
Vitamin D	200 IU/5 mcg	Silica	No guidelines available
Vitamin E	10 IU/7 mg	Zinc	11 mcg
Vitamin K	60 mcg	Total omega-3 essential fatty acids	No guidelines available
Betacarotene	800 mcg	Total omega-6 essential fatty acids	No guidelines available
Bioflavonoids	No guidelines available	DHA	220 mg
Biotin	30 mcg	EPA	220 mg
Choline	440 mg	Evening primrose oil	No guidelines available
Inositol	No guidelines available	Probiotics (mixed strains)	No guidelines available

REFERENCES

Abrahamsson TR et al. Probiotics in prevention of IgE-associated eczema: a double-blind, randomized, placebo-controlled trial. J Allergy Clin Immunol 119.5 (2007): 1174–1180.

Adam B et al. Magnesium, zinc and iron levels in pre-eclampsia. J Matern Fetal Med 10.4 (2001): 246–250.

Aharoni A et al. Hair chromium content of women with gestational diabetes compared with nondiabetic pregnant women. Am J Clin Nutr 55.1 (1992): 104–107.

Ahmed R. Magnesium sulphate as an anticonvulsant in the management of eclampsia. J Coll Physicians Surg Pak 14.10 (2004): 605–607.

Ainy E et al. Changes in calcium, 25(OH) vitamin D3 and other biochemical factors during pregnancy. J Endocrinol Invest 29.4 (2006): 303–307.

Al MD et al. Maternal essential fatty acid patterns during normal pregnancy and their relationship to the neonatal essential fatty acid status. Br J Nutr 74.1 (1995): 55–68.

Alfaleh K, Bassler D. Probiotics for prevention of necrotizing enterocolitis in preterm infants. Cochrane Database Syst Rev 1 (2008): CD005496.

Allen LH. Vitamin B12 metabolism and status during pregnancy, lactation and infancy. Adv Exp Med Biol 352 (1994): 173–186.

Almeras L et al. Developmental vitamin D deficiency alters brain protein expression in the adult rat: implications for neuropsychiatric disorders. Proteomics 7.5 (2007): 769–780.

Andrade-Cetto A. Ethnobotanical study of the medicinal plants from Tlanchinol, Hidalgo, Mexico. Journal of Ethnopharmacology 122.1 (2009):163–171.

Australian Government, Department of Health and Ageing. National Health and Medical Research Council (NHMRC) and the New Zealand Ministry of Health (MoH). Nutrient Reference Values for Australia and New Zealand. Commonwealth of Australia, 2006. Available: https://www.nhmrc.gov.au/_files_nhmrc/publications/attachments/n35.pdf 5/8/2014.

Awang DV. Maternal use of ginseng and neonatal androgenization. JAMA 265.14 (1991): 1828.

Bamford DS et al. Br J Pharmacol 40 (1970): 161P

Barker DJ. The developmental origins of adult disease. J Am Coll Nutr 23.(6 Suppl) (2004): 588S–595S.

Barker DJ. The origins of the developmental origins theory. J Intern Med 261.5 (2007): 412–417.

Becker DV et al. Iodine supplementation for pregnancy and lactation — United States and Canada: Recommendations of the American Thyroid Association. Thyroid 16.10 (2006): 949–951.

Belew C. Herbs and the childbearing woman: Guidelines for midwives. Journal of Nurse-Midwifery 44(3) (1999): 231–252.

Belizan JM et al. Long-term effect of calcium supplementation during pregnancy on the blood pressure of offspring: follow up of a randomised controlled trial. BMJ 315(7103) (1997): 281–285.

Berbel P et al. Iodine supplementation during pregnancy: a public health challenge. Trends Endocrinol Metab 18.9 (2007): 338–343.

Berry RJ et al Prevention of neural-tube defects with folic acid in China. China–U.S. Collaborative Project for Neural Tube Defect Prevention. N Engl J Med 341.20 (1999): 1485–1490.

Biselli JM et al. Genetic polymorphisms involved in folate metabolism and elevated plasma concentrations of homocysteine: maternal risk factors for Down syndrome in Brazil. Genet Mol Res 7.1 (2008): 33–42.

Boeke CE et al. Choline intake during pregnancy and child cognition at age 7 years. Am J Epidemiol 177.12 (2013): 1338–1347.

Bondevik GT et al. Anaemia in pregnancy: possible causes and risk factors in Nepali women. Eur J Clin Nutr 54.1 (2000): 3–8.

Bonham MP et al. Habitual fish consumption does not prevent a decrease in LCPUFA status in pregnant women (the Seychelles Child Development Nutrition Study). Prostaglandins Leukotrienes and Essential Fatty Acids 78.6 (2008): 343–350.

Borrelli F et al. Effectiveness and safety of ginger in the treatment of pregnancy-induced nausea and vomiting. Obstet Gynecol 105.4 (2005): 849–856.

Boskovic R et al Pregnancy outcome following high doses of Vitamin E supplementation. Reprod Toxicol 20.1 (2005): 85–88.

Bothwell TH. Iron requirements in pregnancy and strategies to meet them. Am J Clin Nutr 72.(1 Suppl) (2000): 257S–264S.

Botto LD et al. Periconceptional multivitamin use and the occurrence of conotruncal heart defects: results from a population-based, case-control study. Pediatrics 98.5 (1996): 911–917.

Boyles AL et al. Folate and one-carbon metabolism gene polymorphisms and their associations with oral facial clefts. Am J Med Genet A 146A.4 (2008): 440–449.

Brown AS et al. Elevated prenatal homocysteine levels as a risk factor for schizophrenia. Arch Gen Psychiatry 64.1 (2007): 31–39.

Browne JC et al. Fish consumption in pregnancy and omega-3 status after birth are not associated with postnatal depression. Journal of Affective Disorders 90.2–3 (2006): 131–139.

Bryant B et al. Drugs in Pregnancy. Pharmacology for Health Professionals. Sydney: Mosby, 2003.

Buppasiri P et al. Calcium supplementation (other than for preventing or treating hypertension) for improving pregnancy and infant outcomes. Cochrane Database of Systematic Reviews 10 (2011).

Burn J, Withell E. A principle in raspberry leaves which relaxes uterine muscle. Lancet 5 (1941): 1–3.

Byg KE et al. Erythropoiesis: Correlations between iron status markers during normal pregnancy in women with and without iron supplementation. Hematology 4(6) (2000): 529–539.

Candito M et al. Nutritional and genetic determinants of vitamin B and homocysteine metabolisms in neural tube defects: a multicenter case-control study. Am J Med Genet A 146A.9 (2008): 1128–1133.

Casanueva E, Viteri FE. Iron and oxidative stress in pregnancy. J Nutr 133.(5 Suppl 2) (2003): 1700S–1708S.

Casanueva E et al. Iron and folate status before pregnancy and anemia during pregnancy. Ann Nutr Metab 47.2 (2003): 60–63.

Casanueva E et al. Weekly iron as a safe alternative to daily supplementation for nonanemic pregnant women. Arch Med Res 37(5) (2006): 674–682.

Casey BM et al. Subclinical Hypothyroidism and Pregnancy Outcomes. Obstet Gynecol 105(2) (2005): 239–245.

Caulfield LE et al. Potential contribution of maternal zinc supplementation during pregnancy to maternal and child survival. Am J Clin Nutr 68 (2 Suppl) (1998): 499S–508S.

Cederberg J et al. Combined treatment with vitamin E and vitamin C decreases oxidative stress and improves fetal outcome in experimental diabetic pregnancy. Pediatr Res 49.6 (2001): 755–762.

Cetin I, Koletzko B. Long-chain omega-3 fatty acid supply in pregnancy and lactation. Curr Opin Clin Nutr Metab Care 11.3 (2008): 297–302.

Chaiyakunapruk N et al. The efficacy of ginger for the prevention of postoperative nausea and vomiting: a meta-analysis. Am J Obstet Gynecol 194 (2006): 95–99.

Challa A et al. Breastfeeding and vitamin D status in Greece during the first 6 months of life. Eur J Pediatr 164(12) (2005): 724–729.

Chow G et al. Dietary Echinacea purpurea during murine pregnancy: effect on maternal hemopoiesis and fetal growth. Biol Neonate 89.2 (2006): 133–138.

Cochrane WA. Overnutrition in prenatal and neonatal life: a problem? Can Med Assoc J 93.17 (1965): 893–899.

Coppede F et al. Polymorphisms in folate and homocysteine metabolizing genes and chromosome damage in mothers of Down syndrome children. Am J Med Genet A 143A.17 (2007): 2006–2015.

Cox SE et al. Vitamin A supplementation increases ratios of proinflammatory to anti-inflammatory cytokine responses in pregnancy and lactation. Clin Exp Immunol 144.3 (2006): 392–400.

Cui X et al. Maternal vitamin D depletion alters neurogenesis in the developing rat brain. International Journal of Developmental Neuroscience 25(4) (2007): 227–232.

Czeizel AE. Periconceptional folic acid containing multivitamin supplementation. Eur J Obstet Gynecol Reprod Biol 78.2 (1998): 151–161.

Czeizel AE, Dudas I. Prevention of the first occurrence of neural-tube defects by periconceptional vitamin supplementation. N Engl J Med 327.26 (1992): 1832–1835.

Czeizel AE, Vargha P. Periconceptional folic acid/multivitamin supplementation and twin pregnancy. Am J Obstet Gynecol 191 3 (2004): 790–794.

Daaboul J et al. Vitamin D deficiency in pregnant and breast-feeding women and their infants. J Perinatol 17.1 (1997): 10–14.

Dahle LO et al (1995). The effect of oral magnesium substitution on pregnancy-induced leg cramps. Am J Obstet Gynecol 173(1): 175–180.

Dante, G et al. Herb remedies during pregnancy: a systematic review of controlled clinical trials, J. Mat-Fet and Neo Med 26.3 (2013): 306–312.

Dawson EB et al. Blood cell lead, calcium, and magnesium levels associated with pregnancy-induced hypertension and preeclampsia. Biol Trace Elem Res 74.2 (2000): 107–116.

de Pee S et al. The High Prevalence of Low Hemoglobin Concentration among Indonesian Infants Aged 3–5 Months Is Related to Maternal Anemia. J. Nutr. 132.8 (2002): 2215–2221.

De-Regil LM et al. Effects and safety of periconceptional folate supplementation for preventing birth defects. Cochrane Database of Systematic Reviews 10 (2010): CD007950.

De-Regil LM et al. Vitamin D supplementation for women during pregnancy. Cochrane Database of Systematic Reviews 2 (2012): CD008873.

Delange F. The role of iodine in brain development. Proc Nutr Soc 59.1 (2000): 75–79.

Delange, F. Iodine requirements during pregnancy, lactation and the neonatal period and indicators of optimal iodine nutrition. Public Health Nutr 10.12A (2007): 1571–1583.

Devereux G et al. Low maternal vitamin E intake during pregnancy is associated with asthma in 5-year-old children. Am J Respir Crit Care Med 174.5 (2006): 499–507.

Diplock AT et al. Functional food science and defence against reactive oxidative species. Br J Nutr 80 Suppl 1 (1998): S77–112.

Dodds L et al. Effect of homocysteine concentration in early pregnancy on gestational hypertensive disorders and other pregnancy outcomes. Clin Chem 54.2 (2008): 326–334.

Donnay S et al. Position statement of the working group on disorders related to iodine deficiency and thyroid dysfunction of the Spanish Society of Endocrinology and Nutrition. Endocrinología y Nutrición (2013): S1575-0922.

Dougoua JJ et al. Safety and efficacy of chastetree (Vitex agnus castus) during pregnancy and lactation, Can J Clin Pharmacol 15.1 (2008):e74–e79.

Duley L, Henderson-Smart D (2003). Magnesium sulphate versus diazepam for eclampsia. Cochrane Database Syst Rev(4): CD000127.

Duley L, Henderson-Smart D (2003). Magnesium sulphate versus phenytoin for eclampsia. Cochrane Database Syst Rev(4): CD000128.

Duley L et al. Magnesium sulphate and other anticonvulsants for women with pre-eclampsia. Cochrane Database Syst Rev(2) (2003): CD000025.

Dunstan JA et al. Cognitive assessment of children at age 2(1/2) years after maternal fish oil supplementation in pregnancy: a randomised controlled trial. Arch Dis Child Fetal Neonatal Ed 93.1 (2008): F45–50.

Emamghorashi F, Heidari T. Iron status of babies born to iron-deficient anaemic mothers in an Iranian hospital. East Mediterr Health J 10.6 (2004): 808–814.

Ersino G et al. Clinical assessment of goiter and low urinary iodine concentration depict presence of severe iodine deficiency in pregnant Ethiopian women: a cross-sectional study in rural Sidama, southern Ethiopia. Ethiop Med J. 51.2 (2013): 133–141.

Ettinger AS et al. Influence of maternal bone lead burden and calcium intake on levels of lead in breast milk over the course of lactation. Am J Epidemiol 163.1 (2006): 48–56.

Eyles D et al. Vitamin d3 and brain development. Neuroscience 118.3 (2003): 641–653.

Felter HW, Lloyd JU. King's American dispensatory, 18th edn, 3rd rev. vol 1, Eclectic Medical Publications, USA, 1905, reprinted 1983.

Feron F et al Developmental Vitamin D3 deficiency alters the adult rat brain. Brain Res Bull 65.2 (2005): 141–148.

Forster D et al. Herbal medicine use during pregnancy in a group of Australian women. BMC Pregnancy and Childbirth 6.1 (2006): 21.

Forster DA et al. The use of folic acid and other vitamins before and during pregnancy in a group of women in Melbourne, Australia. Midwifery 2007.

Freeman MP, Sinha P. Tolerability of omega-3 fatty acid supplements in perinatal women. Prostaglandins, Leukotrienes and Essential Fatty Acids 77.3–4 (2007): 203–208.

Freeman MP et al. Omega-3 fatty acids and supportive psychotherapy for perinatal depression: A randomized placebo-controlled study. J Affect Disord 110.1–2 (2008): 142–148.

Freyer AM Drug-prescribing challenges during pregnancy Obstetr, Gynaecol Repr Med, Review 18.7 (2008): 180–186.

Gaber KR et al. Maternal vitamin B12 and the risk of fetal neural tube defects in Egyptian patients. Clin Lab 53.1–2 (2007): 69–75.

Gale CR et al. Maternal vitamin D status during pregnancy and child outcomes. Eur J Clin Nutr 62.1 (2008): 68–77.

Gallo M et al. Pregnancy outcome following gestational exposure to echinacea: a prospective controlled study. Arch Intern Med 160.20 (2000): 3141–3143.

Goddijn-Wessel TA et al. Hyperhomocysteinemia: a risk factor for placental abruption or infarction. Eur J Obstet Gynecol Reprod Biol 66.1 (1996): 23–29.

Grantham-McGregor S, Ani C. A review of studies on the effect of iron deficiency on cognitive development in children. J Nutr 131.2S-2 (2001): 649S–668S.

Greer FR et al. Improving the vitamin K status of breastfeeding infants with maternal vitamin K supplements. Pediatrics 99.1 (1997): 88–92.

Grieve M. A modern herbal. New York, Dover, 1971.

Groenen P M et al. Marginal maternal vitamin B12 status increases the risk of offspring with spina bifida. Am J Obstet Gynecol 191.1 (2004): 11–17.

Grubesic RB. Children aged 6 to 60 months in Nepal may require a vitamin A supplement regardless of dietary intake from plant an animal food sources. Food Nutr Bull 25.3 (2004): 248–255.

Gunton JE et al. Serum chromium does not predict glucose tolerance in late pregnancy. Am J Clin Nutr 73.1 (2001): 99–104.

Gupta S et al. The role of placental oxidative stress and lipid peroxidation in preeclampsia. Obstet Gynecol Surv 60(12) (2005): 807–816.

Haddow JE et al. Maternal Thyroid Deficiency during Pregnancy and Subsequent Neuropsychological Development of the Child. N Engl J Med 341.8 (1999): 549–555.

Hambidge KM et al. The role of zinc in the pathogenesis and treatment of acrodermatitis enteropathica. Prog Clin Biol Res 14 (1977): 329–342.

Hambidge KM et al. Acute effects of iron therapy on zinc status during pregnancy. Obstet Gynecol 70.4 (1987): 593–596.

Hammerman C, Kaplan M. Probiotics and neonatal intestinal infection. Curr Opin Infect Dis 19.3 (2006): 277–282.

Handwerker SM et al. Ionized serum magnesium and potassium levels in pregnant women with preeclampsia and eclampsia. J Reprod Med 40.3 (1995): 201–208.

Hatton DC et al. Gestational calcium supplementation and blood pressure in the offspring. Am J Hypertens 16.10 (2003): 801–805.

Hatun S et al (2005). Vitamin D deficiency in early infancy. J. Nutr. 135(2): 279–282.

Henry A, Crowther C. Patterns of medication use during and prior to pregnancy: the MAP study. Aust N Z J Obstet Gynaecol 40.2 (2000): 165–172.

Hess H M et al. Herbs during pregnancy. Drugs during pregnancy and lactation, 2nd edn. Oxford: Academic Press, 2007, pp 485–501.

Hibbeln JR. Seafood consumption, the DHA content of mothers' milk and prevalence rates of postpartum depression: a cross-national, ecological analysis. J Affect Disord 69.1–3 (2002): 15–29.

Hibbeln JR et al. Maternal seafood consumption in pregnancy and neurodevelopmental outcomes in childhood (ALSPAC study): an observational cohort study. Lancet 369.9561 (2007): 578–585.

Hofmeyr GJ, Atallah, AN et al. Calcium supplementation during pregnancy for preventing hypertensive disorders and related problems. Cochrane Database Syst Rev 3 (2006): CD001059.

Hofmeyr GJ, Lawrie TA et al. Calcium supplementation during pregnancy for preventing hypertensive disorders and related problems. Cochrane Database of Syst Rev 8 (2010): CD001059.

Hofmeyr GJ et al. Dietary calcium supplementation for prevention of pre-eclampsia and related problems: a systematic review and commentary. Bjog 114.8 (2007): 933–943.

Hollis BW. Circulating 25-Hydroxyvitamin D Levels Indicative of Vitamin D Sufficiency: Implications for Establishing a New Effective Dietary Intake Recommendation for Vitamin D. J. Nutr. 135.2 (2005): 317–322.

Hollis BW. Vitamin D requirement during pregnancy and lactation. J Bone Miner Res 22 Suppl 2 (2007): V39–44.

Hollis BW, Wagner CL. Assessment of dietary vitamin D requirements during pregnancy and lactation. Am J Clin Nutr 79(5) (2004): 717–726.

Hollyer T et al. The use of CAM by women suffering from nausea and vomiting during pregnancy. BMC Complement Altern Med 2 (2002): 5.

Horrocks LA, Yeo YK. Health benefits of docosahexaenoic acid (DHA). Pharmacol Res 40.3 (1999): 211–225.

Hubner U et al. Low serum vitamin B12 is associated with recurrent pregnancy loss in Syrian women. Clin Chem Lab Med (2008).

Huiming Y et al. Vitamin A for treating measles in children. Cochrane Database Syst Rev 4 (2005): CD001479.

Huurre A et al. Impact of maternal atopy and probiotic supplementation during pregnancy on infant sensitization: a double-blind placebo-controlled study. Clin Exp Allergy (2008).

Hypponen E et al. Does vitamin D supplementation in infancy reduce the risk of pre-eclampsia? Eur J Clin Nutr 61.9 (2007): 1136–1139.

Iannotti LL et al. Maternal zinc supplementation and growth in Peruvian infants. Am J Clin Nutr 8.1 (2008): 154–160.

Ilhan N et al. The changes of trace elements, malondialdehyde levels and superoxide dismutase activities in pregnancy with or without preeclampsia. Clin Biochem 35.5 (2002): 393–397.

Jamigorn, M, Phupong V. Acupressure and vitamin B6 to relieve nausea and vomiting in pregnancy: a randomized study. Arch Gynecol Obstet 276.3 (2007): 245–249.
Javaid MK et al. Maternal vitamin D status during pregnancy and childhood bone mass at age 9 years: a longitudinal study. Lancet 367.9504 (2006): 36–43.
Jewell D, Young G. Interventions for nausea and vomiting in early pregnancy. Cochrane Database Syst Rev. 4 (2003): CD000145.
Jishage K-i et al. alpha-Tocopherol Transfer Protein Is Important for the Normal Development of Placental Labyrinthine Trophoblasts in Mice. J. Biol. Chem. 276.3 (2001): 1669–1672.
Johansen AM et al. Maternal dietary intake of vitamin A and risk of orofacial clefts: a population-based case-control study in Norway. Am J Epidemiol 167.10 (2008): 1164–1170.
Jones TK, Lawson BM. Profound neonatal congestive heart failure caused by maternal consumption of blue cohosh herbal medication. J Pediatr 132.3–1 (1998): 550–552.
Jovanovic L, Peterson M. Chromium supplementation for women with gestational diabetes mellitus. The Journal of Trace Elements in Experimental Medicine 12.2 (1999): 91–97.
Jovanovic-Peterson L, Peterson CM. Vitamin and mineral deficiencies which may predispose to glucose intolerance of pregnancy. J Am Coll Nutr 15(1) (1996): 14–20.
Judkins A, Eagleton C. Vitamin D deficiency in pregnant New Zealand women. N Z Med J 119.1241 (2006): U2144.
Kalliomaki M et al. Probiotics in primary prevention of atopic disease: a randomised placebo-controlled trial. Lancet 357.9262 (2001): 1076–1079.
Kalliomaki M et al. Probiotics and prevention of atopic disease: 4-year follow-up of a randomised placebo-controlled trial. Lancet 361.9372 (2003): 1869–1871.
Keeler RF. Lupin alkaloids from teratogenic and nonteratogenic lupins. III. Identification of anagyrine as the probable teratogen by feeding trials. J Toxicol Environ Health 1.6 (1976): 887–898.
Keeler RF et al. Lupin alkaloids from teratogenic and nonteratogenic lupins. IV. Concentration of total alkaloids, individual major alkaloids, and the teratogen anagyrine as a function of plant part and stage of growth and their relationship to crooked calf disease. J Toxicol Environ Health 1(6) (1976): 899–908.
Kennelly EJ et al. Detecting potential teratogenic alkaloids from blue cohosh rhizomes using an in vitro rat embryo culture. J Nat Prod 62.10 (1999): 1385–1389.
Keppen LD et al. Zinc deficiency acts as a co-teratogen with alcohol in fetal alcohol syndrome. Pediatr Res 19.9 (1985): 944–947.
King JC. Determinants of maternal zinc status during pregnancy. Am J Clin Nutr 71.(5 Suppl) (2000): 1334S–1343S.
Kirke PN et al. Maternal plasma folate and vitamin B12 are independent risk factors for neural tube defects. Q J Med 86.11 (1993): 703–708.
Kisters K et al. Membrane, intracellular, and plasma magnesium and calcium concentrations in preeclampsia. Am J Hypertens 13.7 (2000): 765–769.
Koren G et al. Maternal ginseng use associated with neonatal androgenisation. JAMA 264.22 (1990): 2866.
Koutkia P et al. Vitamin D intoxication associated with an over-the-counter supplement. N Engl J Med 345.1 (2001): 66–67.
Kovacs CS, Kronenberg HM. Maternal-fetal calcium and bone metabolism during pregnancy, puerperium, and lactation. Endocr Rev 18(6) (1997): 832–872.
Kukkonen K et al. Probiotics and prebiotic galacto-oligosaccharides in the prevention of allergic diseases: a randomized, double-blind, placebo-controlled trial. J Allergy Clin Immunol 119.1 (2007): 192–198.
Lassi ZS et al. Folic acid supplementation during pregnancy formaternal health and pregnancy outcomes. Cochrane Database Syst Rev 3 (2013): CD006896.
Lee A et al. Therapeutics in pregnancy and lactation. Oxford: Radcliffe Medical Press, 2000.
Levant B et al. Reduced brain DHA Content After a Single Reproductive Cycle in Female Rats Fed a Diet Deficient in N-3 polyunsaturated fatty acids. Biological Psychiatry 60.9 (2006): 987–990.
Levant B et al. Decreased brain docosahexaenoic acid content produces neurobiological effects associated with depression: Interactions with reproductive status in female rats. Psychoneuroendocrinol 33.9 (2008): 1279–1292.
Li Z et al. Folic acid supplements during early pregnancy and likelihood of multiple births: a population-based cohort study. Lancet 361.9355 (2003): 380–384.
Li M et al Are Australian children iodine deficient? Results of the Australian National Iodine Nutrition Study. Med J Aust 184.4 (2006): 165–169.
Livingstone C et al. Vitamin A deficiency presenting as night blindness during pregnancy. Ann Clin Biochem 40.Pt 3 (2003): 292–294.
Looker AC et al. Prevalence of iron deficiency in the United States. JAMA 277.12 (1997): 973–976.
Maats FH, Crowther CA. Patterns of vitamin, mineral and herbal supplement use prior to and during pregnancy. Aust N Z J Obstet Gynaecol 42.5 (2002): 494–496.
MacLennan AH et al. The escalating cost and prevalence of alternative medicine. Prev Med 35.2 (2002): 166–173.
Maghbooli Z et al. Correlation between vitamin D3 deficiency and insulin resistance in pregnancy. Diabetes Metab Res Rev 24.1 (2008): 27–32.
Mahomed K et al. Zinc supplementation for improving pregnancy and infant outcome. Cochrane Database Syst Rev. 2 (2007): CD000230.
Makedos G et al. Homocysteine, folic acid and B12 serum levels in pregnancy complicated with preeclampsia. Arch Gynecol Obstet 275.2 (2007): 121–124.
Makrides M, Crowther CA. Magnesium supplementation in pregnancy. Cochrane Database Syst Rev 4 (2001): CD000937.
Makrides M et al. Marine oil, and other prostaglandin precursor, supplementation for pregnancy uncomplicated by pre-eclampsia or intrauterine growth restriction. Cochrane Database Syst Rev 3 (2006): CD003402.

Marchioni E et al. Iodine deficiency in pregnant women residing in an area with adequate iodine intake. Nutrition 24(5) (2008): 458–461.
Martinez GJ. Traditional practices, beliefs and uses of medicinal plants in relation to maternal–baby health of Criollo women in central Argentina. Midwifery 24.4 (2008): 490–502.
Martinez-Frias ML, Salvador J. Epidemiological aspects of prenatal exposure to high doses of vitamin A in Spain. Eur J Epidemiol 6.2 (1990): 118–123.
Mastroiacovo P et al. High vitamin A intake in early pregnancy and major malformations: a multicenter prospective controlled study. Teratology 59.1 (1999): 7–11.
Matthews A et al. Interventions for nausea and vomiting in early pregnancy. Cochrane Database Syst Rev 9 (2010): CD007575.
Mehendale S et al. Fatty acids, antioxidants, and oxidative stress in pre-eclampsia. International Journal of Gynecology and Obstetrics 100.3 (2008): 234–238.
Melamed N et al. Iron supplementation in pregnancy — does the preparation matter? Arch Gynecol Obstet 276.6 (2007): 601–604.
Miller RK et al. General commentary on drug therapy and drug risks in pregnancy. Drugs during pregnancy and lactation, 2nd edn. Oxford: Academic Press, 2007, pp. 1–26.
Mills JL et al. Vitamin A and birth defects. American Journal of Obstetrics and Gynecology 177.1 (1997): 31–36.
Mills S, Bone K. The Essential Guide to Herbal Safety, Elsevier Churchill Livingstone, USA, 2005.
Milman N et al. Iron supplementation during pregnancy. Effect on iron status markers, serum erythropoietin and human placental lactogen. A placebo controlled study in 207 Danish women. Dan Med Bull 38.6 (1991): 471–476.
Milman N et al. Iron prophylaxis during pregnancy — how much iron is needed? A randomized dose–response study of 20–80 mg ferrous iron daily in pregnant women. Acta Obstet Gynecol Scand 84.3 (2005): 238–247.
Milman N et al. Body iron and individual iron prophylaxis in pregnancy — should the iron dose be adjusted according to serum ferritin? Ann Hematol 85.9 (2006): 567–573.
Mori R et al. Zinc supplementation for improving pregnancy and infant outcome. Cochrane Database Syst Rev 7 (2012): CD000230.
Morley R et al. Maternal 25-hydroxyvitamin D and parathyroid hormone concentrations and offspring birth size. J Clin Endocrinol Metab 91.3 (2006): 906–912.
Morris B et al. Increased chromium excretion in pregnancy is associated with insulin resistance. J Trace Elem Exper Med 13 (2000): 389–396.
Morriss-Kay GM, Sokolova N. Embryonic development and pattern formation. Faseb J 10.9 (1996): 961–968.
Mullen W et al Ellagitannins, flavonoids, and other phenolics in red raspberries and their contribution to antioxidant capacity and vasorelaxation properties. J Agric Food Chem 50 (2002): 5191–5196.
Munger KL et al. Vitamin D intake and incidence of multiple sclerosis. Neurology 62.1 (2004): 60–65.
Munger KL et al. Serum 25-hydroxyvitamin D levels and risk of multiple sclerosis. Jama 296.23 (2006): 2832–2838.
Muthayya S et al. Low maternal vitamin B12 status is associated with intrauterine growth retardation in urban South Indians. Eur J Clin Nutr 60.6 (2006): 791–801.
Nakamura H, Yamamoto T. Mutagen and anti-mutagen in ginger, Zingiber officinale. Mutat Res 103(2) (1982): 119–126.
Nambiar S et al. Hypertension in mother and baby linked to ingestion of Chinese herbal medicine [letter]. West J Med 171 (1999): 152.
Napolitano PG et al. Umbilical cord plasma homocysteine concentrations at delivery in pregnancies complicated by pre-eclampsia. Aust N Z J Obstet Gynaecol 48.3 (2008): 261–265.
Nordeng H, Havnen GC. Use of herbal drugs in pregnancy: a survey among 400 Norwegian women. Pharmacoepidemiol Drug Saf 13(6) (2004): 371–380.
Noumi E, Tchakonang NYC. Plants used as abortifacients in the Sangmelima region of Southern Cameroon. J Ethnopharmacology 76.3 (2001): 263–268.
O'Brien KO et al. Prenatal Iron Supplements Impair Zinc Absorption in Pregnant Peruvian Women. J. Nutr. 130.9 (2000): 2251–2255.
Ochoa-Brust GJ et al. Daily intake of 100 mg ascorbic acid as urinary tract infection prophylactic agent during pregnancy. Acta Obstet Gynecol Scand 86.7 (2007): 783–787.
Oken E et al. Maternal fish consumption, hair mercury, and infant cognition in a U.S. cohort. Environmental Health Perspectives 113.10 (2005): 1376–1380.
Oken E et al. Diet during pregnancy and risk of preeclampsia or gestational hypertension. Ann Epidemiol 17.9 (2007): 663–668.
Olsen SF et al. Fish oil intake compared with olive oil intake in late pregnancy and asthma in the offspring: 16 y of registry-based follow-up from a randomized controlled trial. Am J Clin Nutr 88.1 (2008): 167–175.
Omu AE et al. Magnesium sulphate therapy in women with pre-eclampsia and eclampsia in Kuwait. Med Princ Pract 17.3 (2008): 227–232.
Ortega RM et al. Vitamin A status during the third trimester of pregnancy in Spanish women: influence on concentrations of vitamin A in breast milk. Am J Clin Nutr 66.3 (1997): 564–568.
Othman M et al. Probiotics for preventing preterm labour. Cochrane Database Syst Rev 1 (2007): CD005941.
Paiva Ade A et al. Relationship between the iron status of pregnant women and their newborns. Rev Saude Publica 41.3 (2007): 321–327.
Parsons M et al. Raspberry leaf and its effect on labour: safety and efficacy. Aust Coll Midwives Inc J 12.3 (1999): 20–25.
Pena-Rosas JP, Viteri FE. Effects of routine oral iron supplementation with or without folic acid for women during pregnancy. Cochrane Database Syst Rev 3 (2006): CD004736.
Peña-Rosas JP et al. Daily oral iron supplementation during pregnancy. Cochrane Database Syst Rev 12 (2012): CD004736.

Perez-Lopez FR. Iodine and thyroid hormones during pregnancy and postpartum. Gynecol Endocrinol 23.7 (2007): 414–428.
Perri D et al. Safety and efficacy of echinacea (Echinacea angustifolia, E. purpurea, E. pallida) during pregnancy and lactation. Can J Clin Pharmacol 13.3 (2006): e262–267.
Polyzos NP et al. Combined vitamin C and E supplementation during pregnancy for preeclampsia prevention: a systematic review. Obstet Gynecol Surv 62.3 (2007): 202–206.
Pop VJ. Low concentrations of maternal thyroxin during early gestation: a risk factor of breech presentation? BJOG: Int J Obstetric Gynaecolo 111.9 (2004): 925–930.
Prentice A. Micronutrients and the bone mineral content of the mother, fetus and newborn. J Nutr 133.(5 Suppl 2) (2003): 1693S–1699S.
Preziosi P et al. Effect of iron supplementation on the iron status of pregnant women: consequences for newborns. Am J Clin Nutr 66.5 (1997): 1178–1182.
Qiu C et al. Erythrocyte omega-3 and omega-6 polyunsaturated fatty acids and preeclampsia risk in Peruvian women. Archives of Gynecology and Obstetrics 274.2 (2006): 97–103.
Radhika MS et al. Effects of vitamin A deficiency during pregnancy on maternal and child health. Bjog 109.6 (2002): 689–693.
Ranzini A et al. Use of complementary medicines and alternative therapies among obstetric patients. Obstet Gynecol 97.(4 Suppl 1) (2001): 546.
Rautava S et al. Probiotics during pregnancy and breast-feeding might confer immunomodulatory protection against atopic disease in the infant. J Allergy Clin Immunol 109.1 (2002): 119–121.
Rees AM et al. Omega-3 fatty acids as a treatment for perinatal depression: Randomized double-blind placebo-controlled trial. Australian and New Zealand Journal of Psychiatry 42.3 (2008): 199–205.
Repke JT, Villar J. Pregnancy-induced hypertension and low birth weight: the role of calcium. Am J Clin Nutr 54(1 Suppl) (1991): 237S–241S.
Reveiz L et al. Treatments for iron-deficiency anaemia in pregnancy. Cochrane Database Syst Rev(2) (2007): CD003094.
Rhead WJ, Schrauzer GN. Risks of long-term ascorbic acid overdosage. Nutr Rev 29.11 (1971): 262–263.
Riddle JM. Oral contraceptives and early-term abortifacients during classical antiquity and the middle ages. Past & Present 132.1 (1991): 3–32.
Rogers LK et al. DHA supplementation: current implications in pregnancy and childhood. Pharmacol Res 70.1. (2013):13–19.
Ronnenberg AG et al. Preconception homocysteine and B vitamin status and birth outcomes in Chinese women. Am J Clin Nutr 76.6 (2002): 1385–1391.
Ronnenberg AG et al. Preconception B-vitamin and homocysteine status, conception, and early pregnancy loss. Am J Epidemiol 166.3 (2007): 304–312.
Rossander-Hulten L et al. Competitive inhibition of iron absorption by manganese and zinc in humans. Am J Clin Nutr 54.1 (1991): 152–156.
Rumbold A, Crowther CA. Vitamin C supplementation in pregnancy. Cochrane Database Syst Rev(2) (2005): CD004072.
Rumbold A, Crowther CA. Vitamin E supplementation in pregnancy. Cochrane Database Syst Rev(2) (2005): CD004069.
Rumbold A et al. Vitamin supplementation for preventing miscarriage. Cochrane Database Syst Rev(2) (2005): CD004073.
Rumbold A et al. Antioxidants for preventing pre-eclampsia. Cochrane Database Syst Rev(1) (2008): CD004227.
Rumiris D et al. Lower rate of preeclampsia after antioxidant supplementation in pregnant women with low antioxidant status. Hypertens Pregnancy 25. 3 (2006): 241–253.
Sachan A et al. High prevalence of vitamin D deficiency among pregnant women and their newborns in northern India. Am J Clin Nutr 81.5 (2005): 1060–1064.
Sanders R et al. Intracellular and extracellular, ionized and total magnesium in pre-eclampsia and uncomplicated pregnancy. Clin Chem Lab Med 37.1 (1999): 55–59.
Sanz EJ et al. Selective serotonin reuptake inhibitors in pregnant women and neonatal withdrawal syndrome: a database analysis. Lancet 365.9458 (2005): 482–517.
Schiebinger L. Exotic abortifacients and lost knowledge. The Lancet 371 (2008):718–719.
Scholl TO. Iron status during pregnancy: setting the stage for mother and infant. Am J Clin Nutr 81.5 (2005): 1218S–1222.
Scholl TO et al. Vitamin E: maternal concentrations are associated with fetal growth. Am J Clin Nutr 84.6 (2006): 1442–1448.
Senes M et al. Coenzyme Q10 and high-sensitivity C-reactive protein in ischemic and idiopathic dilated cardiomyopathy. Clin Chem Lab Med 46.3 (2008): 382–386.
Seydoux J et al. Serum and intracellular magnesium during normal pregnancy and in patients with pre-eclampsia. Br J Obstet Gynaecol 99.3 (1992): 207–211.
Shahraki AD. Effects of vitamin E, calcium carbonate and milk of magnesium on muscular cramps in pregnant women. J Med Sci 6.6 (2006): 979–983.
Shamsuddin L et al. Use of parenteral magnesium sulphate in eclampsia and severe pre-eclampsia cases in a rural set up of Bangladesh. Bangladesh Med Res Counc Bull 31.2 (2005): 75–82.
Shaw GM et al. Periconceptional intake of vitamin A among women and risk of neural tube defect-affected pregnancies. Teratology 55.2 (1997): 132–133.
Shearer MJ. Vitamin K metabolism and nutriture. Blood Reviews 6 (1992): 92–104.
Shehata HA, Nelson-Piercy C. Drugs to avoid in pregnancy, Curr Obstet & Gyneco, 10 (2000): 44–52.
Shrim A et al. Pregnancy outcome following use of large doses of vitamin B6 in the first trimester. J Obstet Gynaecol 26.8 (2006): 749–751.

Sills IN et al. Vitamin D deficiency rickets. Reports of its demise are exaggerated. Clin Pediatr (Phila) 33.8 (1994): 491–493.

Simpson M et al. Raspberry leaf in pregnancy: Its safety and efficacy in labor. Journal of Midwifery & Women's Health 46.2 (2001): 51–59.

Sontrop J et al. Depressive symptoms during pregnancy in relation to fish consumption and intake of n-3 polyunsaturated fatty acids. Paediatric and Perinatal Epidemiology 22.4 (2008): 389–399.

Soudamini KK et al. Mutagenicity and anti-mutagenicity of selected spices. Indian J Physiol Pharmacol 39.4 (1995): 347–353.

Specker BL. Do North American women need supplemental vitamin D during pregnancy or lactation? Am J Clin Nutr 59.2 (1994): 484S–490.

Sripramote M, Lekhyananda N. A randomized comparison of ginger and vitamin B6 in the treatment of nausea and vomiting of pregnancy. J Med Assoc Thai 86.9 (2003): 846–853.

Steen MT et al. Neural-tube defects are associated with low concentrations of cobalamin (vitamin B12) in amniotic fluid. Prenat Diagn 18.6 (1998): 545–555.

Steer C et al. THe Methylenetetrahydrofolate Reductase (MTHFR) C677T Polymorphism is Associated with Spinal BMD in Nine-Year-Old Children. J Bone Miner Res (2008).

Su KP et al. Omega-3 fatty acids for major depressive disorder during pregnancy: Results from a randomized, double-blind, placebo-controlled trial. Journal of Clinical Psychiatry 69.4 (2008): 644–651.

Suarez L et al. Maternal Serum B12 Levels and Risk for Neural Tube Defects in a Texas–Mexico Border Population. Annals of Epidemiology 13.2 (2003): 81–88.

Suharno D et al. Supplementation with vitamin A and iron for nutritional anaemia in pregnant women in West Java, Indonesia. Lancet 342.8883 (1993): 1325–1328.

Tannis MJ. Potential toxicities of herbal therapies in the developing fetus. Birth Defects Research Part B: Developmental and Reproductive Toxicology 68.6 (2003): 496–498.

Téllez-Rojo M et al. A randomized controlled trial of calcium supllementation to reduce blood lead levels (and fetal lead exposure) in pregnant women. Epidemiology 17.6 (2006): s123.

Thaver D et al. Pyridoxine (vitamin B6) supplementation in pregnancy. Cochrane Database Syst Rev 2 (2006): CD000179.

Thomas, KJ et al. Use and expenditure on complementary medicine in England: a population based survey. Complement Ther Med 9.1 (2001): 2–11.

Tindle HA et al. Trends in use of complementary and alternative medicine by US adults: 1997–2002. Altern Ther Health Med 11(1) (2005): 42–49.

Trotter M, Hixon BB. Sequential changes in weight, density, and percentage ash weight of human skeletons from an early fetal period through old age. Anat Rec 179.1 (1974): 1–18.

Tsui B et al. A survey of dietary supplement use during pregnancy at an academic medical center. Am J Obstet Gynecol 185.2 (2001): 433–437.

Tytgat GN et al. Contemporary understanding and management of reflux and constipation in the general population and pregnancy: a consensus meeting. Aliment Pharmacol Ther 18.3 (2003): 291–301.

Vaidya B et al. Detection of thyroid dysfunction in early pregnancy: universal screening or targeted high-risk case finding? J Clin Endocrinol Metab 92.1 (2007): 203–207.

Valsecchi L et al. Serum levels of alpha-tocopherol in hypertensive pregnancies. Hypertens Pregnancy 18.3 (1999): 189–195.

van den Broek N et al. Vitamin A supplementation during pregnancy for maternal and newborn outcomes. Cochrane Database Syst Rev, 2010 Issue 11:Art. No.: CD008666. DOI:10.1002/14651858.CD008666.pub2.

van der Meer IM et al. High prevalence of vitamin D deficiency in pregnant non-Western women in The Hague, Netherlands. Am J Clin Nutr 84(2) (2006): 350–353.

Velzing-Aarts FV et al. Umbilical vessels of preeclamptic women have low contents of both n-3 and n-6 long-chain polyunsaturated fatty acids. Am J Clin Nutrit 69.2 (1999): 293–298.

Vieth R et al. Wintertime vitamin D insufficiency is common in young Canadian women, and their vitamin D intake does not prevent it. Eur J Clin Nutr 55(12) (2001): 1091–1097.

Vieth R et al. Efficacy and safety of vitamin D3 intake exceeding the lowest observed adverse effect level. Am J Clin Nutr 73.2 (2001): 288–294.

Villar J, Belizan JM. Same nutrient, different hypotheses: disparities in trials of calcium supplementation during pregnancy. Am J Clin Nutr 71(5 Suppl) (2000): 1375S–1379S.

Villar J et al. Epidemiologic observations on the relationship between calcium intake and eclampsia. Int J Gynaecol Obstet 21.4 (1983): 271–278.

Villar J et al. Calcium supplementation reduces blood pressure during pregnancy: results of a randomized controlled clinical trial. Obstet Gynecol 70.3 (Pt 1) (1987): 317–322.

Villar J et al. Nutritional interventions during pregnancy for the prevention or treatment of maternal morbidity and preterm delivery: an overview of randomized controlled trials. J. Nutr. 133.5 (2003): 1606S–1625.

von Kries R et al. Assessment of vitamin K status of the newborn infant. J Pediatr Gastroenterol Nutr 16.3 (1993): 231–238.

Wacker WE, Parisi AF. Magnesium metabolism. N Engl J Med 278.12 (1968): 658–663.

Waller DP. et al. Lack of androgenicity of Siberian ginseng. JAMA 267.17 (1992): 2329.

Wang X et al. Vitamin C and vitamin E supplementation reduce oxidative stress-induced embryo toxicity and improve the blastocyst development rate. Fertility and Sterility 78.6 (2002): 1272–1277.

Webster WS, Freeman JAD. Is this drug safe in pregnancy? Reprod Toxicol 15.6 (2001): 619–629.

Weidner MS, Sigwart K. Investigation of the teratogenic potential of a zingiber officinale extract in the rat. Reprod Toxicol 15.1 (2001): 75–80.

Werler MM. et al. Maternal vitamin A supplementation in relation to selected birth defects. Teratology 42.5 (1990): 497–503.

West KP et al. Double blind, cluster randomised trial of low dose supplementation with vitamin A or beta carotene on mortality related to pregnancy in Nepal. BMJ 318.7183 (1999): 570–575.
Westney OE et al. Nutrition, genital tract infection, hematologic values, and premature rupture of membranes among African American Women. J Nutr 124.(6 Suppl) (1994): 987S–993S.
Whitehouse, B. Fragarine: an inhibitor of uterine action. BMJ 13 (1941): 370–371.
WHO. The prevalence of anaemia in women: a tabulation of available information, World Health Organization, Geneva, 1992.
WHO. WHO traditional medicine strategy 2002–2005, World Health Organization, Geneva 2002.
Woods SE et al. Serum chromium and gestational diabetes. J Am Board Fam Med 21.2 (2008): 153–157.
Wouters MG et al. Hyperhomocysteinemia: a risk factor in women with unexplained recurrent early pregnancy loss. Fertil Steril 60.5 (1993): 820–825.
Wright ME. A case-control study of maternal nutrition and neural tube defects in Northern Ireland. Midwifery 11.3 (1995): 146–152.
Xue CC et al. Complementary and alternative medicine use in Australia: a national population-based survey. J Altern Complement Med 13.6 (2007): 643–650.
Zeghoud F et al. Subclinical vitamin D deficiency in neonates: definition and response to vitamin D supplements. Am J Clin Nutr 65.3 (1997): 771–778.
Zeisel SH. Nutritional importance of choline for brain development. J Am Coll Nutr 23.(6 Suppl) (2004): 621S–626S.
Zhou SJ et al. Routine iron supplementation in pregnancy has no effect on iron status of children at six months and four years of age. J Pediat 151.4 (2007): 438–440.
Zimmermann MB. The adverse effects of mild-to-moderate iodine deficiency during pregnancy and childhood: a review. Thyroid 17.9 (2007): 829–835.

Alpha lipoic acid

HISTORICAL NOTE Lipoic acid was first identified in bacteria in 1937 (Lodge & Packer 1999). In 1951, its isolation and chemical structure characterisation by Reed saw lipoic acid tentatively classified as a vitamin (Wang et al 2011). It was subsequently found to be endogenously produced in humans from octanoic acid and the sulfur residue of cysteine. By the early 1950s, lipoic acid was understood as an essential cofactor in oxidative metabolism, involved in acyl-group transfer and as a mitochondrial coenzyme in the Krebs cycle (Patel & Packer 2008). Currently used as a medicine in the treatment of diabetic neuropathies in Europe, research has focused on its unique antioxidant properties and their application, mainly in diabetes management, but also in various neuropathologies, as well as in immune and inflammation modulation (Shay et al 2009).

OTHER NAMES

Alpha lipoic acid (ALA), lipoic acid (LA), R-lipoic acid, S-lipoic acid, racemic lipoic acid, rhioctic acid, 6,8-thioctic acid, 1,2-dithiolane-3-valeric acid, dehydrolipoic acid (DHLA), 1,2-dithiolane-3-pentanoic acid.

BACKGROUND AND RELEVANT PHARMACOKINETICS

Chemical structure

ALA is a cyclic disulfide compound endogenously synthetised in the mitochondria from octanoic acid (caprylic acid) using cysteine as a source of sulfur. LA is manufactured in both R- and S-enantiomeric forms, but only the naturally produced R-form conjugates to lysine residues and attaches to a lipoyl protein carrier to act as an essential cofactor in physiolological systems (Wang et al 2011); free LA is only present in very small amounts in the body (Patel & Packer 2008, Shay et al 2009), and is usually found in free form after therapeutic supplementation (Teichert et al 1998).

LA is insoluble in water, but soluble in organic solvents. At physiological pH, LA is anionic and in this form it is commonly called lipoate.

Pharmocokinetics and bioavailability of LA

Most of the research for the bioavailability of ALA comes from studies using oral supplementation, usually made from manufactured racemic ALA.

Although not fully understood, the bioavailability of exogenous LA seems dependent on multiple carrier proteins. In vitro studies show that LA is absorbed through the cell membrane in a pH-dependent manner, through the monocarboxylate and Na^+-dependent multivitamin transporter (Keith et al 2012, Shay et al 2009).

The gastrointestinal uptake of ALA is rapid but variable. A pharmacokinetic study by Teichert et al (1998) showed that humans absorb 20–40% of oral racemic ALA. Additionally, preferential uptake of the R-enantiomer has been established, as plasma concentrations were 40–60% more than those of the L-enantiomer. However it is yet to be established if the S-form prevents polymerisation of ALA, thus increasing overall bioavailability (Breithaupt-Grogler et al 1999, Shay et al 2009).

Bioavailability fluctuates with concomitant absorption of food, suggesting nutrient interaction (Teichert et al 1998). Furthermore, it appears that the salt form has better bioavailability (Carlson et al 2007).

After rapid gastrointestinal uptake, ALA appears quickly in the plasma and generally peaks within 1 hour of administration and then declines rapidly, mainly via renal excretion (Harrison & McCormick 1974, Shay et al 2009). R-LA administered as a salt showed high plasma maximum concentrations and high area under the concentration versus time curve values (Carlson et al 2007). Ninety-eight per cent of radiolabelled LA is excreted within 24 hours (Schupke et al 2001).

Erythrocytes and a number of other cells take up ALA by glucose metabolism (GLUT 4), after which it reduces to DHLA, which is subsequently released in the extracellular environment (Packer & Cadenas 2010). However in adipocytes, it is poorly reduced and shows prooxidant activities (Cho et al 2003, Moini et al 2002a, 2002b, Packer & Cadenas 2010).

Supplemental LA has been shown to accumulate transiently in the liver, heart and skeletal muscles. Bioaccumulation in the brain has been debated (Chng et al 2009); however, in view of the large number of studies demonstrating a therapeutic effect on the brain, DHLA and other ALA metabolites should also be measured to establish their potential therapeutic benefits after oral ingestion of ALA (Shay et al 2009), as in vitro studies suggests that it is rapidly reduced to its DHLA form; catabolism of ALA, which occurs via β-oxidation, produces at least 12 major metabolites (Jones et al 2002).

FOOD SOURCES

ALA is found in various natural sources in the form lipoyllysine, which is protein-bound ALA. While it is ubiquitous in most food and especially in organ meats (liver, kidney) and spinach, with lesser amounts in broccoli floral buds, tomato, garden peas and Brussels sprouts, rice bran and yeast extract, it is only present in very low amounts and poorly bioavailable, thus it is not likely that it is consumed in appreciable amounts (Lodge & Packer 1999, Shay et al 2009, Sen & Packer 2000). Dietary supplements provide the main source of exogenous LA (Shay et al 2009).

DEFICIENCY SIGNS AND SYMPTOMS

ALA is endogenously synthesised, primarily in the liver but also in other tissues. Animal studies have established that it is essential to life. To determine deficiency signs and symptoms, animal models of decreased ALA production have been studied.

No recommended daily intake has been established.

As an endogenous nutrient, little is known about the effects of genetic alteration that modify lipoic acid synthase (LIAS) expression and the reduction in endogenous LA production on disease pathogenesis. A rodent study in which the LIAS gene (homozygous mutation) has been switched off demonstrated that absence of LA is incompatible with life and ends in the early demise of all embryos in early implantation, presumably due to the inability of cells to produce oxidative metabolism. Supplementation of the mother did not alter the outcome (Yi & Maeda 2005). Interestingly, the intraperitoneal (IP) injection of ALA to diabetic pregnant rats did improve fetal and placental outcome, suggesting it can travel through the placenta (Al Ghafli et al 2004).

Heterozygous mutation, impairing synthesis of ALA, showed an important decrease in erythrocyte glutathione levels and abnormal cellular antioxidant capacity (Yi & Maeda 2005).

Other animal models showed that LIAS deficiency resulted in overall cellular abnormality in antioxidant defence, increased inflammation and inflammatory cytokine expression, insulin resistance, mitochondrial dysfunction (Padmalayam et al 2009), and enhanced atherosclerosis formation, especially in males (Yi et al 2010). One case report of a newborn baby homozygous for LIAS deficiency manifested in mitochondrial encephalopathy with neonatal-onset epilepsy, muscular hypotonia, lactic acidosis and increased glycine in urine and plasma (Mayr et al 2011).

MAIN ACTIONS

While de novo endogenous synthesis is considered sufficient for metabolic function, less is understood of ALA's role as an oral nutritional supplement. The growing body of evidence suggests it is bioavailable, safe in moderate doses and displays a range of metabolic and clinical effects (Shay et al 2009).

Mitochondrial energy metabolism

De novo R-LA serves as an essential cofactor for the reduction of NAD to NADH in α-keto acid dehydrogenases (a multienzyme complex which includes pyruvate dehydrogenase) in the Krebs cycle, by catalysing the oxidative carboxylation of α-keto acids (Booker 2004, Rüdiger et al 1972, Shay et al 2009).

Antioxidant

Lipoate has the unique ability of being able to act as an antioxidant in fat and water-soluble tissues and also act as a 'metabolic antioxidant'. Enzymes in human cells accept it as a substrate for reduction. It is promptly taken up by cells and reduced to dihydrolipoate at the expense of cellular-reducing equivalents such as NADH and NADPH. As more of these reducing equivalents are used, the rate of cellular metabolism is sped up to cater for the enhanced demand (Sen & Packer 2000).

Both ALA (oxidised) and DHLA (reduced) act as a potent redox pair and scavenge a number of reactive oxygen species (ROS: hydroxyl radicals and hypochlorous acid). DHLA has been demonstrated to regenerate vitamin C and E in vitro (Bast & Haenen 2008, Biewenga et al 1997). R-LA feeding to rats has also been demonstrated to increase ascorbate levels in hepatocytes and cardiomyocytes subjected to normal aged-related loss (Lykkesfeldt et al 1999, Michels et al 2003, Suh et al 2001). Mechanisms of action appear indirect, by inducing the uptake from blood plasma, or promoting the synthesis of intracellular antioxidants via signal transduction (Shay et al 2009). DHLA increases intracellular glutathione by reducing cystine to cysteine (Han et al 1997, Suh et al 2001) and by enhancing cellular cysteine uptake (Suh et al 2004a).

Its role as an antioxidant and involvement in the broader antioxidant network underlie many of its observed actions in preclinical models.

Glucose uptake and metabolism

Lipoate is known to promote the efficiency of glucose uptake by cultured skeletal muscle cells at a magnitude comparable to that of insulin and has also been shown to retain its ability to stimulate glucose uptake even where L6 myotubes were insulin-resistant (Sen & Packer 2000). In a rat model, Streeper et al (1997) demonstrated that a 10-day administration of R-LA improved significantly glucose uptake, decreased insulin resistance and increased glycogen synthesis and glucose oxidation compared to S-LA; it is important to note that GLUT 4 was slightly decreased by S-LA at doses of 30 mg/kg of body weight in the same study.

A SDZ rat study had demonstrated that 10 days' ALA treatment (30 mg/kg IP) enhanced muscle glucose metabolism and increased gastrocnemius GLUT 4 translocation (Khamaisi et al 1997). R-LA enhanced glucose uptake more rapidly and in larger amounts than S-LA or rac-LA (Estrada et al 1996). In the presence of insulin, ALA's effects were increased by 33% (Henriksen et al 1997). Similar results were observed in rat heart cells (Strödter et al 1995).

Estrada et al (1996) and Moini et al (2002b) demonstrated in vitro PI3K involvement. In vivo studies, while supporting the finding of GLUT4 upregulation, indicated a mechanism independent of PI3K as well (Henriksen et al 1997, Packer & Cadenas 2010). It is important to note a great disparity in in vitro and in vivo study dosage administration, which could explain this difference.

Endothelial function

A number of clinical studies have demonstrated that treatment with ALA significantly improves endothelial function, increases nitric oxide (NO) synthesis and prevents loss in endothelial NO synthase phosphorylation, thus restoring vasodilation in diabetic and impaired-glycaemia patients. Although mechanisms are yet to be explained, it is thought to be acting through the PI3K/Akt signalling pathway (Heinisch et al 2010, Heitzer et al 2001, Sena et al 2008, Sola et al 2005, Xiang et al 2011).

Hypotensive

Oral ALA supplementation tested in a number of hypertensive rat models was shown to normalise systolic blood pressure and aortic superoxide production (Vasdev et al 2000a, 2000b, 2003, 2005). In addition to improving endothelial NO synthesis, ALA is thought to reduce sulfhydryl group denaturation of Ca^{2+} channels in vascular smooth muscles through the regeneration of reduced glutathione and by inhibition of renal and vascular overproduction of endothelin-1, an endothelial vasoconstrictor (Takaoka et al 2001). In vivo research further suggests that long-term treatment with ALA improves baroreflex sensitivity in rats with renovascular hypertension (Queiroz et al 2012).

ALA also appears to prevent the development of glucocorticoid-induced hypertension according to in vivo research, an effect not mediated by mitochondrial superoxide reduction (Ong et al 2013).

Anti-inflammatory

Numerous preclinical studies have demonstrated that LA affects several important inflammatory pathways in vivo, such as inducing a significant increase in cyclic adenosine monophosphate (cAMP) concentration and affecting the cAMP/protein kinase A signalling cascade (Salinthone et al 2010). These effects have also been demonstrated in humans.

In particular, LA, in either racemic or individual S- or R-forms, but not DHLA, is able to stimulate cAMP production in natural killer and T cells (Salinthone et al 2011, Schillace et al 2007), thus having an effect on inflammation, immunomodulation and autoimmunity.

It appears that LA stimulates cAMP production by activating G-protein coupled receptors, such as adenosine, likely to be responsible for the anti-inflammatory action of LA; curiously, LA also activated histamine, but not β-adrenergic receptors. The histamine activation pathway findings have an implication in the safety of long-term intake of LA and warrant further studies, especially in the development of allergies and cancers (Salinthone et al 2011).

LA, but not DHLA, downregulates $CD4^+$ expression in a concentration-dependent manner, potentially inhibiting T-cell activation to antigens, especially in the central nervous system environment, showing potential benefits in the management of multiple sclerosis (MS), and autoimmune pathologies (Marracci et al 2006).

In a small clinical study, ALA demonstrated an effect on exercise-induced inflammatory response in physically active males. Twenty minutes after a 90-minute exercise trial, ALA intake increased serum interleukin-6 (IL-6) and IL-10 (anti-inflammatory cytokines) and decreased IL-1β (proinflammatory). It also improved muscle regeneration (Zembron-Lacny et al 2013). In MS patients ($n = 20$), LA was shown to stimulate cAMP by 43%, reduce IL-6 and IL-17 (cytokines involved in MS pathogenesis) and inhibit T-cell proliferation by 90% and activation by 40%, demonstrating anti-inflammatory effects (Salinthone et al 2010).

Neuroprotective

ALA demonstrates neuroprotective effects in various test models. This is accomplished via several different mechanisms. As a result, ALA has a potential role in a number of neurodegenerative disorders, including diabetic neuropathies, Alzheimer's dementia, burning-mouth syndrome, amyotrophic lateral sclerosis, seizures, brain injuries and MS (Yamada et al 2011).

Peroxynitrite involvement has been demonstrated in the pathogenesis of various neurodegenerative diseases through DNA strand break; an in vitro study by Jia et al (2009) demonstrated the inhibition of peroxynitrite-mediated DNA damage by ALA, suggesting it may be partly responsible for the neuroprotective action. ALA's ability to promote the expression of antioxidative genes via the PI3K/Akt pathway that upregulates glutathione has also been demonstrated in SH-SY5Y brain cells in vitro (Yamada et al 2011).

In a cryo-injured rat brain model, ALA was shown to stimulate the synthesis of glutathione, decrease cell death, promote angiogenesis and decrease glial cell scar formation (Rocamonde et al 2012). ALA also appears to reduce monocyte migration across the blood–brain barrier effectively, protect its integrity and inhibit cerebral inflammation in a dose-dependent manner (Schreibelt et al 2006).

A number of experimental models demonstrate protective mechanisms in cerebral ischaemic-reperfusion injury when subjects are pretreated before occlusion (Connell et al 2011, Richard et al 2011). ALA was also shown to significantly prevent neuronal oxidative stress induced by a number a pharmacological drugs and environmental poisons in animal models: haloperidol (Perera et al 2011), L-dopa (Abdin & Sarhan 2011), cyanide-induced seizures (Abdel-Zaher et al 2011), dimethoate, glyphosate and zineb (Astiz et al 2012) and morphine-induced tolerance and dependence (Abdel-Zaher et al 2011).

Hepatoprotective

Hepatoprotective activity has been demonstrated in different animal studies, indicating a potential role in chronic liver disease and damage.

A hepatoprotective effect was observed after ALA treatment in lipid peroxidation-induced liver injury, and thioacetamide-induced fibrosis. Treament with ALA resulted in a decrease in serum aspartate transaminase (AST) and alanine transaminase (ALT), decrease in lipid peroxidation, maintenance of antioxidant capacity, and reduction in histomorphological damage to hepatocytes (Kaya-Dagistanli et al 2013, Ning-Ping et al 2011).

Protection from paracetamol- and methotrexate-induced mitochondrial toxicity was demonstrated in rodent experimental models, again with maintenance of antioxidant capacity, inhibition of oxidative stress and protection of hepatocyte morphology (Abdel-Zaher et al 2008, Tabassum et al 2010).

Antiatherosclerotic

Animal models of LA synthase deficiency in apolipoprotein E-deficient animals show they have an increased propensity to develop atherosclerotic plaque, especially male subjects (Yi et al 2010, 2012b). In animal models fed high-fat, hypercholesterolaemic diets, ALA was shown to attenuate and decrease plaque formation, decrease inflammation, decrease T-cell content in plaque, decrease vascular smooth-muscle proliferation and improve lipid profile (Lee et al 2012, Xu et al 2012, Ying et al 2010).

Cardioprotective

Pretreatment of rats with LA reduced infarct size and preserved cardiac function in a study of myocardial ischaemia-reperfusion injury (Deng et al 2013).

OTHER ACTIONS

Metal chelation

ALA chelates transition metals by forming stable complexes with Mn^{2+}, Cu^{2+} and Zn^{2+} (Sigel et al 1978). DHLA, but not ALA, significantly inhibited ascorbate oxidation by Fe(III) and Cu(II) in a concentration-dependent manner through chelation, without removing copper or iron from the active sites of enzymes or altering the activity of copper- and iron-dependent enzymes (Suh et al 2004b).

While administration of ALA in lead-poisoned animal models or in vitro cellular models demonstrated a reduction in lead oxidation of the brain (Pande & Flora 2002), the kidney (Sivaprasad et al 2004), erythrocytes (Caylak et al 2008) and ovarian tissue (Gurer et al 1999), especially in combination with dimercaptosuccinic acid (DMSA, a pharmacological molecule commonly used as an antidote to heavy metal poisoning), it showed no chelation properties in decreasing the lead burden. Other studies showed a similar effect, alone or with DMSA, in cadmium-induced oxidation of rat heart, brain, testis and liver (Sumathi et al 1996), in arsenic-induced oxidation of rat brain (Shila et al 2005) and in in vitro human glial cells (Cheng et al 2007).

Signal transduction

ALA is involved in the reduction and oxidation of the thiol/disulfide bonds in transcription factors, and as such has been demonstrated to modulate cell signalling via NF-κB, AMPK and PI3K/Akt signalling (Packer & Cadenas 2010).

Cataract protection

ALA inhibited the development and progression of naphthalene and proton-induced cataract in healthy and diabetic rats (Chen et al 2010, Davis et al 2010, Kojima et al 2007). It also showed the ability to penetrate the human aqueous after topical application, showing a potential use of LA's antioxidant capacity in ophthalmology (Cagini et al 2010).

Cancer

Prevention

ALA has exhibited antimutagenic and anticlastogenic activities in tumorigenic animal and human cell models, including breast, melanoma, ovarian epithelial and colon cancers, through the inhibition of inflammatory mediators, the inhibition of NF-κB activity and DNA fragmentation and inhibition of metastasis (Goraca et al 2011).

Treatment

Four cases of pancreatic cancer patients undergoing a long-term treatment of 300–600 mg intravenous (IV) ALA twice a week, oral naltrexone (4.5 g/day) in addition to dietary modification, selenium (200 mcg bd) and silymarin (300 mg qd) were reported to have improved survival outcomes. These results warrant further investigation given the general poor prognosis of pancreatic cancer patients (Berkson et al 2009).

ALA also demonstrated neuroprotection from chemotherapy side effects (paclitaxel, cisplatin, frataxin and methotrexate) in human cell models of cancer and in vivo animal models (Dadhania et al 2010, Melli et al 2009, Tabassum et al 2010). Current clinical trials are underway.

Neuromodulation

LA improved the status of dopamine, serotonin and adrenaline in rodent's aged brain (Arivazhagan & Panneerselvan 2002).

Radioprotection

Report of a Russian open trial of the treatment of children exposed to radiation from the Chernobyl disaster is often stated as the basis of the radioprotective effects of ALA.

A small number of recent published in vitro and in vivo studies seem to support the potential role of ALA in radioprotection. These studies report protection of cerebellar structure and cognitive function in γ-irradiated rodents (Manda et al 2008), increased protection in cell membrane and DNA stability, as well as increased survival time in lethally radiated mice (Ramachandran & Nair 2011) and maintenance of haemogloblin integrity and rheology in irradiated blood bags for transfusion (Desouky et al 2011).

CLINICAL USE

Most clinical research has been conducted in diabetic populations and people with disease states where an antioxidant, neuroprotective and/or anti-inflammatory mechanism of action may have benefits.

Diabetes

Oral and injectable forms of LA have been investigated in diabetes as a means of enhancing insulin sensitivity and either preventing or treating chronic complications which occur years after the onset of disease, such as polyneuropathy, nephropathy and retinopathy. Many of these complications are the result of an overabundance of ROS produced by the mitochondrial transport chain as a result of a sustained hyperglycaemic state.

ALA was approved in Germany several years ago in the treatment of diabetic neuropathy and as a dietary supplement for patients affected by diabetic retinopathy (Nebbioso et al 2013). It is covered by medical insurance (Mijnhout et al 2012).

Insulin resistance

Increase in insulin sensitivity is primarily achieved through diet, exercise, weight loss and improvement of lean:fat body mass ratio and, lastly, pharmacological intervention if glycaemic control cannot be achieved and maintained.

Several clinical trials have investigated the effect of parenterally-administered LA to diabetic subjects. A study by Jacob et al (cited in Evans & Goldfine 2000) showed insulin-mediated metabolic clearance rates (MCR) of glucose improved by at least 30% in subjects with type 2 diabetes (well controlled with diet alone or with glibenclamide) at doses of 500 mg ALA/500 mL NaCl/day infusion for 10 days. A second study by the same group (Jacob et al 1996), using a dose of 1000 mg ALA/500 mL NaCl for 10 days, reported improvement in glucose infusion rates of 47%, MCR by 55% and insulin sensitivity by 57%. No effects were observed on fasting glucose and insulin levels.

More recently, a study by Zhang et al (2011) investigated 22 obese subjects with impaired glucose tolerance (IGT) (obese-IGT), 13 of whom underwent 2-week ALA treatment, 600 mg intravenously once daily. This short-term treatment significantly improved insulin sensitivity and plasma lipid profile. More specifically, the insulin sensitivity index was impressively enhanced by 41% and significant reductions were seen for plasma levels of free fatty acids, triglyceride, total cholesterol, low-density lipoprotein cholesterol, small dense lipoprotein cholesterol, oxidised lipoprotein cholesterol, and very-low-density lipoprotein cholesterol ($P < 0.01$). At the same time, both plasma oxidative products (malondialdehyde, 8-iso-prostaglandin) and inflammatory markers (tumour necrosis factor-alpha, IL-6) were remarkably decreased ($P < 0.01$), while adiponectin was increased ($P < 0.01$) (Zhang et al 2011).

Oral ALA supplementation has also been investigated in several studies and produced inconsistent results regarding effects on insulin sensitivity (de Oliveira et al 2011, Jacob et al 1999, Yan et al 2013).

Four weeks' treatment with oral ALA was found to improve insulin sensitivity in patients with type 2 diabetes according to this early randomised, placebo-controlled study involving 74 volunteers with type 2 diabetes (Jacob et al 1999). Patients were randomised to either placebo or active treatment in various doses of 600 mg once daily, twice daily (1200 mg) or three times daily (1800 mg); however no dose effect was observed. In contrast, no change in insulin sensitivity was reported in this double-blind randomised controlled trial (RCT) of 102 patients with type 2 diabetes which compared 4 months of treatment with 600 mg/day LA ($n = 26$); 800 mg/day α-tocopherol ($n = 25$); 800 mg/day α-tocopherol + 600 mg/day LA ($n = 25$) and placebo ($n = 26$). In this study, no treatment arm resulted in a significant change to the lipid profile or insulin sensitivity of patients (de Oliveira et al 2011).

Yan et al (2013) performed a double-blinded, randomised, cross-over trial involving 103 patients without cardiovascular disease, hypertension, diabetes or any other inflammatory diseases, to investigate whether oral ALA administration lowers the risk of cardiovascular disease by decreasing the level of oxidative stress markers or improving insulin sensitivity (Homeostatic Model Assessment of Insulin Resistance [HOMA-IR] levels, a method used to assess insulin resistance and beta-cell function). Treatment with oral ALA (1200 mg/day) over 8 weeks produced no significant difference in HOMA or oxidative biomarkers between the two groups. Interestingly, at this treatment dose, ALA was associated with significantly lower body mass index (BMI), weight and waist circumference after 8 weeks. There were no significant differences in the incidence of side effects between ALA and placebo.

Overall, it appears that oral supplementation of ALA may not be as effective as intravenous intake, possibly due to the short plasma half-life and limitations on maximal plasma levels achieved with oral dose forms (Evans & Goldfine 2000, Yan et al 2013). Enteric coating, sustained-release forms, timing of administration and form of LA used are also considerations that may influence future results.

Diabetic polyneuropathy

Diabetic polyneuropathy represents a considerable morbidity of long-term uncontrolled diabetes and occurs in about one-third of people. Symptoms of pain have been reported to occur in 13–34% of patients with diabetes, with the risk of painful neuropathic symptoms considerably higher in type 2 diabetes than in type 1 diabetes (Boulton et al 2013). Persistent hyperglycaemia leading to increased synthesis of ROS in the mitochondria and subsequent oxidative damage to endothelium and neuronal cells are part of the aetiology.

The use of ALA as a treatment for diabetic neuropathies has been studied since the 1950s, with numerous clinical trials of variable quality published (McIlldulff & Rutkove 2011). In the last decade, several meta-analyses have been published, with results most consistent for injectable forms of ALA (300–600 mg daily) as a method of reducing symptoms; however the use of high oral doses (600–1200 mg/day) also appears to provide symptomatic relief and, possibly, slow disease progression.

An early meta-analysis from 2004 which analysed four RCTs concluded that 3 weeks of parenterally administered ALA (600 mg/day) provided a significant decrease in pain scores (Ziegler et al 2004). A similar conclusion was reached in a meta-analyis by McIlldulff and Rutkove (2011), which included the ALADIN, SYDNEY, ORPIL, SYDNEY II and ALADIN III trials (n = 1160; level 2b evidence). Once again, authors reported that parenterally-administered ALA was associated with a clinically meaningful improvement on symptom scores compared to placebo, at IV doses of 600 mg/day for at least 3 weeks. Oral supplementation also produced a significant improvement in symptoms and impairment at doses of 600 mg, 1200 mg and 1800 mg/day over periods ranging from 3 weeks to 2 years. Side effects were described as dose-dependent, as an oral dose of 600 mg/day over 2 years was well tolerated; however the higher dose of 1200 mg/day was associated with an increase in side effects (nausea, vomiting and vertigo). This was particularly notable in the ALADIN study, whereby rates of adverse events were 32.6% for ALA 1200 mg/day, 18.2% for ALA 600 mg/day, 13.6% for ALA 100 mg/day and 20.7% for placebo. It is important to note that some of the studies selected did not exclude diet control, hypoglycaemic medication, insulin or recent antioxidant use, or the inclusion of some type 1 diabetes patients, which may have influenced the results.

In 2012, a new meta-analysis evaluated four level 1b RCTs (n = 653) with combined results for both oral and IV effects of LA for symptomatic control of neuropathies (pain, burning, paraesthesiae, numbness). All studies reported a reduction in total symptom scores; however, equivocal results were reported in trials using oral dose forms (Mijnhout et al 2012). Another 2012 meta-analysis, this time evaluating intravenous treatment only, concluded that treatment with 300–600 mg daily for 2–4 weeks was safe, and improved both nerve conduction velocity and neuropathic symptoms (Han et al 2012).

The NATHAN study, not reported in earlier meta-analyses, was a large multicentre, double-blind, RCT that evaluated the efficacy of oral ALA (600 mg/day) taken over 4 years by volunteers with mild to moderate diabetic distal symmetric sensorimotor polyneuropathy. The primary end point was a composite score (Neuropathy Impairment Score-Lower Limbs [NIS-LL] and seven neurophysiological tests), which was not significantly different for ALA compared to placebo after 4 years. However, change from baseline was significantly better with ALA than placebo for NIS (P = 0.028), NIS-LL (P = 0.05) and NIS-LL muscular weakness subscore (P = 0.045). Importantly, more patients showed a clinically meaningful improvement and fewer showed progression of NIS (P = 0.013) and NIS-LL (P = 0.025) with ALA than with placebo. Treatment was well tolerated, although the rates of serious adverse events were higher on ALA (38.1%) than on placebo (28.0%).

The most recent meta-analysis (Xu et al 2013) considered results from a larger cohort of 1106 patients with diabetic neuropathy in a series of 15 China-based trials, which demonstrated significant efficacy of a combined therapy of LA (300–600 mg IV) and methylcobalamin (500–1000 mg IV or intramuscularly) once a day for 2–4 weeks. The combination was shown to be more effective than monotherapy of LA or methylcobalamin. However, the authors recognised methodological quality issues and the small size sample, emphasising the need for larger, well-designed, multicentre RCTs.

Diabetic nephropathy

Administration of LA reduces diabetic nephropathy in animal models through mitonchondrial protection, glomerular histological changes and decrease in ROS generation (Wang et al 2013, Yi et al 2011). Protection of β cells, decrease in cholesterol levels, decrease in albuminuria, serum urea and creatinine, and amelioration of proteinuria have also been noted in these models (Obrosova et al 2003, Wang et al 2013, Winiarska et al 2008, Yi et al 2011). A rodent model of LIAS deficiency was shown to accelerate the development of nephropathy and treatment with ALA improved kidney metabolic regulation and antioxidant capacity (Yi et al 2012a).

In a small clinical study, oral ALA administration (600 mg/day) to diabetic patients (type 1 diabetes $n = 20$; type 2 diabetes $n = 15$) over a period of 18 months has shown a significant decrease in thrombomodulin and unchanged urea/creatinine ratio compared to a control group, demonstrating a slowing of kidney damage (Morcos et al 2001). Larger and better-designed studies are needed to confirm these findings.

Diabetic retinopathy

ALA is used as a dietary supplement to slow down the progression of diabetic retinopathy. ALA prevents microvascular damage and preserves pericyte coverage of retinal capillaries in addition to improving insulin sensitivity, thereby providing a theoretical basis for its use (Nebbioso et al 2013).

IN COMBINATION

One randomised study of 32 diabetic volunteers with pre-retinopathy and good metabolic control found that oral treatment with ALA at 400 mg/day (in association with genistein and vitamins) resulted in an increase in plasma antioxidant capacity after 30 days and significant increases in the electrophysiological response, as measured by electroretinography, suggesting a protective effect on retinal cells by strengthening the plasma antioxidant barrier (Nebbioso et al 2012).

In contrast, a randomised study examining the effects of ALA on macular oedema in patients with type 2 diabetes found an oral dose of 600 mg daily taken over 2 years did not produce a significant improvement in blood levels of glycated haemoglobin, visual acuity or any reduction in retinal thickness compared to placebo (Haritoglou et al 2011). Further clinical research is required, ideally with larger doses taken in divided daily doses. Alternatively, a combination of substances with antioxidant effects, such as the one used in the study by Nebbioso et al (2012), might have more promise.

Age-related macular degeneration (AMD)

A randomised study of 62 patients (50–75 years old) with early and intermediate dry form of AMD showed that treatment with ALA produced a significant increase in serum superoxide dismutase activity, suggesting that ALA may have a possible preventive effect in the development of AMD through an antioxidant mechanism (Sun et al 2012).

Peripheral neuropathic pain (sciatic nerve pain)

A double-blind RCT compared acetyl-L-carnitine (ALC: 1180 mg/day) to ALA (600 mg/day) over a 60-day treatment period in 64 consecutive patients (mean age 61 years; range 29–85 years) with acute backache and moderate sciatica associated with a herniated disc (Memeo & Loiero 2008). Treatment with ALA produced significantly greater mean improvement than ALC from baseline for NIS-LL, Neuropathy Symptoms and Change in the Lower Limbs and Total Symptom Score scores ($P < 0.05$ for all comparisons). Additionally, a significant reduction in analgesic requirements was reported for more patients taking ALA than ALC (71.0% vs 45.5%, respectively; $P < 0.05$).

Cardiac autonomic neuropathy and platelet reactivity

Cardiac neuropathy and platelet reactivity are complications in diabetes which increase the risk of cardiovascular events (Mollo et al 2012). One in vitro study investigating the mechanisms of LA's antiplatelet activity found it significantly inhibited platelet aggregation in a dose-dependent manner and suggested the mechanisms were linked to an increase in cAMP formation, followed by thromboxane A_2 inhibition, Ca^{2+} mobilisation and protein kinase C activation (Lai et al 2010).

One small clinical study looked at platelet reactivity in type 1 diabetes patients ($n = 56$) who were randomly assigned a 600 mg oral LA dose daily or a placebo for 5 weeks and found LA significantly reduced platelet activation. Mechanisms remain unclear, as markers of oxidative stress (8-iso-prostaglandin $F_{2\alpha}$) and inflammation (C-reactive protein) were unchanged (Mollo et al 2012).

In the Deutsche Kardiale Autonome Neuropathie (DEKAN), ALA supplementation (oral ALA, 800 mg daily for 4 months) in 73 type 2 diabetic patients showed modest improvement in heart rate variability, a validated tool in the assessment of cardiac neuropathy (Coleman et al 2001).

HIV/AIDS

Supplementation with ALA (300 mg three times daily) may positively impact patients with HIV and AIDS by restoring blood total glutathione level and improving functional reactivity of lymphocytes to T-cell mitogens, according to a placebo-controlled RCT (Jariwalla et al 2008). The mean blood total glutathione level in ALA-supplemented subjects was significantly elevated and the lymphocyte proliferation response was significantly enhanced or stabilised after 6 months compared to progressive decline in the placebo group (ALA vs placebo: $P < 0.001$ with phytohaemagglutinin; $P = 0.02$ with anti-CD3 monoclonal antibody). A positive correlation was seen between blood total glutathione level and lymphocyte response to anti-CD3 stimulation. There was no change in CD4 count over 6 months.

One study showed that antioxidant supplementation (with ALA + *N*-acetyl cysteine) may have a protective role on mitochondrial function, with limited effects on the reversal of clinical lipodystrophic abnormalities in HIV-1-infected patients (Milazzo et al 2010).

Multiple sclerosis

MS is a chronic inflammatory disease of the central nervous system, characterised mainly as an autoimmune neurodegenerative disorder. Excessive oxidative stress or a loss of the antioxidant/oxidant balance may contribute to its development or be a consequence of disease (Ferreira et al 2013). Additionally, transmigration of activated immune cells across the blood–brain barrier plays a significant role in MS pathogenesis as it leads to the development of new inflammatory lesions in MS. As such, it is not surprising that ALA has been investigated as a potential treatment in this disease.

ALA has been proven to be an effective treatment in the management of MS in experimental autoimmune encephalomyelitis (EAE) rats, the accepted model for MS. In these models, ALA was shown to decrease the migration of encephalitogenic T cells to the spinal cord through the inhibition of intercellular adhesion molecule 1 and vascular cell adhesion molecule-1. In vitro, ALA has been shown to activate cAMP-activated protein kinase A (an enzyme involved in immunomodulation and neuroprotection); this pathway is believed to be central in the pathogenesis of MS (Chaudhari et al 2006, Marracci et al 2002, Morini et al 2004, Salinthone et al 2010, Schreibelt et al 2006). Oral ALA supplementation (1200 mg/day) taken by MS volunteers resulted in increased cAMP levels in peripheral blood mononuclear cells 4 hours after ingestion and, on average, cAMP levels in 20 subjects were 43% higher than baseline (Salinthone et al 2010).

A small, double-blind, placebo-controlled, dose-finding trial (n = 37) found a significant dose relationship between ALA plasma levels and inhibition of metalloprotein 9 and intracellular adhesion molecules also involved in MS pathogenesis. Effects were noted after 2 weeks at doses of oral 1200 mg/day and were significantly better than a 600 mg/day dose; however, there was a significant individual variability in ALA peak serum — potentially an effect of the administration of ALA with food in this study (Yadav et al 2005). A more recent double-blind randomised controlled study testing the effect of oral ALA (1200 mg/day) in 52 MS patients (relapsing-remitting) over 12 weeks showed a significant increase in total antioxidant capacity (P = 0.004) compared to placebo but no change in malondialdehyde levels or the activities of superoxide dismutase or glutathione peroxidase (Khalili et al 2014).

MS is a common aetiology of optic neuritis and is often a presenting sign. A small animal study (n = 14) demonstrated protection against axonal loss and degeneration with ALA (100 mg/kg) reducing $CD4^+$ and $CD11b^+$ T cell, inflammation and demyelination in an EAE mice model (Chaudhari et al 2011).

A study by Yadav et al (2010) compared the pharmacokinetics of a 1200 mg single dose of three different formulations of racemic LA in 24 MS patients (formula A: 1200 mg tablet, excipients unknown; formula B: 300 mg gelatine capsule, cellulose and ascorbyl palmitate and silica; formula C: 600 mg capsule, pine cellulose and ascorbyl acid) against three different doses in rats (20 mg, 50 mg, 100 mg). The MS patients taking the capsule formulas B and C achieved C_{max} and area under the concentration curve (AUC) equivalent to subcutaneous 50 mg/kg in mice, the therapeutic dose in experimental MS mice models. As a result, the authors suggest 1200 mg as a therapeutic dose for further clinical trials. The tablet formulation showed the lowest AUC and clearance, and widest patient intervariability. The authors recognised that the postprandial administration, chosen to decrease potential gastric side effects, rather than the manufacturer-recommended fasting intake, may have influenced the pharmacokinetics of the tablet.

A placebo-controlled study is currently underway in the United States to determine whether oral ALA 1200 mg/day can slow the progression of MS over time.

Weight loss

According to a randomised, double-blind study involving 360 obese participants (BMI ≥ 30 kg/m^2 or 27–30 kg/m^2 plus hypertension, diabetes mellitus or hypercholesterolaemia), active treatment with 1800 mg/day of racemic ALA over 20 weeks led to significantly more weight loss than placebo. Weight loss was significantly greater with 1800 mg/day of ALA compared to placebo from week 4. Additionally, there was a significant difference between the groups with regard to percentage of subjects who achieved a ≥5% reduction in baseline body weight (21.6% vs 10.0%, $P < 0.01$). No significant changes were observed in triglyceride concentrations and triglyceride/high-density lipoprotein cholesterol ratios. The significant difference in weight loss was also reported for the group with BMI 27–30 kg/m^2 plus additional risk factors. Subjects with diabetes receiving 1800 mg/day ALA showed a mean 0.38% reduction from baseline in haemoglobin A_{1C} level ($P < 0.05$) but there was no change in blood pressure or fasting plasma glucose and cholesterol concentrations. Mild and transient urticaria and itching were experienced in ALA groups; however, overall incidence of side effects was similar to the placebo group (Koh et al 2011).

Oral ALA (1200 mg/day) was associated with significantly lower BMI, weight and waist circumference after 8 weeks in another double-blinded, randomised trial, conducted by Yan et al (2013), involving 103 patients without cardiovascular disease, hypertension, diabetes or any other inflammatory disease. There were no significant differences in incidence of side effects between ALA treatment and placebo.

Weight loss in schizophrenia

A case series of a 12-week ALA trial in 5 schizophrenia patients treated with atypical antipsychotic drugs found that treatment resulted in a mean weight loss of 3.16 kg ($P = 0.043$) and, on average, BMI showed a significant reduction ($P = 0.028$) over the 12 weeks (Kim et al 2008). No change was seen to the Brief Psychiatric Rating Scale and the Montgomery-Asberg Depression Rating Scale.

A small open study was more recently published, whereby ALA (1200 mg/day) taken for 10 weeks by 12 non-diabetic schizophrenic patients produced a significant weight loss during the intervention (–2.2 kg ± 2.5 kg). Treatment with ALA was well tolerated and particularly effective for individuals taking strongly antihistaminic antipsychotics (–2.9 kg ± 2.6 kg vs –0.5 kg ± 1.0 kg) (Ratliff et al 2013).

Migraine prophylaxis

An RCT using ALA in migraine prophylaxis was steered by the Belgian Headache Society and included five Belgian centres, which recruited 54 migraineurs (43 migraine without aura, 11 with aura; mean age 38 ± 8 years; 7 males) (Magis et al 2007). ALA (600 mg/day) was taken for 3 months and was found to reduce migraine attack frequency compared to placebo ($P = 0.06$). Within-group analyses showed a significant reduction of attack frequency ($P = 0.005$), headache days ($P = 0.009$) and headache severity ($P = 0.03$) in patients treated with ALA whereas these outcome measures remained unchanged in the placebo group. The treatment was well tolerated with no adverse effects reported.

Before any firm conclusion can be drawn, a larger clinical trial is now necessary.

OTHER USES

Alzheimer's disease (AD)

ALA, with its proven antioxidant, anti-inflammatory, neuroprotective, metal-chelating and glycaemic regulation activities, is showing potential in the treatment of AD and worthy of further investigation.

AD is characterised by neurofibrillary tangles and amyloid plaques leading to neuronal loss. Its pathophysiology is thought to involve progressive cholinergic deficit, a chronic inflammatory oxidative process leading to mitochondrial dysfunction. Recent preliminary studies are showing insulin abnormality and resistance in AD patients, including impaired cerebral glucose metabolism, leading to neuron toxicity (Maczureck et al 2008).

The first indication that ALA may be beneficial in AD and related dementias came from a serendipitous case of a 74-year-old woman with signs of cognitive impairment and diabetic polyneuropathy treated with an anticholinesterase inhibitor drug and 600 mg LA daily for her neuropathy. Since 1997, when treatment first began, several tests have been performed which show no substantial decline in cognitive function and neurological tests show unusually slow progress of her cognitive impairment (Maczureck et al 2008).

Since then, studies in rodents have shown a protective effect of cognitive deficits (Wang & Chen 2007) and chronic feeding of ALA in conjunction with *N*-acetyl cysteine showed improvement in cognition in aged subjects (Farr et al 2003).

A small open pilot trial (*n* = 9) of patients with AD were given 600 mg oral ALA daily, 30 minutes before breakfast in conjunction with standard treatment of acetylcholinesterase inhibitors over a period of 371 days. The treatment provided stabilisation in cognition compared to pretreatment decline in cognition. The size of this pilot study increased to 48 patients for up to 48 months, providing similar results. The need for well-designed RCTs is warranted to confirm these findings (Maczureck et al 2008).

Polycystic ovary syndrome (PCOS)

Although generally associated with high BMI, about 20% of women presenting with PCOS are of normal weight. Some studies have suggested that insulin resistance in PCOS is a result of genetic predisposition to a defective insulin-signalling pathway (and resulting compensatory hyperinsulinaemia), rather than dependent on BMI. In normoinsulaemic lean PCOS women, the use of insulin-reducing and sensitising drugs was shown to improve free testosterone and androstenedione serum values, suggesting insulin-related hyperandrogenism (Baptiste et al 2010); improving this resistance has been recognised as essential to improve metabolic and reproductive outcomes (Marshall & Dunaif 2012).

A pilot trial administering controlled-release lipoic acid 600 mg twice daily to 6 non-obese PCOS patients with no other comorbidity, including insulin resistance, and ingesting an isocaloric diet showed improvement in their insulin sensitivity, a decrease in their triglyceride and increase in low-density lipoprotein molecular size (Masharani et al 2010).

Hepatoprotection

A small trial (*n* = 24) of patients undergoing liver resection showed decreased serum AST and ALT (used in combination in the diagnosis of liver damage) and histomorphological damage to hepatocytes when 600 mg of IV ALA was administered 15 minutes before resection compared to the group administered IV NaCl (Dünschede et al 2006).

ALA (300 mg/day) has been investigated in alcoholic liver disease in a 6-month RCT (*n* = 40), which found that only those participants abstaining from alcohol showed significant improvement in AST and gamma-glutamyl transaminase (which is raised in chronic alcohol toxicity) values and histological biopsy with use (Marshall et al 1982). These results are problematic as the number of abstainers was not even in both groups, and the dose used was low. Hepatoprotective effects have been shown in animal studies in recent studies (Kaya-Dagistanli et al 2013, Foo et al 2011).

Hypertension

A cross-over double-blind study tested whether adding oral ALA to the angiotensin-converting enzyme inhibitor quinapril would potentiate regulation of blood pressure, endothelial function and proteinuria in obese diabetic patients with stage 1 hypertension. Patients were randomised to receive either quinapril (40 mg/day) alone or quinapril (40 mg/day) and LA (600 mg/day) for 6 weeks. Biomarkers of obesity and endothelial-dependent flow-mediated dilation were improved in the group of combination quinapril and ALA (Khan et al 2010). Another study noted a reduction in blood pressure, proteinuria and endothelial function (Rahman et al 2012).

Kwashiorkor

A small longitudinal clinical pilot study comparing the standard World Health Organization treatment protocol to one of three groups supplemented with reduced glutathione, LA or *N*-acetyl cysteine to a healthy control group showed that reduced glutathione and LA both positively increased recovery and survival, and correlated with erythrocyte gluthatione concentration — a predictive value of survival (Becker et al 2005).

Burning-mouth syndrome

Three small clinical trials showed significant results in decreasing symptoms of burning-mouth syndrome with dosages of 600 mg daily for 1–2 months. However, the placebo groups in these studies also reported high levels, although non-significant, of symptomatic improvements, especially in the double-blind trial, compared to the open-label trials (Zakrzewska et al 2009); Crow and Gonzalez (2013) report three subsequent studies with similar dosage in which LA does not yield statistical significance over placebo, possibly due to the large variation in pain response in both groups.

Carpal tunnel syndrome — in combination

A study compared the efficacy of LA (600 mg/day) in combination with γ-linolenic acid 360 mg/day to a vitamin B complex (B_6 150 mg; B1 100 mg; B_{12} 500 mcg/1 daily) for 90 days in 112 subjects with moderate to severe carpal tunnel syndrome. The LA/γ-linolenic group scored significant improvement in symptoms, confirmed by electromyography, compared to the B vitamin group (Di Geronimo et al 2009).

Erectile dysfunction

With the classical causes of erectile dysfunction including diabetes mellitus, hypertension, obesity, hyperlipidaemia and cardiovascular conditions, and the pathophysiological mechanisms understood to involve oxidative stress, especially due to advanced glycosylated end products, and alteration of vascular and endothelial function through dysregulation of NO synthase (Shamloul & Ghanem 2012), a theoretical basis exists for the use of LA for this condition.

An animal study also demonstrated that the neurectomy associated with prostatectomy resulted in a loss of NO synthase-containing nerve fibres and in significant oxidative stress; treatment with LA (65 mg/kg/day IP) showed improvement in cavernous tissue regeneration (Alan et al 2010). No clinical trials are available at this time.

Wound healing

Human trials show that hyperbaric oxygen therapy increases IL-6 and ROS production. In a small double-blind randomised study, supplementation with LA (600 mg/day) in patients undergoing hyperbaric oxygen therapy for various conditions, with the inclusion criterion of leg ulcers older than 30 days, showed an

80% reduction or remission of the lesions at 40 days of treatment compared to the placebo group (Alleva et al 2005).

Glaucoma

Glaucoma is a progressive neurodegenerative condition in which the retinal ganglia and optic nerve are damaged due to increased intraocular pressure, leading to loss of vision. ALA has demonstrated a protective effect on retinal neurons in vitro and in animal models (Koriyama et al 2013). A small Russian study reported an improvement in visual function after 4 weeks of treatment with 150 mg/day of ALA in patients with glaucoma (Cotlier & Weinreb 2008).

Photoageing of skin

The low molecular weight of ALA, combined with its solubility characteristics, suggests the possibility of LA being absorbed by the skin and having pharmacological activities. Swift penetration through the epidermis has been demonstrated in a hairless mouse model and, after 4 hours, distribution to the dermis and subcutaneous tissue underneath. This was further explored in a 12-week RCT (n = 33) with a 5% ALA cream, which was applied twice daily to half the face and placebo cream to the other. Self-assessment, clinician assessment, standardised photography and laser profilometry before and after the period of treatment were used to evaluate effects. The ALA-enriched cream significantly improved profilometry in photoageing of facial skin.

According to photographic evaluations, ALA cream was shown to improve the appearance of fine lines ($P < 0.031$), decrease pigmentation ($P < 0.007$), decrease under-eye bags and puffiness ($P < 0.09$) and decrease pore size ($P < 0.08$). The clinical evaluation also reported a significant improvement in fine lines ($P = 0.01$). Additionally, self-assessment showed that 78% of subjects claimed the active side showed improvement, compared to 31% who claimed the placebo treatment was better ($P < 0.002$).

Amanita spp. mushroom poisoning

The use of thioctic acid in *Amanita* spp. has been a treatment of choice in Europe since the 1960s, often alongside silymarin or silibin. Intravenous doses of 300 mg/24 h with 10% glucose in saline for up to 6 days have been used (Becker et al 1976). However, usage of ALA remains controversial, with some reports of inefficacy (Enjalbert et al 2002, Tong et al 2007), mostly because of the inability to carry out blinded RCTs in mushroom poisoning ethically (Klein et al 1989). ALA is not currently used as an *Amanita* spp. antidote in Australia (Roberts et al 2013).

DOSAGE RANGE

As LA absorption decreases with food intake, it is recommended that LA be ingested 30–60 minutes before meals or 120 minutes after; however, side effects are more likely on an empty stomach (Gleiter et al 1996, McIlduff & Rutkove 2011, Shay et al 2009).

According to clinical studies, oral doses for ALA are:

- Diabetes and peripheral neuropathies: 600–1200 mg/day.
- Cardiac autonomic neuropathy in type 2 diabetes patients: 800 mg/day.
- MS: 1200 mg/day.
- AD: 600 mg/day in conjunction with *N*-acetyl cysteine.
- PCOS: 600 mg twice daily.
- Hypertension: 600 mg/day.
- Burning-mouth syndrome: 200–600 mg/day — efficacy uncertain.

- Carpal tunnel syndrome: 600 mg/day.
- Wound healing: 300 mg twice daily.
- Weight loss: 1800 mg/day.
- Migraine prevention: 600 mg/day.
- Sciatic nerve pain: 600 mg/day.
- Glaucoma: 150 mg/day.

Safety and dosage have not been studied in children.

TOXICITY

The maximum tolerated dose of ALA in human subjects has not been well defined; however, based on the observation that the oral lethal dose (LD_{50}) for rats and mice is 1130 and 502 mg/kg, respectively, it is assumed that human beings can tolerate several grams of ALA daily. The IP LD_{50} is 200 and 160 mg/kg for rats and mice, respectively (Biewenga et al 1997).

ADVERSE REACTIONS

Clinical trials testing oral ALA, at concentrations as high as 1800 mg/day for 6 months and as high as 1200 mg/day for 2 years, have not identified any serious adverse effects. Similarly, a clinical trial of obese volunteers found a daily dose of 1200 mg/day or 1800 mg/day over 20 weeks was well tolerated, with the most common side effects reported as itchiness and urticaria, although the overall incidence of side effects was no different from the placebo group (Koh et al 2011).

Overall, the most common side effects of oral supplementation tend to appear when used at doses of 1200 mg and above and include nausea, vomiting, rashes, tingling and itching sensations and headaches.

Topically, ALA has been used safely for up to 12 weeks at 5% concentration. Side effects can include mild rash and local irritation, stinging and burning sensations.

Intravenously, ALA has been used at doses of 600 mg and 1200 mg daily, with side effects reported at 1200 mg. Local irritations have been reported at the injection site.

A case was reported of a 63-year-old man with multiple pathologies and taking multiple medications who was administrated 600 mg/day of LA to treat diabetic neuropathy. He developed low-grade fever, nausea and fatigue and elevated serum transaminase. Discontinuation resulted in elimination of symptoms and return to normal of liver enzymes. A second attempt at treatment led to the return of symptoms and abnormal transaminase. The report investigated other potential aetiologies of liver injuries. While the authors recognise the case as unique and ALA as generally safe, they recommended liver enzyme monitoring in conjunction with ALA treatment (Ridruejo et al 2011). However the case report does not examine potential LA contamination or a drug–LA interaction as a potential aetiology for the liver enzyme abnormalities.

SIGNIFICANT INTERACTIONS

When controlled studies are not available, interactions are based on evidence of pharmacological activity, case reports and other evidence and are largely theoretical.

Copper

ALA is a metal chelator and binds to copper in vivo — separate doses by 3 h.

Manganese

ALA is a metal chelator and binds to manganese in vivo — separate doses by 3 h.

Zinc

ALA is a metal chelator and binds to zinc in vivo — separate doses by 3 h.

Hypoglycaemic agents

Theoretically, concomitant use may affect glucose control and require medication dosage changes — observe.

Vitamin E, vitamin C, coenzyme Q10 and glutathione

ALA reconstitutes these antioxidants from their oxidised form to their unoxidised form as part of the antioxidant cycle in humans — beneficial interaction.

Warfarin

ALA reduces platelet reactivity in vitro (Lai et al 2010). It is uncertain whether the effect is clinically significant — observe patients taking these agents together.

Levothyroxine

Uncertain interaction exists. When co-administered, ALA may suppress the conversion of thyroxine to triiodothyronine — decrease total cholesterol, triglycerides, albumin and total protein (Segermann et al 1991).

CONTRAINDICATIONS AND PRECAUTIONS

Age is believed to affect bioavailability markedly, with older age associated with reduced bioavailability of oral supplements (Keith et al 2012).

Insulin autoimmune syndrome is a condition that develops in individuals not previously injected with pharmacological insulin; it appears to be drug-induced in about 50% of cases, especially drugs from the sulfhydryl group. In East Asians, especially Japanese, and Native Americans, there is a high expression of a human leucocyte antigen genotype that confers susceptibility to this syndrome. A number of cases have been reported in Japan after intake of ALA. Anti-insulin antibody titres reduce after ALA discontinuation (Ishida et al 2007). The case of an Italian Caucasian woman was also reported in 2011 (Bresciani et al 2011).

ALA supplementation in pigeons and mice has caused fatal toxicity in thiamine-deficient subjects (20 mg/kg, a high dose). A theoretical basis exists for caution in prescribing LA to alcoholics, Wernicke–Korsakoff patients and other thiamine-depleting conditions. ALA does not, however, deplete thiamine in healthy or deficient individuals (Gal & Razevska 1960).

PREGNANCY USE

A study of diabetic rats injected intraperitoneally with ALA improved survival of their embryos, showing that is likely that ALA can cross the placenta. It also showed a decreased rate of neural tube defects (Al Ghafli et al 2004).

While ALA appears essential to fetal rat formation as an essential mitochondrial enzyme (Yi & Maeda 2005), no clinical trials of supplementation exist in human pregnancy or lactation.

Practice points/Patient counselling

- ALA is endogenously synthesised in the human body and is essential for cellular metabolism. It acts as an antioxidant, regenerates vitamins C and E and glutathione in the body, chelates metal ions and repairs oxidised proteins.
- ALA can be safely used in supplementary form at doses under 1200 mg for up to 2 years for a wide range of diseases.
- Meta-analysis supports its use in type 2 diabetes and diabetic neuropathy.
- There is preliminary clinical evidence suggesting a role in PCOS, MS, AD, hypertension, carpal tunnel syndrome, wound healing and glaucoma, although further research is required. Effects are uncertain in burning-mouth syndrome.
- Supplemental forms are often manufactured in a racemic form, but some trials show a greater efficacy with L-enantiomer.

PATIENTS' FAQs

What will this nutrient do for me?

LA supplementation is used in type 2 diabetes, diabetic neuropathy, hypertension, carpal tunnel syndrome, PCOS, MS and AD. ALA confers antioxidant and neuroprotective effects as well as improving glycaemia.

When will it start to work?

It depends on the dose and indication for use.

Are there any safety issues?

LA should be used with caution in people of East Asian and Native American origin; thiamine deficiency and alcoholics; patients with cancer, high homocysteine, liver impairment, thyroid disorders; people treated for diabetes or glycaemic impairment. There are also several drug interactions that should be considered before use.

REFERENCES

Abdel-Zaher A et al. The potential protective role of alpha-lipoic acid against acetaminophen-induced hepatic and renal damage. Toxicology 243 (2008): 261–270.

Abdel-Zaher A et al. Alpha-lipoic acid protect against potassium cyanide-induced seizures and mortality. Experimental and Toxicologic Pathology 23 (2011): 161–165.

Abdin A, Sarhan N. Intervention of mitonchondrial dysfunction-oxidative stress-dependent apoptosis as a possible neuroprotective mechanism od α-lipoic acid against rotenone induce parkinsonism and L-dopa toxicity. Neuroscience research 71 (2011): 387–395.

Alan C et al. Biochemical changes in cavernosal tissue caused by single sided cavernosal nerve resection and the effect of alpha-lipoic acid on these changes. Actas Urológicas Españolas 34.10 (2010): 874–881.

Alleva R et al. α-lipoic acide supplementation inhibits oxidative damage, accelerating chronic wound healing in patients undergoing hyperbaric oxygen therapy. Biochem Biophys Res Commun 333 (2005): 404–410.

Al Ghafli MH et al. Effect of alpha-lipoic acid supplementation on maternal diabetes-induced growth retardation and congenital abnormality in rat fetuses. Mol Cell Biochem 261.1/2 (2004): 123–35.

Arivazhagan P. et al. Effect of DL-alpha-lipoic acid on the status of lipid peroxidation and anti-oxidant enzymes in various brain regions of aged rats. Exp Gerontology 37.6 (2002): 803–11.

Astiz M et al. The oxidative damage and inflammation casued by pesticides are reverted in rat brains. Neurochemistry International 61 (2012): 1231–1242.

Baptiste CG et al. Insulin and hyperandrogenism in women with polycystic ovarian syndrome. The Journal of Steroid Biochemistry and Molecular Biology 122.1–3 (2010): 42–52.

Bast A, Haenen GR. Lipoic acid: a multifunctional antioxidant. BioFactors 17.1–4 (2008): 207–213.

Becker CE et al. Diagnosis and treatment of *Amanita phalloides*-type mushroom poisoning — Use of thioctic acid. West J Med 125 (1976): 100–109.

Becker K et al. Effects of antioxidants on glutathione levels and clinical recovery from the malnutrition syndrome kwashiorkor-a pilot study. Redox Rep 10.4 (2005): 215–26.

Berkson BM et al. Revisiting the ALA/N (α-lipoic acid/ low dose naltrexone) protocol for people with metastatic and non-metastatic pancreatic cancer: a report of 3 new cases. Integrative Cancer Therapies 8.4 (2009): 416–422.

Biewenga GP et al. The pharmacology of the antioxidant lipoic acid. Gen Pharmac. 29.3 (1997): 315–331.

Booker SJ. Uncovering the pathway of lipoic acid biosynthesis. Chemistry and Biology 11 (2004): 10–12.

Boulton, A.J., et al. 2013. Whither pathogenetic treatments for diabetic polyneuropathy? Diabetes Metab Res. Rev., 29, (5) 327–333.

Breithaupt-Grogler K et al. Dose-proportionality of oral thioctic acid — coincidence of assessments via pooled plasma and individual data. Eur J Pharm Sci 8 (1999):57–65.

Bresciani E et al. Insulin autoimmune syndrome induced by α-lipoic acid in a Caucasian woman: case report. Diabetes Care 34.9 (2011): e146.

Cagini C et al. Study of alpha-lipoic acid penetrationin the human aqueous after topical administration. Clin Experiment Opthalmol 38.6 (2010): 572–576.

Carlson DA et al. The plasma pharmacokinetics of R-(+)-lipoic acid deministered as sodium R-(+) lipoate to healthy human subjects. Alter Med Rev 12 (2007) 343–51.

Caylak E et al. Antioxidant effect of methionine, α-lipoic acid, *N*-acetylcysteine and homocysteine on lead-induced oxidative stress to erythrocytes in rats. Experimental and toxicologic pharmacology 60 (2008): 208–294.

Chaudhari P et al. Lipoic aicd inhibits expression of ICAM-1 and VCAM-1 by CNS endothelial cells and T cells migration into the spinal cordin experiemental autoimmune encephalomyelitis. Journal of Neuroimmunology 175 (2006): 87–96.

Chaudhari P et al. Lipoic acid decreases inflammation and confers neuroprotection in experimental autoimmune optic neuritis. J Neuroimmunology 233 (2011): 90–96.

Chen Y et al. Alpha-lipoic acid alters post-translational modificationand protects the chaperone activity of lens alpha-crystallin in naphthaline-induced cataract. Curr Eye Res 35.7 (2010): 620–630.

Cheng et al. Protection against arsenic trioxide-induced autophagic cell death in U118 human gliama cells by use of lipoic acid. Food and chemical toxicology 45 (2007): 1027–1038.

Chng HT et al. Distribution study of orally administrated lipoic acid in rat brain tissues. Brain research 1251 (2009): 80–86.

Cho KJ et al. Alpha-lipoic acid decreases thiol reactivity of the insulin receptor and protein tyrosine phosphatase 1B in 3T3-L1 adipocytes. Biochem Pharmacol 66 (2003): 849–858.

Coleman MD et al. The therapeutic use of lipoic acid in diabetes: a current perspective. Environ Toxicol Pharmacol 10 (2001): 167–172.

Connell BJ et al. Lipoic acid protects against reperfusion injury in the early stages of cerebral ischemia. Brain Res 1375 (2011): 128–136.

Cotlier E, Weinreb R. The potential value of natural antioxidative treatment in glaucoma. Survey of Ophthalmology 53.5 (2008): 479–505.

Crow HC, Gonzalez Y. Burning mouth syndrome. Oral Maxillofacial Surg Clin N Am. 25 (2013): 67–76.

Dadhania VP et al. Intervention of alpha-lipoic acidameliorates methotrexate-induced oxidative stress and genotoxicity; a study in rat intestine. Chemico-Biological Interactions 183.1 (2010): 85–97.

Davis JG et al. Dietary supplements reduce the caractogenic potential of proton and HZE — particle radiation in rats. Radiat Res (2010) 173(3): 353–361.

Deng C et al. α-lipoic acid reduces infarct size and preserve cardiac functions in rat myocardial ischemia/reperfusion injury through activation of PI3K/Akt/Nrf2 pathway. PLoSone 8.3 (2013): e58371.

de Oliveira, A.M., et al. 2011. The effects of lipoic acid and α-tocopherol supplementation on the lipid profile and insulin sensitivity of patients with type 2 diabetes mellitus: A randomized, double-blind, placebo-controlled trial. *Diabetes Research and Clinical Practice*, 92, (2) 253–260.

Desouky OS et al. Impact evaluation of α-lipoic acid in gamma-irradiated erythrocytes. Radiation physics and chemistry 80(2011): 446–452.

Di Geronimo G et al. Treatment of Tunnel carpal syndrome with alpha-lipoic acid. European Review for Medical and Pharcological Sciences 13 (2009): 133–139.

Dünschede F et al. Reduction of ischemia reperfusion injury after liver resection and hepatic inflow occlusion by alpha-lipoic acid in humans. World J Gastroenterol 12.42 (2006): 6812–7.

Enjalbert F et al. Treatment of amatoxin poisoning: 20 retrospective analyis. J Toxicol Clin Toxicol 40.6 (2002): 715–57.

Estrada et al. Stimulation of glucose uptake by the natural enzyme alpha-lipoic acid/thioctic acid: participation of elements of the insulin signaling pathway. Diabetes 45 (1996): 1798–804.

Evans JL Goldfine ID. α-lipoic acid: A multifunctional antioxidant that improve insulin sensitivity in patient with type 2 diabetes. Diabetes Technology and Research 2.3 (2000): 401–413.

Farr SA et al. The antioxidants α-lipoic acid and N-acetylcysteine reverse memory impairement and brain oxidative stress in aged SAMP8 mice. Journal of Neurochemistry 84 (2003): 1173–1183.

Ferreira, B., et al. 2013. Glutathione in multiple sclerosis. Br J Biomed. Sci., 70, (2) 75–79.

Foo NP et al. α-lipoic acid inhibits liver fibrosis through the attenuation of ROS-triggered signaling in hepatic stellate cells activated by PDGF and TGF-β. Toxicology 182.1/2 (2011): 39–46.

Gal E, Razevska DE. Studies on the in-vivo metabolism of lipoic acid. The fate of DL lipoic acid S- in normal and thiamine deficient rats. Archives of Biochemistry and Biophysics 89 (1960): 253–261.

Gleiter CH et al. Influence of food on the bioavailability of thioctic acid eniantomers. Eu J Clin Pharmacol. 50 (1996): 513–514.

Goraca A et al. Lipoic acid — biological activity and therapeutic potential. Pharmacological Report 63 (2011): 849–858.

Gurer et al. Antioxidant effects of α-lipoic acid in lead toxicity. Free radical toxicity and medicine 27.1/2 (1999): 75–81.

Han D et al. Lipic acid increases de novo synthesis of glutathione by improving cytine utilazation. Biofactors. 6 (1997): 321–38.

Han T et al. A systematic reiew and meta analysis of α-lipoic acid in the treatment of diabetic neuropathy. Eur J Endocrinil 167.4 (2012): 465–71.

Haritoglou, C., et al. 2011. Alpha-lipoic acid for the prevention of diabetic macular edema. Ophthalmologica, 226, (3) 127–137.
Harrison EH, McCormick DB. The metabolism of dl-(1,6–14C) lipoic acid in the rat. Arch Biochem Biophys 160 (1974): 514–522.
Heinisch BB et al. Alpha-lipoic acid improves vascular endothelial functions in patients with type 2 diabetes: a placebo-controlled randomized trial. Eur J Clin Invest 40.2 (2010): 148–54.
Heitzer T et al. Beneficial effecs of alpha-lipoic acid and ascorbic acid on endothelium-dependent, nitric oxide-mediated vasodialtion in diabetic patients: relation to parameters of oxidative stress. Free Radic Bio Med 31 (2001): 53–61.
Henriksen et al. Stimulation by alpha-lipoic acid of glucose transport activity in skeletal muscle of lean and obese Zucker rats. Life sci 61 (1997): 805–12.
Ishida Y et al. α-lipoic acid and insulin autoimmune syndrome. Diabetes care. 30.9 (2007): 2240–2241.
Jacob S et al. Improvement of insulin-stimulated glucose-disposal in type 2 diabetes after repeated parenteral administration of thioctic acid. Experimental and Clinical Endocrinology and Diabetes. 104 (1996): 284–288.
Jacob S et al. Oral adminstration of rac-α-lipoic acid modulates insulin sensitivity in patients with type-2 diabetes mellitus: a placebo-controlled pilot trial. Free radical Biology and Medicine 27.3/4 (1999): 309–314.
Jariwalla, R.J., et al. 2008. Restoration of blood total glutathione status and lymphocyte function following alpha-lipoic acid supplementation in patients with HIV infection. J Altern. Complement Med, 14, (2) 139–146.
Jia Z et al. Alpha-lipoic acid potently inhibits peroxynitrite-mediated DNA strand breakage and hydroxyl radical formation: implications for the neuroprotective effects of alpha-lipoic acid. Mol cell Biochem 323.2 (2009): 131–138.
Jones W et al. Uptake, recycling and antioxidant action of α-lipoic acid in endothelial cells. Free radical medicine and biology 33.1 (2002): 83–93.
Kaya-Dagistanli F et al. The effects of alpha lipoic acid on liver cell damages and apoptosis induced by polyunsaturated fatty acids. Food and Chemical Toxicology 53 (2013): 84–93.
Keith et al. Age and gender dependant bioavailability of R- and R/S-α-lipoic acid: a pilot study. Pharmacological Research 66 (2012): 199–206.
Khalili M et al. Effect of lipoic acid consumption on oxidative stress among multiple sclerosis patients: A randomized controlled clinical trial. Nutr. Neurosci 17 (1) 2014: 16–20.
Khamaisi M et al. Lipoic acid reduces glycemia and increases GLUT4 content in streptozotocin-diabetic rats. Metabolism 47.6 (1997): 763–768.
Khan BV et al. Quinapril and lipoic acid improve endothelial function and reduce markers of inflammation: Results of Quinapril and lipoic acid in the metabolic syndrome (QUALITY) study. Journal of the American College of Cardiology. 55.10 (2010): A54-E510.
Kim, E., et al. 2008. A preliminary investigation of alpha-lipoic acid treatment of antipsychotic drug-induced weight gain in patients with schizophrenia. J Clin. Psychopharmacol., 28, (2) 138–146.
Klein AS et al. *Amanita* poisoning: Treatment and the role of transplantation. The American Journal of Medicine 86 (1989): 187–193.
Koh EH et al. Effect of alpha-lipoic acid on body weight in obese subjects. The American Journal of Medicine 124.1 (2011): 85.e1–85.e8.
Kojima M et al. Efficacy of alpha-lipoic acid against diabetic cataract in rats. Jpn J Ophthalmol 51.1 (2007): 10–13.
Koriyama Y et al. Protective effect of lipoic acid against oxidative stress is mediated by Keap1/Nrf2 dependant heme oxigenase-1 induction in the RGC-5 cell line. Brain Research 1499 (2013): 145–157.
Lai YS et al. Antiplatelet activity of alpha-lipoic acid. J Agric Food Chem 58.15 (2010): 8596–608.
Lee WR et al. Alpha-lipoic acid attenuates athesclerotic lesions and inhibits proliferation of vascular smooth muscles through targeting the Ras/MEK/ERK signaling pathway. Mol Biol Rep 39.6 (2012): 6857–66.
Lodge JK, Packer L. Natural sources of lipoic acid in plant and animal tissues. in Packer L et al (eds) Antioxidant food supplements in human health. San Diego, CA: Academic Press (1999): 121–134.
Lykkesfeldt J et al. Age-associated decline in ascorbic acid concentration, recycling, and biosynthesis in rat hepatocytes — reversal with (R)-alpha-lipoic acid supplementation. Faseb J. 13.2 (1999): 411–418.
Maczureck A et al. Lipoic acid as an anti-inflammatory and neuroprotective treatment for Alzheimer's disease. Advanced Drug Delivery Review 60 (2008): 1463–1470.
Magis, D., et al. 2007. A randomized double-blind placebo-controlled trial of thioctic acid in migraine prophylaxis. Headache, 47, (1) 52–57.
Manda K et al. Memory impairment, oxidative stress and apoptosis induced by space radiation: ameliorative potential of α-lipoic acid. Behavioural Brain Research 187.2 (2008): 387–395.
Marracci GH et al. α lipoic acid inhibits T cell migration in the spinal cord and suppresses and treats experimental autoimmune encephalomyelitis. J Neuroimmunol. 131 (2002): 104–114.
Marracci GH et al. Lipoic acid downmodulates CD4 from human T lymphocytes by dissociation of p56lck. Biochemical and Biophysical Research Communications 344 (2006): 963–971.
Marshall AW et al. Treatment of liver-related disease with thioctic acid: a six-month randomized controlled trial. Gut 23.12 (1982): 1088–1093.
Marshall JC, Dunaif A. All women with PCOS should be treated for insulin resistance. Fertil Steril 97.1 (2012): 18–22.
Masharani U et al. Effects of controlled-release alpha lipoic acid in lean, non-diabetic patients with polycystic ovary syndrome. J diabetis Sci Technol 4.2 (2010) 359–364.
Mayr J et al. Lipoic acid synthase deficiency causes neonatal-onset epilepsy, defective mitochondrial energy metabolism, and glycine elevation. Am J Hum Genet 89.6 (2011): 792–797.
McIlldufF CE Rutkove SB Critical appraisal of the use of alpha lipoic acid (thioctic acid) in the treatment of symptomatic diabetic neuropathy. Therapeutics and clinical risk management 7 (2011): 377–385.
Melli G et al. Alpha-lipoic acid prevents mitochondrial damage and neurotoxicity in experimental chemotherapy neuropathy. Exp Neurol 214.2 (2009): 276–284.

Memeo, A. & Loiero, M. 2008. Thioctic acid and acetyl-L-carnitine in the treatment of sciatic pain caused by a herniated disc: a randomized, double-blind, comparative study. Clin. Drug Investig., 28, (8) 495–500.
Michels AJ et al. Age-related decline of sodium-dependant ascorbic acid transport in isolated rat hepatocytes. Arch Biochem Biophys 410 (2003): 112–120.
Mijnhout GS et al. Alpha-lipoic acid for symptomatic peripheral neuropathy in patients with diabetes : a meta-analysis of randomized controlled trials. International Journal of Endocrinology 2012 (2012) 456279.
Milazzo, L., et al. 2010. Effect of antioxidants on mitochondrial function in HIV-1-related lipoatrophy: a pilot study. AIDS Res. Hum. Retroviruses, 26, (11) 1207–1214.
Moini H et al. Antioxidant and proxidant activity of α-lipoic acid and dihydrolipoic acid. Toxicology and applied pharmacology 182 (2002a): 84–90.
Moini H et al. R-alpha lipoic acid action on cell redox status, the insulin receptor, and glucose uptake in 3T3-L1 adipocytes. Arch Biochem Biophys 397 (2002b): 384–391.
Mollo R et al. Effect of alpha-lipoic acid on platelet reactivity in type I diabetic patients. Diabetes Care 35.2 (2012): 196–197.
Morcos M et al. Effect of α-lipoic acid on the progression of endothelial cell damage and albuminuria in patients with diabetes mellitus: an exploratory study. Diabetic Research and Clinical Practice. 52.3 (2001): 175–183.
Morini M et al. Alpha lipoic acid is effective in prevention and treatment of experimental autoimmune encephalomyelitis. J. Neuroimmunology. 148.1/2 (2004): 146–153.
Nebbioso M et al. Oxidative stress in preretinopathic diabetes subjects and antioxidants. Diabetic Technology and Therapeutics. 14–3 (2012): 1–7.
Nebbioso, M., et al. 2013. Lipoic acid in animal models and clinical use in diabetic retinopathy. Expert. Opin. Pharmacother 14–13: 1829–38.
Ning-Ping F et al. α-lipoic acid inhibits liver fibrosis through the attenuation of ROS- triggered signaling in hepatic stellate cells activated by PDGF and TGF-β. Toxicology 182.1/2 (2011): 39–46.
Obrosova IG et al. Early oxidative stress in the diabetic kidney effect of DL-α-lipoic acid. Free Radical Biology and Medicine 34.2 (2003): 186–195.
Ong SLH et al. The effect of alpha lipoic acid on mitondrial superoxide and glucocorticoid-induced hypertension. Oxidative medicine and cellular longevity 2013 (2013): 517045.
Packer L, Cadenas E. Lipoic acid metabolism and redox regulation of transcription and cell signaling. J Clin Biochem Nutr. 48.1 (2010): 26–32.
Padmalayam E et al. Lipoic acid synthase (LASY): a novel role in inflammation, mitochondrial function and insulin resistance. Diabetes 58.3 (2009): 600–608.
Pande M Flora SJS. Lead induced oxidative damage and its response of combined administration of α-lipoic acid and succimers in rats. Toxicology 177 (2002): 187–196.
Patel M, Packer L. "Discovery and molecular structure" in Packer L, Cadenas E (eds) Lipoic acid: Energy production, antioxidant activity and health effects. CRC Press. Boca Raton, Florida (2008): 3–11.
Perera J et al. Neuroprotective effects of alpha lipoic acid on haloperidol-induced oxidative stress in the rat brain. Cell Biosci 1 (2011): 12.
Queiroz, T.M., et al. 2012. Alpha-lipoic acid reduces hypertension and increases baroreflex sensitivity in renovascular hypertensive rats. Molecules., 17, (11) 13357–13367.
Rahman ST et al. The impact of lipoic acid on endothelial function and proteinuria in quinapril-treated diabetic patient with stage I hypertension: results form the QUALITY study. J Cardiovasc Pharmacol Ther 17.2 (2012): 139–45.
Ramachandran L, Nair CK. Protection against genotoxic damages following total body exposure in mice by lipoic acid. Mutation Research 724 (2011): 52–58.
Ratliff, J.C., et al. 2013. An open-label pilot trial of alpha-lipoic acid for weight loss in patients with schizophrenia without diabetes. Clin Schizophr Relat Psychoses 1–13.
Richard M et al. Cellular mechanisms by which lipoic acid confers protection during the early stages of cerebral ischemia: a possible role for calcium. Neuroscience Research 69 (2011): 299–307.
Ridruejo E, et al. Thioctic acid-induced cholestatic hepatitis. Ann Pharmacother 45.7 (2011): 7–8.
Roberts DM et al. Amanita phalloides poisoning and treatment with silibin in the Australian Capital Territory and New South Wales. Med J Aust 198.1 (2013): 43–47.
Rocamonde B et al. Neuroprotection of lipoic acid treatment promotes angiogenesis and reduces the glial scar formation after brain injury. Neuroscience 224 (2012): 102–115.
Rüdiger HW et al. Lipoic acid dependency of human branched chain α-ketoacid oxidase. Biochim Biophys Acta 264 (1972): 220–223.
Salinthone S et al. Lipoic acid attenuates inflammation via camp ad protein kinase A signaling. PLoS ONE 5.9 (2010): e13058.
Salinthone S et al. Lipoic acid stimulates camp production via G-coupled receptor-dependent and independent mechanisms. Journal of nutritional biochemistry 22 (2011): 681–690.
Schillace RV et al. Lipoic acid stimulate camp production in T lymphocytes and NK cells. Biochemical and Biophysical Research Communication. 354 (2007): 259–264.
Schreibelt G et al. Lipoic acid affects cellular migration into the central nervous system and stabilizes blood-brain barrier integrity. The Journal of Immunology 177.4 (2006): 2630–2637.
Schupke H et al. New metabolic pathways of alpha lipoic acid. Drug Metab Dispos 29 (2001): 855–862.
Segermann J et al. Effect of alpha-lipoic acid on the peripheral conversion of thyroxine to triiodothyronine and on serum lipid-, protein- and glucose levels. Arzneimittleforschung 41.12 (1991): 1294–98.
Sen C.K. & Packer, L. 2000. Thiol homeostasis and supplements in physical exercise. Am J Clin. Nutr., 72, (2 Suppl) 653S-669S.
Sena CM et al. Effect of alpha-lipoic acid on endothelial function in aged diabetic and high-fat fed rats. Br J Pharmacol 153 (2008): 894–906.
Shamloul R Ghanem H. Erectile dysfunction. The Lancet 381 (2012): 153–165.

Shay KP et al. Lipoic acid as a dietary supplement: molecular mechanisms and therapeutic potential. Biochem Biophys Acta 1790.10 (2009): 1149–1160.
Shila S et al. Brain regional response in antioxidant systems to α-lipoic acid in arsenic intoxicated rats. Toxicology 210 (2005): 25–36.
Sigel H et al. Stability and structure of binary and ternary complexes of α-lipoate and lipoate derivatives in Mn2+, Cu2+ and Zn2+ in solution. Archives of biochemistry and biophysics 187.1 (1978): 208–214.
Sivaprasad TR et al. Therapeutic efficacy of lipoic acid in combination with dimercaptosuccinic acid against lead-induced renal tubular defects and on isolated brush-border enzyme activities. Chemico-biological interactions 147 (2004): 259–271.
Sola S et al. Irbesartan and lipoic acid improve endothelial function and reduce markers of inflammation in the metabolic syndrome: results of the ISLAND study. Molecular cardiology 111 (2005): 343–348.
Streeper RS et al. Differential effects of lipoic acid stereoisomers on glucose metabolism in insulin-resistant skeletal muscle. Am J physiolol 273 (1997): E185–91.
Strödter D et al. The influence of thioctic acid on metabolism and function of the diabetic heart. Diabetic Res Clin Prac. 29 (1995): 19–26.
Suh JH et al. Oxidative stress in the ageing rat heart is reversed by dietary supplementation with (R)-(alpha)-lipoic acid. Faseb J 15.3 (2001): 700–706.
Suh JH et al. (R)-alpha-lipoic acid reverses the age-related loss in GHS redox status in post-mitotic tissues: evidence for increased cysteine requirement for GSH redox status in post-mitotic tissues: evidence for increased cysteine requirement for GSH synthesis. Arch Biochem Biophys 423 (2004a): 126–135.
Suh JH et al. Dehydrolipoic acid lowers the redox activity of transition metal ions but does not remove them from the active sites of enzymes. Redox rep 9.1 (2004b) 57–61.
Sumathi L et al. Effect of DL α-lipoic acid on tissue redox state in acute cadmium-challenged tissues. Nutritional biochemistry 7 (1996): 85–92.
Sun YD et al. 2012. Effect of (R)-alpha-lipoic acid supplementation on serum lipids and antioxidative ability in patients with age-related macular degeneration. Ann. Nutr. Metab, 60, (4) 293–297.
Tabassum H et al. Protective effect of lipoic acid against methotrexate-induced oxidative stress in liver mitochondria. Food and Chemical toxicology 48 (2010): 1973–1979.
Takaoka M et al. Effects of alpha-lipoic acid on deoxycorticosterone acete-salt-induced hypertension in rats. Eur J Pharmacol 424 (2001): 121–129.
Teichert J et al. Investigations on the pharmacokinetics of alpha-lipoic acid in healthy volunteers. Int J Clin Pharmacol Ther 36 (1998): 625–628.
Tong et al. Comparative treatment of α-amanitin poisoning with N-acetyl-cysteine, benzylpenicillin, Cimetidine, thioctic acid, and sylibin in a murine model. Annals of Emmergency Medicine 50.3 (2007): 282–288.
Vasdev S et al. Dietary lipoic acid supplementation prevents fructose-induces hypertension in rats. Nutr Metab Cardiovasc Dis 10 (2000a): 339–46.
Vasdev S et al. Dietary alpha-lipoic acid supplementation lowers blood pressure in spontaneously hypertensive rats. J Hypers 18 (2000b): 567–573.
Vasdev S et al. Salt-induced hypertension in WKY rats: prevention by alpha-lipoic acid supplementation. Mol Cell Biochem 254 (2003): 319–326.
Vasdev S et al. Dietary lipoic acid supplementation attenuates hypertension in Dahl salt sensitive rats. Moll Cell Biochem 275 (2005): 135–141.
Wang L et al. The protective effect of α-lipoic acid on mitochondria in the kidney of diabetic rats. Int J Clin Exp Med 6.2 (2013): 90–97.
Wang MY et al. Activity assay of lipoamidase, an expected modulator of metabolic fate of externally administered lipoic acid. Inflammation and Regeneration 31.1 (2011): 88–94.
Wang SJ, Chen HH. Pre-synaptic mechanisms underlying the alpha-lipoic acid facilitation of glutamate exocytosis in rat cerebral cortex nerve terminals. Neurochem Int 50–1 (2007): 51–60.
Winiarska K et al. Lipoic acid ameliorates oxidative stress and renal injury in alloxan diabetic rabbits. Biochimie 90.3 (2008): 450–459.
Xiang et al. α-lipoic acid can improve endothelial dysfunction in subjects with impaired fasting glucose. Metabolism clinical and experimental 60 (2011): 480–485.
Xu J et al. Flaxseed oil and alpha-lipoic acid combination reduces atherosclerotis risk factors in rats fed a high-fat diet. Lipids Health Dis 11 (2012): 148.
Xu Q et al. Meta-analysis of methylcobalamin alone and in combination with lipoic acid in patients with diabetic peripheral neuropathy. Diabetes Res Clin Pract 101–2 (2013): 99–105.
Yadav V et al. Lipoic acid in multiple sclerosis: a pilot study. Multiple Sclerosis 11 (2005): 159–165.
Yadav V et al. Pharmacokinetics study of lipoic acid in multiple sclerosis: Comparing mice and human pharmacokinetic parameters. Mult Scler 16.4 (2010): 387–397.
Yamada T et al. α-lipoic acid (LA) enantiomers protect SH-SY5Y cells against glutathione depletion. Neurochemistry International 59 (2011): 1003–1009.
Yan W et al. Effect of oral ALA supplementation on oxidative stress and insulin sensitivity among overweight/obese adults: A double-blinded randomized, controlled cross over intervention trial. International Journal of cardiology 167 (2013): 602–3.
Yi X et al. Genetic reduction of lipoic acid synthase expression moderately increases atherosclerosis in male, but not female, apolipoprotein E-deficient mice. Atherosclerosis 211.2 (2010): 424–30.
Yi X et al. α-lipoic acid protects diabetic apolipoprotein E deficient mice from nephropathy. Journal of Diabetes and Its Complications 25 (2011): 193–201.
Yi X et al. Reduced expression of α-lipoic acid synthase accelerates diabetic nephropathy. J AM Soc Nephrol 23.1 (2012a): 103–111.
Yi X et al. Reduced alpha-lipoic acid synthase gene expression exacerbates atherosclerosis in diabetic apolipoprotein E-deficient mice. Atherosclerosis 223.1 (2012b): 17–143.

Yi X, Meada N. Endogenous production of lipoic acid is essential for mouse development. Molecular and cellular biology 25.18 (2005): 8387–92.
Ying Z et al. Lipoic acid effects on established atherosclerosis. Life Sci 86.3/4 (2010): 95–102.
Zakrzewska JM et al. Intervention for the treatment of burning mouth syndrome. Cochrane Oral Health Group. Cochrane Database of Systematic Reviews 1 (2009).
Zembron-Lacny A et al. Physical activity and lipoic acid modulate inflammatory response through changes in thiol redox status. J Physiol Biochem 69–3 (2013): 397–404.
Zhang, Y., et al. 2011. Amelioration of lipid abnormalities by alpha-lipoic acid through antioxidative and anti-inflammatory effects. Obesity. (Silver. Spring), 19, (8) 1647–1653.
Ziegler D et al. Treatment of symptomatic polyneuropathy with the antioxidant α-lipoic acid: a meta-analysis. Diabet Med 21.2 (2004): 114–121.

Andrographis

HISTORICAL NOTE Andrographis has long been used in traditional medicine systems in numerous countries. It has been included in the pharmacopoeias of India, Korea and China, possibly because it grows abundantly in India, Pakistan and various parts of Southeast Asia. In traditional Chinese medicine, andrographis is considered a 'cold' herb and is used to rid the body of heat, as in fevers and acute infections, and to dispel toxins from the body. In Ayurvedic medicine it is used as a bitter tonic, to stimulate digestion and as a treatment for a wide range of conditions such as diabetes and hepatitis. It is still a common household remedy and found in more than half the combination tonics used to treat liver conditions in India. In recent years, andrographis has gained popularity in Western countries as a treatment for upper respiratory tract infections and influenza.

COMMON NAMES

Andrographis, chirayata, chiretta, green chiretta, Indian echinacea, kalmegh, king of bitters

BOTANICAL NAME/FAMILY

Andrographis paniculata (family Acanthaceae)

PLANT PARTS USED

Leaves, aerial parts

CHEMICAL COMPONENTS

The main active constituent group is considered to be the bitter diterpenoid lactones known as andrographolides. This group includes andrographolide (AP1), 14-deoxy-11,12-didehydroandrographolide (AP3) and neoandrographolide (AP4) (Lim et al 2012). Other constituents found in the plant roots include flavonoids, diterpenoids, phenylpropanoids, oleanolic acid, beta-sitosterol and beta-daucosterol (Xu & Wang 2011). Constituents identified in the aerial parts include flavonoids, alkanes, ketones, aldehydes, lactones, diterpene glucosides, ditriterpenoids and diterpene dimers (Akbar 2011).

Clinical studies show that andrographis is well absorbed, with peak plasma concentrations reached after 1.5–2 hours and a half-life of 6.6 hours (Panossian et al 2000).

MAIN ACTIONS

The mechanism of action of andrographis has not been significantly investigated in clinical studies, so results from in vitro and animal tests provide most of the evidence for this herbal medicine.

Immunomodulation

A number of immunomodulatory actions have been identified with andrographis and its derivatives (Jayakumar et al 2013). One of the main constituents responsible for the immunostimulant activity is andrographolide, which has an effect on the stimulation and proliferation of immunocompetent cells and the production of key cytokines and immune markers in vitro (Panossian et al 2002).

In vitro and in vivo research demonstrates that andrographolide has the ability to interfere with T-cell proliferation, cytokine release and maturation of dendritic cells, as well as to substantially decrease the antibody response in delayed-type hypersensitivity (Iruretagoyena et al 2005). Additionally, andrographolide demonstrated a capacity to inhibit T-cell and antibody responses in experimental autoimmune encephalomyelitis in mice, and to protect against myelin sheath damage (Iruretagoyena et al 2005).

Andrographolide has been demonstrated to inhibit production of interleukin-12 (IL-12) and tumour necrosis factor-alpha (TNF-alpha) in lipopolysaccaride-stimulated mice macrophages, which appeared to relate to suppression of the ERK1/2 signalling pathway (Qin et al 2006). It has also been found to decrease interferon-gamma (IFN-gamma) and IL-2 production and therefore display an immunosuppressive effect. As a result, Burgos et al (2005) concluded that andrographis may be useful for autoimmune disease, especially where high levels of IFN-gamma are present, for example in multiple sclerosis and rheumatoid arthritis. Interestingly, andrographolide exerted antigrowth and proapoptotic effects in a study utilising rheumatoid arthritis fibroblast-like synoviocytes (Yan et al 2012).

Immunostimulatory activity of andrographolide in phytohaemagglutinin-stimulated human peripheral blood lymphocytes has been reported with laboratory studies (Kumar et al 2004).

Other pharmacologically active constituents are also present, as demonstrated by a study that found that the immunostimulant activity of the whole extract is greater than that of the isolated andrographolide constituent alone. Investigation with a combination of the whole extract and *Eleutherococcus senticosus* in the formula Kan Jang demonstrated a more profound effect (Panossian et al 2002).

Anticancer activity

In vivo and in vitro experiments have demonstrated the possible benefits of andrographolide and its derivatives on various cancer cells via multiple mechanisms. According to a recent review, Lim et al (2012) identified anticancer mechanisms, including inhibition of Janus tyrosine kinases-signal transducers, inhibition of activators of phosphatidylinositol 3-kinase, transcription and NF-κB signalling pathways, suppression of growth factors, cyclins, cyclin-dependent kinases, heat shock protein 90 and metalloproteins. Andrographolide has also been shown to induce tumour-suppressor proteins p53 and p21, leading to inhibition of cancer cell proliferation, survival, metastasis and angiogenesis (Lim et al 2012). Andrographolide increases apoptosis of prostate cancer cells and human leukaemic cells and increases cell cycle arrest (Cheung et al 2005, Geethangili et al 2008, Kim et al 2005, Zhao et al 2008, Zhou et al 2006). It also inhibits the proliferation of human cancer cells and increases IL-2 induction in human peripheral blood lymphocytes in vitro (Kumar et al 2004, Rajagopal et al 2003). A cytotoxic effect of andrographolide on HepG1 human hepatoma cells was observed in a laboratory study which was attributed primarily to the induction of cell cycle arrest via alteration of cellular redox status (Li et al 2007).

In vivo results show that andrographolide increases IL-2, IFN-gamma and T-cell activity (Sheeja et al 2007). In certain circumstances, andrographolide has been found to decrease IFN-gamma and IL-2 and may have an immunosuppressive effect (see Immunomodulation, above).

Andrographis and andrographolide may also inhibit angiogenesis and cancer cell adhesion (Jiang et al 2007, Sheeja et al 2007). Antiangiogenesis and chemotherapeutic potential of andrographolide have been shown in a lung tumour mouse model. In this study, andrographolide significantly reduced expression of hVEGF-A165 compared with a control group and also decreased tumour formation (Tung et al 2013).

Halogenated di-spiropyrrolizidino oxindole derivatives of andrographolide were more cytotoxic than andrographolide in some cancer cells, according to a recent study conducted in human cancer cell lines. One of the derivatives (CY2) induced death of a number of different types of cancer cells, involving cell rounding, nuclear fragmentation and an increase in percentage of apoptotic cells, cell cycle arrest at G1 phase, reactive oxygen species (ROS) generation and involvement of the ROS-dependent mitochondrial pathway (Dey et al 2013).

Antimicrobial

Aqueous extract of *Andrographis paniculata* has demonstrated antibacterial and antifungal activity in vitro. In various laboratory studies, activity was shown against *Bacillus subtilis, Escherichia coli, Pseudomonas aeruginosa, Staphylococcus aureus* and *Candida albicans* (Singha et al 2003, Voravuthikunchai & Limsuwan 2006). An ethanolic extract of *A. paniculata* demonstrated potent inhibitory activity against both Gram-positive and Gram-negative bacteria according to an in vitro study (Mishra et al 2009).

The andrographolides from andrographis have displayed antiviral activity against herpes simplex virus type 1 in vitro (Wiart et al 2005). Inhibitory activity against the dengue virus serotype 1 has also been demonstrated in a laboratory study using a methanolic extract of andrographis (Tang et al 2012).

Cardiovascular effects

Several in vivo studies have suggested a potential role for andrographis in cardiovascular disease. Antihypertensive effects have been demonstrated in animal models, which appear to be related to relaxation of vascular smooth muscle and a decrease in heart rate (Jayakumar et al 2013, Yoopan et al 2007). According to a recent review, early animal studies have shown that andrographis may reduce restenosis after angioplasty and may prevent myocardial reperfusion injury (Jayakumar et al 2013). In a study using rat hearts, a dichloromethane extract of andrographis significantly reduced coronary perfusion pressure by up to 24.5 ± 3.0 mmHg at a 3 mg dose and heart rate was also significantly decreased at this dose (Awang et al 2012). Andrographis has demonstrated hypolipidaemic action in an experimental rat model: a significant reduction ($P < 0.05$) in triglycerides, low-density lipoprotein cholesterol and blood glucose levels was observed after administration of a purified andrographolide extract (Nugroho et al 2012).

Hypoglycaemic

Andrographis has demonstrated significant hypoglycaemic activity in vitro and in various diabetic animal models.

In vitro tests reveal that andrographis has a strong dose-dependent action on insulin production in vitro (Wibudi et al 2008) and inhibits alpha-glucosidase (Subramanian et al 2008) and increases glucose uptake via the phospholipase C/protein kinase C pathway (Hsu et al 2004), all of which may contribute to the hypoglycaemic effect.

Hypoglycaemic and lipid lowering have also been observed in vivo in a model of type 2 diabetes. Administration of either andrographis or andrographolide extracts for 5 days significantly reduced preprandial and postprandial blood glucose levels in a dose-dependent manner. The effect was similar to that observed for metformin (90 mg/kg body weight) (Nugroho et al 2012). Similarly, oral administration of aqueous extract of andrographis to streptozotocin-induced diabetic rats resulted in a significant decrease in blood glucose levels at a dose of 400 mg/kg. This was accompanied by an antioxidant effect with an increase in superoxide dismutase and catalase activity (Dandu & Inamdar 2009). One in vivo study in alloxan-induced diabetic rats demonstrated significantly reduced blood glucose levels as compared to placebo (Reyes et al 2006). The authors commented that andrographis may restore impaired oestrous cycle in this model. A previous animal trial concluded that andrographolide (1.5 mg/kg) lowers plasma glucose by enhancing glucose utilisation in diabetic rats (Yu et al 2003).

Hepatoprotective

Hepatoprotective activity of andrographis has been identified in vitro and in vivo using various toxic liver insults and is mainly attributed to the andrographolide constituent. A significant dose-dependent protective action has been shown against paracetamol-induced hepatotoxicity in rats. Experimental rat models have also identified a protective action for andrographis and its constituents against liver toxicity induced by galactosamine, carbon tetrachloride and tertbutylhydroperoxide. Several mechanisms have been identified (Ghosh et al 2011, Jayakumar et al 2013). Pretreatment of mice for 7 days with andrographolide and another andrographis metabolite, arabinogalactan proteins, produced a protective effect against ethanol-induced toxicity to liver and kidney tissue. In this study, at doses of 500 mg/kg body weight andrographolide and 125 mg/kg body weight arabinogalactan proteins respectively, the results were comparable to that seen with silymarin 500 mg/kg body weight. Silymarin is an established heptoprotective agent and was used as a comparator substance in this animal study (Singha et al 2007).

Antipyretic and anti-inflammatory

Antipyretic activity with andrographis has been demonstrated in animal models (Mandal et al 2001, Suebsasana et al 2009).

Anti-inflammatory activity has also been observed in vitro and in vivo with andrographis, which is primarily associated with andrographolide (Jayakumar et al 2013).

Andrographolide has been shown to reduce production of cytokines, chemokines, adhesion molecules, nitric oxide and lipid mediators (Lim et al 2012) as well as IL-1beta, IL-6, prostaglandin E_2 and thromboxane B_2, and the allergic mediator leukotriene B_4 (Chandrasekaran et al 2010). A decreased induction of nitric oxide synthetase and cyclooxygenase-2 has been observed in laboratory studies, probably via inhibition of the NF-κB signalling pathway (Lee et al 2011, Lim et al 2012).

A. paniculata extract completely inhibited inflammation induced by carageenan in mice, compared to controls (Sheeja et al 2006). In vitro data from the same study showed that andrographis inhibited superoxide (32%), hydroxyl radicals (80%), lipid peroxidation (80%) and nitric oxide (42.8%). These antioxidant mechanisms are likely to contribute to the herb's anti-inflammatory effect.

Antiplatelet activity

Research has demonstrated that andrographis inhibits platelet-activating factor (PAF)-induced human platelet aggregation and also appears to confer additional antiplatelet activity, for which several mechanisms may be involved (Jayakumar et al 2013, Lu et al 2011, 2012, Thisoda et al 2006). A number of compounds appear to be involved in these actions. Thisoda et al (2006) identified andrographolide (AP1) and 14-deoxy-11,12 didehydroandrographolide (AP3) as key antiplatelet constituents. More recently, an additional four flavonoids were isolated that inhibit thrombin and PAF-induced platelet aggregation (Wu et al 2008).

OTHER ACTIONS

Anti-HIV activity

Andrographolide derivatives have been shown to possess anti-HIV activity in vitro. Inhibition of gp120-mediated cell fusion of HL2/3 cells with TZM-bl cells was observed. There is potential for future research in this area (Uttekar et al 2012).

Snake antivenom activity

Andrographis ethanolic extracts have been shown to exhibit neutralising effects on cobra venom. Andrographis was shown to prolong survival time in an animal study, but did not prevent death (Premendran et al 2011).

CLINICAL USE

Andrographis is most commonly used for its effects on immune function and inflammation, such as the treatment and prevention of upper respiratory tract infections (URTIs), while use in non-infective conditions such as ulcerative colitis and rheumatoid arthritis has also been investigated.

Upper respiratory tract infections and the common cold

A. paniculata has become popular as a treatment for URTIs. It is most often used in combination with other herbal medicines, in particular Siberian ginseng and sometimes echinacea. The fixed combination known as Kan Jang contains a standardised extract from *Andrographis paniculata* SHA-10 and *Eleutherococcus senticosus* and has been used for more than 20 years in Scandinavia as a herbal medicinal product in uncomplicated URTI (Gabrielian et al 2002). Clinical studies confirm that treatment with andrographis either by itself or in combination with Siberian ginseng (as in Kan Jang) is beneficial in cases of uncomplicated acute URTIs, providing some symptom relief within several days; however maximal effects appear by day 5.

Clinical evidence indicates that treatment with andrographis reduces the severity of cough, expectoration, nasal discharge, headache, fever, sore throat, malaise/fatigue, sinus pain and sleep disturbances. The dose of andrographis used in various studies has differed, but the majority have used a dose standardised to 60 mg andrographolide/day (Coon & Ernst 2004, Kligler et al 2006, Poolsup et al 2004, Saxena 2010).

A systematic review (Kligler et al 2006) of seven clinical trials (n = 879) concluded that evidence for the effectiveness of andrographis in the treatment of URTI is encouraging. At the time, the authors also made the comment that most of the studies have been done in conjunction with a major manufacturer of the product and further independent testing was required (Kligler et al 2006). Similar positive conclusions were drawn in two earlier systematic reviews. Coon and Ernst (2004) conducted a review that included seven double-blind randomised controlled trials (RCTs) and concluded that, collectively, the data suggest that andrographis is superior to placebo in alleviating symptoms of uncomplicated URTI, and has only mild, infrequent adverse effects. In five of the seven trials, the daily dose was equivalent to 60 mg of andrographolide, which was administered for 3–8 days. Another review of four RCTs confirmed that *A. paniculata*, either by itself or in combination with *E. senticosus* (Kan Jang), is effective for the treatment of uncomplicated acute URTI (Poolsup et al 2004).

More recently, the efficacy of a standardised extract of andrographis (KalmCold) was confirmed in a multicentre, double-blind RCT involving 223 adults with uncomplicated URTIs (Saxena 2010). Treatment with KalmCold (100 mg andrographis/capsule, standardised to 31.3% andrographolide), taken twice daily for a period of 5 days, resulted in a significant decrease in symptoms by day 5 compared to the placebo group for cough, expectoration, nasal discharge, headache, fever, sore throat, malaise/fatigue and sleep disturbances ($P \leq 0.05$); however no improvement in the symptom of earache was observed in either group. The overall efficacy of andrographis 200 mg/day (equivalent to approximately 60 mg andrographolide/day) as KalmCold was 2.1 times higher than placebo in reducing symptoms of URTIs (Saxena 2010).

Andrographis (as Kan Jang) may also reduce the incidence of the common cold according to the available evidence. A double-blind RCT of 107 healthy school children found that treatment with Kan Jan tablets (100 mg standardised to 5.6 mg andrographolide/tablet) taken twice daily for 5 days a week for a period of 3 months reduced the risk of developing a cold by approximately 50% after 2 months when compared to placebo. In the third month, the percentage occurrence of the common cold was 30% in the andrographis-treated group, compared to an occurrence of 62% in the placebo group. This represented a 2.1 times lower risk of the common cold in the group taking Kan Jang ($P < 0.05$) (Caceres et al 1997).

Comparisons between andrographis and echinacea in the treatment of the common cold in children

One study has compared andrographis to echinacea. However this was in the form of Kan Jang which also included Siberian ginseng, making a direct comparison difficult. An RCT involving 133 children with uncomplicated common cold compared the effectiveness of Kan Jang to Immunal (containing *Echinacea purpurea* [L.] extract), when both were used as adjuncts to standard treatment (Spasov et al 2004). The children were randomised to one of three groups. Group 1 received Kan Jang (2 tablets three times daily for 10 days) plus standard care; group 2 received Immunal (10 drops three times daily for 10 days) plus standard care; and group 3 received standard care only, including gargles and paracetamol as required. Adjuvant treatment with Kan Jang was shown to be significantly more effective than adjuvant treatment with Immunal or standard treatment alone. The group taking Kan Jang experienced less severe symptoms, in particular nasal congestion and volume of nasal secretion. Recovery time was also faster in the Kan Jang group than in the Immunal group as well as there being less need for additional standard treatment. Additionally, Kan Jang treatment was well tolerated and no side effects or adverse reactions were reported.

Pharyngotonsillitis

A clinical benefit of andrographis in the treatment of pharyngotonsillitis was reported in one early RCT involving 152 volunteers (Thamlikitkul et al 1991). Symptoms of sore throat and fever were reduced at a dose of 6 g/day of a non-standardised andrographis preparation after 3 days. No subsequent research appears to have been conducted for this indication to confirm these results.

Ulcerative colitis

Two RCTs have found benefits for andrographis treatment in mild to moderate ulcerative colitis.

The efficacy of *Andrographis paniculata* (HMPL-004) in the treatment of mild to moderate ulcerative colitis was assessed in a double-blind RCT (n = 224) (Sandborn et al 2013). Two different strengths of andrographis (1200 mg, or 1800 mg per day) were compared to placebo over 8 weeks. By the end of the treatment period, a clinical response was achieved in 60% of patients receiving andrographis 1800 mg/day (P = 0.02), compared to 45% taking the 1200 mg dose and 40% of those taking placebo (P = 0.6 andrographis 1200 mg vs placebo) (Sandborn et al 2013). Therefore, only the higher strength was significantly superior to placebo whereas the lower dose of andrographis was not effective. Interestingly, the lower dose of andrographis 1200 mg (HMPL-004) daily was as effective as slow-release mesalazine (4500 mg/day) after 8 weeks in another multicentre RCT involving 120 patients with mild to moderate ulcerative colitis (Tang et al 2011).

Rheumatoid arthritis

Anti-inflammatory and immunomodulating effects have been observed in laboratory and animal studies providing the basis of investigation into the effects of andrographis in rheumatoid arthritis. To date, only one clinical study has been published, producing promising results.

Treatment with andrographis tablets (standardised to 30 mg andrographolide/tablet) three times a day for 14 weeks significantly reduced joint tenderness, number of swollen or tender joints and total grade of swollen or tender joints compared to placebo in a double-blind RCT involving 60 patients with active rheumatoid arthritis (Burgos et al 2009). A reduction in rheumatoid factor IgA and C4 was also observed. Of note, participants were not permitted to take non-steroidal anti-inflammatory drugs during the study and paracetamol was only used in cases of severe pain. Joint pain intensity decreased in the andrographis treatment group compared to the placebo group, but the difference was not statistically significant (Burgos et al 2009).

OTHER USES

Familial Mediterranean fever — in combination

A standardised fixed combination (ImmunoGuard) of *Andrographis paniculata*, *Eleutherococcus senticosus*, *Schisandra chinensis* and *Glycyrriza glabra* was shown to be effective for the treatment of familial Mediterranean fever (FMF) in children (3–15 years), according to a small double-blind, randomised, placebo-controlled study (Amaryan et al 2003).

The herbal combination treatment significantly reduced the frequency, severity and duration of attacks compared to placebo. The treatment formulation included andrographis 50 mg/tablet (equivalent to 4 mg standardised andrographolide), which was given as four tablets three times a day for 1 month (Amaryan et al 2003). This herbal combination product, ImmunoGuard, has been shown to raise serum nitric oxide levels in FMF patients during attack-free periods and to have a normalising effect on blood levels of both nitric oxide and IL-6 during FMF attack periods (Panossian et al 2003).

HIV infection

A phase I clinical trial involving non-medicated HIV-positive patients and healthy controls found that oral andrographolides taken for 6 weeks at increasing doses produced no significant benefits and a high incidence of adverse effects, causing the trial to be stopped prematurely (Calabrese et al 2000). A recent in vitro study concluded that andrographolide derivatives may still hold promise as a potential agent in the prevention of HIV (Uttekar et al 2012).

Cancer (in combination)

An integrative treatment approach was investigated in 20 patients with various end-stage cancers. The patients were given a daily combination of six different immunoactive nutraceutical products plus *Andrographis paniculata* (500 mg twice daily) for 6 months. After 6 months, 16 of the 20 patients were still alive, with a statistically significant increase in both natural killer function and TNF-alpha levels. Haemoglobin, haematocrit and glutathione levels were all greatly increased (See et al 2002). Although these results are interesting, it is difficult to examine the direct effect of *A. paniculata*, as so many other nutritional supplements were given concurrently.

Spermatogenesis

Early studies with andrographis have reported antifertility effects in animal models at high doses (Jayakumar et al 2013). The only clinical studies investigating this further have used the herbal combination Kan Jang which contains andrographis and Siberian ginseng, making it difficult to ascertain the effect of andrographis alone.

A phase I clinical study investigated the effects of three different strengths of Kan Jang (combination of *Andrographis paniculata* and *Eleutherococcus senticosus*) on spermatogenesis and fertility in 14 healthy men aged between 18 and 35 years (Mkrtchyan et al 2005). The men were randomised into one of five groups to receive one of the following: (1) Kan Jang equivalent to 60 mg andrographolide; (2) Kan Jang equivalent to 120 mg andrographolide; (3) Kan Jang equivalent to 180 mg andrographolide; (4) a ginseng mixture; or (5) a valerian extract. The study confirmed no significant negative effects of Kan Jang on male sperm or fertility even at doses corresponding to three times the standard daily dose and only a positive trend towards the number of active spermatozoids in the whole ejaculate (Mkrtchyan et al 2005).

Traditional uses

The herb is traditionally given as a restorative and tonic in convalescence and used as a choleretic to stimulate bile production and flow, which improves appetite and digestion. It is often used in combination with aromatic herbs, such as peppermint, for stronger digestive effects and to prevent gastrointestinal discomfort at higher doses. It has also been used in traditional cultures for protection against snake bites, to treat fever, dysentery, cholera, gonorrhoea, diabetes, influenza and dyspepsia.

DOSAGE RANGE

The majority of clinical trials have been conducted using products standardised to the andrographolide fraction.

Upper respiratory tract infection

- Symptomatic treatment: 100 mg twice daily of a standardised andrographis extract providing 60 mg andrographolide per day — maximal effects by day 5.
- Prevention: Kan Jang 200 mg (equivalent to standardised extract of 11.2 mg/day of andrographolide) taken daily for 2 months has been used to prevent incidence of the common cold.
- Ulcerative colitis (mild to moderate): 1200–1800 mg/daily of andrographis (HMPL-004) — maximal effects reported by week 8.
- Rheumatoid arthritis: andrographis tablets (standardised to 30 mg andrographolide/tablet) taken three times daily for at least 3 months.

Toxicity

Animal tests suggest low toxicity (Mills & Bone 2000). Dose-related toxicity leading to termination of a study occurred at doses of 5–10 mg/kg/day of andrographolide (Calabrese et al 2000). This dose was 6–12 times higher than the standard dosage range used in all other studies.

ADVERSE REACTIONS

Generally well tolerated with adverse effects infrequent and mild at usual recommended doses. Unpleasant chest sensation, headache, fatigue, urticaria, gastrointestinal discomfort, nausea, vomiting and metallic taste have been reported at high doses (Coon & Ernst 2004).

SIGNIFICANT INTERACTIONS

No specific drug–herb interactions have been reported, therefore interactions are theoretical and based on evidence of pharmacological activity with uncertain clinical significance.

Anticoagulants

Increased risk of bruising and bleeding is theoretically possible, because andrographolide and other constituents in andrographis inhibit PAF-induced platelet aggregation. However andrographis used together with warfarin did not produce any significant effects on the pharmacokinetics of warfarin, and had even less effect on its pharmacodynamics in vivo (Hovhannisyan et al 2006). Caution should still be exercised until further research is available.

Antiplatelet drugs

Additive effects are theoretically possible, as andrographis has been shown to inhibit platelet aggregation in animal and laboratory research — patients should be observed for increased bruising or bleeding.

Barbiturates

Additive effects are theoretically possible, according to an animal study (Mandal et al 2001).

Hypoglycaemic agents

A hypoglycaemic effect has been observed in animal studies (Nugroho et al 2012, Wibudi et al 2008). Additive effects are theoretically possible.

Cytochrome p450 enzyme metabolism

Andrographolide was shown to induce the CYP1A1 enzyme pathway in laboratory studies; however, the clinical significance of this is unknown (Chatuphonprasert et al 2011, Jaruchotikamol et al 2007). Another in vitro study has demonstrated an inhibitive effect of andrographis extract and andrographolide on CYP3A and 2C9 pathways (Pekthong et al 2008). Further research is required before clinical relevance can be determined.

Immunosuppressants

Immunomodulatory activity has been observed with andrographis in vitro and in vivo (Jayakumar et al 2013). Clinical significance of use in combination with immunosuppressive drugs is not clear, but caution is advised.

CONTRAINDICATIONS AND PRECAUTIONS

Inhibition of platelet aggregation has been observed in vitro (Thisoda et al 2006). While it is uncertain whether the effect is clinically relevant, it is advised to suspend use 1 week prior to high-risk surgery, such as neurosurgery, where a small bleed can have serious consequences.

Doses equivalent to or higher than 5 mg/kg/day of the constituent andrographolide should be avoided due to a risk of significant adverse effects (Calabrese et al 2000).

PREGNANCY USE

There is insufficient reliable evidence available to determine safety.

PATIENTS' FAQs

What will this herb do for me?

Human studies confirm that it is effective in reducing symptoms of the common cold and uncomplicated URTIs. New research also suggests it can reduce symptoms in ulcerative colitis and possibly rheumatoid arthritis. It reduces the risk of developing the common cold when taken with Siberian ginseng for at least 2 months.

When will it start to work?

During an acute infection, effects may be seen within 3–4 days of starting the correct dose and maximal symptom-relieving effects are seen by day 5. Used together with Siberian ginseng, it can reduce the risk of developing a cold when used for at least 2 months. Symptom relief in ulcerative colitis develops within 8 weeks and a minimum of 3 months is required to achieve benefits in rheumatoid arthritis.

Are there any safety issues?

Andrographis is not recommended in pregnancy or lactation. This herb is well tolerated but may interact with certain medications.

Practice points/Patient counselling

- Several clinical studies suggest that andrographis, both as a stand-alone treatment and in combination with Siberian ginseng, is a useful symptomatic treatment in cases of common cold and uncomplicated URTIs, with significant symptom relief experienced after 3 days' use.

- It may also reduce the risk of the common cold when used daily for several months.
- New clinical research shows it can reduce symptoms in mild to moderate ulcerative colitis within 8 weeks and may also improve symptoms in rheumatoid arthritis when taken for at least 3 months.
- Preclinical experiments suggest that andrographis may be useful in cases of hepatotoxicity (paracetamol, alcohol), to reduce myocardial reperfusion injury, improve blood glucose management in diabetes, and in hypertension.
- Traditionally, the herb is used to increase bile production and relieve symptoms of dyspepsia and flatulence, loss of appetite and general debility.
- Because of the extreme bitterness of the herb, solid-dose forms may be better tolerated than liquid preparations.

REFERENCES

Akbar S. *Andrographis paniculata*: A review of pharmacological activities and clinical effects. Alternative Medicine Review. 16.1 (2011):66–77.

Amaryan G et al. Double-blind, placebo-controlled, randomized, pilot clinical trial of ImmunoGuard: a standardized fixed combination of *Andrographis paniculata* Nees, with *Eleutherococcus senticosus* Maxim, *Schizandra chinensis* Bail. and *Glycyrrhiza glabra* L. extracts in patients with familial Mediterranean fever. Phytomedicine 10.4 (2003): 271–285.

Awang K et al. Cardiovascular activity of labdane diterpenes from *Andrographis paniculata* in isolated rat hearts. Journal of Biomedicine and Biotechnogy. (2012): 2012;ID 876458.

Burgos RA et al. Andrographolide inhibits IFN-gamma and IL-2 cytokine production and protects against cell apoptosis. Planta Med 71.5 (2005): 429–434.

Burgos RA et al. Efficacy of an *Andrographis paniculata* composition for the relief of rheumatoid arthritis symptoms: a prospective randomized placebo-controlled trial. Clin Rheumatol 28.8 (2009): 931–46.

Caceres DD et al Prevention of common colds with *Andrographis paniculata* dried extract. A pilot double blind trial. Phytomedicine 4.2 (1997):101–104.

Calabrese C et al. A phase I trial of andrographolide in HIV positive patients and normal volunteers. Phytother Res 14.5 (2000): 333–338.

Chandrasekaran CV, et al. Effect of an extract of *Andrographis paniculata* leaves on inflammatory and allergic mediators in vitro. J Ethnopharmacol. 129.2 (2010):203–7.

Chatuphonprasert W et al. Different AhR binding sites of diterpenoid ligands from *Andrographis paniculata* caused differential CYP1A1 induction in primary culture in mouse hepatocytes. Toxicology in Vitro. 25.8 (2011):1757–63.

Cheung HY et al. Andrographolide isolated from *Andrographis paniculata* induces cell cycle arrest and mitochondrial-mediated apoptosis in human leukemic HL-60 cells. Planta Med 71.12 (2005): 1106–1111.

Coon JT, Ernst E. *Andrographis paniculata* in the treatment of upper respiratory tract infections: a systematic review of safety and efficacy. Planta Med 70.4 (2004): 293–298.

Dandu AM, Inamdar NM. Evaluation of beneficial effects of antioxidant properties of aqueous leaf extract of *Andrographis paniculata* in STZ-induced diabetes. Pakistan Journal of Pharmaceutical Sciences. 22.1 (2009):49–52.

Dey SK et al. Cytotoxic activity and apoptosis-inducing potential of di-spiropyrrolidino and di-spiropyrrolizino oxindole andrographolide derivatives. PLoS One 8.3 (2013).

Gabrielian, E.S.,et al. 2002. A double blind, placebo-controlled study of *Andrographis paniculata* fixed combination Kan Jang in the treatment of acute upper respiratory tract infections including sinusitis. Phytomedicine, 9, (7) 589–597.

Geethangili M et al. Cytotoxic constituents from *Andrographis paniculata* induce cell cycle arrest in jurkat cells. Phytother Res 22.10 (2008): 1336–1341.

Ghosh N et al. Recent advances in herbal medicine for treatment of liver diseases. Pharmaceutical Biology 19.9 (2011):970–988.

Hovhannisyan AS et al. The effect of Kan Jang extract on the pharmacokinetics and pharmacodynamics of warfarin in rats. Phytomedicine 13.5 (2006): 318–323.

Hsu JH et al. Activation of alpha1A-adrenoceptor by andrographolide to increase glucose uptake in cultured myoblast C2C12 cells. Planta Med 70.12 (2004): 1230–1233.

Iruretagoyena MI et al. Andrographolide interferes with T cell activation and reduces experimental autoimmune encephalomyelitis in the mouse. J Pharmacol Exp Ther 312.1 (2005): 366–372.

Jaruchotikamol A et al. Strong synergistic induction of CYP1A1 expression by andrographolide plus typical CYP1A inducers in mouse hepatocytes. Toxicol Appl Pharmacol 224.2 (2007): 156–162.

Jayakumar T et al. Experimental and clinical pharmacology of *Andrographis paniculata* and its major bioactive phytoconstituent andrographolide. Evidence-based Complementary and Alternative Medicine. (2013); 2013: 846740.

Jiang CG et al. Andrographolide inhibits the adhesion of gastric cancer cells to endothelial cells by blocking E-selectin expression. Anticancer Res 27 (4B) (2007): 2439–2447.

Kim TG, et al. Morphological and biochemical changes of andrographolide-induced cell death in human prostatic adenocarcinoma PC-3 cells. In Vivo 19.3 (2005): 551–557.

Kligler B et al. *Andrographis paniculata* for the treatment of upper respiratory infection: a systematic review by the natural standard research collaboration. Explore (NY) 2.1 (2006): 25–29.

Kumar RA et al. Anticancer and immunostimulatory compounds from *Andrographis paniculata*. J Ethnopharmacol 92.23 (2004): 291–295.

Lee KC et al. Andrographolide acts as an anti-inflammatory agent in LPS-stimulated RAW264.7 macrophages by inhibiting STAT3-mediated suppression of the NF-kB pathway. J Ethnopharmacol (2011) 135: 678–684.

Li J et al. Andrographolide induces cell cycle arrest at G2/M phase and cell death in HepG2 cells via alteration of reactive oxygen species. Eur J Pharmacol 568.1–3 (2007):31–44.

Lim JC et al. Andrographolide and its analogues: versatile bioactive molecules for combating inflammation and cancer. Clin Exp Pharmacol Physiol 39 (3) (2012):300–10.

Lu WJ et al. A novel role of andrographolide, an NK-kB inhibitor, on inhibition of platelet activation: the pivotal mechanisms of endothelial nitric oxide synthase/cyclic GMP. Journal of Molecular Medicine. 89.12 (2011):1263–1271.

Lu J et al. Suppression of NF-kB signaling by andrographolide with a novel mechanism in human platelets: regulatory roles of the p38 MAPK-hydroxyl radical0-ERK2 cascade. Biochemical Pharmacology 84 (2012):914–924.

Mandal SC, et al. Studies on psychopharmacological activity of *Andrographis paniculata* extract. Phytother Res 15.3 (2001): 253–256.

Mills S, Bone K. Principles and practice of phytotherapy. London: Churchill Livingstone, 2000.

Mishra U et al. Antibacterial activity of ethanol extract of *Andrographis paniculata*. Indian Journal of Pharmaceutical Sciences. 74.4 (2009):436–438.

Mkrtchyan AV et al. A phase I clinical study of *Andrographis paniculata* fixed combination Kan Jang versus ginseng and valerian on the semen quality of healthy male subjects. Phytomedicine 12.6–7 (2005): 403–409.

Nugroho AE et al. Antidiabetic and antihiperlipidemic effect of *Andrographis paniculata* (Burm. f) Nees and andrographolide in high-fructose-fat-fed rats. Indian J Pharmacol 44.3 (2012):377–81.

Panossian A et al. Pharmacokinetic and oral bioavailability of andrographolide from *Andrographis paniculata* fixed combination Kan Jang in rats and human. Phytomedicine 7.5 (2000): 351–364.

Panossian A et al. Effect of andrographolide and Kan Jang (fixed combination of extract SHA-10 and extract SHE-3) on proliferation of human lymphocytes, production of cytokines and immune activation markers in the whole blood cells culture. Phytomedicine 9.7 (2002): 598–605.

Panossian A et al. Plasma nitric oxide level in functional Mediterranean fever and its modulations by ImmunoGuard. Nitric Oxide 9 (2003): 103–110.

Pekthong DH et al. Differential inhibition of rat and human hepatic cytochrome P450 by *Andrographis paniculata* extract and andrographolide. J Ethnopharmacol 115.3 (2008): 432–440.

Poolsup N et al. *Andrographis paniculata* in the symptomatic treatment of uncomplicated upper respiratory tract infection: systematic review of randomized controlled trials. J Clin Pharm Ther 29.1 (2004): 37–45.

Premendran SJ et al. Anti-cobra venom activity of plant *Andrographis paniculata* and its comparison with polyvalent anti-snake venom. Journal of Natural Science, Biology, and Medicine 2.2 (2011):198–204.

Qin LH et al. Andrographolide inhibits the production of TNF-alpha and interleukin-12 in lipopolysaccharide-stimulated macrophages: role of mitogen-activated protein kinases. Biological & Pharmaceutical Bulletin 29.2 (2006):220–4.

Rajagopal S et al. Andrographolide, a potential cancer therapeutic agent isolated from *Andrographis paniculata*. J Exp Ther Oncol 3.3 (2003): 147–158.

Reyes BA et al. Anti-diabetic potentials of *Momordica charantia* and *Andrographis paniculata* and their effects on estrous cyclicity of alloxan-induced diabetic rats. J Ethnopharmacol 105.1–2 (2006): 196–200.

Sandborn WJ et al. *Andrographis paniculata* extract (HMPL-004) for active ulcerative colitis. Am J Gastroenterol 108.1 (2013):90–8.

Saxena RC. A randomized double blind placebo controlled clinical evaluation of extract of *Andrographis paniculata* (KalmCold) in patients with uncomplicated upper respiratory tract infection. Phytomedicine. 17(3–4) (2010):178–185.

See D, et al. Increased tumor necrosis factor alpha (TNF-alpha) and natural killer cell (NK) function using an integrative approach in late stage cancers. Immunol Invest 31.2 (2002): 137–153.

Sheeja K, et al. Antioxidant and anti-inflammatory activities of the plant *Andrographis paniculata* Nees. Immunopharmacol Immunotoxicol 28.1 (2006): 129–140.

Sheeja K, et al. Antiangiogenic activity of *Andrographis paniculata* extract and andrographolide. Int Immunopharmacol 7.2 (2007): 211–221.

Singha PK, et al. Antimicrobial activity of *Andrographis paniculata*. Fitoterapia 74.78 (2003): 692–694.

Singha PK, et al. Protective activity of andrographolide and arabinogalactan proteins from *Andrographis paniculata* Nees. against ethanol-induced toxicity in mice. J Ethnopharmacol 111.1 (2007): 13–21.

Spasov AA et al. Comparative controlled study of *Andrographis paniculata* fixed combination, Kan Jang and an Echinacea preparation as adjuvant, in the treatment of uncomplicated respiratory disease in children. Phytother Res 18.1 (2004): 47–53.

Subramanian R, et al. In vitro alpha-glucosidase and alpha-amylase enzyme inhibitory effects of *Andrographis paniculata* extract and andrographolide. Acta Biochim Pol 55.2 (2008): 391–398.

Suebsasana S et al. Analgesic, antipyretic, anti-inflammatory and toxic effects of andrographolide derivatives in experimental animals. Archives of Pharmacal Research 32.9 (2009):1191–1200.

Tang T et al. Randomised clinical trial: herbal extract HMPL-004 in active ulcerative colitis – a double-blind comparison with sustained release mesalazine. Aliment Pharmacol Ther 33.2 (2011):194–202.

Tang LI et al. Screening of anti-dengue activity in methanolic extracts of medicinal plants. BMC Complementary and Alternative Medicine. 12.3 (2012).

Thamlikitkul V et al. Efficacy of *Andrographis paniculata* nees for pharyngotonsillitis in adults. J Med Assoc Thai 74.10 (1991): 437–442.
Thisoda P et al. Inhibitory effect of *Andrographis paniculata* extract and its active diterpenoids on platelet aggregation. Eur J Pharmacol 553.1–3 (2006): 39–45.
Tung YT et al. Therapeutic potential of andrographolide isolated from the leaves of *Andrographis paniculata* Nees for treating lung adenocarcinoma. Evid Based Complement Alternat Med. (2013):305898
Uttekar MM et al. Anti-HIV activity of semisynthetic derivatives of andrographolide and computational study of HIV-1 gp120 protein binding. European Journal of Medicinal Chemistry. 56 (2012) :368–74.
Voravuthikunchai SP; Limsuwan S. Medicinal plant extracts as anti-*Escherichia coli* 0157:H7 agents and their effects on bacterial cell aggregation. Journal of Food protection 69.10 (2006):2336–2341.
Wiart CK et al. Antiviral properties of ent-labdene diterpenes of *Andrographis paniculata* nees, inhibitors of herpes simplex virus type 1. Phytother Res 19 (12) (2005): 1069–1070.
Wibudi A et al. The traditional plant, *Andrographis paniculata* (Sambiloto), exhibits insulin-releasing actions in vitro. Acta Med Indones 40.2 (2008): 63–68.
Wu TS et al. Flavonoids and ent-labdane diterpenoids from *Andrographis paniculata* and their antiplatelet aggregatory and vasorelaxing effects. J Asian Nat Prod Res 10.1–2 (2008): 17–24.
Xu C, Wang ZT. [Chemical constituents from roots of *Andrographis paniculata*.] Yao Xue Xue Bao 46 (3) (2011):317–21
Yan J et al. Andrographolide induces cell cycle arrest and apoptosis in human rheumatoid arthritis fibroblast-like synoviocytes. Cell Biol Toxicol. 28.1 (2012):47–56.
Yoopan NP et al. Cardiovascular effects of 14-deoxy-11, 12-didehydroandrographolide and *Andrographis paniculata* extracts. Planta Med 73.6 (2007): 503–511.
Yu BC et al. Antihyperglycemic effect of andrographolide in streptozotocin-induced diabetic rats. Planta Med 69.12 (2003): 1075–1079.
Zhao F et al. Anti-tumor activities of andrographolide, a diterpene from *Andrographis paniculata*, by inducing apoptosis and inhibiting VEGF level. J Asian Nat Prod Res 10.5 (2008): 473–479.
Zhou J et al. Critical role of pro-apoptotic Bcl-2 family members in andrographolide-induced apoptosis in human cancer cells. Biochem Pharmacol 72.2 (2006): 132–144.

Astragalus

HISTORICAL NOTE Astragalus was first recorded in *Shen Nong's Materia Medica* about two thousand years ago and was believed to stimulate immune function and have antioxidant effects and other benefits in the treatment of viral infections and cardiovascular disease (Zhang et al 2007). The roots of astragalus are still considered among the most important and popular Chinese herbs for invigorating vital energy, health promotion and strengthening Qi. Western herbalists began using astragalus in the 1800s in various tonics and the gummy sap (tragacanth) is still used as an emulsifier, food thickener and antidiarrhoeal agent. Today, Western herbalists use astragalus as an immunomodulating agent, adaptogen and in the management of cardiovascular disease.

Clinical note — Polysaccharides and immunity

Plant polysaccharides are known for their ability to enhance host defence responses. Several types of immunomodulators have been identified, most recently botanically sourced polysaccharides isolated from mushrooms, algae, lichens and higher plants. These polysaccharides tend to have a broad spectrum of therapeutic properties and relatively low toxicity. One of the primary mechanisms responsible for immunomodulation involves non-specific induction of the immune system, which is thought to occur via macrophage stimulation and modulation of the complement system. According to one report, polysaccharides isolated from 35 plant species among 20 different families have been shown to increase macrophage cytotoxic activity against tumour cells and microorganisms, activate phagocytic activity, increase reactive oxygen species and nitric oxide production, and enhance secretion of cytokines and chemokines, such as tumour necrosis factor-alpha (TNF-alpha), inteleukin-1beta (IL-1beta), IL-6, IL-8, IL-12, interferfon-gamma (IFN-gamma) and IFN-beta2 (Schepetkin & Quinn 2006). These effects have a major influence on the body's ability to respond rapidly and potently to a diverse array of pathogens, giving the polysaccharides wide clinical application.

COMMON NAME

Astragalus

OTHER NAMES

Astragali, beg kei, bei qi, hwanggi, huang-qi, milk vetch, goat's horn, green dragon, Mongolian milk, ogi, Syrian tragacanth

BOTANICAL NAME/FAMILY

Astragalus membranaceus (family Fabaceae)

PLANT PART USED

Root

CHEMICAL COMPONENTS

Astragalus is a chemically complex herb and contains over 60 components, including beta-sitosterol, glycosides (astragalosides I–VII, soyasaponin, daucosterin), polysaccharides (astroglucans A–C), saponins such as cycloastragenol, astragalosides, isoflavones and other flavonoids, plant acid, choline, betaine, rumatakenin, formonetin, amino acids (including gamma-aminobutyric acid), monomeric lectin and various microelements (Duke 2003, Li & Wang 2005, Mills & Bone 2000, Yan et al 2010).

MAIN ACTIONS

Evidence about mechanisms of action is mainly derived from in vitro and animal studies.

Immune modulation

Studies using various experimental models indicate that astragalus and its saponins, polysaccharides and flavonoids have immune-modulating activity by stimulating macrophage activity and enhancing B- and T-cell activity (Chu et al 1988, Jin et al 1994, Kuo et al 2009, Lonkova 2010, Shen et al 2008, Sugiura et al 1993, Sun et al 2008). Astragalus enhances lymphocyte blastogenesis in vitro (Sun et al 1983). Immunostimulant effects have also been observed in the presence of immunosuppressive therapy in vivo (Jin et al 1999).

Although usually administered in the oral form, research has also been undertaken with injectable forms. A study conducted with both normal and immunosuppressed mice found that astragalus administration increased antibody responses and T-helper cell activity (Zhao et al 1990). A flavonoid identified in the stem and leaves of astragalus is believed to be one of the main constituents responsible for immune modulation (Jiao et al 1999) and, more recently, several studies have identified that astragalus polysaccharide also exerts significant biological effects, including increasing cellular and humoral immune responses in vivo (Guo et al 2004).

Other in vitro and animal studies reveal that astragalus polysaccharides increase beneficial gut flora and decrease harmful gut bacteria, suggesting beneficial immune effects within the gastrointestinal tract (Guo et al 2003).

A 2009 animal model observed a switch to Th-1-dominant immune regulation along with increased exercise tolerance in chronic fatigue rats (Kuo et al 2009), which suggests potential benefit for the use of astragalus in postviral syndrome and chronic fatigue.

Hypotensive and positive inotrope

Several constituents from *Astragalus* spp. have demonstrated effects on heart contractility, heart rate and blood pressure. In particular, 3-nitropropionic acid has been shown to decrease blood pressure and induce bradycardia when administered as an intravenous (IV) preparation in normotensive rats or renal hypertensive dogs (Castillo et al 1993). Another compound, astragaloside IV, demonstrated positive inotropic activity in patients with congestive heart failure (Luo et al 1995).

Recent research indicates that astragalus improves endothelial function by increasing the bioavailability of nitric oxide and decreasing reactive oxygen species production (Zhang et al 2007).

Antioxidant

In vivo studies have found that astragalus raises superoxide dismutase activity in the brain and liver, thus demonstrating an indirect antioxidant activity (Jin et al 1999). The constituent astragaloside IV (20 and 40 mg/kg) prevented the formation of cerebral infarction after induced focal ischaemia in an animal model, most likely due to its antioxidant and anti-inflammatory actions (Luo et al 2004). Recent in vitro experiments with astragalus polysaccharides also suggest they are potent free radical scavengers of hydroxyl radicals as well as hydrogen peroxide (Niu 2011).

Anticarcinogenic effects

Both in vitro and animal studies indicate that astragalus may have a role as adjunctive therapy in the treatment of some cancers. In vivo studies have shown that astragalus extract exerts anticarcinogenic effects in carcinogen-treated mice, mediated through activation of cytotoxic activity and the production of cytokines (Kurashige et al 1999). An extract of the root (90 and 180 mg/kg) prevented the development of preneoplastic lesions and delayed hepatic cancer in chemically-induced hepatocarcinogenesis in a rat model (Cui et al 2003). The saponin, astragaloside IV, can increase the fibrinolytic potential of cultured human umbilical vein endothelial cells by downregulating the expression of plasminogen activator inhibitor type 1 (Zhang et al 1997).

Another constituent (astragalan) increased the secretion of TNF-alpha and TNF-beta (Zhao & Kong 1993). More recent research attributes some of the antiproliferative effects of astragalus to lectins which inhibit the growth of tumour cells and induce apoptosis (L Huang et al 2012).

An animal study using a combination of *Astragalus membranaceus* and *Ligustrum lucidum* demonstrated antitumour effects by augmenting phagocyte and lymphokine-activated killer cell activities (Lau et al 1994). Via gene suppression, the saponin, astragaloside II, exerted antitumour effects, in both in vivo and in vitro experimental models on multi-drug-resistant hepatocellular carcinoma cell lines (C Huang et al 2012).

Hypoglycaemic

There is a growing body of experimental evidence demonstrating activities of relevance in insulin resistance and its comorbidities.

A meta-analysis of nine in vivo studies on rats published from 2005 to 2007 found that astragalus significantly lowers fasting blood glucose levels (Zhang et al 2009). In vivo and in vitro experimentation of polysaccharides of astragalus corroborates these findings and hypothesises that this effect is achieved via downregulation of gene expression and gene splicing for enzymes that regulate insulin signalling at a subcellular level (Mao et al 2009). These findings are significant within the context of emerging models of pathological understanding of non-insulin-dependent diabetes, which suggest that stress created at a subcellular level by hyperglycaemia perpetuates dysregulated insulin signalling and sensitivity.

Other rodent models demonstrate lowered blood glucose, and preservation of pancreatic beta cells when compared with controls (C Li et al 2011); improved insulin sensitivity in skeletal muscle (Liu 2010, Zou et al 2009); and restoration of defective hypoglycaemia (Zou et al 2010) with astragalus treatment.

In a diabetic hamster model with concomitant cardiomyopathy, astragalus polysaccharides reduced serum glucose, glycosylated serum protein and myocardial enzymes and lipid levels increased genetic expression for GLUT-4 transporters, suggesting that astragalus may have a significant role in diabetes and comorbid cardiomyopathy (W Chen et al 2012).

Hepatoprotective actions

Astragalus has hepatoprotective qualities against paracetamol, carbon tetrachloride and D-galactosamine poisoning (Zhang et al 1990). Increases in liver glutathione levels observed as a result of the herbal treatment may be partly responsible. Studies have identified the constituent betaine as an important contributor to this activity.

Renal protective

Alone and in combination, astragalus demonstrated reno-protective effects in animal models by reducing proteinuria and by protecting the microstructure of the kidney architecture (Li & Zhang 2009, Song et al 2009, Wojcikowski et al 2009).

Neuroprotective

A decoction of astragalus produced neuroprotective effects in rats with experimentally induced cerebral ischaemia, and memory enhancement has been observed in vivo (Jin et al 1999).

OTHER ACTIONS

Astragalus is also thought to have adaptogenic activity. It has shown weak oestrogenic activity in vitro when compared with other Chinese herbs and controls (17-beta-oestradiol). This could partially explain its traditional use in menopause.

Traditional action

Of note is a recent in vivo study (in rats) exploring the basis for meridian tropism theory in traditional Chinese medicine (TCM), the premise of which is that particular principles in plants have an affinity for specific tissues, organs and meridians, thus influencing the therapeutic application of herbal medicines in TCM. The results produced by Chang et al (2012) confirmed that astragaloside IV was mainly distributed to the liver, kidney, lung, spleen and heart, which reflects the traditional use of astragalus and may provide experimental validity for the application of meridian tropism.

Hypocholesterolaemic

A specific astragalus polysaccharide, extracted from *Astragalus membranaceus*, possessed hydroxyl radicals and hydrogen peroxide scavenging activities, and showed a chelating effect on ferrous ions in vitro (Niu 2011). This suggests that astragalus may have a cholesterol-lowering effect and reduces the risk of cardiovascular diseases.

Digestive effects

Astragalus strengthens the movement and muscle tone of the small intestine (especially the jejunum) in animal tests, which may account for its clinical application in a variety of common digestive symptoms (Yang 1993).

Improved sperm motility

An aqueous extract of *Astragalus membranaceus* was tested in vitro and found to have a significant stimulatory effect on sperm motility (Hong et al 1992). Astragalus has shown a significant effect on human sperm motility in vitro when compared with controls (Liu et al 2004).

Cytochrome 1A2 inhibition

An experimental model found astragaloside IV inhibited the activity of the cytochrome enzyme CYP1A2 in a rat model, suggesting that astragalus may affect the pharmacokinetics of co-administered medicines and that caution should be exercised, especially in medicines with a narrow therapeutic window (Zhang et al 2013).

CLINICAL USE

Astragalus is a popular Chinese herbal medicine and has been the subject of many clinical trials, mainly published in foreign-language peer-reviewed journals. To provide a more complete description of the evidence available, secondary sources have been used when necessary. As a reflection of clinical practice, astragalus is sometimes tested in combination with other herbal medicines, and also administered by injection in some countries. In these instances the preparation or route of administration is stated in this review.

Viral infection

Owing to its immunomodulatary actions, astragalus is widely used for preventing and treating various viral infections. A popular use is as a preventive treatment against common colds and influenza. To date, scientific evidence is scant to confirm effectiveness, although one review stated that astragalus has been tested in clinical trials in China, reducing the incidence and shortening the duration of the common cold (Murray 1995).

A 2013 systematic review found that astragalus reduced the incidence of upper respiratory tract infections in children with nephrotic syndrome, a very common complication in this patient group (Zhou et al 2013).

Viral myocarditis

The effect of astragalus on heart function has been the subject of several investigations and, most recently, a Cochrane systematic review, which analysed studies of Chinese herbs used in viral myocarditis. It concluded that astragalus significantly improves cardiac function, arrhythmia and creatinine kinase levels (Liu et al 2012). The review assessed data from 20 randomised controlled trials (RCTs) that used a variety of single preparations of astragalus as well as combination therapy across a range of dosage forms from decoction to injection. Where possible, comparable studies were included in a meta-analysis which revealed that astragalus injection had a significant positive effect on patients with abnormal electrocardiograms, especially the S-T segment. The authors concluded that the studies which met the inclusion criteria for the review were overall of poor quality in terms of design, reporting and methodology.

Cardiovascular disease

Congestive heart failure

Some of the clinical signs and symptoms recognised as indicators for this medicine by TCM practitioners suggest that the herb may be useful for congestive heart failure. Recent positive results obtained in clinical studies have reinforced this possibility.

Two clinical trials investigated continuous IV administration of astragalus. One study, involving 19 patients, found that after 2 weeks' continuous administration of astragaloside IV, major symptoms were alleviated in 15 patients. Treatment produced a positive inotropic effect and improved left ventricular modelling and ejection function (Luo et al 1995). The second study, involving 38 patients with congestive heart failure who were administered astragalus 24 g IV for 2 weeks, found that 13.6% had significantly shortened ventricular late potentials (Shi et al 1991).

IN COMBINATION

Huang-qi, a traditional Chinese medicine combination of astragalus root, licorice root and zizyphus fruit, has historically and prolifically been used and studied for the treatment of congestive heart failure. However a systematic review of 62 RCTs and quasi-RCT human trials found that, while the results seem promising for huang-qi injections, the overall methodological quality of the studies was poorly described (Fu et al 2011).

Angina pectoris

Two clinical studies have suggested that astragalus may be an effective treatment for angina pectoris. One study used Doppler echocardiography to study the action of astragalus on left ventricular function in 20 patients with angina pectoris. Treatment resulted in increased cardiac output after 2 weeks, but no improvement in left ventricular diastolic function (Lei et al 1994). One Chinese study reported 92 patients with ischaemic heart disease who were successfully treated with astragalus as measured by electrocardiogram readings. Results obtained with the herb were considered superior to those obtained with nifedipine (Li et al 1995).

Stroke

Astragalus membranaceus has an established history of use in China to assist recovery after stroke. Several clinical trials have been undertaken in China to explore the mechanism of action and to measure the effect; however they have not met the standards of the International Conference on Harmonization and Good Clinical Practice guidelines, and they used positive controls (C Chen et al 2012). A more robust trial with a sample size of 68 subjects has demonstrated that, when stroke patients are administered astragalus within 24 hours of the stroke, their functional independent outcome measures, such as dressing, eating and bladder control, were significantly improved when compared to controls at 4 and 12 weeks after the event. The researchers speculate that this may be due to the anti-inflammatory and antioxidant actions of astragalus, therefore reducing oedema (C Chen et al 2012). However inflammatory biomarkers such as erythrocyte sedimentation rate and C-reactive protein were not consistently measured after 7 days.

Cancer

Astragalus is used in cancer patients to enhance the effectiveness of chemotherapy and reduce associated side effects. It is additionally used to enhance immune function.

Few details are available of clinical studies looking at the potential for astragalus to alter patient survival outcomes, as most information has been published in non-English journals. However, two clinical studies are worth mentioning: they suggest that intravenously administered astragalus may have potential benefit as adjunctive therapy when given with chemotherapy. In one randomised study of 120 cancer patients receiving chemotherapy, IV astragalus extract was administered daily (20 mL in 250 mL normal saline), and tumour growth was slowed compared to controls (Duan & Wang 2002). Four treatment cycles were administered lasting 21 days each. Unfortunately, no further details are available about this study.

Another randomised study investigated IV astragalus in 60 patients with advanced non-small-cell lung cancer (Zou & Liu 2003). This time 2–3 treatment cycles were given of 21–18 days each. The mean remission rate was 5.4 months in the herbal-treated group vs 3.3 months in the untreated group, and the 1-year survival rate was 46.75% with herbal treatment vs 30.0% without. All differences were considered statistically significant. Once again, further details are not available in English.

Colorectal cancer

According to a 2005 Cochrane systematic review, astragalus may be a useful adjunct to chemotherapy in colorectal cancer as it reduces treatment side effects. The review assessed various Chinese herbal medicines taken in combination with chemotherapy for colorectal cancer for their ability to reduce common side effects of chemotherapy, such as nausea, vomiting, sore mouth, diarrhoea, hepatotoxicity, myelosuppression and immunosuppression (Taixiang et al 2005). Four trials were analysed: adjunctive treatment with astragalus was compared with chemotherapy alone in three trials, and with two other Chinese herbal treatments in the fourth trial. Overall, herbal treatment resulted in a significant reduction in the proportion of patients who experienced nausea and vomiting when decoctions of huang-qi (astragalus) compounds were given in addition to chemotherapy. There was also a decrease in the rate of leucopenia (white blood cell count $< 3 \times 10^9$/L) and increased proportions of T-lymphocyte subsets: CD3, CD4 and CD8 with no significant effects on immunoglobulins G, A or M. The authors concluded that astragalus may stimulate immunocompetent cells and decrease chemotherapy side effects; however a definitive conclusion could not be made because of the studies' methodological limitations. Additionally, no evidence of harm was identified with use of the Chinese herbal treatment in these studies.

Prostate cancer (in combination)

Although no human studies could be located, encouraging results were obtained from an in vitro study investigating the effects of a proprietary product known as Equiguard on prostate cancer cells. It is prepared according to TCM principles and contains standardised extracts of nine herbs: herb *Epimedium brevicornum maxim* (stem and leaves), *Radix Morindae officinalis* (root), *Fructus rosae laevigatae* Michx (fruit), *Rubus chingii* Hu (fruit), *Schisandra chinensis* (Turz.) Baill (fruit), *Ligustrum lucidum* Ait (fruit), *Cuscuta chinensis* Lam (seed), *Psoralea corylifolia* L. (fruit) and *Astragalus membranaceus* (root). It is used in TCM to restore Qi in the urogenital region. The product was shown to significantly reduce cancer cell growth, induce apoptosis, suppress expression of the androgen receptor and lower intracellular and secreted prostate-specific antigen (Hsieh et al 2002).

Chronic kidney disease

Astragalus is one of the most commonly prescribed Chinese herbs in chronic kidney disease. Pharmacological studies have confirmed that different constituents in the herb have effects which could be valuable in chronic kidney disease such as antioxidant, diuretic and anti-inflammatory effects, and studies in rat models indicate that astragalus decreases glomerular hyperperfusion and improves kidney function (Li & Wang 2005).

A meta-analysis of 14 RCTs involving 524 Chinese patients with primary nephrotic syndrome showed that treatment with astragalus for 1–3 months could increase the therapeutic effect of prednisone and immunosuppressants (reported in Li & Wang 2005). Herbal treatment decreased proteinuria and increased levels of total cholesterol and albumin. Although further details are unavailable, these results are encouraging.

A 2011 meta-analysis measuring the clinical effect of astragalus injection in diabetic nephropathy corroborated these results (M Li et al 2011). The pooled results from 25 clinical studies that included 945 patients and 859 control subjects demonstrated that astragalus injection, when compared with controls, provided greater renal protection and systemic improvement by reducing serum urea nitrogen, serum creatinine, urine protein and urine microalbumin; and increasing serum albumin in patients with diabetic nephropathy compared with controls (Okuda et al 2012).

A Cochrane systematic review compared the efficacy of pharmaceutical treatments and TCM for preventing infections in nephrotic syndrome in adults (Wu et al 2012). While the authors concluded that huang-qi granules (astragalus) may have positive effects on the prevention of infection in children with nephrotic syndrome, the methodological quality of all studies was poor, and there was no compelling evidence on the effectiveness of the intervention.

The efficacy of astragalus injection for hypertensive-induced renal damage was examined by systematic review of five RCTs comparing astragalus to placebo and antihypertensives (Sun et al 2012). Although the individual studies were considered to have poor methodological quality, the pooled data indicate that astragalus has protective effects for this patient group.

Glucose regulation

In a randomised trial of pregnant women with gestational diabetes (n = 84), the treatment group, who received insulin plus astragalus, had better outcomes for malondialdehyde, superoxide dismutase, renal function and blood lipids compared to the control group who received insulin alone (Liang et al 2009).

Adaptogenic tonic – traditional use

Within traditional Chinese herbal medicine, astragalus is used to invigorate and tonify Qi and the blood, as an adaptogen, for severe blood loss, fatigue, anorexia, organ prolapse, chronic diarrhoea, shortness of breath, sweating and to enhance recuperation (Mills & Bone 2000).

> ***Clinical note — The concept of an adaptogen is foreign to Western medicine but often used in traditional medicine***
>
> The term 'adaptogen' was first coined by N. Lazarev in the Soviet Union in the mid 20th century, although the concept has been used for centuries in traditional herbal systems. Adaptogens are considered natural bioregulators that increase the ability of the organism to adapt to environmental factors and to avoid damage from such factors. Herbal medicines with adaptogenic activity are used when extremes of physical or emotional activity are present, environmental influences are severe or allostatic load has developed over time. The aim of treatment is to improve the patient's endurance and ability to deal with these changes in a healthy way, and for abnormal parameters to shift towards normal. The best-known example of a plant adaptogen is ginseng (*Panax ginseng*), but others are also well established, such as *Schisandra chinensis*, *Eleutherococcus senticosus* (Siberian ginseng), *Astragalus membranaceus* and *Withania somnifera* (see Siberian ginseng).

Cholesterol reduction (in combination with other herbs)

A randomised, double-blind clinical trial compared the effects of a traditional Chinese herbal medicine combination known as jian yan ling (which includes astragalus as a main ingredient) to a placebo in 128 hyperlipidaemic patients. After 3 months' treatment it was found that total cholesterol, triglyceride, apoproteins and lipoprotein-a levels were significantly reduced in the treatment group compared with placebo.

Asthma (in combination with other herbs and minerals)

A herbal combination of *Astragalus membranaceus, Codonopsis pilulosa* and *Glycyrrhiza uralensis* was investigated in an open study for effects on airway responsiveness. Twenty-eight patients with asthma were treated with the herbal combination for 6 weeks, after which values for forced vital capacity, forced expiratory volume and peak expiratory flow were all higher than at baseline (Wang et al 1998).

In a 6-week randomised, double-blinded placebo-controlled trial of a proprietary preparation of astragalus and zinc, the intensity of rhinorrhoea was significantly improved in seasonal allergic rhinitis in 48 patients (Matkovic 2010).

Memory deficits (in combination with other herbs)

In TCM, invigorating Qi and warming Yang are believed to have a beneficial therapeutic effect on some brain diseases, such as senile dementia. Some studies have been conducted to determine the outcome of following this ancient principle.

DOSAGE RANGE

- Dried root: 2–30 g/day.
- Liquid extract (1:2) or solid-dose equivalent: 4.5–8.5 mL/day.
- Decoction: 8–12 g divided into two doses daily on an empty stomach.

TOXICITY

Animal studies have shown that the herb has a wide safety margin.

ADVERSE REACTIONS

None known.

SIGNIFICANT INTERACTIONS

Interactions are theoretical and based on the herb's pharmacodynamic effects; therefore clinical significance is unclear and remains to be confirmed. There is some evidence that a component in astragalus inhbits CYP1A2 in vivo but no human studies have tested whether the effect is clinically significant for astragalus extract. Meanwhile, clinicians should supervise patients taking drugs with a narrow therapeutic index chiefly metabolised by CYP1A2 to avoid drug interactions.

Aciclovir

Possibly enhances antiviral activity against herpes simplex type 1 (Stargrove et al 2008) — adjunctive use may be beneficial.

Immunosuppressant medication

Reduced drug activity is theoretically possible, as immunostimulant activity has been demonstrated — use caution.

Positive inotropic drugs

Additive effects are theoretically possible with intravenous administration of astragalus, based on positive inotropic activity identified in clinical studies. The clinical significance of these findings for oral dose forms is unknown — observe patients using high-dose astragalus preparations.

Cyclophosphamide

Adjunctive treatment with astragalus may have beneficial effects in regard to improving patient wellbeing and reducing adverse effects associated with treatment, such as nausea and vomiting — only use combination under professional supervision.

Practice points/Patient counselling

- Astragalus is widely used as an immunostimulant medicine to reduce the incidence of the common cold and influenza and is sometimes used to improve immune responses to other viral infections, such as herpes simplex type 1.
- It is also used to enhance recuperation and reduce fatigue, and reduce the side effects of chemotherapy while improving immune function.
- Astragalus is a commonly prescribed Chinese herb in chronic kidney disease.
- According to TCM practice it is widely used to invigorate and tonify Qi and the blood, and as an important adaptogen.
- Some evidence suggests it enhances digestion, improves heart function in viral myocarditis, lowers cholesterol and fasting blood sugar and has hepatoprotective activity.
- Under the TCM system, astragalus is not used during periods of acute infection.
- In clinical practice it is often used in combination with other herbs, such as *Bupleurum chinense*, *Scutellaria baicalensis* and *Codonopsis pilulosa*. As such, most clinical trials have tested combination formulas.
- Astragalus injections are protective against chronic kidney conditions such as diabetic nephropathy and renal hypertenstion.
- Astragalus may improve the contractility of the heart muscle and prolong the S-T segment in patients with viral myocarditis.
- Astragalus root by oral and nasopharyngeal administration improves functional outcomes in stroke patients, when administered within 24 h of the stroke.

CONTRAINDICATIONS AND PRECAUTIONS

According to the principles of TCM, astragalus should not be used during the acute stages of an infection.

PREGNANCY USE

Safety is unknown, although no evidence of fetal damage has been reported in animal studies (Mills & Bone 2005). There were no reported safety concerns in the trial by Liang et al (2009) of pregnant women with gestational diabetes.

PATIENTS' FAQs

What will this herb do for me?

Astragalus appears to have numerous biological effects, such as digestive and immune system modulation, as a hypoglycaemic agent and cardiac tonic. Research suggests that it may have a role to play in recovery from viral infection, in chronic kidney disease and as an adjunct to chemotherapy treatment for cancer.

When will it start working?

This will depend on the indication and dose; some studies have shown that effects can begin within 2 weeks.

Are there any safety issues?

Overall the herb appears to be safe, although it has the potential to interact with some medicines. Professional supervision is advised for people receiving chemotherapy and considering using this herb.

REFERENCES

Castillo C et al. An analysis of the antihypertensive properties of 3-nitropropionic acid, a compound from plants in the genus *Astragalus*. Arch Inst Cardiol Mex 63.1 (1993): 11–6.

Chang Y et al. The experimental study of *Astragalus membranaceus* on meridian tropsim: The distribution study of astragaloside IV in rat tissues. J of Chromat 911 (2012): 71–75.

Chen CC, et al. Chinese Herb *Astragalus membranaceus* Enhances Recovery of Hemorrhagic Stroke: Double-Blind, Placebo-Controlled, Randomized Study. Evid Based Complement Alternat Med. 2012;2012:708452.

Chen W et al. Improvement of myocardial glycolipid metabolic disorder in diabetic hamster with *Astragalus* polysaccharides treatment. Mol Biol Rep. 2012 Jul;39(7):7609–15.

Chu DT, et al. Immunotherapy with Chinese medicinal herbs. I. Immune restoration of local xenogeneic graft-versus-host reaction in cancer patients by fractionated *Astragalus membranaceus* in vitro. J Clin Lab Immunol 25.3 (1988): 119–23.

Cui R et al. Suppressive effect of *Astragalus membranaceus* Bunge on chemical hepatocarcinogenesis in rats. Cancer Chemother. Pharmacol 51.1 (2003): 75–80.

Duan P, Wang ZM. Clinical study on effect of Astragalus in efficacy enhancing and toxicity reducing of chemotherapy in patients of malignant tumor. Zhongguo Zhong Xi Yi Jie He Za Zhi 22.7 (2002): 515–17.

Duke JA. Dr Duke's phytochemical and ethnobotanical databases. US Department of Agriculture, Agricultural Research Service, National Germplasm Resources Laboratory. Beltsville Agricultural Research Center, Beltsville, MD Online. Available www.ars-grin.gov/duke March 2003.

Fu S, et al. (2011) Huangqi injection (a traditional Chinese patent medicine) for chronic heart failure: a systematic review. PLoS ONE 6(5): e19604.

Guo FC et al. In vitro fermentation characteristics of two mushroom species, an herb, and their polysaccharide fractions, using chicken cecal contents as inoculum. Poult Sci 82.10 (2003): 1608–15.

Guo FC et al. Effects of mushroom and herb polysaccharides on cellular and humoral immune responses of *Eimeria tenella*-infected chickens. Poult Sci 83.7 (2004): 1124–32.

Hong CY, et al. *Astragalus membranaceus* stimulates human sperm motility in vitro. Am J Chin Med 20.3–4 (1992): 289–94.

Hsieh TC et al. Effects of herbal preparation Equiguard™ on hormone-responsive and hormone-refractory prostate carcinoma cells: mechanistic studies. Int J Oncol 20.4 (2002): 681–9.

Huang C, et al. Reversal of P-glycoprotein-mediated multidrug resistance of human hepatic cancer cells by Astragaloside II. J Pharm Pharmacol. 2012 Dec;64(12):1741–50.

Huang L et al. *Astragalus membranaceus* lectin (AML) induces caspase-dependent apoptosis in human leukemia cells. Cell Proliferation 45.1 (2012):15–21.

Jiao Y, et al. Influence of flavonoid of *Astragalus membranaceus*'s stem and leaves on the function of cell mediated immunity in mice. Zhongguo Zhong Xi Yi Jie He Za Zhi 19.6 (1999): 356–8.
Jin R et al. Effect of shi-ka-ron and Chinese herbs on cytokine production of macrophage in immunocompromised mice. Am J Chin Med 22.3–4 (1994): 255–66.
Jin R et al. Studies on pharmacological junctions of hairy root of *Astragalus membranaceus*. Zhongguo Zhong Yao Za Zhi 24.10 (1999): 619–21, 639.
Kurashige S, et al. Effects of astragali radix extract on carcinogenesis, cytokine production, and cytotoxicity in mice treated with a carcinogen, N-butyl-N-butanolnitrosoamine. Cancer Invest 17.1 (1999): 30–5.
Kuo Y, et al. . *Astragalus membranaceus* flavonoids (AMF) ameliorate chronic fatigue syndrome induced by food intake restriction plus forced swimming. J of Ethnopharm 122.1 (2009): 28–34.
Lau BH et al. Chinese medicinal herbs inhibit growth of murine renal cell carcinoma. Cancer Biother 9.2 (1994): 153–61.
Lei ZY, et al. Action of *Astragalus membranaceus* on left ventricular function of angina pectoris. Zhongguo Zhong Xi Yi Jie He Za Zhi 14.4 (1994): 195, 199–202.
Li SQ, et al. Clinical observation on the treatment of ischemic heart disease with *Astragalus membranaceus*. Zhongguo Zhong Xi Yi Jie He Za Zhi 15.2 (1995): 77–80.
Li X, Wang H. Chinese Herbal Medicine in the Treatment of Chronic Kidney Disease. Advances in Chronic Kidney Disease 12 (3) (2005): 276–81.
Li S, Zhang Y. Characterization and renal protective effect of a polysaccharide from *Astragalus membranaceus*. Carbo Polymers 78.2 (2009): 343–348.
Li C et al. Inhibitory effect of Astragalus polysaccharides on apoptosis of pancreatic beta-cells mediated by Fas in diabetes mellitus rats. Zhong Yao Cai. 2011; Oct;34(10):1579–82.
Li M, et al. Meta-analysis of the clinical value of *Astragalus membranaceus* in diabetic nephropathy. J Ethnopharmacol. 2011;133(2):412–9.
Liang HY et al. Clinical evaluation of the antioxidant activity of astragalus in women with gestational diabetes. Nan Fang Yi Ke Da Xue Xue Bao. 2009 Jul;29(7):1402–4.
Liu J et al. Effects of several Chinese herbal aqueous extracts on human sperm motility in vitro. Andrologia 36.2 (2004): 78–83.
Liu M, et al. Astragalus polysaccharide improves insulin sensitivity in KKAy mice: Regulation of PKB/GLUT4 signaling in skeletal muscle. Journal of Ethnopharmacology. 127.8 (2010): 32–37.
Liu JP, et al. Herbal medicines for viral myocarditis. Cochrane Database of Syst Rev 11. (2012): CD003711.
Lonkova, I. Biotechnological production of valuable plant pharmaceuticals: anticancer agents. Advances in Bulgarian Science (2010) 1: 5.
Luo HM, et al. Nuclear cardiology study on effective ingredients of *Astragalus membranaceus* in treating heart failure. Zhongguo Zhong Xi Yi Jie He Za Zhi 15.12 (1995): 707–9.
Luo Y et al. Astragaloside IV protects against ischemic brain injury in a murine model of transient focal ischemia. Neurosci Lett 363.3 (2004): 218–23.
Mao XX, et al. Hypoglycemic effect of polysaccharide enriched extract of Astragalus membranaceus in diet induced insulin resistant C57BL/6J mice and its potential mechanism. Phytomedicine 2009: 16, 416–425.
Matkovic Z. Efficacy and safety of *Astragalus membranaceus* in the treatment of patients with seasonal allergic rhinitis. Phyto Research 24.2(2010): 175–181.
Mills S, Bone K. Principles and practice of phytotherapy. London: Churchill Livingstone, 2000.
Mills S, Bone K. The essential guide to herbal safety. Edinburgh: Churchill Livingstone, 2005.
Murray M. The healing power of herbs. Rocklin CA: Prima Health, 1995.
Niu Y. Structural analysis and bioactivity of a polysaccharide from the roots of *Astragalus membranaceus* (Fisch) Bge. var. mongolicus (Bge.) Hsiao. Food Chemistry 128.3 (2011): 620–626.
Okuda M et al. Beneficial effect of *Astragalus membranaceus* on estimated glomerular filtration rate in patients with progressive chronic kidney disease. HK J of Neph 14.1(2012): 17–23.
Schepetkin IA, Quinn MT. Botanical polysaccharides: Macrophage immunomodulation and therapeutic potential. Int Immunopharmacol 6 (2006): 317–33.
Shen H, et al. *Astragalus membranaceus* prevents airway hyperreactivity in mice related to Th2 response inhibition. J of Ethnopharm 116.2 (2008): 363–369.
Shi HM, et al. Primary research on the clinical significance of ventricular late potentials (VLPs), and the impact of mexiletine, lidocaine and *Astragalus membranaceus* on VLPs. Zhong Xi Yi Jie He Za Zhi 11.5 (1991): 259, 265–7.
Song J et al. A combination of Chinese herbs, *Astragalus membranaceus* var. mongholicus and *Angelica sinensis*, improved renal microvascular insufficiency in 5/6 nephrectomized rats. Vasc Pharm 50.5 (2009): 185–193.
Stargrove M, et al. Herb, nutrient and drug interactions. St Louis: Mosby, 2008.
Sugiura H et al. Effects of exercise in the growing stage in mice and of *Astragalus membranaceus* on immune functions. Nippon Eiseigaku Zasshi 47.6 (1993): 1021–31.
Sun Y et al. Preliminary observations on the effects of the Chinese medicinal herbs *Astragalus membranaceus* and *Ligustrum lucidum* on lymphocyte blastogenic responses. J Biol Response Mod 2.3 (1983): 227–37.
Sun Y et al. Polysaccharides from *Astragalus membranaceus* promote phagocytosis and superoxide anion (O2–) production by coelomocytes from sea cucumber *Apostichopus japonicus* in vitro. Comp Biochem and Phys Part C: 147.3 (2008): 293–298.
Sun T, et al. *Astragalus* injection for hypertensive renal damage: a systematic review. Evid Based Complement Alternat Med. 2012;2012:929025.
Taixiang W, et al. Chinese medical herbs for chemotherapy side effects in colorectal cancer patients. Cochrane Database Syst Rev 1 (2005): CD004540.
Wang H, et al. The effect of herbal medicine including *Astragalus membranaceus* (fisch) bge, Codonopsis pilulosa and Glycyrrhiza uralensis fisch on airway responsiveness. Zhonghua Jie He He Hu Xi Za Zhi 21.5 (1998): 287–8.
Wojcikowski K, et al. Beneficial effect of *Astragalus membranaceus* on estimated glomerular filtration rate in patients with progressive chronic kidney disease. Phyto Research 24.6 (2009): 875–884.

Wu HM, et al. Interventions for preventing infection in nephrotic syndrome. Cochrane Database Syst Rev. 2012 Apr 18;4:CD003964.
Yan Q, et al. Characterisation of a novel monomeric lectin (AML) from *Astragalus membranaceus* with anti-proliferative activity. Food Chemistry 122.3 (2010): 589–595.
Yang DZ [Effect of Astragalus membranaceus on myoelectric activity of small intestine.] Zhongguo Zhong Xi Yi Jie He Za Zhi. 1993;13: 582, 616–7.
Zhang ZL, et al. Hepatoprotective effects of astraglus root. J Ethnopharmacol 30.2 (1990): 145–9.
Zhang WJ, et al. Regulation of the fibrinolytic potential of cultured human umbilical vein endothelial cells: astragaloside IV downregulates plasminogen activator inhibitor-1 and upregulates tissue-type plasminogen activator expression. J Vasc Res 34.4 (1997): 273–80.
Zhang BQ et al. Effects of *Astragalus membranaceus* and its main components on the acute phase endothelial dysfunction induced by homocysteine. Vascular Pharmacology 46.4 (2007): 278–85.
Zhang J et al. Systematic review of the renal protective effect of *Astragalus membranaceus* (root) on diabetic nephropathy in animal models. Journal of Ethnopharmacology. 2009, 126(2):189–196.
Zhang YH et al, Astragaloside IV inhibited the activity of CYP1A2 in liver microsomes and influenced theophylline pharmokinetics in rats. J Pharm Pharmacol 65.1(2013): 149–55.
Zhao K S et al. Enhancement of the immuneresponse in mice by *Astragalus membranaceus* extracts. Immunopharmacology 20.3 (1990): 225–33.
Zhao KW, Kong HY. Effect of Astragalan on secretion of tumor necrosis factors in human peripheral blood mononuclear cells. Zhongguo Zhong Xi Yi Jie He Za Zhi 13.5 (1993): 259, 263–5.
Zhou C et al. Astragalus in the Prevention of Upper Respiratory Tract Infection in Children with Nephrotic Syndrome: Evidence-Based Clinical Practice (Review). Evidence-Based Comp and Alt Med 2013 (2013): 352130.
Zou YH, Liu XM. Effect of astragalus injection combined with chemotherapy on quality of life in patients with advanced non-small cell lung cancer. Zhongguo Zhong Xi Yi Jie He Za Zhi 23.10 (2003): 733–5.
Zou F et al 2009. Astragalus polysaccharides alleviates glucose toxicity and restores glucose homeostasis in diabetic states via activation of AMPK. Acta Pharmacol Sin. 2009 Dec;30(12):1607–15.
Zou F et al. *Radix astragali* (huangqi) as a treatment for defective hypoglycemia counterregulation in diabetes. Am J Chin Med. 2010;38(6):1027–38.

Black cohosh

HISTORICAL NOTE Native Americans first used black cohosh many centuries ago, mainly as a treatment for female reproductive problems, including pain during childbirth, uterine colic and dysmenorrhoea, and also for fatigue, snakebite and arthritis. It was widely adopted by European settlers, eventually becoming a very popular treatment in Europe for gynaecological conditions. It was also a favourite of the Eclectic physicians in North America, who also used it for female reproductive conditions, myalgia, neuralgia and rheumatic conditions.

COMMON NAME

Black cohosh

OTHER NAMES

Baneberry, black snakeroot, bugbane, rattle-root, rattle-top, rattleweed, squaw-root, traubensilberkerze, wanzenkraut

BOTANICAL NAME/FAMILY

Cimicifuga racemosa now known as *Actaea racemosa* Linnaeus (family Ranunculaceae)

PLANT PARTS USED

Rhizome and root

> ***Clinical note — Selective oestrogen receptor modulators (SERMs)***
> These are compounds that, in contrast to pure oestrogen agonists or antagonists, have a mixed and selective pattern of oestrogen agonist–antagonist activity, which largely depends on the tissue targeted. The therapeutic aim of using these substances is to produce oestrogenic actions in those tissues in which it would be beneficial (e.g. bone, brain, liver), and have either no activity or antagonistic activity in tissues, such as breast and endometrium, where oestrogenic actions (like cellular proliferation) might be deleterious. They are a relatively new class of pharmacologically active agents and are being used by women who cannot tolerate pharmaceutical HRT or are unwilling to use it. The most actively studied SERMs are tamoxifen and raloxifen (Hernandez & Pluchino 2003).

CHEMICAL COMPONENTS

Black cohosh contains numerous triterpene glycosides, including cimicifugoside, actein and 27-deoxyactein, *N*-methylcytosine and other quinolizidine alkaloids, phenolic acids, including isoferulic and fukinolic acid, salicylic acids, resins, fatty acids and tannins.

Until recently, the isoflavone formononetin was believed to be a pharmacologically important constituent of the herb; however, testing of numerous samples has failed to detect it in any sample, including the commercial products Remifemin (Schaper & Brummer GmbH & Co. KG, Salzgitter, Germany) and CimiPure (Kennelly et al 2002).

MAIN ACTIONS

Hormone modulation

The hormonal effects of black cohosh are believed to be the result of complex synergistic actions of several components, particularly the triterpene glycosides. Experimental and clinical evidence confirms that black cohosh does not contain natural oestrogens and does not exert significant oestrogenic activity, although some components may exert selective oestrogen receptor modulation. This has been confirmed in studies involving women where no oestrogenic effects on mammary glands or the endometrium were observed (Wuttke et al 2014).

Preclinical studies to determine how black cohosh works have yielded conflicting results, but several hypotheses have been proposed. It acts either (1) as a selective oestrogen receptor modulator (SERM); (2) through serotonergic pathways; (3) as an antioxidant; or (4) on inflammatory pathways (Ruhlen et al 2008). There is evidence to support all these actions.

One study suggests that black cohosh works as a SERM, augmented by central nervous effects (Viereck et al 2005). Results from studies found that it has SERM activity with a lower potency but comparable efficacy to that of 17 beta-oestradiol (Bolle et al 2007). It has no action in the uterus, but beneficial effects in the hypothalamopituitary unit and in bone (Seidlova-Wuttke et al 2003). This has been confirmed in a double-blind, randomised, multicentre study (Wuttke et al 2003). In that study, the standardised black cohosh extract BNO 1055 was equipotent with conjugated oestrogens in reducing menopausal symptoms, had beneficial effects on bone metabolism and significantly increased vaginal superficial cells; however, it did not exert uterotrophic activity. Most recently, a 2013 systematic review concluded that black cohosh does not appear to influence circulating levels of oestradiol, FSH or LH, nor to exert oestrogenic effects on breast, endometrial or vaginal tissues. However, it does appear to display oestrogenic activity on bone by stimulating bone formation and inhibiting bone breakdown (Fritz et al 2013). This validates the understanding of black cohosh as a SERM.

Overall, it is generally agreed that black cohosh reduces LH secretion in menopausal women. This has been confirmed in a human study and is believed to be the result of at least three different active constituents acting synergistically (Duker et al 1991). Reductions in LH have also been demonstrated in PCOS patients experiencing infertility (Kamel 2013).

Anti-inflammatory

Animal studies have identified some anti-inflammatory activity (Hirabayashi et al 1995). More recently, black cohosh extracts have demonstrated *in vitro* anti-inflammatory activity by inhibiting IL-6 and TNF-α, IFN-γ (Schmid et al 2009a) and nitric oxide (Schmid et al 2009b).

Serotonergic

In vitro tests identified compounds in a black cohosh methanol extract that were capable of strong binding to the 5-HT_{1A}, 5-HT_{1D}, and 5-HT_7 receptor subtypes (Burdette et al 2003). Further investigation by these authors found that the components functioned as a partial agonist of the 5-HT_7 receptor. Further investigation has identified triterpenoids and phenolic acids which bind weakly to the 5-HT_7 receptor and a new constituent, $N\omega$-methylserotonin, which demonstrates strong 5-HT_7 receptor binding affinity, together with induction of cAMP and inhibition of serotonin re-uptake (Powell et al 2008). As 5-HT_7 receptors are present in the hypothalamus, it has been speculated that serotonergic activity in the hypothalamic thermoregulatory centres may be responsible for the reduction of hot flushes, although the precise mechanism of action remains unclear.

Dopaminergic

It is suggested that the effects of *A. racemosa* may be due to dopaminergic activity, because black cohosh extract BNO 1055 displayed dopaminergic activity with a D_2-receptor assay (Jarry et al 2003). Considering that dopaminergic drugs reduce some symptoms (e.g. hot flushes) associated with menopause, this theory is feasible; however, further studies are required to explain why black cohosh is devoid of the typical side effects associated with dopaminergic drugs (Borrelli & Ernst 2008).

Cytochromes and P-glycoprotein

Clinical studies have found no indication that Black cohosh affects CYP 3A, 1A2, 2E1 or 2D6 (Gurley et al 2005, 2006a, 2006b, 2008, 2012, Izzo 2012, Pang et al 2011).

Extremely high doses of black cohosh (1090 mg equivalent to 0.2% triterpene glycosides, twice daily for 28 days) demonstrated a minor inhibitory effect on CYP2D6; however, these results are unlikely to be clinically significant due to the high doses and negligible effect. Other studies have demonstrated that recommended doses (40 mg and 80 mg) did not modulate P-gp or CYP3A activity (Borrelli & Ernst 2008, Gurley et al 2006b, Shord et al 2009).

OTHER ACTIONS

Black cohosh serves as an agonist and competitive ligand for the mu-opioid receptor (Rhyu et al 2006), which provides some rationale for the herb's traditional reputation as a treatment for painful conditions such as dysmenorrhoea and arthritis.

A dose-dependent antihypertensive effect was identified for a triterpene found in black cohosh (actein) in animal tests. The clinical significance of this finding for humans using black cohosh root is unknown (Genazzani & Sorrentino 1962). *In vitro* research has demonstrated endothelium-independent vasorelaxation probably due to calcium channel activity (Kim et al 2011), suggesting possible benefit for vascular conditions.

Black cohosh is traditionally thought to act as a tonic and nervous system restorative medicine and to exert antispasmodic and anti-inflammatory activity.

CLINICAL USE

Most clinical research has investigated the use of various black cohosh preparations as either stand-alone treatments or in combination with other herbal medicines, notably St John's wort in the treatment of menopausal symptoms. More recently, investigation has begun to determine whether black cohosh has a role in female infertility.

Menopausal symptoms

Most clinical research on black cohosh has focused on its potential to prevent or decrease the severity of various menopausal symptoms. It can be described as the non-oestrogenic alternative treatment used for menopausal symptoms. Most trials test the commercial preparation of black cohosh known as Remifemin, which is standardised to contain triterpene glycosides (0.8–1.2 mg/tablet), and the extract BNO 1055, an aqueous ethanolic extract (58% vol/vol), sold as Klimadynon and Menofem (Bionorica AG, Neumarkt, Germany). There has also been some investigation with other black cohosh preparations, mainly in the United States. Overall, results from clinical studies have been positive for reducing the frequency of hot flushes, most consistently with the German/Swiss preparations and less consistently with US American black cohosh products. This is likely to be due to great variations in test dose, with lower doses appearing more effective, and differences in herbal extract quality and chemical profile. It may also be because the identity of many American black cohosh preparations is often unknown and they are on the market as food supplements. It was previously shown that many of them contain Asian *Cimicifuga* species, for which no clinical data are available. Importantly, the HPLC profiles of these Asian species look quite different from those of the species that grew originally in America, whereas the German/Swiss products contain extracts of original black cohosh rhizomes that stem from field-planted crops grown under rigidly controlled conditions (Wuttke et al 2014). Unlike hormone replacement therapy, the effect on menopausal symptoms is due to the presence of dopaminergic, adrenergic and serotonergic compounds and not oestrogen.

Systematic reviews and meta-analyses

Given the number of clinical trials conducted with black cohosh in alleviating menopausal symptoms, there have been a number of systematic reviews and meta-analyses of the evidence.

One of the early reviews was published in 1998 which discussed eight clinical trials and concluded that black cohosh (Remifemin) was a safe and effective alternative to HRT for menopausal patients in whom HRT is contraindicated (Lieberman 1998). Symptoms responding to treatment with black cohosh included hot flushes, vaginal thinning and drying, night sweats, sleep disturbances, anxiety and depression. In 2005, a systematic review, including randomised, controlled trials, open trials and comparison group studies, found that the evidence to date suggests that black cohosh is safe and effective for reducing menopausal symptoms, primarily hot flushes and possibly mood disorders (Geller & Studee 2005). Later reviews by the same research team showed that black cohosh significantly reduced depression and anxiety in all studies reviewed (Geller & Studee 2007). Another more recent systematic review identified seven randomised controlled trials of black cohosh and concluded that it may be beneficial in the treatment of menopausal vasomotor symptoms in some women (Cheema et al 2007).

A 2008 update of a previous systematic review evaluated the clinical evidence for or against the efficacy of black cohosh in alleviating menopausal symptoms. Seventy-two clinical trials were identified, but only six of these, with a total of 1163 peri- and postmenopausal women, met the inclusion criteria. With one exception, the results for each of these trials were positive; yet the authors concluded that the efficacy of black cohosh in reducing menopause symptoms is currently not supported by full conclusive evidence, citing small sample size as a limitation in establishing statistical significance (Borrelli & Ernst 2008). Similarly, a review of 16 eligible studies suggested that there were methodological flaws in many studies making a definitive conclusion difficult. Methodological issues included: lack of uniformity of the drug preparation used, variable outcome measures and lack of a placebo group (Palacio et al 2009).

A 2010 systematic review examined nine RCTs and compared black cohosh preparations to placebo in perimenopausal and postmenopausal women (excluding those with a history of breast cancer) for the frequency of vasomotor symptoms. Seven of these trials demonstrated a significant decrease in frequency of vasomotor symptoms in the treatment group and the combined improvement in these symptoms was 24% (95% CI) in the black cohosh group compared to placebo. Again, this review noted the significant heterogeneity of the trials. Black cohosh was found to be more efficacious in treating menopausal symptoms when given in combination with other botanicals such as St John's wort compared with black cohosh alone (Shams et al 2010). In contrast, a 2012 Cochrane review concluded that stand alone treatment with black cohosh was not superior to placebo for reducing the frequency of hot flushes in peri- and postmenopausal women. The authors analysed results of 16 RCTs involving 2027 women, but cautioned that a definitive conclusion could not be made due to the high level of heterogeneity between the studies. Additionally, due to insufficient data they were unable to pool the results for other menopause-related conditions, such as night sweats, bone health, vulvovaginal symptoms, quality of life and sexuality (Leach & Moore 2012).

A review by Wuttke et al (2014) makes the point that most placebo-controlled clinical trials have demonstrated amelioration of climacteric complaints, particularly hot flushes, and these positive effects have been seen mainly with German/Swiss preparations, whereas three out of four placebo controlled trials using US supplements have produced negative results (Geller et al 2009, Newton et al 2006, Pockaj et al 2006). A difference in dosage is one likely reason as the German/Swiss medications contained 2 × 20 mg CR (*Cimicifuga racemosa*) drug (4–8 mg extract), whereas two negative US American studies administered 15–25-fold the amounts used in the European trials and the third, a more moderate over-dosage. In contrast, the positive American trial used a preparation with a standardised amount of triterpenes (2.5%) which yielded a significant reduction of menopausal symptoms not seen when a triterpene-free extract was given.

There is also concern about the quality and herbal authenticity of US CR products as it has previously been shown that many contain Asian Cimicifuga species which have quite different constituent profiles (based on HPLC comparisons) compared to the CR species that originally grew in America. This is particularly of concern when products are not manufactured in countries that enforce strict GMP conditions.

B

Interestingly, since then another positive study has been published which used a European black cohosh extract (Ze450) in 442 unselected ambulatory female outpatients with menopausal complaints under daily practice conditions (Drewe et al 2013). For the first 3 months, doctors were advised to treat patients with 13 mg/day (high dose, HD) and to continue over additional 6 months either with this treatment or to switch to 6.5 mg/day CR (low dose, LD). The choice of treatment and its dose, however, was fully at the discretion of the doctor. After 3 months treatment with HD, symptom severity (Kupperman Menopause Index, KMI) decreased significantly ($p < 0.001$) from baseline values. Continuation of treatment with HD or LD decreased total KMI and its sub-item scores further (HD, LD: $p < 0.001$). However, more patients (84.9%) responded to HD than to LD (78.4%) and showed an improvement of symptoms ($p = 0.011$).

IN COMBINATION

A number of studies have been conducted investigating the combination of black cohosh and St John's wort for the treatment of symptoms of menopause with mood symptoms. One double-blind, randomised study of 301 women found that 16 weeks of herbal treatment produced a significant 50% reduction in the Menopause Rating Scale score compared with 20% for placebo and a significant 42% reduction in the Hamilton Depression Rating Scale compared with only 13% in the placebo group (Uebelhack et al 2006). Another large-scale ($n = 6141$), prospective, controlled open-label observational study supports the effectiveness and tolerability of black cohosh combined with St John's wort for alleviating menopausal mood symptoms (Briese et al 2007). In another double-blind, randomised, placebo-controlled, multicentre study, 89 peri- or postmenopausal women experiencing menopause symptoms were treated with a combination of St John's wort and black cohosh extract (Gynoplus) or a matched placebo. Hot flushes were significantly lower and HDL levels increased in the Gynoplus group (Chung et al 2007).

It is therefore no surprise that two systematic reviews have concluded that black cohosh is more efficacious in treating menopausal symptoms when given in combination with St John's wort, compared to black cohosh alone (Shams et al 2010, Laakmann et al 2012).

Comparison studies

Numerous comparison studies have been conducted utilising various pharmaceutical agents. One pilot study demonstrated that BNO 1055 is able to reduce oestrogen deficiency symptoms to the same degree as conjugated oestrogens (Wuttke et al 2006b). A randomised, double-blind, controlled 3-month study to investigate the efficacy–safety balance of black cohosh (Remifemin) in comparison with tibolone in 244 symptomatic menopausal Chinese women gave remarkable results. The efficacy of both treatments was similar and statistically significant. The safety for both groups was also good. However, the tolerability profile was greatly in favour of the herbal treatment with a significantly lower incidence of adverse events (Bai et al 2007).

An RCT of 120 healthy women with menopausal symptoms found, when compared with fluoxetine, black cohosh was more effective for treating hot flushes and night sweats by the third month, whereas fluoxetine was more effective for reducing mood change according to the Beck's Depression Scale (Beck et al 2003). Monthly scores for hot flushes and night sweats decreased significantly in both groups; however, black cohosh reduced monthly scores for hot flushes and night sweats to a greater extent than did fluoxetine. At the end of the sixth month of treatment, black cohosh reduced the hot flush score by 85%, compared with a 62% result for fluoxetine (Oktem et al 2007).

Wuttke et al (2003) conducted a double-blind, randomised, multicentre study which compared the effects of BNO 1055 (40 mg/day) to conjugated oestrogens (0.6 mg/day) and placebo on climacteric complaints, bone metabolism and endometrium (Wuttke et al 2003). The study involved 62 postmenopausal women who took their allocated treatment for 3 months. BNO 1055 proved to be equipotent to conjugated oestrogens and superior to a placebo in reducing climacteric symptoms, and both active treatments produced beneficial effects on bone metabolism. Vaginal superficial cells increased with both active treatments; however, BNO 1055 had no effect on endometrial thickness, which was significantly increased by conjugated oestrogens.

Commission E has approved the use of this herb as a treatment for menopausal symptoms (Blumenthal et al 2000). Similarly, the World Health Organization (WHO) recognises its use for the 'treatment of climacteric symptoms such as hot flushes, profuse sweating, sleeping disorders and nervous irritability'. The North American Menopause Society recommends black cohosh, in conjunction with lifestyle approaches, as a treatment option for women with mild menopause-related symptoms (North American Menopause Society 2004). In herbal practice generally, menopausal symptoms are usually addressed using a combination of herbs, supplements and dietary and lifestyle advice.

Weight gain

Rat models demonstrate that BNO 1055 black cohosh extract decreases enhanced pituitary LH secretion, attenuates body weight gain and intraabdominal fat accumulation, lowers fasting plasma insulin and has no effects on uterine mass. The effects on plasma lipids are complex and are characterised by an increase of LDL cholesterol and decrease of triglyceride levels, which is in contrast to the effects of oestrogen (Rachon et al 2008). There has been no investigation of these effects in human trials.

Osteoporosis prevention

Black cohosh demonstrates osteoprotective effects comparable to oestrogen, although through a different mechanism of increasing osteoblast activity (Wuttke et al 2006a), mediated via an oestrogen receptor-dependent mechanism (Chan et al 2008). One experimental study has shown that a triterpenoid glycoside isolated from black cohosh (25-acetyl-cimigenol xylopyranoside) both blocks the osteoclastogenesis enhanced by cytokines in vitro and attenuates TNF-alpha-induced bone loss in vivo (Qiu et al 2007). These results demonstrate that black cohosh can offer effective prevention of postmenopausal bone loss.

Breast cancer protection

A number of in vitro studies on black cohosh show that it is cytotoxic to human breast cancer cells and inhibits the conversion of oestrone sulphate to active oestradiol in breast cancer cells (Rice et al 2007), and suppresses tumour cell invasion without affecting cell viability (Hostanska et al 2007). One in vitro study found that black cohosh enhances the action of some chemotherapy agents, most notably tamoxifen (Al-Akoum et al 2007). The triterpene glycoside, actein, induced a stress response and apoptosis in human breast cancer cells (Einbond et al 2006, 2007, 2008). A recent in vitro study suggests that a herbal combination, Avlimil (which includes black cohosh, licorice, red raspberry, red clover and kudzu), exhibits both stimulatory and inhibitory effects on the growth of oestrogen-dependent breast tumour (MCF-7) cells. This casts doubt on the safety of Avlimil for women with oestrogen-dependent breast cancer (Ju et al 2008).

A randomised study (Hernandez & Pluchino 2003) was performed with 136 young premenopausal breast cancer survivors experiencing hot flushes as a result of tamoxifen therapy. When BNO 1055 (Menofem/Klimadynon, corresponding to 20 mg of herbal drug) was used together with tamoxifen for 12 months, the number and severity of hot flushes were reduced, with almost 50% of subjects becoming free of hot flushes, and severe hot flushes were reported by only 24% compared with 74% for those using tamoxifen alone.

In contrast, a previous double-blind, placebo-controlled study (n = 85) failed to detect significant improvements with black cohosh for hot flush frequency or severity when used by patients with breast cancer for 2 months who were also taking tamoxifen (Jacobson et al 2001). Unfortunately, the authors of that study did not specify which black cohosh product was used or the dosage, making a comparison with the previous study difficult.

A 2013 systematic review on the efficacy of black cohosh in breast cancer found that black cohosh does not appear to influence circulating levels of oestradiol, FSH or LH, nor to exert oestrogenic effects on breast, endometrial or vaginal tissues. However, it does appear to display oestrogenic activity on bone by stimulating bone formation and inhibiting bone breakdown (Fritz et al 2013).

Premenstrual syndrome and dysmenorrhoea

Commission E has approved the use of black cohosh as a treatment in these conditions (Blumenthal et al 2000). Randomised clinical studies are still required to confirm efficacy in these conditions.

Menstrual migraine

IN COMBINATION

An RCT of 49 women with menstrual migraines tested placebo against a herbal combination consisting of 60 mg soy isoflavones, 100 mg dong quai and 50 mg black cohosh, with each component standardised to its primary alkaloid (Burke et al 2002). Over the course of the study, the average frequency of menstrually associated migraine episodes was significantly reduced in the active treatment group.

Primary and secondary infertility

Several RCTs have been conducted in the last few years investigating the use of a commercial black cohosh preparation (Klimadynon) as an adjunctive treatment for women with unexplained infertility, both producing promising results (Shahin et al 2008, 2009). One RCT has also been conducted with women diagnosed with polycystic ovarian syndrome (PCOS) and primary or secondary infertility.

Cimicifuga racemosa in conjunction with clomiphene citrate was investigated in a 2008 RCT (n = 119) in women under 35 years with primary or secondary unexplained infertility who were previously unsuccessful in achieving pregnancy after clomiphene citrate cycles. Both groups received clomiphene citrate (150 mg/day from days 3 to 7) and the treatment group also received *Cimicifuga racemosa* (Klimadynon 120 mg/day from days 1 to 12). In the treatment group, there were higher levels of oestradiol (274.5 ± 48.5 vs. 254.6 ± 20.6, NS) and LH concentrations, although these were considered non-significant. There was however a statistically significant increase in endometrial thickness (8.9 ± 1.4 mm vs. 7.5 ± 1.3 mm, $P < 0.001$), serum progesterone (13.3 ± 3.1 ng/mL vs. 9.3 ± 2.0 ng/mL, $P < 0.01$) and clinical pregnancy rate (36.7% vs. 13.6%, $P < 0.01$) (Shahin et al 2008).

A follow-up trial in the same population group (n = 134) compared *Cimicifuga racemosa* (CR) (Klimadynon 120 mg/day from days 1 to 12) to ethinyl oestradiol

(EO) (100 mcg/day from days 1 to 12) in conjunction with clomiphene citrate (150 mg/day from day 3 to 7) (Shahin et al 2009). Although changes to clinical pregnancy rates did not reach statistical significance, these were higher in the black cohosh group (21.1% CR vs. 14.0% EO). The treatment group needed significantly fewer days for follicular maturation (13.55 ± 0.99 vs. 11.65 ± 0.98, $P < 0.001$), had a thicker endometrium (7.66 ± 0.68 vs. 8.08 ± 0.59, $P < 0.001$), higher luteal-phase serum progesterone (10.52 ± 0.89 vs. 12.15 ± 1.99, $P < 0.001$) and higher oestradiol concentration at the time of human chorionic gonadotrophin injection (245.10 ± 15.24 vs. 277.0 ± 27.73, $P < 0.001$).

A 2012 prospective RCT compared *Cimicifuga racemosa* as a stand-alone treatment to clomiphene citrate in 100 women aged 21–27 with polycystic ovarian syndrome (PCOS) and primary or secondary infertility (Kamel 2013). Both groups received black cohosh (Klimadynon 20 mg/day for 10 days) or clomiphene citrate (100 mg/day for 5 days) from the second day of the cycle for three consecutive cycles. Again, although the change in pregnancy rate was not statistically significant, more women taking *Cimicifuga racemosa* became pregnant (7 vs. 4 pregnancies; $P = 0.1$). Remarkable hormonal differences were noted in the black cohosh group, particularly in LH level and FSH/LH ratio, with a marked reduction in the LH level (first cycle 8.5 ± 0.28 vs. 8.9 ± 0.55; $P = 0.0001$) which was significant in all three treatment cycles. This confirms the understanding of black cohosh as a hypothalamic-pituitary-ovarian axis modulator. Progesterone was also statistically higher in the Klimadynon group, especially in the first cycle (10.12 ± 0.14 vs. 9.54 ± 0.15 ng/mL, $P = 0.0001$) along with endometrial thickness (first cycle: 8.34 vs. 6.89 mm; second cycle: 9.67 vs. 6.34 mm; third cycle: 9.11 vs. 7.32 mm; $P = 0.0004$). This study suggests that black cohosh has potential as an alternative to clomiphene citrate for ovulation induction in women with PCOS-related infertility.

Prostate cancer

Two in vitro studies suggest that black cohosh may have theoretical usefulness in the treatment of prostate cancer (Hostanska et al 2005, Jarry et al 2005, Seidlova-Wuttke et al 2006). Further research is now required to determine whether black cohosh may play a role in the prevention or treatment of prostate cancer.

OTHER USES

Black cohosh has been used traditionally to treat a variety of other female reproductive disorders and inflammatory disorders, especially menopausal arthritis and diarrhoea. It has also been used to promote menstruation. The British Herbal Pharmacopoeia states it is indicated in ovarian dysfunction and ovarian insufficiency.

SAFETY

Evidence now confirms that black cohosh does not pose a risk in women with breast cancer, nor increase its incidence or recurrence. Four hundred postmenopausal women with symptoms related to oestrogen deficiency were enrolled into a prospective, open-label, multinational, multicentre study to investigate endometrial safety and the tolerability and efficacy of the black cohosh extract, BNO 1055. Low dose treatment (40 mg) for 52 weeks showed no case of hyperplasia or more serious adverse endometrial outcome occurred (Raus et al 2006). This finding is supported by the HALT study (Reed et al 2008).

A population-based case-control study consisting of 949 breast cancer cases and 1524 controls was used to evaluate the relationship between phyto-oestrogens and breast cancer risk. Use of black cohosh was found to have a significant breast cancer protective effect. This association was similar among women who reported use of either black cohosh or Remifemin (Rebbeck et al 2007). Another smaller trial demonstrated that Remifemin does not cause adverse effects on breast tissue. A total of 65 healthy, naturally postmenopausal women completed a trial with 40 mg black cohosh daily. Mammograms were performed, and breast cells were collected by percutaneous fine needle aspiration biopsies at baseline and after 6 months (Hirschberg et al 2007). A systematic review was conducted about the safety and efficacy of black cohosh in patients with cancer. There is laboratory evidence of antiproliferative properties but no confirmation from clinical studies for a protective role in cancer prevention. Black cohosh appears to be safe in breast cancer patients (Walji et al 2007).

A pharmacoepidemiological, observational, retrospective cohort study examined breast cancer patients to investigate the influence of Remifemin on recurrence-free survival after breast cancer, including oestrogen-dependent tumours. Remifemin was not found to be associated with an increase in the risk of recurrence but was associated with prolonged disease-free survival. After 2 years following initial diagnosis, 14% of the control group had developed a recurrence, while the Remifemin group reached this proportion after 6.5 years, demonstrating a protractive effect of black cohosh on the rate of recurrence of breast cancer for women with a history of breast cancer who had used Remifemin, compared to women who had not (Zepelin et al 2007).

In regards to safety, a 2013 systematic review of black cohosh in breast cancer found that the current evidence does not demonstrate an increased risk or recurrence of breast cancer in women with or without a history. Of the four studies investigating risk, two found no significant association with the use of black cohosh and two reported reduced risk, including a study that combined black cohosh with tamoxifen. When considering hormones, black cohosh does not appear to influence circulating levels of oestradiol, FSH or LH, nor to exert oestrogenic effects on breast, endometrial or vaginal tissues (Fritz et al 2013).

DOSAGE RANGE

- Decoction or powdered root: 0.3–2 g three times daily.
- Tincture (1:10): 2–4 mL three times daily.
- Fluid extract (1:1) (g/mL): 0.3–2 mL three times daily.
- Perimenopausal symptoms: 40–160 mg per day.
- Infertility: 20–120 mg per day.

Many practitioners have used black cohosh long term without safety concerns.

TOXICITY

Overdose has produced nausea and vomiting, vertigo and visual disturbances.

Idiosyncratic hepatic reactions

Rare, spontaneous hepatotoxicity has been reported in at least 42 case reports worldwide with treatment by *Cimicifugae racemosae rhizoma* (Levitsky et al 2005, Nisbet & O'Connor 2007, Teschke & Schwarzenboeck 2009, Whiting et al 2002). As a result, several safety reviews have been conducted to evaluate the available data and determine what risk exists with the use of this herb. A 2008 safety review of black cohosh products was conducted by the Dietary Supplement Information Expert Committee of the US Pharmacopeia's Council of Experts. All the reports of liver damage were assigned possible causality, and none were probable or certain causality. The clinical pharmacokinetic and animal toxicological information did not reveal unfavourable information about black cohosh. The Expert Committee determined that in the United States black cohosh products should be labelled to include a cautionary statement, a change from their decision of 2002, which required no such statement (Mahady et al 2008).

Assessment of the 42 cases by European Medicines Agency (EMEA) has shown a possible or probable causality in only four out of 42 patients. A diagnostic algorithm has been applied in the four patients with suspected BC (black cohosh) hepatotoxicity using several methods to allow objective assessment, scoring and scaling of the probability in each case. Due to incomplete data, the case of one patient was not assessable. For the remaining three patients, quantitative evaluation showed no causality for BC in any patient regarding the observed severe liver disease (Teschke & Schwarzenboeck 2009).

In Australia in February 2006, the TGA announced that based on the appraisal of case reports, a causal association between black cohosh and serious hepatitis exists; however, the incidence is very low considering its widespread use. As a result, products available in Australia containing black cohosh have to carry label warnings informing consumers of the risk. The conclusion made by the TGA is considered controversial by some experts because numerous confounding factors were present in many of the case reports, such as the use of multiple ingredient preparations, concurrent use of at least one pharmaceutical medicine and the presence of other medical conditions.

A 2008 study evaluated the effects of black cohosh extract on liver morphology and on levels of various hepatic function indices in an experimental model finding that at high doses, well above the recommended dosage, black cohosh appears quite safe (Mazzanti et al 2008).

More recently, Teschke (2010) investigated data from 69 spontaneous or published case reports of suspected black cohosh-induced hepatotoxicity and found confounding variables such as uncertainty about the quality and authenticity of the black cohosh product, dose or insufficient adverse event description, missing or inadequate evaluation of a clear temporal association, the possible presence of other medications or comorbidities and lack of de-challenge or re-exposure. A clear causal relationship between black cohosh and hepatotoxicity was not found.

A 2011 meta-analysis investigated the potential hepatotoxicity of black cohosh (Remifemin) from published RCTs in peri- and postmenopausal women. Liver function data (AST, ALT and γ-GT) from 1020 women was compared at baseline and after taking black cohosh (40–128 mg/day) for 3 to 6 months. No significant difference between the treatment and reference groups was found (Naser et al 2011).

ADVERSE REACTIONS

Black cohosh is a well tolerated treatment. A 2012 Cochrane systematic review of 16 RCTs involving 2027 women found no significant difference in incidence of adverse effects between black cohosh and placebo groups (Leach & Moore 2012). The adverse effects associated with black cohosh tend to be rare, mild and reversible. The most common adverse effects reported are gastrointestinal symptoms, musculoskeletal and connective tissue disorders such as rashes (Borrelli & Ernst 2008). According to data from clinical studies and spontaneous reporting programs, large doses can cause headache, tremors or giddiness in some people (Huntley & Ernst 2003).

A few rare but serious adverse events, including hepatic and circulatory conditions, have been reported, but without a clear causality relationship in most instances (see above).

SIGNIFICANT INTERACTIONS

Cisplatin

Black cohosh decreased the cytotoxicity of cisplatin in an experimental breast cancer model — while the clinical significance of this finding is unknown, it is recommended that patients taking cisplatin should avoid black cohosh until safety can be confirmed.

Clomiphene citrate

RCTs in women with infertility have demonstrated improved pregnancy rates, hormone profiles, follicular maturation and endometrial thickness when taking black cohosh in conjunction with clomid treatment when used during the follicular phase (Shahin et al 2008, Shahin et al 2009). Beneficial interaction possible under professional supervision.

Doxorubicin

Black cohosh increased the cytotoxicity of doxorubicin in an experimental breast cancer model — while the clinical significance of this finding is unknown, it is recommended patients taking doxorubicin avoid black cohosh until safety can be confirmed.

Docetaxel

A trial used mouse breast cancer cell line to test whether black cohosh altered the response of cancer cells to radiation and to four drugs commonly used in cancer therapy. The black cohosh extracts increased the cytotoxicity of doxorubicin and docetaxel and decreased the cytotoxicity of cisplatin, but did not alter the effects of radiation or 4-hydroperoxycyclophosphamide (4-HC), an analogue of cyclophosphamide which is active in cell culture. This evidence may be applicable to humans, so it is advisable that patients undergoing cancer therapy should be made aware that use of black cohosh could alter their response to the agents commonly used to treat breast cancer (Rockwell et al 2005).

CONTRAINDICATIONS AND PRECAUTIONS

There is some controversy over the use of black cohosh in women with a history of breast cancer. Results from a 2002 study testing the safety of black cohosh in an in vitro model for oestrogen-dependent breast tumours found that the herbal extract significantly inhibited tumour cell proliferation, oestrogen-induced proliferation and enhanced the antiproliferative effects of tamoxifen (Bodinet & Freudenstein 2002). This finding is supported in a more recent in vitro study that showed black cohosh having a cytotoxic effect on both oestrogen-sensitive and oestrogen-insensitive breast cancer cells and a synergism with tamoxifen for inhibition of cancerous cell growth (Al-Akoum et al 2007). A 2013 systematic review of black cohosh in breast cancer found that the current evidence does not demonstrate an increased risk or recurrence of breast cancer in women with or without a history (Fritz et al 2013). As with all medicines, a risk-versus-benefit conversation should take place with patients.

Practice points/Patient counselling

- In general, clinical trials support the use of black cohosh for relieving menopausal symptoms, with most consistent benefits reported for the European extracts.

- It appears that 4–12 weeks continuous treatment are required for adequate menopausal symptom relief and it can be used successfully with St John's wort.
- Black cohosh is also used in the treatment of premenstrual syndrome and dysmenorrhoea and is Commission E-approved for these uses; however, controlled studies are not available to confirm its efficacy.
- Black cohosh has many different actions, including selective oestrogen receptor modulator activity, serotonergic, dopaminergic, anti-inflammatory and analgesic activity.
- Black cohosh should be used only under professional supervision by people with oestrogen-dependent tumours, or during pregnancy.
- Black cohosh is well tolerated with few side effects; however, rare case reports of idiosyncratic hepatic reactions have been described. Until safety can be confirmed, avoid prescribing black cohosh in conjunction with medications that are potentially hepatotoxic or in patients with liver disease.

PREGNANCY USE

Although it has been used to assist in childbirth, black cohosh is not traditionally recommended in pregnancy, particularly during the first trimester although it has been used in the final weeks of pregnancy to aid in delivery. Safety in lactation remains to be confirmed; however, it is usually avoided because of its hormonal effects (Dugoua et al 2006).

PATIENTS' FAQs

What will this herb do for me?

Black cohosh may be an effective treatment for menopausal symptoms in most women, especially those with mild to moderate symptoms. The European extracts give the most consistently positive results for reducing the frequency of hot flushes. Effects are also good when combined with the herb St John's wort. It may also be useful in the treatment of premenstrual syndrome and prevention of period cramping. Black cohosh can also be considered in women with unexplained or PCOS-related infertility.

When will it start to work?

Studies suggest that benefits are seen within 4–12 weeks for the treatment of menopausal symptoms.

Are there any safety issues?

Black cohosh is well tolerated with few side effects. It should only be used under professional supervision by people undergoing chemotherapy, receiving treatment for oestrogen-dependent tumours or during pregnancy.

Due to rare case reports of idiosyncratic hepatic reactions, avoid prescribing black cohosh in conjunction with medications that are potentially hepatotoxic or in patients with liver disease, until safety can be confirmed.

REFERENCES

Al-Akoum M, Dodin S, Akoum A. Synergistic cytotoxic effects of tamoxifen and black cohosh on MCF-7 and MDA-MB-231 human breast cancer cells: an in vitro study. Can J Physiol Pharmacol 85.11 (2007): 1153–1159.

Bai W et al. Efficacy and tolerability of a medicinal product containing an isopropanolic black cohosh extract in Chinese women with menopausal symptoms: a randomized, double blind, parallel-controlled study versus tibolone. Maturitas 58.1 (2007): 31–41.

Beck V et al. Comparison of hormonal activity (estrogen, androgen and progestin) of standardized plant extracts for large scale use in hormone replacement therapy. J Steroid Biochem Mol Biol 84.2–3 (2003): 259–68.
Blumenthal M, Goldberg A, Brinckmann J (eds). Herbal medicine: expanded Commission E monographs. Austin, TX: Integrative Medicine Communications, 2000.
Bodinet C, Freudenstein J. Influence of Cimicifuga racemosa on the proliferation of estrogen receptor-positive human breast cancer cells. Breast Cancer Res Treat 76.1 (2002): 1–10.
Bolle P et al. Estrogen-like effect of a Cimicifuga racemosa extract sub-fraction as assessed by in vivo, ex vivo and in vitro assays. J Steroid Biochem Mol Biol 107.3–5 (2007): 262–269.
Borrelli F, Ernst E. Black cohosh (Cimicifuga racemosa) for menopausal symptoms: a systematic review of its efficacy. Pharmacol Res 58.1 (2008): 8–14.
Briese V et al. Black cohosh with or without St. John's wort for symptom-specific climacteric treatment — results of a large-scale, controlled, observational study. Maturitas 57.4 (2007): 405–414.
Burdette JE et al. Black cohosh acts as a mixed competitive ligand and partial agonist of the serotonin receptor. J Agric Food Chem 51.19 (2003): 5661–5670.
Burke BE, Olson RD, Cusack BJ. Randomized, controlled trial of phytoestrogen in the prophylactic treatment of menstrual migraine. Biomed Pharmacother 56.6 (2002): 283–288.
Chan BY et al. Ethanolic extract of Actaea racemosa (black cohosh) potentiates bone nodule formation in MC3T3-E1 preosteoblast cells. Bone 43.3 (2008): 567–573.
Cheema D, Coomarasamy A, El-Toukhy T. Non-hormonal therapy of post-menopausal vasomotor symptoms: a structured evidence-based review. Arch Gynecol Obstet 276.5 (2007): 463–469.
Chung DJ et al. Black cohosh and St. John's wort (GYNO-Plus) for climacteric symptoms. Yonsei Med J 48.2 (2007): 289–294.
Drewe J, Zimmermann C, Zahner C. The effect of a Cimicifuga racemosa extracts Ze 450 in the treatment of climacteric complaints — an observational study. Phytomedicine, 20.8–9 (2013): 659–666.
Dugoua JJ et al. Safety and efficacy of black cohosh (Cimicifuga racemosa) during pregnancy and lactation. Can J Clin Pharmacol 13.3 (2006): e257–261.
Duker EM et al. Effects of extracts from Cimicifuga racemosa on gonadotropin release in menopausal women and ovariectomized rats. Planta Med 57.5 (1991): 420–424.
Einbond LS et al. Actein and a fraction of black cohosh potentiate antiproliferative effects of chemotherapy agents on human breast cancer cells. Planta Med 72.13 (2006): 1200–1206.
Einbond LS et al. The growth inhibitory effect of actein on human breast cancer cells is associated with activation of stress response pathways. Int J Cancer 121.9 (2007): 2073–2083.
Einbond LS et al. Growth inhibitory activity of extracts and compounds from Cimicifuga species on human breast cancer cells. Phytomedicine 15.6–7 (2008): 504–511.
Fritz H et al. Black Cohosh and Breast Cancer: A Systematic Review. Integr Cancer Ther. 2013 Mar 25 [Epub ahead of print]
Geller SE, Studee L. Botanical and dietary supplements for menopausal symptoms: what works, what does not. J Womens Health (Larchmt) 14.7 (2005): 634–649.
Geller SE, Studee L. Botanical and dietary supplements for mood and anxiety in menopausal women. Menopause 14.3 (Pt 1) (2007): 541–549.
Geller SE et al. Safety and efficacy of black cohosh and red clover for the management of vasomotor symptoms: a randomized controlled trial. Menopause 16.6 (2009): 1156–1166.
Genazzani E, Sorrentino L. Vascular action of actein: active constituent of Actaea racemosa L. Nature 194 (1962): 544–5 (as cited in Micromedex Thomsen 2003. www.micromedex.com).
Gurley BJ et al. In vivo effects of goldenseal, kava kava, black cohosh, and valerian on human cytochrome P450 1A2, 2D6, 2E1, and 3A4/5 phenotypes. Clin. Pharmacol. Ther., 77.5 (2005): 415–426.
Gurley B et al. Assessing the clinical significance of botanical supplementation on human cytochrome P450 3A activity: comparison of a milk thistle and black cohosh product to rifampin and clarithromycin. J Clin Pharmacol 46 (2006a): 201–213.
Gurley BJ et al. Effect of milk thistle (Silybum marianum) and black cohosh (Cimicifuga racemosa) supplementation on digoxin pharmacokinetics in humans. Drug Metab Dispos 34.1 (2006b): 69–74.
Gurley BJ et al. Clinical assessment of CYP2D6-mediated herb-drug interactions in humans: effects of milk thistle, black cohosh, goldenseal, kava kava, St. John's wort, and Echinacea. Mol Nutr Food Res 52.7 (2008) 755–763.
Gurley BJ, Fifer EK, Gardner Z. Pharmacokinetic herb -drug interactions (part 2): drug interactions involving popular botanical dietary ssupplements and their clinical relevance. Planta Med 78.13 (2012): 1490–1514.
Hernandez MG, Pluchino S. Cimicifuga racemosa for the treatment of hot flushes in women surviving breast cancer. Maturitas 44 (Suppl 1) (2003): S59–65.
Hirabayashi T et al. Inhibitory effect of ferulic acid and isoferulic acid on murine interleukin-8 production in response to influenza virus infections in vitro and in vivo. Planta Med 61.3 (1995): 221–6 (as cited in Micromedex Thomsen 2003. www.micromedex.com).
Hirschberg AL et al. An isopropanolic extract of black cohosh does not increase mammographic breast density or breast cell proliferation in postmenopausal women. Menopause 14.1 (2007): 89–96.
Hostanska K et al. Apoptosis of human prostate androgen-dependent and -independent carcinoma cells induced by an isopropanolic extract of black cohosh involves degradation of cytokeratin (CK) 18. Anticancer Res 25.1A (2005): 139–147.
Hostanska K et al. Inhibitory effect of an isopropanolic extract of black cohosh on the invasiveness of MDA-mB 231 human breast cancer cells. In Vivo 21.2 (2007): 349–355.
Huntley A, Ernst E. A systematic review of the safety of black cohosh. Menopause 10.1 (2003): 58–64.
Izzo AA. Interactions between herbs and conventional drugs: overview of the clinical data. Med Princ Pract 21.5 (2012): 404–428.
Jacobson JS et al. Randomized trial of black cohosh for the treatment of hot flashes among women with a history of breast cancer. J Clin Oncol 19.10 (2001): 2739–2745.

Jarry H et al. In vitro effects of the Cimicifuga racemosa extract BNO 1055. Maturitas 44 (Suppl 1) (2003): S31–38.
Jarry H et al. Cimicifuga racemosa extract BNO 1055 inhibits proliferation of the human prostate cancer cell line LNCaP. Phytomedicine 12.3 (2005): 178–182.
Ju YH, Doerge DR, Helferich WG. A dietary supplement for female sexual dysfunction, Avlimil, stimulates the growth of estrogen-dependent breast tumors (MCF-7) implanted in ovariectomized athymic nude mice. Food Chem Toxicol 46.1 (2008): 310–320.
Kamel HH. Role of phyto-oestrogens in ovulation induction in women with polycystic ovarian syndrome. Eur J Obstet Gynecol Reprod Biol 168.1 (2013): 60–63.
Kennelly EJ et al. Analysis of thirteen populations of black cohosh for formononetin. Phytomedicine 9.5 (2002): 461–467.
Kim EY, Lee YJ, Rhyu MR. Black cohosh (*Cimicifuga racemosa*) relaxes the isolated rat thoracic aorta through endothelium-dependentand -independent mechanisms. J Ethnopharmacol 138.2 (2011): 537–542.
Laakmann E et al. Efficacy of Cimicifuga racemosa, Hypericum perforatum and Agnus castus in the treatment of climacteric complaints: a systematic review. Gynecol Endocrinol 28.9 (2012):703–9.
Leach MJ, Moore V. Black cohosh (Cimicifuga spp.) for menopausal symptoms. Cochrane Database Syst Rev 12.9 (2012): CD007244.
Levitsky J et al. Fulminant liver failure associated with the use of black cohosh. Dig Dis Sci 50.3 (2005): 538–539.
Lieberman S. A review of the effectiveness of Cimicifuga racemosa (black cohosh) for the symptoms of menopause. J Womens Health 7.5 (1998): 525–529.
Mahady GB et al. United States Pharmacopeia review of the black cohosh case reports of hepatotoxicity. Menopause 15.4 Pt 1 (2008): 628–638.
Mazzanti G et al. Effects of Cimicifuga racemosa extract on liver morphology and hepatic function indices. Phytomedicine 15.11 (2008): 1021–1024.
Naser B et al. Suspected black cohosh hepatotoxicity: no evidence by meta-analysis of randomized controlled clinical trials for isopropanolic black cohosh extract. Menopause 18.4 (2011): 366–375.
Newton KM et al. Treatment of vasomotor symptoms of menopause with black cohosh, multibotanicals, soy, hormone therapy, or placebo: a randomized trial. Ann Intern Med 145.12 (2006): 869–879.
Nisbet BC, O'Connor RE. Black cohosh-induced hepatitis. Del Med J 79.11 (2007): 441–444.
North American Menopause Society. Treatment of menopause-associated vasomotor symptoms: position statement of The North American Menopause Society. Menopause 11 (2004): 11–33.
Oktem M et al. Black cohosh and fluoxetine in the treatment of postmenopausal symptoms: a prospective, randomized trial. Adv Ther 24.2 (2007): 448–461.
Palacio C, Masri G, Mooradian AD. Black cohosh for the management of menopausal symptoms: a systematic review of clinical trials. Drugs Aging 26.1 (2009): 23–26.
Pang X et al. Pregnane X receptor-mediated induction of Cyp3a by black cohosh. Xenobiotica 41.2 (2011): 112–123
Pockaj BA et al. Phase III double-blind, randomized, placebo-controlled crossover trial of black cohosh in the management of hot flashes: NCCTG Trial N01CC1. J Clin Oncol 24.18 (2006): 2836–2841.
Powell SL et al. In vitro serotonergic activity of black cohosh and identification of N(omega)-methylserotonin as a potential active constituent. J Agric Food Chem 56.24 (2008):11718–11726.
Qiu SX et al. A triterpene glycoside from black cohosh that inhibits osteoclastogenesis by modulating RANKL and TNFalpha signaling pathways. Chem Biol 14.7 (2007): 860–869.
Rachon D et al. Effects of black cohosh extract on body weight gain, intra-abdominal fat accumulation, plasma lipids and glucose tolerance in ovariectomized Sprague-Dawley rats. Maturitas 60.3–4 (2008): 209–215.
Raus K et al. First-time proof of endometrial safety of the special black cohosh extract (Actaea or Cimicifuga racemosa extract) CR BNO 1055. Menopause 13.4 (2006): 678–691.
Rebbeck TR et al. A retrospective case-control study of the use of hormone-related supplements and association with breast cancer. Int J Cancer 120.7 (2007): 1523–1528.
Reed SD et al. Vaginal, endometrial, and reproductive hormone findings: randomized, placebo-controlled trial of black cohosh, multibotanical herbs, and dietary soy for vasomotor symptoms: the Herbal Alternatives for Menopause (HALT) Study. Menopause 15.1 (2008): 51–58.
Rhyu MR et al. Black cohosh (Actaea racemosa, Cimicifuga racemosa) behaves as a mixed competitive ligand and partial agonist at the human mu opiate receptor. J Agric Food Chem 54.26 (2006): 9852–9857.
Rice S, Amon A, Whitehead SA. Ethanolic extracts of black cohosh (Actaea racemosa) inhibit growth and oestradiol synthesis from oestrone sulphate in breast cancer cells. Maturitas 56.4 (2007): 359–367.
Rockwell S, Liu Y, Higgins SA. Alteration of the effects of cancer therapy agents on breast cancer cells by the herbal medicine black cohosh. Breast Cancer Res Treat 90.3 (2005): 233–239.
Ruhlen RL, Sun GY, Sauter ER. Black cohosh: insights into its mechanism/s of action. Integrative Medicine Insights 3 (2008): 21–32.
Schmid D et al. Aqueous extracts of Cimicifugas racemosa and phenolcarboxylic constituents inhibit production ofproinflammatory cytokines in LPS-stimulated human whole blood. Can J Physiol Pharmacol 87.11 (2009a): 963–972.
Schmid D et al. Inhibition of inducible nitric oxide synthesis by Cimicifuga racemosa (Actaea racemosa, black cohosh) extractsin LPS-stimulated RAW 264.7 macrophages. J Pharm Pharmacol 61.8 (2009b): 1089–1096.
Seidlova-Wuttke D et al. Evidence for selective estrogen receptor modulator activity in a black cohosh (Cimicifuga racemosa) extract: comparison with estradiol-17beta. Eur J Endocrinol 149 (2003): 351–362.
Seidlova-Wuttke D, Thelen P, Wuttke W. Inhibitory effects of a black cohosh (Cimicifuga racemosa) extract on prostate cancer. Planta Med 72.6 (2006): 521–526.
Shahin AY et al. Adding phytoestrogens to clomiphene induction in unexplained infertility patients — a randomized trial. Reprod Biomed Online 16.4 (2008): 580–588.

Shahin AY, Ismail AM, Shaaban OM. Supplementation of clomiphene citrate cycles with *Cimicifuga racemosa* or ethinyl oestradiol — a randomized trial. Reprod Biomed Online 19.4 (2009): 501–507.
Shams T et al. Efficacy of black cohosh-containing preparations on menopausal symptoms: a meta-analysis. Altern Ther Health Med 16.1 (2010): 36–44.
Shord SS, Shah K, Lukose A. Drug-botanical interactions: a review of the laboratory, animal, and human data for 8 common botanicals. Integr Cancer Ther 8.3 (2009): 208–227.
Teschke R. Black cohosh and suspected hepatotoxicity: inconsistencies, confounding variables, and prospective use of a diagnostic causality algorithm. A critical review. Menopause 17.2(2010): 426–440.
Teschke R, Schwarzenboeck A. Suspected hepatotoxicity by Cimicifugae racemosae rhizoma (black cohosh, root): critical analysis and structured causality assessment. Phytomedicine 16.1 (2009): 72–84.
Uebelhack R et al. Black cohosh and St John's wort for climacteric complaints: a randomized trial. Obstet Gynecol 107 (2006): 247–255.
Verhoeven MO et al. Effect of a combination of isoflavones and Actaea racemosa Linnaeus on climacteric symptoms in healthy symptomatic perimenopausal women: a 12-week randomized, placebo-controlled, double-blind study. Menopause 12 (2005): 412–420.
Viereck V, Emons G, Wuttke W. Black cohosh: just another phytoestrogen? Trends Endocrinol Metab 16.5 (2005): 214–221.
Walji R et al. Black cohosh (Cimicifuga racemosa [L.] Nutt.): safety and efficacy for cancer patients. Support Care Cancer 15.8 (2007): 913–921.
Whiting PW, Clouston A, Kerlin P. Black cohosh and other herbal remedies associated with acute hepatitis. Med J Aust 177 (2002): 440–443.
Wuttke W, Seidlova-Wuttke D, Gorkow C. The Cimicifuga preparation BNO 1055 vs conjugated estrogens in a double-blind placebo-controlled study: effects on menopause symptoms and bone markers. Maturitas 44 (Suppl 1) (2003): S67–77.
Wuttke W, Gorkow C, Seidlova-Wuttke D. Effects of black cohosh (Cimicifuga racemosa) on bone turnover, vaginal mucosa, and various blood parameters in postmenopausal women: a double-blind, placebo-controlled, and conjugated estrogens-controlled study. Menopause 13.2 (2006a): 185–196.
Wuttke W, Raus K, Gorkow C. Efficacy and tolerability of the Black cohosh (Actaea racemosa) ethanolic extract BNO 1055 on climacteric complaints: a double-blind, placebo- and conjugated estrogens-controlled study. Maturitas 55(Supplement 1) (2006b): S83–91.
Wuttke W et al. The non-estrogenic alternative for the treatment of climacteric complaints: Black cohosh (Cimicifuga or Actaea racemosa). J Steroid Biochem Mol Biol 139 (2014): 302–310.
Zepelin HH et al. Isopropanolic black cohosh extract and recurrence-free survival after breast cancer. Int J Clin Pharmacol Ther 45.3 (2007): 143–154.

Brahmi

HISTORICAL NOTE Brahmi is the Sanskrit name for the herb *Bacopa monniera* and has been used in Ayurvedic medicine as a nerve tonic since time immemorial. Under this system, *B. monniera* is classified under 'Medhya rasayana', that is, medicinal plants rejuvenating intellect and memory, and has been used in India for almost 3000 years. The ancient classical Ayurvedic treatises recommend it for the promotion of memory, intelligence and general performance. Over time, it has earned a reputation as an important brain tonic (Williamson 2002).

COMMON NAME

Brahmi

OTHER NAMES

Bacopa, herb of grace, herpestis herb, Indian pennywort, jalanimba, jalnaveri, sambrani chettu, thyme-leave gratiola, keenmind, Nira-Brahmi, Sambrani Chettu

Centella asiatica (gotu kola) and *Merremia gangetica* have also been referred to by the name brahmi, but most authorities associate brahmi with *Bacopa monniera*.

The name brahmi is derived from the word 'Brama', the mythical 'creator' in the Hindu pantheon. Because the brain is the centre for creative activity, any compound that improves brain health is called brahmi (Russo & Borrelli 2005).

BOTANICAL NAME/FAMILY

Bacopa monniera (family Scrophulariaceae)

PLANT PARTS USED

Dried whole plant or herb, mainly leaves and stems (aerial parts)

CHEMICAL COMPONENTS

Dammarene-type saponins (bacosides [A, B, C] and bacosaponines [D, E, F], based on the bacogenins A1–A5, are considered the most important) and alkaloids (brahmine, herpestine), flavonoids (luteolin-7-glucoside, glucuronyl-7-apigenin and glucuronyl-7-luteolin), phytosterols (Chakravarty et al 2003) and luteolin, phenylethanoid glycosides, monnierasides I–III and plantainoside B have been isolated (Adams et al 2007).

Standardised extract BacoMind has been shown to contain bacoside A_3, bacopaside I, bacopaside II, jujubogenin isomer of bacopasaponin C, bacosine, luteolin, apigenin and β-sitosterol D-glucoside (Dutta et al 2008).

The commercial extract KeenMind is standardised for bacosides A and B (no less than 55% of combined bacosides). Each capsule contains 150 mg *B. monniera* extract (20 : 1), equivalent to 3 g dried herb.

MAIN ACTIONS

Information about the mechanisms of action of brahmi chiefly comes from in vitro and animal tests using various experimental models, although an increasing number of clinical trials are now available. Some studies have investigated the effects of an Ayurvedic herbal combination known as brahmi rasayan, which consists of 10 parts bacopa, two parts cloves, one part cardamom, one part *Piper longum* and 40 parts sucrose.

Antioxidant

Brahmi has potent antioxidant activity, which appears to be a result of both direct free radical scavenging activity and increasing the activity of endogenous antioxidant systems (Bhattacharya et al 2000, Tripathi et al 1996). Administration of bacoside A reduced the effects of cigarette smoke in an animal model by increasing lactate dehydrogenase and its isoenzymes (Anbarasi et al 2005a). Bacoside A has also been shown to reduce creatine kinase in brain and cardiac tissue (Anbarasi et al 2005b), and prevent expression of hsp70 and neuronal apoptosis (Anbarasi et al 2006), thus preventing smoke-induced damage. An extract of brahmi provided protection against DNA damage in both animal cells (Russo et al 2003a) and human cells (Russo et al 2003b) in vitro. Dose-related increases in superoxide dismutase, catalase and glutathione peroxidase activities in several important regions of the brain have been demonstrated in animal models (Bhattacharya et al 2000) and it has been shown to induce the activity of superoxide dismutase and catalase in the liver (Kar et al 2002). Additionally, brahmi enhances antioxidant activity to protect against reactive oxygen species-induced damage in diabetic rats (Kapoor et al 2009).

Neuroprotective

Bacopa has demonstrated neuroprotective activity in a number of animal models, chiefly mediated by an antioxidant mechanism (Saini et al 2012). In particular, antioxidant effects have been observed for bacopa in areas of the brain that are key memory areas, such as hippocampus, frontal cortex and striatum (Bhattacharya et al 2000).

In one study, bacopa significantly protected lipids and proteins from oxidative stress-induced damage caused by aluminium. The protective antioxidant effect was described as similar to L-deprenyl (Jyoti et al 2007). In another experiment, bacopa improved memory functions in hypobaric conditions which induce hypoxia, most likely due to neuroprotective activity, antioxidant and mitochondria-stabilising effects (Hota et al 2009). Antioxidant activity and attenuation of oxidative damage were further confirmed for an oral bacopa extract in a study using a colchicine-induced dementia model (Saini et al 2012).

Administration of bacoside A prevented the structural and functional impairment of mitochondria upon exposure to cigarette smoke in vivo (Anbarasi et al 2005c). From the results, it was suggested that chronic cigarette smoke exposure induces damage to the mitochondria and that bacoside A protects the brain from this damage by maintaining the structural and functional integrity of the mitochondrial membrane.

In an Alzheimer's dementia model, bacopa extract significantly reduced beta-amyloid levels when administered prior to beta-amyloid deposition (Dhanasekaran et al 2004). The neuroprotective effect was specific for beta amyloid-induced cell death but not glutamate-induced excitotoxicity (Limpeanchob et al 2008). Bacopa extracts contain polyphenols and sulfhydryl compounds that demonstrate dose-dependent antioxidant activity, which reduces divalent metals, decreases the formation of lipid peroxides and inhibits lipoxygenase activity (Dhanasekaran et al 2007).

Cognitive or nootropic effects — multiple mechanisms

Cognitive and nootropic effects are not merely due to antioxidant activity and neuroprotection, as demonstrated in an experimental model of Alzheimer's dementia whereby the cognitive-enhancing effect of *Bacopa monniera* was not well correlated with its neuroprotection (Uabundit et al 2010).

Evidence shows that cognitive activation is due to a combination of mechanisms, which include serotonergic and cholinergic systems together with antioxidant and mitochondrial stabilisation activities. Further research with experimental models indicates that bacopa enhances synaptic plasticity (Preethi et al 2012). The saponins bacoside A and B are considered to be the most important active constituents responsible for enhancing cognitive function (Russo & Borelli 2005, Singh & Dhawan 1982).

Effects on the cholinergic system include the modulation of acetylcholine release, choline acetylase activity and muscarinic cholinergic receptor binding (Das et al 2002). Results from a double-blind, placebo-controlled trial using brahmi (300 mg/day) support this view, as one of the major effects seen was on speed of early information processing, a function predominantly modulated by the cholinergic system (Stough et al 2001). *Bacopa monniera* (120 mg/kg oral) significantly reversed diazepam-induced (1.75 mg/kg intraperitoneal) amnesia in an animal study (Saraf et al 2008), thereby confirming previous reports of cholinergic activity (Dhanasekaran et al 2007).

Research in animal models provides evidence of activation of the serotonergic system (Charles et al 2011). In one study, the level of serotonin (5-HT) increased in rat brains while dopamine decreased significantly. Based on this observation, the learning and memory enhancement effects are likely to be due to upregulation of serotonin-synthesising enzyme tryptophan hydroxylase-2 expression which could enhance 5-HT synthesis and also upregulated SERT (serotonin transporter) expression, which would enhance transportation of 5-HT and subsequent activation of the 5-HT_{3A} receptor during hippocampus-dependent learning. The characterised *Bacopa monniera* leaf extract used in this study contained 31.27% bacosides, i.e. bacopaside I (0.9%), bacoside A3 (9.47%), bacopaside II (17.15%), jujubogenin of bacopasaponin C (0.38%) and bacopasaponin C (3.37%). High-performance liquid chromatography analysis confirmed the presence of bioactive compounds in the serum of treated rats.

Clinical note — what is a nootropic agent?

Giurgen first coined the phrase when describing a proposed class of pharmacologically active substances that improve cognition or intelligence without side effects and which should protect the brain from damage (Stough et al 2011). This is in contrast to pharmaceutical cognitive activators such as amphetamine or modafinil that only improve cognition and are accompanied by side effects and therefore cannot be described as true nootropic agents. Bacopa is a good example of a nootropic agent due to its cognitive-enhancing and neuroprotective activities and excellent safety profile.

Antidepressant activity

A rodent model of depression found that an extract of brahmi produced significant antidepressant activity comparable to that of imipramine after 5 days of oral administration (Sairam et al 2002).

Serotonergic activity identified in animal models provides a mechanistic basis for the antidepressant activity.

Antiulcer effects

Significant antiulcer activity for the fresh juice from the whole plant of *Bacopa monniera* has been demonstrated in an animal model of aspirin-induced gastric ulceration (Rao et al 2000). The study found that brahmi had a beneficial influence on the natural mucosal defensive factors, such as enhanced mucin secretion, mucosal glycoprotein production and decreased cell shedding, thereby reducing ulceration (Rao et al 2000). A follow-up in vivo study in various gastric ulcer models further confirmed brahmi's ability to increase the body's natural defence factors and showed that *B. monniera* is effective for both the prophylaxis and the treatment of gastric ulcers (Sairam et al 2001). In addition, brahmi was shown to reduce lipid peroxidation. An in vitro study demonstrated that *B. monniera* significantly inhibited *Helicobacter pylori*, and the effect was comparable to that of bismuth subcitrate, a known *H. pylori* growth inhibitor (Goel et al 2003).

Anti-inflammatory effects

Several different mechanisms are responsible for the observed anti-inflammatory activity of brahmi. Inhibition of cyclooxygenase-2, 5-lipoxygenase (5-LOX) and 15-LOX and downregulation of tumour necrosis factor-alpha were demonstrated in one study testing a methanolic extract of *B. monniera*. The activity was found for both ethyl acetate and bacoside fractions (Viji & Helen 2008). Channa et al (2006) also identified anti-inflammatory activity but reported that this was mediated by prostaglandin E_2 inhibition, inhibition of histamine, serotonin and bradykinin release (Channa et al 2006).

The anti-inflammatory activity of bacopa was found to be comparable to indomethacin without causing an associated gastric irritation (Jain et al 1994). Several constituents are thought to be responsible for the anti-inflammatory action, chiefly the triterpene, betulinic acid, saponins and flavonoids.

OTHER ACTIONS

Adaptogen

A standardised extract of *B. monniera* possesses adaptogenic effects in an animal model, which were found to be comparable to *Panax quinquefolium* (Rai et al 2003). The neuropharmacological adaptogenic activity of brahmi was identified by significant normalisation of stress-induced changes in plasma corticosterone, and monoamine levels and dopamine in cortex and hippocampus regions of the brain (Sheikh et al 2007).

Antinociceptive activity

Previously, brahmi rasayan (an Ayurvedic herbal combination containing brahmi) demonstrated antinociceptive activity in animal experiments (Shukia et al 1987). An interaction with the GABAergic system is believed to be involved. More recent research confirms antinociceptive activity specifically for *Bacopa monniera* (Bhaskar & Jagtap 2011). Research using an aqueous extract in an experimental model indicates that the endogenous adrenergic, serotonergic and opioidergic systems are involved in the analgesic mechanism of action of the herb.

Mast cell stabilisation

The methanolic fraction of brahmi exhibits potent mast cell-stabilising activity in vitro, which was found to be comparable to that of disodium cromoglycate (Samiulla et al 2001).

Increased thyroid hormone levels

Results from animal experiments have found that brahmi increases thyroxine concentrations by 41% without enhancing hepatic lipid peroxidation (Kar et al 2002).

Antispasmodic effect on smooth muscle

A spasmolytic effect on smooth muscle has been demonstrated in vivo, and is predominantly due to inhibition of calcium influx into the cell (Dar & Channa 1999). Bronchodilatory effects have also been demonstrated, most likely due to the same mechanism (Channa et al 2003).

Anticlastogenic effect

An in vitro study identified significant anticlastogenic effects of the standardised extract of BacoMind on human lymphocytes due to the herb's antioxidant activity (Dutta et al 2008).

Hepatoprotective

Bacoside A was hepatoprotective against D-galactosamine-induced liver injury in rat studies. Researchers found that bacoside A reduced alanine transaminase, aspartate transaminase, alkaline phosphatase, gamma-glutamyl transpeptidase, lactate dehydrogenase and 5'ND enzyme levels and restored the decreased levels of vitamins C and E reduced by D-galactosamine in both liver and plasma (Sumathi & Nongbri 2008).

Cholesterol-lowering activity

According to a study using an experimental model of hypercholesterolaemia, feeding test animals an ethanolic extract of whole plant material (*Bacopa monniera*) for 45 days resulted in a significant reduction in levels of total cholesterol (TC), triglycerides, low-density lipoproteins (LDL), very-low-density lipoprotein (VLDL), atherogenic index, LDL : high-density lipoprotein (HDL) ratio and TC : HDL ratio and significantly increased the level of HDL (Kamesh & Sumathi 2012).

Anticonvulsant activity

Using an experimental epileptic model, Matthew et al (2012) demonstrated that *Bacopa monniera* and bacoside A treatment reverses epilepsy-associated changes to near controls. The effect appears to be mediated via GABA-A receptors and attributed to the bacoside A constituent (Mathew et al 2010, 2011).

Clinical note — Scientific investigation of Ayurvedic medicines in India

Modern-day interest in many Ayurvedic herbs, such as brahmi, really started in 1951 when the then Prime Minister of India set up the Central Drug Research centre in Lucknow. The goal of this initiative was to encourage scientists to investigate many of the traditional Ayurvedic herbs in a scientific way, and to determine their potential as contemporary drugs or as potential sources for newer drugs.

CLINICAL USE

Brahmi has been subject to many in vitro and animal studies, which indicate that the herb and several of its key constituents have significant pharmacological activity. Increasingly, clinical studies are being published which provide a scientific basis for its use in practice. Most clinical research has been conducted with standardised bacopa extracts and focused on its effects on memory and learning, overall supporting its traditional reputation as a 'brain tonic'.

Improving cognitive function — learning, memory, intelligence

In Ayurvedic medicine, bacopa is used to improve cognitive function and increase intelligence. Over time, it has developed an excellent reputation, prompting scientific researchers to investigate the activity of bacopa more closely.

The evidence available from clinical studies indicates a significant effect on various aspects of memory and learning when bacopa extract is taken long-term. Less is known about the acute neurocognitive effects as there is less research to draw on and the two available clinical trials have produced inconsistent results (Downey et al 2013, Nathan et al 2001).

The bacopa extract known as KeenMind has been the subject of most studies, although there is evidence that other extracts, including BacoMind, also have significant effects.

Healthy adults

A double-blind, placebo-controlled trial using a dose of 300 mg bacopa (KeenMind) over 12 weeks in 46 healthy volunteers aged between 18 and 60 years found that it significantly improved the speed of visual information processing, learning rate and memory consolidation and that it has a significant anxiolytic effect (Stough et al 2001).

Another study of the same design tested brahmi (KeenMind) in 76 adults aged 45–60 years taken for over 3 months (Roodenrys et al 2002); significant improvements in a test for new information retention was observed, but there were no changes in the rate of learning.

More recently, a 90-day double-blind placebo-controlled study demonstrated that bacopa (300 mg/day: KeenMind) produced significantly improved performance on the 'working memory' factor, more specifically spatial working memory accuracy and accuracy in the rapid visual information processing task compared to placebo (Stough et al 2008). Additionally, those receiving active treatment reported significantly greater incidence of increased energy. The only significant increase in side effects was for incidence of diarrhoea and reduction in the number of dreams. While 107 people were originally enrolled in the study, there were 45 withdrawals, a similar amount from both groups (23 and 22), so only 62 people were considered sufficiently compliant with treatment and included in the final analysis.

Older adults

In 2008, Calabrese et al demonstrated that whole-plant standardised dry extract of *Bacopa monniera* (300 mg/day) safely enhanced cognitive performance in the aged in a double-blind, randomised, placebo-controlled study. The trial involved 54 volunteers aged 65 years or older, without clinical signs of dementia, who received placebo or herbal treatment for 12 weeks. The group receiving active herbal treatment also experienced a reduction in anxiety, whereas anxiety increased in the placebo group.

A double-blind, placebo-controlled randomised study was conducted in India involving 40 volunteers aged over 55 years and complaining of memory impairment (Ranghav et al 2008). The subjects received either 125 mg of an ethanolic standardised bacopa extract (containing 55% bacosides) or placebo twice a day for a period of 12 weeks followed by a placebo period of another 4 weeks (total duration of the trial 16 weeks). Active treatment produced a significant improvement in calculating ability, logical memory and paired associate learning compared to the placebo group.

Calculating ability was significantly improved by the end of week 8 and became highly significant at the end of week 12 and was maintained for a further 4 weeks after treatment withdrawal. Logical memory and recall of story improved by the end of week 4 onwards with active treatment and, once again, remained for 4 weeks after treatment ceased. Paired associate learning improved by week 8.

In 2010, results from a 12-week, randomised, double-blind, placebo-controlled trial using a brahmi extract known as BacoMind (300 mg/day: Natural Remedies) were published (Morgan & Stevens 2010). The study involved 81 healthy participants aged over 55 years of age. This comprehensive study measured audio-verbal and visual memory performance together with subjective memory performance using a battery of validated measures. Treatment with bacopa significantly improved memory acquisition and retention in healthy older people — specifically verbal learning, memory acquisition and delayed recall — when compared to controls.

Acute effects in healthy people

Whether bacopa has acute effects is uncertain as current clinical trials have produced inconsistent results. Nathan et al (2001) found no significant change in cognitive function 2 hours after ingesting 300 mg of a bacopa extract (standardised to 55% combined bacosides A and B). The double-blind, placebo-controlled trial of 38 healthy volunteers (ages 18–60) found no effects on working and short-term memory, memory consolidation, information processing, executive processes, problem solving or motor responsiveness.

In contrast, acute neurocognitive effects were identified in a double-blind, placebo-controlled, crossover study utilising bacopa extract (KeenMind) and involving 24 healthy participants (Downey et al 2013). Two doses of bacopa (320 mg and 640 mg) were compared to each other and placebo for effects on participants' performance on six repetitions of the Cognitive Demand Battery (CDB). The standard treatment dose of 320 mg improved performance on the first, second and fourth repetition of the CDB but had no effects on cardiovascular parameters, task-induced rating of stress or fatigue.

Children

Less research has been conducted with children; however the available evidence is promising. A single-blind open clinical study reported memory- and learning-enhancing effects and improved reaction time in children after 12 weeks of treatment (Sharma et al 1987). In this study children were given bacopa syrup three times daily (350 mg/dose) over 3 months. A small, randomised, double-blind trial of 36 children diagnosed with attention-deficit hyperactivity disorder (ADHD) showed that 12 weeks' treatment with fresh whole-plant extract of bacopa (50 mg twice daily) improved logical memory impairment (Negi et al 2000).

An Israeli study utilising a patented herbal and nutritional combination produced significant improvements to attention, cognition and impulse control in a larger double-blind, placebo-controlled study of 120 children with newly diagnosed ADHD (Katz et al 2010). After 4 months of treatment, the group showed substantial, statistically significant improvement in the four subscales and overall test of variables of attention scores, compared with no improvement in the control group, which persisted in an intention-to-treat analysis. The treatment being evaluated consisted of a patented blend of nutritive, food-grade herbs, prepared as a highly stable, dilute ethanol extract called Nurture & Clarity. Bacopa was one of the main herbal ingredients, but not the sole ingredient. Others in the treatment included *Paeoniae alba, Withania somnifera, Centella asiatica, Spirulina platensis* and *Mellissa officinalis,* together with a range of vitamins.

Anxiety

Bacopa has traditionally been used in Ayurvedic medicine to treat anxiety, and preliminary evidence is promising.

A placebo-controlled, randomised study of healthy subjects found that 300 mg of brahmi (KeenMind) daily reduced the anxiety compared with placebo, an effect most pronounced after 12 weeks compared to 5 weeks of treatment (Stough et al 2001). A reduction in anxiety was also reported by Calabrese et al (2008) in a double-blind, randomised, placebo-controlled study which tested whole-plant standardised dry extract of *Bacopa monniera* (300 mg/day) over 12 weeks. The trial of 54 volunteers aged 65 years or older, without clinical signs of dementia, found that active treatment reduced anxiety whereas anxiety increased in the placebo group.

OTHER USES

Traditional uses

Bacopa has been traditionally used as a brain tonic and is commonly recommended to improve memory and heighten learning capacity. It is also used as a nerve tonic to treat anxiety, nervous exhaustion or debility and is prescribed to enhance rehabilitation after any injury causing nervous deficit, such as stroke. Other traditional uses include promoting longevity, and treating diarrhoea and asthma. It is used as an anti-inflammatory, analgesic, anxiolytic and antiepileptic agent, with some support for these uses provided by in vitro and in vivo studies.

Irritable bowel syndrome

An Ayurvedic herbal combination consisting of *Aegle marmelos correa* and *Bacopa monniera* successfully treated 65% of patients with irritable bowel syndrome under double-blind, randomised conditions (Yadav et al 1989). Herbal treatment was particularly useful in the diarrhoea-predominant form of irritable bowel syndrome, compared with the placebo. Follow-up reviews 6 months after the trial found that relapse rates were the same among all test subjects. Although encouraging, it is not certain to what extent brahmi was responsible for these results.

DOSAGE RANGE

- Dried aerial parts of herb: 5–10 g/day.
- Fluid extract (1 : 2) or equivalent oral dose form: 5–13 mL/day in divided doses.
- Standardised extract (BacoMind or KeenMind) 300 mg/day.

For children aged 6 years and older: 350 mg of dried plant extract in a syrup form was administered three times daily.

According to clinical studies

- Cognitive activator effects: 300 mg/day.

Positive results obtained in one controlled study have found that 5–12 weeks' use is required before clinical effects are observed (Stough et al 2001).

TOXICITY

The LD_{50} data for an ethanolic extract of bacopa is 17 g/kg (oral) (Mills & Bone 2005).

Animal studies indicate that LD_{50} of standardised extract (BacoMind) is 2400 mg/kg body weight with no observed adverse effect limit of 500 mg/kg body weight after 90 days (Allan et al 2007).

ADVERSE REACTIONS

The most common side effects are minor gastrointestinal disturbances, nausea, abdominal cramps, increased stool frequency and diarrhoea (Morgan & Stevens 2010, Pravina et al 2007). Less frequent side effects include sleepiness, headache, palpitations, dry mouth, thirst and fatigue, insomnia and vivid dreams or lack of dreams.

SIGNIFICANT INTERACTIONS

Controlled studies are not available, so interactions are based on evidence of activity and are largely theoretical and speculative.

Cholinergic drugs

Cholinergic activity has been identified for brahmi, therefore increased drug activity is theoretically possible — observe patient, although a beneficial interaction is possible under professional supervision.

Serotonergic drugs

Serotonergic activity has been identified for bacopa extracts, therefore there is a theoretical increased risk of serotonin syndrome when bacopa is used together with selective serotonin reuptake inhibitor and serotonin-noradrenaline reuptake inhibitor medicines — the clinical significance of the interaction is unclear. Caution until further investigation can confirm.

Practice points/Patient counselling

- Brahmi is an Ayurvedic herb that has been used for several thousand years as a brain tonic, to enhance intellect, treat psychiatric illness, epilepsy and insomnia and as a mild sedative.
- There is now good evidence that bacopa exerts cognitive and nootropic activity via multiple mechanisms, including activation of the serotonergic and cholinergic systems, antioxidant and mitochondrial stabilisation activities and enhancement of synaptic plasticity.
- Human studies have shown that brahmi (KeenMind, BacoMind, whole-plant extract) has a significant effect on various aspects of learning and memory when used long-term; effects with short-term use or single doses are less well investigated. There is also evidence of anxiolytic activity according to clinical studies.
- Brahmi has potent antioxidant activity, which appears to be a result of both direct free radical scavenging activity and increasing endogenous antioxidant systems in the brain and liver.
- Anticholinesterase, antidepressant, antiulcer, antispasmodic, anti-inflammatory, antihistamine, neuroprotective, antinociceptive activities and lipid-lowering actions have been demonstrated in animal studies. Elevated thyroxine levels have also been observed.

CONTRAINDICATIONS AND PRECAUTIONS

Caution is advised in hyperthyroidism, as bacopa has been shown to significantly elevate thyroxine levels in vivo. The clinical significance of this finding is unknown.

Brahmi may cause gastrointestinal symptoms in people with coeliac disease, fat malabsorption syndrome, vitamins A, D, E or K deficiency, dyspepsia or pre-existing cholestasis due to the high saponins content of the herb (Mills & Bone 2005).

PREGNANCY USE

Brahmi is recommended as a tonic for anxiety in pregnancy according to traditional Ayurvedic medicine; however, insufficient information is available to confirm safety during pregnancy.

PATIENTS' FAQs

What will this herb do for me?

Brahmi has a long history of use as a brain tonic. Results from scientific studies demonstrate that it will enhance aspects of learning, memory and cognitive function with long-term use and is also likely to reduce anxiety,

B

When will it start to work?
Studies indicate that 5–12 weeks' continual use is required for benefits on cognitive function to become apparent. Acute effects may also be possible, but there is less evidence to be certain.

Are there any safety issues?
Information from traditional sources suggests that brahmi is well tolerated at the usual therapeutic doses and the most common side effects relate to gastrointestinal disturbances which are mild and reversible, such as nausea, frequent bowel motions and abdominal cramping. Clinical studies have not confirmed drug interactions so cautions are theoretical.

REFERENCES

Adams M, et al. Plants traditionally used in age-related brain disorders. A survey of ethnobotanical literature. J Ethnopharmacol 113.3 (2007): 363–81.

Allan JJ et al. Safety evaluation of a standardized phytochemical composition extracted from *Bacopa monnieri* in Sprague-Dawley rats. Food Chem Toxicol 45.10 (2007): 1928–1937.

Anbarasi K, et al. Protective effect of bacoside A on cigarette smoking-induced brain mitochondrial dysfunction in rats. J Environ Pathol Toxicol Oncol 24.3 (2005a): 225–34.

Anbarasi K, et al. Lactate dehydrogenase isoenzyme patterns upon chronic exposure to cigarette smoke: protective effects of bacoside A. Environmental Toxicology and Pharmacology 20 (2005b): 345–350.

Anbarasi K et al. Creatine kinase isoenzyme patterns upon chronic exposure to cigarette smoke: protective effect of bacoside A. Vascul Pharmacol 42.2 (2005c): 57–61.

Anbarasi K et al. Cigarette smoking induces heat shock protein 70 kDa expression and apoptosis in rat brain: modulation by bacoside A. Neuroscience 138.4 (2006): 1127–1135.

Bhaskar, M. & Jagtap, A.G. 2011. Exploring the possible mechanisms of action behind the antinociceptive activity of *Bacopa monniera*. Int. J Ayurveda.Res., 2, (1) 2–7.

Bhattacharya SK et al. Antioxidant activity of *Bacopa monniera* in rat frontal cortex, striatum and hippocampus. Phytother Res 14.3 (2000): 174–179.

Calabrese C et al. Effects of a standardized *Bacopa monnieri* extract on cognitive performance, anxiety, and depression in the elderly: a randomized, double-blind, placebo-controlled trial. J Altern Complement Med 14.6 (2008): 707–713.

Chakravarty AK, et al. Bacopasides III-V: three new triterpenoid glycosides from *Bacopa monniera*. Chem Pharm Bull (Tokyo) 51 (2003): 215–2117.

Channa S et al. Broncho-vasodilatory activity of fractions and pure constituents isolated from *Bacopa monniera*. J Ethnopharmacol 86.1 (2003): 27–35.

Channa S et al. Anti-inflammatory activity of *Bacopa monniera* in rodents. J Ethnopharmacol 104 (2006): 296–289.

Charles, P.D., et al. 2011. *Bacopa monniera* leaf extract up-regulates tryptophan hydroxylase (TPH2) and serotonin transporter (SERT) expression: implications in memory formation. J Ethnopharmacol., 134, (1) 55–61

Dar A, Channa S. Calcium antagonistic activity of *Bacopa monniera* on vascular and intestinal smooth muscles of rabbit and guinea-pig. J Ethnopharmacol 66.2 (1999): 167–174.

Das A et al. A comparative study in rodents of standardized extracts of *Bacopa monniera* and Ginkgo biloba. Anticholinesterase and cognitive enhancing activities. Pharmacol Biochem Behav 73.4 (2002): 893–900.

Dhanasekaran M et al. *Bacopa monniera* extract reduces beta-amyloid deposition in doubly transgenic PSAPP Alzheimer's disease mouse model. Neurology 63.8 (2004): 1545–8.

Dhanasekaran M et al. Neuroprotective mechanisms of ayurvedic antidementia botanical *Bacopa monniera*. Phytother Res 21.10 (2007): 965–969.

Downey, L.A., et al. 2013. An Acute, double-blind, placebo-controlled crossover study of 320 mg and 640 mg doses of a special extract of *Bacopa monnieri* (CDRI 08) on sustained cognitive performance. Phytother. Res. 27: 1407–1413.

Dutta D et al. In vitro safety evaluation and anticlastogenic effect of BacoMind™ on human lymphocytes. Biomed Environ Sci 21.1 (2008): 7–23.

Goel RK et al. In vitro evaluation of *Bacopa monniera* on anti-*Helicobacter pylori* activity and accumulation of prostaglandins. Phytomedicine 10.6–7 (2003): 523–527.

Hota SK et al. *Bacopa monniera* leaf extract ameliorates hypobaric hypoxia induced spatial memory impairment. Neurobiol Dis 34.1 (2009): 23–39.

Jain P et al. Anti-inflammatory effects of an Ayurvedic preparation, Brahmi Rasayan, in rodents. Indian J Exp Biol 32 (1994): 633–636.

Jyoti A, et al. *Bacopa monniera* prevents from aluminium neurotoxicity in the cerebral cortex of rat brain. J Ethnopharmacol 111.1 (2007): 56–62.

Kamesh, V. & Sumathi, T. 2012. Antihypercholesterolemic effect of *Bacopa monniera* Linn. on high cholesterol diet induced hypercholesterolemia in rats. Asian Pac. J Trop. Med, 5 (12) 949–955.

Kapoor R, et al. *Bacopa monnieri* modulates antioxidant responses in brain and kidney of diabetic rats. Environmental Toxicology and Pharmacology 27.1 (2009): 62–69.

Kar A, et al. Relative efficacy of three medicinal plant extracts in the alteration of thyroid hormone concentrations in male mice. J Ethnopharmacol 81.2 (2002): 281–285.

Katz, M., et al. 2010. A compound herbal preparation (CHP) in the treatment of children with ADHD: a randomized controlled trial. J Atten. Disord., 14, (3) 281–291.

Limpeanchob N et al. Neuroprotective effect of *Bacopa monnieri* on beta-amyloid-induced cell death in primary cortical culture. J Ethnopharmacol 120.1 (2008): 112–1117.

Mathew, J., et al. 2010. Behavioral deficit and decreased GABA receptor functional regulation in the cerebellum of epileptic rats: effect of *Bacopa monnieri* and bacoside A. Epilepsy Behav., 17, (4) 441–447.

Mathew, J., et al. 2011. Behavioral deficit and decreased GABA receptor functional regulation in the hippocampus of epileptic rats: effect of *Bacopa monnieri*. Neurochem.Res., 36, (1) 7–16.

Mathew, J., et al. 2012. Decreased GABA receptor in the cerebral cortex of epileptic rats: effect of *Bacopa monnieri* and Bacoside-A. J Biomed.Sci., 19, 25.

Mills S, Bone K. The essential guide to herbal safety. Edinburgh: Churchill Livingstone, 2005.

Morgan A, Stevens J. Does *Bacopa monnieri* improve memory performance in older persons? Results of a randomized, placebo-controlled, double-blind trial. J Altern Complement Med 2010;16:753–9.

Nathan PJ et al. The acute effects of an extract of *Bacopa monniera* (Brahmi) on cognitive function in healthy normal subjects. Hum Psychopharmacol 16.4 (2001): 345–351.

Negi, K.S., et al. 2000. Clinical evaluation of memory enhancing properties of Memory Plus in children with attention deficit hyperactivity disorder. Indian J Psychiatry, 42, (SUPPL.) 42–50

Pravina K et al. Safety evaluation of BacoMind™ in healthy volunteers: a phase 1 study. Phytomedicine 14.5 (2007): 301–308.

Preethi, J., et al. 2012. Participation of microRNA 124-CREB pathway: a parallel memory enhancing mechanism of standardised extract of *Bacopa monniera* (BESEB CDRI-08). Neurochem. Res., 37, (10) 2167–2177.

Rai D et al. Adaptogenic effect of *Bacopa monniera* (Brahmi). Pharmacol Biochem Behav 75.4 (2003): 823–830.

Ranghav, S., et al. Randomized controlled trial of standardized *Bacopa monniera* extract in age-associated memory impairment. Indian J Psychiatry. 48[4], 238–242. 2008.

Rao CV, et al. Experimental evaluation of *Bacopa monnieri* on rat gastric ulceration and secretion. Indian J Physiol Pharmacol 44.4 (2000): 435–441.

Roodenrys S et al. Chronic effects of Brahmi (*Bacopa monnieri*) on human memory. Neuropsychopharmacology 27.2 (2002): 279–281.

Russo A, Borrelli F. *Bacopa monniera*, a reputed nootropic plant: an overview. Phytomedicine 12 (2005): 305–317.

Russo A et al. Nitric oxide-related toxicity in cultured astrocytes: effect of *Bacopa monniera*. Life Sci 73.12 (2003a): 1517–26.

Russo A et al. Free radical scavenging capacity and protective effect of *Bacopa monniera* L. on DNA damage. Phytother Res 17.8 (2003b): 870–5.

Saini, N., et al. 2012. Neuroprotective effects of *Bacopa monnieri* in experimental model of dementia. Neurochem. Res., 37, (9) 1928–1937.

Sairam K et al. Prophylactic and curative effects of *Bacopa monniera* in gastric ulcer models. Phytomedicine 8.6 (2001): 423–430.

Sairam K et al. Antidepressant activity of standardized extract of *Bacopa monniera* in experimental models of depression in rats. Phytomedicine 9.3 (2002): 207–211.

Samiulla DS, et al. Mast cell stabilising activity of *Bacopa monnieri*. Fitoterapia 72.3 (2001): 284–285.

Saraf MK et al. *Bacopa monniera* ameliorates amnesic effects of diazepam qualifying behavioral-molecular partitioning. Neuroscience 155.2 (2008): 476–484.

Sharma R, et al. Efficacy of *Bacopa monniera* in revitalizing intellectual functions in children. J Res Edu Indian Med. 1987;1:12

Sheikh N et al. Effect of *Bacopa monniera* on stress induced changes in plasma corticosterone and brain monoamines in rats. J Ethnopharmacol 111.3 (2007): 671–6776.

Shukia B, et al. Effect of Brahmi Rasayan on the central nervous system. J Ethnopharmacol 21.1 (1987): 65–74.

Singh HK, Dhawan BN. Effect of *Bacopa monniera* Linn. (brahmi) extract on avoidance responses in rat. J Ethnopharmacol 5.2 (1982): 205–214.

Stough C et al. The chronic effects of an extract of *Bacopa monniera* (Brahmi) on cognitive function in healthy human subjects. Psychopharmacology (Berl) 156.4 (2001): 481–484.

Stough C, et al. Examining the nootropic effects of a special extract of *Bacopa monniera* on human cognitive functioning: 90 day double-blind placebo-controlled randomized trial. Phytother Res 2008;22:1629–34.

Stough, C., et al. 2011. Improving general intelligence with a nutrient-based pharmacological intervention. Intelligence, 39, (2–3) 100–107.

Sumathi T, Nongbri A. Hepatoprotective effect of bacoside-A, a major constituent of *Bacopa monniera*. Phytomedicine 15.10 (2008): 901–9005.

Tripathi YB et al. *Bacopa monniera* Linn. as an antioxidant: mechanism of action. Indian J Exp Biol 34.6 (1996): 523–526.

Uabundit, N., et al. 2010. Cognitive enhancement and neuroprotective effects of *Bacopa monnieri* in Alzheimer's disease model. J Ethnopharmacol., 127, (1) 26–31.

Viji V, Helen A. Inhibition of lipoxygenases and cycloxygenase-2 enzymes by extracts isolated from *Bacopa monniera*. J Ethnopharmacol 118.2 (2008): 305–311.

Williamson EM. Major herbs of Ayurveda. Dabur Research Foundation and Dabur Ayurvet Ltd. London: Churchill Livingstone, 2002.

Yadav SK et al. Irritable bowel syndrome: therapeutic evaluation of indigenous drugs. Indian J Med Res 90 (1989): 496–503.

Calcium

BACKGROUND AND RELEVANT PHARMACOKINETICS

In the context of both biosphere and biology (plant and animal) calcium plays a leading role. Its abundance in the environment (e.g. limestone, marble, coral) is reflected, in part, in the human body, with calcium being the most abundant mineral in the body. Calcium homeostasis reflects a balancing act between requirements for proper function and the organism's need to protect against excess cellular calcium levels and associated toxicity. This balance has ramifications not only for our own physiology, but also in terms of levels and bioavailability of dietary calcium.

Three hormones regulate calcium status in the body — calcitriol (active vitamin D), parathyroid hormone (PTH) and calcitonin. Calcitriol increases intestinal absorption of dietary calcium when blood levels are low. In addition, PTH signals the kidneys to reduce calcium loss, produce more calcitriol and also activate osteoclasts that release bone calcium. Calcitonin is secreted by the thyroid gland when calcium levels become too high and opposes the action of PTH, thereby returning calcium levels back to normal.

Calcium, found in the diet or supplements, exists in salt form, from which it must be released for absorption to occur. Adequate hydrochloric acid levels are required to solubilise the majority of these calcium ions, failing which calcium salts entering the higher pH environment of the small intestine are more likely to precipitate and be rendered insoluble (Wahlqvist 2002). Low or moderate calcium intakes (≤400 mg/day) are absorbed via active transport mechanisms that are influenced by vitamin D. When intake is high, active transport mechanisms become saturated, leading to greater passive absorption. Although most absorption occurs in the small intestine, the large intestine may also be responsible for up to 4% of absorption and provides compensatory mechanisms for those individuals with compromised small intestine absorption (Groff & Gropper 2009).

Calcium's bioavailability from both food and supplements shows substantial variation, and may be influenced by other foods present in the gastrointestinal tract. Phytates (in wholegrains, nuts and seeds), oxalates, all types of fibres, unabsorbed dietary fatty acids and other divalent minerals all potentially compromise its absorption, while lactose (especially in children) and other sugars, as well as protein and the presence of vitamin D, all enhance uptake (Groff & Gropper 2009).

Calcium salts differ in the amount of elemental calcium, which may have clinical implications and affect dose selection. Calcium carbonate contains the highest amount of elemental calcium by weight (40%), calcium citrate (21%), calcium lactate (14%) and calcium gluconate (9%) (Kopic & Geibel 2013). In addition to having variable calcium fractions, the different calcium salts have widely divergent water solubility, which may also affect absorption and bioavailability. For example, calcium citrate dissolves 17 times more readily than calcium carbonate in water. However, 86% of calcium carbonate will still dissolve in a slightly more acidic environment (pH 5.5), which is higher than a normal maximum stomach pH of 4.5. Researchers in this area have not reached consensus as to whether the difference in water solubility is clinically relevant, provided the stomach pH is sufficiently acidic to dissolve the calcium supplement and allow for absorption (Kopic & Geibel 2013).

Besides the variation in absorption due to gastric pH, other dietary components and type of calcium salt, there are differences between individuals in their calcium absorption efficiency which can be up to 60% variance; the underlying mechanisms, although unclear, may be linked to vitamin D receptor (VDR) polymorphisms (Heaney & Weaver 2003). Consistent with this, our understanding of the magnitude of vitamin D's influence upon calcium absorption continues to broaden, including the life-stage-dependent bioavailability of this mineral. The age-associated decline in calcium absorption (children absorb ≈75% compared with ≤30% in adults) (Groff & Gropper 2009) has now been linked to vitamin D via reduced available calcitriol and decreased intestinal VDR levels, producing vitamin D resistance (Groff & Gropper 2009, Pattanaungkul et al 2000). Similarly, the decreasing bioavailability associated with (peri)menopause and the increased absorption evident early in pregnancy (Prentice 2003) are attributed largely to vitamin D-mediated effects. Calcium absorption, however, is described as being generally inefficient, with a substantial amount of calcium remaining unabsorbed in the lumen (Heaney & Weaver 2003).

Distribution results in 99% of absorbed calcium being deposited in bones. The remainder of the absorbed calcium is present in teeth and the intracellular or extracellular fluids. Calcium is excreted in faeces, sweat and urine.

FOOD SOURCES

Good dietary sources of calcium include dairy products, fortified soy products, fish with bones (especially salmon and sardines), tofu, broccoli, collard greens, mustard greens, bok choy, clams and black strap molasses. Certain brands of soy milk, fruit juice, breakfast cereal and bread are also fortified with calcium, which provides an alternative for people who don't eat dairy products. People with limited dairy intake may still need to consider supplementation to ensure they meet RDI levels.

DEFICIENCY SIGNS AND SYMPTOMS

Optimal calcium intake is essential during every stage of life and insufficient intake in childhood years can have ramifications later in life.

While there is little information available about the prevalence of deficiency across the general Australian population, a Melbourne study of 1045 women aged 20–92 years in 2000 revealed that approximately 76% of women consumed calcium at levels less than the recommended daily intake (RDI), and an additional 14% demonstrated a grossly inadequate intake of less than 300 mg/day (Pasco et al 2000). Dietary calcium intake has been found to be inadequate and below Estimated Average Requirement (EAR) in the majority of elderly Australian women (Meng et al 2010). These figures are similar to those obtained by larger studies in the United States (Groff & Gropper 2009). Calculating the prevalence of calcium deficiency is partly hampered by physiological preservation of 'non-osseous' calcium for critical roles in exchange for the 'expendable' reserves in bone and, therefore, the slow development of overt deficiency features. Consequently, calcium deficiency is insidious in its early stages and potentially irreversible in the latter, making preventive optimisation the only successful pathway in all patients perceived to be at an increased risk. In addition to this, long-term suboptimal calcium has been linked to an increased risk of a range of other morbidities, including preeclampsia and colorectal cancer.

Deficiency signs and symptoms include:

- tetany: muscle pain, spasms and paraesthesias
- rickets
- osteomalacia
- increased neuromuscular irritability
- altered heart rate

- ambulatory developmental delays in children
- osteoporosis and increased risk of fractures
- bone pain and deformity
- tooth discolouration and increased decay
- hypertension
- increased risk of preeclampsia
- increased risk of colon cancer (controversial).

There are many situations and conditions in which the risk of hypocalcaemia may be increased.

Primary deficiency

Primary deficiency occurs as a result of inadequate dietary intake, with greatest risk seen in populations with increased calcium requirements e.g. children, adolescents, pregnant and lactating women, postmenopausal women (particularly those taking hormone replacement therapy [HRT] [Wahlqvist 2002]), people experiencing rapid weight loss or patients receiving total parenteral nutrition (TPN).

Secondary deficiency

Calcium absorption is impaired in achlorhydria (more common in the elderly), intestinal inflammation and any malabsorptive disorder accompanied by steatorrhoea (Wilson et al 1991). Increased faecal calcium loss occurs with higher intakes of fibre and in fat malabsorption, while renal excretion has been shown in some studies to be increased in those patients ingesting a high protein diet (Kerstetter et al 1998).

Factors that compromise vitamin D status or activity will also affect calcium status), e.g. oral and inhaled corticosteroids (Beers & Berkow 2003, Pattanaungkul et al 2000, Prince et al 1997, Rossi et al 2005).

Other conditions that can predispose to hypocalcaemia include hypoparathyroidism (a deficiency or absence of PTH), idiopathic hypoparathyroidism (an uncommon condition in which the parathyroid glands are absent or atrophied), pseudohypoparathyroidism (characterised not by deficiency of PTH, but by target organ resistance to its action), magnesium depletion, renal tubular disease, renal failure, acute pancreatitis, hypoproteinaemia, septic shock or the use of certain medicines such as anticonvulsants (phenytoin, phenobarbitone) and rifampicin, and corticosteroids (Beers & Berkow 2003, Rossi et al 2005).

MAIN ACTIONS

Calcium is an essential mineral required for the proper functioning of numerous intracellular and extracellular processes, including muscle contraction, nerve conduction, beating of the heart, hormone release, blood coagulation, energy production and maintenance of immune function. It also plays a role in intracellular signalling and is involved in the regulation of many enzymes.

Bone and teeth mineralisation

Calcium is found in bone where it is mainly complexed with other ions in the form of hydroxyapatite crystals. Approximately 1% of calcium in bone can be freely exchanged into the extracellular fluid in order to buffer changes in calcium balance.

Muscle contraction

Calcium plays a major role in muscle contraction. Ionised serum calcium helps to initiate both smooth and skeletal muscle contraction and in particular, the regulation of rhythmic contraction of the heart muscle in combination with sodium and potassium. During exercise, one cause of muscle fatigue is the impaired activity of calcium in muscle cells (Insel et al 2013).

Blood clotting

Calcium is required in order for blood to clot. It is involved in several steps of the blood clotting cascade and is required for the production of fibrin, the protein that gives structure to blood clots (Insel et al 2013).

Nerve conduction

Calcium is required for nerve cells to transmit signals. The strength of the signal is proportional to the number of calcium ions crossing the nerve cell membrane (Insel et al 2013).

Altered membrane functions

Calcium fluxes across membranes, both within the cell and across the plasma membrane, and acts as a vehicle for the signal transduction necessary for neurotransmitter and hormone function. It also selectively alters cell wall permeability to regulate passage of fluids in and out of cells.

OTHER ACTIONS

Regulates various enzyme systems responsible for muscle contraction, fat digestion and protein metabolism.

CLINICAL USE

Many of the indications for calcium supplements are conditions thought to arise from a gross or marginal deficiency; however, some are based on the concept of 'beyond-repletion' calcium therapy.

Calcium deficiency

Traditionally, calcium supplementation has been used to treat deficiency or prevent deficiency in high-risk conditions or people with increased calcium requirements such as pregnant and lactating women. Acute severe hypocalcaemic states are treated initially with intravenous infusion of calcium salts. In chronic cases, oral calcium supplements are often combined with vitamin D supplements to improve absorption and utilisation.

Rickets and osteomalacia

A deficiency of either calcium or vitamin D can produce these bone disorders. (See *Vitamin D* monograph for further information.)

Infants

The percentage and type of fats within an infant formula and their ability to bind calcium salts and increase excretion has been shown to influence the bone mineral content (BMC) of infants. One hundred 8-week-old infants given formulas considered to be more similar to breastmilk and less likely to form calcium soaps in the gut showed increased BMC after only 1 month's treatment compared with those infants on standard formula (Kennedy et al 1999).

Bone mineral density (BMD), osteoporosis prophylaxis and reducing fracture risk

Calcium supplements are prescribed widely to promote bone health, including the treatment and prevention of osteoporosis, a major cause of morbidity and mortality in older people (Hennekens & Barice 2011). RCTs assessing BMD generally show a beneficial effect of calcium treatment in both men and women (typically a 1%–2% absolute difference between the treatment and control groups over 2–3 years), which results in a sustained reduction in bone loss of 50%–60%. The effect appears to be greatest for people whose baseline dietary calcium intake is low (Sanders et al 2009).

Adequate calcium intake is particularly important to consider in at-risk populations because osteoporosis-related fractures can lead to early disability and death. Ensuring adequate calcium intake alone is not sufficient and vitamin D status is also important as both contribute to bone density and associated protective effects. Sufficient trace minerals such as manganese, zinc and copper and weight-bearing exercise is also suggested and the use of anti-resorptive drugs together with mineral supplementation may be required in high risk groups or those with pre-existing osteoporosis.

The lifetime risk of fracture is highest in white women, and decreases successively among Hispanic, Asian and African-American people. For white women, it occurs 20% for the spine, 15% for the wrist and 18% for the hip, with an exponential increase in risk beyond the age of 50 years. Within 12 months after a hip fracture, approximately 13% of people die, with most survivors losing their previous independence. Calcium supplementation, together with vitamin D, may reduce vertebral and non-vertebral fractures (Vestergaard et al 2011). This is supported by a 2010 meta-analysis of seven randomised studies of vitamin D or calcium and vitamin D which included 68,517 participants (mean age 69.9 years, range 47–107 years, 14.7% men) (Abrahamsen 2010). The study found that calcium and vitamin D given together significantly reduced hip fractures and total fractures, and probably vertebral fractures, irrespective of age, sex or previous fractures. The protective effect is modest for combined therapy, whereas no significant effects were seen for vitamin D alone in doses of 10–20 microg/day for preventing fractures. Recently, a question has arisen as to whether calcium supplementation may in fact increase hip fracture risk; however, the issue has not been resolved and deserves further investigation.

Based on these findings, calcium could be considered a low potency anti-resorptive agent which should be taken in sufficient doses together with adequate vitamin D to produce any benefits.

The position statement from Osteoporosis Australia, the Endocrine Society of Australia and the Australian and New Zealand Bone and Mineral Society states that the balance of evidence remains in favour of combined calcium and vitamin D supplementation in elderly men and women for the prevention of fractures and calcium is regarded as an integral component of anti-resorptive regimens (Sanders et al 2009).

Children and adolescents

Most, but not all, RCTs involving children and adolescents using either dairy-supplemented foods or calcium supplementation have demonstrated some benefit at one or more of the BMD sites measured (Sanders et al 2009). However, a meta-analysis of 19 RCTs showed that there was no effect on BMD in children at the femoral neck or lumbar spine, and only a small benefit on total body BMD and upper limb BMD that was unlikely to substantially reduce adult fracture risk (Winzenberg et al 2006). The upper limb was the only site where a sustained BMD benefit was demonstrated after cessation of calcium supplementation. More studies are required in children with low calcium intakes and in peripubertal children.

The benefits of long-term supplementation may be greatest in children with pre-existing deficiency according to a meta-analysis of 21 RCTs (Huncharek et al

2008b). This study found no effect for calcium supplementation in individuals with (near)adequate calcium intake at baseline but found a significantly increased BMC (35–49 g) in individuals with a preexisting deficiency taking long-term treatment.

The same year, Lambert et al (2008) undertook an 18-month study of calcium-deficient adolescent girls (average age 12 years), increasing their mean daily intake by 555 mg in the treatment group which yielded a significantly increased BMC and BMD and reduced bone turnover markers in the treatment group compared with a placebo (Lambert et al 2008).

A more recent meta-analysis investigating whether weight-bearing exercises done by prepubertal children improves BMC found that the effect was strongest when done alongside a high calcium intake and only weak otherwise (Behringer et al 2014). Numerous studies, including one by Stear et al in 2003 of 144 pubertal girls, have confirmed a synergistic relationship between mechanical load through physical activity, calcium status and bone calcium accumulation; however, it is important to note that physical activity has a positive effect on BMD only at high calcium intakes, with no effect at calcium intakes of less than 1000 mg/day (Harkness & Bonny 2005).

The results of one long-term study has suggested that skeletal stature may be a determinant in whether long-term benefits are more likely with supplementation during puberty. The placebo-controlled study (n = 354 pubertal girls) used calcium supplements (670 mg/day) over a 7-year period and reported significant increases in BMD during growth spurts in the supplemented group; however, these gains did not uniformly persist into late adolescence and only girls of tall stature received long-lasting benefits. Interestingly, the placebo group exhibited a 'catch-up' in bone mineral accretion subsequent to the pubertal growth spurt (Matkovic et al 2005).

A second study introduces other issues regarding the impact of variable calcium status in adolescents. This RCT of 144 prepubertal girls used 850 mg/day of calcium over 1 year. After follow-up some 7 years later, in addition to positive effects on BMD outcomes, an inverse relationship became apparent between calcium supplementation and age of menarche. The authors speculate that higher calcium intake prior to menarche may favourably impact on long-term BMD through this dual mechanism (Chevalley et al 2005).

Postmenopausal women

Bone mass remains relatively stable during early adulthood but changes dramatically after menopause. For about the first 5 years after menopause, women lose bone at the rate of about 2%–3% per year and then continue to lose about 1% of bone mass per year to the end of life. During this time, there is a decline in intestinal calcium absorption and an increase in urinary calcium excretion (Sanders et al 2009).

Numerous studies have confirmed a role for calcium in bolstering BMD in late postmenopausal women where results are more consistent than for perimenopausal women (Sanders et al 2009). Clinical studies have assessed its efficacy as a sole agent against placebo, in comparison with steroid hormones, antiresorptive drugs and as part of combination therapy. While increased calcium intake provides some benefits it should be accompanied by sufficient vitamin D status for optimal results. In addition, a protein rich-diet together with weight-bearing exercise are considered the key pillars for osteoporosis prevention among postmenopausal women (Bischoff-Ferrari 2012). Adequate levels of trace minerals such as zinc, copper and manganese are also recommended (Strause et al 1994).

The efficacy of supplementation with calcium is not only dependent on vitamin D status but also baseline calcium levels as women with poor dietary intakes tend to achieve significant improvements over placebo, with more modest or no effect evident in groups with higher intakes at baseline (Daniele et al 2004, Fardellone et al 1998).

In a recent RCT trial of 159 postmenopausal women, calcium 1200 mg daily was shown to reduce the parathyroid hormone and bone turnover markers (cross-linked C-telopeptide and procollagen type 1 N-terminal propeptide) after 6 months (Aloia et al 2013). This provides some rationale for the long-term use of calcium supplements for osteoporosis prevention.

Men

While bone mineral density remains stable throughout adulthood, men start to lose bone density about the age of 50 years, although at a slower rate than women. By the age of 60 years, the rate of bone loss is similar for men and women as calcium absorption decreases over time (Sanders et al 2009).

The overwhelming majority of calcium studies for bone health have been conducted in postmenopausal women and often their results have simply been extrapolated to produce clinical protocols for men regarding osteoporosis prevention and management. The few studies conducted in male populations have produced inconsistent results, possibly due to differences in dosage and also vitamin D status of participants. For example, one study showed no benefit at 600 mg/day, while yielding BMD improvements secondary to higher doses (1200 mg/day) comparable with postmenopausal women (Reid et al 2008).

The elderly

A number of large studies have investigated the preventive effect of calcium alone or in combination with vitamin D in the elderly. Studies by Chapuy et al (1992, 1994, 2002), Dawson-Hughes et al (1997) and Larsen et al (2004) demonstrate a significant reduction in fracture risk (≤16%), while a meta-analysis of 29 RCTs conducted in 63,897 individuals 50 years of age or older over an average of 3.5 years also concluded that calcium alone (≥1200 mg/day) or in combination with vitamin D (≥800 IU/day) reduced the risk of fracture by 12–24% and reduced bone loss by 0.54% at the hip and 1.19% at the spine (Tang et al 2007).

More recently, a meta-analysis of over 68,000 participants (mean age 69.9 years) concluded that calcium combined with vitamin D significantly but modestly reduced hip fractures and total fractures, and probably vertebral fractures, irrespective of age, sex or previous fractures (2010).

In general, the greatest improvements are noted specifically in the elderly, institutionalised, underweight and calcium deficient.

Glucocorticoid (GC)-induced osteoporosis

Glucocorticoid-induced osteoporosis is the leading cause of osteoporosis in young adults and the most common cause of secondary osteoporosis. GCs induce rapid bone loss and increase the risk of fracture; however, the fracture risk is higher than expected based on bone mineral density values suggesting excess bone fragility is multifactorial (Soen 2013). GCs have a negative impact on bone through direct effects on bone cells and indirect effects on calcium absorption (Warriner & Saag 2013).

The use of GCs is widespread in medicine as they are used in almost all medical specialties. They are also used long-term by various patient groups such as those with severe asthma or rheumatological disease. In regards to rheumatological disease, morbidity secondary to the use of GCs represents an important aspect of the management as the incidences of vertebral and non-vertebral fractures are elevated, ranging from 30% to 50% of the individuals on GC for over 3 months

(Pereira et al 2012). The risk or fracture is also elevated among asthmatics receiving inhaled and/or systemic glucocorticoids, with one report indicating approximately one in six people with asthma developed fractures over 5 years. The interaction with calcium plays a small role in this process, with GCs directly inhibiting vitamin D-mediated intestinal absorption of calcium. High vitamin D doses (50,000 IU twice weekly) in combination with 1.5 g calcium daily can overcome this interference (Wilson et al 1991), whereas treatment with calcium alone or in combination with etidronate may not be effective (Campbell et al 2004).

Supplementation during pregnancy and lactation

The NHMRC nutrient reference value recommendations for calcium intakes for pregnant women (ages 14–18 years) are 1300 mg/day and 1000 mg/day for older women (19–50 years). If the woman avoids dairy in her usual diet (e.g. lactose intolerant) and does not consume alternative high calcium food (e.g. calcium enriched soya milk), calcium supplementation is recommended at 1000 mg/day. Sufficient calcium intake is important as deficiency is associated with preeclampsia and intrauterine growth restriction. Supplementation may reduce both the risk of low birth weight and the severity of preeclampsia (Hovdenak & Haram 2012).

Evidence from 1997 found that approximately 40% of primiparous Australian women failed to meet the RDI for calcium. Considered a critical nutrient during pregnancy with at least a two-fold increase in requirements observed, its metabolism during gestation significantly changes from as early as 12 weeks, with doubling of both absorption and excretion, followed by additional losses through lactation, which can account for reductions in maternal bone mineral content of 3–10% (Prentice 2003).

Prevention of hypertension and preeclampsia

Gestational hypertensive disorders are the second leading cause of maternal deaths worldwide. Both epidemiological and clinical studies have shown that an inverse relationship exists between calcium intake and development of hypertension in pregnancy (Imdad & Bhutta 2012).

A 2012 systematic review analysing results from 15 RCTs confirmed that calcium supplementation during pregnancy is associated with a significant reduction in risk of gestational hypertensive disorders and pre-term birth and an increase in birthweight (85 gm) without any associated increased risk of kidney stones. Pooled analysis showed that calcium supplementation during pregnancy reduced risk of preeclampsia by 52% and that of severe preeclampsia by 25%. There was no effect on incidence of eclampsia. Importantly, there was a significant reduction for risk of maternal mortality/severe morbidity by 20% and a 24% reduction in risk of pre-term birth with calcium supplementation during pregnancy (Imdad & Bhutta 2012).

Trials that included a 1996 meta-analysis of studies involving calcium and hypertension in pregnancy have shown a substantial mean reduction in both systolic blood pressure (SBP) and diastolic blood pressure (DBP), which was also confirmed by more recent reviews (Atallah et al 2002, Bucher et al 1996).

Further reviews of studies involving over 15,000 women, however, have supported calcium's preventive role with researchers demonstrating significant risk reduction in both low-risk (RR 0.48) and high-risk women (RR 0.22), hence concluding calcium supplementation should be recommended for those women with a low calcium intake who are at risk of developing gestational hypertension (Crowther et al 1999, Hofmeyr et al 2003, 2006, 2007).

There is currently no unanimous explanation for calcium's protective effect (Villar et al 2003). While the antagonistic relationship between calcium and lead has been previously hypothesised to be involved (Sowers et al 2002), recent evidence of calcium's lack of effect on platelet count, plasma urate and proteinuria, in spite of reducing preeclamptic incidence, implies that high-dose calcium effectively lowers blood pressure without influencing the condition's underlying pathology (Hofmeyr et al 2008).

A small number of studies have investigated the effects of calcium in combination with other nutrients, including antioxidant and omega-3 oils in this population. One randomised, placebo-controlled, double-blind study involving a sample of 48 primigravidas, using a combination of 600 mg/day calcium and 450 mg/day of conjugated linoleic acid (CLA) from weeks 18–22 until delivery, resulted in a significantly reduced incidence of pregnancy-induced hypertension (8% vs 42% of the control group) (Herrera et al 2005). Further studies are warranted to elicit the individual impact of both nutrients and to determine the superiority of sole or combination treatment.

Leg cramps

Calcium supplements are commonly prescribed in pregnancy when leg cramps are a problem. A Cochrane review of five trials involving 352 women taking various supplements for the treatment of leg cramps in pregnancy included only one placebo-controlled trial of calcium. From this, researchers concluded that any improvement in cramps in those groups treated solely with calcium was likely to be due to a placebo effect, with significant findings limited to the groups taking other nutrients (Young & Jewell 2013).

Lead toxicity

Increased blood lead levels may occur during pregnancy and lactation as a result of bone resorption to accommodate the calcium needs of the developing fetus or nursing infant. Lead exposure is considered a potential risk to fetal and infant health and may affect fetal neurodevelopment and growth. Ninety-five per cent of lead is stored in the bone and, if mobilised, can be transferred to the fetus and infant via cord blood and breast milk (Ettinger et al 2007). Several studies suggest a low placental barrier to lead, with 79% of the mobilised lead from maternal bone passed to the infant (Dorea & Donangelo 2005). While a number of studies have indicated lead levels in the breast milk of Australian women appear to be well within a safe range, recent data from a study conducted by Ettinger et al (2004) revealed that even low lead content in human milk appears to be highly influential on the lead levels of infants in their first month of life. A separate review published in 2005 discussed additional related trends, such as increased lead concentrations in cord blood during winter months, because of lower vitamin D status (Dorea 2004).

Dietary calcium supplementation of 1200 mg/day commencing in the first trimester was associated with modest reductions in blood lead during pregnancy and may reduce risk of fetal exposure, according to the findings of a RCT of 670 pregnant women (Ettinger et al 2009).

A RCT of 617 lactating women supplemented with high-dose calcium carbonate found that the women in the calcium group showed significant reductions in blood lead levels. Those subjects who showed improved compliance and also had baseline higher bone lead content produced an overall reduction of 16.4% (Hernandez-Avila et al 2003). Similar positive findings came from a study in Mexico of 367 lactating women; however, the maximal reduction in lead concentrations reached only 10% (Ettinger et al 2006). When considered together, these results suggest that calcium supplementation may represent an important interventional strategy, albeit with a modest effect, for reducing infant lead exposure.

Neonatal benefits

Calcium supplementation during pregnancy has been postulated to have prolonged benefits in the offspring, as indicated in a study of nearly 600 children aged 5–9 years whose mothers had previously participated in a calcium trial during their pregnancy. The children demonstrated reduced SBP, compared with the children whose mothers had taken placebo, with significance reached particularly for those in the upper BMI bracket (Belizan et al 1997). More recent reviews, while still demonstrating some association between gestational calcium supplementation and reduced blood pressure and incidence of hypertension in the offspring (particularly older children e.g. 7 years), highlight the weakness of the evidence to date, including small sample sizes, methodological issues and the fact that most of the studies have been conducted in developed countries where calcium intake is more likely to be adequate (Bergel & Barros 2007, Hiller et al 2007).

Dyspepsia

A first-line over-the-counter (OTC) treatment for heartburn, indigestion and dyspepsia has often been an antacid, based on calcium carbonate in combination with magnesium and aluminium salts. Calcium, alone or in combination with the other ingredients, neutralises stomach acid allowing for immediate short-term symptomatic relief (Kopic & Giebel 2013, Sulz et al 2007). There have been case-reports of milk-alkali syndrome associated with excessive prolonged use of calcium carbonate products, especially for dyspepsia, however the incidence appears rare (Kopic & Giebel 2013, Bailey et al 2008, Picolos et al 2004, Nabhan et al 2004, Beall & Scofield 1995). Long-term use of calcium carbonate as an antacid has largely been superseded by use of H_2-antagonists or proton pump inhibtors, thus the milk-alkali risk is possibly also of less clinical relevance than it was several years ago.

Prevention of cancer

Interest in a relationship between dairy consumption and cancer incidence continues to grow, with evidence of both protective and contributory effects dependent upon both cancer type and timing of exposure. The consumption of dairy products, however, represents a mix of numerous variables and biological pathways that potentially convey these underlying actions, from which calcium's role is difficult to extricate (van der Pols et al 2007). An interventional study of calcium (1400–1500 mg/day), alone or with vitamin D_3 (1100 IU/day) compared to placebo over 4 years, offers more specific information regarding calcium's role in cancer (Lappe et al 2007). The study, conducted in 1179 women of more than 55 years, was primarily designed to assess effects on fracture incidence; however, upon further analysis also demonstrated significant risk reduction (RR 0.40) for all cancer incidence among the calcium and vitamin D group. When the analysis was restricted to only those cancers diagnosed after the first year of treatment, the RR became 0.23. While the group receiving calcium alone also demonstrated a reduced risk, the researchers speculate that this may not be robust and conclude that vitamin D is the key variable in reduced incidence of all cancer.

Prevention of colorectal cancer and recurrence of adenomatous polyps

Currently, the gold standard for measuring risk reduction by an intervention in colorectal cancer investigates the incidence of recurrence of adenomatous polyps following removal of all colonic polyps by polypectomy; further analyses evaluate reduction of total adenomatous polyps and reduction of advanced polyps as defined by size and the presence of severe dysplasia.

Low calcium intake has been associated with a higher risk of colorectal cancer (Kim et al 2013). A meta-analysis of 10 cohort studies showed a reduction in risk of colorectal cancer in those with a higher calcium intake (Cho et al 2004). Reasonably consistent evidence suggests that calcium supplementation of 1200 mg/day reduces total adenomas by approximately 20% and advanced adenomas by about 45% (Holt 2008). Calcium supplementation may also significantly prevent risk of recurrence of adenomas 3–4 years after initial removal, according to findings of a meta-analysis of three trials (*n* = 1485) (Shaukat et al 2005). Further to this, a 2008 Cochrane review examining the effect of supplementary calcium on the incidence of colorectal cancer and the incidence or recurrence of adenomatous polyps included two double-blind, placebo-controlled trials with a pooled population of 1346 subjects. Doses of supplementary elemental calcium used were 1200–2000 mg/day for 3–4 years. Reviewers concluded that, while the evidence to date appears promising and suggests a moderate degree of prevention against colorectal adenomatous polyps, more research with similar findings is required before this can be translated into any preventive protocol (Weingarten et al 2008).

Interestingly, some studies show that calcium's protective effect against recurrent adenomas is largely restricted to individuals with baseline serum 25-hydroxy vitamin D above the median (≈ 29 ng/mL). These data, together with other research findings, strongly point to the importance of both calcium and vitamin D for reducing colorectal cancer risk and altering adenoma recurrence (Mizoue et al 2008, Grau et al 2003, Holt 2008, Oh et al 2007).

Interactions between calcium and other variables in colorectal carcinogenesis have also been explored, revealing gender-specific results; protective in males but not in females in most (Ishihara et al 2008, Jacobs et al 2007, Ryan-Harshman & Aldoori 2007), but not all, studies. Further research, including re-analysis of the Women's Health Initiative (WHI) findings pertaining to colorectal cancer incidence, has elucidated oestrogen's critical modifying effect upon calcium, whereby the higher oestrogen levels of both menstruating and postmenopausal women taking HRT negate calcium's otherwise protective effect (Ding et al 2008). Explanations for this phenomenon include oestrogen's influence upon calcium distribution: removing it from circulation for bone deposition and competition for binding evident between vitamin D and oestrogen (Ding et al 2008, Oh et al 2007).

Early hypotheses regarding calcium's general protective effects focused on its ability to bind bowel-irritating substances secreted into bile. This notion is further supported by a number of studies demonstrating enhanced chemoprotection when high doses of calcium have been combined with dietary factors such as reduced fat and increased carbohydrate, fibre and fluid intakes (Hyman et al 1998, Rozen et al 2001, Schatzkin & Peters 2004).

One significant development in our understanding has been the discovery of human parathyroid calcium-sensing receptors in the human colon epithelium, which function to regulate epithelial proliferation and differentiation. New in vitro studies suggest that expression of these receptors may be induced by the presence of extracellular calcium and vitamin D, therefore promoting greater differentiation of the epithelial cells (Chakrabarty et al 2005, Holt 2008) and inducing apoptosis (Miller et al 2005). The effect of the calcium-sensing receptor (CASR) gene on development of colorectal cancer has also been investigated, with in vitro studies suggesting that CASR may mediate the pro-cell proliferative effects of low intestinal calcium concentration. Results from a recent case-controlled study involving 1235 participants showed that low calcium intake was associated with an increase in colorectal cancer risk; however, this did not appear to relate directly to CASR polymorphism (Kim et al 2013).

Clear parameters for dosing are not yet available, with some studies showing no further benefit above 700–800 mg/day of total calcium, while other studies suggest an ongoing inverse dose-dependent relationship without cutoff (Schatzkin & Peters 2004). Current evidence for a combined protective role of calcium, either dietary or supplemental, and vitamin D, particularly in men and postmenopausal women not taking HRT, is strong and further elucidation of the independent and combined effects of these nutrients will assist in the development of preventive protocols.

Other cancers

Ongoing research regarding calcium's potential role in a range of other cancers suggests a possible protective effect against breast and ovarian cancers (Genkinger et al 2006, McCullough et al 2005, 2008); however, the research remains preliminary and largely of epidemiological design. A greater body of evidence has developed regarding the interplay between calcium and prostate cancer, with initial findings touting a positive association between dairy product consumption, total dietary calcium intake (especially >1500 mg/day) and risk. The results of ongoing extensive, prospective epidemiological research involving hundreds of thousands of men, however, have been conflicting, both confirming (Ahn et al 2008, Gao et al 2005) and negating (Huncharek et al 2008a, Park et al 2007a, 2007b) earlier evidence. Two important details have recently emerged regarding the potential interaction between calcium and prostate cancer risk with several studies consistently demonstrating that calcium derived from supplements does not convey a greater risk (Ahn et al 2008, Baron et al 2005, Park et al 2007a) and limiting calcium as a risk factor only when consumed as dairy products, while greater non-dairy calcium intake appears to lower the risk (Allen et al 2008, Park et al 2007b). A prospective study of serum calcium adds to the riddle, revealing that results in the highest tertile typically more than 9 years prior to diagnosis were strongly associated with increased risk of fatal prostate cancer (Skinner & Schwartz 2008); however, such results may be indicative of calcium dysregulation rather than high intakes.

Hypertension

Ongoing broad-scale international epidemiological data, including prospective studies, link low dietary calcium intake with a slightly increased risk of hypertension (Alonso et al 2005, Elliott et al 2008, Geleijnse et al 2005, Wang et al 2008), in particular raised systolic blood pressure. Conversely, increased dietary calcium, typically in the form of low-fat dairy products, has been shown to be independently protective (RR 0.87 for highest quintile of calcium intake) (Alonso et al 2005, Wang et al 2008). One study identified that high dietary calcium was associated with SBP/DBP reductions of −2.42/−1.48 mmHg, after controlling for other known risk factors (Elliott et al 2008). This effect was more pronounced when accompanied by increased magnesium and phosphorus consumption. Interestingly, neither high-fat dairy products nor calcium supplements convey protection (Wang et al 2008).

Additional findings attracting attention include epidemiological links between markers of low calcium status or calcium metabolism abnormalities, hypertension and insulin resistance. Supporting the possible link between these phenomena are the results of a Japanese study of 34 non-diabetic hypertensive and 34 non-diabetic normotensive women. Multiple group assessments revealed statistically significant increased urinary calcium, lower BMD, depressed serum calcium and elevated circulating PTH in the hypertensive sample (Gotoh et al 2005).

Underlying mechanisms for calcium's protective effect are speculated to involve reduced calcium influx into cells, inhibiting vascular smooth muscle cell constriction, reduced activity of the renin–angiotensin system and improved Na/K balance (Wang et al 2008).

A 2006 Cochrane review of 13 RCTs involving 485 volunteers found that calcium supplementation significantly reduced SBP (mean difference: −2.5 mmHg), but not DBP (mean difference: −0.8 mmHg) compared with controls (Dickinson et al 2006). The authors temper their conclusion, stating that the quality of included trials was poor and the heterogeneity between trials means there is a tendency to overestimate treatment effects. Earlier, an extensive systematic review, updated in 1999 to include 42 randomised comparative trials, showed modest reductions in both SBP and DBP (−2 mmHg and −1 mmHg, respectively) with 1–2 g/day calcium over a 4–14-week intervention (Griffith et al 1999). Dietary calcium appeared to have a larger effect than supplementation, a finding reiterated in more recent studies (Wang et al 2008). The clinical significance of these small effects has been questioned and the recommendation of calcium as a therapy for all types of hypertension appears premature (Kawano et al 1998), particularly in light of more recent negative findings from the WHI, which investigated the effects of 1 g of calcium together with 400 IU of vitamin D over a median follow-up period of 7 years in postmenopausal women (Margolis et al 2008). Some studies have proposed that it is only a particular hypertensive subset that is calcium responsive. A number of researchers, for example, have hypothesised a physiological correlation between 'salt sensitive' hypertension and responsiveness to calcium treatment (Coruzzi & Mossini 1997, Resnick 1999). The link may be that sodium excess encourages calcium losses. This theory is further supported by an epidemiological study demonstrating that, while blood pressure was inversely correlated with dietary calcium, further analysis revealed sodium intake to be the primary influence, increasing pressures while concomitantly reducing BMD (Woo et al 2008).

Premenstrual syndrome

Of all the vitamins and minerals used in the treatment of premenstrual syndrome (PMS), calcium supplements show overwhelmingly positive results.

One of the earliest trials to show that calcium supplementation can alleviate symptoms in PMS was conducted in 1989 (Thys-Jacobs et al 1989). A randomised, double-blind, crossover trial involving 33 women with confirmed PMS compared the effects of daily 1000 mg calcium carbonate with placebo over 6 months. Results showed that 73% of women reported improved symptoms while taking calcium supplementation, whereas 15% preferred placebo. The premenstrual symptoms responding significantly to calcium supplementation were mood changes, water retention and premenstrual pain. Menstrual pain was also significantly alleviated.

In 1993, the *American Journal of Obstetrics and Gynecology* published a study that compared the effects of calcium (587 mg or 1336 mg) and manganese (1.0 mg or 5.6 mg) on menstrual symptoms. Ten women with normal menstrual cycles were observed over four 39-day periods during the trial (Penland & Johnson 1993). The researchers found that increasing calcium intake reduced mood, concentration and behavioural symptoms generally and reduced water retention during the premenstrual phase. Additionally, menstrual pain was reduced.

A more recent large, double-blind, placebo-controlled, randomised parallel-group study was conducted in the United States and supports the previous findings

(Thys-Jacobs et al 1998). Four hundred and sixty-six premenopausal women with confirmed moderate to severe PMS were randomly assigned to receive either 1200 mg elemental calcium (from calcium carbonate) or placebo for three menstrual cycles. Symptoms were documented daily by the subjects based on 17 core symptoms and four symptom factors (negative affect, water retention, food cravings and pain). Additionally, adverse effects and compliance were monitored daily. During the luteal phases of both the second and the third treatment cycles, a significantly lower mean symptom score was observed in the calcium group. By the third treatment cycle, calcium treatment resulted in a 48% reduction in total symptom score compared with baseline, whereas placebo achieved a 30% reduction. Furthermore, all four symptom factors responded in the calcium-treated group.

A 1999 review of multiple trials investigating calcium supplementation as an effective therapy for PMS has found overwhelming positive results (Ward & Holimon 1999).

The only RCT to be conducted in recent years was published in 2009 and once again produced positive results. The double-blind RCT compared 500 mg of calcium carbonate twice daily to placebo taken for 3 months by young female college students (mean age 21.4 ± 3.6 years) with diagnosed PMS. Active treatment resulted in significant improvements to early tiredness, appetite changes and depressive symptoms compared to placebo (Ghanbari et al 2009).

Some researchers in this area have hypothesised that part of the PMS aetiology lies in calcium dysregulation in the luteal phase and have highlighted the dramatic similarities between symptoms of PMS and hypocalcaemia (Thys-Jacobs 2000). Recent data from the Nurses' Health Study II support this theory, with evidence of low calcium and vitamin D levels in PMS populations when compared to controls (Bertone-Johnson et al 2005).

Weight loss

Evidence suggests that higher calcium intake may be associated with a lower body weight. This has been seen in several epidemiological studies and also some, but not all, studies using calcium supplementation (Onakpoya et al 2011, Tremblay & Gilbert 2011, Christensen et al 2009, Barba & Russo 2006, Garcia-Lorad et al 2007, Bueno et al 2008, Zhu et al 2013).

A relationship between low calcium intake and obesity was observed in an epidemiological study involving 1459 adults in Brazil, where the prevalence of participants that were overweight was higher in those with a low calcium intake, especially when less than 398.5 mg/day (Bueno et al 2008). Similarly, a negative relationship between calcium intake and BMI was reported in a study of 647 Spanish men and women (Garcia-Lorad et al 2007).

A meta-analysis of seven RCTs reported that calcium supplementation in overweight and obese individuals results in a small, but significant reduction in body weight (0.74 kg) and body fat (0.93 kg) compared to placebo. This review excluded studies that had been conducted for less than 6 months or that included subjects that were of a normal weight (Onakpoya et al 2011).

A prolific researcher in this area is Zemel (2004, Zemel et al 2004, 2005a, 2005b), having published three small trials investigating the effects of dietary and supplemental calcium in patients for weight maintenance or weight loss. These trials have consistently yielded positive results, demonstrating that in addition to enhanced weight loss on isocaloric and identical macronutrient profiles, with or without energy restriction, a diet providing high calcium levels of 1100–1200 mg/day results in central fat loss and corresponding improvements in blood pressure, insulin sensitivity and retention of lean tissue. Australian researchers Bowen and colleagues have also demonstrated similar results (Bowen et al 2004). Zemel et al conclude that dietary calcium and, in particular, dairy-based foods are the most effective form of calcium for weight loss and that results are significant within 12 weeks.An early review by Teegarden (2003), bringing together trials dating back 10 years to the first rat studies and updated in 2005, while acknowledging the promising data in relation to increased consumption of dairy products and weight management which had emerged over the intervening 2 years, noted the limitations of the current body of evidence that required addressing to elucidate the full extent of calcium's effect on weight. A more recent meta-analysis of 13 RCTs investigating calcium interventions ranging between 610 mg and 2400 mg/day over a period of 12 weeks–36 months failed to demonstrate a positive effect on weight loss for either calcium supplements or dairy products; however, once again methodological concerns were raised (Trowman et al 2006). In particular, this meta-analysis included RCTs designed to investigate the effects of calcium on bone health and only one of the included RCTs was specifically designed and powered to see if calcium supplementation altered fat loss. As Astrup (2008) notes in an editorial piece, this point is highly relevant, because a body fat loss of ≈1 kg/year may be extremely important in the prevention of weight gain and obesity, but large study groups are required in a randomised trial to obtain the statistical power necessary to detect such an effect (Astrup 2008).

In spite of this, studies have continued to emerge yielding positive findings in postmenopausal women as part of the WHI study (calcium and vitamin D treatment reducing risk of weight gain by 11%) (Caan et al 2007) and in overweight and obese type 2 diabetic patients (>8% more weight loss in those consuming calcium in the highest compared with the lowest tertile) (Shahar et al 2007). Additionally, one small study demonstrated an augmenting effect of calcium (1200 mg together with 400 IU vitamin D/day) over 15 weeks on weight loss-induced beneficial changes to blood lipids and lipoproteins (Major et al 2007). Most recently, an RCT involving 53 subjects showed that calcium (600 mg elemental/day) plus vitamin D_3 (125 IU/day) supplementation for 12 weeks promoted loss of body fat and visceral fat (Zhu et al 2013).

Although the underlying mechanism of action remains unclear, there is general acceptance that high calcium intake, particularly in the form of dairy products, and more recently calcium-fortified soy (Lukaszuk et al 2007), depresses PTH levels and $1,25(OH)_2D$, which in turn decreases intracellular calcium, thereby potentially inhibiting lipogenesis and stimulating lipolysis (Major et al 2007, McCarty & Thomas 2003, Schrager 2005, Zemel et al 2004). Additional proposed actions include promoting faecal fat loss and fat oxidation (Christensen et al 2009, Gonzalez et al 2012, Tremblay & Gilbert 2011), as well as by decreasing energy intake and facilitating appetite control (Tremblay & Gilbert 2011) and promoting satiety (Kabrnova-Hlavata et al 2008).

Christensen et al (2009) performed a meta-analysis of 15 RCTs that assessed the effect of calcium on faecal fat loss, The authors concluded that an increase in dietary calcium by about 1240 mg/day has the potential to increase faecal fat excretion by about 5.2 g/day, which is enough to be relevant for prevention of weight gain, or re-gain (Christensen et al 2009). Another meta-analysis investigating mechanisms by which calcium intake may affect weight reported that a high calcium intake appears to increase rate of fat oxidation, however the magnitude of effect appears relatively weak (Gonzalez et al 2012).

Nephrolithiasis

In spite of previous concerns regarding a causal relationship between dietary or supplemental calcium intake and the recurrence of oxalate stones, recent studies demonstrate that this fear appears unfounded. Collectively, the evidence points more towards a protective effect for increased dietary calcium, in relation to both urinary oxalate concentrations (Taylor & Curhan 2004) and reduced stone formation (Goldfarb 2009). The current view is that, rather than being a contributing factor for oxalate stones, dietary calcium, through its binding of oxalate in the gut, can minimise recurrence, as substantiated by other studies (Curhan et al 1997, Liebman & Chai 1997).

One study comprised 120 men with recurrent calcium oxalate stones due to idiopathic hypercalciuria and who were randomly assigned to either a low-calcium diet or low-animal protein, low-salt normal-calcium diet and assessed for changes in frequency of stone formation. Results clearly showed reduced oxalate excretion in those on a normal calcium intake, as well as a greater decrease in calcium oxalate saturation (Borghi et al 2002). In another study of 14 healthy men, assessment of the influence of dietary calcium on the given amount of oxalate demonstrated that with the inclusion of additional calcium (1121 mg) urinary oxalate levels increased in the control but not in the treatment group (Hess et al 1998).

OTHER USES

Hyperlipidaemia

Only a very few studies investigating calcium intake and serum lipids in postmenopausal women have been described and these showed significant increases in high-density lipoprotein and high-density lipoprotein to low-density lipoprotein ratio (Challoumas et al 2013).

For example, a randomised, placebo-controlled crossover trial of 56 patients with mild–moderate hypercholesterolaemia on a controlled low-cholesterol diet, calcium carbonate supplementation was shown to significantly reduce LDL levels by 4.4%, with additional 4.1% increases in HDL levels. No other effects on other blood lipids or blood pressure were observed (Bell et al 1992). Another small study demonstrated an augmenting effect of calcium (1200 mg together with 400 IU vitamin D/day) over 15 weeks on weight loss-induced beneficial changes to blood lipids and lipoproteins, with significantly greater reductions in total HDL, LDL:HDL and LDL levels (Major et al 2007).

Clinical note — Is calcium supplementation a risk for increased vascular events?

Recently, concern has emerged regarding a potential increase in cardiovascular events associated with long-term high-dose calcium supplementation. This was largely triggered by the results of a New Zealand RCT investigating the effect of calcium supplements (1000 mg/day elemental calcium as calcium citrate) administered to 1471 postmenopausal women, with an average age 74 years, over 5 years. Concomitant vitamin D supplements were not given to participants in this trial (Bolland et al 2008). The primary outcome of this study was bone density; however, the researchers also hypothesised that a secondary effect of the treatment would be a reduction in cardiovascular (CV) events, based on existing observational studies highlighting calcium's positive effect on blood lipids and blood pressure (Nainggolan 2008). However, secondary analysis of the data revealed that the women taking calcium supplements experienced an increase in CV events rather than the expected decrease in CV event. In the calcium-treated group, there was a statistically significant higher rate of verified myocardial infarction (MI) ($P = 0.05$), and a non-significant increase in all vascular events ($P = 0.08$) and stroke ($P = 0.21$), compared to those taking placebo. While the authors concluded that their study does not unequivocally demonstrate causality, it did suggest that high calcium intakes may have an adverse effect on vascular health (Bolland et al 2008).

The same authors subsequently conducted a meta-analysis of 15 RCT of calcium ≥500 mg vs placebo, concluding that in the absence of vitamin D, calcium supplements were associated with a significant increase in MI ($P = 0.035$) and non-significant increase in composite end point of MI, stroke or sudden death ($P = 0.057$) or death ($P = 0.18$) (Bolland et al 2010). In addition, this research group conducted a re-analysis of data from a sub-group in the Women's Health Initiative Calcium Vitamin D study (WHI CaD) and concluded that calcium, with or without vitamin D, modestly increased risk of CV events, especially for MI (Bolland et al 2011).

While these findings have caused substantial alarm and led to much speculation, the evidence suggesting cardiovascular harm needs to be balanced against the body of opposing evidence that reports that calcium does not significantly increase cardiovascular event risk.

Daily supplementation with calcium carbonate 1000 mg plus vitamin D 400 IU for 7 years showed neither an increase nor a decrease in coronary or cerebrovascular events in a large-scale study (WHI CaD) involving 36,282 postmenopausal women aged 50–79 years (Hsia et al 2007). Another prospective study (EPIC-Heidelberg) that involved almost 24,000 participants with an 11-year follow-up found no significant association between calcium intake and risk of stroke or cardiovascular mortality. Interestingly, a trend towards a decrease in MI risk was observed in those with a moderately high dairy calcium intake (mean = 820 mg/day), especially in women. By contrast, a statistically significant increase in MI was found in the group taking supplemental calcium in the absence of vitamin D; however, this may not be clinically meaningful as it translated to only 20 cases of MI in the calcium users, out of 24,000 participants (Li et al 2012). Results from the NHANES III study ($n = 20{,}024$) reported that there was no clear association for CVD death and intake of dietary or supplemental calcium (van Hemelrijk et al 2013). Another large prospective study involving 388,229 men and women aged 50–71 years, with a 12-year follow-up, reported that supplemental calcium intake was not associated with increased CVD or cerebrovascular death in women, although an increase CV risk was observed in men taking supplemental calcium (>1000 mg/day), who were also smokers (Xiao et al 2013).

Further to this, a 5-year study of 1460 older women suggested that supplementation with calcium carbonate (1200 mg/day) may reduce risk of hospitalisation and mortality in patients with pre-existing atherosclerotic CVD (Lewis et al 2011). It has been proposed that high calcium intake may increase risk of vascular calcification, or carotid atherosclerosis, although this effect was not demonstrated in recent studies (Lewis et al 2013, Kim et al 2012). In addition, there is some evidence that calcium may have a beneficial role in terms of cardiovascular disease by modestly reducing blood pressure and improving serum lipid profiles (Guessous et al 2011). In addition, a review of studies involving over 70,000 people concluded that mortality was reduced with vitamin D plus calcium (odds ratio, 0.94; 95% CI, 0.88–0.99), but not with vitamin D alone (odds ratio, 0.98; 95% CI, 0.91–1.06) (Rejnmark et al 2012).

While it is difficult at this stage to either confirm or refute the association between calcium supplementation and cardiovascular disease, there are a few factors for consideration:

- No RCTs have been conducted to specifically examine the effects of calcium supplementation on CVD morbidity and mortality; concerns have been raised due to secondary data analysis
- Current data does not support an association between dietary or supplemental calcium intake and an increased risk of stroke, cerebrovascular disease, cardiovascular disease or cardiovascular death
- Increased dietary intake of calcium has not been associated with an increase in risk of myocardial infarction
- Supplemental calcium may possibly be associated with an increased risk of myocardial infarction, but this appears to be limited to calcium given alone, without vitamin D.
- Known benefits of combined calcium and vitamin D therapy for reducing risk of osteoporotic fractures needs to be balanced against unproven risk of MI when making treatment decisions for an individual patient, and research now indicates that calcium and vitamin D reduce mortality in the elderly.

Dry eye

A controlled double-masked study of petrolatum ointment containing 10% w/w calcium carbonate applied on the lower lid twice daily for 3 months resulted in significant improvements in all criteria assessed. However, significance over placebo was only found in ocular surface staining, therefore determination of the action of petrolatum needs to be established and controlled in future studies to identify the therapeutic value of calcium (Tsubota et al 1999).

Fluorosis

Calcium has been shown to reduce the clinical manifestations of fluorosis in children exposed to contaminated water (Gupta et al 1996).

DOSAGE RANGE

Australian RDIs

- Infants
  1–3 years: 500 mg/day.
  4–8 years: 700 mg/day.
- Children
  9–11 years: 1000 mg/day.
  12–18 years: 1300 mg/day.
- Adults
  <70 years: 1000 mg/day.
  >70 years: 1300 mg/day.
- Pregnancy: 1000–1300 mg/day.
- Lactation: 1000–1300 mg/day.

According to clinical studies

- Osteoporosis prophylaxis: 1500 mg/day in combination with vitamin D and accessory nutrients (e.g. zinc, manganese, copper and fluoride) and/or antiresorptive agents
- Premenstrual syndrome: 1200–1600 mg/day; however, 500 mg calcium carbonate twice daily for 3 months is also effective
- Prevention of preeclampsia: 2000 mg/day.
- Increased BMD in children with low intake: 100 mg/day.
- Supplementation during pregnancy to increase mineral accretion in fetus: 2000 mg/day for last trimester.
- Allergic rhinitis: 100 mg/day.
- Hyperacidity: 500–1500 mg/day as required.
- Hyperlipidaemia: 400 mg three times daily.
- Hypertension: 1000–2000 mg/day.
- Dry eye: 10% w/w calcium carbonate in petrolatum base applied twice daily.
- Fluorosis in children: 250 mg/day.
- Prevention of colorectal cancer: 1200 mg/day.
- Weight loss: 1000–1200 mg/day long term.

ADVERSE REACTIONS

Oral administration of calcium supplements may cause gastrointestinal discomfort, nausea, constipation and flatulence.

Hypercalcaemia

Increased serum calcium may be associated with anorexia, nausea and vomiting, constipation, hypotonia, depression and occasionally lethargy and coma. Prolonged hypercalcaemic states, especially if associated with normal or elevated serum phosphate, can precipitate ectopic calcification of blood vessels, connective tissues around joints, gastric mucosa, cornea and renal tissue (Wilson et al 1991).

SIGNIFICANT INTERACTIONS

Calcium carbonate when taken as an antacid alters the absorption and excretion of a wide range of drugs. Please refer to a drug interaction guide for specific concerns. Only those interactions encountered with oral administration of calcium supplements will be included in this section.

Antacids, including H_2 antagonists and proton pump inhibitors

Use of drugs that raise gastric pH may reduce calcium absorption, especially that of calcium carbonate or calcium phosphate as these salts require an acidic environment for solubilisation before calcium can be absorbed. Aluminium- and magnesium-containing antacids may increase urinary excretion of calcium.

Bisphosphonates

Bisphosphonates (e.g. alendronate) are indicated for the treatment of osteoporosis; however, they commonly cause hypocalcaemia as an adverse effect, which reduces drug effectiveness in maintaining bone mineral density. Adequate intake of both calcium and vitamin D is essential for those taking bisphosphonates, however the drug must be taken on an empty stomach, at least 30 minutes before calcium supplementation.

Caffeine

Caffeine increases urinary excretion of calcium and may affect calcium absorption — ensure adequate calcium intake and monitor for signs and symptoms of deficiency in those with high caffeine intake.

Calcium channel blockers

Calcium supplements can have an antagonistic effect on the desired action of calcium channel blockers that could precipitate the re-emergence of arrhythmias — avoid high-dose supplements unless under professional supervision.

Cardiac glycosides (e.g. digoxin)

Administered concurrently, high-dose calcium may potentiate digoxin toxicity — use this combination with caution unless under medical supervision.

Corticosteroids

Long-term use of corticosteroids, especially oral formulations, may lead to reduced intestinal calcium absorption, increased calcium excretion and inhibtion of osteoblasts, leading to drug-induced osteoporosis — ensure adequate calcium intake and monitor for signs and symptoms of deficiency. Consider supplementation with long-term drug therapy.

Excess dietary fat

This increases urinary excretion of calcium — ensure adequate calcium intake and monitor for signs and symptoms of deficiency.

Excess fibre, including guar gum

May simply delay or decrease absorption of calcium — separate doses by at least 2 hours.

Iron

Concurrent administration of calcium with iron may reduce absorption of both minerals. Separate supplemental or dietary intake of minerals by at least 2 hours.

Levothyroxine

Calcium administered concurrently may reduce drug absorption, while levothyroxine may block absorption of calcium, e.g. calcium carbonate — separate doses by at least 4 hours.

Lysine

Additive effects may occur as lysine enhances intestinal absorption and reduces renal excretion of calcium — potentially beneficial interaction.

Magnesium

Magnesium decreases calcium absorption as they compete for the same absorption pathway, however it is unclear if this mineral interaction is clinically significant — it is advisable to separate doses by at least 2 hours.

Oestrogen and progesterone

Calcium supplementation in combination with these hormones will have an additive effect on minimising bone resorption in postmenopausal women — potential beneficial interaction, so consider increasing intake.

Phosphorus

Excess intake (soft drinks, meat consumption) can increase urinary excretion of calcium — ensure adequate calcium intake and monitor for signs and symptoms of deficiency.

Quinolone antibiotics

Drug bioavailability may be reduced by concurrent administration with calcium supplements, reducing drug efficacy and increasing risk of developing bacterial resistance — quinolones should be taken either 2 hours before or 4–6 hours after calcium.

Tetracyclines

Calcium supplements form complexes with these antibiotics and render 50% or more insoluble, therefore reducing the efficacy of the drug and absorption of calcium — separate doses by at least 2 hours.

Thiazide diuretics

These diuretics decrease urinary excretion of calcium. Monitor serum calcium and look for signs of hypercalcaemia, such as anorexia, polydipsia, polyuria, constipation and muscle hypertonia when using high-dose calcium supplements. Contributing risk factors are the presence of hyperparathyroidism or concurrent use of vitamin D.

Zinc

Concurrent administration of calcium and zinc may reduce absorption of both minerals, however it is unclear if this is clinically significant. Calcium supplementation has been shown in some studies to increase faecal losses of zinc (McKenna et al 1997) — ensure adequate zinc intake and monitor for signs and symptoms of deficiency.

CONTRAINDICATIONS AND PRECAUTIONS

People with hyperparathyroidism, chronic renal impairment or kidney disease, sarcoidosis or other granulomatous diseases should only take calcium supplements under medical supervision. Calcium supplementation is contraindicated in hypercalcaemia.

PREGNANCY USE

The safety of calcium supplementation during pregnancy in doses up to 2000 mg elemental calcium per day is well established in clinical trials.

Practice points/Patient counselling

- Calcium is an essential mineral required for the proper functioning of numerous intracellular and extracellular processes, including muscle contraction, nerve conduction, beating of the heart, hormone release, blood coagulation, energy production and maintenance of immune function.
- Low-calcium states are associated with several serious diseases such as colorectal cancer, osteoporosis types I and II, hypertension, preeclampsia and eclampsia.

- Although supplementation is traditionally used to correct or avoid deficiency states, research has also shown a role in the prevention of osteoporosis, pre-eclampsia and management of numerous disease states and research now indicates that calcium and vitamin D reduces mortality in the elderly.
- Clinical studies show that calcium supplementation has benefits in symptomatic relief in premenstrual syndrome, reducing the risk of fracture (when combined with vitamin D), reducing the risk of preeclampsia and improving birthweight, weight loss and reducing incidence of some cancers.
- Calcium can interact with numerous drugs and should be used with caution by people with renal disease or hyperparathyroid conditions.

PATIENTS' FAQs

What will this supplement do for me?

Calcium is essential for health and wellbeing. Although used to prevent or treat deficiency states, and primarily associated with BMD, it is also beneficial in a wide range of conditions such as prevention of preeclampsia, premenstrual syndrome, reducing the risk of bone fractures (with vitamin D), aiding in weight loss, maintenance of fetal growth, treatment of lead toxicity. It is considered to be a critical nutrient in pregnancy, and may actually reduce mortality in the elderly when taken with vitamin D.

When will it start to work?

This will depend on the indication it is being used to treat; however, in most instances long-term administration is required (i.e. months to years).

Are there any safety issues?

In very high doses, calcium supplements can cause some side effects, including constipation, but generally calcium is considered safe and has a wide therapeutic range. High-dose supplements should not be used by people taking some medications. Caution should also be exercised with high doses in individuals with pre-existing cardiovascular disease. (See *Significant interactions* above for specific information.)

REFERENCES

Abrahamsen B et al. Patient level pooled analysis of 68 500 patients from seven major vitamin D fracture trials in US and Europe. BMJ 340 (2010).

Ahn J et al. Serum vitamin D concentration and prostate cancer risk: a nested case-control study. J Natl Cancer Inst 100.11 (2008): 796–804.

Allen NE et al. Animal foods, protein, calcium and prostate cancer risk: the European Prospective Investigation into Cancer and Nutrition. Br J Cancer 98.9 (2008): 1574–1581.

Aloia JF et al. Calcium and vitamin D supplementationa in postmenopausal women. Journal of Clinical Endocrinology and Metabolism 98.11 (2013).

Alonso A et al. Low-fat dairy consumption and reduced risk of hypertension: the Seguimiento Universidad de Navarra (SUN) cohort. Am J Clin Nutr 82.5 (2005): 972–979.

Astrup A. The role of calcium in energy balance and obesity: the search for mechanisms. Am J Clin Nutr 88.4 (2008) 873–874.

Atallah AN et al. Calcium supplementation during pregnancy for preventing hypertensive disorders and related problems. Cochrane Database Syst Rev 1 (2002): CD001059.

Bailey CS et al. Excessive calcium ingestion leading to milk-alkali syndrome. Annals of Clinical Biochemistry. 45 (Pt 5) (2008): 527–529.

Barba G, Russo P. Dairy foods, dietary calcium and obesity: a short review of the evidence. Nutrition, Metabolism & Cardiovascular Diseases. 16 (2006): 445–451.

Baron JA et al. Risk of prostate cancer in a randomized clinical trial of calcium supplementation. Cancer Epidemiol Biomarkers Prev 14.3 (2005): 586–589.

Beall DP, Scofield RH. Milk-alkali syndrome associated with calcium carbonate consumption. Report of 7 patients with parathyroid hormone levels and an estimate of prevalence among patients hospitalized with hypercalcemia. Medicine. 74.2 (1995): 89–96.

Beers MH, Berkow R (eds). The Merck Manual of Diagnosis and Therapy, 17th edn. Rahway, NJ: Merck, 2003.

C

Behringer M et al. Effects of weight-bearing activities on bone mineral content and density in children and adolescents: a meta-analysis. J Bone Miner Res, 29.2 (2014) 467–478.

Belizan JM et al. Long-term effect of calcium supplementation during pregnancy on the blood pressure of offspring: follow up of a randomised controlled trial. BMJ 315.7103 (1997): 281–285.

Bell L et al. Cholesterol-lowering effects of calcium carbonate in patients with mild to moderate hypercholesterolemia. Arch Intern Med 152.12 (1992): 2441–2444.

Bergel E, Barros AJ. Effect of maternal calcium intake during pregnancy on children's blood pressure: a systematic review of the literature. BMC Pediatr 7 (2007): 15.

Bertone-Johnson ER et al. Calcium and vitamin D intake and risk of incident premenstrual syndrome. Arch Intern Med 165.11 (2005): 1246–1252.

Bischoff-Ferrari HA Which vitamin D oral supplement is best for postmenopausal women? Curr Osteoporos Rep 10.4 (2012): 251–257.

Bolland MJ et al. Calcium supplements with or without vitamin D and risk of cardiovascular events: reanalysis of the Women's Health Initiative limited access dataset and meta-analysis. BMJ 2011 doi 10.1136/bmj.d2040

Bolland MJ et al. Effect of calcium on risk of myocardial infarction and cardiovascular events:meta-analysis. BMJ 341 (2010): c3691.

Bolland MJ et al. Vascular events in healthy older women receiving calcium supplementation: randomised controlled trial. BMJ 336.7638 (2008): 262–266.

Borghi L et al. Comparison of two diets for the prevention of recurrent stones in idiopathic hypercalciuria. N Engl J Med 346.2 (2002): 77–84.

Bowen J, Noakes M, Clifton P. A high dairy protein, high-calcium diet minimizes bone turnover in overweight adults during weight loss. J Nutr 134 (2004): 568–573.

Bucher HC et al. Effect of calcium supplementation on pregnancy-induced hypertension and preeclampsia. JAMA 275 (1996): 1113–11117.

Bueno MB et al. Dietary calcium intake and overweight: An epidemiologic view. Nutrition 24 (2008):1110–1115.

Caan B et al. Calcium plus vitamin D supplementation and the risk of postmenopausal weight gain. Arch Intern Med 167.9 (2007): 893–902.

Campbell IA et al. Five year study of etidronate and/or calcium as prevention and treatment for osteoporosis and fractures in patients with asthma receiving long term oral and/or inhaled glucocorticoids. Thorax 59 (2004): 761–768.

Chakrabarty S et al. Calcium sensing receptor in human colon carcinoma: interaction with Ca(2+) and 1,25-dihydroxyvitamin D(3). Cancer Res 65.2 (2005): 493–498.

Challoumas D et al. Effects of calcium intake on the cardiovascular system in postmenopausal women. Atherosclerosis 231.1 (2013): 1–7

Chapuy MC et al. Combined calcium and vitamin D3 supplementation in elderly women: confirmation of reversal of secondary hyperparathyroidism and hip fracture risk: the Decalyos II study. Osteoporosis Int 13 (2002): 257–264.

Chapuy MC et al. Effect of calcium and cholecalciferol treatment for 3 years on hip fractures in elderly women. BMJ 308 (1994): 1081–1082.

Chapuy MC et al. Vitamin D3 and calcium to prevent hip fractures in elderly women. N Engl J Med 327 (1992): 1637–1642.

Chevalley T et al. Interaction between calcium intake and menarcheal age on bone mass gain: an eight-year follow-up study from prepuberty to postmenarche. J Clin Endocrinol Metab 90.1 (2005): 44–51.

Cho E et al. Dairy foods, calcium, and colorectal cancer: a pooled analysis of 10 cohort studies. J Natl Cancer Institute. 96.13 (2004):1015–1022.

Christensen R et al. Effects of calcium from dairy and dietary supplements on faecal fat excretion: a meta-analysis of randomized controlled trials. Obesity Review. 10 (2009):475–486.

Coruzzi P, Mossini G. Central hypervolemia does not invariably modulate calcium excretion in essential hypertension. Nephron 75 (1997): 368–369.

Crowther CA et al. Calcium supplementation in nulliparous women for the prevention of pregnancy-induced hypertension, preeclampsia and preterm birth: an Australian randomized trial: FRACOG and the ACT Study Group. Aust N Z J Obstet Gynaecol 39.1 (1999): 12–118.

Curhan GC et al. Comparison of dietary calcium with supplemental calcium and other nutrients as factors affecting the risk for kidney stones in women. Ann Intern Med 126 (1997): 497–504.

Daniele ND et al. Effect of supplementation of calcium and vitamin D on bone mineral density and bone mineral content in peri- and post-menopause women A double-blind, randomized, controlled trial. Pharmacol Res 50.6 (2004): 637–641.

Dawson-Hughes B et al. Effect of calcium and vitamin D supplementation on bone density in men and women 65 years of age or older. N Engl J Med 337 (1997): 670–676.

Dickinson HO et al. Calcium supplementation for the management of primary hypertension in adults. Cochrane Database Syst Rev 2 (2006): CD004639.alendula

Ding EL et al. Interaction of estrogen therapy with calcium and vitamin D supplementation on colorectal cancer risk: reanalysis of Women's Health Initiative randomized trial. Int J Cancer 122.8 (2008): 1690–1694.

Dorea JG, Donangelo CM. Early (in uterus and infant) exposure to mercury and lead. Clin Nutr (2005): [Epub ahead of print].

Dorea JG. Mercury and lead during breast-feeding. Br J Nutr 92 (2004): 21–40.

Elliott P et al. Dietary phosphorus and blood pressure: international study of macro- and micro-nutrients and blood pressure. Hypertension 51.3 (2008): 669–675.

Ettinger AS et al. Effect of breast milk lead on infant blood lead levels at 1 month of age. Environ Health Perspect 112.14 (2004): 1381–1385.

Ettinger AS et al. Effects of calcium supplementation on blood levels in pregnancy: a randomised placebo-controlled trial. Environ Health Perspect 117.1 (2009): 26–31.

Ettinger AS et al. Influence of maternal bone lead burden and calcium intake on levels of lead in breast milk over the course of lactation. Am J Epidemiol 163.1 (2006): 48–56.
Ettinger AS. Hu H, Avila MH. Dietary calcium supplementation to lower blood lead levels in pregnancy and lactation. J Nutr Biochem 18.3 (2007) :172–178.
Fardellone P et al. Biochemical effects of calcium supplementation in postmenopausal women: influence of dietary calcium intake. Am J Clin Nutr 67 (1998): 1273–1278.
Gao X, LaValley MP, Tucker KL. Prospective studies of dairy product and calcium intakes and prostate cancer risk: a meta-analysis. J Natl Cancer Inst 97.23 (2005): 1768–1777.
Garcia-Lorda P et al. Dietary calcium and body mass index in a Mediterranean population. In J Vitam Nutri Res. 77.1 (2007): 34–40.
Geleijnse JM, Grobbee DE, Kok FJ. Impact of dietary and lifestyle factors on the prevalence of hypertension in Western populations. J Hum Hypertens 19 (Suppl 3) (2005): S1–S4.
Genkinger JM et al. Dairy products and ovarian cancer: a pooled analysis of 12 cohort studies. Cancer Epidemiol Biomarkers Prev 15.2 (2006): 364–372.
Ghanbari Z et al. Effects of calcium supplement therapy in women with premenstrual syndrome. Taiwan J Obstet Gynecol 48.2 (2009): 124–129.
Goldfarb DS. Prospects for dietary therapy of recurrent nephrolithiasis. Adv Chronic Kidney Dis 16.1 (2009): 21–29.
Gonzalez JT, Rumbold PL, Stevenson EJ. Effect of calcium intake on fat oxidation in adults: a meta-analysis of randomized, controlled trials. Obes Rev. 13.10 (2012): 848–887.
Gotoh M et al. High blood pressure, bone-mineral loss and insulin resistance in women. Hypertens Res 28.7 (2005): 565–570.
Grau MV et al. Vitamin D, calcium supplementation, and colorectal adenomas: results of a randomized trial. J Natl Cancer Inst 95.23 (2003): 1765–1771.
Griffith LE et al. The influence of dietary and nondietary calcium supplementation on blood pressure: an updated metaanalysis of randomised controlled trials. Am J Hypertens 1291 (1999): 84–92.
Groff JL, Gropper SS. Advanced nutrition and human metabolism. Wadsworth, Belmont, CA, 2009.
Guessous I et al. Calcium, vitamin D and cardiovascular disease. Kidney Bloo Pres Res. 34 (2011): 404–417.
Gupta SK et al. Reversal of fluorosis in children. Acta Paediatr Jpn 38.5 (1996): 5113–5119.
Harkness LS, Bonny AE. Calcium and vitamin D status in the adolescent: key roles for bone, body weight, glucose tolerance, and estrogen biosynthesis. J Pediatr Adolesc Gynecol 18.5 (2005): 305–311.
Heaney RP, Weaver CM. Calcium and vitamin D. Endocrinol Metab Clin North Am 32.1 (2003): 181–188.
Hennekens CH, Barice EJ. Calcium supplements and risk of myocardial infarction: a hypothesis formulated but not yet adequately tested. Am J Med, 124.12 (2011): 1097–1098.
Hernandez-Avila M et al. Dietary calcium supplements to lower blood lead levels in lactating women: a randomized placebo-controlled trial. Epidemiology 14.2 (2003): 206–212.
Herrera JA et al. Calcium plus linoleic acid therapy for pregnancy-induced hypertension. Int J Gynecol Obstet 91.3 (2005): 221–227.
Hess B et al. High-calcium intake abolishes hyperoxaluria and reduces urinary crystallization during a 20-fold normal oxalate load in humans. Nephrol Dial Transplant 13 (1998): 2241–2247.
Hiller JE et al. Calcium supplementation in pregnancy and its impact on blood pressure in children and women: follow up of a randomised controlled trial. Aust N Z J Obstet Gynaecol 47.2 (2007): 115–121.
Hofmeyr GJ et al. Calcium supplementation during pregnancy for preventing hypertensive disorders is not associated with changes in platelet count, urate, and urinary protein: a randomized control trial. Hypertens Pregnancy 27.3 (2008): 299–304.
Hofmeyr GJ et al. Calcium supplementation to prevent pre-eclampsia: a systematic review. S Afr Med J 93.3 (2003): 224–228.
Hofmeyr GJ, Atallah AN, Duley L. Calcium supplementation during pregnancy for preventing hypertensive disorders and related problems. Cochrane Database Syst Rev 3 (2006): CD001059.
Hofmeyr GJ, Duley L, Atallah A. Dietary calcium supplementation for prevention of pre-eclampsia and related problems: a systematic review and commentary. BJOG 114.8 (2007): 933–943.
Holt PR. New insights into calcium, dairy and colon cancer. World J Gastroenterol 14.28 (2008): 4429–4433.
Hovdenak N, Haram K. Influence of mineral and vitamin supplements on pregnancy outcome. Eur J Obstet Gyneco Reprod Biol, 164.2 (2012): 127–132.
Hsia J et al. Calcium/vitamin D supplementation and cardiovascular events. Circulation. 115 (2007): 846–854.
Huncharek M et al. Dairy products, dietary calcium and vitamin D intake as risk factors for prostate cancer: a meta-analysis of 26,769 cases from 45 observational studies. Nutr Cancer 60.4 (2008a): 421–441.
Huncharek M et al Impact of dairy products and dietary calcium on bone-mineral content in children: results of a meta-analysis. Bone 43.2 (2008b): 312–321.
Hyman J et al. Dietary and supplemental calcium and the recurrence of colorectal adenomas. Cancer Epidemiol Biomarkers Prev 7.4 (1998): 291–295.
Imdad A, Bhutta ZA Effects of calcium supplementation during pregnancy on maternal, fetal and birth outcomes. Paediatr Perinat Epidemiol 26 (Suppl 1) (2012): 138–152.
Insel P et al. Discovering Nutrition; Jones and Burlington MA: Bartlett Learning, 2013.
Ishihara J et al. Dietary calcium, vitamin D, and the risk of colorectal cancer. Am J Clin Nutr 88.6 (2008): 1576–1583.
Jacobs ET, Thompson PA, Martínez ME. Diet, gender, and colorectal neoplasia. J Clin Gastroenterol 41.8 (2007): 731–746.
Kabrnova-Hlavata K et al. Calcium intake and the outcome of short-term weight management. Physiol Res 57.2 (2008): 237–45.
Kawano Y et al. Calcium supplementation in patients with essential hypertension assessment by office, home and ambulatory blood pressure. J Hypertens 16.11 (1998): 1693–1699.

Kennedy K et al. Double-blind, randomized trial of a synthetic triacylglycerol in formula-fed term infants: effects on stool biochemistry, stool characteristics, and bone mineralization. Am J Clin Nutr 70.5 (1999): 920–927.

Kerstetter JE et al. Dietary protein affects intestinal calcium absorption. Am J Clin Nutr 68 (1998): 859–865.

Kim JH et al. Increased dietary calcium intake is not associated with coronary artery calcification. International Journal of Cardiology. 157.3 (2012):429–431

Kim K-Z et al. Association between CASR polymorphisms, calcium intake, and colorectal cancer risk. PLoS ONE 8.3 (2013): e59628.

Kopic S, Geibel JP. Gastric acid, calcium absorption, and their impact on bone health. Physiol Rev 93 (2013): 189–268.

Lambert HL et al. Calcium supplementation and bone mineral accretion in adolescent girls: an 18-mo randomized controlled trial with 2-y follow-up. Am J Clin Nutr 87.2 (2008): 455–462.

Lappe JM et al. Vitamin D and calcium supplementation reduces cancer risk: results of a randomized trial. Am J Clin Nutr 85.6 (2007): 1586–1591.

Larsen ER, Mosekilde L, Foldspang A. Vitamin D and calcium supplementation prevents osteoporotic fractures in elderly community dwelling residents: a pragmatic population-based 3-year intervention study. J Bone Miner Res 19 (2004): 370–378.

Lewis JR et al. Calcium supplementation and the risks of atherosclerotic vascular disease in older women: results of a 5-year RCT and a 4.5-year follow-up. J Bone Miner Res. 26.1 (2011): 35–41.

Lewis JR et al. The effects of 3 years of calcium supplementation on common carotid artery intimal medial thickness and carotid atherosclerosis in older women: an ancillary study of the CAIFOS randomized controlled trial. J Bone Miner Res (2013).

Li K et al. Associations of dietary calcium intake and calcium supplementation with myocardial infarction and overall cardiovascular mortality in the Heidelberg cohort of the European Prospective Investigation into Cancer and Nutrition study (Epic-Heidelberg). Heart. 98 (2012): 920–925.

Liebman M, Chai W. Effect of dietary calcium on urinary oxalate excretion after oxalate loads. Am J Clin Nutr 65 (1997): 1453–1459.

Lukaszuk JM et al. Preliminary study: soy milk as effective as skim milk in promoting weight loss. J Am Diet Assoc 107.10 (2007): 1811–18114.

Major GC et al. Supplementation with calcium + vitamin D enhances the beneficial effect of weight loss on plasma lipid and lipoprotein concentrations. Am J Clin Nutr 85.1 (2007): 54–59.

Margolis KL et al. Effect of calcium and vitamin D supplementation on blood pressure: the Women's Health Initiative Randomized Trial. Hypertension 52.5 (2008): 847–855.

Matkovic V et al. Calcium supplementation and bone mineral density in females from childhood to young adulthood: a randomized controlled trial. Am J Clin Nutr 81.1 (2005): 175–188.

McCarty MF, Thomas CA. PTH excess may promote weight gain by impeding catecholamine-induced lipolysis-implications for the impact of calcium, vitamin D, and alcohol on body weight. Med Hypotheses 61.5–6 (2003): 535–542.

McCullough ML et al. Dairy, calcium, and vitamin D intake and postmenopausal breast cancer risk in the Cancer Prevention Study II Nutrition Cohort. Cancer Epidemiol Biomarkers Prev 14.12 (2005): 2898–2904.

McCullough ML et al. Vitamin D and calcium intake in relation to risk of endometrial cancer: a systematic review of the literature. Prev Med 46.4 (2008): 298–302.

McKenna AA et al. Zinc balance in adolescent females consuming a low- or high-calcium diet. Am J Clin Nutr 65 (1997): 1460–1464.

Meng X et al. Calcium intake in elderly Australian women is inadequate. Nutrients. 2 (2010):1036–1043.

Miller EA et al. Calcium, vitamin D, and apoptosis in the rectal epithelium. Cancer Epidemiol Biomarkers Prev 14.2 (2005): 525–528.

Mizoue T et al. Calcium, dairy foods, vitamin D, and colorectal cancer risk: the Fukuoka Colorectal Cancer Study. Cancer Epidemiol Biomarkers Prev 17.10 (2008): 2800–2807.

Nabhan FA et al. Milk-alkali syndrome from ingestion of calcium carbonate in a patient with hypoparathyroidism. Endocr Pract. 10.4 (2004): 372–375.

Nainggolan L. Calcium supplements increase vascular events? Medscape web MD Available: www.theheart.org.

Oh K et al. Calcium and vitamin D intakes in relation to risk of distal colorectal adenoma in women. Am J Epidemiol 165.10 (2007): 1178–1186.

Onakpoya IJ et al. Efficacy of calcium supplementation for management of overweight and obesity: systematic review of randomized clinical trials. Nutri Rev 69.6 (2011): 335–343.

Park SY et al. Calcium, vitamin D, and dairy product intake and prostate cancer risk: the Multiethnic Cohort Study. Am J Epidemiol 166.11 (2007a): 1259–1269.

Park Y et al. Calcium, dairy foods, and risk of incident and fatal prostate cancer: the NIH-AARP Diet and Health Study. Am J Epidemiol 166.11 (2007b): 1270–1279.

Pasco JA et al. Calcium intakes among Australian women: Geelong Osteoporosis Study. Aust N Z J Med 30.1 (2000): 21–27.

Pattanaungkul S et al. Relationship of intestinal calcium absorption to 1,25-dihydroxyvitamin D [1,25(OH)2D] levels in young versus elderly women: evidence for age-related intestinal resistance to 1,25(OH)2D action. J Clin Endocrinol Metab 85.11 (2000): 4023–4027.

Penland JG, Johnson PE. Dietary calcium and manganese effects on menstrual cycle symptoms. Am J Obstet Gynecol 168 (1993): 1417–1423.

Pereira RM et al. Guidelines for the prevention and treatment of glucocorticoid-induced osteoporosis. Rev Bras Reumatol 52.4 (2012): 580–593.

Picolos M et al. Milk-alkali syndrome in pregnancy. Obstet & Gynecology. 104.5 (pt2) (2004):1201–1204.

Prentice A. Micronutrients and the bone mineral content of the mother, fetus and newborn. J Nutr 133 (2003): 1693–1699.

Prince RL et al. The pathogenesis of age-related osteoporotic fracture: effects of dietary calcium deprivation. J Clin Endocrinol Metab 82.1 (1997): 260–264.
Reid IR et al. Randomized controlled trial of calcium supplementation in healthy, nonosteoporotic, older men. Arch Intern Med 168.20 (2008): 2276–2282.
Rejnmark L et al. Vitamin D with calcium reduces mortality: Patient level pooled analysis of 70,528 patients from eight major vitamin D trials. J Clin Endocrinol Metabol 97.8 (2012): 2670–2681.
Resnick LM. The role of dietary calcium in hypertension: a hierarchal overview (Review). Am J Hypertens 12 (1999): 99–112.
Rossi GA, Cerasoli F, Cazzola M. Safety of inhaled corticosteroids: room for improvement. Pulm Pharmacol Ther (2005) [Epub ahead of print].
Rozen P et al. Calcium supplements interact significantly with long-term diet while suppressing rectal epithelial proliferation of adenoma patients. Cancer 91.4 (2001): 833–840.
Ryan-Harshman M, Aldoori W. Diet and colorectal cancer: review of the evidence. Can Fam Physician 53.11 (2007): 1913–1920.
Sanders KM et al. Calcium and bone health: position statement for the Australian and New Zealand Bone and Mineral Society, Osteoporosis Australia and the Endocrine Society of Australia. Med J Aust 190.6 (2009): 316–320.
Schatzkin A, Peters U. Advancing the calcium–colorectal cancer hypothesis (Editorial). J Natl Cancer Inst 96.12 (2004): 893–894.
Schrager S. Dietary calcium intake and obesity evidence-based clinical practice. J Am Board Fam Pract 18 (2005): 205–210.
Shahar DR et al. Does dairy calcium intake enhance weight loss among overweight diabetic patients? Diabetes Care 30.3 (2007): 485–489.
Shaukat A, Scouras N, Schunemann HJ. Role of supplemental calcium in the recurrence of colorectal adenomas: a metaanalysis of randomized controlled trials. Am J Gastroenterol. 100.2 (2005): 390–394.
Skinner HG, Schwartz GG. Serum calcium and incident and fatal prostate cancer in the National Health and Nutrition Examination Survey. Cancer Epidemiol Biomarkers Prev 17.9 (2008): 2302–2305.
Soen, S. [The effects of glucocorticoid on bone architecture and strength]. Clin Calcium 23.7 (2013): 993–999.
Sowers M et al. Blood lead concentrations and pregnancy outcomes. Arch Environ Health 57.5 (2002): 489–495.
Stear SJ et al. Effect of a calcium and exercise intervention on the bone mineral status of 16–18-year-old adolescent girls. Am J Clin Nutr 77.4 (2003): 985–992.
Strause L et al. Spinal bone loss in postmenopausal women supplemented with calcium and trace minerals. J Nutr 124 (1994): 1060–1064.
Sulz MC et al. Comparison of two antacid preparations on intragastric acidity-a two-centre open randomised cross-over placebo-controlled trial. Digestion 75 (2007): 69–73.a
Tang BM et al. Use of calcium or calcium in combination with vitamin D supplementation to prevent fractures and bone loss in people aged 50 years and older: a meta-analysis. Lancet 370.9588 (2007): 657–666.
Taylor EN, Curhan GC. Role of nutrition in the formation of calcium-containing kidney stones. Nephron Physiol 98.2 (2004): 55–63.
Teegarden D. Calcium intake and reduction in weight or fat mass. J Nutr 133 (2003): 249–51S.
Thys-Jacobs S et al. Calcium carbonate and the premenstrual syndrome: effects on premenstrual and menstrual symptoms. Premenstrual Syndrome Study Group. Am J Obstet Gynecol 179.2 (1998): 444–452.
Thys-Jacobs S et al. Calcium supplementation in premenstrual syndrome: a randomized crossover trial. J Gen Intern Med 4 (1989): 183–189.
Thys-Jacobs S. Micronutrients and the premenstrual syndrome: the case for calcium. J Am Coll Nutr 19.2 (2000): 220–227.
Tremblay A, Gilbert JA. Human obesity: is sufficient calcium/dairy intake part of the problem? J Am Coll Nutri 20 (5 Suppl 1)(2011):449S–53S.
Trowman R et al. A systematic review of the effects of calcium supplementation on body weight. Br J Nutr 95.6 (2006): 1033–1038.
Tsubota K et al. New treatment of dry eye: the effect of calcium ointment through eyelid skin delivery. Br J Ophthalmol 83.7 (1999): 767–770.
van der Pols JC et al. Childhood dairy intake and adult cancer risk: 65-y follow-up of the Boyd Orr cohort. Am J Clin Nutr 86.6 (2007): 1722–1729.
Van Hemelrijck M et al. Calcium intake and serum concentration in relation to risk of cardiovascular death in NHANES III. PLoS One 10.8 (2013).
Vestergaard P et al. Fracture prevention in postmenopausal women. Clin Evid 2011.
Villar J et al. Nutritional interventions during pregnancy for the prevention or treatment of maternal morbidity and preterm delivery: an overview of randomized controlled trials. J Nutr 133 (Suppl) (2003): 1606–25.
Wahlqvist ML (ed). Food and nutrition: Australasia, Asia and the Pacific 2nd edn. Sydney: Allen & Unwin, 2002.
Wang L et al. Dietary intake of dairy products, calcium, and vitamin D and the risk of hypertension in middle-aged and older women. Hypertension 51.4 (2008): 1073–1079.
Ward MW, Holimon TD. Calcium treatment for premenstrual syndrome. Ann Pharmacother 33.12 (1999): 1356–1358.
Warriner AH, Saag KG. Glucocorticoid-related bone changes from endogenous or exogenous glucocorticoids. Curr Opin Endocrinol Diabetes Obes 20.6 (2013): 510–516.
Weingarten MA et al. Dietary calcium supplementation for preventing colorectal cancer and adenomatous polyps (Review). Cochrane Database Syst Rev 4 (2008): CD003548.
Wilson JD et al. Harrison's principles of internal medicine, 12th edn. New York: McGraw-Hill, 1991.
Winzenberg TM et al. Calcium supplementation for improving bone mineral density in children. Cochrane Database Syst Rev 2 (2006): CD005119.

Winzenberg T et al. Effects of calcium supplementation on bone density in healthy children: meta-analysis of randomised controlled trials. BMJ 333.7572 (2006): 775.

Woo J et al. Dietary intake, blood pressure and osteoporosis. J Hum Hypertens (2008 Dec 18) [Epub ahead of print].

Xiao Q et al. Dietary and Supplemental Calcium Intake and Cardiovascular Disease Mortality: The National Institutes of Health–AARP Diet and Health Study. JAMA Intern Med 173.8 (2013): 639–646.

Young GL, Jewell D. Interventions for leg cramps in pregnancy. Cochrane Database Syst Rev 1 (2013): CD000121.

Zemel MB et al. Calcium and dairy acceleration of weight and fat loss during energy restriction in obese adults. Obes Res 12 (2004): 582–590.

Zemel MB et al. Dairy augmentation of total and central fat loss in obese subjects. Int J Obes (Lond) 29.4 (2005a): 391–397.

Zemel MB et al. Effects of calcium and dairy on body composition and weight loss in African-American adults. Obes Res 13.7 (2005b): 218–225.

Zemel MB. Role of calcium and dairy products in energy partitioning and weight management. Am J Clin Nutr 79.5 (2004): 907S–912S.

Zhu W et al. Calcium plus vitamin D3 supplementation facilitated fat loss in overweight and obese college students with very low calcium consumption: a randomized controlled trial. Nutrition Journal 12.8 (2013).

Chaste tree

HISTORICAL NOTE Chaste tree fruits and leaves were a popular remedy in ancient Greece and Rome to promote celibacy. Leaves of the chaste tree were worn by vestal virgins in ancient Rome as a symbol of chastity. In the 17th century it was written that the chaste tree is a 'remedy for such as would willingly live chaste' (Gerard 1975). The dried fruits of the chaste tree have a peppery taste and smell and were used in place of pepper in monasteries to 'check violent sexual desires', hence one of its common names, monk's pepper. The berries have also been used to reduce fever and headaches, stimulate perspiration and dispel wind. However, since ancient times the chaste tree has primarily been used for a variety of gynaecological purposes, primarily to treat menstrual abnormalities and mastalgia, to aid in expulsion of the placenta after birth, to facilitate lactation and to promote menstruation. A commercial preparation of chaste tree has been available in Germany for over 50 years and it is still commonly used for menstrual irregularities.

OTHER NAMES

Vitex agnus castus, chasteberry, monk's pepper, gattilier, hemp tree, Keusch-Lamm-Fruechte, wild pepper.

BOTANICAL NAME/FAMILY

Vitex agnus-castus (family Labiatae)

PLANT PART USED

Dried, ripened or fresh ripe fruits (berries)

CHEMICAL COMPONENTS

Vitex agnus-castus contains many different chemical constituents: 10 flavonoids (including luteolin-like flavonoids casticin, orientin, isovitexin), five terpenoids (viteagnusins A–E), three neolignans and four phenolic compounds, as well as one glyceride, essential fatty acids (linoleic acid) and the essential oils cineole, limonene and sabinene. The phenolic and flavonoid compounds confer antioxidant and antimicrobial activity. Apigenin, 3-methylkaempferol, luteolin and casticin are weak ligands of delta and mu-opioid receptors, exhibiting dose-dependent receptor binding (Chen et al 2011, Ono et al 2008, Sarikurkcu et al 2009, Stojkovic et al 2011). Casticin is a potent immunomodulatory and cytotoxic compound (Mesaik et al 2009). Several secondary metabolites exhibit significant anti-inflammatory and lipo-oxygenase inhibition activity (Choudhary et al 2009).

MAIN ACTIONS

Vitex displays multiple mechanisms of action identified through in vitro and experimental model research.

One major area of activity is the pituitary–hypothalamic axis.

Decreases prolactin release

The most thoroughly studied mechanism for vitex is its interaction with dopamine receptors in the anterior pituitary. Several studies have indicated that vitex acts on dopamine D_2 receptors and decreases prolactin levels (Berger et al 2000, Halaska et al 1998, Jarry et al 1994, Meier & Hoberg 1999, Meier et al 2000, Milewicz et al 1993, Sliutz et al 1993, Wuttke et al 2003). It is likely that this mechanism is responsible for the symptom-relieving effects seen with vitex in mastodynia and hyperprolactinaemia (Meier & Hoberg 1999, Milewicz et al 1993, Wuttke et al 1997) and provides some rationale for its use by herbalists in disorders complicated by hyperprolactinaemia, such as amenorrhoea, mastalgia or polycystic ovarian syndrome.

Results from one study involving healthy males propose that this effect is dose-dependent, as lower doses (120 mg) were found to increase secretion and higher doses (204–480 mg) were found to decrease secretion (Merz et al 1996).

A study using the vitex extract BNO 1095 (70% ethanol, 30% H_2O extract, Bionorica, Neumarkt, Germany) identified that the major dopaminergic compounds are the clerodadienols, which act as potent inhibitors of prolactin release; however, other active compounds of lesser activity were also identified (Wuttke et al 2003). Dopaminergic bicyclic diterpenes have also been isolated that inhibit cAMP formation and prolactin release in rat pituitary cell cultures (Jarry et al 2006).

Oestrogen receptor binding

Vitex contains oestrogenic compounds, the flavonoids penduletin and apigenin. There are inconsistent results on whether vitex competitively binds to oestrogen receptors alpha and beta in vitro (Cavieres & Castillo 2011, Jarry et al 2003, Liu et al 2001, Wuttke et al 2003).

Increases progesterone levels

In vitro research has found that vitex stimulates progesterone receptor expression (Liu et al 2001), significantly increases plasma progesterone and total oestrogen levels and significantly reduces luteinising hormone (LH) and plasma prolactin (Ibrahim et al 2008). A randomised controlled trial of women with hyperprolactinaemia showed that vitex extract (20 mg daily) normalises progesterone levels after 3 months' treatment (Milewicz et al 1993).

Opioid receptors

Recent research reported that a methanol extract of vitex had affinity to the mu-opioid and delta-opioid (but not kappa-opioid) receptors (Webster et al 2011). Of note, the mu-opiate receptor is the primary action site for beta-endorphin in vivo, a peptide which assists in regulating the menstrual cycle through inhibition of the hypothalamus–pituitary–adrenal axis.

Cytotoxic activity

Cytotoxic activity has been reported for an ethanolic extract of the dried ripe fruit of vitex against various human cancer cell lines (Imai et al 2009, Ohyama et al 2003, 2005, Weisskopf et al 2005). The extract increased intracellular oxidative stress and mitochondrial damage, leading to apoptosis. In vitro studies demonstrate that vitex extract inhibits the proliferation of human prostate epithelial cell lines via apoptosis (Weisskopf et al 2005) and induces apoptosis in human colon carcinoma cell lines (Imai et al 2009).

OTHER ACTIONS

Conflicting results have been obtained in studies with regard to the effect on follicle-stimulating hormone (FSH), LH and testosterone levels. In vivo research suggests that vitex significantly decreases LH and testosterone levels (Nasri et al 2007). However, one clinical study found that vitex extract did not alter FSH or LH levels, whereas another showed that it increased LH release (Lauritzen et al 1997, Milewicz et al 1993). Inconsistent clinical results may be due to variations in chemical constituent levels present in the different test herbal products.

In vivo research on male rats demonstrated osteoprotective effects (Sehmisch et al 2009).

CLINICAL USE

Although double-blind studies have recently been conducted with chasteberry, uncontrolled trials go back to the 1940s, when a product known as Agnolyt was tested. The product was developed and patented by Dr Gerhard Madaus in Germany and contained *Vitex agnus-castus*. Several different vitex products have been investigated to date, including: Agnolyt (standardised to 3.5–4.2 mg of dried chasteberry extract), *Vitex agnus-castus* L. extract Ze440 (each 20 mg tablet standardised for casticin and agnuside), Femicur (contains 1.6–3.0 mg of dried extract per capsule) and Mastodynon (53% v/v ethanol), a homeopathic preparation. The BNO 1095 extract contains 4.0 mg of dried ethanolic (70%) extract of vitex (corresponding to 40 mg of herbal drug) and is found in Agnucaston/Cyclodynon (Bionorica, Neumarkt, Germany).

Premenstrual syndrome

Vitex is an effective and well-tolerated treatment for mild, moderate and severe premenstrual syndrome (PMS) according to numerous clinical trials (Atmaca et al 2003, Berger et al 2000, Dittmar 1992, He et al 2009, Lauritzen et al 1997, Loch et al 2000, Schellenberg 2001, Schellenberg et al 2012, Zamani et al 2012). According to these studies, the PMS symptoms that respond best to treatment are breast tenderness, irritability, depressed mood, anger, mood changes, headache and constipation. The most studied extract investigated in PMS is Ze440 and, more recently, BNO 1095 extract (see Clinical note).

A recent systematic review evaluated the evidence for the efficacy and safety of vitex extracts from randomised controlled trials investigating women's health. Of the 12 trials included in this review, eight investigated PMS. Seven of the eight trials found vitex extracts to be superior to placebo (five of six studies), pyridoxine (one study) and magnesium oxide (one study). Additionally, adverse events with vitex were mild and generally infrequent (van Die et al 2013). A Cochrane review investigating the use of *Vitex agnus-castus* for the treatment of PMS symptoms is currently underway (Shaw et al 2011).

The most recent double blind study was conducted with 162 women and tested three different doses: Ze 440 (8, 20 and 30 mg) over three menstrual cycles. Improvement in the total symptom score (TSS) in the 20 mg group was significantly higher than in the placebo and 8 mg treatment group. The highest dose of 30 mg did not significantly decrease symptom severity compared to the 20 mg treatment, providing a rationale for the usage of 20 mg daily as the effective dose (Schellenberg et al 2012).

Two prospective randomised double-blind placebo-controlled studies investigating efficacy of vitex extract (BNO 1095) in the treatment of Chinese women suffering moderate to severe PMS (n = 67 and n = 217, respectively) found that vitex significantly ameliorated all symptoms except abdominal cramping, and especially improved negative affect (depressed mood) and fluid retention. In the treatment arm, there was a significantly greater decrease in depressive symptoms in the luteal phase and PMS self-assessment compared to placebo after two menstrual cycles, with the differences between placebo and active treatment groups becoming even more significant after 3 months' treatment. This further supports the use of vitex in PMS and indicates that full benefit requires at least three menstrual cycles to become established. Of note, these studies found a placebo effect of 50%, but still a significantly greater effect of vitex (He et al 2009, Ma et al 2010).

A multicentre, randomised, controlled, double-blind study investigating the effects of vitex (Ze440) for PMS involved 170 women and was published in the *British Medical Journal* (Schellenberg 2001). Of the group, 13% were also taking oral contraceptive pills (OCP). Treatment with a 20-mg tablet of dry extract of chasteberry taken daily resulted in a significant improvement of PMS symptoms, particularly headache, breast fullness, irritability, anger and mood changes. Over 50% of women in the active treatment group achieved at least a 50% reduction in symptoms. Similar results were obtained in a 2006 prospective, open, non-comparative study of 121 women with moderate to severe PMS who took vitex (BNO 1095) over three menstrual cycles. Assessment using the validated PMS diary and the premenstrual tension syndrome score showed that the severity of PMS symptoms consistently decreased during treatment (Prilepskaya et al 2006).

Another three-arm double-blind study of women with premenstrual dysphoric disorder (n = 108), compared 20–40 mg fluoxetine, 20 mg vitex or multivitamin placebo for 6 months. Women in both treatment arms showed significant improvement on the Hamilton Depression Rating Scale ($P < 0.001$ and $P < 0.05$ respectively) compared with placebo, and the vitex group demonstrated no side effects (Ciotta et al 2012).

Previously, a number of open studies had generally produced positive results for vitex as a symptomatic treatment in PMS. One multicentre, open-label study showed that daily treatment with a 20-mg tablet of vitex (Ze440) over three menstrual cycles significantly reduced the Moor menstrual distress self-assessment questionnaire (MMDQ), with 46% of women experiencing a 50% reduction in the MMDQ. Treatment also reduced the duration of PMS symptoms from 7.5 days to 6 days and was as effective for women taking OCP as for those who were not (Berger et al 2000). Once treatment was stopped, PMS symptoms gradually returned to baseline within three further cycles.

The largest multicentre trial was an open study of 1634 women with PMS, which found that treatment with vitex (Femicur) for three menstrual cycles decreased the number of PMS symptoms in 93% of subjects (Loch et al 2000). Symptoms completely resolved in 40% of subjects and 94% overall rated vitex treatment as well tolerated. An early study using vitex (Agnolyt) in 1542 women

C

with PMS reported an improvement in symptoms with an average dose of 42 drops daily taken for an average of 25 days (Dittmar 1992, as reported in Ulbricht & Basch 2005). According to Ulbricht and Basch (2005), three earlier uncontrolled studies produced inconclusive results.

An open-label clinical trial of 100 women with PMS and migraine headaches was conducted using 40 mg/day vitex extract over a 3-month period. Sixty-six women reported a dramatic reduction of PMS symptoms, 26 a mild reduction, with no effect in eight of the trial participants. Forty-two women experienced greater than 50% reduction in frequency of premenstrual migraine. No patients reported side effects. While this was not a placebo-controlled trial, it points to vitex being a safe and effective treatment for women with premenstrual migraine headaches: the frequency and duration of migraine attacks were reduced (Ambrosini et al 2013).

Clinical note — The opiate system and PMS

The opiate system consists of mu, delta and kappa opiate receptors and endogenous opiate peptides such as beta-endorphin (Webster et al 2006). The opiate system plays an essential role in regulating tonic pain perception, mood, appetite and other functions. PMS is characterised by a reduction of opiate activity and the severity of symptoms such as anxiety, food cravings and physical discomfort is inversely proportional to the amount of decline in beta-endorphin levels in the luteal phase. Based on recent research, the symptom-relieving effects of vitex in PMS may be due to direct activation of analgesic and mood-regulatory pathways via opiate receptor activation and/or reversal of the loss of opiate inhibition in the luteal phase.

Clinical note — Ze440 extract

The naming of the Ze440 extract (Premular in Australia) is derived from the name Zeller, the 150-year-old Swiss company manufacturing it, combined with a unique number ascribed during the initial studies. In order to ensure that products deliver consistent results, Ze440 is measured by both composition and consistency from batch to batch. To promote product uniformity, every batch is grown, harvested and manufactured into tablets under controlled conditions and is extracted in a standardised method that ensures consistent and high levels of the important lipophilic compound casticin and an established marker compound, the iridoid glycoside, named agnuside. A daily dose of 20 mg (equivalent to one tablet) has demonstrated effectiveness (Schellenberg et al 2012).

IN COMBINATION

A 2008 Australian study investigated the effects of a combination of *Vitex agnus-castus* (equivalent to 1000 mg dry fruit) and *Hypericum perforatum* (St John's wort) on PMS-like symptoms in a small subpopulation of late perimenopausal women participating in a double-blind, placebo-controlled, randomised trial on menopausal symptoms. Of 100 volunteers recruited to the larger study, 14 late perimenopausal women who had menstruated at least once within the last 12 weeks of the treatment phase provided data for PMS-like symptoms. This herbal combination was found to be superior to placebo for total PMS-like symptoms and the subclusters, PMS-D (depression) and PMS-C (cravings) (van Die et al 2009a).

Comparison to SSRI drugs

A systematic review of herbal treatments for alleviating premenstrual symptoms looked at four clinical trials of vitex and found it had significant efficacy for relieving physical symptoms of PMS, but lesser effectiveness compared with fluoxetine for treating the psychological symptoms of premenstrual dysphoric disorder and a similar incidence to placebo of self-limiting minor adverse reactions (nausea, headaches) (Dante & Facchinetti 2011). In 2003, a randomised 8-week study involving 42 women compared the effects of 20–40 mg daily of fluoxetine, a selective serotonin reuptake inhibitor (SSRI), and 20–40 mg of vitex extract and found no statistically significant difference between the groups with respect to the rate of responders (Atmaca et al 2003). More specifically, patients with premenstrual dysphoric disorder responded well to both treatments; however, fluoxetine was more effective for psychological symptoms such as depression and irritability, whereas the herbal extract was more effective for diminishing physical symptoms such as breast tenderness, cramps, food cravings and swelling. Unfortunately, the authors did not report the type of vitex extract used in the study.

Comparison to vitamin B_6

Although vitamin B_6 (pyroxidine) is a popular treatment for PMS symptoms, the results from a double-blind comparative study have found that vitex (Agnolyt) is as effective, and possibly more so (Lauritzen et al 1997). The randomised, double-blind study of 175 women compared vitex, pyridoxine and placebo. In the study, 77% of women receiving vitex reported symptom alleviation compared with 61% with pyridoxine (200 mg/day), which was considered a small but significant difference. Additionally, doctors' assessments were more likely to rate treatment with vitex as 'excellent' compared with pyridoxine.

Commission E approves the use of vitex for PMS.

Mastalgia

Mastalgia is considered to relate to latent and increased basal prolactin levels; therefore, agents that reduce prolactin levels are anticipated to reduce symptoms. Vitex is a popular treatment for cyclical mastalgia as it interacts with dopamine D_2 receptors to reduce prolactin levels.

In two randomised, double-blind studies, vitex (Mastodynon) effectively reduced premenstrual mastalgia (Halaska et al 1998, Wuttke et al 1997, Wuttke et al 2003). Subjects completed a visual analogue scale and rated their breast pain from 0 (lowest breast pain) to 10 (extremely strong breast pain). Active treatment reduced the mastalgia score by 35–40%, an effect significantly stronger than that of placebo (25%). One of these studies also demonstrated that treatment with vitex reduced serum prolactin levels (Wuttke et al 1997, as reported in Wuttke et al 2003). According to Halaska et al (1998), symptom relief was experienced after the first month of treatment, with continued improvements experienced after the second and third months.

Commission E approves the use of vitex for this indication.

Irregularities of the menstrual cycle

Vitex is used to normalise menstruation in women with shortened, lengthened or infrequent menstruation, particularly when low progesterone and luteal-phase defects are suspected. In practice, vitex has also been used traditionally to treat both amenorrhoea and menorrhagia. Herbalists speculate that beneficial effects obtained in practice may be due to the herb's ability to reduce elevated prolactin levels in these conditions. This is particularly indicated where chronic stress is also present, as this has an effect on the hypothalamus–pituitary axis, resulting in elevated prolactin levels (Mills 2000, Trickey 1998). While the use of vitex in all these indications has not yet been tested under double-blind conditions, one randomised controlled trial of women with luteal-phase defect due to latent hyperprolactinaemia demonstrated that vitex extract (20 mg daily) effectively reduced prolactin levels and normalised luteal-phase length and progesterone levels after treatment for 3 months (Milewicz et al 1993).

Commission E approves the use of vitex for this indication.

Menopause

Vitex has only recently been utilised for menopause-related complaints. Based on pharmacological studies and clinical research, there is emerging support for its role in the alleviation of menopausal symptoms (van Die et al 2009c). While evidence from rigorous randomised controlled trials is lacking for the use of vitex as an individual herb in this context, further investigation is warranted.

IN COMBINATION

Vitex has been studied as part of several different polyherbal treatments for effectiveness in treating menopausal symptoms. The use of herbal combinations reflects real-world practice but makes it difficult to assess the value of vitex as a stand-alone treatment for this indication. To date, these studies using combination herbal therapy, including vitex, have produced mixed results.

A systematic review assessed the effectiveness of a combination of vitex and St John's wort versus placebo and found no significant differences in measured end points, including vasomotor symptoms, somatic complaints, sleep disorders, sexual disorders or mental disorders, with side effects comparable between the two (Laakmann et al 2012). It has been suggested, however, that some of the symptoms typically attributed to menopause may be more related to PMS in some women and, in these cases, the vitex and St John's wort combination could provide some relief (van Die et al 2009b).

Vitex (200 mg daily), in combination with other herbs, notably black cohosh, produced a significantly superior mean reduction in menopausal symptoms compared to placebo according to a 2007 randomised controlled study (Rotem & Kaplan 2007). The study of 50 healthy pre- and postmenopausal women found herbal treatment improved menopausal symptoms gradually and, after 3 months of treatment, there was a 73% decrease in hot flushes and a 69% reduction in frequency of night sweats, accompanied by a decrease in their intensity and a significant benefit in terms of sleep quality. Importantly, hot flushes ceased completely in 47% of women in the study group, compared with only 19% in the placebo group. No changes were detected for vaginal epithelium or levels of relevant hormones (oestradiol, FSH), liver enzymes or thyroid-stimulating hormone in either group.

Poor lactation

Vitex has been used since ancient times as a galactagogue to promote milk production, especially in the first 10 days after delivery.

Currently, there are no double-blind studies to confirm its efficacy; however, an early uncontrolled study provides some support for the use of vitex in lactation, finding a favourable effect on milk production in 80% of women (Noack 1943). Results from a small study of males suggest that increases in prolactin may be possible with low-dose vitex (120 mg daily), whereas higher doses (480 mg daily) result in decreased levels (Merz et al 1996).

Fertility disorders

Vitex is used in practice with other herbal medicines to enhance fertility in women with progesterone deficiency or luteal-phase defects. Currently, no large studies have been published to evaluate the effectiveness of this approach; however, a double-blind, randomised, placebo-controlled study of 96 women with fertility disorders (38 with secondary amenorrhoea, 31 with luteal insufficiency and 27 with idiopathic infertility) used the vitex product Mastodynon, with encouraging results (Gerhard et al 1998). Treatment of 30 drops was administered twice daily for 3 months and resulted in women with amenorrhoea or luteal insufficiency achieving pregnancy more than twice as often as the placebo group, with 15 women conceiving during the study period ($n = 7$ with amenorrhoea, $n = 4$ with idiopathic infertility, $n = 4$ with luteal insufficiency). Although promising, this study has been criticised for pooling of diverse conditions, unclear reporting of results and variable significance (Ulbricht & Basch 2005).

Acne vulgaris

An open study of 117 subjects (male and female) with different forms of acne found that, after 6 weeks' treatment with a 0.2% dried extract of *Vitex agnus-castus* and a topical disinfectant, 70% of cases experienced total resolution, with the highest success rates reported for acne vulgaris, follicularis and excoriated acne (Amann 1975). A group that was not treated with the herb took 30–50% longer to achieve similar results. Although encouraging, it is difficult to determine the contribution of vitex treatment to these results. Until controlled studies using vitex as a stand-alone treatment are conducted, the herb's role in this condition is still uncertain.

OTHER USES

Vitex is used to aid the expulsion of the placenta after birth. It is also used to treat fibroids, to normalise hormones following the use of OCP and in cases of premature ovarian failure. Studies on rats suggest that the dopaminergic agonist action of vitex may be useful to reduce or control epileptic seizures (Saberi et al 2008).

DOSAGE RANGE

General guide

- Liquid extract (1:2): 1–2.5 mL in the morning.
- Dried fruit: 1.5–3 g in the morning.
- Dry fruit flesh (solid-dose form): 1000–1800 mg/day.
- Manufacturers have recommended vitex preparations be taken daily as a single dose upon rising, before breakfast, throughout the menstrual cycle.

According to clinical studies

PMS

- Ze440 extract (Premular) 20 mg daily.
- Femicur 40 mg daily.

Cyclic mastalgia

- Mastodynon 60 drops daily or one tablet daily.

Menstrual irregularities

- 20 mg daily (extract unknown).

Infertility

- Mastodynon 30 drops twice daily.

C

Practice points/Patient counselling

- Clinical trials support the use of vitex in mild, moderate and severe PMS. It is particularly suited to treating common PMS symptoms, such as mood changes and irritability, breast tenderness, headaches and constipation. According to the available evidence, it is more effective than pyridoxine treatment and has a similar response rate to fluoxetine.
- It may also be effective in the treatment of menstrual irregularities and mastalgia.
- Vitex is also used to relieve perimenopausal symptoms, enhance fertility in women with progesterone deficiency or luteal-phase defects, aid the expulsion of the placenta after birth, reduce fibroids and normalise hormones following the use of oral contraceptives.
- Traditionally, it is described as a galactagogue (i.e. a medicine able to increase milk production in lactation) and is used in low doses for this indication.
- A mechanism of action has not been conclusively identified, but it appears to inhibit prolactin release by selective stimulation of pituitary dopamine D_2 receptors, to increase progesterone levels and works via the opiate system.

ADVERSE REACTIONS

A systematic review of the herb's safety, published in 2005, analysed data from six electronic databases, postmarketing surveillance studies, spontaneous reporting schemes (including the World Health Organization), herbalist organisations and manufacturers (Daniele et al 2005). The review concluded that vitex is a safe herbal medicine and any adverse effects associated with its use tend to be mild and reversible. The most common adverse effects are nausea, headache, dizziness, tiredness, mild gastrointestinal disturbances, dry mouth, menstrual disorders, acne, pruritus and erythematous rash. Additionally, no drug interactions have been reported. More recently, a 2009 placebo-controlled study of 202 women with moderate to severe PMS found no significant difference between incidence of adverse effects in the placebo- or vitex-treated groups (He et al 2009). Headache was reported as one of the more common side effects experienced by both groups, but was attributed to the PMS itself and not treatment.

SIGNIFICANT INTERACTIONS

Controlled studies are not available, so interactions are based on evidence of activity and are largely theoretical and speculative.

Dopamine antagonists

An antagonistic interaction is theoretically possible — observe patients.

Oral contraceptives

There has been speculation about the effectiveness of vitex when OCP are being taken. Several clinical studies involving women taking oral contraceptives have confirmed the herb still reduces PMS symptoms and does not affect OCP.

CONTRAINDICATIONS AND PRECAUTIONS

People with tumours sensitive to oestrogen or progesterone should avoid using this herb until safety can be established. It has been suggested that the ability of vitex to reduce prolactin levels may inhibit medical investigations and may mask diagnosis and proper treatment of prolactinoma (Gallagher et al 2008).

PREGNANCY USE

Vitex is not traditionally recommended in pregnancy. In practice, some herbalists use it during the first 10 weeks of pregnancy in cases of difficult conception.

PATIENTS' FAQs

What will this herb do for me?

Vitex is used to relieve common symptoms of PMS, such as irritability, mood swings, breast tenderness, headache and constipation. It is also used in combination with other herbal medicines to enhance fertility, relieve menopausal symptoms, regulate irregular menstruation, improve acne and promote milk production in new mothers.

When does it start to work?

Most trials show that treatment for at least three menstrual cycles may be required before symptom relief is experienced in PMS.

Are there any safety issues?

In cases of irregular menstruation, investigation for serious pathology should be undertaken before use of this herb.

REFERENCES

Amann W. Acne vulgaris and *Agnus castus* (Agnolyt). Z Allgemeinmed 51.35 (1975): 1645–1648.

Ambrosini, A., et al. (2013). Use of *Vitex agnus-castus* in migrainous women with premenstrual syndrome: an open-label clinical observation. Acta Neurol Belg, 113(1), 25-29.

Atmaca M, et al. Fluoxetine versus *Vitex agnus castus* extract in the treatment of premenstrual dysphoric disorder. Hum Psychopharmacol 18.3 (2003): 191–195.

Berger D et al. Efficacy of *Vitex agnus castus* L. extract Ze 440 in patients with pre-menstrual syndrome (PMS). Arch Gynecol Obstet 264.3 (2000): 150–153.

Cavieres, M., & Castillo, R. (2011). Evaluation of the estrogenicity of *Vitex agnus castus*. Toxicology Letters, 205 Supplement, S250.

Chen, S.-N., et al. (2011). Phytoconstituents from *Vitex agnus-castus* fruits. Fitoterapia, 82, 528-533.

Choudhary, M., et al. (2009). Antiinflammatory and lipoxygenase inhibitory compounds from *Vitex agnus-castus*. Phytotherapy Research, 23(9), 1336-1339.

Ciotta, L., et al. (2012). Long-term treatment with *Vitex agnus castus* (VAC) in premenstrual dysphoric disorders (PMDD). International Journal of Gynecology & Obstetrics, 119(Supplement 3), S605.

Daniele C et al. *Vitex agnus castus*: a systematic review of adverse events. Drug Saf 28.4 (2005): 319–332.

Dante, G., & Facchinetti, F. (2011). Herbal treatments for alleviating premenstrual symptoms: a systematic review. Journal of Psychosomatic Obstetrics & Gynecology, 32(1), 42-51.

Dittmar FW. Premenstrual syndrome: treatment with a phytopharmaceutical. TW Gynakologie 5.1(1992): 60–68.

Gallagher, J., et al. (2008). A prolactinoma masked by a herbal remedy. European Journal of Obstetrics, Gynecology and Reproductive Biology, 137(2), 257-258.

Gerard J. The herbal, or general history of plants. The complete 1633 edition as revised and enlarged by Thomas Johnson. New York: Dover Publications, 1975.

Gerhard II et al. Mastodynon(R) bei weiblicher Sterilitat. Forsch Komplementarmed 5.6 (1998): 272–278.

Halaska M et al. [Treatment of cyclical mastodynia using an extract of *Vitex agnus castus*: results of a double-blind comparison with a placebo.] Ceska Gynekol 63.5 (1998): 388–392.

He Z et al. Treatment for premenstrual syndrome with *Vitex agnus castus*: a prospective, randomized, multi-center placebo controlled study in China. Maturitas 63.1 (2009): 99–103.

Ibrahim, N., et al. (2008). Gynecological efficacy and chemical investigation of *Vitex agnus-castus* L. fruits growing in Egypt. Natural Product Research, 22(6), 537-546.

Imai, M., et al. (2009). Cytotoxic effects of flavonoids against a human colon cancer derived cell line, COLO 201: A potential natural anti-cancer substance. Cancer Letters, 276(1), 74-80.

Jarry H et al. In vitro prolactin but not LH and FSH release is inhibited by compounds in extracts of *Agnus castus*: direct evidence for a dopaminergic principle by the dopamine receptor assay. Exp Clin Endocrinol 102.6 (1994): 448–454.

Jarry H et al. Evidence for estrogen receptor beta-selective activity of *Vitex agnus-castus* and isolated flavones. Planta Med 69.10 (2003): 945–947.

C

Jarry H et al. In vitro assays for bioactivity-guided isolation of endocrine active compounds in *Vitex agnus-castu.* Maturitas 55 (Supplement 1) (2006): S26–S36.

Laakmann, E., et al. (2012). Efficacy of *Cimicifuga racemosa, Hypericum perforatum* and *Agnus castus* in the treatment of climacteric complaints: a systematic review. Gynecological Endocrinology, 28(9), 703-709.

Lauritzen C et al. Treatment of premenstrual tension syndrome with *Vitex agnus castus*: controlled, double-blind study versus pyridoxin. Phytomedicine 4 (1997): 183–189.

Liu J et al. Evaluation of estrogenic activity of plant extracts for the potential treatment of menopausal symptoms. J Agric Food Chem 49.5 (2001): 2472–2479.

Loch EG, et al. Treatment of premenstrual syndrome with a phytopharmaceutical formulation containing *Vitex agnus castus*. J Womens Health Gend Based Med 9.3 (2000): 315–320.

Ma, L., et al. (2010). Treatment of moderate to severe premenstrual syndrome with *Vitex agnus castus* (BNO 1095) in Chinese women. Gynecological Endocrinolfog, 26(8), 612-616.

Meier B, Hoberg E. Agni-casti fructus: an overview of new findings in phytochemistry, pharmacology and biological activity. Zeitschr Phytother 20.3 (1999): 140–158.

Meier B et al. Pharmacological activities of *Vitex agnus-castus* extracts in vitro. Phytomedicine 7.5 (2000): 373–381.

Merz PG et al. The effects of a special *Agnus castus* extract (BP1095E1) on prolactin secretion in healthy male subjects. Exp Clin Endocrinol Diabetes 104.6 (1996): 447–453.

Mesaik, M., et al. (2009). Isolation and immunomodulatory properties of a flavonoid, casticin from *Vitex agnus-castus*. Phytotherapy Research, 23(11), 1516-1520.

Milewicz A et al. *Vitex agnus castus* extract in the treatment of luteal phase defects due to latent hyperprolactinemia: results of a randomized placebo-controlled double-blind study. Arzneimittelforschung 43.7 (1993): 752–756.

Mills SB. Principles and practice of phytotherapy: modern herbal medicine. Sydney: Churchill Livingstone, 2000.

Nasri, S., et al. (2007). The effects of *Vitex agnus castus* extract and its interaction with dopaminergic system on LH and testosterone in male mice. Pakistan Journal of Biological Sciences, 10(14), 2300-2307.

Noack M. Dtsch Med Wochenschr (1943): 204. Available at: www.phytotherapies.org.

Ohyama K et al. Cytotoxicity and apoptotic inducibility of *Vitex agnus-castus* fruit extract in cultured human normal and cancer cells and effect on growth. Biol Pharm Bull 26.1 (2003): 10–1118.

Ohyama K et al. Human gastric signet ring carcinoma (KATO-III) cell apoptosis induced by *Vitex agnus-castus* fruit extract through intracellular oxidative stress. Int J Biochem Cell Biol 37.7 (2005): 1496–1510.

Ono, M., et al. (2008). Five new diterpenoids, viteagnusians A-Z, from the fruit of *Vitex angus-castus*. Chemical & Pharmaceutical Bulletin, 56(11), 1621-1624.

Prilepskaya VN et al. *Vitex agnus castus*: successful treatment of moderate to severe premenstrual syndrome. Maturitas 55 (Supplement 1) (2006): S55–S63.

Rotem C, Kaplan B. Phyto-female complex for the relief of hot flushes, night sweats and quality of sleep: randomized, controlled, double-blind pilot study. Gynecol Endocrinol 23.2 (2007): 117–122.

Saberi M, et al. The antiepileptic activity of *Vitex agnus castus* extract on amygdala kindled seizures in male rats. Neurosci Lett 441.2 (2008): 193–196.

Sarikurkcu, C., et al. (2009). Studies on the antioxidant activity of essential oil and different solvent extracts of *Vitex agnus castus* L. fruits from Turkey. Food and Chemical Toxicology, 47, 2479-2483.

Schellenberg R. Treatment for the premenstrual syndrome with agnus castus fruit extract: prospective, randomised, placebo controlled study. BMJ 322.7279 (2001): 134–137.

Schellenberg, R., et al. (2012). Dose-dependent efficacy of the *Vitex agnus castus* extract Ze 440 in patients suffering from premenstrual syndrom. Phytomedicine, 19(14), 1325-1331.

Sehmisch, S., et al. (2009). *Vitex agnus castus* as prophylaxis for osteopenia after orchidectomy in rats compared with estradiol and testosterone supplementation. Phytotherapy Research, 23(6), 851-858.

Shaw, S., et al. (2011). *Vitex agnus castus* for premenstrual syndrome (Protocol). Cochrane Database of Systematic Reviews.

Sliutz G et al. Agnus castus extracts inhibit prolactin secretion of rat pituitary cells. Horm Metab Res 25.5 (1993): 253–255.

Splitt G et al. Behandlung zyklusabhangiger Brustschmerzen mit einem Agnus castus-haltigen Arzneimittel: Ergebnisse einer randomisierten, plazebokontrollierten Doppelblindstudie. Geburtsh u Frauenheilk 57 (1997): 569–574.

Stojkovic, C., Sokovic, M., Glamoclija, J., et al. (2011). Chemical composition and antimicrobial activity of *Vitex agnus-castus* L. fruits and leaves essential oils. Food Chemistry, 128, 1017-1022.

Trickey R. Women, hormones & the menstrual cycle. St Leonards, NSW. Australia: Allen & Unwin, 1998.

Ulbricht C, Basch E. Chasteberry. Missouri: Mosby, 2005:136–43.

van Die, M., et al. (2009a). Effects of a Combination of *Hypericum perforatum* and *Vitex agnus-castus* on PMS-Like Symptoms in Late-Perimenopausal Women: Findings from a Subpopulation Analysis. The Journal of Alternative and Complementary Medicine, 15(9), 1045-1048.

van Die, M., et al. (2009b). Effects of a combination of *Hypericum perforatum* and *Vitex agnus-castus* on PMS-like symptoms in late-perimenopausal women: findings from a subpopulation analysis. Journal of Alternative & Complementary Medicine, 15(9), 1045-1048.

van Die, M., et al. (2009c). *Vitex agnus-castus* (Chaste-Tree = Berry) in the Treatment of Menopause-Related Complaints. The Journal of Alternative and Complementary Medicine, 15(8), 853-862.

van Die, M. D., Burger, H. G., Teede, H. J., et al. (2013). *Vitex agnus-castus* Extracts for Female Reproductive Disorders: A Systematic Review of Clinical Trials. Planta Med, 79(8), 562-575.

Webster DE et al. Activation of the mu-opiate receptor by *Vitex agnus-castus* methanol extracts: implication for its use in PMS. J Ethnopharmacol (2006): 106: 216-221.

Webster, D., et al. (2011). Opiodergic mechanisms underlying the actions of *Vitex agnus-castus* L. Biochemical Pharmacology, 81(1), 170-177.

Weisskopf M et al. A *Vitex agnus-castus* extract inhibits cell growth and induces apoptosis in prostate epithelial cell lines. Planta Med 71.10 (2005): 910–916.
Wuttke W et al. Chaste tree (*Vitex agnus-castus*): pharmacology and clinical indications. Phytomedicine 10.4 (2003): 348–357.
Zamani, M., et al. (2012). Therapeutic Effect of *Vitex agnus castus* in Patients with Premenstrual Syndrome. Acta Medica Iranica, 50(2), 101-106.

Chondroitin

OTHER NAMES

Chondroitin sulfate, chondroitin sulfuric acid, chondroitin 4-sulfate, chondroitin 4- and 6-sulfate

BACKGROUND AND RELEVANT PHARMACOKINETICS

Chondroitin sulfate is an amino sugar polymer, made up of glucuronic acid and galactosamine, that is in the class of large polymers known as glucosaminoglycans or mucopolysaccharides. These compounds act as the flexible connecting matrix between the protein filaments in cartilage and connective tissue (Liesegang 1990) as well as being a major component of the extracellular matrix in the brain (Kwok et al 2012). It has been found that serum levels of chondroitin sulfate are increased in patients with both rheumatoid arthritis and osteoarthritis (OA) and this may provide the basis for systemic detection of OA (Pothacharoen et al 2006).

Chondroitin sulfate molecules represent a heterogeneous population, the structure of which varies with source, manufacturing processes, presence of contaminants and other factors (Lauder 2009). There are also differences in the absorption and bioavailability of chondroitin formulations due to differences in molecular mass, charge density and cluster of disulfated disaccharides of the parental molecules (Volpi 2003). This has led to a call for reference standards with high specificity, purity and well-known physicochemical properties for use in accurate and reproducible quantitative analyses (Volpi 2007).

Chondroitin is generally manufactured from natural sources, such as shark and bovine (usually tracheal) cartilage and may have a molecular weight that varies from 10 to 50 kDa, depending on the product's source or preparation (Ross 2000). Low-molecular-weight chondroitin appears to be absorbed orally in both animals and humans (Adebowale et al 2002, Du et al 2004) and displays accumulation after multiple dosing (Adebowale et al 2002). Chondroitin is concentrated in the intestine, liver, kidneys, synovial fluid and cartilage (Conte et al 1995) and the elimination half-life is about 5–6 hours, with 40–50% being excreted in the urine (Conte et al 1991, Ronca & Conte 1993). Oral chondroitin is absorbed as several metabolites, and as the active moiety has not yet been identified it is difficult to establish bioequivalence between different products (Volpi 2003).

CHEMICAL COMPONENTS

Chondroitin sulfate is a linear polymer of two alternating sugars, alpha-D-*N*-acetylgalactosamine and beta-D-glucuronic acid, with the sulfate moiety being a covalent part of the molecule and not a counter ion, as is the case with glucosamine sulfate (Ross 2000).

FOOD SOURCES

Chondroitin is naturally present in the gristle in meat. As a supplement it is generally produced from natural sources, such as shark or bovine (usually tracheal) cartilage and it can also be manufactured in the laboratory using various methods. The purity and content of products have been questioned in the United States, where it is regarded as a nutritional supplement and its quality is unregulated (Consumer-lab 2009).

MAIN ACTIONS

Chondroprotective effect

A review of chondroitin sulfate in the pathophysiology of OA suggests that chondroitin exerts its antiarthritic effects via the stimulation of proteoglycan synthesis and reduction of chondrocyte catabolic activity. It does this by inhibiting the synthesis of proteolytic enzymes as well as via anti-inflammatory activity and actions on osteoblasts in subchondral bone, with modulation of osteoprotegerin/receptor activator of NF-κB ligand ratio in favour of reduced bone resorption (Martel-Pelletier et al 2010). Chondroitin appears to protect cartilage by providing it with the raw material required for repair, as well as inhibiting the enzymes in synovial fluid, such as elastase and hyaluronidase, that damage joint cartilage. It improves chondrocyte nutrition by increasing hyaluronic acid production in articular cells (Raoudi et al 2005) and hence, the fluid content of the extracellular matrix (Sasada et al 2005), which not only acts as a shock absorber but also brings nutrients into the cartilage (Krane & Goldring 1990).

In vitro studies have shown that low-dose combinations of glucosamine hydrochloride and chondroitin sulfate stimulate collagen and non-collagenous protein synthesis by ligament cells, tenocytes and chondrocytes (Lippiello 2007). An overall chondroprotective effect of chondroitin has also been demonstrated in different animal models. In a rabbit model oral or intramuscular chondroitin sulfate was shown to protect articular cartilage from experimental chymopapain injury (Uebelhart et al 1998a) and inhibit the destruction of the cartilage extracellular matrix (Sumino et al 2005). In a dog model, chondroitin sulfate was seen to stimulate articular cartilage and decrease or delay the alterations of degenerative joint disease (Melo et al 2008). In other animal models, co-administration with glucosamine was shown to prevent both biochemical and histological alterations and provide pain reduction (Silva et al 2009).

It has been suggested that at least some of the chondroprotective action of chondroitin sulfate is due to the provision of a source of additional inorganic sulfur which is essential for glycosaminoglycan synthesis, as well as being a structural component of glutathione and other key enzymes, coenzymes and metabolites that play fundamental roles in cellular homeostasis and control of inflammation (Nimni et al 2006). This is supported by the finding that the chondroprotective action of chondroitin is potentiated by high-sulfur mineral water (Caraglia et al 2005).

Urinary chondroitin sulfate and keratan sulfate excretion is reported to reflect the turnover rates of cartilage matrix proteoglycans, leading to the suggestion that the measurement of these compounds could provide an objective means of evaluating and monitoring joint diseases (Baccarin et al 2012). Furthermore, it has been found that technetium-99m-chondroitin sulfate accumulates in cartilage tissue, either by acting as a substrate for proteoglycan synthesis or by adsorption to cartilage, suggesting that this compound could serve to target and radioimage OA (Sobal et al 2009).

Anti-inflammatory

Chondroitin exerts an anti-inflammatory action with an inhibitory effect over complement (Pipitone 1991). In an in vitro study of bovine cartilage, chondroitin alone, and in combination with glucosamine, was found to regulate gene expression and synthesis of nitric oxide and prostaglandin E_2, suggesting a basis for its anti-inflammatory properties (Chan et al 2005). Chondroitin sulfate has been found to increase the levels of antioxidant enzymes and reduce inflammation and cirrhosis of liver tissue in an ovariectomised rat model, suggesting that it enhances antioxidant activity (Ha 2004). It has been suggested that chondroitin's multiple anti-inflammatory effects in chondrocytes and synoviocytes are primarily due to a common mechanism, through the inhibition of NF-κB nuclear translocation (Iovu et al 2008). Chondroitin sulfate has also been shown to inhibit the production of prostaglandin E_2 and matrix metalloproteinases in osteoblasts, leading to the suggestion that chondroitin's action in OA is not only due to effects on cartilage but may also be due to effects on subchondral bone (Pecchi et al 2012).

Based on in vitro and in vivo evidence, it is suggested that the antioxidant and anti-inflammatory effects of chondroitin contribute to neuro-protective properties (Egea et al 2010). A recent review further suggests that chondroitin improves moderate to severe psoriasis and experimental and clinical data suggest chondroitin might be a useful therapeutic agent in inflammatory diseases such as inflammatory bowel disease, atherosclerosis, Parkinson's and Alzheimer's disease, multiple sclerosis, amyotrophic lateral sclerosis, rheumatoid arthritis and systemic lupus erythematosus (Vallieres & du Souich 2010).

Viscoelastic agent

Chondroitin sulfate is a viscoelastic agent and, together with similar substances such as sodium hyaluronate and hydroxypropyl methylcellulose, is used in ophthalmic surgery to protect and lubricate cells and tissues (Larson et al 1989, Liesegang 1990).

OTHER ACTIONS

There are suggestions from laboratory studies and uncontrolled human trials that chondroitin may have potential antiatherogenic properties (Morrison 1969, 1971, Morrison & Enrick 1973).

A review of the potential therapeutic applications of chondroitin sulfate/dermatan sulfate suggest that chondroitin sulfate may have potential applications in parasitic and viral infections, regenerative medicine and development of anti-tumour therapies (Yamada & Sugahara 2008).

CLINICAL USE

Osteoarthritis: symptom control and retarding disease progression

There are now a number of reviews and meta-analyses of clinical data (Bruyere & Reginster 2007, Hochberg 2010, Monfort et al 2008, Uebelhart 2008, Vangsness et al 2009), including a critical appraisal of five separate meta-analyses (Monfort et al 2008), which indicate that oral chondroitin sulfate is a valuable and safe symptomatic treatment for OA disease (Kubo et al 2009). Chondroitin sulfate appears to produce a slow but gradual reduction of the clinical symptoms of OA. Multiple human clinical trials lasting from a few weeks to 3 years have shown that chondroitin sulfate can significantly alleviate symptoms of pain and improve function in patients with OA of the knee, finger and hip (Bourgeois et al 1998, Bucsi & Poor 1998, Fioravanti et al 1991, Lazebnik & Drozdov 2005, Mazieres et al 2001, Morreale et al 1996, Oliviero et al 1991, Rovetta 1991, Uebelhart 2008, Zegels et al 2013) and that these effects last months after the cessation of treatment (Mazieres et al 2005), as well as being evident with intermittent treatment (Uebelhart et al 2004).

There is also evidence from double-blind clinical trials that chondroitin can reverse, retard or stabilise the pathology of OA (Volpi 2005), as evidenced by stabilisation of the joint space (Uebelhart et al 1998b), less progression of erosions (Rovetta et al 2002, Verbruggen et al 1998) and improved articular cartilage thickness (Pipitone et al 1992, Raynauld et al 2012) and interarticular space, as observed by X-rays (Conrozier 1998, Michel et al 2005, Uebelhart et al 2004). A subanalysis of patients involved in the Glucosamine/Chondroitin Arthritis Intervention Trial (GAIT) study (see below and Glucosamine monograph) further suggests that chondroitin sulfate may have differential effects on OA symptoms depending on the degree of radiographic involvement, and that chondroitin may provide improvements in knee pain in patients with relatively early radiographic disease (Clegg et al 2005). These results are supported by a more recent controlled trial that found that chondroitin sulfate, but not paracetamol, reduced synovitis and clinical symptoms of OA with a carry-over effect and high safety profile (Monfort et al 2012). In contrast to the above findings, a 24-month, double-blind, placebo-controlled study of 572 patients conducted as part of the GAIT study did not demonstrate reductions in joint space narrowing, although there was a trend for improvement in knees with Kellgren/Lawrence grade 2 radiographic OA. The authors state, however, that power of this study was diminished by the limited sample size, variance of joint space width measurement and a smaller than expected loss in joint space (Sawitzke et al 2008).

Clinical Note

In 2014 the European Society for Clinical and Economic Aspects of Osteoporosis and Osteoarthritis (ESCEO) gathered an international task force of 13 members to determine clinical management of patients with OA. They concluded that the first step in patients with OA and pain is to use either glucosamine sulfate ± chondroitin sulphate or paracetamol on a regular basis, while NSAIDS should only be used as an advanced step, if response is not adequate. They recommended that the safer, more sensible approach is not to use paracetamol due to its side effects and questionable efficacy on pain with chronic use, but to recommend chronic symptomatic, slow-acting dugs for osteoarthritis such as chondroitin sulphate. For chondroitin, the effect size on pain is clinically significant and there are benefits on joint structure changes in patients with mild-to-moderate disease using prescription chondroitin 4&6 sulfate. (Bruyere et al 2014). Interestingly, they noted that US groups are reluctant to recommend dietary supplements due to quality issues, whereas there is less concern in Europe as pharmaceutical grade preparations are used.

Comparisons with NSAIDs

Although chondroitin appears to be at least as effective as non-steroidal anti-inflammatory drugs (NSAIDs) in treating the symptoms of OA (Fioravanti et al 1991, Morreale et al 1996), it has a slower onset of action, taking 2–4 months to establish an effect (Leeb et al 2000, Morreale et al 1996). Chondroitin may, however, provide benefits that persist after treatment is stopped (Mazieres et al 2001, Morreale et al 1996). A cost-effectiveness analysis suggests that chondroitin sulfate in the treatment for OA has less cost and better gastrointestinal tolerability compared than NSAIDs and that, for every 10,000 cases treated, 2666 cases of gastrointestinal adverse events (including 90 serious adverse events) will have been avoided (Rubio-Terres & Grupo del estudio 2010).

Combined use of chondroitin sulfate and glucosamine sulfate

Chondroitin and glucosamine are frequently marketed together in combination products and some studies suggest that this combination is effective in treating symptoms (Das & Hammad 2000, Leffler et al 1999, McAlindon et al 2000, Miller & Clegg 2011, Nguyen et al 2001) or reducing joint space narrowing (Rai et al 2004, Fransen et al 2014). These findings are supported by an in vitro study on horse cartilage that found that a combination of glucosamine and chondroitin was more effective than either product alone in preventing articular cartilage glycosaminoglycan degradation (Dechant et al 2005), as well as an in vivo study on rats that found that the combined treatment prevented the development of cartilage damage and was associated with a reduction in interleukin-1-beta and matrix metalloprotease-9 synthesis (Chou et al 2005). The GAIT trial (see above and Glucosamine monograph) provides evidence that glucosamine hydrochloride and chondroitin are more effective when given in combination than when either substance is given alone, with the combined treatment being more effective than the cyclooxygenase-2 inhibitor, celecoxib, for treating moderate to severe arthritis compared with chondroitin alone (Clegg et al 2006). A substudy of the GAIT trial on the pharmacokinetics of glucosamine and chondroitin sulfate when taken separately or in combination suggests that pain relief following ingestion of chondroitin probably does not depend on simultaneous or prior intake of glucosamine and that any effect on joint pain probably does not result from ingested chondroitin reaching the joint space but rather from changes in cellular activities in the gut lining or in the liver, where concentrations of ingested chondroitin, or its breakdown products, could be substantially elevated following oral ingestion (Jackson et al 2010). More recently, a large double-blind, placebo-controlled, randomised study (n = 605) conducted in Australia concluded that 2 years of treatment with glucosamine sulfate 1500 mg/day, taken together with chondroitin sulfate 800 mg/day, resulted in significant and clinically relevant joint structure modification (Fransen et al 2014). The same effect was not seen for stand-alone chondroitin sulfate or glucosamine sulfate.

A small randomised controlled trial has suggested that the addition of high-molecular-weight hyaluronate to glucosamine and chondroitin may provide additional benefits to the use of glucosamine and chondroitin alone (Bucci et al 2005).

Topical preparations

A topical preparation containing chondroitin with glucosamine and camphor has been shown to reduce pain from OA of the knee in one randomised controlled trial (Cohen et al 2003).

OTHER USES

Heart disease

There are suggestions that chondroitin in doses of up to 10 g/day may have antiatherogenic actions and beneficial effects on serum lipid levels and may be useful for reducing the risk of myocardial infarction (Morrison 1969, 1971, Morrison & Enrick 1973, Morrison et al 1969).

Snoring

The results of a pilot crossover study of seven subjects suggest that chondroitin sulfate instilled into the nostril at bedtime may reduce snoring (Lenclud et al 1998).

Ophthalmic surgery and dry eyes

Chondroitin sulfate is used as a viscoelastic substance to protect and lubricate cells and tissues during ophthalmic surgery, as well as to preserve corneas before transplantation (Larson et al 1989, Liesegang 1990). In a double-blind, crossover study of 20 subjects, 1% chondroitin sulfate was found to be as effective as polyvinyl alcohol artificial tear formulation and 0.1% hyaluronic acid in reducing itching, burning and foreign-body sensation in people with keratoconjunctivitis sicca (Limberg et al 1987).

Psoriasis

It has been found that some patients with psoriasis experience a significant clinical and histological improvement in their psoriatic lesions after taking chondroitin to treat their OA (Verges et al 2004, 2005), and this has been confirmed in a clinical trial which suggests that chondroitin could represent a special benefit in patients with both pathologies, since NSAIDs have been reported to induce or exacerbate psoriasis (Moller et al 2010).

Interstitial cystitis

Evidence from community-based clinical practice studies along with small randomised controlled trials suggests that intravesical chondroitin sulfate may play a role in the treatment of interstitial cystitis (Berger 2011, Gentile et al 2011, Nickel et al 2009, 2010, 2012).

DOSAGE RANGE

- Oral doses of chondroitin range from 800 to 1200 mg/day in either single or divided doses. Intramuscular, intravenous and topical forms are also available.
- A 4–5-month trial is generally used in order to determine whether it is effective for an individual patient.
- A dose-finding study in patients with knee OA suggests that administration of 800 mg of chondroitin sulfate orally had nearly the same effect as 1200 mg/day, while the use of a sequential 3-month administration mode, twice a year, was also shown to provide the same results as continuous treatment (Uebelhart 2008). More recently a double-blind randomised placebo-controlled trial found no significant difference in efficacy, security or tolerability between a single oral daily dose of 1200 mg and three divided doses of 400 mg (Zegels et al 2013).

ADVERSE REACTIONS

Chondroitin is generally deemed to be extremely safe, with the incidence of adverse reactions being comparable to placebo in studies lasting from 2 months to 6 years (Bourgeois et al 1998, Bucsi & Poor 1998, Hathcock & Shao 2007, Leeb et al 2000, McAlindon et al 2000, Uebelhart et al 1998b, Vangsness et al 2009).

Oral chondroitin may cause mild gastrointestinal disturbance. While there is a theoretical risk of anticoagulant activity, this has not been demonstrated in clinical trials (Chavez 1997) and chondroitin has been assessed as having a complete absence of adverse effects and an observed safe level at doses of up to 1200 mg/day (Hathcock & Shao 2007).

SIGNIFICANT INTERACTIONS

Controlled studies are not available; therefore, interactions are based on evidence of activity and are largely theoretical and speculative.

Anticoagulants

Additive effect theoretically possible — observe patient.

Non-steroidal anti-inflammatory drugs

Chondroitin may enhance drug effectiveness, suggesting a beneficial interaction is possible — drug dosage may require modification.

CONTRAINDICATIONS AND PRECAUTIONS

Due to theoretical anticoagulant activity, chondroitin should be used with caution in people with clotting disorders.

Some forms of chondroitin are produced from bovine (usually tracheal) cartilage, so it is theoretically possible that it may be a source of transmission of bovine spongiform encephalopathy (mad-cow disease) and other diseases. This transmission has not been demonstrated and is deemed unlikely.

PREGNANCY USE

Insufficient reliable information is available to advise on safety in pregnancy.

Practice points/Patient counselling

- Chondroitin is a naturally-occurring building block of joint tissue and cartilage. Supplements are made from shark cartilage or bovine tracheal cartilage.
- Chondroitin is an effective symptomatic treatment in OA and considered to improve the disability associated with the condition. It appears to slow disease progression when used long-term with positive results most consistently reported when it is used with glucosamine sulphate together. Its symptom-relieving effects occur after several weeks as it is a slow-acting substance.
- It is considered extremely safe and may reduce the need for NSAIDs, which can have serious side effects. In 2014, the European Society for Clinical and Economic Aspects of Osteoporosis and Osteoarthritis (ESCEO) recommended that chondroitin sulfate, glucosamine sulfate or paracetamol be used before NSAIDS in OA.
- Taking chondroitin in conjunction with glucosamine for treating arthritis provides the best results when being used long-term for delaying disease progression.
- Patients undergoing anticoagulant therapy or with clotting disorders should have their blood clotting monitored while taking chondroitin.

PATIENTS' FAQs

What will this supplement do for me?

Multiple scientific studies have shown that chondroitin sulfate reduces the symptoms of OA and may also slow down further progression of the condition. When used long term for slowing the progression of OA, it should be used together with glucosamine. Some people find that they do not require NSAIDs as often when taking chondroitin sulfate.

When will it start to work?

Symptom relief takes 2–4 months to reach maximal effect, but protection effects on the joints occur only with long-term use of several years.

Are there any safety issues?

Generally considered a very safe treatment and far safer than pharmaceutical anti-inflammatory drugs; however, it should be used with caution by people with clotting disorders or taking anticoagulants.

REFERENCES

Adebowale A et al. The bioavailability and pharmacokinetic of glucosamine hydrochloride and low molecular weight chondroitin sulfate after single and multiple doses to beagle dogs. Biopharm Drug Dispos 23.6 (2002): 217–225.

Baccarin, R. Y., et al. (2012). Urinary glycosaminoglycans in horse osteoarthritis. Effects of chondroitin sulfate and glucosamine. Res Vet Sci, 93(1), 88–96.

Berger, R E. (2011). Re: Prevention of Recurrent Urinary Tract Infections by Intravesical Administration of Hyaluronic Acid and Chondroitin Sulphate: A Placebo-Controlled Randomised Trial. The Journal of Urology, 186(1), 132.

Bourgeois P et al. Efficacy and tolerability of chondroitin sulfate 1200 mg/day vs chondroitin sulfate 3 × 400 mg/day vs placebo. Osteoarthritis Cartilage 6 (Suppl A) (1998): 25–30.

Bruyere O, Reginster JY. Glucosamine and chondroitin sulfate as therapeutic agents for knee and hip osteoarthritis. Drugs and Aging 24.7 (2007): 573–580.

Bucci LR et al. P196 Comparison between glucosamine with chondroitin sulfate and glucosamine with chondroitin sulfate and hyaluronate for symptoms of knee osteoarthritis. Osteoarthritis Cartilage 13 (Suppl 1) (2005): S99.

Bucsi L, Poor G. Efficacy and tolerability of oral chondroitin sulfate as a symptomatic slow-acting drug for osteoarthritis (SYSADOA) in the treatment of knee osteoarthritis. Osteoarthritis Cartilage 6 (Suppl A) (1998): 31–36.

Caraglia M et al. Alternative therapy of earth elements increases the chondroprotective effects of chondroitin sulfate in mice. Exp Mol Med 37.5 (2005): 476–481.

Chan PS et al. Glucosamine and chondroitin sulfate regulate gene expression and synthesis of nitric oxide and prostaglandin E2 in articular cartilage explants. Osteoarthritis Cartilage 13.5 (2005): 387–394.

Chavez ML. Glucosamine sulfate and chondroitin sulfates. Hosp Pharm 32.9 (1997): 1275–1285.

Chou MM et al. Effects of chondroitin and glucosamine sulfate in a dietary bar formulation on inflammation, interleukin-1-beta, matrix metalloprotease-9, and cartilage damage in arthritis. Exp Biol Med (Maywood) 230.4 (2005): 255–262.

Clegg DO et al. P145 Chondroitin sulfate may have differential effects on OA symptoms related to degree of radiographic involvement. Osteoarthritis Cartilage 13 (Suppl 1) (2005): S76–S77.

Clegg DO et al. Glucosamine, chondroitin sulfate, and the two in combination for painful knee osteoarthritis. N Engl J Med 354.8 (2006): 795–808.

Cohen M et al. A randomized double blind, placebo controlled trial of a topical cream containing glucosamine sulfate, chondroitin sulfate, and camphor for osteoarthritis of the knee. J Rheumatol 30 (2003): 523–528.

Conrozier T. Anti-arthrosis treatments: efficacy and tolerance of chondroitin sulfates (CS 4&6). Presse Med 27.36 (1998): 1862–1865.

Consumer-lab. Product review: glucosamine and chondroitin. Available online: www.consumerlab.com/reviews/Joint_Supplements_Glucosamine_Chondroitin_and_MSM/jointsupplements February 2009.

Conte A et al. Metabolic fate of exogenous chondroitin sulfate in man. Arzneimittelforschung 41.7 (1991): 768–772.

Conte A et al. Biochemical and pharmacokinetic aspects of oral treatment with chondroitin sulfate. Arzneimittelforschung 45.8 (1995): 918–925.

Das A Jr, Hammad TA. Efficacy of a combination of FCHG49 glucosamine hydrochloride, TRH122 low molecular weight sodium chondroitin sulfate and manganese ascorbate in the management of knee osteoarthritis. Osteoarthritis Cartilage 8.5 (2000): 343–350.

Dechant JE et al. Effects of glucosamine hydrochloride and chondroitin sulphate, alone and in combination, on normal and interleukin-1 conditioned equine articular cartilage explant metabolism. Equine Vet J 37.3 (2005): 227–231.

Du J, et al. The bioavailability and pharmacokinetics of glucosamine hydrochloride and chondroitin sulfate after oral and intravenous single dose administration in the horse. Biopharm Drug Dispos 25.3 (2004): 109–116.

Egea, J., et al. (2010). Antioxidant, antiinflammatory and neuroprotective actions of chondroitin sulfate and proteoglycans. Osteoarthritis Cartilage, 18 Suppl 1(0), S24–27.

Fioravanti A et al. Clinical efficacy and tolerance of galactosoaminoglucuronoglycan sulfate in the treatment of osteoarthritis. Drugs Exp Clin Res 17.1 (1991): 41–44.

Fransen M et al. Glucosamine and chondroitin for knee osteoarthritis: a double-blind randomised placebo-controlled clinical trial evaluating single and combination regimens. Ann Rheum Dis (2014) [Epub ahead of print].

Gentile, B., et al. (2011). UP-01.074 Recurrent Bacterial Cystitis, Bladder Instillation with a Combined Solution of Sodium Halurate and Chondroitin Sulfate (IALURIL): One Year of Follow-Up. Urology, 78(3), S209.

Ha BJ. Oxidative stress in ovariectomy menopause and role of chondroitin sulfate. Arch Pharm Res 27.8 (2004): 867–872.

Hathcock JN, Shao A. Risk assessment for glucosamine and chondroitin sulfate. Regul Toxicol Pharmacol 47.1 (2007): 78–83.

Hochberg, M. C. (2010). Structure-modifying effects of chondroitin sulfate in knee osteoarthritis: an updated meta-analysis of randomized placebo-controlled trials of 2-year duration. Osteoarthritis Cartilage, 18 Suppl 1(0), S28–31.
Iovu M, et al. Anti-inflammatory activity of chondroitin sulfate. Osteoarthritis Cartilage 16 (Suppl 3) (2008): S14–S118.
Jackson, C. G., et al. (2010). The human pharmacokinetics of oral ingestion of glucosamine and chondroitin sulfate taken separately or in combination. Osteoarthritis Cartilage, 18(3), 297–302.
Krane SM, Goldring MB. Clinical implications of cartilage metabolism in arthritis. Eur J Rheumatol Inflamm 10.1 (1990): 4–9.
Kubo, M., et al. (2009). Chondroitin sulfate for the treatment of hip and knee osteoarthritis: current status and future trends. Life Sci, 85(13-14), 477–483.
Kwok, J. C., et al. (2012). Chondroitin sulfate: a key molecule in the brain matrix. Int J Biochem Cell Biol, 44(4), 582–586.
Larson RS et al. Viscoelastic agents. Contact Lens Assoc Ophthalmol J 15.2 (1989): 151–160.
Lauder RM. Chondroitin sulphate: a complex molecule with potential impacts on a wide range of biological systems. Complement Ther Med 17.1 (2009): 56–62.
Lazebnik LB, Drozdov VN. Efficacy of chondroitin sulphate in the treatment of elderly patients with gonarthrosis and coxarthrosis. Ter Arkh 77.8 (2005): 64–69.
Leeb BF et al. A metaanalysis of chondroitin sulfate in the treatment of osteoarthritis. J Rheumatol 27.1 (2000): 205–211.
Leffler CT et al. Glucosamine, chondroitin, and manganese ascorbate for degenerative joint disease of the knee or low back: a randomized, double-blind, placebo-controlled pilot study. Mil Med 164.2 (1999): 85–91.
Lenclud CCP et al. Effects of chondroitin sulfate on snoring characteristics: a pilot study. Curr Ther Res 59.4 (1998): 234–243.
Liesegang TJ. Viscoelastic substances in ophthalmology. Surv Ophthalmol 34.4 (1990): 268–293.
Limberg MB et al. Topical application of hyaluronic acid and chondroitin sulfate in the treatment of dry eyes. Am J Ophthalmol 103.2 (1987): 194–197.
Lippiello L. Collagen synthesis in tenocytes, ligament cells and chondrocytes exposed to a combination of glucosamine HCl and chondroitin sulfate. Evid Based Complement Alternat Med 4.2 (2007): 219–224.
Martel-Pelletier, J., et al. (2010). Effects of chondroitin sulfate in the pathophysiology of the osteoarthritic joint: a narrative review. Osteoarthritis Cartilage, 18 Suppl 1(0), S7–11.
Mazieres B et al. Chondroitin sulfate in osteoarthritis of the knee: a prospective, double blind, placebo controlled multicenter clinical study. J Rheumatol 28.1 (2001): 173–181.
Mazieres B, et al. P140 Chondroitin sulfate in the treatment for knee osteoarthritis: a randomized, double blind, multicenter, placebo-controlled trial. Osteoarthritis Cartilage 13 (Suppl 1) (2005): S74.
McAlindon TE et al. Glucosamine and chondroitin for treatment of osteoarthritis: a systematic quality assessment and meta analysis. JAMA 283.11 (2000): 1469–1475.
Melo EG et al. [Chondroitin sulfate and sodium hyaluronate in the treatment of the degenerative joint disease in dogs. Histological features of articular cartilage and synovium.] Arq Bras Med Vet Zootec 60.1 (2008): 83–92.
Michel BA et al. Chondroitins 4 and 6 sulfate in osteoarthritis of the knee: a randomized, controlled trial. Arthritis Rheum 52.3 (2005): 779–786.
Miller, K. L., & Clegg, D. O. (2011). Glucosamine and chondroitin sulfate. Rheum Dis Clin North Am, 37(1), 103–118.
Moller, I., et al. (2010). Effectiveness of chondroitin sulphate in patients with concomitant knee osteoarthritis and psoriasis: a randomized, double-blind, placebo-controlled study. Osteoarthritis Cartilage, 18 Suppl 1(0), S32–40.
Monfort J, et al. Chondroitin sulphate for symptomatic osteoarthritis: critical appraisal of meta-analyses. Curr Med Res Opin 24.5 (2008): 1303–1308.
Monfort, J., et al. (2012). Chondroitin sulfate and not acetaminophen effectively reduces synovitis in patients with knee osteoarthritis: results from a pilot study. Osteoarthritis and Cartilage, 20(0), S283–S284.
Morreale P et al. Comparison of the antiinflammatory efficacy of chondroitin sulfate and diclofenac sodium in patients with knee osteoarthritis. J Rheumatol 23.8 (1996): 1385–1391.
Morrison LM. Response of ischemic heart disease to chondroitin sulfate-A. J Am Geriatr Soc 17.10 (1969): 913–923.
Morrison LM. Reduction of ischemic coronary heart disease by chondroitin sulfate A. Angiology 22.3 (1971): 165–174.
Morrison LM, Enrick NL. Coronary heart disease: reduction of death rate by chondroitin sulfate-A. Angiology 24.5 (1973): 269–287.
Morrison LM et al. The prevention of coronary arteriosclerotic heart disease with chondroitin sulfate A: preliminary report. Exp Med Surg 27.3 (1969): 278–289.
Nguyen P et al. A randomized double-blind clinical trial of the effect of chondroitin sulfate and glucosamine hydrochloride on temporomandibular joint disorders: a pilot study. Cranio 19.2 (2001): 130–139.
Nickel JC et al. A real-life multicentre clinical practice study to evaluate the efficacy and safety of intravesical chondroitin sulphate for the treatment of interstitial cystitis. BJU Int 103.1 (2009): 56–60.
Nickel, J. C., et al. (2010). A multicenter, randomized, double-blind, parallel group pilot evaluation of the efficacy and safety of intravesical sodium chondroitin sulfate versus vehicle control in patients with interstitial cystitis/painful bladder syndrome. Urology, 76(4), 804–809.
Nickel, J. C., et al. (2012). Second multicenter, randomized, double-blind, parallel-group evaluation of effectiveness and safety of intravesical sodium chondroitin sulfate compared with inactive vehicle control in subjects with interstitial cystitis/bladder pain syndrome. Urology, 79(6), 1220–1224.
Nimni ME, et al. Chondroitin sulfate and sulfur containing chondroprotective agents: is there a basis for their pharmacological action? Curr Rheum Rev 2.2 (2006): 137–149.

Oliviero U et al. Effects of the treatment with matrix on elderly people with chronic articular degeneration. Drugs Exp Clin Res 17.1 (1991): 45–51.
Pecchi, E., et al. (2012). A potential role of chondroitin sulfate on bone in osteoarthritis: inhibition of prostaglandin E(2) and matrix metalloproteinases synthesis in interleukin-1beta-stimulated osteoblasts. Osteoarthritis Cartilage, 20(2), 127–135.
Pipitone V. Chondroprotection with chondroitin sulfate. Drugs Exp Clin Res 17.1 (1991): 3–7.
Pipitone V et al. A multicenter, triple-blind study to evaluate galactosaminoglucuronoglycan sulfate versus placebo in patients with femorotibial gonarthritis. Curr Ther Res 52.4 (1992): 608–638.
Pothacharoen P et al. Raised chondroitin sulfate epitopes and hyaluronan in serum from rheumatoid arthritis and osteoarthritis patients. Osteoarthritis Cartilage 14.3 (2006): 299–301.
Rai J et al. Efficacy of chondroitin sulfate and glucosamine sulfate in the progression of symptomatic knee osteoarthritis: a randomized, placebo-controlled, double blind study. Bull Postgrad Inst Med Educ Res Chandigarh 38.1 (2004): 18–22.
Raoudi M et al. P152 Effect of chondroitin sulfate on hyaluronan synthesis and expression of udp-glucose dehydrogenase and hyaluronan synthases in synoviocytes and articular chondrocytes. Osteoarthritis Cartilage 13 (Suppl 1) (2005): S79–S80.
Raynauld, J. P., et al. (2012). Prediction of Total Knee Replacement in a 6-Month Multicentre Clinical Trial with Chondroitin Sulfate in Knee Osteoarthritis: Results from a 4-Year Observation. Osteoarthritis and Cartilage, 20(0), S175–S175.
Ronca G, Conte A. Metabolic fate of partially depolymerized shark chondroitin sulfate in man. Int J Clin Pharmacol Res 13 (Suppl) (1993): 27–34.
Ross I. A submission to the Complementary Medicines Evaluation Committee concerning chondroitin sulfate. Canberra: Complementary Healthcare Council of Australia, 2000.
Rovetta G. Galactosaminoglycuronoglycan sulfate (matrix) in therapy of tibiofibular osteoarthritis of the knee. Drugs Exp Clin Res 17.1 (1991): 53–57.
Rovetta G et al. Chondroitin sulfate in erosive osteoarthritis of the hands. Int J Tissue React 24.1 (2002): 29–32.
Rubio-Terres, C., & Grupo del estudio, Vectra. (2010). [An economic evaluation of chondroitin sulfate and non-steroidal anti-inflammatory drugs for the treatment of osteoarthritis. Data from the VECTRA study.] Reumatol Clin, 6(4), 187–195.
Sasada T et al. Role of chondroitin sulfate on mechanical behavior of articular cartilage. Report of Chiba Institute of Technology 52 (2005): 91–97.
Sawitzke AD et al. The effect of glucosamine and/or chondroitin sulfate on the progression of knee osteoarthritis: a report from the glucosamine/chondroitin arthritis intervention trial. Arthritis Rheum 58.10 (2008): 3183–3191.
Silva FS Jr et al. Combined glucosamine and chondroitin sulfate provides functional and structural benefit in the anterior cruciate ligament transection model. Clin Rheumatol 28.2 (2009): 109–117.
Sobal, G., et al. (2009). Uptake of 99mTc-labeled chondroitin sulfate by chondrocytes and cartilage: a promising agent for imaging of cartilage degeneration? Nucl Med Biol, 36(1), 65–71.
Sumino T et al. P163 Effect of long term oral administration of glucosamine hydrochloride and chondroitin sulfate on the progression of cartilage degeneration in a guinea pig model of spontaneous osteoarthritis. Osteoarthritis Cartilage 13 (Suppl 1) (2005): S84.
Uebelhart D. Clinical review of chondroitin sulfate in osteoarthritis. Osteoarthritis Cartilage 16 (Suppl 3) (2008): S19–S21.
Uebelhart D et al. Protective effect of exogenous chondroitin 4,6-sulfate in the acute degradation of articular cartilage in the rabbit. Osteoarthritis Cartilage 6 (Suppl A) (1998a): 6–13.
Uebelhart D et al. Effects of oral chondroitin sulfate on the progression of knee osteoarthritis: a pilot study. Osteoarthritis Cartilage 6 (Suppl A) (1998b): 39–46.
Uebelhart D et al. Intermittent treatment of knee osteoarthritis with oral chondroitin sulfate: a one-year, randomized, double-blind, multicenter study versus placebo. Osteoarthritis Cartilage 12.4 (2004): 269–276.
Vallieres, M., & du Souich, P. (2010). Modulation of inflammation by chondroitin sulfate. Osteoarthritis Cartilage, 18 Suppl 1(0), S1–6.
Vangsness CT Jr, et al. A review of evidence-based medicine for glucosamine and chondroitin sulfate use in knee osteoarthritis. Arthroscopy 25.1 (2009): 86–94.
Verbruggen G, et al. Chondroitin sulfate: S/DMOAD (structure/disease modifying anti-osteoarthritis drug) in the treatment of finger joint OA. Osteoarthritis Cartilage 6 (Suppl A) (1998): 37–38.
Verges J et al. Clinical and histopathological improvement of psoriasis in patients with osteoarthritis treated with chondroitin sulfate: report of 3 cases. Med Clin (Barc) 123.19 (2004): 739–742.
Verges J et al. P156 Chondroitin sulfate: a novel symptomatic treatment for psoriasis. Report of eleven cases. Osteoarthritis Cartilage 13 (Suppl 1) (2005): S81.
Volpi N. Oral absorption and bioavailability of ichthyic origin chondroitin sulfate in healthy male volunteers. Osteoarthritis Cartilage 11.6 (2003): 433–441.
Volpi N. Chondroitin sulphate for the treatment of osteoarthritis. Curr Med Chem Anti-Inflamm Anti-Allergy Agents 4.3 (2005): 221–234.
Volpi N. Analytical aspects of pharmaceutical grade chondroitin sulfates. J Pharm Sci 96.12 (2007): 3168–3180.
Yamada S, Sugahara K. Potential therapeutic application of chondroitin sulfate/dermatan sulfate. Curr Drug Discov Technol 5.4 (2008): 289–301.
Zegels, B., et al. (2013). Equivalence of a single dose (1200 mg) compared to a three-time a day dose (400 mg) of chondroitin 4&6 sulfate in patients with knee osteoarthritis. Results of a randomized double blind placebo controlled study. Osteoarthritis Cartilage, 21(1), 22–27.

Chromium

HISTORICAL NOTE Shortly after its discovery in 1959, chromium's importance and role in insulin sensitivity and glucose control was observed in vitro (Schwarz & Mertz 1959). Its importance was confirmed in 1977 when a woman on long-term total parenteral nurtrition (TPN), without chromium, developed symptoms of diabetes that could not be controlled by insulin. After further investigation it was noted that she was deficient in chromium and when < 50 mcg was added to her TPN solution, symptoms resolved. This led to the US FDA listing chromium as an essential trace nutrient. However, problems in elucidating the effects of chromium supplementation persist, due to a lack of practical methods for diagnosing deficiency (Mertz 1998). Over the years researchers have focused on investigating the effects of chromium supplementation on insulin sensitivity and management and prevention of type 2 diabetes (and to a lesser extent PCOS and other presentations) and cardiovascular disease (Hummel et al 2007), and more recently, mental health and atypical depression (Arthur 2008).

BACKGROUND AND RELEVANT PHARMACOKINETICS

Absorption of chromium occurs by passive diffusion and is inversely related to dietary intake (e.g. from a dose of 10 mcg, 2% is absorbed; from a dose of 40 mcg, 0.5% is absorbed) (Anderson & Kozlovsky 1985). Absorption may be inhibited by zinc (Hahn & Evans 1975) and phytates, and enhanced by oxalate (Bryson & Goodall 1983) and ascorbic acid (Offenbacher 1994). Unfortunately, much of the current information is based on chromium chloride, which is an inorganic and poorly absorbed form, so effects may vary for different forms (Arthur 2008). For example, the complexation of picolinic acid with chromium increases its bioavailability (Press et al 1990). Nicotinic acid is a metabolite of tryptophan that also improves the absorption of chromium (Arthur 2008).

Chromium is transported around the systemic circulation primarily by transferrin (Campbell et al 1997), therefore potentially competing with iron and other microminerals that use this transport mechanism, and accumulates in kidney, muscle and liver (Hepburn & Vincent 2003). It is excreted primarily in urine, but small amounts are lost in hair, perspiration and faeces.

CHEMICAL COMPONENTS

Chromium exists mostly in two valence states in nature: hexavalent chromium (chromium (VI)) and trivalent chromium (chromium (III)). The hexavalent form is toxic and poses a significant risk mainly via occupational exposure. It is recognised as a potent carcinogen to animals and humans, orally, often as a result of water contamination from industry (Kirman et al 2013, Sedman et al 2006) or when inhaled (Haney 2012). Trivalent chromium is an essential trace element in the human body and approved as a supplement.

Supplemental forms used in trials include organic chromium complexes, such as chromium picolinate and chromium nicotinate/polynicotinate (niacin-bound chromium [NBC]), and inorganic salts such as chromium chloride. While a number of different commercial trivalent chromium supplements exist the best evidence is for the picolinate and polynicotinate forms (Preuss et al 2008).

The picolinate form has been plagued by some controversy over the years — relating to both questions over its effects on iron levels and DNA damage (see below).

Clinical note — Problems testing for chromium deficiency

Currently, testing for chromium deficiency is a serum assay. This is problematic as it is unclear whether serum levels correlate with tissue levels. Previous studies have shown that subjects with widely varying serum chromium levels respond favourably to chromium supplementation, suggesting that this marker is misleading (Bahijri 2000). As a consequence, serum tests should not be solely relied upon, leaving the diagnosis of deficiency up to a practitioner's clinical judgement. Other tests have been proposed, such as toenail chromium concentration (Ayodele & Ajala 2009, Guallar et al 2005) and urinary chromium response to glucose load (Bahijri & Mufti 2002), as conditions that increase circulating glucose and insulin concentrations increase urinary chromium output (Vincent 2004); however, further research is required to confirm the validity of these tests. The recent development and change towards a more sensitive and accurate whole blood test (Cieslak et al 2013) may be better than serum testing; however, there still remains some uncertainty as to whether this newer test provides an accurate reflection of tissue levels.

FOOD SOURCES

The chromium content of food is geochemically dependent and Australian soils appear to vary widely in chromium content, thus dietary sources are likely to vary in chromium content due to growing location together with processing methods. In particular, Australian soils appear to be low in chromium, unlike some other locations such as USA (Thor et al 2011). Recommended dietary sources of chromium in Australia include Brewer's yeast, wholegrain breads and cereals, processed meat products and chocolate products (Ashton et al 2003). Other sources documented in the international literature include organ meat, cheese, green beans, broccoli, egg yolk, nuts, poultry, spices, tea, beer, wine (Arthur 2008).

DEFICIENCY SIGNS AND SYMPTOMS

Primary deficiency

Symptoms of weight loss, glucose intolerance and neuropathy have been noted in patients on TPN deficient in chromium (Verhage et al 1996). Deficiency may also be a precursor to the development of insulin resistance, and thus associated with hyperglycaemia, hypoglycaemia and obesity. Up to 90% of US diets have been found to be below the minimum suggested adequate daily intake for chromium of 50 mcg/day (Anderson & Kozlovsky 1985); as previously mentioned, Australian foods have been found to contain lower levels of this mineral (Ashton 2003), suggesting that the average Australian diet is likely to be lower.

Animal studies suggest that maternal chromium deficiency prior to and during gestation may also have detrimental effects in the offspring such as increased body weight, central obesity and overall percentage of body fat, together with impaired glycaemia (Padmavathi et al 2011). It remains to be tested whether the same results occur in humans.

Secondary deficiency

Factors that may exacerbate deficiency, generally by increasing requirements for or urinary excretion of chromium, include pregnancy, excessive exercise, infection, physical trauma and stress (Anderson 1986). Diets high in simple sugars have been found to increase urinary chromium excretion up to 30-fold, thereby increasing the risk of deficiency (Kozlovsky et al 1986). Corticosteroids also increase urinary losses of chromium (Kim et al 2002).

MAIN ACTIONS

Most of chromium's main actions are ultimately related to its role in glycaemic control and regulation and secondary benefits for antioxidant systems.

Important cofactor

Chromium is an essential trace mineral required for carbohydrate, lipid, protein and corticosteroid metabolism (Kim et al 2002).

Improves blood sugar control

Trivalent chromium is an essential trace element for normal carbohydrate metabolism and insulin sensitivity (Wilson & Gondy 1995), aiding the ability of insulin to transport glucose into cells. In particular, chromium improves the ability of insulin to bind to cells by enhancing skeletal muscle Glut4 translocation; enhancing beta-cell sensitivity; increasing the number of insulin receptors; and activating insulin receptor kinase, thus increasing insulin sensitivity; it also appears to reduce the cholesterol ratio in plasma membrane, improving insulin sensitivity (Anderson 1997, Hua 2012, Penumathsa 2009, Wang 2009). Additionally, in vitro studies have shown that chromium inhibits the secretion of TNF-alpha, a cytokine known to reduce the sensitivity and action of insulin, and that this appears to be mediated by its antioxidant effects (Jain & Kannan 2001). In vitro studies also show that chromium chloride prevents the increase in protein glycosylation and oxidative stress caused by high levels of glucose in erythrocytes (Jain et al 2006).

Lipid-lowering activity

Although the mechanism of action is yet to be fully explained, studies show that chromium supplementation may decrease triglyceride levels, total and LDL-cholesterol and modestly increase HDL-cholesterol (Bahijri 2000, Lee & Reasner 1994, Press et al 1990, Preuss et al 2000, Sundaram 2013b). In a study by Cefalu (2010), chromium decreased and modulated peripheral tissue lipids in insulin-resistant subjects with improved insulin response post-chromium supplementation. Another in vitro study suggested chromium may have a role in modulating cellular cholesterol accumulation induced by hyperinsulinaemia; mechanisms are thought to involve the upregulation of HDL-C (Sealls et al 2011).

Antihypertensive, cardioprotective

In rats with sugar-induced hypertension, niacin-bound chromium lowers systolic blood pressure, at least in part due to its effects on the renin-angiotensin system (Perricone et al 2008). Niacin-bound chromium and chromium phenylalanine also demonstrated improvement in cardiac contractile function and protection in ischaemic-reperfusion injury in a diabetic rat model (Hua 2012).

Antidepressant/neurotransmitter effects

According to McCarty (1994), a large proportion of unipolar depressive patients may also have insulin resistance, indicating that people with diabetes may have an increased risk of depression. Increased brain insulin levels, secondary to elevated cortisol or insulin resistance, influences the normal functioning of catecholaminergic neurons, contributing to a depressive state (McCarty 1994). The reputed antidepressant effects of chromium may be explained by improvements in insulin sensitivity (Davidson et al 2003) and related increases in tryptophan availability and/or noradrenaline release (McLeod & Golden 2000). Chromium has also been shown to lower the cortisol response to challenge with 5-hydroxy-L-tryptophan (5-HTP) and decrease the sensitivity of 5-HT_{2A} receptors (Attenburrow et al 2002). Influences on serotonergic pathways have also been reported in animal studies using chromium picolinate (Khanam & Pillai 2006) and potassium channels are thought to be involved. Chromium chloride in a rodent model of depression showed antagonistic activities to glutamanergic NMDA and AMPA receptors, as well as a 5-HT_{1A} agonistic effect, resulting in antidepressant effects (Piotrowska 2008).

OTHER ACTIONS

Immunomodulation

A review detailing the effects of chromium on the immune system found that chromium has both immunostimulatory and immunosuppressive effects, as shown by its effects on T- and B-lymphocytes, macrophages and cytokine production (Shrivastava et al 2002).

Bone density protection

It has been suggested that modulation of insulin by chromium may have positive effects on bone density, reducing bone resorption and promoting collagen production by osteoblasts (McCarty 1995). One placebo-controlled study using chromium picolinate (equivalent to 200 mcg chromium/day for 60 days) has shown a 47% reduction in the urinary hydroxyproline : creatinine ratio, indicating a decrease in calcium excretion and a potential role in the prevention of osteoporosis (Evans et al 1995).

Antioxidant

A placebo-controlled trial using 1000 mcg/day of chromium (in yeast form) for 6 months found chromium to be an effective treatment in reducing oxidative stress in people with type 2 diabetes (T2DM) and severe hyperglycaemia (HbA_{1C} > 8.5%); however, the authors noted that it may act as a pro-oxidant in euglycaemic people (Cheng et al 2004).

A similar randomised study confirmed chromium's antioxidant capacity in a similar cohort; chromium (1000 mcg in yeast form), alone or in combination with vitamin C (1000 mg) and vitamin E (800 IU), reduced oxidation markers after 6 months in 30 T2DM subjects with similar Cr and oxidation markers plasma baseline values (Lai 2008).

The histadinate form of chromium may be superior to picolinate for antioxidant activity according to in vivo research with a diabetic model, notably by decreasing cerebral levels of NF-κB and 4-HNE, two inflammatory markers found in diabetic subjects (Sahin et al 2012).

Anti-inflammatory

In diabetic rats, chromium supplementation can lower the risk of vascular inflammation. Chromium niacinate appears to be more effective than the picolinate form in lowering blood levels of pro-inflammatory cytokines (TNF-alpha, IL-6) and C-reactive protein, and in reducing oxidative stress and lipid levels (Jain et al 2007).

Increases dehydroepiandrosterone (DHEA)

In a placebo-controlled trial, chromium picolinate (equivalent to 200 mcg chromium/day for 60 days) increased DHEA by 24% in postmenopausal women (Evans et al 1995).

Hepatoprotection

In alloxan-induced diabetic rats with mild chronic hepatic injury, supplementation with chromium picolinate prevented and ameliorated histopathological damage, elevation in AST and ALT, as well as LFABP, a biomarker of hepatic injury (Fan 2013).

CLINICAL USE

Supplemental forms used in trials include organic chromium complexes, such as chromium picolinate and chromium nicotinate, and inorganic salts such as chromium chloride. Chromium is known to improve insulin sensitivity and metabolic markers, and as such its clinical applications reflect this central action; it is used in conditions associated with insulin resistance such as T2DM, gestational diabetes (GDM), polycystic ovarian syndrome (PCOS), obesity and syndrome X. It is also used in practice to curb sugar cravings and stabilise blood sugar levels. More recently, it is attracting interest as a potential treatment in mental health disorders, depression in particular.

Deficiency states: prevention and treatment

Although frank demonstrable chromium deficiency is uncommon (Vincent 2004) and is mostly described in relation to the use of TPN with inadequate chromium levels, subclinical deficiency states in the USA and Australia are thought to be more prevalent (Anderson & Kozlovsky 1985, Ashton 2003); however, it is difficult to detect chromium deficiency via pathology testing so true estimates remain unknown. Chromium supplementation is used in cases ***at risk*** of deficiency, such as long-term corticosteroid use (Kim et al 2002), patients with evidence of impaired insulin sensitivity, people with a high sugar intake (Kozlovsky et al 1986) or those suspected to be deficient after a thorough clinical history has been taken.

Diabetes

Subjects with diabetes (both T1DM & T2DM) appear to have lower tissue levels of chromium and a correlation exists between low circulating levels of chromium and incidence of T2DM (Hummel et al 2007). Additionally, insulin resistance has been associated with higher rates of chromium excretion (Bahijri & Alyssa 2011) and a study of people with T2DM of less than 2 years' duration found they had lower chromium plasma levels (33%) and increased chromium excretion (100%) compared with healthy controls (Morris et al 1999). While still controversial, a number of studies and reviews suggest that chromium supplementation may facilitate insulin signalling and therefore improve systemic insulin sensitivity. A review of 15 clinical studies involving a total of 1690 subjects (1505 of which received chromium picolinate) reported significant improvement in at least one outcome of glycaemic control. The pooled data showed substantial reductions in both hyperglycaemia and hyperinsulinaemia (Broadhurst & Domenico 2006).

Type 2 diabetes mellitus (T2DM)

Results have shown that chromium supplementation appears to be more effective in patients with T2DM than in those with T1DM (Ravina & Slezack 1993, Wang & Cefalu 2010).

In 2013, a meta-analysis of seven RCTs comparing chromium supplementation (>250 mcg/day for at least 3 months) to placebo on glucose and lipid profiles in patients with T2DM concluded that chromium significantly reduced fasting blood sugar compared to the placebo ($P < 0.0001$), but had no significant effects on glycated haemoglobin, total cholesterol (TC), high-density lipoprotein cholesterol (HDL-C), low-density lipoprotein cholesterol (LDL-C), very low-density lipoprotein cholesterol (VLDL-C), triglyceride (TG) or body mass index (BMI) (Abdollahi et al 2013).

Despite this conclusion, not all studies have produced positive results and several researchers have sought to identify the best responders. It is accepted that chromium supplementation given to human subjects in documented deficiency states experience improved glucose levels. However, it also appears that a clinical response to chromium (i.e. decreased glucose and improved insulin sensitivity) may be more likely in insulin-resistant individuals with T2DM who have more elevated fasting glucose and haemoglobin A(1C) levels (Wang & Cefalu 2010).

In support of this, a more recent study seeking to evaluate the metabolic and physiological differences in responders and non-responders found that a clinical response to a dose of 1000 mcg was correlated to baseline values of poorer insulin sensitivity, high glycosylated haemoglobin (HbA_{1C}) and high fasting blood glucose (Cefalu 2010). Furthermore, in a double-blind RCT of 31 non-obese, normoglycaemic subjects, those with the highest serum chromium at the start experienced a worsening of their insulin sensitivity after treatment with chromium (500 mcg twice daily for 16 weeks) compared to placebo (Marashani et al 2012).

Some study findings suggest that improvements are dose-related but may also be affected by treatment duration, initial chromium status (Ghosh et al 2002, Amato et al 2000, Masharani et al 2012) and age. A controlled trial of elderly T2DM patients (average age 73 years) reported that supplementation with chromium (200 mcg twice daily) for 3 weeks improved fasting blood glucose, HbA_{1C}, and total cholesterol levels (Rabinovitz et al 2004), suggesting lower doses may be effective in older patients. Another study (single blind prospective) in 40 newly diagnosed T2DM subjects (ages 35–67 years) supplemented with 9 g of a chromium-containing brewer's yeast for 3 months also yielded improvements of glycaemia, reducing glycosylated haemoglobin and fasting blood glucose values as well as improving their lipid profile (Sharma 2011).

The most promising RCT to date tested chromium picolinate at doses of 200 and 1000 mcg/day in subjects with T2DM who were instructed to maintain their current medications, diet and lifestyle habits. HbA_{1C} values improved significantly in the higher treatment group after 2 months and in both groups after 4 months' treatment. Fasting glucose was lower in the 1000 mcg group after 2 and 4 months (4-month values: 7.1 ± 0.2 mmol/L vs placebo 8.8 ± 0.3 mmol/L). Two-hour glucose values were also significantly lower in the 1000 mcg group after both 2 and 4 months (4-month values: 10.5 ± 0.2 mmol/L vs placebo 12.3 ± 0.4 mmol/L). Fasting and 2-hour insulin values decreased significantly in both groups receiving supplemental chromium after 2 and 4 months. Plasma total cholesterol also decreased in the subjects receiving 1000 mcg chromium after 4 months (Anderson et al 1997). In another study T2DM patients taking sulfonylurea agents, chromium picolinate supplementation (equivalent to 1000 mcg chromium) for 6 months significantly improved insulin sensitivity and glucose control; and attenuated bodyweight gain and visceral fat accumulation compared with the placebo (Martin et al 2006).

Studies using chromium nicotinic acid have proven more promising with higher doses of nicotinic acid (100 mg/day) (Urberg & Zemel 1987) than those with low-dose nicotinic acid (1.8 mg) (Thomas & Gropper 1996), demonstrating a synergistic effect with chromium (200 mcg/day).

It appears the picolinate form of chromium is crucial in obtaining improvements of glycaemic parameters.

Type 1 diabetes mellitus (T1DM)

As chromium appears to improve insulin sensitivity rather than secretion its therapeutic potential in T1DM is limited (Edmondson 2002). One study did show reduced requirements for insulin in 33.6% of patients with T1DM taking 200 mcg chromium/day (Ravina & Slezack 1993), and another showed a 30% reduction in insulin requirements in 71% of subjects at the same dose (Ravina et al 1995), but it is unclear which patients might respond to treatment. No further studies have been done on this population.

Gestational diabetes mellitus (GDM)

Pregnancy can be described as an increased insulin resistant state, which may result in GDM if the pancreas is unable to increase insulin levels to maintain blood glucose balance (Jovanovic & Peterson 1996). While chromium serum measurement in pregnancy yielded inconclusive results (Sundararaman 2012, Wood 2008), it appears that chromium excretion is elevated in normal pregnancy, potentially contributing to the insulin resistance (Morris et al 2000). The beneficial effect of chromium on insulin sensitivity provides a theoretical basis for its use in this condition. A small placebo-controlled trial using 4 or 8 mcg/kg of chromium daily in GDM found a significant dose-dependent improvement in fasting insulin, 1-hour insulin and glucose, and postprandial glucose levels after 8 weeks supplementation (Jovanovic et al 1999).

Corticosteroid-induced diabetes mellitus

Human trials have shown that corticosteroid use significantly increases urinary chromium excretion. Supplementation with chromium picolinate (equivalent to 600 mcg chromium/day) in patients experiencing steroid-induced diabetes resulted in decreased fasting blood glucose values (from >13.9 mmol/L to <8.3 mmol/L). Furthermore, hypoglycaemic medications were also reduced by 50% in all patients within 1 week (Ravina et al 1999).

Antiretroviral medication-induced dysglycaemia

In a study of people with HIV (n = 56) and evidence of elevated glucose, altered lipids or body-fat redistribution secondary to antiretroviral medication, supplementation with chromium nicotinate (400 mcg daily) for 16 weeks significantly decreased insulin, triglycerides and total body fat mass; however, blood glucose, HbA_{1C}, HDL and LDL values remained unchanged (Aghdassi 2010).

Prevention of long-term diabetic complications

Both QTc interval prolongation and chronic hyperinsulinaemia have been associated with atherosclerosis progression and increased cardiovascular morbidity in patients with T2DM. In a crossover trial of 60 subjects, chromium picolinate (1000 mcg/day) for 3 months was shown to reduce both QTc interval duration and plasma insulin levels (Vrtovec et al 2005), probably by reducing the adrenergic activation of the sympathetic nervous system due to hyperinsulinaemia. Benefits were most significant in obese patients with higher peripheral insulin resistance (Vrtovec et al 2005).

In a retrospective study of patients hospitalised with uncontrolled acute hyperglycaemia non- responsive to intravenous insulin, treatment with intravenous chromium chloride at 20 mcg/hour for 10 to 15 hours decreased insulin needs and improved glucose control at 12 and 24 hours post-treatment (Drake 2012).

Animal studies have found that chromium supplementation in mice with T2DM reduces the symptoms of hyperglycaemia and improves the renal function by recovering renal chromium concentration (Mita et al 2005, Mozaffari et al

2005, 2012, Selcuk 2012), which may hold promise for human trials investigating the potential role of chromium in reducing the incidence of diabetic nephropathy.

Hypoglycaemia

Eight patients with reactive hypoglycaemia were given chromium chloride (equivalent to 200 mcg chromium) for 3 months in a double-blind crossover study. Chromium supplementation significantly improved blood sugar regulation, insulin binding to receptors and red blood cells, and alleviated symptoms of hypoglycaemia (Anderson et al 1987).

A double-blind crossover study using chromium chloride (equivalent to 200 mcg/day elemental chromium) for 8 weeks found a significant improvement in glycaemic control in subgroups where the 2-hour glucose level was >10% above or below the fasting level (Bahijri 2000). In these subgroups chromium supplementation resulted in a 2-hour mean not significantly different to the fasting mean, suggesting an amphoteric effect on glycaemic control.

Hyperlipidaemia

It has been suggested that some of the potential benefits of HRT on total and LDL-cholesterol and total: HDL-cholesterol ratio may be related to its ability to improve chromium status (Bureau et al 2002, Roussel et al 2002), and trials yielding both positive and negative results for supplemental chromium in hyperlipidaemia have been reported. In a systematic review of 41 trials, 18 studies, with a total 655 participants, reported lipid data for participants with either T2DM or glucose intolerance (Balk 2007). Overall, chromium supplementation was not found to exert a statistically significant effect on lipid levels in either group, although brewer's yeast supplementation did result in a statistically significant increase in HDL cholesterol (+0.21 mmol/L) compared to chromium picolinate.

Currently, it is unclear what circumstances or conditions and type of subjects are most likely to respond to treatment, so in practice a treatment trial period is often used to establish usefulness in individual patients.

A placebo-controlled trial using chromium tripicolinate (equivalent to 200 mcg chromium/day) for 42 days found a reduction in total cholesterol, LDL and apolipoprotein B (the major protein of the LDL fraction) with a slight increase in HDL and a significant increase in apolipoprotein A1 (the major protein of the HDL fraction) (Press et al 1990). Another RCT of 40 hypercholesterolaemic subjects found that chromium polynicotinate (equivalent to 200 mcg elemental chromium) twice daily for 2 months decreased total (10%) cholesterol and LDL-cholesterol (14%) (Preuss et al 2000).

Another double-blind RCT of young, non-obese adults taking chromium nicotinate (equivalent to 220 mcg elemental chromium) for 90 days found no statistically significant differences in lipid levels (total cholesterol, HDL-cholesterol, LDL-cholesterol, triglycerides) at this dose compared to the placebo; however, this dose is lower than used in most successful studies (Wilson & Gondy 1995).

Lipid-lowering activity does not appear to be significant in people with T2DM according to a meta-analysis of seven RCTs that tested chromium supplementation (>250 mcg/day) taken for at least 3 months (Abdollahi et al 2013).

Obesity

As chromium has a role in maintaining carbohydrate and lipid metabolism, it has been suggested that chromium supplementation may positively impact body composition, including reducing fat mass and increasing lean body mass (Vincent 2003).

A meta-analysis of RCTs concluded that chromium picolinate elicited a relatively small effect compared with placebo for reducing body weight (Pittler et al 2003). One study, however, did show promising results using 200 mcg niacin-bound chromium TIDS (600 mcg/day) with moderate exercise. At these high doses, while overall reduction in body weight was similar for both the chromium and the placebo groups, total fat loss was more significant in the chromium group, suggesting a muscle-sparing effect (Crawford et al 1999). More recent RCTs using chromium picolinate (equivalent to 200 mcg and 1000 mcg/day) were unable to reproduce these effects (Lukaski et al 2007).

A more recent meta analysis of 20 RCTs concurred with Pittler's findings, and found a small but significant difference in weight loss (1 kg) over placebo for studies lasting at least 16 weeks, but not in studies of shorter duration (Onakpoya et al 2013).

Atypical depression

The anti-depressant activity of chromium has been noted in a small number of rodent and human studies (Khanam & Pillai 2006, Komorowski et al 2012), however mechanisms are poorly understood (Iovieno et al 2011). Preclinical studies provide a biological basis for its use in depression, chiefly relating to neurotransmitter synthesis and release (McCarty 1994, Liu & Lin 1997) with decreases seen for serotonergic 5-HT_{2A} receptor expression and increased receptor sensitivity (Attenburrow et al 2002, Piotrowska et al 2008), antagonistic effects on NMDA and AMPA glutamanergic receptors (Piotrowska et al 2008) and antagonist effects on the dopamine and noradrenergic pathway (Piotrowska et al 2013).

In humans, a case series and a single blind trial conducted by McLeod and colleagues (1999, 2000) have shown that supplementation with chromium 400–600 mcg/day alone or in conjunction with sertraline or nortriptyline antidepressant led to the improvement of symptoms of patients with various treatment-resistant mood disorders.

A small placebo-controlled double-blind study of chromium picolinate (600 mcg/day) for 8 weeks was conducted in 15 patients with DSM-IV major depressive disorder, atypical type. Seven (70%) of 10 patients receiving chromium picolinate and none of the placebo group responded to treatment. Six subjects in the chromium group also experienced remission compared with none in the placebo group. However, only a moderate difference was detected in the Hamilton Depression Scale at the end of treatment for a small number of patients (Davidson et al 2003). A replication of the Davidson study by Docherty and colleagues (2005) with a larger cohort (n = 113) demonstrated similar significant improvements compared to the placebo. The study highlighted that patients with carbohydrate cravings, increased appetite and hyperphagia and diurnal mood variation responded particularly well. While these studies have limitations because they include patients with varied depressive pathologies, they provide encouraging evidence for further studies (Iovieno et al 2011).

OTHER USES

Chromium is also used in the following conditions, based on a theoretical understanding of its pharmacological actions.

Exercise aid — not effective

Chromium has demonstrated an ability to enhance insulin-mediated glucose uptake in cultured cells; however, human supplementation does not appear to exert such benefits. In a small RCT, 16 overweight men were randomised to receive chromium picolinate (equivalent to 600 mcg chromium/day) for 4 weeks before being subjected to supramaximal cycling exercises to deplete glycogen stores, followed by high glycaemic index carbohydrate feedings. At this dose, supplementation did not appear to improve glycogen synthesis during the recovery phase (Volek et al 2006).

In addition, studies in female athletes have shown no effect on body composition or muscle strength following supplementation with 500 mcg chromium picolinate daily during 6 weeks of resistance training (Livolsi et al 2001). In a clinical trial of older women a high-dose chromium picolinate supplement did not affect body composition, skeletal muscle size or maximal strength above that of resistance training alone (Campbell et al 2002). A meta-analysis of trials of dietary supplements for enhancing lean muscle mass and strength during resistance training did not support the use of chromium for this purpose (Nissen & Sharp 2003).

POLYCYSTIC OVARIAN SYNDROME (PCOS)

The relationship between PCOS and insulin resistance provides a theoretical basis for the use of chromium in this condition. A small study has found that chromium picolinate (200 mcg/day) appears to improve glucose tolerance but not ovulatory frequency in women with polycystic ovary syndrome (Lucidi et al 2005). Larger studies are required to investigate the potential benefits of chromium supplementation in this population.

Critical care

It is reported that up to 67% of critical care patients present on admission to intensive care with acute insulin resistance and blood sugar control may have better outcomes with intra-venous (IV) chromium (Surani et al 2012). Surani reports a case study of a 62-year-old diabetic, hypercholesterolaemic woman presenting to ICU with cardiac arrest and respiratory failure secondary to aspiration pneumonia and septic shock presenting with acute insulin resistance and requiring 7000 units of insulin over 12 hours, successfully stabilised with an IV infusion of chromium chloride at the rate of 3 mcg/hr (100 mcg in 1 L of saline infused at 30 mL/hr) and leading to the cessation of the insulin infusion.

Clinical note — Does chromium picolinate cause cancer?

There has been some concern in the past arising from in vitro studies suggesting chromium picolinate exerts clastogenic effects in hamster ovarian cells (Stearns et al 1995a, 2002) and possible DNA damage (Levina & Lay 2008, Speetjens et al 1999). While some recent reviews seem to maintain the controversy (Jana 2009, Wise 2012, Golubnitschaja 2012), this genotoxicity has been refuted by a number of authors, suggesting the doses tested were several thousand times higher than equivalent human doses (McCarty 1997, Salmon 1996) and that chromium has a relatively short half-life so that the accumulated doses suggested by researchers (Stearns et al 1995a) were not clinically relevant (Hepburn & Vincent 2003). Furthermore, in vivo evidence from animals and humans suggests that under normal circumstances trivalent chromium (Cr III) has only restricted access to cells, which would limit or prevent genotoxic effects. A recent rodent study by Komorowski (2008) showed no DNA deletions, chromosome gaps or breaks after a single megadose of 7,500 mg/kg. A 2-year study in rats and mice fed CrPic daily at doses three to five times higher than those commonly recommended showed a general lack of toxicity, except in male rats which developed preputial gland adenomas at the highest doses. The reasons for this remain unclear (Stout 2009). Another study showed no histopathological changes or DNA damage in the kidney of male rats supplemented chromium picolinate (100 mg/kg diet), despite accumulation in the kidney (Mozaffari 2012). Therefore, supplementation at low to moderate doses is not currently considered to be detrimental (Eastmond et al 2008). It should also be noted that picolinic acid appears to be the source of the concern and other forms of chromium have not been implicated (Bagchi et al 2002, Stearns et al 1995b).

Osteoporosis

Effects on bone resorption, calcium excretion and collagen production suggest a role in the prevention of osteoporosis (Evans et al 1995, McCarty 1995); however, there are no controlled trials to determine clinical effectiveness.

DOSAGE RANGE

The ESADDI is 50–200 mcg/day. The most common doses studied include 200, 400, 600 and 1000 mcg daily. Doses in the upper range appear to produce more convincing trial results.

- Glycaemic control — 200–1000 mcg for at least 1 to 3 months.

Australian adequate intake

- Women: 25 mcg/day.
- Men: 35 mcg/day.

Chromium picolinate is the best absorbed form (Press et al 1990); chromium nicotinate, which also improves absorption (Arthur 2008), may have a better safety profile and the synergistic effects with nicotinic acid (providing a minimum of 100 mg) may have further benefits in some conditions, especially with regard to lipid profiles and anti-inflammatory effects (Jain et al 2007).

ADVERSE REACTIONS

It is important to differentiate between hexavalent chromium (Cr IV) and trivalent chromium (Cr III) when discussing the potential toxicity of chromium. Cr IV is used in industry and is highly toxic, whereas Cr III is approved for use as a supplement and does not attract the same concerns. Recent in vitro studies suggest a possibility that Cr III may oxidise to Cr V, a potential carcinogen (Shrivastava et al 2005); however, this requires confirmation from in vivo studies.

Irritability and insomnia have been reported with chromium yeast supplementation (Schrauzer et al 1992).

A follow-up survey found no side effects for doses up to 1000 mcg/day of chromium picolinate at 1 year (Cheng et al 1999).

Of five anecdotal adverse reports attributed to chromium picolinate and reviewed by Lamson and Plaza (2002), only one reporting transient and vague symptoms was considered to be a possible adverse reaction (Huszonek 1993). Three could not be validated by the reviewers due to concurrent medications (Cerulli et al 1998, Martin & Fuller 1998, Wasser et al 1997), and another involved the inappropriate use of potassium dichromate, a strong oxidising agent known to elicit reactions in a majority of people (Fowler 2000). A case report exists of toxic hepatitis and greatly elevated hepatic chromium levels (>10-fold normal) after 5 months' ingestion of chromium polynicotinate in combination with vegetable extracts (Lanca et al 2002). Whether chromium supplementation was responsible for this incident is currently unclear.

No adverse effects on iron status

As chromium competes with iron for binding to transferrin it has been suggested that high-dose chromium supplementation may adversely affect iron status. While some studies support this (Ani & Moshtaghie 1992), others show that serum iron concentrations and serum ferritin concentrations are unaffected by chromium picolinate supplementation (Campbell et al 1997, Lukaski et al 2007). Iron does not use all available transferrin binding sites and therefore this situation is unlikely under normal conditions.

SIGNIFICANT INTERACTIONS

Corticosteroids

Corticosteroids increase urinary losses of chromium, and chromium supplementation has been shown to aid in recovery from steroid-induced diabetes mellitus. Therefore a beneficial interaction may be possible (Kim et al 2002).

Hypoglycaemic medicines

Chromium may reduce requirements for hypoglycaemic agents (Ravina & Slezack 1993, Ravina et al 1995). While a beneficial interaction is possible, this combination should be used with caution and drug requirements monitored and adjusted if necessary by a healthcare professional.

Hormone replacement therapy

Women receiving HRT appear to have improved chromium status (Bureau et al 2002, Roussel et al 2002) and the addition of trivalent chromium to 17-beta-oestradiol may enhance IL-6 inhibition in experimental models (Jain et al 2004). Whether this alters chromium requirements is unknown.

Lipid-lowering medicines

Additive effects are theoretically possible as some clinical studies have indicated lipid-lowering effects. Observe patients taking this combination and monitor drug requirements.

CONTRAINDICATIONS AND PRECAUTIONS

Hypersensitivity to chromium.

PREGNANCY USE

Oral ingestion of doses typically found in the diet are likely to be safe. Taken under professional supervision, supplements are also likely to be safe and may be beneficial in the prevention and treatment of gestational diabetes (Jovanovic & Peterson 1996, Jovanovic et al 1999).

Practice points/Patient counselling

- Chromium is an essential trace mineral required for carbohydrate, lipid, protein and corticosteroid metabolism.
- Dietary intakes are generally below the minimum suggested safe and adequate levels, and factors such as high-sugar diets, corticosteroid use, excessive

exercise, infection, physical trauma and psychological stress further increase the risk of deficiency.

- Chromium supplements are used in the management of T2DM, hypoglycaemia, gestational diabetes and hyperlipidaemia. It appears chromium supplementation taken by people with T2DM for at least 3 months can reduce fasting glucose levels, but have no significant effect on lipids.
- It is also used in the treatment of obesity, atypical depression, polycystic ovary syndrome, to curb sugar cravings and improve osteoporosis.
- Supplemental forms used in trials include organic chromium complexes, such as chromium picolinate and chromium nicotinate, and inorganic salts such as chromium chloride.

PATIENTS' FAQs

What will this supplement do for me?

Chromium is essential for health and wellbeing. It reduces fasting glucose levels in people with T2DM when taken as a supplement for at least 3 months. It may also have benefits in gestational diabetes, hypoglycaemia and elevated cholesterol and triglyceride levels in some people, although scientific research has produced mixed results. In practice, it is also used to curb sugar cravings.

When will it start to work?

Effects in T2DM take at least 3 months.

Are there any safety issues?

Used under professional supervision, chromium supplements are considered safe.

REFERENCES

Abdollahi M et al. Effect of chromium on glucose and lipid profiles in patients with type 2 diabetes; a meta-analysis review of randomized trials. J Pharm Pharmaceut Sci 16.1 (2013): 99–114.

Aghdassi E et al. In patients with HIV-infection, chromium supplementation improves insulin resistance and other metabolic abnormalities: a randomized, double-blind, placebo controlled trial. Curr HIV Res 8.2(2010): 113–120.

Amato P et al. Effects of chromium picolinate supplementation on insulin sensitivity, serum lipids, and body composition in healthy, nonobese, older men and women. J Gerontol A Biol Sci Med Sci 55.5 (2000): M260–M263.

Anderson RA et al. Effects of supplemental chromium on patients with symptoms of reactive hypoglycemia. Metabolism 36.4 (1987): 351–355.

Anderson RA et al. Elevated intakes of supplemental chromium improve glucose and insulin variables in individuals with type 2 diabetes. Diabetes 46.11 (1997): 1786–1791.

Anderson RA, Kozlovsky AS. Chromium intake, absorption and excretion of subjects consuming self-selected diets. Am J Clin Nutr 41.6 (1985): 1177–1183.

Anderson RA. Chromium metabolism and its role in disease processes in man. Clin Physiol Biochem 4 (1986): 31–41 [cited in Salmon B. The truth about chromium. What science knows won't kill you. Let's Live Apr 1996].

Anderson RA. Nutritional factors influencing the glucose/insulin system: chromium. J Am Coll Nutr 16.5 (1997): 404–410.

Ani M, Moshtaghie AA. The effect of chromium on parameters related to iron metabolism. Biol Trace Elem Res Jan–Mar 32 (1992): 57–64.

Arthur R. Chromium. J Compl Med 7.4 (2008): 33–42.

Ashton, J.F. (2003) The Chromium content of some Australian foods. Food Australia 55.5 (2003): 201–204.

Attenburrow MJ et al. Chromium treatment decreases the sensitivity of 5-HT2A receptors. Psychopharmacology (Berl) 159.4 (2002): 432–436.

Ayodele JT, Ajala IC. Chromium and copper in toenails of some Kano inhabitants. Journal of Public Health and Epidemiology 1.2 (2009): 46–52.

Bagchi D et al. Cytotoxicity and oxidative mechanisms of different forms of chromium. Toxicology 180.1 (2002): 5–22.

Bahijri SM, Alyssa EM. Increased insulin resistance is associated with increased urinary excretion of chromium in non-diabetic, normotensive Saudi adults. J Clin Biochem Nutr 49.3 (2011): 164–168.

Bahijri SM, Mufti AM. Beneficial effects of chromium in people with type 2 diabetes, and urinary chromium response to glucose load as a possible indicator of status. Biol Trace Elem Res 85.2 (2002): 97–109.

Bahijri SM. Effect of chromium supplementation on glucose tolerance and lipid profile. Saudi Med J 21.1 (2000): 45–50.
Balk EM et al. Effect of chromium supplementation on glucose metabolism and lipids: a systematic review of randomized controlled trials. Diabetes Care 30.8 (2007): 2154–2163.
Broadhurst CL, Domenico P. Clinical studies on chromium picolinate supplementation in diabetes mellitus–a review. Diabetes Technol Ther 8.6 (2006): 677–687.
Bryson WG, Goodall CM. Differential toxicity and clearance kinetics of chromium III or IV in mice. Carcinogenesis 4 (1983): 1535–1539.
Bureau I et al. Trace mineral status in post menopausal women: impact of hormonal replacement therapy. J Trace Elem Med Biol 16.1 (2002): 9–13.
Campbell WW et al. Chromium picolinate supplementation and resistive training by older men: effects on iron-status and hematologic indexes. Am J Clin Nutr 66.4 (1997): 944–949.
Campbell WW et al. Effects of resistive training and chromium picolinate on body composition and skeletal muscle size in older women. Int J Sport Nutr Exerc Metab 12.2 (2002): 125–135.
Cefalu SD et al. Characterization of the metabolic and physiologic response to chromium supplementation in subjects with type 2 diabetes mellitus. Metabolism 59.5 (2010): 755–762.
Cerulli J et al. Chromium picolinate toxicity. Ann Pharmacother 32 (1998): 428–431.
Cheng HH et al. Antioxidant effects of chromium supplementation with type 2 diabetes mellitus and euglycemic subjects. J Agric Food Chem 52.5 (2004): 1385–1389.
Cheng N et al. Follow-up survey of people in China with type-II diabetes mellitus consuming supplemental chromium. J Trace Elem Exper Med 12 (1999): 55–60.
Cieslak W et al. Highly sensitive measurement of whole blood chromium by inductively coupled plasma mass spectrometry. Clinical Biochemistry 46 (2013): 266–270.
Crawford V, Scheckenbach R, Preuss HG. Effects of niacin-bound chromium supplementation on body composition in overweight African-American women. Diabetes Obes Metab 1.6 (1999): 331–337.
Davidson JR et al. Effectiveness of chromium in atypical depression: a placebo-controlled trial. Biol Psychiatry 53.3 (2003): 261–264.
Docherty JP et al. A double-blind, placebo-controlled, exploratory trial of chromium picolinate in atypical depression: effect on carbohydrate cravings. J. Psychiatr. Pract. 11 (2005): 302–314.
Drake TC. Chromium infusion in hospitalized patients with severe insulin resistance: a retrospective analysis. Endocr Prat 18.3 (2012): 394–398.
Eastmond DA et al. Trivalent chromium: assessing the genotoxic risk of an essential trace element and widely used human and animal nutritional supplement. Crit Rev Toxicol 38.3 (2008): 173–190.
Edmondson C. Can chromium be used for diabetes? Drug Utilization Rev 18.11 (2002): 5.
Evans GW, Swensen G, Walters K. Chromium picolinate decreases calcium excretion and increases dehydroepiandrosterone [DHEA] in postmenopausal women. FASEB J 9 (1995): A449.
Fan W et al. Role of liver fatty acid binding protein in hepatocellular injury: effect of CrPic treatment. Journal of inorganic chemistry 124 (2013): 46–53.
Fowler JF Jr. Systemic contact dermatitis caused by oral chromium picolinate. Cutis 65 (2000): 116.
Ghosh D et al. Role of chromium supplementation in Indians with type 2 diabetes mellitus. J Nutr Biochem 13.11 (2002): 690–697.
Golubnitschaja O, Yeghiazaryan K. Opinion controversy to chromium picolinate therapy's safety and therapy: ignoring 'anectodes" of case reports or recognizing individual risks and new guidelines urgency to introduce innovation by predictive diagnosis. EPMA J 3.1 (2012): 11.
Guallar E et al. Low toenail chromium concentration and increased risk of nonfatal myocardial infarction. Am J Epidemiol 162.2 (2005): 157–164.
Hahn CJ, Evans GW. Absorption of trace minerals in zinc-deficient rats. Am J Physiol 228 (1975): 1020–1023.
Haney JT et al. Development of a cancer-based chronic inhalation reference value for hexavalent chromium based on a nonlinear-threshold carcinogenic assessment. Regul Toxicol Pharmacol 64.3(2012): 466–480.
Hepburn DD, Vincent JB. Tissue and subcellular distribution of chromium picolinate with time after entering the bloodstream. J Inorg Biochem 94.1–2 (2003): 86–93.
Hua Y et al. Molecular mechanisms of chromium in alleviating insulin resistance. J Nutr Biochem 23.4 (2012): 313–319.
Hummel M et al. Chromium in metabolic and cardiovascular disease. Horm Metab Res 39.10 (2007): 743–751.
Huszonek J. Over-the-counter chromium picolinate. Am J Psychiatry 150 (1993): 1560–1561.
Iovieno N et al. Second-tier natural antidepressants: Review and critique. Journal of Affective Disorders 130 (2011): 343–357.
Jain SK et al. Effect of chromium niacinate and chromium picolinate supplementation on lipid peroxidation, TNF-alpha, IL-6, CRP, glycated hemoglobin, triglycerides, and cholesterol levels in blood of streptozotocin-treated diabetic rats. Free Radic Biol Med 43.8 (2007): 1124–1131.
Jain SK et al. Protective effects of 17beta-estradiol and trivalent chromium on interleukin-6 secretion, oxidative stress, and adhesion of monocytes: relevance to heart disease in postmenopausal women. Free Radic Biol Med 37.11 (2004): 1730–1735.
Jain SK et al. Trivalent chromium inhibits protein glycosylation and lipid peroxidation in high glucose-treated erythrocytes. Antioxid Redox Signal 8.1–2 (2006): 238–241.
Jain SK, Kannan K. Chromium chloride inhibits oxidative stress and TNF-alpha secretion caused by exposure to high glucose in cultured U937 monocytes. Biochem Biophys Res Commun 289.3 (2001): 687–691.
Jana M et al. Chromium picolinate induced apoptosis of lymphocytes and the signalling mechanisms thereof. Toxicology and applied pharmacology 237.3 (2009): 331–344.
Jovanovic L, Gutierrez M, Peterson CM. Chromium supplementation for women with gestational Diabetes mellitus. J Trace Elem Exp Med 12 (1999): 91–97.

Jovanovic L, Peterson CM. Vitamin and mineral deficiencies which may predispose to glucose intolerance of pregnancy. J Am Coll Nutr 15.1 (1996): 14–20.
Khanam R, Pillai KK. Effect of chromium picolinate on modified forced swimming test in diabetic rats: involvement of serotonergic pathways and potassium channels. Basic Clin Pharmacol Toxicol 98.2 (2006): 155–159.
Kim DS et al. Effects of chromium picolinate supplementation on insulin sensitivity, serum lipids, and body weight in dexamethasone-treated rats. Metabolism 51.5 (2002): 589–594.
Kirman CR et al. Physiologically based pharmacokinetics for humans orally exposed to chromium. Chemico-Biological Interactions 204.1 (2013): 13–27.
Komorowski JR et al. Chromium picolinate does not produce chromosome damage. Toxicology in vitro 22 (2008): 819–826.
Komorowski JR et al. Chromium picolinate modulates serotonergic properties and carbohydrate metabolism in a rat model of diabetes. Biol Trace Elem Res 149.1 (2012): 50–56.
Kozlovsky AS et al. Effects of diets high in simple sugars on urinary chromium losses. Metabolism 35.6 (1986): 515–5118.
Lai MH. Antioxidant effects and insulin resistance improvement of chromium combined with vitamin C and E supplementation for type 2 daibetes mellitus. J Clin Biochem Nutr 43 (2008): 191–198.
Lamson DW, Plaza SM. The safety and efficacy of high-dose chromium. Alt Med Rev 7.3 (2002): 218–235.
Lanca S et al. Chromium-induced toxic hepatitis. Eur J Int Med 13.8 (2002): 518–520.
Lee NA, Reasner CA. Beneficial effect of chromium supplementation on serum triglyceride levels in type 2 diabetes. Diabetes Care 17.12 (1994): 1449–1452.
Levina A, Lay PA. Chemical properties and toxicity of chromium(III) nutritional supplements. Chem Res Toxicol 21.3 (2008): 563–571.
Liu, P.S., Lin, M.K. Biphasic effects of chromium compounds oncatecholamine secretion from bovine adrenal medullary cells. Toxicology 117 (1997) 45–53.
Livolsi JM, Adams GM, Laguna PL. The effect of chromium picolinate on muscular strength and body composition in women athletes. J Strength Cond Res 15.2 (2001): 161–166.
Lucidi RS et al. The effect of chromium supplementation on insulin resistance and ovarian/menstrual cyclicity in women with polycystic ovary syndrome. Fertil Steril 84 (Suppl 1) (2005): S427–S428.
Lukaski HC et al. Chromium picolinate supplementation in women: effects on body weight, composition, and iron status. Nutrition 23.3 (2007): 187–195.
Marashani U et al. Chromium supplementation in non-obese non-diabetic subjects is associated with a decline in insulin sensitivity. BMC Endocr Disord 12.31 (2012).
Martin J et al. Chromium picolinate supplementation attenuates body weight gain and increases insulin sensitivity in subjects with type 2 diabetes. Diabetes Care 29.8 (2006): 1826–1832.
Martin WR, Fuller RE. Suspected chromium picolinate-induced rhabdomyolysis. Pharmacotherapy 18 (1998): 860–862.
Masharani U et al. Chromium supplementation in non-obese non-diabetic subjects is associated with a decline in insulin sensitivity. BMC Endocrine Disorders 12.31 (2012).
McCarty MF. Anabolic effects of insulin on bone suggest a role for chromium picolinate in preservation of bone density. Med Hypotheses 45.3 (1995): 241–246.
McCarty MF. Enhancing central and peripheral insulin activity as a strategy for the treatment of endogenous depression: an adjuvant role for chromium picolinate? Med Hypotheses 43.4 (1994): 247–252.
McCarty MF. Subtoxic intracellular trivalent chromium is not mutagenic: implications for safety of chromium supplementation. Med Hypotheses 49.3 (1997): 263–269.
McLeod MN, Golden RN. Chromium treatment of depression. Int J Neuropsychopharmacol 3.4 (2000): 311–14.
McLeod MN, Gaynes BN, Golden RN. Chromium potentiation of antidepressant pharmacotherapy for dysthymic disorder in 5 patients. J. Clin. Psychiatry 60 (1999) 237–240.
Mertz W. Chromium research from a distance: from 1959 to 1980. J Am Coll Nutr 17.6 (1998): 544–547.
Mita Y et al. Supplementation with chromium picolinate recovers renal Cr concentration and improves carbohydrate metabolism and renal function in type 2 diabetic mice. Biol Trace Elem Res 105.1–3 (2005): 229–248.
Morris BW et al. Chromium homeostasis in patients with type II (NIDDM) diabetes. J Trace Elem Med Biol 13.1–2 (1999): 57–61.
Morris BW et al. Increased chromium excretion in pregnancy is associated with insulin resistance. J Trace Elem Exp Med 13 (2000): 389–396.
Mozafarri M S et al. Renal and glycemic effects of high dose chromium picolinate in *db/db* mice: assessment of DNA damage. J Nutrit Biochem 23.8 (2012): 977–985.
Mozaffari MS et al. Effects of chronic chromium picolinate treatment in uninephrectomized rat. Metabolism 54.9 (2005): 1243–1249.
Nissen SL, Sharp RL. Effect of dietary supplements on lean mass and strength gains with resistance exercise: a meta-analysis. J Appl Physiol 94.2 (2003): 651–659.
Offenbacher EG. Promotion of chromium absorption by asccorbic acid. Trace Elem Electrolytes 11 (1994): 178.
Onakpoya I et al. Chromium supplementation in overweight and obesity: a systematic review and meta-analysis of randomized clinical trials. Obesity Reviews 14 (2013): 496–507.
Padmavathi IJN et al. Impact of maternal chromium restriction on glucose tolerance, plasma insulin and oxidative stress in WNIN rat offspring. Journal of molecular endocrinology 47 (2011): 261–271.
Penumathsa SV et al. Niacin bound chromium treatment induces myocardial glut4 translocation and caveolar interaction via Akt, AMPK and eNOS phosphorylation in streptozotocin induced diabetic rats after ischemia-reperfusion injury. BBA 1792.1 (2009): 39–48.
Perricone NV et al. Blood pressure lowering effects of niacin-bound chromium(III) (NBC) in sucrose-fed rats: renin-angiotensin system. J Inorg Biochem 102.7 (2008): 1541–1548.

Piotrowska A et al. Antidepressant-like effect of chromium chloride in the mouse forced swim test: involvement of glutamatergic and serotonergic receptors. Pharmacological Report 60 (2008): 991–995.

Piotrowska A et al. involvement of the monoaminergic system in the antidepressant-like activity of chromium chloride in the force swim test. Journal of Physiology and Pharmacology 64(2013): 493–498.

Pittler MH, Stevinson C, Ernst E. Chromium picolinate for reducing body weight: meta-analysis of randomized trials. Int J Obes Relat Metab Disord 27.4 (2003): 522–529.

Press RI, Geller J, Evans GW. The effect of chromium picolinate on serum cholesterol and apolipoprotein fractions in human subjects. West J Med 152.1 (1990): 41–45.

Preuss HG et al. Comparing metabolic effects of six different commercial trivalent chromium compounds. J Inorg Biochem 102.11 (2008): 1986–90.

Preuss HG et al. Effects of niacin-bound chromium and grape seed proanthocyanidin extract on the lipid profile of hypercholesterolemic subjects: a pilot study. J Med 31.5–6 (2000): 227–246.

Rabinovitz H et al. Effect of chromium supplementation on blood glucose and lipid levels in type 2 diabetes mellitus elderly patients. Int J Vitam Nutr Res 74.3 (2004): 178–182.

Ravina A et al. Clinical use of the trace element chromium III in the treatment of diabetes mellitus. J Trace Elem Exp Med 8 (1995): 183–190.

Ravina A et al. Reversal of corticosteroid-induced diabetes mellitus with supplemental chromium. Diabet Med 16.2 (1999): 164–167.

Ravina A, Slezack L. Chromium in the treatment of clinical diabetes mellitus. Harefuah 125.5–6 (1993): 142–45, 191 [in Hebrew].

Roussel AM et al. Beneficial effects of hormonal replacement therapy on chromium status and glucose and lipid metabolism in postmenopausal women. Maturitas 42.1 (2002): 63–69.

Sahin K et al. The effects of chromium picolinate and chromium histidinate administration on NF-κB and Nrf2/HO-1 pathway in the brain of diabetic rats. Bio Trace Elem Res 150.3 (2012): 291–96.

Salmon B. The truth about chromium: What science knows won't kill you. Let's Live (Apr 1996).

Schrauzer GN, Shrestha KP, Arce MF. Somatopsychological effects of chromium supplementation. J Nutr Med 3.1 (1992): 43–48.

Schwarz K, Mertz W. Chromium(III) and the glucose tolerance factor. Arch Biochem Biophys 85 (1959): 292–295.

Sealls W Penque BA Elmendorf JS. Evidence that chromium modulates cellular cholesterol homeostasis and ABCA1 functionality impaired by hyperinsulinemia. Arterioscler Thromb Vasc Biol 31.5 (2011): 1139–1140.

Sedman RM et al. Review of the evidence regardingthe carcinogenicity of hexavalent chromium in drinking water. J Environ Sci Health C Environ Carcinog Ecotoxicol Rev 24.1 (2006): 155–82.

Selcuk M et al. chromium picolinate and chromium histidinate protect against renal dysfunction by modulation of NF-κB pathway in high-fat diet fed rats and streptozotocin–induced diabetic rats. Nutrition and Metabolism 9 (2012): 30.

Sharma S et al. Beneficial effects of chromium supplementation on glucose, HbA1C, and lipid variables in individuals with newly onset type-2 diabetes. Journal of Trace Elements in Medicine and Biology 25 (2011): 149–153.

Shrivastava HY et al. Cytotoxicity studies of chromium(III) complexes on human dermal fibroblasts. Free Rad Biol Med 38.1 (2005): 58–69.

Shrivastava R et al. Effects of chromium on the immune system. FEMS Immunol Med Microbiol 34.1 (2002): 1–7.

Speetjens JK et al. The nutritional supplement chromium(III) tris(picolinate) cleaves DNA. Chem Res Toxicol 12.6 (1999): 483–487.

Stearns DM et al. Chromium(III) picolinate produces chromosome damage in Chinese hamster ovary cells. FASEB J 9.15 (1995a): 1643–1648.

Stearns DM et al. Chromium(III) tris(picolinate) is mutagenic at the hypoxanthine (guanine) phosphoribosyltransferase locus in Chinese hamster ovary cells. Mutat Res 513.1–2 (2002): 135–142.

Stearns DM, Belbruno JJ, Wetterhahn KE. A prediction of chromium (III) accumulation in humans from chromium dietary supplements. FASEB J 9.15 (1995b): 1650–1657.

Stout MD et al. Chronic toxicity and carcinogenicity studies of chromium picolinate monohydrate administered in feed to F344N rats and B6C3F1 mice for 2 years. Food Chem Toxicol 47.4 (2009): 729–733.

Sundaram B et al. Anti-atherogenic effects of chromium picolinate in streptozotocin-induced experimental diabetes. J Diabetes 5.1 (2013b): 43–50.

Sundararaman PG et al. Serum chromium levels in gestational diabetes. Indian J Endocrinol Metab 16.1 (2012): S70–73.

Surani SR et al. Severe insulin resistance treatment with intravenous chromium in septic shock patient. World J Diabetes 3.9 (2012): 170–173.

Thomas VL, Gropper SS. Effect of chromium nicotinic acid supplementation on selected cardiovascular disease risk factors. Biol Trace Elem Res 55.3 (1996): 297–305.

Thor MY et al. Evaluation of the comprehensiveness and reliability of the chromium composition of foods in the literature. J Food Compost Anal. 24.8 (2011): 1147–1152 [pubmed]

Urberg M, Zemel MB. Evidence for synergism between chromium and nicotinic acid in the control of glucose tolerance in elderly humans. Metabolism 36.9 (1987): 896–899.

Verhage AH, Cheong WK, Jeejeebhoy KN. Neurologic symptoms due to possible chromium deficiency in long-term parenteral nutrition that closely mimic metronidazole-induced syndromes. J Parenter Enteral Nutr 20.2 (1996): 123–127.

Vincent J. The potential value and toxicity of chromium picolinate as a nutritional supplement, weight loss agent and muscle development agent. Sports Med 33.3 (2003): 213–230.

Vincent JB. Recent advances in the nutritional biochemistry of trivalent chromium. Proc Nutr Soc 63.1 (2004): 41–47.

Volek JS et al. Effects of chromium supplementation on glycogen synthesis after high-intensity exercise. Med Sci Sports Exerc 38.12 (2006): 2102–2109.

Vrtovec M et al. Chromium supplementation shortens QTc interval duration in patients with type 2 diabetes mellitus. Am Heart J 149.4 (2005): 632–636.
Wang, Y, Yao M, Effects of chromium picolinate on glucose uptake in insulin-resistant 3T3-L1 adipocytes involve activation of p38 MAPK, J Nutritional Biochemistry 20 (2009): 982–991.
Wang ZQ, Cefalu WT. Current concepts about chromium supplementation in type 2 diabetes and insulin resistance. Curr Diab Rep, 10.2 (2010): 145–151.
Wasser WG, Feldman NS, Agnati VD. Chronic renal failure after ingestion of over-the-counter chromium picolinate. Ann Intern Med 126 (1997): 410.
Wilson BE, Gondy A. Effects of chromium supplementation on fasting insulin levels and lipid parameters in healthy, non-obese young subjects. Diabetes Res Clin Pract 28.3 (1995): 179–184.
Wise SS, Wise SP. Chromium and genomic stability. Mutation Research 733 (2012): 78–82.
Woods SE et al. Serum chromium and gestational diabetes. J Am Board Fam Med 21.2 (2008): 153–157.

Coenzyme Q10

OTHER NAMES

Ubiquinone, ubidecarenone, ubiquinol

BACKGROUND AND RELEVANT PHARMACOKINETICS

Coenzyme Q10 (CoQ10) is an endogenous enzyme cofactor produced in humans from tyrosine through a cascade of reactions that itself requires eight vitamin coenzymes: tetrahydrobiopterin, vitamins B_6, C, B_2, B_{12}, folic acid, niacin and pantothenic acid (Folkers et al 1990). CoQ10 is also a fat-soluble antioxidant vitamin that plays an indispensable role in intracellular energy production.

Absorption occurs in the small intestine and tends to be poor, and is influenced by the presence of food and drink. CoQ10 is better absorbed in the presence of a fatty meal and is primarily bound to VLDL and LDL cholesterol and transported to the systemic circulation via the lymphatic system. As such, serum levels of CoQ10 depend mostly on the amount of CoQ10-containing lipoproteins in circulation.

After incorporation into lipoproteins in the liver, CoQ10 is subsequently concentrated in various tissues, including the adrenal glands, spleen, kidneys, lungs and myocardium. Physical activity markedly reduces muscle tissue levels of CoQ10, which do not correlate to serum levels, suggesting that they are independently regulated (Laaksonen et al 1995, Overvad et al 1999).

CHEMICAL COMPONENTS

The basic structure of ubiquinones is a benzoquinone head and terpinoid tail. The number of isoprenoid units in the tail portion varies among coenzymes. CoQ10 contains one quinine group and 10 isoprenyl units (Overvad et al 1999). Ubiquinones have been found in microorganisms, plants and animals but the CoQ10 form is the most common type found in mammals and humans.

FOOD SOURCES

Meat and fish products are the most concentrated sources of CoQ10, although lesser quantities are found in boiled broccoli, cauliflower, nuts, spinach and soy. Dietary intake of CoQ10 is approximately 3–5 mg per day (Potgieter et al 2013).

DEFICIENCY SIGNS AND SYMPTOMS

No recommended daily intake (RDI) levels have been established, but there has been some speculation as to possible deficiency signs and symptoms. These include fatigue, muscle aches and pains and chronic gum disease.

Based on biopsy and/or serum samples, it has been observed that relative CoQ10 deficiency is associated with:

- congestive heart failure (Sole & Jeejeebhoy 2002, Spigset 1994a, Molyneux et al 2008)
- cardiomyopathy (Mortensen et al 1990, Senes et al 2008)
- hypertension (Karlsson et al 1991)
- ischaemic heart disease (Karlsson et al 1991, Lee et al 2012a, 2012b, 2012c)
- hyperthyroidism (Bianchi et al 1999)
- breast cancer (Folkers et al 1997)
- cystic fibrosis (Laguna et al 2008)
- pancreatic insufficiency (Laguna et al 2008)
- depression (Maes et al 2009)
- fibromyalgia (Cordero et al 2012, Miyamae et al 2013)
- septic shock (Dupic et al 2011, Donnino et al 2011)
- chronic fatigue syndrome (Maes et al 2009)
- mitochondrial myopathy (Sacconi et al 2010).

At this stage, it is still unclear whether an observation of relative deficiency in a particular disease state can be interpreted as part of the aetiology of that disease, or whether lowered levels are a consequence of disease.

A deficiency state may result from:

- impaired or reduced synthesis due to nutritional deficiencies, advancing age or medication use.
- interactions with drugs — there is clinical evidence that lovastatin, pravastatin and simvastatin reduce CoQ10 status in humans, which may, in part, explain the incidence of side effects, particularly myopathy, associated with their use (Bargossi et al 1994a, 1994b, Folkers et al 1990, Mortensen et al 1997). Clinical evidence also suggests that use of gemfibrozil and other fibric acid derivatives reduce CoQ10 levels (Aberg et al 1998). The clinical significance and long-term consequences of decreased CoQ10 synthesis due to chronic use of lipid-lowering drugs remains to be tested.

  In vitro evidence suggests that other drugs, such as clonidine, hydralazine, hydrochlorothiazide, methyldopa, metoprolol and propranolol, may also decrease endogenous production of CoQ10 (Kishi et al 1975). Other sources cite tricyclic antidepressants as further medicines that can reduce CoQ10 status (Pelton et al 1999). Whether this evidence translates to significant clinical outcomes, remains to be seen.
- inadequate intake or biosynthesis to meet increased requirements resulting from illness or excess physical exertion.
- genetic defects — deficiencies of CoQ10 have been associated with four major clinical phenotypes: (1) encephalomyopathy characterised by a triad of recurrent myoglobinuria, brain involvement and ragged-red fibres; (2) infantile multisystemic disease, typically with prominent nephropathy and encephalopathy; (3) cerebellar ataxia with marked cerebellar atrophy; and (4) pure myopathy (Quinzii et al 2008).

MAIN ACTIONS

Antioxidant

CoQ10 is a powerful antioxidant that buffers the potential adverse consequences of free radicals produced during oxidative phosphorylation in the inner mitochondrial membrane (Young et al 2007). It also binds to a site in the inner mitochondrial membrane that inhibits the mitochondrial permeability transition pore (MPTP).

Being a vital electron and proton carrier, CoQ10 supports adenosine triphosphate (ATP) synthesis in the mitochondrial inner membrane and stabilises cell membranes, preserving cellular integrity and function. It also reconstitutes vitamin E into its antioxidant form by transforming vitamin E radicals to their reduced (active) form (Kaikkonen et al 2002).

Clinical note — Improving bioavailability

Absorption of compounds from the gastrointestinal tract is one of the important determinants of oral bioavailability. The absorption of oral CoQ10 is slow and limited due to its hydrophobicity and large molecular weight (Ochiai et al 2007). Research indicates that intestinal absorption of CoQ10 is enhanced when taken with food. To further improve bioavailability, specialty formulations have been produced by various manufacturers. Ochiai et al (2007) report that an emulsified form of CoQ10 had superior intestinal absorption and achieved a higher peak concentration than for a suspension formulation. Zmitek et al (2008) found that the water solubility and bioavailability of CoQ10 was increased significantly with the use of an inclusion complex with beta-cyclodextrin. This complex is widely used as Q10Vital in the food industry. PureSorb-Q40 (water-soluble type CoQ10 powder) is reported in single-dose human and rat studies to have a greater absorption rate and absorbed volume of CoQ10, even taken postprandially, than those of regular CoQ10, which is lipid-soluble and generally taken in the form of soft gel capsules (Nuku et al 2007). Ullmann et al (2005) tested the bioavailability of DSM Nutritional Products Ltd (Kaiseraugst, Switzerland). CoQ10 10% TG/P (all-Q), a new tablet-grade formulation, with CoQ10 Q-Gel Softsules based on the Bio-Solv technology (Tishcon Corp., Salisbury, MD; marketed by Epic4Health, Smithtown, NY) and Q-SorB (Nature's Bounty, Bohemia, NY). They conducted a crossover study, which showed a bioequivalence between Q-Gel and all-Q, and both preparations were found to have better bioavailability properties than Q-SorB.

Recently, CoQ10 producers in Kaneka, Japan, have synthesised ubiquinol (the reduced form of CoQ10) in an attempt to achieve better bioavailability and higher plasma concentrations with lower oral doses. This form is now available in Australia for over-the-counter use. Single-blind, placebo-controlled studies with healthy subjects testing single oral doses of 150 or 300 mg/day and longer term (4 weeks) oral administration of 90, 150 or 300 mg/day confirmed significant absorption of ubiquinol from the gastrointestinal tract (Hosoe et al 2007). Additionally, no safety concerns were noted on standard laboratory tests for safety or on assessment of adverse events for doses of up to 300 mg for up to 2 weeks after treatment completion.

Cardioprotective

CoQ10 supplementation offers myocardial protection during cardiac surgery, as indicated by clinical trials that observed improved postoperative cardiac function and reduced myocardial structural damage with presurgery administration of CoQ10. Studies with animal models have found that CoQ10 improves preservation of mitochondrial ATP-generating capacity after ischaemia and reperfusion (Pepe et al 2007). Treated animals demonstrate improved myocardial contractile function, increased coronary flow, reduced release of creatine kinase and malondialdehyde in the cardiac effluent. Recent RCTs have found supplementation of 150 mg daily of CoQ10 reduced the inflammatory marker interleukin-6 by 14% (Lee et al 2012a), reduced lipid peroxidation (plasma malondialdehyde) and increased endogenous antioxidant activity (superoxide dismutase and catalase) in patients with coronary heart disease (Lee et al 2012a, 2012b). However, it did not have any effect on homocysteine or highly sensitive C-reactive protein (Lee et al 2012c). Recently, in vitro evidence has suggested CoQ10 protects LDL cholesterol from oxidation, which may have benefits in atherosclerosis (Ahmadvand et al 2013).

Doxorubicin — induced cardiotoxicity

Irreversible oxidative damage to cardiac mitochondria is believed to account for the dose-related cardiomyopathy induced by anthracyclines. Tests in animal models have demonstrated that CoQ10 protects against doxorubicin cardiotoxicity, possibly via antioxidant activity and protection of mitochondrial function (Combs et al 1977, Folkers et al 1978). Clinical studies provide some support for the use of oral CoQ10 and indicate that adjunctive treatment provides protection against cardiotoxicity or liver toxicity during cancer therapy; however, further studies are required to prove this association conclusively and confirm safety (Roffe et al 2004).

Antihypertensive

In the 1970s, Yamagami et al (1975, 1976) observed a deficiency in CoQ10 in patients with hypertension and suggested that correction of the deficiency could result in hypotensive effects. Small studies were initially conducted with hypertensive patients identified as CoQ10-deficient.

Since then, numerous studies have been conducted. In 2007, a meta-analysis was published which evaluated 12 clinical trials (*n* = 362) and found that oral CoQ10 has the potential in hypertensive patients to lower systolic blood pressure by up to 17 mmHg and diastolic blood pressure by up to 10 mmHg without significant side effects (Rosenfeldt et al 2007). Interestingly, most trials fail to identify the subjects' baseline CoQ10 plasma levels and determine whether oral administration restored levels to within the normal range. It has been suggested that CoQ10 supplementation is associated with a decrease in total peripheral resistance, possibly because of action as an antagonist of vascular superoxide, either scavenging or suppressing its synthesis (McCarty 1999).

More specifically, suspected mechanisms of action include: increased antioxidant activity reducing free-radical damage to the endothelial lining and increasing nitric oxide bioavailability (Graham et al 2009); increasing superoxide dismutase-1 which scavenges superoxide anion, which reacts with nitric oxide impairing endothelium-derived relaxation (Kedziora-Kornatowska et al 2010), reduced aldosterone secretion (Louis et al 1965), improved angiotensin II-induced oxidative stress and endothelial dysfunction and reduced angiotensin II-induced upregulation of intercellular adhesion molecule 1 (ICAM-1) and vascular cell adhesion molecule 1 (VCAM-1) (Tsuneki et al 2013).

Immunostimulant activity

Several models of immune function have demonstrated the immunostimulant activity of CoQ10 (Folkers & Wolaniuk 1985), and immunomodulating activity of CoQ10 (Bessler et al 2010).

Endothelial function

The vascular endothelium is the interface between the blood and vascular smooth muscle in arteries and is easily damaged by oxidative stress, resulting in impaired endothelial function. Substances with antioxidant and anti-inflammatory activity, such as CoQ10, have been studied for beneficial effects on endothelial function. A recent meta-analysis (n = 194) found CoQ10 supplementation (150–300 mg/daily) taken for 4 to 12 weeks was associated with a significant improvement in endothelial function compared to placebo, as assessed peripherally by flow-mediated dilation (FMD) of the brachial artery (Gao et al 2012). The improvement measured by FMB was a clinically significant 1.7%, which may translate to 10–25% reduction in residual cardiovascular risk for these patients. FMD is designated as an endothelium-dependent process that reflects vasorelaxation. CoQ10 supplementation was not found to improve nitrate-mediated dilation, suggesting no effect on endothelium-independent vasorelaxation. Of the study participants, 33% were women, 44% had diabetes, 34.5% had hypertension and 28% had established coronary artery disease, indicating activity in patients with and without overt cardiovascular disease. The studies included in this meta-analysis were Watts et al 2002, Tiano et al 2008, Hamilton et al 2009 and Dai et al 2011.

Recently, several in vitro studies have examined the mechanisms of CoQ10 on endothelial function using human umbilical vein endothelial cells. CoQ10 was found to prevent the oxidative stress and subsequent endothelial dysfunction induced by angiotensin II (Tsuneki et al 2013) and by the expression of oxidised low-density lipoprotein receptor (via suppressing NADPH oxidase activation) (Tsai et al 2011). In another study examining CoQ10 on the effects of oxidised LDL cholesterol on endothelial dysfunction, it was found to suppress inflammation and oxidative damage by protecting the activity of superoxide dismutase and catalase, reducing the increase in intracellular calcium and attenuating changes to nitric oxide synthase (Tsai et al 2012).

Neuroprotective

Oxidative stress, resulting in glutathione loss and oxidative DNA and protein damage, has been implicated in many neurodegenerative disorders, including Alzheimer's disease, Parkinson's disease and Huntington's disease (Young et al 2007). Of relevance in Alzheimer's disease, CoQ10 inhibits the formation of beta-amyloid protein in vitro (Ono et al 2005) and clinically, lower levels of CoQ10 have been found in the cortex of the brain in Parkinson's patients (Hargreaves et al 2008). Experimental studies in animal models suggest that CoQ10 may protect against neuronal damage that is produced by ischaemia, atherosclerosis and toxic injury. Though most have tended to be pilot studies, there are published preliminary clinical trials showing that CoQ10 may offer promise in many brain disorders.

Regulates genomic expression

CoQ10 targets the expression of multiple genes, especially those involved in cell signalling, intermediary metabolism and transport (Groneberg et al 2005, Pepe et al 2007) and inflammation (Schmelzer et al 2008, Sohet et al 2009). These mechanisms may account for some of the pharmacological effects observed with CoQ10 supplementation.

OTHER ACTIONS

Tissue protection

A protective effect of coenzyme Q10 against acute paracetamol hepatotoxicity, mostly via antioxidant, anti-inflammatory and antiapoptotic effects, has been demonstrated in vivo (Fouad & Jresat 2012). Additionally, pretreatment of test animals with coenzyme CoQ10 for 6 days protected against acute cisplatin nephrotoxicity, reducing the induced adverse effects on antioxidant defences, lipid peroxidation, tumour necrosis factor-alpha and nitric oxide concentration (Fouad et al 2010).

CoQ10 affects the transport activity of P-gp according to an in vitro test, although the clinical significance of this remains to be established (Itagaki et al 2008).

Recently, a possible antidepressant activity was identified for CoQ10 in vivo. Test animals treated with CoQ10 (25, 50, 100 and 150 mg/kg/day, for 3 weeks) found CoQ10 reduced the hippocampal DNA damage induced by chronic restraint stress in an experimental model of depression, possibly via antioxidant mechanisms and activity within the mitochondria (Aboul-Fotouh 2013).

CLINICAL USE

Cardiovascular diseases

In 1972, Folkers and Littaru from Italy documented a deficiency of CoQ10 in human heart disease (Ernster & Dallner 1995). Since those early reports, a steady stream of research articles has been published and clinical experience in its use as an adjunct to conventional treatment in various forms of heart disease has accumulated. Data from laboratory studies have also accumulated and generally provide a supportive basis for its use.

A review by Langsjoen and Langsjoen of over 34 controlled studies and additional open studies concluded that CoQ10 supplementation goes beyond the correction of a simple deficiency state with strong evidence to show that it has the potential to reduce the risk of cardiovascular disease by the maintenance of optimal cellular and mitochondrial function in cardiomyocytes.

Although investigation into specific cardiovascular diseases has been undertaken, the results of an open study of 424 patients suggested that CoQ10 may have widespread benefits. The study found that CoQ10 supplementation produced clinically significant improvements in cardiac function and reduced medication requirements in patients with a range of cardiovascular disorders, including ischaemic cardiomyopathy, dilated cardiomyopathy, primary diastolic dysfunction, hypertension, mitral valve prolapse and valvular heart disease (Langsjoen et al 1994).

A review by Langsjoen & Langsjoen (1999) of more than 34 controlled studies and additional open studies concluded that CoQ10 supplementation goes beyond the correction of a simple deficiency state, with strong evidence to show that it has the potential to reduce the risk of cardiovascular disease by the maintenance of optimal cellular and mitochondrial function in cardiomyocytes. Furthermore, a recent meta-analysis confirms that CoQ10 supplementation is associated with a significant improvement in endothelial function as measured by FMD, which may translate to 10–25% reduction in residual cardiovascular risk in people both with and without established cardiovascular disease (Gao et al 2012).

Congestive heart failure (CHF)

The potential of CoQ10 as a therapeutic agent is of great interest because it is a safe and well tolerated supplement and CHF causes significant morbidity and mortality and currently has no known cure. CoQ10 has been reported to improve symptoms of congestive heart failure (CHF) and quality of life (QOL), and to reduce hospitalisation, and is used as standard therapy for CHF in some parts of Europe, Russia and Japan.

At the cellular level, oxidative stress, mitochondrial dysfunction and energy starvation are believed to play important roles in the aetiology of CHF (Overvad et al 1999). As such, it has been suggested that low CoQ10 levels identified in patients with CHF may play a role in disease development (Jeejeebhoy et al 2002), and that restoring myocyte nutrition with vitamin supplementation, including CoQ10, produces significant improvement (Sole & Jeejeebhoy 2002). Furthermore, an inverse relationship has been found between the severity of CHF and CoQ10 levels in blood from endocardial biopsies. Some evidence suggests that decreased myocardial function is associated with decreased CoQ10 myocardial tissue concentrations and observational studies have reported that the plasma CoQ10 concentration was an independent predictor of mortality in patients with CHF (Fotino et al 2013).

Recently, the CORONA study by McMurray et al (2010) showed that while low coenzyme Q10 was a marker of greater disease severity, it is very unlikely to have utility as a clinically important prognostic biomarker in heart failure. They observed that people with lower baseline serum coenzyme Q10 levels were found to have risk factors associated with more advanced disease and poorer prognosis such as being older, more severe heart failure (higher NYHA functional class), lower EF and lower estimated glomerular filtration rate; however, multivariate analysis did not find serum coenzyme Q10 to be an independent prognostic variable (McMurray et al 2010). These results are in contrast to those published by Molyneux et al (2008), who had previously identified that plasma CoQ10 concentration in people with CHF was an independent predictor of mortality.

Clinical studies

A meta-analysis of studies published prior to 2012 examined whether CoQ10 supplementation could improve the ejection fraction (EF) and/or New York Heart Association (NYHA) classification of people with congestive heart failure (Fotino et al 2013). The analysis included 13 placebo-controlled clinical trials (seven crossover and six parallel-arm) involving a total of 395 subjects, with several additional studies not included in an earlier meta-analysis (Berman et al 2004). The included studies had a duration of 4–28 weeks, testing a dose of CoQ10 from 60–300 mg daily. Importantly, baseline EF ranged from 22% to 46% and the baseline NYHA functional class ranged from 2.3 to 3.4.

From the limited number of studies available, the changes in EF for CoQ10 compared with placebo ranged from −3.0% to 17.8% (mean 3.67%) and the pooled mean net change in NYHA classification was −0.30, which meant a slight, but non-significant improvement in NYHA heart failure classification. Additional post hoc analysis by a subgroup found positive effects in crossover trials, study duration less than 12 weeks, conducted prior to 1994 (which tended to include less sick patients) using doses less than 100 mg daily, and in those with a milder stage of CHF (baseline EF ≥ 30%). The authors stated that due to the small number of studies with NYHA classification, use of various different CoQ10 formulations and doses and lack of information about adjunctive medications used and comorbidities, results should be viewed cautiously and the study may have been under-powered to detect a true effect.

The finding regarding changes to EF largely supports the conclusion made in an earlier meta-analysis (Sander et al 2006). The primary outcome measure was EF and secondary outcome measures were cardiac output (CO), cardiac index (CI), stroke volume (SV) and stroke index (SI). The analyses used data from 11 eligible trials (randomised, double-blind, placebo-controlled) and CoQ10 doses ranging from 60 to 200 mg/day with treatment periods ranging from 1 to 6 months. Overall, there was a significant 3.7% net improvement in EF ($P < 0.00001$).

Interestingly, more profound effects on EF were observed for patients not receiving angiotensin-converting enzyme inhibitors (6.74% net improvement). To put the degree of EF improvement into perspective, the beta-blocker drug, metoprolol, is associated with an average increase in EF of 7.4% (range 3–16%), whereas carvedilol is associated with an increase of 5% (3–11%). CoQ10 also significantly increased the cardiac output by an average of 0.28 L/min. When a less conservative meta-analysis model was used, cardiac index, stroke volume and stroke index were also significantly improved. Sander et al (2006) used data from clinical trials by Hofman-Bang et al 1995, Judy et al 1986, Keogh et al 2003, Khatta et al 2000, Langsjoen et al 1985, Morisco et al 1994, Munkholm et al 1999, Permanetter et al 1992, Pogessi et al 1991, Serra et al 1991 and Watson et al 1999.

The largest controlled trial in adult cardiomyopathy and CHF was reported in 1993 and not included in the 2013 meta-analysis (Morisco et al 1993). It involved 641 patients with CHF New York Heart Association (NYHA) classes III and IV. The double-blind, placebo-controlled study used a dose of 2 mg CoQ10 per kg daily over 1 year and found that active treatment significantly improved arrhythmias and episodes of pulmonary oedema, as well as reducing the number of hospitalisations and overall mortality rate. The same researchers conducted a smaller double-blind, crossover study that again produced positive results. Oral CoQ10 (150 mg/day) taken for 4 weeks significantly improved EF, stroke volume and cardiac output in chronic heart failure patients (Morisco et al 1994).

Although CoQ10 is generally studied in heart failure patients (NYHA class II and III), a double-blind, placebo-controlled, randomised study published in 2004 (Berman et al) describes its effects in end-stage heart failure among patients awaiting heart transplantation. The study of 32 subjects compared Ultrasome CoQ10 (60 mg/day) to placebo over 3 months as an adjunct to conventional therapy. Significant improvements in functional status, clinical symptoms and QOL were reported for CoQ10; however, no significant changes in the echocardiography parameters (dimensions and contractility of cardiac chambers) or atrial natriuretic factor and tumour necrosis factor (ANF and TNF) blood levels were observed.

While the overall body of evidence generally supports the use of CoQ10 in mild heart failure, not every trial has produced positive results. One theory proposes that the most profound effects on myocardial function occur when supplementation is given shortly after the diagnosis of CHF and before the development of irreversible myocyte loss and fibrosis. Some commentators have suggested that the sample sizes, severity and duration of disease, treatment dose and duration of treatment may have contributed to the inconsistent results observed (Langsjoen 2000). An important issue that often fails to be considered is the measurement of plasma and myocyte CoQ10 concentrations and whether supplementation has achieved levels that are within the range likely to produce clinical results.

Langsjoen and Langsjoen (2008) reported that patients with CHF, NYHA class IV, often fail to achieve adequate plasma CoQ10 levels on supplemental ubiquinone at dosages up to 900 mg/day. These patients often have plasma total CoQ10 levels of less than 2.5 microgram/mL and limited clinical improvement. Interestingly, the 2013 meta-analysis reported that CHF patients had a baseline blood CoQ10 concentration ranging from 0.61 to 1.01 mcg/mL and those receiving CoQ10 supplementation had a pooled mean net increase in blood CoQ10 concentration of 1.4 mcg/mL, suggesting some may have had plasma levels at less than the optimal range (Fotino et al 2013).

One theory proposed to explain this discrepancy is that critically ill patients have intestinal oedema, which reduces oral CoQ10 absorption. To test this hypothesis, seven patients with advanced CHF were identified (mean EF 22%) with subtherapeutic plasma CoQ10 levels with mean level of 1.6 microgram/mL on an average dose of 450 mg of ubiquinone daily (150–600 mg/day) (Langsjoen & Langsjoen 2008). The doses of all patients were increased by an average of 580 mg/day of ubiquinol (450–900 mg/day) with follow-up plasma CoQ10 levels, clinical status and EF measurements by echocardiography. At these higher doses, mean plasma CoQ10 levels increased from 1.6 microgram/mL (0.9–2.0 microgram/mL) up to 6.5 microgram/mL (2.6–9.3 microgram/mL) with a subsequent mean improvement in EF from 22% (10–35%) to 39% (10–60%). Substantial clinical improvements were also reported with higher dosing as patients' NYHA class improving from a mean of IV to a mean of II (I–III).

Stocker and Macdonald make the observation that a major change in the treatment of CHF in the mid-1990s with the increase in prescription of β-blockers may account for the less impressive results obtained in CoQ10 studies conducted after this period compared to earlier ones (as reported by Fotino et al 2013). They suggest it is possible that there is an incremental benefit of CoQ10 when added to treatment that includes angiotensin-converting enzyme inhibitors but no or less incremental benefit of CoQ10 in addition to angiotensin-converting enzyme inhibitors plus β-blockers (Stocker & Macdonald 2013). To test the theory, a future study utilising CoQ10 with adjunctive beta-blockade would be necessary, but as they point out, funding such an expensive study without patent protection for CoQ10 will be near impossible.

Mortality and CHF

Ultimately, whether CoQ10 has a significant effect on EF or NYHA classifications is relatively less important than whether it affects mortality. To this end, the Q-SYMBIO trial has been conducted, a randomised, double-blind, multicentre trial with CoQ10 as adjunctive treatment of CHF, with focus on SYMptoms, BIOmarker status and long-term outcome (hospitalisations/mortality) (Stocker & Macdonald 2013). Most recently, the preliminary results were presented at the 7th International Coenzyme Q10 Association Meeting in Seville, Spain (SA Mortensen, unpublished data, 2012 reported by Stocker and Macdonald). At completion, 422 patients with CHF were recruited and those receiving CoQ10 (2 mg/kg/day) experienced a significantly reduced all-cause mortality at 2 years compared with placebo. This important trial makes a major addition to the evidence base supporting a role of CoQ10 in the management of CHF.

Paediatric myopathy

The potential role of CoQ10 in paediatric idiopathic dilated cardiomyopathy has been investigated in a small double blind RCT. Thirty-eight subjects (<18 years) using standard treatment were given additional placebo or 2 mg/kg/daily of CoQ10 in divided doses which were increased to the maximum dose of 10 mg/kg/daily or until side effects occurred. After 6 months of treatment, those receiving CoQ10 supplementation had improved cardiac performance with ι-ejection fraction, heart rate and grading of diastolic dysfunction (measured by electrocardiogram) reaching statistical significance. Additionally, the cardiac failure index score was reduced in those receiving treatment compared to the controls and CoQ10 was well tolerated (Kocharian et al 2009).

Haemodialysis

In a prospective, double-blind, placebo-controlled, crossover study, haemodialysis patients were given CoQ10 200 mg/day during 8 weeks, with a 4-week washout period. There was no significant improvement in left ventricle diastolic functions compared with placebo; however, it did improve left ventricle hypertrophy (Turk et al 2013).

IN COMBINATION

A randomised, double-blind, placebo-controlled trial the addition of a supplement containing water-soluble CoQ10 (320 mg) terclatrate and creatine (340 mg) on exercise tolerance and health-related quality of life in 67 patients with stable chronic heart failure was examined. After 8 weeks, exercise tolerance measured by peak oxygen consumption and health-related quality of life (physical component) were significantly improved compared to placebo (Fumagalli et al 2011).

Hypertension

CoQ10 has been studied both as stand-alone and adjunctive treatment in hypertension. In 2007, a meta-analysis was published which evaluated 12 clinical trials (n = 362) consisting of three randomised controlled trials, one crossover study and eight open label studies (Rosenfeldt et al 2007). In the randomised controlled trials (n = 120), systolic blood pressure in the treatment group decreased by 16.6 mmHg (12.6–20.6, $P < 0.001$), with no significant change in the placebo group. Diastolic blood pressure in the treatment group was also significantly reduced after treatment by 8.2 mmHg (6.2–10.2, $P < 0.001$), with no significant change in the placebo group. In the crossover study (n = 18), systolic blood pressure decreased by 11 mmHg and diastolic blood pressure by 8 mmHg with no significant change in the placebo group. In the open label studies (n = 214), mean systolic blood pressure decreased by 13.5 mmHg (9.8–17.1, $P < 0.001$) with active treatment and mean diastolic blood pressure significantly decreased by 10.3 mmHg (8.4–12.3, $P < 0.001$). Previously, a review of eight studies concluded that supplemental CoQ10 results in a mean decrease in systolic blood pressure of 16 mmHg and in diastolic blood pressure of 10 mmHg (Rosenfeldt et al 2003). The effect on blood pressure has been reported within 10 weeks of treatment at doses usually starting at 100 mg daily.

A 2009 Cochrane review of CoQ10 in the treatment of essential hypertension reported that despite a clinically significant greater reduction in blood pressure in the treatment group receiving 100–120 mg daily for 4–12 weeks (systolic by 11 mmHg and diastolic by 7 mmHg) compared to the placebo group, caution is needed in interpreting the findings due to the limited available data and the possibility of bias (Ho et al 2009). The review analysed results from one crossover study and two RCTs which met the inclusion criteria (n = 96) (Digiesi 1994, Singh 1999, Yamagami 1976) and were also included in the earlier meta-analysis by Rosenfeldt et al 2007).

In conjunction

The effect of CoQ10 in patients with metabolic syndrome and inadequately controlled hypertension (n = 30) was examined in a randomised, double blind, placebo-controlled, crossover trial. Subjects received either 100 mg CoQ10 twice daily or placebo for 12 weeks in addition to their antihypertensive medication, and were then changed over to the alternative treatment following a 4-week washout period. Plasma levels of CoQ10 increased 3.7 fold following treatment, however, there was no significant reduction in clinic or 24-hour ambulatory blood pressure compared to placebo, though there was a non-statistically significant trend towards reduction in 24-hour blood pressure, and a reduction in daytime diastolic blood pressure loads (the proportion of 24-hour blood pressure readings increased above 90 mmHg and ≥ 85 mmHg in diabetics) (Young et al 2012).

Cardiac surgery

The use of CoQ10 supplementation before cardiac surgery has been studied since the early 1980s. Since that time, growing evidence has suggested that

CoQ10 can reduce reperfusion injury after coronary artery bypass surgery, reduce surgical complications, accelerate recovery times and, possibly, shorten hospital stays (Chello et al 1996, Chen et al 1994, Judy et al 1993, Rosenfeldt et al 2002, Taggart et al 1996, Tanaka et al 1982, Zhou et al 1999). In general, the studies that achieved positive results had provided supplements for 1–2 weeks prior to surgery. One study observed that continuing to administer CoQ10 for 30 days after surgery hastened the recovery course to 3–5 days without complications, compared with a 15–30-day recovery period for a control group, which did experience complications (Judy et al 1993, Rosenfeldt et al 2002).

A randomised, double-blind trial investigated the effects of preoperative high-dose CoQ10 therapy (300 mg/day) in patients undergoing elective cardiac surgery (mainly coronary artery bypass graft surgery (CABG) or valve replacement) (Rosenfeldt et al 2005). Approximately 2 weeks of active treatment resulted in significantly increased CoQ10 levels in the serum, atrial myocardium and mitochondria compared with placebo, but no significant change in the duration of hospital stay. Active treatment also improved subjective assessment of physical QOL (+13%) compared with placebo; however, the authors point out that physical QOL does not necessarily indicate improved cardiac pump function and further studies are required with larger sample sizes to clarify the role of CoQ10 in QOL.

More recently, a prospective, randomised trial involving patients undergoing CABG compared coenzyme Q10 supplementation (150–180 mg/day) taken for 7 to 10 days prior to surgery as an adjunct to standard care to a cohort receiving standard care only. Compared to the control group, those receiving CoQ10 experienced shorter hospital stays (7.1 vs 10.3 days) and better clinical outcomes, such as fewer reperfusion arrhythmias, greater spontaneous return of heartbeat and normal sinus rhythm after clamping, lower total inotropic medication requirements (dopamine and adrenaline). Interestingly, no significant difference in plasma levels of total antioxidants was observed between the groups until 24 hours after aortic clamp release, where it was significantly higher than baseline ($P < 0.05$) for CoQ10 treatment (Makhija et al 2008).

The use of CoQ10 as preoperative treatment may hold special significance for older patients, who generally experience poorer recovery of cardiac function after cardiac surgery than their younger counterparts. One explanation gaining support is that the aged myocardium has less homeostatic reserve and so is more sensitive to both aerobic and physical stress and less well equipped to deal with cardiac surgery. Two studies have confirmed this theory, demonstrating an age-related deficit in myocardial performance after aerobic and ischaemic stress and the capacity of CoQ10 treatment to correct age-specific diminished recovery of function (Rosenfeldt et al 1999).

Besides improving cardiac resilience, CoQ10 has been found to reduce skeletal muscle reperfusion injury after clamping and declamping by reducing the degree of peroxidative damage (Chello et al 1996).

IN COMBINATION

CoQ10 supplementation has been utilised as part of a multi-component metabolic treatment in a double-blind, randomised, placebo-controlled trial of 117 elective CABG and valve surgery patients at The Alfred Hospital (Melbourne, Australia) (Leong et al 2010). Treatment was commenced while on the waiting list for surgery (approximately 2 months) and continued for 1 month after surgery. Active treatment consisted of CoQ10 (Blackmore's CoQ10; 300 mg/day), magnesium orotate, alpha lipoic acid, omega-3 EFAs and selenium which was taken for a mean of 76 ± 7.5 days and resulted in increased antioxidant levels preoperatively so that the adverse effect of surgery on redox status was attenuated. Active treatment also reduced plasma troponin I, 24 hours postoperatively from 1.5 (1.2–1.8) mcg/L, to 2.1 (1.8–2.6) mcg/L ($P = 0.003$) and shortened the mean length of postoperative hospital stay by 1.2 days from 8.1 (7.5–8.7) to 6.9 (6.4–7.4) days ($P = 0.004$) and reduced associated hospital costs.

As a result of these positive findings, the Integrative Cardiac Wellness Program was established at The Alfred Hospital in 2008, whereby metabolic therapy is provided to all elective cardiothoracic patients prior to surgery. Metabolic therapy consists of: CoQ10 225 mg/day; R,S alpha-lipoic acid 225 mg/day; magnesium orotate 1500 mg/day (as FIT Bioceutical's Cardionutrients) and omega-3 EFAs 3000 mg/day (as FIT Bioceuticals Ultra-Clean). Supplements are commenced after visiting the surgery pre-admission clinic, continued until the day before surgery and resumed on the ward, once solids are recommenced. A clinical audit of 337 elective cardiothoracic surgical patients in the program was recently undertaken, which found that coronary artery bypass patients had a relative reduction of 42% for positive inotropic requirements post-surgery compared to controls ($P < 0.001$) and valve repair/replacement patients, a 40% relative reduction ($P = 0.02$). Multivariate analysis was used to compare them to a historical control group receiving standard care only in the previous 3 years at the same hospital (Braun et al 2013).

Angina pectoris

Based on the observation of relative CoQ10 deficiency in patients with ischaemic heart disease, and in animal models showing that it prevents reperfusion injury, several randomised clinical trials have been performed in angina pectoris. The doses used have varied from 60 mg to 600 mg daily, and the time frames for use varied from 4 days to 4 weeks. Overall, CoQ10 appears to delay signs of oxygen deficiency in the myocardium, increases patients' stamina on a treadmill or during exercise and delays the onset of angina (Overvad et al 1999), as well as reducing glyceryl trinitrate consumption (Kamikawa et al 1985).

Statin drug use

The mechanism of action of the statin group of drugs is inhibition of 3-hydroxy-3-methylglutaryl-coenzyme A (HMG-CoA) reductase, an enzyme involved in the biosynthesis of cholesterol from acetyl-CoA. Inhibition of this enzyme also adversely affects the intrinsic biosynthesis of CoQ10, as demonstrated in laboratory animals and humans and reduces plasma and myocardial levels of CoQ10 (Bargossi et al 1994b, Folkers et al 1990, Rosenfeldt et al 2005).

This fact, plus the role of CoQ10 in mitochondrial energy production, which is required in muscle function, has prompted the hypothesis that statin-induced CoQ10 deficiency is involved in the pathogenesis of statin myopathy and long-term statin use may actually impair cardiac function.

At least nine observational studies and six RCTs have demonstrated that statins reduce plasma/serum levels of CoQ10 by 16–54% (Marcoff & Thompson 2007). This could be related to the fact that statins lower plasma LDL levels, and CoQ10 is mainly transported in LDL; however, a decrease is also found in platelets and in lymphocytes of statin-treated patients and, therefore, it could truly depend on inhibition of CoQ10 synthesis (Littarru & Langsjoen 2007). Additionally, studies have also demonstrated that co-administration of oral CoQ10 can still effectively raise serum levels when taken together with statin drugs (Bargossi et al 1994, Silver et al 2004).

Reduced muscle CoQ10 concentrations are of greater concern because they may be associated with impaired cardiac function and, theoretically, increased risk of myopathy and possibly side effects such as physical fatigue. The results obtained by Folkers et al (1990), Silver et al (2004) and Paiva et al (2005) provide support for an association between statin use and reduced intramuscular CoQ10 levels, whereas other studies find no change to intramuscular CoQ10 concentrations (Laaksonen et al 1994, 1995, 1996), increased risk of cardiovascular disease or impaired left ventricular systolic or diastolic function in hypercholesterolaemic subjects (Colquhoun et al 2005, Stocker et al 2006). Further investigation is required to determine whether long-term reductions of CoQ10 as a result of chronic statin therapy increases the risk of myopathy and whether subpopulations at risk, such as patients with familial hypercholesterolaemia, heart failure or who are over 65 years of age, may benefit from CoQ10 supplementation (Levy & Kohlhaas 2006).

Statin-induced myalgia

The decreased formation of coenzyme Q10 (CoQ10) within the body due to statin use is suspected of contributing to the incidence of statin-associated muscle pain (myalgia), one of the possible side effects of statins. The question of whether supplemental CoQ10 can help prevent or treat statin myopathy is regularly asked by clinicians.

In recent years, several intervention studies have been performed whereby CoQ10 supplementation has been tested in volunteers also taking statin medication and experiencing myalgia.

A 2012 study examined the effect of CoQ10 supplementation (Q max 30 mg twice daily) on statin-associated myopathy in 28 patients. After 6 months, serum CoQ10 levels had substantially increased (194%), subjective muscle pain reduced by almost 54% and muscle weakness by 44% (Zlatohlavek et al 2012). Similarly, positive results were obtained in a controlled double-blind randomised trial, which demonstrated 100 mg CoQ10 daily produced a 40% reduction in pain severity and 38% in pain interference with daily activities compared to a control group receiving 400 IU of vitamin E (Caso et al 2007).

In contrast, a 3-month placebo-controlled, randomised trial found no difference in the reduction of muscle pain between CoQ10 (60 mg twice daily) or placebo in patients who had developed myalgia within 2 months of starting or increasing statins. Interestingly, both the groups demonstrated significant reduction in pain after one month, suggesting a substantial placebo effect. The endpoints measured in this trial were the 10 cm visual analogue scale and the McGill pain questionnaire (Bookstaver et al 2012). Additionally, Young et al (2007) found no change in the myalgia score compared to placebo in a group receiving 200 mg CoQ10 for 12 weeks (Caso et al 2007).

It is difficult to explain the reasons for these inconsistent results; however some of the following factors should be considered. As there was no measurement of CoQ10 levels (serum or muscle) at baseline or at the end of treatment it is not possible to know if there were any differences between the study groups at baseline, if there was any change in levels by the end of the study, and therefore if the bioavailability or dose of CoQ10 used may have been factors.

There is another placebo controlled study currently being conducted in the USA to test whether CoQ10 supplementation is beneficial for reducing pain intensity in statin-induced myalgic patients (Parker et al 2013). In practice, a 3-month trial of supplemental CoQ10 can be safely considered for patients with fatigue, mild muscle soreness or slightly impaired concentration while taking long-term statins and with other risk factors for low CoQ10, such as advanced age, low meat intake or multisystem diseases.

C

Statin-induced cognitive impairment

Cognitive problems are also identified among some patients reporting statin adverse events. Brain tissue shares with muscle tissue a high mitochondrial vulnerability and both are the dominant organs clinically affected in CoQ10-deficiency mitochondrial syndromes (Golomb & Evans 2008). Whether the cognitive side effects reported by statin users are due to CoQ10 depletion or responds to CoQ10 treatment is not well explored. To date, a study with aged dogs that had undergone long-term statin use demonstrated significant cognitive deficits with statin use compared to age-matched controls. In addition, poorer cognition was associated with lower parietal cortex CoQ10, and statin use was associated with a significant reduction in serum CoQ10 (Martin et al 2011). Human trials are now warranted to determine whether CoQ10 supplementation improves cognitive function in long-term statin users.

Statin use and CoQ10 supplementation

Overall, whether supplementation is effective as a treatment in statin-associated myalgia remains unclear because test results are inconsistent. Due to the low risk nature of CoQ10, a 3-month trial is worth considering in people presenting with statin-associated myalgia or generalised muscle pain and who cannot be satisfactorily treated with other agents.

It is also worth considering for people reporting fatigue, poor concentration and headaches in association with long-term statin use. Particularly consider it for those with a family history of heart failure, elevated cholesterol levels, and who are over 65 years of age and taking statin drugs long-term (Levy & Kohlhaas 2006). A trial of therapy may also be worthwhile in patients reporting fatigue, malaise, cognitive impairment and headaches as possible side effects to statin treatment.

Arrhythmias

A small open study of 27 volunteers showed that CoQ10 exerts antiarrhythmic effects in some individuals (Fujioka et al 1983).

Hypercholesterolemia

Oral CoQ10 reduces cholesterol levels, according to two clinical trials. One small 10-week open study of 26 subjects with essential hypertension study found that an oral dose of 50 mg CoQ10 taken twice daily also reduced total serum cholesterol levels with a modest increase in serum HDL cholesterol (Digiesi et al 1994). A reduction in total cholesterol was also seen in a 2013 randomised, double-blind, placebo-controlled study of 64 people with type 2 diabetes. A dose of CoQ10 (200 mg/day) significantly reduced total cholesterol, LDL-cholesterol and improved glycaemic control compared to placebo in the 12-week trial (Kolahdouz et al 2013).

Sports supplement/ergogenic aid

Because CoQ10 is essential for energy metabolism and reduces oxidative stress, researchers have speculated that it may improve athletic performance. Clinical studies investigating the effects of CoQ10 supplementation on physical capacity generally show negative results. One theory as to the differences in study results is due to great variations in serum CoQ10 levels resulting from differences in dosage and also individual responses to treatment. Nine earlier studies used test doses of CoQ10 which varied from 60 mg to 150 mg daily over time periods of 28 days to 8 weeks. Of these eight studies, only two produced positive results. One was a double-blind, crossover trial which produced positive results on both objective and subjective parameters of physical performance (Ylikoski et al 1997). In that study 94% of athletes felt that CoQ10 had improved their performance and recovery times, compared with the 33% receiving placebo. Most recently, another double-blind, placebo-controlled, crossover study of healthy people found that oral CoQ10 (300 mg/day) taken for 8 days improved subjective fatigue sensation and physical performance during fatigue-inducing workload trials (Mizuno et al 2008).

Of the others, one study found that 150 mg CoQ10 taken over 2 months had no effect on maximal oxygen consumption, lactate thresholds or forearm blood flow, although it did improve the subjective perceived level of vigour (Porter et al 1995). Another study demonstrated that CoQ10 did not alter physiological or metabolic parameters measured as part of cardiopulmonary exercise testing; however, it did extend the time and the workload required to reach muscular exhaustion (Bonetti et al 2000). Five further clinical trials produced negative results.

One retrospective study found that muscle CoQ10 levels were positively related to exercise capacity and/or marathon performance, suggesting that runners with the highest levels performed better than those with lower levels (Karlsson et al 1996).

More recent studies also demonstrate mixed results, though the majority of studies are negative. Whether negative results are due to insufficient dose or treatment time frames or differences in baseline CoQ10 levels remains to be clarified.

In another double-blind RCT of trained and untrained subjects, a single dose of CoQ10 (200 mg) resulted in raised plasma levels and significantly correlated with higher muscle CoQ10 levels, maximal oxygen consumption and treadmill time to exhaustion. After supplementation for 2 weeks, there was an increase in plasma CoQ10 levels and a non-significant trend towards increased time to exhaustion (Cooke et al 2008). In a study where 18 elite kendo athletes were given either 300 mg CoQ10 or placebo for 20 days, the active treatment group had reduced exercise-induced muscular injury with lower levels of creatine kinase, myoglobin and lipid peroxides compared with the corresponding values in the placebo group (Kon et al 2008). Similarly, the increase in lipid peroxidation induced by repeated bouts of supramaximal exercises was partially prevented following 8 weeks of CoQ10 supplementation (100 mg) in a randomised, double-blind, crossover study involving 15 sedentary men (Gul et al 2011). Recently, a small, randomised, double-blind, crossover study involving 15 healthy sedentary men found supplementation with 100 mg CoQ10 increased mean power during repeated bouts of supramaximal exercises, suggesting possible benefits in performance; however, while fatigue indexes decreased, they did not significantly differ from placebo (Gokbel et al 2010). A study by Ostman et al (2012) also failed to show any benefit from 8 weeks of supplemental CoQ10 (90 mg) daily on exercise capacity, muscle damage or oxidative stress in a small randomised, double-blind, controlled study involving moderately trained healthy men.

Postpolio syndrome

One randomised, double-blind study tested whether adding oral CoQ10 to resistance training would further improve muscle strength and endurance as well as functional capacity and health-related quality of life (Skough et al 2008). All 14 patients (8 women and 6 men) with postpolio syndrome in the 12-week study undertook muscular resistance training 3 days/week and were randomised to receive either CoQ10 200 mg/day or placebo. For all patients, muscle strength, muscle endurance and quality of life regarding mental health increased statistically significantly, but there was no significant difference between the CoQ10 and placebo groups.

Chronic obstructive pulmonary disease (COPD)

Patients with COPD have increased oxidative stress, which increases further during periods of exacerbation, so the investigation of supplements with antioxidant activity has been of interest in this cohort (Tanrikulu et al 2011). At least two clinical trials have investigated the use of CoQ10 supplementation in COPD (Fujimoto et al 1993, Satta et al 1991). In one study, 20 patients with COPD were randomly assigned CoQ10 (50 mg) or placebo as part of their pulmonary rehabilitation program (Satta et al 1991). Treatment resulted in a 13% increase in maximum oxygen consumption and a 10% increase in maximum expired volume — both significant improvements. A dose of CoQ10 (90 mg) daily over 8 weeks was studied in a smaller trial of patients with COPD (Fujimoto et al 1993). Significantly elevated serum CoQ10 levels were associated with improved hypoxaemia at rest, but pulmonary function was unchanged.

IN COMBINATION

A double-blind, placebo-controlled study found that supplementation of CoQ10 (Q-Ter) and creatine in COPD patients with chronic respiratory failure (in long term O_2 therapy) during the stable phase of the disease significantly increased lean body mass, exercise tolerance as measured by the 6-minute walk test, reduced severity of dyspnoea, improved quality of life and decreased exacerbations. Treatment consisted of Creatine 340 mg + 320 mg Coenzyme Q-Ter (Eufortyn), Scharper Therapeutics SRL taken for 2 months while diet and lifestyle remained unchanged and the study involved 55 volunteers (Marinari et al 2013).).

Cystic fibrosis

Pancreatic insufficiency and a diminished bile acid pool cause malabsorption of important essential nutrients and other dietary components in cystic fibrosis (CF) (Papas et al 2008). Of particular significance is the malabsorption of fat-soluble antioxidants such as carotenoids, tocopherols and CoQ10. Despite supplementation, CF patients are often deficient in these compounds, resulting in increased oxidative stress, which may contribute to adverse health effects. Papas et al (2008) conducted a pilot study to evaluate the safety of a novel micellar formulation (CF-1) of fat-soluble nutrients and antioxidants, which included CoQ10 (30 mg/10 mL), alpha-tocopherol (200 IU), beta-carotene (30 mg), gamma tocopherol (94 mg), vitamin D_3 (400 IU) and other tocopherols (31 mg). Ten CF subjects aged 8–45 years were given 10 mL of the formulation orally daily for 56 days after a 21-day washout period in which subjects stopped supplemental vitamin use, except for a standard multivitamin. No serious adverse effects, laboratory abnormalities or elevated nutrient levels (above normal) were identified for the treatment. Supplementation with CF-1 significantly increased CoQ10, beta-carotene and gamma tocopherol from baseline in all subjects and improvements in antioxidant plasma levels were associated with reductions in airway inflammation in CF patients.

Periodontal disease

Dry mouth is associated with ageing and may also contribute to diseases such as periodontal disease. CoQ10 is used both topically and internally for the treatment of chronic periodontal disease. Topical application has been shown to improve adult periodontitis (Hanioka et al 1994) and a small open study has shown that oral CoQ10 supplementation can produce dramatic results within 5–7 days, making location of baseline biopsy sites impossible (Wilkinson et al 1975).

Supplemental CoQ10 (100 mg ubiquinol or ubiquinone) taken for 1 month was found to significantly increase salivary secretion and salivary CoQ10 concentration in patients with dry mouth compared to placebo. The authors suggest the effects were due to improving the decreased energy production and reducing oxidative stress in salivary glands (Ryo et al 2011).

Parkinson's disease

Parkinson's disease (PD) is a neurodegenerative disorder characterised by progressive loss of dopaminergic neurons within the substantia nigra pars compacta. The pathogenesis of PD remains obscure, but there is increasing experimental and clinical data that points to a defect of the mitochondrial respiratory chain, oxidative damage and inflammation as major pathogenetic factors in PD, inducing degeneration of nigrostriatal dopaminergic neurons (Beal 2003, Ebadi et al 2001, Gotz et al 2000, Storch 2007).

It has been theorised that restoration of mitochondrial respiration and reduction of oxidative stress by CoQ10 could induce neuroprotective effects against the dopaminergic cell death in PD and could also enhance dopaminergic dysfunction (Storch 2007). As a result, CoQ10 might exert both neuroprotective and symptomatic effects in PD. Current data from controlled clinical trials are not sufficient to answer conclusively whether CoQ10 is neuroprotective in PD or has significant symptomatic effects, as results are inconsistent. The data are presented here.

A number of preclinical studies using in vitro and in vivo models of PD have demonstrated that CoQ10 can protect the nigrostriatal dopaminergic system, and levels of CoQ10 have been reported to be decreased in blood and platelet mitochondria from subjects with PD (Shults 2005, Mischley et al 2012), as well as reduced brain CoQ10 status (Hargreaves 2008).

As a result, several clinical intervention studies have been conducted to determine whether CoQ10 supplementation can provide benefits for people with PD. An early randomised, placebo-controlled, double-blind study compared three different doses of CoQ10 (300 mg, 600 mg or 1200 mg) with placebo in 80 subjects with early PD. After 9 months of treatment, subjects taking 1200 mg CoQ10 daily experienced significant improvements in disability compared with the placebo group. CoQ10 was also well tolerated at the dosages studied (Shults et al 2002). In 2003, results were published of a double-blind, placebo-controlled study, which showed that even a relatively low dose of CoQ10 (360 mg/day) taken for a short period (4 weeks) produced a significant mild benefit on PD symptoms and significantly improved visual function compared with placebo (Muller et al 2003).

The safety and tolerability of high-dose CoQ10 in subjects with PD was investigated in an open study of 17 patients (Shults et al 2004). The study used an escalating dosage of 1200, 1800, 2400 and 3000 mg/day administered together with vitamin E (alpha-tocopherol) 1200 IU/day and failed to identify any serious adverse effects with CoQ10 administration. It also identified that plasma CoQ10 levels reached a plateau at 2400 mg/day, suggesting that higher treatment doses are not required.

In 2007, a multicentre, randomised, double-blind, placebo-controlled, stratified, parallel-group, single-dose trial was conducted which used nanoparticular CoQ10, as it has been shown to provide symptomatic effects in patients with mid-stage PD without motor fluctuations (Storch et al 2007). The study of 131 volunteers with PD without motor fluctuations and a stable anti-parkinsonian treatment were randomly assigned to receive placebo or nanoparticular CoQ10

(100 mg three times a day) for a treatment period of 3 months. This form and dose of CoQ10 led to plasma levels similar to 1200 mg/day of standard formulations; however, no significant changes to the Unified Parkinson's Disease Rating Scale (UPDRS) were observed with CoQ10 after stratification for L-dopa dosing in this group of people with mid-stage PD.

More recently, a 2011 Cochrane review examined the efficacy and safety of coenzyme Q10 in patients with early and midstage Parkinson's disease. Four randomised, double-blind, placebo-controlled trials (Muller 2003, Shults 2002, Storch 2007, The NINDS NET-PD 2007) involved a total of 452 patients, with CoQ10 doses ranging from 300 mg to 2400 mg/day. Positive effects were identified in activities of daily life in Unified Parkinson's Disease Rating Scale and the Schwab and England scale for Q10 at 1200 mg/day for 16 months versus placebo. There were no differences in the withdrawals from adverse effects between treatment and placebo groups, although there was a mildly increased relative risk ratio for pharyngitis and diarrhoea (Liu et al 2011).

A large phase III trial comparing placebo and 1200 and 2400 mg of CoQ10 daily was recently published that found no effect for oral CoQ10 supplementation on slowing the progression of disease (Beal et al 2014).

Another form of parkinsonism is progressive supranuclear palsy. A short-term double-blind, randomised, placebo-controlled, phase II trial was conducted in patients with progressive supranuclear palsy, a disease which causes down-gaze palsy with progressive rigidity and imbalance. Impairment of mitochondrial ETC complex I activity is thought to play a role in its pathogenesis suggesting a possible role for CoQ10 in its treatment. Twenty-one patients received either CoQ10 at a dose of 5 mg/kg/day or placebo. After 6 weeks, magnetic resonance spectroscopy showed a statistically significant increase in oxidative phosphorylation in the occipital cortex with an increase in the ratio of high-energy to low-energy phosphates, and an increase in motor and neuropsychological dysfunction measured by the PSP rating scale and the Frontal Assessment Battery (Stamelou et al 2008).

Alzheimer's dementia

Similar to Parkinson's disease, mitochondrial dysfunction and oxidative damage appear to play a role in the pathogenesis of Alzheimer's dementia and, therefore, CoQ10 supplementation has been investigated as a possible treatment. Currently, evidence is limited to test tube and animal studies and is far from definitive.

CoQ10 was shown to inhibit beta-amyloid formation in vitro (Ono et al 2005) and in an animal model of AD (Dumont et al 2011, Choi et al 2012, Yang et al 2008, Yang et al 2010), activate the phosphatidylinositol 3-kinase pathway involved in neuronal cell survival and adult neurogenesis (Choi et al 2013), and protect against brain mitochondrial dysfunction induced by a neurotoxic beta-peptide in a study using brain mitochondria isolated from diabetic rats (Moreira et al 2005). McDonald et al (2005) conducted two studies with test animals and found that supplemental CoQ10 (123 mg/kg/day) taken with alpha-tocopherol acetate (200 mg/kg/day) improved age-related learning deficits; however, supplementation of CoQ10 alone at this dose, or higher doses of 250 or 500 mg/kg/day, failed to produce comparable effects.

Haemodialysis

Increased oxidative stress is associated with various complications in haemodialysis (HD) patients (Sakata et al 2008). Due to its antioxidant activity, CoQ10 was administered for 6 months to 36 HD patients. Treatment was found to partially reduce oxidative stress as measured by a decrease of oxygen radical absorbing capacity (ORAC) and Trolox equivalent antioxidant capacity (TEAC).

Migraine

There is now good supportive evidence to recommend the use of CoQ10 supplementation as a preventive treatment for migraine headache. Due to its relatively good safety profile when compared to pharmaceutical migraine treatments, a 3-month trial can be considered for prevention.

Research began over a decade ago to determine whether CoQ10 could affect the course of migraine attacks and reduce their frequency, largely because migraine was starting to become known as a disorder with an underlying mitochondrial dysfunction component.

An open-labelled trial investigated the effects of oral CoQ10 supplementation (150 mg/day) over 3 months in 32 volunteers with a history of episodic migraine with or without aura. CoQ10 significantly reduced both the frequency of attacks and the number of days with migraine after 3 months' treatment (Rozen et al 2002). In 2005, Sandor et al investigated the effects of CoQ10 (300 mg/day) taken over 3 months in 42 migraine subjects in a double-blind, randomised, placebo-controlled study; 47.6% of CoQ10-treated patients responded to treatment compared with 14.4% for placebo, experiencing a (50% or less) reduction in migraine frequency (number needed to treat, 3). Active treatment was superior to placebo for reducing attack frequency, headache days and days with nausea in the third treatment month and was well tolerated.

In 2007, Hershey et al assessed 1550 paediatric patients (mean age 13.3 ± 3.5, range 3–22 yrs) attending a tertiary care centre with frequent headaches for CoQ10 deficiency (Hershey et al 2007). Of these patients, 32.9% were below the reference range. Patients with low CoQ10 were recommended to start 1 to 3 mg/kg/day of CoQ10 in liquid gel capsule formulation as part of their multidisciplinary treatment plan. Those patients who returned for follow-up (mean, 97 days) demonstrated significantly increased total CoQ10 levels and significant improvements for headache disability and headache frequency (19.2 ± 10.0 to 12.5 ± 10.8). In a subsequent, placebo-controlled, double-blind, crossover, add-on trial, 120 paediatric and adolescent migraine patients were given either CoQ10 (100 mg/day) or placebo for 32 weeks. Migraine frequency, severity and duration improved in both groups by the end of the study; however, the treatment group had significant early improvement in frequency in the first 4 weeks (Slater et al 2011).

In 2012, the Canadian Headache Society made a strong recommendation for the use of CoQ10 supplementation as a preventive treatment in migraine (Pringsheim et al 2012). This was based on a comprehensive search strategy to identify randomised, double-blind, controlled trials of drug treatments for migraine prophylaxis and relevant Cochrane reviews and then grading the evidence according to criteria developed by the US Preventive Services Task Force.

Fibromyalgia

Fibromyalgia presents with a range of symptoms including chronic pain, allodynia, fatigue, joint stiffness and migraines. Oxidative stress and mitochondrial dysfunction are thought to play a role in its pathogenesis, with some academics suggesting CoQ10 deficiency as part of the pathophysiology of fibromyalgia (Alcocer-Gomez et al 2013). This theory has gained momentum as a result of the observation that, compared to healthy controls, several studies have identified lower levels of CoQ10 in fibromyalgia patients (Cordero et al 2009, 2012, Miyamae et al 2013), as well as increased levels of oxidative stress and decreased ATP production (Cordero et al 2009, 2012). Cordero et al identified a significant correlation between high oxidative stress (measured as low CoQ10 or catalase levels, and high levels of lipid peroxidation) with headache symptoms experienced by fibromyalgia subjects.

Futhermore, in fibromyalgia subjects given CoQ10 (300 mg/day for 12 weeks), the level of oxidative stress decreased to similar levels to the controls, and the levels of CoQ10, ATP and catalase significantly increased, although they were still lower than controls. Supplementation also improved clinical symptoms and headaches measured by tender points, Fibromyalgia Impact Questionnaire, visual analogue scales and the Headache Impact Test scores (Cordero et al 2012). A small case series involving four patients who met the American College of Rheumatology (ACR) Diagnostic Criteria of 1990 and 2010 for FM found that all were CoQ10-deficient. Treatment with CoQ10 resulted in an improvement in clinical symptoms as assessed by three different methods (Alcocer-Gomez et al 2013).

In a study involving young patients with fibromyalgia (14.7 ± 2.9 years), CoQ10 100 mg/day for 12 weeks similarly increased CoQ10 levels and decreased the ratio of ubiquinone-10 to total coenzyme Q10. Cholesterol metabolism was also improved with treatment (decreased free cholesterol and cholesterol esters) as well as fatigue (measured by the Chalder Fatigue Scale); however, subjective pain intensity (assessed by VAS) and health-related QOL did not change (Miyamae et al 2013).

Further investigation with doubled-blind, placebo-controlled clinical trials is warranted.

Male infertility

Several studies have recently examined the role of coenzyme Q10 in the treatment of male infertility, with most reporting positive results. Potentially beneficial mechanisms include its role as an antioxidant, improving mitochondrial activity and energy production, all of which influence spermatogenesis and motility.

The level of seminal plasma coenzyme Q10 and oxidative stress was examined in patients with different types of male infertility in a case-controlled study. Compared to the age-matched healthy controls, those with infertility had lower seminal levels of CoQ10 and lower CoQ10 was associated with higher levels of oxidative stress (measured by malondialdehyde (MDA) (Abdul-Rasheed et al 2010). A randomised, placebo-controlled study examined the seminal levels and antioxidants effects of CoQ10 in infertile men with idiopathic oligoasthenoteratozoospermia. After 3 months of 200 mg CoQ10 supplementation daily, the levels of CoQ10 increased in the treatment group, as did the activity of seminal antioxidants catalase and superoxide dismutase while the marker of oxidative stress, seminal plasma 8-isoprostane, decreased. There was significant correlation found between the reduction in seminal oxidative stress and improved sperm morphology (Nadjarzadeh et al 2013).

Several clinical trials have suggested treatment with CoQ10 improves sperm parameters and may increase the pregnancy rate in those with male infertility. In a placebo-controlled, double-blind, randomised trial, men with idiopathic infertility receiving 200 mg/day of CoQ10 for 6 months had significantly increased seminal plasma and sperm levels of CoQ10 and increased sperm motility. The greatest response was seen in those with the lowest baseline CoQ10 and sperm motility levels (Balercia et al 2009). Similarly, in a study by Safarinejad et al (2009) involving 212 infertile men (aged 21–42 years) with idiopathic oligoasthenoteratospermia, 300 mg/day of CoQ10 for 26 weeks led to a significant increase in sperm density (increase of 21.5% versus 1.3%) and motility (increase of 30.7% versus 2%), as well as a decrease in serum follicle-stimulating hormone (suggesting better spermatogenesis) and increase in inhibin B (reflecting better Sertoli's cell function); however, there was no difference in the pregnancy rate compared to placebo. Interestingly, at the 56 week follow-up (30 weeks post-treatment) sperm count, motility and morphology were still higher in the CoQ10 treated group compared to placebo, although it was not statistically significant. More recently, Safarinejad has conducted two additional studies. Using the same study design as above, 200 mg ubiquinol/day was given to 114 infertile men with idiopathic oligoasthenoteratozoospermia for 26 weeks. Compared to the placebo group (n = 114), active treatment improved several sperm parameters including sperm density, sperm motility (35.8% versus 25.4%) and sperm morphology (17.6% versus 14.8%). As in the 2009 study, serum follicle-stimulating hormone decreased while inhibin B levels increased. Sperm parameters had decreased again at the 12-week follow-up post-treatment; however, there was still a statistically significant improvement from the placebo group for sperm density and motility (Safarinejad et al 2012b). An open label prospective study was conducted with 287 infertile men with idiopathic oligoasthenoteratospermia who had previously undergone at least two failed infertility treatments. They received CoQ10 300 mg (Nutri Q10) twice daily for 12 months. Compared to baseline, blood and seminal CoQ10 levels increased at 3 months and remained steady for the remainder of the study. Sperm parameters significantly increased concentration by 114%, progressive motility by 105%, and morphology by 79%. There was also a pregnancy rate of 34.1% achieved within a 8.4 ± 4.7 months (Safarinejad 2012).

In contrast, a double-blind, placebo-controlled clinical trial (n = 47) found 200 mg CoQ10 for 3 months did not significantly change sperm concentration, motility and morphology in infertile men with idiopathic oligoasthenoteratozoospermia, although total antioxidant capacity of seminal plasma significantly increased (Nadjarzadeh et al 2011). As this study was shorter than those reporting positive results, the shorter treatment timeframe may have been a factor.

OTHER USES

Cancer

Currently, controlled studies are not available to determine the clinical effectiveness of CoQ10 in cancer; however, there have been several case reports of CoQ10 (390 mg/day) successfully reducing metastases or eliminating tumours entirely (Lockwood et al 1994, 1995). This supports numerous recent in vitro and animal studies that also suggest a protective role for CoQ10 against cancer development (Bahar et al 2010, Fouad et al 2012, Kim & Park 2010, Mizushina et al 2008). An in vivo study found that CoQ10 enhances the effects of immunochemotherapy (Kokawa et al 1983).

Studies investigating the plasma level of CoQ10 in those with cancer have reported variable correlation. In postmenopausal women, higher CoQ10 levels were found to be associated with an increased risk of breast cancer (Chai et al 2010), while a moderate amount was associated with reduced risk of prostate cancer in men (Chai et al 2011). Furthermore, compared to placebo, supplementation with CoQ10 for 12 weeks significantly lowered PSA levels from baseline in men with PSA levels below 2.5 ng/L, and there was a strong correlation between serum CoQ10 and PSA (Safarinejad et al 2012a).

Reducing cardiotoxic effects of anthracyclines

There is some evidence that CoQ10 supplementation protects the mitochondria of the heart from anthracycline-induced damage. A systematic review of six studies (three randomised), in which patients in five of the six studies received anthracyclines, concluded that CoQ10 provides some protection against cardiotoxicity or liver toxicity during cancer treatment; however, weaknesses in design and reporting made it difficult to reach a definitive conclusion (Roffe et al 2004). Despite the high level of heterogeneity, it appeared that CoQ10 had a stabilising effect on the heart. Importantly, CoQ10 was not shown to interfere with standard treatments in the clinical trials reviewed and no adverse effects were reported in any single study for CoQ10 administration.

Sample sizes in the studies ranged from 19 to 88 patients and one study included children. The methods researchers used to measure patient tolerance to anthracyclines and other cancer treatments were heart function and toxicity in five studies, and hair loss and liver enzymes in one study. The dose of CoQ10 investigated in the trials ranged from 90 mg/day to 240 mg/day. The lack of adverse effect by CoQ10 on cytotoxicity of doxorubicin was also supported by a recent in vitro study using breast cancer cell lines treated with doxorubicin at a range of CoQ10 concentrations (Greenlee et al 2012).

Reducing side effects of tamoxifen

Tamoxifen is a common treatment used by those with breast cancer and is associated with some adverse effects, such as increasing oxidative stress and causing hypertriglyceridaemia. A study examining the effects of Coenzyme Q10 (100 mg) supplementation in addition to tamoxifen in breast cancer patients found it counteracted the effects of tamoxifen on raising triglycerides and increasing angiogenesis (increasing potential tumour metastasis) (Sachdanandam 2008). Similarly, in a study examining postmenopausal women with breast cancer treated with tamoxifen, the addition of CoQ10 combined with niacin and riboflavin for 90 days reduced oxidative stress and improved antioxidant status.

Several animal and in vitro studies have suggested a protective effect of CoQ10 from chemotherapy-induced organ toxicity (Celebi et al 2013, da Silva Machado et al 2013, El-Sheikh et al 2012, Sato et al 2013).

Mitochondrial myopathy

An open multicentre study involving 44 volunteers with mitochondrial myopathies showed that treatment with CoQ10 (2 mg/kg daily) over 6 months decreased post-exercise lactate levels by at least 25% in 16 patients. Of those responding, a further 3 months' treatment with either CoQ10 or placebo produced no significant differences (Bresolin et al 1990). A more recent randomised, double-blind, crossover trial involving 30 patients with mitochondrial disease (mostly due to MELAS, chronic external progressive encephalopathy and mitochondrial DNA deletions) tested a high dose of oral CoQ10 (1200 mg/day). After 60 days of treatment, plasma CoQ10 levels were increased 5.5-fold, the post-exercise rise in lactate was reduced and the cycle aerobic capacity (measured by oxygen consumption in lean body mass) was increased, There was no effect on other measurements including grip strength, or resting lactate production during a non-ischaemic isometric forearm exercise protocol (Glover et al 2010).

Age-related macular degeneration (in combination)

Mitochondrial dysfunction is likely to play a role in the pathophysiology of age-related macular degeneration (Littarru & Tiano 2005). The level of CoQ10 in the retina has been shown to decrease with age by approximately 40% and the reduction in antioxidant protection and ATP synthesis may contribute to age-associated eye diseases, such as macular degeneration (Qu et al 2009). Further potential benefits of CoQ10 for eye health include in vitro evidence of its ability to protect lens epithelial cells from light-induced damage (Kernt et al 2010) and retinal cells from radiation-induced apoptosis (Lulli et al 2012a, Lulli et al 2012b).

As a result, researchers are investigating therapeutic agents, such as CoQ10, which affect mitochondrial function.

Metabolic therapy consisting of a combination of omega-3 fatty acids, CoQ10 and acetyl-L-carnitine may have potential benefits as a treatment for early age-related macular degeneration by improving mitochondrial dysfunction, specifically improving lipid metabolism and ATP production in the retinal pigment epithelium, improving photoreceptor turnover and reducing generation of reactive oxygen species (Feher et al 2007). According to a pilot study and a randomised, placebo-controlled, double-blind clinical trial, both central visual field and visual acuity slightly improved after 3–6 months of treatment with the metabolic combination; however, the difference was not statistically significant when compared to the baseline or to controls. Treatment produced an improvement in fundus alterations as the drusen-covered area decreased significantly compared to baseline readings or controls, and was most marked in the less-affected eyes. Interestingly, a prospective case study on long-term treatment confirmed these observations. Visual function remained stable and, generally, drusen regression continued for years and for some intermediate and advanced cases, significant regression of drusen was found with treatment.

Friedreich's ataxia

Decreased mitochondrial respiratory chain function and increased oxidative stress and iron accumulation play significant roles in the disease mechanism of Friedreich's ataxia (FRDA), raising the possibility that energy enhancement and antioxidant therapies may be an effective treatment (Cooper & Schapira 2007). Therapeutic avenues for patients with FRDA are beginning to be explored; in particular, targeting antioxidant protection, enhancement of mitochondrial oxidative phosphorylation and iron chelation. The use of quinone therapy (ubiquinone and idebenone) has been the most extensively studied to date, with clear benefits demonstrated using evaluations of both disease biomarkers and clinical symptoms (Mariotti et al 2003).

A 4-year follow-up on 10 Friedreich's ataxia patients treated with CoQ10 (400 mg/day) and vitamin E (2100 IU/day) showed a substantial improvement in cardiac and skeletal muscle bioenergetics and heart function, which was maintained over the test period and some clinical feature of disease (Hart et al 2005). Comparison with cross-sectional data from 77 patients with FRDA indicated the changes in total International Cooperative Ataxia Rating Scale and kinetic scores over the trial period were better than predicted for seven patients, but the posture and gait and hand dexterity scores progressed as predicted.

In a more recent pilot study involving 50 subjects, the potential for high dose CoQ10 and vitamin E to modify the clinical progression of Friedreich's ataxia was investigated. Patients were randomly assigned to either high- or low-dose CoQ10 and vitamin E. At baseline, both groups had low serum CoQ10 and vitamin E, which significantly increased in both groups over the course of the 2-year trial. There was improvement in the International Cooperative Ataxia Rating Scale (ICARS) in 49% of patients when compared to cross-sectional data, but the response did not differ between the high- and low-dose groups. Serum CoQ10 levels were the best predictor of positive clinical response to treatment with CoQ10/vitamin E (Cooper et al 2008).

Tinnitus and hearing loss

CoQ10 has been considered in hearing impairment due to its ability to act as an antioxidant and inhibit oxidative stress in the inner ear and reduce damage induced by noise (Hirose et al 2008).

In patients with a low plasma CoQ10 concentration, CoQ10 supply may decrease the tinnitus expression in chronic tinnitus aurium according to a 16-week prospective, non-randomised clinical trial (*n* = 20) (Khan et al 2007). CoQ10 was tested in this population because of its antioxidant activity.

IN COMBINATION

A controlled prospective study (*n* = 120) examined the effects of CoQ10 in addition to steroid treatment in patients diagnosed with sudden sensorineural hearing loss. The CoQ10 was administered at a dose of 200 mg three times daily for 5 days and then 100 mg three times daily for another 10 days. After 3 months, the CoQ10 group had a non-statistically-significant additional benefit in hearing improvement compared to the steroid treatment alone (78.3% compared to 71.7%), but had a significantly better improvement in speech discrimination (Ahn et al 2010). This was supported by a more recent study in patients with presbycusis, a disorder with progressive bilateral symmetrical age-related sensorineural hearing loss. Patients (*n* = 60) were given either a water-soluble form of CoQ10 (Q-TER, 160 mg), vitamin E (50 mg) or placebo for 30 days. All patients receiving the CoQ10 had improvement in hearing, which was significant at most frequencies compared to the vitamin E group. No differences were found in those receiving the placebo treatment (Salami et al 2010).

Myelodysplastic syndromes

The myelodysplastic syndromes (MDS) are a collection of haematopoietic disorders with varying degrees of mono- to trilineage cytopenias and bone marrow dysplasia. In recent years, much progress has been made in the treatment of MDS and there are now several therapeutic compounds used with varying levels of success; however, side effects make them unattractive for patients (Galili et al 2007).

Galili et al tested CoQ10 supplementation in MDS patients with low- to intermediate-2-risk disease. A variety of responses were observed in 7 of 29 patients. Sequencing mitochondrial DNA (mtDNA) from pretreatment bone marrows showed multiple mutations, some resulting in amino acid changes, in 3 in 5 non-responders, 1 in 4 responders and in two control samples. Based on these observations, it appears that CoQ10 may be of clinical benefit in a subset of MDS patients, but responders cannot be easily preselected on the basis of either the conventional clinical and pathological characteristics or mtDNA mutations.

Huntington's chorea

A randomised, double-blind study involving 347 patients with early Huntington's chorea showed that a dose of CoQ10 (600 mg/day) taken over 30 months produced a trend towards slow decline as well as beneficial trends in some secondary measures; however, changes were not significant at this dosage level (Huntington's Study Group, 2001).

In a more recent 20-week open-label study by the same group, the effect on blood levels and safety of high dose CoQ10 supplementation was tested. Subjects (8 healthy and 20 with Huntington's disease) were supplemented with 1200 mg CoQ10 for 4 weeks, with the dose increasing by 1200 mg every 4 weeks to the maximum of 3600 mg/day. Blood levels of CoQ10 increased steadily from baseline 1.26 ± 1.27 mcg/mL to a peak of 7.49 ± 4.09 mcg/mL at a dose of 3600 mg at 12 weeks, and then declined again to 6.78 ± 3.36 mcg/mL at the same dose at week 20. The most common adverse effects reported were gastrointestinal symptoms. Most symptoms developed at the initial dosage of 1200 mg/day, with no new symptoms occurring at the 2400 mg dose although two new cases occurred at the 3600 mg dose. It is possible that a smaller initial dose may reduce initial symptoms. The authors suggest that 2400 mg provides the best balance between increased blood levels and tolerability (Huntington Study Group, 2010).

Preeclampsia

Teran et al (2009) conducted a randomised, double-blind, placebo-controlled trial involving 235 pregnant women at increased risk of preeclampsia. Women who received 100 mg of CoQ10 twice daily from week 20 until delivery had significantly reduced risk of developing preeclampsia compared to the placebo group (14.4% versus 25.6%). Possible mechanisms of action include reducing oxidative stress and improving endothelial function, but further research is required to clarify the outcomes.

Diabetes

In 2009, the observation was made that plasma CoQ10 was significantly lower in a cohort of 28 people with type 2 diabetes compared to healthy controls and there was a negative correlation between plasma CoQ10 and glycosylated haemoglobin (El-ghoroury et al 2009). Soon after, a small open-label study found that volunteers with type 2 diabetes given 200 mg ubiquinol daily for 12 weeks, in addition to their existing hypoglycaemic medication, improved their glycosylated haemoglobin readings. No significant differences were seen for blood pressure, lipid profile, oxidative stress or inflammatory markers. Furthermore, five healthy volunteers who received 200 mg ubiquinol daily for 4 weeks had improved insulinogenic index and ratio of proinsulin to insulin, suggesting that CoQ10 may improve glucose control via increasing insulin secretion (Mezawa et al 2012). In 2013, a randomised, double-blind, placebo-controlled study of 64 people with type 2 diabetes, CoQ10 (200 mg/day) significantly reduced total cholesterol, LDL-cholesterol and improved glycaemic control compared to placebo (Kolahdouz et al 2013). Treatment was taken for 12 weeks, resulting in serum HbA_{1C} concentration decreasing in the CoQ10-treated group (8 ± 2.28% vs 8.61 ± 2.47%) with no significant changes seen for placebo.

Peyronie's disease

Peyronie's disease is an acquired idiopathic localised fibrosis of the penis which causes the penis to curve and associated sexual dysfunction. Safarinejad et al investigated the effects of CoQ10 supplementation in the treatment of early chronic Peyronie's disease in 186 patients. Treatment with CoQ10 300 mg/day for 24 weeks significantly reduced plaque size and penile curvature, improved erectile function (International Index of Erectile Function increasing by 117.1 versus 8.6%) and slowed disease progression compared to the placebo group (Safarinejad 2010).

DOSAGE RANGE

According to clinical studies

- Generally 100–150 mg/day has been used for conditions such as congestive cardiac failure (Mortensen et al 1990), hypertension, neurological disease, performance enhancement, periodontal disease (Wilkinson et al 1975).
- As preparation for cardiac surgery: 100–300 mg/day for 2 weeks before surgery followed by 100–225 mg/day for 1 month after surgery has been used (Judy et al 1993, Rosenfeldt et al 2002, 2005, Braun et al 2013).
- Adjunct to chemotherapy (anthracyclines) 90–240 mg/day, but evidence is not definitive.

- Angina pectoris: 60–600 mg daily.
- Chronic obstructive pulmonary disease: 50–90 mg daily.
- Cholesterol lowering: 200 mg daily (in type 2 diabetes).
- Congestive heart failure: 60–200 mg/day or 2 mg/kg/day for reducing mortality.
- Dry mouth: 100 mg/day.
- Fibromyalgia: 100–300 mg/day.
- Huntington's chorea: 600 mg daily.
- Hypertension: 100–120 mg/day.
- Male infertility: 200–600 mg/day.
- Migraine: 150–300 mg daily.
- Parkinson's disease: 1200 mg/day.
- Peyronie disease: 300 mg/day.
- Type 2 diabetes: 200 mg daily ubiquinol for improved glycosylated Hb levels.
- Sports supplement: 60–300 mg/day — inconsistent results.
- Statin-associated myalgia: 60–200 mg/day — inconsistent results.

ADVERSE REACTIONS

CoQ10 appears relatively safe and non-toxic and is extremely well tolerated. Dizziness, nausea, epigastric discomfort, anorexia, diarrhoea, photophobia, irritability and skin rash occur in less than 1% of patients. This tends to occur with higher doses (> 200 mg/day).

SIGNIFICANT INTERACTIONS

When controlled studies are not available, interactions are based on evidence of pharmacological activity, case reports and other evidence and are largely theoretical.

Beta-adrenergic antagonists

Induces CoQ10 depletion — beneficial interaction with co-administration (Stargrove et al 2008).

Doxorubicin

Tests in animal models have demonstrated that CoQ10 protects against doxorubicin cardiotoxicity (Combs et al 1977, Folkers et al 1978) and clinical studies provide some support for the use of oral CoQ10, and indicate that adjunctive treatment provides some protection against cardiotoxicity or liver toxicity during cancer therapy; however, further studies are required to prove this association conclusively (Roffe et al 2004). Furthermore, in vivo results indicate that CoQ10 has no significant effect on the pharmacokinetics of doxorubicin and the formation of the cytotoxic metabolite, doxorubicinol (Combs et al 1977, Zhou & Chowbay 2002) — potentially beneficial interaction with co-administration under professional supervision.

Phenothiazines

CoQ10 reduces adverse effect this drug class has on CoQ10-related enzymes, NADH oxidase and succinoxidase — beneficial interaction with co-administration (Stargrove et al 2008).

Statin drugs

Currently, it is still not clear whether CoQ10 supplementation should be considered a necessary adjunct to all patients taking statin drugs; however, there are no known risks to this supplement and there is some anecdotal and clinical trial evidence of its effectiveness (Marcoff & Thompson 2007). Consequently, CoQ10 can be tested in patients requiring statin treatment, who develop statin myalgia, headache, fatigue or malaise as statin-induced side effects. It may also prove useful for patients considered at risk of deficiency, in particular, patients with a family history of heart failure, elevated cholesterol levels and who are older than 65 years and taking statin drugs long term (Levy & Kohlhaas 2006) — possible beneficial interaction with co-administration, particularly with the antioxidant effects of superoxide dismutase (Okello et al 2009).

Sulfonylureas

CoQ10 reduces adverse effect this drug class has on CoQ10-related enzymes, NADH oxidase and low CoQ10 levels have been observed in people with diabetes — beneficial interaction with co-administration (Stargrove et al 2008).

Tamoxifen

Concomitant use of CoQ10 reduced triglyceride levels in one study — potentially beneficial.

Theophylline

An animal study suggests significant changes to the pharmacokinetics of theophylline, such as time to peak concentration, half-life and distribution following treatment with CoQ10. While there is very limited research, there may be possible interactions (Baskaran et al 2008).

Timolol

Eye drops — oral CoQ10 reduced the vascular side effects of timolol without affecting eye pressure (Takahashi 1989) — beneficial interaction with co administration.

Tricyclic antidepressants

CoQ10 reduces adverse effect this drug class has on CoQ10-related enzymes, NADH-oxidase and succinoxidase — beneficial interaction with co-administration (Stargrove et al 2008).

Warfarin

There are three case reports suggesting that CoQ10 may decrease the international normalised ratio (INR) in patients previously stabilised on anticoagulants (Spigset 1994b). However, a double-blind crossover study involving 24 outpatients on stable long-term warfarin found that oral CoQ10 (100 mg) daily had no significant effect on INR or warfarin levels (Engelson et al 2003). One observational study suggested an increase in minor bleeding events but not INR (Shalansky et al 2007). Observe patients using high CoQ10 doses and taking warfarin.

Vitamin E

Reconstitutes oxidised vitamin E to its unoxidised form — beneficial interaction with co-administration.

CONTRAINDICATIONS AND PRECAUTIONS

Insufficient reliable evidence — unknown.

C

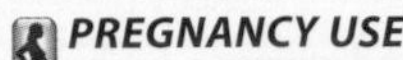

PREGNANCY USE

Since this is an endogenously produced substance that has been tested in preeclampsia without serious negative outcomes, it is likely to be safe in this population during the final trimester.

Practice points/Patient counselling

- CoQ10 is a safe antioxidant vitamin used in supplement form for a wide range of diseases.
- Meta-analyses provide support for its use in congestive heart failure and hypertension.
- Clinical evidence further supports the use of presurgical supplementation in cardiac surgery, as it improves recovery and has cardioprotective activity.
- Clinical evidence supports its use in the prevention of migraine headache.
- There is also some clinical evidence suggesting a role in fibromyalgia, dry mouth, type 2 diabetes, Huntington's chorea, mitochondrial myopathy, COPD, periodontal disease, haemodialysis, Friedreich's ataxia, tinnitus, age-related macular degeneration, cystic fibrosis, male infertility and reducing cardiotoxicity and liver toxicity associated with anthracyclines, although further research is required.
- Whether CoQ10 may slow the progression of PD is unclear.
- Several common medicines, such as statins, have been found to reduce serum CoQ10 status. It is still unclear whether CoQ10 should be considered a necessary adjunct to statin drugs; however, there are no known risks to this supplement and there is some anecdotal and clinical trial evidence of its effectiveness. In particular, it may be useful in patients who develop statin myalgia, headache, fatigue or malaise and those considered at risk of deficiency, such as people of advanced age and vegetarians..

PATIENTS' FAQs

What will this vitamin do for me?

CoQ10 is an antioxidant vitamin used in every cell of the body. It is necessary for healthy function and can improve heart function, lower blood pressure and reduce angina. Taken before cardiac surgery, it has been shown to reduce complications and hasten recovery in some studies. It may also provide benefits in preventing migraine headache, Huntington's chorea, mitochondrial myopathy, COPD, type 2 diabetes, chronic obstructive airways disease, periodontal disease, haemodialysis, Friedreich's ataxia, tinnitus, age-related macular degeneration, cystic fibrosis and reducing cardiotoxicity and liver toxicity associated with anthracyclines, although further research is required to definitively confirm effect. Whether it is helpful in Parkinson's disease is not clear. People taking statin drugs long term and experiencing mild side effects could safely take a 3-month trial of CoQ10 and see whether it helps them.

When will it start to work?

This depends on the indication. For heart conditions and to reduce migraine, 10–12 weeks may be required. To delay the progression of PD, one study found that effects started after 9 months' use.

Are there any safety issues?

Medical monitoring is required in patients taking warfarin and starting high-dose CoQ10 supplements; however, even high-dose supplements are well tolerated and considered safe.

REFERENCES

Abdul-Rasheed OF et al. Coenzyme Q10 and oxidative stress markers in seminal plasma of Iraqi patients with male infertility. Saudi Med J 31.5 (2010): 501–506.

Aberg F et al. Gemfibrozil-induced decrease in serum ubiquinone and alpha- and gamma-tocopherol levels in men with combined hyperlipidaemia. Eur J Clin Invest 28.3 (1998): 235–242.

Aboul-Fotouh S. Coenzyme Q10 displays antidepressant-like activity with reduction of hippocampal oxidative/nitrosative DNA damage in chronically stressed rats. Pharmacol Biochem Behav 104 (2013): 105–112.

Ahmadvand H et al. Effects of coenzyme Q10 on LDL oxidation in vitro. Acta Med Iran 51.1 (2013): 12–18.

Ahn JH et al. Coenzyme Q10 in combination with steroid therapy for treatment of sudden sensorineural hearing loss: a controlled prospective study. Clin Otolaryngol 35.6 (2010): 486–489.

Alcocer-Gomez E et al. Effect of coenzyme Q10 evaluated by 1990 and 2010 ACR Diagnostic Criteria for Fibromyalgia and SCL-90-R: Four case reports and literature review. Nutrition 29.11–12 (2013): 1422–1425.

Bahar M et al. Exogenous coenzyme Q10 modulates MMP-2 activity in MCF-7 cell line as a breast cancer cellular model. Nutr J 9 (2010): 62.

Balercia G et al. Coenzyme Q10 treatment in infertile men with idiopathic asthenozoospermia: a placebo-controlled, double-blind randomized trial. Fertil Steril 91.5 (2009): 1785–1792.

Bargossi AM et al. Exogenous CoQ10 preserves plasma ubiquinone levels in patients treated with 3-hydroxy-3-methylglutaryl coenzyme A reductase inhibitors. Int J Clin Lab Res 24.3 (1994a): 171–176.

Bargossi AM et al. Exogenous CoQ10 supplementation prevents plasma ubiquinone reduction induced by HMG-CoA reductase inhibitors. Mol Aspects Med 15 (Suppl) (1994b): S187–193.

Baskaran R et al. The effect of coenzyme Q10 on the pharmacokinetic parameters of theophylline. Arch Pharm Res 31(7) (2008): 938–944.

Beal MF et al. A randomized clinical trial of high-dosage coenzyme Q10 in early Parkinson disease: no evidence of benefit. JAMA Neurol 71.5 (2014): 543–552.

Beal MF. Mitochondria, oxidative damage, and inflammation in Parkinson's disease. Ann N Y Acad Sci 991 (2003): 120–131.

Berman M et al. Coenzyme Q10 in patients with end-stage heart failure awaiting cardiac transplantation: a randomized, placebo-controlled study. Clin Cardiol 27 (2004): 295–299.

Bessler, H., Bergman, M., et al. Coenzyme Q10 decreases TNF-alpha and IL-2 secretion by human peripheral blood mononuclear cells. J Nutr Sci Vitaminol (Tokyo) 1 (2010): 77–81.

Bianchi G et al. Oxidative stress and anti-oxidant metabolites in patients with hyperthyroidism: effect of treatment. Horm Metab Res 31.11 (1999): 620–624.

Bonetti A et al. Effect of ubidecarenone oral treatment on aerobic power in middle-aged trained subjects. J Sports Med Phys Fitness 40.1 (2000): 51–57.

Bookstaver DA et al. Effect of coenzyme Q10 supplementation on statin-induced myalgias. Am J Cardiol 110.4 (2012): 526–529.

Braun L et al. A wellness program for cardiac surgery improves clinical outcomes. Advances in Integrative Medicine 1.1 (2013): 32–37.

Bresolin N et al. Ubidecarenone in the treatment of mitochondrial myopathies: a multi-center double-blind trial. J Neurol Sci 100.1–2 (1990): 70–78.

Caso G et al. Effect of coenzyme q10 on myopathic symptoms in patients treated with statins. Am J Cardiol 99.10 (2007): 1409–1412.

Celebi N et al. Protective effect of coenzyme Q10 in paclitaxel-induced peripheral neuropathy in rats. Neurosciences (Riyadh) 18(2) (2013): 133–137.

Chai W et al. Plasma coenzyme Q10 levels and postmenopausal breast cancer risk: the multiethnic cohort study. Cancer Epidem Biomar 19.9 (2010): 2351–2356.

Chai W et al. Plasma coenzyme Q10 levels and prostate cancer risk: the multiethnic cohort study. Cancer Epidem Biomar 20.4 (2011): 708–710.

Chello M et al. Protection by coenzyme Q10 of tissue reperfusion injury during abdominal aortic cross-clamping. J Cardiovasc Surg (Torino) 37.3 (1996): 229–235.

Chen YF et al. Effectiveness of coenzyme Q10 on myocardial preservation during hypothermic cardioplegic arrest. J Thorac Cardiovasc Surg 107 (1994): 242–247.

Choi H et al. Coenzyme Q10 protects against amyloid beta-induced neuronal cell death by inhibiting oxidative stress and activating the P13K pathway. Neurotoxicology 33.1 (2012): 85–90.

Choi, H et al. Coenzyme Q10 restores amyloid beta-inhibited proliferation of neural stem cells by activating the PI3K Pathway. Stem Cells Dev. 1.22 (2013): 2112–2120.

Colquhoun DM et al. Effects of simvastatin on blood lipids, vitamin E, coenzyme Q10 levels and left ventricular function in humans. Eur J Clin Invest 35 (2005): 251–258.

Combs AB et al. Reduction by coenzyme Q10 of the acute toxicity of adriamycin in mice. Res Commun Chem Pathol Pharmacol 18.3 (1977): 565–568.

Cooke M et al. Effects of acute and 14-day coenzyme Q10 supplementation on exercise performance in both trained and untrained individuals. J Int Soc Sports Nutr 5 (2008): 8.

Cooper JM et al. Coenzyme Q10 and vitamin E deficiency in Friedreich's ataxia: predictor of efficacy of vitamin E and coenzyme Q10 therapy. Eur J Neurol 15.12 (2008): 1371–1379.

Cooper JM, Schapira AH. Friedreich's ataxia: coenzyme Q10 and vitamin E therapy. Mitochondrion 7 (Suppl) (2007): S127–S135.

Cordero MD et al. Oxidative stress correlates with headache symptoms in fibromyalgia: coenzyme Q(10) effect on clinical improvement. PLoS One 7(4) (2012): e35677.

da Silva Machado C et al. Coenzyme Q10 protects Pc12 cells from cisplatin-induced DNA damage and neurotoxicity. Neurotoxicology 36C (2013): 10–16.

Dai Y-L et al. Reversal of mitochondrial dysfunction by coenzyme Q10 supplement improves endothelial function in patients with ischaemic left ventricular systolic dysfunction: a randomized controlled trial. Atherosclerosis 216.2 (2011): 395–401.

Digiesi V et al. Coenzyme Q10 in essential hypertension. Mol Aspects Med 15 (Suppl) (1994): S257–S263.

Donnino MW et al. Coenzyme Q10 levels are low and may be associated with the inflammatory cascade in septic shock. Crit Care. Aug 9 15.4 (2011): R189.

Dumont, M et al. Coenzyme Q10 decreases amyloid pathology and improves behavior in a transgenic mouse model of Alzheimer's disease. J Alzheimer's Disease 27.1 (2011): 211–223.

Dupic, L et al. Coenzyme Q!0 deficiency in septic shock patients. Critical Care. 15 (2011):194.

Ebadi M et al. Ubiquinone (coenzyme q10) and mitochondria in oxidative stress of parkinson's disease. Biol Signals Recept 10.3–4 (2001): 224–253.

El-ghoroury EA et al. Malondialdehyde and coenzyme Q10 in platelets and serum in type 2 diabetes mellitus: correlation with glycemic control. Blood Coagul Fibrinolysis, 20.4 (2009): 248–251.

El-Sheikh AA et al. Effect of coenzyme-q10 on Doxorubicin-induced nephrotoxicity in rats. Adv Pharmacol Sci 2012 (2012): 981461.

Engelson J et al. Effect of coenzyme Q10 and Ginkgo biloba on warfarin dosage in patients on long-term warfarin treatment: a randomized, double-blind, placebo-controlled cross-over trial. Ugeskr Laeger 165.18 (2003): 1868–1871.

Ernster L, Dallner G. Biochemical, physiological and medical aspects of ubiquinone function. Biochim Biophys Acta 1271.1 (1995): 195–204.

Feher J et al. [Metabolic therapy for early treatment of age-related macular degeneration]. Orv Hetil 148.48 (2007): 2259–2268.

Folkers K et al. Activities of vitamin Q10 in animal models and a serious deficiency in patients with cancer. Biochem Biophys Res Commun 234.2 (1997): 296–299.

Folkers K et al. Lovastatin decreases coenzyme Q levels in humans. Proc Natl Acad Sci U S A 87.22 (1990): 8931–8934.

Folkers K, Choe JY, Combs AB. Rescue by coenzyme Q10 from electrocardiographic abnormalities caused by the toxicity of adriamycin in the rat. Proc Natl Acad Sci U S A 75.10 (1978): 5178–5180.

Folkers K, Wolaniuk A. Research on coenzyme Q10 in clinical medicine and in immunomodulation. Drugs Exp Clin Res 11.8 (1985): 539–545.

Fotino AD et al. Effect of coenzyme Q(1)(0) supplementation on heart failure: a meta-analysis. Am J Clin Nutr 97.2 (2013): 268–275.

Fouad AA et al. Coenzyme Q10 treatment ameliorates acute cisplatin nephrotoxicity in mice. Toxicology 274(1–3) (2010): 49–56.

Fouad AA, Jresat I. Hepatoprotective effect of coenzyme Q10 in rats with acetaminophen toxicity. Environ Toxicol Pharmacol 33.2 (2012): 158–167.

Fujimoto S et al. Effects of coenzyme Q10 administration on pulmonary function and exercise performance in patients with chronic lung diseases. Clin Invest 71.8 (Suppl) (1993): S162–S166.

Fujioka T et al. Clinical study of cardiac arrhythmias using a 24-hour continuous electrocardiographic recorder (5th report): antiarrhythmic action of coenzyme Q10 in diabetics. Tohoku J Exp Med 141 (Suppl) (1983): 453–463.

Fumagalli S et al. Coenzyme Q10 terclatrate and creatine in chronic heart failure: a randomized, placebo-controlled, double-blind study. Clin Cardiol 34(4) (2011): 211–217.

Galili N et al. Clinical response of myelodysplastic syndromes patients to treatment with coenzyme Q10. Leuk Res 31.1 (2007): 19–26.

Gao L et al. Effects of coenzyme Q10 on vascular endothelial function in humans: a meta-analysis of randomized controlled trials. Atherosclerosis, 221.2 (2012): 311–316.

Glover EI et al. A randomized trial of coenzyme Q10 in mitochondrial disorders. Muscle Nerve 42.5 (2010): 739–748.

Gokbel H et al. The effects of coenzyme Q10 supplementation on performance during repeated bouts of supramaximal exercise in sedentary men. J Strength Cond Res 24.1 (2010): 97–102.

Golomb BA, Evans MA. Statin adverse effects: a review of the literature and evidence for a mitochondrial mechanism. Am J Cardiovasc Drugs 8.6 (2008): 373–418.

Gotz ME et al. Altered redox state of platelet coenzyme Q10 in Parkinson's disease. J Neural Transm 107.1 (2000): 41–48.

Graham D et al. Mitochondria-targeted antioxidant MitoQ10 improves endothelial function and attenuates cardiac hypertrophy. Hypertension 54(2) (2009): 322–328.

Greenlee H et al. Lack of effect of coenzyme q10 on doxorubicin cytotoxicity in breast cancer cell cultures. Integr Cancer Ther 11(3) (2012): 243–250.

Groneberg DA et al. Coenzyme Q10 affects expression of genes involved in cell signalling, metabolism and transport in human CaCo-2 cells. Int J Biochem Cell Biol 37 (2005): 1208–1218.

Gul I et al. Oxidative stress and antioxidant defense in plasma after repeated bouts of supramaximal exercise: the effect of coenzyme Q10. J Sports Med Phys Fitness 51.2 (2011): 305–312.

Hamilton SJ et al. Coenzyme Q10 improves endothelial dysfunction in statin-treated type 2 diabetic patients. Diabetes Care. 32.5 (2009): 810–812.

Hanioka T et al. Effect of topical application of coenzyme Q10 on adult periodontitis. Mol Aspects Med 15 (Suppl) (1994): S241–S248.

Hargreaves IP et al. The coenzyme Q10 status of the brain regions of Parkinson's disease patients. Neurosci Lett 447.1 (2008): 17–19.
Hart PE et al. Antioxidant treatment of patients with Friedreich ataxia: four-year follow-up. Arch Neurol 62.4 (2005): 621–626.
Hershey AD et al. Coenzyme Q10 deficiency and response to supplementation in pediatric and adolescent migraine. Headache 47.1 (2007): 73–80.
Hirose Y et al. Effect of water-soluble coenzyme Q10 on noise-induced hearing loss in guinea pigs. Acta Otolaryngol 128(10) (2008): 1071–1076.
Ho MJ et al. Blood pressure lowering efficacy of coenzyme Q10 for primary hypertension. Cochrane Database Syst Rev(4) (2009): CD007435.
Hofman-Bang C et al. Coenzyme Q10 as an adjunctive in the treatment of chronic congestive heart failure. The Q10 Study Group. J Card Fail 1.2 (1995): 101–107.
Hosoe K et al. Study on safety and bioavailability of ubiquinol (Kaneka QH) after single and 4-week multiple oral administration to healthy volunteers. Regul Toxicol Pharmacol 47.1 (2007): 19–28.
Huntington Study Group Pre et al. Safety and tolerability of high-dosage coenzyme Q10 in Huntington's disease and healthy subjects. Mov Disord 25.12 (2010): 1924–1928.
Huntington's Study Group. A randomized, placebo-controlled trial of coenzyme Q10 and remacemide in Huntington's disease. Neurology 57.3 (2001): 397–404.
Itagaki S et al. Interaction of coenzyme Q10 with the intestinal drug transporter P-glycoprotein. J Agric Food Chem 56.16 (2008): 6923–6927.
Jeejeebhoy F et al. Nutritional supplementation with MyoVive repletes essential cardiac myocyte nutrients and reduces left ventricular size in patients with left ventricular dysfunction. Am Heart J 143.6 (2002): 1092–1100.
Judy WV et al. Double-blind-double crossover study of coenzyme Q10 in heart failure. In: Folkers K, Yamamura Y (eds). Biomedical and Clinical Aspects of Coenzyme Q. Vol 5, Amsterdam: Elsevier, 1986: 315–323.
Judy WV et al. Myocardial preservation by therapy with coenzyme Q10 during heart surgery. Clin Invest 71.8 (Suppl) (1993): S155–S161.
Kaikkonen J et al. Coenzyme Q10: absorption, antioxidative properties, determinants, and plasma levels. Free Radic Res 36.4 (2002): 389–397.
Kamikawa T et al. Effects of coenzyme Q10 on exercise tolerance in chronic stable angina pectoris. Am J Cardiol 56.4 (1985): 247–251.
Karlsson J et al. Muscle fibre types, ubiquinone content and exercise capacity in hypertension and effort angina. Ann Med 23.3 (1991): 339–344.
Karlsson J et al. Muscle ubiquinone in healthy physically active males. Mol Cell Biochem 156.2 (1996): 169–172.
Kedziora-Kornatowska K et al. Effects of coenzyme Q10 supplementation on activities of selected antioxidative enzymes and lipid peroxidation in hypertensive patients treated with indapamide. A pilot study. Arch Med Sci 6.4 (2010): 513–518.
Keogh A et al. Randomised double-blind, placebo-controlled trial of coenzyme Q10 therapy in class II and III systolic heart failure. Heart Lung Circ 12 (2003): 135–141.
Kernt M et al. Coenzyme Q10 prevents human lens epithelial cells from light-induced apoptotic cell death by reducing oxidative stress and stabilizing BAX / Bcl-2 ratio. Acta Ophthalmol 88.3 (2010): e78–86.
Khan M et al. A pilot clinical trial of the effects of coenzyme Q10 on chronic tinnitus aurium. Otolaryngol Head Neck Surg 136.1 (2007): 72–77.
Khatta M et al. The effect of coenzyme Q10 in patients with congestive heart failure. Ann Intern Med 132 (2000): 636–640.
Kim JM, Park E. Coenzyme Q10 attenuated DMH-induced precancerous lesions in SD rats. J Nutrit Sci Vitaminology, 56.2 (2010): 139–144.
Kishi H et al. Bioenergetics in clinical medicine. III. Inhibition of coenzyme Q10-enzymes by clinically used anti-hypertensive drugs. Res Commun Chem Pathol Pharmacol 12.3 (1975): 533–540.
Kocharian A et al. Coenzyme Q10 improves diastolic function in children with idiopathic dilated cardiomyopathy. Cardiol Young 19.5 (2009): 501–506.
Kokawa T et al. Coenzyme Q10 in cancer chemotherapy: experimental studies on augmentation of the effects of masked compounds, especially in the combined chemotherapy with immunopotentiators. Gan To Kagaku Ryoho 10.3 (1983): 768–774.
Kolahdouz MR et al. The effect of coenzyme Q10 supplementation on metabolic status of type 2 diabetic patients. Minerva Gastroenterol Dietol 59.2 (2013): 231–236.
Kon M et al. Reducing exercise-induced muscular injury in kendo athletes with supplementation of coenzyme Q10. Br J Nutr 100.4 (2008): 903–909.
Laaksonen R et al. Decreases in serum ubiquinone concentrations do not result in reduced levels in muscle tissue during short-term simvastatin treatment in humans. Clin Pharmacol Ther 57.1 (1995): 62–66.
Laaksonen R et al. Serum ubiquinone concentrations after short- and long-term treatment with HMG-CoA reductase inhibitors. Eur J Clin Pharmacol 46.4 (1994): 313–317.
Laaksonen R et al. The effect of simvastatin treatment on natural antioxidants in low-density lipoproteins and high-energy phosphates and ubiquinone in skeletal muscle. Am J Cardiol 77.10 (1996): 851–854.
Laguna TA et al. Decreased total serum coenzyme-Q10 concentrations: a longitudinal study in children with cystic fibrosis. J Pediatr 153.3 (2008): 402–407.
Langsjoen PH et al. Usefulness of coenzyme Q10 in clinical cardiology: a long-term study. Mol Aspects Med 15 (Suppl) (1994a): S165–S175.
Langsjoen PH, Langsjoen AM. Overview of the use of CoQ10 in cardiovascular disease. Biofactors 9 (1999): 273–284.
Langsjoen PH, Langsjoen AM. Supplemental ubiquinol in patients with advanced congestive heart failure. Biofactors 32.1–4 (2008): 119–128.

C

Langsjoen PH, Vadhanavikit S, Folkers K. Effective treatment with coenzyme Q10 of patients with chronic myocardial disease. Drugs Exp Clin Res 11.8 (1985): 577–579.

Langsjoen PH. Lack of effect of coenzyme Q on left ventricular function in patients with congestive heart failure. J Am Coll Cardiol 35.3 (2000): 816–8117.

Lee BJ et al. Coenzyme Q10 supplementation reduces oxidative stress and increases antioxidant enzyme activity in patients with coronary artery disease. Nutrition 28.3 (2012b): 250–255.

Lee BJ et al. Effects of coenzyme Q10 supplementation on inflammatory markers (high-sensitivity C-reactive protein, interleukin-6, and homocysteine) in patients with coronary artery disease. Nutrition 28.7–8 (2012a): 767–772.

Lee BJ et al. The relationship between coenzyme Q10, oxidative stress, and antioxidant enzymes activities and coronary artery disease. Sci World J 2012 (2012c): 792756.

Leong JY et al. Perioperative metabolic therapy improves redox status and outcomes in cardiac surgery patients: a randomised trial. Heart Lung Circ 19.10 (2010): 584–591.

Levy HB, Kohlhaas HK. Considerations for supplementing with coenzyme Q10 during statin therapy. Ann Pharmacother 40.2 (2006): 290–294.

Littarru GP, Langsjoen P. Coenzyme Q10 and statins: biochemical and clinical implications. Mitochondrion 7 (Suppl) (2007): S168–S174.

Littarru GP, Tiano L. Clinical aspects of coenzyme Q10: an update. Curr Opin Clin Nutr Metab Care 8.6 (2005): 641–646.

Liu J et al. Coenzyme Q10 for Parkinson's disease. Cochrane Database Syst Rev (12) (2011): CD008150.

Lockwood K et al. Partial and complete regression of breast cancer in patients in relation to dosage of coenzyme Q10. Biochem Biophys Res Commun 199.3 (1994): 1504–1508.

Lockwood K et al. Progress on therapy of breast cancer with vitamin Q10 and the regression of metastases. Biochem Biophys Res Commun 212.1 (1995): 172–177.

Louis F et al. Effects of ubiquinone and related substances on secretion of aldosterone and cortisol. Am J Physiol 208 (1965): 1275–1280.

Lulli M et al. Coenzyme Q10 instilled as eye drops on the cornea reaches the retina and protects retinal layers from apoptosis in a mouse model of kainate-induced retinal damage. Invest Ophthalmol Vis Sci 53.13 (2012b): 8295–8302.

Lulli M et al. Coenzyme Q10 protects retinal cells from apoptosis induced by radiation in vitro and in vivo. J Radiat Res 53.5 (2012a): 695–703.

Maes M et al. Coenzyme Q10 deficiency in myalgic encephalomyelitis/chronic fatigue syndrome (ME/CFS) is related to fatigue, autonomic and neurocognitive symptoms and is another risk factor explaining the early mortality in ME/CFS due to cardiovascular disorder. Neuro Endocrinol Lett 30.4 (2009): 470–476.

Makhija N et al. The role of oral coenzyme Q10 in patients undergoing coronary artery bypass graft surgery. J Cardiothorac Vasc Anesth 22.6 (2008): 832–839.

Marcoff L, Thompson PD. The role of coenzyme Q10 in statin-associated myopathy: a systematic review. J Am Coll Cardiol 49.23 (2007): 2231–2237.

Marinari S et al. Effects of nutraceutical diet integration, with coenzyme Q10 (Q-Ter multicomposite) and creatine, on dyspnea, exercise tolerance, and quality of life in COPD patients with chronic respiratory failure. Multidiscip Respir Med 8.1 (2013): 40.

Mariotti C et al. Idebenone treatment in Friedreich patients: one-year-long randomized placebo-controlled trial. Neurology 60.10 (2003): 1676–1679.

Martin SB et al. Coenzyme Q10 and cognition in atorvastatin treated dogs. Neurosci Lett 501.2 (2011): 92–95.

McCarty MF. Coenzyme Q versus hypertension: does CoQ decrease endothelial superoxide generation? Med Hypotheses 53.4 (1999): 300–304.

McDonald SR et al. Concurrent administration of coenzyme Q10 and alpha-tocopherol improves learning in aged mice. Free Radic Biol Med 38 (2005): 729–736.

McMurray JJ et al. (2010). Coenzyme Q10, rosuvastatin, and clinical outcomes in heart failure: a pre-specified substudy of CORONA (controlled rosuvastatin multinational study in heart failure). J Am Coll Cardiol 56(15): 1196–1204.

Mezawa M et al. The reduced form of coenzyme Q10 improves glycemic control in patients with type 2 diabetes: an open label pilot study. Biofactors 38.6 (2012): 416–421.

Mischley LK et al. Coenzyme Q10 deficiency in patients with Parkinson's disease. J Neurol Sci 318(1–2) (2012): 72–75.

Miyamae T et al. Increased oxidative stress and coenzyme Q10 deficiency in juvenile fibromyalgia: amelioration of hypercholesterolemia and fatigue by ubiquinol-10 supplementation. Redox Rep 18.1 (2013): 12–19.

Mizuno K et al. Antifatigue effects of coenzyme Q10 during physical fatigue. Nutrition 24.4 (2008): 293–299.

Mizushina Y et al. Coenzyme Q10 as a potent compound that inhibits Cdt1–geminin interaction. Biochimica et Biophysica Acta (BBA)-General Subjects, 1780.2 (2008): 203–213.

Molyneux SL et al. Coenzyme Q10: an independent predictor of mortality in chronic heart failure. J Am Coll Cardiol 52.18 (2008): 1435–1441.

Moreira PI et al. CoQ10 therapy attenuates amyloid beta-peptide toxicity in brain mitochondria isolated from aged diabetic rats. Exp Neurol 196 (2005): 112–119.

Morisco C et al. Noninvasive evaluation of cardiac hemodynamics during exercise in patients with chronic heart failure. Effects of short-term coenzyme Q10 treatment. Mol Aspects Med 15 (Suppl) (1994): S155–S163.

Morisco C, Trimarco B, Condorelli M. Effect of coenzyme Q10 therapy in patients with congestive heart failure: a long-term multicenter randomized study. Clin Invest 71 (1993): S134–S136.

Mortensen SA et al. Coenzyme Q10: clinical benefits with biochemical correlates suggesting a scientific breakthrough in the management of chronic heart failure. Int J Tissue React 12.3 (1990): 155–162.

Mortensen SA et al. Dose-related decrease of serum coenzyme Q10 during treatment with HMG-CoA reductase inhibitors. Mol Aspects Med 18 (Suppl) (1997): S137–S144.

Muller T et al. Coenzyme Q10 supplementation provides mild symptomatic benefit in patients with Parkinson's disease. Neurosci Lett 341 (2003): 201–204.

Munkholm H, Hansen HH, Rasmussen K. Coenzyme Q10 treatment in serious heart failure. Biofactors 9.2–4 (1999): 285–289.

Nadjarzadeh A et al. Effect of Coenzyme Q10 supplementation on antioxidant enzymes activity and oxidative stress of seminal plasma: a double-blind randomised clinical trial. Andrologia 46.2 (2013): 177–183.

Nadjarzadeh, A., Sadeghi, M. R., et al. (2011). Coenzyme Q10 improves seminal oxidative defense but does not affect on semen parameters in idiopathic oligoasthenoteratozoospermia: a randomized double-blind, placebo controlled trial. J Endocrinol Invest 34(8): e224–228.

Nuku K et al. Safety assessment of PureSorb-Q40 in healthy subjects and serum coenzyme Q10 level in excessive dosing. J Nutr Sci Vitaminol (Tokyo) 53.3 (2007): 198–206.

Ochiai A et al. Improvement in intestinal coenzyme q10 absorption by food intake. Yakugaku Zasshi 127.8 (2007): 1251–1254.

Okello E et al. Combined statin/coenzyme Q10 as adjunctive treatment of chronic heart failure. Med Hypoth 73.3 (2009): 306–308.

Ono K et al. Preformed beta-amyloid fibrils are destabilized by coenzyme Q10 in vitro. Biochem Biophys Res Commun 330 (2005): 111–116.

Ostman B et al. Coenzyme Q10 supplementation and exercise-induced oxidative stress in humans. Nutrition 28.4 (2012): 403–417.

Overvad K et al. Coenzyme Q10 in health and disease. Eur J Clin Nutr 53.10 (1999): 764–770.

Paiva H et al. High-dose statins and skeletal muscle metabolism in humans: a randomized, controlled trial. Clin Pharmacol Ther 78.1 (2005): 60–68.

Papas KA et al. A pilot study on the safety and efficacy of a novel antioxidant rich formulation in patients with cystic fibrosis. J Cyst Fibros 7.1 (2008): 60–67.

Parker BA et al. A randomized trial of coenzyme Q10 in patients with statin myopathy: rationale and study design. J Clin Lipidol 7.3 (2013): 187–193.

Pelton R et al. Drug-induced nutrient depletion handbook 1999–2000. Lexi-Comp (1999).

Pepe S et al. Coenzyme Q10 in cardiovascular disease. Mitochondrion 7 (Suppl) (2007): S154–S167.

Permanetter B et al. Ubiquinone (coenzyme Q10) in the long-term treatment of idiopathic dilated cardiomyopathy. Eur Heart J 13.11 (1992): 1528–1533.

Pogessi L et al. Effect of coenzyme Q10 on left ventricular function in patients with dilative cardiomyopathy. Curr Ther Res 49 (1991): 878–886.

Porter DA et al. The effect of oral coenzyme Q10 on the exercise tolerance of middle-aged, untrained men. Int J Sports Med 16.7 (1995): 421–427.

Potgieter M et al. Primary and secondary coenzyme Q10 deficiency: the role of therapeutic supplementation. Nutrition Reviews 71.3 (2013): 180–188.

Pringsheim T et al. Canadian Headache Society guideline for migraine prophylaxis. Can J Neurol Sci 39 (2 Suppl 2) (2012): S1–S59.

Qu J et al. Coenzyme Q10 in the human retina. Invest Ophthalmol Vis Sci 50.4 (2009): 1814–1818.

Quinzii CM et al. Human CoQ10 deficiencies. Biofactors 32.1–4 (2008): 113–118.

Roffe L et al. Efficacy of coenzyme Q10 for improved tolerability of cancer treatments: a systematic review. J Clin Oncol 22.21 (2004): 4418–4424.

Rosenfeldt F et al. Coenzyme Q10 improves the tolerance of the senescent myocardium to aerobic and ischemic stress: studies in rats and in human atrial tissue. Biofactors 9.2–4 (1999): 291–299.

Rosenfeldt F et al. Coenzyme Q10 therapy before cardiac surgery improves mitochondrial function and in vitro contractility of myocardial tissue. J Thorac Cardiovasc Surg 129 (2005): 25–32.

Rosenfeldt F et al. Systematic review of effect of coenzyme Q10 in physical exercise, hypertension and heart failure. Biofactors 18 (2003): 91–100.

Rosenfeldt F et al. The effects of ageing on the response to cardiac surgery: protective strategies for the ageing myocardium. Biogerontology 3 (2002): 37–40.

Rosenfeldt FL et al. Coenzyme Q10 in the treatment of hypertension: a meta-analysis of the clinical trials. J Hum Hypertens 21.4 (2007): 297–306.

Rozen TD et al. Open label trial of coenzyme Q10 as a migraine preventive. Cephalalgia 22.2 (2002): 137–141.

Ryo, K., Ito, A., et al. (2011). Effects of coenzyme Q10 on salivary secretion. Clin Biochem 44(8–9): 669–74.

Sacconi S et al. Coenzyme Q10 is frequently reduced in muscle of patients with mitochondrial myopathy. Neuromuscul Disord 20.1 (2010): 44–48.

Sachdanandam P. Antiangiogenic and hypolipidemic activity of coenzyme Q10 supplementation to breast cancer patients undergoing Tamoxifen therapy. Biofactors 32.1–4 (2008):151–159.

Safarinejad MR et al. Effects of EPA, gamma-linolenic acid or coenzyme Q10 on serum prostate-specific antigen levels: a randomised, double-blind trial. Br J Nutr (2012): 1–8.

Safarinejad MR et al. Effects of the reduced form of coenzyme Q10 (ubiquinol) on semen parameters in men with idiopathic infertility: a double-blind, placebo controlled, randomized study. J Urol 188(2) (2012b): 526–531.

Safarinejad MR. Efficacy of coenzyme Q10 on semen parameters, sperm function and reproductive hormones in infertile men. J Urol 182.1 (2009): 237–248.

Safarinejad MR. Safety and efficacy of coenzyme Q10 supplementation in early chronic Peyronie's disease: a double-blind, placebo-controlled randomized study. Int J Impot Res 22.5 (2010): 298–309.

Safarinejad MR. The effect of coenzyme Q(1)(0) supplementation on partner pregnancy rate in infertile men with idiopathic oligoasthenoteratozoospermia: an open-label prospective study. Int Urol Nephrol 44(3) (2012): 689–700.

Sakata T et al. Coenzyme Q10 administration suppresses both oxidative and antioxidative markers in hemodialysis patients. Blood Purif 26.4 (2008): 371–378.

Salami A et al. Water-soluble coenzyme Q10 formulation (Q-TER((R))) in the treatment of presbycusis. Acta Otolaryngol 130.10 (2010): 1154–1162.
Sander S et al. The impact of coenzyme Q10 on systolic function in patients with chronic heart failure. J Card Fail 12.6 (2006): 464–472.
Sandor PS et al. Efficacy of coenzyme Q10 in migraine prophylaxis. a randomized controlled trial. Neurology 64 (2005): 713–715.
Sato Y et al. Emulsification Using Highly Hydrophilic Surfactants Improves the Absorption of Orally Administered Coenzyme Q10. Biolog and Pharmaceut Bulletin 36.12 (2013): 2012–2017.
Satta A et al. Effects of ubidecarenone in an exercise training program for patients with chronic obstructive pulmonary diseases. Clin Ther 13.6 (1991): 754–757.
Schmelzer C et al. Functions of coenzyme Q10 in inflammation and gene expression. Biofactors 32.1–4 (2008): 179–183.
Senes M et al. Coenzyme Q10 and high-sensitivity C-reactive protein in ischemic and idiopathic dilated cardiomyopathy. Clin Chem Lab Med 46.3 (2008): 382–386.
Serra G et al. Evaluation of coenzyme Q10 in patients with moderate heart failure and chronic stable effort angina. In: Folkers K, Yamamura Y (eds). Biomedical and Clinical Aspects of Coenzyme Q. Vol 6, Amsterdam: Elsevier, 1991: 327–338.
Shalansky S et al. Risk of warfarin-related bleeding events and supratherapeutic international normalized ratios associated with complementary and alternative medicine: a longitudinal analysis. Pharmacotherapy, 27.9 (2007): 1237–1247.
Shults CW et al. Effects of coenzyme Q10 in early Parkinson disease: evidence of slowing of the functional decline. Arch Neurol 59.10 (2002): 1541–1550.
Shults CW et al. Pilot trial of high dosages of coenzyme Q10 in patients with Parkinson's disease. Exp Neurol 188 (2004): 491–494.
Shults CW. Therapeutic role of coenzyme Q(10) in Parkinson's disease. Pharmacol Ther 107 (2005): 120–130.
Silver MA et al. Effect of atorvastatin on left ventricular diastolic function and ability of coenzyme Q10 to reverse that dysfunction. Am J Cardiol 94 (2004): 1306–1310.
Singh RB et al. Effect of hydrosoluble coenzyme Q10 on blood pressure and insulin resistance in hypertensive patients with coronary artery disease. J Hum Hypertens 13 (1999): 203–208.
Skough K et al. Effects of resistance training in combination with coenzyme Q10 supplementation in patients with post-polio: a pilot study. J Rehabil Med 40.9 (2008): 773–775.
Slater SK et al. c. Cephalalgia 31.8 (2011): 897–905.
Sohet FM et al. Coenzyme Q10 supplementation lowers hepatic oxidative stress and inflammation associated with diet-induced obesity in mice. Biochem Pharmacol 78.11 (2009): 1391–400.
Sole MJ, Jeejeebhoy KN. Conditioned nutritional requirements: therapeutic relevance to heart failure. Herz 27.2 (2002): 174–178.
Spigset O. Coenzyme Q10 (ubiquinone) in the treatment of heart failure. Are any positive effects documented? Tidsskr Nor Laegeforen 114.8 (1994a): 939–942.
Spigset O. Reduced effect of warfarin caused by ubidecarenone. Lancet 344 (1994b): 1372–1373.
Stamelou M et al. Short-term effects of coenzyme Q10 in progressive supranuclear palsy: a randomized, placebo-controlled trial. Mov Disord 23(7) (2008): 942–949.
Stargrove M et al. Herb, nutrient and drug interactions. St Louis: Mosby, 2008.
Stocker R et al. Neither plasma coenzyme Q10 concentration, nor its decline during pravastatin therapy, is linked to recurrent cardiovascular disease events: a prospective case-control study from the LIPID study. Atherosclerosis 187.1 (2006): 198–204.
Stocker R, Macdonald P. The benefit of coenzyme Q10 supplements in the management of chronic heart failure: a long tale of promise in the continued absence of clear evidence. Am J Clin Nutr 97.2 (2013): 233–234.
Storch A et al. Randomized, double-blind, placebo-controlled trial on symptomatic effects of coenzyme Q(10) in Parkinson disease. Arch Neurol 64.7 (2007): 938–944.
Storch A. [Coenzyme Q10 in Parkinson's disease. Symptomatic or neuroprotective effects?]. Nervenarzt 78.12 (2007): 1378–1382.
Taggart DP et al. Effects of short-term supplementation with coenzyme Q10 on myocardial protection during cardiac operations. Ann Thorac Surg 61 (1996): 829–833.
Takahashi N et al. Effect of coenzyme Q10 on hemodynamic response to ocular timolol. J Cardiovasc Pharmacol 14.3 (1989): 462–468.
Tanaka J et al. Coenzyme Q10: the prophylactic effect on low cardiac output following cardiac valve replacement. Ann Thorac Surg 33.2 (1982): 145–151.
Tanrikulu AC et al. Coenzyme Q10, copper, zinc, and lipid peroxidation levels in serum of patients with chronic obstructive pulmonary disease. Bio Trace Elem Res 143.2 (2011): 659–667.
Teran E et al. Coenzyme Q10 supplementation during pregnancy reduces the risk of pre-eclampsia. Int J Gynaecol Obstet 105.1 (2009): 43–45.
Tiano L et al. Coenzyme Q10 and oxidative imbalance in Down syndrome: biochemical and clinical aspects. Biofactors 32(1–4) (2008): 161–167.
Tsai KL et al. A novel mechanism of coenzyme Q10 protects against human endothelial cells from oxidative stress-induced injury by modulating NO-related pathways. J Nutr Biochem 23.5 (2012): 458–468.
Tsai, K. L., Chen, L. H., et al. (2011). Coenzyme Q10 suppresses oxLDL-induced endothelial oxidative injuries by the modulation of LOX-1-mediated ROS generation via the AMPK/PKC/NADPH oxidase signaling pathway. Mol Nutr Food Res 55 Suppl 2: S227–40.
Tsuneki H et al. Protective effects of coenzyme Q10 against angiotensin II-induced oxidative stress in human umbilical vein endothelial cells. European J Pharmacol 701.1 (2013): 218–227.
Turk S et al. Coenzyme Q10 supplementation and diastolic heart functions in hemodialysis patients: A randomized double-blind placebo-controlled trial.Hemodialysis International, 17.3 (2013): 374–381.

Ullmann U et al. A new Coenzyme Q10 tablet-grade formulation (all-Q) is bioequivalent to Q-Gel and both have better bioavailability properties than Q-SorB. J Med Food 8.3 (2005): 397–399.
Watson PS et al. Lack of effect of coenzyme Q on left ventricular function in patients with congestive heart failure. J Am Coll Cardiol 33.6 (1999): 1549–1552.
Watts GF et al. Coenzyme Q(10) improves endothelial dysfunction of the brachial artery in type II diabetes mellitus. Diabetologia 45 (2002): 420–426.
Wilkinson EG et al. Bioenergetics in clinical medicine. II. Adjunctive treatment with coenzyme Q in periodontal therapy. Res Commun Chem Pathol Pharmacol 12.1 (1975): 111–123.
Yamagami T, Shibata N, Folkers K. Bioenergetics in clinical medicine: studies on coenzyme Q10 and essential hypertension. Res Commun Chem Pathol Pharmacol 11 (1975): 273–288.
Yamagami T, Shibata N, Folkers K. Bioenergetics in clinical medicine. VIII. Adminstration of coenzyme Q10 to patients with essential hypertension. Res Commun Chem Pathol Pharmacol 14 (1976): 721–727.
Yang X et al. Coenzyme Q10 reduces β-amyloid plaque in an APP/PS1 transgenic mouse model of Alzheimer's disease. J Mol Neurosci 41.1 (2010): 110–113.
Yang, X et al. Coenzyme Q10 attenuates β-amyloid pathology in the aged transgenic mice with Alzheimer Presenilin 1 mutation. J Mol Neurosci 34.2 (2008): 165–171.
Ylikoski T et al. The effect of coenzyme Q10 on the exercise performance of cross-country skiers. Mol Aspects Med 18 (Suppl) (1997): S283–S290.
Young AJ et al. Coenzyme Q10: a review of its promise as a neuroprotectant. CNS Spectr 12.1 (2007): 62–68.
Young JM et al. A randomized, double-blind, placebo-controlled crossover study of coenzyme Q10 therapy in hypertensive patients with the metabolic syndrome. Am J Hypertens 25.2 (2012): 261–270.
Zhou M et al. Effects of coenzyme Q10 on myocardial protection during cardiac valve replacement and scavenging free radical activity in vitro. J Cardiovasc Surg (Torino) 40 (1999): 355–361.
Zhou Q, Chowbay B. Effect of coenzyme Q10 on the disposition of doxorubicin in rats. Eur J Drug Metab Pharmacokinet 27.3 (2002): 185–192.
Zlatohlavek L et al. The effect of coenzyme Q10 in statin myopathy. Neuro Endocrinol Lett 33 (2012): 98–101.
Zmitek J et al. Relative bioavailability of two forms of a novel water-soluble coenzyme Q10. Ann Nutr Metab 52.4 (2008): 281–287.

Cranberry

HISTORICAL NOTE Native American Indians used cranberries as both a food and a treatment for bladder and kidney diseases. In the mid-1800s, German scientists suggested that cranberry juice had antibacterial activity, supporting its use as a treatment for bladder infections. Recent investigation has confirmed its usefulness in the prevention of urinary tract infections.

OTHER NAMES

Kronsbeere, marsh apple, moosbeere, preisselbeere

BOTANICAL NAME/FAMILY

Vaccinium oxycoccus, *Vaccinium macrocarpon* (family Ericaceae)

PLANT PART USED

Fruit

CHEMICAL COMPONENTS

Catechin, flavone glycosides, fructose, organic acids, proanthocyanidins, vitamin C. Cranberry has a high flavonol content (100–263 mg/kg) (Hakkinen et al 1999) — higher than commonly consumed fruits and vegetables.

C

MAIN ACTIONS

Bacteriostatic and antiadhesive activity

The adhesion of pathogenic organisms to a tissue surface is required to initiate most infectious diseases (Sharon & Ofek 2002). Various in vitro and in vivo studies have identified that cranberry has antiadhesion properties relevant to several different strains of bacteria, including *Escherichia coli, Staphylococcus aureus, Helicobacter pylori, Streptococcus pneumoniae* and *Streptococcus mutans*.

The proanthocyanidins in cranberry are potent inhibitors of *E. coli* adhesion, thereby influencing the initiation of disease without exerting bactericidal activity. One in vitro study found that cranberry juice inhibited adhesion of 46 different *E. coli* isolates by 75% (Sobota 1984): when administered to mice for 14 days, adherence of *E. coli* to uroepithelial cells was inhibited by 80%. Significant inhibition of adherence was also observed in samples of human urine 1–3 hours after subjects drank a cranberry drink. A water-soluble extract was found to be most effective in its antimicrobial inhibition of seven bacterial strains, including *E. coli, Listeria monocytogenes* and *Salmonella typhimurium* (Côté et al 2011).

The morphology of *E. coli* is changed when grown in the presence of cranberry juice or extract (Johnson et al 2008). It appears that the antiadhesion effects are a result of irreversible inhibition of the expression of P-fimbriae of *E. coli* (Ahuja et al 1998). Electron micrographic evidence suggests that cranberry juice acts either on the cell wall, preventing proper attachment of the fimbrial subunits, or as a genetic control, preventing the expression of normal fimbrial subunits, or both (Gupta et al 2007). Of the cranberry constituents, it appears that the sugars in conjunction with organic acids cause osmotic stress and the anthocyanins and phenolics lead to the disintegration of the outer membrane when tested against *E. coli* (Lacombe et al 2010). Furthermore, cranberry juice has been shown to disrupt bacterial ligand-uroepithelial cell receptor binding (Liu et al 2008). This inhibitory effect has been seen with *Staphylococcus aureus* (Magarinos et al 2008, Su et al 2012), *E. coli* and uroepithelial tissues, but also in the adhesion of *Helicobacter pylori* to human gastrointestinal cells (Burger et al 2002) and in the co-aggregation of oral bacteria and *Streptococcus mutans* counts in saliva (Sharon & Ofek 2002, Weiss et al 1998).

New research on human bronchial cells found a 90% adhesion inhibition for *Streptococcus pneumoniae* (a common cause of pneumonia, meningitis and otitis media) with cranberry juice (Huttunen et al 2011). Two studies have looked at the effect of cranberry extracts on biofilm production, which can cause infections with catheter use and corneal infections caused by contact lens use. Both studies found a reduction in growth of biofilm with Gram-positive bacteria, specifically *Staphylococcus* spp. (LaPlante et al 2012, Leshem et al 2011).

Antioxidant

Cranberries consistently rank highly among common fruits with antioxidant activity. In particular, the polyphenolic compounds in cranberry display substantial antioxidant capacity. In vitro tests with whole fruit and isolated flavonol glycosides found in cranberry showed free radical scavenging activity comparable or superior to that of vitamin E (Yan et al 2002). In vivo studies demonstrate that cranberry juice increases plasma antioxidant status (Villarreal et al 2007). A small human trial demonstrated that a single 240-mL serving of cranberry juice increased plasma antioxidant capacity significantly greater than controls receiving an equivalent amount of vitamin C in solution (Vinson et al 2008).

Increases excretion of oxalic acid and uric acid

According to an open study, a dose of 330 mL cranberry juice can increase the excretion of oxalic acid and uric acid (Kessler et al 2002).

Alterations to urinary pH

Earlier hypotheses that cranberry juice prevents urinary tract infection (UTI) by acidification of urine or by its hippuric acid content have not been substantiated. Results from human studies are contradictory, but overall suggest no significant change in urinary pH at doses less than 330 mL daily. A crossover study of 27 patients with indwelling urinary catheters and chronic bacteriuria showed no change in urinary pH (Nahata et al 1982); the results of a double-blind study of 153 women were the same (Avorn et al 1994). One small, open study involving 12 healthy subjects found that 330 mL of cranberry juice reduced the urinary pH (Kessler et al 2002).

Chemoprotective

Studies employing mainly in vitro tumour models show that cranberry extracts and compounds inhibit the growth and proliferation of several types of tumour, including lymphoma, bladder, breast, colon, prostate, ovaries, oesophageal, lung, oral squamous cell carcinoma and gastric cancer cells (Chatelain et al 2008, Ferguson et al 2006, Hochman et al 2008, Kim et al 2012, Kresty et al 2008, Liu et al 2009, MacLean et al 2011, Prasain et al 2008, Singh et al 2009, Sun & Hai Liu 2006, Vu et al 2012). The flavonoid components may act in a complementary fashion to limit carcinogenesis by inducing apoptosis in tumour cells (Neto et al 2008).

Cytochromes

Although some studies with animal models have suggested effects on various cytochromes, human studies have found that cranberry juice has no significant effect on CYP 2C9, 1A2 or 3A4 (Greenblatt et al 2006, Grenier et al 2006, Lilja et al 2007, Mohammed Abdul et al 2008, Ushijima et al 2009).

Before we can definitively conclude that cranberry juice has no effect on CYP3A4, it must be noted that a human study testing five commercial cranberry juices has identified substantial interbrand variations in ability to inhibit intestinal (but not hepatic) CYP3A, ranging from 34% to abolishment (Ngo et al 2009). Further testing indicates that three triterpenes are able to inhibit CYP3A in humans, suggesting it may be the natural variation in concentration of these constituents between products which is responsible for the inconsistent results seen between in vivo and clinical trials to date (Kim et al 2011a).

OTHER ACTIONS

Preliminary research with in vitro tests and those using animal models are identifying many different actions which are worthy of further exploration.

Antiviral activity

A non-specific antiviral effect has been demonstrated in vitro for a commercially produced cranberry fruit juice drink (Lipson et al 2007).

Antifungal activity

A recent in vitro study of cranberry proanthocyanidin fractions on human fungi, *Candida* spp. and *Cryptococcus neoformans* reported antifungal activity (Patel et al 2011).

ACE inhibitor

Cranberry powders have been shown in vitro to have a limited inhibitory activity on alpha-amylase and to significantly impact angiotensin 1-converting enzyme (ACE) (Pinto Mda et al 2010).

Lipid lowering and anti-inflammatory

According to a rat study, cranberry powder may modify serum lipids and reduce inflammatory markers (Kim et al 2011b).

CLINICAL USE

Prevention of UTI

A number of controlled clinical trials support the use of cranberry products (solid-dose form and juice) in the prevention of UTIs in women experiencing recurrent infections; however, the heterogeneity of studies makes a clear interpretation difficult. There is emerging evidence to suggest that cranberry juice with high concentrations of Type A proanthocyanidin may be more effective than other forms; however further studies are required to assess this (Afshar et al 2012).

A significant preventive effect was concluded in a 2012 systematic review and meta-analysis of 10 randomised controlled trials (RCTs) which included 1494 subjects (Wang et al 2012). Wang et al reported that, on subgroup analysis, cranberry-containing products seemed to be more effective in several subgroups, including women with recurrent UTIs (relative risk [RR] 0.53), female populations (RR 0.49), children (RR 0.33), cranberry juice drinkers (RR 0.47) and subjects using cranberry-containing products more than twice daily (RR 0.58). While the conclusion was positive, authors cautioned that the results should be interpreted in the context of substantial heterogeneity across the studies.

In contrast, a 2012 Cochrane review evaluated data from RCTs and also quasi-RCTs of cranberry products for the prevention of UTIs in all populations (n = 4473) and concluded that there is no statistically significant difference between cranberry and placebo for the prevention of UTIs (Jepson et al 2012). The effects of cranberry/cranberry-lingonberry juice versus placebo, juice, lactobacillus, antibiotics or water were evaluated in 13 studies (with amounts ranging from 30 mL to 1000 mL), and cranberry tablets versus placebo in nine studies (daily dose range from 400 mg to 2000 mg); one study evaluated both juice and tablets. Overall, cranberry products did not significantly reduce the incidence of UTIs at 12 months compared with placebo/control. Cranberry products showed a small benefit in some of the smaller studies for women with recurrent UTIs; however no significant benefit was seen in the elderly, pregnant women, children with recurrent UTIs, cancer patients, those with neuropathic bladder or spinal injury or people requiring catheterisation. Only one study reported a significant result for the outcome of symptomatic UTIs. One study (McMurdo et al 2009) showed that cranberry treatment was as effective as an antibiotic. Beerepoot et al (2011) did not get the same result. Gurley (2011) suggests the negative result with Beerepoot was because he used a cranberry treatment whereby the quantity of type-A proanthocyanidins used amounted to only 9 mg/g, making the amount of free proanthocyanidins reaching the urinary tract of study participants less than 1 mg/day. Side effects were common in all studies, and dropouts/withdrawals in several of the studies were high (Jepson et al 2012).

Why the conflicting conclusions?

The systematic review and meta-analysis completed by Wang et al, also in 2012, reported conflicting results, possibly due to the significant heterogeneity of the trials, making the literature difficult to evaluate in a meaningful way. The Wang review confirmed the findings of the earlier 2008 Cochrane review, concluding that cranberry products were effective especially for women with recurrent UTIs. It excluded the Barbosa-Cesnik RCT of women with recurrent UTIs (Barbosa-Cesnik et al 2011), as they inadvertently used ascorbic acid in the placebo. As this in itself may reduce UTIs, it may have masked the effects of cranberry, especially as the authors expected the placebo arm to have 30% recurrence of UTIs and the rate was only 14%. The study also used the lowest threshold of bacteria in the urine to determine a UTI (Wang et al 2012). Gurley (2011) reports that the amount of type A procyanidin present in the test extracts needs to be of a sufficient quantity to have an effect, as they tend to have very poor bioavailability and some studies, such as Beerepoot et al (2011), use extracts with insufficient amounts.

Since these two reviews were published, further RCTs have also been published.

A clear protective effect and significant decrease in the rate of relapse were seen amongst women aged aged over 50 years taking cranberry juice in a double-blind RCT by Takahashi et al (2013). The study involved 118 women aged 20–79, given 125 mL of cranberry juice to drink daily before going to sleep over a 24-week period. In a subgroup analysis of women aged over 50 years, relapse of UTI was observed in 16 of 55 (29.1%) patients drinking cranberry juice compared with 31 of 63 (49.2%) in the placebo group.

In 2012, an RCT of 176 premenopausal women with a history of UTIs found cranberry juice (120–240 mL/day) demonstrated a potentially protective effect with a hazard ratio for UTI of 0.68 compared with placebo, but it was not statistically significant. In addition, researchers found that the group ingesting cranberry juice had reduced infection with P-fimbriated *E. coli* strains, which suggests benefits from cranberry juice therapy are possible and confirms the antiadhesion mechanism clinically. One major limitation of this study was that it was underpowered to show a significant effect of cranberry on the cumulative rate of UTI, as they did not achieve the necessary sample size (Stapleton et al 2012).

A concentrated cranberry liquid blend (UTI-Stat with Proantinox) was tested for safety, tolerability and maximal tolerated dose in 28 women with a history of recurrent UTI and an average age of 46 years. A secondary outcome was UTI recurrence.The secondary end points demonstrated that 2 (9.1%) of 23 women reported a recurrent UTI, a rate considered superior to their historical data. At 12 weeks, there was a significant reduction in worry about recurrent infection and increased quality of life in regard to the physical functioning domain and role limitations from physical health domain, as measured by the Medical Outcomes Study short-form 36-item questionnaire ($P = 0.0097$). A lower American Urological Association Symptom Index indicating greater quality of life was also significant ($P = 0.045$) (Efros et al 2010).

Another RCT with 137 women aged 45 years or older, who had experienced cystitis at least twice in the past year and been treated with antibiotics, were given a 500 mg cranberry capsule (Cran-Max, Buckton Scott Health Products, UK) at bedtime for a period of 6 months or 100 mg of the antibiotic trimethoprim. Overall, 28% of women experienced a UTI during the study (25 in the cranberry group and 14 in the trimethoprim group), with median time to recurrence of 84.5 days for the cranberry group and 91 days for the trimethoprim group. Trimethoprim was more effective at reducing UTIs in older women in this study but it was not statistically significant and compared with cranberry the trimethoprim conferred only 7 extra UTI-free days. Cranberry may be a cheaper, better-tolerated option for recurrent UTI treatment in older women and does not carry the risk of antimicrobial antibiotic resistance (McMurdo et al 2009).

Renal transplant patients

A small retrospective trial of 82 renal transplant patients receiving cranberry juice (2 × 50 mL/day) found the annual number of UTI episodes was reduced by 63.9% (Pagonas et al 2012).

Spinal cord injuries

Patients with spinal cord injuries are a high-risk group for catheter-associated UTIs, so cranberry products are popular in this group. One double-blind, factorial-design, RCT of 305 people with spinal cord injuries showed no significant UTI-free period compared to placebo when taking 800 mg of cranberry tablets twice daily (Lee et al 2007), while another randomised, double-blind, placebo-controlled, crossover trial in 47 patients with spinal cord injury demonstrated a significant reduction in the frequency of UTIs (Hess et al 2008). An open pilot study involving 15 volunteers with spinal cord injuries showed that three glasses of cranberry juice daily significantly reduced the adhesion of Gram-negative and Gram-positive bacteria to uroepithelial cells (Reid 2002). Treatment using catheter device with proanthocyanidin solutions has also been shown to inhibit adhesion of bacteria to non-biological particles such as PVC (Eydelnant & Tufenkji 2008). While these results are promising, a 2010 review of five studies of spinal cord injury patients reported that there is limited evidence that cranberry may be helpful in preventing or treating UTIs and suggests that more rigorous research is required (Opperman 2010).

Radiotherapy and UTI prevention

Bladder infections are a common side effect of radiotherapy for prostate cancer. This controlled trial of 370 patients who were receiving radiotherapy for prostate cancer in an Italian hospital were given a 200 mg enteric-coated tablet (VO370 or Monoselect Macrocarpon) containing standardised cranberry extract titrated as 30% proanthocyanidins. This trial took place over 6–7 weeks and a significant reduction was found in the number of UTIs and recurrent UTIs in the treatment group vs controls. Good compliance and only two gastric complaints were reported. It was also found to help reduce urinary symptoms of dysuria, nocturia, urinary frequency and urgency (Bonetta & Di Pierro 2012).

Gynaecological surgery and UTI prevention

The short-term use of cranberry capsules produced no statistically significant difference in UTI incidence in a cohort of 286 women undergoing gynaecological surgery. The treatment group received cranberry capsules for 4 days prior to surgery and 5 days postoperatively (Cadkova et al 2009).

Children

Catheterisation and renal disease

Cranberry use is popular for children with renal disease. An anonymous survey of 117 parents of children seen in a hospital paediatric nephrology clinic identified that 29% gave cranberry products to their children to treat as well as prevent diverse renal problems (Super et al 2005). Most parents felt that it was beneficial and only one reported an adverse reaction (nausea).

Two studies conducted in children managed by clean intermittent catheterisation found no clinical or statistical difference in the number of symptomatic UTIs observed in either the cranberry or the placebo group (Foda et al 1995, Schlager et al 1999). Foda et al used a dose of 5 mL/kg/day of cranberry cocktail for 6 months and the dose used by Schlager et al was 2 oz (≈55 g) of cranberry concentrate.

Recurrent UTIs in children

There has been a recent Cochrane systematic review and a meta-analysis by Wang et al, both published in 2012 and both reporting different conclusions. The Cochrane review found no significant difference of cranberry compared to placebo in children with recurrent UTIs (RR 0.48, 95% confidence interval [CI] 0.19–1.22); whereas the Wang meta-analysis concluded benefit for children (RR 0.33; 95% CI 0.16–0.69). The Cochrane review included three studies, one RCT (Ferrara et al 2009) of 84 girls randomised to cranberry (50 mL daily), *Lactobacillus* or control for 6 months, and reported that daily cranberry drink significantly reduced recurrent UTIs in children. Also in the Cochrane review was a study by Salo et al (2012) which was a randomised placebo-controlled trial with 263 children recruited in seven hospitals in Finland reported no significant difference in the number of children with recurrent UTIs, although there was a non-significant reduction, with 20 children (16%) in the cranberry group and 28 (22%) in the placebo group experiencing a recurrent UTI (difference −6%; 95% CI −16 to 4%; $P = 0.21$). The cranberry juice dose was 5 mL/kg up to 300 mL per day. Although cranberry did not significantly reduce the number of children with a UTI, the authors reported a significant reduction in the number of times a child got a UTI and also the number of days the child needed to take antibiotics.

The third study (Uberos et al 2010) mentioned in the Cochrane review was dismissed as it was unclear about whether they were testing for a UTI or just a positive culture. Uberos et al did report that cranberry syrup was equally effective to trimethoprim for recurrent UTIs in their population of 192 children.

The Wang meta-analysis included only the Ferrara study for children with recurrent UTIs and report that the current data support the use of cranberry products in children with UTIs, although suggest that more trials are needed. Overall the differences in the two meta-analyses appear to be that Wang did not include either the Salo et al (2012) or the Uberos et al (2010) trials. The difference in the individual trial results may be explained by the variety of cranberry products used and the dosage levels (for children, dosage may need to be adjusted by body weight), although in general the trend on all the trials is towards benefit for children with recurrent UTIs.

A later RCT looked at a cranberry juice with high concentrations of proanthocyanidin and compared that to regular cranberry juice for 1 year. There were 40 children in the study and the incidence of infection in the treatment group of high proanthocyanidins was 0.4 per patient per year and 1.15 in the placebo group, showing a 65% reduction in the risk of UTIs in non-febrile children (Afshar et al 2012). This high-proanthocyanidin-containing cranberry juice shows promise and further investigation is warranted.

Treatment of UTI

Although cranberry may be a viable adjunctive treatment in UTI when antibiotic resistance is encountered, there is no reliable evidence that it is an effective sole treatment in diagnosed UTI (Ulbricht & Basch 2005). One study of pregnant women demonstrated comparable effects of daily cranberry juice mixture to those of placebo for asymptomatic bacteriuria and symptomatic UTIs; however, the results were not statistically significant and more than one-third of participants withdrew from the study because of gastrointestinal upset (Wing et al 2008). In another study, cranberry exhibited only weak antimicrobial activity in urine specimens of symptom-free subjects after ingestion of a single dose (Lee et al 2010).

Nephroprotection

Cranberries have an antioxidant function and may prevent infection-induced oxidative renal damage. Animal studies suggest that cranberries might be used clinically as a beneficial adjuvant treatment to prevent damage due to pyelonephritis in children with vesicoureteric reflux (Han et al 2007).

OTHER USES

Gout

Cranberry juice has been used to treat gout. Evidence of increased uric acid excretion in humans provides a theoretical basis for the indication, although studies in patients with gout are not available to confirm effectiveness (Kessler et al 2002).

Oral hygiene

The antiadhesion effect of cranberry on oral microbial flora has been demonstrated in vitro (Bodet et al 2008, Koo et al 2006, Polak et al 2013, Yamanaka et al 2007). More specifically, cranberry polyphenol fraction significantly decreased the hydrophobicity of oral streptococci in a dose-dependent manner, suggesting that it may reduce bacterial adherence to the tooth surface (Yamanaka-Okada et al 2008). It has been shown in vitro to prevent biofilm formation and reduce adherence of *Candida albicans* and so may have a role in the prevention or treatment of oral candidiasis (Feldman et al 2012). The same research group also found the synergy of cranberry proanthocyanidins and licochalcone A inhibited *Porphyromonas gingivalis* growth and biofilm formation, offering potential in the treatment and prevention of periodontal disease (Feldman & Grenier 2012).

Prevention and treatment of *Helicobacter* infection

Cranberry inhibits the adhesion of *H. pylori* to human gastrointestinal cells in vitro (Matsushima et al 2008); however, very little clinical evidence is available to confirm significance in humans (Burger et al 2002). A multicentre, randomised controlled, double-blind trial found that regular intake of cranberry juice or a probiotic inhibited *H. pylori* in a trial of 295 children (Gotteland et al 2008). Another double-blind, randomised clinical study was carried out in 177 patients with *H. pylori* infection to investigate the possible additive effect of cranberry juice to triple therapy with omeprazole, amoxicillin and clarithromycin. Overall, there was no statistically significant difference; however, analysis by gender showed that the eradication rate was higher in females taking cranberry, but not in males (Shmuely et al 2007).

Cardioprotection

Consumption of 250 mL cranberry juice daily is associated with decreasing markers of oxidative stress (Ruel et al 2008) and a significant increase in plasma high-density lipoprotein (HDL) cholesterol concentration (Ruel et al 2006). A small study of 30 abdominally obese, healthy, middle-aged men who consumed increasing doses of cranberry juice, up to 500 mL/day over 12 weeks, found a significant reduction in plasma matrix metalloproteinase-9, a substance which can accelerate atherosclerotic progression (Ruel et al 2009). The same authors recruited 35 overweight men in an RCT using an intervention of 500 mL/day of low-calorie cranberry juice or placebo juice. In a 4-week trial there was no significant difference in the cardiometabolic parameters but some benefit was noted in the augmentation index measuring arterial stiffness (Ruel et al 2013). These potential cardioprotective effects (which may be useful in reducing hypertension and atherosclerotic plaque vulnerability) need larger studies to confirm the findings. In addition, cranberry extract increases cholesterol uptake and the synthesis of low-density lipoprotein (LDL) receptors (Chu & Liu 2005), suggesting that accelerated cholesterol excretion may occur in vivo (McKay & Blumberg 2007). An oestrogen-deficient animal model found improvements in cholesterol parameters and endothelial function and suggested that cranberry juice consumption may be a useful food for postmenopausal women (Yung et al 2013).

Type 2 diabetes

Some studies have suggested that consumption of a low-calorie cranberry juice is associated with a favourable glycaemic response (Wilson et al 2008a, 2008b). In a double-blind RCT, 60 males with type 2 diabetes, some of whom were taking oral hypoglycaemic drugs, were asked to drink one cup of cranberry juice daily for 12 weeks or placebo. A significant decrease in serum glucose and apolipoprotein B and a significant increase in serum apolipoprotein A-1 and paraoxonase 1 activity in the cranberry juice group resulted. The authors concluded that cranberry juice may assist in the management of type 2 diabetic males to reduce cardiovascular disease risk factors (Shidfar et al 2012). However, a randomised, placebo-controlled, double-blind study of 16 males and 14 females demonstrated that a 500 mg capsule of cranberry extract had a neutral effect on glycaemic control in type 2 diabetics who were on oral glucose-lowering medication. This same study found, however, that cranberry supplements are effective in reducing atherosclerotic cholesterol profiles, including LDL cholesterol and total cholesterol levels, as well as total:HDL cholesterol ratio in people with type 2 diabetes (Lee et al 2008). A study of 13 participants with type 2 diabetes, attempting to find palatable options for food choices, found that raw cranberries and sweetened dried cranberries containing less sugar and with polydextrose added as a bulking agent significantly improved glycaemic control when compared to sweetened dried cranberries alone or white bread (Wilson et al 2010).

Prostate health

A trial of 42 men at risk of prostate disease (with negative prostate biopsy) with UTIs, elevated prostate-specific antigen (PSA) and chronic non-bacterial prostatitis were prescribed cranberry powder (1500 mg) for 6 months, with the control group receiving no treatment. The treatment group showed benefits with statistically significant improvement in International Prostate Symptom Score, quality of life, urination parameters and lower total PSA levels (Vidlar et al 2009, 2010). More research is required to confirm these promising findings.

Urinary deodorising activity

Cranberry juice and solid-dose forms are popular in nursing homes as urinary deodorising agents in older adults with incontinence. Although no clinical study is available to confirm efficacy, numerous anecdotal reports suggest that it is useful when used on a regular basis.

DOSAGE RANGE

Preventing UTI

According to clinical studies

- Adults: 120–400 mL daily or 400–500 mg capsule 1–3 times daily.
- Children: 15 mL/kg or up to 300 mL daily.

In practice, much higher doses are being used in an attempt to achieve quicker results (e.g. cranberry capsules or tablets 10,000 mg/day for prevention).

Recent studies reveal that cranberry extract regimens containing 72 mg of type-A proanthocyanidins produced significant bacterial anti-adhesion activity in human urine, therefore the dose of bioavailable type-A proanthocyanidins is important to consider (Gurley 2011).

ADVERSE REACTIONS

At high doses (3 L or greater), gastrointestinal discomfort and diarrhoea can occur (Ulbricht & Basch 2005).

SIGNIFICANT INTERACTIONS

The composition of bioactive components of cranberry juice can vary substantially and there is potential for drug interaction (Ngo et al 2009).

CYP3 A substrates

Whether cranberry juice inhibits the metabolism of drugs chiefly metabolised by CYP3A isoenzymes appears to be dependent on the concentration of three triterpenes (maslinic acid, corosolic acid and ursolic acid) in the juice (Kim et al 2011a). These have been identified as the important constituents responsible for inhibiting intestinal CYP3A and most likely explain the interbrand differences seen in various clinical and preclinical trials.

Caution — monitor patients taking high-strength cranberry preparations and medicines chiefly metabolised by CYP3A. Special care should be taken if the medicines have a narrow therapeutic index.

Proton pump inhibitors

Cranberry juice increases the absorption of vitamin B_{12} when used concurrently with proton pump inhibitor medicines (Saltzman et al 1994) — beneficial interaction.

Warfarin

There are a small number of case reports suggesting that cranberry juice may increase the international normalised ratio (INR) in patients taking warfarin; however, clinical pharmacokinetic studies have found no clinically relevant interaction between cranberry and warfarin (Ansell et al 2008, Pham & Pham 2007), changes to the anticoagulant activity of warfarin or a significant effect on the activities of CYP2C9, CYP1A2 or CYP3A4 (Lilja et al 2007). Other clinical studies have found a daily glass of cranberry juice has no significant effect on INR compared to placebo (Ansell et al 2009) and two glasses of cranberry juice daily do not change prothrombin times (Mellen et al 2010). Ansell et al (2009) conducted an RCT with 30 patients on stable warfarin anticoagulation (international normalised ratio [INR], 1.7–3.3) and found 240 mL of CJ had no effect on plasma S- or R-warfarin plasma levels, thereby excluding a pharmacokinetic interaction.

An earlier study suggests that a pharmacodynamic interaction is more likely (Mohammed Abdul et al 2008).

In regard to the case reports, a systematic review concluded that the suggested drug interactions were questionable and that moderate consumption of cranberry juice was unlikely to affect coagulation (Zikria et al 2010).

Until the interaction can be better understood, patients taking warfarin with cranberry juice should continue to monitor their INR changes and signs and symptoms of bleeding.

CONTRAINDICATIONS AND PRECAUTIONS

People with diabetes should take care when using commercially prepared cranberry juices because of the high sugar content.

If symptoms of UTI become more severe while cranberry is being administered, other treatments may be required and medical advice is recommended.

Cranberries contain oxalates and theoretically this could encourage kidney stone formation. People with a history of oxalate kidney stones should therefore limit their intake of cranberry juice.

PREGNANCY USE

Women experience UTIs with greater frequency during pregnancy. A systematic review of the literature for evidence on the use, safety and pharmacology of cranberry, focusing on issues pertaining to pregnancy and lactation, found that there is no direct evidence of safety or harm to the mother or fetus as a result of consuming cranberry during pregnancy. A survey of 400 pregnant women did not uncover any adverse events when cranberry was regularly consumed. In lactation, the safety or harm of cranberry is unknown (Dugoua et al 2008). Recent trials have not shown evidence for benefit of cranberry juice in preventing UTIs in pregnant women so, although it has a good safety profile, its benefit may be limited.

Practice points/Patient counselling

- Cranberry preparations are widely used to prevent minor UTIs.
- Overall, clinical testing suggests that cranberry products, particularly the juice, with high concentrations of type-A proanthocyanidin may have some benefits for UTI prevention in certain populations.
- It may be more effective to take the cranberry products more than twice daily.
- Cranberry exerts bacteriostatic effects by reducing bacterial adhesion to host tissues.
- Overall, evidence suggests no significant alteration to urinary pH at doses less than 330 mL daily.
- Cranberry products have also been used to treat gout and to deodorise urine in people with incontinence.
- Preliminary research suggests a possible role in preventing conditions such as *Helicobacter pylori* infection, dental plaque formation and periodontal disease, managing glucose control in type 2 diabetes, prostate health and reducing cardiovascular risk among type 2 diabetics.
- Patients taking warfarin and regular cranberry intake should have their INR monitored.

PATIENTS' FAQS

What will this herb do for me?

Cranberry products, in particular the juice, with high concentrations of proanthocyanidin, may reduce the risk of developing UTI in some populations.

When will it start to work?

Studies using 1–2 glasses of cranberry juice suggest that 4–8 weeks' continual use is required.

Are there any safety issues?

If fever or pain exists or symptoms of UTI become more severe, seek medical advice. People taking warfarin together with cranberry should monitor their INR for changes. People taking concentrated cranberry juice should also check with their healthcare provider if also taking medication to avoid drug interactions.

REFERENCES

Afshar, K et al. 2012. Cranberry juice for the prevention of pediatric urinary tract infection: a randomized controlled trial. J Urol, 188, 1584–7.

Ahuja S, et al. Loss of fimbrial adhesion with the addition of *Vaccinium macrocarpon* to the growth medium of P-fimbriated *Escherichia coli*. J Urol 159.2 (1998): 559–562.

Ansell, J., et al. 2008. A randomized, double-blind trial of the interaction between cranberry juice and warfarin. Journal of Thrombosis and Thrombolysis, 25, 112–112.

Avorn J et al. Reduction of bacteriuria and pyuria after ingestion of cranberry juice. JAMA 271.10 (1994): 751–754.

Barbosa-Cesnik, C, et al. 2011. Cranberry juice fails to prevent recurrent urinary tract infection: results from a randomized placebo-controlled trial. Clin Infect Dis, 52, 23–30.

Beerepoot MA, ter RG, Nys S, van der Wal WM, de Borgie CA, de Reijke TM, et al. Cranberries vs antibiotics to prevent urinary tract infections: a randomized double-blind noninferiority trial in premenopausal women. Arch Intern Med 171(14) (2011): 1270–1278.

Bodet C et al. Potential oral health benefits of cranberry. Crit Rev Food Sci Nutr 48.7 (2008): 672–680.

Bonetta, A. & Di Pierro, F. 2012. Enteric-coated, highly standardized cranberry extract reduces risk of UTIs and urinary symptoms during radiotherapy for prostate carcinoma. Cancer Manag Res, 4, 281–6.

Burger O et al. Inhibition of *Helicobacter pylori* adhesion to human gastric mucus by a high-molecular-weight constituent of cranberry juice. Crit Rev Food Sci Nutr 42.3 (Suppl) (2002): 279–284.

Cadkova, I., et al. 2009. [Effect of cranberry extract capsules taken during the perioperative period upon the post-surgical urinary infection in gynecology.] Ceska Gynekol, 74, 454–8.

Chatelain K et al. Cranberry and grape seed extracts inhibit the proliferative phenotype of oral squamous cell carcinomas. Evid Based Complement Altern Med (2008); 2011: 467691.

Chu YF, Liu RH. Cranberries inhibit LDL oxidation and induce LDL receptor expression in hepatocytes. Life Sci 77 (2005): 1892–1901.

Côté, J., et al. 2011. Antimicrobial effect of cranberry juice and extracts. Food Control, 22, 1413–1418.

Dugoua JJ et al. Safety and efficacy of cranberry (*Vaccinium macrocarpon*) during pregnancy and lactation. Can J Clin Pharmacol 15.1 (2008): e80–e86.

Efros, M., et al. 2010. Novel Concentrated Cranberry Liquid Blend, UTI-STAT With Proantinox, Might Help Prevent Recurrent Urinary Tract Infections in Women. Urology, 76, 841–845.

Eydelnant IA, Tufenkji N. Cranberry derived proanthocyanidins reduce bacterial adhesion to selected biomaterials. Langmuir 24.18 (2008): 10273–10281.

Feldman, M. & Grenier, D. 2012. Cranberry proanthocyanidins act in synergy with licochalcone A to reduce *Porphyromonas gingivalis* growth and virulence properties, and to suppress cytokine secretion by macrophages. J Appl Microbiol, 113, 438–47.

Feldman, M., et al. 2012. Cranberry proanthocyanidins inhibit the adherence properties of *Candida albicans* and cytokine secretion by oral epithelial cells. BMC Complement Altern Med, 12, 6.

Ferrara P et al. Cranberry juice for the prevention of recurrent urinary tract infections: a randomized controlled trial in children. Scand J Urol Nephrol 43.5 (2009): 369–372.

Ferguson PJ et al. In vivo inhibition of growth of human tumor lines by flavonoid fractions from cranberry extract. Nutr Cancer 56.1 (2006): 86–94.

Foda MM et al. Efficacy of cranberry in prevention of urinary tract infection in a susceptible pediatric population. Can J Urol 2.1 (1995): 98–102.

Gotteland M et al. Modulation of *Helicobacter pylori* colonization with cranberry juice and *Lactobacillus johnsonii* La1 in children. Nutrition 24.5 (2008): 421–426.

Greenblatt, D.J., et al. 2006. Interaction of flurbiprofen with cranberry juice, grape juice, tea, and fluconazole: in vitro and clinical studies. Clin.Pharmacol.Ther., 79, (1) 125–133.

Grenier, J., et al. 2006. Pomelo juice, but not cranberry juice, affects the pharmacokinetics of cyclosporine in humans. Clin.Pharmacol.Ther., 79, (3) 255–262.

Gupta K et al. Cranberry products inhibit adherence of P-fimbriated *Escherichia coli* to primary cultured bladder and vaginal epithelial cells. J Urol 177.6 (2007): 2357–2360.

Gurley B. Cranberries as Antibiotics? Comment on 'Cranberries vs Antibiotics to Prevent Urinary Tract Infections: A Randomized Double-Blind Noninferiority Trial in Premenopausal Women' Arch Intern Med 171.14 (2011): 1279–1280.

Hakkinen SH et al. Content of the flavonols quercetin, myricetin, and kaempferol in 25 edible berries. J Agric Food Chem 47.6 (1999): 2274–2279.

Han CH et al. Protective effects of cranberries on infection-induced oxidative renal damage in a rabbit model of vesico-ureteric reflux. BJU Int 100.5 (2007): 1172–1175.

Hess MJ et al. Evaluation of cranberry tablets for the prevention of urinary tract infections in spinal cord injured patients with neurogenic bladder. Spinal Cord 46.9 (2008): 622–626.

Hochman N et al. Cranberry juice constituents impair lymphoma growth and augment the generation of antilymphoma antibodies in syngeneic mice. Nutr Cancer 60.4 (2008): 511–517.

Huttunen, S., et al. 2011. Inhibition activity of wild berry juice fractions against *Streptococcus pneumoniae* binding to human bronchial cells. Phytother Res, 25, 122–7.

Jepson, R. G., et al. 2012. Cranberries for preventing urinary tract infections. Cochrane Database Syst Rev, 10, CD001321.

Johnson BJ et al. Impact of cranberry on *Escherichia coli* cellular surface characteristics. Biochem Biophys Res Commun 377.3 (2008): 992–994.

Kessler T, et al. Effect of blackcurrant-, cranberry- and plum juice consumption on risk factors associated with kidney stone formation. Eur J Clin Nutr 56.10 (2002): 1020–1023.

Kim, E., et al. 2011a. Isolation and identification of intestinal CYP3A inhibitors from cranberry (*Vaccinium macrocarpon*) using human intestinal microsomes. Planta Med, 77, 265–70.

Kim, M. J., et al. 2011b. Effects of freeze-dried cranberry powder on serum lipids and inflammatory markers in lipopolysaccharide treated rats fed an atherogenic diet. Nutr Res Pract, 5, 404–11.

Kim, K. K., et al. 2012. Anti-angiogenic activity of cranberry proanthocyanidins and cytotoxic properties in ovarian cancer cells. Int J Oncol, 40, 227–35.

Koo H et al. Influence of cranberry juice on glucan-mediated processes involved in *Streptococcus mutans* biofilm development. Caries Res 40.1 (2006): 20–27.

Kresty LA, et al. Cranberry proanthocyanidins induce apoptosis and inhibit acid-induced proliferation of human esophageal adenocarcinoma cells. J Agric Food Chem 56.3 (2008): 676–680.

Lacombe, A., et al. 2010. Antimicrobial action of the American cranberry constituents; phenolics, anthocyanins, and organic acids, against *Escherichia coli* O157:H7. Int J Food Microbiol, 139, 102–7.

Laplante, K. L., et al. 2012. Effects of cranberry extracts on growth and biofilm production of *Escherichia coli* and *Staphylococcus* species. Phytother Res, 26, 1371–4.

Lee BB et al. Spinal-injured neuropathic bladder antisepsis (SINBA) trial. Spinal Cord 45.8 (2007): 542–550.

Lee IT et al. Effect of cranberry extracts on lipid profiles in subjects with type 2 diabetes. Diabet Med 25.12 (2008): 1473–7.

Lee YL et al. Anti-microbial activity of urine after ingestion of cranberry: a pilot study. Evid Based Complement Alternat Med (2010); 7: 227–232.

Leshem, R., et al. 2011. The effect of nondialyzable material (NDM) cranberry extract on formation of contact lens biofilm by *Staphylococcus epidermidis*. Invest Ophthalmol Vis Sci, 52, 4929–34.

Lilja JJ, et al. Effects of daily ingestion of cranberry juice on the pharmacokinetics of warfarin, tizanidine, and midazolam—probes of CYP2C9, CYP1A2, and CYP3A4. Clin Pharmacol Ther 81.6 (2007): 833–839.

Lipson SM et al. Antiviral effects on bacteriophages and rotavirus by cranberry juice. Phytomedicine 14.1 (2007): 23–30.

Liu Y et al. Cranberry changes the physicochemical surface properties of *E. coli* and adhesion with uroepithelial cells. Colloids Surf B Biointerfaces 65.1 (2008): 35–42.

Liu, M., et al. 2009. Cranberry phytochemical extract inhibits SGC-7901 cell growth and human tumor xenografts in Balb/c nu/nu mice. J Agric Food Chem, 57, 762–8.

MacLean, M. A., et al. 2011. North American cranberry (*Vaccinium macrocarpon*) stimulates apoptotic pathways in DU145 human prostate cancer cells in vitro. Nutr Cancer, 63, 109–20.

Magarinos HL et al. In vitro inhibitory effect of cranberry (*Vaccinium macrocarpon* Ait.) juice on pathogenic microorganisms. Prikl Biokhim Mikrobiol 44.3 (2008): 333–336.

Matsushima M et al. Growth inhibitory action of cranberry on *Helicobacter pylori*. J Gastroenterol Hepatol 23 (Suppl 2) (2008): S175–S180.

McKay DL, Blumberg JB. Cranberries (*Vaccinium macrocarpon*) and cardiovascular disease risk factors. Nutr Rev 65.11 (2007): 490–502.

McMurdo, M. E. T., et al. 2009. Cranberry or trimethoprim for the prevention of recurrent urinary tract infections? A randomized controlled trial in older women. Journal of Antimicrobial Chemotherapy, 63, 389–395.

Mellen, C. K., et al. 2010. Effect of high-dose cranberry juice on the pharmacodynamics of warfarin in patients. Br J Clin Pharmacol, 70, 139–42.

Mohammed Abdul MI et al. Pharmacodynamic interaction of warfarin with cranberry but not with garlic in healthy subjects. Br J Pharmacol 154.8 (2008): 1691–1700.

Nahata MC et al. Effect of urinary acidifiers on formaldehyde concentration and efficacy with methenamine therapy. Eur J Clin Pharmacol 22.3 (1982): 281–284.

Neto CC, et al. Anticancer activities of cranberry phytochemicals: an update. Mol Nutr Food Res 52 (Suppl 1) (2008): S18–S27.

Ngo N et al. Identification of a cranberry juice product that inhibits enteric CYP3A-mediated first-pass metabolism in humans. Drug Metab Dispos 37.3 (2009): 514–522.

Opperman, E. A. 2010. Cranberry is not effective for the prevention or treatment of urinary tract infections in individuals with spinal cord injury. Spinal Cord, 48, 451–6.

Pagonas, N., et al. 2012. Prophylaxis of Recurrent Urinary Tract Infection After Renal Transplantation by Cranberry Juice and L-Methionine. Transplantation Proceedings, 44, 3017–3021.

Patel, K. D., et al. 2011. Proanthocyanidin-rich extracts from cranberry fruit (*Vaccinium macrocarpon* Ait.) selectively inhibit the growth of human pathogenic fungi *Candida* spp. and *Cryptococcus neoformans*. J Agric Food Chem, 59, 12864–73.

Pham DQ, Pham AQ. Interaction potential between cranberry juice and warfarin. Am J Health Syst Pharm 64.5 (2007): 490–494.

Pinto Mda, S., et al. 2010. Potential of cranberry powder for management of hyperglycemia using in vitro models. J Med Food, 13, 1036–44.

C

Polak, D., et al. 2013. The Protective Potential of Non-Dialysable Material Fraction of Cranberry Juice on the Virulence of P. Gingivalis and F. Nucleatum Mixed Infection. J Periodontol 84: 1019–1025.

Prasain JK et al. Effect of cranberry juice concentrate on chemically-induced urinary bladder cancers. Oncol Rep 19.6 (2008): 1565–1570.

Reid G. The role of cranberry and probiotics in intestinal and urogenital tract health. Crit Rev Food Sci Nutr 42.3 (Suppl) (2002): 293–300.

Ruel G et al. Favourable impact of low-calorie cranberry juice consumption on plasma HDL-cholesterol concentrations in men. Br J Nutr 96.2 (2006): 357–364.

Ruel G et al. Low-calorie cranberry juice supplementation reduces plasma oxidized LDL and cell adhesion molecule concentrations in men. Br J Nutr 99.2 (2008): 352–359.

Ruel, G., et al. 2009. Plasma matrix metalloproteinase (MMP)-9 levels are reduced following low-calorie cranberry juice supplementation in men. J Am Coll Nutr, 28, 694–701.

Ruel, G., et al. 2013. Evidence that cranberry juice may improve augmentation index in overweight men. Nutrition Research, 33, 41–49.

Salo J et al. Cranberry juice for the prevention of recurrences of urinary tract infections in children: a randomized placebo-controlled trial. Clin Infect Dis 54.3 (2012): 340–346.

Saltzman JR et al. Effect of hypochlorhydria due to omeprazole treatment or atrophic gastritis on protein-bound vitamin B12 absorption. J Am Coll Nutr 13.6 (1994): 584–591.

Schlager TA et al. Effect of cranberry juice on bacteriuria in children with neurogenic bladder receiving intermittent catheterization. J Pediatr 135.6 (1999): 698–702.

Sharon N, Ofek I. Fighting infectious diseases with inhibitors of microbial adhesion to host tissues. Crit Rev Food Sci Nutr 42.3 (Suppl) (2002): 267–272.

Shidfar, F., et al. 2012. The effects of cranberry juice on serum glucose, apoB, apoA-I, Lp(a), and Paraoxonase-1 activity in type 2 diabetic male patients. J Res Med Sci, 17, 355–60.

Shmuely H et al. Effect of cranberry juice on eradication of *Helicobacter pylori* in patients treated with antibiotics and a proton pump inhibitor. Mol Nutr Food Res 51.6 (2007): 746–751.

Singh AP et al. Cranberry proanthocyanidins are cytotoxic to human cancer cells and sensitize platinum-resistant ovarian cancer cells to paraplatin. Phytother Res 23.8 (2009): 1066–1074.

Sobota AE. Inhibition of bacterial adherence by cranberry juice: potential use for the treatment of urinary tract infections. J Urol 131.5 (1984): 1013–10116.

Stapleton, A. E., et al. 2012. Recurrent urinary tract infection and urinary *Escherichia coli* in women ingesting cranberry juice daily: a randomized controlled trial. Mayo Clin Proc, 87, 143–50.

Su, X., et al. 2012. Antibacterial effects of plant-derived extracts on methicillin-resistant *Staphylococcus aureus*. Foodborne Pathog Dis, 9, 573–8.

Sun J, Hai Liu R. Cranberry phytochemical extracts induce cell cycle arrest and apoptosis in human MCF-7 breast cancer cells. Cancer Lett 241.1 (2006): 124–134.

Super EA et al. Cranberry use among pediatric nephrology patients. Ambul Pediatr 5.4 (2005): 249–252.

Takahashi, S., et al. 2013. A randomized clinical trial to evaluate the preventive effect of cranberry juice (UR65) for patients with recurrent urinary tract infection. J Infect Chemother 19: 112–117.

Uberos J et al. Urinary excretion of phenolic acids by infants and children: a randomised double-blind clinical assay. Clin Med Insights Pediatr 6 (2012): 67–74.

Ulbricht CE, Basch EM. Natural standard herb and supplement reference. St Louis: Mosby, 2005.

Ushijima, K., et al. 2009. Cranberry juice suppressed the diclofenac metabolism by human liver microsomes, but not in healthy human subjects. Br J Clin.Pharmacol., 68, (2) 194–200.

Vidlar, A., et al. 2009. C10 Beneficial effects of cranberries on prostate health: Evidence from a randomized controlled trial. European Urology Supplements, 8, 660.

Vidlar, A., et al. 2010. The effectiveness of dried cranberries (*Vaccinium macrocarpon*) in men with lower urinary tract symptoms. Br J Nutr, 104, 1181–9.

Villarreal A et al. Cranberry juice improved antioxidant status without affecting bone quality in orchidectomized male rats. Phytomedicine 14.12 (2007): 815–820.

Vinson JA et al. Cranberries and cranberry products: powerful in vitro, ex vivo, and in vivo sources of antioxidants. J Agric Food Chem 56.14 (2008): 5884–5891.

Vu, K. D., et al. 2012. Effect of different cranberry extracts and juices during cranberry juice processing on the antiproliferative activity against two colon cancer cell lines. Food Chemistry, 132, 959–967.

Wang, C. H., et al. 2012. Cranberry-containing products for prevention of urinary tract infections in susceptible populations: a systematic review and meta-analysis of randomized controlled trials. Arch Intern Med, 172, 988–96.

Weiss EI et al. Inhibiting interspecies coaggregation of plaque bacteria with a cranberry juice constituent. J Am Dent Assoc 129.12 (1998): 1719–1723: [published erratum J Am Dent Assoc 130.1(1999): 36 and 130.3 (1999): 332].

Wilson T et al. Favorable glycemic response of type 2 diabetics to low-calorie cranberry juice. J Food Sci 73.9 (2008a): H241–5.

Wilson T et al. Human glycemic response and phenolic content of unsweetened cranberry juice. J Med Food 11.1 (2008b): 46–54.

Wilson, T., et al. 2010. Glycemic responses to sweetened dried and raw cranberries in humans with type 2 diabetes. J Food Sci, 75, H218–23.

Wing DA et al. Daily cranberry juice for the prevention of asymptomatic bacteriuria in pregnancy: a randomized, controlled pilot study. J Urol 180.4 (2008): 1367–1372.

Yamanaka A et al. Inhibitory effect of cranberry polyphenol on biofilm formation and cysteine proteases of *Porphyromonas gingivalis*. J Periodontal Res 42.6 (2007): 589–592.

Yamanaka-Okada A et al. Inhibitory effect of cranberry polyphenol on cariogenic bacteria. Bull Tokyo Dent Coll 49.3 (2008): 107–112.

Yan X et al. Antioxidant activities and antitumor screening of extracts from cranberry fruit (*Vaccinium macrocarpon*). J Agric Food Chem 50.21 (2002): 5844–5849.
Yung, L. M., et al. 2013. Chronic cranberry juice consumption restores cholesterol profiles and improves endothelial function in ovariectomized rats. Eur J Nutr 52: 1145–1155.
Zikria, J., et al. 2010. Cranberry juice and warfarin: when bad publicity trumps science. Am J Med, 123, 384–92.

Devil's claw

HISTORICAL NOTE The botanical name *Harpagophytum* means 'hook plant' in Greek, after the hook-covered fruits of the plant. Devil's claw is native to southern Africa and has been used traditionally as a bitter tonic for digestive disturbances, febrile illnesses and allergic reactions, and to relieve pain (Mills & Bone 2000). It has been used in Europe for the treatment of rheumatic conditions for over 50 years, and was first cited in the literature by Zorn at the University of Jena, Germany, who described his observations on the antiphlogistic and anti-arthritic effects after administration of oral aqueous extracts prepared from the secondary roots of *H. procumbens* in patients suffering from arthritides (Chrubasik et al 2006).

COMMON NAMES

Devil's claw root, grapple plant, harpagophytum, wood spider

BOTANICAL NAME/FAMILY

Harpagophytum procumbens (family Pedaliaceae)

The closely related *H. zeyheri* and *H. procumbens* are collectively known as devil's claw and have been used interchangeably. However, *H. zeyheri* has a lower concentration of the biologically active constituents. Sometimes it is included in raw materials and products as an adulterant of *H. procumbens*, the preferred species of commerce (Mncgwangi et al 2014).

Plant Part Used

Dried tuber/roots. Forms used include dried raw materials, aqueous and ethanol extracts, aqueous-ethanol extracts standardised for harpagocide content, and powdered dry herb tablets (Mncgwangi et al 2012).

Chemical Components

The major active constituent is considered to be the bitter iridoid glycoside, harpagoside (8-cinnamoyl harpagide), which should constitute not less than 1.2% of the dried herb (Georgiev et al 2013). Other iridoid glycosides include harpagide, procumbide, 8-O-(p-coumaroyl)-harpagide and verbascoside, and a newly discovered minor constituent, tentatively identified as methoxypagoside (Karioti et al 2011). About 50% of the herb consists of sugars. There are also triterpenes, phytosterols, plant phenolic acids, flavonol glycosides and phenolic glycosides. *Harpagophytum zeyheri*, which has a lower level of active compounds, may be partially substituted for *H. procumbens* in some commercial preparations (Stewart & Cole 2005). The extraction solvent (e.g. water, ethanol) has a major impact on the active principle of the products (Chrubasik 2004a), and a concentrated aqueous maceration blended with methanol was found to be most efficient for optimal extraction of harpagoside (El Babili et al 2012). When administering *H. procumbens* extract topically it was found that higher penetration of all compounds occurred from an ethanol/water preparation (Abdelouahab & Heard 2008b), and the hydro-alcoholic tincture of devil's claw is very stable when tested over a 6 month period, with levels of marker iridoids not falling below 90% of their initial concentration (Karioti et al 2011).

MAIN ACTIONS

Anti-inflammatory/analgesic

There is good in vitro and in vivo pharmacological evidence of the anti-inflammatory and analgesic properties of devil's claw, although some negative findings have also been reported (McGregor et al 2005). Overall, greatest activity appears to be in semi-chronic rather than acute conditions.

Devil's claw exerted significant analgesic effects against thermally and chemically-induced nociceptive pain stimuli in mice and significant dose-related reduction of experimentally-induced acute inflammation in rats (Mahomed & Ojewole 2004), as well as reducing pain and inflammation in Freund's adjuvant-induced arthritis in rats (Andersen et al 2004). Results from a study in mice suggest that the opioid system is involved in the antinociceptive effects of *H. procumbens* extract (Uchida et al 2008).

The iridoids, particularly harpagoside, are thought to be the main active constituents responsible for the anti-inflammatory activity; however, in vitro evidence suggests that the anti-inflammatory effect may in part be due to antioxidant activity (Denner 2007, Grant et al 2009, Langmead et al 2002), and it is particularly rich in water-soluble antioxidants (Betancor-Fernandez et al 2003). A study administering *H. procumbens* extract intraperitoneally to rats found that the anti-inflammatory response does not depend on the release of adrenal corticosteroids (Catelan et al 2006).

Contradictory evidence exists as to whether devil's claw affects prostaglandin (PG) synthesis. Early in vitro and in vivo and clinical studies suggest that it does not inhibit PG synthesis (Whitehouse et al 1983, Moussard et al 1992); however, more recent investigations have suggested that its anti-inflammatory and analgesic activities are due to suppression of PGE_2 synthesis and nitric oxide production and that the herb may suppress expressions of COX-2 and iNOS (Jang et al 2003). Harpagoside alone has been shown to suppress COX-2 and iNOS at both the mRNA and the protein level in vitro due to a suppression of NF-kappaB activation, although no influence on COX-1 was noted (Huang et al 2006). In vitro research shows that harpagoside and 8-O-(p-coumaroyl)-harpagide exhibit a greater reduction in COX-2 expression than verbascoside and that harpagide on the other hand causes a significant increase in COX-2 expression (Abdelouahab & Heard 2008a). Methanolic extracts of devil's claw have been shown to inhibit COX-2 in vivo (Kundu et al 2005, Na et al 2004), and more recently an ethanol extract of devil's claw was found to inhibit the expression of COX-2 and PGE_2 when applied to freshly excised porcine skin, although no significant effect on 5-LOX or iNOS was noted (Quitas & Heard 2009).

Inhibition of leukotriene synthesis has been observed in vitro, which appears to relate to the amount of harpagoside present (Loew et al 2001, Anauate et al 2010). A study using subcritical and supercritical CO_2 extracts (15 to 30% harpagoside) showed almost total inhibition of 5-lipoxygenase biosynthesis at 51.8 mg/mL of extract, whereas the conventional extract (2.3% harpagoside) did not inhibit the enzyme significantly (Gunther et al 2006).

In vivo experiments have determined that the method of administration of devil's claw affects its anti-inflammatory properties. Intraperitoneal and intraduodenal administration was shown to reduce carrageenan-induced oedema, whereas oral administration had no effect, suggesting that exposure to stomach acid may reduce its anti-inflammatory activity (Soulimani et al 1994). This is supported by a study that found a loss of anti-inflammatory activity after acid treatment (Bone & Walker 1997). In addition, harpagoside inhibits release of the inflammatory mediator RANTES (Regulated on Activation, Normal T cell Expressed and Secreted) by stimulated human bronchial epithelial (BEAS-2B) cells, indicating that it has potential utility for treating respiratory disorders (Boeckenholt et al 2012). It also ameliorates dopaminergic neurodegeneration and movement disorder in a mouse model of Parkinson's disease by elevating the glial cell line-derived neurotrophic factor (Sun et al 2012).

In vitro studies on rat mesangial cells suggest that devil's claw may be used as an anti-inflammatory agent in the treatment of glomerular inflammatory diseases (Kaszkin et al 2004a). Devil's claw extract produced a concentration-dependent suppression of nitrite formation in rat mesangial cells in vitro due to an inhibition of iNOS expression through interference with the transcriptional activation of iNOS. It was found that this activity was due to harpagoside, together with other constituents that possibly have strong anti-oxidant activity (Kaszkin et al 2004b).

It has been suggested that the suppression of inflammatory cytokine synthesis, demonstrated in vitro and vivo (Fiebich et al 2001, Spelman et al 2006), could explain its therapeutic effect in arthritic inflammation (Kundu et al 2005). Fiebich and co-workers found that a 60% ethanolic extract decreases the expression of IL-1-beta, IL-6 and TNF-alpha (Fiebich et al 2001). A follow up study by the same authors found a dose-dependent inhibition of release of TNF-α, interleukin (IL)-6, IL-1-beta and prostaglandin E_2 (PGE_2) in addition to inhibiting the induction of pro-inflammatory gene expression in human monocytes (Fiebich et al 2012). Another study showed that devil's claw extract inhibits inflammation in the chronic stage of adjuvant-induced arthritis, and the same study showed that devil's claw extract displays potent inhibitory activity against IL-1β, IL-6, and TNF-α production in mouse macrophages. Harpagoside also inhibited production of these inflammatory cytokines without cytotoxicity (Inaba et al 2010).

Chondroprotective

In vitro data suggest that the active principles of *H. procumbens* inhibit not only inflammatory mediators but also mediators of cartilage destruction, such as matrix metalloproteinases, NO and elastase (Boje et al 2003, Schulze-Tanzil et al 2004). A study using an animal model confirmed a chondroprotective effect in which the tissue inhibitor of metalloproteinase-2 is involved (Chrubasik et al 2006).

Hypoglycaemic

Devil's claw extract produced a dose-dependent, significant reduction in the blood glucose concentrations of both fasted normal and fasted diabetic rats (Mahomed & Ojewole 2004).

OTHER ACTIONS

Traditional uses include dyspepsia, fever, blood diseases, urinary tract infections, postpartum pain, sprains, sores, ulcers and boils (Mncwangi et al 2012). Recent research with animal models indicates an analgesic effect on acute postoperative and chronic neuropathic pain (Lim et al 2014). In vitro and in vivo evidence suggests that harpagoside may exhibit cardiac affects and lower blood pressure, heart rate and reduce arrhythmias (Fetrow & Avila 1999). As an extremely bitter herb, devil's claw is thought to increase appetite and bile production. Diterpenes extracted from the roots and seeds of devil's claw exhibited selective antiplasmodial (Clarkson et al 2003) and antibacterial activity (Weckesser et al 2007) in vitro, which may have future relevance in view of the increasing resistance to conventional antimalarials and antibiotics. One study showed that aqueous devil's claw extract can markedly delay the onset, as well as reduce the average duration, of convulsion in mice. Although not conclusive, it seems that the extract produces its anticonvulsant activity by enhancing GABAergic neurotransmission and/or facilitating GABAergic action in the brain (Mahomed & Ojewole 2006).

CLINICAL USE

Arthritis

Devil's claw is mainly used to reduce pain and inflammation in practice, with a focus on musculoskeletal conditions. Overall, evidence from clinical trials suggests that devil's claw is effective in the treatment of arthritis; however, additional well-designed, long term studies are required in order to determine effects of its long-term administration in chronic models of joint inflammation and the minimum effective doses, safety and optimal administration routes must be thoroughly determined (Georgiev et al 2013, DiLorenzo et al 2013).

An observational study of 6 months' use of 3–9 g/day of an aqueous extract of devil's claw root reported significant benefit in 42–85% of the 630 people suffering from various arthritic complaints (Bone & Walker 1997). In a 12-week uncontrolled multicentre study of 75 patients with arthrosis of the hip or knee, a strong reduction in pain and the symptoms of osteoarthritis were observed in patients taking 2400 mg of devil's claw extract daily, corresponding to 50 mg harpagoside (Wegener & Lupke 2003). Similar results were reported in a 2-month observational study of 227 people with osteoarthritic knee and hip pain and non-specific low back pain, where both the generic and the disease-specific outcome measures improved by week 4 and further by week 8 (Chrubasik et al 2002). A double-blind study of 89 subjects with rheumatic complaints used powdered devil's claw root (2 g/day) for 2 months, which also provided significant pain relief, whereas another double-blind study of 100 people reported benefit after 1 month (Bone & Walker 1997). A case report suggests that devil's claw relieved strong joint pain in a patient with Crohn's disease (Kaszkin et al 2004b). A single group open study of 8 weeks duration involving 259 patients showed statistically significant improvements in patient assessment of global pain, stiffness and function, and significant reductions in mean pain scores for hand, wrist, elbow, shoulder, hip, knee and back pain. Moreover, quality of life scores significantly increased and 60% of patients either reduced or stopped concomitant pain medication (Warnock et al 2007).

Comparison studies

Comparisons with standard treatment have also been investigated. In 2000, encouraging results of a randomised double-blind study comparing the effects of treatment with devil's claw 2610 mg/day with diacerein 100 mg/day were published (Leblan et al 2000). The study involved 122 people with osteoarthritis of the hip and/or knee and was conducted over 4 months. It found that both treatment groups showed similar considerable improvements in symptoms of osteoarthritis; however, those receiving devil's claw required fewer rescue analgesics.

One double-blind, randomised, multicentre clinical study of 122 patients with osteoarthritis of the knee and hip found that treatment with Harpadol (6 capsules/day, each containing 435 mg of cryoground powder of *H. procumbens*) given over

4 months was as effective as diacerein (an analgesic) 100 mg/day (Chantre et al 2000). However, at the end of the study, patients taking Harpadol were using significantly fewer NSAIDs and had a significantly lower frequency of adverse events. In a 6-week study of only 13 subjects, similar benefits for devil's claw and indomethacin were reported (Newall et al 1996). A preliminary study comparing the proprietary extract Doloteffin with the COX-2 inhibitor rofecoxib reported a benefit with the herbal treatment but suggested that larger studies are still required (Chrubasik et al 2003b).

Previously reviews have concluded that there is moderate evidence of the effectiveness of *H. procumbens* in the treatment of osteoarthritis of the spine, hip and knee; however it is suggested, as with many herbal medicines, that evidence of effectiveness is not transferable from product to product and that the evidence is more robust for products that contain at least 50 mg of harpagoside in the daily dosage (Chrubasik et al 2003a, Gagnier et al 2004, Long et al 2001, Lopez 2012). Two reviews have concluded that 'data from higher quality studies suggest that devil's claw appeared effective in the reduction of the main clinical symptom of pain' (Brien et al 2006) and that the evidence of effectiveness was 'strong' for at least 50 mg of harpagoside as the daily dose, with extracts of devil's claw resulting in pain relief for 60% of patients with an osteoarthritic hip or knee, or nonspecific lower back pain (Chrubasik JE et al 2007). Nevertheless, two other reviews concluded that there was only 'limited evidence' (Ameye & Chee 2006) and 'insufficient reliable evidence' regarding the long term effectiveness of devil's claw (Gregory et al 2008), however this may be as the result of lack of continuity in clinical testing and the definition of 'physical impairment'. Different measures of physical impairment have been used in the clinical trials (including the Arhus low back pain index, the Schober test and the Waddell scale), and this may be a reason for varied results rather than a lack of effectiveness of the extracts (Chrubasik 2008).

The herb is Commission E approved as supportive therapy for degenerative musculoskeletal disorders (Blumenthal et al 2000) and approved for painful osteoarthritis by the European Scientific Cooperative on Phytotherapy (ESCOP 2003).

Back pain

Three reviews looking at the treatment of low back pain concluded that there is strong evidence for short-term improvements in pain and reduction in rescue medication for devil's claw treatment, standardised to 50 and 100 mg harpagoside as daily doses (Chrubasik et al 2007, Gagnier 2008, Gagnier et al 2006, 2007). The reliability and quality of some of these clinical trials have been investigated in detail by different research groups (Brien et al 2006, Chrubasik et al 2003a, Gagnier et al 2004, 2007). All reviews of clinical studies conclude that Harpagophytum extracts show strong evidence of efficacy and reliability in the treatment of lower back pain.

Eight weeks treatment with devil's claw extract LI 174, known commercially as Rivoltan, significantly decreased back pain and improved mobility in a double-blind RCT of 117 people (Laudahn & Walper 2001) although another double blind RCT using the same product found that pain relief was established more quickly, after 4 weeks amongst subjects with muscle stiffness (Gobel et al 2001). Similar results were reported in two double-blind studies of 118 people (Chrubasik et al 1996) and 197 people (Chrubasik et al 1999) with chronic lower back pain.

Devil's claw appears to compare favourably to conventional treatments. A 6-week double-blind study of 88 subjects comparing devil's claw to rofecoxib found equal improvements in both groups (Chrubasik et al 2003b). A follow-up of the subjects from that study who were all given devil's claw for 1 year found that it was well tolerated and improvements were sustained (Chrubasik et al

2005). In an open, prospective study, an unspecific lower back pain treatment with *Harpagophytum* extract and conventional therapy were found to be equally effective (Schmidt et al 2005).

Dyspepsia

Traditionally, devil's claw has also been used to treat dyspepsia and to stimulate appetite (Fisher & Painter 1996). The bitter principles in the herb provide a theoretical basis for its use in these conditions, although controlled studies are not available to determine effectiveness. The herb is Commission E (Blumenthal et al 2000) and ESCOP (2003) approved for dyspepsia and loss of appetite.

OTHER USES

Use in oncology

There is a case report that two Stage IIIA follicular lymphoma patients demonstrated objective tumour regression after taking 500 mg daily doses of devil's claw without cytotoxic therapy, which was confirmed by computed tomography (CT) scans. This result was presumably as a result of COX-2 inhibition, which has been implicated in lymphomagenesis. Although this case report introduces a possible use of the herb, it is unknown as to whether the regression was spontaneous (as has been observed in up to 16% of lymphoma patients) or due to devil's claw, and further studies are warranted (Wilson 2009).

Traditional use

Traditionally, the herb is also used internally to treat febrile illnesses, allergic reactions and to induce sedation, and topically for wounds, ulcers, boils and pain relief (Fisher & Painter 1996, Mills & Bone 2000), as well as for diabetes, hypertension, indigestion and anorexia (Van Wyk 2000).

DOSAGE RANGE

Musculoskeletal conditions

- Dried root or equivalent aqueous or hydroalcoholic extracts: 2–6 g daily for painful arthritis; 4.5–9 g daily for lower back pain.
- Liquid extract (1 : 2): 6–12 mL/day.
- Tincture (1 : 5): 2–4 mL three times daily.

It is suggested that devil's claw extracts with at least 50 mg harpagoside in the daily dosage should be recommended for the treatment of pain, and dosages corresponding to 30–100 mg harpagosides have been used in clinical trials (Chrubasik 2004a, 2004b, Street & Prinsloo 2012).

Digestive conditions (e.g. dyspepsia)

- Dosages equivalent to 1.5 g/day dried herb are used (Blumenthal et al 2000). It is suggested that devil's claw preparations be administered between meals, when gastric activity is reduced.

TOXICITY

The acute LD_{50} of devil's claw was more than 13.5 g/kg according to one study (Bone & Walker 1997). In a recent review of 28 clinical trials only a few reports on acute toxicity were found, whereas no reports on chronic toxicity had been reported. The review concluded that more studies for long-term treatment are needed (Vlachojannis et al 2008). An earlier review looking at 14 clinical trials had come to the same conclusion (Brien et al 2006).

ADVERSE REACTIONS

Devil's claw is a well tolerated treatment. In a recent review of 28 clinical trials it was found that only minor adverse events, mainly mild gastrointestinal symptoms (e.g. diarrhoea), occur in 3% of the patients. The incidence of adverse effects in the treatment groups was never higher than in the placebo groups for all 28 trials (Vlachojannis et al 2008).

SIGNIFICANT INTERACTIONS

Devil's claw was previously found to moderately inhibit cytochrome P450 enzymes (CYP2C9, 2C19, 3A4) in vitro (Unger & Frank 2004); however a subsequent study found no significant interactions when testing 10 different commercial devil's claw preparations (Modari et al 2011). An in vitro study found commercial preparations of devil's claw and pure harpagoside upregulated P-glycoprotein in a dose-dependent manner (Romiti et al 2009); however the effect has not been tested in vivo. In contrast to NSAIDs, devil's claw does not affect platelet function (Izzo et al 2005).

Warfarin

Rare case reports suggest that devil's claw may potentiate the effects of warfarin, but the reports are mostly inconclusive (Argento et al 2000, Heck et al 2000, Izzo et al 2005). Clinical testing would be required to confirm a possible interaction.

Anti-arrhythmic drugs

Theoretical interaction exists when the herb is used in high doses; however, clinical testing is required to determine significance — observe patients taking concurrent antiarrhythmics (Fetrow & Avila 1999).

Practice points/Patient counselling

- Devil's claw reduces pain and inflammation and is a useful treatment in arthritis and back pain, according to controlled studies.
- The anti-inflammatory action appears to be different to that of NSAIDs and has not been fully elucidated. There is also preliminary evidence of a chondroprotective effect.
- Preliminary research suggests that it is best to take devil's claw between meals, on an empty stomach.
- Devil's claw appears to be relatively safe but should not be used in pregnancy and should be used with caution in people with ulcers or gallstones or in those taking warfarin.

CONTRAINDICATIONS AND PRECAUTIONS

Use cautiously in patients with gastric and duodenal ulcers, gallstones or acute diarrhoea, as devil's claw may cause gastric irritation (Blumenthal et al 2000).

PREGNANCY USE

Devil's claw is not recommended in pregnancy, as it has exhibited oxytocic activity in animals.

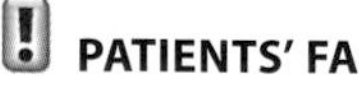

PATIENTS' FAQs

What will this herb do for me?

Devil's claw is a useful treatment for arthritis and back pain. It may also increase appetite and improve digestion and dyspepsia.

D

When will it start to work?

Results from studies suggest that pain-relieving effects will start within 4–12 weeks reaching maximum pain relief after 3–4 months (Chrubasik S et al 2007, Thanner et al 2008).

Are there any safety issues?

Devil's claw should be used cautiously by people with gallstones, diarrhoea, stomach ulcers and those taking the drug warfarin. It is also not recommended in pregnancy.

REFERENCES

Abdelouahab N, Heard C. Effect of the major glycosides of Harpagophytum procumbens (Devil's Claw) on epidermal cyclooxygenase-2 (COX-2) in vitro. J Nat Prod 71.5 (2008a): 746–749.

Abdelouahab N, Heard CM. Dermal and transcutaneous delivery of the major glycoside constituents of Harpagophytum procumbens (Devil's Claw) in vitro. Planta Med 74.5 (2008b): 527–531.

Ameye LG, Chee WS. Osteoarthritis and nutrition. From nutraceuticals to functional foods: a systematic review of the scientific evidence. Arthritis Res Ther 8.4 (2006): R127.

Andersen ML et al. Evaluation of acute and chronic treatments with Harpagophytum procumbens on Freund's adjuvant-induced arthritis in rats. J Ethnopharmacol 91.2–3 (2004): 325–330.

Anauate, MC et al. Effect of Isolated Fractions of Harpagophytum Procumbens D.C. (devil's Claw) on COX-1, COX-2 Activity and Nitric Oxide Production on Whole-blood Assay. Phyto Res 24.9 (2010): 1365–369.

Argento AE et al. Oral anticoagulants and medicinal plants: An emerging interaction. Ann Ital Med Intern 15.2 (2000): 139–143.

Betancor-Fernandez A et al. Screening pharmaceutical preparations containing extracts of turmeric rhizome, artichoke leaf, devil's claw root and garlic or salmon oil for antioxidant capacity. J Pharm Pharmacol 55.7 (2003): 981–986.

Blumenthal M, Goldberg A, Brinckmann J (eds). Herbal medicine: expanded Commission E monographs. Austin, TX: Integrative Medicine Communications, 2000.

Boeckenholt, C et al. Effect of silymarin and harpagoside on inflammation reaction of BEAS-2B cells, on ciliary beat frequency (CBF) of trachea explants and on mucociliary clearance (MCC). Planta Med. 78 (2012): 761–766.

Boje K, Lechtenberg M, Nahrstedt A. New and known iridoid- and phenylethanoid glycosides from Harpagophytum procumbens and their in vitro inhibition of human leukocyte elastase. Planta Med 69 (2003): 820–825.

Bone K, Walker M. Devil's claw. MediHerb Professional Review. Australia: Mediherb Pty Ltd (February 1997).

Brien S, Lewith GT, McGregor G. Devil's Claw (Harpagophytum procumbens) as a treatment for osteoarthritis: a review of efficacy and safety. J Altern Complement Med 12.10 (2006): 981–993.

Catelan SC et al. The role of adrenal corticosteroids in the anti-inflammatory effect of the whole extract of Harpagophytum procumbens in rats. Phytomedicine 13.6 (2006): 446–451.

Chantre P et al. Efficacy and tolerance of Harpagophytum procumbens versus diacerhein in treatment of osteoarthritis. Phytomedicine 7.3 (2000): 177–183.

Chrubasik JE et al. Potential molecular basis of the chondroprotective effect of Harpagophytum procumbens. Phytomedicine 13.8 (2006): 598–600.

Chrubasik JE, Roufogalis BD, Chrubasik S. Evidence of effectiveness of herbal antiinflammatory drugs in the treatment of painful osteoarthritis and chronic low back pain. Phytother Res 21.7 (2007): 675–683.

Chrubasik S. Devil's claw extract as an example of the effectiveness of herbal analgesics. Der Orthopade 33.7 (2004a): 804–808.

Chrubasik S. Salix and Harpagophytum for chronic joint and low back pain: From evidence-based view herbal medicinal products are recommended. Schweiz Z Ganzheits Med 16.6 (2004b): 355–359.

Chrubasik S et al. Effectiveness of Harpagophytum procumbens in treatment of acute low back pain. Phytomedicine 3.1 (1996): 1–110.

Chrubasik S et al. Effectiveness of Harpagophytum extract WS 1531 in the treatment of exacerbation of low back pain: a randomized, placebo-controlled, double-blind study. Eur J Anaesthesiol 16.2 (1999): 118–129.

Chrubasik S et al. Comparison of outcome measures during treatment with the proprietary Harpagophytum extract doloteffin in patients with pain in the lower back, knee or hip. Phytomedicine 9.3 (2002): 181–194.

Chrubasik S et al. The quality of clinical trials with Harpagophytum procumbens. Phytomedicine 10.6–7 (2003a): 613–623.

Chrubasik S et al. A randomized double-blind pilot study comparing Doloteffin(R) and Vioxx(R) in the treatment of low back pain. Rheumatology 42.1 (2003b): 141–148.

Chrubasik S et al. A 1-year follow-up after a pilot study with Doloteffin(R) for low back pain. Phytomedicine 12.1–2 (2005): 1–9.

Chrubasik S et al. Patient-perceived benefit during one year of treatment with Doloteffin. Phytomedicine 14.6 (2007): 371–376.

Chrubasik C et al. Impact of herbal medicines on physical impairment. Phytomedicine 15 (2008): 536–539.

Clarkson C et al. In vitro antiplasmodial activity of abietane and totarane diterpenes isolated from Harpagophytum procumbens (Devil's Claw). Planta Med 69.8 (2003): 720–724.

Denner SS. A review of the efficacy and safety of devil's claw for pain associated with degenerative musculoskeletal diseases, rheumatoid, and osteoarthritis. Holist Nurs Pract 21.4 (2007): 203–207.

Di Lorenzo C et al. Plant food supplements with anti-inflammatory properties: A Systematic Review (II). Crit Rev in Food Sc Nutr 53:5 (2013): 507–516.

ESCOP. European Scientific Co-operative on Phytomedicine, 2nd edn. Stuttgart: Thieme, 2003.
El Babili F et al. Anatomical study of secondary tuberized roots of *Harpagophytum procumbens* DC and quantification of harpagoside by highperformance liquid chromatography method. Pharmacogn Mag. 8.30 (2012): 175–180.
Fetrow CW, Avila JR. Professionals' handbook of complementary and alternative medicines. Springhouse, PA: Springhouse Publishing, 1999.
Fiebich BL et al. Inhibition of TNF-alpha synthesis in LPS-stimulated primary human monocytes by Harpagophytum extract SteiHap 69. Phytomedicine 8.1 (2001): 28–30.
Fiebich BL et al. Molecular targets of the anti-inflammatory Harpagophytum procumbens (devil's claw): inhibition of TNFa and COX-2 gene expression by preventing activation of AP-1. Phytother Res 26.6 (2012): 806–11.
Fisher C, Painter G. Materia Medica for the Southern hemisphere. Auckland: Fisher-Painter Publishers, 1996.
Gagnier JJ et al. Harpgophytum procumbens for osteoarthritis and low back pain: a systematic review. BMC Complement Altern Med 4 (2004): 13.
Gagnier JJ et al. Herbal medicine for low back pain. Cochrane Database Syst Rev 2 (2006): CD004504.
Gagnier JJ et al. Herbal medicine for low back pain: a Cochrane review. Spine 32.1 (2007): 82–92.
Gagnier JJ Evidence-informed management of chronic low back pain with herbal, vitamin, mineral, and homeopathic supplements. The Spine Journal 8 (2008): 70–79.
Georgiev MI et al Harpagoside: from Kalahari Desert to pharmacy shelf. Phytochemistry Aug (2013): 8–15.
Gobel HA et al. Effects of Harpagophytum procumbens LI 174 (devil's claw) on sensory, motor and vascular muscle reagibility in the treatment of unspecific back pain. Schmerz 15.1 (2001): 10–118.
Grant L et al. The inhibition of free radical generation by preparations of Harpagophytum procumbens in vitro. Phytother Res 23.1 (2009): 104–110.
Gregory PJ, Sperry M, Wilson AF. Dietary supplements for osteoarthritis. Am Fam Physician 77.2 (2008): 177–184.
Gunther M, Laufer S, Schmidt PC. High anti-inflammatory activity of harpagoside-enriched extracts obtained from solvent-modified super- and subcritical carbon dioxide extractions of the roots of Harpagophytum procumbens. Phytochem Anal 17.1 (2006): 1–7.
Heck AM et al. Potential interactions between alternative therapies and warfarin. Am J Health-System Pharm 57.13 (2000): 1221–1227: quiz 1228–30.
Huang TH et al. Harpagoside suppresses lipopolysaccharide-induced iNOS and COX-2 expression through inhibition of NF-kappaB activation. J Ethnopharmacol 104 (2006): 149–155.
Inaba K et al. Inhibitory effects of devil's claw (secondary root of Harpagophytum procumbens) extract and harpagoside on cytokine production in mouse macrophages. J Nat Med 64 (2010): 219–222.
Izzo AA et al. Cardiovascular pharmacotherapy and herbal medicines: the risk of drug interaction. Int J Cardiol 98.1 (2005): 1–114
Jang MH et al. Harpagophytum procumbens suppresses lipopolysaccharide-stimulated expressions of cyclooxygenase-2 and inducible nitric oxide synthase in fibroblast cell line L929. J Pharmacol Sci 93.3 (2003): 367–371.
Karioti A et al. Analysis and stability of the constituents of Curcuma longa and Harpagophytum procumbens tinctures by HPLC-DAD and HPLC–ESI-MS. J Pharma Biomed Anal 55 (2011): 479–486.
Kaszkin M et al. Downregulation of iNOS expression in rat mesangial cells by special extracts of Harpagophytum procumbens derives from harpagoside-dependent and independent effects. Phytomedicine 11.7–8 (2004a): 585–595.
Kaszkin M et al. High dosed Harpagophytum special extract for maintenance of remission in patients with Crohn's disease: A case report. Arztezeitschr Naturheilverfahr 45.2 (2004b): 102–106.
Kundu JK et al. Inhibitory effects of the extracts of Sutherlandia frutescens (L.) R. Br. and Harpagophytum procumbens DC. on phorbol ester-induced COX-2 expression in mouse skin: AP-1 and CREB as potential upstream targets. Cancer Lett 218.1 (2005): 21–31.
Langmead L et al. Antioxidant effects of herbal therapies used by patients with inflammatory bowel disease: an in vitro study. Aliment Pharmacol Ther 16.2 (2002): 197–205.
Laudahn D, Walper A. Efficacy and tolerance of Harpagophytum extract LI 174 in patients with chronic non-radicular back pain. Phytother Res 15.7 (2001): 621–624.
Leblan D, Chantre P, Fournie B. Harpagophytum procumbens in the treatment of knee and hip osteoarthritis: Four-month results of a prospective, multicenter, double-blind trial versus diacerhein. Joint Bone Spine 67.5 (2000): 462–467.
Lim DW et al. Analgesic effect of Harpagophytum procumbens on postoperative and neuropathic pain in rats. Molecules 19.1 (2014): 1060–1068.
Loew D et al. Investigations on the pharmacokinetic properties of Harpagophytum extracts and their effects on eicosanoid biosynthesis in vitro and ex vivo. Clin Pharmacol Ther 69.5 (2001): 356–364.
Long L, Soeken K, Ernst E. Herbal medicines for the treatment of osteoarthritis: a systematic review. Rheumatology 40 (2001): 779–4693.
Lopez H. Nutritional Interventions to Prevent and Treat Osteoarthritis. Part II: Focus on Micronutrients and Supportive Nutraceuticals. Phys Med Rehab 4 (2012) S:155–68.
Mahomed IM, Ojewole JAO. Analgesic, antiinflammatory and antidiabetic properties of Harpagophytum procumbens DC (Pedaliaceae) secondary root aqueous extract. Phytother Res 18.12 (2004): 982–989.
Mahomed IM, Ojewole JA. Anticonvulsant activity of Harpagophytum procumbens DC [Pedaliaceae] secondary root aqueous extract in mice. Brain Res Bull 69.1 (2006): 57–62.
McGregor GB et al. Devil's claw (Harpagophytum procumbens): An anti-inflammatory herb with therapeutic potential. Phytochem Rev 4.1 (2005): 47–53.
Mills S, Bone K. Principles and practice of phytotherapy. London: Churchill Livingstone, 2000.
Moussard CD et al. A drug used in traditional medicine, Harpagophytum procumbens: no evidence for NSAID-like effect on whole blood eicosanoid production in human. Prostaglandins Leukot Essent Fatty Acids 46.4 (1992): 283–286.

Mncwangi N et al. Devil's Claw—A review of the ethnobotany, phytochemistry and biological activity of Harpagophytum procumbens. J Ethnopharmacology 143 (2012): 755–771.
Mncgwangi N et al. Mid-infrared spectroscopy and short wave infrared hyperspectral imaging—A novel approach in the qualitative assessment of Harpagophytum procumbens and H. zeyheri (Devil's Claw). Phytochemistry Letters 7 (2014):143–149.
Modari M et al. The interaction potential of herbal medicinal products: a luminescence-based screening platform assessing effects on cytochrome P450 and its use with devil's claw (*Harpagophyti radix*) preparations. J Pharm Pharmacol 63 (2011) 429–438.
Na HK et al. Inhibition of phorbol ester-induced COX-2 expression by some edible African plants. Oxford: BioFactors 21.1–4 (2004): 149–353.
Newell CA, Anderson LA, Phillipson JD. Herbal medicines: A guide for health care professionals. London, UK: The Pharmaceutical Press, 1996.
Quitas NA, Heard CM A novel ex vivo skin model for the assessment of the potential transcutaneous anti-inflammatory effect of topically applied Harpagophytum procumbens extract. Int J Pharm. 376.1–2 (2009):63–8.
Romiti, N et al Effects of Devil's Claw (Harpagophytum procumbens) on the multidrug transporter ABCB1/P-glycoprotein. Phytomedicine 16.12 (2009): 1095–100.
Schmidt A et al. Effectiveness of Harpagophytum procumbens in treatment of unspecific low back pain. Physikal Med Rehabilitationsmed Kurortmed 15.5 (2005): 317–321.
Schulze-Tanzil G, Hansen C, Shakibaei M. Effect of a Harpagophytum procumbens DC extract on matrix metalloproteinases in human chondrocytes in vitro. Arzneimittelforschung 54 (2004): 213–220.
Soulimani R et al. The role of stomachal digestion on the pharmacological activity of plant extracts, using as an example extracts of Harpagophytum procumbens. Can J Physiol Pharmacol 72.12 (1994): 1532–1536.
Spelman K et al. Modulation of cytokine expression by traditional medicines: a review of herbal immunomodulators. Altern Med Rev 11.2 (2006): 128–150.
Stewart KM, Cole D. The commercial harvest of devil's claw (Harpagophytum spp.) in southern Africa: The devil's in the details. J Ethnopharmacol 100.3 (2005): 225–236.
Street RA, Prinsloo G. Commercially important medicinal plants of South Africa: A Review. J Chemistry (2013) Article ID 205048.
Sun, X et al. Harpagoside attenuates MPTP/MPP(+) induced dopaminergic neurodegeneration and movement disorder via elevating glial cell line derived neurotrophic factor. J. Neurochem. 120 (2012):1072–1083.
Thanner J et al. Retrospective evaluation of biopsychosocial determinants and treatment response in patients receiving devil's claw extract (doloteffin(R)). Phytother Res 23.5 (2008): 742–744.
Uchida S et al. Antinociceptive effects of St. John's wort, Harpagophytum procumbens extract and Grape seed proanthocyanidins extract in mice. Biol Pharm Bull 31.2 (2008): 240–245.
Unger M, Frank A. Simultaneous determination of the inhibitory potency of herbal extracts on the activity of six major cytochrome P450 enzymes using liquid chromatography/mass spectrometry and automated online extraction. Rapid Commun in Mass Spectrometry 18.19 (2004): 2273–2281.
Van Wyk BE, Gericke N. People's plants: a guide to useful plants of Southern Africa. Pretoria: Briza Publications, 2000.
Vlachojannis J, Roufogalis BD, Chrubasik S. Systematic review on the safety of Harpagophytum preparations for osteoarthritic and low back pain. Phytother Res 22.2 (2008): 149–152.
Warnock M et al. Effectiveness and safety of Devil's Claw tablets in patients with general rheumatic disorders. Phytother Res 21.12 (2007): 1228–1233.
Weckesser S et al. Screening of plant extracts for antimicrobial activity against bacteria and yeasts with dermatological relevance. Phytomedicine 14.7–8 (2007): 508–516.
Wegener T, Lupke N-P. Treatment of patients with arthrosis of hip or knee with an aqueous extract of devil's claw (Harpagophytum procumbens DC). Phytother Res 17.10 (2003): 1165–1172.
Whitehouse LW et al. Devil's claw (Harpagophytum procumbens): no evidence for anti-inflammatory activity in the treatment of arthritic disease. Can Med Assoc J 129.3 (1983): 249–251.
Wilson KS. Regression of follicular lymphoma with Devil's Claw: coincidence or causation? Curr Onc 16.4 (2009): 67–70.

Echinacea

HISTORICAL NOTE Echinacea was first used by Native American Sioux Indians centuries ago as a treatment for snakebite, colic, infection and external wounds, among other things. It was introduced into standard medical practice in the United States during the 1800s as a popular anti-infective medication, which was prescribed by eclectic and traditional doctors until the 20th century. Remaining on the national list of official plant drugs in the United States until the 1940s, it was produced by pharmaceutical companies during this period. With the arrival of antibiotics, echinacea fell out of favour and was no longer considered a 'real' medicine for infection. Its use has re-emerged, probably because we are now in a better position to understand the limitations of antibiotic therapy and because there is growing public interest in self-care. The dozens of clinical trials conducted overseas have also played a role in its renaissance.

COMMON NAME

Echinacea

OTHER NAMES

Echinacea angustifolia — American coneflower, black sampson, black susans, coneflower, echinaceawurzel, Indian head, kansas snakeroot, purple coneflower, purpursonnenhutkraut, racine d'echinacea, *Rudbeckia angustifolia* L., scurvy root, snakeroot

E. purpurea — *Brauneria purpurea* (L.) Britt., combflower, purple coneflower, red sunflower

Rudbeckia purpurea L. — *E. pallida*, *Brauneria pallida* (Nutt.) Britt., pale coneflower, *Rudbeckia pallida* Nutt.

BOTANICAL NAME/FAMILY

Echinacea species (family Asteraceae [Compositae])

The name 'echinacea' generally refers to several different plants within the genus — *E. purpurea*, *E. pallida* and *E. angustifolia*.

PLANT PARTS USED

Root, leaf and aerial parts

CHEMICAL COMPONENTS

The most important constituents with regard to pharmacological activity are the polysaccharides, caffeic acid derivatives, alkylamides, essential oils and polyacetylenes, although there are other potentially active constituents, as well as a range of vitamins, minerals, fatty acids, resins, glycoproteins and sterols (Pizzorno & Murray 2006). Cynarin, a potential immunosuppressant and CD28 ligand, was also identified in *E. purpurea* (Dong et al 2006). Constituent concentrations vary depending on the species, plant part and growing conditions. With regard to the final chemical composition of an echinacea-containing product, the drying and extraction processes further alter chemical composition. Therefore, the pharmacological effects of an echinacea product depend very much on which constituents are present and their relative ratios. This is outlined further in the following sections.

Pharmacokinetics

The absorption of *E. purpurea* alkylamides from lozenges is rapid and linear (Guiotto et al 2008).

A clinical study with healthy volunteers showed that, following ingestion of tablets containing ethanolic echinacea extract, alkylamides were detectable in plasma 20 minutes after ingestion, whereas caffeic acid derivatives were not detectable in the plasma at any time after tablet ingestion (Matthias et al 2005a). A further study by the same authors showed that there was no significant difference in the bioavailability of alkylamides from a liquid and solid oral dosage form of an echinacea product (mixture of *E. purpurea* and *E. angustifolia*), with T_{max} reached at 20 and 30 minutes, respectively (Matthias et al 2007b). Two other studies reported that, 30–45 minutes following administration of *E. purpurea* products (Echinaforce tincture, tablets, spray) containing milligram amounts of alkylamides, plasma concentrations of alkylamides of about 0.07–0.40 ng/mL were recorded (Woelkart et al 2006, 2008b), and effects on the immune markers were observed 23 hours after oral administration (Woelkart et al 2006).

E

Furthermore, tetraene alkylamides, present in *E. angustifolia* and *E. purpurea*, are metabolised by CYP450 enzymes (Matthias et al 2005b). In addition, the metabolism of tetraene alkylamides can be significantly decreased by monoene alkylamides that are only found in *E. angustifolia* (Matthias et al 2005b). A recent study found that the human CYP450 enzymes involved in the metabolism of one of the most abundant alkylamides, *N*-isobutyldodeca-2E,4E,8Z,10Z-tetraenamide, are CYP2E1, CYP2C9 and CYP1A2 (Toselli et al 2010).

MAIN ACTIONS

Due to the wide assortment of chemical constituents found in echinacea, it has varied pharmacological effects.

Immunomodulator

Experimental results suggest that echinacea functions more as a modulator of the immune response rather than as a straightforward immune stimulant. This is well illustrated by a recent study conducted by Ritchie et al (2011), which showed that the response to treatment with the product Echinaforce was dependent on subjects' baseline constitution. For example, echinacea treatment induced an additional formation of antiviral interferon-gamma, chemotactic molecules (interleukin-8 [IL-8]) or monocyte chemoattractant protein-1 in subjects with a low initial production at baseline (from +18 to +49%). In contrast, subjects with higher levels of these factors at baseline experienced no further increase after treatment (Ritchie et al 2011). Similarly, volunteers reporting higher stress levels or higher susceptibility to cold infections have reacted to echinacea treatment with improved immune responses (Schapowal 2013).

The immunomodulator activity of echinacea has been the subject of countless studies and appears to be the result of multiple mechanisms.

Overall, the fresh-pressed leaf juice of *E. purpurea* and alcoholic extracts of the roots of *E. pallida*, *E. angustifolia* and *E. purpurea* have been shown to act mainly on non-specific cellular immunity (Blumenthal et al 2000). It was reported that no one single constituent is responsible for the herb's immunomodulating action, with the most important elements being polysaccharides, glycoproteins, alkamides and flavonoids (Ernst 2002). More recent research indicates that the water-soluble compounds (such as polysaccharides) rather than lipophilic constituents are chiefly responsible for the immunostimulatory activity (Pillai et al 2007).

Macrophage activation has been well demonstrated, as has stimulation of phagocytosis (Barrett 2003, Bauer et al 1988, Groom et al 2007, Pugh et al 2008, Zhai et al 2009a). Orally administered root extracts of echinacea have produced stronger effects on phagocytosis than aerial parts, with *E. purpurea* roots producing the greatest effect, followed by that of *E. angustifolia* and *E. pallida* (Pizzorno & Murray 2006).

The activation of polymorphonuclear leucocytes and natural killer (NK) cells and increased numbers of T-cell and B-cell leucocytes have also been reported for echinacea (Groom et al 2007, Zhai et al 2007a).

Echinacea stimulates cytokine (Altamirano-Dimas et al 2007, Brush et al 2006, Dong et al 2006, 2008, Farinacci et al 2009, Sharma et al 2006, Zhai et al 2007a, Zwickey et al 2007) and chemokine production (Wang et al 2006, 2008).

Moreover, various echinacea species stimulate nitric oxide (NO) production in vitro (Classen et al 2006, Sullivan et al 2008).

Contradictory results were obtained for tumour necrosis factor-alpha (TNF-alpha) production, possibly due to the different preparations used producing different effects. In one study, echinacea significantly increased TNF-alpha production (Senchina et al 2006), whereas no effects on TNF-alpha were observed for all echinacea species in another study (McCann et al 2007), and in a third study, NF-κB expression and TNF-alpha levels decreased in non-stimulated macrophages following echinacea treatment (Matthias et al 2007a).

In lipopolysaccharide-stimulated (endotoxin) cells, echinacea inhibited NF-κB, TNF-alpha, NO and cytokine production, with different alkylamides exerting different effects (Matthias et al 2007a, 2008, Raduner et al 2006, Sasagawa et al 2006, Stevenson et al 2005, Woelkart et al 2006, Zhai et al 2007a). Another study found that the *E. purpurea* root extract (polysaccharide-rich) increased specific surface biomarkers whereas the leaf extract (alkylamide-rich) inhibited their expression. Moreover, IL-6 and TNF-alpha production was increased due to the root extract, but unchanged following exposure to the leaf extract (Benson et al 2010).

Similarly, a more recent study found that different alkylamides either suppressed or stimulated influenza A-induced secretion of cytokines, chemokines and prostaglandin E_2 from RAW264.7 macrophage-like cells (Cech et al 2010). Unidentified constituents from echinacea have been shown to stimulate inositol-1,4,5-trisphosphate receptor and phospholipase C mediation of cytosolic Ca^{2+} levels in non-immune mammalian cells (Wu et al 2010).

Anti-inflammatory

Studies indicate that alcohol extracts of all three echinacea species (*E. angustifolia*, *E. purpurea* and *E. pallida*) exert significant anti-inflammatory activity (Raso et al 2002, Zhai et al 2009a). The result is due to multiple constituents acting with multiple mechanisms. The alkylamide fraction inhibits inducible nitric oxide synthase (iNOS) and the caffeic acid fraction enhances arginase activity (Zhai et al 2009a). In vivo tests further identify anti-inflammatory effects also for *E. angustifolia* and *E. pallida* when applied topically (Speroni et al 2002, Tragni et al 1985, Tubaro et al 1987).

A recent study reports on the selective induction of pro- and anti-inflammatory cytokines by low-dose *E. purpurea* (Kapai et al 2011). Similarly, anti-inflammatory effects have been identified for the essential oils of *E. purpurea* extract, with pro-inflammatory cytokines such as IL-2, IL-6 and TNF-alpha being reduced in the blood of treated mice (Yu et al 2013).

COX-1/COX-2

Alkylamides from the roots of *E. purpurea* partially inhibit both cyclooxygenase-1 (COX-1) and COX-2 isoenzymes, thus decreasing prostaglandin E_2 levels (Clifford et al 2002, LaLone et al 2007, Raman et al 2008). Several alkylamides isolated from a CO_2 extract of the roots of *E. angustifolia* have been shown to inhibit COX-2-dependent prostaglandin E_2 formation, although COX-2 mRNA and protein expression were not inhibited, but rather increased (Hinz et al 2007).

A 2009 study further confirmed that certain alkylamides and ketones present in various *Echinacea* species were the key anti-inflammatory contributors inhibiting prostaglandin E_2 production (LaLone et al 2009).

Cannabinoid and TRPV1 receptor interaction

The alkamides from echinacea also modulate TNF-alpha mRNA expression in human monocytes/macrophages via the cannabinoid type 2 (CB2) receptor, thus identifying a possible mode of action for its immunomodulatory activity (Raduner et al 2006, Woelkart & Bauer 2007). Two alkylamides, which bind to the CB2 receptor more strongly than endogenous cannabinoids and activate it, have been classified as a new class of cannabinomimetics (Gertsch et al 2006). It was found that some of the alkylamides in echinacea self-assemble into micelles in aqueous solution, which then determines their binding to the CB2 receptor (Raduner et al 2007). In a subsequent study, Chicca et al (2009) showed that ethanolic *E. purpurea* root and herb extracts and specific *N*-alkylamides within produce synergistic pharmacological effects on the endocannabinoid system in vitro by simultaneously targeting the CB2 receptor, endocannabinoid transport and degradation. In contrast, ketoalkenes from *E. pallida* did not interact with cannabinoid receptors (Egger et al 2008).

Ethanol extracts from echinacea roots showed potent agonist activity on TRPV1, a mammalian pain receptor. The compounds involved in the TRPV1 receptor activation differ from those involved in the inhibition of prostaglandin E_2 production (Birt et al 2008).

Antiviral activity

Four different *Echinacea* species (*E. angustifolia, E. purpurea, E. tennesseensis* and *E. pallida)* increase the amount of iNOS protein, but to varying degrees. The results suggest that any potential antiviral activities of *Echinacea* spp. extracts are not likely to be mediated through large inductions of type 1 interferon, but may involve iNOS (Senchina et al 2010). *E. purpurea* extract Echinaforce inhibited the induction of multiple proinflammatory cytokines by respiratory viruses (Sharma et al 2009). The same authors showed in a three-dimensional tissue model of normal human airway epithelium that this specific *E. purpurea* extract, Echinaforce, reversed rhinovirus type 1A (RV1A)-stimulated mucopolysaccharide inclusion in goblet cells, RV1A-induced mucin secretion and the RV1A-stimulated secretion of proinflammatory cytokines (Sharma et al 2010).

Herpes simplex virus

Extracts of eight taxa of the genus *Echinacea* were found to have antiviral activity against herpes simplex virus type 1 (HSV-1) in vitro when exposed to visible and ultraviolet A light (Binns et al 2002). Antiviral activity was confirmed for *E. purpurea* extracts in 2008, with evidence suggesting that polyphenolic compounds other than the known HIV inhibitor, cichoric acid, may also be involved (Birt et al 2008). A 2010 study found that hydroalcoholic *E. pallida* extracts interfere with free HSV-1 or HSV-2 and pressed juice is able to interact with HSV-1 or HSV-2 inside and outside the cell, as well as to protect cells against viral infection, probably by interfering with virus attachment (Schneider et al 2010). Another study in mice showed that *E. purpurea* polysaccharide reduces the latency rate in HSV-1 infections when supplied prior to infection (Ghaemi et al 2009).

Antibacterial activity

An in vitro study showed that Echinaforce inhibits the proliferation of *Propionibacterium acnes* and decreases bacterial-induced inflammation (Sharma et al 2011).

Antiadhesive activity against *Campylobacter jejuni* was found for two different *Echinacea* species, with *E. purpurea* extract displaying a higher activity than *E. angustifolia*. The extracts used were of the MediHerb brand (Bensch et al 2011). The standardised extract of *E. purpurea* (Echinaforce) readily inactivated *Streptococcus pyogenes*, *Haemophilus influenzae* and *Legionella pneumophila* and also reversed their proinflammatory responses. *Staphylococcus aureus* (methicillin-resistant and sensitive strains) and *Mycobacterium smegmatis* were less sensitive to the bactericidal effects of *Echinacea*; however, their proinflammatory responses were still completely reversed. In contrast, some other pathogens tested, including *Candida albicans*, were relatively resistant (Sharma et al 2010).

Cytochromes and P-glycoprotein

Earlier research suggested caution when using echinacea with anticancer and antiretroviral agents (Meijerman et al 2006, van den Bout-van den Beukel et al 2006), due to possible effects on drug-metabolising and transporting enzymes. However, most of the warnings were based on in vitro studies, which now appear to have little or no clinical relevance in vivo (Heinrich et al 2008, Huntimer et al 2006, Izzo 2012, Unger 2010). Moreover, recent research found no pharmacokinetic interactions between echinacea and different antiretrovirals and warfarin (Abdul et al 2010, Hermann & von Richter 2012).

In fact, clinical studies found that echinacea has no clinically significant effect on CYP1A2, CYP2D6, CYP2E1 or CYP3A4 activity (Gurley et al 2004). This was demonstrated for the *E. purpurea* extract Echinaforce (Modarai et al 2011) and 400 mg of powdered dried root of *E. purpurea* taken four times daily for 8 days (Gorski et al 2004). Moreover, studies by Gurley et al found no effects on CYP2D6 in healthy volunteers after echinacea (*E. purpurea)* use for 14 days (Gurley et al 2008a).

To further confirm no clinically significant effects of *E. purpurea* on CYP3A4, two more recent studies using a dose of 500 mg three times daily found no change to the pharmacokinetics of lopinavir-ritonavir (CYP3A4 substrates) in healthy people (Penzak et al 2010) and darunavir-ritonavir in HIV patients (Moltó et al 2011).

In another study investigating echinacea 1275 mg, four times daily (capsules containing a mixture of 600 mg of *E. angustifolia* roots and 675 mg of *E. purpurea* root; standardised to contain 5.75 mg of total alkylamides per tablet) with warfarin in 12 healthy male subjects (single oral dose of 25 mg warfarin or received this dose after 14 days of pretreatment with echinacea) significantly reduced plasma concentrations of S-warfarin and no change for R-warfarin were reported. Warfarin pharmacodynamics, platelet aggregation and baseline were not significantly affected by echinacea (Abdul et al 2010).

Differences between in vitro and clinical results were also found among studies investigating effects on P-glycoprotein, indicating that the effect on P-glycoprotein is not clinically significant (Hellum & Nilsen 2008). A 14-day clinical trial of 18 healthy volunteers detected no significant alteration to digoxin pharmacokinetics for *E. purpurea* extract consisting of 195 mg aerial, root and seed parts, and 72 mg *E. angustifolia* root parts which were standardised to contain 2.2 mg isobutylamides per capsule (Gurley et al 2008b).

Clinical note — Echinacea and cannabinoid receptors

Alkylamides found in echinacea show a structural similarity with anandamide, an endogenous ligand of cannabinoid receptors. CB1 and CB2 receptors belong to G-protein-coupled receptors. CB2 receptors are believed to play an important role in various processes, including metabolic dysregulation, inflammation, pain and bone loss. Compounds such as cannabinoids, which act on these receptors, are becoming more and more popular as they represent new targets for drug discovery. A well-known plant cannabinoid is delta-9-tetrahydrocannabinol, a constituent of *Cannabis sativa*.

OTHER ACTIONS

Antioxidant

Free radical scavenging activity can be attributed to numerous antioxidant constituents found in echinacea, such as vitamin C, beta-carotene, flavonoids, selenium and zinc. One in vitro study reported that the antioxidant activity exerted by echinacea tincture was significantly greater than that observed for *Ginkgo biloba* (Masteikova et al 2007).

Anaesthetic

The alkylamides exert a mild anaesthetic activity, which is typically experienced as a tingling sensation on the tongue (Pizzorno & Murray 2006).

Apoptosis

Apoptosis, or programmed cell death, is a physiological, active cellular suicide process that can be modulated by various stimuli, including hormones, cytokines, growth factors and some chemotherapeutic agents. Research has been undertaken with the three clinically used *Echinacea* spp., several key constituents and different herbal fractions to investigate mechanisms of action, strength of activity and specificity of effect.

The *n*-hexane extracts of all three *Echinacea* spp. exert cytotoxic effects on human pancreatic and colon cancer cells in a concentration- and time-dependent manner, with *E. pallida* being the most active species (Aherne et al 2007). The effects were partially due to apoptosis by significantly increasing caspase-3/7 activity (Chicca et al 2007, 2008). Cytotoxic effects of the *n*-hexane extract of *E. angustifolia* on lung cancer cells have also been reported (Ramirez-Erosa et al 2007). However, in comparison to other herbal medicines such as wild yam and dichora root, echinacea exhibits only weak tumoricidal effects (Mazzio & Soliman 2009).

Isolated hydroxylated polyacetylenes and polyenes (more hydrophilic) from *E. pallida* are less cytotoxic than the more hydrophobic compounds (Pellati et al 2006).

It has been shown that the effects of isolated constituents on cell proliferation vary. In cervical and breast cancer cells treated with doxorubicin and *E. purpurea* extract or isolated echinacea constituents (i.e. cynarin, chicoric acid), the ethyl acetate fraction of echinacea extract and chicoric acid increased breast cancer cell growth and cynarin enhanced the growth of cervical cancer cells. However, cynarin showed antiproliferative effects on breast cancer cells (Huntimer et al 2006).

Chemoprevention

Several experimental studies with mice have found that treatment with echinacea reduces the incidence of tumour development (Brousseau & Miller 2005, Hayashi et al 2001, Miller 2005). Most research has been conducted with *E. purpurea*. In a study with gamma-irradiated mice, *E. purpurea* was able to show radioprotection (use before radiation) as well as radio-recovery effectiveness (Abouelella et al 2007). One study reported that *E. angustifolia* can stimulate mammary epithelial cell differentiation (Starvaggi Cucuzza et al 2008).

An animal study showed that the administration of *E. purpurea* extract to rats with hyperplasia for 4 and 8 weeks gradually and significantly reduced the prostate mass and reversed the degenerative changes in the structure of the prostate gland (Skaudickas et al 2009).

Immunological adjuvants

In vitro studies in human lymphocytes activated with different lectins showed that using *E. purpurea* root extract in addition to individual lectins increased lymphoproliferation, which would suggest adjuvant activity (Chaves et al 2007). In mice, no adjuvant activity was detected for lipophilic, neutral and acidic extracts of echinacea (Gaia Herbs) (Ragupathi et al 2008).

Antifungal activity

Hexane extracts of echinacea have phototoxic antimicrobial activity against fungi (Binns et al 2000). The extracts inhibited growth of yeast strains of *Saccharomyces cerevisiae*, *Candida shehata*, *C. kefyr*, *C. albicans*, *C. steatulytica* and *C. tropicalis*. A recent study reports on antifungal activities of echinacea against *S. cerevisiae* and *Cryptococcus neoformans* by disrupting the fungal cell wall structure (Mir-Rashed et al 2010).

Antiparasitic

Aqueous extracts of echinacea showed activity against gastrointestinal nematodes in goats and pigs (Lans et al 2007). Four preparations of echinacea, with distinct chemical compositions, inhibited the proliferation of *Leishmania donovani*, *Leishmania major* and *Trypanosoma brucei* and at least one extract seems to reverse the proinflammatory activity of *L. donovani* (Canlas et al 2010).

Anxiolytic

The anxiolytic potential of five different echinacea preparations (*E. purpurea*: two different root and one herb extract; *E. angustifolia:* two different root extracts) were tested in a rat model. Three of these decreased anxiety but two of them had a very narrow effective dose range. One extract, *E. purpurea* root extract (70% ethanol v/v), decreased anxiety within a wide dose range (3–8 mg/kg) in three different tests of anxiety. These findings suggest for the first time that certain preparations have a considerable anxiolytic potential (Haller et al 2010).

Hypoglycaemic

Alkylamides and fatty acids isolated from an *n*-hexane extract of the flowers of *E. purpurea* were found to activate peroxisome proliferator-activated receptor gamma without stimulating adipocyte differentiation. This suggests that these compounds have the potential to manage insulin resistance and type 2 diabetes (Christensen et al 2009).

CLINICAL USE

Clinical trials using echinacea have used various preparations, such as topical applications, homeopathic preparations, injectable forms and oral dose forms, characteristics that should be noted when reviewing the data available. Overall, the majority of clinical studies performed in Europe have involved a commercial product known as Echinacin (Madaus, Germany), which is a hydrophilic product prepared from the stabilised juice of fresh *E. purpurea* tops (aerial parts). However, other preparations have also been tested, such as the fresh plant tincture of the whole plant of *E. purpurea* and several preparations manufactured by an Australian company, Mediherb. Due to the different species, plant parts and extraction processes used, the chemical constituent profiles of the different preparations will vary, which may partly account for the differences in test results.

Upper respiratory tract infections

Clinical studies investigating the use of various echinacea preparations in the treatment of upper respiratory tract infections (URTIs) have produced inconsistent results due to the use of different extracts and plant parts, *Echinacea* species, populations and study designs, making interpretation difficult. Overall, the most consistently positive results are obtained from preparations containing *E. purpurea* and *E. angustifolia* for reducing symptoms and possibly the duration of infection, when used as soon as symptoms arise. However, supportive evidence has also accumulated for the use of echinacea as a preventive approach.

In 2000, a Cochrane review was published that had assessed the evidence available from 16 clinical trials (eight treatment and eight prevention) involving a total of 3396 subjects (Melchart et al 2000), and it concluded that some echinacea preparations may be better than placebo, with a majority of studies reporting favourable effects.

Certain facets of quality of life improve with echinacea treatment during an URTI, according to a 2006 review, suggesting that treatment provides symptom relief and improved wellbeing (Gillespie & Coleman 2006). A more recent Cochrane systematic review (Linde et al 2009) evaluated data from 16 trials (up to October 2007). While reviewers reported that evaluation was difficult because of the heterogeneity of preparations tested and variability of trial approaches, it was concluded that preparations based on the aerial parts of *E. purpurea* might be effective for the early treatment of colds in adults, although results are not completely consistent. Also, beneficial effects of other echinacea preparations (i.e. from *E. angustifolia* and *E. pallida*) may exist, but independently replicated rigorous randomised controlled trials (RCTs) are lacking (Linde et al 2009) and further research is needed (Woelkart et al 2008b).

A review including evidence until August 2009 concluded that there is moderate evidence to support the use of *E. purpurea* for treatment of the common cold (Nahas & Balla 2011). Treatment should be commenced at the first signs of infection (Schoop et al 2006a, Woelkart et al 2008a).

Since then a large placebo-controlled trial (n = 719) testing an echinacea preparation made from the roots of *E. purpurea* and *E. angustifolia* (tablets containing the equivalent of 675 mg *E. purpurea* root standardised to 2.1 mg alkamides and 600 mg *E. angustifolia* root standardised to 2.1 mg alkamides: MediHerb brand) failed to find that treatment decreased the severity and duration of the common cold compared to placebo (Barrett et al 2010). Frequency of adverse effects did not differ between the placebo and echinacea group.

Commission E approves the use of *E. purpurea* herb as an immune system support in cases of respiratory and lower urinary tract infection, and *E. pallida* root as supportive treatment in influenza-like infections (Blumenthal et al 2000).

Prevention

According to a 2009 Cochrane systematic review, the beneficial effects of echinacea preparations for the prevention of URTIs may also exist, but require further investigation (Linde et al 2009). Since then, two new RCTs have been published confirming *E. purpurea* preparations are effective at reducing the incidence of the common cold (Jawad et al 2012, Tiralongo et al 2012).

An Australian study published by Tiralongo et al (2012) used a standardised echinacea tablet, known as Echinacea Premium, by MediHerb, which contained 112.5 mg *Echinacea purpurea* 6:1 extract (equivalent to 675 mg dry root) and 150 mg *Echinacea angustifolia* 4:1 extract (equivalent to 600 mg dry root), standardised to 4.4 mg alkylamides. The prevention study did not use artificial rhinovirus inoculation, unlike previous studies, choosing to test the treatment effectiveness in preventing respiratory symptoms in air travellers. The RCT included 175 adults travelling overseas on a long-haul, economy flight for a period of 1–5 weeks. Treatment with the echinacea preparation before and during travel reduced the incidence of respiratory symptoms during travel compared to placebo (Tiralongo et al 2012).

A much larger RCT (n = 755 healthy adults) found that compliant prophylactic use of *E. purpurea* (Echinaforce, produced by Bioforce, Switzerland, containing an alcoholic extract of *E. purpurea*, 95% herb and 5% roots) over a 4-month period reduced the total number of cold episodes, cumulated episode days and painkiller-medicated episodes, inhibited virally confirmed colds and especially prevented enveloped virus infections ($P < 0.05$). Preventive effects increased with therapy compliance and adherence to the protocol (Jawad et al 2012).

Additionally, the treatment was considered well tolerated, with adverse event incidence similar to placebo and no induction of allergic reactions, leucopenia or autoimmune diseases (Schapowal 2013).

Previously, a 2006 meta-analysis by Schoop et al concluded that the odds of experiencing a clinical cold were 55% higher with placebo than with pressed *Echinacea purpurea* juice or hydroethanolic *E. angustifolia* extract following inoculation with rhinovirus. Schoop et al concluded that *E. purpurea* (pressed juice) and *E. angustifolia* (alcoholic extract) show the most promise as preventive treatment, although further investigation is still required to confirm this (Schoop et al 2006b). A 2007 meta-analysis published in *Lancet Infectious Diseases* was also positive and concluded that echinacea products from all species were beneficial in significantly decreasing the incidence (by 58%) and duration (by 1.4 days) of the common cold (Shah et al 2007b).

Athletes

Echinacea has been used to prevent exercise-induced immunosuppression (Gleeson et al 2001). Standardised *E. purpurea* extract (Echinaforce Forte) was effective in the prophylaxis, as well as treatment, of athletes in an open-label study (n = 80) (Ross 2010, Schoop et al 2006a). It is believed that echinacea attenuates mucosal immune suppression known to occur with intensive exercise and can reduce the duration of URTIs that exercising people incur (Hall et al 2007).

Interestingly, a double-blind study of 24 healthy men (20–28 years of age) showed that oral echinacea supplementation resulted in significant increases in erythropoietin, VO_{2max} and running economy (Whitehead 2012).

Paediatric studies

Four randomised studies published after 2000 were conducted with children and generally produced disappointing results (Cohen et al 2004, Spasov et al 2004, Taylor et al 2003, Weber et al 2005). A short review by Koenig and Roehr (2006) has also concluded that there is currently no evidence for the efficacy of *E. purpurea* in the treatment of URTI in children (Koenig & Roehr 2006). A 2008 clinical study with 60 children aged 12–60 months suggests that treating cold with *E. purpurea* in otitis-prone young children does not decrease the risk of acute otitis media, but is associated with a borderline increased risk of having at least one episode of acute otitis media during a 6-month follow-up compared to placebo (Wahl et al 2008).

No clear evidence of benefit in children was also reported in the most recent Cochrane reviews (Fashner et al 2012, Linde et al 2009).

Clinical note — Common cold symptoms: What is usual?

The pathogenesis of the common cold involves a complex interplay between replicating viruses and the host's inflammatory response (Heikkinen & Jarvinen 2003). The onset of cold symptoms after viral incubation varies considerably and depends on the causative virus. In experimental rhinovirus infections, the onset of symptoms has been reported to occur as soon as 10–12 hours after intranasal inoculation. Generally, the severity of the symptoms increases rapidly, peaks within 2–3 days of infection and decreases soon after. The mean duration of the common cold is 7–10 days, but in a proportion of patients some symptoms can still be present after 3 weeks. Symptoms typically start with a sore throat, which is soon accompanied by nasal stuffiness and discharge, sneezing and cough. The soreness of the throat usually disappears quickly, whereas the initial watery rhinorrhoea becomes thicker and more purulent over time and can be accompanied by fever, most usually in children. Other symptoms associated with the cold syndrome include hoarseness, headache, malaise and lethargy.

Acute sore throat

A multicentre, randomised, double-blind, double-dummy-controlled trial (n = 154) found that an echinacea/sage preparation is as efficacious and well tolerated as a chlorhexidine/lignocaine spray in the treatment of acute sore throat (Schapowal et al 2009).

Wound healing

Several uncontrolled clinical studies support the topical use of echinacea to enhance wound healing. A trial involving 4598 people investigated the effects of a preparation consisting of the juice of the aerial parts of *E. purpurea* on various wounds, burns, skin infections and inflammatory skin conditions (Kinkel et al 1984). Topical application of echinacea produced an 85% overall success rate, and the key constituent responsible for enhancing wound healing appears to be echinacoside (Speroni et al 2002).

Preclinical research with a mice model provides some support for its role. An alcoholic extract of *E. pallida* reversed stress-delayed wound healing in mice, but had no apparent wound-healing effect for the non-stressed mice when compared to controls (Zhai et al 2009b).

Commission E approves the external use of *E. purpurea* herb for poorly healing wounds and chronic ulcerations (Blumenthal et al 2000).

Genital herpes *(Condyloma acuminata)*

Human papillomavirus is the most common cause of sexually transmitted disease. It is associated with immunosuppression and shows a marked tendency to recur.

A prospective, double-blind, placebo-controlled, crossover trial conducted over 1 year investigated the effects of an extract of the plant and root of *E. purpurea* (Echinaforce 800 mg twice daily) on the incidence and severity of genital herpes outbreaks in 50 patients (Vonau et al 2001). Treatment was taken for 6 months, then crossed over to the alternative treatment for an additional 6 months. The entry criteria specified a minimum of four recurrences during the previous 12 months or prior to suppressive aciclovir. The study found no statistically significant benefit compared with placebo after 6 months of therapy. It is important to note that, during the study, 15 people dropped out, thereby reducing the sample size, which was considered insufficient by the authors.

IN COMBINATION

A preventive effect against recurrence was found in a more recent RCT for a herbal combination consisting of echinacea, uncaria, tabebuja, papaya, grapefruit and andrographis (*Andrographis paniculata*). In this study, 261 patients allocated to surgical excision were divided into two groups, with one receiving additional treatment with the herbal combination in a dose of three tablets per day for 1 month postoperatively or no additional treatment after surgery. Over a 6-month follow-up period, the group receiving the herbal combination experienced a significantly reduced incidence of recurrence of anal condylomata (7.2% [10/139] compared to 27.1% [33/122] in the control group which received no additional treatment: $P < 0.0001$) (Mistrangelo et al 2010).

Reducing chemotherapy side effects

Results from a small, open, prospective study of subjects with advanced gastric cancer suggest that intravenous administration of a polysaccharide fraction isolated from *E. purpurea* may be effective in reducing chemotherapy-induced leucopenia (Melchart et al 2002). Test subjects had advanced gastric cancer and were undergoing palliative chemotherapy with etoposide, leucovorin and 5-fluorouracil. The median number of leucocytes 14–16 days after chemotherapy was 3630/mcL (range 1470–5770 mcL) in the patients receiving herbal treatment compared with 2370/mcL (870–3950 mcL) in the patients of the historical control group (P = 0.015).

Radiation-associated leucopenia

Equivocal evidence exists for the use of echinacea in radiation-induced leucopenia, according to a small number of randomised studies (Ulbricht & Basch 2005). The product tested was Esberitox, which contains ethanolic extracts of three herbs, including root of echinacea. A study investigated the radioprotective properties of *E. purpurea* tablets (two 275 mg echinacea tablets twice daily) in a group of radiation workers who were identified as carrying dicentric chromosomes in their lymphocytes. After the 2-week treatment, lymphocyte chromosome aberration frequency dropped significantly, and the number of apoptotic cells increased, indicating that echinacea treatment may be beneficial for the prevention of adverse health effects in workers exposed to ionising radiation (Joksić et al 2009).

Halitosis

A study with healthy volunteers suggests that a palatal adhesive tablet containing echinacea may serve as an effective means of treatment for patients complaining of oral malodour, because it resulted in a significant reduction in both oral malodour scores and volatile sulfide compound levels. The reduction in volatile sulfide compound levels was significantly higher than with zinc and chlorhexidine (Sterer et al 2008).

Recurrent candidiasis

The herb is used to treat recurrent candidiasis, chiefly because of its antifungal and immunostimulant properties. Controlled studies are unavailable to determine effectiveness in this condition.

OTHER USES

Echinacea has also been used to treat urinary tract infections, allergies, acne and abscesses, and as adjunctive therapy in cancer (Mills & Bone 2000). Based on the herb's antiviral activity against HSV-1 in vitro, it is also used in the treatment of herpes infections. In practice, it is prescribed with other herbs to treat common infections and to prevent infections generally.

A recent study reported on preliminary results suggesting that Polinacea could be used to improve the immune response to influenza vaccine (Di Pierro et al 2012). The extract is made from the roots of *E. angustifolia* standardised to the complex polysaccharide IDN5405, the phenylethanoid echinacoside and substantial lack of alkamide. This follows a previous study showing that this preparation modulates bovine peripheral blood mononuclear cell proliferation (Wu et al 2009).

It may have potential as a topical cream for improving skin hydration and reducing wrinkles, according to a small study with 10 healthy people aged 25–40 years; however it showed low storage stability (Yotsawimonwat et al 2010).

DOSAGE RANGE

General guide

- Dried herb: 3 g/day of either *E. angustifolia* or *E. purpurea.*
- Liquid extract (1:2): 3–6 mL/day of either *E. angustifolia* or *E. purpurea.*

This dose may be increased to 10–20 mL/day in acute conditions.

Treatment is usually started at the first sign of URTI and continued for 7–14 days.

Specific guide

- *E. angustifolia* dried root: 1–3 g/day.
- *E. purpurea* dried root: 1.5–4.5 g/day.
- *E. purpurea* dried aerial parts: 2.5–6.0 g/day.
- *E. purpurea* expressed juice of fresh plant: 6–9 mL/day.

It appears that the cold-pressed juice and ethanolic extract of the aerial parts of *E. purpurea* and the hydroethanolic extracts from the roots of *E. angustifolia* are the most studied preparation for URTIs.

Doses according to clinical trials

URTI: Treatment

- 10.2 g of dried echinacea root during the first 24 hours and 5.1 g during each of the next 4 days. One tablet contained: 675 mg *E. purpurea* root and 600 mg *E. angustifolia* root standardised to 2.1 mg alkamides (MediHerb brand, produced by Integria Healthcare).
- 4000 mg of extract/day taken as 0.9 mL five times a day, Echinaforce, produced by Bioforce, Switzerland (alcoholic extract of *E. purpurea*, 95% herb and 5% roots, 5 mg/100 g, standardised to contain 5 mg/100 g of dodecatetraenoic acid isobutylamide)

Prevention

- 3825 mg dry root equivalent/day, taken as one tablet three times a day for 6 weeks. One tablet contained: 675 mg *E. purpurea* root and 600 mg *E. angustifolia* root standardised to 2.1 mg alkamides (MediHerb brand, produced by Integria Healthcare).

- 2400 mg of extract/day taken as 0.9 mL three times a day for 1 month, Echinaforce, produced by Bioforce, Switzerland (alcoholic extract of *E. purpurea*, 95% herb and 5% roots, 5 mg/100 g, standardised to contain 5 mg/100 g of dodecatetraenoic acid isobutylamide).
- Two tablets per day, over 8 weeks; each 750-mg tablet contained 1200 mg of tincture mass of Echinaforce, which corresponded to 18.6 mg dry mass of *E purpurea* (drug extract ratio of the 95% herb = 1 : 12; ratio of the 5% root = 1 : 11).

Protection from radiation

- Two 275 mg *E. purpurea* tablets twice daily for 2 weeks (brand not specified).

Genital herpes

- Echinaforce 800 mg twice daily for 1 year.

ADVERSE REACTIONS

Echinacea is well tolerated. A recent analysis of systematic reviews noted only minor adverse effects for *Echinacea* spp. (Posadzki 2013). Short-term use of echinacea is associated with a good safety profile, with a slight risk of transient, reversible and self-limiting gastrointestinal symptoms and rashes (Huntley et al 2005). However, cases of allergic reactions have been reported, resulting in pruritus, urticaria, angio-oedema and anaphylaxis (Mullins 1998, Mullins & Heddle 2002), especially in people with known plant allergies (Tiralongo et al 2012). Hypereosinophilia has been reported, and various authors suggest that the allergic reaction observed is an IgE-mediated hypersensitivity reaction (Maskatia & Baker 2010, Mullins & Heddle 2002).

Overall, echinacea is safe for asthmatics and only in rare instances has been associated with allergic reactions or disease exacerbation (Huntley et al 2005).

It is unclear whether children are more prone to rashes with *E. purpurea* than adults. One study found that rash occurred in 7.1% of children using echinacea compared with 2.7% taking placebo (Taylor et al 2003), whereas a more recent study failed to identify allergic responses or adverse reactions in children with echinacea use (Saunders et al 2007).

There is no clear evidence from basic science or human studies to show that echinacea causes liver toxicity (Ulbricht & Basch 2005). Echinacea (8000 mg/day) taken over 28 days resulted in an increase in serum erythropoietin levels at days 7, 14 and 21, but did not significantly alter red blood cell, haemoglobin and haematocrit levels (Whitehead et al 2007). A single 350-mg dose of *E. purpurea* had no effect on electrocardiographic and blood pressure measurements (Shah et al 2007a).

One clinical study has reported that 1 g *E. purpurea* administered over 10 days altered the gastrointestinal microflora by significantly increasing total aerobic bacteria and bacteria belonging to the *Bacteroides* genus, but not significantly changing the number of enteric bacteria, enterococci, lactobacilli, bifidobacteria or total anaerobic bacteria (Hill et al 2006). Moreover, a review reported several ocular adverse effects due to *E. purpurea* (Santaella & Fraunfelder 2007). A recent review states that echinacea contributes to dry eye (Askeroglu et al 2013). One case report exists where it is believed that an ethanolic extract of *E. pallida*, taken 10–20 days before, may have induced or exacerbated severe thrombotic thrombocytopenic purpura in a healthy 32-year-old man (Liatsos et al 2006).

SIGNIFICANT INTERACTIONS

Cyclophosphamide

Echinacea appears to increase the immunostimulatory effect of low-dose cyclophosphamide, which may be detrimental in autoimmune disease where low doses are used (Stargrove et al 2008) — the clinical significance of this observation is unknown — avoid until safety can be assured.

Immunosuppression agents (e.g. cyclosporine)

Theoretically, there may be an antagonistic pharmacodynamic interaction with immunosuppressive medication, but the clinical relevance is unclear. Exercise caution when using immunosuppressive agents and echinacea concurrently.

Myelosuppressive chemotherapeutic agents

Use of echinacea between treatment cycles may theoretically improve white cell counts, reduce dose-limiting toxicities on myelopoeisis and improve patient's quality of life — potentially beneficial interaction under professional supervision.

Etoposide

One recent case study of a 61-year-old man undergoing chemoradiation with cisplatin and etoposide reports on a probable interaction with echinacea resulting in profound thrombocytopenia requiring platelet transfusion. The authors postulated an interaction via the CYP3A4 enzyme, with echinacea being an inhibitor of CYP3A4 in vitro and etoposide being a substrate of CYP3A4 (Bossaer & Odle 2012). However clinical research casts doubt on this given that various echinacea extracts had no effect on CYP3A4 in human studies (see section on cytochromes and P-glycoprotein, above).

CONTRAINDICATIONS AND PRECAUTIONS

Contraindicated in people with allergies to the Asteraceae (Compositae) family of plants (e.g. chamomile, ragweed).

Commission E warns against using echinacea in cases of autoimmune disorders, such as multiple sclerosis, systemic lupus erythematosus and rheumatoid arthritis, as well as tuberculosis or leucocytosis (Blumenthal et al 2000). A recent review identifies echinacea as one of the herbs with the largest number of documented contraindications, adding multiple sclerosis, tuberculosis and HIV infection to the above list. However, most references used in this review to support this claim were older than 2004 and were not critically evaluated (Tsai et al 2012). As highlighted by Lee and Werth (2004), most contraindications are based on theoretical considerations and case reports with a questionable causal relationship; however, this warning does not appear to be warranted. For example, Boullata and Nace (2000) recommended the avoidance of echinacea use in patients with autoimmune disease, but this recommendation was only seen as the 'extrapolation from experimental observations of echinacea's effects on the immune system' by other authors (Logan & Ahmed 2003).

Moreover, no adverse effects were reported when echinacea was consumed by mice afflicted with autoimmune (type 1) diabetes for up to 18 weeks. Instead, a consistent, long-lasting immunostimulation of only NK cells was observed, thus warranting further research (Delorme & Miller 2005). In addition, recent human studies reported safe and effective systemic echinacea treatment of low-grade autoimmune idiopathic uveitis, resulting in longer steroid-free treatment periods for patients on echinacea treatment (Neri et al 2006).

In practice, echinacea has been successfully used by herbalists in autoimmune disease without mishap (Mills & Bone 2005).

Duration of use

Based on evidence that parenterally administered echinacea reversibly depresses immune parameters, Commission E has recommended that echinacea should not be used for more than 8 weeks. However, in a study in which it was taken orally for up to 6 months, no changes in immune parameters were detected (Vonau et al 2001). As such, no conclusive evidence demonstrates that long-term use is detrimental.

PREGNANCY USE

Oral use of echinacea has generally been considered safe in pregnancy when used in recommended doses (Mills & Bone 2005). This was substantiated by preliminary results from a prospective study of 206 women who had inadvertently taken echinacea during their pregnancy; the study found that gestational use was not associated with an increased risk for major malformations (Gallo et al 2000). Moreover, a review concluded that echinacea is non-teratogenic when used during pregnancy, but that caution should prevail when using echinacea during lactation until further high-quality human studies can determine its safety (Perri et al 2006).

Studies in animal models have reported that echinacea preparations derived from *E. purpurea* produce unwanted effects in pregnant animals, such as interference with embryonal angiogenesis (Barcz et al 2007), alteration of maternal haemopoiesis, fetal growth and a reduction in number of viable fetuses (Chow et al 2006). Due to the high rate of false positives obtained in such animal studies and problems with extrapolating data to humans from these models, the clinical significance of these findings remains unknown.

Practice points/Patient counselling

- Different types of echinacea have demonstrated immunomodulating, anti-inflammatory, antifungal, antiviral and antioxidant activity.
- Overall, clinical studies support the use of echinacea in URTIs, such as bacterial sinusitis, common cold, influenza-like viral infections and streptococcal throat. Current evidence supports its use as acute treatment in URTIs, with some evidence supporting its use as prophylactic treatment.
- Several uncontrolled clinical studies support the topical use of echinacea to enhance wound healing.
- Echinacea is also used to treat urinary tract infections, allergies, acne and abscesses, as adjunctive therapy in cancer, herpesvirus infections and candidiasis.
- Although controversy still exists over which part of the plant and which particular plant has the strongest pharmacological activity, it appears that the cold-pressed juice and ethanolic extracts of the *E. purpurea* plant and *E. angustifolia* root are the most-studied preparations for URTIs.

E

PATIENTS' FAQs

What will this herb do for me?

Echinacea stimulates immune function and also has antifungal (candida), antiviral (herpes) and anti-inflammatory activity. Human studies support its use as an acute treatment and preventive medicine for URTIs in adults. It may also be useful as an adjunct to reduce chemotherapy and radiation-associated side effects. Topically it seems to be useful for chronic wounds and sore throats.

When will it start to work?

As an acute treatment for URTI, echinacea should be started when the first signs and symptoms of infection appear.

Are there any safety issues?

Echinacea is well tolerated, although allergic reactions are possible in rare cases. Patients being treated for autoimmune diseases should be cautious due to echinacea's immune-stimulating effects. Interactions with some immunosuppressant medicines may occur.

REFERENCES

Abdul MI, et al. Pharmacokinetic and pharmacodynamic interactions of echinacea and policosanol with warfarin in healthy subjects. Br J Clin Pharmacol. 2010 May;69(5):508–15.

Abouelella AM et al. Phytotherapeutic effects of *Echinacea purpurea* in gamma-irradiated mice. J Vet Sci 8.4 (2007): 341–51.

Aherne SA, et al. Effects of plant extracts on antioxidant status and oxidant-induced stress in Caco-2 cells. Br J Nutr 97.2 (2007): 321–8.

Altamirano-Dimas M et al. Modulation of immune response gene expression by echinacea extracts: results of a gene array analysis. Can J Physiol Pharmacol 85.11 (2007): 1091–8.

Askeroglu U, et al. Pharmaceutical and herbal products that may contribute to dry eyes. Plast Reconstr Surg. 2013 Jan;131(1):159–67.

Barcz E et al. Influence of *Echinacea purpurea* intake during pregnancy on fetal growth and tissue angiogenic activity. Folia Histochem Cytobiol 45 (Suppl 1) (2007): S35–9.

Barrett B. Medicinal properties of *Echinacea*: a critical review. Phytomedicine 10.1 (2003): 66–86.

Barrett B, et al. Echinacea for treating the common cold: a randomized trial. Ann Intern Med. 2010 Dec 21;153(12):769–77

Bauer VR et al. Immunologic in vivo and in vitro studies on Echinacea extracts. Arzneimittelforschung 38.2 (1988): 276–81.

Bensch K et al. Investigations into the anti-adhesive activity of herbal extracts against *Campylobacter jejuni*. Phytotherapy Research 2011;25(8):1125–32

Benson JM, et al. *Echinacea purpurea* extracts modulate murine dendritic cell fate and function. Food Chem Toxicol. 2010 May;48(5):1170–7.

Binns SE et al. Light-mediated antifungal activity of Echinacea extracts. Planta Med 66.3 (2000): 241–4.

Binns SE et al. Antiviral activity of characterized extracts from *Echinacea* spp. (Heliantheae: Asteraceae) against herpes simplex virus (HSV-1). Planta Med 68.9 (2002): 780–3.

Birt DF et al. Echinacea in infection. Am J Clin Nutr 87.2 (2008): 488S–92S.

Blumenthal M, et al. (eds). Herbal medicine: expanded commission E monographs. Austin, TX: Integrative Medicine Communications, 2000.

Bossaer JB, Odle BL. Probable etoposide interaction with Echinacea. J Diet Suppl. 2012 Jun;9(2): 90–5.

Boullata JI, Nace AM. Safety issues with herbal medicine. Pharmacotherapy 20.3 (2000): 257–69.

Brousseau M, Miller SC. Enhancement of natural killer cells and increased survival of aging mice fed daily Echinacea root extract from youth. Biogerontology 6.3 (2005): 157–63.

Brush J et al. The effect of *Echinacea purpurea, Astragalus membranaceus* and *Glycyrrhiza glabra* on CD69 expression and immune cell activation in humans. Phytother Res 20.8 (2006): 687–95.

Canlas J, et al. Echinacea and trypanasomatid parasite interactions: growth-inhibitory and anti-inflammatory effects of Echinacea. Pharm Biol. 2010 Sep;48(9):1047–52.

Cech NB, et al. Echinacea and its alkylamides: effects on the influenza A-induced secretion of cytokines, chemokines, and PGE_2 from RAW 264.7 macrophage-like cells. Int Immunopharmacol. 2010 Oct;10(10):1268–78.

Chaves F et al. Effect of *Echinacea purpurea* (Asteraceae) aqueous extract on antibody response to Bothrops asper venom and immune cell response. Rev Biol Trop 55.1 (2007): 113–19.

Chicca A et al. Cytotoxic effects of Echinacea root hexanic extracts on human cancer cell lines. J Ethnopharmacol 110.1 (2007): 148–53.

Chicca A et al. Cytotoxic activity of polyacetylenes and polyenes isolated from roots of *Echinacea pallida*. Br J Pharmacol 153.5 (2008): 879–85.

Chicca A, et al. Synergistic immunomopharmacological effects of N-alkylamides in *Echinacea purpurea* herbal extracts. Int Immunopharmacol. 2009 Jul;9(7–8):850–8.

Chow G, et al. Dietary *Echinacea purpurea* during murine pregnancy: effect on maternal hemopoiesis and fetal growth. Biol Neonate 89.2 (2006): 133.

Christensen KB, et al. Activation of PPARgamma by metabolites from the flowers of purple coneflower (*Echinacea purpurea*). J Nat Prod. 2009 May 22;72(5):933–7.

Classen B et al. Immunomodulatory effects of arabinogalactan-proteins from Baptisia and Echinacea. Phytomedicine 13.9–10 (2006): 688–94.

Clifford LJ et al. Bioactivity of alkamides isolated from *Echinacea purpurea* (L.) Moench. Phytomedicine 9.3 (2002): 249–53.

Cohen HA et al. Effectiveness of an herbal preparation containing echinacea, propolis, and vitamin C in preventing respiratory tract infections in children: a randomized, double-blind, placebo-controlled, multicenter study. Arch Pediatr Adolesc Med 158.3 (2004): 217–21.

Delorme D, Miller SC. Dietary consumption of Echinacea by mice afflicted with autoimmune (type I) diabetes: effect of consuming the herb on hemopoietic and immune cell dynamics. Autoimmunity 38.6 (2005): 453–61.

Di Pierro F, et al. Use of a standardized extract from *Echinacea angustifolia* (Polinacea) for the prevention of respiratory tract infections. Altern Med Rev. 2012 Mar;17(1):36–41.

Dong GC et al. Immuno-suppressive effect of blocking the CD28 signaling pathway in T-cells by an active component of Echinacea found by a novel pharmaceutical screening method. J Med Chem 49.6 (2006): 1845–54.

Dong GC et al. Blocking effect of an immuno-suppressive agent, cynarin, on CD28 of T-cell receptor. Pharm Res 26.2 (2008): 375–81.

Egger M et al. Synthesis and cannabinoid receptor activity of ketoalkenes from Echinacea pallida and nonnatural analogues. Chemistry 14.35 (2008): 10978–84.

Ernst E. The risk-benefit profile of commonly used herbal therapies: Ginkgo, St. John's Wort, Ginseng, Echinacea, Saw Palmetto, and Kava. Ann Intern Med 136.1 (2002): 42–53.

Farinacci M, et al. Modulation of ovine neutrophil function and apoptosis by standardized extracts of *Echinacea angustifolia, Butea frondosa* and *Curcuma longa.* Vet Immunol Immunopathol 128.4 (2009): 366–73.

Fashner J, et al., Treatment of the common cold in children and adults., Am Fam Physician. 2012 Jul 15;86(2):153–9.

Gallo M et al. Pregnancy outcome following gestational exposure to echinacea: a prospective controlled study. Arch Intern Med 160.20 (2000): 3141–3.

Gertsch J, et al. New natural noncannabinoid ligands for cannabinoid type-2 (CB2) receptors. J Recept Signal Transduct Res 26.5–6 (2006): 709–30.

Ghaemi A, et al. *Echinacea purpurea* polysaccharide reduces the latency rate in herpes simplex virus type-1 infections. Intervirology. 2009;52(1):29–34.

Gillespie EL, Coleman CI. The effect of Echinacea on upper respiratory infection symptom severity and quality of life. Conn Med 70.2 (2006): 93–7.

Gleeson M, et al. Nutritional strategies to minimise exercise-induced immunosuppression in athletes. Can J Appl Physiol 26 (Suppl) (2001): S23–35.

Gorski JC et al. The effect of echinacea (*Echinacea purpurea* root) on cytochrome P450 activity in vivo. Clin Pharmacol Ther. 2004 Jan;75(1):89–100.

Groom SN, et al. The potency of immunomodulatory herbs may be primarily dependent upon macrophage activation. J Med Food 10.1 (2007): 73–9.

Guiotto P et al. Pharmacokinetics and immunomodulatory effects of phytotherapeutic lozenges (bonbons) with *Echinacea purpurea* extract. Phytomedicine 15.8 (2008): 547–54.

Gurley BJ et al. In vivo assessment of botanical supplementation on human cytochrome P450 phenotypes: *Citrus aurantium, Echinacea purpurea,* milk thistle, and saw palmetto. Clin Pharmacol Ther 76.5 (2004): 428–40.

Gurley BJ et al. Clinical assessment of CYP2D6-mediated herb–drug interactions in humans: effects of milk thistle, black cohosh, goldenseal, kava kava, St. John's wort, and Echinacea. Mol Nutr Food Res 52.7 (2008a): 755–63.

Gurley BJ, et al. Gauging the clinical significance of P-glycoprotein-mediated herb–drug interactions: comparative effects of St. John's wort, Echinacea, clarithromycin, and rifampin on digoxin pharmacokinetics. Mol Nutr Food Res. (2008b) Jul;52(7):772–9.

Hall H, et al. *Echinacea purpurea* and mucosal immunity. Int J Sports Med 28.9 (2007): 792–7.

Haller J. et al. The Effect of Echinacea Preparations in Three Laboratory Tests of Anxiety: Comparison with Chlordiazepoxide. Phytother. Res. 24: 1605–1613 (2010).

Hayashi I et al. Effects of oral administration of *Echinacea purpurea* (American herb) on incidence of spontaneous leukemia caused by recombinant leukemia viruses in AKR/J mice. Nihon Rinsho Meneki Gakkai Kaishi 24.1 (2001): 10–20.

Heikkinen T, Jarvinen A. The common cold. Lancet 361.9351 (2003): 51–9.

Heinrich M, et al. Herbal extracts used for upper respiratory tract infections: are there clinically relevant interactions with the cytochrome P450 enzyme system? Planta Med 74.6 (2008): 657–60.

Hellum BH, Nilsen OG. In vitro inhibition of CYP3A4 metabolism and P-glycoprotein-mediated transport by trade herbal products. Basic Clin Pharmacol Toxicol 102.5 (2008): 466–75.

Hermann R, von Richter O. Clinical evidence of herbal drugs as perpetrators of pharmacokinetic drug interactions. Planta Med. 2012 Sep;78(13):1458–77.

Hill LL et al. *Echinacea purpurea* supplementation stimulates select groups of human gastrointestinal tract microbiota. J Clin Pharm Ther 31.6 (2006): 599–604.

Hinz B, et al. Alkamides from Echinacea inhibit cyclooxygenase-2 activity in human neuroglioma cells. Biochem Biophys Res Commun 360.2 (2007): 441–6.

Huntimer ED, et al. Proliferative activity of *Echinacea angustifolia* root extracts on cancer cells: Interference with doxorubicin cytotoxicity. Chem Biodivers 3.6 (2006): 695–703.

Huntley AL, et al. The safety of herbal medicinal products derived from *Echinacea* species: a systematic review. Drug Saf 28.5 (2005): 387–400.

E

Izzo AA. Interactions between herbs and conventional drugs: overview of the clinical data. Med Princ Pract. 2012;21(5):404–28.
Jawad M, et al. Safety and efficacy profile of *Echinacea purpurea* to prevent common cold episodes: a randomized, double-blind, placebo-controlled trial. Evid Based Complement Alternat Med. 2012:841315.
Joksić G, et al. Biological effects of *Echinacea purpurea* on human blood cells. Arh Hig Rada Toksikol. 2009 Jun;60(2):165–72.
Kapai NA, et al. Selective cytokine-inducing effects of low dose Echinacea. Bull Exp Biol Med. 2011 Apr;150(6):711–3.
Kinkel HJ, et al. Effect of Echinacin ointment in healing of skin lesions. Med Klin 1984; 79: 580–4; as cited in Micromedex Thomson 2003. www.micromedex.com.
Koenig K, Roehr CC. Does treatment with *Echinacea purpurea* effectively shorten the course of upper respiratory tract infections in children? Arch Dis Child 91.6 (2006): 535–7.
LaLone CA et al. Echinacea species and alkamides inhibit prostaglandin E(2) production in RAW264.7 mouse macrophage cells. J Agric Food Chem 55.18 (2007): 7314–22.
LaLone CA, et al. Endogenous levels of Echinacea alkylamides and ketones are important contributors to the inhibition of prostaglandin E2 and nitric oxide production in cultured macrophages. J Agric Food Chem. 2009 Oct 14;57(19):8820–30.
Lans C et al. Ethnoveterinary medicines used to treat endoparasites and stomach problems in pigs and pets in British Columbia, Canada. Vet Parasitol 148.3–4 (2007): 325–40.
Lee AN, Werth VP. Activation of autoimmunity following use of immunostimulatory herbal supplements. Arch Dermatol 140.6 (2004): 723–7.
Liatsos G et al. Severe thrombotic thrombocytopenic purpura (TTP) induced or exacerbated by the immunostimulatory herb Echinacea. Am J Hematol 81.3 (2006): 224.
Linde K et al. Echinacea for preventing and treating the common cold. Cochrane Database Syst Rev 1 (2009): CD000530.
Logan JL, Ahmed J. Critical hypokalemic renal tubular acidosis due to Sjogren's syndrome: association with the purported immune stimulant echinacea. Clin Rheumatol 22.2 (2003): 158–9.
Maskatia ZK, Baker K. Hypereosinophilia associated with echinacea use. South Med J. 2010 Nov;103(11): 1173–4.
Masteikova R et al. Antioxidative activity of Ginkgo, Echinacea, and Ginseng tinctures. Medicina (Kaunas) 43.4 (2007): 306–9.
Matthias A et al. Bioavailability of Echinacea constituents: Caco-2 monolayers and pharmacokinetics of the alkylamides and caffeic acid conjugates. Molecules 10.10 (2005a): 1242–51.
Matthias A et al. Cytochrome P450 enzyme-mediated degradation of Echinacea alkylamides in human liver microsomes. Chem Biol Interact 155 (2005b): 62–70: 1–2.
Matthias A et al. Alkylamides from echinacea modulate induced immune responses in macrophages. Immunol Invest 36.2 (2007a): 117–30.
Matthias A et al. Comparison of Echinacea alkylamide pharmacokinetics between liquid and tablet preparations. Phytomedicine 14.9 (2007b): 587–90.
Matthias A et al. Echinacea alkylamides modulate induced immune responses in T-cells. Fitoterapia 79.1 (2008): 53–8.
Mazzio EA, Soliman KF. In vitro screening for the tumoricidal properties of international medicinal herbs. Phytother Res 23.3 (2009): 385–98.
McCann DA et al. Cytokine- and interferon-modulating properties of *Echinacea* spp. root tinctures stored at –20 degrees C for 2 years. J Interferon Cytokine Res 27.5 (2007): 425–36.
Meijerman I, et al. Herb–drug interactions in oncology: focus on mechanisms of induction. Oncologist 11.7 (2006): 742–52.
Melchart D et al. Echinacea for preventing and treating the common cold. Cochrane Database Syst Rev 2 (2000): CD000530.
Melchart D et al. Polysaccharides isolated from *Echinacea purpurea* herba cell cultures to counteract undesired effects of chemotherapy: a pilot study. Phytother Res 16.2 (2002): 138–42.
Miller SC. Echinacea: a miracle herb against aging and cancer? Evidence in vivo in mice. Evid Based Complement Altern Med 2.3 (2005): 309–14.
Mills S, Bone K. Principles and practice of phytotherapy. London: Churchill Livingstone, 2000.
Mills S, Bone K. The essential guide to herbal safety. St Louis, MO: Churchill Livingstone, 2005.
Mir-Rashed N, et al. Disruption of fungal cell wall by antifungal Echinacea extracts. Med Mycol. 2010 Nov;48(7):949–58.
Mistrangelo M, et al. Immunostimulation to reduce recurrence after surgery for anal condyloma acuminata: a prospective randomized controlled trial. Colorectal Dis. 2010 Aug;12(8):799–803.
Modarai M, et al. Safety of herbal medicinal products: echinacea and selected alkylamides do not induce CYP3A4 mRNA expression. Evid Based Complement Alternat Med. 2011;2011:213021.
Moltó J, et al. Herb–drug interaction between *Echinacea purpurea* and darunavir-ritonavir in HIV-infected patients. Antimicrob Agents Chemother. 2011 Jan;55(1):326–30.
Mullins RJ. Echinacea-associated anaphylaxis. Med J Aust 168.4 (1998): 170–171.
Mullins RJ, Heddle R. Adverse reactions associated with echinacea: the Australian experience. Ann Allergy Asthma Immunol 88.1 (2002): 42–51.
Nahas R, Balla A. Complementary and alternative medicine for prevention and treatment of the common cold. Can Fam Physician. 2011 Jan;57(1):31–6.
Neri PG et al. Oral *Echinacea purpurea* extract in low-grade, steroid-dependent, autoimmune idiopathic uveitis: a pilot study. J Ocul Pharmacol Ther 22.6 (2006): 431–6.
Pellati F et al. Isolation and structure elucidation of cytotoxic polyacetylenes and polyenes from Echinacea pallida. Phytochemistry 67.13 (2006): 1359–64.

Penzak SR, et al. *Echinacea purpurea* significantly induces cytochrome P450 3A activity but does not alter lopinavir-ritonavir exposure in healthy subjects. Pharmacotherapy. 2010 Aug;30(8):797–805.

Perri D et al. Safety and efficacy of echinacea (*Echinacea angustafolia, E. purpurea* and *E. pallida*) during pregnancy and lactation. Can J Clin Pharmacol 13.3 (2006): e262–7.

Pillai S et al. Use of quantitative flow cytometry to measure ex vivo immunostimulant activity of echinacea: the case for polysaccharides. J Altern Complement Med 13.6 (2007): 625–34.

Pizzorno J, Murray M. Textbook of natural medicine. St Louis: Elsevier, 2006.

Posadzki P, (2013) "http://www.ncbi.nlm.nih.gov/pubmed?term=Posadzki%20P%5BAuthor%5D&cauthor=true&cauthor_uid=23472485"

Pugh ND et al. The majority of in vitro macrophage activation exhibited by extracts of some immune enhancing botanicals is due to bacterial lipoproteins and lipopolysaccharides. Int Immunopharmacol 8.7 (2008): 1023–32.

Raduner S et al. Alkylamides from *Echinacea* are a new class of cannabinomimetics: Cannabinoid type 2 receptor-dependent and -independent immunomodulatory effects. J Biol Chem 281.20 (2006): 14192–206.

Raduner S et al. Self-assembling cannabinomimetics: supramolecular structures of N-alkyl amides. J Nat Prod 70.6 (2007): 1010–15.

Ragupathi G et al. Evaluation of widely consumed botanicals as immunological adjuvants. Vaccine 26.37 (2008): 4860–5.

Raman P, et al. Lipid peroxidation and cyclooxygenase enzyme inhibitory activities of acidic aqueous extracts of some dietary supplements. Phytother Res 22.2 (2008): 204–12.

Ramirez-Erosa I et al. Xanthatin and xanthinosin from the burrs of *Xanthium strumarium* L. as potential anticancer agents. Can J Physiol Pharmacol 85.11 (2007): 1160–72.

Raso GM et al. In-vivo and in-vitro anti-inflammatory effect of *Echinacea purpurea* and *Hypericum perforatum*. J Pharm Pharmacol 54.10 (2002): 1379–83.

Ritchie, M.R., et al. 2011. Effects of Echinaforce(R) treatment on ex vivo-stimulated blood cells. Phytomedicine, 18, (10) 826–831 available from: PM:21726792

Ross SM. A standardized Echinacea extract demonstrates efficacy in the prevention and treatment of colds in athletes. Holist Nurs Pract. 2010 Mar-Apr;24(2):107–9.

Santaella RM, Fraunfelder FW. Ocular adverse effects associated with systemic medications: recognition and management. Drugs 67.1 (2007): 75–93.

Sasagawa M et al. Echinacea alkylamides inhibit interleukin-2 production by Jurkat T cells. Int Immunopharmacol 6.7 (2006): 1214–21.

Saunders PR, et al. *Echinacea purpurea* L. in children: safety, tolerability, compliance, and clinical effectiveness in upper respiratory tract infections. Can J Physiol Pharmacol 85.11 (2007): 1195–9.

Schapowal, A. 2013. Efficacy and safety of Echinaforce(R) in respiratory tract infections. Wien.Med Wochenschr., 163, (3–4) 102–105.

Schapowal A, et al. Echinacea/sage or chlorhexidine/lidocaine for treating acute sore throats: a randomized double-blind trial. Eur J Med Res. 2009 Sep 1;14(9):406–12.

Schneider S, et al Anti-herpetic properties of hydroalcoholic extracts and pressed juice from *Echinacea pallida*. Planta Med. 2010 Feb;76(3):265–72

Schoop R, et al. Open, multicenter study to evaluate the tolerability and efficacy of Echinaforce Forte tablets in athletes. Adv Ther 23.5 (2006a): 823–33.

Schoop R et al. Echinacea in the prevention of induced rhinovirus colds: a meta-analysis. Clin Ther 28.2 (2006b): 174–83.

Senchina DS et al. Phenetic comparison of seven Echinacea species based on immunomodulatory characteristics. Econ Bot 60.3 (2006): 205–11.

Senchina DS, et al. Effects of Echinacea extracts on macrophage antiviral activities. Phytother Res. 2010 Jun;24(6):810–6.

Shah SA et al. Effects of echinacea on electrocardiographic and blood pressure measurements. Am J Health Syst Pharm 64.15 (2007a): 1615–18.

Shah SA et al. Evaluation of echinacea for the prevention and treatment of the common cold: a meta-analysis. Lancet Infect Dis 7.7 (2007b): 473–80.

Sharma M et al. Echinacea extracts modulate the pattern of chemokine and cytokine secretion in rhinovirus-infected and uninfected epithelial cells. Phytother Res 20.2 (2006): 147–52.

Sharma M, et al. Induction of multiple pro-inflammatory cytokines by respiratory viruses and reversal by standardized Echinacea, a potent antiviral herbal extract. Antiviral Res. 2009 Aug;83(2):165–70.

Sharma SM, et al Bactericidal and anti-inflammatory properties of a standardized Echinacea extract (Echinaforce): dual actions against respiratory bacteria. Phytomedicine. 2010 Jul;17(8–9):563–8

Sharma M, et al. The potential use of Echinacea in acne: control of *Propionibacterium acnes* growth and inflammation. Phytother Res. 2011 Apr;25(4):517–21.

Skaudickas D, et al. The effect of *Echinacea purpurea* (L.) Moench extract on experimental prostate hyperplasia. Phytother Res. 2009 Oct;23(10):1474–8.

Spasov AA et al. Comparative controlled study of *Andrographis paniculata* fixed combination, Kan Jang and an Echinacea preparation as adjuvant, in the treatment of uncomplicated respiratory disease in children. Phytother Res 18.1 (2004): 47–53.

Speroni E et al. Anti-inflammatory and cicatrizing activity of *Echinacea pallida* Nutt. root extract. J Ethnopharmacol 79.2 (2002): 265–72.

Stargrove M, et al. Herb, nutrient and drug interactions. St Louis: Mosby, Elsevier, 2008.

Starvaggi Cucuzza L et al. Effect of *Echinacea augustifolia* extract on cell viability and differentiation in mammary epithelial cells. Phytomedicine 15.8 (2008): 555–62.

Sterer N et al. Oral malodor reduction by a palatal mucoadhesive tablet containing herbal formulation. J Dent 36.7 (2008): 535–9.

Stevenson LM et al. Modulation of macrophage immune responses by Echinacea. Molecules 10.10 (2005): 1279–85.

Sullivan AM et al. Echinacea-induced macrophage activation. Immunopharmacol Immunotoxicol 30.3 (2008): 553–74.

Taylor JA et al. Efficacy and safety of echinacea in treating upper respiratory tract infections in children: a randomized controlled trial. JAMA 290.21 (2003): 2824–30.

Tiralongo, E., et al. Randomised, double blind, placebo controlled trial of *Echinacea* supplementation in air-travellers, eCAM, 2012;2012:417267.

Toselli F, et al. Metabolism of the major Echinacea alkylamide N-isobutyldodeca-2E,4E,8Z,10Z-tetraenamide by human recombinant cytochrome P450 enzymes and human liver microsomes. Phytother Res. 2010 Aug;24(8):1195–201.

Tragni E et al. Evidence from two classic irritation tests for an anti-inflammatory action of a natural extract, Echinacina B. Food Chem Toxicol 23.2 (1985): 317–19.

Tsai HH et al Evaluation of documented drug interactions and contraindications associated with herbs and dietary supplements: a systematic literature review. Int J Clin Pract. 2012 Nov;66(11):1056–78.

Tubaro A et al. Anti-inflammatory activity of a polysaccharidic fraction of *Echinacea angustifolia*. J Pharm Pharmacol 39.7 (1987): 567–9.

Ulbricht CE, Basch EM. Natural standard herb and supplement reference. St Louis: Mosby, 2005.

Unger M. Pharmacokinetic drug interactions by herbal drugs: Critical evaluation and clinical relevance. Wien Med Wochenschr. 2010 Dec;160(21–22):571–7.

Van den Bout-van den Beukel CJ et al. Possible drug-metabolism interactions of medicinal herbs with antiretroviral agents. Drug Metab Rev 38.3 (2006): 477–514.

Vonau B et al. Does the extract of the plant *Echinacea purpurea* influence the clinical course of recurrent genital herpes? Int J STD AIDS 12.3 (2001): 154–8.

Wahl RA et al. *Echinacea purpurea* and osteopathic manipulative treatment in children with recurrent otitis media: a randomized controlled trial. BMC Complement Altern Med 8 (2008): 56.

Wang CY et al. Modulatory effects of *Echinacea purpurea* extracts on human dendritic cells: a cell- and gene-based study. Genomics 88.6 (2006): 801–8.

Wang CY et al. Genomics and proteomics of immune modulatory effects of a butanol fraction of *Echinacea purpurea* in human dendritic cells. BMC Genomics 9 (2008): 479.

Weber W et al. *Echinacea purpurea* for prevention of upper respiratory tract infections in children. J Altern Complement Med 11.6 (2005): 1021–6.

Whitehead MT Running economy and maximal oxygen consumption after 4 weeks of oral echinacea supplementation. J Strength Cond Res. 2012 Jul;26(7):1928–33.

Whitehead MT et al. The effect of 4 wk of oral echinacea supplementation on serum erythropoietin and indices of erythropoietic status. Int J Sport Nutr Exerc Metab 17.4 (2007): 378–90.

Woelkart K, Bauer R. The role of alkamides as an active principle of echinacea. Planta Med 73.7 (2007): 615–23.

Woelkart K et al. Bioavailability and pharmacokinetics of *Echinacea purpurea* preparations and their interaction with the immune system. Int J Clin Pharmacol Ther 44.9 (2006): 401–8.

Woelkart K, et al. Echinacea for preventing and treating the common cold. Planta Med 74.6 (2008a): 633–7.

Woelkart K et al. Pharmacokinetics of the main alkamides after administration of three different *Echinacea purpurea* preparations in humans. Planta Med 74.6 (2008b): 651–6.

Wu H, et al. Effects of a standardized purified dry extract from *Echinacea angustifolia* on proliferation and interferon gamma secretion of peripheral blood mononuclear cells in dairy heifers. Res Vet Sci. 2009 Dec;87(3):396–8.

Wu L, Rowe EW, Jeftinija K, et al. Echinacea-induced cytosolic Ca^{2+} elevation in HEK293. BMC Complement Altern Med. 2010 Nov 23;10:72.

Yotsawimonwat S, et al. Skin improvement and stability of *Echinacea purpurea* dermatological formulations. Int J Cosmet Sci. 2010 Apr 1 (epub ahead of print).

Yu D, et al. Anti-inflammatory effects of essential oil in *Echinacea purpurea* L. Pak J Pharm Sci. 2013 Mar;26(2):403–8.

Zhai Z et al. Alcohol extracts of Echinacea inhibit production of nitric oxide and tumor necrosis factor-alpha by macrophages in vitro. Food Agric Immunol 18.3–4 (2007a): 221–36.

Zhai Z et al. Echinacea increases arginase activity and has anti-inflammatory properties in RAW 264.7 macrophage cells, indicative of alternative macrophage activation. J Ethnopharmacol 122.1 (2009a): 976–85.

Zhai Z, et al. Alcohol extract of *Echinacea pallida* reverses stress-delayed wound healing in mice. Phytomedicine. 2009b Jun;16(6–7):669–78.

Zwickey H et al. The effect of *Echinacea purpurea, Astragalus membranaceus* and *Glycyrrhiza glabra* on CD25 expression in humans: a pilot study. Phytother Res 21.11 (2007): 1109–12.

E

Feverfew

HISTORICAL NOTE Feverfew has been used traditionally to treat migraine (Shrivastava et al 2006). Feverfew has been used for centuries as a febrifuge, with the common plant name being derived from the Latin term 'febrifugia' which means to 'drive out fevers' (Knight 1995). Feverfew has been used for centuries in Europe to treat headaches, arthritis, coughs and colds, atonic dyspepsia, worm infestation and menstrual disorders, and used as an emmenagogue and anthelmintic agent. In the 1970s it was 'rediscovered' by the medical establishment and subjected to clinical studies, which produced encouraging results that suggested feverfew was an effective prophylactic medicine for migraine headache. The ancient Greeks called it parthenium because legend has it that it was used to save the life of a worker who had fallen from the Parthenon during its construction (Setty & Sigal 2005).

Clinical note — Natural variations in parthenolide content

The amount of parthenolide present in commercial preparations of feverfew leaves varies significantly, with some exhibiting levels as high as 1.7% dry weight and others as low as 0.01% to non-detectable (Cutlan et al 2000). The study by Cutlan et al measured the parthenolide content in plants produced from seeds taken from over 30 different sources and germinated under identical conditions. According to this study, feverfew collected from the wild and distributed by botanical gardens or US Department of Agriculture seed banks yielded plants with the highest mean parthenolide value, and plants with yellow leaves also had significantly higher parthenolide levels than those with green leaves.

OTHER NAMES

Altamisa, bachelor's button, camomilegrande, featherfew, featherfoil, chrysanthemum parthenium, mutterkraut, matrem, midsummer daisy, tanaceti parthenii herba/folium

BOTANICAL NAME/FAMILY

Tanacetum parthenium (family [Asteraceae] Compositae)

PLANT PART USED

Leaf

CHEMICAL COMPONENTS

The leaves and flowering tops contain many monoterpenes and sesquiterpenes as well as sesquiterpene lactones (chrysanthemolide, chrysanthemonin, 10-epi-canin, magnoliolide and parthenolide), reynosin, santamarin, tanaparthins and other compounds. Until recently, the sesquiterpene lactone parthenolide was thought to be the major biologically active constituent. However, in vitro and in vivo research suggests that others are also present (Brown et al 1997, Pugh & Sambo 1988). A study from the early 1990s (Heptinstall et al 1992) found that feverfew grown in the United Kingdom contained a high level of parthenolide in leaves, flowering tops and seeds but had lower levels in stalks and roots. The level of parthenolide in powdered-leaf material fell during storage. Melatonin has been detected in leaf samples of feverfew (1.37–2.45 mcg/g) and in a commercially available product (0.57 mcg/g) (Murch et al 1997).

MAIN ACTIONS

Anti-inflammatory and analgesic

Parthenolide has been shown to have multiple effects on target cells, ranging from phosphorylation to transcriptional inhibition activities (Mathema et al 2012). Several in vivo studies have identified anti-inflammatory and antinociceptive activity for feverfew extracts and parthenolide. When feverfew extracts were orally administered, or pure parthenolide was injected intraperitoneally, significant dose-dependent, anti-inflammatory and antinociceptive effects were observed in animal models (Jain & Kulkarni 1999). Similarly, when feverfew extracts and parthenolide from *Tanacetum vulgare* were administered orally in a rat model, gastric ulcer index was significantly reduced (Tournier et al 1999).

The mechanisms responsible for these effects are not well elucidated. Jain and Kulkarni (1999) demonstrated that the antinociceptive effect was not mediated through the opiate pathway and was not associated with sedation. With regard to the anti-inflammatory effect, several mechanisms appear to be responsible.

In vitro studies have found evidence of cyclooxygenase (COX) and lipoxygenase (LOX) inhibition (Capasso 1986, Pugh & Sambo 1988, Sumner et al 1992), while other tests reveal no effect on COX (Collier et al 1980, Makheja & Bailey 1982). Preincubation of intact rat and human leucocytes for 10 minutes with crude chloroform extracts of fresh feverfew leaves caused a dose-dependent and potent inhibition of their capacity to generate COX and LOX pathways (Sumner et al 1992).

Inhibition of phospholipase A_2 has also been suggested (Heptinstall 1988, Sumner et al 1992). Direct binding and inhibition of I-kappa B kinase beta, an important subunit involved in cytokine-mediated signalling, has been demonstrated for parthenolide in in vitro studies (Kwok et al 2001). Parthenolide also inhibits nitric oxide production, an important regulator and inducer of various inflammatory states (Wong & Menendez 1999). More recently, results from an in vivo study confirm that parthenolide inhibits proinflammatory cytokine responses, although the authors propose that proinflammatory mediators, including chemokines (MIP-2), plasma enzyme mediators (complement, kinin and clotting systems) and lipid mediators (COX, prostaglandins, platelet-activating factor), are also likely to be involved (Smolinski & Pestka 2003). Parthenolide acts as inhibitor of inflammasomes. Inflammasomes engage and activate caspase-1, which in turn processes the inactive pro-IL-18 and pro-IL-1β into their corresponding active forms of proinflammatory cytokines, IL-18 and IL-1β, respectively (Mathema et al 2012). In an in vitro study, synovial fibroblasts were cultured with and without feverfew extract and subsequently stimulated with interleukin-1 (IL-1), interferon (IFN) and tumour necrosis factor (TNF) to induce expression of intercellular adhesion molecule-1 (ICAM-1). The most potent inhibition of ICAM-1 was seen in cultures stimulated with IL-1 and TNF (46–95% suppression) and less so in cultures stimulated with IFN-gamma (17–39% suppression). One of the major proinflammatory functions of ICAM-1 in vivo is as a cellular ligand for T cells. Feverfew inhibition of ICAM-1 was associated with a decrease in functional T-cell adhesion. Feverfew inhibition of IL-1-induced ICAM-1 was dose-dependent (Piela-Smith & Liu 2001).

Parthenolide suppresses inflammation by inhibiting activity of NF-κB (Mathema et al 2012). The majority of NF-κB activities are related to TNF-alpha and oxidative stress.

In vitro testing has identified that parthenolide-induced reduction in IL-6 secretion is dose-dependent: 29% by 200 nm ($P < 0.001$); 45% by 1 mcm ($P < 0.001$); 98% by 5 mcm ($P < 0.001$). At the highest concentration tested, at 5 mcm, it reduced the secretion of TNF-alpha by 54% ($P < 0.001$) (Magni et al 2012). These combined actions, inhibiting proinflammatory agents and reducing microglial activation, provide a theoretical rationale behind the proposed clinical effects of feverfew in reducing the frequency and severity of acute migraine attacks.

The essential oil constituent of feverfew, chrysanthenyl acetate, inhibits prostaglandin synthetase in vitro and also seems to possess analgesic properties (Pugh & Sambo 1988).

Antispasmodic

The results from several in vitro studies generally indicate that feverfew decreases vascular smooth-muscle spasm (Barsby et al 1992, 1993a, 1993b, Collier et al 1980).

Inhibits serotonin release and binding

Parthenolide and several other sesquiterpene lactone constituents inhibit serotonin release but do not bind to 5-HT_1 receptors, according to in vivo data (Groenewegen & Heptinstall 1990, Marles et al 1992, Weber et al 1997a). Some tests with 5-HT_{2A} receptors show that parthenolide is a low-affinity antagonist (Weber et al 1997b), whereas other tests found no effect on 5-HT_{2A} or 5-HT_{2B} receptors. Feverfew extract potently and directly blocked 5-HT_{2A} and 5-HT_{2B} receptors and neuronally released 5-HT, suggesting that feverfew powder or extracts are more effective than isolated parthenolide (Mittra et al 2000).

Anticancer activity

In the last decade, there has been increasing investigation into the parthenolide constituent from feverfew as an anticancer agent. It displays multiple mechanisms, such as its selectivity to biological and/or epigenetic targets, tumours and cancer stem cells (Ghantous et al 2013), which make it an attractive candidate for further cancer research.

Parthenolide has been shown to withdraw cells from cell cycle or to promote cell differentiation, and finally to induce programmed cell death (Pajak et al 2008). It has an ability to induce apoptosis in a variety of cancer lines, has chemosensitising properties and is non-toxic to normal cells. The potent anticancer activity of parthenolide is in part due to its ability to inhibit transcription factor NF-κB, thereby reducing survival potential in a number of cancer cells (Anderson & Bejcek 2008, Pajak et al 2008, Zunino et al 2007). The effect is specific to tumour cells. Parthenolide-induced generation of reactive oxygen species (ROS) in cancer cells has also been shown to play a role in promoting apoptotic cell death. Interestingly, experiments in animal models indicate that, in non-cancerous cells, parthenolide acts as an antioxidant molecule by increasing levels of intracellular glutathione, resulting in a decrease in ROS. In contrast, an increase in ROS generation in response to parthenolide appears to increase apoptotic cell death in cancer cells. Recently, parthenolide was found to induce apoptosis in cancer cells, through mitochondrial dysfunction. Through this mechanism, it was shown to significantly inhibit tumour growth and angiogenesis in a xenograft model, exhibiting anticancer activity in human colorectal cancer in vitro and in vivo (Kim SL et al 2012).

This proapoptotic action is suggested to occur through the activation of p53 and the increased production of ROS (Mathema et al 2012).

Signal transducer and activator of transcription (STAT) proteins are transcriptional factors responding to extracellular ligands that mediate diverse biological functions, such as cell proliferation, differentiation and apoptosis. Parthenolide shows strong NF-κB and STAT inhibition-mediated transcriptional suppression of proapoptotic genes. Parthenolide induced ROS exclusively in tumour cells. Parthenolide was found to have the unique ability to induce sensitisation to extrinsic as well as intrinsic apoptosis signalling in cancer cells. The proapoptotic activity is not observed in normal cells (Mathema et al 2012). A comparison of parthenolide treatment with that of the standard chemotherapy drug cytosine arabinoside (Ara-C) found it was much more specific to leukaemia cells (Guzman et al 2005), whereas Ara-C killed both leukaemia cells and normal cells to an equivalent extent; parthenolide showed significantly less toxicity to normal haematopoietic cells from bone marrow and cord blood.

Parthenolide is cytotoxic to several breast cancer cell lines, one human cervical cancer cell line (SiHa), prostate tumour-initiating cells isolated from prostate cancer cell lines, as well as primary prostate tumour-initiating cells, glioblastoma cells and pre-B acute lymphoblastic leukaemia lines (Anderson & Bejcek 2008, Kawasaki et al 2009, Wu et al 2006, Zunino et al 2007).

An in vitro and in vivo study of parthenolide in breast cancer found that parthenolide has significant in vivo chemosensitising properties in the metastatic breast cancer setting (Sweeney et al 2005). Parthenolide was effective either alone or in combination with docetaxel in reducing colony formation, inducing apoptosis and reducing the expression of prometastatic genes IL-8 and the antiapoptotic gene GADD45beta1 in vitro. In an adjuvant setting, animals treated with parthenolide and docetaxel combination showed significantly enhanced survival compared with untreated animals or animals treated with either drug. The enhanced survival in the combination arm was associated with reduced lung metastases. In addition, nuclear NF-κB levels were lower in residual tumours and lung metastasis of animals treated with parthenolide, docetaxel or both.

Studies are being conducted with a series of aminoparthenolide analogues, which have been synthesised by a conjugate addition of several primary and secondary amines to the alpha-methylene-gamma-butyrolactone function of the sesquiterpene lactone, parthenolide (Nasim & Crooks 2008).

Metastatic melanoma is a highly life-threatening disease. Parthenolide has been found to inhibit the proliferation of various cancer cells, mainly by inducing apoptosis (Lesiak et al 2010). In this in vitro study, parthenolide reduced the number of viable adherent cells in melanoma cultures. Half maximal inhibitory concentration values were around 4 mcmol/L. Cell death accompanied by mitochondrial membrane depolarisation and caspase-3 activation was observed as the result of parthenolide application (Lesiak et al 2010). In breast cancer cell lines, parthenolide reduced the number of viable MCF-7 and MDA-MB-231 cells, with half maximal inhibitory concentration values between 6 and 9 mcmol/L (Wyrębska et al 2013).

In colorectal cancer cell line COLO205, parthenolide depletes intracellular thiols and increases ROS and cytosolic calcium levels, resulting in cellular stress, which consequently leads to cell apoptosis. Similar effects of parthenolide mediate mitochondrial damage and cell death in human gastric cancer cell line SGC7901, suggesting that parthenolide-induced ROS-mediated apoptosis may be common to many types of cancer cells (Mathema et al 2012).

Parthenolide has been found to selectively affect gene regulation or activity and consequently controls of target cells (Mathema et al 2012).

OTHER ACTIONS

Platelet aggregation inhibition

Evidence is contradictory as to whether feverfew inhibits platelet aggregation. Several in vitro studies and animal models have observed inhibition of platelet aggregation (Heptinstall et al 1988, Jain & Kulkarni 1999, Makheja & Bailey 1982). However, no significant effects were seen in a clinical study of 10 patients receiving feverfew (Biggs et al 1982). Feverfew was found to inhibit secretory activity in platelets. Release of serotonin from platelets induced by various aggregating agents (adenosine diphosphate, adrenaline, arachidonic acid, collagen and U46619) was inhibited. Platelet aggregation was consistently inhibited. It is interesting to note that parthenolide stimulated functional platelet production from human megakaryocyte cell lines as well as from primary mouse and human megakaryocytes in vitro. Parthenolide enhanced platelet production via inhibition of NF-κB signalling in megakaryocytes. Parthenolide significantly reduced the basal NF-κB activity at 6 h. This effect was found to be independent of the parthenolide-induced oxidative stress response. Additionally, parthenolide treatment of human peripheral blood platelets attenuated activation of stimulated platelets (Sahler et al 2011).

Mast cell stabilisation

Tests with rat mast cells indicate that feverfew extract inhibits histamine release, but the mechanism of action is different from cromoglycate and quercetin (Hayes & Foreman 1987). In vivo tests confirm that parthenolide significantly inhibits IgE antigen-induced mast cell degranulation in a dose-dependent manner (Miyata et al 2008). The formation of microtubules is well known to be crucial for IgE antigen-induced degranulation in mast cells, and parthenolide exhibits tubulin/microtubule-interfering activity. The mast cell stabilisation effect is rapid in vivo, as an immediate-type allergic response was induced in test animals and strongly inhibited by parthenolide administration.

Hepatoprotective effects

Parthenolide exhibits potent antifibrotic activity both in vitro and in vivo. The apoptotic and antifibrotic effects of parthenolide have been investigated for its apoptotic effects in test tube studies on hepatic stellate cells and for antifibrotic action on hepatic fibrosis in an in vivo rat model (Kim IH et al 2012). Parthenolide inhibited cell growth and induced apoptotic cell death in a dose-dependent manner in hepatic stellate cells. Parthenolide (at 2 and 4 mg/kg) significantly reduced hepatic fibrosis in thioacetamide-treated rats and decreased expression of transforming growth factor-beta-1.

Bone regulation effects

Parthenolide shows potential in bone-destructive disorders associated with osteoclast-mediated bone resorption (Kim SL et al 2012).

Osteoclasts, which are bone-resorbing multinucleated giant cells differentiated from haematopoietic stem cells upon stimulation by two essential cytokines, receptor activator of NF-κB ligand (RANKL) and macrophage colony-stimulating factor (M-CSF), play a central role in bone-destructive disorders. RANKL promotes osteoclast formation from osteoclast precursors while M-CSF supports proliferation and survival of precursor cells during osteoclast differentiation. In a mouse model, parthenolide suppressed RANKL-mediated osteoclast differentiation in bone marrow macrophages. In addition, parthenolide inhibited mRNA expression of osteoclast-associated receptor, tartrate-resistant acid phosphatase, dendritic cell-specific transmembrane protein and cathepsin K by RANKL, suggesting that parthenolide inhibits the bone-resorbing activity of mature osteoclasts. Parthenolide inhibits differentiation and bone-resolving activity of osteoclast by RANKL.

> ***Clinical note — Migraine***
>
> Migraine is a common episodic familial headache disorder characterised by a combination of headache and neurological, gastrointestinal and autonomic symptoms. It has a 1-year prevalence of approximately 18% in women, 6% in men and 4% in children before puberty (Silberstein 2004). Several underlying mechanisms are considered responsible for the onset of migraine.
>
> One of the genes linked to migraine is associated with dysfunction in P-type neuronal calcium channels, which mediate 5-HT and excitatory neurotransmitter release. This dysfunction can impair release of 5-HT and predispose patients to migraine attacks or impair their self-aborting mechanism (Silberstein 2004). Additionally, nitric oxide may be involved in the initiation and maintenance of migraine headache (Ferrari 1998). Migraine aura is now thought to be caused by neuronal dysfunction, not ischaemia, and headache begins while cortical blood flow is reduced.
>
> In clinical practice, the three goals of migraine-preventive therapy are to reduce attack frequency, severity and duration, improve responsiveness to treatment of acute attacks, improve function and reduce disability. Ultimately, choice of treatment should be based on efficacy, adverse effects and coexisting conditions, with a full therapeutic trial taking 2–6 months.

CLINICAL USE

Migraine headache

Currently available research investigating the use of feverfew for migraine prophylaxis is promising, especially with the dried feverfew leaf formulations, whereas ethanolic extracts have produced inconsistent results.

Ideally, more research into the most effective formulation and dosage regimen is required to provide more consistent results. In particular, further work is needed to determine which other constituents, beside parthenolide, are important for producing the desired clinical effect, whether by pharmacodynamic or pharmacokinetic interaction with parthenolide or as stand-alone active constituents (Saranitzky et al 2009).

Traditionally, feverfew has been used in the treatment and prevention of headaches. Its growing popularity in the United Kingdom, in the 1970s and 1980s, prompted researchers to investigate its usefulness under controlled trial conditions. The first double-blind study investigating feverfew in migraine prophylaxis was published in 1985 and involved 17 patients who had been chewing fresh feverfew leaves on a daily basis (Johnson et al 1985). Therapeutic effect was maintained when capsules containing freeze-dried feverfew powder were continued, whereas those allocated placebo capsules experienced a significant increase in the frequency and severity of headache, nausea and vomiting during the early months of withdrawal.

Since then, numerous clinical studies have been conducted to determine the role of feverfew in the prevention of migraine headache.

In 2000, Ernst and Pittler published a systematic review of six randomised, placebo-controlled, double-blind trials of feverfew as a prophylactic treatment and concluded that the evidence favours feverfew as an effective preventive treatment against migraine headache, and is generally well tolerated. One of the studies in the systematic review noted a 24% reduction in the number of attacks during feverfew treatment but found no significant alteration in the duration of individual attacks. There was a non-significant tendency ($P = 0.06$) towards milder headaches with feverfew and a significant reduction ($P < 0.02$) in nausea and vomiting accompanying the attacks (Murphy et al 1988).

A Cochrane systematic review of five placebo-controlled, randomised, double-blind trials ($n = 343$) concluded that there was insufficient evidence to determine whether feverfew was superior to placebo in reducing migraine frequency or incidence, severity of nausea or severity of migraines (Pittler & Ernst 2004). A closer look at the studies reveals that results were mixed, methodological quality varied and various dosage regimens, administration forms and extracts were used. One study used three different dosing regimens for a CO_2 extract, two studies used an alcoholic and CO_2 extract, three studies used dried feverfew leaves for 8–24 weeks and one study used an alcoholic extract for 8 weeks. Interpretation of test results is made even more difficult when one considers the naturally occurring chemical variations among the preparations.

The authors have offered several explanations for the inconsistent clinical findings and point out that previous negative studies used extracts standardised for parthenolide concentration; however, it is possible that other compounds found in whole-leaf preparations may also be important for pharmacological activity. In vivo studies support this view (Mittra et al 2000). Others have also suggested that the alcoholic extracts may not contain the same amount of adjunctive compounds necessary for action or, conversely, the alcoholic extract may contain greater concentrations of compounds which reduce the action of parthenolide (Saranitzky et al 2009). It is also possible that the negative results obtained by some studies may be due to underdosing.

Since then, positive results were obtained for a CO_2 extract of feverfew (with enriched parthenolide) in a randomised, double-blind, placebo-controlled, multicentre study of 170 patients with frequent migraine headache (Diener et al 2005). Active treatment with feverfew (MIG-99) at a dose of 6.25 mg, three times daily, significantly reduced the frequency of migraine headache episodes, the number of migraine headache days and migraine duration over a 16-week period. More specifically, migraine frequency decreased from 4.8 to 2.9 attacks per month in the MIG-99 group and to 3.5 attacks for placebo ($P = 0.046$). The prophylactic effect was most pronounced in the first 2 months and then appeared to stabilise. The treatment was very well tolerated. Participants included in this study needed to have experienced migraine headaches for at least 1 year, have an average of 4–6 migraine attacks in the month before commencing treatment and a duration of attack between 4 and 72 hours. All prophylactic migraine treatment was ceased at least 4 weeks prior to study commencement.

IN COMBINATION

A number of trials have tested feverfew in combination with other herbs and nutritional supplements. Shrivastava et al (2006) tested a combination of feverfew (600 mg/day) and willow bark (600 mg/day), known as Mig-RL, in a 12-week prospective study for the prophylaxis of migraine and the combination was shown to significantly reduce attack frequency and severity. The combination was selected because previous in vitro studies identified that feverfew and willow bark inhibit binding to 5-$HT_{2A/2C}$ receptors and the combination of willow bark with feverfew further inhibited 5-HT_{1D} receptors, whereas feverfew on its own did not. Combination herbal treatment significantly reduced migraine attack frequency by 57.2% at 6 weeks ($P < 0.029$) and by 61.7% at 12 weeks ($P < 0.025$) in nine of 10 patients, with 70% of patients having a reduction of at least 50%. Attack intensity was reduced by 38.7% at 6 weeks ($P < 0.005$) and by 62.6% at 12 weeks ($P < 0.004$) in all of the 10 patients, with 70% of patients having a reduction of at least 50%. Attack duration decreased by 67.2% at 6 weeks ($P < 0.001$) and by 76.2% at 12 weeks ($P < 0.001$) in all of the 10 patients. Two patients were excluded for reasons unrelated to treatment. Self-assessed general health, physical performance, memory and anxiety also improved by the end of the study. The treatment was well tolerated and no adverse events occurred (Shrivastava et al 2006).

The combination of feverfew with ginger (GelStat Migraine) in a sublingually administered fluid was evaluated as an acute treatment in an open-label study involving 29 patients with 1-year history of migraine meeting International Headache Society diagnostic criteria of 2–8 migraines per month and ≤15 headache days per month, with or without aura. People ingested the test substance during the early mild headache phase of an oncoming migraine. Herbal treatment was found to totally relieve pain in 48% of people within 2 hours and a further 34% reported pain had remained mild and not worsened. Of the group, 59% were satisfied with their response to GelStat Migraine therapy (Cady et al 2005). Of note, the product is marketed as a homeopathic product and contains extremely small amounts of both herbs.

In 2011, a randomised, multicentre study of 60 patients found that 2 hours after acute treatment with sublingual feverfew/ginger, 32% of subjects receiving active medication and 16% of subjects receiving placebo were pain-free ($P = 0.02$). At 2 hours, 63% of subjects receiving feverfew/ginger found pain relief (pain-free or mild headache) vs 39% for placebo ($P = 0.002$) and pain severity was significantly less with the feverfew/ginger combination (Cady et al 2011). All subjects in this study had <15 headache days per month and were not experiencing medication overuse headache.

Feverfew (100 mg) combined with riboflavin (400 mg) and magnesium (300 mg) was compared to stand-alone riboflavin (25 mg) treatment in a randomised, double-blind study of migraine sufferers (Maizels et al 2004). Both treatments showed a significant reduction in number of migraines, migraine days and migraine index in the 3-month trial, which was greater than responses for placebo in other trials of migraine prophylaxis. When treatment responses were compared, no significant differences were seen between the groups, indicating that feverfew at this low dose is ineffective.

Women patients ($n = 22$) with headache who were treated with acupuncture for 10 weeks showed significant improvements in symptoms, migraine disability assessment score (MIDAS; quantifies headache-related disability over a 3-month period) and overall health-related quality of life (Ferro et al 2012). When feverfew (150 mg/day taken at bedtime) was combined with acupuncture ($n = 23$), the results were better than in patients who received acupuncture ($n = 22$) or feverfew alone ($n = 23$). There was a substantial mean reduction from baseline in the visual analogue scale (rated from 0 [pain-free] to 10 [unbearable pain]) outcome measure in both treatment groups. However, the combination of acupuncture and feverfew was statistically significantly more effective than acupuncture or feverfew alone in reducing the mean of score of pain on the visual analogue scale.

Arthritic conditions

Although traditionally used as a treatment for inflammatory joint conditions, the results of a randomised, double-blind study involving 41 patients with symptoms of rheumatoid arthritis found no difference between chopped dried feverfew (70–86 mg) or placebo after 6 weeks' treatment (Pattrick et al 1989).

OTHER USES

Dermatology

Feverfew may protect the skin from the numerous external aggressions encountered daily by the skin as well as reduce the damage to oxidatively challenged skin (Martin et al 2008). Parthenolide-free feverfew extract is being investigated in various dermatological conditions. It has been found to protect the skin against inflammation and ultraviolet (UV)-induced damage (Finkey et al 2005). When the parthenolide-free feverfew extract was topically applied, it significantly reduced loss of cell viability, increase in proinflammatory mediator release and induction of DNA damage induced by solar-simulated UV radiation in a human epidermal model. It also exhibited potent antioxidant activity in vitro and has been shown to dismutate superoxide, thereby protecting cells from the pro-oxidant depletion of endogenous skin antioxidants.

In the next phase of testing, a clinical study was conducted with an emollient containing the parthenolide-free feverfew extract, which confirmed that treatment significantly reduced the erythema effects of acute UVB exposure by up to 60% compared to placebo. Assessment was done by a blinded clinical grader and a chroma meter. These results suggest that topical application of parthenolide-depleted feverfew extract (PD-feverfew) can protect skin from UV-induced damage and from oxidative damage and help to repair damaged DNA.

In another study, PD-feverfew extract was found to possess free radical scavenging activity against a wide range of ROS and with greater activity than vitamin C (Martin et al 2008). In vitro, PD-feverfew attenuated the formation of UV-induced hydrogen peroxide and reduced proinflammatory cytokine release. It also restored cigarette smoke-mediated depletion of cellular thiols. In vivo, topical PD-feverfew reduced UV-induced epidermal hyperplasia, DNA damage and apoptosis. This suggests that feverfew has the ability to scavenge free radicals, preserve endogenous antioxidant levels, reduce DNA damage and induce DNA repair enzymes, which can help repair damaged DNA.

Oncology

Parthenolide has demonstrated potent antitumour activity in a variety of experimental models (in vitro and in vivo), and its mechanisms of action are becoming better elucidated. The positive results obtained in these preliminary studies indicate that it may have potential in the treatment of cancer; however, no clinical studies have been published to date to determine its efficacy in humans.

DOSAGE RANGE

- Dried leaf: 50–200 mg daily.
- Fresh plant tincture (1 : 1): 0.7–2.0 mL/day.
- Dried plant tincture (1 : 5): 1–3 mL/day.
- Prevention of migraine headaches (based on clinical studies): 125–600 mg/day of powder, standardised to contain a minimum parthenolide content of 0.2%, or 400 mcg, which should be taken for at least 4 months. It is still controversial as to whether ethanolic standardised extracts are best for migraine prophylaxis or not.
- According to a large 2005 randomised controlled trial: a commercial CO_2 extract of *Tanacetum parthenium* (MIG-99) 6.25 mg taken three times daily

TOXICITY

Unknown, although no major safety issues have been identified (Ernst & Pittler 2000).

ADVERSE REACTIONS

According to a Cochrane systematic review of five studies (Pittler & Ernst 2004), feverfew is well tolerated and adverse events are generally mild and reversible. Symptoms were most frequently reported by long-term users and were predominantly mouth ulceration and gastrointestinal symptoms. Contact dermatitis, mouth soreness and lip swelling have also been reported when leaves are chewed. People allergic to the Asteraceae (Compositae) family of plant, or feverfew in particular, should avoid feverfew products that contain parthenolide, as it is this component which is thought to be the main inducer of the allergic response (Sharma & Sethuraman 2007).

SIGNIFICANT INTERACTIONS

Controlled studies are not available; therefore, interactions are based on evidence of activity and are largely theoretical and speculative.

Anticoagulants

Theoretically, feverfew may increase bruising and bleeding; however, although feverfew inhibits platelet aggregation in vitro and in vivo, no effects were seen in a clinical study (Biggs et al 1982) — observe patients taking this combination.

CONTRAINDICATIONS AND PRECAUTIONS

Hypersensitivity to plants in the daisy (Asteraceae/Compositae) family (e.g. chamomile, ragweed).

PREGNANCY USE

Feverfew is contraindicated in pregnancy. An in vitro and in vivo preliminary screen using a rat model suggested that feverfew consumption may have detrimental effects in pregnancy, a finding which needs to be more fully explored in larger studies (Yao et al 2006). Feverfew-treated animals had reduced litter sizes, a greater proportion of smaller fetuses than the control group and increased pre-implantation loss, indicating maternal and embryonic effects. However, it should be noted that the doses used were 59 times the accepted human dose, and therefore the clinical relevance of the findings are unclear. A full reproductive toxicity study is warranted to determine whether the observed effects are clinically significant.

Practice points/Patient counselling

- Currently available research investigating the use of feverfew for migraine prophylaxis is promising, especially with the dried feverfew-leaf formulations, whereas ethanolic extracts have produced inconsistent results.
- A study with a commercial CO_2 extract of *Tanacetum parthenium* (MIG-99) showed it reduced the frequency, severity and duration of migraine headache in chronic sufferers.
- Tincture or solid-dose preparations may be better tolerated than chewing the fresh leaves, which have been associated with mouth ulcers and lip swelling in some individuals.

- Traditionally, feverfew has also been used to treat coughs and colds, fevers, atonic dyspepsia, worm infestation, menstrual disorders, nervous debility, joint pain and headaches.
- Parthenolide-free feverfew shows promise as a dermatological and UV-protective agent when used topically.
- Many preliminary studies with parthenolide confirm that it has potent anti-tumour activity; however, it has not yet been tested in humans.
- Use is contraindicated in pregnancy until safety can be better established.

PATIENTS' FAQs

What will this herb do for me?

Evidence suggests that feverfew may reduce the frequency and severity of migraine headaches when dried-leaf preparations are used, whereas results with ethanolic extracts are inconsistent. Topical application with parthenolide-free feverfew cream shows promise as a dermatological preparation to reduce redness after sun exposure and help heal damaged skin.

When will it start to work?

Of those studies producing positive results, it appears that benefits in migraine occur within 2 months of use; however, in practice, some patients experience benefits within the first 4 weeks.

Are there any safety issues?

Feverfew should not be used in pregnancy or by people with Asteraceae (Compositae) allergy.

REFERENCES

Anderson KN, Bejcek BE. Parthenolide induces apoptosis in glioblastomas without affecting NF-kappaB. J Pharmacol Sci 106.2 (2008): 318–20.

Barsby RW et al. Feverfew extracts and parthenolide irreversibly inhibit vascular responses of the rabbit aorta. J Pharm Pharmacol 44.9 (1992): 737–40.

Barsby RW, et al. A chloroform extract of the herb feverfew blocks voltage-dependent potassium currents recorded from single smooth muscle cells. J Pharm Pharmacol 45.7 (1993a): 641–5.

Barsby RW et al. Feverfew and vascular smooth muscle: extracts from fresh and dried plants show opposing pharmacological profiles, dependent upon sesquiterpene lactone content. Planta Med 59.1 (1993b): 20–5.

Biggs MJ et al. Platelet aggregation in patients using feverfew for migraine. Lancet 2.8301 (1982): 776.

Brown AM et al. Pharmacological activity of feverfew (*Tanacetum parthenium* (L.) Schultz-Bip.): assessment by inhibition of human polymorphonuclear leukocyte chemiluminescence in-vitro. J Pharm Pharmacol 49.5 (1997): 558–61.

Cady RK et al. Gelstat Migraine (sublingually administered feverfew and ginger compound) for acute treatment of migraine when administered during the mild pain phase. Med Sci Monit 11.9 (2005): I65–9.

Cady, R.K., et al. 2011. A double-blind placebo-controlled pilot study of sublingual feverfew and ginger (LipiGesic M) in the treatment of migraine. Headache, 51, (7) 1078–1086.

Capasso F. The effect of an aqueous extract of *Tanacetum parthenium* L. on arachidonic acid metabolism by rat peritoneal leucocytes. J Pharm Pharmacol 38.1 (1986): 71–2.

Collier HO et al. Extract of feverfew inhibits prostaglandin biosynthesis. Lancet 2.8200 (1980): 922–3.

Cutlan AR et al. Intra-specific variability of feverfew: correlations between parthenolide, morphological traits and seed origin. Planta Med 66.7 (2000): 612–17.

Diener HC et al. Efficacy and safety of 6.25 mg t.i.d. feverfew CO2-extract (MIG-99) in migraine prevention: a randomized, double-blind, multicentre, placebo-controlled study. Cephalalgia 25.11 (2005): 1031–41.

Ernst E, Pittler MH. The efficacy and safety of feverfew (*Tanacetum parthenium* L.): an update of a systematic review. Public Health Nutr 3.4A (2000): 509–14.

Ferrari MD. Migraine. Lancet 351.9108 (1998): 1043–51.

Ferro EC et al. The combined effect of acupuncture and *Tanacetum parthenium* on quality of life in women with headache: randomised study. Acupunct Med 30.4 (2012): 252–7.

Finkey MB et al. Parthenolide-free feverfew extract protects the skin against UV damage and inflammation. J Am Acad Dermatol 52.3 (2005): 93.

Ghantous A et al. Parthenolide: from plant shoots to cancer roots. Drug Discov Today (2013) May 17. S1359–6446.

Groenewegen WA, Heptinstall S. A comparison of the effects of an extract of feverfew and parthenolide, a component of feverfew, on human platelet activity in-vitro. J Pharm Pharmacol 42.8 (1990): 553–7.

Guzman ML et al. The sesquiterpene lactone parthenolide induces apoptosis of human acute myelogenous leukemia stem and progenitor cells. Blood 105.11 (2005): 4163–9.
Hayes NA, Foreman JC. The activity of compounds extracted from feverfew on histamine release from rat mast cells. J Pharm Pharmacol 39.6 (1987): 466–70.
Heptinstall S. Feverfew: an ancient remedy for modern times? J R Soc Med 81.7 (1988): 373–4.
Heptinstall S et al. Inhibition of platelet behaviour by feverfew: a mechanism of action involving sulphydryl groups. Folia Haematol Int Mag KlinMorpholBlutforsch 115.4 (1988): 447–9.
Heptinstall S et al. Parthenolide content and bioactivity of feverfew (*Tanacetum parthenium* (L.) Schultz-Bip.). Estimation of commercial and authenticated feverfew products. J Pharm Pharmacol 44.5 (1992): 391–5.
Jain NK, Kulkarni SK. Antinociceptive and anti-inflammatory effects of *Tanacetum parthenium* L. extract in mice and rats. J Ethnopharmacol 68.1–3 (1999): 251–9.
Johnson ES et al. Efficacy of feverfew as prophylactic treatment of migraine. BMJ (Clin Res Ed) 291.6495 (1985): 569–73.
Kawasaki BT et al. Effects of the sesquiterpene lactone parthenolide on prostate tumor-initiating cells: an integrated molecular profiling approach. Prostate 69.8 (2009): 827–37.
Kim IH et al. Parthenolide-induced apoptosis of hepatic stellate cells and anti-fibrotic effects in an in vivo rat model. Exp Mol Med 44.7 (2012): 448–56.
Kim SL et al. Parthenolide suppresses tumor growth in a xenograft model of colorectal cancer cells by inducing mitochondrial dysfunction and apoptosis. Int.J Oncol 41.4 (2012): 1547–1553.
Knight DW. Feverfew: chemistry and biological activity. Nat. Prod. Rep 12.3 (1995): 271–276.
Kwok BH et al. The anti-inflammatory natural product parthenolide from the medicinal herb Feverfew directly binds to and inhibits IkappaB kinase. Chem Biol 8.8 (2001): 759–66.
Lesiak K et al. Parthenolide, a sesquiterpene lactone from the medical herb feverfew, shows anticancer activity against human melanoma cells in vitro. Melanoma Res 20.1 (2010):21–34.
Magni P et al. Parthenolide inhibits the LPS-induced secretion of IL-6 and TNF-alpha and NF-kappaB nuclear translocation in BV-2 microglia. Phytother Res 26.9 (2012) 1405–1409.
Maizels M, et al. A combination of riboflavin, magnesium, and feverfew for migraine prophylaxis: a randomized trial. Headache 44.9 (2004): 885–90.
Makheja AN, Bailey JM. A platelet phospholipase inhibitor from the medicinal herb feverfew (*Tanacetum parthenium*).Prostaglandins Leukot Med 8.6 (1982): 653–60.
Marles RJ et al. A bioassay for inhibition of serotonin release from bovine platelets. J Nat Prod 55.8 (1992): 1044–56.
Martin K et al. Parthenolide-depleted Feverfew (*Tanacetum parthenium*) protects skin from UV irradiation and external aggression. Arch Dermatol Res 300.2 (2008): 69–80.
Mathema VB et al. Parthenolide, a sesquiterpene lactone, expresses multiple anti-cancer and anti-inflammatory activities. Inflammation 35.2 (2012): 560–5.
Mittra S et al. 5-hydroxytryptamine-inhibiting property of feverfew: role of parthenolide content. Acta Pharmacol Sin 21.12 (2000): 1106–14.
Miyata N et al. Inhibitory effects of parthenolide on antigen-induced microtubule formation and degranulation in mast cells. Int Immunopharmacol 8.6 (2008): 874–80.
Murch SJ et al. Melatonin in feverfew and other medicinal plants. Lancet 350.9091 (1997):1598–9.
Murphy JJ et al. Randomised double-blind placebo-controlled trial of feverfew in migraine prevention. Lancet 2.8604 (1988): 189–92.
Nasim S, Crooks PA. Antileukemic activity of aminoparthenolide analogs. Bioorg Med ChemLett 18.14 (2008): 3870–3.
Pajak B, et al. Molecular basis of parthenolide-dependent proapoptotic activity in cancer cells. Folia HistochemCytobiol 46.2 (2008): 129–35.
Pattrick M, et al. Feverfew in rheumatoid arthritis: a double blind, placebo controlled study. Ann Rheum Dis 48.7 (1989): 547–9.
Piela-Smith T, Liu X. Feverfew extracts and sesquiterpene lactone parthenolide inhibit intercellular adhesion molecule-1 expression in human synovial fibroblasts. Cell Immunol, 209 (2001), 89–96.
Pittler M, Ernst E. Feverfew for preventing migraine. Cochrane Database Syst Rev 1 (2004): CD 002286.
Pugh WJ, Sambo K. Prostaglandin synthetase inhibitors in feverfew. J Pharm Pharmacol 40.10 (1988): 743–5.
Sahler J et al. The Feverfew plant-derived compound, parthenolide enhances platelet production and attenuates platelet activation through NF-κB inhibition. Thromb Res 127.5 (2011):426–34.
Saranitzky E et al. Feverfew for migraine prophylaxis: a systematic review. J Diet Suppl 6.2 (2009): 91–103.
Setty AR, Sigal LH. Herbal medications commonly used in the practice of rheumatology: mechanisms of action, efficacy, and side effects. Semin Arthritis Rheum 34.6 (2005):773–84.
Sharma VK, Sethuraman G. Parthenium dermatitis. Dermatitis 18.4 (2007): 183–90.
Shrivastava R, et al. *Tanacetum parthenium* and *Salix alba* (Mig-RL) combination in migraine prophylaxis: a prospective, open-label study. Clin Drug Investig 26.5 (2006): 287–96.
Silberstein SD. Migraine. Lancet 363.9406 (2004): 381–91.
Smolinski AT, Pestka JJ. Modulation of lipopolysaccharide-induced proinflammatory cytokine production in vitro and in vivo by the herbal constituents apigenin (chamomile), ginsenoside Rb1 (ginseng) and parthenolide (feverfew). Food ChemToxicol 41.10 (2003): 1381–90.
Sumner H et al. Inhibition of 5-lipoxygenase and cyclo-oxygenase in leukocytes by feverfew. Involvement of sesquiterpene lactones and other components. Biochem Pharmacol, 43.11 (1992), 2313–2320.
Sweeney CJ et al. The sesquiterpene lactone parthenolide in combination with docetaxel reduces metastasis and improves survival in a xenograft model of breast cancer. Mol Cancer Ther 4.6 (2005): 1004–12.
Tournier H et al. Effect of the chloroform extract of *Tanacetum vulgare* and one of its active principles, parthenolide, on experimental gastric ulcer in rats. J Pharm Pharmacol 51.2 (1999): 215–19.

F

Weber JT et al. Rabbit cerebral cortex 5HT1a receptors. Comp Biochem Physiol C Pharmacol Toxicol Endocrinol 117.1 (1997a): 19–24.
Weber JT et al. Activity of Parthenolide at 5HT2A receptors. J Nat Prod 60.6 (1997b): 651–3.
Wong HR, Menendez IY. Sesquiterpene lactones inhibit inducible nitric oxide synthase gene expression in cultured rat aortic smooth muscle cells. BiochemBiophys Res Commun 262.2 (1999): 375–80.
Wu C et al. Antiproliferative activities of parthenolide and golden feverfew extract against three human cancer cell lines. J Med Food 9.1 (2006): 55–61.
Wyrębska A et al. Apoptosis-mediated cytotoxic effects of parthenolide and the new synthetic analog MZ-6 on two breast cancer cell lines. Mol Biol Rep 40.2 (2013):1655–63.
Yao M, et al. A reproductive screening test of feverfew: is a full reproductive study warranted? Reprod Toxicol 22.4 (2006): 688–93.
Zunino SJ, et al. Parthenolide induces significant apoptosis and production of reactive oxygen species in high-risk pre-B leukemia cells. Cancer Lett 254.1 (2007): 119–27.

Fish oils

BACKGROUND AND RELEVANT PHARMACOKINETICS

One of the two human essential fatty acids (EFAs) EFAs is alpha-linolenic acid (ALA or 18:3ω-3), which, due to the position of its first double bond, is classified as an omega-3 (ω-3) EFA. Although mammals have the ability to introduce double bonds into most positions of the fatty-acid chain in fat metabolism, therefore producing various unsaturated metabolites, they lack the capacity to insert double bonds at the ω-3 and ω-6 positions. Consequently, linoleic acid (LA) and ALA, which already have the double bond at the ω-3 or ω-6 position, respectively, are considered essential and must be consumed in the diet. When the EFAs are consumed in this precursor state they follow a pathway of further elongation and desaturation via the action of delta-6- and delta-5-desaturase until they form the 'active' fatty acids: eicosapentaenoic acid (20:5ω-3) (EPA) and docosahexaenoic acid (DHA) (22:6ω-3), also referred to as the ω-3 long-chain polyunsaturated fats (ω-3 LCPUFAs).

Fish oils, also known as marine oils, are rapidly absorbed from the gastrointestinal tract and compete with arachidonic acid (AA) for incorporation into phospholipids, particularly of platelets, erythrocytes, neutrophils, monocytes and liver cells (Simopoulos 1999). When stimulated, the cell membranes release polyunsaturated fatty acids (PUFAs), which are then converted into 20-carbon eicosanoids, which have profound and extensive physiological effects. The most active of these metabolites are prostaglandins, prostacyclins and thromboxanes, which affect blood chemistry, muscle contraction, immune function and inflammation. Dietary fats not used in this way are stored in adipose tissue and ultimately oxidised to produce energy. The fatty-acid cell membrane profile of different tissues will have varying ratios of EPA and DHA, but generally DHA is considered the major component of phospholipids in the retina, brain, male reproductive tissue and myocardium (Groff & Gropper 2004).

Supplements based on fish liver oils, such as cod and halibut, contain EPA and DHA together with high levels of vitamins A and D. As such, they have additional actions and safety issues besides those found with traditional marine lipid supplements. This review will focus on the research surrounding those fish oils that are not liver extractions.

CHEMICAL COMPONENTS

Dietary fish contains a number of nutrients important for health, such as several B vitamins, vitamin E, calcium, magnesium and potassium, and are an excellent source of protein with a low saturated fat content. Importantly, they also contain the two PUFAs: EPA and DHA. EPA has 20 carbon atoms and five double bonds, and DHA has 22 carbon atoms and six double bonds. Both are derived from ALA and are considered conditionally essential. The EPA and DHA found in whole fish are predominantly esterified in the *sn*-2 position of triacylglycerols and glyercophospholipids; however, when found in supplements, most commonly exist as ethyl esters (Visioli et al 2003). This minor chemical distinction may explain the speculated superior bioavailability of these fats when derived from the diet as opposed to supplements.

FOOD SOURCES

Most dietary EPA and DHA are consumed in the form of fish or seafood. Deep-sea cold-water fish, such as salmon, mackerel, halibut and herring, provide the most concentrated sources. Current Australian estimates of intake indicate inadequate consumption according to World Health Organization (WHO) standards (Meyer et al 2003).

DEFICIENCY SIGNS AND SYMPTOMS

Based on epidemiological studies, low levels of ω-3 LCPUFAs are associated with:

- fetal alcohol syndrome (DHA) (Horrocks & Yeo 1999)
- attention-deficit hyperactivity disorder (ADHD) (DHA) (Horrocks & Yeo 1999)
- learning deficits (DHA) (Horrocks & Yeo 1999)
- cystic fibrosis (DHA) (Horrocks & Yeo 1999)
- phenylketonuria (DHA) (Horrocks & Yeo 1999)
- cardiovascular disease (CVD), including an increased risk of sudden death due to heart disease (Siscovick et al 2003)
- inflammatory disorders
- rheumatoid arthritis (RA) (Navarro et al 2000)
- unipolar depression (DHA) (Horrocks & Yeo 1999)
- senile dementia.

In addition to these symptoms, lack of dietary EFAs has been implicated in the development or aggravation of numerous diseases such as breast cancer, prostate cancer, RA, asthma, pre-eclampsia, depression and schizophrenia (Yehuda et al 2005).

Clinical note — Are ALA-rich oils a worthy substitute for fish oils?

Both EPA and DHA are derived from ALA, so food sources containing ALA are seen as indirect dietary sources. ALA is commonly found in non-hydrogenated canola oil, linseed oil, soybean oil, flaxseed, pumpkin and walnuts. Studies investigating the effects of ALA supplementation have not consistently produced the same positive results as for fish oils, most likely due to inefficient conversion of ALA into EPA and DHA. This is reportedly poor in healthy individuals, with only 5–10% of ALA converted to EPA and 2–5% of ALA converted to DHA (Davis & Kris-Etherton 2003). Consequently, the few foods that contain both EPA and DHA in their preformed state offer a significant advantage over other sources. The most concentrated dietary source of both EPA and DHA is deepsea oily fish.

Primary deficiency

Full-term babies fed a skim-milk formula low in ALA are at risk of primary deficiency. In the past, patients fed long-term with fat-free total parenteral nutrition solutions were at risk, but fat emulsions are now in general use and prevent deficiency. Studies have demonstrated lower plasma levels of EPA and DHA in vegetarians and vegans, suggesting they may be at risk of deficiency; however, the findings of a cross-sectional study comparing the dietary intakes and plasma levels of 196 meat-eating, 231 vegetarian and 232 vegan men in the United Kingdom did not suggest that there is cause for alarm (Rosell et al 2005). Vegans and vegetarians had significantly lower levels of these fatty acids; however, they remained steady and there is evidence of some conversion of ALA into EPA and DHA.

There is much discussion regarding the inadequate intake of EPA and DHA generally in the Western diet. Australian data, based on dietary intake records from the 1995 National Nutrition Survey, have estimated the average daily intake of EPA and DHA to be 0.008 g and 0.015 g, respectively. If correct, this indicates that the majority of Australians are failing to meet recommended amounts (Meyer et al 2003).

Secondary deficiency

People with fat malabsorption syndromes, serious trauma or burns are at risk of reduced PUFA levels (Beers & Berkow 2003). A secondary deficiency may also manifest as a result of abnormal or compromised activity of the delta-6 and delta-5 desaturase enzymes, for example in diabetics, patients with a variety of metabolic disorders and individuals with increased dietary saturated fats and *trans* fatty acids, alcoholics and the elderly (Davis & Kris-Etherton 2003, Houston 2005).

MAIN ACTIONS

As precursors of eicosanoids, PUFAs found in fish oils exert a wide influence over many important physiological processes.

Cardiovascular effects

Fish oils exert myriad different effects on the heart and vessels, demonstrated in both experimental models and human studies. It is speculated that the clinical effects attributed to ω-3 PUFAs are due to the summation of many small pharmacological effects, adding up to a larger protective effect on mortality and/or cardiovascular events.

Prevent malignant cardiac arrhythmias

Dietary fish or fish oil intake has been shown to prevent cardiac arrhythmias and associated sudden death in numerous animal studies (Billman et al 1997, 1999, Kang & Leaf 1996, 2000, McLennan et al 1988, 1990), in vitro and more recently in human clinical trials (Jung et al 2008). This has been achieved using intakes below those required to alter plasma lipids or blood pressure. It appears that the myocardial membrane phospholipid content increases in DHA but not always EPA, with fish intake. The preferential accumulation of DHA affords protection against ventricular fibrillation induced under a variety of conditions, such as ischaemia and reperfusion (McLennan 2001).

Inadequate DHA in myocyte membranes has been reported to be associated with altered sodium, calcium and potassium ion channel functions, mitochondrial function and increased arrhythmia susceptibility with an increased prevalence of sudden cardiac death (Jung et al 2008, Siscovick et al 2003). One in vivo study suggests that fish oils electrically stabilise myocytes, increasing the electrical impulse required to produce an action potential by approximately 50% and prolonging the refractory time by 150% (Kang & Leaf 2000).

Triglyceride (TG)-lowering activity

Fish oil supplements effectively reduce TG levels, as demonstrated in human studies. This is of particular interest, given only moderate elevations in TG levels have been associated with a progressively increased risk of ischaemic heart disease, independently of other major risk factors, including high-density lipoprotein (HDL) cholesterol (Jeppesen et al 1998). A significant plasma TG-lowering activity has also been demonstrated for a highly potent form of ω-3 fatty acids, available as Lovaza in the United States (previously Omacor) (Kar 2014).

Lipoprotein effects

Both ω-6 and ω-3 LCPUFAs can inhibit the expression of genes involved in fatty-acid and TG synthesis (Jung et al 2008). Dietary ω-3 LCPUFAs, in particular, and their metabolites, through this mechanism are reported to increase beta-oxidation and inhibit adipogenesis. Ultimately, this may result in reduced substrate for TG synthesis and thus explain ω-3 PUFAs' profound TG-lowering effects.

Concerns raised previously about increased LCPUFAs in lipoproteins increasing the susceptibility to oxidation of the low-density lipoproteins (LDLs) have recently been moderated, with a demonstrable difference between EPA and DHA. While increased levels of EPA (4.8 g/day) did increase the LDL susceptibility to damage, DHA supplementation (4.9 g/day) had no effect on the oxidation process (Mesa et al 2004). Concurrent supplementation with antioxidants however appears prudent with high doses of ω-3 PUFAs.

Improved endothelial function

Studies have indicated that fish oils can improve endothelial relaxation by enhancing nitric oxide- (NO) and non-NO-induced vasodilation (Holub 2002).

A double-blind study conducted by Mori et al (2000) showed that, relative to placebo, DHA, but not EPA, enhances vasodilator mechanisms and attenuates constrictor responses in forearm microcirculation.

Reducing resting heart rate

Regular ω-3 LCPUFA intake can lower resting heart rate by up to 5 beats/min in patient and healthy populations, in healthy individuals during exercise without compromising maximum heart rate and during exercise recovery in post myocardial infarction (MI) patients (McLennan 2014).

Reduce blood pressure

Three meta-analyses have concluded that fish oils exert a significant blood pressure-lowering effect in hypertensive people; however, the effects can only be described as modest, between 2 and 5 mmHg (Geleijnse et al 2002, Miller et al 2014, Morris et al 1993). Hypotensive activity appears to be dose-dependent and DHA may have greater effect than EPA. Alternatively, a 2006 Cochrane review found no significant changes to systolic or diastolic blood pressure with ω-3 LCPUFA consumption (Hooper et al 2006). The review assessed studies that used both plant- and fish-based ω-3 fatty acids, dietary sources and supplements.

While the mechanism is unknown, current theories include EPA stimulation of prostacyclin synthesis and increased NO production — both vasodilators. An additional action may be improved autonomic nervous system function, and inhibition of adrenal activation (Din et al 2004, Ross 2005); however, these are inconsistent with the attribution of action to DHA. In addition to the actions improving endothelial function generally, other posited mechanisms for a hypotensive effect include: blunting of the renin–angiotensin–aldosterone system via reduced adrenal aldosterone synthesis, altered AA metabolism, modulation of calcium release and influx into vascular smooth-muscle cells and activation of vascular adenosine triphosphate-sensitive potassium channels (Jung et al 2008).

Clinical interest — Do fish oil supplements pose a significant bleeding risk?

A search through Medline reveals several case reports where bleeding episodes are attributed to fish oil ingestion (Buckley et al 2004, Jalili & Dehpour 2007, McClaskey & Michalets 2007). In each case, the person affected was elderly and also taking warfarin. One was a report of an elderly man taking high-dose ω-3 fatty acids (6 g/day) with both aspirin and warfarin who developed a subdural haematoma after a minor fall (McClaskey & Michalets 2007). Another case is reported of a 67-year-old woman taking warfarin for 1.5 years who doubled the fish oil dose from 1000 to 2000 mg/day, causing an associated elevation in international normalised ratio (INR) from 2.8 to 4.3 within 1 month (Buckley et al 2004). A third case was of a 65-year-old male who had been taking warfarin for 6 months and then was recommended trazodone and fish oils, causing his INR to rise to 8.06 (Jalili & Dehpour 2007).

Although these case reports would lead us to believe that ω-3 fatty acids interact with warfarin and increase the risk of bleeding, several intervention studies have come to a different conclusion. One randomised study of 511 patients taking either aspirin (300 mg/day) or warfarin (INR aimed at 2.5–4.2) found that a dose of 4 g/day of fish oils did not increase the number of bleeding episodes, bleeding time or any parameters of coagulation and fibrinolysis (Eritsland et al 1995). A smaller placebo-controlled study by Bender et al (1998) of patients receiving chronic warfarin therapy found that fish oil doses of 3–6 g/day produced no statistically significant difference in INR between the placebo lead-in and treatment period within each group. There was also no difference in INR between groups.

More recently, Harris (2007) examined 19 clinical studies which used doses of fish oils varying from 1 g/day to 21 g/day in patients undergoing major vascular surgery (coronary artery bypass grafting, endarterectomy) or femoral artery puncture for either diagnostic cardiac catheterisation or percutaneous transluminal coronary angioplasty. Of note, in 16 studies patients were taking aspirin and in three studies patients were taking heparin. The review concluded that the risk for bleeding was virtually non-existent. Frequent comments accompanying the studies were 'no difference in clinically significant bleeding noted' or 'no patient suffered from bleeding complications'. The same conclusion was reached in a 2008 review which stated that no published studies have reported clinically significant bleeding episodes amongst patients treated with antiplatelet drugs and fish oils (3–7 g/day) (Harris et al 2008). In 2014, a clinical audit of over 900 cardiac surgery patients at the Alfred Hospital found that those taking 3 g of fish oils daily in the week before surgery did not have a significantly increased risk of major haemorrhage or re-admission due to bleeding, once again demonstrating the lack of risk for fish oil supplements in this population (Braun et al 2014).

Overall, when we consider the body of evidence available regarding ω-3 fatty acid supplementation, it is clear that the benefits for cardioprotection far outweigh the risk of bleeding. This not only applies to patients taking aspirin but also those patients about to undergo coronary artery bypass surgery or percutaneous transluminal coronary angioplasty. While the evidence suggests that fish oils in low to moderate doses do not increase bleeding risk with warfarin, a general caution should still apply to patients taking high doses with antiplatelet or anticoagulant medication.

Reduce and possibly reverse atherogenesis

Ω-3 fatty acids alter eicosanoid synthesis and inhibit smooth-muscle cell proliferation, suggesting a role in reducing atherosclerotic development (Holub 2002). One controlled study demonstrated that fish oil ingestion had a clinically significant influence on atherosclerosis (von Schacky et al 2001). This randomised, double-blind study of 223 patients found that a dose of 1.5 g ω-3 fatty acids reduced progression and increased regression of established coronary artery disease as assessed by coronary angiography. The content of diets and relevant risk factors were examined through a health survey on the inhabitants in a fishing village ($n = 261$) and in a farming village ($n = 209$) in Japan (Yamada et al 2000). Pulse wave velocity of the aorta, intima media thickness (IMT) of the carotid artery and atherosclerotic plaques as obtained by ultrasonography were used as measures of atherosclerosis. The fish consumption of both males and females in the fishing village was about 1.8 and 1.6 times higher, respectively, than that reported in the farming village ($P < 0.0001$). Dietary consumption of EPA and DHA was significantly higher in the fishing village versus the farming village ($P < 0.001$). Pulse wave velocity and IMT were significantly lower in the fishing village than in the farming village in males ($P < 0.01$ and $P < 0.001$, respectively). IMT was significantly lower in females ($P < 0.001$). There was an eightfold difference in the average number of plaques in the common carotid arteries in males ($P < 0.0001$) and a fivefold difference in females between the villages ($P < 0.0001$).

Antithrombotic and antiplatelet

Dietary ω-3 PUFAs enhance antiaggregatory and antiadhesive platelet activity by inducing increased production of prostacyclin I_3 and suppressing synthesis of the chemotactic platelet adhesion-promoting substances, leukotriene B_4 and thromboxane A_2 (Jung et al 2008, Kinsella 1987). A meta-analysis of randomised controlled trials (RCTs) ($n = 15$) with 409 participants found daily supplementation with ω-3 PUFA significantly reduced adenosine diphosphate (ADP)-induced platelet aggregation compared with placebo ($P = 0.02$) (Gao et al 2013). Independently of this, ω-3 LCPUFAs reduce levels of several coagulating factors (e.g. VII and X, and fibrinogen) (Jung et al 2008).

Platelet aggregation studies and flow cytometric analyses of platelet activation and platelet–leucocyte aggregates were determined at baseline and after 4 weeks of a moderate dose of ω-3 (DHA 520 mg and EPA 120 mg) supplementation in 40 healthy subjects and 16 patients with a history of CVD. In healthy subjects, ω-3 PUFA significantly reduced ADP-induced platelet aggregation, as measured by maximum amplitude of platelet aggregation ($P = 0.036$) and velocity of aggregation ($P = 0.014$), as well as adrenaline-induced platelet aggregation (maximum slope, $P = 0.013$; lag time to platelet aggregation, $P = 0.002$). ω-3 PUFA also reduced P-selectin expression ($P = 0.049$) on platelets and platelet–monocyte aggregates ($P = 0.022$). There were fewer changes in platelet aggregation and activation found in subjects with CVD. Nevertheless, there was a reduction in the velocity of AA-induced platelet aggregation (P = 0.009) and increased lag time to platelet aggregation for U46619-induced platelet aggregation. ω-3 PUFA had a greater effect on platelet aggregation and activation in healthy subjects and the findings of this study support the recommendation of a higher dose of ω-3 PUFA in patients with CVD who are already receiving antiplatelet medication than in healthy people with CVD (P = 0.018) (McEwen et al 2013).

In animal models of arterial thrombosis, fish oil-enriched diets have been shown to have an antithrombotic effect; however, there is evidence suggesting that this is most likely to occur when associated with reduced saturated fat intake (Hornstra 1989).

Clinical observations of Eskimos have found lowered platelet counts, inhibition of platelet aggregation and prolonged bleeding times compared with age- and sex-matched Danes. However, intervention studies using fish oil supplements have produced conflicting results (Hellsten et al 1993, Kristensen et al 1989, Radack et al 1990) and, more recently, a review of clinical studies concluded that there was no clinically significant effect on bleeding with usual therapeutic doses (Harris 2007).

Anti-inflammatory

Fish oils induce a series of chemical changes in the body that ultimately exert an anti-inflammatory action. They partially replace AA in inflammatory cell membranes, and compete with it for the enzymes cyclo-oxygenase and lipoxygenase, leading to reduced production of proinflammatory metabolites such as 2-series prostaglandins and 4-series leukotrienes (Calder 2002, 2003, Cleland et al 2003). Resolvins are compounds that reduce cellular inflammation by inhibiting the production and transportation of inflammatory cells and chemicals. EPA-derived lipid mediator resolvin E1 has potent anti-inflammatory and pro-resolution actions both in vitro and in vivo. In addition, EPA-derived and DHA-derived products such as resolvin D1 and protectin D1 have potent anti-inflammatory and pro-resolution properties (Seki et al 2009).

Besides this, ω-3 PUFAs suppress the production of proinflammatory cytokines, and reduce the expression of cell adhesion molecules, critical in recruiting circulating leucocytes to the vascular endothelium (Calder 2002, Din et al 2004). According to new research, it appears that anti-inflammatory activity may vary among different sources of fish oils due to variations in EPA/DHA content (Bhattacharya et al 2007).

Neurological effects

Fatty acids are major components of the brain and are found in high concentrations in two structural components: the neuronal membrane and the myelin sheath. About 50% of the neuronal membrane is composed of fatty acids (one-third from ω-3 LCPUFAs), while in the myelin sheath lipids constitute about 70% (Yehuda et al 2005). The lipid component has a relatively high turnover, in contrast to the protein component, which is fundamentally stable. The de novo synthesis of PUFA is very low within the brain (Chen & Bazinet 2014). The supply of PUFA to the brain is via the blood, either from exogenous PUFA obtained through diet or from endogenous liver synthesis of PUFA from dietary precursors. Brain DHA levels are 250–300-fold higher than EPA compared to about four-, five-, 14- and 86-fold higher levels of DHA versus EPA in plasma, erythrocyte, liver and heart, respectively. EPA enters the brain at a broadly similar rate to DHA and is rapidly and extensively β-oxidised upon entry into the brain (Chen & Bazinet 2014).

ω-3 fatty acids play an active role in neuronal membrane function, fluidity and control of neuronal growth factors. They also potentially influence each step in biogenic amine function, including neurotransmitter synthesis, degradation, release, reuptake and binding (Bruinsma & Taren 2000). Studies indicate that dietary PUFAs may influence noradrenergic and serotonergic neurotransmission and receptor function in the nervous system and, thereby, have a direct effect on function, mood and behaviour. Other actions at the neuronal cell membrane include suppression of the phosphatidyl-associated signal transduction pathways, blocking of the calcium ion influx through L-calcium channels and direct inhibition of protein kinase C, which are similar actions to those exhibited by some pharmaceutical mood stabilisers.

Prenatal and postnatal neurological development

DHA plays an important, if not critical, role in the growth and functional development of the brain during the third trimester and the early postnatal period when maximal growth occurs (Horrocks & Yeo 1999). Given that 15% of brain growth occurs during infancy, much attention has been paid to the consequences of variable ω-3 levels during late pregnancy and early infancy. It also plays an important role in retinal development, where DHA constitutes 60% of total PUFAs.

Chemopreventive effects

Marine fatty acids, particularly EPA and DHA, have been consistently shown to inhibit the proliferation of breast and prostate cancer cell lines in vitro and to reduce the risk and progression of these tumours in animal experiments (Bagga et al 2002, Terry et al 2003). Similar effects have also been observed for colorectal and prostate cancers (Calder et al 1998, Llor et al 2003, Stoll 2002).

Chemopreventive actions demonstrated by ω-3 LCPUFAs include suppression of neoplastic transformation, cell growth inhibition and enhanced apoptosis and antiangiogenicity (Rose & Connolly 1999). The proposed mechanisms for these are extensive, including the suppression of ω-6 eicosanoid synthesis; influences on transcription factor activity, gene expression and signal transduction pathways; effects on oestrogen metabolism; increased or decreased production of free radicals and reactive oxygen species, and influences on both insulin sensitivity and membrane fluidity (Larsson et al 2004). Ongoing research is attempting to elucidate the specific chemopreventive mechanisms of fish oils with the individual cancer cell lines.

CLINICAL USE

Thousands of studies have been conducted in various populations to determine the clinical consequences of regular fish consumption and fish oil supplementation. Initially, interest was focused on CVD but in recent years this has extended to other areas such as neurological conditions, neonatal and childhood health and development and mental health. While the plethora of studies published have begun to clarify the potential benefits of increasing intakes of ω-3 EFAs and fish on a regular basis, some are inconsistent with the general body of evidence, an issue which needs to be resolved.

There are multiple factors which could account for the sometimes inconsistent results that are seen. Some studies have focused on ω-3 fatty acids intake as a whole and included both vegetable and marine-based sources; however, in light of the lack of bioequivalence and clinical efficacy between the ω-3 precursors (e.g. ALA) and their long-chain derivatives (e.g. EPA/DHA), the results of these studies are likely to be confounded. Similarly, prospective studies investigating the effects of ω-3 PUFAs may be producing inconsistent results due to improper placebo selection (e.g. olive oil) (Pizzorno & Murray 2006). This was most recently seen in a large RCT comparing ω-3 EFAs to olive oil (placebo) and both groups experiencing a reduction in cardiovascular risk factors (Roncaglioni et al 2013). It is also important to note that few studies or reviews have considered the effect of variations in ω-3 : ω-6 ratio, which may be important, and the ratio of EPA : DHA being administered. McLennan (2014) suggests that dietary fish tends to have a greater amount of DHA than EPA whereas many studies use supplements containing EPA > DHA, which means they don't replicate the usual dietary sources which tend to show multiple health benefits. In regard to cardiovascular benefits, this could be important, as the human myocardium selectively incorporates DHA over EPA. De (2011) further suggests that the great variation in dietary fish intakes between populations could be another influence, as people with low baseline levels of ω-3 EFAs are more likely to experience a range of benefits with supplementation compared to those who already have high dietary intakes. Finally, the role of mercury in fish needs to be taken into account as research suggests it counteracts the benefits of ω-3 PUFAS on sudden cardiac death and MI and possibly other outcomes. Unfortunately, few studies consider participants' mercury levels when analysing results (see Clinical note p. 379).

Prevention of morbidity and mortality of cardiovascular disease

Consuming fatty fish at least twice per week reduces the risk of developing cardiovascular disease. In addition, a reduced risk of all-cause mortality, cardiovascular death, sudden death, and myocardial infarction is often reported in population studies. This is largely based on research conducted over the last three decades, which has linked fish and fish oils to CV health. Benefits have also been reported in people with pre-existing CV disease. This association was first recognised when significantly lower death rates from acute MI were found among Greenland's Inuit population, despite only moderate differences between the Inuits' blood cholesterol levels and those of other populations (Holub 2002). A high dietary ω-3 LCPUFA intake in the form of marine mammals (seal, whale) and various fish was thought to be responsible for the protective effect (Bang et al 1980).

In 1989, results from the first large, randomised, clinical trial investigating the effects of fatty fish consumption on survival and risk of secondary MI confirmed a link to cardiovascular health (Burr et al 1989). The Diet and Reinfarction Trial (DART) found that a modest intake of two to three portions weekly of fatty fish reduced mortality in men who had previously experienced an MI and produced a relative reduction in total mortality of 29% during the 2-year follow-up, attributed mainly to a reduction in deaths from coronary heart disease (CHD). Increased consumption of fish (relative risk [RR] = 0.66 for five or more times per week) was further confirmed in the Nurses Study as significantly reducing risk in both CHD and CHD-related mortality independent of the cardiovascular status (Hu et al 2002).

Since then, 25 studies involving a total of 280,000 participants have identified an inverse association between fish consumption and morbidity or mortality from CHD. Blood levels of ω-3 fatty acids also appear to correlate inversely with death from cardiovascular causes and total mortality (De 2011). Similar findings were reached in another 2011 review which concluded that prospective observational studies and adequately powered RCTs provide strong concordant evidence of the benefits of ω-3 PUFA, most consistently for CHD mortality and sudden cardiac death (Mozaffarian & Wu 2011). More specifically, both epidemiological and interventional approaches have clearly demonstrated that individuals with a diet rich in fish (30–35 g/day) or supplemented with EPA and DHA (up to 665 mg/day) show a 30–50% reduction in CHD and CHD-related mortality compared to individuals who did not eat fish (Russo 2009). It appears that, while some level of primary CVD prevention occurs, secondary prevention effects are more notable.

These protective effects are achieved via multiple mechanisms which include lowering plasma TGs, resting heart rate and blood pressure and possibly also improvements to myocardial filling and efficiency and lowering inflammation. There is also evidence that ω-3-PUFAs have the ability to protect vascular endothelial cells by decreasing oxidative stress, halting atherosclerotic events and preventing vascular inflammatory and adhesion cascades (Balakumar & Taneja 2012). The effects have been succinctly described as both intrinsic and extrinsic. Intrinsic effects refer to effects on cardiac function dependent upon membrane incorporation at <1 g/day; extrinsic effects are indirect cardiac effects through vascular disease which require EPA + DHA doses >3 g/day (McLennan 2014).

F

Not surprisingly, in 2004, the US Food and Drug Administration (FDA) reported that it would allow products containing ω-3 fatty acids to claim that eating the product may reduce the risk of heart disease. The FDA based its decision on the wealth of scientific evidence that suggests a correlation between ω-3 fatty acids such as EPA and DHA and a reduced risk of coronary artery disease. The FDA subsequently approved ω-3 fatty acids as a treatment to reduce plasma TGs (Frishman et al 2009).

The largest study is known as the GISSI trial, which involved 11,324 survivors of MI, demonstrating that a low-dose fish oil supplement (1 g/day) significantly reduced the risk of all-cause death, non-fatal MI and non-fatal stroke compared to vitamin E (300 mg/day) (Stone 2000). The group receiving ω-3 EFAs experienced a 15% reduction in the composite primary end point of death, non-fatal MI or non-fatal stroke ($P < 0.02$), with a 20% reduction in the rate of death from any cause ($P < 0.01$) and a 45% reduction in the rate of sudden death, an end point adjudicated by a committee whose members were unaware of the group assignments ($P < 0.001$), whereas the incidence of MI was not significantly reduced. Vitamin E provided no additional benefit. The effect on significantly reducing total mortality was evident early on, within 3 months (RR 0.59), and the rate of sudden death after only 4 months (RR 0.47) (De 2011). The effect was highly significant at 3.5 years, the end of the study, when it accounted for 59% of the ω-3 PUFA advantage in mortality. The reduction observed in all-cause mortality and in cardiovascular mortality resulted mainly from the prevention of sudden cardiac death by the ω-3 LCPUFAs. (Marchioli et al 2002).

The Japan Eicosapentaenoic Acid Lipid Intervention (JELIS) study followed afterwards and was a very large open-label study testing the long-term use of isolated EPA (1800 mg/day) in addition to statin therapy for the prevention of major coronary events in Japanese patients with hypercholesterolaemia. At a mean follow-up of 4.6 years a 19% relative reduction in major coronary events ($P = 0.01$) was observed with the combination therapy compared to statins alone and there was also a significant reduction in stroke (Tanaka et al 2008, Yokoyama 2009). Non-fatal coronary events were also significantly reduced in the EPA group, but sudden death from cardiac causes and death from coronary causes were not. Importantly, the reduction in events associated with EPA was similar in patients with and those without a history of coronary artery disease, but it was significant only in the former group, with a very low number needed to treat (De 2011). The JELIS study involved a total of 18,645 patients with total cholesterol levels ≥6.5 mmol/L who were randomly assigned to 1800 mg of EPA per day with statins or statins alone. A later analysis comparing people with good adherence (>80% of dose) to others found that, in good adherers with previous coronary artery disease, EPA substantially reduced the risk compared with statin alone (hazard ratio 0.55, $P < 0.014$). Furthermore, the clinical benefit of EPA + statin was significantly larger in patients with good adherence than in those with poor adherence ($P = 0.041$) (Origasa et al 2010). De Caterina (2011) suggests that the high dietary intake of fish amongst the Japanese population may account for the lack of effect on death from cardiac causes in this trial as a result of high baseline levels.

More recently, a 2013 double-blind study which compared fish oils (1 g/day) to placebo (olive oil) in people with multiple cardiovascular risk factors or atherosclerotic vascular disease but not MI found no change to the end points of cumulative rate of death, non-fatal MI and non-fatal stroke. Interestingly, at 1 year the event rate was found to be lower than anticipated so the researchers revised the primary end point to death from cardiovascular causes or admission to hospital for cardiovascular causes. They concluded that daily treatment with ω-3 fatty acids did not reduce cardiovascular mortality and morbidity as compared to the placebo group (Roncaglioni et al 2013). Unlike the GISSI trial, which used vitamin E as a comparator, this study used olive oil, a choice which must be questioned as it was obviously active because both groups experienced lower event rates than expected and, by the end of the trial, the overall cardiovascular risk profile had improved in both groups.

Unfortunately, the authors of these three studies did not report on the ratio of EPA:DHA used in their ω-3 EFA capsules or baseline EPA + DHA measures, thereby limiting further comparisons and interpretation.

Meta-analyses

In 2002, a high-quality systematic review of 11 RCTs on the effect of fish-based dietary or supplemental ω-3 fatty acids on cardiovascular morbidity and mortality in people with CHD found a strongly significant benefit (Bucher et al 2002); however, a 2006 Cochrane review came to a different conclusion (Hooper et al 2006). The review assessed 48 studies that compared at least 6 months of ω-3 fats (vegetable- and fish-based) with placebo or control and used data involving 36,913 participants. Meta-analysis of the studies assessing the effects of increased ω-3 fats on total mortality or combined cardiovascular events found strongly significant statistical heterogeneity. When randomised studies considered to be at medium or high risk of bias were removed, there was no significant effect of ω-3 fats on total mortality (RR 0.87; 95% confidence interval [CI] 0.73–1.03, with significant heterogeneity), whereas the cohort studies suggested significant protection (RR 0.65; 95% CI 0.48–0.88, no significant heterogeneity).

It is important to note that, until the publication of the DART-2 trial in 2003 (Burr et al 2003), the evidence showed that ω-3 from oily fish or supplements reduced the risks of fatal MI, sudden death and overall mortality among people with existing disease. Inclusion of the DART-2 trial in the Cochrane review had a major influence on the conclusion, as removing it produced RRs similar to those in the Bucher review (fatal MI: RR 0.70, 95% CI 0.54–0.91; sudden death: RR 0.68, 95% CI 0.42–1.10; overall mortality: RR 0.83, 95% CI 0.75–0.91). The DART-2 trial included 3114 men with stable angina and tested the hypothesis that the main benefit of ω-3 fat is derived from its antiarrhythmic action in the presence of chronic disease. Surprisingly, it did not confirm this, showing an excess of sudden and total cardiac deaths most clearly in participants taking fish oil capsules rather than eating oily fish. Authors of the Cochrane review report that something about the DART-2 study is different from the other included studies; however, further investigation has failed to clarify the issue. It is possible that, based on this latest review, the effect of ω-3 fats on CVD is smaller than previously thought or that effects in people who have had an MI are protective, but the effects in men with angina and no MI are not.

More recently, a 2013 meta-analysis of 11 double-blind RCTs for investigating the cardiovascular-preventive effects of ω-3 EFA supplementation (at least 1 g/

day) for at least 1 year in patients with existing CVD concluded that there were significant protective effects observed for cardiac death (RR 0.68; 95% CI 0.56–0.83), sudden death (RR 0.67; 95% CI 0.52–0.87) and MI (RR 0.75; 95% CI 0.63–0.88) (Casula et al 2013). The review, involving 15,348 patients with a history of CVD, also found no statistically significant association for all-cause mortality (RR 0.89; 95% CI 0.78–1.02) and stroke (RR 1.31; 95% CI 0.90–1.90).

Congestive heart failure

The current body of evidence indicates modest benefits for fish oils in patients with chronic heart failure. One of the first major studies was published in 2005: this was a large epidemiology study of 4738 adults aged over 65 years that showed 20% reduced incidence of heart failure associated with the consumption of tuna or other broiled or baked fish (but not fried), delivering estimated intakes of ω-3 LC-PUFA as low as 260 mg/day (Mozaffarian et al 2005). In 2008, a large, double-blind, placebo-controlled trial involving 6975 patients with CHF New York Heart Association class II–IV (GISSI-HF) demonstrated that the use of 1 g of ω-3 EFAs was associated with a statistically significant 9% reduction in all-cause mortality and cardiac-cause hospitalisations, with specific improvement in the proportion of subjects with low (<40%) ejection fraction (Tavazzi et al 2008).

More recently, a large cohort trial which recruited 12,500 patients with multiple CVD risk factors reported a 35% reduction in hospitalisations from heart failure as the only physiologically and clinically meaningful outcome from treatment with 850 mg/day EPA + DHA over 5 years (Risk and Prevention Study Collaborative Group 2013). These outcomes reflect improved myocardial function in clinical populations.

EPA levels appear to be more important than DHA levels in patients with CHF, according to a 2013 study which tested baseline levels of ω-3 EFAs in patients with CHF enrolled in the GISSI-HF study. An average difference of 43% was seen between patients with the lowest and highest consumptions of dietary fish ($P < 0.0001$). Baseline EPA but not DHA was inversely related to C-reactive protein, pentraxin-3, adiponectin, natriuretic peptide and troponin levels and 3 months of supplementation raised their levels of PUFA by 43%, independently of dietary fish consumption. Additionally, increases in EPA levels were associated with decreased pentraxin-3. Importantly, low EPA levels were inversely related to total mortality in patients with chronic heart failure (Masson et al 2013).

Patients with implantable cardioverter defibrillators (ICDs)

At least three double-blind RCTs have been conducted in patients with ICDs exploring whether ω-3 EFAs can reduce ventricular tachycardia. In one study, a dose of 2.6 g/day of combined EPA and DHA demonstrated significantly increased 'time to first ICD event' for ventricular tachycardia, fibrillation or death (Jung et al 2008). However, not all studies have produced such positive results, with some suggesting that the ω-3 LCPUFAs are ineffective in this patient group (Jenkins et al 2008, Nair & Connolly 2008).

Clinical note — The ω-3 : ω-6 balance: implications in cardiovascular disease and cancer

In recent years, attention has been drawn to the importance of not only ω-3 fatty acid intake but also its relation to concurrent ω-6 fatty acid intake (Simopoulos 2008). When there is increased ω-3 LCPUFAs in the diet and in our bodies, a shift in AA metabolism occurs, which results in the production of metabolites that have beneficial effects on cardiovascular physiology and cancer incidence and promotion (Leaf 2002). For example, when EPA is available to compete with AA, production of thromboxane A_2 (a potent vasoconstrictor and platelet activator) is reduced and production of thromboxane B_3 results, which is only weakly active. Additionally, several forms of research implicate ω-6 PUFAs as stimulating processes that promote human cancer development and progression, whereas ω-3 LCPUFAs have the opposite effect (Weisburger 1997). Once again, competition with AA is thought to be involved, although several other protective mechanisms have also been identified. Overall, it seems that, in order to obtain maximal cardiovascular and chemopreventive benefits, intake of ω-3 LCPUFAs should be increased and intake of ω-6 PUFAs must be reduced.

It has been estimated that the ratio of ω-6 to ω-3 EFAs in the Western diet is some 15:1 to 20:1 or higher, whereas the optimal ratio appears to be closer to 2:1 or 1:1 (Leaf 2002, Simopoulos 1999, 2008).

Elevated triglyceride levels

DHA and EPA supplementation significantly reduces TG levels in both normo- and hyperlipidaemic individuals and is used as sole therapy in cases of elevation or as adjunctive therapy with cholesterol-lowering medication when indicated. ω-3 LCPUFAs reduce TG concentrations in a dose-dependent manner, with intakes approximating 4 g/day lowering serum TGs by 25–30% in hyperlipidaemic patients at baseline (Balk et al 2006, Din et al 2004, Jung et al 2008). Studies have emerged using ω-3 LCPUFA in combination with statins for the treatment of hyperlipidaemia (Barter & Ginsberg 2008). While LDL reduction is the primary target of statins, fish oil co-supplementation both enhances this action and produces additional beneficial changes in other lipid parameters (e.g. HDL, TGs and lipoprotein particle size).

Overall, it appears that the smallest amount of ω-3 LCPUFAs required to lower serum TG levels significantly is approximately 1 g/day, as provided by a fish diet (Weber & Raederstorff 2000).

In the United States in 2004, the FDA approved Omacor as an ω-3 fatty acid prescription for adults with severe hypertriglyceridaemia (>5.65 mmol/L). Each 1 g capsule contains 465 mg (46%) EPA ethyl esters, 375 mg (38%) DHA ethyl esters and approximately 60 mg (6%) other ω-3 fatty acid ethyl esters. The remaining part is mainly composed of ω-6 fatty acids along with 4 mg α-tocopherol (Nicholson et al 2013). In 2007 the name was changed to Lovaza. Evidence to support its use as an effective therapy for elevated TGs is derived from clinical trials involving patients suffering from dyslipidaemia, familial combined hyperlipidaemia and CHD and studies examining its effects in combination with statin therapy (atorvastatin, simvastatin). A dose of 4 g daily was used in all studies, taken as a single dose or as two capsules twice daily. The reduction in TGs ranged from 19.1% to 45%; however, changes in LDL and HDL cholesterol were inconsistent and often insignificant (Nicholson et al 2013).

Hypertension

According to three meta-analyses, fish oils have a significant but modest dose-dependent effect on blood pressure in hypertension (Geleijnse et al 2002, Miller et al 2014, Morris et al 1993). The DHA component is likely to have stronger effects than EPA.

The most recent meta-analysis analysed results from 70 RCTs and confirmed that fish oils significantly reduce blood pressure, most notably amongst hypertensive patients but also to a modest extent amongst normotensive people (Miller et al 2014). More specifically, compared with placebo, EPA + DHA reduced systolic blood pressure (−1.52 mmHg; 95% CI −2.25 to −0.79) and diastolic blood pressure (−0.99 mmHg; 95% CI −1.54 to −0.44). The strongest effects of EPA + DHA were observed amongst untreated hypertensive subjects (systolic blood pressure = −4.51 mmHg, 95% CI −6.12 to −2.83; diastolic blood pressure = −3.05 mmHg, 95% CI −4.35 to −1.74), although blood pressure also was lowered among normotensive subjects but to a very modest extent only (systolic blood pressure = −1.25 mmHg, 95% CI −2.05 to −0.46; diastolic blood pressure = −0.62 mmHg, 95% CI −1.22 to −0.02). Doses of at least 2 g/day are required to achieve the effect.

Prior to cardiac surgery

While many secondary CHD prevention trials require months of treatment before the benefits of ω-3 fatty acid supplementation are detected, a clinical study with cardiothoracic surgical patients suggests acute benefits within weeks. Calo et al (2005) conducted a randomised, placebo-controlled study which found that patients taking 2 g/day of fish oils for at least 5 days prior to coronary artery bypass grafting and until discharge had a significantly reduced incidence of postoperative atrial fibrillation. Specifically, 15.2% of patients receiving fish oils experienced postoperative atrial fibrillation compared with 33.3% of patients who were not taking the supplement. In addition, hospital length of stay was significantly reduced by 1 day. Except for a single case of allergy, no adverse effects were observed.

A meta-analysis of 21 high-quality RCTs and subgroup analysis of trials using intravenously administered fish oil-enhanced lipid emulsions found that active treatment was associated with a significant reduction in the length of hospital stay (mean = −2.14 days, 95% CI = −3.02 to −1.27), infections (odds ratio [OR] = 0.53, 95% CI = 0.35–0.81), alanine aminotransferase (mean = −6.35 U/L, 95% CI = −11.75 to −0.94), gamma-glutamyl transferase (mean = −11.01 U/L, 95% CI = −20.77 to −1.25) and total bilirubin (mean = −2.06 micromol/L, 95% CI = −3.6 to −0.52), as well as a non-significant change in mortality and postoperative medical cost (Li et al 2014).

Intermittent claudication

A 2007 Cochrane review of six studies involving 313 subjects suffering from intermittent claudication and treated with ω-3 LCPUFAs (typical dose 1.8 g EPA and 1.2 g DHA per day) over weeks to years found that, in spite of some haematological improvements (e.g. reduced viscosity), there were no demonstrable improvements in clinical outcomes (Sommerfield et al 2007). A more recent 2013 Cochrane systematic review came to a similar conclusion, stating that ω-3 fatty acids appear to have little benefit in this condition (Campbell et al 2013). A closer look at the studies reveals there is relatively little research looking at long-term use of fish oils as a stand-alone treatment for this indication and further research is required to better explore this potential treatment option.

Clinical note — Would you like methylmercury (MeHg) or organohalogen pollutants (OHPs) with that?

In aquatic environments, inorganic mercury, either naturally occurring or as an industrial byproduct (e.g. coal-fired power plants, waste incinerators), is converted into MeHg by microorganisms present in sediment or within the intestine of fish themselves (Dórea 2006). The MeHg, which is the most hazardous dietary form, then accumulates in the aquatic food chain, making fish the primary source of exposure for most individuals (FSANZ 2004). There has been increasing public awareness and concern regarding MeHg exposure secondary to fish consumption. This has been partly in response to the health warnings issued by Food Standards Australia and New Zealand (FSANZ) in March 2004 regarding maximal intake of selected fish species during pregnancy and childhood (Bambrick & Kjellstrom 2004). Interestingly, while the main public concern relates to neurodevelopmental toxicity, some data show a relationship between increasing MeHg exposure and CVD, in particular MI (Stern 2005). Postulated mechanisms include the oxidative stress and reactive oxygen species observed with in vitro exposures to MeHg, as well as impaired calcium homeostasis and kidney function.

MeHg concentrations in fish and shellfish species, which represent 80–90% of the mercury present, range from <0.1 ppm for shellfish, such as oysters and mussels, to multiple parts per million in large predatory fish such as tuna, marlin, swordfish and shark. Consequently, MeHg intake depends on the species and age of fish consumed, as well as the quantity eaten. Previous American data determined that adults consumed an average of 18 mcg MeHg/day, with 80–90% coming from fish and shellfish (Mahaffey et al 2004).

Inorganic mercury is readily excreted in the urine, whereas MeHg accumulates in erythrocytes across a wide range of exposures (Mahaffey et al 2004). Multiple international studies assessing MeHg exposure levels have revealed that approximately 10% of blood samples were high. American studies have identified populations at greater risk, among them a subpopulation consuming a substantial amount of fish in pursuit of health benefits. Blood MeHg analysis revealed blood mercury levels up to 90 mcg/L (Hightower & Moore 2003). This is concerning, given levels >5 mcg/L have been reported as potentially detrimental in women of child-bearing age.

Some researchers propose that the potentially cardiotoxic effects of MeHg are countered by the presence of the ω-3 oils also found within fish, and interestingly, there is some overlap between those species with the highest concentrations of both (Bambrick & Kjellstrom 2004). However, there is also concern that the converse is true and MeHg could counteract the health-giving benefits of fish.

While fish oil supplements are not a major source of mercury and as such there is no need to restrict their intake (Bays 2007, FSANZ 2004, Levine et al 2005, Schaller 2001), OHPs such as polychlorinated biphenyls, dioxins and organochlorine pesticides, widely used in flame retardants, pesticides, paints and electrical equipment prior to their ban in the 1980s in most countries (Bays 2007), may be present in these products. OHPs also accumulate in the aquatic food chain and are lipophilic carcinogens as well as being associated with other health risks (Dórea 2006). Data across the board confirm significantly higher OHPs in farmed fish and the supplements produced from these (Jacobs et al 1998, 2004) compared with wild harvested samples. These higher levels are attributed most consistently with use of contaminated feed (Domingo & Bocio 2007, Dórea 2006, Easton et al 2002, Jacobs et al 2002, Melanson et al 2005).

A UK study analysing the OHP content of 21 commercially available fish (both whole-body fish and cod liver oil) and vegetable oil dietary supplements in 2004 found that levels in all fish oil products had increased dramatically in brands tested 8 years previously (Jacobs et al 1998, 2004). For example, OHP levels in cod liver oils, which originally ranged from 0 to 13 ng/g, were found to contain 15–34 ng/g in the most recent analysis. The findings of an American study contrast with this, however, with OHP levels below the level of detection in five over-the-counter fish oil products (Melanson et al 2005). There are no published data on Australian products.

There remains little doubt that the discriminating inclusion of fish is an important part of a healthy diet. Recent research suggests that high exposure to mercury may reduce the benefits of long-chain ω-3 PUFA on sudden cardiac death (Virtanen et al 2012). It also reduces the benefits of fish oils on preventing MI, according to a Scandinavian study involving over 500 volunteers. It was identified that a small increase in fish consumption (increasing serum PUFA by 1%) would prevent 7% of MI, despite a small increase in mercury (Wennberg et al 2012). However, the higher the hair–mercury, the more the benefits on preventing MI were counteracted. Thus, MI risk may be reduced by the consumption of fish high in PUFAs and low in methylmercury.

F

Neurological effects

There is evidence that alterations to ω-3 fatty acid metabolism and the composition of the phospholipids in serum and membranes are involved in the pathogenesis of some neurological disorders (Ulbricht & Basch 2005). Also, several epidemiological studies have reported low-plasma DHA status in individuals with schizophrenia, ADHD, dyslexia, personality disorder, depression and bipolar disorder (BD) (Riediger et al 2009). As a result, there has been much interest in understanding the effects of supplemental ω-3 fatty acids in neurological development, cognitive function, behavioural problems and other neurological conditions.

Cognitive function

Low-serum DHA level is considered a significant risk factor for the development of Alzheimer's dementia (Conquer et al 2000). Additionally, both DHA and total ω-3 LCPUFAs are significantly lower in cognitively impaired but non-demented people and people with other dementias. One of the first interventional studies was a small RCT of 4.3 g/day DHA in 20 elderly nursing-home residents, assessing the efficacy of fish oil in the treatment of vascular dementia. DHA supplementation resulted in a small improvement in dementia-rating scores within 3 months of treatment (Terano et al 1994).

Dietary factors influence the association between physical activity and cognitive performance. Executive and memory functions were investigated in 344 participants. High levels of DHA relative to AA mitigated the effects of lower levels of physical activity on cognitive performance. The combination of higher AA:DHA ratios with lower physical activity was associated with markedly decreased performance. In contrast, there were no significant associations between serum AA:DHA ratio levels and cognitive function (Leckie et al 2014).

The results from numerous animal studies, demonstrating neuroprotection and slowing of neurodegeneration from the ω-3 LCPUFAs, appear promising (Hashimoto et al 2005, Mucke & Pitas 2004); however, more clinical trials are required to determine the clinical implications of these positive findings.

Alzheimer's dementia

Epidemiological studies have shown that dementia and CVD may share several common risk factors, including high intakes of dietary total fat, high saturated fat, high ω-6 : ω-3 fatty acid ratio and low fish intake (Riediger et al 2009). Considering ω-3 fatty acids possess anti-inflammatory properties and inflammatory markers have been located in the brain of patients with Alzheimer's disease, it seems reasonable to suggest that ω-3 fatty acids may delay the onset of Alzheimer's disease by reducing brain inflammatory state. This may be one of the reasons behind prevention of Alzheimer's disease/dementia by adequate DHA/EPA intake suggested by the Framingham heart study (Kalmijn 2000, Kalmijn et al 2004), the Rotterdam study (Kalmijn et al 1997) and the 2003 prospective study by Morris et al (2003), although later follow-up of the Rotterdam study found no association (Engelhart et al 2002).

In 2005, a review of the evidence prepared for the US Department of Health and Human Services concluded that there is a significant correlation between fish consumption and reduced incidence of Alzheimer's disease. Total ω-3 LCPUFA and DHA consumption correlated with this risk reduction; however, ALA and EPA did not (MacLean et al 2004). A Cochrane review came to a similar conclusion, reporting that there is a growing body of evidence from biological, observational and epidemiological studies to suggest a protective effect of ω-3 LCPUFAs against dementia; however, further research is required before firm conclusions can be made (Lim et al 2006). A study investigating supplementation with 1.8 g/day of fish oils over 24 weeks in subjects with either mild to moderate Alzheimer's disease or mild cognitive impairment yielded greatest benefits in individuals suffering only mild cognitive impairment (Chiu et al 2008). Further studies using higher doses, larger sample sizes and only subjects mildly affected by the condition are recommended.

Brain trauma injury

Brain trauma injury is characterised by significant neuroinflammation. Acute administration of ω-3 PUFA after injury and dietary exposure before or after injury have the potential to improve neurological outcomes in traumatic brain injury and spinal cord injury. The mechanisms include decreased neuroinflammation and oxidative stress, neurotrophic support and activation of cell survival pathways (Michael-Titus & Priestley 2014). A paper by Sears et al (2013) reported a case where ω-3 supplementation was given (10.8 g of EPA and 5.4 g of DHA) in two divided doses on a daily basis. The patient was a 26-year-old male exposed to a carbon monoxide and methane gas atmosphere for 41 hours following an explosion at a coal mine. When rescued, his breathing was laboured, and he had significant neurological, cardiovascular and renal dysfunction (being the classic symptoms of carbon monoxide poisoning), dehydration and rhabdomyolysis. Magnetic resonance imaging scans indicated significant cytotoxic cell injury and demyelination. He emerged from the coma after 3 weeks. He spent the next 2 months in a rehabilitation facility, at which time the ω-3 fatty acid supplementation was continued for another 2 months. He steadily improved over time. He was released into home care nearly 3 months after the explosion. Six years after the explosion he was functionally normal and had fathered two young children (Sears et al 2013). Although this is a single case report, ω-3 PUFAs show potential in brain trauma injury and are worthy of further investigation.

Autism spectrum disorder (ASD)

Two studies have found evidence of low levels of EPA and DHA in autistic patients (Curtis & Patel 2008). A moderately sized epidemiological study of women with children with ASD (n = 317) revealed that pregnant mothers with the lowest ω-3 intake had a significant increase in offspring ASD risk as compared with the remaining distribution (n = 17,728; RR = 1.53). The data obtained from online survey research from 861 parents of autistic children also suggest that consumption of a formula devoid in DHA and AA during infancy is associated with an OR of 4.41 for autism generally and 12.96 for regressive autism, compared with breastfed infants (Schultz et al 2006). However, the heavy reliance upon self-reporting in addition to the non-random sample leaves these results open to scrutiny. Given all this epidemiological evidence, surprisingly few studies have investigated the effects of ω-3 LCPUFAs in autistic individuals. One study conducted in a sample of 12 children, employing 5 g/day of ω-3 LCPUFAs over 6 weeks, produced significant remission of hyperactivity (Amminger et al 2007); however another using comparable doses in adults failed to demonstrate efficacy on any behavioural parameter (Politi et al 2008). The paucity of ω-3 studies in ASD is striking and has been commented on by reviewers (Frye et al 2013), including the Cochrane review which failed to find a single study that met their inclusion criteria in this area (Tan et al 2012).

While theories abound about the potential role of aberrant LCPUFA metabolism in ASD (Das 2013) as an explanation for the higher incidence in boys, secondary to hormonal differences in fat metabolism (Field 2014), other reviewers argue there isn't a plausible biological mechanism by which ω-3 could be implicated (Prior & Galduroz 2012).

F

Pregnancy, breastfeeding and infants

The three big focus points in ω-3 research for improved offspring health are in the areas of reduced adulthood obesity, prevention of atopy in at-risk individuals (≥1 atopic primary family member) and improved cognitive outcomes.

Animal studies suggest that changes in peri- and early postnatal ω-3 intake can affect the development of adulthood obesity (Bagley et al 2013); however, attempts to replicate these findings in humans have so far produced negative findings in both early infancy and even adolescence (Hauner et al 2013, Rytter et al 2011).

Prevention of atopy in at-risk infants

Cross-sectional studies measuring breast milk ω-3 content in new mothers found an inverse relationship between LCPUFA levels and positive skin prick test responses in infants at 12 months (Soto-Ramirez et al 2012), while maternal and infant phospholipid ω-3 were inversely correlated with non-atopic persistent infant wheezing and positive skin prick test at 6 years old (Pike et al 2012). These later cross-sectional studies suggest ≤50% reduced incidence.

Pregnancy ω-3 interventions in high-risk mothers for allergic offspring have demonstrated a protective effect against immunoglobulin E (IgE) sensitisation; however, an absolute reduction in atopic incidence is less certain (Dunstan et al 2008, Furuhjelm et al 2011, Noakes et al 2012, Storro et al 2010). There have been several RCTs with positive findings, such as a significantly reduced incidence of food allergy (2% vs 15%) and atopic eczema (8% vs 24%) in 1-year-old infants whose mothers consumed high-dose ω-3 (1.6 g/day EPA and 1.1 g/day DHA) from week 25 to 3–4 months postpartum compared with those receiving placebo (Furuhjelm et al 2008). A follow-up study of this original cohort found the decreased incidence was sustained at 2-years-old and higher maternal and infant ω-3 levels were associated with less IgE-associated disease and reduced severity of the allergic phenotype (Furuhjelm et al 2011). One of the strengths of this study was the comprehensive diagnosis of food allergy — a combination of clinical picture assessment, IgE antibody assays and skin prick test.

A large Mexican RCT of 869 pregnant women administered 400 mg/day DHA from the third trimester to delivery observed a significant protective effect of DHA treatment on respiratory symptoms (phlegm and nasal discharge) following adjustment for potential confounders, among infants of atopic mothers (Escamilla-Nunez et al 2014). Interestingly, however, there was no significant difference in cord blood IgE levels between the treatment and placebo groups (Hernandez et al 2013). A large Norwegian study adopted a multipronged approach to reducing asthma in offspring, advising pregnant women in the treatment group to increase their ω-3 intake, stop parental smoking and reduce exposure to damp environments during the first 2 years of life (Dotterud et al 2013). The combined effect was a significantly reduced incidence of asthma compared with controls but only in girls (OR 0.41).

One of the longest longitudinal studies in this area to date is a 16-year follow-up investigation of offspring born to women supplemented with 2.7 g/day fish oils from week 30 until delivery as part of an RCT (Olsen et al 2008). Children born to mothers in the fish oil group demonstrated a 63% reduction in asthma diagnoses and 87% reduction in the prevalence of allergic asthma. In line with these findings, it has been suggested that longer follow-up may be necessary to accurately ascertain the impact of ω-3 interventions on offspring allergy incidence (Almqvist et al 2007, Marks et al 2006).

In regard to infants' diets, the results of a prospective, longitudinal study from Sweden of 4921 infants' diets, exposure patterns and eczema diagnoses have found a protective effect for early introduction of fish (Alm et al 2009). Infants introduced to fish prior to 9 months of age demonstrated reduced rates of eczema at 1 year (OR 0.76). This finding flies in the face of previous primary prevention strategies whereby many child health authorities have encouraged delaying the introduction of fish in order to reduce allergy.

Cognitive development

Although numerous studies of mothers and infants have demonstrated that consuming greater amounts of EFAs had a positive effect on the subsequent cognitive development and IQ of their young offspring (Cohen et al 2005, Helland et al 2003, Williams et al 2001), the Evidence Report/Technology Assessment prepared for the Agency of Healthcare Research and Quality of the US Department of Health and Human Services concludes that, based on the small number of current well-designed studies, there is no conclusive evidence of any benefit (Moher 2005). The report observes that studies demonstrating a positive relationship between ω-3 LCPUFAs and cognition are those that assessed children under 1 year of age, whereas in studies of older children a significant statistical relationship is not sustained. Despite the conclusions of this report, several studies with longer follow-up periods have demonstrated both improved eye and hand coordination (Dunstan et al 2008) and IQ at 4 years old (Helland et al 2003), but not at 7 years old (Helland et al 2008). The latter is an Australian study, following up on 98 women who were supplemented with 2.2 g DHA and 0.1 g EPA per day or placebo from 20 weeks' gestation. Children's eye and hand coordination scores correlated with ω-3 LCPUFA levels in cord blood red blood cells (RBC) and inversely correlated with ω-6 LCPUFA at 2½ years of age.

Other studies investigating fish oil supplementation during lactation have produced mixed findings, including possible negative outcomes only in male offspring (impaired working memory and inhibitory control, increased diastolic blood pressure at 7 years old). However, these figures all come from the same small study (n = 122) of Danish mothers administered either 1.5 g/day of fish or olive oil for 4 months during lactation and these conclusions were based on only 36 children in the treatment group who were assessed at 7 years old (Asserhoj et al 2009, Cheatham et al 2011). Therefore, additional research is necessary before any firm conclusions can be drawn.

According to the WHO and Food and Agriculture Organization (FAO), pregnant women should take at least 2.6 g of ω-3 EFAs, incorporating 100–300 mg of DHA, daily to look after the needs of the fetus (Bambrick & Kjellstrom 2004). Postnatal deficiencies have been associated with reduced visual acuity, poor neurodevelopment and ill effects on behaviour. Breastfed infants generally receive sufficient DHA if the maternal diet is adequate, but it is not known whether formula-fed infants receive adequate amounts if their formula does not contain PUFAs.

F

Clinical note — What determines infants' ω-3 inheritance?

Many expectant mothers are aware that one 'breast is best' argument relates to an improved fatty-acid profile in breast milk compared with formula milk. Adding to this is a study by Meldrum et al (2012), investigating the efficacy of direct high-dose fish oil supplementation of infants from birth to 6 months, which found that even in supplemented infants, the ω-3 content of the breast milk was the stronger determinant of infant RBC DHA, in spite of total daily exposure being approximately a third of that provided by the supplement. While this result may be the consequence of methodological error, there is speculation that this underscores the superior bioavailability of LCPUFAs in breast milk.

Consistent evidence points to a correlation between ω-3 intake during pregnancy (dietary or supplements) and breast milk ω-3 concentrations (Urwin et al 2012), but what else influences the infant's ω-3 inheritance? Breast milk DHA levels are at their highest in the early postpartum period and progressively decline over the first month of lactation (Weiss et al 2013). However, other variables that dictate how much is available to begin with include birth order (levels decline with each subsequent pregnancy) and multiple versus single pregnancies (Al et al 2000). Additionally, there is growing interest in genetic variations with the FADS1/2 gene clusters which code for the desaturases and how this impacts on ω-3 status of mother and infant. Molto Puigment (2010) found that, while plasma DHA levels rose in mothers regardless of genotype, their breast milk DHA changed. Women homozygous for a mutation, with reduced efficacy of these enzymes, demonstrated limited incorporation into breast milk. The results of another interesting but very small study suggest that women with atopic eczema had lower ω-3 breast milk levels compared with non-atopic mothers and even atopic mothers who were free from eczema, in spite of comparable intake (Johansson et al 2011). The key take-home message currently seems to be that, while good ω-3 intake during pregnancy and lactation is sensible, intake and breast milk concentrations will not perfectly correlate due to a range of other variables we are just starting to identify.

Prevention and treatment of postpartum depression (PPD)

The rationale for considering ω-3 EFAs as potential risk reducers in PPD relates to consistent evidence of maternal DHA depletion and increasing inflammation throughout pregnancy. However, in spite of evidence of decreased DHA in the frontal cortex correlated with lower serotonin in pregnant animals (Chen et al 2012) and several international cross-sectional epidemiological studies suggesting that higher seafood intake (reflected especially in higher breast milk DHA content) is protective against PPD (Jans et al 2010, Kendall-Tackett 2010), interventional studies in humans have not produced consistently positive findings.

A large Australian study of 2399 pregnant women randomised to DHA-rich fish oil (800 mg DHA and 100 mg EPA/day) or placebo found a non-significant reduction in the percentage of women with high levels of depressive symptoms overall and in the subgroup of women with previously diagnosed depression (Makrides et al 2010). Criticisms of this study include the lack of dietary ω-3 assessment, the inclusion of individuals with depression at baseline, the use of self-rated depression scales only and the reliance on high-dose DHA with nominal EPA. A systematic review published the same year, which didn't include the trial by Makrides, examined seven studies of EPA/DHA administration in pregnancy for the prevention of PPD (four studies sampled healthy individuals and in three studies individuals were depressed at baseline) and found the pooled mean effect size was non-significant and indicated no or a small pre- to posttreatment decrease in perinatal depression.

More recently, 126 women in early pregnancy at high risk of depression were randomised in a trial to receive EPA-rich or DHA-rich fish oil or placebo throughout pregnancy. While fatty-acid analyses revealed increased ω-3 levels in the DHA-rich group particularly, demonstrating an inverse relationship between DHA levels and depression-rating scores evident at 34–36 weeks, overall there were no statistically significant differences in the mean depression scores among the groups at entry or at any of the study visits and no statistically significant differences among the groups in the proportion of women who started antidepressant medications (Mozurkewich et al 2013). In summary, these findings have led researchers, and the latest Cochrane review on nutritional prevention of PPD, to currently conclude that fish oil is not effective (Miller et al 2013). In spite of these findings, Goren and Tewksbury (2011) reiterate the numerous benefits of adequate DHA during pregnancy (e.g. fetal neurocognitive development, reduced cardiovascular risks) and encourage pregnant women to continue supplementing high-dose DHA during the third trimester.

Preventing depression

After adjusting for several confounding factors, Kamphuis et al (2006) reported that every 50 mg/day increase in ω-3 fatty acid intake was correlated with a 7% risk reduction of depressive symptoms in elderly men. It has been suggested that the balance between ω-6 and ω-3 EFA influences the metabolism of biogenic amines, an interaction that may be relevant to changes in mood and behaviour (Bruinsma & Taren 2000). In several observational studies, low concentrations of ω-3 LCPUFAs predicted impulsive behaviours and greater severity of depression. Additionally, early research by Horrobin and Bennett (1999) revealed that almost all studies on depression have found increased prostaglandin G_2 series or related thromboxanes and there is evidence that the older antidepressants (monoamine oxidase inhibitors and tricyclic antidepressants) either inhibit prostaglandin synthesis or are powerful antagonists of their actions. The findings of a number of studies showing a correlation between low erythrocyte ω-3 EFAs and suicide attempts go one step further. One demonstrated an eightfold difference in suicide attempt risk between the lowest and highest RBC EPA quartiles (Huan et al 2004). Belgian researchers have also speculated about seasonal variations in EFA status that correlate with seasonal patterns of suicide (De Vriese et al 2004); however, studies on larger populations of depressed people are required to confirm this link.

Several international cross-sectional studies have found a correlation between ω-3 intake and rates of depression, including that depression rates are 10 times higher in countries with limited seafood intake and PPD 10–50 times higher (Kendall-Tackett 2010). In countries with traditionally high seafood consumption, such as Finland, individuals who consume smaller amounts were found to have a 31% higher chance of developing depression, even when other risk factors were controlled for. Noaghiul and Hibbeln (2003) postulated that countries where individuals consumed less than ≈ 450–680 g of seafood per person per week demonstrated the highest rates of affective disorders.

Superior epidemiological evidence comes from longitudinal rather than cross-sectional studies of ω-3 intake in healthy individuals and subsequent depression diagnoses. Four such trials were included in a recent review (Sanhueza et al 2013). While two of these did not find any association between fish consumption and depression incidence, the other two found that an inverse relationship was only seen with intermediate intake which equated to ≈0.16% of the total energy intake or 1.17 g/day (energy-adjusted) and produced a significant risk reduction of 35–40% in depression. The loss of apparent protection with the highest fish intake remains unexplained, possibly an issue of excess exposure to the contaminants found in certain fish (see Would you like methylmercury (MeHg) or organohalogen pollutants (OHPs) with that?). However, it is noteworthy that a similar phenomenon was evident with ω-3 supplementation (Peet & Horrobin 2002).

Treating depression

In spite of widespread epidemiological data correlating ω-3 status with a range of depressive disorders, including major depression, PPD and seasonal affective disorder, and extensive evidence of the role of inflammation in depression (Kendall-Tackett 2010), there are relatively few interventional studies and those published are typically compromised by small sample size and possess heterogeneous designs, particularly with regard to the composition and dose of the intervention itself (Grenyer et al 2007). More recent reviews have focused on eliminating the confounding issue of variable ω-3 forms and dose. These reviews (Martins 2009, Ross et al 2007, Sublette et al 2011) appear to have reached a consensus regarding the superiority of EPA over DHA in depressed individuals. Sublette et al (2011) in particular postulate that interventions providing >60% EPA and a minimum of 200–2200 mg EPA in excess of DHA were significantly more effective. Although DHA is more prevalent in the brain and possesses actions that would suggest it would be helpful in depression, several theories are proposed why this doesn't translate into clinical findings, including that oral DHA supplementation has not conclusively been shown to increase brain DHA levels. Secondly, it is EPA that directly competes with AA for conversion to eicosanoids and therefore may have the most relevant anti-inflammatory action.

Trials published since these reviews include a small, double-blind randomised study ($n = 66$) of mildly depressed elderly individuals (mean age 80 years) administered low-dose EPA and DHA (180 mg and 120 mg/day, respectively) over 6 months to Iranian nursing-home patients with extremely low dietary ω-3, e.g. three fish meals over 6 months. Using self-assessment via the Geriatric Depression Scale-15, 40.7% of subjects in the treatment group demonstrated improved mood compared with only 27.6% of placebo, which was a significant difference (Tajalizadekhoob et al 2011). In young healthy adults (aged 18–35 years) also with low baseline ω-3 intake, EPA-rich (EPA 300 mg and DHA 200 mg/day) and DHA-rich (450 mg and EPA 90 mg/day) supplements were compared with placebo for improving cognition and, as a secondary assessment, mood, via the Depression Anxiety Stress Scale and Bond-Lager visual analogue (Jackson et al 2012). Treatment with fish oils at these doses failed to produce any mood or cognitive benefits, which the authors argue may be illustrative that baseline ω-3 levels need to be lower and functional impairment evident in order to benefit from fish oil supplementation. However, the results could also be explained by inadequate unopposed EPA according to the work of Sublette et al (2011). Most recently, a randomised double-blind placebo-controlled study of 152 patients preparing for interferon treatment revealed that those treated with EPA 2 weeks before interferon treatment started reported significantly lower rates of depression (10%) compared with both DHA-supplemented individuals (28%) and subjects taking placebo (30%) (Su et al 2014).

Bipolar disorder

Interest in the role and therapeutic potential of ω-3 in BD is substantial and has moved beyond the epidemiological associations to more sophisticated investigations, i.e. fatty-acid levels present in specific brain regions of BD sufferers, genetic variations in expression of LCPUFA metabolic enzymes (Igarashi et al 2010). Proposed mechanisms of action include their capacity to increase cell membrane fluidity (altering receptor numbers and dampening signal transduction pathways), reduce brain inflammation, antagonise phosphoinositide protein kinase C and, to a small extent, inhibit reuptake of serotonin and dopamine, which would all be beneficial in BD depression (Sarris et al 2011). Additionally, some researchers have found a correlation between individuals' LCPUFA levels and BD severity (DHA and depression; EPA and mania) (Clayton et al 2009). It is also noteworthy that many of the medications prescribed in BD (e.g. lithium, valproate) reduce turnover of AA and therefore are postulated to be anti-inflammatory (Goren & Tewksbury 2011).

Poor methodological quality as well as heterogeneous design have plagued ω-3 interventional studies, however, as illustrated by the Cochrane review which based their negative conclusion on the results of one study (Frangou et al 2006), while >23 others failed to meet their inclusion criteria (Montgomery & Richardson 2008).

A broader review by Sarris et al (2011) notes that, of nine adjunctive ω-3 trials in BD, seven were randomised, double-blind and placebo-controlled and four of these demonstrated a statistically significant positive effect on reducing depression. While generally ω-3 oils have not demonstrated significantly superior results to placebo in the management of mania, Sarris et al comment that all studies are in favour of fish oils over placebo in this respect; however, small sample sizes could explain the lack of statistically significant findings. Again, particular note is made of the differences in ω-3 preparations, which range from high-dose EPA alone, EPA:DHA blends, to flaxseed oil and with dosage variations, e.g. up to 3400 mg DHA and 6000 mg ethyl-EPA. One of the open-label studies also included by Sarris is a small Australian study ($n = 18$) of juvenile BD, in which subjects stable on pharmaceutical medications then took ω-3 (360 mg/day EPA 1560 mg/day DHA) for 6 weeks, producing a 50% reduction in depression ratings, and again a non-significant improvement in mania (Clayton et al 2009).

Addiction/abstinence

A study in polysubstance abusers (Buydens-Branchey et al 2008), using 2.25 g EPA and 500 mg DHA administered over 3 months to 24 individuals, resulted in decreased anger and anxiety scores, corresponding with plasma increases in both EPA and DHA. A randomised double-blind placebo-controlled study of abstinent alcoholics revealed that 3 weeks of supplementation with fish oil (60 mg/day EPA and 252 mg/day DHA) produced lower basal salivary cortisol levels compared with placebo, accompanied by lower depression and anxiety ratings. At the end of intervention, amplitude and duration of stress-evoked cortisol response did not differ between groups; however, the peak of cortisol response was temporally anticipated in supplemented subjects (Barbadoro et al 2013).

An animal study which injected rats with amphetamine and fed subgroups different dietary fats (soybean, hydrogenated vegetable fats or fish oil) found that fish oils largely attenuated the detrimental effects on brain structure, mitochondrial activity and vitamin C levels typically seen with chronic amphetamine exposure. The researchers hypothesise that this action could be similar to the protective effects of ω-3 oils in other forms of mania (Trevizol et al 2001).

Aggressive and impulsive behaviour

Animal studies demonstrate increased aggression test scores in rats and other species deprived of ω-3 LCPUFAs during either gestation or early life. This has been linked to deficits in neuronal arborisation and multiple indices of synaptic pathology, including deficits in serotonin and mesocorticolimbic dopamine neurotransmission (Hibbeln et al 2006, Liu & Raine 2006). Human data also support this proposition, whereby preterm delivery is associated with deficits in fetal cortical DHA accrual, and children/adolescents born preterm exhibit deficits in cortical grey-matter maturation, neurocognitive deficits, particularly in the realm of attention, impulsivity and increased risk of ADHD and schizophrenia (Hibbeln et al 2006, McNamara & Carlson 2006). While there is strong support for the biological basis for a relationship between ω-3 LCPUFAs and aggressive and impulsive behaviour (Garland & Hallahan 2006), the results of interventional studies have been somewhat mixed.

DHA has been used to reduce aggressive behaviour in children and adolescents. One placebo-controlled study of 42 college students showed that DHA supplementation (1.5–1.8 g/day) prevented an increase in aggression towards others at times of mental stress (Hamazaki et al 1996); however, there was no effect on aggressive behaviour under non-stressful conditions (Hamazaki et al 1998). A 2005 randomised, placebo-controlled clinical trial looked at 166 Japanese children aged 9–12 years administered 3.6 g DHA and 840 mg per week via both supplements and fortified foods over a period of 3 months (Itomura et al 2005). While reducing aggression in girls, concomitant with improved EPA:AA RBC ratios, the same effect was not evident in boys. Impulsivity amongst female subjects was also significantly reduced in the treatment group.

Other small successful studies for anger reduction have been conducted in abstaining polysubstance abusers (2.25 g EPA, 500 mg DHA administered over 3 months) (Buydens-Branchey et al 2008), borderline personality disorder (1 g/day ethyl EPA over 8 weeks) (Zanarini et al 2003) and borderline personality disorder in adolescents at high risk of psychosis (1.2 g/day ω-3 over 12 weeks) (Amminger et al 2013). In a separate study, however, individuals exhibiting recurrent self-harm, scores for impulsivity, aggression and hostility remained unchanged, in spite of decreased depression and suicidality scores, when treated with 1.2 g EPA and 900 mg DHA per day over 12 weeks (Hallahan et al 2007). New research has found a relationship between AA/EPA + DHA RBC ratios and individuals' vulnerability to anger with interferon treatment. Marked anger and irritability are common adverse effects of interferon that can compromise compliance and success of the treatment, therefore co-administration of ω-3 LCPUFA may represent an effective way to reduce the likelihood of this occurrence (Lotrich et al 2013).

Anxiety

In spite of consistent animal evidence that decreased ω-3 LCPUFA leads to chronic mild stress-induced anxiety (Vinot et al 2011), limited well-designed studies have been conducted in patients with anxiety disorders as a stand-alone diagnosis rather than a comorbidity, e.g. BD, substance abuse (Goren & Tewksbury 2011).

Animal studies of both supplemental ω-3 during the perinatal period and, more recently, adulthood confirm a moderate anxiolytic action (Vinot et al 2011) and new mechanisms such as improved neural plasticity and endocannibinoid activity have been elucidated (Larrieu et al 2011). A placebo-controlled, double-blind 12-week RCT compared ω-3 (2085 mg EPA and 348 mg DHA) supplementation with placebo on proinflammatory cytokine production and anxiety symptoms in medical students (n = 68) for 12 weeks. ω-3 supplementation produced a 20% reduction in anxiety symptoms ($P = 0.04$), as measured by the Beck Anxiety Inventory, and a 14% decrease in stimulated interleukin-6 production ($P = 0.04$). ω-3 PUFA also had a borderline effect on serum tumour necrosis factor-alpha (TNF-α) (7% decrease, $P = 0.06$). At the completion of the study, plasma levels of EPA and DHA were approximately sixfold and ½-fold higher compared to levels prior to supplementation. The levels of EPA and DHA in peripheral blood mononucleated cells (PBMCs) also increased but were not as dramatic in increase: threefold and 1/3-fold, respectively, for EPA and DHA. Supplementation with the placebo oil resulted in no changes of either plasma or PBMC EPA and DHA. There was no significant change in depressive symptoms (Kiecolt-Glaser et al 2011). Further human studies of anxiety disorders are needed to confirm these findings.

Attention-deficit hyperactivity disorder

It has been reported that many children with ADHD have EFA deficiency (mainly ω-3 fatty acid), with a high correlation between severity of symptoms and severity of deficiency (Yehuda et al 2005). Deficiency may be due to insufficient dietary intake or inefficient conversion of EFA to LCPUFAs. Several studies have investigated the effects of supplemental fatty acids in ADHD with mixed results; however, interpretation of findings is difficult because of the use of different treatments, measurements and subject selection (Richardson & Puri 2000). Although the evidence is hampered by small samples and other methodological issues, at this time ω-3 LCPUFAs do not appear to be effective in ADHD (Goren & Tewksbury 2011).

Schizophrenia

Schizophrenic patients have been frequently found to have low LCPUFAs (Peet 2003, 2006). Some studies have found higher saturated and monounsaturated fat in red cells at the expense of LCPUFAs of both the ω-3 and ω-6 families (Kemperman et al 2006). The evidence linking LCPUFAs with this condition was so persuasive it generated the 'membrane phospholipid theory of schizophrenia'; however, while most evidence points to increased LCPUFA turnover, a consensus on the exact nature of this disturbance is still pending (Atker et al 2012). Interestingly, an in vitro study of cells exposed to H_2O_2 as a model of the high oxidative stress seen in schizophrenia found that respiridone and fish oils together reduced lipid peroxidation and free Ca^{2+} while simultaneously increasing glutathione, glutathione peroxidase and vitamin C levels (Altinkilic 2010).

A key researcher in the area of EFAs and psychiatry also points to the significant overlap between core features of the metabolic syndrome and established physiological aberrations evident in schizophrenia, including visceral adiposity, insulin resistance, dyslipidaemias, increased inflammatory markers and reduced ω-3 LCPUFAs in cell membranes (Peet 2006). Importantly, these similarities predate the introduction of the novel antipsychotics, which are known to be diabesogenic. Schizophrenic patients demonstrate a two- to fourfold increased risk of type 2 diabetes mellitus (T2DM) and two to three times greater risk of coronary artery disease mortality, which cannot be entirely related to secondary lifestyle behaviours.

In a 2003 review, four out of five placebo-controlled, double-blind trials of EPA in the adjunctive treatment of schizophrenia have produced positive results with a typical effective dose of 2 g/day of EPA for a minimum of 3 months (Peet 2003). An updated Cochrane review of six studies, involving 353 subjects, has similarly concluded that ethyl-EPA may exert positive effects when added to standard medication; however, more large well-designed, conducted and reported studies are needed (Joy et al 2006). Since this time another systematic review has reached similar conclusions (Akter et al 2012), with small sample sizes (n = 16–122), short intervention duration (6–16 weeks) and heterogeneous LCPUFA interventions hampering more robust findings. The authors note, however, with suggestive positive effects in this cohort and an excellent safety profile, many clinicians may opt to add ω-3 into their schizophrenic patient management.

A new area of research opening up is psychosis prevention in high-risk individuals. One randomised double-blind placebo-controlled study of 81 adolescents classified as being at ultra-high risk of psychosis, treated with either fish oils (480 mg/day DHA, 700 mg/day EPA, 7.6 mg vitamin E) or placebo over 12 weeks, found that, while 27.5% of the control group transitioned to their first psychotic episode, only 4.9% of those taking fish oil did (Amminger et al 2010). Impressively, these benefits were sustained following cessation of the intervention throughout the year of follow-up. Early treatment of psychosis is considered to be a major determinant of overall outcomes and, compared to the risks associated with long-term antipsychotic medications, ω-3 supplements are an appealing alternative.

Cancer

It is well established that dietary fat has an influence on human cancer development and progression. Several forms of research implicate ω-6 PUFAs as catalysts, whereas ω-3 LCPUFAs have the opposite effect and have been shown to inhibit development and progression (Leitzmann et al 2004, Weisburger 1997). Therefore, it is the ratio of ω-3 to ω-6 PUFAs intake that appears to be an important factor influencing cancer incidence and progression.

This observation is supported by both animal and epidemiological studies. The largest to date involved 24 European countries and identified a significant inverse correlation with fish and fish oil consumption, when expressed as a proportion of total or animal fat, for both male and female colorectal cancer and for female breast cancer (Caygill et al 1996). Importantly, the protective effects were only detected in countries with a high animal fat intake, suggesting that fish oil protects against the promotional effects of animal fat in carcinogenesis.

Breast and prostate cancers

Increased intake of ω-3 fatty acids associated with decreased ω-6, resulting in a higher ω-3/ω-6 ratio compared with the western diet, are inversely associated with breast cancer risk, as shown by Yang et al in their meta-analysis (de Lorgeril and Salen 2014). A 2003 review found that overall it remains unclear as to whether dietary fish or fish oil consumption exerts a protective effect against the development of breast and prostate cancers (Terry et al 2003). The assessment of EPA and DHA intake and their relation to ω-6 fatty acid intake and cancer incidence still requires further examination before conclusions can be confidently made. An updated review conducted by the same researchers in 2004 (Terry et al 2004) reached a similar conclusion; however, they also observed that those studies that assess ω-3 intake concomitant with the ω-6 consumption were most likely to yield a statistically significant inverse relationship between fish oils and breast and prostate cancers. Once again this reinforces the understanding that due to interrelated metabolism and actions the fats should not be viewed independently.

A prospective cohort study in the United States of 47,866 men aged 40–75 years with no cancer history were assessed using a 131-item semiquantitative food frequency questionnaire administered annually over 14 years, as part of the Health Professionals Follow-Up study. Nutrient intake data from this trial suggest an association between ALA and advanced prostate cancer, but an inverse relationship with the ALA metabolites, EPA and DHA. Earlier studies investigating the relationship between ALA and prostate cancer have had mixed results while the inverse relationship with EPA/DHA appears to be largely supported. Again the authors demonstrate that ratios of ω-3 : ω-6 appear to be highly influential in conveyed risk (Leitzmann et al 2004).

More recently, an association was confirmed between consuming salted or smoked fish and an increased risk of advanced prostate cancer, whereas fish oil consumption may be protective against progression of prostate cancer in elderly men (Torfadottir et al 2013). Interestingly, serum PSA concentrations from 6018 men (from the 2003–2010 National Health and Nutrition Examination Survey), matched with dietary intake of fish, found little evidence for ω-3PUFA consumption in influencing PSA levels (Patel et al 2014). Emerging data further suggest ω-3 PUFAs may slow the growth of many tumours, including prostate (Masko et al 2013).

Colorectal cancer

Epidemiological evidence investigating associations between fish intake and colorectal cancer have produced mixed findings (Caygill et al 1996, Daniel et al 2009), with the most recent prospective cohort study (Cancer Prevention Study-II Nutrition Cohort) involving over 99,000 individuals failing to demonstrate a protective effect of increased ω-3 intake. In fact, increased consumption of ALA was associated with increased risk in women. Contrastingly, higher marine ω-3 intake did appear protective. The latter finding is consistent with the results of other large prospective studies on this issue (Hall et al 2008).

Other sources of evidence attribute both EPA and DHA and their main dietary source, fish oil, with antineoplastic effects in colorectal cancer (Llor et al 2003). Fish oil supplementation, in one study, providing 4.1 g EPA and 3.6 g DHA per day in patients with sporadic adenomatous colorectal polyps, was reported to reduce the percentage of cells in the S-phase in the upper crypt of the rectal mucosa (Anti et al 1992). The evidence to date, as reviewed in 2004 by Roynette et al, suggests a primary preventive effect with some residual ambiguity over the safety of ω-3 LCPUFA with respect to secondary tumour formation.

One study has investigated the effects of ω-3 LCPUFA parenteral supplementation postoperatively on clinical outcomes and immunomodulation in colorectal cancer patients using a randomised, double-blind design (Liang et al 2008). Treatment effect comparisons revealed that those treated with ω-3 LCPUFAs had significantly lower serum interleukin, TNF-alpha and increased ratios of $CD4^+$/$CD8^+$. These patients also tended towards shorter postoperative hospital stays. Consequently, the authors conclude that such a treatment regimen may have beneficial effects on lowering the magnitude of inflammatory responses and modulating the immune response in this patient group.

The results of an in vitro study have demonstrated synergistic inhibition of proliferating colon cancer cells using a combination of lycopene and EPA (Tang et al 2009). The results of other in vitro studies attribute the protective effects of ω-3 LCPUFAs with DHA rather than EPA (Kato et al 2007). Both animal studies and RCTs are now required to clarify the 'active' fatty acid and confirm these findings.

Diabetes

Increasing the intake of ω-3 LCPUFA has been shown to be both preventive in a healthy population and beneficial in people with diabetes (Montori et al 2000, Nettleton et al 2005, Sirtori & Galli 2002, Sirtori et al 1997). A recent systematic review and meta-analysis revising results from 24 studies, including 24,509 type 2 diabetes patients and 545,275 participants overall, found marine ω-3 PUFA to have beneficial effects on the prevention of type 2 diabetes in Asian populations (Zheng et al 2012). Alternately, no clear association was found between ω-3 EFAS and type 2 diabetes in a review of 16 studies comprising 540,184 individuals (Wu et al 2012). In addition, no major harms or benefits of fish/seafood or EPA+DHA on development of DM were observed, but there was suggestion of modestly lower risk with ALA.

While the preventative effect of ω-3 EFAS on diabetes is still being investigated, ω-3EFAs do provide other benefits for people with established diabetes. Diets higher in fish and ω-3 PUFA may reduce cardiovascular risk in diabetes by inhibiting platelet aggregation, improving lipid profiles and reducing cardiovascular mortality (McEwen et al 2010). Two meta-analyses found that fish oil supplementation lowers plasma TG levels in type 2 diabetic subjects; however, a possible rise in plasma LDL cholesterol may occur (Balk et al 2006, Montori et al 2000). Although an increase in LDL cholesterol was noted after ω-3 supplementation, the levels of LDL were not significantly increased in subgroup analyses of hypertriglyceridaemic patients, high (greater than 2 g of EPA and DHA daily) or low ω-3 PUFA doses and in trials lasting longer than 2 months (Hartweg et al 2008). The rise in plasma LDL cholesterol has been speculated to be the result of enhanced conversion of very LDLs and studies in primates suggest that ω-3 LCPUFA-enriched LDLs do not convey the same atherogenic potential (Jung et al 2008). Additionally, no significant effect occurs on glycaemic control, total cholesterol or HDL cholesterol. In addition, studies reveal an average of 7.4% increase in HDL levels concomitant with a 25% reduction in TGs in response to 1020 mg EPA and 700 mg DHA supplementation over 6 months (Sirtori et al 1998). Such findings are supported by the results of other trials in patients with diabetes (Nettleton et al 2005).

In a randomised study, serum phospholipid ω-3 PUFA levels were found to be significantly decreased in patients with type 2 diabetes and non-alcoholic fatty liver disease ($n = 51$; $P < 0.05$). In addition, serum ω-3 levels were negatively related with insulin resistance. Homeostasis model assessment method (HOMA-IR) levels were higher in patients with type 2 diabetes and non-alcoholic fatty liver disease than in the type 2 diabetes ($n = 50$), non-alcoholic fatty liver disease ($n = 45$) and healthy control groups ($n = 42$; $P < 0.05$). Furthermore, Pearson analysis showed that the ω-3 PUFA level was negatively correlated with HOMA-IR ($r = -0.491$), total cholesterol ($r = -0.376$), TGs ($r = -0.462$) and LDL cholesterol ($r = -0.408$), all $P < 0.05$ (Lou et al 2014).

The effect of fish on endothelial function was investigated in 23 postmenopausal women with type 2 diabetes. Participants were assigned to two 4-week periods of either a fish-based diet (ω-3 PUFAs ≥ 3.0 g/day) or a control diet in a randomised crossover design. Endothelial function was measured with reactive hyperaemia using strain-gauge plethysmography and peak forearm blood flow, duration of reactive hyperaemia and flow debt repayment (FDR). This was then compared with the serum levels of fatty acids and their metabolites. In the fish-first group, the peak forearm blood flow response and FDR increased markedly after the fish-based diet period (4 weeks), and these effects were sustained after the control diet period (8 weeks). In addition, the durations of reactive hyperaemia and FDR increased significantly, and the peak forearm blood flow showed improvement. Conversely, in the control diet-first group, the peak forearm blood flow response, duration of reactive hyperaemia and FDR were unchanged after the control diet period (4 weeks) (Kondo 2014).

Furthermore, the anti-inflammatory properties of ω-3 PUFA, such as the reduction of prostaglandin E_2, leukotrienes (B_4 and E_4), thromboxane B_2 and C-reactive protein, may be of beneficial use in patients with diabetes and CVD. Large trials are suggested to assess the therapeutic potential of ω-3 PUFA as an anti-inflammatory agent in patients with diabetes and CVD (McEwen et al 2010). Despite the potential benefits associated with ω-3 LCPUFAs, a 2008 Cochrane review of 23 RCTs involving 1075 individuals concluded there is currently insufficient evidence to recommend high-dose fish oils to T2DM patients for cardiovascular benefits (Hartweg et al 2008).

Weight reduction

Animal studies illustrate the potential for ω-3 as disease modifiers in obesity via anti-inflammatory mechanisms such as activation of peroxisome proliferator-activated receptors, lowering levels of TNF-α produced by adipocytes and therefore attenuating secondary insulin resistance (Pedersen et al 2011), and that ω-3 interventions consistently reduce body weight and fat mass (Munro & Garg 2013). The results of ω-3 interventions in humans, however, are very mixed. Some positive findings include attenuating negative PUFA changes associated with weight loss regimes (Hlavatý et al 2008) and improving insulin resistance in overweight subjects (Ramel et al 2008), and possible reduced incidence of obesity, increased ease of weight loss and maintenance of body weight in this population (Nettleton et al 2005). One study found that overweight and obese subjects consuming >1300 mg/day ω-3 LCPUFAs compared with those consuming <240 mg/day demonstrated significantly increased satiety 2 hours postprandially, which correlated with increased ω-3 : ω-6 (Parra et al 2008). In contrast there are numerous interventional studies which have failed to produce these anticipated outcomes, including a recent small Australian trial (n = 33) conducted over 12 weeks (Munro & Garg 2013). Speculation regarding such inconsistent results includes the heterogeneous nature of the supplements, with highly variable DHA and EPA ratios and dose, the possible need for longer treatment periods and the perennial issue of human dietary compliance. A new finding in animal research may shed some light on this, with evidence that background diet exerts a crucial influence on the ability of fish oil to protect against obesity development and adipose tissue inflammation (Hao et al 2012). In fact, in this study of mice the beneficial effects of ω-3 intake in mice were significantly diminished or completely abrogated by a simultaneous intake of high-glycaemic index carbohydrates. Another Australian study posits the question of whether other nutrients in fish beyond LCPUFAs contribute to positive weight- and insulin-lowering effects, with a small human trial showing statistically greater adiponectin increases with high dietary ω-3 versus comparable EPA/DHA from supplements (Neale et al 2012). Finally, preliminary research investigating ω-3's effect on lowering endocannibinoid levels in obese rats and humans suggests that krill oil may be superior for this application (Banni et al 2011). Further human studies investigating these issues are necessary.

Polycystic ovarian syndrome (PCOS)

Evidence of fish oil's ability to improve insulin sensitivity has led to several small investigations in PCOS populations. One study of 45 non-obese PCOS sufferers administered 1.5 g of ω-3 for 6 months found that body mass index, insulin and HOMA levels decreased significantly, in addition to hormonal improvements e.g.

lower serum LH, testosterone and higher SHBG. Glucose levels themselves however didn't change and TNF-α levels showed a significant increase (Oner & Muderris 2013). Similar results were obtained in another study of 61 PCOS patients administered 720 mg/day EPA and 480 mg/DHA or placebo over 8 weeks. Again statistically significant improvements were evident on multiple parameters (TGs, HDLs, HOMA) but the inflammatory marker, this time CRP, was unchanged (Mohammadi et al 2012). Interestingly, in a study of PCOS patients which included those with healthy body mass index, favourable lipid changes were lessened. Several of these studies illustrate the androgen-lowering effect of high-dose ω-3 (Oner & Muderris 2013, Phelan et al 2011) which is hypothesised to be the result of reduced ω-6 : ω-3 rather than a direct effect of ω-3 (Phelan et al 2011).

Inflammatory diseases

Numerous clinical trials have investigated the effects of fish oil supplementation in several inflammatory and autoimmune diseases, such as RA, Crohn's disease, ulcerative colitis, lupus erythematosus and migraine headaches (Belluzzi 2002, Belluzzi et al 1996, Miura et al 1998, Simopoulos 2002). Although not all trials have produced positive results, many of the placebo-controlled trials reveal significant benefit in chronic disease, including decreased disease activity and sometimes reduced requirement for anti-inflammatory medicines (Adam et al 2003).

Rheumatoid arthritis

Of the inflammatory diseases, the use of fish oil supplementation is most widely seen and supported in RA. RCTs, meta- and mega-analysis of RCTs indicate reduction in tender joint counts, pain intensity, morning stiffness and decreased use of non-steroidal anti-inflammatory drugs with fish oil supplementation in long-standing RA (Adam et al 2003, Cleland et al 2003, Goldberg & Katz 2007, James et al 2010, Kremer 2000, Miles & Calder 2012, Ulbricht & Basch 2005, Volker et al 2000). Since non-steroidal anti-inflammatory drugs confer cardiovascular risk and there is increased cardiovascular mortality in RA, an additional benefit of fish oil in RA may be reduced cardiovascular risk via direct mechanisms and decreased non-steroidal anti-inflammatory drug use. Interestingly, fish oil has been shown to slow the development of RA in animal models and to reduce disease severity (Miles & Calder 2012).

Generally, supplements are taken daily as adjuncts to standard therapy, with clinical effects appearing after 12 weeks. A dose ranging from 30 mg to 40 mg/kg of EPA and DHA daily has been used successfully, although some studies have found a minimum of 3 g/day is required. Results from a double-blind, crossover study suggest that the beneficial effects obtained from fish oil capsules are further enhanced when combined with an anti-inflammatory diet providing less than 90 mg/day of AA (Adam et al 2003).

Symptomatic relief with ω-3 LCPUFAs in RA was more recently confirmed in a meta-analysis of 17 RCTs assessing the pain-relieving effects in RA patients or joint pain secondary to inflammatory bowel disease and dysmenorrhoea (Goldberg & Katz 2007). Supplementation for 3–4 months significantly reduced patient-reported joint pain intensity, minutes of morning stiffness, number of painful and/or tender joints and non-steroidal anti-inflammatory drug consumption. Significant effects were not detected, however, for doctor-assessed pain or Ritchie articular index. These papers, together with other authoritative reviews, conclude that, based on high-level evidence, ω-3 LCPUFAs are an attractive adjunctive treatment for joint pain associated with RA and have a beneficial follow-on effect on cardiovascular morbidity and mortality pertinent to this population (Proudman et al 2008).

Although the anti-inflammatory activity of fish oil supplementation is thought to be chiefly responsible for symptom-relieving effects, there is also evidence that ω-3 LCPUFAs can modulate expression and activity of degradative factors that cause cartilage destruction (Curtis et al 2000). A 2005 randomised study found that fish oil supplements (3 g/day), whether taken alone or in combination with olive oil (9.6 mL), produced a statistically significant improvement ($P < 0.05$) compared to placebo on several clinical parameters (Berbert et al 2005). Significant improvements were observed for joint pain intensity, right and left handgrip strength after 12 and 24 weeks, duration of morning stiffness, onset of fatigue, Ritchie's articular index for pain joints after 24 weeks, ability to bend down to pick up clothing from the floor and getting in and out of a car after 24 weeks. The group using a combination of oils showed additional improvements with respect to duration of morning stiffness after 12 weeks, patient global assessment after 12 and 24 weeks, ability to turn taps on and off after 24 weeks and rheumatoid factor after 24 weeks. In addition, this group showed a significant improvement in patient global assessment compared with fish oils alone after 12 weeks.

Based on these results, it appears that, while fish oils will not improve all parameters of RA, overall they have demonstrated symptomatic relief in the majority and result in significantly reduced use of anti-inflammatory and corticosteroid use, a fact that MacLean et al (2004) acknowledge and which is confirmed by a 2005 review by Stamp et al and meta-analysis by Goldberg and Katz (2007). There appears to be little evidence of sustained improvements following cessation of the supplements.

A 2008 paper from the Joint Nutrition Society notes that, in addition to modifying the lipid mediator profile, ω-3 LCPUFAs exert effects on other aspects of immunity relevant to RA, such as antigen presentation, T-cell reactivity and inflammatory cytokine production (Calder 2008).

Reducing incidence of RA

A large prospective cohort study ($n = 57,053$) investigating the association between dietary factors and risk of RA found that each increase in intake of 30 g fatty fish (≥8 g fat/100 g fish) per day was associated with 49% reduction in the risk of RA ($P = 0.06$); however, a medium intake of fatty fish (3–7 g fat/100 g fish) was associated with significantly increased risk of RA (Pedersen et al 2005). No associations were found between risk of RA and intake of a range of other dietary factors, including long-chain fatty acids, olive oil, vitamins A, C, D and E, zinc, selenium, iron and meat. The authors caution that, due to the limited number of patients who developed RA during follow-up, it is not yet possible to make firm conclusions.

Asthma

Ω-3 LCPUFAs exhibit anti-inflammatory activity and epidemiological evidence has demonstrated an inverse relationship between fish intake, asthma risk and improved lung function (Wong 2005). Evidence suggests this protective effect may extend back as far as adequate fetal ω-3 LCPUFA exposure (Salam et al 2005).

A 2002 Cochrane review of nine RCTs conducted between 1986 and 2001 concluded that ω-3 LCPUFA supplementation demonstrated no consistent effect on any of the analysable outcomes: forced expiratory volume in 1 s, peak flow rate, asthma symptoms, asthma medication use or bronchial hyperreactivity (Woods et al 2002). However, one of the RCTs involving children showed that, when fish oil supplementation was combined with dietary changes, positive results were obtained, as evidenced by improved peak flow and reduced asthma medication use.

An interesting crossover study of 72 asthmatic children aged 7–10 years involved five randomised phases of treatment each lasting 6 weeks: placebo; ω-3 (300 mg/day combined EPA and DHA); zinc (15 mg/day); vitamin C (200 mg/day); combination of all nutrients (Biltagi et al 2009). While the ω-3 LCPUFA supplementation was associated with improved lung function and a reduction in both sputum production and markers of airway inflammation, these positive effects were significantly augmented when combined with zinc and vitamin C, suggesting that a broader nutritional approach to inflammation and oxidation control results in greatest clinical outcomes.

The equivocal nature of ω-3 LCPUFAs interventions, as documented by a 2005 review (Wong 2005), may be clarified in future with the identification of a subtype of asthma more likely to respond to EFA manipulation.

Another interesting paper reports on three patients with disabling salicylate intolerance producing urticaria, asthma and anaphylactic reactions who, following administration of 10 g/day fish oils for 6–8 weeks, experienced complete or virtually complete resolution of symptoms (Healy et al 2008). Treatment response was so effective corticosteroids could be discontinued; however, symptoms reappeared following fish oil dose reduction.

The focus for fish oils in asthma has broadened to include other populations such as athletes. One randomised, double-blind, crossover study of 16 non-atopic asthmatic patients with documented exercise-induced broncoconstriction compared the effects of 3.2 g of EPA and 2.0 g DHA per day and placebo capsules for 3 weeks. During treatment with fish oils, subjects demonstrated improved pulmonary function to below the diagnostic exercise-induced bronco-constriction threshold, which was associated with a concurrent reduction in bronchodilator use. Measurement of leukotriene B_4 and B_5 levels also confirmed a significant reversal of the inflammatory picture (Mickleborough et al 2006).

Clinical note — Oils ain't oils

Arguably the biggest ongoing methodological sticking point in ω-3 research is the heterogeneous nature of the interventions used, which has hindered comparisons, meta-analyses and consensus about their therapeutic actions. While the inferiority of plant-based ω-3 EFAs has now been established (see Are ALA-rich oils a worthy substitute for fish oils?), new questions over different forms — e.g. fish versus supplements, supplemental forms, e.g. TGs, ethyl esters, ratios of EPA to DHA and sources, e.g. krill, algal — have arisen and there is a focused effort to clarify differences in the behaviour and bioavailability of each, such that researchers can better understand disparate outcomes of RCTs and, most importantly, identify superior ways of improving ω-3.

Fish versus fish oil supplements

Underpinning interest and excitement about ω-3s, particularly in the context of CVD prevention, stemmed from epidemiological studies of high fish-consuming populations. Early on an assumption was made that these benefits were entirely attributable to the ω-3 fatty acids. More recently, however, this has been questioned, with increasing speculation that EPA/DHA may interact with other nutrients, e.g. taurine, selenium, astaxanthin, within fish and/or that dietary fish may displace other unhealthy food choices and therefore may be superior to supplementation with fish oils (Brazionis et al 2012, Deckelbaum & Torrejon 2012, Harvard Heart Letter 2011, He 2009). Some researchers reason that this explains the disparate and somewhat disappointing results of fish oil interventions in some RCTs compared with studies of increasing fish intake in the prevention of CVD, especially fatal CHD (He 2009). An interesting small crossover Australian study found that fish consumption (150 g of Atlantic salmon twice a week) significantly reduced blood pressure and waist circumference when compared with fish oil (1.2 g/day 6 days/week) in spite of comparable changes in ω-3 index (Brazionis et al 2012). The current consensus is: eat low mercury-containing fish where possible and if not possible, take supplements; however, more research in other conditions is necessary.

Triglycerides versus ethyl esters

Several studies confirm improved bioavailability from fish oils presented as TGs (either natural or re-esterified) over ethyl esters, including a long-term study (6 months) of moderate intake (1.01 g EPA and 0.67 g DHA) and its effects on RBC levels in healthy individuals (Neubronner et al 2011). Another debate is the impact of the position of the LCPUFAs along the glycerol backbone in these TGs; this differs between natural TGs and chemically re-esterified TGs. However, a small study found that EPA bioavailability at least was significantly greater from the re-esterified TGs than the NTGs (Wakil et al 2010). Other similar studies reviewing DHA uptake, however, are inconsistent.

Comparing krill, algal and fish oil

Pressing issues of non-sustainability of both wild harvesting and aquaculture together with increasing contaminants in fish and their products have motivated researchers to search for alternative sources to meet our increasing ω-3 demand (Racine & Deckelbaum 2007, Robert 2006). Two key emerging areas are algal and krill oil (*Euphausia superba*). Microalgae, such as *Crypthecodinium cohnii* and *Schizochytrium* spp., represent part of the coastal food chain as a primary food source for shellfish, contain no contaminants (Arterburn et al 2000, Doughman et al 2007) and are currently commercially developed as sustainable crops (Doughman et al 2007, Whelan & Rust 2006). Krill is by far the most dominant member of the Antarctic zooplankton in terms of biomass, which also makes it attractive as a more sustainable crop (Ulven et al 2011); however, both algal and krill oil are produced at significantly higher production costs (Deckelbaum & Torrejon 2012) and differ chemically and behaviourally from fish oil, e.g. both algal and krill oil contain the astaxanthin not found in fish oil. Also, algal oil predominates in DHA and initial human studies have confirmed both bioequivalence and comparable clinical efficacy with other DHA sources such as salmon (Arterburn et al 2000, Doughman et al 2007). However, some conditions respond preferentially to higher EPA levels (see Depression), which would limit the application of these products. Attempts to produce high EPA forms have been unsuccessful to date (Deckelbaum & Torrejon 2012).

In contrast, krill oil has a lower yield per gram of LCPUFAs compared with fish oil but its ratio of EPA:DHA is greater. Additionally, LCPUFAs in fish oils are presented as either TGs or ethyl esters; however, 30–65% found in krill oil are incorporated into phospholipids. This phospholipid form appears to favour increased bioavailability and several studies have found that krill oil can produce comparable or superior improvements in ω-3 levels in spite of lower actual EPA and DHA content (approximately 68% of that used in fish oil comparator studies) (Banni et al 2011, Ramprasath et al 2013, Schuchardt et al 2011, Ulven et al 2011). Preliminary evidence suggests that krill oil may offer a therapeutic advantage over fish oil in the treatment of metabolic syndrome and weight loss (Banni et al 2011, Vigerust et al 2013); however the vast majority of RCTs performed to date with PUFAs have used fish oils.

F

Atopic dermatitis and eczema

In a sample of adult patients (n = 53), randomised to 5.4 g/day DHA or isoenergetic saturated fats for 20 weeks, active fish oil treatment produced significant clinical improvements which correlated with increases in plasma DHA (Koch et al 2008); however, due to the small sample size, larger studies are required to confirm these preliminary results.

Previously, a double-blind multicentre study involving 145 patients with moderate to severe atopic dermatitis showed that ω-3 LCPUFAs (6 g/day) improved clinical symptom scores by 30% after 4 months' treatment (Soyland et al 1994). The results were confirmed by patients' subjective scoring. An earlier, 12-week, prospective, double-blind study produced similar results, with a dose of 10 g/day (fish oil) improving overall severity of atopic dermatitis and reducing scaling (Bjorneboe et al 1989). A 2012 Cochrane review that included all four studies concluded that two trials suggest a moderate effect on reducing severity in adults; however, further research is needed (Bath-Hextall et al 2012).

OTHER USES

Fish oil supplements are also used in the management of acute respiratory distress syndrome, psoriasis, multiple sclerosis, osteoporosis and dysmenorrhoea and in children with dyslexia.

DOSAGE RANGE

- Fish should be considered part of a healthy diet for everybody and be consumed at least twice a week. Care should be taken to avoid intake of fish known or suspected to contain higher levels of mercury.
- Additional administration of ω-3 LCPUFA supplements should be considered in specific groups.
- Fish meals should consist of deep-sea oily fish, whereas fried or processed fish containing partially hydrogenated fats and salted or pickled fish should be avoided.

Cardiovascular disease

Secondary prevention trials after MI indicate that consumption of 0.5–1.8 g/day of EPA and DHA from fish or fish oil supplements may be beneficial. Intake of marine-derived ω-3 fatty acids can be increased through diet or with fish oil supplements.

- An expert US panel of nutrition scientists has recommended an intake of 0.65 g/day, whereas the British Nutrition Foundation's recommendation is 1.2 g/day (Din et al 2004).

- National Heart Foundation/Cardiac Society of Australia and New Zealand: >2 servings/week.
- Patients who have experienced coronary artery bypass surgery with venous grafts: 4 g/day of ω-3 LCPUFAs.
- Moderate hypertension: 4 g/day of fish oils.
- Elevated TG levels: 1–4.6 g/day of fish oils; Lovaza 4 g/day.

Other conditions

- Aggression induced by mental stress: DHA supplementation, 1.5–1.8 g/day.
- Anger and anxiety reduction in polysubstance abuse withdrawers: 2.25 g EPA, 500 mg DHA and 250 mg other ω-3 per day.
- Asthma prevention in pregnancy: 2.7 g/day from week 20 gestation until delivery.
- Asthma treatment in children: 300 mg combined EPA and DHA with 15 mg zinc and 200 mg vitamin C per day.
- Atopic dermatitis: 6 g/day fish oils or 5.4 g/day DHA.
- Autism: 5 g/day (limited evidence to support).
- BD: 1 g/day EPA.
- Colorectal cancer: 4.1 g EPA + 3.6 g DHA daily.
- Dementia: DHA supplementation, 4.32 g/day.
- Depression: 1 g/day EPA or a combined supplement with ≥60% EPA.
- Exercise-induced asthma in non-atopic individuals: 3.2 g EPA + 2.0 g DHA daily.
- High blood pressure: 3–5.6 g/day.
- Intermittent claudication: 1.8 g EPA and 1.2 g DHA per day (limited evidence to support).
- Pregnancy: According to the WHO and FAO, the pregnant woman should take at least 2.6 g of ω-3 EFAs, incorporating 100–300 mg of DHA daily to look after the needs of the fetus.
- Psychosis prevention in high-risk individuals: 480 mg/day DHA, 700 mg/day EPA for 12 weeks.
- RA: 30–40 mg/kg body weight of EPA and DHA daily.
- Schizophrenia: 2 g/day EPA for a minimum of 3 months.
- Weight reduction and improved insulin sensitivity: 660 mg EPA and 440 mg DHA/day.

ADVERSE REACTIONS

Fish oil supplementation is generally safe and well tolerated. The few side effects reported are usually mild and can include gastrointestinal discomfort and loose bowels, halitosis and a fishy odour of the skin and urine.

Studies using Lovaza (previously Omacor) report the main side effects as belching, indigestion, taste aversions, fishy taste, infection and flu-like symptoms. Reports have also shown that it may increase levels of alanine aminotransferase; in addition ratio of LDL:apolipoprotein B may increase after pharmacological doses of ω-3 (Nicholson et al 2013).

SIGNIFICANT INTERACTIONS

Antiplatelet agents

Theoretically, concomitant use with antiplatelet agents may increase the risk of bleeding; however, multiple clinical studies have found no clinically significant effect on bleeding and one study has suggested that the combined effects may be beneficial (Engstrom et al 2001) — no clinically significant interaction expected at therapeutic doses.

Anticoagulants

Clinical studies of surgical patients taking warfarin have not found a clinically significant increase in bleeding. According to one clinical study, bleeding time is increased at very high doses of 12 g/day. Usual therapeutic doses, which tend to fall below this dosage, appear safe in this population, although care should still be taken. Very high doses >12 g should be used only under professional supervision to ensure no adverse outcomes.

Non-steroidal anti-inflammatory drugs

Additional anti-inflammatory effects are theoretically possible with concurrent use of fish oil supplements, suggesting a beneficial interaction. Drug dosage may require modification.

Pravastatin

Low-dose pravastatin combined with fish oil supplementation is more effective than pravastatin alone for changing the lipid profile after renal transplantation, according to one clinical study — potential beneficial interaction.

CONTRAINDICATIONS AND PRECAUTIONS

One area of concern is the growing problem of heavy-metal contamination found in fish, specifically mercury. In areas where contamination is possible, fish oil supplements may represent a safer option. According to the *Australia New Zealand Food Standards Code*, fish with higher levels of mercury include: marlin, swordfish, southern bluefin tuna, barramundi, ling, orange roughy, rays and shark. Fish considered to have lower levels of mercury include: mackerel, silver wahoo, Atlantic salmon, canned salmon and canned tuna in oil, herrings and sardines.

People with bleeding disorders should take fish oil supplements under medical supervision.

PREGNANCY USE

Fish oils appear to be safe during pregnancy at dietary doses and are likely to have benefits.

Practice points/Patient counselling

- As precursors of eicosanoids, PUFAs found in fish oils exert a wide influence over many important physiological processes.
- They have demonstrated anti-inflammatory, immunological, neurological, antiplatelet and chemopreventive effects, and a range of beneficial actions within the cardiovascular system.
- Daily ingestion of at least 1 g EPA and DHA (equivalent to fish eaten at least twice weekly) may result in a reduction in total mortality, cardiovascular mortality and morbidity and incidence of dementia and depression.

- Trials generally support the use of supplements in a range of inflammatory and autoimmune diseases such as RA and atopic dermatitis, elevated TGs, hypertension and other cardiovascular conditions, poor cognitive function and diabetes. Preliminary research suggests a possible role in depression.
- People with bleeding disorders should take fish oil supplements under medical supervision.

PATIENTS' FAQs

What will this supplement do for me?

Regular consumption of fish oils may reduce total mortality, cardiovascular mortality and morbidity, dementia, depression and possibly diabetes and various cancers. Additionally, beneficial effects have been demonstrated in a wide variety of conditions.

When will it start to work?

This will depend on the dosage taken and indication for use.

Are there any safety issues?

People with bleeding disorders should take fish oil supplements under medical supervision.

REFERENCES

Adam O et al. Anti-inflammatory effects of a low arachidonic acid diet and fish oil in patients with rheumatoid arthritis. Rheumatol Int 23.1 (2003): 27–36.

Alm B et al. Early introduction of fish decreases the risk of eczema in infants. Arch Dis Child 94.1 (2009): 11–15.

Almqvist C et al. CAPS team. Omega-3 and omega-6 fatty acid exposure from early life does not affect atopy and asthma at age 5 years. J Allergy Clin Immunol 119.6 (2007): 1438–1444.

Amminger GP et al. Omega-3 fatty acids supplementation in children with autism: a double-blind randomized, placebo-controlled pilot study. Biol Psychiatry 61.4 (2007): 551–553.

Anti M et al. Effect of omega-3 fatty acids on rectal mucosal cell proliferation in subjects at risk for colon cancer. Gastroenterology 103 (1992): 883–891.

Arterburn LM et al. A combined subchronic (90-day) toxicity and neurotoxicity study of a single-cell source of docosahexaenoic acid triglyceride (DHASCO oil). Food Chem Toxicol 38.1 (2000): 35–49.

Bagga D et al. Long-chain n-3 to n-6 polyunsaturated fatty acid ratios in breast adipose tissue from women with and without breast cancer. Nutr Cancer 42.2 (2002): 180–185.

Balakumar, P. & Taneja, G. 2012. Fish oil and vascular endothelial protection: bench to bedside. Free Radic.Biol. Med, 53, (2) 271–279.

Balk EM et al. Effects of omega-3 fatty acids on serum markers of cardiovascular disease risk: a systematic review. Atherosclerosis 189.1 (2006): 19–30.

Bambrick HJ, Kjellstrom TE. Good for your heart but bad for your baby? Revised guidelines for fish consumption in pregnancy. Med J Aust 181.2 (2004): 61–62.

Bang HO, et al. The composition of the Eskimo food in north western Greenland. Am J Clin Nutr 33.12 (1980): 2657–2661.

Barter P, Ginsberg HN. Effectiveness of combined statin plus omega-3 fatty acid therapy for mixed dyslipidemia. Am J Cardiol 102.8 (2008): 1040–1045.

Bays HE. Safety considerations with omega-3 fatty acid therapy. Am J Cardiol 99.6A (2007): 35C–43C.

Beers MH, Berkow R (eds), The Merck manual of diagnosis and therapy, 17th edn. Rahway, NJ: Merck, 2003.

Belluzzi A et al. Effect of an enteric-coated fish-oil preparation on relapses in Crohn's disease. N Engl J Med 334.24 (1996): 1557–1560.

Belluzzi A. N-3 fatty acids for the treatment of inflammatory bowel diseases. Proc Nutr Soc 61.3 (2002): 391–395.

Bender NK et al. Effects of marine fish oils on the anticoagulation status of patients receiving chronic warfarin therapy. J Thromb Thrombolysis 5.3 (1998): 257–261.

Berbert AA et al. Supplementation of fish oil and olive oil in patients with rheumatoid arthritis. Nutrition 21.2 (2005): 131–136.

Bhattacharya A et al. Different ratios of eicosapentaenoic and docosahexaenoic omega-3 fatty acids in commercial fish oils differentially alter pro-inflammatory cytokines in peritoneal macrophages from C57BL/6 female mice. J Nutr Biochem (2007); 18: 23–30.

Billman GE, et al. Prevention of ischemia-induced cardiac sudden death by n-3 polyunsaturated fatty acids in dogs. Lipids 32.11 (1997): 1161–1168.

Billman GE, et al. Prevention of sudden cardiac death by dietary pure omega-3 polyunsaturated fatty acids in dogs. Circulation 99.18 (1999): 2452–2457.

Biltagi MA et al. Omega-3 fatty acids, vitamin C and Zn supplementation in asthmatic children: a randomized self-controlled study. Acta Paediatr 2009; 98: 737–742.

Bjorneboe A et al. Effect of n-3 fatty acid supplement to patients with atopic dermatitis. J Intern Med Suppl 225.731 (1989): 233–236.
Braun L et al. A wellness program for cardiac surgery improves clinical outcomes. Adv in Integrat Med 1.1 (2014): 32–37.
Bruinsma KA, Taren DL. Dieting, essential fatty acid intake, and depression. Nutr Rev 58.4 (2000): 98–108.
Bucher HC et al. N-3 polyunsaturated fatty acids in coronary heart disease: a meta-analysis of randomized controlled trials. Am J Med 112.4 (2002): 298–304.
Buckley MS, et al. Fish oil interaction with warfarin. Ann Pharmacother 38.1 (2004): 50–52.
Burr ML et al. Effects of changes in fat, fish, and fibre intakes on death and myocardial reinfarction: diet and reinfarction trial (DART). Lancet 2.8666 (1989): 757–761.
Burr ML et al. Lack of benefit of dietary advice to men with angina: results of a controlled trial. Eur J Clin Nutr 57.2 (2003): 193–200.
Buydens-Branchey L, et al. Associations between increases in plasma n-3 polyunsaturated fatty acids following supplementation and decreases in anger and anxiety in substance abusers. Prog Neuropsychopharmacol Biol Psychiatry 32.2 (2008): 568–575.
Calder PC. Dietary modification of inflammation with lipids. Proc Nutr Soc 61.3 (2002): 345–358.
Calder PC. N-3 polyunsaturated fatty acids and inflammation: from molecular biology to the clinic. Lipids 38.4 (2003): 343–352.
Calder PC. Session 3: Joint Nutrition Society and Irish Nutrition and Dietetic Institute Symposium on 'Nutrition and autoimmune disease' PUFA, inflammatory processes and rheumatoid arthritis. Proc Nutr Soc 67.4 (2008): 409–418.
Calder PC et al. Dietary fish oil suppresses human colon tumour growth in athymic mice. Clin Sci (Lond) 94.3 (1998): 303–311.
Calo L et al. N-3 Fatty acids for the prevention of atrial fibrillation after coronary artery bypass surgery: a randomized, controlled trial. J Am Coll Cardiol 45.10 (2005): 1723–1728.
Campbell, A., et al. 2013. Omega-3 fatty acids for intermittent claudication. Cochrane Database Syst Rev., 7, CD003833.
Casula, M., et al. 2013. Long-term effect of high dose omega-3 fatty acid supplementation for secondary prevention of cardiovascular outcomes: A meta-analysis of randomized, placebo controlled trials [corrected]. Atheroscler. Suppl, 14, (2) 243–251.
Caygill CP et al. Fat, fish, fish oil and cancer. Br J Cancer 74.1 (1996): 159–164.
Chen CT and Bazinet RP. β-Oxidation and rapid metabolism, but not uptake regulate brain eicosapentaenoic acid levels. Prostaglandins, Leukotrienes and Essential Fatty Acids (PLEFA) (in press).
Chiu CC et al. The effects of omega-3 fatty acids monotherapy in Alzheimer's disease and mild cognitive impairment: a preliminary randomized double-blind placebo-controlled study. Prog Neuropsychopharmacol Biol Psychiatry 32.6 (2008): 1538–1544.
Cleland LG et al. The role of fish oils in the treatment of rheumatoid arthritis. Drugs 63.9 (2003): 845–853.
Cohen JT et al. A quantitative analysis of prenatal intake of n-3 polyunsaturated fatty acids and cognitive development. Am J Prev Med 29.4 (2005): 366: e1–e12.
Conquer JA et al. Fatty acid analysis of blood plasma of patients with Alzheimer's disease, other types of dementia, and cognitive impairment. Lipids 35.12 (2000): 1305–1312.
Curtis CL et al. N-3 fatty acids specifically modulate catabolic factors involved in articular cartilage degradation. J Biol Chem 275.2 (2000): 721–724.
Curtis LT, Patel K. Nutritional and environmental approaches to preventing and treating autism and attention deficit hyperactivity disorder (ADHD): a review. J Altern Complement Med 14.1 (2008): 79–85.
Daniel CR et al. Dietary intake of omega-6 and omega-3 fatty acids and risk of colorectal cancer in a prospective cohort of U.S. men and women. Cancer Epidemiol Biomarkers Prev 18.2 (2009): 516–525.
Davis BC, Kris-Etherton PM. Achieving optimal essential fatty acid status in vegetarians: current knowledge and practical implications. Am J Clin Nutr 78.3 (2003): 640–6S.
De, C.R. 2011. N-3 fatty acids in cardiovascular disease. N. Engl. J Med, 364, (25) 2439–2450.
de Lorgeril M, Salen P. Helping women to good health: breast cancer, omega-3/omega-6 lipids, and related lifestyle factors. BMC Med 12.54 (2014): PM:24669767.
De Vriese SR, et al. In humans, the seasonal variation in poly-unsaturated fatty acids is related to the seasonal variation in violent suicide and serotonergic markers of violent suicide. Prostaglandins Leukot Essent Fatty Acids 71.1 (2004): 13–18.
Din JN, et al. Omega 3 fatty acids and cardiovascular disease: fishing for a natural treatment. BMJ 328 (2004): 30–35.
Domingo J. Omega-3 fatty acids and the benefits of fish consumption: is all that glitters gold? Environ Int 33.7 (2007): 993–998.
Domingo J, Bocio A. Levels of PCDD/PCDFS and PCBS in edible marine species and human intake: a literature review. Environ Int 33.3 (2007): 397–405.
Dórea J. Fish meal in animal feed and human exposure to persistent bioaccumulative and toxic substances. J Food Prot 69.11 (2006): 2777–2785.
Doughman S, et al. Omega-3 fatty acids for nutrition and medicine: considering microalgae oil as a vegetarian source of EPA and DHA. Curr Diabetes Rev 3.3 (2007): 198–203.
Dunstan JA et al. Cognitive assessment of children at age 2½ years after maternal fish oil supplementation in pregnancy: a randomised controlled trial. Arch Dis Child Fetal Neonatal Ed 93.1 (2008): F45–F50.
Easton M, et al. Preliminary examination of contaminant loadings in farmed salmon, wild salmon and commercial salmon feed. Chemosphere 46.7 (2002): 1053–1074.
Engelhart MJ et al. Diet and risk of dementia: Does fat matter? The Rotterdam Study. Neurology 59.12 (2002): 1915–1921.
Engstrom K, et al. Effect of low-dose aspirin in combination with stable fish oil on whole blood production of eicosanoids. Prostaglandins Leukot Essent Fatty Acids 64.6 (2001): 291–297.

F

Eritsland J et al. Long-term effects of n-3 polyunsaturated fatty acids on haemostatic variables and bleeding episodes in patients with coronary artery disease. Blood Coagul Fibrinolysis 6.1 (1995): 17–22.

Food Standards Australia New Zealand (FSANZ). www.foodstandards.gov.au (accessed 18-03-04).

Foran J et al. Quantitative analysis of the benefits and risks of consuming farmed and wild salmon. J Nutr 135.11 (2005): 2639–2643.

Frangou S, et al. Efficacy of ethyl-eicosapentaenoic acid in bipolar depression: randomised double-blind placebo-controlled study. Br J Psychiatry 188 (2006): 46–50.

Frishman WH, et al. Alternative and complementary medicine for preventing and treating cardiovascular disease. Dis Mon 55.3 (2009): 121–192.

FSANZ. Mercury in Fish. Canberra: FSANZ, 2004.

Gao L et al. Influence of omega-3 polyunsaturated fatty acid-supplementation on platelet aggregation in humans: A meta-analysis of randomized controlled trials. Atherosclerosis. 226.2 (2013): 328–334.

Garland MR, Hallahan B. Essential fatty acids and their role in conditions characterised by impulsivity. Int Rev Psychiatry 18.2 (2006): 99–105.

Geleijnse JM et al. Blood pressure response to fish oil supplementation: metaregression analysis of randomized trials. J Hypertens 20.8 (2002): 1493–1499.

Goldberg RJ, Katz J. A meta-analysis of the analgesic effects of omega-3 polyunsaturated fatty acid supplementation for inflammatory joint pain. Pain 129.1–2 (2007): 210–223.

Grenyer BF et al. Fish oil supplementation in the treatment of major depression: a randomised double-blind placebo-controlled trial. Prog Neuropsychopharmacol Biol Psychiatry 31.7 (2007): 1393–1396.

Groff J, Gropper S. Advanced nutrition and human metabolism. Belmont USA: Wadsonworth Thomsen Learning, 2004.

Hall MN et al. A 22-year prospective study of fish, n-3 fatty acid intake, and colorectal cancer risk in men. Cancer Epidemiol Biomarkers Prev 17.5 (2008): 1136–1143.

Hallahan B et al. Omega-3 fatty acid supplementation in patients with recurrent self-harm. Single-centre double-blind randomised controlled trial. Br J Psychiatry 190 (2007): 118–122.

Hamazaki T et al. The effect of docosahexaenoic acid on aggression in young adults: A placebo-controlled double-blind study. J Clin Invest 97.4 (1996): 1129–1133.

Hamazaki T et al. Docosahexaenoic acid does not affect aggression of normal volunteers under nonstressful conditions: a randomized, placebo-controlled, double-blind study. Lipids 33.7 (1998): 663–667.

Harris WS. Expert opinion: omega-3 fatty acids and bleeding — cause for concern? Am J Cardiol 99.6A (2007): 44C–46C.

Harris WS et al. Omega-3 fatty acids and coronary heart disease risk: clinical and mechanistic perspectives. Atherosclerosis 197.1 (2008): 12–24.

Hartweg J et al. Omega-3 polyunsaturated fatty acids (PUFA) for type 2 diabetes mellitus. Cochrane Database Syst Rev 23; (1) (2008): CD003205.

Hashimoto M et al. Chronic administration of docosahexaenoic acid ameliorates the impairment of spatial cognition learning ability in amyloid beta-infused rats. J Nutr 135.3 (2005): 549–555.

Healy E et al. Control of salicylate intolerance with fish oils. Br J Dermatol 159.6 (2008): 1368–1369.

Helland IB et al. Maternal supplementation with very-long chain n-3 fatty acids during pregnancy and lactation augments children's IQ at 4 years of age. Pediatrics 111.1 (2003): e39–e44.

Helland IB et al. Effect of supplementing pregnant and lactating mothers with n-3 very-long-chain fatty acids on children's IQ and body mass index at 7 years of age. Pediatrics 122.2 (2008): e472–e479.

Hellsten G et al. Effects on fibrinolytic activity of corn oil and a fish oil preparation enriched with omega-3-polyunsaturated fatty acids in a long-term study. Curr Med Res Opin 13.3 (1993): 133–139.

Hibbeln JR, et al. Omega-3 fatty acid deficiencies in neurodevelopment, aggression and autonomic dysregulation: opportunities for intervention. Int Rev Psychiatry 18.2 (2006): 107–118.

Hightower JM, Moore D. Mercury levels in high-end consumers of fish. Environ Health Perspect 111 (2003): 604–608.

Hlavatý P et al. Change in fatty acid composition of serum lipids in obese females after short-term weight-reducing regimen with the addition of n-3 long chain polyunsaturated fatty acids in comparison to controls. Physiol Res 57 (Suppl 1) (2008): S57–S65.

Holub BJ. Clinical nutrition: 4. Omega-3 fatty acids in cardiovascular care. Can Med Assoc J 166.5 (2002): 608–615.

Hooper L et al. Risks and benefits of omega 3 fats for mortality, cardiovascular disease, and cancer: systematic review. BMJ 332.7544 (2006): 752–760.

Hornstra G. Influence of dietary fish oil on arterial thrombosis and atherosclerosis in animal models and in man. J Intern Med (Suppl) 225.731 (1989): 53–59.

Horrobin DF, Bennett CN. Depression and bipolar disorder: relationships to impaired fatty acid and phospholipid metabolism and to diabetes, cardiovascular disease, immunological abnormalities, cancer, ageing and osteoporosis. Possible candidate genes. Prostaglandins Leukot Essent Fatty Acids 60.4 (1999): 217–234.

Horrocks LA, Yeo YK. Health benefits of docosahexaenoic acid (DHA). Pharmacol Res 40.3 (1999): 211–225.

Houston MC. Nutraceuticals, vitamins, antioxidants, and minerals in the prevention and treatment of hypertension. Progr Cardiovasc Dis 47.6 (2005): 396–449.

Hu FB et al. Fish and omega-3 fatty acid intake and risk of coronary heart disease in women. JAMA 287 (2002): 1815–1821.

Huan M et al. Suicide attempt and n-3 fatty acid levels in red blood cells: A case control study in China. Biol Psychiatry 56.7 (2004): 490–496.

Itomura M et al. The effect of fish oil on physical aggression in schoolchildren — a randomized, double-blind, placebo-controlled trial. J Nutr Biochem 16.3 (2005): 163–171.

Jackson, P. A., et al. (2012). No effect of 12 weeks' supplementation with 1 g DHA-rich or EPA-rich fish oil on cognitive function or mood in healthy young adults aged 18–35 years. British Journal Of Nutrition, 107(8), 1232–1243.

Jacobs M et al. Organochlorine residues in fish oil dietary supplements: comparison with industrial grade oils. Chemosphere 37.9–12 (1998): 1709–1721.
Jacobs M, et al. Investigation of selected persistent organic pollutants in farmed Atlantic salmon (*Salmo salar*), salmon aquaculture feed, and fish oil components of the feed. Environ Sci Technol 36.13 (2002): 2797–2805.
Jacobs M et al. Time Trend Investigation of PCBs, PBDEs, and organochlorine pesticides in selected n-3 polyunsaturated fatty acid rich dietary fish oil and vegetable oil supplements; nutritional relevance for human essential n-3 fatty acid requirements. J Agric Food Chem 52.6 (2004): 1780–1788.
Jalili M, Dehpour AR. Extremely prolonged INR associated with warfarin in combination with both trazodone and omega-3 fatty acids. Arch Med Res 38.8 (2007): 901–904.
James, M., et al. 2010. Fish oil and rheumatoid arthritis: past, present and future. Proc.Nutr.Soc., 69, (3) 316–323.
Jans, L. A., et al. (2010). The efficacy of n-3 fatty acids DHA and EPA (fish oil) for pernatal depression. British Journal of Nutrition, 104(11), 1577–1585.
Jenkins DJ et al. Fish-oil supplementation in patients with implantable cardioverter defibrillators: a meta-analysis. CMAJ 178.2 (2008): 157–164.
Jeppesen J et al. Triglyceride concentration and ischemic heart disease: an eight-year follow-up in the Copenhagen Male Study. Circulation 97.11 (1998): 1029–1036.
Joy CB, et al. Polyunsaturated fatty acid supplementation for schizophrenia. Cochrane Database Syst Rev 3 (2006): CD001257.
Jung UJ et al. N-3 Fatty acids and cardiovascular disease: mechanisms underlying beneficial effects. Am J Clin Nutr 87.6 (2008): 2003S–2009S.
Kalmijn S. Fatty acid intake and the risk of dementia and cognitive decline: a review of clinical and epidemiological studies. J Nutr Health Aging 4.4 (2000): 202–207.
Kalmijn S et al. Dietary fat intake and the risk of incident dementia in the Rotterdam Study. Ann Neurol 42.5 (1997): 776–782.
Kalmijn S et al. Dietary intake of fatty acids and fish in relation to cognitive performance at middle age. Neurology 62.2 (2004): 275–280.
Kamphuis MH et al. Depression and cardiovascular mortality: a role for n-3 fatty acids? Am J Clin Nutr 84.6 (2006): 1513–1517.
Kang JX, Leaf A. The cardiac antiarrhythmic effects of polyunsaturated fatty acid. Lipids 31 (Suppl) (1996): S41–S44.
Kang JX, Leaf A. Prevention of fatal cardiac arrhythmias by polyunsaturated fatty acids. Am J Clin Nutr 71. (1 Suppl) (2000): 202–27S.
Kar, S. 2014. Omacor and omega-3 fatty acids for treatment of coronary artery disease and the pleiotropic effects. Am J Ther., 21, (1) 56–66.
Kato T, et al. Docosahexaenoic acid (DHA), a primary tumor suppressive omega-3 fatty acid, inhibits growth of colorectal cancer independent of p53 mutational status. Nutr Cancer 58.2 (2007): 178–187.
Kemperman RF et al. Low essential fatty acid and B-vitamin status in a subgroup of patients with schizophrenia and its response to dietary supplementation. Prostaglandins Leukot Essent Fatty Acids 74.2 (2006): 75–85.
Kendall-Tackett, K. (2010). Long-chain omega-3 fatty acids and women's mental health in the perinatal period and beyond. Journal of Midwifery & Women's Health, 55(6), 561–567.
Kiecolt-Glaser JK et al. Omega-3 supplementation lowers inflammation and anxiety in medical students: A randomized controlled trial. Brain, Behavior, and Immunity. 25.8 (2011): 1725–1734.
Kinsella JE. Effects of polyunsaturated fatty acids on factors related to cardiovascular disease. Am J Cardiol 60.12 (1987): 23G–32G.
Koch C et al. Docosahexaenoic acid (DHA) supplementation in atopic eczema: a randomized, double-blind, controlled trial. Br J Dermatol 158.4 (2008): 786–792.
Kondo K. A fish-based diet intervention improves endothelial function in postmenopausal women with type 2 diabetes mellitus: A randomized crossover trial. Metabolism. 63.7 (2014): 930–940.
Kremer JM. N-3 fatty acid supplements in rheumatoid arthritis. Am J Clin Nutr 71.(1 Suppl) (2000): 349S–351S.
Kristensen SD, et al. Dietary supplementation with n-3 polyunsaturated fatty acids and human platelet function: a review with particular emphasis on implications for cardiovascular disease. J Intern Med (Suppl) 225.731 (1989): 141–150.
Larsson SC et al. Dietary long-chain n-3 fatty acids for the prevention of cancer: a review of potential mechanisms. Am J Clin Nutr 79.6 (2004): 935–945.
Leaf A. On the reanalysis of the GISSI-Prevenzione. Circulation 105.16 (2002): 1874–1875.
Leckie RL et al. Omega-3 fatty acids moderate effects of physical activity on cognitive function. Neuropsychologia. 59 (2014): 103–111.
Leitzmann MF et al. Dietary intake of n-3 and n-6 fatty acids and the risk of prostate cancer. Am J Clin Nutr 80.1 (2004): 204–216.
Levine KE et al. Determination of mercury in an assortment of dietary supplements using an inexpensive combustion atomic absorption spectrometry technique. J Autom Methods Manag Chem 2005 (2005): 211–216.
Li, N.N., et al. 2014. Does intravenous fish oil benefit patients post-surgery? A meta-analysis of randomised controlled trials. Clin Nutr., 33, (2) 226–239.
Liang B et al. Impact of postoperative omega-3 fatty acid-supplemented parenteral nutrition on clinical outcomes and immunomodulations in colorectal cancer patients. World J Gastroenterol 14.15 (2008): 2434–2439.
Lim WS et al. Omega 3 fatty acid for the prevention of dementia. Cochrane Database Syst Rev 1 (2006): CD005379.
Liu J, Raine A. The effect of childhood malnutrition on externalizing behavior. Curr Opin Pediatr 18.5 (2006): 565–570.
Llor X et al. The effects of fish oil, olive oil, oleic acid and linoleic acid on colorectal neoplastic processes. Clin Nutr 22.1 (2003): 71–79.

Lou DJ et al. Serum phospholipid omega-3 polyunsaturated fatty acids and insulin resistance in type 2 diabetes mellitus and non-alcoholic fatty liver disease. J Diabetes Complications. 2014 (epub ahead of print).
MacLean CH et al. Effects of omega-3 fatty acids on lipids and glycemic control in type II diabetes and the metabolic syndrome and on inflammatory bowel disease, rheumatoid arthritis, renal disease, systemic lupus erythematosus, and osteoporosis. Evid Rep Technol Assess (Summ) 89 (2004): 1–4.
Mahaffey KR, et al. Blood organic mercury and dietary mercury intake: National Health and Nutrition Examination Survey, 1999 and 2000. Environ Health Perspect 112.5 (2004): 562–570.
Makrides, M., et al. (2010). Effect of DHA supplementation during pregnancy on maternal depression and neurodevelopment of young children: a randomized controlled trial. JAMA 304(15), 1675–1683.
Marchioli R et al. Early protection against sudden death by n-3 polyunsaturated fatty acids after myocardial infarction: time-course analysis of the results of the Gruppo Italiano per lo Studio della Sopravvivenza nell'Infarto Miocardico (GISSI)-Prevenzione. Circulation 105 (2002): 1897–1903.
Marks GB et al. Prevention of asthma during the first 5 years of life: a randomized controlled trial. J Allergy Clin Immunol 118.1 (2006): 53–61.
Masko EM et al. The Relationship Between Nutrition and Prostate Cancer: Is More Always Better? Eur Urol 63.5 (2013): 810–820.
Masson, S., et al. 2013. Plasma n-3 polyunsaturated fatty acids in chronic heart failure in the GISSI-Heart Failure Trial: relation with fish intake, circulating biomarkers, and mortality. Am Heart J, 165, (2) 208–215.
McClaskey EM, Michalets EL. Subdural hematoma after a fall in an elderly patient taking high-dose omega-3 fatty acids with warfarin and aspirin: case report and review of the literature. Pharmacotherapy 27.1 (2007): 152–160.
McEwen B et al. Effect of omega-3 fish oil on cardiovascular risk in diabetes. Diabetes Educ. 36.4 (2010): 565–84.
McEwen BJ et al. Effects of omega-3 polyunsaturated fatty acids on platelet function in healthy subjects and subjects with cardiovascular disease. Semin Thromb Hemost. 39.1 (2013): 25–32.
McLennan PL. Myocardial membrane fatty acids and the antiarrhythmic actions of dietary fish oil in animal models. Lipids 36 (Suppl) (2001): S111–S114.
McLennan, P.L. 2014a. Cardiac physiology and clinical efficacy of dietary fish oil clarified through cellular mechanisms of omega-3 polyunsaturated fatty acids. Eur J Appl. Physiol, 114, (7) 1333–1356.699892.
McLennan, P.L. 2014b. Cardiac physiology and clinical efficacy of dietary fish oil clarified through cellular mechanisms of omega-3 polyunsaturated fatty acids. Eur J Appl. Physiol, 114, (7) 1333–1356.
McLennan PL, et al. Dietary fish oil prevents ventricular fibrillation following coronary artery occlusion and reperfusion. Am Heart J 116.3 (1988): 709–717.
McLennan PL, et al. Reversal of the arrhythmogenic effects of long-term saturated fatty acid intake by dietary n-3 and n-6 polyunsaturated fatty acids. Am J Clin Nutr 51.1 (1990): 53–58.
McNamara RK, Carlson SE. Role of omega-3 fatty acids in brain development and function: potential implications for the pathogenesis and prevention of psychopathology. Prostaglandins Leukot Essent Fatty Acids 75.4–5 (2006). 329–349.
Melanson S et al. Measurement of organochlorines in commercial over-the-counter fish oil preparations: implications for dietary and therapeutic recommendations for omega-3 fatty acids and a review of the literature. Arch Pathol Lab Med 129.1 (2005): 74–77.
Mesa MD et al. Effects of oils rich in eicosapentaenoic and docosahexaenoic acids on the oxidizability and thrombogenicity of low-density lipoprotein. Atherosclerosis 175.2 (2004): 333–343.
Meyer BJ et al. Dietary intakes and food sources of omega-6 and omega-3 polyunsaturated fatty acids. Lipids 38.4 (2003): 391–398.
Michael-Titus AT and Priestley JV. Omega-3 fatty acids and traumatic neurological injury: from neuroprotection to neuroplasticity? Trends in Neurosciences. 37.1 (2014): 30–38.
Mickleborough TD et al. Protective effect of fish oil supplementation on exercise-induced bronchoconstriction in asthma. Chest 129.1 (2006): 39–49.
Miles, E.A. & Calder, P.C. 2012. Influence of marine n-3 polyunsaturated fatty acids on immune function and a systematic review of their effects on clinical outcomes in rheumatoid arthritis. Br J Nutr., 107 Suppl 2, S171–S184.
Miller, B. J., et al. (2013). Dietary supplements for preventing postnatal depression. Cochrane Database Syst Rev, 10, CD009104.
Miller PE et al. Long-chain omega-3 fatty acids eicosapentaenoic acid and docosahexaenoic acid and blood pressure: a meta-analysis of randomized controlled trials. Am J Hypertens. 27.7 (2014): 885–96.
Miura S et al. Modulation of intestinal immune system by dietary fat intake: relevance to Crohn's disease. J Gastroenterol Hepatol 13.12 (1998): 1183–1190.
Moher D. Effects of omega-3 fatty acids on child and maternal health. Rockville, MD: US Department of Health and Human Services, 2005.
Montgomery P, Richardson AJ. Omega-3 fatty acids for bipolar disorder. Cochrane Database Syst Rev 2 (2008): CD005169.
Montori VM et al. Fish oil supplementation in type 2 diabetes: a quantitative systematic review. Diabetes Care 23.9 (2000): 1407–1415.
Mori TA et al. Differential effects of eicosapentaenoic acid and docosahexaenoic acid on vascular reactivity of the forearm microcirculation in hyperlipidemic, overweight men. Circulation 102.11 (2000): 1264–1269.
Morris MC, et al. Does fish oil lower blood pressure? A meta-analysis of controlled trials. Circulation 88.2 (1993): 523–533.
Morris MC et al. Consumption of fish and n-3 fatty acids and risk of incident Alzheimer disease. Arch Neurol 60.7 (2003): 940–946.
Mozaffarian D et al. Fish intake and risk of incident heart failure. J Am Coll Cardiol 45.12 (2005): 2015–2021.
Mozaffarian D, Rimm E. Fish intake, contaminants, and human health: evaluating the risks and the benefits. JAMA 296.15 (2006): 1885–1899.
Mozaffarian, D. & Wu, J.H. 2011. Omega-3 fatty acids and cardiovascular disease: effects on risk factors, molecular pathways, and clinical events. J Am Coll. Cardiol., 58, (20) 2047–2067.

Mozurkewich, E. L., et al. (2013). The Mothers, Omega-3, and Mental Health Study: a double-blind, randomized controlled trial. American Journal of Obstetrics & Gynecology, 208(4), 313.e311–319.

Mucke L, Pitas RE. Food for thought: essential fatty acid protects against neuronal deficits in transgenic mouse model of AD. Neuron 43.5 (2004): 596–599.

Nair GM, Connolly SJ. Should patients with cardiovascular disease take fish oil? CMAJ 178.2 (2008): 181–182.

Navarro E et al. Abnormal fatty acid pattern in rheumatoid arthritis. A rationale for treatment with marine and botanical lipids. J Rheumatol 27.2 (2000): 298–303.

Nettleton JA, et al. N-3 long-chain polyunsaturated fatty acids in type 2 diabetes: a review. J Am Diet Assoc 105.3 (2005): 428–440.

Nicholson, T., et al. 2013. The role of marine n-3 fatty acids in improving cardiovascular health: a review. Food Funct., 4, (3) 357–365.

Noaghiul, S., & Hibbeln, J. R. (2003). Cross-national comparisons of seafood consumption and rates of bipolar disorders. Am J Psychiatry, 160(12), 2222–2227.

Olsen SF et al. Fish oil intake compared with olive oil intake in late pregnancy and asthma in the offspring: 16 y of registry-based follow-up from a randomized controlled trial. Am J Clin Nutr 88.1 (2008): 167–175.

Origasa, H., et al. 2010. Clinical importance of adherence to treatment with eicosapentaenoic acid by patients with hypercholesterolemia. Circ.J, 74, (3) 510–517.

Parra D et al. A diet rich in long chain omega-3 fatty acids modulates satiety in overweight and obese volunteers during weight loss. Appetite 51.3 (2008): 676–680.

Patel D et al. Omega-3 polyunsaturated fatty acid intake through fish consumption and prostate specific antigen level: Results from the 2003 to 2010 national health and examination survey. Prostaglandins, Leukotrienes and Essential Fatty Acids (PLEFA) 91.4 (2014): 155–160.

Pedersen M et al. Diet and risk of rheumatoid arthritis in a prospective cohort. J Rheumatol 32.7 (2005): 1249–1252.

Peet, M., & Horrobin, D. F. (2002). A dose-ranging study of the effects of ethyl-eicosapentaenoate in patients with ongoing depression despite apparently adequate treatment with standard drugs. Arch Gen Psychiatry, 59(10), 913–919.

Peet M. Eicosapentaenoic acid in the treatment of schizophrenia and depression: rationale and preliminary double-blind clinical trial results. Prostaglandins Leukot Essent Fatty Acids 69.6 (2003): 477–485.

Peet M. The metabolic syndrome, omega-3 fatty acids and inflammatory processes in relation to schizophrenia. Prostaglandins Leukot Essent Fatty Acids 75.4–5 (2006): 323–327.

Pizzorno J, Murray M. Textbook of natural medicine. St Louis: Elsevier, 2006.

Politi P et al. Behavioral effects of omega-3 fatty acid supplementation in young adults with severe autism: an open label study. Arch Med Res 39.7 (2008): 682–685.

Proudman SM, et al. Dietary omega-3 fats for treatment of inflammatory joint disease: efficacy and utility. Rheum Dis Clin North Am 34.2 (2008): 469–479.

Racine R, Deckelbaum R. Sources of the very-long-chain unsaturated omega-3 fatty acids: eicosapentaenoic acid and docosahexaenoic acid. Curr Opin Clin Nutr Metab Care 10.2 (2007): 123–128.

Radack K, et al. The comparative effects of n-3 and n-6 polyunsaturated fatty acids on plasma fibrinogen levels: a controlled clinical trial in hypertriglyceridemic subjects. J Am Coll Nutr 9.4 (1990): 352–357.

Ramel A et al. Beneficial effects of long-chain n-3 fatty acids included in an energy-restricted diet on insulin resistance in overweight and obese European young adults. Diabetologia 51.7 (2008): 1261–1268.

Richardson AJ, Puri BK. The potential role of fatty acids in attention-deficit/hyperactivity disorder. Prostaglandins Leukot Essent Fatty Acids 63.1–2 (2000): 79–87.

Riediger ND et al. A systemic review of the roles of n-3 fatty acids in health and disease. J Am Diet Assoc 109.4 (2009): 668–679.

Risk and Prevention Study Collaborative Group (2013) n-3 Fatty acids in patients with multiple cardiovascular risk factors. N Engl J Med 368(19):1800–1808.

Robert SS. Production of eicosapentaenoic and docosahexaenoic acid-containing oils in transgenic land plants for human and aquaculture nutrition. Mar Biotechnol (NY) 8.2 (2006): 103–109.

Roncaglioni, M.C., et al. 2013. N-3 fatty acids in patients with multiple cardiovascular risk factors. N. Engl. J Med, 368, (19) 1800–1808.

Rose DP, Connolly JM. Omega-3 fatty acids as cancer chemopreventive agents. Pharmacol Ther 83.3 (1999): 217–244.

Rosell MS et al. Long-chain n-3 polyunsaturated fatty acids in plasma in British meat-eating, vegetarian, and vegan men. Am J Clin Nutr 82.2 (2005): 327–334.

Ross CM. Fish oil, adrenal activation, and cardiovascular health [Letter]. Thromb Res 116.3 (2005): 273.

Roynette CE et al. N-3 polyunsaturated fatty acids and colon cancer prevention. Clin Nutr 23.2 (2004): 139–151.

Russo GL. Dietary n-6 and n-3 polyunsaturated fatty acids: from biochemistry to clinical implications in cardiovascular prevention. Biochem Pharmacol 77.6 (2009): 937–946.

Salam MT et al. Maternal fish consumption during pregnancy and risk of early childhood asthma. J Asthma 42.6 (2005): 513–518.

Sanhueza, C., et al. (2013). Diet and the risk of unipolar depression in adults: systematic review of cohort studies. Journal of Human Nutrition & Dietetics, 26(1), 56–70.

Schaller JL. Mercury and fish oil supplements. Med Gen Med 3.2 (2001): 20.

Schultz ST et al. Breastfeeding, infant formula supplementation, and autistic disorder: the results of a parent survey. Int Breastfeed J 1 (2006): 16.

Sears B et al. Therapeutic uses of high-dose omega-3 fatty acids to treat comatose patients with severe brain injury. PharmaNutrition. 1.3 (2013): 86–89.

Seki H et al. Omega-3 PUFA derived anti-inflammatory lipid mediator resolvin E1. Prostaglandins & Other Lipid Mediators. 89.3–4 (2009): 126–130.

Simopoulos AP. Essential fatty acids in health and chronic disease. Am J Clin Nutr 70.(3 Suppl) (1999): 56–9S.

F

Simopoulos AP. Omega-3 fatty acids in inflammation and autoimmune diseases. J Am Coll Nutr 21.6 (2002): 495–505.
Simopoulos AP. The importance of the omega-6/omega-3 fatty acid ratio in cardiovascular disease and other chronic diseases. Exp Biol Med (Maywood) 233.6 (2008): 674–688.
Sirtori CR et al. N-3 fatty acids do not lead to an increased diabetic risk in patients with hyperlipidemia and abnormal glucose tolerance: Italian Fish Oil Multicenter Study. Am J Clin Nutr 65.6 (1997): 1874–1881.
Sirtori CR et al. One-year treatment with ethyl esters of n-3 fatty acids in patients with hypertriglyceridemia and glucose intolerance: reduced triglyceridemia, total cholesterol and increased HDL-C without glycemic alterations. Atherosclerosis 137.2 (1998): 419–427.
Sirtori CR, Galli C. N-3 fatty acids and diabetes. Biomed Pharmacother 56.8 (2002): 397–406.
Siscovick DS, et al. The fish story: a diet-heart hypothesis with clinical implications: n-3 polyunsaturated fatty acids, myocardial vulnerability, and sudden death. Circulation 107.21 (2003): 2632–2634.
Sommerfield T, et al. Omega-3 fatty acids for intermittent claudication. Cochrane Database Syst Rev 4 (2007): CD003833.
Soyland E et al. Dietary supplementation with very long-chain n-3 fatty acids in patients with atopic dermatitis: A double-blind, multicentre study. Br J Dermatol 130.6 (1994): 757–764.
Stamp LK, et al. Diet and rheumatoid arthritis: A review of the literature. Semin Arthritis Rheum 35.2 (2005): 77–94.
Stern AH. A review of the studies of the cardiovascular health effects of methylmercury with consideration of their suitability for risk assessment. Environ Res 98.1 (2005): 133–142.
Stoll BA. N-3 fatty acids and lipid peroxidation in breast cancer inhibition. Br J Nutr 87.3 (2002): 193–198.
Stone NJ. The Gruppo Italiano per lo Studio della Sopravvivenza nell' Infarto Miocardio (GISSI)-Prevenzione Trial on fish oil and vitamin E supplementation in myocardial infarction survivors. Curr Cardiol Rep 2.5 (2000): 445–451.
Tacon A, Metian M. Aquaculture feed and food safety. Ann N Y Acad Sci 1140 (2008): 50–59.
Tajalizadekhoob, Y. et al. (2011). The effect of low-dose omega 3 fatty acids on the treatment of mild to moderate depression in the elderly: a double-blind, randomized, placebo-controlled study. European Archives of Psychiatry & Clinical Neuroscience, 261(8), 539–549.
Tanaka, K., et al. 2008. Reduction in the recurrence of stroke by eicosapentaenoic acid for hypercholesterolemic patients: subanalysis of the JELIS trial. Stroke, 39, (7) 2052–2058.
Tang FY et al. Concomitant supplementation of lycopene and eicosapentaenoic acid inhibits the proliferation of human colon cancer cells. J Nutr Biochem (2009); 20: 426–434.
Tavazzi L et al. Effect of n-3 polyunsaturated fatty acids in patients with chronic heart failure (the GISSI-HF trial): a randomised, double-blind, placebo-controlled trial. Lancet 372.9645 (2008): 1223–1230.
Terano T et al. Docosahexanoic acid supplementation improves the moderately severe dementia from thrombotic cerebrovascular disease. Lipids 34 (Suppl) (1994): S345–S346.
Terry PD, et al. Intakes of fish and marine fatty acids and the risks of cancers of the breast and prostate and of other hormone-related cancers: a review of the epidemiologic evidence. Am J Clin Nutr 77.3 (2003): 532–543.
Terry PD, et al. Long-chain (n-3) fatty acid intake and risk of cancers of the breast and the prostate: recent epidemiological studies, biological mechanisms, and directions for future research. J Nutr 134 (2004): 3412–320S.
Torfadottir JE et al. Consumption of fish products across the lifespan and prostate cancer risk. PLoS.One 8.4 (2013): e59799.
Ulbricht CE, Basch EM. Natural standard herb and supplement reference. St Louis: Mosby, 2005.
Visioli F et al. Dietary intake of fish vs. formulations leads to higher plasma concentrations of n-3 fatty acids. Lipids 38.4 (2003): 415–418.
Virtanen JK et al. Serum long-chain n-3 polyunsaturated fatty acids, mercury, and risk of sudden cardiac death in men: a prospective population-based study. PLoS.One 7.7 (2012): e41046.
Volker D et al. Efficacy of fish oil concentrate in the treatment of rheumatoid arthritis. J Rheumatol 27.10 (2000): 2343–2346.
von Schacky C, et al. The effect of n-3 fatty acids on coronary atherosclerosis: results from SCIMO, an angiographic study, background and implications. Lipids 36 (Suppl) (2001): S99–102.
Weber P, Raederstorff D. Triglyceride-lowering effect of omega-3 LC-polyunsaturated fatty acids: a review. Nutr Metab Cardiovasc Dis 10.1 (2000): 28–37.
Weisburger JH. Dietary fat and risk of chronic disease: mechanistic insights from experimental studies. J Am Diet Assoc 97.(7 Suppl) (1997): S16–S23.
Wennberg M et al. Myocardial infarction in relation to mercury and fatty acids from fish: a risk-benefit analysis based on pooled Finnish and Swedish data in men. Am J Clin Nutr 96.4 (2012): 706–713.
Whelan J, Rust C. Innovative dietary sources of n-3 fatty acids. Annu Rev Nutr 26 (2006): 75–103.
Williams C et al. Stereo acuity at age 3–5 years in children born full term is associated with pre-natal and post-natal dietary factors: a report from a population-based cohort study. Am J Clin Nutr 73 (2001): 316–322.
Wong KW. Clinical efficacy of n-3 fatty acid supplementation in patients with asthma. J Am Diet Assoc 105.1 (2005): 98–105.
Woods RK, et al. Dietary marine fatty acids (fish oil) for asthma in adults and children. Cochrane Database Syst Rev 3 (2002): CD001283.
Wu JH et al. Omega-3 fatty acids and incident type 2 diabetes: a systematic review and meta-analysis. Br J Nutr 107(Suppl 2) (2012): S214–S227.
Yamada T et al. Atherosclerosis and ω-3 fatty acids in the populations of a fishing village and a farming village in Japan. Atherosclerosis. 153.2 (2000): 469–481.
Yehuda S, et al. Essential fatty acids and the brain: from infancy to aging. Neurobiol Aging 26.(Suppl 1) (2005): 98–102.

Yokoyama, M. 2009. [Japan EPA Lipid Intervention Study (JELIS). Randomized clinical trial involving primary and secondary prevention of cardiovascular events with EPA in hypercholesterolemia.] Nihon Ronen Igakkai Zasshi, 46, (1) 22–25.

Zheng JS et al. Marine N-3 polyunsaturated fatty acids are inversely associated with risk of type 2 diabetes in Asians: a systematic review and meta-analysis. PLoS.One 7.9 (2012): e44525.

F

Folate

HISTORICAL NOTE Folic acid was isolated from spinach leaves in 1941 and synthesised in 1946; hence, its name comes from the Latin *folium*, which means leaf.

OTHER NAMES

Folacin, vitamin B_9, folic acid, pteroylmonoglutamic acid (PGA)

BACKGROUND AND RELEVANT PHARMACOKINETICS AND CHEMICAL COMPONENTS

Folate is the generic term for a large family of chemically similar trace compounds that fall within the vitamin B group. Folic acid is the most oxidised and stable form and the one characteristically used in supplements and food fortification. Folate found in animal sources is present in a 'free form' and is readily absorbed; however, aside from the organ meats, animal products are notoriously poor sources. Folate found in plant foods exists in conjugated forms, which require deconjugation by zinc-dependent enzymes in the gut prior to absorption. (Kelly 1998). This step is inhibited by chronic alcohol ingestion and some foods, including oranges and legumes (Gropper et al 2009). Secondary to this difference, the average bioavailability of natural folate is half that of the synthetic form (e.g. 55–66% versus ≈ 100% (Carmel et al 2006, Kelly 1998). Small amounts of folate are endogenously produced by bacteria in the intestines, but this appears to be predominantly lost via the faeces (Gropper et al 2009).

Dietary folate and synthetic folic acid alike then undergo complex conversion into folate's active forms, e.g. tetrahydrofolate (THF). This occurs via a multistep pathway now proposed to occur solely within the liver (Wright et al 2007). In contrast, a less common supplemental form of folate — folinic acid (5-formyltetrahydrofolate or 5-formylTHF), as an intermediate folate metabolite — bypasses some of these steps to readily form 5,10-methylenetetrohydrofolate (5,10-formylTHF) (Kelly 1998, McGuire et al 1987, Priest et al 1991).

Secretion into the bile of the THF derivatives and their subsequent reabsorption through the enterohepatic circulation enable redistribution throughout the body. Distribution of folate appears to be regulated via an unknown mechanism, ensuring increased availability to those tissues demonstrating rapid cell division (Gropper et al 2009). Although many of the biochemical pathways in which folate is involved act to regenerate the nutrient, there is still a significant amount that is broken down and eliminated, chiefly in the urine.

Clinical note — Food fortification with folate: still not enough for pregnant women?

In 1997, voluntary folic acid fortification of foods was introduced in Australia and New Zealand to improve the folate status, particularly of pregnant women. Following this, a study evaluating mean serum folate levels in over 20,000 Australian women aged 14–45 years found that although concentrations had increased by 19%, the prevalence of poor folate status in this age group had only reduced from 8.5% to 4.1% (Metz et al 2002). Several state-based studies since 1997 have shown a variety of improvements in a range of measures, including haematological markers, folate awareness and supplementation rates among Australian women (Brown et al 2011, Chan et al 2008, du Plessis et al 2008, Hickling et al 2005) and corresponding reductions in NTD births have varied from 17% to 40%; however, some researchers suggest that this decrease occurred in the first 2 years following fortification and the launch of awareness campaigns, and that there has been no further reduction since this time (du Plessis et al 2008). Unsurprisingly, an economic evaluation of the Australian mandatory fortification determined that while it was a cost-effective approach offering substantial long-term benefits with respect to life years gained and quality-adjusted life years, mandatory supplementation alone would be insufficient to achieve folate status required for NTD prevention (Rabovskaja et al 2013). Although fortification programs, including mandatory fortification of bread flour in Australia and New Zealand (FSANZ 2007), provide some measure of protection for women of reproductive age, supplementation is still required. Unfortunately, widespread public health campaigns have had limited success and many women remain unaware of the need to take supplements prior to pregnancy, or are aware but still fail to use supplements (du Plessis et al 2008, Metz et al 2002). In Australia, only 36% and 46% of new mothers in Victoria and New South Wales, respectively, took folate supplements in 2006, with even lower rates reported for women of low socio-economic or non-English speaking backgrounds (Watson et al 2006) and women aged 20–24 years. The last group also experiences the highest rate of NTD births (du Plessis et al 2008).

Clinical note — A challenge to the perceived safety and superiority of synthetic folic acid?

Given its relative stability in processing and enhanced bioavailability, synthetic folic acid in food fortificants and supplements has long been regarded as more reliable than natural dietary sources for ensuring folate adequacy (Kelly 1998). This, in turn, has led to widening implementation of mandatory folate fortification programs aimed at the prevention of neural tube defects (NTDs). Recently, however, the safety of increased exposure to synthetic folic acid has been thrown into question. Individuals who consume high doses (≥400 mcg/day) exhibit unmetabolised folic acid in their blood, a form that does not naturally occur in human physiology (Kelly 1998, Lucock 2004, 2006, Sauer et al 2009, Smith et al 2008, Sweeney et al 2007, Troen et al 2006, Wright et al 2007). While this will eventually be hepatically converted into a natural folate derivative, there is speculation regarding the interim effects, with evidence of competition between the unmetabolised folic acid and the main active folate form methyl-THF at receptors and their subsequent downregulation on cell surfaces (Sauer et al 2009, Smith et al 2008). Particular at-risk groups identified by researchers include those individuals taking anti-folate medications, folate-replete cancer patients and elderly patients with B_{12} deficiency (Smith et al 2008, Wright et al 2007), while others question the long-term safety for the unborn fetus (Kelly 1998). Until further research is conducted in this area, the implications remain unclear.

FOOD SOURCES

Good dietary sources of folate are fresh green leafy vegetables, such as cabbage and spinach, asparagus, broccoli, sprouts, mushrooms, legumes, nuts and fortified cereals and organ meats.

Food preparation and processing can destroy up to 100% of the naturally occurring folate, as it is sensitive to light and air but especially heat; therefore, raw foods, as well as fortified foods, are considered superior sources, which in Australia provide 100 mcg per serve (Gropper et al 2009, Hickling et al 2005).

DEFICIENCY

Folate deficiency is not uncommon and can develop within just 4 months of an inadequate diet (Carmel et al 2006, Gropper et al 2009, Wilson et al 1991).

In light of folate's fundamental role in DNA synthesis, deficiency of this nutrient will predictably impact most on those cells and tissues that exhibit a high turnover (e.g. blood and the cells in the gastrointestinal tract), which also applies to those stages of development with increased rates of growth, such as pregnancy and fetal tissue development.

Signs and symptoms of deficiency

- Macrocytic/megaloblastic anaemia
- Fatigue
- Psychological symptoms such as irritability and depression (Reynolds 2002)
- Headache
- Hair loss
- Nausea
- Insomnia (Pelton et al 2000)
- Peripheral neuropathy
- Myelopathy (Okada et al 2014)
- Tendon hyperreflexivity
- Diarrhoea
- Weight loss
- Cerebral disturbances (Botez 1976), cerebral cortex atrophy and cognitive decline
- Increased blood levels of homocysteine

Primary deficiency

This develops in response to inadequate dietary intake and can be caused by a diet generally lacking in fresh, lightly cooked vegetables. Risk is increased in patients with *MTHFR* gene polymorphisms, in people receiving total parenteral nutrition (TPN), chronic alcoholics, phenylketonuria patients on restricted diets, patients with sickle cell anaemia and the institutionalised elderly (Carmel et al 2006, Wahlqvist 2002).

Folate enzyme polymorphisms

Single allele substitution in the gene encoding for the *N*5,10-methylenetetrahydrofolate reductase enzyme, responsible for converting folate into its methylated 'active' form, results in several possible polymorphisms. Individuals who are homozygous for the *MTHFR* C677T polymorphism (2–16% white populations) convert the active folate form at only 30% of the normal capacity, while the *MTHFR* A1298C genotype produces an enzyme with 60% of the unaffected enzyme activity (Gilbody et al 2007). Homozygotes for either polymorphism are at a significantly increased risk of folate deficiency and cannot maintain adequacy with recommended dietary intake levels (NHMRC 2006).

Secondary deficiency

Secondary deficiency is caused by compromised absorption, increased excretion or increased demands or losses. Inadequate absorption can occur in malabsorption syndromes such as coeliac and Crohn's disease, with long-term use of certain medications such as phenytoin, sulfasalazine, cimetidine, antacids and oral contraceptive pill (OCP), in congenital malabsorption states and in blind loop syndrome (Beers & Berkow 2003), especially when combined with suboptimal dietary intake (Carmel et al 2006). In chronic kidney disease, down-regulation of folate transporters in the intestine, heart, liver and brain can lead to reduced intestinal absorption of folate (Bukhari et al 2011). Significantly impaired absorption has also been observed in HIV patients (Revell et al 1991).

Besides impaired absorption, inadequate use can occur with concurrent vitamin B_{12} or C deficiency, smoking (Gabriel et al 2006, Okumura & Tsukamoto 2011) or acute or chronic alcoholism (Hamid & Kaur 2007). A genetic variation in folate requirement has also been identified, as a congenital enzyme deficiency exists in approximately 13% of the Western population (Ma et al 1996). In these cases, total or partial absence of the enzyme responsible for the final step in converting folate to its major active metabolite (methylenetetrahydrofolate reductase) results in decreased plasma levels (Kumar & Clarke 2002). Therefore, these individuals have a higher folate requirement than others without this congenital enzyme deficiency and display increased susceptibility to folate deficiency.

A number of pharmaceutical drugs, such as folic acid antagonists (e.g. methotrexate), can affect status by interfering with absorption, use and conversion to its active forms. In such cases, oral folic acid supplements are sometimes given to reduce side effects, although it may marginally reduce drug efficacy (Kumar & Clarke 2002, Strober & Menon 2005). Oral isotretinoin treatment may induce folic acid deficiency, although the mechanisms underlying this observation remain unclear (Karadag et al 2011).

Additionally, there are several subpopulations with increased demands for folic acid, such as pregnant and lactating women, the elderly and patients with malignancies, haemolytic anaemias such as sickle cell disease, chronic exfoliative skin disorders or achlorhydria (Gropper et al 2009). Extra losses have also been reported in haemodialysis patients.

The chronic use of alcohol during pregnancy may be associated with reduced folate transport to the fetus (Hutson et al 2012). The ratio of serum folate in maternal blood compared to umbilical cord blood at time of delivery was significantly lower in pregnancies with chronic and heavy alcohol exposure ($P = 0.014$), further emphasising the need for abstinence from alcohol during pregnancy.

Excess folic acid

Adults and children with phenylketonuria may be at risk of receiving folic acid at higher doses than daily recommendations as a result of high folic acid content in protein substitutes (Stølen et al 2013). These patients should be individually monitored for nutrient status, as the effects of very high doses, in particular in children, is uncertain.

MAIN ACTIONS

Folate's actions are all secondary to its ability to donate methyl groups and its central role, therefore, in one-carbon metabolism.

F

Coenzyme

As a key methyl donor, folate is involved in a variety of reactions important for the metabolism of amino acids and nucleic acids.

DNA and RNA synthesis

Folate plays an essential part in the production of purines and pyrimidines that make up DNA, making it a critical nutrient in relation to cell division and repair of genetic material, and is generally required for genomic stability. Subsequently, folate plays an indirect role in the synthesis of transfer RNA.

Production of the active form of B_{12}

Folate and B_{12} are intrinsically linked; for example, the conversion of B_{12} into methylcobalamin is dependent upon the presence of a THF derivative.

Reduction of homocysteine levels

Folate, via B_{12} activation, donates a methyl group to homocysteine facilitating its recycling back to methionine. Together with vitamin B_6, necessary for homocysteine catabolism, folate effectively lowers homocysteine levels.

Synthesis of S-adenosyl-l-methionine (SAMe)

Following regeneration of methionine from homocysteine, the methyl group donated by folate is then taken up by SAMe, enabling it to become a carbon donor in multiple transmethylation reactions throughout the body, including neurotransmitter synthesis (Hendler & Rorvik 2001).

Amino acid metabolism

Folate is involved in the synthesis of some of the non-essential amino acids such as serine and glycine. It is also required for the conversion of histidine into glutamate (Gropper et al 2009).

CLINICAL USE

The conditions for which folate is indicated as a potential treatment are primarily due to an existing deficiency, through either primary or secondary pathways. Research has focused particularly on those conditions in which folate deficiency is a consequence of medication use and the benefits of improved folate status.

Prevention and treatment of deficiency

Commonly, folic acid supplements are used to correct identifiable deficiency states, such as macrocytic anaemia, or given as preventive treatment to those patients at risk of deficiency, such as in malabsorption syndromes or taking long-term folate antagonist medication. Increased oral intake of folate has been found to be effective, even in cases of malabsorption due to the passive diffusion evident with pharmacological doses (Carmel et al 2006).

Preconception and during pregnancy

Neural tube defects

Poor folate status either 1 month before conception or during the first trimester of pregnancy is an independent risk factor for NTD in the newborn. One study has suggested that the increased risk could be as high as 10-fold (Daly et al 1995). Despite a wealth of scientific evidence and global health promotion campaigns, it would appear many pregnant women still fail to meet folate intake requirements (Manniën et al 2013, Timmermans et al 2008). It is estimated that, worldwide, only 25% of folic acid-preventable spina bifida and anencephaly are currently being prevented through folic acid fortification (Youngblood et al 2013). Interestingly, a study from Northern Ireland found that women who had been pregnant previously were less likely to follow folate intake recommendations compared to women in their first pregnancy ($P = 0.001$), highlighting the need to emphasise supplementation irrespective of previous pregnancy experience (McNulty et al 2011).

The continued supplementation of 400 mcg folic acid daily in the second and third trimester of pregnancy has been found to increase maternal and placental cord blood folate status, and prevent the increase in homocysteine concentration that otherwise occurs in late pregnancy (McNulty et al 2013). The clinical implication on pregnancy outcomes or early childhood development requires further investigation.

Intervention trials for pregnancy have routinely used 400 mcg folic acid/day; however, there is some suggestion that routine ingestion of only 100 mcg folate from fortified food would prevent the majority of NTDs. Studies have also been conducted on women with a previous NTD birth, with benefits demonstrated at doses of 4 mg/day. There is a general consensus among researchers and health authorities that due to the inconsistent nature of natural food sources, taking a supplement or incorporating fortified foods is the most reliable way to increase levels sufficiently (Cuskelly et al 1996). A maternal red blood cell folate concentration >906 nmol/L is thought to be optimal for lowering risk (Pietrzik et al 2007).

The prevalence of NTD-affected pregnancies has been reported as up to 75% higher in obese women and up to threefold higher for women who are severely obese (Rasmussen et al 2008, Stothard et al 2009). An observational study found obese women to have lower serum folate levels but increased red blood cell folate concentrations, which may be due to body mass index and tissue type affecting the distribution of folate (Tinker et al 2012).

Other neonatal outcomes

While a number of other birth defects besides NTD have been attributed to folate deficiency in recent times, including Down syndrome (Eskes 2006) and cleft lip and/or palate (CL/P), a 2010 Cochrane review concluded that there was no statistically significant evidence of any effects of folate supplementation on prevention of cleft palate, cleft lip, congenital cardiovascular defects, miscarriage or other birth defects (De-Regil et al 2010).

A more recent case-control study from the Netherlands found that regular folic acid supplementation during 0–12 weeks after conception was associated with increased risk of cleft formation in the offspring (OR 1.72, 95% CI 1.19–2.49) (Rozendaal et al 2013). Despite this, available evidence surrounding the role of folic acid in non-NTD birth defects is still contradictory (Bean et al 2011, Hollis et al 2013); as such, the role that supplementation has in the aetiology of these conditions still remains unclear.

Data from numerous studies have suggested that supplementation with folic acid prior to conception and during early pregnancy may reduce autism spectrum disorder (ASD) risk (Berry 2013, Schmidt et al 2012). Analysis of the Norwegian Mother and Child Cohort Study (*n* = 85,176) found that the maternal supplementation from 4 weeks before to 8 weeks after the start of pregnancy was associated with a lower risk of autistic disorder, the most severe form of ASD, in children (adjusted OR 0.61, 95% CI 0.41–0.90) (Surén et al 2013). Using the same data, another study identified that folic acid supplementation or dietary folate did not protect against spontaneous pre-term delivery; pre-conceptional folic acid supplementation starting more than 8 weeks before conception was associated with an increased risk of pre-term delivery (hazard ratio 1.19, 95% CI 1.05–1.34) (Sengpiel et al 2013).

Higher folate levels are linked to the prevention of miscarriages, decreased risk of intrauterine growth retardation, increased birth weight in the offspring of smoking mothers (Sram et al 2005) and increased rates of twin pregnancies, from both natural and in vitro fertilisation (IVF) conception (Haggarty et al 2006). Folic acid supplementation may modify some of the adverse effects of maternal smoking on neonatal outcomes and fetal growth, particularly during the first trimester, although no effect on risk of preterm birth or on risk of 'small size for gestational age' at birth (Bakker et al 2011).

A recent Cochrane review concluded that folic acid supplementation was associated with an improved mean birth weight (mean difference (MD) 135.75, 95% CI: 47.85–223.68) and with a reduction in megaloblastic anaemia incidence (RR 0.21, 95% CI 0.11–0.38) (Lassi et al 2013). Conversely, this review also found that folic acid supplementation had no conclusive benefit on pregnancy outcomes such as preterm birth (RR 1.33, 95% CI 0.73–1.38), stillbirths/neonatal deaths (RR 1.33, 95% CI 0.96–1.85) or some haematological parameters including pre-delivery anaemia (RR 0.62, 95% CI 0.35–1.10), mean pre-delivery haemoglobin level (MD –0.03, 95% CI –0.25–0.19), mean pre-delivery serum folate levels (standardised mean difference 2.03, 95% CI 0.80–3.27) and mean pre-delivery red cell folate levels (SMD 1.59, 95% CI –0.07–3.26).

A large population-based cohort study (*n* = 193,554) found that daily supplementation with 400 mcg folic acid did not prevent preeclampsia or gestational hypertension in Chinese women (Li et al 2013). Periconception folate supplementation was found to be associated with lower uteroplacental vascular resistance and higher blood pressures during pregnancy in a population-based cohort study (*n* = 5993) (Timmermans et al 2011). These observed effects were small and remained within normal physiological ranges, and did not correlate with risk of preeclampsia or gestational hypertension.

A case-control study in Chinese mothers found that folic acid supplementation was associated with significantly reduced risk of congenital heart defects (Li et al 2013). Supplementing with folic acid for a longer period of time appeared to be more effective in reducing the risk of heart defects. Similarly, a prelimary study found that mothers with the *MDR1* 3435T allele who did not use folic acid during the 4 weeks prior to conception until 10 weeks post-conception were at an increased risk of congenital heart defects in their offspring (OR 2.8, 95% CI 1.2–6.4) (Obermann-Borst et al 2011). Further studies are suggested to clarify this finding. Interestingly, several studies have failed to demonstrate a significant relationship between the *MTHFR* C677T genotype and CL/P (Boyles et al 2008, Butali et al 2013, Chevrier et al 2007); however, this may be confounded by concurrent folic acid supplementation in some individuals.

Childhood diseases

There is a small amount of evidence suggesting folic acid supplementation during early pregnancy may increase the risk of asthma and allergic diseases (Håberg et al 2009, Hollingsworth et al 2008). Despite this, a 2013 systematic review and meta-analysis concluded that there was no evidence of an association between maternal folic acid supplementation and increased risk of asthma in children (RR 1.01, 95% CI 0.78–1.30) (Crider et al 2013). Due to limitations of current studies, further high-quality studies may be of benefit (Ownby et al 2009).

OCP-induced folate deficiency

Long-term use of the oral contraceptive pill (OCP) (>5 years) has historically been associated with a progressive decrease in serum folate levels, of up to 40%, which could feasibly result in changes to cognition and mood, increased risk of macrocytic anaemia and increased risk of NTD in newborns once use has ceased. Results from some studies suggest this last concern may be unfounded (Lussanaa et al 2003, Sütterlin et al 2003).

There are a number of proposed mechanisms for folate depletion with OCP use, including concurrent depletion of B_{12}, which is involved in the regeneration pathway of THF (Bielenberg 1991), and impaired folate resorption (Sütterlin et al 2003).

Hyperhomocysteinaemia

Together with vitamins B_{12} and B_6, folic acid has been shown to reduce high plasma levels of homocysteine (Hcy). Of the three, folate appears to have the strongest effect (Voutilainen et al 2001). A randomised dose-response clinical trial found that for adults with existing folate deficiencies, there was a trend towards reduced homocysteine levels with increasing folic acid dose (Anderson et al 2010). Supplementation in healthy adults with adequate folate status did not appear to reduce homocysteine.

Although elevated Hcy has been implicated as a risk for cardiovascular disease (including atherosclerosis and coronary artery disease), cerebrovascular disease, peripheral vascular disease and venous thromboembolism (Clarke et al 1991, den Heijer et al 1996, Malinow et al 1989, Selhub et al 1995), exudative age-related macular degeneration (Nowak et al 2005), noise-related hearing loss (Gok et al 2004), cognitive dysfunction, posttraumatic stress disorder (Jendricko et al 2008), breast cancer incidence in postmenopausal women (Gatt et al 2007) and adverse pregnancy outcomes (Bjorke Monsen & Ueland 2003) including postnatal depression (Behzadi et al 2008), clinical trials are ongoing to determine the clinical relevance of these associations.

Bone health and fracture risk

Elevated Hcy has been identified as a strong risk factor for osteoporotic fractures (Abrahamsen et al 2006, Green et al 2007, McLean et al 2008, Rejnmark et al 2008). While a significant association between the *MTHFR* C677T polymorphism and fractures has also been demonstrated, this is only significant when coupled with low reported intake of folate, B_{12}, B_2 and B_6 (Abrahamsen et al 2006). This has led some researchers to conclude that the response rate to folate treatment among an osteoporotic population is likely to be as little as 2% (Abrahamsen et al 2006). This may explain the lack of positive effect on bone turnover seen in an RCT of hyperhomocysteinaemic (>5 mmol/L) older patients treated with 1 mg folate, 500 mcg B_{12} and 10 mg B_6 treated for 2 years, in spite of significant Hcy lowering (Green et al 2007). Similarly, 800 mcg daily folic acid supplemented for 4 months in 31 women with Hcy > 10 micromol/L failed to identify any significant effect on bone turnover markers compared to placebo despite lowering of Hcy ($P = 0.007$) (Keser et al 2013).

Cardiovascular protection and treatment

In spite of two early meta-analyses which concluded that risk of ischaemic heart disease could be reduced by 16% following a decrease in Hcy of 3 mmol/L (Homocysteine Study Collaboration 2002, Wald et al 2002), there are few folate interventional studies in established hyperhomocysteinaemic cardiovascular populations and recent studies have produced mixed findings.

In patients with kidney disease, two recent meta-analyses have yielded conflicting conclusions concerning the effect of folic acid supplementation on cardiovascular disease. A 2013 meta-analysis (9 RCTs, $n = 8234$) determined that folic acid supplementation reduced the risk of cardiovascular disease in patients with kidney disease, in patients with folate deficiency, diabetes or advanced and end-stage renal disease (RR 0.85, 95% CI 0.77–0.94) (Qin et al 2013a). Conversely, a 2012 systematic review and meta-analysis (11 RCTs, $n = 10{,}951$) determined that folic acid-based homocysteine lowering does not reduce cardiovascular events in patients with kidney disease (RR 0.97, 95% CI 0.92–1.03) and thus should not be used solely for CVD prevention in this population (Jardine et al 2012).

An interesting trial investigating the benefits of combined B vitamins (5 mg folic acid and high-dose B complex, both administered twice weekly) to patients with a history of cardiovascular events has revealed that those participants whose Hcy decreased within the first 3 months demonstrated significantly reduced cardiovascular risk over the next 5 years; however, no protection was conveyed for slower responders (Siragusa et al 2007). While another small study of B vitamins in hyperhomocysteinaemic elderly subjects failed to improve blood pressure (McMahon et al 2007), elevated Hcy secondary to impaired kidney function in this population group cannot be excluded as a confounding variable.

Alzheimer's dementia and impaired cognitive function in the elderly

Findings such as the prevalence of folate deficiency in the elderly, increasing Hcy levels with age, evidence of an inverse relationship between total plasma Hcy levels and cognitive function and preliminary evidence of correlation between Hcy and plasma amyloid peptide levels in Alzheimer patients (Aisen et al 2008) have attracted attempts to link the phenomena, providing an explanation for neurodegenerative disorders.

In spite of this, and a large number of investigations of B vitamins, very few have restricted participation to only hyperhomocysteinaemic individuals, which may partly explain their negative findings. The Folic Acid and Carotid Intima-Media Thickness (FACIT) trial, however, administered 800 mcg/day over 3 years to participants with elevated baseline Hcy (≥ 13 mmol/L), producing a mean increase in serum folate of 576% and 26% reduction in plasma Hcy (Durga et al 2007). Treated subjects demonstrated significant improvements in three of the six cognitive testing domains (memory, information processing speed and sensorimotor speed), leading the authors to conclude that folic acid is an effective agent for improving cognitive function that tends to decline with age.

In patients with organic brain disease including Alzheimer's and vascular dementia, again only one study has restricted participation to hyperhomocysteinaemic individuals, administering 5 mg folic acid together with 1 mg B_{12} daily over 2 months (Nilsson et al 2001). As this stands alone in its positive findings, it is suggestive that Hcy is a key indicator of likelihood for response to B vitamin supplementation (Nilsson et al 2001).

It is important to note that hyperhomocysteinaemic patients suffering dementia do not typically co-present with macrocytic anaemia, as might be expected (McCaddon et al 2004). Therefore, the neurological and haematological features of B_{12} and folate deficiency are often unrelated in these patients.

Diabetes mellitus

An RCT (n = 48) of overweight and obese men with type 2 diabetes mellitus found that folic acid supplementation (5 mg daily for 8 weeks) significantly reduced HbA_{1C} by 8% (P = 0.005), reduced serum insulin by 16.2% (P = 0.02), reduced insulin resistance by 20.5% (P = 0.04) and reduced plasma homocysteine by 21.2% (P = 0.000) (Gargari et al 2011).

More recently, a systematic review and meta-analysis of 4 studies (n = 183) also found that daily supplementation of 5 mg folic acid in patients with type II diabetes mellitus significantly reduced plasma total homocysteine levels (Sudchada et al 2012). However, the meta-analysis concluded that the effect of folic acid on HbA_{1C} levels was not found to be significant and that further large-scale studies with larger sample sizes would be required to accuracy determine any effect of folic acid in type 2 diabetes mellitus.

Renal transplant recipients

Combination vitamin B treatment (folate, B_{12} and B_6) may be of benefit in renal transplant patients, according to an RCT of 56 renal transplant patients, which found that vitamin supplementation with folic acid (5 mg/day), vitamin B_6 (50 mg/day) and vitamin B_{12} (400 mcg/day) for 6 months reduced the progression of atherosclerosis, as evidenced by a significant decrease in carotid intima-media thickness. Additionally, a significant decrease in homocysteine levels was observed (Marcucci et al 2003).

Restenosis after percutaneous coronary intervention

An RCT found that treatment with vitamin B_{12} (cyanocobalamin 400 mcg/day), folic acid (1 mg/day) and vitamin B_6 (pyridoxine hydrochloride 10 mg/day) for 6 months significantly decreased the incidence of major adverse events, including restenosis, after percutaneous coronary intervention (Schnyder et al 2002). By contrast, one trial demonstrated an increased risk of in-stent restenosis in those patients intravenously administered 1 mg of folic acid, 5 mg of vitamin B_6 and 1 mg of vitamin B_{12} followed by daily oral doses of 1.2 mg of folic acid, 48 mg of vitamin B_6 and 60 mcg of vitamin B_{12} for 6 months (Lange et al 2004). Further research with more consistent study designs is required to elucidate the true effects.

Idiopathic recurrent miscarriage (IRM)

Maternal hyperhomocysteinaemia and poor folate status are risk factors for recurrent embryo loss and for first early embryo loss (George et al 2002). There has also been conflicting evidence in relation to the role of *MTHFR* polymorphisms and pregnancy, although many studies point towards increased risk of recurrent spontaneous abortion. One explanation for the discrepant results may be that the numbers of study participants have been relatively small (Zetterberg 2004). Although researchers encourage the periconceptional use of both folate and B_{12} to reduce these risks, there is a lack of interventional studies in this area other than one investigation of combined aspirin (100 mg/day) and folic acid (5 mg/alternate days) throughout gestation, on top of initial (12 weeks) prednisone and progesterone treatment (Tempfer et al 2006). This treatment yielded higher live birth rate compared with no treatment in women with IRM.

Cardiovascular disease protection and treatment independent of homocysteine status

In the absence of a causal relationship between Hcy and cardiovascular disease, what remains most promising for folate are studies illustrating its protective effects, mediated through other mechanisms. This has led some researchers to suggest that folate deficiency may be the primary cause of an increased vascular risk and that elevated Hcy levels should principally be considered an indicator of low folate status rather than a pathogenetic marker (Verhaar et al 2002). Demonstrations of in vitro antioxidant activity, effects on co-factor availability and direct and indirect interactions with the endothelial NO synthase enzyme have been proposed as plausible mechanisms, through which folate may prevent endothelial dysfunction (Antoniades et al 2007, Das 2003, Verhaar et al 2002).

Several meta-analyses have been conducted that assess the impact of folate alone or in combination on cardiovascular and all-cause mortality, including in individuals with preexisting cardiovascular or kidney disease, and have concluded that the treatments conveyed no significant benefits (Bazzano et al 2002, Bleys et al 2006, Leung et al 2010, Yang et al 2012). This was confirmed in a recent meta-analysis (n = 27,418) which concluded that folic acid supplementation had no significant effect on coronary revascularisation, coronary artery bypass grafting, percutaneous coronary intervention, coronary restenosis or total revascularisation (Qin et al 2014).

Combined B vitamins failed to reduce cardiovascular risk in high-risk women (Albert et al 2008), improve mortality and cardiovascular event frequency in patients with coronary artery disease (Ebbing et al 2008), failed to protect against cardiovascular events over 40 months (Bønaa et al 2006) and failed to prevent vascular events in patients with a stroke history after 3.9 years (Potter et al 2008).

On a more promising note, 51 heart transplant recipients who took 15 mg/day of methyltetrahydrofolate for 1 year following transplantation were found at their 7-year follow-up to have reduced all-cause mortality with a relative risk (RR) 0.53 when compared to the placebo group (Potena et al 2008).

Stroke

Several studies show the cardiovascular protective effects of folic acid, including the predictive value of low folate status on stroke risk (Bazzano et al 2002, Verhaar et al 2002).

Primary prevention with folic acid was found to effectively reduce the risk of stroke in a large-scale meta-analysis (n = 16,841; RR 0.82) (Wang et al 2007). The greatest beneficial effect was seen in subjects who received folic acid for longer than 3 years. A more recent 2012 meta-analysis of 26 RCTs similarly suggested there may be a modest benefit of folic acid supplementation in stroke prevention (Yang et al 2012).

Carotid intima-media thickness

Several studies have observed a beneficial effect of folic acid supplementation on markers of atherosclerosis, such as carotid intima-media thickness (Ntaios et al 2010, Vianna et al 2007).

A 2012 meta-analysis of 10 RCTs (n = 2052) found that folic acid supplementation was effective in reducing the progression of carotid intima-media thickness, a measure of atherosclerosis progression ($P < 0.001$) (Qin et al 2012). In particular, subjects with chronic kidney disease or high cardiovascular risk appeared to benefit from folic acid supplementation.

Hypertension and glucose control

In a multi-centre RCT, the combination of folic acid (400 mcg or 800 mcg) with enalapril (10 mg), an ACE inhibitor, was no more effective than enalapril alone in reducing blood pressure over 8 weeks (Mao et al 2008). The same study found that in subjects with hyperglycaemia, the combination of enalapril and 800 mcg folic acid significantly reduced fasting plasma glucose compared to enalapril alone and enalapril with 400 mcg ($P < 0.015$). Conversely, 8-week folic acid supplementation (400 mcg/day) in elderly women ($n = 122$) resulted in increased overnight fasting blood glucose concentrations (baseline: 84.8 ± 1.0 mg/dL; at 8 weeks: 98.2 ± 5.2 mg/dL, $P < 0.01$) (Chmurzynska et al 2013). When this cohort was stratified by *MTHFR* genotype, significant differences in HDL-cholesterol before and after supplementation were observed, with levels almost 10% lower in T-allele carriers than in CC homozygous subjects ($P < 0.05$).

Another small study, employing high-dose folate (10 mg/day) in patients with a recent history of acute myocardial infarction, demonstrated improved endothelial function (Moens et al 2007). These positive findings were independent of Hcy levels at baseline or changes to Hcy throughout the trial.

Cognitive decline, dementia and Alzheimer's disease prevention or treatment independent of homocysteine status

Independent of Hcy, folate is implicated in cognition and neurodegeneration due to its ability to improve nitric oxide levels in the brain and facilitate synthesis of neurotransmitters (Malouf & Grimley Evans 2008). Additionally, atrophy of the cerebral cortex results from folate deficiency. Despite an abundance of epidemiological evidence and a limited number of studies showing a positive correlation between folate status and dementia, the role of folic acid supplementation in cognition remains unclear.

A 2008 Cochrane review examining the effects of folic acid supplementation, with or without vitamin B_{12}, concluded that there was no consistent evidence that folate had any beneficial effect on cognitive function of healthy or cognitively impaired subjects (Malouf & Grimley Evans 2008). This was corroborated by a 2010 meta-analysis which found no effect of folic acid, with or without other B vitamins, on cognitive function within 3 years of the start of treatment.

Of the evidence available, including trials examined by the Cochrane review, a 2002 review has estimated that 71% of acute hospital admissions with severe folate deficiency have organic brain syndrome, compared with 31% of controls (Reynolds 2002). Low baseline serum folate also predicted dementia in a sample of 625 individuals followed over 2.4 years (Kim et al 2008), with onset of dementia significantly associated with exaggerated declines in folate and B_{12} and increases in Hcy, which may, however, have been the result of concomitant weight loss. In spite of this knowledge, the results of studies investigating supplemental folic acid have been equivocal and warrant closer examination of the disparate methodologies.

A review by Balk et al in 2007, which sub-analysed folic-acid-only treatments (three RCTs, using 750 mcg to 15 mg/day over 5–10 weeks) in elderly patients who were either healthy or cognitively impaired, found that while folic acid was not universally effective, there was evidence to suggest that patients with low baseline folate (<3 ng/mL) may significantly benefit.

Several studies investigating folic acid, either alone or in combination with other B vitamins, for slowing cognitive decline in Alzheimer's disease have failed to demonstrate an effect, independent of the hyperhomocysteinaemic population (Aisen et al 2008). One small study using 1 mg folic acid/day in conjunction with cholinesterase inhibitors over 6 months did, however, point towards an additive effect on patients' function (rather than cognition per se) regardless of Hcy (Connelly et al 2008); however, a similar study using higher doses of combined B vitamins failed to produce any statistically significant benefits (Sun et al 2007).

Anticonvulsant-induced folate deficiency

Anticonvulsant medications such as phenytoin, carbamazepine and valproate reduce serum folate status. Individual studies have estimated an incidence of 15% folate deficiency in this group, compared with 2% for control groups (Froscher et al 1995). However, the figure may be as high as 97% with long-term phenytoin therapy (Rivey et al 1984). This may be due to increased use of folate in drug metabolism and/or decreased mucosal absorption (Berg et al 1992, Pelton et al 2000). Often, folic acid supplements are recommended to avoid deficiency, but this requires close supervision to ensure drug efficacy is not substantially reduced (Rivey et al 1984). A series of published case reports documenting NTD births to women supplemented with folic acid 5 mg/day while on anticonvulsants has thrown into question whether this commonly recommended dose is sufficient or whether concomitant administration of other B vitamins, especially B_6, may be necessary (Candito et al 2007).

Psychiatric illness

Over the past three decades, a vast number of case reports, open studies and, to a lesser extent, case-control studies have been published on the topic of psychopathology and folate deficiency. Many report a high incidence of serum folate deficiency in patients with symptoms of depression and various psychiatric disorders, particularly in geriatric populations (Reynolds 2002). For instance, one review identified that rates of deficiency varied between 8% and 50% in patients with various psychiatric disorders, including depression and schizophrenia (Young & Ghadirian 1989). Two large studies, involving over 350 patients diagnosed with acute psychiatric presentations, identified low folate levels or frank deficiency (31% and 12% respectively). The patients with the most marked deficiency were also the group with the highest percentage of inpatients (Carney et al 1990). Another study of similar design found that 30% of 224 newly admitted psychiatric patients had low serum folate (<3.5 ng/mL) compared to just 2.4% of controls, and that patients with low folate were 3.5-fold more likely to present with depressive features (Lerner et al 2006). Disturbingly, the researchers also identified a significant trend between folate deficiency and hospital readmissions.

Depression

Aetiological role

It has been estimated that 15–38% of depressed people are folate deficient (Alpert & Fava 1997, Lerner et al 2006). Studies have also demonstrated that low dietary folate consumption (<256 mcg/day) (Tolmunen et al 2004), low serum folate (<3.5 ng/mL) (typically co-occurring with B_{12} deficiency) (Gilbody et al 2007, Lerner et al 2006) and an *MTHFR* C677T genotype (OR 1.36) are all independently associated with an increased risk of depression (Gilbody et al 2007, Kelly et al 2004). One study found that while folic acid supplementation did not reduce the risk of depression during and up to 8 months after pregnancy, it appeared to protect against depression for up to 21 months postpartum (Lewis et al 2012). This effect was more pronounced in those with the MTHFR C677T TT genotype ($P = 0.01$). The lesser-studied *MTHFR* A1298C genotype (although more active than the C677T genotype, but still 40% underactive) also demonstrates a weak positive relationship with depression incidence; however, more studies are required (Gilbody et al 2007). Following on from these findings, serum folate has also been negatively correlated with depression severity and duration in some, but not all, studies (Kim et al 2008). One proposed explanation for these inconsistencies is that low folate and elevated Hcy are only found in a sub-group of depressed patients; in particular, those who experience increased anger and hostility as part of their depression (Fraguas et al 2006).

Additional studies also highlight an association between antenatal and postnatal depression and elevated Hcy or low folate levels but not serum B_{12} nor dietary intake of these two nutrients (Abou-Saleh et al 1999, Miyake et al 2006) and depression in antenatal and postnatal patients, with Hcy naturally peaking in the third trimester (Abou-Saleh et al 1999, Behzadi et al 2008). The link between folate and B_{12} and depression has been hypothesised to be via Hcy and independent of this, due to its methylation role generally (Bottiglieri 2005, Coppen & Bolander-Gouaille 2005, Das 2008, Gilbody et al 2007, Lerner et al 2006, Roberts et al 2007, Tiemeier et al 2002).

Therapeutic role

Given the volume of evidence linking folate with depression, it is surprising that so few clinical trials have been conducted. A Cochrane systematic review of three RCTs involving 247 depressed people suggested that, on the limited evidence available, folate shows potential as an augmenting agent, but speculated that its effectiveness might be restricted to folate-deficient patients (Taylor et al 2003). The studies included in this review used 500 mcg folic acid, 15 mg or 50 mg of methyltetrahydrofolate once daily and lasted from 8 weeks to 6 months.

More recent studies, particularly in the elderly, who exhibit high rates of both folate deficiency and depression, have investigated the effects of broad-scale nutritional supplementation (meeting recommended daily intakes (RDIs) for all essential micronutrients) over a 6-month period with promising results. Red cell folate and serum B_{12} values rose in supplemented individuals in accordance with significantly reduced scores on depression scales (Gariballa & Forster 2007). Prophylactic treatment of non-depressed elderly men with 2 mg folic acid, 25 mg B_6 and 400 mcg B_{12}, in another study, however, failed to reduce depression incidence over 2 years (Ford et al 2008).

Improves response to standard antidepressants

Research investigating folate's adjunctive role in depression treatment has escalated in recent years and there is now evidence of an impaired fluoxetine response in patients with low folate levels, with response rates dropping from 44.7% in subjects with normal serum folate to only 7.1% of deficient patients (<2.5 ng/mL) (Papakostas et al 2004a, 2004b), as well as a potentiating effect when only 500 mcg/day of folic acid is added to fluoxetine (Coppen & Bailey 2000). Reduced folate levels have also been associated with reduced response to sertraline (Alpert et al 2003). Poor folate status negatively impacts response time (+1.5 weeks) (Papakostas et al 2005) and relapse rates during continuation of fluoxetine (42.9% relapse in patients with low folate levels versus 3.2%) (Papakostas et al 2004a, 2004b), independent of B_{12} and Hcy levels.

Schizophrenia

Folate has been implicated in schizophrenic aetiology since the 1950s with one-carbon metabolism abnormalities proposed as a distinct hypothesis at a similar time (Regland 2005). With current knowledge linking the two, there has been renewed interest in the role of folate in this disorder. In particular, folate deficiency fits with the neurodevelopmental theory, implicating malnutrition amongst other environmental stressors during gestation in the subsequent susceptibility to neurological disorders of offspring (Applebaum et al 2004, Gilbody et al 2007, Haidemenos et al 2007, Muntjewerff & Blom 2005). Specifically, elevated Hcy in the third trimester has been associated with significantly elevated risk. This theory is supported in part by the parallel increases in NTD births and schizophrenia incidence in populations affected by famine (Muntjewerff & Blom 2005). Further evidence of folate's role comes from elevated Hcy and a high incidence of the *MTHFR* C677T genotype which are frequently, but not consistently, found in this patient group (Kemperman et al 2006, Regland 2005). A meta-analysis of links between this folate polymorphism and schizophrenia found an odds ratio of 1.44 (Gilbody et al 2007).

Several studies in adult schizophrenic patients have reported increased rates of active folate deficiency. One, in addition to this, demonstrated an inverse relationship between serum folate and degree of negative symptoms and a positive association between Hcy and extra-pyramidal symptoms (Goff et al 2004). There have been several case reports of successful treatment using 15–30 mg folate together with B_{12} injections (1 mg every 10 days) and *N*-acetylcysteine (200 mg twice daily) (Regland 2005), as well as a study which administered a combination of 2 mg folic acid, 25 mg B_6 and 400 mcg B_{12} to schizophrenic patients with baseline Hcy > 15 mmol, which produced improvements in both clinical features and neuropsychological test performance (Levine et al 2006).

Other neurological and psychiatric presentations

Significantly decreased red cell folate (not serum) has been documented in both phases of bipolar disorder (Hasanah et al 1997), as well as frequently found in patients chronically treated with lithium (Coppen & Bolander-Gouaille 2005). There is also preliminary evidence of mildly elevated Hcy in post-traumatic stress disorder (PTSD) sufferers; however, more thorough investigation is required to confirm this tentative association (Jendricko et al 2008).

A 2011 Cochrane review determined that there are insufficient high-quality data to determine the effect of folic acid on fragile X-syndrome patients (Rueda & Ballesteros 2011).

Chemopreventative role

Epidemiological, animal and human studies all suggest that folate status may affect the risk of developing cancers in selected tissues; however, the exact nature of this relationship continues to elude researchers (Bollheimer et al 2005, Powers 2005). One current theory points to the negative synergism between ageing and folate inadequacy, producing aberrations in one-carbon transfer such as gene hypomethylation, implicated in potentially carcinogenic genomic changes (Jang et al 2005). Despite the wealth of studies available concerning folate and cancer risk, recent meta-analyses of over 50,000 subjects concluded that folic acid supplementation did not substantially increase or decrease incidence of site-specific cancer during the first five years of treatment (RR 1.06, $P = 0.10$) (Vollset et al 2013). This large-scale study also found no significant effect of folic acid supplementation on the incidence of cancer within the breast, prostate, lung, large intestine or any other specific site. Conversely, a meta-analysis by Qin and colleagues (2013) found that folic acid supplementation was associated with a significantly reduced risk of melanoma (RR 0.47) although no significant effect was observed with total cancer incidence, colorectal cancer, prostate cancer, lung cancer, breast cancer or haematological malignancy (Qin et al 2013b).

Previously, high folate intake was purported to have an almost universally protective effect. An extensive review of the role of the *MTHFR* C677T polymorphism in cancer risk concluded that, in spite of the poor folate status associated with this polymorphism, however, many studies identify it as protective against a range of cancers (Sharp & Little 2004). In addition to this, a group of Swedish researchers have demonstrated that the relationship between serum folate and colorectal cancer follows a bell-shaped curve distribution (Van Guelpen et al 2006). Speculation regarding the role of additional co-factors involved in folate activity has also emerged (Powers 2005).

Folate's actions, however, still constitute a plausible cancer risk modulator, due to its critical role in the production, methylation and repair of DNA, regulation of cell turnover and suppression of excessive proliferation (Choi & Mason 2000, 2002).

Colon cancer

The link between folate status and colorectal cancer was first suggested as a result of 1990s epidemiological findings. Subsequent rodent studies further strengthened the theory, when chemically induced colorectal carcinogenesis was shown to be enhanced under dietary folate deprivation and reduced with folate administration (Cravo et al 1992, Kim et al 1996). The *MTHFR* C677T genotype has been identified as a risk factor (OR 1.34), compounded by dietary folate below median intakes (Murphy et al 2008). Based on a recent systematic review and meta-analysis, folate may be associated with a protective effective against colorectal cancer (Kennedy et al 2011); however, this is not yet definitive as some studies show no effects. A 2013 meta-analysis of RCTs concluded that long-term folic acid use (3.5 years) did not increase or decrease the occurrence of new colorectal adenomas in patients with history of adenoma (RR any adenoma 0.98; RR advanced adenoma 1.06) (Figueiredo et al 2013). Similarly, in subjects with a history of colorectal cancer, a 2008 multicentre RCT found 0.5 mg/day folate did not reduce the risk of colorectal adenoma recurrence (RR any adenoma 1.07; RR advanced adenoma 0.98) (Logan et al 2008). Additionally, a large placebo-controlled RCT (n = 5442) of women at high risk of cardiovascular disease found that use of B-vitamins, including folate, was not associated with the prevention of colorectal adenoma, with no apparent benefit or harm being identified (Song et al 2012).

Breast cancer

While the epidemiological evidence with respect to dietary folate and breast cancer risk has produced equivocal results, more consistent evidence points to low folate intake as a risk factor only when combined with increased alcohol consumption (Larsson et al 2007, Mahoney et al 2007). This negative synergy is further supported by evidence that maintaining adequate folate intake, usually via supplementation, can reduce or eliminate the excess risk due to increased alcohol consumption (Mahoney et al 2007). A comparable detrimental additive effect has been demonstrated between the *MTHFR* genotype and low folate intake (OR 2.80) (Suzuki et al 2008).

Cervical cancer

Folate deficiency may increase the risk of cervical cancer in individuals infected with high risk human papiloma virus (HR-HPV) (Piyathilake et al 2004). Evidence suggests a diet rich in fruit and vegetables generally (OR 0.52), and folate independently (OR 0.55), reduces the risk of developing cervical cancer (Ghosh et al 2008); however, much of the other evidence pertaining to a protective relationship has been ambiguous and results from intervention studies on cervical cancer have been inconsistent (Henao et al 2005, Kwanbunjan et al 2005, Sedjo et al 2003). The most surprising finding is that the *MTHFR* genotype appears protective against cervical cancer (Shekari et al 2008), enhanced further by a concomitant low intake of B_2 (Piyathilake et al 2007).

The most promising RCT involved 47 patients taking an OCP who demonstrated mild to moderate intraepithelial dysplasia. A dose of 10 mg folic acid daily over 3 months resulted in significantly lower biopsy scores in the treatment group and a significant reduction in cytology scores from baseline (Butterworth et al 1982). Other studies have shown that folic acid treatment does not alter the course of disease in patients with pre-established cervical dysplasia (Childers et al 1995).

Other cancers

A protective role for folate in the prevention of a growing number of other cancers, e.g. prostate (Marchal et al 2008), lung (Suzuki et al 2007), pancreas (Suzuki et al 2008) and nervous system cancers (Milne et al 2012, Sirachainan et al 2008), has been tentatively made. Due to the limited or, in some cases, conflicting evidence that is available, more research is required to validate these preliminary findings (Rycyna et al 2013).

In a case-control study, maternal folic acid supplementation before and during pregnancy may reduce the risk of childhood acute leukaemia (OR 0.4) (Amigou et al 2012). This study also suggested that genotypes homozygous for any of the MTHFR polymorphisms or carrying both MTRR variant alleles may also be a risk factor for developing acute leukaemia; however, this study had some limitations thus further research is recommended.

Periodontal disease

A series of RCTs have shown that rinsing with a solution of folate (5 mg/dose) twice daily alleviates gingival inflammation in all age groups and in pregnant and non-pregnant women (Pack 1984, Thomson & Pack 1982). Treatment results in a significant reduction in inflammation without altering plaque levels or folate serum status and appears to be more successful than oral supplements (Vogel et al 1976).

Preliminary evidence suggests that topical folate may also have a role in controlling gingival hyperplasia associated with long-term phenytoin use (Drew et al 1987).

Methotrexate toxicity

Methotrexate is a cytotoxic drug with folate antagonist properties. In part, its efficacy is dependent on this effect, but severe deficiency symptoms such as macrocytic anaemia are sometimes induced (Lambie & Johnson 1985). Co-administration of folic acid or folinic acid has been investigated as preventive treatment, with both forms capable of reducing drug side effects (Ortiz et al 1998, Strober & Menon 2005). A 2013 Cochrane review found a statistically significant and clinically important reduction in the incidence of GI adverse effects, hepatic dysfunction and methotrexate discontinuation in methotrexate patients with rheumatoid arthritis receiving folic or folinic acid (Shea et al 2013). A trend towards a reduction in stomatitis was observed; however, this did not reach statistical significance.

Sickle cell anaemia

In the past, folate supplements were recommended to patients with sickle cell anaemia, but more recent studies show that clinically significant folate deficiency occurs in a very small percentage of these patients and other nutrients may be indicated (Reed et al 1987).

Vitiligo

Although a number of uncontrolled studies testing combination treatments have been promising, folate has never been assessed as a sole treatment. As such, it is difficult to determine its role in the treatment of this condition. In previous studies, a combination of oral folic acid and vitamin B_{12}, together with increased sun exposure, has produced response rates in the vicinity of 50% (Juhlin & Olsson 1997). A controlled study by a different group of researchers found that exposure to a specific band width of UV radiation produced repigmentation in 92% of subjects, irrespective of vitamin supplementation (Tjioe et al 2002).

Erectile dysfunction

The combination of folic acid (5 mg daily) with tadalafil (10 mg every other day) was found to be more effective in improving sexual function than tadalafil alone (10 mg every other day) in an RCT of 83 patients with type 2 diabetes mellitus (Hamidi Madani et al 2013). Due to limitations in study design, including failure to obtain baseline serum folate levels or serum testosterone levels, more research into the clinical implication of this finding is recommended.

DOSAGE RANGE

Australian RDI (NHMRC 2006)

- 400 mcg/day for adults; up to 1 mg/day in deficiency states.
- Up to 600 mcg/day is recommended as the Suggested Dietary Target to reduce chronic disease risk in adults.
- 600 mcg/day in pregnancy.
- 500 mcg/day during lactation.

According to clinical studies

- Preconception care or early pregnancy supplementation: 400–600 mcg/day.
- Preconception and pregnancy supplementation in women with a previous NTD birth: 4 mg/day.
- Idiopathic recurring miscarriage: aspirin (100 mg/day) and folic acid (5 mg/alternate days) throughout gestation plus prednisone and progesterone treatment for first 12 weeks.
- Anticonvulsant-induced deficiency: 15 mg/day (under supervision).
- Prevention of cervical cancer: 800–10,000 mcg/day.
- Prevention of breast cancer in high alcohol consumers: 400 mcg/day.
- Alzheimer's dementia in the presence of elevated Hcy: 800 mcg/day.
- Alzheimer's dementia with normal Hcy: 1 mg/day in combination with cholinesterase inhibitors.
- Cognitive decline in elderly with folate deficiency: 750 mcg/day.
- Depression: minimum of 2 mg or sufficient dose to reduce elevated homocysteine as stand-alone treatment.
- Depression as an augmenting agent with standard antidepressants: 500 mcg/day.
- Acute psychiatric presentation: 15–30 mg methylfolate daily in combination with standard psychotropic treatment.
- Hyperhomocysteinaemia: 500–5000 mcg/day.
- Cardiovascular protection in patients with elevated Hcy: 5 mg/day with high-dose B complex.

- Cardiovascular protection in heart transplant recipients or patients with recent history of MI: 10–15 mg/day.
- Methotrexate toxicity: 5 mg/week.
- OCP-induced folate deficiency: 2 mg/day.
- Periodontal disease: rinse mouth with a solution of folate (5 mg/dose) twice daily.
- Prevention of restenosis after percutaneous coronary intervention: 1 mg in combination with vitamin B_{12} (400 mcg) and vitamin B_6 (10 mg) daily.
- Schizophrenia with marked negative symptoms: 2 mg/day in combination with 25 mg/day B_6 and 400 mcg/day B_{12}.
- Sickle cell anaemia: 1 mg/day.
- Ulcerative colitis: 15 mg/day.
- Vitiligo: 2–10 mg/day.

ADVERSE REACTIONS

Adverse reactions appear to be limited to oral doses greater than 5 mg/day. Reactions include a generalised urticaria associated with an allergic response, nausea, flatulence and bitter taste in the mouth, irritability and excitability.

One study found high-dose folic acid supplementation in children aged 6–30 months was associated with an increased risk of persistent diarrhoea (Taneja et al 2013).

SIGNIFICANT INTERACTIONS

Antacids

Reduce folic acid absorption — separate doses by 2–3 hours.

Anticonvulsants (phenytoin)

Reduced folate levels frequently develop with long-term use, but macrocytic anaemia is rare (Lambie & Johnson 1985). Supplementation can reduce toxicity, which is a beneficial interaction, although medical supervision is advised.

Cholestyramine (e.g. Questran)

Reduced folate absorption — observe patient for signs and symptoms of folate deficiency and separate doses by at least 4 hours.

Gastric acid inhibitors (proton-pump inhibitors)

Reduced folic acid absorption — separate doses by 2–3 hours.

Methotrexate

Methotrexate is a folate antagonist drug. Folate supplementation can reduce toxicity, which is a beneficial interaction; however, it may reduce the efficacy of methotrexate (Al-Dabagh et al 2013) — medical supervision advised.

Oral contraceptives

Folate levels are reduced with long-term use of the OCP, particularly those with high oestrogen content; therefore, increased intakes may be required for women undertaking long-term use.

Pancreatin

Reduced folate absorption (Kelly 1998) — separate doses by 2–3 hours.

Pyrimethamine (e.g. maloprim)

Impairs the use of folate and, as such, supplementation with folinic acid may be beneficial.

Sulfasalazine

Folic acid can reduce drug absorption — separate doses by 2–3 hours.

Trimethoprim

Trimethoprim is a folate antagonist drug. Supplementation can reduce toxicity, which is a beneficial interaction — medical supervision advised.

Zinc

At high doses (>15 mg/day), minor zinc depletion may develop (Carmel et al 2006, Kelly 1998) — observe patients for signs and symptoms of zinc deficiency.

Practice points/Patient counselling

- Folate is involved in a number of important biochemical pathways required for health and wellbeing, in particular development and cell growth.
- Folate supplements are often given to correct deficiencies or prevent deficiency in people at risk, such as those with malabsorption syndromes (e.g. coeliac disease and Crohn's disease), long-term use of certain medications such as phenytoin, sulfasalazine, cimetidine, antacids and the OCP, in congenital malabsorption states and blind loop syndrome, chronic alcoholism, HIV infection, the institutionalised elderly, pregnant and lactating women.
- It is considered to be the most important supplement to be taken by women in the weeks leading up to conception and during the first 12 weeks of pregnancy, in order to significantly reduce the risk of NTD in newborns. Food fortification is not considered sufficient.
- Both tablet and multivitamin softgel capsules have similar bioavailability profiles, with both peak level and total serum folate similar between each dosage form. Time to peak concentration appears slower in softgel capsules compared to tablets (Maki et al 2012).
- Other uses for folic acid supplements include reducing homocysteine levels (often in combination with vitamins B_{12} and B_6), reducing primary cardiovascular disease risk and cancer risk in general, periodontal disease (as a topical application), depression, schizophrenia and other psychiatric presentations and vitiligo.

CONTRAINDICATIONS AND PRECAUTIONS

Use of folate supplements may mask a B_{12} deficiency state by correcting an apparent macrocytic anaemia without altering progression of neurological damage. It is recommended that patients be screened for vitamin B_{12} deficiency.

PREGNANCY USE

According to the Australian Drug Evaluation Committee (1999), folate is considered to be safe to take during both pregnancy and lactation. Retrospective analysis of a trial of folate in pregnancy in the 1960s has suggested a possible increase in all-cause mortality and breast cancer in pregnant women taking 5 mg/day folate; however, this finding could be due to a number of factors unrelated to folate (Bland 2005, Charles et al 2004). The only context requiring special consideration is those pregnant women taking anticonvulsant medication (see Significant interactions).

F

PATIENTS' FAQs

What will this supplement do for me?

Folic acid is essential for health and wellbeing. Supplements have a critical role in preventing NTD in newborns and may also reduce the risk of primary cardiovascular disease and improve brain function in Alzheimer's dementia and non-Alzheimer's dementia and depression. It can also reduce the toxic effects of some medicines and may reduce the risk of developing some forms of cancer.

When will it start to work?

This depends on the indication.

Are there any safety issues?

The major concern with high doses of folate is that they may mask an underlying vitamin B_{12} deficiency and allow it to progress unnoticed, which means that a vitamin B_{12} deficiency should be excluded. It also interacts with some drugs in both a potentially harmful and a beneficial way. High doses should not be used in patients with a history of bowel polyps or adenomas.

REFERENCES

Abou-Saleh MT et al. The role of pterins and related factors in the biology of early postpartum depression. Eur Neuropsychopharmacol 9.4 (1999): 295–300.

Abrahamsen B et al. MTHFR c.677C > T polymorphism as an independent predictor of peak bone mass in Danish men–results from the Odense Androgen Study. Bone 38.2 (2006): 215–2119.

Aisen PS et al. High-dose B vitamin supplementation and cognitive decline in Alzheimer disease: a randomized controlled trial. JAMA 300.15 (2008): 1774–1783.

Albert CM et al. Effect of folic acid and B vitamins on risk of cardiovascular events and total mortality among women at high risk for cardiovascular disease: a randomized trial. JAMA 299.17 (2008): 2027–2036.

Al-Dabagh A et al. The effect of folate supplementation on methotrexate efficacy and toxicity in psoriasis patients and folic acid use by dermatologists in the USA. Am J Clin Dermatol 14.3 (2013): 155–161.

Alpert JE, Fava M. Nutrition and depression: the role of folate. Nutr Rev 55.5 (1997): 145–149.

Alpert M. et al. Prediction of treatment response in geriatric depression from baseline folate level: interaction with an SSRI or a tricyclic antidepressant. J Clin Psychopharmacol 23 (2003): 309–313.

Amigou A et al. Folic acid supplementation, MTHFR and MTRR polymorphisms, and the risk of childhood leukemia: the ESCALE study (SFCE). Cancer Causes Control 23.8 (2012): 1265–1277.

Anderson CA et al. Effects of folic acid supplementation on serum folate and plasma homocysteine concentrations in older adults: a dose-response trial. Am J Epidemiol 172.8 (2010): 932–941.

Antoniades C et al. Homocysteine lowering: any use in atherosclerosis? Hellenic J Cardiol 48.5 (2007): 249–251.

Applebaum J et al. Homocysteine levels in newly admitted schizophrenic patients. J Psychiatr Res 38.4 (2004): 413–4116.

Australian Drug Evaluation Committee. Prescribing medicines in pregnancy, 4th edn. Canberra: TGA Publications, 1999.

Bakker R et al. Folic acid supplements modify the adverse effects of maternal smoking on fetal growth and neonatal complications. J Nutr 141.12 (2011): 2171–2179.

Balk EM et al. Vitamin B6, B12, and folic acid supplementation and cognitive function: A systematic review of randomized trials. Arch Intern Med 167.1 (2007): 21–30.

Bazzano LA et al. Dietary intake of folate and risk of stroke in US men and women: NHANES1 epidemiological follow-up study. Stroke 33 (2002): 1183–1189.

Bean LJ et al. Lack of maternal folic acid supplementation is associated with heart defects in Down syndrome: a report from the National Down Syndrome Project. Birth Defects Res A Clin Mol Teratol 91.10 (2011): 885–893.

Beers MH, Berkow R (eds), The Merck manual of diagnosis and therapy, 17th edn. Whitehouse, NJ: Merck, 2003.

Behzadi AH, Behbahani AS, Ostovar N. Therapeutic effects of folic acid on ante partum and postpartum depression. Med Hypotheses 71.2 (2008): 313–14.

Berg MJ et al. Phenytoin pharmacokinetics: before and after folic acid administration. Epilepsia 33.4 (1992): 712–720.

Berry RJ. Maternal prenatal folic acid supplementation is associated with a reduction in development of autistic disorder. J Pediatr 163.1 (2013): 302–306.

Bielenberg J. Folic acid and vitamin deficiency caused by oral contraceptives. Med Monatsschr Pharm 14.8 (1991): 244–247.

Bjorke Monsen AL, Ueland PM. Homocysteine and methylmalonic acid in diagnosis and risk assessment from infancy to adolescence. Am J Clin Nutr 78.1 (2003): 7–21.

Bland JM. Taking folate in pregnancy and risk of maternal breast cancer. What's in a name? BMJ 330 (2005): 600.

Bleys J et al. Vitamin-mineral supplementation and the progression of atherosclerosis: a meta-analysis of randomized controlled trials. Am J Clin Nutr 84.4 (2006): 880–887.

Bollheimer LC et al. Folate and its preventative potential in colorectal carcinogenesis. How strong is the biological and epidemiological evidence? Crit Rev Oncol Hematol 55 (2005): 13–36.

Bønaa K et al. Homocysteine lowering and cardiovascular events after acute myocardial infarction. N Engl J Med 354 (2006): 1578–1588.

Botez MI. Folate deficiency and neurological disorders in adults. Med Hypotheses 2 (1976): 135–240.

Bottiglieri T. Homocysteine and folate metabolism in depression. Progr Neuro-psychopharmacol Biol Psychiatry 29 (2005): 1103–1112.

Boyles AL et al. Folate and one-carbon metabolism gene polymorphisms and their associations with oral facial clefts. Am J Med Genet A 146A.4 (2008): 440–449.

Brown RD et al. The impact of mandatory fortification of flour with folic acid on the blood folate levels of an Australian population. Med J Aust 194.2 (2011): 65–67.

Bukhari FJ et al. Effect of chronic kidney disease on the expression of thiamin and folic acid transporters. Nephrol Dial Transplant 26.7 (2011): 2137–2144.

Butali A et al. Folic acid supplementation use and the MTHFR C677T polymorphism in orofacial clefts etiology: An individual participant data pooled-analysis. Birth Defects Res A Clin Mol Teratol. 97.8 (2013): 509–514.

Butterworth CE Jr. et al. Improvement in cervical dysplasia associated with folic acid therapy in users of oral contraceptives. Am J Clin Nutr 35.1 (1982): 73–82.

Candito M et al. Plasma vitamin values and antiepileptic therapy: case reports of pregnancy outcomes affected by a neural tube defect. Birth Defects Res A Clin Mol Teratol 79.1 (2007): 62–64.

Carmel R et al. Folic acid. in: Shils M (ed), Modern nutrition in health and disease. Baltimore: Lippincott Williams & Wilkins, 2006, pp 470–481.

Carney MW et al. Red cell folate concentrations in psychiatric patients. J Affect Disord 19.3 (1990): 207–213.

Chan AC et al. Folate awareness and the prevalence of neural tube defects in South Australia, 1966–2007. Med J Aust 189.10 (2008): 566–569.

Charles D et al. Taking folate in pregnancy and risk of maternal breast cancer. BMJ 329 (2004): 1375–1376.

Chevrier C et al. Fetal and maternal MTHFR C677T genotype, maternal folate intake and the risk of nonsyndromic oral clefts. Am J Med Genet A 143.3 (2007): 248–257.

Childers JM et al. Chemoprevention of cervical cancer with folic acid: phase III Southwest Oncology Group Intergroup study. Cancer Epidemiol Biomarkers Prev 4.2 (1995): 155–159.

Chmurzynska A et al. Elderly women: Homocysteine reduction by short-term folic acid supplementation resulting in increased glucose concentrations and affecting lipid metabolism (C677T *MTHFR* polymorphism). Nutrition 29.6 (2013): 841–844.

Choi SW, Mason JB. Folate and carcinogenesis: an integrated scheme. J Nutr 130 (2000): 129–132.

Choi SW, Mason JB. Folate status: effects on pathways of colorectal carcinogensis. J Nutr 132 (2002): 2413–18S.

Clarke R et al. Hyperhomocysteinemia: an independent risk factor for vascular disease. N Engl J Med 324 (1991): 1149–1155.

Connelly PJ et al. A randomised double-blind placebo-controlled trial of folic acid supplementation of cholinesterase inhibitors in Alzheimer's disease. Int J Geriatr Psychiatry 23.2 (2008): 155–160.

Coppen A, Bailey J. Enhancement of the antidepressant action of fluoxetine by folic acid: A randomised, placebo controlled trial. J Affect Disord 60.2 (2000): 121–130.

Coppen A, Bolander-Gouaille C. Treatment of depression: time to consider folic acid and vitamin B12. J Psychopharmacol 19.1 (2005): 59–65.

Cravo ML et al. Folate deficiency enhances the development of colonic neoplasia in dimethylhydrazine-treated rats. Cancer Res 52.18 (1992): 5002–5006.

Crider KS et al. Prenatal folic acid and risk of asthma in children: a systematic review and meta-analysis. Am J Clin Nutr 98.5 (2013): 1272–1281.

Cuskelly GJ, McNulty H, Scott JM. Effect of increased dietary folate on red-cell folate: implications for the prevention of neural tube defects. Lancet 47.9002 (1996): 657–659.

Daly LE et al. Folate levels and neural tube defects. Implications for prevention. JAMA 274 (1995): 1698–1702.

Das U. Folic acid says NO to vascular diseases. Nutrition 19.7–8 (2003): 686–692.

Das UN. Folic acid and polyunsaturated fatty acids improve cognitive function and prevent depression, dementia, and Alzheimer's disease–but how and why? Prostaglandins Leukot Essent Fatty Acids 78.1 (2008): 11–119.

De-Regil LM et al. Effects and safety of periconceptional folate supplementation for preventing birth defects. Cochrane DB Syst Rev 10 (2010): CD007950.

den Heijer M et al. Hyperhomocysteinemia as a risk factor for deep-vein thrombosis. N Engl J Med 334 (1996): 759–762.

Drew HJ et al. Effect of folate on phenytoin hyperplasia. J Clin Periodontal 14.6 (1987): 350–356.

du Plessis L et al. What has happened with neural tube defects and women's understanding of folate in Victoria since 1998? Med J Aust 189.10 (2008): 570–574.

Durga J et al. Effect of 3-year folic acid supplementation on cognitive function in older adults in the FACIT trial: a randomised, double blind, controlled trial. Lancet 369.9557 (2007): 208–216.

Ebbing M et al. Mortality and cardiovascular events in patients treated with homocysteine-lowering B vitamins after coronary angiography: a randomized controlled trial. JAMA 300.7 (2008): 795–804.

Eskes T. Abnormal folate metabolism in mothers with Down syndrome offspring: review of the literature. Eur J Obstet Gynecol Reprod Biol 124 (2006): 130–133.

Figueiredo JC et al. Folic acid and prevention of colorectal adenomas: a combined analysis of randomized clinical trials. Int J Cancer 129.1 (2013): 192–203.

Ford AH et al. Vitamins B12, B6, and folic acid for onset of depressive symptoms in older men: results from a 2-year placebo-controlled randomized trial. J Clin Psychiatry 69.8 (2008): 1203–1209.

Fraguas R Jr. et al. Anger attacks in major depressive disorder and serum levels of homocysteine. Biol Psychiatry 60.3 (2006): 270–274.

Froscher W et al. Folate deficiency, anticonvulsant drugs, and psychiatric morbidity. Clin Neuropharmacol 18.2 (1995): 165–182.

FSANZ. Consideration of mandatory fortification with folic acid. Canberra: Food Standards Australia New Zealand, 2007.

Gabriel HE et al. Chronic cigarette smoking is associated with diminished folate status, altered folate form distribution, and increased genetic damage in the buccal mucosa of healthy adults. Am J Clin Nutr 83.4 (2006): 835–841.

Gargari BP et al. Effect of folic acid supplementation on biochemical indices in overweight and obese men with type 2 diabetes. Diabetes Res Clin Pract 94.1 (2011): 33–38.

Gariballa S, Forster S. Effects of dietary supplements on depressive symptoms in older patients: a randomised double-blind placebo-controlled trial. Clin Nutr26.5 (2007): 545–551.

Gatt A et al. Hyperhomocysteinemia in women with advanced breast cancer. Int J Lab Hematol 29.6 (2007): 421–425.

George L et al. Plasma folate levels and risk of spontaneous abortion. JAMA 288.15 (2002): 1867–1873.

Ghosh C et al. Dietary intakes of selected nutrients and food groups and risk of cervical cancer. Nutr Cancer 60.3 (2008): 331–341.

Gilbody S, Lewis S, Lightfoot T. Methylenetetrahydrofolate reductase (MTHFR) genetic polymorphisms and psychiatric disorders: a HuGE review. Am J Epidemiol 165.1 (2007): 1–13.

Goff DC et al. Folate, homocysteine, and negative symptoms in schizophrenia. Am J Psychiatry 161.9 (2004): 1705–1708.

Gok U et al. Comparative analysis of serum homocysteine, folic acid and vitamin B12 levels in patients with noise-induced hearing loss. Auris Nasus Larynx 31.1 (2004): 19–22.

Green TJ et al. Lowering homocysteine with B vitamins has no effect on biomarkers of bone turnover in older persons: a 2-y randomized controlled trial. Am J Clin Nutr 85.2 (2007): 460–464.

Gropper S, Smith J, Groff J. Advanced nutrition and human metabolism, 4th edn. Belmont, CA: Wadsworth Thomson Learning, 2009.

Håberg SE et al. Folic acid supplements in pregnancy and early childhood respiratory health. Arch Dis Child 94.3 (2009): 180–184.

Haggarty P et al. Effect of B vitamins and genetics on success of in-vitro fertilisation: prospective cohort study. Lancet 367 (2006): 1513–15119.

Haidemenos A et al. Plasma homocysteine, folate and B12 in chronic schizophrenia. Prog Neuropsychopharmacol Biol Psychiatry 31.6 (2007): 1289–1296.

Hamid A, Kaur J. Long-term alcohol ingestion alters the folate-binding kinetics in intestinal brush border membrane in experimental alcoholism. Alcohol 41.6 (2007): 441–446.

Hamidi Madani A et al. Assessment of the efficacy of combination therapy with folic acid and tadalafil for the management of erectile dysfunction in men with type 2 diabetes mellitus. J Sex Med 10.4 (2013): 1146–1150.

Hasanah CI et al. Reduced red-cell folate in mania. J Affect Disord 46.2 (1997): 95–99.

Henao O et al. Women with polymorphisms of methylenetetrahydrofolate reductase (MTHFR) and methionine synthase (MS) are less likely to have cervical intraepithelial neoplasia (CIN) 2 or 3. Int J Cancer 113.6 (2005): 991–997.

Hendler SS, Rorvik D (eds), PDR for nutritional supplements. Montvale, NJ: Medical Economics, 2001.

Hickling S et al. Impact of voluntary folate fortification on plasma homocysteine and serum folate in Australia from 1995 to 2001: a population based cohort study. J Epidemiol Community Health 59 (2005): 371–376.

Hollingsworth JW et al. In utero supplementation with methyl donors enhances allergic airway disease in mice. J Clin Invest 118.10 (2008): 3462–3469.

Hollis ND et al. Preconception folic acid supplementation and risk for chromosome 21 nondisjunction: a report from the National Down Syndrome Project. Am J Med Genet A 161A.3 (2013): 438–444.

Homocysteine Study Collaboration. Homocysteine and risk of ischemic heart disease and stroke: a meta-analysis. JAMA 288.16 (2002): 2015–2022.

Hutson JR et al. Folic acid transport to the human fetus is decreased in pregnancies with chronic alcohol exposure. PLoS One 7.5 (2012): e38057.

Jang H, Mason JB, Choi SW. Genetic and epigenetic interactions between folate and aging in carcinogenesis. J Nutr 135 (12 Suppl) (2005): 2967S–2971S.

Jardine MJ et al. The effect of folic acid based homocysteine lowering on cardiovascular events in people with kidney disease: systematic review and meta-analysis. BMJ 344 (2012): e3533.

Jendricko T et al. Homocysteine and serum lipids concentration in male war veterans with posttraumatic stress disorder. Prog Neuropsychopharmacol Biol Psychiatry (2008 Nov 14): [Epub ahead of print].
Juhlin L, Olsson MJ. Improvement of vitiligo after oral treatment with vitamin B12 and folic acid and the importance of sun exposure. Acta Derm Venereol 77.6 (1997): 460–462.
Karadag AS et al. Effect of isotretinoin treatment on plasma holotranscobalamin, vitamin B12, folic acid, and homocysteine levels: non-controlled study. Int J Dermatol 50.12 (2011): 1564–1569.
Kelly C et al. The MTHFR C677T polymorphism is associated with depressive episodes in patients from Northern Ireland. J Psychopharmacol 18.4 (2004): 567–571.
Kelly GS. Folate supplemental forms and therapeutic applications. Altern Med Rev 3 (1998): 208–220.
Kemperman R et al. Low essential fatty acids and B-vitamin status in a subgroup of patients with schizophrenia and its response to dietary supplementation. Prostaglandins Leukot Essent Fatty Acids 74 (2006): 75–85.
Kennedy DA et al. Folate intake and the risk of colorectal cancer: A systematic review and meta-analysis. Cancer Epidemiol 35.1 (2011): 2–10.
Keser I et al. Folic acid and vitamin B_{12} supplementation lowers plasma homocysteine but has no effect on serum bone turnover markers in elderly women: a randomized, double-blind, placebo-controlled trial. Nutr Res 33.3 (2013): 211–219.
Kim JM et al. Changes in folate, vitamin B12 and homocysteine associated with incident dementia. J Neurol Neurosurg Psychiatry 79.8 (2008): 864–868.
Kim YI et al. Dietary folate protects against the development of macroscopic colonic neoplasia in a dose responsive manner in rats. Gut 39.5 (1996): 732–740.
Kumar P, Clarke M. Clinical medicine, 5th edn. London: WB Saunders, 2002.
Kwanbunjan K et al. Low folate status as a risk factor for cervical dysplasia in Thai women. Nutr Res 25 (2005): 641–654.
Lambie DG, Johnson RH. Drugs and folate metabolism. Drugs 30.2 (1985): 145–155.
Lange H et al. Folate therapy and in-stent restenosis after coronary stenting. N Engl J Med 350 (2004): 2673–2681.
Larsson SC, Giovannucci E, Wolk A. Folate and risk of breast cancer: a meta-analysis. J Natl Cancer Inst 99.1 (2007): 64–76.
Lassi ZS et al. Folic acid supplementation during pregnancy for maternal health and pregnancy outcomes. Cochrane DB Syst Rev (2013) Issue 3 Art:CD006896.
Lerner V et al. Vitamin B12 and folate serum levels in newly admitted psychiatric patients. Clin Nutr 25 (2006): 60–67.
Leung J et al. Folic Acid Supplementation and Cardiac and Stroke Mortality among Hemodialysis Patients. J Ren Nutr 20.5 (2010): 293–302.
Levine J et al. Homocysteine-reducing strategies improve symptoms in chronic schizophrenic patients with hyperhomocysteinemia. Biol Psychiatry 60.3 (2006): 265–269.
Lewis SJ et al. Folic acid supplementation during pregnancy may protect against depression 21 months after pregnancy, an effect modified by MTHFR C677T genotype. Eur J Clin Nutr 66.1 (2012): 97–103.
Li X et al. The association between periconceptional folic acid supplementation and congenital heart defects: A case–control study in China. Prev Med 56.6 (2013): 385–389.
Li Z et al. Folic acid supplementation during early pregnancy and the risk of gestational hypertension and preeclampsia. Hypertension 61.4 (2013): 873–879.
Logan RFA et al. Aspirin and folic acid for the prevention of recurrent colorectal adenomas. Gastroenterol 134.1 (2008): 29–38.
Lucock M. Is folic acid the ultimate functional food component for disease prevention? BMJ 328.7433 (2004): 211–214.
Lucock MD. Synergy of genes and nutrients: the case of homocysteine. Curr Opin Clin Nutr Metab Care 9.6 (2006): 748–756.
Lussanaa F et al. Blood levels of homocysteine, folate, vitamin B6 and B12 in women using oral contraceptives compared to non-users. Thromb Res 112.1–2 (2003): 37–41.
Ma J et al. Methylenetertahydrofolate reductase polymorphism, plasma folate, homocysteine, and risk of myocardial infarction in US physicians. Circulation 94.10 (1996): 2410–24116.
Mahoney MC. et al. Breast cancer risk reduction and counseling: lifestyle, chemoprevention, and surgery. J Natl Compr Canc Netw 5.8 (2007): 702–710.
Maki KC et al. Absorption of Folic Acid from a Softgel Capsule Compared to a Standard Tablet. J Acad Nutr Diet 112.7 (2012):1062–1067.
Malinow MR et al. Prevalence of hyperhomocyst(e)inemia in patients with peripheral arterial occlusive disease. Circulation 79 (1989): 1180–1188.
Malouf R, Grimley Evans J. Folic acid with or without vitamin B12 for the prevention and treatment of healthy elderly and demented people. Cochrane Database Syst Rev 8.4 (2008): CD004514.
Manniën J et al. Factors associated with not using folic acid supplements preconceptionally. Public Health Nutr (2013) [Epub ahead of print].
Mao G et al. Efficacy of folic acid and enalapril combined therapy on reduction of blood pressure and plasma glucose: A multicenter, randomized, double-blind, parallel-controlled, clinical trial. Nutrition 24.11–12 (2008): 1088–1096.
Marchal C et al. Association between polymorphisms of folate-metabolizing enzymes and risk of prostate cancer. Eur J Surg Oncol 34.7 (2008): 805–810.
Marcucci R et al. Vitamin supplementation reduces the progression of atherosclerosis in hyperhomocysteinemic renal-transplant recipients. Transplantation 75.9 (2003): 1551–1555.
McCaddon A et al. Absence of macrocytic anaemia in Alzheimer's disease. Clin Lab Haematol 26.4 (2004): 259–263.
McGuire BW et al. Absorption kinetics of orally administered leucovorin calcium. NCI Monogr 5 (1987): 47–56.

McLean RR et al. Plasma B vitamins, homocysteine, and their relation with bone loss and hip fracture in elderly men and women. J Clin Endocrinol Metab 93.6 (2008): 2206–2212.

McMahon JA et al. Lowering homocysteine with B vitamins has no effect on blood pressure in older adults. J Nutr 137.5 (2007): 1183–1187.

McNulty B et al. Impact of continuing folic acid after the first trimester of pregnancy: findings of a randomized trial of Folic Acid Supplementation in the Second and Third Trimesters. Am J Clin Nutr 98.1 (2013): 92–98.

McNulty B et al. Women's compliance with current folic acid recommendations and achievement of optimal vitamin status for preventing neural tube defects. Hum Reprod 26.6 (2011): 1530–1536.

Metz J et al. Changes in serum folate concentrations following voluntary food fortification in Australia. Med J Aust 176.2 (2002): 90–91.

Milne E et al. Maternal use of folic acid and other supplements and risk of childhood brain tumors. Cancer Epidemiol Biomarkers Prev 21.11 (2012): 1933–1941.

Miyake Y et al. Dietary folate and vitamins B12, B6, and B2 intake and the risk of postpartum depression in Japan: the Osaka Maternal and Child Health Study. J Affect Disord 96.1–2 (2006): 133–138.

Moens AL et al. Effect of folic acid on endothelial function following acute myocardial infarction. Am J Cardiol 99.4 (2007): 476–481.

Muntjewerff J-W, Blom H. Aberrant folate status in schizophrenic patients: what is the evidence? Prog Neuro-psychopharmacol Biol Psychiatry 29.7 (2005): 1133–1139.

Murphy G et al. Folate and MTHFR: risk of adenoma recurrence in the Polyp Prevention Trial. Cancer Causes Control 19.7 (2008): 751–758.

NHMRC (National Health and Medical Research Council). Nutrient reference values for Australia and New Zealand. Canberra: Department of Health and Ageing, 2006.

Nilsson K, Gustafson L, Hultberg B. Improvement of cognitive functions after cobalamin/folate supplementation in elderly patients with dementia and elevated plasma homocysteine. Int J Geriatr Psychiatry 16.6 (2001): 609–614.

Nowak M et al. Homocysteine, vitamin B12, and folic acid in age-related macular degeneration. Eur J Ophthalmol 15.6 (2005): 764–767.

Ntaios G et al. The effect of folic acid supplementation on carotid intima-media thickness in patients with cardiovascular risk: A randomized, placebo-controlled trial. Int J Cardiol 143.1 (2010): 16–19.

Obermann-Borst SA et al. General maternal medication use, folic acid, the *MDR1*C3435T polymorphism, and the risk of a child with a congenital heart defect. Am J Obstet Gynecol 204.3 (2011): 236.e1–236.e8.

Okada A et al. Slowly progressive folate-deficiency myelopathy: Report of a case. J Neurol Sci 336.1–2 (2014): 273–275.

Okumura K & Tsukamoto H. Folate in smokers. Clin Chim Acta 412.7–8 (2011): 521–526.

Ortiz Z et al. The efficacy of folic acid and folinic acid in reducing methotrexate gastrointestinal toxicity in rheumatoid arthritis. A meta-analysis of randomized controlled trials. J Rheumatol 25.1 (1998): 36–43.

Ownby DR. et al. Has mandatory folic acid supplementation of foods increased the risk of asthma and allergic disease? J All Clin Immunol 123.6 (2009): 1260–1261.

Pack ARC. Folate mouthwash: effects on established gingivitis in odontal patients. J Clin Periodontol 11.9 (1984): 619–628.

Papakostas G et al. Serum folate, vitamin B12, and homocysteine in major depressive disorder. Part 1: predictors of clinical response in fluoxetine-resistant depression. J Clin Psychiatry 65.8 (2004a): 1090–5.

Papakostas G et al. Serum folate, vitamin B12, and homocysteine in major depressive disorder. Part 2: predictors of relapse during the continuation phase of pharmacotherapy. J Clin Psychiatry 65.8 (2004b): 1096–8.

Papakostas G et al. The relationship between serum folate, vitamin B12, and homocysteine levels in major depressive disorder and the timing of improvement with fluoxetine. Int J Neuro-psychopharmacol 8.4 (2005): 523–528.

Pelton R et al. Drug-induced nutrient depletion handbook 1999–2000. Hudson, OH: Lexi-Comp, 2000.

Pietrzik K et al. Calculation of red blood cell folate steady state conditions and elimination kinetics after daily supplementation with various folate forms and doses in women of childbearing age. Am J Clin Nutr 86.5 (2007): 1414–14119.

Piyathilake C et al. Folate is associated with the natural history of high-risk human papillomaviruses. Cancer Res 64 (2004): 8788–8793.

Piyathilake CJ et al. Protective association of MTHFR polymorphism on cervical intraepithelial neoplasia is modified by riboflavin status. Nutrition 23.3 (2007): 229–235.

Potena L et al. Long-term effect of folic acid therapy in heart transplant recipients: follow-up analysis of a randomized study. Transplantation 85.8 (2008): 1146–1150.

Potter K et al. The effect of long-term homocysteine-lowering on carotid intima-media thickness and flow-mediated vasodilation in stroke patients: a randomized controlled trial and meta-analysis. BMC Cardiovasc Disord 8 (2008): 24.

Powers HJ. Interaction among folate, riboflavin, genotype, and cancer, with reference to colorectal and cervical cancer. J Nutr 135 (2005): 2960–6S.

Priest DG et al. Pharmacokinetics of leucovorin metabolites in human plasma as a function of dose administered orally and intravenously. J Natl Cancer Inst 83.24 (1991): 1806–1812.

Qin X et al. Effect of folic acid supplementation on the progression of carotid intima-media thickness: A meta-analysis of randomized controlled trials. Atherosclerosis 222.2 (2012): 307–313.

Qin X et al. Homocysteine-lowering therapy with folic acid is effective in cardiovascular disease prevention in patients with kidney disease: A meta-analysis of randomized controlled trials. Clin Nutr 32.5 (2013a): 722–727.

Qin X et al. Folic acid supplementation and cancer risk: a meta-analysis of randomized controlled trials. Int J Cancer 133.5 (2013b): 1033–1041.

Qin X et al. Folic acid supplementation with and without vitamin B6 and revascularization risk: A meta-analysis of randomized controlled trials. Clin Nutr (2014) http://dx.doi.org/10.1016/j.clnu.2014.01.006.

Rabovskaja V et al. The Cost-Effectiveness of Mandatory Folic Acid Fortification in Australia. J Nutr 143.1 (2013): 59–66.
Rasmussen SA et al. Maternal obesity and risk of neural tube defects: a metaanalysis. Am J Obstet Gynecol 198.6 (2008): 611–619.
Reed JD et al. Nutrition and sickle cell disease. Am J Hematol 24.4 (1987): 441–455.
Regland B. Schizophrenia and single-carbon metabolism. Prog Neuro-psychopharmacol Biol Psychiatry 29 (2005): 1124–1132.
Rejnmark L et al. Dietary intake of folate, but not vitamin B2 or B12, is associated with increased bone mineral density 5 years after the menopause: results from a 10-year follow-up study in early postmenopausal women. Calcif Tissue Int 82.1 (2008): 1–111.
Revell P et al. Folic acid absorption in patients infected with human immunodeficiency virus. J Intern Med 230 (1991): 227–231.
Reynolds EH. Folic acid, ageing, depression and dementia. BMJ 324 (2002): 1512–15115.
Rivey MP, Schottelius DD, Berg MJ. Phenytoin-folic acid: a review. Drug Intell Clin Pharm 18.4 (1984): 292–301.
Roberts SH et al. Folate augmentation of treatment — evaluation for depression (FolATED): protocol of a randomised controlled trial. BMC Psychiatry 7 (2007): 65.
Rozendaal AM et al. Periconceptional folic acid associated with an increased risk of oral clefts relative to non-folate related malformations in the Northern Netherlands: a population based case-control study. Eur J Epidemiol 28.11 (2013): 875–887.
Rueda J-R & Ballesteros J. Folic acid for fragile X syndrome. Coch DB Syst Rev 5 (2011): CD008476.
Rycyna KJ et al. Opposing Roles of Folate in Prostate Cancer. Urology 82.6 (2013): 1197–1203.
Sauer J, Mason JB, Choi SW. Too much folate: a risk factor for cancer and cardiovascular disease? Curr Opin Clin Nutr Metab Care12 (2009): 30–6.
Schmidt RJ et al. Maternal periconceptional folic acid intake and risk of autism spectrum disorders and developmental delay in the CHARGE (CHildhood Autism Risks from Genetics and Environment) case-control study. Am J Clin Nutr 96.1 (2012): 80–89.
Schnyder G et al. Effect of homocysteine-lowering therapy with folic acid, vitamin B12, and vitamin B6 on clinical outcome after percutaneous coronary intervention: the Swiss Heart study: a randomized controlled trial. JAMA 288.8 (2002): 973–979.
Sedjo R et al. Folate, vitamin B12, and homocysteine status. findings of no relation between human papillomavirus persistence and cervical dysplasia. Nutrition 19.6 (2003): 497–502.
Selhub J et al. Association between plasma homocysteine concentrations and extracranial carotid-artery stenosis. N Engl J Med 332 (1995): 286–291.
Sengpiel V et al. Folic acid supplementation, dietary folate intake during pregnancy and risk for spontaneous preterm delivery: a prospective observational cohort study. BMC Pregnancy Childbirth 13.160 (2013). doi 10.1186/1471-2393-13-160.
Sharp L, Little J. Polymorphisms in genes involved in folate metabolism and colorectal neoplasia: a HuGE review. Am J Clin Epidemiol 159.5 (2004): 423–443.
Shea B et al. Folic acid and folinic acid for reducing side effects in patients receiving methotrexate for rheumatoid arthritis. Cochrane DB Syst Rev (2013) Issue 5 Art CD000951.
Shekari M et al. Impact of methylenetetrahydrofolate reductase (MTHFR) codon (677) and methionine synthase (MS) codon (2756) on risk of cervical carcinogenesis in North Indian population. Arch Gynecol Obstet 278.6 (2008): 517–524.
Sirachainan N et al. Folate pathway genetic polymorphisms and susceptibility of central nervous system tumors in Thai children. Cancer Detect Prev 32.1 (2008): 72–78.
Siragusa S et al. The risk of recurrent cardiovascular events in patients with increased plasma homocysteine levels is reduced by short but not long-term therapy with folate and B vitamins. Thromb Res 121.1 (2007): 51–53.
Smith AD, Kim YI, Refsum H. Is folic acid good for everyone? Am J Clin Nutr 87.3 (2008): 517–533.
Song Y et al. Effect of combined folic acid, vitamin B(6), and vitamin B(12) on colorectal adenoma. J Natl Cancer Inst 104.20 (2012): 1562–1575.
Sram R et al. The impact of plasma folate levels of mothers and newborns on intrauterine growth retardation and birth weight. Mutat Res 591 (2005): 302–310.
Stølen LH et al. High Dietary Folic Acid and High Plasma Folate in Children and Adults with Phenylketonuria. JIMD Rep (2013) [epub ahead of print] doi: 10.1007/8904_2013_260.
Stothard KJ et al. Maternal overweight and obesity and the risk of congenital anomalies. A systematic review and meta-analysis. JAMA 301.6 (2009): 636–650.
Strober B, Menon K. Folate supplementation during methotrexate therapy for patients with psoriasis. J Am Acad Dermatol 53 (2005): 652–659.
Sudchada P et al. Effect of folic acid supplementation on plasma total homocysteine levels and glycemic control in patients with type 2 diabetes: A systematic review and meta-analysis. Diabetes Res Clin Pr 98.1 (2012): 151–158.
Sun Y et al. Efficacy of multivitamin supplementation containing vitamins B6 and B12 and folic acid as adjunctive treatment with a cholinesterase inhibitor in Alzheimer's disease: a 26-week, randomized, double-blind, placebo-controlled study in Taiwanese patients. Clin Ther 29.10 (2007): 2204–2214.
Surén P et al. Association between maternal use of folic acid supplements and risk of autism in children. JAMA 309.6 (2013): 570–577.
Sütterlin M et al. Serum folate and vitamin B12 levels in women using modern oral contraceptives (OC) containing 20 μg ethinyl estradiol. Eur J Obstet Gynecol Reprod Biol 107.1 (2003): 57–61.
Suzuki T et al. Alcohol drinking and one-carbon metabolism-related gene polymorphisms on pancreatic cancer risk. Cancer Epidemiol Biomarkers Prev 17.10 (2008): 2742–2747.
Suzuki T et al. Impact of one-carbon metabolism-related gene polymorphisms on risk of lung cancer in Japan: a case control study. Carcinogenesis 28.8 (2007): 1718–1725.

Sweeney MR, McPartlin J, Scott J. Folic acid fortification and public health: report on threshold doses above which unmetabolised folic acid appear in serum. BMC Public Health 22.7 (2007): 41.

Taneja S et al. Folic acid and vitamin B-12 supplementation and common infections in 6–30-mo-old children in India: a randomized placebo-controlled trial. Am J Clin Nutr 98.3 (2013): 731–737.

Taylor MJ et al. Folate for depressive disorders. Cochrane Database Syst Rev 2 (2003).

Tempfer CB et al. A combination treatment of prednisone, aspirin, folate, and progesterone in women with idiopathic recurrent miscarriage: a matched-pair study. Fertil Steril 86.1 (2006): 145–148.

Thomson ME, Pack ARC. Effects of extended systemic and topical folate supplementation on gingivitis of pregnancy. J Clin Periodontol 9.3 (1982): 275–280.

Tiemeier H et al. Vitamin B12, folate, and homocysteine in depression: the Rotterdam Study. Am J Psychiatry 159.12 (2002): 2099–2101.

Timmermans S et al. Determinants of folic acid use in early pregnancy in a multi-ethnic urban population in The Netherlands: The Generation R study. Prev Med 47.4 (2008): 427–432.

Timmermans S et al. Folic acid is positively associated with uteroplacental vascular resistance: The Generation R Study. Nutr Metab Cardiovas 21.1 (2011): 54–61.

Tinker SC et al. Does obesity modify the association of supplemental folic acid with folate status among nonpregnant women of childbearing age in the United States? Birth Defects Res Part A Clin Mol Teratol 94.10 (2012): 749–755.

Tjioe M et al. Treatment of vitiligo with narrow band UVB (311 nm) for one year and the effect of addition of folic acid and vitamin B12. Acta Derm Venereol 82.5 (2002): 369–372.

Tolmunen T et al. Dietary folate and the risk of depression in Finnish middle-aged men: a prospective follow-up study. Psychother Psychosom 73.6 (2004): 334–339.

Troen AM et al. Unmetabolized folic acid in plasma is associated with reduced natural killer cell cytotoxicity among postmenopausal women. J Nutr 136.1 (2006): 189–194.

Van Guelpen B et al. Low folate levels may protect against colorectal cancer. Gut 55.10 (2006): 1461–1466.

Verhaar MC, Stroes E, Rabelink TJ. Folates and cardiovascular disease. Arterioscler Thromb Vasc Biol 22 (2002): 6.

Vianna AC et al. Uremic hyperhomocysteinemia: a randomized trial of folate treatment for the prevention of cardiovascular events. Hemodial Int 11.2 (2007): 210–216.

Vogel RI et al. The effect of folic acid on gingival health. J Periodontol 47.11 (1976): 667–668.

Vollset SE et al. Effects of folic acid supplementation on overall and site-specific cancer incidence during the randomised trials: meta-analyses of data on 50,000 individuals. Lancet 381.9871 (2013): 1029–1036.

Voutilainen S et al. Low dietary folate intake is associated with an excess incidence of acute coronary events. Circulation 103 (2001): 2674–2680.

Wahlqvist ML (ed), Food and nutrition, 2nd edn. Sydney: Allen & Unwin, 2002.

Wald DS, Law M, Morris JK. Homocysteine and cardiovascular disease: evidence on causality from a meta-analysis. BMJ 325.7374 (2002): 1202.

Wang X et al. Efficacy of folic acid supplementation in stroke prevention: a meta-analysis. Lancet 369.9576 (2007): 1876–1882.

Watson L, Brown S, Davey M. Use of periconceptional folic acid supplements in Victoria and New South Wales. Australia. Aust NZ J Public Health 30.1 (2006): 42–49.

Wilson JD et al. Harrison's principles of internal medicine, 12th edn. New York: McGraw-Hill, 1991.

Wright AJ, Dainty JR, Finglas PM. Folic acid metabolism in human subjects revisited: potential implications for proposed mandatory folic acid fortification in the UK. Br J Nutr 98.4 (2007): 667–675.

Yang H-T et al. Efficacy of folic acid supplementation in cardiovascular disease prevention: An updated meta-analysis of randomized controlled trials. Eur J Int Med 23.8 (2012): 745–754.

Young SN, Ghadirian AM. Folic acid and psychopathology. Prog Neuro-psychopharmacol Biol Psychiatry 13.6 (1989): 841–863.

Youngblood ME et al. 2012 Update on global prevention of folic acid–preventable spina bifida and anencephaly. Birth Defects Res A Clin Mol Teratol 97.10 (2013): 658–663.

Zetterberg H. Methylenetetrahydrofolate reductase and transcobalamin genetic polymorphisms in human spontaneous abortion: biological and clinical implications. Reprod Biol Endocrinol 2.7 (2004): 1–8.

Garlic

HISTORICAL NOTE Garlic has been used as both a food and a medicine since antiquity. Legend has it that garlic was used in ancient Egypt to increase workers' resistance to infection and later used externally to prevent wound infection. Other ancient civilisations have also used it medicinally. Sanskrit records document the use of garlic approximately 5000 years ago and the Chinese have been using it for over 3000 years. One of the uses of garlic was as a treatment for tumours, a use that extends back to the Egyptian Codex Ebers of 1550 BC (Hassan 2004). Louis Pasteur was one of the first scientists to confirm that garlic had antimicrobial properties. Garlic was used to prevent gangrene and treat infection in both world wars. Traditionally, garlic has been used as a warming and blood-cleansing herb to prevent and treat colds, flu, coughs and menstrual pain and to expel worms and other parasites.

COMMON NAME

Garlic

OTHER NAMES

Ail, ajo, allium, camphor of the poor, da-suan, knoblauch, la-juan, poor man's treacle, rustic treacle, stinking rose

BOTANICAL NAME/FAMILY

Allium sativum (family Liliaceae)

PLANT PART USED

Bulb, and oil from the bulb

CHEMICAL COMPONENTS

Garlic bulbs contain organosulfur compounds (OSCs), protein (mainly alliinase), amino acids (such as arginine, lysine, threonine and tryptophan), fibre, lipids, phytic acid, saponins, beta-sitosterol and small quantities of vitamins and minerals, such as vitamin C, vitamin E, beta-carotene, chromium, iron and selenium (Duke 2003). Of the numerous constituents present, it is the alliin component and resultant degradation products, such as allicin and ajoene, that produce much of the herb's pharmacological activity. These are formed when garlic is crushed or chewed and alliin is exposed to the enzyme alliinase. According to Commission E, 1 mg of alliin produces 0.458 mg of allicin (Blumenthal 2000). Allicin is unstable and degrades to various sulfides depending on the conditions. Steam distillation converts water-soluble thiosulfanates to lipid-soluble diallyl sulfides (DAS), whereas oil maceration results in the production of ajoenes and vinyl-dithines (Stargrove et al 2008).

The pharmacological actions of the herb are due to its organosulfur components: alliin, allyl cysteine, allyl disulfide and allicin (Chung 2006). In garlic oil, there are three major OSCs: diallyl trisulfide (DATS), DAS and diallyl disulfide (DADS) (Liu et al 2006). In aged garlic the sulfur compounds are metabolites of γ-glutamylcysteine; including water-soluble S-allylcysteine (SAC) and its metabolites S-allylmercaptocysteine (SAMC) and S-methylcysteine (Tsai et al 2012).

MAIN ACTIONS

Antioxidant

Garlic and many of its constituents have strong antioxidant activity and is capable of directly scavenging free radicals, and indirectly enhancing endogenous antioxidant systems such as glutathione, superoxide dismutase (SOD), catalase and glutathione peroxidase (Arhan et al 2009). This has been demonstrated in vitro and in vivo (Arhan et al 2009, Hassan et al 2010).

When tested individually, the four main chemical classes of garlic, allyl disulfide, alliin, allicin and allyl cysteine, have been shown to exhibit different patterns of antioxidant activity. Alliin scavenges superoxide via the oxanthine oxidase system; alliin, allyl cysteine and allyl disulfide act as hydroxyl scavengers; and allyl disulfide prevents lipid peroxidation (Chung 2006). SAC has also been shown to scavenge reactive oxygen and nitrogen species, including superoxide anion, hydrogen peroxide, hydroxyl radical and peroxynitrite anion (Medina-Campos et al 2007).

According to in vitro tests, garlic prevents cadmium- and arsenic-induced oxidative damage by inducing endogenous antioxidant defence mechanisms (Chowdhury et al 2008, Ola-Mudathir et al 2008, Suru 2008). A later study demonstrated the protective effects of DADS from garlic on human osteoblasts exposed to cigarette smoke (Ehnert et al 2012).

In vivo studies suggest protection from radiofrequency electromagnetic radiation associated with mobile phone use via the reduction of protein oxidation (Avci et al 2012), and cardioprotection with aged garlic on doxorubicin-induced cardiotoxicity (Alkreathy et al 2010, 2012). Large doses of garlic (500 mg/kg) improved sperm viability and partially preserved seminiferous tubule histological organisation after 28 days when compared to controls, most likely due to an antioxidant mechanism (Asadpour et al 2013).

Antioxidant activity and lower levels of oxidative stress have further been demonstrated in several clinical studies for garlic supplementation. One study used a dose of garlic 0.1 g/kg/day for 1 month; this was shown to induce a significant reduction in erythrocyte malondialdehyde (an indicator of oxidative stress) and significantly increase levels of SOD and glutathione peroxidase (Avci et al 2008). Similarly, oral garlic (250 mg/day) taken for 2 months caused a significant reduction in markers of lipid peroxidation in people with essential hypertension compared to normotensive controls (Dhawan & Jain 2005).

Protection against ischaemic and reperfusion injury

Prophylactic administration of garlic protects against renal and hepatic ischaemia/reperfusion injury in vitro and in a rat model (Kabasakal et al 2005, Sener et al 2005) prevents ischaemic and perfusion injuries after testicular torsion and detorsion in rats (Unsal et al 2006). More recently, pre-feeding mice with garlic attenuated oxidative damage in isoproterenol-induced myocardial infarction (MI) via the nitric oxide (NO) signalling pathway (Khatua et al 2012).

Anti-inflammatory activity

Fresh garlic extracts and garlic oil exert anti-inflammatory action in various models. Mechanisms of action identified include a direct action upon Toll-like receptor-mediated signalling pathway, inhibiting NF-kappa activation (Youn et al 2008), modification of the expression of cyclooxygenase (COX) activity (Thomson et al 2000) and suppression of inducible nitric oxide synthase (iNOS) and NO production (Liu et al 2006). The sulfur compounds Z- and E-aejones and their sulfonyl analogues have been shown to suppress lipopolysaccharide-promoted NO and prostaglandin E_2-mediated NF-κB-induced expression of iNOS/COX-2 genes (D Lee et al 2012). Lee et al investigated the anti-inflammatory action of DAS in articular chondrocytes and synovial fibroblasts harvested from patients undergoing joint replacement for osteoarthritis. Incubation with DAS inhibited the upregulation of COX-2 expression in synovial cells and chondrocytes and ameliorated crystal-induced synovitis through the inhibition of NF-κB (Lee et al 2009). Mice infected with malaria (*Plasmodium yoelli* 17XL) then treated with allicin 3 mg or 9 mg/kg had increased inflammatory mediators tumour necrosis factor, interferon-gamma, interleukin-12 (IL-12), p70, and NO; and immune cells, $CD4^+$ T cells, dendritic cells and macrophages were significantly higher in the treatment group, resulting in longer survival in a dose-dependent manner (Feng et al 2012).

Inhibits platelet aggregation and antithrombotic effects

In vitro studies indicate that garlic inhibits platelet aggregation through multiple mechanisms, including inhibition of COX activity and thromboxane A_2 formation, via the suppression of intraplatelet Ca^{2+} mobilisation and by increasing cAMP and cGMP levels. The antioxidant action of garlic also increased platelet-derived NO, and interaction with glycoprotein IIb/IIIa receptors reduces platelets' ability to bind to fibrinogen (Allison et al 2006, Chan et al 2007, Rahman 2007).

Importantly, the method of garlic preparation can influence its antiplatelet activity in humans (Lawson et al 1992, Rahman & Billington 2000), yet microwaving, oven heating at 200°C or submersion in boiling water for 3 min has shown no reduction in inhibition of platelet aggregation as compared to raw garlic (Cavagnaro et al 2007).

The clinical significance of the in vitro findings is hard to determine, as a double-blind, placebo-controlled crossover study of 14 volunteers concluded that solvent-extracted garlic oil had minimal or no effect on platelet aggregation. Researchers found that administration of garlic 9.9 g over 4 h exerted little or no effect on both collagen and adenosine 5'-diphosphate (ADP)-induced aggregation. Adrenaline-induced aggregation did, however, exert a slight but significant ($P < 0.05$; 12) reduction (Wojcikowski et al 2007).

Stimulates fibrinolysis

A significant increase in fibrinolysis has been observed in several clinical tests for both raw and fried garlic, which appears to be dose-dependent (Bordia et al 1998, Chutani & Bordia 1981, Gadkari & Joshi 1991). A recent controlled animal study found a statistically significant decrease in plasma fibrinogen and increase in clotting time in treatment groups receiving doses of raw garlic 750 and 1000 mg/kg, respectively, in comparison to that of 500 mg/kg (Gorinstein et al 2006). Odourless garlic has been shown to stimulate fibrinolytic activity via accelerated tissue plasminogen activator-mediated plasminogen activation and to inhibit the formation of thrombin, leading to suppression of coagulation (Fukao et al 2007).

Antiatherosclerotic activity

Evidence from in vitro, animal and human research has shown that garlic supplementation significantly reduces the atherosclerotic process (Campbell et al 2001, Durak et al 2002, Ferri et al 2003, Koscielny et al 1999, Kwon et al 2003, Orekhov et al 1995, Tsai et al 2012). Early research demonstrated that garlic significantly decreases accumulation of aortic tissue cholesterol, fatty-streak formation and the size of atherosclerotic plaque in vivo (Campbell et al 2001).

The adherence of leucocytes/monocytes to endothelium is also implicated in early-stage atherogenesis. In vitro studies have shown that incubation with garlic compounds significantly inhibits the oxidation of low-density lipoprotein (LDL) (Lau 2006), prevents adhesion of monocytes to IL-1alpha-stimulated endothelial cells (Rassoul et al 2006), suppresses oxidised LDL-mediated leucocyte adhesion to human endothelial cells (Lei et al 2008) and inhibits the uptake of oxidised LDL and CD36 expression (homocysteine-induced) by human macrophages (Morihara et al 2011).

A critical review conducted on in vitro studies established that garlic inhibits enzymes involved in lipid synthesis, platelet aggregation and oxidisation of LDL, while increasing antioxidant status (Rahman & Lowe 2006). Results from several published animal studies further exhibit antiatherogenic effects and have investigated the mechanisms responsible (Durak et al 2002, Ferri et al 2003, Kwon et al 2003). One in vivo study found that garlic activated antioxidant systems and decreased peroxidation in aortic tissue (Durak et al 2002), whereas ajoene inhibited smooth-muscle cell proliferation in another (Ferri et al 2003). The administration of 9 mg/kg of pure allicin in an animal model was found to reduce atherosclerotic plaque, Cu^{2+} binding to LDL, macrophages and the inhibition of LDL and oxidised LDL degradation. Allicin was also found to directly bind to lipoproteins, suggesting a further mechanism of action (Gonen et al 2005).

Similar results have been obtained using ultrasound techniques. Koscielny et al (1999) conducted a long-term randomised, double-blind, placebo-controlled trial involving 152 volunteers to determine whether garlic powder supplements (Kwai 900 mg daily) directly alter plaque volumes in carotid and/or femoral arteries. After 4 years' treatment, garlic intake significantly reduced the expected increase in arteriosclerotic plaque volume by 5–18%, with a slight regression also observed. A subsequent re-evaluation of the results found that significant effects were limited to women (Siegel & Klussendorf 2000).

In a multifactor prognostic evaluation of high-risk patients assessing risk of coronary heart disease (CHD), MI and sudden death, prolonged administration of Allicor containing 150 mg of dehydrated garlic powder in a slow-release form significantly reduced multifactor risk of CHD in both genders. However, reduced risk of MI and sudden death was achieved significantly in men, but not in women. A pilot study suggests that incremental benefits were identified when evaluating the role of garlic therapy in coronary artery calcification with patients also on concomitant statin therapy (Budoff 2006).

A published review suggested that the antiatherosclerotic action of garlic, while dose-dependent, is a valuable component in an atherosclerosis-preventing diet (Gorinstein et al 2007). A need for the standardisation of garlic products has been called for, to enable the opportunity to evaluate and draw conclusions from research findings (El-Sabban & Abouazra 2008).

A possible role for garlic in the prevention of cerebrovascular damage has been postulated through a reduction in levels of beta-amyloid and apoptosis, associated with the pathogenesis of Alzheimer's disease (Borek 2006). S-allyl-L-cysteine, an OSC purified from aged garlic extract (AGE), exerted an antiamyloidogenic activity in vitro, protecting against amyloid-beta-induced neuronal cell death, inhibiting amyloid-beta fibril formation and defibrillating amyloid-beta preformed fibrils (Gupta & Rao 2007, Gupta et al 2009, Imai et al 2007, Ishige et al 2007).

Reduces serum cholesterol levels

Two recent meta-analyses confirm that long-term garlic treatment modestly reduces total cholesterol levels (Ried et al 2013, Zeng et al 2012). Garlic powder capsules (mainly Kwai) are the most studied preparation; however the AGE preparations appear to have slightly stronger cholesterol-lowering activity than other forms.

A critical review published in 2006 suggests that garlic and its constituents exert a capacity to inhibit the enzymes involved in cholesterol and fatty acid synthesis, particularly mono-oxygenase and 3-hydroxy-3-methyl-glutaryl-CoA reductase (Rahman & Lowe 2006).

A 75% inhibition of cholesterol synthesis was achieved in garlic-treated human hepatoma cells without any evidence of cytotoxicity. Results indicated that compounds containing allyl-disulfide or allyl-sulfhydryl have the strongest inhibitory effect, likely to be through mediation of sterol 4-alpha-methyl oxidase (Singh & Porter 2006). Administration of high-dose (500 mg/kg) raw garlic extract to rats showed a significant (38%) reduction in triglycerides and cholesterol (Thomson et al 2006).

The capacity for modulating lipids may be attributed to the release of allicin through enzyme activation. A clinical crossover study involving 50 renal transplant patients involved the ingestion of one garlic clove daily for 2 months, either by swallowing or chewing. The swallowing route achieved a significant reduction in systolic blood pressure (SBP) and malondialdehyde (MDA) but no change in lipid parameters. However, chewing garlic achieved a reduction in cholesterol and a significant reduction in triglycerides, MDA and systolic and diastolic blood pressures, but no changes in high-density lipoprotein (HDL) or LDL (Jabbari et al 2005).

The metabolic activity of garlic has been studied in an obese rat model which compared three interventions to controls (garlic, exercise, garlic plus exercise). While all groups showed positive effects on cholesterol lowering, obesity and inflammation, the combination of garlic plus exercise group showed the greatest effects ($P < 0.001$) (Seo et al 2012).

Garlic's beneficial effects on serum lipids have been shown to decline following cessation of treatment, suggesting that long-term supplementation is required. A reduction in cholesterol and triglycerides and an increase in HDL were achieved in 30 participants with elevated blood cholesterol ingesting 5 g of raw garlic twice daily for 42 days. However, following a 42-day washout period, cholesterol and triglycerides increased and HDL decreased (Mahmoodi et al 2006). This study was repeated in 30 participants with blood cholesterol >245 mg/dL, with decreases in total blood cholesterol ($P < 0.001$) and triglycerides ($P < 0.01$), while HDL-C was increased ($P < 0.01$); these results were again reversed after a 42-day washout period (Hosseini et al 2013). Earlier clinical evidence also supports these results (Bordia et al 1998, Sobenin et al 2005).

Hypoglycaemic activity

Animal studies have shown that garlic and its constituents exhibit a hypoglycaemic action (Hattori et al 2005, Jelodar et al 2005) and produce significant changes in glucose tolerance and insulin secretion (Liu et al 2005, Padiya et al 2011). An antioxidant isolated from garlic, S-allyl cysteine sulfoxide, was found to stimulate insulin secretion from beta cells in rats (Augusti & Sheela 1996). Oral administration of garlic extract for 14 days significantly decreased serum glucose in streptozotocin-induced diabetic rats but not in normal rats. The garlic extract was also compared to that of glibenclamide, a known antidiabetic drug, and was found to be more effective (Eidi et al 2006). A similar study using garlic oil found no effect on oral glucose tolerance acutely, but did report significantly improved oral glucose tolerance at 4, 8, 12 and 16 weeks (Liu et al 2006). A study in a diabetic animal model showed garlic 100 mg/kg significantly reduced blood glucose levels and increased serum insulin levels in dogs when compared to controls. The effect was comparable to metformin (Mosallanejad et al 2013). A similar study in rabbits testing several doses of garlic extract in both normal and diabetic test animals found that the highest dose (350 mg/kg) had the strongest effect and significantly lowered blood glucose compared to controls in both cohorts. Levels of triglycerides and cholesterol also significantly reduced in both groups compared to controls, 4 h after administration. When compared to metformin, garlic had greater lipid-lowering activity whereas metformin was superior for hypoglycaemic activity (Sher et al 2012).

Antihypertensive activity

Numerous clinical studies have identified mild to moderate antihypertensive activity with various garlic preparations when used for at least 12 weeks (Andrianova et al 2002, Dhawan & Jain 2005, Ried et al 2013, Silagy & Neil 1994, Stabler et al 2012, Tsai et al 2012). Although the mechanism of action has not been fully elucidated, evidence from in vivo research suggests that both the renin–angiotensin system and the NO system are responsible for this activity (Al-Qattan et al 2006, Mohamadi et al 2000). A controlled animal study found that both raw and aged garlic produced a reduction in induced elevated SBP compared to control. A reduction in pulse pressure was also achieved in the aged garlic-treated group (Harauma & Moriguchi 2006). Rats receiving a conjugate of allicin and captopril (allylmercaptocaptopril) showed a greater reduction in blood pressure and improved cardiac hypertrophy than those receiving captopril alone. Allylmercaptocaptopril improved, whereas captopril impaired, fasting glucose tolerance (Ernsberger et al 2007). A similar study compared the effect of a fresh garlic homogenate (125–250 mg/kg) and its bioactive sulfur compound S-allylcysteine sulfoxide (SACS) in potentiating antihypertensive and cardioprotective activities of captopril (30 mg/kg) in rats. The combined treatment of garlic plus captopril was more effective than either alone and significantly reduced SBP, cholesterol, triglycerides and glucose in a dose-dependent manner (Asdaq & Inamdar 2010). In particular, a synergistic effect was seen for the blood pressure-lowering activity.

G

Enhances microcirculation

Jung et al (1991) found that, 5 hours after the administration of garlic powder (Kwai: total dose 900 mg garlic powder), a significant increase in capillary skin perfusion (55%) occurred in healthy volunteers, whereas Kiesewetter et al (1993a) showed a 48% increase with a dose of 800 mg garlic.

Antimicrobial and immune-enhancing activities

Garlic and its components have been demonstrated in vitro to exert a direct and indirect activity against various pathogens, including bacteria (both Gram-negative and Gram-positive), fungi and parasites. Antimicrobial sensitivity tests conducted on *Escherichia coli*, *Shigella* spp., *Salmonella* spp. and *Proteus mirabilis* found that no isolates were resistant to garlic; moreover, Gram-negative isolates were found to be highly sensitive to garlic in comparison to ciprofloxacin and ampicillin (Eja et al 2007).

Multiple chemical components in garlic demonstrate immunomodulating activity, including garlic sulfur compounds, lectins ASA I and II, agglutinins, proteins and fructans (Chandrashekar & Venkatesh 2009, Clement & Venkatesh 2010, Clement et al 2010, Chandrashekar et al 2011).

Allicin was initially believed to be chiefly responsible for the antimicrobial activity of garlic. Research found it to exert antibacterial activity against a wide range of Gram-negative and Gram-positive bacteria, including multidrug-resistant enterotoxicogenic strains of *Escherichia coli*, *Staphylococcus aureus*, *Mycobacterium tuberculosis*, *Proteus* spp., *Streptococcus faecalis* and *Pseudomonas aeruginosa*; antifungal activity, particularly against *Candida albicans*; antiparasitic activity against some of the major human protozoan parasites such as *Cryptosporidium parvum, Trichomonas vaginalis, Entamoeba histolytica* and *Giardia lamblia* and antiviral activity (Ankri & Mirelman 1999, Davis 2005, Gaafar et al 2012, Ibrahim 2013, Tessema et al 2006). Allicin has been found to exert an antimalarial action in vitro and in vivo (Coppi et al 2006, Feng et al 2012) and to significantly enhance the effect of amphotericin B against *Candida albicans* in vitro and in vivo, mediated through oxidative damage to *C. albicans* (An et al 2008, 2009). Additionally, in vitro investigations have identified the capacity of allicin to activate macrophage activity (Dong et al 2011, Ghazanfari et al 2006) and inhibit macrophage apoptosis (Cho et al 2006).

Ajoene, another important antimicrobial constituent, has been attributed to more biological activities in vitro and in vivo, including antifungal and antiparasitic actions (Ledezma & Apitz-Castro 2006), with greater antiviral activity than that of allicin, according to one in vitro test (Weber et al 1992), plus an interesting anti-leech effect (Eftekhari et al 2012).

The role of garlic in oral hygiene and the pathogenesis of dental disease has been investigated. All isolates of *Streptococcus mutans* identified in human carious teeth were sensitive to garlic extract, suggesting a role for garlic in mouthwashes for the prevention of dental caries (Fani et al 2007). This antimicrobial effect against streptococci was found to continue for 2 weeks posttreatment (Groppo et al 2007). Garlic extract was also found to significantly kill *Porphyromonas gingivalis* and its protease enzymes, indicating a role in the treatment of periodontitis (Bakri & Douglas 2005). A randomised trial of 56 patients found garlic paste to be as effective as that of clotrimazole solution in suppressing signs of oral candidiasis (Sabitha et al 2005).

Helicobacter pylori infection

Several in vitro and in vivo tests have shown that garlic has activity against *H. pylori* (Chung et al 1998, Jonkers et al 1999, O'Gara et al 2000); however, results from clinical studies are equivocal. Two studies found that a combination of garlic and omeprazole produced synergistic effects against *H. pylori* (Cellini et al 1996, Jonkers et al 1999). A rapid anti-*H. pylori* action of garlic oil was observed in artificial gastric juice, suggesting it as a useful treatment (O'Gara et al 2008).

Antineoplastic and chemopreventive effects

Garlic was first used over 3500 years ago in Egypt for the treatment of cancer. Garlic, and, in particular, its OSCs, including allicin, DAS, DADS, DATS and ajoene, have been investigated for their chemoprotective actions (Shukla & Kalra 2007). Many review articles have identified the multiple mechanisms by which garlic's compounds exert anticarcinogenic properties.

Garlic OSCs demonstrate a capacity to modulate detoxification enzyme systems often responsible for the activation of carcinogens (Yang et al 2001); for example, DAS and its metabolites have been found to competitively inhibit the metabolism of cytochrome P450 2E1 substrates in vitro (Brady et al 1991). This inhibitory activity has been shown in rat nasal mucosa (Hong et al 1991) and hepatocytes (Brady et al 1991). In addition, garlic OSCs increase the expression of phase II enzymes by enhancement of detoxification of activated carcinogenic intermediates such as quinine reductase and glutathione transferases (Bianchini & Vainio 2001, Rose et al 2005). Phase II enzyme modulation by OSCs has been reported in forestomach and lung cancer in mice (Singh et al 1998), and hepatoma cells (Chen et al 2004). Further investigations have established garlic OSCs' capacity to upregulate gene expression of glutathione S-transferase.

Garlic OSCs have been shown to suppress neoplastic cell formation by inhibition of cell cycle progression, leading to cellular accumulation in the G2/M phase (Frantz et al 2000, Zheng et al 1997). Human colon cancer cells treated with DADS have not only been seen to arrest the G2/M phase: concomitant alterations were also seen to DNA repair and cellular adhesion factors (Knowles & Milner 2003), with increases in cyclin B1 expression and p53 expression leading to cellular apoptosis (Jo et al 2008, Song et al 2009). DATS also induced apoptosis in primary colorectal cancer cells via mitochondrial-signalling pathways (Yu et al 2012), while treatment with DATS was reported to be more effective in arresting the G2/M phase of the cell cycle than DADS or DAS in human prostate cells (Xiao et al 2005). However DADS induced apoptosis in prostate cancer cells through modulation of the insulin growth factor pathway and the resulting inhibition of Akt phosphorylation, which resulted in reduced expression of antiapoptotic molecules and increased expression of proapoptotic signalling molecules (Arunkumar et al 2012). In human cervical cell cancer lines (Ski) DAS caused apoptosis via p53-induced cell cycle arrest and mitochondrial disruption (Chiu et al 2013).

Treatment with garlic and its compounds has been shown to display characteristics of mitotic arrest, exhibiting alterations to tubulin network and chromatin condensation (Herman-Antosiewicz & Singh 2005). Treatment of human colon cells with garlic-derived compound SAMC resulted in depolymerisation of microtubules and cytoskeleton disruption (Xiao et al 2005). Similarly, DATS treatment induced rapid microtubule disassembly and cell cycle arrest in human colon cancer cells (Hosono et al 2008).

Garlic and its constituents have demonstrated actions that modify apoptopic pathways mostly through regulation of antiapoptotic Bcl-2 and proapoptotic Bax and Bac proteins (Herman-Antosiewicz et al 2007). For example, modification to transcription ratios of Bax/Bcl-2 proteins following treatment with OSCs has induced apoptosis in neuroblastoma and lung cancer cells (Hong et al 2000), breast cancer cell lines (Nakagawa et al 2001) and prostate cancer cells (Arunkumar et al 2012, Xiao et al 2004). Another mechanism shown to induce cellular apoptosis following treatment with OSCs is the induction of reactive oxygen species (ROS) generation (Song et al 2009, Sriram et al 2008). DATS has been shown to induce ROS, reduce cell viability, increase apoptosis and inhibit cell migration in human breast cancer cells, but not in normal breast tissue cells (Chandra-Kuntal et al 2013). It has also been shown to induce ROS-related mitochondrial membrane disruption in hepatic cancer cells (Kim et al 2012). Additionally regulation of Akt-Bad (protein kinase B) pathway (Arunkumar et al 2012, Xiao & Singh 2006) and increased free intracellular calcium (Lin et al 2006) have been demonstrated. Malignant cells appear to be more sensitive to OSC-mediated apoptosis than normal cells (Chandra-Kuntal et al 2013, Powolny & Singh 2008). Garlic OSCs' protective qualities include increased histone acetylation by the inhibition of histone deacetylase, leading to cancer cell growth inhibition; for example, treatment of rodent erythroleukaemia and human leukaemia cells with DADS increases H4 and H3 histone acetylations (Lea & Randolph 2001). Increased acetylation has also been reported with treatment of OSCs in human colon cancer cells (Druesne et al 2004), breast cancer cells (Altonsy et al 2012) and prostate cancer cells (Arunkumar et al 2007). Similar research has been repeated in many different human cancer cell lines (Tsai et al 2012).

Finally, in vitro studies in human and animal cell lines indicate garlic and/or its constituents' ability to inhibit angiogenesis and metastasis. In human colon cancer cells, AGE was shown to inhibit angiogenesis by reducing endothelial cell motility, inhibiting tube formation, proliferation and invasion (Matsuura et al 2006). Administration of alliin exerted a dose-dependent inhibition of fibroblast growth factor-2-induced human endothelial cell tube formation and angiogenesis (Mousa & Mousa 2005). Similarly, treatments with DATS, DADS and DAS have been shown to inhibit capillary-like tube formation, cellular proliferation and migration (Thejass & Kuttan 2007). DADS was also found to inhibit angiogenesis by inhibiting the activation of matrix metalloproteinase (Thejass & Kuttan 2007). In human breast tumour cells, SAC reduced cell adhesion and invasion through expression of E-cadherin and reduced expression of matrix metalloproteinase-2 (Gapter et al 2008). In animal studies, intravenous administration of ajoene significantly inhibited lung metastasis of melanoma cells (Taylor et al 2006) and AGE inhibited sarcoma cell migration (Hu et al 2002). A mouse model of inserted fibrosarcoma showed treatment with AGE reduced tumour progression and significantly improved survival with $CD4^+/CD8^+$ T-cell modulation (Fallah-Rostami et al 2013).

There are many published reviews confirming garlic and its constituents' chemoprotective capacity in various human cancer cell lines (Herman-Antosiewicz et al 2007, Moriarty et al 2007, Nagini 2008, Powolny & Singh 2008, Seki et al 2008, Shukla & Kalra 2007). It is suggested that future research should focus on pharmacokinetics and pharmacodynamics in humans (Powolny & Singh 2008).

OTHER ACTIONS

Hepatoprotective effects

AGE has a glutathione-sparing effect in the liver and specifically elevates reduced glutathione content, thereby enhancing endogenous protective mechanisms, according to in vitro tests (Wang et al 1999). The protective effects of a single simultaneous dose of garlic oil have been demonstrated on acute ethanol-induced fatty liver in mice, by significantly inhibiting elevation of MDA levels, restoring glutathione levels and enhancing SOD, glutathione reductase and glutathione S-tranferase activities (Zeng et al 2008). More recent studies with organosulfur components from garlic have also demonstrated hepatoprotective effects in vivo (D'Argenio et al 2013, Xiao et al 2013) and a small clinical trial demonstrated a dose-dependent protective effect of a garlic oil and diphenyl-dimethyldicarboxylate (DDM) supplement, as measured by aspartate aminotransferase and alanine aminotransferase levels in patients with chronic hepatitis, with the greatest benefit seen in doses of 75–100 mg of DDB and 100–150 mg of garlic oil (M Lee et al 2012).

Homocysteine-lowering action

AGE exhibits homocysteine-lowering action that indicates its potential for the treatment of cardiovascular disease (Yeh & Yeh 2006). A pilot study conducted in patients with cardiovascular disease showed that pretreatment for 6 weeks with AGE significantly reduced the effects of acute hyperhomocysteinaemia (Weiss et al 2006). It is postulated that the homocysteine-lowering action of AGE is due to its ability to inhibit CD36 expression and OxLDL uptake in macrophages involved in the formation of atherosclerotic lesions (Ide et al 2006).

Inhibits CYP 2E1 and induces P-glycoprotein

According to in vitro and animal studies, garlic and some of its components may affect various cytochromes (Engdal et al 2009, Fisher et al 2007, Greenblatt et al 2006); however, human research has not produced the same findings (Cox et al 2006, Dalvi 1992, Foster et al 2001, Gurley et al 2002, 2005) and now confirmed that it is only clinically relevant for cytochrome 2E1 and P-glycoprotein with no effects on CYP3A4.

Researchers using human volunteers found that garlic oil reduced CYP2E1 activity by 39%, but had no effect on CYP1A2, CYP2D6 or CYP3A4 activity (Gurley et al 2002). The lack of a clinically significant effect on CYP1A2, CYP2D6 and CYP3A4 activity was confirmed in a later study of 12 elderly healthy volunteers receiving garlic oil for 28 days, followed by a 30-day washout period. Garlic oil had a mild inhibitory effect on CYP2E1 activity (by approximately 22%) (Gurley et al 2005). Additionally, tests with allicin found no effect on CYP3A4 in women receiving docetaxel treatment (Cox et al 2006).

More recently, a clinical study further confirmed no significant effect on CYP3A4 for oral ingestion of garlic extract by human volunteers but a significant induction of P-glycoprotein (Hajda et al 2010). Specifically, the ingestion of garlic extract increased expression of duodenal P-glycoprotein to 131% (95% confidence interval [CI] 105–163%) and negatively correlated with changes to the average area under the plasma concentration curve of saquinavir, which decreased to 85% (95% CI 66–109%).

Another clinical study identified that co-administration of garlic did not significantly alter warfarin pharmacokinetics or pharmacodynamics in healthy volunteers who had taken a single dose of 25 mg warfarin administered after 2 weeks of pretreatment with garlic (Mohammed Abdul et al 2008).

Quality of life

A small open-label study observed the effect of a Japanese garlic extract supplement (Aomori) 500 mg daily on 17 active workers with significant improvements in self-assessed stress, sleep quality, fatigue, dehydroepiandrosterone sulfate and cortisol awakening response, as measurements of improved quality of life (Ohiro et al 2013).

G

CLINICAL USE

The use of garlic to treat a variety of conditions is supported by several authorities. Treatment of atherosclerosis, arterial vascular disease, blood lipids, respiratory tract infections and catarrhal conditions has been indicated by the European Scientific Cooperative on Phytotherapy (ESCOP). Treatment of hyperlipidaemia and age-related vascular changes with garlic is supported by the expert German panel, the Commission E, while the World Health Organization (WHO) also reports that there are sufficient clinical data to indicate the use of garlic in hyperlipidaemia, age-dependent atherosclerosis and mild hypertension. Many different dietary forms and commercial preparations of garlic have been tested in clinical trials and several meta-analyses have been published to further aid our understanding of its role in practice.

Cardiovascular disease

Epidemiological studies show an inverse correlation between garlic consumption and progression of CVD in general (Rahman & Lowe 2006). Several intervention studies have also been published producing promising results for various forms of garlic treatment.

A double-blind, placebo-controlled study of 167 patients with hyperlipidaemia demonstrated that Allicor was effective in reducing the 10-year absolute multifactorial risk of cardiovascular diseases (Sobenin et al 2005). Garlic was also found to reduce the 10-year risk of acute MI and sudden death in a double-blind, placebo-controlled study of 51 patients with coronary artery disease receiving Allicor for a 12-month period (Sobenin et al 2007).

Previously, Koscielny et al (1999) conducted a long-term randomised, double-blind, placebo-controlled trial involving 152 volunteers to determine whether garlic powder supplements (Kwai 900 mg daily) directly alter plaque volumes in carotid and/or femoral arteries. After 4 years' treatment, garlic intake significantly reduced the expected increase in arteriosclerotic plaque volume by 5–18%, with a slight regression also observed. A subsequent re-evaluation of the results found that significant effects were limited to women (Siegel & Klussendorf 2000).

In a multifactor prognostic evaluation of high-risk patients assessing risk of CHD, MI and sudden death, prolonged administration of Allicor significantly reduced multifactor risk of CHD in both genders. However, reduced risk of MI and sudden death was achieved significantly in men, but not in women (Sobenin et al 2005).

Long-term use of AGE (1200 mg/day) appears to retard calcification of coronary arteries according to a placebo-controlled, double-blind, randomised pilot study involving high-risk patients while on a stable course of statin and aspirin therapy (Budoff 2006). Active treatment slowed down progression of disease, as the study showed that patients on placebo (with statin baseline therapy) progressed at a rate of 22.2% per year compared to those also taking AGE, who had a reduced progression to 7.5%.

IN COMBINATION

In 2009 Budoff et al reported on a well-designed double-blind randomised controlled trial (RCT) of 65 intermediate-risk patients taking statin medication and presenting with subclinical atherosclerosis coronary artery disease. Subjects were treated with a capsule containing 250 mg of AGE, B_{12} 100 mcg, folic acid 300 mcg, B_6 12.5 mg and l-arginine 100 mg or placebo daily for 1 year. The treatment group achieved significantly favourable changes in oxidative biomarkers, vascular factors and reduced progression of atherosclerosis. In 2012, results of an RCT once again found that coronary artery calcification could be significantly decreased with AGE (1200 mg/day), this time used together with coenzyme Q10 (120 mg/day) for 1 year. The placebo-controlled study involved 65 intermediate-risk firemen and found both coronary artery calcium and C-reactive protein significantly decreased with active treatment compared to placebo ($P = 0.01$). Interestingly, only 24.4% of participants were on statin drugs (Zeb et al 2012).

Hypertension

The current clinical evidence indicates that garlic treatment has a slow-onset blood pressure-reducing effect when taken for approximately 12 weeks; however, it is difficult to quantify the size of effect. It has been tested as a stand-alone treatment or used together with standard antihypertensive medication to produce further reductions in blood pressure. Based on current clinical and preclinical research, the effectiveness of treatment is primarily determined by its content of SAC and ability to yield allicin, although other compounds may also be important.

An early meta-analysis reported in 1994 analysing results from seven trials using Kwai 600–900 mg daily showed a mean reduction of 7.7 mmHg for SBP and 5 mmHg for diastolic blood pressure (DBP) (Silagy & Neil 1994). Isolating the results of the two placebo-controlled trials involving hypertensive patients, the reduction in SBP was 11.1 mmHg and 6.5 mmHg reduction in DBP with garlic treatment.

In 2000, the Agency for Health Care Research and Quality analysed results from 27 randomised, placebo-controlled trials and reported that results were mixed, with occasional small reductions reported (Mulrow et al 2000).

In contrast, in 2008 Reinhart et al analysed 10 clinical trials, reporting that garlic reduced blood pressure in patients with an elevated SBP, but not in those with normal SBP. The same year, Ried et al (2008) conducted a meta-analysis of 11 randomised placebo-controlled trials ($n = 1298$) and concluded that garlic preparations are superior to placebo in reducing SBP and DBP in normotensive people and those with hypertension (Ried et al 2008).

In 2012, a Cochrane systematic review confirmed that garlic treatment reduces blood pressure when compared to placebo; however, the magnitude of this effect cannot be accurately quantified. The review analysed the results of two studies ($n = 87$) which met the entry criteria of being randomised, blinded, controlled to treatment, including intention-to-treat data and involving only participants with primary hypertension. One of the included studies reported that 12 weeks of treatment with 200 mg garlic powder (Kwai) three times daily reduced supine

SBP by 10–12 mmHg and DBP by 5–9 mmHg and significantly reduced standing SBP by 21 mmHg (from 171 to 150 mmHg) and DBP by 11 mmHg (from 101 to 90 mmHg) (Auer et al 1990). The other study found that 12 weeks' treatment with two capsules of 100 mg high-potency garlic powder taken three times daily produced a statistically significant mean reduction in supine SBP of 16 mmHg (from 178 to 162 mmHg) and supine DBP of 15 mmHg (from 100 to 85 mmHg). Treatment also produced a statistically significant mean reduction in standing SBP of 16 mmHg (from 174 to 158 mmHg) and standing DBP of 16 mmHg (from 99 to 83 mmHg) (Stabler et al 2012).

Due to the limited data available, the Cochrane systematic review was unable to determine whether garlic treatment reduced all-cause mortality, cardiovascular events or cerebrovascular events in hypertensive patients (Stabler et al 2012).

Since then, three further randomised trials have been published. An RCT of 50 participants with uncontrolled hypertension taking standard treatment were given additional AGE 960 mg (standardised to 2.4 mg SAC) or placebo and found active treatment produced a significant reduction in SBP after 12 weeks for people with baseline SBP > 140 mmHg ($P = 0.036$). There was no significant reduction seen across the whole treatment group, which also consisted of people with SBP < 140 mmHg (Ried et al 2010).

In 2013 the same authors published results of a double-blind, randomised trial comparing three different dosages (240/480/960 mg containing 0.6/1.2/2.4 mg SAC) of AGE (Kyolic aged garlic; extract: High Potency Everyday Formula 112; Wakunaga/Wagner) plus regular treatment in 79 subjects with uncontrolled systolic hypertension. Similar to previous studies, SBP was significantly lowered after 12 weeks of treatment by 11.8 ± 5.4 mmHg compared with placebo ($P = 0.006$). The effect was only seen in the groups taking at least 480 mg daily. Interestingly, the hypotensive effect did not occur in all patients and ranged from −40 mmHg to +5 mmHg across all groups; however this study was unable to predict responder characteristics. Mild gastrointestinal side effects were reported, mainly in the highest-dose group (Ried et al 2013).

A traditional Japanese garlic homogenate (300 mg/day)-supplemented diet was compared to placebo in a randomised, double-blind study involving 81 participants with prehypertension or mild hypertension. Once again, treatment for 12 weeks induced significant reductions in SBP (−6.6 mmHg to −7.5 mmHg) and DBP (−4.6 mmHg to −5.2 mmHg) compared to placebo with no major side effects. Importantly, the effect was only clinically relevant in subjects with hypertension (Nakasone et al 2013).

Hyperlipidaemia

The most recent meta-analyses confirm that long-term garlic treatment modestly reduces total cholesterol levels. Garlic powder capsules (mainly Kwai) are the most-studied preparation; however the AGE preparations appear to have slightly stronger cholesterol-lowering activity than the powder forms.

In 2000, a meta-analysis of 13 clinical trials concluded that garlic reduces total cholesterol levels significantly more than placebo; however, the effects can only be described as modest (Stevinson et al 2001). The same year, a systematic review and meta-analysis were published by the Agency for Health Care Research and Quality, which analysed results from 44 studies with lipid outcomes (Mulrow et al 2000). Most studies involved fewer than 100 volunteers and randomisation techniques were unclear in 82% of the studies. Pooled data from the placebo-controlled trials reporting changes in total cholesterol levels found a significant average reduction in total cholesterol levels of 7.2 mg/dL after 4–6 weeks, using any form of garlic, and a reduction of 17.1 mg/dL at 8–12 weeks. Results at

20–24 weeks were not significant and thought to be due to low statistical power, fewer long-term studies or a time-dependent effect of garlic.

Two meta-analyses have been published more recently. The first, in 2012, analysed results from 26 RCTs and did not discriminate between preparation or dose, finding that total cholesterol and triglycerides were significantly reduced ($P = 0.001$), with the most marked outcomes seen in people with higher triglyceride levels and long-term interventions. The most-studied preparation was garlic powder, mainly Kwai brand, with doses ranging from 600 to 900 mg, whereas four studies used garlic oil and three studies used AGE. The duration of treatment ranged from 2 weeks to 1 year and no other lipid parameters were affected. Further, the review surmises that total cholesterol is most affected by aged garlic and powdered garlic, while triglycerides were most affected by powdered preparations (Zeng et al 2012).

In 2013, Ried et al published a meta-analysis of 37 RCTs ($n = 2,298$) which produced similar results: a significant cholesterol-lowering effect of garlic preparations compared with placebo and that the cholesterol-lowering treatment effect was more pronounced in trials of longer duration. The best effects were obtained when the intervention was used for longer than 12 weeks. More specifically, interventions >2 months in those with total cholesterol >200 mg/dL (~5.2 mmol/L) had significant reductions in total cholesterol by 17 ± 6 mg, reduction in LDL cholesterol by 9 ± 6 mg/dL, only marginal improvements in HDL cholesterol (1.5 ± 1.3 mg/dL) and no significant improvement in triglycerides. Subgroup analysis by single type of garlic preparation suggested a greater cholesterol-lowering effect for AGE than for garlic powder, and a borderline effect for garlic oil, The effect of garlic on HDL cholesterol levels was significant but small and most pronounced for garlic oil and the effect on triglycerides was non-significant overall (Ried et al 2013).

Comparative studies

Two clinical studies have compared different garlic preparations with pharmaceutical cholesterol-lowering medicines. Garlic taken as 300 mg three times daily (Kwai) produced similar lipid-lowering effects to 200 mg Bezafibrate (a hypolipidaemic fibrate) three times daily in subjects with primary hyperlipidaemia (Holzgartner et al 1992), whereas Clofibrate 500 mg was more effective than an essential oil extract of 50 g raw garlic (Arora & Arora 1981). The administration of 600 mg of fish oil with 500 mg of garlic pearls (garlic oil) per day to 16 hypercholesterolaemic subjects with a total cholesterol above 220 mg/dL for 60 days was found to reduce total cholesterol, LDL, serum triglyceride and very-low-density lipoprotein (Jeyaraj et al 2005).

Commission E approves the use of garlic as an adjunct to dietary changes in the treatment of hyperlipidaemia (Blumenthal 2000).

Clinical note — Not all garlic preparations are the same

One of the difficulties encountered when interpreting the research available for garlic is comparing the effects of different preparations, which often have not been tested for the presence of important constituents or allicin-releasing potential. It is known that fresh garlic and dried garlic powder contain alliin. When cut, crushed, chewed or dehydrated, the enzyme allinase is rapidly released, which allows the biotransformation of alliin to active organo-sulfur compounds. Some other forms may only contain alliin, and not the necessary alliinase component, thus compromising allicin-releasing potential. An example of the manufacturing process affecting potency has been suggested for a commercial garlic product known as Kwai, which has often been used in cholesterol research (Lawson et al 2001). According to a 2001 experiment, substantial differences were found between tablets manufactured before 1993 (the years when all but one of the positive trials were conducted) and those manufactured after 1993 (the years when all of the negative trials were conducted). Kwai products manufactured after 1993 released only one-third as much allicin as older preparations. Those preparations from before 1993 disintegrated more slowly, protecting alliinase from acid exposure and inactivation.

Diabetes mellitus (plus hyperlipidaemia)

Garlic may be of benefit to people with diabetes, according to the available clinical research; however mixed results hamper the interpretation of results.

In the 1990s, one double-blind study reported that 800 mg garlic powder taken daily for a period of 4 weeks reduced blood glucose concentrations by 11.6% (Kiesewetter et al 1993b); however, another study using a higher dose of 3 g/day over 26 weeks found no effects (Ali & Thomson 1995).

Ten years later, a 12-week, placebo-controlled, single-blind, randomised study found that treatment with a garlic tablet (Garlex: Bosch Pharmaceuticals, 300 mg, containing 1.3% allicin) twice daily, together with a diet and exercise plan, resulted in a significant reduction in total cholesterol of 28 mg/dL (12.03%) compared to placebo (Ashraf et al 2005). The study involved 70 patients with type 2 diabetes and newly diagnosed dyslipidaemia.

The metabolic action of Allicor (INAT-Farma, Russia) was investigated in a 4-week, double-blind, placebo-controlled study of 60 type 2 diabetic patients taken off their hypoglycaemic medication. Active treatment resulted in better metabolic control compared to placebo as measured by several parameters. In particular, a significant decrease in serum triglyceride levels was observed after 3 weeks of treatment, and by the end of the study the difference from baseline levels accounted for 36% ($P < 0.05$). Additionally, fasting blood glucose levels decreased and were maintained at the mean levels below 7.0 mmol/L during the whole study period whereas they began to rise in the placebo group (Sobenin et al 2008). Allicor contains 150 mg of dehydrated garlic powder in a slow-release form and the dose used was 300 mg twice daily.

In contrast, a short-term double-blind placebo-controlled crossover trial of 26 people with type 2 diabetes found no change in endothelial function, vascular inflammation, insulin resistance or oxidative stress when 1200 mg of AGE was added to usual treatment for 4 weeks followed by a 4-week washout period (Atkin 2011).

In the past few years, several more clinical studies have been published, one comparing garlic to metformin and others adding garlic to metformin treatment to see if further benefits develop.

A single-blind placebo-controlled, escalating dose study was conducted with 210 people with type 2 diabetes comparing the effects of garlic 300, 600, 900, 1200, 1500 mg, metformin and placebo for 24 weeks. Results showed significant effects ($P < 0.005$) for both fasting blood sugar and HbA_{1C} with the higher garlic doses (1200 and 1500 mg) compared to placebo, both being comparable to metformin (Phil et al 2011).

Adjunctive therapy to metformin

An RCT involving 60 participants taking metformin 500 mg twice daily compared the addition of garlic 300 mg three times daily or placebo over a 24-week test period. Results showed that adding garlic to the treatment induced an improvement in both glycaemic control and cholesterol markers ($P < 0.005$) compared to placebo (Ashraf et al 2011). Most recently an open-label study of 60 obese patients with type 2 diabetes compared the effects of stand-alone metformin 500 mg twice daily to metformin and garlic 250 mg twice daily for 12 weeks. Combination treatment resulted in significantly improved postprandial blood glucose levels ($P < 0.001$), total cholesterol, triglycerides, LDL ($P < 0.05$), adenosine deaminase ($P < 0.01$) and C-reactive protein ($P < 0.05$); however changes in HbA_{1C} were not significantly different between the two groups (Kumar et al 2013).

Antiplatelet effects

Antiplatelet effects of garlic are well recognised, but the dose at which this becomes significant remains uncertain. Results from a 1996 double-blind study have identified a dose of 7.2 g/day of AGE as significantly inhibiting platelet aggregation and adhesion (Steiner et al 1996). In contrast, a double-blind, placebo-controlled crossover study of 14 volunteers concluded that solvent-extracted garlic oil had minimal or no effect on platelet aggregation. Researchers found that administration of garlic 9.9 g over 4 hours exerted little or no effect on both collagen and ADP-induced aggregation. Adrenaline-induced aggregation did, however, exert a slight but significant ($P < 0.05$; 12) reduction (Wojcikowski et al 2007).

Peripheral arterial occlusive disease

In 2000, Mulrow et al reported on two double-blind placebo-controlled trials in participants with atherosclerotic lower-extremity disease. One study of 64 participants showed that pain-free walking distance increased by approximately 40 m with standardised dehydrated garlic (Kwai 800 mg daily), compared with approximately 30 m with placebo over 12 weeks. The other study of 100 participants (Mulrow et al 2000) showed that a combination treatment of garlic oil macerate/soya lecithin/hawthorn oil/wheatgerm oil significantly increased the maximum walking distance (114%) compared to placebo (17%) ($P < 0.05$). A 2008 Cochrane review found only one study meeting quality criteria and having a diagnosis of peripheral vascular atherosclerosis. The study included 78 participants, with garlic powder coated tablets 200 mg twice a day being no better than placebo for measured outcomes of walking distance and subjective symptoms after 12 weeks (Jepson et al 2008).

Infection

Garlic oil is effective against numerous bacteria, viruses and fungi, including *Staphylococcus aureus*, methicillin-resistant *Staphylococcus aureus* and several species of *Candida*, *Aspergillus* and *Cryptococcus neoformans* in vitro (Davis et al 1994, Tsao & Yin 2001, Yoshida et al 1987). As such, it has been used both internally and externally to treat various infections and prevent wound infection.

Tinea pedis, tinea corporis, tinea cruris

A trial comparing the effects of three different strengths of ajoene cream (0.4%, 0.6% and 1%) with 1% terbinafine applied twice daily found the cure rate to be 72% for 0.6% ajoene, 100% for 1% ajoene and 94% for 1% terbinafine after 60 days (Ledezma et al 2000).

Vaginitis

Taken internally as a 'natural antibiotic' or applied topically in a cream base, garlic is used to treat vaginitis. The considerable antibacterial activity of garlic provides a theoretical basis for its use in this condition, but controlled studies are not available to determine its effectiveness.

Common cold prevention

A 12-week, double-blind, randomised study involving 146 people demonstrated that allicin-containing garlic preparations significantly reduce the incidence of colds and accelerate recovery compared with placebo (Josling 2001). More specifically, the number of symptom days in the placebo group was 5.01 compared with 1.52 days in the garlic-treated group. Additionally, garlic reduced the incidence of developing a second cold, whereas placebo did not. These results were similar to those reported in a randomised, double-blind, placebo-controlled parallel intervention study of 120 participants given AGE 2.56 g/day for 90 days. At day 45 γδ T-cell and natural killer cell proliferation were significantly increased, and at day 90 there was no change in cold and flu incidence between the two groups; however the treatment group had fewer symptoms (21%), fewer sick days (58%) and fewer days lost from school/work (58%) than placebo (Nantz et al 2012).

G

Helicobacter pylori infection

It has been suggested that gastrointestinal lesions, such as gastric ulcers, duodenal ulcers and gastric cancers, are strongly associated with *H. pylori* infection (Scheiman & Cutler 1999). Medical treatment consisting of 'triple therapy' has a high eradication rate, yet is associated with side effects and has started to give rise to antibiotic resistance. Since garlic intake has been associated with a lowered incidence of stomach cancer, researchers have started investigating whether garlic has activity against *H. pylori*. Several in vitro and in vivo tests have shown garlic to be effective against *H. pylori* (see section on Main actions, above). However, to date only a few small clinical trials have been conducted, with disappointing and controversial results (Aydin et al 2000, Graham et al 1999, McNulty et al 2001).

A small pilot study of dyspeptic patients with confirmed *H. pylori* infection found that treatment with 4 mg garlic oil capsules taken four times daily with meals for 14 days did not alter symptoms or lead to *H. pylori* eradication (McNulty et al 2001). Another small study using garlic oil 275 mg three times a day (allicin 800 mcg/capsule) either as stand-alone treatment or in combination with omeprazole (20 mg twice daily) found that both treatments produced similar results (Aydin et al 2000). These results were confirmed in another small clinical study (Graham et al 1999).

Protective effects against cancer

Whether long-term garlic consumption reduces the risk of cancer is uncertain. A 2001 critical review of the epidemiological evidence suggests a preventive effect for garlic consumption in stomach and colorectal cancers, but not other cancers (Fleischauer & Arab 2001). With regard to gastric cancer protection, case-control studies suggested a protective effect for raw and/or cooked garlic when eaten at least once a week, whereas protective effects against colorectal cancer seem to require at least two servings of garlic per week. A similar view was reported in a 2003 review by Ernst, which stated that the weight of evidence to support the use of allium vegetables, such as garlic, in cancer is clearly positive. However, a 2009 review of 19 human studies evaluated the evidence supporting a relationship between garlic intake and a reduction in risk of different cancers with respect to food labelling. No evidence was found to suggest that garlic consumption reduced the risk of gastric, breast, lung or endometrial cancer, with very limited evidence supporting a reduction in risk of colon, prostate, oesophageal, larynx, oral, ovary or renal cell cancers due to garlic consumption (Kim & Kwon 2009). This has been reinforced by a 2012 systematic review of RCTs that found no benefit in reducing risk of cancer (Ernst & Posadzki 2012). Additionally, a report on the Nurses' study and Health Professional follow-up study, which followed 76,208 women and 45,592 men for up to 24 years, found no benefit in either dietary garlic or garlic supplement use (Meng et al 2013). Data collected included those using up to one clove of garlic (or equivalent) per day and only 6% of participants used supplements, not enough to perform statistical analysis, and no information on dosage or preparation was collected.

In addition, the Cancer Prevention Study-II investigating colorectal cancer risk in the nutrition cohort of 42,824 men and 56,876 women, whose garlic use was tracked for 7 years, indicated at best a weak protective effect in women, and a slight increase in risk for men (McCullough et al 2012).

Intervention study in colorectal cancer

A preliminary double-blind, randomised clinical trial in patients with colorectal adenomas — precancerous lesions of the large bowel — produced promising results with the use of high-dose AGE 2.4 mL/day (Tanaka et al 2006). The study of 51 patients measured the number and size of adenomas at baseline and at 6 and 12 months and found that AGE significantly suppressed both the size and the number of colon adenomas in patients after 1 year of treatment ($P = 0.04$). In comparison, the number of adenomas increased linearly in the control group from the beginning.

A systematic review of scientific evidence from all studies conducted over the last decade that examined the effects of garlic on colorectal cancer was conducted. Five of eight case-control/cohort studies suggested that a high intake of raw/cooked garlic produced a chemoprotective effect. Review of 11 animal studies showed a significant anticarcinogenic effect of garlic. Overall, the authors concluded that there was consistent scientific evidence derived from RCT animal studies, despite heterogeneity of human epidemiological studies (Ngo et al 2007).

Endometrial cancer

Analysis of data from a multicentre, case-control study of 454 endometrial cancer cases and 908 controls found a moderately protective role for allium vegetables on the risk of endometrial cancer, with a significant inverse trend identified for high intakes of garlic (Galeone et al 2008). Topical application of garlic-derived ajoene to tumours of 21 patients with either nodular or superficial basal cell carcinoma resulted in reduction in tumour size in 17 patients. Chemical assays prior to and posttreatment showed a significant decrease in the expression of the apoptosis suppression protein Bcl-2 (Tilli et al 2003).

OTHER USES

Some early research suggests that garlic may prevent the incidence of altitude sickness (Fallon et al 1998, Kim-Park & Ku 2000) and reduce mosquito numbers (Jarial 2001).

A small Indian trial randomly assigned 41 patients with hepatopulmonary syndrome to receive garlic oil capsules (1–2 $g/m^2/day$) or placebo in divided doses over a period of 18 months, with monthly evaluations. After 9 months there was a 24.7% increase in baseline arterial oxygen levels ($P < 0.001$) compared to a 7.4% increase in placebo. There was a 28.4% decrease in the alveolar-arterial oxygen gradient ($P < 0.001$) and a 10.7% reduction in placebo, which was significantly better than placebo ($P < 0.001$). Hepatopulmonary syndrome was reversed in 66.7% of patients in the treatment group compared to 5% in placebo (intention to treat) and at 18-month follow-up two had died in the treatment group compared to seven in the placebo group (De Binay et al 2010). This is an interesting study looking at a condition widely believed to be associated with increased NO production in liver cirrhosis.

DOSAGE RANGE

General guide

- Fresh garlic: 2–5 g/day (ensure it is bruised, crushed or chewed).
- Dried powder: 0.4–1.2 g/day.
- AGEs have been studied in amounts ranging from 2.4 to 7.2 g/day.
- Oil: 2–5 mg/day.
- Garlic preparations that will provide 4–12 mg alliin daily.
- Fluid extract (1 : 1): 0.5–2 mL three times daily.

According to clinical studies

- Type 2 diabetes: Allicor 300 mg twice daily.
- Hypertension: AGE: 480–960 mg standardised to SAC 4.8 mg/day in divided doses and taken for at least 12 weeks to see maximal results.
- Hyperlipidaemia: 600–900 mg/day.
- Hyperglycaemia: 1200–1500 mg/day.
- Fungal infection: topical 0.4–0.6% ajoene cream applied twice daily.
- Occlusive arterial disease: 600–800 mg/day.

It is important to be aware of the thiosulfinate content, in particular the allicin-releasing ability, of any commercial product to ensure efficacy.

ADVERSE REACTIONS

Internal use

Side effects tend to be limited to mild gastrointestinal side effects such as bloating, reflux, flatulence, garlic odour and breath. A dose–response study with hypertensive subjects found 32% of people using AGE at a dose of 960 mg daily experienced mild gastrointestinal side effects compared to 15% taking 480 mg daily. These effects were minimised by taking the garlic treatment in the morning (Ried et al 2013). Others have reported garlic odour and breath, allergic reactions, nausea, abdominal discomfort and diarrhoea (Berthold & Sudhop 1998). These side effects are more common when garlic is taken on an empty stomach and at doses greater than 1 g.

Headache, myalgia and fatigue were reported in one study using a dose of 900 mg garlic powder (standardised to 1.3% alliin) (Holzgartner et al 1992).

A meta-analysis of 37 RCTs investigating garlic for lipid lowering found no changes in liver function, biochemistry or haematology with use (Ried et al 2013).

Topical use

An ajoene 0.6% gel produces a transient burning sensation after application, according to one study (Ledezma et al 1999). Garlic has been classified as a type 1 allergen with various reactions, including contact dermatitis, urticaria, asthma, pemphigus and anaphylaxis, being reported. DADS, allylpropyl disulfide and allylmercaptin have been identified as allergens (Tsai et al 2012).

SIGNIFICANT INTERACTIONS

Saquinavir, darunavir and ritonavir

Ritonavir toxicity has been reported in AIDS patients co-administering with garlic, most likely due to P-glycoprotein inhibition by allicin in garlic (Tsai et al 2012) — avoid using concurrently (Piscitelli et al 2002).

Anticoagulants

Theoretically, a pharmacodynamic interaction is possible when using garlic at high doses (>7 g), in excess of usual dietary amounts; however, results from clinical studies cast doubt on this proposition. Published clinical studies have identified no significant action of enteric-coated or aged garlic on warfarin pharmacodynamics or pharmacokinetics. A double-blind, randomised, placebo-controlled pilot study of 48 patients demonstrated that the concomitant use of garlic containing 14.7 mg/day of SAC and warfarin showed no adverse effects (Macan et al 2006). An open-label, three-treatment, randomised, crossover clinical trial involving 12 healthy males, investigating potential effects of garlic and cranberry on warfarin (25 mg single dose), found that two garlic tablets daily containing 2000 mg of fresh garlic bulb equivalent to 3.71 mg of allicin per tablet did not significantly alter warfarin's pharmacokinetics or pharmacodynamics (Mohammed Abdul et al 2008). Use caution with doses >7 g/day.

Antiplatelet drugs

Theoretically, a pharmacodynamic interaction is possible when using garlic at high doses in excess of usual dietary amounts, although a small clinical study involving 10 adult participants showed garlic had no effect on platelet function (Beckert et al 2007). Observe.

Antihypertensive agents

Theoretically, potentiation effects are possible when using garlic at high doses in excess of usual dietary amounts — this can be used as adjunctive therapy to produce beneficial results — observe.

Antihyperlipidaemic agents

Theoretically, potentiation effects are possible when using garlic at high doses in excess of usual dietary amounts — this can be used as adjunctive therapy to produce beneficial results — observe.

Helicobacter pylori triple therapy

Additive effects are theoretically possible. While it is prudent to observe the patient for adverse reactions, the interaction may be beneficial.

Hepatotoxic drugs

Garlic may exert hepatoprotective activity against liver damage induced by drugs, according to in vitro tests, which suggest a beneficial interaction.

Paracetamol

In vivo protection from garlic and ajoene on paracetamol-induced hepatotoxicity has been observed (Hsu et al 2006) — beneficial interaction.

Hydrochlorothiazide
Co-administration may require a reduction in the dose of hydrochlorothiazide due to a pharmacokinetic interaction raising drug serum levels (Asdaq & Inamdar 2009). Cautious use under medical supervision.

CONTRAINDICATIONS AND PRECAUTIONS

Patients with bleeding abnormalities should avoid high doses of garlic. Although usual dietary intakes are likely to be safe prior to major surgery, suspend the use of high-dose garlic supplements 1 week before, as there is a theoretical increased risk of bleeding.

Avoid if known allergy to sulfurous vegetables. If being used as part of a topical application, a test patch is advised before more widespread application.

G

Practice points/Patient counselling

- Garlic is both a food and a therapeutic medicine capable of significant and varied pharmacological activity.
- It has antioxidant, antimicrobial, modest antiplatelet, antithrombotic, anti-atherosclerotic and vasoprotective activities.
- Human research confirms that some garlic preparations lower total cholesterol levels and blood pressure and possibly blood glucose levels in people with type 2 diabetes.
- It also enhances microcirculation and may have anti-inflammatory and immunostimulant activities.
- Garlic is used as a treatment for many common infections, to reduce the incidence of colds, to improve peripheral circulation and to manage hyperlipidaemia and hypertension.
- Topical garlic preparations have been used to treat common fungal infections.
- Several important drug interactions are possible with garlic (see significant interactions, above).

PREGNANCY USE

Garlic is not recommended at doses greater than usual dietary intakes in the first trimester until safety can be confirmed. A small trial in 100 pre-eclamptic primigravida women prescribed 800 mg of a dried garlic powder supplement throughout the third trimester reported no side effects or unexpected birth outcomes (Ziaei et al 2001).

PATIENTS' FAQs

What will this herb do for me?
Garlic has many different actions in the body and is used to treat conditions such as elevated blood pressure and cholesterol levels, poor peripheral circulation, higher than normal blood glucose levels and common infections such as the

common cold, flu and athlete's foot. Research suggests that it may be effective in all of these conditions; however, in some cases, the effect is small.

When will it start to work?

This varies greatly, depending on the reason for use. For example, garlic has been shown to improve microcirculation within 5 hours of ingestion, whereas slowing down of the atherosclerotic process or cancer-protective effects are likely to require several years' continuous use.

Are there any safety issues?

When garlic is taken at doses above the usual dietary levels, it may interact with a number of medications. Also, it should not be taken by people with bleeding disorders.

REFERENCES

Ali M, Thomson M. Consumption of a garlic clove a day could be beneficial in preventing thrombosis. Prostaglandins Leukot Essent Fatty Acids 53.3 (1995): 211–212.

Alkreathy, H., et al. Aged garlic extract protects against doxorubicin-induced cardiotoxicity in rats. Food and chemical toxicology 48 (2010) 951–956.

Alkreathy, H.M., et al. Mechanisms of cardioprotective effect of aged garlic extract against doxorubicin induced cardiotoxicity. Integrative Cancer Therapies 11.4 (2012): 364–370.

Allison GL, Lowe GM, Rahman K. Aged garlic extract may inhibit aggregation in human platelets by suppressing calcium mobilization. J Nutr 136 (3 Suppl) (2006): 789S–792S.

Al-Qattan KK et al. Nitric oxide mediates the blood-pressure lowering effect of garlic in the rat two-kidney, one-clip model of hypertension. J Nutr 136 (3 Suppl) (2006): 774S–776S.

Altonsy, M. O., T. N. Habib, and S. C. Andrews. Diallyl Disulfide-Induced Apoptosis in a Breast-Cancer Cell Line (MCF-7) may be caused by Inhibition of Histone Deacetylation. Nutrition and cancer 64.8 (2012): 1251–60.

An M et al. Allicin enhances the oxidative damage effect of amphotericin B against *Candida albicans*. Int J Antimicrob Agents 33.3 (2008): 258–263

An, MM et al. Allicin enhances the oxidative damage effect of amphotericin B against *Candida albicans*. International journal of antimicrobial agents 33.3 (2009): 258–263.

Andrianova IV, Fomchenkov IV, Orekhov AN. [Hypotensive effect of long-acting garlic tablets allicor (a double-blind placebo-controlled trial)]. Ter Arkh 74.3 (2002): 76–78.

Ankri S, Mirelman D. Antimicrobial properties of allicin from garlic. Microbes Infect 1.2 (1999): 125–129.

Arhan M et al. Hepatic oxidant/antioxidant status in cholesterol-fed rabbits: effects of garlic extract. Hepatol Res 39.1 (2009): 70–77.

Arora RC, Arora S. Comparative effect of clofibrate, garlic and onion on alimentary hyperlipemia. Atherosclerosis 39.4 (1981): 447–452.

Arunkumar A et al. Induction of apoptosis and histone hyperacetylation by diallyl disulfide in prostate cancer cell line PC-3. Cancer Lett 251.1 (2007): 59–67.

Arunkumar, R., et al. Effect of Diallyl Disulfide on Insulin-Like Growth Factor Signaling Molecules Involved in Cell Survival and Proliferation of Human Prostate Cancer Cells in Vitro and in Silico Approach through Docking Analysis. Phytomedicine 19.10 (2012): 912–23.

Asadpour, R., et al. Comparison of the Protective Effects of Garlic (*Allium sativum* L) Extract, Vitamin E and N Acetyl Cystein on Testis Structure and Sperm Quality in Rats Treated with Lead Acetate. Revue de Medecine Veterinaire 164.1 (2013): 28–33.

Asdaq, S. M. B., and M. N. Inamdar. The potential for interaction of hydochlorothiazide with Garlic in Rats. Chemico-biological Interactions 181 (2009):472–79.

Asdaq, S. M. & Inamdar, M. N. Potential of garlic and its active constituent, S-allyl cysteine, as antihypertensive and cardioprotective in presence of captopril. Phytomed. 17 (2010) 1016–26.

Ashraf R et al. Effects of garlic on dyslipidemia in patients with type 2 diabetes mellitus. J Ayub Med Coll Abbottabad 17.3 (2005): 60–64.

Ashraf, R., et al. Garlic (*Allium sativum*) supplementation with standard antidiabetic agent provides better diabetic control in type 2 diabetes patients. Pak J Pharm Sci. 24.4 (2011): 565–70.

Atkin, M. The effects of garlic upon endothelial function, vascular inflammation, oxidative stress and insulin resistance in patients with type 2 diabetes at high cardiovascular risk: a double blind randomised placebo controlled trial. Dissertation. University of Portsmouth, 2011.

Auer, W., Eiber, A., Hertkorn, E., et al. 1990. Hypertension and hyperlipidaemia: garlic helps in mild cases. Br J Clin. Pract. Suppl, 69, 3–6.

Augusti KT, Sheela CG. Antiperoxide effect of S-allyl cysteine sulfoxide, an insulin secretagogue, in diabetic rats. Experientia 52.2 (1996): 115–120.

Avci A et al. Effects of garlic consumption on plasma and erythrocyte antioxidant parameters in elderly subjects. Gerontology 54.3 (2008): 173–176

Avci, B., et al. Oxidative Stress Induced by 1.8 GHz Radio Frequency Electromagnetic Radiation and Effects of Garlic Extract in Rats. International journal of radiation biology 88.11 (2012): 7

Aydin A et al. Garlic oil and *Helicobacter pylori* infection. Am J Gastroenterol 95.2 (2000): 563–564.

Bakri IM, Douglas CW. Inhibitory effect of garlic extract on oral bacteria. Arch Oral Biol 50.7 (2005): 645–651.

Beckert BW et al. The effect of herbal medicines on platelet function: an in vivo experiment and review of the literature. Plast Reconstr Surg 120.7 (2007): 2044–2050.

Berthold HK, Sudhop T. Garlic preparations for prevention of atherosclerosis. Curr Opin Lipidol 9.6 (1998): 565–569.

Bianchini F, Vainio H. Allium vegetables and organosulfur compounds: do they help prevent cancer? Environ Health Perspect 109.9 (2001): 893–902.

Blumenthal M. Herbal medicine — expanded Commission E monographs. Newton: American Botanical Council, 2000.

Bordia A, Verma SK, Srivastava KC. Effect of garlic (*Allium sativum*) on blood lipids, blood sugar, fibrinogen and fibrinolytic activity in patients with coronary artery disease. Prostaglandins Leukot Essent Fatty Acids 58.4 (1998): 257–263.

Borek C. Garlic reduces dementia and heart-disease risk. J Nutr 136 (3 Suppl) (2006): 810S–812S.

Brady JF et al. Inhibition of cytochrome P-450 2E1 by diallyl sulfide and its metabolites. Chem Res Toxicol 4.6 (1991): 642–647.

Budoff M. Aged garlic extract retards progression of coronary artery calcification. J Nutr 136 (3 Suppl) (2006): 741S–744S.

Budoff, M. J., et al. Aged garlic extract supplemented with B vitamins, folic acid and L-arginine retards the progression of subclinical atherosclerosis: a randomized clinical trial. Preventive Medicine, 49(2), (2009). 101–107.

Campbell JH et al. Molecular basis by which garlic suppresses atherosclerosis. J Nutr 131.3s (2001): 1006S–1009S.

Cavagnaro PF et al. Effect of cooking on garlic (*Allium sativum* L.) antiplatelet activity and thiosulfinates content. J Agric Food Chem 55.4 (2007): 1280–1288.

Cellini L et al. Inhibition of *Helicobacter pylori* by garlic extract (*Allium sativum*). FEMS Immunol Med Microbiol 13.4 (1996): 273–277.

Chan KC, Yin MC, Chao WJ. Effect of diallyl trisulfide-rich garlic oil on blood coagulation and plasma activity of anticoagulation factors in rats. Food Chem Toxicol 45.3 (2007): 502–507.

Chandra-Kuntal, K., J. Lee, and S. V. Singh. Critical Role for Reactive Oxygen Species in Apoptosis Induction and Cell Migration Inhibition by Diallyl Trisulfide, a Cancer Chemopreventive Component of Garlic. Breast cancer research and treatment 138.1 (2013): 69–79.

Chandrashekar, P.M. Venkatesh, Y. P. Identification of the protein components displaying immunomodulatory activity in aged garlic extract. Journal of ethnopharmacology 124.3 (2009): 384–390.

Chandrashekar, P. M., Prashanth, K. V. H., and Venkatesh, Y. P. Isolation, structural elucidation and immunomodulatory activity of fructans from aged garlic extract. Phytochemistry 72.2 (2011): 255–264.

Chen C et al. Induction of detoxifying enzymes by garlic organosulfur compounds through transcription factor Nrf2: effect of chemical structure and stress signals. Free Radic Biol Med 37.10 (2004): 1578–1590.

Chiu, T. -H, et al. Diallyl Sulfide Promotes Cell-Cycle Arrest through the p53 Expression and Triggers Induction of Apoptosis Via Caspase- and Mitochondria-Dependent Signaling Pathways in Human Cervical Cancer Ca Ski Cells. Nutrition and cancer 65.3 (2013): 505–14.

Cho SJ, Rhee DK, Pyo S. Allicin, a major component of garlic, inhibits apoptosis of macrophage in a depleted nutritional state. Nutrition 22.11–12 (2006): 1177–1184.

Chowdhury R et al. In vitro and in vivo reduction of sodium arsenite induced toxicity by aqueous garlic extract. Food Chem Toxicol 46.2 (2008): 740–751.

Chung LY. The antioxidant properties of garlic compounds: allyl cysteine, alliin, allicin, and allyl disulfide. J Med Food 9.2 (2006): 205–213.

Chung, J. G., et al. Effects of garlic compounds diallyl sulfide and diallyl disulfide on arylamine N-acetyltransferase activity in strains of *Helicobacter pylori* from peptic ulcer patients. The American journal of Chinese medicine 26.03–04 (1998): 353–364.

Chutani SK, Bordia A. The effect of fried versus raw garlic on fibrinolytic activity in man. Atherosclerosis 38.3–4 (1981): 417–421.

Clement, F, Venkatesh YP. Dietary garlic (*Allium sativum*) lectins, ASA I and ASA II, are highly stable and immunogenic. International immunopharmacology 10.10 (2010): 1161–1169.

Clement F, Pramod SN, Venkatesh YP. Identity of the immunomodulatory proteins from garlic (*Allium sativum*) with the major garlic lectins or agglutinins. International Immunopharmacology 10.3 (2010): 316–324.

Coppi A et al. Antimalarial activity of allicin, a biologically active compound from garlic cloves. Antimicrob Agents Chemother 50.5 (2006): 1731–1737.

Cox MC et al. Influence of garlic (*Allium sativum*) on the pharmacokinetics of docetaxel. Clin Cancer Res 12.15 (2006): 4636–4640.

Dalvi RR. Alterations in hepatic phase I and phase II biotransformation enzymes by garlic oil in rats. Toxicol Lett 60.3 (1992): 299–305.

D'Argenio, G., et al. Garlic Extract Attenuating Rat Liver Fibrosis by Inhibiting TGF-β1. Clinical Nutrition 32.2 (2013): 252–8.

Dae Yun Seo, et al. Aged garlic extract enhances exercise-mediated improvement of metabolic parameters in high fat diet induced obese rats. Nutr Res Pract 6.6 (2012): 513–519.

Davis SR. An overview of the antifungal properties of allicin and its breakdown products – the possibility of a safe and effective antifungal prophylactic. Mycoses 48.2 (2005): 95–100.

Davis LE, Shen J, Royer RE. In vitro synergism of concentrated *Allium sativum* extract and amphotericin B against *Cryptococcus neoformans*. Planta Med 60.6 (1994): 546–549.

De Binay K., et al. The role of garlic in hepatopulmonary syndrome: a randomized controlled trial. Canadian Journal of Gastroenterology 24.3 (2010): 183.

Dhawan V, Jain S. Garlic supplementation prevents oxidative DNA damage in essential hypertension. Mol Cell Biochem 275.1–2 (2005): 85–94.

Dong, Q., et al. Stimulation of IFN-γ Production by Garlic Lectin in Mouse Spleen Cells: Involvement of IL-12 via Activation of p38 MAPK and ERK in Macrophages. Phytomedicine 18.4 (2011): 309–16.

Druesne N et al. Diallyl disulfide (DADS) increases histone acetylation and p21(waf1/cip1) expression in human colon tumor cell lines. Carcinogenesis 25.7 (2004): 1227–1236.

Duke Dr. Dr Duke's phytochemical and ethnobotanical database. Available online at: http://www.ars-grin. gov/duke/ (accessed 2003).

Durak I et al. Effects of garlic extract on oxidant/antioxidant status and atherosclerotic plaque formation in rabbit aorta. Nutr Metab Cardiovasc Dis 12.3 (2002): 141–147.

Eftekhari, Z., et al. Evaluating the Anti-Leech (*Limnatis nilotica*) Activity of Methanolic Extract of *Allium sativum* L. Compared with Levamisole and Metronidazole. Comparative Clinical Pathology 21.6 (2012): 1219–22.

Ehnert, S., et al. Diallyl-disulphide is the effective ingredient of garlic oil that protects primary human osteoblasts from damage due to cigarette smoke. Food Chemistry 132.2 (2012): 724–729.

Eidi A, Eidi M, Esmaeili E. Antidiabetic effect of garlic (*Allium sativum* L.) in normal and streptozotocin-induced diabetic rats. Phytomedicine 13.9–10 (2006): 624–629.

Eja ME et al. A comparative assessment of the antimicrobial effects of garlic (*Allium sativum*) and antibiotics on diarrheagenic organisms. Southeast Asian J Trop Med Public Health 38.2 (2007): 343–348.

El-Sabban F, Abouazra H. Effect of garlic on atherosclerosis and its factors. East Mediterr Health J 14.1 (2008): 195–205.

Engdal S, Klepp O, Nilsen OG. Identification and exploration of herb-drug combinations used by cancer patients. Integr Cancer Ther 8.1 (2009): 29–36.

Ernsberger P et al. Therapeutic actions of allylmercaptocaptopril and captopril in a rat model of metabolic syndrome. Am J Hypertens 20.8 (2007): 866–874.

Ernst, E. The current position of complementary/alternative medicine in cancer. European Journal of Cancer 39.16 (2003): 2273–2277.

Ernst, E., and P. Posadzki. Can Garlic-Intake Reduce the Risk of Cancer? A Systematic Review of Randomised Controlled Trials. Focus on Alternative and Complementary Therapies 17.4 (2012): 192–6.

Fallah-Rostami, F., et al. "Immunomodulatory Activity of Aged Garlic Extract Against Implanted Fibrosarcoma Tumor in Mice." North American Journal of Medical Sciences 5.3 (2013): 207–12.

Fallon MB et al. Garlic prevents hypoxic pulmonary hypertension in rats. Am J Physiol 275.2 (Pt 1) (1998): L283–L287.

Fani MM, Kohanteb J, Dayaghi M. Inhibitory activity of garlic (*Allium sativum*) extract on multidrug-resistant *Streptococcus mutans*. J Indian Soc Pedod Prev Dent 25.4 (2007): 164–168.

Feng, Y., et al. Allicin Enhances Host Pro-Inflammatory Immune Responses and Protects Against Acute Murine Malaria Infection. Malaria Journal 11 (2012) 10–1186.

Ferri N et al. Ajoene, a garlic compound, inhibits protein prenylation and arterial smooth muscle cell proliferation. Br J Pharmacol 138.5 (2003): 811–8118.

Fisher CD et al. Induction of drug-metabolizing enzymes by garlic and allyl sulfide compounds via activation of constitutive androstane receptor and nuclear factor E2 related factor 2. Drug Metab Dispos 35.6 (2007): 995–1000.

Fleischauer AT, Arab L. Garlic and cancer: a critical review of the epidemiologic literature. J Nutr 131.3s (2001): 1032S–1040S.

Foster BC et al. An in vitro evaluation of human cytochrome P450 3A4 and P-glycoprotein inhibition by garlic. J Pharm Pharm Sci 4.2 (2001): 176–184.

Frantz DJ et al. Cell cycle arrest and differential gene expression in HT-29 cells exposed to an aqueous garlic extract. Nutr Cancer 38.2 (2000): 255–264.

Fukao H et al. Antithrombotic effects of odorless garlic powder both in vitro and in vivo. Biosci Biotechnol Biochem 71.1 (2007): 84–90.

Gaafar, MR. Efficacy of *Allium sativum* (garlic) against experimental cryptosporidiosis. Alexandria Journal of Medicine 48.1 (2012): 59–66.

Gadkari JV, Joshi VD. Effect of ingestion of raw garlic on serum cholesterol level, clotting time and fibrinolytic activity in normal subjects. J Postgrad Med 37.3 (1991): 128–131.

Galeone C et al. Allium vegetables intake and endometrial cancer risk. Public Health Nutr (2008): 1–4.

Gapter LA, Yuin OZ, Ng KY. S-Allylcysteine reduces breast tumor cell adhesion and invasion. Biochem Biophys Res Commun 367.2 (2008): 446–451.

Ghazanfari T, Hassan ZM, Khamesipour A. Enhancement of peritoneal macrophage phagocytic activity against *Leishmania major* by garlic (*Allium sativum*) treatment. J Ethnopharmacol 103.3 (2006): 333–337.

Gonen A et al. The antiatherogenic effect of allicin: possible mode of action. Pathobiology 72.6 (2005): 325–334.

Gorinstein S et al. Dose-dependent influence of commercial garlic (*Allium sativum*) on rats fed cholesterol-containing diet. J Agric Food Chem 54.11 (2006): 4022–4027.

Gorinstein S et al. The atherosclerotic heart disease and protecting properties of garlic: contemporary data. Mol Nutr Food Res 51.11 (2007): 1365–1381.

Graham DY, Anderson SY, Lang T. Garlic or jalapeno peppers for treatment of *Helicobacter pylori* infection. Am J Gastroenterol 94.5 (1999): 1200–1202.

Greenblatt DJ, Leigh-Pemberton RA, von Moltke LL. In vitro interactions of water-soluble garlic components with human cytochromes p450. J Nutr 136 (3 Suppl) (2006): 806S–809S.

Groppo FC et al. Antimicrobial activity of garlic against oral streptococci. Int J Dent Hyg 5.2 (2007): 109–115.

Gupta VB, Rao KS. Anti-amyloidogenic activity of S-allyl-L-cysteine and its activity to destabilize Alzheimer's beta-amyloid fibrils in vitro. Neurosci Lett 429.2–3 (2007): 75–80.

Gupta VB, Indi SS, Rao KS. Garlic extract exhibits antiamyloidogenic activity on amyloid-beta fibrillogenesis: relevance to Alzheimer's disease. Phytother Res 23.1 (2009): 111–115.

Gurley BJ et al. Cytochrome P450 phenotypic ratios for predicting herb–drug interactions in humans. Clin Pharmacol Ther 72.3 (2002): 276–287.

Gurley BJ et al. Clinical assessment of effects of botanical supplementation on cytochrome P450 phenotypes in the elderly: St John's wort, garlic oil, Panax ginseng and Ginkgo biloba. Drugs Aging 22.6 (2005): 525–539.

Hajda, J., Rentsch, K.M., Gubler, C., et al. 2010. Garlic extract induces intestinal P-glycoprotein, but exhibits no effect on intestinal and hepatic CYP3A4 in humans. Eur.J Pharm.Sci., 41, (5) 729–735.

Harauma A, Moriguchi T. Aged garlic extract improves blood pressure in spontaneously hypertensive rats more safely than raw garlic. J Nutr 136 (3 Suppl) (2006): 769S–73S.
Hassan HT. Ajoene (natural garlic compound): a new anti-leukaemia agent for AML therapy. Leuk Res 28.7 (2004): 667–671.
Hassan A., et al. Garlic oil as a modulating agent for oxidative stress and neurotoxicity induced by sodium nitrite in male albino rats. Food and Chemical Toxicology 48 (2010): 1980–1985.
Hattori A et al. Antidiabetic effects of ajoene in genetically diabetic KK-A(y) mice. Tokyo: J Nutr Sci Vitaminol, 51.5 (2005): 382–40.
Herman-Antosiewicz A, Singh SV. Checkpoint kinase 1 regulates diallyl trisulfide-induced mitotic arrest in human prostate cancer cells. J Biol Chem 280.31 (2005): 28519–28528.
Herman-Antosiewicz A, Powolny AA, Singh SV. Molecular targets of cancer chemoprevention by garlic-derived organosulfides. Acta Pharmacol Sin 28.9 (2007): 1355–1364.
Holzgartner H, Schmidt U, Kuhn U. Comparison of the efficacy and tolerance of a garlic preparation vs. bezafibrate. Arzneimittelforschung 42.12 (1992): 1473–1477.
Hong JY et al. Metabolism of carcinogenic nitrosamines by rat nasal mucosa and the effect of diallyl sulfide. Cancer Res 51.5 (1991): 1509–1514.
Hong YS et al. Effects of allyl sulfur compounds and garlic extract on the expression of Bcl-2, Bax, and p53 in non small cell lung cancer cell lines. Exp Mol Med 32.3 (2000): 127–134.
Hosono T et al. Alkenyl group is responsible for the disruption of microtubule network formation in human colon cancer cell line HT-29 cells. Carcinogenesis 29.7 (2008): 1400–1406.
Hosseini, E., Bahrami, A.M., Razmjo, M. Study of the effects of raw garlic consumption on lipids and some blood biochemical factors in hyperlipdemic individuals. Global Veterinaria 10.1 (2013): 9–12.
Hsu CC et al. Protective effect of s-allyl cysteine and s-propyl cysteine on acetaminophen-induced hepatotoxicity in mice. Food and Chemical Toxicology 44.3 (2006): 393–397.
Hu X et al. Attenuation of cell migration and induction of cell death by aged garlic extract in rat sarcoma cells. Int J Mol Med 9.6 (2002): 641–643.
Ibrahim, A. N. Comparison of in Vitro Activity of Metronidazole and Garlic-Based Product (Tomex®) on *Trichomonas vaginalis*. Parasitology research 112.5 (2013): 2063–7
Ide N, Keller C, Weiss N. Aged garlic extract inhibits homocysteine-induced CD36 expression and foam cell formation in human macrophages. J Nutr 136 (3 Suppl) (2006): 755S–758S.
Imai T et al. Amyloid beta-protein potentiates tunicamycin-induced neuronal death in organotypic hippocampal slice cultures. Neuroscience 147.3 (2007): 639–651.
Ishige K et al. Role of caspase-12 in amyloid beta-peptide-induced toxicity in organotypic hippocampal slices cultured for long periods. J Pharmacol Sci 104.1 (2007): 46–55.
Jabbari A et al. Comparison between swallowing and chewing of garlic on levels of serum lipids, cyclosporine, creatinine and lipid peroxidation in renal transplant recipients. Lipids Health Dis 4 (2005): 11.
Jarial MS. Toxic effect of garlic extracts on the eggs of *Aedes aegypti* (Diptera: Culicidae): A scanning electron microscopic study. J Med Entomol 38.3 (2001): 446–450.
Jelodar GA et al. Effect of fenugreek, onion and garlic on blood glucose and histopathology of pancreas of alloxan-induced diabetic rats. Indian J Med Sci 59.2 (2005): 64–69.
Jepson, R.G. et al. Garlic for peripheral arterial occlusive disease. John Wiley and Sons, The Cochrane Library Issue 3 (2008)
Jeyaraj S et al. Effect of combined supplementation of fish oil with garlic pearls on the serum lipid profile in hypercholesterolemic subjects. Indian Heart J 57.4 (2005): 327–331.
Jo HJ et al. Diallyl disulfide induces reversible G2/M phase arrest on a p53-independent mechanism in human colon cancer HCT-116 cells. Oncol Rep 19.1 (2008): 275–280.
Jonkers D et al. Antibacterial effect of garlic and omeprazole on *Helicobacter pylori*. J Antimicrob Chemother 43.6 (1999): 837–839.
Josling P. Preventing the common cold with a garlic supplement: a double-blind, placebo-controlled survey. Adv Ther 18.4 (2001): 189–193.
Jung EM et al. Influence of garlic powder on cutaneous microcirculation. A randomized placebo-controlled double-blind cross-over study in apparently healthy subjects. Arzneimittelforschung 41.6 (1991): 626–630.
Kabasakal L et al. Protective effect of aqueous garlic extract against renal ischemia/reperfusion injury in rats. J Med Food 8.3 (2005): 319–326.
Khatua, T. N., et al. Garlic provides protection to mice heart against isoproterenol-induced oxidative damage: Role of nitric oxide. Nitric Oxide 27 (2012):9–17.
Kiesewetter H et al. Effects of garlic coated tablets in peripheral arterial occlusive disease. Clin Investig 71.5 (1993a): 383–386.
Kiesewetter H, Jung F, Jung EM, et al. Effect of garlic on platelet aggregation in patients with increased risk of juvenile ischaemic attack. Eur J Clin Pharmacol 45.4 (1993b): 333–336.
Kim JY, Kwon O. Garlic intake and cancer risk: an analysis using the Food and Drug Administration's evidence-based review system for the scientific evaluation of health claims. Am J Clin Nutr 89.1 (2009): 257–264.
Kim, H. J., et al. Hexane Extracts of Garlic Cloves Induce Apoptosis through the Generation of Reactive Oxygen Species in Hep3B Human Hepatocarcinoma Cells. Oncology reports 28.5 (2012): 1757–63.
Kim-Park S, Ku DD. Garlic elicits a nitric oxide-dependent relaxation and inhibits hypoxic pulmonary vasoconstriction in rats. Clin Exp Pharmacol Physiol 27.10 (2000): 780–786.
Knowles LM, Milner JA. Diallyl disulfide induces ERK phosphorylation and alters gene expression profiles in human colon tumor cells. J Nutr 133.9 (2003): 2901–2906.
Koscielny J et al. The antiatherosclerotic effect of *Allium sativum*. Atherosclerosis 144.1 (1999): 237–249.
Kwon MJ et al. Cholesteryl ester transfer protein activity and atherogenic parameters in rabbits supplemented with cholesterol and garlic powder. Life Sci 72.26 (2003): 2953–2964.

Kumar, R., et al. Antihyperglycemic, antihyperlipidemic, anti-inflammatory and adenosine deaminase – lowering effects of garlic in patients with type 2 diabetes mellitus with obesity Diabetes, Metabolic Syndrome and Obesity: Targets and Therapy 6 (2013): 49–56.

Lau BH. Suppression of LDL oxidation by garlic compounds is a possible mechanism of cardiovascular health benefit. J Nutr 136 (3 Suppl) (2006): 765S–768S.

Lawson LD, Ransom DK, Hughes BG. Inhibition of whole blood platelet-aggregation by compounds in garlic clove extracts and commercial garlic products. Thromb Res 65.2 (1992): 141–156.

Lawson LD, Wang ZJ, Papadimitriou D. Allicin release under simulated gastrointestinal conditions from garlic powder tablets employed in clinical trials on serum cholesterol. Planta Med 67.1 (2001): 13–118.

Lea MA, Randolph VM. Induction of histone acetylation in rat liver and hepatoma by organosulfur compounds including diallyl disulfide. Anticancer Res 21.4A (2001): 2841–2845.

Ledezma E, Apitz-Castro R. [Ajoene the main active compound of garlic (*Allium sativum*): a new antifungal agent.] Rev Iberoam Micol 23.2 (2006): 75–80.

Ledezma, E et al. Ajoene in the topical short-term treatment of tinea cruris and tinea corporis in humans. Arzneimittelforschung 49.06 (1999): 544–547.

Ledezma E et al. Efficacy of ajoene in the treatment of tinea pedis: a double-blind and comparative study with terbinafine. J Am Acad Dermatol 43.5 Pt 1 (2000): 829–832.

Lee HS et al. Inhibition of cyclooxygenase 2 expression by diallyl sulfide on joint inflammation induced by urate crystal and IL-1beta. Osteoarthritis Cartilage 17.1 (2009): 91–99.

Lee, D. Y., et al. Anti-Inflammatory Activity of Sulfur-Containing Compounds from Garlic. Journal of Medicinal Food 15.11 (2012a): 992–9.

Lee, M. H., Y. M. Kim, and S. G. Kim. Efficacy and Tolerability of Diphenyl-Dimethyldicarboxylate Plus Garlic Oil in Patients with Chronic Hepatitis. International journal of clinical pharmacology and therapeutics 50.11 (2012b): 778–86.

Lei YP et al. Diallyl disulfide and diallyl trisulfide suppress oxidized LDL-induced vascular cell adhesion molecule and E-selectin expression through protein kinase A- and B-dependent signaling pathways. J Nutr 138.6 (2008): 996–1003.

Lin HL et al. The role of Ca2+ on the DADS-induced apoptosis in mouse-rat hybrid retina ganglion cells (N18). Neurochem Res 31.3 (2006): 383–393.

Liu CT et al. Effects of garlic oil and diallyl trisulfide on glycemic control in diabetic rats. Eur J Pharmacol 516.2 (2005): 165–173.

Liu KL et al. DATS reduces LPS-induced iNOS expression, NO production, oxidative stress, and NF-kappaB activation in RAW 264.7 macrophages. J Agric Food Chem 54.9 (2006): 3472–3478.

Macan H et al. Aged garlic extract may be safe for patients on warfarin therapy. J Nutr 136 (3 Suppl) (2006). 793S–795S.

Mahmoodi M et al. Study of the effects of raw garlic consumption on the level of lipids and other blood biochemical factors in hyperlipidemic individuals. Pak J Pharm Sci 19.4 (2006): 295–298.

Matsuura N et al. Aged garlic extract inhibits angiogenesis and proliferation of colorectal carcinoma cells. J Nutr 136 (3 Suppl) (2006): 842S–846S.

McCullough, M. L., et al. "Garlic Consumption and Colorectal Cancer Risk in the CPS-II Nutrition Cohort." Cancer Causes and Control 23.10 (2012): 1643–51.

McNulty CA et al. A pilot study to determine the effectiveness of garlic oil capsules in the treatment of dyspeptic patients with *Helicobacter pylori*. Helicobacter 6.3 (2001): 249–253.

Medina-Campos ON et al. S-allylcysteine scavenges singlet oxygen and hypochlorous acid and protects LLC-PK(1) cells of potassium dichromate-induced toxicity. Food Chem Toxicol 45.10 (2007): 2030–2039.

Meng, S., et al. No Association between Garlic Intake and Risk of Colorectal Cancer. Cancer Epidemiology 37.2 (2013): 152–5.

Mohamadi A et al. Effects of wild versus cultivated garlic on blood pressure and other parameters in hypertensive rats. Heart Dis 2.1 (2000): 3–9.

Mohammed Abdul MI, Jiang X, Williams, K.M., et al. Pharmacodynamic interaction of warfarin with cranberry but not with garlic in healthy subjects. Br J Pharmacol 154.8 (2008): 1691–1700.

Moriarty RM, Naithani R, Surve B. Organosulfur compounds in cancer chemoprevention. Mini Rev Med Chem 7.8 (2007): 827–838.

Morihara, N., Nagatoshi, I., Weiss, N. Aged garlic extract inhibits homocysteine-induced scavenger receptor CD36 expression and oxidized low-density lipoprotein cholesterol uptake in human macrophages in vitro. J of ethnopharm. 134 (2011): 711–716.

Mosallanejad, B., et al. A Comparison between Metformin and Garlic on Alloxan-Induced Diabetic Dogs. Comparative Clinical Pathology 22.2 (2013): 169–74.

Mousa AS, Mousa SA. Anti-angiogenesis efficacy of the garlic ingredient alliin and antioxidants: role of nitric oxide and p53. Nutr Cancer 53.1 (2005): 104–110.

Mulrow C et al. Garlic: effects on cardiovascular risks and disease, protective effects against cancer, and clinical adverse effects. Evid Rep Technol Assess (Summ) 20 (2000): 1–4.

Nagini S. Cancer chemoprevention by garlic and its organosulfur compounds-panacea or promise? Anticancer Agents Med 8.3 (2008): 313–321.

Nakagawa H et al. Growth inhibitory effects of diallyl disulfide on human breast cancer cell lines. Carcinogenesis 22.6 (2001): 891–897.

Nakasone, Y., et al. Effect of a Traditional Japanese Garlic Preparation on Blood Pressure in Prehypertensive and Mildly Hypertensive Adults. Experimental and Therapeutic Medicine 5.2 (2013): 399–405.

Nantz, M. P., et al. Supplementation with aged garlic extract improves both nk and γδ-t cell function and reduces the severity of cold and flu symptoms: a randomized, double-blind, placebo-controlled nutrition intervention. Clinical Nutrition 31.3 (2012): 337–44

Ngo SN et al. Does garlic reduce risk of colorectal cancer? A systematic review. J Nutr 137.10 (2007): 2264–2269.

O'Gara EA, Hill DJ, Maslin DJ. Activities of garlic oil, garlic powder, and their diallyl constituents against *Helicobacter pylori*. Appl Environ Microbiol 66.5 (2000): 2269–2273.

O'Gara EA et al. The effect of simulated gastric environments on the anti-*Helicobacter* activity of garlic oil. J Appl Microbiol 104.5 (2008): 1324–1331.

Ohiro, A., et al. Effects of the "Aomori Garlic Extract"-Containing Dietary Supplement on the Stress, Quality of Sleep, Fatigue, and Quality of Life in Active Workers. Japanese Pharmacology and Therapeutics 41.3 (2013): 281–7.

Ola-Mudathir KF et al. Protective roles of onion and garlic extracts on cadmium-induced changes in sperm characteristics and testicular oxidative damage in rats. Food Chem Toxicol 46.12 (2008): 3604–3611.

Orekhov AN et al. Direct anti-atherosclerosis-related effects of garlic. Ann Med 27.1 (1995): 63–65.

Padiya, R., et al. Garlic improves insulin sensitivity and associated metabolic syndromes in fructose fed rats. Nutrition and metabolism (2011); 8: 53.

Phil, R. A. M., et al. Effects of garlic on blood glucose levels and HbA1c in patients with type 2 diabetes mellitus. J. of Med. Plants Research 5.13 (2011): 2922–28.

Piscitelli SC et al. The effect of garlic supplements on the pharmacokinetics of saquinavir. Clin Infect Dis 34.2 (2002): 234–238.

Powolny AA, Singh SV. Multitargeted prevention and therapy of cancer by diallyl trisulfide and related *Allium* vegetable-derived organosulfur compounds. Cancer Lett 269.2 (2008): 305–314.

Rahman K. Effects of garlic on platelet biochemistry and physiology. Mol Nutr Food Res 51.11 (2007): 1335–1344.

Rahman K, Billington D. Dietary supplementation with aged garlic extract inhibits ADP-induced platelet aggregation in humans. J Nutr 130.11 (2000): 2662–2665.

Rahman K, Lowe GM. Garlic and cardiovascular disease: a critical review. J Nutr 136 (3 Suppl) (2006): 736S–740S.

Rassoul F et al. The influence of garlic (*Allium sativum*) extract on interleukin 1alpha-induced expression of endothelial intercellular adhesion molecule-1 and vascular cell adhesion molecule-1. Phytomedicine 13.4 (2006): 230–235.

Reinhart KM et al. Effects of garlic on blood pressure in patients with and without systolic hypertension: a meta-analysis. Ann Pharmacother 42.12 (2008): 1766–1771.

Ried K et al. Effect of garlic on blood pressure: a systematic review and meta-analysis. BMC Cardiovasc Disord 8 (2008): 13.

Ried, K., O. R. Frank, and N. P. Stocks. Aged Garlic Extract Lowers Blood Pressure in Patients with Treated but Uncontrolled Hypertension: A Randomised Controlled Trial. Maturitas 67.2 (2010): 144–50.

Ried, K., et al. Aged garlic extract reduces blood pressure in hypertensives: a dose-response trial. European journal of clinical nutrition 67.1 (2013): 64–70.

Ried, K., et al. Effect of garlic on serum lipids: an updated meta-analysis. Nutr Rev 71.5 (2013): 282–299

Rose P et al. Bioactive S-alk(en)yl cysteine sulfoxide metabolites in the genus Allium: the chemistry of potential therapeutic agents. Nat Prod Rep 22.3 (2005): 351–368.

Sabitha P et al. Efficacy of garlic paste in oral candidiasis. Trop Doct 35.2 (2005): 99–100.

Scheiman JM, Cutler AF. *Helicobacter pylori* and gastric cancer. Am J Med 106.2 (1999): 222–226.

Seki T et al. Anticancer effects of diallyl trisulfide derived from garlic. Asia Pac J Clin Nutr 17 (Suppl 1) (2008): 249–252.

Sener G et al. Chronic nicotine toxicity is prevented by aqueous garlic extract. Plant Foods Hum Nutr 60.2 (2005): 77–86.

Seo, D Y, et al. Aged garlic extract enhances exercise-mediated improvement of metabolic parameters in high fat diet-induced obese rats. Nutrition research and practice 6.6 (2012): 513–519.

Sher, A., et al. Effect of Garlic Extract on Blood Glucose Level and Lipid Profile in Normal and Alloxan Diabetic Rabbits. Advances in Clinical and Experimental Medicine 21.6 (2012): 705–11.

Shukla Y, Kalra N. Cancer chemoprevention with garlic and its constituents. Cancer Lett 247.2 (2007): 167–181.

Siegel G, Klussendorf D. The anti-atheroslerotic effect of *Allium sativum*: statistics re-evaluated. Atherosclerosis 150.2 (2000): 437–438.

Silagy CA, Neil HA. A meta-analysis of the effect of garlic on blood pressure. J Hypertens 12.4 (1994): 463–468.

Singh DK, Porter TD. Inhibition of sterol 4alpha-methyl oxidase is the principal mechanism by which garlic decreases cholesterol synthesis. J Nutr 136.(3 Suppl) (2006): 759S–764S.

Singh SV et al. Differential induction of NAD(P)H:quinone oxidoreductase by anti-carcinogenic organosulfides from garlic. Biochem Biophys Res Commun 244.3 (1998): 917–920.

Sobenin IA et al. [Allicor efficacy in lowering the risk of ischemic heart disease in primary prophylaxis.] Ter Arkh 77.12 (2005): 9–13.

Sobenin IA et al. [Use of allicor to lower the risk of myocardial infarction.] Klin Med (Mosk) 85.3 (2007): 25–28.

Sobenin IA et al. Lipid-lowering effects of time-released garlic powder tablets in double-blinded placebo-controlled randomized study. J Atheroscler Thromb 15.6 (2008): 334–338.

Song JD et al. Molecular mechanism of diallyl disulfide in cell cycle arrest and apoptosis in HCT-116 colon cancer cells. J Biochem Mol Toxicol 23.1 (2009): 71–79.

Sriram N et al. Diallyl sulfide induces apoptosis in Colo 320 DM human colon cancer cells: involvement of caspase-3, NF-kappaB, and ERK-2. Mol Cell Biochem 311.1–2 (2008): 157–165.

Stabler, S. N., et al. Garlic for the prevention of cardiovascular morbidity and mortality in hypertensive patients., Cochrane Database of Systematic Reviews, no. 8, Article ID CD007653, 2012

Stargrove M, Treasure J, McKee D. Herb, nutrient and drug interactions. St Louis: Mosby, Elsevier, 2008.

Steiner M et al. A double-blind crossover study in moderately hypercholesterolemic men that compared the effect of aged garlic extract and placebo administration on blood lipids. Am J Clin Nutr 64.6 (1996): 866–870.

Stevinson C, Pittler MH, Ernst E. Garlic for treating hypercholesterolemia. A meta-analysis of randomized clinical trials. Ann Intern Med 133.6 (2001): 420–429.

Suru SM. Onion and garlic extracts lessen cadmium-induced nephrotoxicity in rats. Biometals 21.6 (2008): 623–633.

Tanaka S et al. Aged garlic extract has potential suppressive effect on colorectal adenomas in humans. J Nutr 136. (3 Suppl) (2006): 821S–826S.

Taylor P et al. Ajoene inhibits both primary tumor growth and metastasis of B16/BL6 melanoma cells in C57BL/6 mice. Cancer Lett 239.2 (2006): 298–304.

Tessema B et al. An in vitro assessment of the antibacterial effect of garlic (*Allium sativum*) on bacterial isolates from wound infections. Ethiop Med J 44.4 (2006): 385–389.

Thejass P, Kuttan G. Inhibition of angiogenic differentiation of human umbilical vein endothelial cells by diallyl disulfide (DADS). Life Sci 80.6 (2007): 515–521.

Thomson M, Mustafa T, Ali M. Thromboxane-B(2) levels in serum of rabbits receiving a single intravenous dose of aqueous extract of garlic and onion. Prostaglandins Leukot Essent Fatty Acids 63.4 (2000): 217–221.

Thomson M et al. Including garlic in the diet may help lower blood glucose, cholesterol, and triglycerides. J Nutr 136 (3 Suppl) (2006): 800S–802S.

Tilli CM et al. The garlic-derived organosulfur component ajoene decreases basal cell carcinoma tumor size by inducing apoptosis. Arch Dermatol Res 295.3 (2003): 117–123.

Tsai, C-W., et al. Garlic: health benefits and actions. Biomedicine (2012) 17–29.

Tsao SM, Yin MC. In-vitro antimicrobial activity of four diallyl sulphides occurring naturally in garlic and Chinese leek oils. J Med Microbiol 50.7 (2001): 646–649.

Unsal A et al. Protective role of natural antioxidant supplementation on testicular tissue after testicular torsion and detorsion. Scand J Urol Nephrol 40.1 (2006): 17–22.

Wang BH et al. Treatment with aged garlic extract protects against bromobenzene toxicity to precision cut rat liver slices. Toxicology 132.2–3 (1999): 215–225.

Weber ND et al. In vitro virucidal effects of *Allium sativum* (garlic) extract and compounds. Planta Med 58.5 (1992): 417–423.

Weiss N et al. Aged garlic extract improves homocysteine-induced endothelial dysfunction in macro- and microcirculation. J Nutr 136 (3 Suppl) (2006): 750S–754S.

Wojcikowski K, Myers S, Brooks L. Effects of garlic oil on platelet aggregation: a double-blind placebo-controlled crossover study. Platelets 18.1 (2007): 29–34.

Xiao D, Singh SV. Diallyl trisulfide, a constituent of processed garlic, inactivates Akt to trigger mitochondrial translocation of BAD and caspase-mediated apoptosis in human prostate cancer cells. Carcinogenesis 27.3 (2006): 533–540.

Xiao D et al. Diallyl trisulfide-induced apoptosis in human prostate cancer cells involves c-Jun N-terminal kinase and extracellular-signal regulated kinase-mediated phosphorylation of Bcl-2. Oncogene 23.33 (2004): 5594–5606.

Xiao D et al. Diallyl trisulfide-induced G(2)-M phase cell cycle arrest in human prostate cancer cells is caused by reactive oxygen species-dependent destruction and hyperphosphorylation of Cdc 25 C. Oncogene 24.41 (2005): 6256–6268.

Xiao, J et al. Garlic-derived S-allylmercaptocysteine is a hepato-protective agent in non-alcoholic fatty liver disease in vivo animal model. European journal of nutrition 52.1 (2013): 179–191.

Yang CS et al. Mechanisms of inhibition of chemical toxicity and carcinogenesis by diallyl sulfide (DAS) and related compounds from garlic. J Nutr 131.3s (2001): 1041S–1045S.

Yeh YY, Yeh SM. Homocysteine-lowering action is another potential cardiovascular protective factor of aged garlic extract. J Nutr 136 (3 Suppl) (2006): 745S–749S.

Yoshida S et al. Antifungal activity of ajoene derived from garlic. Appl Environ Microbiol 53.3 (1987): 615–6117.

Youn HS et al. Garlic (*Allium sativum*) extract inhibits lipopolysaccharide-induced Toll-like receptor 4 dimerization. Biosci Biotechnol Biochem 72.2 (2008): 368–375.

Yu, C. -S, et al. Diallyl Trisulfide Induces Apoptosis in Human Primary Colorectal Cancer Cells. Oncology reports 28.3 (2012): 949–54.

Zeb, I., et al. Aged Garlic Extract and Coenzyme Q10 have Favorable Effect on Inflammatory Markers and Coronary Atherosclerosis Progression: A Randomized Clinical Trial. Journal of Cardiovascular Disease Research 3.3 (2012): 185–90.

Zeng T et al. The anti-fatty liver effects of garlic oil on acute ethanol-exposed mice. Chem Biol Interact 176.2–3 (2008): 234–242.

Zeng, T., et al. A Meta-Analysis of Randomized, Double-Blind, Placebo-Controlled Trials for the Effects of Garlic on Serum Lipid Profiles. Journal of the science of food and agriculture 92.9 (2012): 1892–902.

Zheng S et al. Initial study on naturally occurring products from traditional Chinese herbs and vegetables for chemoprevention. J Cell Biochem Suppl 27 (1997): 106–112.

Ziaei, S. et al. The effect of garlic tablet on plasma lipids and platelet aggregation in nulliparous pregnants at high risk of preeclampsia. European Journal of Obstetrics & Gynecology and Reproductive Biology 99.2 (2001): 201–206.

Ginger

HISTORICAL NOTE Ginger has been used as both a food and a medicine since ancient times. Confucius wrote about it in his Analects, the Greek physician Dioscorides listed ginger as an antidote to poisoning, as a digestive, and as being warming to the stomach in De Materia Medica, and the Koran, the Talmud and the Bible all mention ginger. Records suggest that ginger was highly valued as an article of trade and in 13th- and 14th-century England, one pound of ginger was worth the same as a sheep (Rosengarten 1969). Ginger is still extremely popular in the practice of phytotherapy, particularly in traditional Chinese medicine (TCM), which distinguishes between the dried and fresh roots. It is widely used to stimulate circulation, treat various gastrointestinal disorders and as a stimulant heating agent.

OTHER NAMES

African ginger, Indian ginger, Jamaica ginger, common ginger, rhizoma zingiberis, shokyo (Japanese).

BOTANICAL NAME/FAMILY

Zingiber officinale Roscoe (family Zingiberaceae)

PLANT PART USED

Rhizome

CHEMICAL COMPONENTS

The ginger rhizome contains an essential oil and resin known collectively as oleoresin. The composition of the essential oil varies according to the geographical origin, but the chief constituents, sesquiterpene hydrocarbons, which are responsible for the characteristic aroma, are fairly constant.

The oleoresin contains:

- Sesquiterpenes: zingiberene, ar-curcumene, beta-sesquiphellandrene and beta-bisabolene.
- Pungent phenolic compounds: gingerols and their corresponding degradation products, shogaols, zingerone and paradol. Zingerone and shogaols are found in small amounts in fresh ginger and in larger amounts in dried or extracted products (Govindarajan 1982).
- Other constituents: diarylheptanoids galanolactone (diterpenoid), 6-gingesulfonic acid, monoacyldigalactosylglycerols (Awang 1992, Bhattarai et al 2001, Charles et al 2000, Govindarajan 1982, Kikuzaki et al 1991, WHO 2003, Yamahara et al 1992, Yoshikawa et al 1992, 1993).

PHARMACOKINETICS

Metabolites of [6]-, [8]- and [10]-gingerol as well as [6]-shogaol have been detected as glucuronide and sulfate conjugates in the plasma of healthy human volunteers after oral ingestion of 100 mg–2 gram doses of ginger (Zick et al 2008). A clinical study estimated the half-life of [6]-, [8]- and [10]-gingerol as well as [6]-shogaol and their metabolites to be 1–3 hours in human plasma (Yu et al 2011).

MAIN ACTIONS

Anti-emetic

Ginger has demonstrated anti-emetic activity in both experimental models and human studies. It appears that several key constituents are responsible, which exert several different mechanisms. In vivo studies have demonstrated [6]-, [8]- and [10]-gingerol as well as [6]-shogaol exert anti-emetic activity (Abdel-Aziz et al 2006, Kawai et al 1994), most likely by acting on the 5-HT_3 receptor ion-channel complex, either by binding directly to a modulatory site distinct from the serotonin binding site or indirectly via underlying muscarinic receptors. Specific constituents of ginger volatile oil including terpinolene, beta-pinene and alpha-phellandrene were also found to induce an antispasmodic effect via interaction with the 5-HT_3 receptor channel system in rat ileum (Riyazi et al 2007). Galactone has also been identified as a serotonin-receptor antagonist (Huang et al 1991, Mustafa et al 1993, Yamahara et al 1990). Such mechanisms of action also explain the inhibitory effect of ginger on serotonin-induced diarrhoea and antispasmodic effect on visceral and vascular smooth muscle.

Ginger has been shown to blunt gastric dysrhythmias and nausea evoked by acute hyperglycaemia in humans. The anti-arrhythmic and anti-emetic effects are thought to be due to a blockade of prostaglandins rather than inhibition of their release (Gonlachanvit et al 2003). Ginger has also been shown to reduce radiation-induced gastrointestinal distress and emesis in rat models, which is thought to be due at least in part to its antioxidant properties and the ability to scavenge free radicals and inhibit lipid peroxidation (Sharma et al 2005). Ginger extract displayed comparable radioprotection against radiation-induced taste aversion (CTA) when compared to dexamethasone and ondansetron in male and female rats. The most effective concentration was 1000 microgram/mL of ginger extract, which exerted free radial scavenging of hydroxyl ions and nitric oxide and modulation of CTA (Haksar et al 2006).

Gastrointestinal activity

Ginger exerts several effects in the gastrointestinal tract, which lead to an improvement in gastrointestinal symptoms. It stimulates the flow of saliva, bile and gastric secretions (Platel & Srinivasan 1996, 2001; Yamahara et al 1985), and has been shown to increase gastrointestinal motility in several animal models and human studies (Gupta & Sharma 2001, Micklefield et al 1999, Phillips et al 1993). In a double-blind RCT involving 24 healthy volunteers, ginger was found to accelerate gastric emptying and stimulate antral contractions (Wu et al 2008), a result that was confirmed in a follow-up double blind RCT using 1.2 g ginger root (Hu et al 2011). Ginger has also been observed to have prokinetic activity in mice in vivo and antispasmodic activity in vitro (Ghayur & Gilani 2005). These findings appear to support the traditional use of ginger in the treatment of gastrointestinal discomfort, colic, diarrhoea and bloating, and its use as a carminative agent. New insight into the mechanisms of the antidiarrhoeal action of a decoction of ginger root indicates that it may modify bacterial as well as host cell metabolism, reducing colonisation of epithelial cells (Daswani et al 2010). In vitro studies confirm cholinergic agonistic activity on postsynaptic M3 receptors, as well as suggesting an inhibitory effect on presynaptic muscarinic autoreceptors; the [6]-gingerol constituent displayed the strongest antispasmodic activity (Ghayur et al 2008).

Anti-ulcer activity

A number of in vivo studies have identified anti-ulcer activity for ginger extract and several of its isolated constituents. The orally administered acetone extract of ginger at a dose of 1000 mg/kg and zingiberene, the main terpenoid in this extract, at 100 mg/kg significantly inhibited gastric lesions by 97.5% and 53.6%, respectively. Additionally, the pungent principle, [6]-gingerol at 100 mg/kg, significantly inhibited gastric lesions by 54.5%. These results suggest that both zingiberene and [6]-gingerol are important constituents responsible for ginger's anti-ulcer activity (Yamahara et al 1988). Other constituents demonstrating anti-ulcer properties in gastric ulcer models in rats include beta-sesquiphellandrene, beta-bisabolene, ar-curcumene and shogaol (Sertie et al 1992, Yoshikawa et al 1994). Furthermore, an animal study showed that ginger was able to protect against indomethacin-induced gastric ulceration when administered at 100, 200 and 400 mg/kg, and was comparable in efficacy to the study's reference drug, ranitidine (Anoiske et al 2009).

Helicobacter pylori has been identified as a major causative factor in gastric ulcers. In vitro studies have established ginger extract containing gingerols effectively inhibited the growth of 19 strains of *H. pylori* including CagA+ strains (Mahady et al 2003, 2005). While ginger is effective in inhibiting *H. pylori*, its ability to prevent bacterial adhesion to the stomach tissue is limited (O'Mahony et al 2005).

In addition to direct anti-ulcer activity, ginger exerts synergistic effects with the antibiotic clarithromycin in inhibiting different *H. pylori* isolates independent of the organisms' susceptibility to clarithromycin (Nostro et al 2006). Ginger-free phenolic and ginger hydrolysed phenolic fractions were found to be potent inhibitors of gastric cell proton potassium ATPase and *H. pylori*, exhibiting a six-to-eight-fold better potency over lansoprazole (Siddaraju & Dharmesh 2007).

Hypolipidaemic

Ginger demonstrates significant lipid lowering activity in several animal models and, more recently, a double-blind clinical trial.

High doses of an aqueous extract of ginger (500 mg/kg) significantly reduced serum cholesterol according to an animal study that used oral doses of a raw aqueous extract of ginger administered daily for a period of 4 weeks (Thomson et al 2002). Treatment with ginger methanol and ethyl acetate extracts (250 mg/kg) for 8 weeks also resulted in a significant reduction in lipid levels in vivo (Goyal & Kadnur 2006). Similarly, methanolic and ethyl acetate extracts of dried ginger rhizome significantly reduced fructose-elevated lipid levels and body weight in vivo (Kadnur & Goyal 2005). Reductions in lipid levels were further reported for ethanolic extract of ginger (200 mg/kg for 20 days) by using a streptozocin-induced diabetic rat model. In addition, herbal treatment effectively reduced serum glucose (Bhandari et al 2005).

Effects on triglyceride levels are more difficult to determine, as one study demonstrated that 250 microgram ginger extract/day reduced serum triglyceride levels by 27% in mice (Fuhrman et al 2000), whereas another study using a high dose of 500 mg/kg found no significant effects (Thomson et al 2002).

An ex vivo study found that 250 mcg/day of a standardised ginger extract significantly reduced plasma cholesterol, triglycerides and LDL cholesterol levels, the LDL basal oxidative state, as well as LDL cholesterol and serum cholesterol's susceptibility to oxidation and aggregation, compared with placebo. Ginger also reduced aortic atherosclerotic lesions by 44% in atherosclerotic mouse aorta (Fuhrman et al 2000).

According to a double-blind controlled clinical trial study of 85 volunteers, ginger (3 g/day) demonstrates clinically significant lipid lowering effects compared to controls. After 45 days of treatment, triglyceride and cholesterol levels were reduced, as well as a reduction in LDL levels and an increase in HDL levels (Alizadeh-Navaei et al 2008).

Glycaemic response

Ginger improves insulin sensitivity and reduces serum glucose levels in vivo (Al-Amin et al 2006, Goyal & Kandur 2006). The mechanisms underlying these actions are associated with the inhibition of key enzymes controlling carbohydrate metabolism, an insulinotropic effect rather than hypoglycaemic (Islam & Choi 2008), increased insulin release/sensitivity (Goyal & Kandur 2006), resulting in enhanced glucose uptake in peripheral adipose and skeletal muscle tissues. Significant lipid lowering activity further contributes to improving the insulin resistant condition (Li et al 2012).

Gingerols have been identified as the main constituent group responsible for improving insulin sensitivity. In an assay for aldose reductase inhibitors within ginger, five active compounds were isolated and two were found to be inhibitors of recombinant human aldose reductase (Kato et al 2006).

Anti-inflammatory and analgesic

The anti-inflammatory and analgesic effects reported for ginger are attributed to multiple constituents exerting several different mechanisms.

An acetone extract containing gingerols, shogaols and minor compounds like gingerenone A, [6]-gingerdiol, hexahydrocurcumin and zingerone has been shown synergistically to produce dose-dependent anti-inflammatory effects (Schuhbaum & Franz 2000). Other studies have identified the gingerols and diarylheptanoids and gingerdione as the key compounds responsible (Flynn et al 1986, Kiuchi et al 1992).

Investigations on macrophages in vitro found that [6]-shogaol and [6]-gingerol inhibit the expression of inflammatory iNOS and COX-2 proteins (Pan et al 2008). [6]-Gingerol has also been shown to inhibit catalytic activity of iNOS in murine macrophages via attenuation of NF-kappaB-mediated iNOS gene expression (Aktan et al 2006). [6]-Gingerol proved to be useful in treatment of inflammation by selectively inhibiting the production of inflammatory cytokines of murine peritoneal macrophages without interfering with the antigen-presenting function of the macrophages (Tripathi et al 2007). Ginger extract inhibited interleukin (IL)-12, tumour necrosis factor (TNF)-alpha, IL-1-beta in lipopolysaccharide-stimulated macrophages and significantly reduced T-cell proliferation (Tripathi et al 2008).

Ginger has been found to modulate the arachidonic acid cascade, as COX-1 and -2 and lipoxygenase inhibition has been shown in vitro (Kobayashi et al 1987) and high oral doses of an aqueous extract of ginger (500 mg/kg) significantly lowered serum PGE_2 and thromboxane B_2 levels in rats (Thomson et al 2002). A hydroalcoholic extract of ginger exerted anti-inflammatory and attenuated COX metabolites in rat trachea hyperactivity for 90 minutes and 48 hours after exposure to lipopolysaccharide (LPS). Ginger reduced serum levels of prostaglandin (PGE_2) and thromboxane (TXA_2) post LPS exposure (Aimbire et al 2007). Ginger also suppresses leukotriene biosynthesis by inhibiting 5-lipoxygenase, thus distinguishing ginger from non-steroidal anti-inflammatory drugs (NSAIDs). Additionally, ginger extract has been shown to inhibit thromboxane synthase (Langner et al 1998) and a ginger extract (EV.EXT 77) has been found to inhibit the induction of several genes involved in the inflammatory response. These include genes encoding cytokines, chemokines and the inducible enzyme COX-2, thus providing evidence that ginger modulates biochemical pathways activated in chronic inflammation (Grzanna et al 2005). A positive response to ginger administration was also demonstrated in an arthritic animal model whereby a significant reduction in inflammatory cytokines occurred that was superior to indomethacin (Ramadan et al 2011).

Gingerol and [8]-gingerol have been found to evoke capsaicin-like intracellular Ca^{2+} transients and ion currents in vitro and it has been suggested that gingerols represent a novel class of naturally occurring vanilloid receptor agonists that contribute to ginger's medicinal properties (Dedov et al 2002). This is supported by the finding that topical application of ginger creams or compresses produce an analgesic capsaicin-like effect on the release of the immunoreactive substance P from primary afferent neurons (Onogi et al 1992). In animal models of chemically induced inflammation, ginger extract reduced oedema that was partly caused by serotonin-receptor antagonism (Penna et al 2003) and has been shown to reduce inflammation in a non-dose dependent manner, and display equivalent efficacy to indomethacin (Anosike et al 2009). Additionally, ginger oil has shown anti-inflammatory activity, significantly suppressing both paw and joint swelling in severe adjuvant arthritis in rats (Sharma et al 1994).

G

In an animal model of rheumatoid arthritis, both crude ginger extract and gingerols were efficacious in preventing streptococcal cell wall-induced arthritis. However, the crude ginger extract, which also contained essential oils, was more effective in preventing both joint inflammation and attenuating cellular destruction (Funk et al 2009).

Antiplatelet

It has been suggested that gingerols and their derivatives represent a potential new class of platelet activation inhibitors, with synthetic gingerols being found to inhibit the arachidonic acid-induced platelet release reaction in vitro in a similar dose range as aspirin possibly due to an effect on COX activity in platelets (Koo et al 2001, Lu 2005, Nurtjahja-Tjendraputra et al 2003, Tjendraputra et al 2001).

Powdered ginger exerted an antiplatelet activity when taken in very high doses of at least 10 g, according to one human study (Bordia et al 1997). A randomised double-blind study found that doses up to 2 g of dried ginger had no effect on bleeding time, platelet aggregation or platelet count (Lumb 1994). This lack of effect has been demonstrated in healthy volunteers (Janssen et al 1996) and those with type 1 diabetes mellitus or coronary artery disease (Bordia et al 1997).

Antimicrobial and antiparasitic

Ginger extract, several of its main constituents and essential oil of ginger exhibit antimicrobial activity in vitro and in vivo. Ginger extract has been shown to have an antibacterial effect against *Staphylococcus aureus*, *Streptococcus pyogenes*, *Streptococcus pneumoniae* and *Haemophilus* collected from throat swabs of infected individuals. The minimum inhibitory concentration of ginger ranged from 0.0003 to 0.7 mcg/mL, and the minimum bactericidal concentration ranged from 0.135 to 2.04 mcg/mL (Akoachere et al 2002). Recent in vitro studies confirmed ginger compounds were effective against *Penicillium* spp., *Escherichia coli, Bacillus subtilis* and *Staphylococcus aureus*, with minimal inhibitory concentrations of the oleoresin and essential oil 2 mg/mL and 869.2 mg/mL, respectively (Bellik 2014). The anti-*H. pylori* effects of ginger have also been shown to inhibit *H. pylori* $CagA^+$ strains in vitro (Mahady et al 2003). Essential oils of ginger have also been shown to have antimicrobial activity against Gram-positive and Gram-negative bacteria in vitro (Martins et al 2001).

Various ginger extracts have demonstrated significant larvicidal potential against larvae of the dengue fever mosquito vector, *Aedes aegypti*. The application of ginger alcoholic and oil-based extracts resulted in complete mortality with no pupal or adult emergence (Kalaivani et al 2012, Kumar et al 2012).

Ginger constituents

[10]-Gingerol and [12]-gingerol successfully inhibited oral bacteria associated with periodontitis. Ethanol and *n*-hexane extracts of ginger have demonstrated antibacterial activities against the bacteria *Porphyromonas gingivalis*, *Porphyromonas endodontalis* and *Prevotella intermedia*, associated with periodontal disease, effectively inhibited the growth of these anaerobic Gram-negative bacteria (Park et al 2008). Intraperitoneally administered ginger exerted a dose-dependent antimicrobial activity against *Pseudomonas aeruginosa*, *Salmonella typhimurium*, *Escherichia coli* and *Candida albicans* (Jagetia et al 2003).

Gingerols demonstrated antibacterial activity against *Bacillus subtilis* and *Escherichia coli* in vitro (Yamada et al 1992). [10]-Gingerol was found to potentiate the antibacterial actions of aminoglycosides in vancomycin-resistant enterococci, bacitracin and polymixin B suggesting [10]-gingerol increases membrane permeability of enterococcal cells promoting an enhanced influx of aminoglycosides (Nagoshi et al 2006).

Ginger has also shown antischistosomal activity. Gingerol (5.0 ppm) completely abolished the infectivity of *Schistosoma* spp (blood flukes) in animal studies (Adewunmi et al 1990). Gingerol and shogaol exhibited potent molluscicidal activity in vivo. Shogaol and gingerol have demonstrated anti-nematode activities; 6.25 mcg/mL 6-shogaol destroyed *Anisakis* larvae within 16 hours in vitro, whereas the anti-nematodal medication pyrantel pamoate had no lethal effect at 1 mg/mL (Goto et al 1990).

Antifungal and antiviral

Ginger constituents have demonstrated antifungal and antiviral activity. Shogaol and zingerone strongly inhibited *Salmonella typhi*, *Vibrio cholerae* and *Trícophyton violaceum*. Aqueous extracts have also been shown to be effective against *Trichomonas vaginalis* (Henry & Piggott 1987). Several sesquiterpenes, but especially beta-sesquiphellandrene, isolated from ginger have also been shown to have antirhinoviral activity in vitro (Denyer et al 1994).

Essential oils of ginger have been shown to have activity yeasts and filamentous fungi in vitro (Martins et al 2001). Such oils have exhibited virucidal activity against aciclovir-sensitive and resistant strains of herpes simplex-1 reducing plaque formation significantly (Schnitzler et al 2007). A further in vitro study has indicated a dose-dependent virucidal activity against herpes simplex-2 is possible by interaction with the viral envelope (Koch et al 2008).

Antioxidant

Various investigations have confirmed that ginger displays strong in vitro and in vivo antioxidant properties. Orally administered ginger significantly lowered levels of free radicals and raised the activities of endogenous antioxidants, superoxide dismutase and catalase and had a sparing effect on vitamins C and E (Jeyakumar et al 1999). Ginger has been found to protect against lipid peroxidation in the liver (Ahmed et al 2008) and kidney (Asnani & Verma 2007). Ginger root aqueous extract taken orally (500 mg/kg/day) reduced testicular toxicity, including the restoration of sperm function, testicular steroidogenesis and reproductive organo-somatic indices in an animal model, effects which were attributed to the antioxidant activity of ginger (Morakinyo et al 2010).

An in vivo and in vitro research has shown [6]-gingerol to be effective in reducing ultraviolet B (UVB)-induced intracellular reactive oxygen species (ROS), UVB-induced expression of COX-2 and inhibited the translocation of NF-kappaB from cytosol to cell nucleus. Moreover, topical application of [6]-gingerol prior to UVB exposure on hairless mice inhibited COX-2 mRNA, and protein and NF-kappaB translocation (Kim et al 2007).

Immunomodulation

In vitro and in vivo research suggests that ginger extract exerts some degree of immunomodulatory activity (Ahui et al 2008, Imanishi et al 2006, Tripathi et al 2008).

Ginger exerted an immunosuppressive in vitro lymphocyte proliferation analysis, an effect modulated through IL-2 production (Wilasrusmee et al 2002). Ginger oil has also been shown to have immunomodulatory activity in mice, with dose-dependent inhibition of T lymphocyte proliferation and IL-1-alpha secretion and reduced delayed type of hypersensitivity response in vivo (Zhou et al 2006).

Hepatoprotective

Experimental models of alcohol-induced liver damage previously showed that ginger has significant hepatoprotective effects comparable to those of silymarin (Bhandari et al 2003). The effect appears to be mediated by an antioxidative mechanism. Reversal of ethanol-induced liver damage was achieved following the treatment with 1% ginger for 4 weeks. The hepatoprotective action was mediated by preventing a decline in antioxidant status (Mallikarjuna et al 2008). Pretreatment with an ethanol extract of ginger exerted a protective effect against carbon tetrachloride and paracetamol-induced acute liver damage in rats, with attenuation of serum and liver marker enzymes (Yemitan & Izegbu 2006). In a similar study ginger exerted significant declines in the activities of serum transaminases and alkaline phosphatase and restoration of hepatic oxidative status post administration of a single dose (Ajith et al 2007). More recently, two animal studies comparing ginger to silymarin (an active constituent in St Mary's thistle), oral extracts of ginger were found to attenuate carbon tetrachloride-induced damage of the liver. The first study involved the use of methanolic extract, resulting in reductions of the inflammatory enzymes alkaline phosphatase (ALP) and gamma-glutamyl transpeptidase (GGT) and also showed no symptoms of morbidity or mortality in dosages of up to 5000 mg/kg in rats (Atta et al 2010). In the second, ethanolic extract of ginger significantly increased glutathione, superoxide dismutase and protein levels in addition to reduced aspartate and alanine amintransferases (AST and ALT), GGT and bilirubin levels and markedly reduced necrosis and collagen deposition fibrosis (Motawi et al 2011).

Nephroprotection

Ginger prevented the decline in renal antioxidant status by increasing glutathione-S-transferase activity in an experimental model of nephrotoxicity (Ajith et al 2008). Ginger exhibited a significant dose-dependent nephroprotective role in experimentally induced acute renal damage when administered as a stand-alone treatment (250 mg/kg) and when used in combination with vitamin E (Ajith et al 2007).

Chemoprotective

The inhibitory effects of ginger and its constituents in tumour development have previously been demonstrated in animal models and human cell lines with activity observed against human breast cancer (Lee et al 2008), ovarian cancer (Rhode et al 2007), gastric cancer (Ishiguro et al 2007) and pancreatic cancer (Park et al 2006).

Antitumour properties have been isolated to several key constituents of ginger including [6]-gingerol, [6]-paradol, shogaols, zerumbone and zingerone and are partly due to an antioxidative and anti-inflammatory mechanism (Kim et al 2005).

Application of ginger or its constituents achieved induction of apoptosis in cancerous cells resulting in suppression of proliferation (Lee & Surh 1998) and apoptosis resulting in cell transformation (Bode et al 2001). The apoptotic effect of ginger constituents was also demonstrated in human promyelocytic leukaemia cells (Wei et al 2005), and an ethanolic extract of ginger also demonstrated cytotoxic activity against cultured non-hormone-dependent cancer cell lines, arresting development in the sub-G1 phase (Sabli et al 2012) The modulation of proteins involved in apoptosis has also been demonstrated in in vivo and in vitro prostate cancer models (Shukla et al 2007). [6]-Gingerol administration exerted actions of cell cycle arrest and induction of apoptosis in suppression of hepatoma cells (Yagihashi et al 2008). [6]-Gingerol was also found to exert a direct suppressive effect on colon cancer cell growth and inhibit angiogenesis by reduction in tumour blood supply (Brown et al 2008). [6]-Shogaol has been found to effectively induce apoptotic cell death in human hepatoma p53 mutant cells by way of an intracellular oxidative stress mediated cascade which ultimately leads to cell death (Chen et al 2007), and the same constituent was shown to be a potent inhibitor of MDA-MB-231 breast cancer cell invasion, possibly by down-regulating transcription by targeting the NF-kappaB activation cascade (Ling et al 2010).

Reduction of lipid peroxidation and increased antioxidant activity was attributed to suppression of colon carcinogenesis by ginger in male Wistar rats (Manju & Nalini 2005). Differing types of tumours exhibit high NF-kappaB activity sustaining angiogenesis and cell proliferation gingerols were found to display properties inhibiting the activation of NF-kappaB (Kim et al 2009, Takada et al 2005).

The activity seen in test tube and animal models may have clinical significance according to a double blind RCT. The trial involved 33 participants with normal risk of colorectal cancer who were given ginger powder (2 g/day) for 28 days. Colon biopsy results showed that compared to placebo, ginger significantly reduced prostaglandin E_2 and the eicosanoid 5-hydroxyeicosatetraenoic normalised to arachidonic acid, indicating that ginger extract may have an inhibitory effect on colon tissue cyclooxygenase and lipoxygenase enzymes in humans (Zick et al 2011).

Clinical note — Ginger and moxibustion — a clinical perspective

Moxibustion as a part of acupuncture has been well noted in TCM and is widely accepted as a useful complementary and alternative medicine therapy (Okada & Kawakita 2009). Indirect moxibustion utilises ginger slices placed at specific acupuncture points to insulate the skin from burning moxa sticks and provides therapeutic effects via thermal stimulation and sympathetic vibration (Shen et al 2006).

A review of 587 acupuncture and moxibustion randomised controlled papers from 1978 to 2007 conducted by Du et al (2009) demonstrated the growing indications for, and applications of, the use of moxibustion and acupuncture. Clinical trials have shown ginger-partitioned moxibustion to be therapeutically effective in the treatment of child diarrhoea (Liu et al 2003), cervical vertigo (Xiaoxiang 2006), poststroke urination disorders (Liu & Wang 2006), leucopenia induced by chemotherapy (Zhao et al 2007) and rheumatoid arthritis (Xie & Lei 2008).

OTHER ACTIONS

Antihistamine

Shogaols and certain gingerols exhibit dose-dependent inhibition of drug-induced histamine release from rat peritoneal mast cells in vitro (Yamahara et al 1995).

Anxiolytic

A combination of ginger and *Ginkgo biloba* has been shown to reduce anxiety in an animal model (elevated plus-maze test). The effect was similar to diazepam (Hasenohrl et al 1996). A highly non-polar fraction of a ginger extract has been shown to possess anticonvulsant, anxiolytic and antiemetic activities in animals (Vishwakarma et al 2002).

G

> ***Clinical note — Morning sickness***
> Nausea and vomiting are the most common symptoms experienced in early pregnancy, with nausea affecting between 70% and 85% of women. About half of pregnant women experience vomiting (Jewell & Young 2002). Hyperemesis gravidarum is more severe and affects between 0.3% and 2% of all pregnant women. It is a multifactorial disease in which pregnancy-induced hormonal changes associated with concurrent gastrointestinal dysmotility and possible *Helicobacter pylori* infection function as contributing factors (Eliakim et al 2000).

Antifibrotic

Supplementation with 5 g ginger not only prevented a decrease, but also significantly increased fibrinolytic activity in 30 healthy adult volunteers who consumed 50 g fat in a meal in an open clinical study (Verma & Bordia 2001).

Positive inotrope

Gingerols and shogaols isolated from ginger have positive inotropic activity, as demonstrated on isolated heart muscle (Shoji et al 1982, Yamahara et al 1995). The effect of gingerol seems to be rather specific to SR Ca^{2+}–ATPase activity (Kobayashi et al 1987).

Thermogenic

Ginger helps to maintain body temperature and inhibit serotonin-induced hypothermia in vivo (Huang et al 1991, Kano et al 1991). However, the addition of a ginger-based sauce to a meal did not produce any significant effect on metabolic rate in humans (Henry & Piggott 1987).

Hypotensive

Aqueous ginger extract has been shown to lower blood pressure via stimulation of muscarinic receptors and blockade of Ca^{2+} channels in guinea pig atria (Ghayur et al 2005). The calcium channel blocking effect of ginger has been demonstrated in acetycholine (ACh)-induced airway constriction of mouse lung tissue. Pretreatment with a 70% aqueous methanolic crude extract of ginger 30 minutes prior to ACh administration achieved significant reduction in airway contraction and Ca^{2+}. Similar results were achieved with verapamil, indicating comparable modes of action. Concomitant use of both ginger extract and verapamil achieved the same outcome as when each was used alone (Ghayur et al 2008).

CLINICAL USE

Although ginger is used in many forms, including fresh ginger used in cooking or chai (Indian spicy tea), pickled or glazed ginger, ethanol extracts and concentrated powdered extracts, preparations made with the root are used medicinally. Depending on the specific solvent used, the resultant preparation will contain different concentrations of the active constituents and may differ markedly from crude ginger. The great majority of research refers specifically to the species *Zingiber officinale*; however, there is the potential for confusion with other species or even with other genera (Canter 2004). Furthermore, there are reported to be wide variations in the quality of commercial ginger supplements with concentrations of gingerols ranging from 0.0 to 9.43 mg/g. As such, the results of specific extracts cannot necessarily be extrapolated to different preparations (Schwertner et al 2006).

Prevention of nausea and vomiting

Many clinical studies have investigated the effects of ginger in the prevention and treatment of nausea and vomiting associated with different circumstances, including pregnancy (Fischer-Rasmussen et al 1990, Keating & Chez 2002, Portnoi et al 2003, Smith et al 2004, Sripramote & Lekhyananda 2003, Vutyavanich et al 2001, Willetts et al 2003), the postoperative period (Arfeen et al 1995, Bone et al 1990, Meyer et al 1995, Phillips et al 1993, Visalyaputra et al 1998), motion sickness (Grontved & Hentzer 1986, Lien et al 2003, Mowrey & Clayson 1982, Schmid et al 1994, Stewart et al 1991) and chemotherapy (Manusirivithaya et al 2004, Meyer et al 1995, Sontakke et al 2003, Ryan et al 2012).

A systematic review of 24 randomised controlled trials (RCTs) covering 1073 patients suggests that results for the treatment of nausea and vomiting in pregnancy are encouraging and generally supportive; however, results for postoperative nausea and vomiting and motion sickness are unclear and daily doses of up to 6 g of ginger seem to have few side effects (Betz et al 2005). More reviews provide further encouragement and suggest that ginger may indeed be effective in nausea associated with pregnancy (Boone & Shields 2005) and the postoperative period (Chaiyakunapruk et al 2006). Similarly a review of four well-controlled, double-blind, randomised clinical studies concluded there was convincing evidence for application of ginger in the treatment of nausea and vomiting of pregnancy (Bryer 2005).

Nausea and vomiting in pregnancy

There is supportive evidence from clinical studies that ginger preparations in pregnancy reduce the duration and severity of nausea and vomiting.

Nausea of pregnancy

There are many studies, including an observational study (Portnoi et al 2003) and at least seven RCTs (Fischer-Rasmussen et al 1990, Keating & Chez 2002, Portnoi et al 2003, Smith et al 2004, Sripramote & Lekhyananda 2003, Vutyavanich et al 2001, Willetts et al 2003), as well as multiple systematic reviews, including a Cochrane review (Matthews et al 2010), that suggest that ginger powder or extract may be safe and effective in treating nausea and vomiting of pregnancy (Boone & Shields 2005, Borrelli et al 2005, Bryer 2005, Dib & El-Saddik 2004, Ernst & Pittler 2000, Jewell 2003). A subsequent review, considering four double-blind RCTs including 504 subjects, suggests that ginger is superior to placebo and as effective as vitamin B_6 in reducing the frequency and intensity of pregnancy-related nausea and vomiting and that there is an absence of significant side effects and adverse pregnancy outcomes; however, the review does mention uncertainty regarding the maximum safe dosage and the need for further research (Ding et al 2013).

In three double-blind, placebo-controlled, randomised trials of ginger for pregnancy-related nausea and vomiting, including one trial on hyperemesis gravidarum, 1 g ginger in divided doses was significantly more effective than placebo in reducing nausea and vomiting (Fischer-Rasmussen et al 1990, Keating & Chez 2002, Vutyavanich et al 2001). In a further double-blind trial of 120 women, 25 mg of the ginger extract EV.EXT 35 (equivalent to 1.5 g of dried ginger) four times daily was useful in patients experiencing nausea and retching, although no significant result was seen for vomiting (Willetts et al 2003).

Comparative studies

A comparative double-blind randomised controlled trial of 170 pregnant women who attended an antenatal clinic with the symptoms of nausea and vomiting in pregnancy found one capsule of ginger (0.5 g ginger powder) twice daily was identical in efficacy to treatment with 50 mg dimenhydrinate twice daily. In addition, ginger treatment resulted in fewer side effects (Pongrojpaw et al 2007). Initial comparative randomised, double-blind controlled trials found ginger to be equivalent to vitamin B_6 in helping to reduce pregnancy-related nausea, dry retching and vomiting (Smith et al 2004, Sripramote & Lekhyananda 2003). However, ginger (650 mg qid) proved more effective than vitamin B_6 (25 mg qid) in a randomised double-blind controlled trial involving 126 pregnant women, with a gestational age of ≤16 weeks who had nausea and vomiting (Chittumma et al 2007). Investigations over a 3-month duration into the efficacy of ginger compared to vitamin B_6 of 70 pregnant women with nausea and a gestational age of ≤17 weeks were randomised to receive either ginger 1 g/day or vitamin B_6 40 mg/day for 4 days. Treatment with ginger (1 g/day) was found to be more effective than vitamin B_6 (40 mg/day) for relieving the severity of nausea, as well as equally effective in decreasing the episodes of vomiting (Ensiyeh & Sakineh 2008). Another clinical trial suggests that ginger at a dose of 250 mg taken four times per day is as effective as the higher dose of B_6 40 mg twice per day for reducing pregnancy-induced nausea (Haji Seid Javadi et al 2013).

Postoperative nausea

Ginger may be useful for the prevention of postoperative nausea; however, not all studies have produced positive results and as the ginger preparations used have not been standardised, it is difficult to directly compare studies. A meta-analysis of five randomised trials (n = 363) found that a fixed dose of at least 1 g of ginger was more effective than placebo for the prevention of postoperative nausea and vomiting (Chaiyakunapruk et al 2006).

Most of the studies on postoperative nausea and vomiting have been conducted on patients undergoing gynaecological surgery. Powdered ginger (2 g) was administered to 239 women undergoing elective caesarean section at term, in order to evaluate the effects on intra- and post-operative nausea and vomiting. Ginger reduced the number of episodes of intraoperative nausea compared to placebo, but had no effect on incidence of nausea, vomiting or pain during or after elective caesarean section (Kalava et al 2013). In two other double-blind RCTs, ginger significantly reduced the incidence of postoperative nausea and vomiting (Bone et al 1990, Phillips et al 1993), although two further studies failed to show any benefit with ginger (Arfeen et al 1995, Eberhart et al 2003). A fifth study of 80 women undergoing gynaecological laparoscopy found that 1 g of ginger taken 1 hour before surgery was significantly superior to placebo in reducing the incidence of nausea 2–4 hours afterwards; however, it failed to show statistical significance for an observed reduction in the incidence and frequency of vomiting (Pongrojpaw & Chiamchanya 2003).

A double-blind RCT of 120 patients who underwent major gynaecological surgery found that a pretreatment with ginger powder (0.5 g) as compared to placebo resulted in lower incidence and frequency of vomiting in the treatment group. Frequency of vomiting was evaluated at 0, 2, 6, 12 and 24 hours postoperatively with the most statistically significant differences between ginger and placebo occurring at the 2- and 6-hour time intervals (Nanthakomon & Pongrojpaw 2006). Similarly a randomised study of 60 inpatients who underwent laparoscopic operations for non-cancer gynaecological conditions found that pretreatment 1 hour prior to surgery with three capsules of ginger (0.5 g of ginger powder per capsule) when compared to placebo significantly prevented vomiting at 6 hours postoperation. The effect was not apparent at 2 hours postoperation (Apariman et al 2006).

Although other types of surgery have not been as extensively studied as gynaecological surgery, there is a report on 6 months of clinical anaesthetic experience that suggests that a nasocutaneously administered 5% solution of essential oil of ginger given pre-operatively, together with conventional therapies, to general anaesthesia patients at high risk for postoperative nausea and vomiting is a safe and cost-effective way of reducing nausea and vomiting post anaesthesia (Geiger 2005).

Another RCT recently showed that inhaled ginger essential oil produced significant benefits by reducing postoperative nausea. The study involving 303 subjects in an ambulatory post anaesthesia care unit were administered three deep inhalations of a gauze pad soaked with saline (placebo), alcohol, ginger essential oil (EO) or a combination of ginger, spearmint, peppermint and cardamom. The ginger EO and the ginger blend showed significant beneficial effects over placebo for nausea severity and a significant reduction in postoperative antiemetic medication was required (Hunt et al 2013).

In the only double-blind, placebo-controlled study of postoperative nausea and vomiting in patients undergoing middle ear surgery, ginger was ineffective and the use of 1 g of ginger 1 hour before surgery was associated with significantly more postoperative nausea and vomiting than the use of ondansetron or placebo (Gulhas et al 2003).

Motion sickness

Commission E approves the use of ginger root for the prevention of motion sickness (Blumenthal et al 2000) and several clinical studies have assessed its effects as either prophylaxis or treatment. An early double-blind, randomised, placebo-controlled study involving 80 naval cadets found that ginger was significantly superior to placebo in reducing symptoms of vomiting and cold sweats due to seasickness. Fewer symptoms of nausea and vertigo were also reported with ginger, but the difference was not statistically significant (Grontved & Hentzer 1986). In another randomised double-blind study of seasickness involving over 1700 tourists on a whale-watching safari 300 km north of the Arctic Circle, 500 mg ginger was found to be as effective for the treatment of motion sickness as several common antiemetic medications (cinnarizine, cyclizine, dimenhydrinate, domperidone, meclizine and scopolamine) with ginger preventing seasickness in 80% of the subjects during the 6-hour boat trip, although the incidence of severe vomiting did not differ significantly between treatment groups (Schmid et al 1994).

At least three studies have had mixed results from experimental models of motion sickness whereby subjects are seated in a rotating chair. The first study involving 28 volunteers found no significant protective effects for powdered ginger (500 mg or 1000 mg) or fresh ginger root (1000 mg) (Stewart et al 1991), whereas a second study involving 36 undergraduate men and women who reported very high susceptibility to motion sickness found that ginger was superior to dimenhydrinate

(Mowrey & Clayson 1982). Another double-blind, randomised, placebo-controlled crossover study showed positive benefits with ginger pretreatment on prolonging time before nausea, shortening recovery time and effectively reducing nausea (Lien et al 2003). This study used pretreatment doses of 1000 mg and 2000 mg, which were also shown to reduce tachygastria and plasma vasopressin.

Chemotherapy-induced nausea and vomiting (CINV)

A review of seven RCTs and crossover trials concluded that ginger may be useful as an adjuvant therapy; however, interpretation is difficult because of mixed results due to methodological differences and the complex aetiology of chemotherapy-induced nausea and vomiting (CINV). Chemotherapy may affect both the central nervous system and the gastrointestinal tract which can influence their development of CINV. Patients may also be affected by sensory input (e.g. smell, sight) or 'anticipatory nausea' as a result of the individual's psychological condition (e.g. fear, anxiety) (Marx et al 2013).

One of the largest most recent placebo-controlled studies was conducted by Ryan et al (2012) which involved 576 cancer patients and showed that supplementation of 0.5, 1.0 and 1.5 g powdered ginger significantly reduced self-assessed acute nausea severity compared to placebo when administered for 3 days prior and 3 days after chemotherapy administration (Ryan et al 2012).

Comparative studies

Powdered ginger root effectively reduced cyclophosphamide-induced nausea and vomiting in a randomised, prospective, crossover double-blind study, with the anti-emetic effect of ginger being equal to metoclopramide (Sontakke et al 2003). Ginger was found to have similar efficacy to metoclopramide in reducing cisplatin-induced emesis in a randomised, double-blinded, crossover study of 48 gynaecological cancer patients receiving chemotherapy (Manusirivithaya et al 2004); however, the current clinical significance of this result is questionable, due to the fact that metoclopramide is no longer used as a stand-alone antiemetic treatment (Marx et al 2013).

Use with other anti-nausea medication

A recent combination study found that 1.5 g/day ginger taken with granisetron plus dexamethasone was more effective at reducing CINV than granisetron plus dexamethasone alone. A significantly lower prevalence of nausea, vomiting and retching was observed in the 6–24 hour post-chemotherapy period (Panahi et al 2012). Another RCT compared ginger root powder capsules or placebo in addition to ondansetron and dexamethasone for chemotherapy-induced nausea and vomiting in children and young adults, undergoing 60 cycles of cisplatin/doxorubicin for bone sarcoma (Pillai et al 2011). Acute moderate to severe vomiting and delayed nausea were reduced by 37–47% in the ginger group compared to placebo, highlighting the potential for ginger to act as an effective add-on therapy.

Nausea and vomiting with antiretroviral treatment

Ginger (500 mg twice daily) was effective in ameliorating antiretroviral-induced nausea and vomiting in a placebo-controlled RCT involving 102 HIV-positive patients (Dabaghzadeh et al 2014).

Musculoskeletal disorders

Ginger is described in Ayurvedic (traditional Indian) and Tibb (traditional Arabian) systems of medicine to be useful in inflammation and rheumatism and this traditional use is supported by modern studies demonstrating ginger's anti-inflammatory activity.

A highly purified and standardised ginger extract (EV.EXT 77) moderately reduced the symptoms of osteoarthritis (OA) of the knee in a double-blind, placebo-controlled, multicentre, parallel-group 6-week study of 261 patients (Altman & Marcussen 2001). Similarly, 250 mg of the ginger extract (Zintona EC) taken four times daily for 6 months was significantly more effective than placebo in reducing pain and disability in 29 OA patients in a double-blind, placebo-controlled, crossover study (Wigler et al 2003).

These studies are supported by an open retrospective study involving 56 patients (28 with RA, 18 with OA, 10 with muscular discomfort) that revealed more than three-quarters experienced varying degrees of relief of pain and swelling from the long-term use of powdered ginger (Srivastava & Mustafa 1992). Further support comes from studies comparing ginger to NSAIDs.

In one double-blind RCT involving 120 patients, 30 mg of an ethanolic ginger extract equivalent to 1 g of ginger and prepared from fresh ginger purchased from a local market in India was found to be significantly more effective than placebo and was as effective as 1.2 g of ibuprofen in the symptomatic treatment of OA (Haghighi et al 2005). In another double-blind crossover study, 170 mg of the ginger extract EV.EXT 33 with a standardised content of hydroxy-methoxy-phenyl compounds given twice daily was found to be significantly more effective than placebo but not as effective as ibuprofen in reducing pain and disability in 75 patients with OA before the crossover period, whereas no statistical difference was seen between ginger and placebo in the analysis after the crossover period. The authors commented that the washout period may have been insufficient to prevent carry-over effects, and that ginger might need to be administered for longer than 3 weeks, and possibly in a higher dosage, to be clinically effective (Bliddal et al 2000).

Topical ginger preparation

In a small pilot study, 10 patients with osteoarthritis applied external ginger compresses over the kidneys for 7 days in a phenomenological approach and found benefits such as improved posture, more comfortable and flexible joint mobility and a positive shift in pain perception (Therkleson 2010).

Post-exercise muscle pain

In a double blind, placebo-controlled clinical trial of healthy volunteers, daily consumption of 2 g of raw or heated ginger for 11 days was found to reduce eccentric exercise-induced muscle pain when compared to placebo (Black et al 2010). In this study, dried powdered ginger was placed in a sealed bottle with deionised water and heated in a water bath for 3 hours and 15 minutes at 100 degrees Celsius. No significant difference in pain reduction effect was found with the heated versus raw ginger (Black et al 2010).

Dysmenorrhoea

Ginger has been used orally to treat dysmenorrhoea and appears to be effective based on available evidence. Due to its ability to inhibit thromboxane synthetase and activate endorphin receptors, the use of ginger has been suggested in treatment of dysmenorrhoea (Backon 1991). A double-blind comparative clinical trial involving 150 participants demonstrated that ginger (250 mg ginger rhizome powder qid for 3 days from the start of their menstrual period) was just as effective as 250 mg mefenamic acid or 400 mg ibuprofen capsules in relieving pain in women with primary dysmenorrhoea (Ozgoli et al 2009). Significant benefits were also seen in a RCT of 120 participants with mild-moderate dysmenorrhoea. Treatment with 500 mg powdered ginger given three times per day for 3–5 days produced a significant improvement in intensity and duration of menstrual pain (Rahnama et al 2012).

Dyspepsia

Ginger stimulates the flow of saliva, bile and gastric secretions and therefore is traditionally used to stimulate appetite, reduce flatulence and colic, gastrointestinal spasms and generally act as a digestive aid. Commission E approves the use of ginger root for the treatment of dyspepsia (Blumenthal et al 2000).

Hyperlipidaemia

A double-blind controlled clinical trial of 85 volunteers with hyperlipidaemia showed ginger treatment (3 g/day) produced a significant lipid-lowering effect compared to controls. Measurement of lipid concentrations before and after 45 days of treatment showed significantly higher mean changes in triglyceride and cholesterol levels for ginger compared to control ($P < 0.05$) as well as significant mean reduction in LDL level and increase in HDL levels compared to controls (Alizadeh-Navaei et al 2008). This initial study shows promising results; however, further controlled human trials are necessary to prove efficacy, a conclusion shared by a review of the pharmacological properties of ginger (Li et al 2012).

G

Migraine

Ginger is used to prevent and treat migraine headache. Its ability to inhibit thromboxane A_2 and exert antihistamine, anti-inflammatory and gastric actions makes it a theoretically attractive choice (Mustafa & Srivastava 1990). This use is supported by an open-label study of 30 migraine sufferers reporting that treatment with a sublingual ginger and feverfew preparation (GelStat MigraineO) in the initial phase of a migraine resulted in most patients being satisfied with the therapy and being pain-free or only having mild headache post-treatment (Cady et al 2005).

IN COMBINATION

In a follow-up randomised pilot study of 60 patients, 221 migraine episodes were treated with sublingual feverfew/ginger (LipiGesic) or placebo, resulting in significant reductions in migraine and headache pain when used as a first line suppressive treatment (Cady et al 2011). Due to the use of a combination product, it is difficult to determine which herb is clinically effective from this study.

Pain

A review of eight RCTs for the treatment of any type of pain raised methodological concerns regarding previous clinical trial designs. Specifically, it concluded that the form of ginger (powder or ethanolic extract) results in variation in active constituent profiles, and this in combination with different therapeutic dosages results in variable levels of efficacy. Administration of over 1 g ginger per day results in amelioration of pain in most trials, whereas less than 510 mg per day does not (Terry et al 2011).

OTHER USES

Ginger cream or compress is used externally for mastitis.

Cognitive function

As a follow-up trial to a successful animal study, a double-blind RCT was conducted which involved 60 healthy middle aged women who received 800 mg ginger per day for 1 month or placebo. When compared to placebo, active treatment resulted in statistically significant improvements in attention, cognitive processing and working memory, including speed of recall and quality of memory (Saenghong et al 2012).

Diabetes

A randomised, double-blind placebo-controlled trial of 88 diabetic participants recently found that 1 g ginger capsules taken three times daily for 8 weeks significantly improved fasting blood sugar, fasting insulin and insulin sensitivity (Mozaffari-Khosravi et al 2014). Animal studies have also shown that ginger may have potential benefits in the treatment of diabetes, indicating that ginger improves insulin sensitivity and reduces serum glucose levels. Further clinical trials are required to confirm the significance of these findings in humans.

Weight loss

Further investigations in animal models and mixed-herbal clinical trials suggest a potential role for ginger in weight loss (Hasani-Ranjbar et al 2009). A significant reduction in body weight and parametrial adipose tissue following oral administration of zingerone in ovariectomised rats indicated that by increasing noradrenaline-induced lipolysis in adipocytes, zingerone may prevent fat storage (Han et al 2008). The anti-obesity action of ginger may be a result of slowed intestinal absorption of dietary fat (Han et al 2008).

Asthma

A possible therapeutic role for gingerol in the treatment of asthma has been indicated through a recent animal model. An aqueous ginger extract enriched in *n*-gingerols was investigated in Th2-mediated pulmonary inflammation where gingerols were found to decrease recruitment of eosinophils to the lungs and suppress Th2 cell response to allergen. Serum IL-4, IL-5 and IgE titres were diminished in ginger-treated mice relative to controls (Ahui et al 2008).

Ulcerative colitis

Recent research has identified a potential role for ginger in attenuating inflammatory bowel disease. In an in vitro study involving ulcerated male Wistar rats, ginger extract was found to be comparable to sulfasalazine in attenuating colonic mucosal injury. The effect of ginger against acetic acid-induced ulcerative colitis has been attributed to its anti-inflammatory and antioxidant properties (El-Abhar et al 2008). Clinical trials are required to determine the significance of this effect in humans.

DOSAGE RANGE

The recommended dose ranges widely from 500 mg to 9 g/day dried root or equivalent; however, a safe maximal dose is 4 g/day. As there are wide variations in the gingerol concentrations in commercial ginger supplements (Schwertner et al 2006), the effective dosage will depend on the preparation and the indication for use.

- Liquid extract (1:2): 0.7–4.0 mL/day.
- Dried root: 1–3 g daily in divided doses.
- Infusion: 4–6 slices of fresh ginger steeped in boiling water for 30 minutes.

According to clinical studies

- Dysmenorrhoea: 250 mg ginger rhizome powder taken four times daily for 3 days from the start of the menstrual period.
- Hyperlipidaemia: 3 g/day.
- Nausea and vomiting of pregnancy: 1–2 g taken daily in divided doses.
- Motion sickness: powdered ginger (500 mg or 1000 mg) or fresh ginger root (1000 mg) up to 2000 mg.
- Osteoarthritis: 250 mg of the ginger extract (Zintona EC) four times daily.

- Prevention of postoperative nausea: 1 g 1 hour prior to surgery.
- Rheumatoid arthritis: 1–2 g/day of powdered ginger.

ADVERSE REACTIONS

Gastric irritation, heartburn and bloating have been reported in clinical trials (Arfeen et al 1995). Contact dermatitis of the fingertips has also been reported (Seetharam & Pasricha 1987) with topical use.

SIGNIFICANT INTERACTIONS

Controlled studies are not available for many interactions; therefore they are based on evidence of activity and are largely theoretical and speculative.

Antibiotics

According to a recent review, ginger may enhance the absorption of antibiotics such as azithromycin, erythromycin and cephalexin when used in doses of between 10 and 30 mg/kg due to the herb's modulating effect on the gastric mucosa; however, the clinical significance of this effect is untested (Kesarwani & Gupta 2013).

Warfarin

Due to the herb's antiplatelet effects there is a theoretical risk of increased bleeding at high doses (>10 g), although this is not evident clinically. There is no evidence of an interaction with warfarin at the usual dietary and therapeutic intakes (Jiang et al 2005, Stenton et al 2001, Vaes & Chyka 2000), and ginger has been shown not to alter prothrombin times in pooled human plasma collected from male volunteers between the ages of 18 and 57 years (Jones et al 2001). A standardised ginger extract, EV.EXT 33, has demonstrated no significant effect on coagulation parameters or on warfarin-induced changes in blood coagulation in rats (Weidner & Sigwart 2000) and three ginger capsules (each containing an extract equivalent to 400 mg of ginger rhizome powder) taken three times daily for 2 weeks had no effect on the pharmacokinetics or pharmacodynamics of a single 25-mg dose of warfarin taken on day 7. Moreover, ginger alone did not affect the International Normalised Ratio (INR), platelet aggregation or the pharmacokinetics or pharmacodynamics of warfarin in healthy human subjects (Jiang et al 2005).

Antiplatelet drugs

Theoretically, increased antiplatelet and anti-inflammatory effects may occur with high-dose ginger preparations, but the clinical significance of this is unknown. Caution should be exercised with doses > 10 g — possible beneficial effect.

Cisplatin

Pretreatment has restored testicular antioxidant parameters and sperm motility in cisplatin-induced damage in an animal model (Amin & Hamza 2006). Clinical implications are uncertain; however, potential benefits may be found upon further testing.

CONTRAINDICATIONS AND PRECAUTIONS

Ginger in high doses is not recommended for children under 6 years of age due to the pungent nature of ginger. However, if the benefits of ginger treatment outweigh the potential for gastric irritation, then it can be used.

Alternatively, ginger lollies or ginger ale is sometimes used and a dose of 250 mg every 4 hours for motion sickness is safe.

Commission E suggests that people with gallstones consult with their doctor before using ginger. People with gastric ulcers or reflux should use this herb with caution. Suspend use of high-dose supplements (>10 g) 1 week before major surgery.

PREGNANCY USE

Although Commission E suggests that ginger is contraindicated in pregnancy, more recent research suggests that ginger is not contraindicated in pregnancy — doses up to 2 g/day of dried ginger root have been used safely.

No adverse effects on pregnancy were observed in multiple studies of ginger for nausea and vomiting (Boone & Shields 2005, Borrelli et al 2005, Bryer 2005, Dib & El-Saddik 2004, Ernst & Pittler 2000, Jewell & Young 2002).

Practice points/Patient counselling

- Ginger is most often used for its antiemetic, anti-inflammatory and gastrointestinal effects.
- There is good clinical support for the use of ginger in the treatment of nausea and vomiting associated with pregnancy and some evidence for its use in motion sickness, the postoperative period and chemotherapy although this is less consistent.
- Ginger is traditionally used for gastrointestinal disorders, including dyspepsia, poor appetite, flatulence, colic, vomiting, diarrhoea and spasms, as well as a diaphoretic in the treatment of the common cold and influenza.
- Ginger is also used as an anti-inflammatory agent for arthritis, although large controlled studies have yet to produce strong support for this use.
- Although antiplatelet effects have been reported, these require very large doses and are not likely to be significant in normal therapeutic doses or dietary intake levels.
- A study of 24 subjects found that ginger did not significantly affect clotting status or pharmacokinetics of warfarin in healthy subjects (Jiang et al 2006).
- Due to the potential seriousness of the proposed interaction, people taking warfarin should use high-dose supplements (>10 g/day) with caution.

PATIENTS' FAQs

What will this herb do for me?

Ginger is a useful treatment for nausea and vomiting associated with pregnancy and may also be of benefit in motion sickness, postoperative nausea and seasickness. It is also useful for treating symptoms of dyspepsia and may have symptom-relieving effects in arthritis, although this is less certain.

When will it start to work?

In the case of dyspepsia and motion sickness prevention, ginger will have an almost immediate effect, with improvement reported within 30 minutes. For motion sickness, 0.5–1.0 g ginger should be taken 30 minutes before travel and repeated 4-hourly. For nausea of pregnancy it should be taken for at least 4 days; however, symptoms should start to reduce within 1 hour of administration.

Are there any safety issues?

Ginger is well tolerated, although it should be used with caution by people with gallstones, gastric ulcers or reflux.

REFERENCES

Abdel-Aziz H et al. Mode of action of gingerols and shogaols on 5-HT3 receptors: binding studies, cation uptake by the receptor channel and contraction of isolated guinea-pig ileum. Eur J Pharmacol 530.1–2 (2006): 136–143.

Adewunmi CO, Oguntimein BO, Furu P. Molluscicidal and antischistosomal activities of Zingiber officinale. Planta Med 56.4 (1990): 374–376.

Ahmed RS et al. Protective effects of dietary ginger (Zingiber officinale Rosc.) on lindane-induced oxidative stress in rats. Phytother Res 22.7 (2008): 902–906.

Ahui ML et al. Ginger prevents Th2-mediated immune responses in a mouse model of airway inflammation. Int Immunopharmacol 8.12 (2008): 1626–1632.

Aimbire F et al. Effect of hydroalcoholic extract of Zingiber officinalis rhizomes on LPS-induced rat airway hyperreactivity and lung inflammation. Prostaglandins Leukot Essent Fatty Acids 77.3–4 (2007): 129–138.

Ajith TA, Hema U, Aswathy MS. Zingiber officinale Roscoe prevents acetaminophen-induced acute hepatotoxicity by enhancing hepatic antioxidant status. Food Chem Toxicol 45.11 (2007): 2267–2272.

Ajith TA et al. Protective effect of Zingiber officinale Roscoe against anticancer drug doxorubicin-induced acute nephrotoxicity. Food Chem Toxicol 46.9 (2008): 3178–3181.

Akoachere JF et al. Antibacterial effect of Zingiber officinale and Garcinia kola on respiratory tract pathogens. East Afr Med J 79.11 (2002): 588–592.

Aktan F et al. Gingerol metabolite and a synthetic analogue Capsarol inhibit macrophage NF-kappaB-mediated iNOS gene expression and enzyme activity. Planta Med 72.8 (2006): 727–734.

Al-Amin ZM et al. Anti-diabetic and hypolipidaemic properties of ginger (Zingiber officinale) in streptozotocin-induced diabetic rats. Br J Nutr 96.4 (2006): 660–666.

Alizadeh-Navaei R et al. Investigation of the effect of ginger on the lipid levels. A double blind controlled clinical trial. Saudi Med J 29.9 (2008): 1280–1284.

Altman RD, Marcussen KC. Effects of a ginger extract on knee pain in patients with osteoarthritis. Arthritis Rheum 44.11 (2001): 2531–2538.

Amin A, Hamza AA. Effects of Roselle and Ginger on cisplatin-induced reproductive toxicity in rats. Asian J Androl 8.5 (2006): 607–612.

Anoiske CA et al. Anti-inflammatory and anti-ulcerogenic activity of the ethanol extract of ginger (*Zingiber officinale*). Afr J of Biochem Res 3.12 (2009): 379–384.

Apariman S et al. Effectiveness of ginger for prevention of nausea and vomiting after gynecological laparoscopy. J Med Assoc Thai 89.12 (2006): 2003–2009.

Arfeen Z et al. A double-blind randomised controlled trial of ginger for the prevention of postoperative nausea and vomiting. Anaesth Intensive Care 23.4 (1995): 449–452.

Asnani V, Verma RJ. Antioxidative effect of rhizome of Zinziber officinale on paraben induced lipid peroxidation: an in vitro study. Acta Pol Pharm 64.1 (2007): 35–37.

Atta AH et al Hepatoprotective effect of methanol extracts of Zingiber officinale and Cichorium intybus Indian J of Pharm Sc 72.5 (2010): 564–70.

Awang DVC. Ginger. Can Pharm J 125.7 (1992): 309–311.

Backon J. Mechanism of analgesic effect of clonidine in the treatment of dysmenorrhea. Med Hypotheses 36.3 (1991): 223–224.

Bellik Y Total antioxidant activity and antimicrobial potency of the essential oil and oleoresin of Zingiber officinale Roscoe. Asian Pac J Trop Dis 4.1 (2014): 40–44.

Betz O et al. Is ginger a clinically relevant antiemetic? A systematic review of randomised controlled trials. Forsch Komplementarmed Klass Naturheilkd 12.1 (2005): 14–23.

Bhandari U et al. Antihepatotoxic activity of ginger ethanol extract in rats. Pharm Biol 41.1 (2003): 68–71.

Bhandari U, Kanojia R, Pillai KK. Effect of ethanolic extract of Zingiber officinale on dyslipidaemia in diabetic rats. J Ethnopharmacol 97.2 (2005): 227–230.

Bhattarai S, Tran VH, Duke CC. The stability of gingerol and shogaol in aqueous solutions. J Pharm Sci 90.10 (2001): 1658–1664.

Black CD et al. Ginger (Zingiber officinale) Reduces Muscle Pain Caused by Eccentric Exercise. Journal of Pain 11.9 (2010): 894–903.

Bliddal H et al. A randomised, placebo-controlled, cross-over study of ginger extracts and ibuprofen in osteoarthritis. Osteoarthritis Cartilage 8.1 (2000): 9–12.

Blumenthal M, Goldberg A, Brinckmann J (eds). Herbal medicine: expanded commission E monographs. Austin, TX: Integrative Medicine Communications, 2000.

Bode AM et al. Inhibition of epidermal growth factor-induced cell transformation and activator protein 1 activation by [6]-gingerol. Cancer Res 61.3 (2001): 850–853.

Bone ME et al. Ginger root: a new antiemetic: the effect of ginger root on postoperative nausea and vomiting after major gynaecological surgery. Anaesthesia 45.8 (1990): 669–671.

Boone SA, Shields KM. Treating pregnancy-related nausea and vomiting with ginger. Ann Pharmacother 39.10 (2005): 1710–1713.

Bordia A, Verma SK, Srivastava KC. Effect of ginger (Zingiber officinale Rosc.) and fenugreek (Trigonella foenum-graecum L.) on blood lipids, blood sugar and platelet aggregation in patients with coronary artery disease. Prostaglandins Leukot Essent Fatty Acids 56.5 (1997): 379–384.

Borrelli F et al. Effectiveness and safety of ginger in the treatment of pregnancy-induced nausea and vomiting. Obstet Gynecol 105.4 (2005): 849–856.

Brown AC et al. Ginger's (Zingiber officinale Roscoe) inhibition of rat colonic adenocarcinoma cells proliferation and angiogenesis in vitro. Phytother Res 23.5 (2008): 640–645.

Bryer E. A literature review of the effectiveness of ginger in alleviating mild-to-moderate nausea and vomiting of pregnancy. J Midwifery Womens Health 50.1 (2005): e1–e3.

Cady RK et al. Gelstat Migraine (sublingually administered feverfew and ginger compound) for acute treatment of migraine when administered during the mild pain phase. Med Sci Monitor Int Med J Exp Clin Res 11.9 (2005): PI65–PI69.

Cady RK et al A double-blind placebo-controlled pilot study of sublingual feverfew and ginger (LipiGesic M) in the treatment of migraine. Headache 51.7 (2011): 1078–86.

Canter PH. Ginger: do we know what we are talking about? Focus Altern Complement Ther 9.3 (2004): 184–185.

Chaiyakunapruk N et al. The efficacy of ginger for the prevention of postoperative nausea and vomiting: a meta-analysis. Am J Obstet Gynecol 194.1 (2006): 95–99.

Charles R et al. New gingerdione from the rhizomes of Zingiber officinale. Fitoterapia 71.6 (2000): 716–718.

Chen CY et al. 6-shogaol (alkanone from ginger) induces apoptotic cell death of human hepatoma p53 mutant Mahlavu subline via an oxidative stress-mediated caspase-dependent mechanism. J Agric Food Chem 55.3 (2007): 948–954.

Chittumma P et al. Comparison of the effectiveness of ginger and vitamin B6 for treatment of nausea and vomiting in early pregnancy: a randomized double-blind controlled trial. J Med Assoc Thai 90.1 (2007): 15–20.

Dabaghzadeh F et al. Ginger for prevention of antiretroviral-induced nausea and vomiting: a randomized clinical trial. Expert Opin Drug Saf 13.7 (2014): 859–866.

Daswani PG et al Antidiarrhoeal activity of Zingiber officinale (Rosc). Current Science 98.2 (2010): 222–229.

Dedov VN et al. Gingerols: a novel class of vanilloid receptor (VR1) agonists. Br J Pharmacol 137.6 (2002): 793–798.

Denyer CV et al. Isolation of antirhinoviral sesquiterpenes from ginger (Zingiber officinale). J Nat Prod 57.5 (1994): 658–662.

Dib JG, El-Saddik RA. Ginger for nausea and vomiting in pregnancy. J Pharm Pract Res 34.4 (2004): 305–307.

Ding M et al. The effectiveness and safety of ginger for pregnancy-induced nausea and vomiting:A systematic review. Women Birth 26.1 (2013): e26–30.

Du YH et al. [Preliminary study on disease menu of acupuncture and moxibustion abroad]. Zhongguo Zhen Jiu 29.1 (2009): 53–55.

Eberhart LHJ et al. Ginger does not prevent postoperative nausea and vomiting after laparoscopic surgery. Anesth Analg 96.4 (2003): 995–998.

El-Abhar HS et al. Modulating effect of ginger extract on rats with ulcerative colitis. J Ethnopharmacol 118.3 (2008): 367–372.

Eliakim R, Abulafia O, Sherer DM. Hyperemesis gravidarum: a current review. Am J Perinatol 17.4 (2000): 207–218.

Ensiyeh J, Sakineh MA. Comparing ginger and vitamin B6 for the treatment of nausea and vomiting in pregnancy: a randomised controlled trial. Midwifery (2008).

Ernst E, Pittler MH. Efficacy of ginger for nausea and vomiting: a systematic review of randomized clinical trials. Br J Anaesth 84.3 (2000): 367–371.

Fischer-Rasmussen W et al. Ginger treatment of hyperemesis gravidarum. Eur J Obstet Gynecol Reprod Biol 38.1 (1990): 19–24.

Flynn DL et al. Inhibition of human neutrophil 5-lipoxygenase activity by gingerdione, shogaol, capsaicin and related pungent compounds. Prostaglandins Leukot Med 24.2–3 (1986): 195–198.

Fuhrman B et al. Ginger extract consumption reduces plasma cholesterol, inhibits LDL oxidation and attenuates development of atherosclerosis in atherosclerotic, apolipoprotein E-deficient mice. J Nutr 130.5 (2000): 1124–1131.

Funk JL et al. Comparative effects of two gingerol-containing Zingiber officinale extracts on experimental rheumatoid arthritis (perpendicular). J Nat Prod (2009).

Geiger JL. The essential oil of ginger, Zingiber officinale, and anaesthesia. Int J Aromather 15.1 (2005): 7–14.

Ghayur MN, Gilani AH. Pharmacological basis for the medicinal use of ginger in gastrointestinal disorders. Dig Dis Sci 50.10 (2005): 1889–1897.

Ghayur MN et al. Muscarinic, Ca(++) antagonist and specific butyrylcholinesterase inhibitory activity of dried ginger extract might explain its use in dementia. J Pharm Pharmacol 60.10 (2008): 1375–1383.

Gonlachanvit S et al. Ginger reduces hyperglycemia-evoked gastric dysrhythmias in healthy humans: possible role of endogenous prostaglandins. J Pharmacol Exp Ther 307.3 (2003): 1098–1103.

Goto C et al. Lethal efficacy of extract from Zingiber officinale (traditional Chinese medicine) or [6]-shogaol and [6]-gingerol in Anisakis larvae in vitro. Parasitol Res 76.8 (1990): 653–656.

Govindarajan VS. Ginger: chemistry, technology, and quality evaluation: part 2. Crit Rev Food Sci Nutr 17 (1982): 189–258.

Goyal RK, Kadnur SV. Beneficial effects of Zingiber officinale on goldthioglucose induced obesity. Fitoterapia 77.3 (2006): 160–163.

Grontved A, Hentzer E. Vertigo-reducing effect of ginger root: a controlled clinical study. ORL J Otorhinolaryngol Relat Spec 48.5 (1986): 282–286.

Grzanna R et al. Ginger: an herbal medicinal product with broad anti-inflammatory actions. J Med Food 8.2 (2005): 125–132.

Gulhas N et al. The effect of ginger and ondansetron on nausea and vomiting after middle ear surgery. Anestezi Dergisi 11.4 (2003): 265–268.

Gupta YK, Sharma M. Reversal of pyrogallol-induced delay in gastric emptying in rats by ginger (Zingiber officinale). Methods Find Exp Clin Pharmacol 23.9 (2001): 501–503.

Haghighi M et al. Comparing the effects of ginger (Zingiber officinale) extract and ibuprofen on patients with osteoarthritis. Arch Iran Med 8.4 (2005): 267–271.
Haji Seid Javadi, E et al. Comparing the effectiveness of Vitamin B6 and Ginger in the treatment of pregnancy-induced nausea and vomiting. Obstet Gynecol Int (2013): Article ID 927834.
Haksar A et al. Zingiber officinale exhibits behavioral radioprotection against radiation-induced CTA in a gender-specific manner. Pharmacol Biochem Behav 84.2 (2006): 179–188.
Han LK et al. Effects of zingerone on fat storage in ovariectomized rats. Yakugaku Zasshi 128.8 (2008): 1195–1201.
Hasani-Ranjbar S et al. A systematic review of the efficacy and safety of herbal medicines used in the treatment of obesity. World J Gastroenterol 15.25 (2009): 3073–3085.
Hasenohrl RU et al. Anxiolytic-like effect of combined extracts of Zingiber officinale and ginkgo biloba in the elevated plus-maze. Pharmacol Biochem Behav 53.2 (1996): 271–275.
Henry CJ, Piggott SM. Effect of ginger on metabolic rate. Hum Nutr Clin Nutr 41.1 (1987): 89–92.
Hu ML et al. Effect of ginger on gastric motility and symptoms of functional dyspepsia. World J. Gastroenterol.17.1 (2011) 105–10.
Huang QR et al. Anti-5-hydroxytryptamine3 effect of galanolactone, diterpenoid isolated from ginger. Chem Pharm Bull 39.2 (1991): 397–399.
Hunt R et al. Aromatherapy as treatment for postoperative nausea: a randomized trial. Anaesth Analg 117.3 (2013): 597–604.
Imanishi N et al. Macrophage-mediated inhibitory effect of Zingiber officinale Rosc., a traditional oriental herbal medicine, on the growth of influenza A/Aichi/2/68 virus. Am J Chin Med 34.1 (2006): 157–169.
Ishiguro K et al. Ginger ingredients reduce viability of gastric cancer cells via distinct mechanisms. Biochem Biophys Res Commun 362.1 (2007): 218–223.
Islam MS, Choi H. Comparative effects of dietary ginger (Zingiber officinale) and garlic (Allium sativum) investigated in a type 2 diabetes model of rats. J Med Food 11.1 (2008): 152–159.
Jagetia GC et al. Influence of ginger rhizome (Zingiber officinale Rosc.) on survival, glutathione and lipid peroxidation in mice after whole-body exposure to gamma radiation. Radiat Res 160.5 (2003): 584–592.
Janssen PL et al. Consumption of ginger (Zingiber officinale Roscoe) does not affect ex vivo platelet thromboxane production in humans. Eur J Clin Nutr 50.11 (1996): 772–774.
Jewell D, Young G. Interventions for nausea and vomiting in early pregnancy. Cochrane Database Syst Rev 1 (2002): CD000145.
Jewell D. Nausea and vomiting in early pregnancy. Am Fam Physician 68.1 (2003): 143–144.
Jeyakumar SM et al. Antioxidant activity of ginger (Zingiber officinale Rosc.) in rats fed a high fat diet. Med Sci Res 27.5 (1999): 341–344.
Jiang X et al. Investigation of the effects of herbal medicines on warfarin response in healthy subjects: a population pharmacokinetic-pharmacodynamic modeling approach. J Clin Pharmacol 46.11 (2006): 1370–1378.
Jiang X et al. Effect of ginkgo and ginger on the pharmacokinetics and pharmacodynamics of warfarin in healthy subjects. Br J Clin Pharmacol 59.4 (2005): 425–432.
Jones SC et al. The development of a human tissue model to determine the effect of plant-derived dietary supplements on prothrombin time. J Herbal Pharmacother 1.1 (2001): 21–34.
Kadnur SV, Goyal RK. Beneficial effects of Zingiber officinale Roscoe on fructose induced hyperlipidemia and hyperinsulinemia in rats. Indian J Exp Biol 43.12 (2005): 1161–1164.
Kano Y et al. Pharmacological properties of galenical preparation. XIV. body temperature retaining effect of the Chinese traditional medicine, goshuyu-to and component crude drugs. Tokyo: Chem Pharm Bull 39.3 (1991): 690–692.
Kalaivani K et al. Biological activity of selected Lamiaceae and Zingiberaceae plant essential oils against the dengue vector Aedes aegypti L. (Diptera: Culicidae). Parasitol Res 110 (2012): 1261–1268.
Kalava A et al. Efficacy of ginger on intraoperative and postoperative nausea and vomiting in elective cesarean section patients. Euro J Obstet Gynecol Repro Biol 169.2 (2013): 184–188.
Kato A et al. Inhibitory effects of Zingiber officinale Roscoe derived components on aldose reductase activity in vitro and in vivo. J Agric Food Chem 54.18 (2006): 6640–6644.
Kawai T et al. Anti-emetic principles of Magnolia obovata bark and Zingiber officinale rhizome. Planta Med 60.1 (1994): 17–20.
Keating A, Chez RA. Ginger syrup as an antiemetic in early pregnancy. Altern Ther Health Med 8.5 (2002): 89–91.
Kesawarni K, Gupta R. Bioavailability enhancers of herbal origin. Asian Pac J Trop Biomed 3.4 (2013): 253–266.
Kikuzaki H et al. Constituents of Zingiberaceae. I. Diarylheptanoids from the rhizomes of ginger (Zingiber officinale Roscoe). Chem Pharm Bull 39.1 (1991): 120–122.
Kim JH et al. [6]-Gingerol suppresses interleukin-1 beta-induced MUC5AC gene expression in human airway epithelial cells. Am J Rhinol Allergy 23.4 (2009): 385–391.
Kim JK et al. [6]-Gingerol prevents UVB-induced ROS production and COX-2 expression in vitro and in vivo. Free Radic Res 41.5 (2007): 603–614.
Kim SO et al. [6]-Gingerol inhibits COX-2 expression by blocking the activation of p38 MAP kinase and NF-kappaB in phorbol ester-stimulated mouse skin. Oncogene 24.15 (2005): 2558–2567.
Kiuchi F et al. Inhibition of prostaglandin and leukotriene biosynthesis by gingerols and diarylheptanoids. Chem Pharm Bull 40.2 (1992): 387–391.
Kobayashi M, Shoji N, Ohizumi Y. Gingerol, a novel cardiotonic agent, activates the Ca^{2+}-pumping ATPase in skeletal and cardiac sarcoplasmic reticulum. Biochim Biophys Acta 903.1 (1987): 96–102.
Koch C et al. Inhibitory effect of essential oils against herpes simplex virus type 2. Phytomedicine 15.1–2 (2008): 71–78.
Koo KL et al. Gingerols and related analogues inhibit arachidonic acid-induced human platelet serotonin release and aggregation. Thromb Res 103.5 (2001): 387–397.
Kumar S et al. Evaluation of 15 local plant species as larvicidal agents against an Indian strain of dengue fever mosquito, *Aedes aegypti* L.(Diptera: Culicidae). Frontiers in Phys. 3 (2012) Art 104.

Langner E et al. Ginger: history and use. Adv Ther 15.1 (1998): 25–44.
Lee E, Surh YJ. Induction of apoptosis in HL-60 cells by pungent vanilloids, [6]-gingerol and [6]-paradol. Cancer Lett 134.2 (1998): 163–168.
Lee HS et al. [6]-Gingerol inhibits metastasis of MDA-MB-231 human breast cancer cells. J Nutr Biochem 19.5 (2008): 313–3119.
Li Y et al. Preventive and protective properties of Zingiber officinale (Ginger) in diabetes mellitus, diabetic complications, and associated lipid and other metabolic disorders: a brief review. Evidence-Based Complementary and Alternative Medicine Volume 2012 (2012): ID 516870.
Lien HC et al. Effects of ginger on motion sickness and gastric slow-wave dysrhythmias induced by circular vection. Am J Physiol Gastrointest Liver Physiol 284.3 (2003): G481–G489.
Ling H et al. 6-Shogaol, an active constituent of ginger, inhibits breast cancer cell invasion by reducing matrix metalloproteinase-9 expression via blockade of nuclear factor-kB activation. British J Pharma 161 (2010): 1763–1777.
Liu HL, Wang LP. [Randomized controlled study on ginger-salt-partitioned moxibustion at shenque (CV 8) on urination disorders poststroke]. Zhongguo Zhen Jiu 26.9 (2006): 621–624.
Liu N et al. [Effect of Zingiber Officinale Rosc on lipid peroxidation in hyperlipidemia rats]. Wei Sheng Yan Jiu 32.1 (2003): 22–23.
Lu CJ. Function of ginger on cerebrovascular disease and its gateway. Chin J Clin Rehab 9.45 (2005): 187–189.
Lumb AB. Effect of dried ginger on human platelet function. Thromb Haemost 71.1 (1994): 110–1111.
Mahady GB et al. Ginger (Zingiber officinale Roscoe) and the gingerols inhibit the growth of Cag A+ strains of Helicobacter pylori. Anticancer Res 23.5A (2003): 3699–3702.
Mahady GB et al. In vitro susceptibility of Helicobacter pylori to botanical extracts used traditionally for the treatment of gastrointestinal disorders. Phytother Res 19.11 (2005): 988–991.
Mallikarjuna K et al. Ethanol toxicity: rehabilitation of hepatic antioxidant defense system with dietary ginger. Fitoterapia 79.3 (2008): 174–178.
Manju V, Nalini N. Chemopreventive efficacy of ginger, a naturally occurring anticarcinogen during the initiation, post-initiation stages of 1,2 dimethylhydrazine-induced colon cancer. Clin Chim Acta 358.1–2 (2005): 60–67.
Manusirivithaya S et al. Antiemetic effect of ginger in gynecologic oncology patients receiving cisplatin. Int J Gynecol Cancer 14.6 (2004): 1063–1069.
Martins AP et al. Essential oil composition and antimicrobial activity of three Zingiberaceae from S.Tome e Principle. Planta Med 67.6 (2001): 580–584.
Marx WM et al. Ginger (Zingiber officinale) and chemotherapy-induced nausea and vomiting: a systematic literature review. Nutrition Reviews 71.4 (2013): 245–254.
Matthews A et al. Interventions for nausea and vomiting in early pregnancy. Cochrane Database Sys Rev 9 (2010):CD007575.
Meyer K et al. Zingiber officinale (ginger) used to prevent 8-Mop associated nausea. Dermatol Nurs 7.4 (1995): 242–244.
Micklefield GH et al. Effects of ginger on gastroduodenal motility. Int J Clin Pharmacol Ther 37.7 (1999): 341–346.
Morakinyo AO et al. Effect of Zingiber officinale (Ginger) on sodium arsenite-induced reproductive toxicity in male rats. Afr. J. Biomed. Res. 13 (2010): 39–45.
Motawi TK et al. *Zingiber officinale* acts as a nutraceutical agent against liver fibrosis. Nutr Metab (Lond). 8 (2011): 40.
Mowrey D, Clayson D. Motion sickness, ginger and psychosis. Lancet 319.8273 (1982): 655–657.
Mozaffari-Khosravi H et al. The effect of ginger powder supplementation on insulin resistance and glycemic indices in patients with Type 2 diabetes: a randomized, double-blind, placebo-controlled trial. Complementary Therapies in Medicine (2014): http://dx.doi.org/10.1016/j.ctim.2013.12.017 online ahead of print.
Mustafa T, Srivastava KC. Possible leads for arachidonic acid metabolism altering drugs from natural products. J Drug Develop 3.1 (1990): 47–60.
Mustafa T et al. Pharmacology of ginger. Zingiber officinale. J Drug Dev 6.11 (1993): 25–39.
Nagoshi C et al. Synergistic effect of [10]-gingerol and aminoglycosides against vancomycin-resistant enterococci (VRE). Biol Pharm Bull 29.3 (2006): 443–447.
Nanthakomon T, Pongrojpaw D. The efficacy of ginger in prevention of postoperative nausea and vomiting after major gynecologic surgery. J Med Assoc Thai 89 (Suppl 4) (2006): S130–S136.
Nostro A et al. Effects of combining extracts (from propolis or Zingiber officinale) with clarithromycin on Helicobacter pylori. Phytother Res 20.3 (2006): 187–190.
Nurtjahja-Tjendraputra E et al. Effective anti-platelet and COX-1 enzyme inhibitors from pungent constituents of ginger. Thromb Res 111.4–5 (2003): 259–265.
Okada K, Kawakita K. Analgesic action of acupuncture and moxibustion: a review of unique approaches in Japan. Evid Based Complement Alternat Med 6.1 (2009): 11–117.
O'Mahony R et al. Bactericidal and anti-adhesive properties of culinary and medicinal plants against Helicobacter pylori. World J Gastroenterol 11.47 (2005): 7499–7507.
Onogi T et al. Capsaicin-like effect of (6)-shogaol on substance P-containing primary afferents of rats: a possible mechanism of its analgesic action. Neuropharmacology 31.11 (1992): 1165–1169.
Ozgoli G et al. Comparison of effects of ginger, mefenamic acid, and ibuprofen on pain in women with primary dysmenorrhea. J Altern Complement Med 15.2 (2009): 129–32.
Pan MH et al. 6-Shogaol suppressed lipopolysaccharide-induced up-expression of iNOS and COX-2 in murine macrophages. Mol Nutr Food Res 52.12 (2008): 1467–1477.
Panahi Y et al. Effect of ginger on acute and delayed chemotherapy-induced nausea and vomiting: a pilot, randomized, open-label clinical trial. Integr Cancer Ther 11.3 (2012): 204–211.
Park YJ et al. [6]-Gingerol induces cell cycle arrest and cell death of mutant p53-expressing pancreatic cancer cells. Yonsei Med J 47.5 (2006): 688–697.

Park M et al. Antibacterial activity of [10]-gingerol and [12]-gingerol isolated from ginger rhizome against periodontal bacteria. Phytother Res 22.11 (2008): 1446–1449.

Penna SC et al. Anti-inflammatory effect of the hydralcoholic extract of Zingiber officinale rhizomes on rat paw and skin edema. Phytomedicine 10.5 (2003): 381–385.

Phillips S et al. Zingiber officinale (ginger): an antiemetic for day case surgery. Anaesthesia 48.8 (1993): 715–7117.

Pillai AK et al. Anti-emetic effect of ginger powder versus placebo as an add-on therapy in children and young adults receiving high emetogenic chemotherapy. Pediatr Blood Cancer 56.2 (2011): 234–8.

Platel K, Srinivasan K. Influence of dietary spices or their active principles on digestive enzymes of small intestinal mucosa in rats. Int J Food Sci Nutr 47.1 (1996): 55–59.

Platel K, Srinivasan K. Studies on the influence of dietary spices on food transit time in experimental rats. Nutr Res 21.9 (2001): 1309–1314.

Pongrojpaw D, Chiamchanya C. The efficacy of ginger in prevention of post-operative nausea and vomiting after outpatient gynecological laparoscopy. J Med Assoc Thailand 86.3 (2003): 244–250.

Pongrojpaw D et al. A randomized comparison of ginger and dimenhydrinate in the treatment of nausea and vomiting in pregnancy. J Med Assoc Thai 90.9 (2007): 1703–1709.

Portnoi G et al. Prospective comparative study of the safety and effectiveness of ginger for the treatment of nausea and vomiting in pregnancy. Am J Obstet Gynecol 189.5 (2003): 1374–1377.

Rahnama et al. Effect of Zingiber officinale R. rhizomes (ginger) on pain relief in primary dysmenorrhea: a placebo randomized trial. BMC Complementary and Alternative Medicine 12.92 (2012).

Ramadan G et al. anti-inflammatory and anti-oxidant properties of Curcuma longa (Turmeric) versus Zingiber officinale (Ginger) rhizomes in rat adjuvant-induced arthritis. Inflammation 34.4 (2011): 291–301.

Rhode J et al. Ginger inhibits cell growth and modulates angiogenic factors in ovarian cancer cells. BMC Complement Altern Med 7 (2007): 44.

Riyazi A et al. The effect of the volatile oil from ginger rhizomes (Zingiber officinale), its fractions and isolated compounds on the 5-HT3 receptor complex and the serotoninergic system of the rat ileum. Planta Med 73.4 (2007): 355–362.

Ryan JL et al. Ginger (Zingiber officinale) reduces acute chemotherapy-induced nausea: a URCC CCOP study of 576 patients. Support Care Cancer 20.7 (2012): 1479–489.

Rosengarten FJ. The book of spices. Wynnewood, PA: Livingston Publishing, 1969.

Sabli F et al Cytotoxic Properties of selected *Etlingera* spp. and *Zingiber* spp. (Zingiberaceae) endemic to Borneo. Pertanika J. Trop. Agric. Sci. 35.3 (2012): 663–671.

Saenghong N et al. Zingiber officinale improves cognitive function of the middle-aged healthy women. Evidence-Based Complementary and Alternative Medicine 2012 (2012): ID 383062.

Schmid R et al. Comparison of seven commonly used agents for prophylaxis of seasickness. J Travel Med 1.4 (1994): 203–206.

Schnitzler P et al. Susceptibility of drug-resistant clinical herpes simplex virus type 1 strains to essential oils of ginger, thyme, hyssop, and sandalwood. Antimicrob Agents Chemother 51.5 (2007): 1859–1862.

Schuhbaum H, Franz G. Ginger: spice and versatile medicinal plant. Z Phytother 21.4 (2000): 203–209 [in German].

Schwertner HA et al. Variation in concentration and labeling of ginger root dietary supplements. Obstet Gynecol 107.6 (2006): 1337–1343.

Seetharam KA, Pasricha JS. Condiments and contact dermatitis of the finger-tips. Indian J Dermatol Venereol Leprol 53.6 (1987): 325–328.

Sertie JAA et al. Preventive anti-ulcer activity of the rhizome extract of Zingiber officinale. Fitoterapia 63.1 (1992): 55–59.

Sharma JN et al. Suppressive effects of eugenol and ginger oil on arthritic rats. Pharmacology 49.5 (1994): 314–3118.

Sharma A et al. Zingiber officinale Rosc. modulates gamma radiation-induced conditioned taste aversion. Pharmacol Biochem Behav 81.4 (2005): 864–870.

Shen X et al. An infrared radiation study of the biophysical characteristics of traditional moxibustion. Complement Ther Med 14.3 (2006): 213–2119.

Shoji N et al. Cardiotonic principles of ginger (Zingiber officinale Roscoe). J Pharm Sci 71.10 (1982): 1174–1175.

Shukla Y et al. In vitro and in vivo modulation of testosterone mediated alterations in apoptosis related proteins by [6]-gingerol. Mol Nutr Food Res 51.12 (2007): 1492–1502.

Siddaraju MN, Dharmesh SM. Inhibition of gastric H^+, K^+-ATPase and Helicobacter pylori growth by phenolic antioxidants of Zingiber officinale. Mol Nutr Food Res 51.3 (2007): 324–332.

Smith C et al. A randomized controlled trial of ginger to treat nausea and vomiting in pregnancy. Obstet Gynecol 103.4 (2004): 639–645.

Sontakke S et al. Ginger as an antiemetic in nausea and vomiting induced by chemotherapy: a randomized, cross-over, double blind study. Indian J Pharmacol 35.1 (2003): 32–36.

Sripramote M, Lekhyananda N. A randomized comparison of ginger and vitamin B6 in the treatment of nausea and vomiting of pregnancy. J Med Assoc Thai 86.9 (2003): 846–853.

Srivastava KC, Mustafa T. Ginger (Zingiber officinale) in rheumatism and musculoskeletal disorders. Med Hypotheses 39.4 (1992): 342–348.

Stenton SB et al. Interactions between warfarin and herbal products, minerals, and vitamins: a pharmacist's guide. Can J Hospital Pharm 54.3 (2001): 184–190.

Stewart JJ et al. Effects of ginger on motion sickness susceptibility and gastric function. Pharmacology 42.2 (1991): 111–120.

Takada Y et al. Zerumbone abolishes NF-kappaB and IkappaBalpha kinase activation leading to suppression of antiapoptotic and metastatic gene expression, upregulation of apoptosis, and downregulation of invasion. Oncogene 24.46 (2005): 6957–6969.

Terry R. et al. The use of ginger (*Zingiber officinale*) for the treatment of pain: a systematic review of clinical trials. Pain Medicine 12 (2011) 1808–1818.

Therkleson T. Ginger compress therapy for adults with osteoarthritis. J Adv Nurs 66.10 (2010), 2225–2233.

Thomson M et al. The use of ginger (Zingiber officinale Rosc.) as a potential anti-inflammatory and antithrombotic agent. Prostaglandins Leukot Essent Fatty Acids 67.6 (2002): 475–478.

Tjendraputra E et al. Effect of ginger constituents and synthetic analogues on cyclooxygenase-2 enzyme in intact cells. Bioorgan Chem 29.3 (2001): 156–163.

Tripathi S et al. Ginger extract inhibits LPS-induced macrophage activation and function. BMC Complement Altern Med 8 (2008): 1.

Tripathi S et al. Effect of 6-gingerol on pro-inflammatory cytokine production and costimulatory molecule expression in murine peritoneal macrophages. J Surg Res 138.2 (2007): 209–213.

Vaes LP, Chyka PA. Interactions of warfarin with garlic, ginger, ginkgo, or ginseng: nature of the evidence. Ann Pharmacother 34.12 (2000): 1478–1482.

Verma SK, Bordia A. Ginger, fat and fibrinolysis. Indian J Med Sci 55.2 (2001): 83–86.

Visalyaputra S et al. The efficacy of ginger root in the prevention of postoperative nausea and vomiting after outpatient gynaecological laparoscopy. Anaesthesia 53.5 (1998): 506–510.

Vishwakarma SL et al. Anxiolytic and antiemetic activity of Zingiber officinale. Phytother Res 16.7 (2002): 621–626.

Vutyavanich T et al. Ginger for nausea and vomiting in pregnancy: Randomized, double-masked, placebo-controlled trial. Obstet Gynecol 97.4 (2001): 577–582.

Wei QY et al. Cytotoxic and apoptotic activities of diarylheptanoids and gingerol-related compounds from the rhizome of Chinese ginger. J Ethnopharmacol 102.2 (2005): 177–184.

Weidner MS, Sigwart K. The safety of a ginger extract in the rat. J Ethnopharmacol 73.3 (2000): 513–520.

WHO. Rhizoma Zingiberis. Geneva: World Health Organization. Available online at: www.who.int/medicines/library/trm/medicinalplants (accessed 15-12-03).

Wigler I et al. The effects of Zintona EC (a ginger extract) on symptomatic gonarthritis. Osteoarthritis Cartilage 11.11 (2003): 783–789.

Wilasrusmee C et al. In vitro immunomodulatory effects of herbal products. Am Surg 68.10 (2002): 860–864.

Willetts KE, Ekangaki A, Eden JA. Effect of a ginger extract on pregnancy-induced nausea: a randomised controlled trial. Aust NZ J Obstet Gynaecol 43.2 (2003): 139–144.

Wu KL et al. Effects of ginger on gastric emptying and motility in healthy humans. Eur J Gastroenterol Hepatol 20.5 (2008): 436–440.

Xiaoxiang Z. Jinger moxibustion for treatment of cervical vertigo — a report of 40 cases. J Tradit Chin Med 26.1 (2006): 17–118.

Xie XX, Lei QH. [Observation on therapeutic effect of the spreading moxibustion on rheumatoid arthritis]. Zhongguo Zhen Jiu 28.10 (2008): 730–732.

Yagihashi S et al. Inhibitory effect of gingerol on the proliferation and invasion of hepatoma cells in culture. Cytotechnology 57.2 (2008): 129–136.

Yamada Y et al. Identification of antimicrobial gingerols from ginger (Zingiber officinale Roscoe). J Antibact Antifungal Agents Jpn 20.6 (1992): 309–311.

Yamahara J et al. Cholagocic effect of ginger and its active constituents. J Ethnopharmacol 13.2 (1985): 217–225.

Yamahara J et al. The anti ulcer effect in rats of ginger constituents. J Ethnopharmacol 23.2–3 (1988): 299–304.

Yamahara J et al. Gastrointestinal motility enhancing effect of ginger and its active constituents. Chem Pharm Bull 38.2 (1990): 430–431.

Yamahara J et al. Stomachic principles in ginger. II. Pungent and anti-ulcer effects of low polar constituents isolated from ginger, the dried rhizoma of Zingiber officinale Roscoe cultivated in Taiwan: the absolute stereostructure of a new diarylheptanoid. Yakugaku Zasshi 112.9 (1992): 645–655 [in Japanese].

Yamahara J et al. Pharmacological study on ginger processing. I. Antiallergic activity and cardiotonic action of gingerols and shogaols. Nat Med 49.1 (1995): 76–83: [in Japanese].

Yemitan OK, Izegbu MC. Protective effects of Zingiber officinale (Zingiberaceae) against carbon tetrachloride and acetaminophen-induced hepatotoxicity in rats. Phytother Res 20.11 (2006): 997–1002.

Yoshikawa M et al. 6-Gingesulfonic acid, a new anti-ulcer principle, and gingerglycolipids A, B and C, three new monoacyldigalactosylglycerols from Zingiberis rhizoma originating in Taiwan. Chem Pharm Bull 40.8 (1992): 2239–2241.

Yoshikawa M et al. Crude drug processing by far-infrared treatment. II. Chemical fluctuation of the constituents during the drying of Zingiberis Rhizoma. Yakugaku Zasshi 113.10 (1993): 712–7117.

Yoshikawa M et al. Stomachic principles in ginger. III: An anti-ulcer principle, 6-gingesulfonic acid, and three monoacyldigalactosylglycerols, gingerglycolipids A, B, and C, from Zingiberis Rhizoma originating in Taiwan. Chem Pharm Bull 42.6 (1994): 1226–1230.

Yu, Y et al Examination of the Pharmacokinetics of Active Ingredients of Ginger in Humans. The AAPS Journal 13.3 (2011) 417–26.

Zhao XX et al. [Multi-central clinical evaluation of ginger-partitioned moxibustion for treatment of leukopenia induced by chemotherapy]. Zhongguo Zhen Jiu 27.10 (2007): 715–720.

Zhou H-L, Deng YM, Xie QM. The modulatory effects of the volatile oil of ginger on the cellular immune response in vitro and in vivo in mice. J Ethnopharmacol 105.1–2 (2006): 301–305.

Zick SM et al. Pharmacokinetics of 6-gingerol, 8-gingerol, 10-gingerol, and 6-shogaol and conjugate metabolites in healthy human subjects. Cancer Epidemiol Biomarkers Prev 17 (2008): 1930–1936.

Zick SM et al Phase II study of the effects of ginger root extract on eicosanoids in colon mucosa in people at normal risk for colorectal cancer. Cancer Prev Res 4.11 (2011): 1929–1937.

Ginkgo biloba

HISTORICAL NOTE *Ginkgo biloba* is one of the world's oldest living tree species, earning it the name 'living fossil'. Its existence can be traced back more than 200 million years and it was commonly found in North America and Europe before the Ice Age. Its place of origin is believed to be remote mountainous valleys of Zhejiang province of eastern China and, up to 350 years ago, knowledge about this plant was restricted to China (Singh et al 2008). Ginkgo was first introduced into Europe in 1690 by the botanist Engelbert Kaempfer, who described it as the 'tree with duck feet'. Ginkgo has been used medicinally for decades and is now one of the most popular therapeutic agents prescribed in Europe by medical doctors. It has been estimated that, in Germany and France, prescriptions for ginkgo make up 1% and 1.3%, respectively, of total prescription sales (Pizzorno & Murray 2006). Also popular in the United States, it was the top-selling herbal medicine in 1999, with sales of US$148 million. Current estimates indicate that the use of *G. biloba* has been growing at a very rapid rate worldwide, at 25% per year in the open-world commercial market (Singh et al 2008). Germany, Switzerland and France have respectively 31%, 8% and 5% of the world commercial market. To meet the demand for ginkgo products, 50 million *G. biloba* trees are grown, especially in China, France and South Carolina, United States, producing 8000 tons of dried leaves each year.

G

COMMON NAME

Ginkgo

In England, it is known as 'maidenhair tree' based on its resemblance to the foliage of the 'maidenhair fern' (*Adiantum*). In Japan, it is known as 'ginkyo' and in France, 'l'arbre aux quarante écus' and 'noyer du Japon' (Singh et al 2008).

OTHER NAMES

Adiantifolia, arbre aux quarante écus, bai guo ye, duck foot tree, fossil tree, ginnan, icho, Japanese silver apricot, kew tree, maidenhair tree, salisburia, silver apricot, tempeltrae, temple balm, yinhsing

BOTANICAL NAME/FAMILY

Ginkgo biloba (family Ginkgoaceae)

PLANT PARTS USED

In modern times only the leaf is used, but traditionally the nut was also used.

CHEMICAL COMPONENTS

Important constituents present in the leaves are the terpene trilactones (i.e. ginkgolides A, B, C and J and bilobalide), many flavonol glycosides (mostly derivatives of quercetin and kaempferol) (Hibatallah et al 1999), biflavones, proanthocyanidins, alkylphenols, simple phenolic acids, 6-hydroxykynurenic acid, 4-*O*-methylpyridoxine and polyprenols (van Beek 2002). *G. biloba* contains more than 30 genuine flavonoids, of which the flavonol glycosides are the most abundant (Singh et al 2008).

There has been some interest in ginkgo alkylphenols (ginkgolic acids) because of their allergenic properties, so most manufacturers limit the concentration of alkylphenols to 5 ppm.

> ***Clinical note — Ginkgo extract used in practice***
> The standardised ginkgo extract is made from dried ginkgo leaves extracted in 60% acetone. Only a fraction of the leaf matter is extracted; 98% is not extracted. Of the 2% extracted, the flavones account for 25%, the ginkgolides 3% and the bilobalide 3%. The remaining 69% is not specified. The drug ratio may vary from 35 : 1 to 67 : 1 (average ratio 50 : 1). This means that, on average, it takes 50 kg dried leaf to produce 1 kg of extract. Standardised ginkgo extract (e.g. EGb 761) must be standardised to 22–27% flavone glycosides, 5–7% terpene lactones (2.8–3.4% ginkgolides A, B and C, and 2.6–3.2% bilobalide). The content of ginkgolic acids must be less than 5 ppm (Blumenthal et al 2000). Although the standardisation is very specific, the compounds are considered to be marker compounds, as the active constituents of *G. biloba* have not been fully identified (unpublished data: Keller K, Chair of the Herbal Medicinal Products Working Group, European Medicines Evaluation Agency. Quality Assurance of Herbal Medicines, March 2001).

MAIN ACTIONS

The many and varied pharmacological actions of ginkgo preparations are related to the presence of several classes of active constituents. Research has mainly been conducted with a standardised ginkgo biloba extract (GBE) and also several of its key constituents, such as ginkgetin. Various preparations have also been tested, including oral, injectable and topical preparations.

Antioxidant

GBE and several of its individual constituents, such as quercetin and kaempferol, have demonstrated significant antioxidant properties in vitro (Hibatallah et al 1999, Sloley et al 2000). Antioxidant activity has further been demonstrated in several different animal models.

Experimental models investigating the effects of ginkgo on reducing ischaemic injury in various tissues have shown positive results, indicating that ginkgo reduces the damage caused by oxidative stress during reperfusion (Liu et al 2007, Schneider et al 2008).

Hepatoprotective effects, via an antioxidant action, have also been seen in an animal study in the treatment of non-alcoholic steatohepatitis (Zhou et al 2010).

A novel study has investigated the effect of *G. biloba* on mobile phone-induced oxidative damage in brain tissue of rats (Ilhan et al 2004). Rats were exposed to the same amount of mobile phone-induced radiation for 7 days, with some also pretreated with *G. biloba*. After exposure, oxidative damage was evident by the: (1) increase in malondialdehyde and nitric oxide (NO) levels in brain tissue; (2) decrease in brain superoxide dismutase and glutathione peroxidase activities; and (3) increase in brain xanthine oxidase and adenosine deaminase activities. *Ginkgo biloba* prevented these alterations and the mobile phone-induced cellular injury in brain tissue histopathologically.

Initial research on apoptosis of human lens epithelial cells when exposed to high glucose suggests that GBE has a protective effect inhibiting this oxidative stress (Wu et al 2008b).

G. biloba's antioxidant action and prevention of mitochondrial degeneration may have some effect on protecting Sertoli and spermatid cells in a rat model with testicular torsion (Kanter 2011).

Topical antioxidant effects have also been investigated. *G. biloba* has been shown to reduce the effects of ultraviolet radiation on skin (Aricioglu et al 2001, Hibatallah et al 1999, Kim 2001, Lin & Chang 1997). When applied topically, ginkgo increases the activity of superoxide dismutase within skin, thereby enhancing the skin's natural defences.

Cardioprotective

Ginkgo reduces the damage caused by oxidative stress during reperfusion according to research with various preclinical models.

One study using a model of myocardial infarction found that pretreatment with GBE EGb 761 reduced ischaemic myocardial injury compared to untreated controls (Schneider et al 2008) and another showed *G. biloba* may provide cardioprotection in preventing diabetic complications of cardiovascular autonomic neuropathy, as seen in diabetes-induced myocardial nervous damage (Schneider et al 2010). Another animal study demonstrated that *G. biloba* phytosomes conferred significant cardiac protection with antioxidant activity and decreased lipid peroxidation (Panda & N 2009).

EGb 761 may have a role in reducing cardiotoxic effects of the antineoplastic drug, Adriamycin, as pretreatment for 10 days prior to drug use resulted in normalisation of cardiac enzymes (having an effect on cardiac malondialdehyde, total antioxidant capacity, tumour necrosis factor-alpha [TNF-alpha] and NO levels) (El-Boghdady 2013b). A recent rat study revealed cardioprotective effects reducing ischaemic free radical damage to the heart mitochondria (Bernatoniene et al 2011). These cardiac benefits found in animal studies did not translate to show a clinical effect in the Ginkgo Evaluation of Memory study assessing *G. biloba*'s effect on cardiovascular disease. This enormous double-blind trial randomised 3069 participants over 75 years (120 mg of *G. biloba* EGb 761 twice daily) with follow-up over 6.1 years; no reduction was found in cardiovascular disease events or mortality (Kuller et al 2010).

Anti-inflammatory

The anti-inflammatory activity of ginkgo has been investigated for the whole extract and an isolated biflavonoid component known as ginkgetin, with both forms demonstrating significant anti-inflammatory activity.

Ginkgo extract

Intravenously administered ginkgo extract produced an anti-inflammatory effect that was as strong as the same dose of prednisolone (i.e. 1 mg GBE = 1 mg prednisolone) in an experimental model. Ginkgo extract was also found to significantly reduce the concentration of prostaglandin E_2, TNF-alpha and NO production in vitro (Ilieva et al 2004). Studies with subcutaneously administered GBE in experimental models have further confirmed significant anti-inflammatory activity, with the addition of antinociceptive effects (Abdel-Salam et al 2004).

Investigation with an animal model of colitis revealed that *G. biloba* (EGb 761) extract reduces markers of inflammation (inducible nitric oxide synthase [iNOS], cyclooxygenase-2 [COX-2] and TNF-alpha) and inflammatory stress (p53 and p53-phosphoserine 15) (Kotakadi et al 2008). In the case of ischaemia-reperfusion injury in a rat model, *G. biloba* was found to inhibit inflammatory cytokines (interleukin-6 [IL-6]) and promote anti-inflammatory cytokines (IL-4) (Bao et al 2010).

Ginkgetin

Ginkgetin showed a stronger anti-inflammatory activity than prednisolone when administered by intraperitoneal injection in an animal model of arthritis.

Histological examination of the knee joints confirmed the effect (Kim et al 1999). When used topically in an animal model of chronic skin inflammation and proinflammatory gene expression, it was found to inhibit ear oedema by approximately 26% and prostaglandin E_2 production by 30% (Lim et al 2006). Histological comparisons revealed that ginkgetin reduced epidermal hyperplasia, inhibited phospholipase A_2 and suppressed COX-2 and iNOS expression (Lim et al 2006).

Vascular effects

Vasodilation

Ginkgo promotes vasodilation and improves blood flow through arteries, veins and capillaries. Increases in microcirculatory blood flow occur rapidly and have been confirmed under randomised crossover test conditions 1 h after administration (Jung et al 1990).

Several mechanisms of action are responsible. Currently, these are considered to be: inhibition of NO release, activation of Ca^{2+}-activated K^+ channels, increased prostacyclin release and an antioxidant and anti-inflammatory effect (Chen et al 1997, 2011a, Koltermann et al 2007, Nishida & Satoh 2003). In 2008, a clinical study by Wu et al investigated the effects of GBE on the distal left anterior descending coronary artery (LAD) blood flow and plasma NO and endothelin-1 (ET-1) levels (Wu et al 2008c). The randomised controlled trial (RCT) of 80 volunteers with coronary artery disease (CAD) used Doppler echocardiography to determine blood flow, which was measured at baseline and after 2 weeks of treatment. A significant improvement in maximal diastolic peak velocity, maximal systolic peak velocity and diastolic time velocity integral was observed for the group treated with GBE compared with controls ($P < 0.01$). Additionally, a significant increase in NO and decrease in ET-1 was observed, suggesting that the observed increase of LAD blood flow might be related to restoration of the delicate equilibrium between NO and ET-1.

Reduces oedema

Various flavonoids, including anthocyanosides and GBE, have been shown to be effective against experimentally induced capillary hyperfiltration (Cohen-Boulakia et al 2000).

Antiplatelet and anticoagulant — no significant effect

Standardised *G. biloba* therapy is not associated with a higher bleeding risk, according to a 2011 meta-analysis of 18 RCTs (Kellermann & Kloft 2011). This level 1 evidence overrides previous speculation based on several case reports suggesting ginkgo biloba can cause bleeding and some evidence that one of its components, ginkgolide B, is a platelet-activating factor antagonist (Smith et al 1996).

Controlled studies have included young healthy volunteers, older adults, people with multiple sclerosis (MS) and people using warfarin or aspirin at the same time as *G. biloba* (Aruna & Naidu 2007, Bal Dit et al 2003, Beckert et al 2007, Carlson et al 2007, Engelsen et al 2003, Gardner et al 2007, Jiang et al 2005, Kohler et al 2004, Lovera et al 2007, Wolf 2006). An escalating-dose study found that 120 mg, 240 mg or 480 mg given daily for 14 days did not alter platelet function or coagulation (Bal Dit et al 2003).

Only one study could be located which demonstrated that EGb 761 (80 mg/day) produced a significant reduction in blood viscosity after 30 days' treatment

(Galduroz et al 2007). When measured again 90 days after commencement of EGb 761 treatment, a further reduction was observed which appeared to stabilise, as no further reduction was observed after 180 days of use.

Alters neurotransmitters

Monoamine oxidase (MAO) inhibition — not in vivo

In vitro tests in rat brains suggest that EGb 761 may exert MAO-A and MAO-B inhibitor activity (Wu & Zhu 1999). Tests with isolated constituents, kaempferol, apigenin and chrysin, have demonstrated these to be potent MAO inhibitors, with greater effect on MAO-A than MAO-B (Sloley et al 2000). A recent rat model showed MAO activity was not affected by EGb 761, suggesting the effect is not significant in vivo (Fehske et al 2009). The lack of significant in vivo MAO-inhibitory activity was confirmed in a human study using positron emission tomography, which found that treatment with *G. biloba* (EGb 761: 120 mg/day) for 1 month did not produce significant changes in brain MAO-A or MAO-B in the 10 participating volunteers (Fowler et al 2000).

Serotonin

An in vitro study found that oral EGb 761 significantly increases the uptake of serotonin, but not dopamine, in cerebral cortex samples from mice (Ramassamy et al 1992) and a later in vivo study identified an antiaggressive effect mediated by 5-HT_{2A} receptors (Shih et al 2000). In contrast, an animal study suggests no change in 5-HT uptake after 14 days of oral treatment with EGb 761 (Fehske et al 2009).

Cholinergic effects

Considering that *G. biloba* appears to be as effective as anticholinesterase drugs, several researchers have investigated whether it exerts cholinergic effects. Evidence from behavioural, in vitro and ex vivo tests with *G. biloba* has shown both direct and indirect cholinergic activities (Das et al 2002, Nathan 2000). The extract appears to increase the rate of acetylcholine turnover and stimulate the binding activity of ligands to muscarinic receptors in the hippocampus (Muller 1989).

Gamma-aminobutyric acid (GABA) receptors

Bilobalide in *G. biloba* is a competitive antagonist for GABA-A receptors according to in vitro tests (Huang et al 2003). The effect is almost as potent as bicuculline and pictrotoxin.

Corticosterone

In vivo tests have found that EGb 761 has stress-alleviating properties mediated through its moderation of corticosterone levels (Puebla-Perez et al 2003).

Dopamine

Chronic, but not acute, treatment with *G. biloba* (EGb 761) significantly increases extracellular dopamine in vivo, which may be one of the mechanisms in improving cognitive function (Yoshitake et al 2010). *G. biloba* (EGb 761) affects the dopaminergic system, which was observed as a reduction in serum prolactin levels in male rats (Yeh et al 2008) and an increase in dopamine and acetylcholine levels in the prefrontal cortex (Kehr et al 2012). *G. biloba*'s dopamine-enhancing effect may be explained by its ability to decrease the uptake of noradrenaline as dopamine clearance in the frontal cortex is mediated by noradrenaline (Fehske et al 2009).

Neuroprotection

G. biloba leaf extract (EGb 761) has demonstrated neuroprotective effects in a variety of studies ranging from molecular and cellular, to animal and human; however not all the cellular and molecular mechanisms have been elucidated (Ao et al 2006, Kaur et al 2013, Smith et al 2002). Of the constituents studied, it appears that the bilobalide constituent is chiefly responsible for this activity, although others are also involved (DeFeudis & Drieu 2000).

Until recently, it was believed that the antioxidant, membrane-stabilising and platelet-activating factor antagonist effects were chiefly responsible for neuroprotection, but effects at the mitochondria may also be important contributing mechanisms. Recent research suggests that *G. biloba* (EGb 761) exerts a multifunctional neuroprotective role associated with activation of the haem oxygenase 1 (HO1) and nuclear factor erythroid 2-related factor 2 (Nrf2), upregulation of vascular endothelial growth factor (VEGF) and downregulation of inflammatory mediators (Tulsulkar & Shah 2012). Another in vivo animal study suggests the neuroprotection may also be a result of antiapoptotic activity and effects on energy metabolism (Mahdy et al 2011).

Beta-amyloid

GBE EGb 761 protects cells against toxicity induced by beta-amyloid in a concentration-dependent manner, according to in vitro tests (Bastianetto & Quirion 2002a, 2002b, Bastianetto et al 2000). In vivo studies have confirmed that ginkgo extract has an antiamyloid aggregation effect (Luo 2006). It appears that ginkgo increases transthyretin RNA levels in mouse hippocampus, which is noteworthy because transthyretin is involved in the transport of beta-amyloid and may provide a mechanism to reduce amyloid deposition in brain (Watanabe et al 2001). There is also evidence that *G. biloba* modulates alpha-secretase, the enzyme that cuts the amyloid precursor protein and prevents amyloidogenic fragments from being produced (Colciaghi et al 2004).

Cerebral ischaemia

There is evidence from experimental and clinical studies that GBE protects cerebral tissues from ischaemia/reperfusion damage and, while the effect has been reported for prophylactic use (Janssens et al 2000, Kaur et al 2013, Peng et al 2003), some research also suggests *G. biloba* exerts significant neuroprotective effects after acute ischaemic stroke (Ma et al 2012, Nada & Shah 2012, Zhang et al 2012b). This was confirmed most recently in a 2013 placebo-controlled RCT of 102 consecutive patients with acute ischaemic stroke which found that treatment with GBE for 4 months produced a significant reduction in poststroke National Institutes of Health Stroke Scale (NIHSS) score compared to placebo, showing improved function (Oskouei et al 2013). The treatment used was *G. biloba* tablets (Gol-Darou, Isfahan, Iran) with a total dose of 120 mg/day (40 mg three times/day),

G. biloba crosses the blood–brain barrier and reaches extracellular concentrations in the brain, allowing efficient interaction with target molecules. The availability of ginkgo in cerebral tissue is high when given before ischaemia, but severely limited after the occurrence of ischaemia, which may explain the greater success seen in animal model research when used prophylactically and mean higher doses are required poststroke (Oskouei et al 2013).

Stabilisation and protection of mitochondrial function

Several in vitro tests have demonstrated that EGb 761 stabilises and protects mitochondrial function (Eckert et al 2005, Janssens et al 2000). These observations are gaining the attention of researchers interested in neurodegenerative diseases, as it is suspected that the mitochondria and the phenomenon of mitochondrial permeability transition play a key role in neuronal cell death and the development of such diseases (Beal 2003, Shevtsova et al 2005). Animal studies are confirming these in vitro findings and it may be that both the ginkgolides and the bilobalide compounds have this mitochondrial protective action on neural function (Eckert 2012).

Immunostimulant

Immunostimulatory activity has been demonstrated in several experimental models (Puebla-Perez et al 2003, Tian et al 2003, Villasenor-Garcia et al 2004).

The beneficial effects of EGb 761 on immune function are based on its antioxidant properties, as well as the cell proliferation-stimulating effect. An in vitro animal study has suggested that nebulised total ginkgo flavone glycosides have a therapeutic effect for asthmatic mice, perhaps through regulating Th1/Th2 imbalance (Chen et al 2008).

Anticancer

Studies conducted with various molecular, cellular and whole-animal models have revealed that leaf extracts of *G. biloba* may have anticancer (chemopreventive) properties that are related to its antioxidant, antiangiogenic and gene-regulatory actions (DeFeudis et al 2003). Both the flavonoid and terpenoid constituents are thought to be responsible for many of these mechanisms, meaning that the whole extract is required for activity. In vitro and in vivo studies have shown GBE inhibits the growth and proliferation of several types of tumour, including colon cancer cells (Chen et al 2011b), gastric precancerous lesions (Jiang et al 2009), pancreatic cancer cells (Zhang et al 2008), liver cancer cells (Hao et al 2009, Wang et al 2011), breast cancer cells (Jiang et al 2011, Park et al 2013) and ovarian cancer BRCA1 gene mutation cells (Jiang et al 2011) and provides protection from cigarette smoke in human lung cells (Hsu et al 2009). An in vitro study identified the kaempferol and quercetin constituents of *G. biloba* as key components inducing apoptosis in oral-cavity cancer cells (Kang et al 2010). Studies in humans have found that ginkgo extracts inhibit the formation of radiation-induced (chromosome-damaging) clastogenic factors and ultraviolet-induced oxidative stress, both effects that may contribute to the overall chemopreventive activity. As a result of these observations, there has been a call by some academics for ginkgo to be more widely investigated and used in the prevention and treatment of cancer (Eli & Fasciano 2006).

OTHER ACTIONS

Antiatherosclerotic

Animal models have found *G. biloba* to be effective against atherosclerosis (Chen et al 2011a, Lim et al 2011, Pierre et al 2008). An in vitro study suggests an antiatherosclerotic effect via downregulation of VEGF (Liu et al 2009) and an in vivo study suggests that *G. biloba* may have a cholesterol-lowering effect via HMG-CoA reductase activity and decreasing cholesterol influx (Xie et al 2009). Another animal model found *G. biloba*'s antiatherosclerotic action was through lipid modulation, reducing vascular lesions and modulation of connexin 43 protein (Wei et al 2013).

Antiviral

Ginkgolic acid inhibits HIV protease activity and HIV infection in vitro (Lu et al 2012). In vitro research also identified anti-influenza action with GBE, but only with pretreatment before cell exposure, suggesting it interferes with the interaction between the virus and erythrocytes (Haruyama & Nagata 2013).

Glycaemia

Some in vitro and animal research has suggested that *G. biloba* may have a beneficial effect on reducing insulin resistance (Cong et al 2011, Zhou et al 2011).

Antiosteoporotic

G. biloba treatment produced a significant reversal in bone loss of the mandible and femur in a glucocorticoid-induced osteoporosis model (Lucinda et al 2010).

Activity on cytochromes and P-glycoprotein

Several studies have investigated *G. biloba* for effects on different cytochromes in test tube and animal models and, more recently, human studies. While early in vitro tests demonstrated that *G. biloba* inhibits CYP 3A4, clinical studies have found no such effect (Budzinski et al 2000, Gurley et al 2002, 2005, 2012, Markowitz et al 2003). In vitro tests have suggested that the effect on cytochromes is biphasic, with low doses of ginkgo extract inducing CYP 1A2 and inhibiting 2D6 and higher doses exhibiting the opposite effect (Hellum et al 2007). Studies investigating ginkgo extract and its various constituents in animal models have identified induction of CYP 3A1, 1A1, 1A2, 2E1, 2B12 for ginkgo, which appears to be largely mediated by the bilobalide constituent, whereas no effect on CYP 2D6, 2C11 or 2C7 has been demonstrated (Deng et al 2008, Ribonnet et al 2011, Taki et al 2009, Tang et al 2007a, Zhao et al 2006).

The question arises of clinical significance and whether the effects observed in animal models also occur in humans to an appreciable degree. To this end, clinical studies have been conducted clarifying the issue (Duche et al 1989, Gurley et al 2002, 2005, Kim et al 2010, Markowitz et al 2003, Tang et al 2007a, Zadoyan et al 2012, Zuo et al 2010). Tests with human volunteers have found no significant effect on CYP 3A4, 2D6 or 1A2 with GBE. Gurley et al (2012) report that 29 drugs mediated by various cytochromes have been evaluated and conclude that there is little risk of herb–drug interactions with *G. biloba* at doses of 240 mg/day or less.

Less is known about the effects of ginkgo on the drug transporter molecule P-glycoprotein (P-gp, also known as ABCB1). In vitro studies have identified induction of P-gp with ginkgo (Hellum & Nilsen 2008, Yeung et al 2008). A human study found no effects on P-gp after a single ginkgo dose (120 mg); however use of 120 mg three times daily (360 mg/day) for 14 days did show significant P-gp inhibition for *G. biloba* (Fan et al 2009). The most common therapeutic dose used is 240 mg daily, suggesting some minor effects are possible clinically. More clinical trials are needed to confirm this finding.

Antiasthmatic

In an asthma mouse study ginkgolide B exhibited a significant effect on regulating the kinase/MAPK pathway and a significant decrease in eosinophil count in bronchoalveolar lavage fluid after treatment (Chu et al 2011). Emerging research demonstrates how GBE may be useful in asthma treatment and acute lung injury by its action of suppressing NF-κB gene expression (Huang et al 2013, Li et al 2008).

CLINICAL USE

G. biloba is a complex herb that contains many different active constituents and works by means of multiple mechanisms. In practice, its therapeutic effect is a result of interactions between constituents and mechanisms, giving it applications in many varied conditions. To date, most of the research conducted in Europe has used a standardised preparation known as EGb 761.

Dementia, memory impairment

G. biloba has been used and studied as a cognitive activator in a variety of populations, such as cognitively intact people and those with cerebral insufficiency, age-related memory impairment, Alzheimer's dementia or multi-infarct dementia and dementia with neuropsychiatric features. It has also been tested in healthy adults with poor memory and others with no cognitive deficits to determine whether treatment can further improve memory. Overall, the evidence suggests that oral ginkgo extract improves cognitive function in people with mild to moderate cognitive impairment when used long-term and it also provides benefits for people with dementia and neuropsychiatric symptoms when used long-term (approximately 6 months). Some benefits may also be possible for various aspects of cognitive function in older adults, such as retrieval of learned material, but results are inconsistent for cognitive function overall. In regard to younger healthy adults, acute dosing appears more successful than chronic use.

While ginkgo biloba demonstrates neuroprotective effects in experimental models, the current evidence indicates long-term use does not protect against the development of dementia.

G

Clinical note — What is cerebral insufficiency?

Cerebral insufficiency is a syndrome characterised by a collection of symptoms, although it is not associated with any clear pathological changes. The 12 symptoms associated with this condition are: (1) difficulties of memory; (2) difficulties of concentration; (3) being absent-minded; (4) confusion; (5) lack of energy; (6) tiredness; (7) decreased physical performance; (8) depressive mood; (9) anxiety; (10) dizziness; (11) tinnitus; and (12) headaches (Kleijnen & Knipschild 1992). Some of these symptoms are also described as early symptoms of dementia and appear to be associated with decreased cerebral blood flow, although frequently no explanation is found.

A 2013 systematic review and meta-analysis of eight RCTs involving people with dementia reported significant, although modest, improvements in both cognitive function and daily activities. All studies used the GBE EGb 761 and two of the studies compared the extract to the drug donepezil and found no significant difference between the two treatments when treating mild to moderate dementia (Brondino et al 2013). Two of the studies included in the Brondino review focused on outpatients ($n = 410$) with mild to moderate dementia and neuropsychiatric symptoms who were treated with *G. biloba* (240 mg daily EGb 761) for 24 weeks; a significant improvement was produced in apathy, sleep, irritability, depression and aberrant motor behaviour and improved wellbeing of their caregivers (Bachinskaya et al 2011, Herrschaft et al 2012). Another trial in the 2013 review was a double-blind RCT of 400 subjects with mild to moderate dementia (Alzheimer's disease or vascular dementia) with neuropsychiatric features testing EGb 761 extract over 22 weeks (Napryeyenko & Borzenko 2007). Active treatment produced a mean −3.2-point improvement in the Specialty Knowledge Test (SKT) with an average deterioration by +1.3 points on placebo ($P < 0.001$). EGb 761 was significantly superior to placebo on all secondary outcome measures, including the Neuropsychiatric Inventory (NPI), and an activities-of-daily-living scale. Treatment results were essentially similar for Alzheimer's disease or vascular dementia subgroups. The drug was well tolerated and adverse events were similar for ginkgo and placebo treatment. A secondary analysis of this Napryeyenko RCT found *G. biloba* (EGb 761 240 mg/day) to be effective for both Alzheimer's disease and vascular dementia for neuropsychiatric symptoms (Napryeyenko et al 2009).

A 2009 Cochrane systematic review of 36 RCTs for ginkgo (any dose) in the treatment of dementia and cognitive decline (any severity) concluded that the results were inconsistent and unreliable but explained that the studies were mainly small, often poorly designed and of less than 3 months' duration, which may explain the inconsistency. All but one study used the EGb 761 extract (dose ranging from 80 to 600 mg/day, with most less than 200 mg daily). The authors reported that, although earlier studies found significant benefits, later studies were inconsistent and they found no difference between the 120 mg and 240 mg standard dosing (Birks & Grimley Evans 2009). This inconsistency may be in part due to reviewers pooling all studies regardless of patient diagnoses, the myriad of different scales and measures used and the fact that some studies are over 20 years old and randomisation and blinding techniques have changed in recent years. As a result, the findings are not straightforward and deserve more detailed description to be better understood. A literature review in 2012 suggested that the evidence for the use of *G. biloba* for cognitive impairment and dementia was not convincing (Roland & Nergard 2012).

However, other meta-analyses, with well-defined parameters, have found *G. biloba* to be clinically effective. One review and meta-analysis included nine well-designed studies between 12 and 52 weeks (n = 2372), all using the standardised extract EGb 761 (once-a-day dose of 240 mg) and found *G. biloba* to be more effective than placebo; with the Alzheimer's disease subgroup experiencing a larger cognitive benefit (Weinmann et al 2010). Another meta-analysis of six RCTs took a bivariate random approach considering the influence of baseline risk and found *G. biloba* to be effective for cognitive function in dementia with 6 months of treatment (Wang et al 2010). Kaschel undertook a literature review in 2009, aiming to discover the differential effects in neuropsychological improvement with *G. biloba* use, hypothesising that there may be certain parts of our memory that improve with this herb. Results from 29 RCTs were analysed, giving psychometric scores in different cognitive domains and 14 cognitive subfunctions. This reviewer suggested there is consistent evidence for long-term use of *G. biloba* in providing benefits for selective attention, fluid intelligence and long-term memory for both verbal and non-verbal material. It does not seem to have much effect on pure speed or on the less age-sensitive area of short-term memory (Kaschel 2009). This selective testing has provided a credible explanation for why there may be inconsistent study results and is perhaps the best way forward for future studies.

Two trials were not included in the recent reviews: the first was a double-blind, parallel-group RCT of 176 subjects with mild to moderate dementia which used low-dose standardised extract of *G. biloba* (120 mg daily) over 6 months, finding no benefits beyond placebo (McCarney et al 2008). The second trial was a larger double-blind RCT of 400 patients with dementia associated with neuropsychiatric features, testing a higher dose of EGb 761 extract (240 mg/day) (Scripnikov et al 2007). The study population included people with probable or possible Alzheimer's disease with cerebrovascular disease or vascular dementia. At this dose, EGb 761 was significantly superior to placebo with respect to the primary outcome (SKT battery) and all secondary outcome variables. While herbal treatment improved outcomes, the placebo group showed evidence of deterioration as measured by the mean composite score (frequency × severity) and the mean caregiver distress score ($P < 0.001$). The largest effects for EGb 761 were found for apathy/indifference, anxiety, irritability/lability, depression/dysphoria and sleep/nighttime behaviour.

Some smaller recent trials report benefit in treating mild cognitive impairment (Dong et al 2012) and one group found that episodic memory of patients with mild cognitive impairment improved (Zhao et al 2012).

Several recent reviews have focused on the role of ginkgo in Alzheimer's disease, producing inconsistent conclusions, which may be due to differences in exclusion criteria and the heterogeneity of the studies making data analysis difficult. A Cochrane systematic review in 2009 found 925 patients from nine Alzheimer's disease and ginkgo trials and suggested no consistent pattern of benefit (Birks & Grimley Evans 2009) and another systematic review suggested results were inconclusive (Fu & Li 2011). However, in 2010, a systematic review of the use of *G. biloba* in Alzheimer's disease found evidence of high-dose *G. biloba* (240 mg/day EGb 761) improving daily living, mood and cognition; the results were statistically significant in three of the four studies within the subgroup analysis. The complete meta-analysis included six quality studies of at least 16 weeks' duration and, although benefit for *G. biloba* was reported, the authors found that no potential effect size could be estimated because of the heterogeneous results and recommend future research focusing on subgroups of Alzheimer's disease. No evidence of harm was found in any of the studies (Janssen et al 2010).

Alzheimer's disease or vascular dementia with neuropsychiatric features

A 2013 review of four RCTs testing EGb 761 in elderly patients ($n = 1294$) with a total score of 9–23 in the SKT cognitive test battery (cognitive domain) and with a composite score of 6 and greater in the NPI (behavioural domain) concluded that active treatment with ginkgo was safe, effective and well tolerated (Ihl 2013). Patients treated with EGb 761 showed improvements of cognitive performance and behavioural symptoms that were associated with advances in activities of daily living and a reduced burden to caregivers, whereas the placebo groups showed only minimal improvements or signs of disease progression. EGb 761 was significantly superior to placebo groups in all mentioned domains ($P < 0.01$) and had similar effects to donepexil. The RCTs compared a dose of EGb 761 2 capsules of 120 mg/day or one capsule of 240 mg/day to placebo while one RCT used donepezil as an active control. The duration of treatment was 22 or 24 weeks.

Use in healthy subjects

Many double-blind studies have investigated the effects of *G. biloba* (120–600 mg/day) on cognitive function in younger and older healthy subjects. Some studies have evaluated the effects of a single dose, whereas others are long-term studies (2 days–13 weeks).

A 2012 meta-analysis of *G. biloba* as a cognitive enhancer in healthy individuals identified 10 RCTs (with 13 data sets) and concluded that, on measures of memory, executive function and attention, there was no significant effect on cognitive function. In the analysis the authors reported all effect sizes as non-significant and found no difference with age of participants, dose, time of trial or type of GBE. In the 13 studies assessing memory, not one of the studies found a significant effect (Laws et al 2012).

Previously, a systematic review of placebo-controlled trials, published in 2007, investigated whether *G. biloba* enhances cognitive function in healthy subjects aged under 60 years (Canter & Ernst 2007). A number of the acute studies included in the analysis used multiple outcomes and reported positive effects on one or more of these at particular time points with particular doses, but these findings were either not replicated or contradicted by other studies. The evidence from long-term studies is largely negative. Of those studies that measured subjective effects, only one of five acute studies and one of six long-term studies reported any significant positive results.

More recently, a benefit was found in 188 healthy middle-aged volunteers who were given placebo or ginkgo 240 mg once daily (EGb 761) for 6 weeks. There was significant improvement on the demanding standardised free-recall test but no benefit in another memory test on recalling a driving route. This confirms previous evidence suggesting a role for *G. biloba* in retrieval of learned material, which is known to be sensitive to ageing (Kaschel 2011).

Overall, tests with younger subjects taking *G. biloba* long-term have failed to show positive effects on memory; however, short-term benefits after acute dosing may be possible for some aspects of memory. Healthy older adults with poorer cognitive performance appear to experience greater benefit than those with higher cognitive function levels. This was confirmed in a 2011 RCT which found a more pronounced and consistent improvement in cognition in subjects with a lower memory function at baseline in mild cognitive impairment (n = 300) who were taking *G. biloba* (240 mg/daily EGb 761) for 12 weeks (Grass-Kapanke et al 2011).

Tests with younger (18–43 years) and older volunteers (55–79 years) produced different results in a 12-week, double-blind, placebo-controlled study (Burns et al 2006). The effects of ginkgo (120 mg/day) were assessed for both groups on a wide range of cognitive abilities, executive function, attention and mood. The older group responded to treatment as long-term memory assessed by associational learning tasks showed significant improvement with ginkgo; however, no other significant differences were found on any other measure. The young adult group (n = 104) failed to respond on any measure, as no significant differences were observed for the treatment or placebo groups. Similarly, no significant effects on mood or any of the cognitive tests employed by Elsabagh et al (2005a) were found for ginkgo (120 mg/day) taken over 6 weeks in a placebo-controlled study of 52 young adults. In contrast, acute treatment of younger subjects with ginkgo (120 mg) significantly improved performance on the sustained-attention task and pattern recognition memory task according to a randomised, double-blind study (Elsabagh et al 2005a). The study of 52 students found no further effects for ginkgo on working memory, planning, mental flexibility or mood.

Kennedy et al (2007b) reported on a re-analysis of data from three methodologically identical, double-blind, crossover studies that each included a treatment of 120 mg ginkgo extract and matched placebo. The analysis found that 120 mg of ginkgo conferred a significant improvement on the 'quality of memory' factor and was most evident at 1 and 4 hours after single-dose treatment, but had a negative effect on performance on the 'speed of attention' factor, which was most evident at 1 and 6 hours after treatment.

Vascular cognitive impairment

One study of 80 patients diagnosed with vascular cognitive impairment compared conventional treatment with antiplatelet medication to treatment with adjunctive *G. biloba* and the antiplatelet medication. The 3-month trial found addition of ginkgo improved the therapeutic effect, with increases in cerebral blood flow and cognitive enhancement observed (Zhang & Xue 2012).

Ginkgo complexed with phospholipids

Some recent data suggest that the complexation of standardised GBE with soy-derived phospholipids may enhance the bioavailability of active components, thereby producing better results. Kennedy et al (2007a) tested two different ginkgo products complexed with either phosphatidylserine or phosphatidylcholine in a placebo-controlled study of younger volunteers. Test subjects were given an acute dose of ginkgo, one of the ginkgo combinations or placebo on separate days (7 days apart). Confirming earlier results, *G. biloba* (120 mg) as sole treatment was not associated with markedly improved performance on the primary outcomes in this younger population; however, administration of GBE complexed with phosphatidylserine resulted in improved secondary memory performance and significantly increased speed of memory task performance across all of the postdose testing sessions. Interestingly, all three herbal treatments were associated with improved calmness. Whether the superior effect obtained for this combination is due to the complexation of the extracts, their mere combination or the separate psychopharmacological actions of the two extracts remains to be tested.

G

Cognitive effects in postmenopausal women

A systematic review of herbal and dietary supplements and their use in menopause for cognitive function included two *G. biloba* studies, both using a low dose of 120 mg/day (Clement et al 2011). In one RCT, 57 postmenopausal women were given a combination of ginkgo at 120 mg and ginseng at 200 mg (Gincosan) over 12 weeks. No significant effects were found in any of the symptoms measured of anxiety and mood and cognitive measures of attention and memory (Hartley et al 2004). The second was a double-blind RCT of 87 postmenopausal women; it was found that 1 week's treatment with ginkgo (120 mg/day) significantly improved mental flexibility in older (mean age 61 years) postmenopausal women beyond placebo. However no significant benefits were seen for younger women with better cognitive performance at baseline and no benefit for any of the women for the cognitive function of memory and sustained attention (Elsabagh et al 2005b). The study tested ginkgo extract (LI 1370, Lichtwer Pharma, Marlow, UK) over 6 weeks (Elsabagh et al 2005b).

Comparisons with anticholinesterase drugs

The type of central nervous system effects produced by EGb 761 in elderly dementia patients is similar to those induced in tacrine responders and those seen after the administration of other 'cognitive activators', according to a small randomised study involving 18 elderly people diagnosed with mild to moderate dementia (possible or probable Alzheimer's disease) (Itil et al 1998). The results also demonstrated that 240 mg EGb produced typical cognitive activator electrocardiogram profiles (responders) in more subjects (8 of 18) than 40 mg tacrine (3 of 18 subjects). Later reviews concluded that ginkgo extract and second-generation cholinesterase inhibitors (donepezil, rivastigmine, metrifonate) should be considered equally effective in the treatment of mild to moderate Alzheimer's dementia (Kasper & Schubert 2009, Wettstein 2000). One double-blind exploratory RCT with 96 outpatients compared *G. biloba*, donepezil or combined treatment over 22 weeks and found no significant differences between them and only superior benefits when they were combined (Yancheva et al 2009).

Commission E approves the use of standardised ginkgo extract in dementia syndromes, including vascular, primary degenerative and mixed types (Blumenthal et al 2000).

Dementia prevention

The many mechanisms attributed to ginkgo make it an ideal candidate for the long-term prevention of many age-related diseases such as dementia. Two clinical trials were published in 2008, which investigated whether treatment with *G. biloba* could significantly reduce the incidence of dementia and, more recently, a large RCT released results in 2012. Overall, the current body of evidence indicates that ginkgo treatment does not protect against the development of dementia or Alzheimer's disease when taken by people over 70 years (DeKosky et al 2008, Dodge et al 2008, Vellas et al 2012).

DeKosky et al (2008) compared the effectiveness of *G. biloba* to placebo in reducing the incidence of all-cause dementia and Alzheimer's disease in elderly individuals with normal cognition and those with mild cognitive impairment. The large randomised, double-blind, placebo-controlled clinical trial involved 3069 community-dwelling subjects aged 75 years or older with normal cognition (n = 2587) or mild cognitive impairment (n = 482). It was conducted at five academic medical centres in the United States between 2000 and 2008, with a median follow-up of 6.1 years. Treatment consisted of a twice-daily dose of 120 mg extract of *G. biloba* and was not shown to reduce the overall incidence rate of either dementia or Alzheimer's disease incidence in elderly individuals. Treatment was well tolerated by this population, as the incidence of side effects was similar for both groups.

In the same year, Dodge et al (2008) published the results of a double-blind study involving 118 cognitively intact older subjects (85 years or older). In the intention-to-treat analysis, there was no reduced risk of progression to clinical dementia among the GBE group; however, in the secondary analysis, where medication adherence level was controlled, the GBE group had a significantly lower risk of progression and a smaller decline in memory scores. Importantly, more stroke and transient ischaemic attack cases were observed among the GBE group; further investigation is required to confirm this finding.

A 5-year double-blind RCT (GuidAge) released results in 2012. This large clinical trial recruited participants aged over 70 years who had consulted their primary care doctor for memory problems; 1404 patients were prescribed a dose of 120 mg twice daily (EGb 761) and 1414 were given placebo. The findings were negative and *G. biloba* did not reduce the incidence of Alzheimer's disease in elderly patients with memory complaints (Vellas et al 2012).

Acute ischaemic stroke

GBE is widely used in the treatment of acute ischaemic stroke in China.

A 2005 Cochrane systematic review identified 14 trials, of which 10 (792 patients) were included (Zeng et al 2005). In those 10 trials, follow-up was performed at 14–35 days after stroke and, in all studies, neurological outcome was assessed, but none of them reported on disability (activities of daily living function) or quality of life and only three trials reported adverse events. Nine of the trials were considered to be of inferior quality. Overall, results from the 10 studies found that GBE was associated with a significant increase in the number of improved patients. Of note, one placebo-controlled trial, assessed to be of good quality, failed to show an improvement in neurological deficit at the end of treatment. A recent review of *G. biloba* confirmed previous Cochrane reviews and concluded that there was no convincing evidence of ginkgo being effective for acute ischaemic stroke (Roland & Nergard 2012).

However, the story is not yet complete, as two more recent studies have shown benefits for ginkgo treatment in ischaemic stroke. A double-blind RCT of 31 patients after an acute ischaemic stroke or a cerebrovascular accident were administered standard pharmacotherapy or standard treatment with the addition of *G. biloba* (1500 mg/day) for 30 days. Blood samples before and after the treatment showed greater antioxidant status and lower inflammatory markers, such as C-reactive protein, which may assist in neuroprotection after a stroke (Thanoon et al 2012). Of more interest is a 2013 placebo-controlled RCT of 102 consecutive patients with acute ischaemic stroke which tested treatment with *G. biloba* tablets (Gol-Darou, Isfahan, Iran) with a total dose of 120 mg/day (40 mg three times/day) over 4 months (Oskouei et al 2013). The primary outcome was a 50% reduction in the 4-month NIHSS, which was used to measure functional outcome. Treatment with ginkgo was significantly superior to placebo and the risk ratio and number needed to treat were 3.16 and 2.50, respectively. In addition, multivariate regression adjusted for age and sex revealed a significant NIHSS decline in the *G. biloba* group compared to the placebo group ($P < 0.05$).

G

Depression

Although studies have investigated the effects of *G. biloba* in cerebral insufficiency, a syndrome that is often characterised by depression and dementia with neuropsychiatric features, no clinical studies are available that have specifically investigated its use in clinical depression.

One randomised, double-blind, placebo-controlled study has investigated its effects in seasonal affective disorder (SAD). GBE PN246, in tablet form (Bio-Biloba), was tested in 27 patients with SAD over 10 weeks or until they developed symptoms, starting in a symptom-free phase about 1 month before symptoms were expected. In this trial, *G. biloba* failed to prevent the development of SAD (Lingaerde et al 1999).

Cieza et al (2003) tested EGb 761 (240 mg/day) on the subjective emotional wellbeing of healthy older subjects (50–65 years) in a randomised, double-blind study. Ginkgo treatment produced a statistically significant difference for the visual analogue scale on mental health and for quality of life, as well as for the Subjective Intensity Scale: Mood score in week 2 compared with placebo. At the end of the study, statistically significant improvement in the EGb 761 group was observed for the variables of depression, fatigue and anger. Several more-recent studies investigating the effects of ginkgo on memory have also measured effects on mood. The double-blind studies found no significant effects for healthy older or younger volunteers (Burns et al 2006, Carlson et al 2007, Elsabagh et al 2005a). Whether ginkgo may have a mood-enhancing effect in a population with diagnosed depression remains to be tested.

Generalised anxiety disorder (GAD)

EGb 761 has demonstrated stress-alleviating and anxiolytic-like activity in preclinical studies, and in a randomised study of 107 patients with GAD ($n = 82$) or adjustment disorder with anxious mood ($n = 25$) (Woelk et al 2007). *G. biloba* was tested in two different doses (480 mg/day and 240 mg/day) against placebo over 4 weeks and found to be significantly superior, with a dose–response trend being identified. Beneficial effects were observed after 4 days of treatment. Additionally, ginkgo treatment was safe and well-tolerated. A review of controlled studies of the use of medicinal plants for GAD found only a small number of studies on *G. biloba* but in those studies ginkgo showed an effect similar to or better than anxiolytic drugs (Faustino et al 2010).

Peripheral vascular diseases

Ginkgo has been used in the treatment of intermittent claudication, Raynaud's syndrome and chilblains (Mouren et al 1994, Pittler & Ernst 2000). This is often based on the known pharmacological actions of ginkgo in improving peripheral circulation and exerting antioxidant and anti-inflammatory activities. While clinical trials have produced inconsistent results, the lack of non-surgical and safe pharmaceutical treatment options means ginkgo biloba is worthy of consideration in practice as a 3-month trial to determine individual response.

Intermittent claudication

A 2013 Cochrane database systematic review included 14 trials with 739 patients and found a non-significant increase of only 64.5 m on a flat treadmill being the absolute claudication distance (ACD) and concluded no significant benefit for patients with peripheral arterial disease. In the 24 weeks subgroup, authors found a significant improvement in ACD with an increase of 85.3 m. Nine trials compared 120–160 mg *G. biloba* daily with placebo and three of the trials used larger doses of 240 mg (Wang et al 2007), 300 mg (Gardner et al 2008) and 320 mg (Mouren et al 1994), with the majority of the trials lasting 12–24 weeks. The authors suggest that a publication bias and exclusion of some 'negative' trials in earlier reviews skewed the results and also suggested that exercise therapy alone has shown a 5–10 times greater benefit than GBE (Nicolai et al 2013).

The earlier trials referred to included a 2004 meta-analysis reporting that ginkgo was more effective than placebo in intermittent claudication (Horsch & Walther 2004). Nine double-blind studies of EGb 761 for intermittent claudication were assessed in a total of 619 patients. A sensitivity analysis of a homogeneous sample in terms of design, treatment duration, inclusion and exclusion criteria and methods of measurement confirms these findings. Most studies have used a dose of 120 mg/day taken in divided doses, although one trial found that 240 mg/day gave better results. It should be recommended as long-term therapy and as an adjunct to exercise for the best results. An earlier randomised study measuring transcutaneous partial pressure of oxygen during exercise showed that a dose of 320 mg/day EGb 761 taken for 4 weeks significantly decreased the amount of ischaemic area by 38%, compared with no change with placebo (Mouren et al 1994).

Commission E approved the use of standardised ginkgo extract for intermittent claudication (Blumenthal et al 2000).

Clinical note — Peripheral arterial disease

Peripheral arterial disease is the chronic obstruction of the arteries supplying the lower extremities. The most frequent symptom is intermittent claudication, which results from poor oxygenation of the muscles of the lower extremities and is experienced typically as an aching pain, cramping or numbness in the calf, buttock, hip, thigh or arch of the foot. Symptoms are induced by walking or exercise and are relieved by rest. Presently, medical treatment revolves around lifestyle changes, such as increased exercise, and surgery as a final option.

Raynaud's syndrome

Whether ginkgo is an effective treatment in Reynaud's syndrome is difficult to ascertain. A review and meta-analysis of complementary medicine and Raynaud's syndrome (Malenfant et al 2009) included only one study on *G. biloba* by Muir et al (2002), which found a non-significant change in duration and severity of symptoms ($P = 0.75$ and 0.23, respectively). This study used a standardised GBE (Seredrin 360 mg daily) taken over a 10-week period which significantly reduced the number of attacks per week (from 13.2 to 5.8) compared with placebo (Muir et al 2002).

Several later studies were published, including an RCT conducted over 8 weeks, with 93 patients, which compared the use of the calcium channel blocker nifedipine with *G. biloba* and found a 50% improvement in the drug group versus a 31% improvement in the ginkgo group (Choi et al 2009). Another RCT conducted during the coldest part of the year involved 41 participants and found no significant differences between EGb 761 (240 mg/day) and placebo after 10 weeks (Bredie & Jong 2012). Whether participants in these last two studies had more severe symptoms than in the previous positive study is unknown

Vertigo, tinnitus, labyrinthitis and sudden deafness

Ginkgo is used to treat these and other symptoms of vestibulocochlear disorders.

Tinnitus

A recent Cochrane review included only four quality trials ($n = 1543$) and they found no evidence to suggest that *G. biloba* was effective in patients whose primary issue was tinnitus, although they did report a small, statistically significant reduction in tinnitus in patients with vascular dementia and Alzheimer's disease (Hilton et al 2013). Two double-blind studies included in the recent Cochrane review have shifted the evidence against the use of *G. biloba* in tinnitus. The first was a large, double-blind, placebo-controlled study involving 1121 people aged between 18 and 70 years with tinnitus and 978 matched controls, which found that 12 weeks of treatment with ginkgo extract, LI 1370 (Lichtwer Pharma, Berlin, Germany), 50 mg three times daily resulted in no significant differences when subjects assessed their tinnitus in terms of loudness and how troublesome it was (Drew & Davies 2001). The second RCT of 66 subjects with tinnitus failed to show benefits with active treatment using a dose of 120 mg extract daily over 12 weeks (Rejali et al 2004). The primary outcome measures used were the Tinnitus Handicap Inventory, the Glasgow Health Status Inventory and the average hearing threshold at 0.5, 1, 2 and 4 kHz. In 2004, Rejali et al conducted a meta-analysis of clinical trials and found that 21.6% of patients with tinnitus reported benefit from *G. biloba* versus 18.4% of patients who reported benefit from a placebo.

Importantly, a 2011 systematic review which looked at the quality of plant extract and dosage levels included results of eight trials (all with EGb 761 with 120–240 mg/day) and excluded trials such as the Rejali study that did not specify the ginkgo preparation and which had a large drop-out rate due to illness. This review found that GBE EGb 761 was superior to placebo and was an effective treatment option for tinnitus. The authors suggest that trials with other GBEs were often of poor methodological quality (von Boetticher 2011).

Salicylate-induced tinnitus

One in vivo study investigating the effects of ginkgo in salicylate-induced tinnitus found a statistically significant decrease in the behavioural manifestation of tinnitus for ginkgo in doses of 25, 50 and 100 mg/kg/day (Jastreboff et al 1997).

Vertigo

Despite being a common disease, there is no effective and side effect-free pharmaceutical agent that has shown efficacy for vertigo, creating interest in well-tolerated treatments such as ginkgo biloba, which displays mechanisms of action which may be relevant, such as antioxidant, neuroprotective, cognitive enhancing, improved perfusion and possibly vigilance enhancing. Research with animal models further indicates EGb 761 has an effect on the vestibular system and vestibular compensation (Hamann 2007).

In 2013, the REVERT registry collected data from 4294 patients with vertigo in 13 countries over 28 months and found that, in real-life medical practice, the most common treatments prescribed were betahistine followed by piracetam, ginkgo biloba and diuretics, and the greatest improvements were seen in the more severely ill, and those with benign paroxysmal positional vertigo or 'other vertigo of peripheral origin' (Agus et al 2013). Although the registry reported that 93% of patients had some improvement in the 6-month follow-up, there were no specific data on the ginkgo subsection.

A systematic review of preclinical studies and five double-blind RCTs investigating the effects of EGb 761 in vestibular and non-vestibular vertigo concluded that ginkgo has benefits in vertiginous syndromes (Hamann 2007). The RCTs used a daily dose between 120 and 160 mg which was taken for 3 months.

Labyrinthitis

A novel guinea pig model has shown that *G. biloba* can minimise cochlear damage on otitis media-induced labyrinthitis (Jang et al 2011). Clinical trials are needed to confirm if this has any clinical relevance.

Sudden deafness

Ginkgo extract was as effective as pentoxifylline in the treatment of sudden deafness, according to one randomised, double-blind study (Reisser & Weidauer 2001). Both treatments equally reduced associated symptoms of tinnitus and produced the same effects on the return to normal of speech discrimination. Subjective assessment suggested that GBE was more beneficial than pentoxifylline. EGb 761 (240 mg/day) has also been shown to accelerate and secure recovery of acute idiopathic sudden sensorineural hearing loss, observable within 1 week of treatment under randomised double-blind test conditions (Burschka et al 2001).

Commission E approves the use of standardised ginkgo extract in these conditions when of vascular origin (Blumenthal et al 2000).

Macular degeneration, glaucoma and retinopathy

With regard to these ophthalmological conditions, ginkgo has numerous properties that should theoretically make it a useful treatment, such as increasing ocular blood flow, antioxidant and platelet-activating factor inhibitor activity, NO inhibition, protecting retinal ganglion cells against apoptosis (Wang et al 2012) and neuroprotective abilities.

Macular degeneration

Although some positive evidence exists, a 2013 Cochrane review has suggested that, overall, there is insufficient evidence currently available to conclude that *G. biloba* treatment is effective in macular degeneration, with further testing required (Evans 2013). Based on its known mechanisms of action, it is a worthy candidate for further research.

Glaucoma

With regard to glaucoma, the little research conducted so far appears promising. Researchers using colour Doppler imaging have observed significantly increased end-diastolic velocity in the ophthalmic artery after treatment with EGb (120 mg/day) in a placebo-controlled, randomised, crossover study (Chung et al 1999).

A randomised, double-blind, crossover study found that EGb 761 (120 mg/day) taken for 4 weeks produces positive effects in normal-tension glaucoma (Quaranta et al 2003). Furthermore, ginkgo treatment did not significantly alter intraocular pressure, blood pressure or heart rate and was well tolerated.

Other more recent studies have confirmed a benefit for normal-tension glaucoma. One RCT of 30 patients, administered 80 mg GBE twice a day over 4 weeks, found that retinal blood flow increased significantly in these normal-tension glaucoma patients (Park et al 2011). A retrospective study of 42 patients with a mean follow-up time of 12.3 years showed that 80 mg GBE twice daily slowed visual field defect damage (Lee et al 2013). These findings were also confirmed in a retrospective study with 332 patients who were compared to controls (n = 97); of the cohort, 132 patients were given bilberry anthocyanins and 103 patients received *G. biloba* (ginkgo leaf extract from SK Chemicals, Gyeonggi-do, Korea) at a dose of one 80-mg tablet twice a day. Both treatments were found to improve visual function in some patients with normal-tension glaucoma (Shim et al 2012).

Chloroquine retinopathy

In vivo tests using electroretinography have identified protective effects against the development of chloroquine-induced retinopathy using *G. biloba* (Droy-Lefaix et al 1992). This has been observed in both acute and chronic chloroquine toxicity of the retina (Droy-Lefaix et al 1995).

Prevention of altitude sickness/acute mountain sickness

Acetazolamide and ginkgo biloba are the two most investigated drugs for the prevention of acute mountain sickness (AMS) (Ke et al 2013). In general, research indicates that ginkgo may be useful as a prophylactic treatment when started 4–5 days prior to ascent to reduce the incidence of AMS (van Patot et al 2009). Considering its excellent safety profile, it is a treatment worthy of consideration.

While many studies have shown that pretreatment with ginkgo extract reduces the incidence of developing AMS, not all studies are positive when compared to placebo. This was most clearly seen in a study which consisted of two RCTs, one of which showed significant results (standardised *Ginkgo biloba* produced by Spectrum Chemical and Laboratory Products, Gardena, CA, United States) and the other did not (*Ginkgo biloba* 24/6/5 from Technical Sourcing International, TSI, Missoula, MT, United States) (Leadbetter et al 2009). The positive study used a dose of 120 mg twice daily starting 4 days before ascent to 4300 m and the other used prophylaxis at the same dose for 3 days.

In the positive study, treatment with 120 mg GBE twice daily significantly reduced both the incidence and the severity of AMS in participants rapidly exposed to high altitude; 68% of participants had AMS in the placebo group, compared to 33% in the GBE group and the number needed to treat was 3. In contrast, no significant effects on AMS incidence or severity were seen with the other ginkgo treatment and AMS developed in 45% of the placebo group compared to 27% taking ginkgo. Of note, the incidence of AMS in both ginkgo groups was still lower than placebo; however, the higher rate of AMS in the placebo group in the positive study may have been responsible for the discrepant results. The authors noted that the studies were underpowered to confirm these suspicions; however, the rates of AMS observed with placebo reflected the rates reported in the literature (50–75%).

A 2012 systematic shortcut review of literature (Seupaul et al 2012) on prophylaxis for AMS suggested that *G. biloba* was not effective; however, this review only included one study with *G. biloba* which was negative and involved 487 healthy Western hikers (Gertsch et al 2004). While the study by Gertsch et al is considered to be the only adequately powered GBE and AMS study published, treatment was not administered until participants reached approximately 4300 m without evidence of AMS, thus skewing the population towards those who are less susceptible to the condition and not being a proper trial design to test prophylaxis (Leadbetter et al 2009).

Numerous other studies not reported in the 2012 systematic review by Seupaul et al have been conducted, with research commencing in the 1990s and generally showing some benefits with ginkgo biloba pretreatment. Roncin et al (1996) involved 44 subjects and found that a dose of 160 mg/day taken for 5 days as prophylactic treatment resulted in 0% of subjects developing the cerebral symptoms of AMS versus 41% of subjects in the placebo group, whereas only 3 subjects (13.6%) in the EGb 761 group developed respiratory symptoms of AMS; 18 (81.8%) in the placebo group developed these symptoms. Besides effectively preventing AMS for moderate altitude (5400 m), the treatment also decreased vasomotor disorders of the extremities. In 2001, Maakestad et al reported on a randomised, double-blind trial of *G. biloba* (120 mg twice daily starting 5 days before ascent) compared to placebo for the prevention of AMS in 40 college students who underwent rapid ascent from 1400 to 4300 m. Using the Lake Louise Symptoms score and Environmental Symptoms Questionnaire as outcomes, *G. biloba* was shown to significantly reduce the incidence of AMS compared to placebo.

In subsequent years, some researchers compared ginkgo to acetazolamide. In 2003, two studies produced conflicting results. The study by Moraga et al (2003) compared prophylaxis with *G. biloba* (80 mg twice daily) versus acetazolamide (250 mg twice daily) versus placebo, which was started 24 hours before rapid ascent to 3700 m. Of 32 subjects enrolled, none of those in the *G. biloba* group developed AMS, compared with 35% of those in the acetazolamide group and 54% of those receiving placebo. Alternatively, ginkgo (120 mg twice daily) started 3 days before ascent produced no significant effects when compared to placebo or acetazolamide in a randomised, double-blind study by Leadbetter and Hackett (2003). The study involved 59 subjects who experienced a rapid ascent to 4300 m. Negative results were also obtained by Chow et al (2005) in a small RCT, showing no benefits over placebo and superiority of acetazolamide.

A study published in 2007 tested a different type of treatment regimen that produced significant benefits. The placebo-controlled study of 36 people found that pretreatment followed by continued treatment with *G. biloba* prevented AMS and was significantly more effective than acetazolamide (Moraga et al 2007). Volunteers were given placebo, acetazolamide (250 mg per dose) or ginkgo (80 mg per dose) every 12 hours starting 24 hours before ascending and continuing throughout the 3-day stay at high altitude. Not a single person treated with ginkgo experienced AMS, compared with 36% taking acetazolamide and 54% taking placebo. While ginkgo did not alter arterial oxygen saturation compared to acetazolamide, a marked increased saturation in arterial oxygen was seen in comparison with the placebo group.

Premenstrual syndrome (PMS)

A double-blind RCT evaluating the effects of EGb 761 in treating congestive symptoms of PMS in a group of 165 women found that treatment over two menstrual cycles (from day 16 until day 5 of the next cycle) was successful. Treatment was particularly effective in reducing breast symptoms, although neuropsychological symptoms were also alleviated (Tamborini & Taurelle 1993). A more recent placebo-controlled RCT with 85 participants has confirmed that *G. biloba* can significantly reduce the severity of PMS symptoms when given at a dose of 40 mg ginkgo extract three times a day from day 16 of the menstrual cycle to day 5 of the next menstrual cycle (Ozgoli et al 2009).

Vitiligo

A dose of 120 mg/day ginkgo extract significantly stopped active progression of depigmentation in slow-spreading vitiligo and induced repigmentation in some treated patients under double-blind, placebo-controlled study conditions (Parsad et al 2003). Although the mechanism of action responsible is unknown, antioxidant activity is thought to be important. An open-label trial of just 12 participants also reported repigmentation with *G. biloba* 120 mg/day given over 12 weeks (Szczurko et al 2011).

Sexual dysfunction/sexual function

Due to its vasodilatory effects, ginkgo has been used in the management of sexual dysfunction in cases where compromised circulation is suspected. One open study has been conducted with subjects experiencing sexual dysfunction associated with antidepressant use (Cohen & Bartlik 1998). Ginkgo extract (average dose 209 mg/day) was found to be 84% effective in treating antidepressant-induced sexual dysfunction, predominantly caused by selective serotonin reuptake inhibitor, in a study of 63 subjects. A relative success rate of 91% was observed for women, compared with 76% for men, and a positive effect was reported on all four phases of the sexual response cycle: desire, excitement (erection and lubrication), orgasm and resolution. Although this was an open trial, the results are encouraging when one considers that the placebo effect is about 25% from past randomised trials of US Federal Drug Administration-approved medications for erectile dysfunction (Moyad 2002).

More recently, a small, triple-blind (investigator, patient, statistician), randomised, placebo-controlled trial of *G. biloba* (240 mg/day for 12 weeks) was undertaken with 24 subjects experiencing sexual impairment caused by antidepressant drugs (Wheatley 2004). The authors report some spectacular individual responses in both groups, but no statistically significant differences, and no differences in side effects.

Meston et al (2008) conducted two studies of women with sexual dysfunction. The first was a single-dose, placebo-controlled study using 300 mg ginkgo extract, which produced a small but significant facilitatory effect on physiological, but not subjective, sexual arousal in 99 sexually dysfunctional women. The second study investigated long-term use of ginkgo (300 mg/day) over 8 weeks, and found that herbal treatment combined with sex therapy significantly increased sexual desire and contentment compared to placebo or ginkgo as sole treatment. A newer study looking at the effect of *G. biloba* on menopausal women's sexual function reported significant improvement in sexual desire, sexual pleasure, orgasm and importance of sex in comparison to previous years. The triple-blind, randomised, placebo-controlled trial included 80 healthy women aged 50–60 years who were given a dose of 120–240 mg *G. biloba* daily (Taavoni et al 2012).

OTHER USES

G. biloba is used for many other indications, including improving connective tissue conditions such as haemorrhoids, common allergies, reducing the effects of exposure to radiation and to prevent some of the complications associated with diabetes. In the United Kingdom and other European countries, the cardioprotective effects of EGb 761 in myocardial ischaemia and reperfusion are currently being investigated in preclinical studies.

Attention-deficit hyperactivity disorder and autism — no effect

A clinical trial in children with attention-deficit hyperactivity disorder (ADHD) found *G. biloba* to be less effective than the drug methylphenidate (Salehi et al 2010). A systematic review of herbal and nutritional products for treating ADHD confirmed no evidence of benefit with ginkgo (Sarris et al 2011). Additionally, *G. biloba* provided no benefits when used as add-on therapy in autism, according to a double-blind clinical trial adding the herb to risperidone therapy (Hasanzadeh et al 2012).

Addiction — no effect

A pilot study for the treatment of cocaine dependence found no benefit to *G. biloba*. In the RCT 10-week trial 44 participants dependent on cocaine took piracetam (4.8 g/day) or ginkgo (120 mg/day) or placebo. The results found that piracetam was associated with more cocaine use and that ginkgo was not superior to placebo (Kampman et al 2003).

Allergic conjunctivitis

An RCT of 60 patients with symptomatic allergic conjunctivitis using a topical GBE with hyaluronic acid ophthalmic solution (Trium) or hyaluronic acid alone found that additional *G. biloba* produced a significant decrease in symptoms of conjunctival hyperaemia, conjunctival discharge and chemosis (Russo et al 2009).

Adjunct in cancer treatment

As a herb with significant antioxidant and neuroprotective activities, ginkgo has been used to reduce the toxic side effects of some chemotherapeutic drugs. Evidence from in vivo studies demonstrates protective effects against nephrotoxicity induced by cisplatin, cardiotoxicity induced by doxorubicin (El Boghdady 2013a, Naidu et al 2002, Ozturk et al 2004), cisplatin-induced ototoxicity (Huang et al 2007), Adriamycin-induced hyperlipidaemic nephrotoxicity (Abd-Ellah & Mariee 2007) and protective effects for testicular tissue after doxorubicin therapy (Yeh et al 2009). An in vitro study produced a protective effect against radiation of human peripheral blood lymphocytes (Esmekaya et al 2011) and another found *G. biloba* may be helpful with cisplatin therapy sensitising ovarian cancer cells to treatment (Jiang et al 2014).

Little clinical research has been conducted thus far to determine its potential use in practice. One recent open-label clinical study enrolled 34 irradiated brain tumour patients who were given *G. biloba* (120 mg/day) for 24 weeks and found some improvement in quality of life and cognitive function (Attia et al 2012). Another trial with low-dose *G. biloba* (60 mg/day EGb 761) found no benefit in reducing cognitive dysfunction, which can often be associated with treatment in women who are undergoing chemotherapy for breast cancer (Barton et al 2013).

Patients (n = 23) undergoing radioiodine therapy for differentiated thyroid cancer were assigned placebo or GBE before and after treatment (120 mg/day for a month). The treated group did not have a significant increase in lymphocytes and ginkgo was found to be protective from possible oxidative and genotoxic damage from the treatment (Dardano et al 2012).

Asthma

Ginkgo shows promise as a treatment for asthma, according to studies using a mouse model of asthma (Babayigit et al 2008) and two clinical studies (Li et al 1997, Tang et al 2007b). Ginkgo significantly reduced airway hyperreactivity and improved clinical symptoms and pulmonary function in asthmatic patients in a placebo-controlled study (Li et al 1997). Platelet-activating factor inhibitor, antioxidant and anti-inflammatory activities are likely to be involved.

Reduced airway inflammation was reported in another study of 75 asthma patients, which compared the effects of fluticasone propionate with fluticasone propionate plus ginkgo (Tang et al 2007b). The addition of ginkgo to treatment resulted in a significant decrease in the infiltration of inflammatory cells such as eosinophils and lymphocytes in the asthmatic airway and relieved airway inflammation.

Cancer prevention

A 2006 review proposes that *G. biloba* should be more widely used as a safe preventive agent for reducing cancer incidence. This recommendation is based on results from numerous in vitro and experimental studies showing that ginkgo affects many factors associated with the incidence and mortality of cancer (Eli & Fasciano 2006). However, a more recent secondary analysis of the Ginkgo Evaluation of Memory study, which is the largest placebo-controlled RCT of ginkgo, evaluated cancer hospitalisations during the 6.1-year follow-up and found no evidence of reduced incidence of cancer. The intervention of 120 mg twice daily of ginkgo extract (EGb 761) was chosen for cognition and not cancer prevention, and the authors also suggested that the follow-up may have been too short to detect benefits with regard to cancer prevention (Biggs et al 2010).

Cardiac surgery support

An RCT of 20 patients undergoing cardiac surgery found the GBE group (0.5 mg/kg Ginaton) increased the production of plasma VEGF, offering some myocardial protection in the perioperative period (Deng et al 2009). Another study with 80 CAD patients found that the GBE group caused an increase in coronary artery blood flow (Wu et al 2008a).

Diabetic nephropathy

Ginkgo had a beneficial effect on vascular endothelial function in patients with early-stage diabetic nephropathy, according to an RCT of 64 patients (Li et al 2009).The known pharmacological mechanisms of ginkgo provide some basis for this finding.

Migraine headache

Ginkgolide B demonstrates anti-inflammatory activity and a reduction of the excitatory effect of glutamate in the central nervous system, which may be of benefit in the treatment of migraine headache with and without aura. Initial studies have been undertaken, often with a combination of nutrients, showing promise in the prevention of migraine.

An open study of 50 women with a history of migraine with typical aura used a product (Migrasoll) containing ginkgolide B from *G. biloba* (60 mg) with coenzyme Q10 (11 mg) and vitamin B_2 (8.7 mg) for 4 months, whereby migraine frequency and duration were reduced, an effect seen after the first 2 months and further enhanced after taking the product for 4 months (D'Andrea et al 2009). Another open-label study with 119 school-aged volunteers with a history of migraine found that treatment with a combination product (ginkgolide B, coenzyme Q10, riboflavin and magnesium) taken twice daily as a prophylactic therapy for 3 months significantly reduced migraine frequency (Esposito & Carotenuto 2011). A similar combination of nutrients with ginkgolide B (80 mg), coenzyme Q10 (20 mg), vitamin B_2 (1.6 mg) and magnesium (300 mg) was given to 30 children twice a day for 3 months. In this open-label prospective trial the children were followed up over a year; combination treatment was shown to be an effective preventive treatment in significantly reducing migraine frequency and reducing analgesic medication after 3 months and at 1-year follow-up (Usai et al 2011).

Multiple sclerosis

MS is a chronic demyelinating neurological disease afflicting young and middle-aged adults, resulting in problems with coordination, strength, cognition, affect and sensation. Several clinical studies have investigated whether ginkgo treatment may help reduce some of these impairments, generally producing disappointing results.

Johnson et al (2006) conducted a randomised, double-blind study which compared the effects of ginkgo (EGb 761: 240 mg/day) to placebo on depression, anxiety, fatigue, symptom severity and functional performance using validated measures for each outcome. Twenty-two people with MS were enrolled in the study. Significantly, more people administered ginkgo showed improvement on four or more measures, with improvements associated with significantly larger effect sizes on measures of fatigue, symptom severity and functionality. The ginkgo group also exhibited less fatigue at follow-up compared with the placebo group and treatment was well tolerated, with no side effects or adverse effects reported.

The cognitive function of people with MS did not significantly improve after 12 weeks of treatment with GBE (120 mg twice a day), according to a randomised, double-blind, placebo-controlled trial (Lovera et al 2007). However, a treatment effect trend, limited to the Stroop test, indicated that ginkgo treatment may have an effect on cognitive domains assessed by this test, such as susceptibility to interference and mental flexibility. People with greater cognitive impairment at the start of the study experienced more improvement with treatment than higher-functioning people. No serious drug-related side effects occurred. A Cochrane systematic review of treatment for memory disorders in MS patients only found the 2007 Lovera study worthy of inclusion and confirmed *G. biloba* was not effective as an intervention in this group (He et al 2011). The same author, Lovera, repeated his earlier study with a RCT of 120 subjects with MS and *G. biloba* (120 mg twice daily) over 12 weeks and confirmed that there were no improvements in cognitive performance (Lovera et al 2012).

Parkinson's disease

There is great interest in the application of safe substances, such as *G. biloba*, in neurodegenerative diseases such as Parkinson's disease because of their neuroprotective and mitochondrial protective effects. Currently, investigation with ginkgo is limited to animal studies of experimentally induced Parkinson's disease, which have shown it to afford some protection against neuronal loss (Ahmad et al 2005, Kim et al 2004) and neuronal damage (Rojas et al 2012).

Schizophrenia — adjunctive treatment

G. biloba given as an adjunct to the atypical antipsychotic medicine clozapine in the treatment of refractory schizophrenia was shown to enhance drug effects on negative symptoms according to a placebo-controlled study involving 42 patients with chronic, treatment-resistant schizophrenia (Doruk et al 2008). Ginkgo was used at a dose of 120 mg/day for 12 weeks. This study has been further validated by a review and meta-analysis conducted in 2010 which included six studies of 466 patients taking ginkgo and 362 people taking placebo. When prescribed in combination with antipsychotic medication, *G. biloba* resulted in statistically significant positive effects with symptoms of chronic schizophrenia (Singh et al 2010). Since the publication of the meta-analysis a further randomised double-blind, placebo-controlled trial found benefit of using GBE (EGb 761) for reducing symptoms of tardive dyskinesia in schizophrenia patients. This trial recruited 157 in a psychiatric hospital in China and the treatment arm were given 240 mg/day of *G. biloba* or placebo for 12 weeks. The authors hypothesise that the improvement may be due to the antioxidant activity of this herb (Zhang et al 2011, 2012a).

Tardive syndromes — including tardive dyskinesias

The American Academy of Neurology in 2013 conducted a broad literature review to make evidence-based recommendations regarding management of tardive syndromes, including tardive dyskinesias (Bhidayasiri et al 2013). They came to the conclusion that clonazepam probably improves tardive dyskinesias and ginkgo biloba probably improves tardive syndromes (both level B) and both should be considered as treatment.

DOSAGE RANGE

The recommended dose varies, depending on indication and condition treated.

General guide

- Dried herb: 9–10 g/day.
- 120–240 mg of a 50:1 standardised extract daily in divided doses (40 mg extract is equivalent to 1.4–2.7 g leaves).
- Fluid extract (1:1): 0.5 mL three times daily.

According to clinical studies

- Asthma: 40 mg three times daily.
- Dementia and memory impairment: 120–240 mg standardised extract daily in divided doses.
- Generalised anxiety disorder: 240–480 mg daily.
- Intermittent claudication, vertigo: 120–320 mg standardised extract daily in divided doses.
- Normal-tension glaucoma: 120–160 mg standardised extract daily.
- MS — to improve energy levels, cognitive function and mood: 120 mg twice daily.
- PMS: 80 mg twice daily, starting on the 16th day of the menstrual cycle until the 5th day of the next cycle.
- Prevention of altitude sickness: 160 mg standardised extract daily, starting 5 days prior to ascent or ginkgo (80 mg per dose) every 12 hours, starting 24 hours before ascending and continuing throughout stay at high altitude.
- Schizophrenia: as an adjunct to clozapine in refractory cases: 120–240 mg daily.
- Raynaud's syndrome: 240–360 mg/day divided into three doses.
- Sexual dysfunction associated with antidepressant drugs: 200 mg standardised extract daily.
- Sexual dysfunction (women): 300 mg daily in conjunction with sex therapy.
- Vitiligo: 120 mg standardised extract daily.

Although some studies report positive effects after 4–6 weeks' continual use, a trial of at least 12 weeks is recommended in chronic conditions.

ADVERSE REACTIONS

In most placebo-controlled studies, there is no difference between the side effect incidence with ginkgo and placebo. Standardised ginkgo leaf extracts have been used safely in trials lasting from several weeks to up to 6 years. In a few cases (less than 0.001%), gastrointestinal upset, headaches and dizziness were reported. Ginkgo does not appear to alter heart rate and blood pressure, change cholesterol and triglyceride levels or increase intraocular pressure in clinical studies (Chung et al 1999).

A 2011 systematic review of bleeding associated with *G. biloba* therapy found no higher bleeding risk associated with standardised GBE in a meta-analysis of 18 RCTs (Kellermann & Kloft 2011); however, rare case reports of subarachnoid haemorrhage, subdural haematoma, intracerebral haemorrhage, subphrenic haematoma, vitreous haemorrhage and postoperative bleeding have been reported.

Crude ginkgo plant parts that may contain concentrations of 5 ppm of the toxic ginkgolic acid constituents should be avoided, as they can induce severe allergic reactions.

Clinical note — Does* Ginkgo biloba *cause significant bleeding and does it interact with warfarin?

The current body of evidence casts doubt on the clinical significance of the proposed interaction between warfarin and ginkgo, revealing that there is little evidence from controlled studies to demonstrate significant platelet inhibition, bleeding or changes to international normalised ratio (INR) with use of ginkgo (especially EGb 761 or phytochemically similar extracts).

Several clinical trials have been published in peer-reviewed journals which demonstrate that *G. biloba* does not have a significant effect on platelet function, two studies showing no interaction with warfarin, one study showing no interaction with aspirin and a further study showing no interaction with clopidogrel (Aruna & Naidu 2007, Bal Dit et al 2003, Beckert et al 2007, Carlson et al 2007, Engelsen et al 2003, Gardner et al 2007, Jiang et al 2005, Kohler et al 2004). Studies have included young healthy volunteers and older adults, using doses up to 480 mg/day of ginkgo and time frames up to 4 months.

The first controlled study was published in 2003. Bal Dit et al conducted a double-blind, randomised, placebo-controlled study of 32 young healthy volunteers to evaluate the effect of three doses of GBE (120, 240 and 480 mg/day for 14 days) on haemostasis, coagulation and fibrinolysis (Bal Dit et al 2003). This escalating dose study found no effect on platelet function or coagulation for any dose tested. A year later, results from a larger randomised, placebo-controlled, crossover study that produced similar results were published (Kohler et al 2004). The study by Kohler et al investigated the effects of ginkgo (2 × 120 mg/day EGb 761) on 29 different coagulation and bleeding parameters. Once again, no evidence of inhibition of blood coagulation and platelet aggregation was detected. In Australia, Jiang et al (2005) investigated the interaction between warfarin and *G. biloba* using a randomised, cross-over study design. The study of 12 healthy males found no evidence that INR or platelet aggregation was affected by *G. biloba*. Engelsen et al (2003) also found no evidence of an interaction between *G. biloba* and warfarin under double-blind, placebo-controlled trial conditions. The study involved patients stable on long-term warfarin and reported no changes to INR values.

In 2007, four more studies were published. Carlson et al (2007) conducted a study of 90 older adults (65–84 years) who were randomly assigned to placebo or a *G. biloba*-based supplement (160 mg/day) for 4 months. No evidence of alteration to platelet function was seen at this dose. Beckert et al (2007) conducted a smaller trial of 10 volunteers who were administered ginkgo for 2 weeks, after which in vivo platelet function was quantified using the PFA-100 assay. The study used aspirin as a control agent and found that platelet function was not affected by *G. biloba*, but was markedly inhibited by the administration of aspirin. No clinically or statistically significant differences were seen in a randomised, double-blind, placebo-controlled trial, which investigated the effects of *G. biloba* (EGb 761, 300 mg/day) on several measures of platelet aggregation among 55 older adults (age 69 ± 10 years) also consuming 325 mg/day aspirin (Gardner et al 2007). Reports of bleeding or bruising were infrequent and similar for both study groups. A study of 10 healthy volunteers investigated the effects of two different doses of *G. biloba* (120 mg and 240 mg) taken together with clopidogrel (75 mg) (Aruna & Naidu 2007). Platelet inhibition with the combination of *G. biloba* and clopidogrel was not statistically significant, compared with individual doses of drugs. Finally, a 2011 randomised, double-blind, placebo-controlled, two-way cross-over trial was conducted on 12 healthy volunteers for 5 weeks. It was found that there was no effect on clotting process alone and *G. biloba* had limited effects on the pharmacokinetics and no effect on the pharmacodynamics of single-dose warfarin in health volunteers (Zhou & Zeng 2011).

G

SIGNIFICANT INTERACTIONS

A small clinical study suggests that *G. biloba* inhibits P-gp, so caution is advised when taking GBE and P-gp substrates together, as drug doses may need to be adjusted. Various cytochromes have been evaluated, and drugs metabolised this way seem to have little risk of herb–drug interactions with *G. biloba* at doses of 240 mg/day or less (Gurley et al 2012).

Adriamycin

Studies with an animal model indicate that ginkgo extract EGb 761 reduces the hyperlipidaemia and proteinuria associated with Adriamycin-induced nephropathy, which might be beneficial to enhance the therapeutic index of Adriamycin (Abd-Ellah & Mariee 2007). Clinical trials have not been conducted to confirm the activity.

Antidepressant drugs

Ginkgo may reduce the sexual dysfunction side effects of these drugs and improve sleep continuity; however, results from clinical studies are mixed — possible beneficial interaction.

Bleomycin

Studies with an animal model indicate that ginkgo extract EGb 761 reduces oxidative stress induced by bleomycin. This may improve drug tolerance; however, clinical studies have not yet been conducted to test this further (Erdogan et al 2006).

Cholinergic drugs

Cholinergic activity has been identified for ginkgo; therefore, combined use may theoretically increase drug activity — observe patients using this combination, although the effects may be beneficial when used under supervision.

Cilostazol

Used for intermittent claudication with peripheral arterial disease. Adjunctive use with *G. biloba* may produce additional benefits based on in vivo studies (Jung et al 2012) — observe.

Cisplatin

As a herb with significant antioxidant activity, ginkgo has also been employed as a means of reducing the nephrotoxic effects of cisplatin, a use supported by two in vivo studies (Gulec et al 2006, Ozturk et al 2004). Other researchers using animal models have indicated that ginkgo may protect against cisplatin-induced ototoxicity (Huang et al 2007). Clinical trials are required to confirm significance — adjunctive use may be beneficial when used under professional supervision.

Clozapine

Ginkgo may enhance the effects of clozapine on negative affect in refractory schizophrenic patients, according to a placebo-controlled study (Doruk et al 2008) — beneficial interaction.

Doxorubicin

In vivo research suggests that ginkgo can prevent doxorubicin-induced cardiotoxicity, suggesting a potentially beneficial interaction, although no human studies are available to confirm clinical significance (Naidu et al 2002).

Haloperidol

In three clinical trials, the effectiveness of haloperidol was enhanced when co-administered with 360 mg of ginkgo daily (Chavez et al 2006) — beneficial interaction under supervision.

Platelet inhibitor drugs

Due to its platelet-activating factor antagonist activity, *G. biloba* may theoretically enhance the effects of these drugs and increase the risk of bruising or bleeding; however, evidence from recent clinical trials and a systematic review has cast doubt on the clinical significance of this activity (Diamond & Bailey 2013, Kim et al 2010, Ryu et al 2009) — observe.

Valproate, Dilantin, Depakote

There is a report of 2 patients using valproate who experienced seizures with ginkgo use (Chavez et al 2006). There is also a report of a patient taking Dilantin, Depakote and ginkgo, together with other herbal medicines, who suffered a fatal breakthrough seizure, with no evidence of non-compliance with anticonvulsant medications (Kupiec & Raj 2005). The autopsy report revealed subtherapeutic serum levels for both anticonvulsants, Depakote and Dilantin; however, it is uncertain whether effects can be attributed to ginkgo — observe patient taking ginkgo with these medicines.

Warfarin

Theoretically, ginkgo may increase bleeding risk when used together with warfarin; however, evidence from controlled clinical studies does not support this conclusion and has failed to identify any clinically significant pharmacodynamic or pharmacokinetic interaction. This conclusion is supported by a systematic review (Bone 2008) — observe.

> ***CONTRAINDICATIONS AND PRECAUTIONS***
>
> If unusual bleeding or bruising occurs, stop use immediately. Although new clinical evidence suggests that *G. biloba* does not affect clotting times, it may be prudent to suspend use for 1 week prior to major surgery in at-risk populations.

Cerebral haemorrhage and epilepsy

Rare case reports have suggested that ginkgo should be used with caution in people with known risk factors for cerebral haemorrhage and epilepsy until further investigation can clarify its safety (Benjamin et al 2001, Granger 2001, Vale 1998).

> ***PREGNANCY USE***
>
> Insufficient reliable evidence in humans to determine safety. In clinical usage there would be no adverse effects expected (Bone 2003).

Practice points/Patient counselling

- *G. biloba* is a complex herb that contains many different active constituents and works by means of multiple mechanisms. Therefore, it has applications in many varied conditions.
- Oral ginkgo extract improves cognitive function in people with mild to moderate cognitive impairment or those people with dementia with neuropsychiatric features, but it is less successful in people with normal cognitive function.
- Long-term use does not protect against the development of dementia.
- It may be an effective treatment in peripheral vascular diseases such as intermittent claudication; however, study findings are not always consistent. Due to the herb's inherent safety, a therapeutic trial may be useful in practice to determine an individual's response.
- Some positive evidence exists for PMS, sudden deafness, tardive syndromes, preventing altitude sickness, ischaemic stroke, SAD and vertigo.
- Largely based on the herb's physiological actions, ginkgo is also used to treat chilblains and haemorrhoids, and prevent macular degeneration, glaucoma, sexual dysfunction, impotence, allergies and asthma, and improve wellbeing.
- The form of ginkgo most often tested and used is a preparation known as EGb 761, which is standardised to 24% ginkgo flavonol glycosides and 6% terpene lactones.
- Overall, *G. biloba* is a very safe herb and is extremely well tolerated.

PATIENTS' FAQs

What will this herb do for me?

Ginkgo is a very popular herbal treatment that increases peripheral circulation, beneficially influences brain chemicals, protects nerve cells from damage and may stimulate immune function and reduce inflammation. Scientific evidence has shown that it may improve cognitive function in people with mild to moderate cognitive impairment when used long-term in sufficient dosage, but it is less successful in people with normal function. It may also improve some aspects of memory in younger people when used short-term. Ginkgo may improve symptoms of intermittent claudication and be useful in treating chilblains, PMS and vitiligo, preventing altitude sickness, vertigo and SAD and possibly sexual dysfunction such as impotence. If taken long-term, it does not protect against the development of dementia in the future.

When will it start to work?

This will depend on the condition treated and the dose used. Generally, *G. biloba* is a slow-acting herb that can take anywhere from 4 weeks to 6 months to exert maximal effects.

Are there any safety issues?

Ginkgo has been extensively studied and appears to be extremely safe with virtually no side effects in healthy people. Some contraindications and interactions are possible, so it is recommended that it should be taken under professional supervision.

REFERENCES

Abd-Ellah MF, Mariee AD. *Ginkgo biloba* leaf extract (EGb 761) diminishes adriamycin-induced hyperlipidaemic nephrotoxicity in rats: association with nitric oxide production. Biotechnol Appl Biochem 46 (2007): 35–40.

Abdel-Salam OM et al. Evaluation of the anti-inflammatory, anti-nociceptive and gastric effects of *Ginkgo biloba* in the rat. Pharmacol Res 49.2 (2004): 133–142.

Agus, S., et al. 2013. Clinical and Demographic Features of Vertigo: Findings from the REVERT Registry. Front Neurol., 4, 48 available from: PM:23675366.

Ahmad M et al. *Ginkgo biloba* affords dose-dependent protection against 6-hydroxydopamine-induced parkinsonism in rats: neurobehavioural, neurochemical and immunohistochemical evidences. J Neurochem 93.1 (2005): 94–104.

Ao Q et al. Protective effects of extract of *Ginkgo biloba* (EGb 761) on nerve cells after spinal cord injury in rats. Spinal Cord 44.11 (2006): 662–667.

Aricioglu A et al. Changes in zinc levels and superoxide dismutase activities in the skin of acute, ultraviolet-B-irradiated mice after treatment with *Ginkgo biloba* extract. Biol Trace Elem Res 80.2 (2001): 175–179.

Aruna D, Naidu MU. Pharmacodynamic interaction studies of *Ginkgo biloba* with cilostazol and clopidogrel in healthy human subjects. Br J Clin Pharmacol 63.3 (2007): 333–338.

Attia, A., et al. 2012. Phase II study of *Ginkgo biloba* in irradiated brain tumor patients: effect on cognitive function, quality of life, and mood. J Neurooncol, 109, 357–63.

Babayigit A et al. Effects of *Ginkgo biloba* on airway histology in a mouse model of chronic asthma. Allergy Asthma Proc 30.2 (2008): 186–2591.

Bachinskaya, N., et al. 2011. Alleviating neuropsychiatric symptoms in dementia: the effects of *Ginkgo biloba* extract EGb 761. Findings from a randomized controlled trial. Neuropsychiatr Dis Treat, 7, 209–15.

Bal Dit SC et al. No alteration in platelet function or coagulation induced by EGb 761 in a controlled study. Clin Lab Haematol 25.4 (2003): 251–253.

Bao, Y. M., et al. 2010. [Effects of *Ginkgo biloba* extract 50 preconditioning on contents of inflammation-related cytokines in myocardium of rats with ischemia-reperfusion injury.] Zhong Xi Yi Jie He Xue Bao, 8, 373–8.

Barton, D. L., et al. 2013. The use of *Ginkgo biloba* for the prevention of chemotherapy-related cognitive dysfunction in women receiving adjuvant treatment for breast cancer, N00C9. Support Care Cancer. 21: 1185–1192.

Bastianetto S, Quirion R. EGb 761 is a neuroprotective agent against beta-amyloid toxicity. Cell Mol Biol (Noisy-le-grand) 48.6 (2002a): 693–7.

Bastianetto S, Quirion R. Natural extracts as possible protective agents of brain aging. Neurobiol Aging 23.5 (2002b): 891–7.

Bastianetto S et al. The *Ginkgo biloba* extract (EGb 761) protects hippocampal neurons against cell death induced by beta-amyloid. Eur J Neurosci 12.6 (2000): 1882–1890.

Beal MF. Bioenergetic approaches for neuroprotection in Parkinson's disease. Ann Neurol 53 (Suppl 3) (2003): S39–S47.

Beckert BW et al. The effect of herbal medicines on platelet function: an in vivo experiment and review of the literature. Plast Reconstr Surg 120.7 (2007): 2044–2050.

Benjamin J et al. A case of cerebral haemorrhage: can *Ginkgo biloba* be implicated? Postgrad Med J 77.904 (2001): 112–1113.

Bernatoniene, J., et al. 2011. The effect of *Ginkgo biloba* extract on mitochondrial oxidative phosphorylation in the normal and ischemic rat heart. Phytother Res, 25, 1054–60.

Bhidayasiri, R., et al. 2013. Evidence-based guideline: treatment of tardive syndromes: report of the Guideline Development Subcommittee of the American Academy of Neurology. Neurology, 81, (5) 463–469 available from: PM:23897874.

Biggs, M. L., et al. 2010. *Ginkgo biloba* and risk of cancer: secondary analysis of the Ginkgo Evaluation of Memory (GEM) Study. Pharmacoepidemiol Drug Saf, 19, 694–8.

Birks, J. & Grimley Evans, J. 2009. *Ginkgo biloba* for cognitive impairment and dementia. Cochrane Database Syst Rev, CD003120.

Blumenthal M, et al. (eds). Herbal medicine expanded commission E monographs. Austin, TX: Integrative Medicine Communications, 2000.

Bone, K. 2003. A Clinical guide to blending liquid herbs, Qld, Australia, Churchill Livingstone.

Bone KM. Potential interaction of *Ginkgo biloba* leaf with antiplatelet or anticoagulant drugs: what is the evidence? Mol Nutr Food Res 52.7 (2008): 764–771.

Bredie, S. J. & Jong, M. C. 2012. No significant effect of ginkgo biloba special extract EGb 761 in the treatment of primary Raynaud phenomenon: a randomized controlled trial. J Cardiovasc Pharmacol, 59, 215–21.

Brondino, N., et al. 2013. A Systematic Review and Meta-Analysis of *Ginkgo biloba* in Neuropsychiatric Disorders: From Ancient Tradition to Modern-Day Medicine. Evid Based Complement Alternat Med, 2013, 915691.

Budzinski JW et al. An in vitro evaluation of human cytochrome P450 3A4 inhibition by selected commercial herbal extracts and tinctures. Phytomedicine 7.4 (2000): 273–282.

Burns NR, et al. *Ginkgo biloba*: no robust effect on cognitive abilities or mood in healthy young or older adults. Hum Psychopharmacol 21.1 (2006): 27–37.

Burschka MA et al. Effect of treatment with *Ginkgo biloba* extract EGb 761 (oral) on unilateral idiopathic sudden hearing loss in a prospective randomized double-blind study of 106 outpatients. Eur Arch Otorhinolaryngol 258.5 (2001): 213–2119.

Canter PH, Ernst E. *Ginkgo biloba* is not a smart drug: an updated systematic review of randomised clinical trials testing the nootropic effects of *G. biloba* extracts in healthy people. Hum Psychopharmacol 22.5 (2007): 265–278.

Carlson JJ et al. Safety and efficacy of a ginkgo biloba-containing dietary supplement on cognitive function, quality of life, and platelet function in healthy, cognitively intact older adults. J Am Diet Assoc 107.3 (2007): 422–432.

Chavez ML, et al. Evidence-based drug: herbal interactions. Life Sci 78.18 (2006): 2146–2157.

Chen X, et al. Extracts of *Ginkgo biloba* and ginsenosides exert cerebral vasorelaxation via a nitric oxide pathway. Clin Exp Pharmacol Physiol 24.12 (1997): 958–959.

Chen, L. L., et al. 2008. [Effect of nebulized TFG on Th1/Th2 imbalance in mouse model with asthma.] Zhongguo Zhong Yao Za Zhi, 33, 1865–8.

Chen, J. S., et al. 2011a. Nrf-2 mediated heme oxygenase-1 expression, an antioxidant-independent mechanism, contributes to anti-atherogenesis and vascular protective effects of *Ginkgo biloba* extract. Atherosclerosis, 214, 301–9.

Chen, X. H., et al. 2011b. Effects of *Ginkgo biloba* extract EGb761 on human colon adenocarcinoma cells. Cell Physiol Biochem, 27, 227–32.

Choi, W. S., et al. 2009. To compare the efficacy and safety of nifedipine sustained release with *Ginkgo biloba* extract to treat patients with primary Raynaud's phenomenon in South Korea; Korean Raynaud study (KOARA study). Clin Rheumatol, 28, 553–9.

Chow T et al. *Ginkgo biloba* and acetazolamide prophylaxis for acute mountain sickness: a randomized, placebo-controlled trial. Arch Intern Med 165.3 (2005): 296–301.

Chu, X., et al. 2011. A novel anti-inflammatory role for ginkgolide B in asthma via inhibition of the ERK/MAPK signaling pathway. Molecules, 16, 7634–48.

Chung HS et al. *Ginkgo biloba* extract increases ocular blood flow velocity. J Ocul Pharmacol Ther 15.3 (1999): 233–240.

Cieza A, et al. [The effect of ginkgo biloba on healthy elderly subjects.] Fortschr Med Orig 121.1 (2003): 5–10.

Clement, Y. N., et al. 2011. Effects of herbal and dietary supplements on cognition in menopause: a systematic review. Maturitas, 68, 256–63.

Cohen AJ, Bartlik B. *Ginkgo biloba* for antidepressant-induced sexual dysfunction. J Sex Marital Ther 24.2 (1998): 139–143.

Cohen-Boulakia F et al. In vivo sequential study of skeletal muscle capillary permeability in diabetic rats: effect of anthocyanosides. Metabolism 49.7 (2000): 880–885.

Colciaghi F et al. Amyloid precursor protein metabolism is regulated toward alpha-secretase pathway by *Ginkgo biloba* extracts. Neurobiol Dis 16.2 (2004): 454–460.

Cong, W.-N., et al. 2011. EGb761, an extract of *Ginkgo biloba* leaves, reduces insulin resistance in a high-fat-fed mouse model. Acta Pharmaceutica Sinica B, 1, 14–20.

D'Andrea, G., et al. 2009. Efficacy of Ginkgolide B in the prophylaxis of migraine with aura. Neurol Sci, 30 Suppl 1, S121–4.

Dardano, A., et al. 2012. The effect of *Ginkgo biloba* extract on genotoxic damage in patients with differentiated thyroid carcinoma receiving thyroid remnant ablation with iodine-131. Thyroid, 22, 318–24.

Das A et al. A comparative study in rodents of standardized extracts of *Bacopa monniera* and *Ginkgo biloba*: anticholinesterase and cognitive enhancing activities. Pharmacol Biochem Behav 73.4 (2002): 893.

DeFeudis FV, Drieu K. *Ginkgo biloba* extract (EGb 761) and CNS functions: basic studies and clinical applications. Curr Drug Targets 1.1 (2000): 25–58.

DeFeudis FV, et al. *Ginkgo biloba* extracts and cancer: a research area in its infancy. Fundam Clin Pharmacol 17.4 (2003): 405–417.

DeKosky ST et al. *Ginkgo biloba* for prevention of dementia: a randomized controlled trial. JAMA 300.19 (2008): 2253–2262.

Deng Y et al. Induction of cytochrome P450s by terpene trilactones and flavonoids of the *Ginkgo biloba* extract EGb 761 in rats. Xenobiotica 38.5 (2008): 465–481.

Deng, Y. K., et al. 2009. [Effect of ginkgo biloba extract on plasma vascular endothelial growth factor during peri-operative period of cardiac surgery.] Zhongguo Zhong Xi Yi Jie He Za Zhi, 29, 40–2.

Diamond, B. J. & Bailey, M. R. 2013. *Ginkgo biloba*: indications, mechanisms, and safety. Psychiatr Clin North Am, 36, 73–83.

Dodge HH et al. A randomized placebo-controlled trial of *Ginkgo biloba* for the prevention of cognitive decline. Neurology 70.19 (Pt 2) (2008): 1809–1817.

Dong, Z. H., et al. 2012. [Effects of ginkgo biloba tablet in treating mild cognitive impairment.] Zhongguo Zhong Xi Yi Jie He Za Zhi, 32, 1208–11.

Doruk A, et al. A placebo-controlled study of extract of ginkgo biloba added to clozapine in patients with treatment-resistant schizophrenia. Int Clin Psychopharmacol 23.4 (2008): 223–227.

Drew S, Davies E. Effectiveness of *Ginkgo biloba* in treating tinnitus: double blind, placebo controlled trial. BMJ 322.7278 (2001): 73.

Droy-Lefaix MT et al. Effect of *Gingko biloba* extract (EGb 761) on chloroquine induced retinal alterations. Lens Eye Toxic Res 9.3–4 (1992): 521–528.

Droy-Lefaix MT et al. Antioxidant effect of a *Ginkgo biloba* extract (EGb 761) on the retina. Int J Tissue React 17.3 (1995): 93–100.

Duche JC et al. Effect of *Ginkgo biloba* extract on microsomal enzyme induction. Int J Clin Pharmacol Res 9.3 (1989): 165–168.

Eckert, A. 2012. Mitochondrial effects of *Ginkgo biloba* extract. Int Psychogeriatr, 24 Suppl 1, S18–20.

Eckert A et al. Stabilization of mitochondrial membrane potential and improvement of neuronal energy metabolism by *Ginkgo biloba* extract EGb 761. Ann NY Acad Sci 1056 (2005): 474–485.

El Boghdady, N. A. 2013a. Antioxidant and antiapoptotic effects of proanthocyanidin and ginkgo biloba extract against doxorubicin-induced cardiac injury in rats. Cell Biochem Funct 13: 344–351.

El-Boghdady, N. A. 2013b. Increased cardiac endothelin-1 and nitric oxide in adriamycin-induced acute cardiotoxicity: protective effect of *Ginkgo biloba* extract. Indian J Biochem Biophys, 50, 202–9.

Eli R, Fasciano JA. An adjunctive preventive treatment for cancer: ultraviolet light and ginkgo biloba, together with other antioxidants, are a safe and powerful, but largely ignored, treatment option for the prevention of cancer. Med Hypotheses 66.6 (2006): 1152–1156.

Elsabagh S et al. Differential cognitive effects of *Ginkgo biloba* after acute and chronic treatment in healthy young volunteers. Psychopharmacology (Berl) 179.2 (2005a): 437–46.

Elsabagh S, et al. Limited cognitive benefits in Stage +2 postmenopausal women after 6 weeks of treatment with *Ginkgo biloba*. J Psychopharmacol 19.2 (2005b): 173–81.

Engelsen J, et al. Effect of coenzyme Q10 and *Ginkgo biloba* on warfarin dosage in patients on long-term warfarin treatment: a randomized, double-blind, placebo-controlled cross-over trial. Ugeskr Laeger 165.18 (2003): 1868–1871.

Erdogan H et al. Effects of *Ginkgo biloba* on plasma oxidant injury induced by bleomycin in rats. Toxicol Ind Health 22.1 (2006): 47–52.

Esmekaya, M. A., et al. 2011. Mutagenic and morphologic impacts of 1.8GHz radiofrequency radiation on human peripheral blood lymphocytes (hPBLs) and possible protective role of pre-treatment with *Ginkgo biloba* (EGb 761). Sci Total Environ, 410–411, 59–64.

Esposito, M. & Carotenuto, M. 2011. Ginkgolide B complex efficacy for brief prophylaxis of migraine in school-aged children: an open-label study. Neurol Sci, 32, 79–81.

Evans, J. R. 2013. *Ginkgo biloba* extract for age-related macular degeneration. Cochrane Database Syst Rev, 1, CD001775.

Fan, L., et al. 2009. Effects of *Ginkgo biloba* extract ingestion on the pharmacokinetics of talinolol in healthy Chinese volunteers. Ann Pharmacother, 43, 944–9.

Faustino, T. T., et al. 2010. [Medicinal plants for the treatment of generalized anxiety disorder: a review of controlled clinical studies.] Rev Bras Psiquiatr, 32, 429–36.

Fehske, C. J., et al. 2009. *Ginkgo biloba* extract (EGb761) influences monoaminergic neurotransmission via inhibition of NE uptake, but not MAO activity after chronic treatment. Pharmacol Res, 60, 68–73.

Fowler JS et al. Evidence that gingko biloba extract does not inhibit MAO A and B in living human brain. Life Sci 66.9 (2000): L141–L146.

Fu, L. M. & Li, J. T. 2011. A systematic review of single Chinese herbs for Alzheimer's disease treatment. Evid Based Complement Alternat Med, 2011, 640284.

Galduroz JC, et al. Gender- and age-related variations in blood viscosity in normal volunteers: a study of the effects of extract of *Allium sativum* and *Ginkgo biloba*. Phytomedicine 14.7–8 (2007): 447–451.

Gardner CD et al. Effect of *Ginkgo biloba* (EGb 761) and aspirin on platelet aggregation and platelet function analysis among older adults at risk of cardiovascular disease: a randomized clinical trial. Blood Coagul Fibrinolysis 18.8 (2007): 787–793.

Gardner CD et al. Effect of *Ginkgo biloba* (EGb 761) on treadmill walking time among adults with peripheral artery disease: a randomized clinical trial. J Cardiopulm Rehabil Prev 28.4 (2008): 258–65.

Gertsch JH et al. Randomised, double blind, placebo controlled comparison of ginkgo biloba and acetazolamide for prevention of acute mountain sickness among Himalayan trekkers: the prevention of high altitude illness trial (PHAIT). BMJ 328.7443 (2004): 797.

Granger AS. *Ginkgo biloba* precipitating epileptic seizures. Age Ageing 30.6 (2001): 523–525.
Grass-Kapanke, B., et al. 2011. Effects of Ginkgo Biloba Special Extract EGb 761® in Very Mild Cognitive Impairment (vMCI). Neuroscience and Medicine, 2, 48–56.
Gulec M et al. The effects of ginkgo biloba extract on tissue adenosine deaminase, xanthine oxidase, myeloperoxidase, malondialdehyde, and nitric oxide in cisplatin-induced nephrotoxicity. Toxicol Ind Health 22.3 (2006): 125–130.
Gurley BJ et al. Cytochrome P450 phenotypic ratios for predicting herb-drug interactions in humans. Clin Pharmacol Ther 72.3 (2002): 276–287.
Gurley BJ et al. Clinical assessment of effects of botanical supplementation on cytochrome P450 phenotypes in the elderly: St John's wort, garlic oil, *Panax ginseng* and *Ginkgo biloba*. Drugs Aging 22.6 (2005): 525–539.
Gurley, B., et al. 2012. Pharmacokinetic Herb-Drug Interactions (Part 2): Drug Interactions Involving Popular Botanical Dietary Supplements and Their Clinical Relevance. Planta Med 2012, 78, 1490–1514.
Hamann, K.F. 2007. [Special ginkgo extract in cases of vertigo: a systematic review of randomised, double-blind, placebo controlled clinical examinations.] HNO, 55, (4) 258–263.
Hao, Y. R., et al. 2009. [*Ginkgo biloba* extracts (EGb761) inhibits aflatoxin B1-induced hepatocarcinogenesis in Wistar rats.] Zhong Yao Cai, 32, 92–6.
Hartley, D. E., et al. 2004. Gincosan (a combination of *Ginkgo biloba* and *Panax ginseng*): the effects on mood and cognition of 6 and 12 weeks' treatment in post-menopausal women. Nutr Neurosci, 7, 325–33.
Haruyama, T. & Nagata, K. 2013. Anti-influenza virus activity of *Ginkgo biloba* leaf extracts. J Nat Med, 67, 636–42.
Hasanzadeh, E., et al. 2012. A double-blind placebo controlled trial of *Ginkgo biloba* added to risperidone in patients with autistic disorders. Child Psychiatry Hum Dev, 43, 674–82.
He, D., et al. 2011. Pharmacologic treatment for memory disorder in multiple sclerosis. Cochrane Database of Systematic Reviews [Online]. Available: http://onlinelibrary.wiley.com/doi/10.1002/14651858.CD008876.pub2/abstract.
Hellum BH, Nilsen OG. In vitro inhibition of CYP3A4 metabolism and P-glycoprotein-mediated transport by trade herbal products. Basic Clin Pharmacol Toxicol 102.5 (2008): 466–475.
Hellum BH, et al. The induction of CYP1A2, CYP2D6 and CYP3A4 by six trade herbal products in cultured primary human hepatocytes. Basic Clin Pharmacol Toxicol 100.1 (2007): 23–30.
Herrschaft, H., et al. 2012. *Ginkgo biloba* extract EGb 761(R) in dementia with neuropsychiatric features: a randomised, placebo-controlled trial to confirm the efficacy and safety of a daily dose of 240 mg. J Psychiatr Res, 46, 716–23.
Hibatallah J, et al. In-vivo and in-vitro assessment of the free-radical-scavenger activity of Ginkgo flavone glycosides at high concentration. J Pharm Pharmacol 51.12 (1999): 1435–1440.
Hilton, M. P., et al. 2013. *Ginkgo biloba* for tinnitus. Cochrane Database Syst Rev, 3, CD003852.
Horsch S, Walther C. *Ginkgo biloba* special extract EGb 761 in the treatment of peripheral arterial occlusive disease (PAOD): a review based on randomized, controlled studies. Int J Clin Pharmacol Ther 42.2 (2004): 63–72.
Hsu, C. L., et al. 2009. *Ginkgo biloba* extract confers protection from cigarette smoke extract-induced apoptosis in human lung endothelial cells: Role of heme oxygenase-1. Pulm Pharmacol Ther, 22, 286–96.
Huang SH et al. Bilobalide, a sesquiterpene trilactone from *Ginkgo biloba*, is an antagonist at recombinant alpha1beta2gamma2L GABA(A) receptors. Eur J Pharmacol 464.1 (2003): 1–8.
Huang X, et al. *Ginkgo biloba* extract (EGb 761) protects against cisplatin-induced ototoxicity in rats. Otol Neurotol 28.6 (2007): 828–833.
Huang, C. H., et al. 2013. *Ginkgo biloba* leaves extract (EGb 761) attenuates lipopolysaccharide-induced acute lung injury via inhibition of oxidative stress and NF-kappaB-dependent matrix metalloproteinase-9 pathway. Phytomedicine 20: 303–309.
Ihl, R. 2013. Effects of *Ginkgo biloba* extract EGb 761 (R) in dementia with neuropsychiatric features: review of recently completed randomised, controlled trials. Int.J Psychiatry Clin Pract., 17 Suppl 1, 8–14.
Ilhan A et al. *Ginkgo biloba* prevents mobile phone-induced oxidative stress in rat brain. Clin Chim Acta 340.1–2 (2004): 153–162.
Ilieva I et al. The effects of *Ginkgo biloba* extract on lipopolysaccharide-induced inflammation in vitro and in vivo. Exp Eye Res 79.2 (2004): 181–187.
Itil TM et al. The pharmacological effects of ginkgo biloba, a plant extract, on the brain of dementia patients in comparison with tacrine. Psychopharmacol Bull 34.3 (1998): 391–397.
Jang, C. H., et al. 2011. Effect of *Ginkgo biloba* extract on endotoxin-induced labyrinthitis. International Journal of Pediatric Otorhinolaryngology, 75, 905–909.
Janssen, I. M., et al. 2010. *Ginkgo biloba* in Alzheimer's disease: a systematic review. Wien Med Wochenschr, 160, 539–46.
Janssens D et al. Protection by bilobalide of the ischaemia-induced alterations of the mitochondrial respiratory activity. Fundam Clin Pharmacol 14.3 (2000): 193–201.
Jastreboff PJ et al. Attenuation of salicylate-induced tinnitus by *Ginkgo biloba* extract in rats. Audiol Neurootol 2.4 (1997): 197–212.
Jiang X et al. Effect of ginkgo and ginger on the pharmacokinetics and pharmacodynamics of warfarin in healthy subjects. Br J Clin Pharmacol 59.4 (2005): 425–432.
Jiang, X. Y., et al. 2009. Interventional effect of *Ginkgo biloba* extract on the progression of gastric precancerous lesions in rats. J Dig Dis, 10, 293–9.
Jiang, W., et al. 2011. Ginkgo may prevent genetic-associated ovarian cancer risk: multiple biomarkers and anticancer pathways induced by ginkgolide B in BRCA1-mutant ovarian epithelial cells. Eur J Cancer Prev, 20, 508–17.

Jiang, W., et al. 2014. Ginkgo may sensitize ovarian cancer cells to cisplatin: antiproliferative and apoptosis-inducing effects of ginkgolide B on ovarian cancer cells. Integr Cancer Ther 13: NP10–NP17.

Johnson SK et al. a pilot randomized controlled trial. The effect of *Ginkgo biloba* on functional measures in multiple sclerosis. NY: Explore 2.1 (2006): 19–24.

Jung F et al. Effect of *Ginkgo biloba* on fluidity of blood and peripheral microcirculation in volunteers. Arzneimittelforschung 40.5 (1990): 589–593.

Jung, I. H., et al. 2012. *Ginkgo biloba* extract (GbE) enhances the anti-atherogenic effect of cilostazol by inhibiting ROS generation. Exp Mol Med, 44, 311–8.

Kampman, K., et al. 2003. A pilot trial of piracetam and ginkgo biloba for the treatment of cocaine dependence. Addict Behav, 28, 437–48.

Kang, J. W., et al. 2010. Kaempferol and quercetin, components of *Ginkgo biloba* extract (EGb 761), induce caspase-3-dependent apoptosis in oral cavity cancer cells. Phytother Res, 24 Suppl 1, S77–82.

Kanter, M. 2011. Protective effects of *Ginkgo biloba* (EGb 761) on testicular torsion/detorsion-induced ischemia-reperfusion injury in rats. Exp Mol Pathol, 91, 708–13.

Kaschel, R. 2009. *Ginkgo biloba*: specificity of neuropsychological improvement — a selective review in search of differential effects. Hum Psychopharmacol, 24, 345–70.

Kaschel, R. 2011. Specific memory effects of *Ginkgo biloba* extract EGb 761 in middle-aged healthy volunteers. Phytomedicine, 18, 1202–7.

Kasper, S. & Schubert, H. 2009. [*Ginkgo biloba* extract EGb 761 in the treatment of dementia: evidence of efficacy and tolerability.] Fortschr Neurol Psychiatr, 77, 494–506.

Kaur, S., et al. 2013. *Ginkgo biloba* extract attenuates hippocampal neuronal loss and cognitive dysfunction resulting from trimethyltin in mice. Phytomedicine, 20, (2) 178–186.

Ke, T., et al. 2013. Effect of acetazolamide and gingko biloba on the human pulmonary vascular response to an acute altitude ascent. High Alt.Med Biol., 14, (2) 162–167.

Kehr, J., et al. 2012. *Ginkgo biloba* leaf extract (EGb 761(R)) and its specific acylated flavonol constituents increase dopamine and acetylcholine levels in the rat medial prefrontal cortex: possible implications for the cognitive enhancing properties of EGb 761(R). Int Psychogeriatr, 24 Suppl 1, S25–34.

Kellermann, A. J. & Kloft, C. 2011. Is there a risk of bleeding associated with standardized *Ginkgo biloba* extract therapy? A systematic review and meta-analysis. Pharmacotherapy, 31, 490–502.

Kennedy DO et al. Acute cognitive effects of standardised *Ginkgo biloba* extract complexed with phosphatidylserine. Hum Psychopharmacol 22.4 (2007a): 199–210.

Kennedy DO et al. Modulation of cognitive performance following single doses of 120 mg *Ginkgo biloba* extract administered to healthy young volunteers. Hum Psychopharmacol 22.8 (2007b): 559–66.

Kim SJ. Effect of biflavones of *Ginkgo biloba* against UVB-induced cytotoxicity in vitro. J Dermatol 28.4 (2001): 193–199.

Kim HK et al. Inhibition of rat adjuvant-induced arthritis by ginkgetin, a biflavone from ginkgo biloba leaves. Planta Med 65.5 (1999): 465–467.

Kim MS et al. Neuroprotective effect of *Ginkgo biloba* L. extract in a rat model of Parkinson's disease. Phytother Res 18.8 (2004): 663–666.

Kim, B. H., et al. 2010. Influence of *Ginkgo biloba* extract on the pharmacodynamic effects and pharmacokinetic properties of ticlopidine: an open-label, randomized, two-period, two-treatment, two-sequence, single-dose crossover study in healthy Korean male volunteers. Clin Ther, 32, 380–90.

Kleijnen J, Knipschild P. *Ginkgo biloba* for cerebral insufficiency. Br J Clin Pharmacol 34.4 (1992): 352–358.

Kohler S, et al. Influence of a 7-day treatment with *Ginkgo biloba* special extract EGb 761 on bleeding time and coagulation: a randomized, placebo-controlled, double-blind study in healthy volunteers. Blood Coagul Fibrinolysis 15.4 (2004): 303–309.

Koltermann A et al. *Ginkgo biloba* extract EGb 761 increases endothelial nitric oxide production in vitro and in vivo. Cell Mol Life Sci 64.13 (2007): 1715–1722.

Kotakadi VS et al. *Ginkgo biloba* extract EGb 761 has anti-inflammatory properties and ameliorates colitis in mice by driving effector T cell apoptosis. Carcinogenesis 29.9 (2008): 1799–1806.

Kuller, L. H., et al. 2010. Does *Ginkgo biloba* reduce the risk of cardiovascular events? Circ Cardiovasc Qual Outcomes, 3, 41–7.

Kupiec T, Raj V. Fatal seizures due to potential herb-drug interactions with *Ginkgo biloba*. J Anal Toxicol 29.7 (2005): 755–758.

Laws, K. R., et al. 2012. Is *Ginkgo biloba* a cognitive enhancer in healthy individuals? A meta-analysis. Hum Psychopharmacol, 27, 527–33.

Leadbetter GW, Hackett P. Comparison of *Ginkgo biloba*, acetazolamide, and placebo for prevention of acute mountain sickness. High Alt Med Biol 3 (2003): 455.

Leadbetter, G., et al. 2009. *Ginkgo biloba* does — and does not — prevent acute mountain sickness. Wilderness Environ Med, 20, 66–71.

Lee, J., et al. 2013. Effect of *Ginkgo biloba* Extract on Visual Field Progression in Normal Tension Glaucoma. J Glaucoma 22: 780–784.

Li MH, et al. Effects of ginkgo leaf concentrated oral liquor in treating asthma. Zhongguo Zhong Xi Yi Jie He Za Zhi 17.4 (1997): 216–2118.

Li, G. H., et al. 2008. [Studies on the effect of *Ginkgo biloba* extracts on NF-kappaB pathway.] Zhong Yao Cai, 31, 1357–60.

Li, X. S., et al. 2009. Effect of Ginkgo leaf extract on vascular endothelial function in patients with early stage diabetic nephropathy. Chin J Integr Med, 15, 26–9.

Lim H et al. Effects of anti-inflammatory biflavonoid, ginkgetin, on chronic skin inflammation. Biol Pharm Bull 29.5 (2006): 1046–1049.

Lim, S., et al. 2011. EGb761, a *Ginkgo biloba* extract, is effective against atherosclerosis in vitro, and in a rat model of type 2 diabetes. PLoS One, 6, e20301.

Lin SY, Chang HP. Induction of superoxide dismutase and catalase activity in different rat tissues and protection from UVB irradiation after topical application of *Ginkgo biloba* extracts. Methods Find Exp Clin Pharmacol 19.6 (1997): 367–371.

Lingaerde O, et al. Can winter depression be prevented by *Ginkgo biloba* extract? A placebo-controlled trial. Acta Psychiatr Scand 100.1 (1999): 62–66.

Liu KX et al. *Ginkgo biloba* extract (EGb 761) attenuates lung injury induced by intestinal ischemia/reperfusion in rats: roles of oxidative stress and nitric oxide. World J Gastroenterol 13.2 (2007): 299–305.

Liu, H. J., et al. 2009. Inhibitions of vascular endothelial growth factor expression and foam cell formation by EGb 761, a special extract of *Ginkgo biloba*, in oxidatively modified low-density lipoprotein-induced human THP-1 monocytes cells. Phytomedicine, 16, 138–45.

Lovera J et al. *Ginkgo biloba* for the improvement of cognitive performance in multiple sclerosis: a randomized, placebo-controlled trial. Mult Scler 13.3 (2007): 376–385.

Lovera, J. F., et al. 2012. *Ginkgo biloba* does not improve cognitive function in MS: a randomized placebo-controlled trial. Neurology, 79, 1278–84.

Lu, J. M., et al. 2012. Ginkgolic acid inhibits HIV protease activity and HIV infection in vitro. Med Sci Monit, 18, BR293–298.

Lucinda, L. M. F., et al. 2010. Evidences of osteoporosis improvement in Wistar rats treated with *Ginkgo biloba* extract: A histomorphometric study of mandible and femur. Fitoterapia, 81, 982–987.

Luo Y. Alzheimer's disease, the nematode Caenorhabditis elegans, and *Ginkgo biloba* leaf extract. Life Sci 78.18 (2006): 2066–2072.

Ma, S., et al. 2012. Neuroprotective effect of ginkgolide K against acute ischemic stroke on middle cerebral ischemia occlusion in rats. J Nat Med, 66, 25–31.

Maakestad K et al. *Ginkgo biloba* reduces incidence and severity of acute mountain sickness. Wilderness Environ Med 12 (2001): 51.

Mahdy, H. M., et al. 2011. The effect of *Ginkgo biloba* extract on 3-nitropropionic acid-induced neurotoxicity in rats. Neurochem Int, 59, 770–778.

Malenfant, D., et al. 2009. The efficacy of complementary and alternative medicine in the treatment of Raynaud's phenomenon: a literature review and meta-analysis. Rheumatology (Oxford), 48, 791–5.

Markowitz JS et al. Multiple-dose administration of *Ginkgo biloba* did not affect cytochrome P-450 2D6 or 3A4 activity in normal volunteers. J Clin Psychopharmacol 23.6 (2003): 576–581.

McCarney R et al. *Ginkgo biloba* for mild to moderate dementia in a community setting: a pragmatic, randomised, parallel-group, double-blind, placebo-controlled trial. Int J Geriatr Psychiatry 23.12 (2008): 1222–1230.

Meston CM, et al. Short- and long-term effects of *Ginkgo biloba* extract on sexual dysfunction in women. Arch Sex Behav 37.4 (2008): 530–547.

Moraga F et al. *Ginkgo biloba* decreases acute mountain sickness at 3700 m. High Alt Med Biol 3 (2003): 453.

Moraga FA et al. *Ginkgo biloba* decreases acute mountain sickness in people ascending to high altitude at Ollague (3696 m) in northern Chile. Wilderness Environ Med 18.4 (2007): 251–257.

Mouren X, et al. Study of the antiischemic action of EGb 761 in the treatment of peripheral arterial occlusive disease by TcPo2 determination. Angiology 45.6 (1994): 413–4117.

Moyad MA. Dietary supplements and other alternative medicines for erectile dysfunction. What do I tell my patients? Urol Clin North Am 29.1 (2002): 11–22: vii.

Muir AH et al. The use of *Ginkgo biloba* in Raynaud's disease: a double-blind placebo-controlled trial. Vasc Med 7.4 (2002): 265–267.

Muller WE. Nootropics, the therapy of dementia between aspiration and reality. Drug News Perspect 2 (1989): 295–300.

Nada, S. E. & Shah, Z. A. 2012. Preconditioning with *Ginkgo biloba* (EGb 761(R)) provides neuroprotection through HO1 and CRMP2. Neurobiol Dis, 46, 180–9.

Naidu MU et al. Protective effect of *Gingko biloba* extract against doxorubicin-induced cardiotoxicity in mice. Indian J Exp Biol 40.8 (2002): 894–900.

Napryeyenko O, Borzenko I. *Ginkgo biloba* special extract in dementia with neuropsychiatric features. A randomised, placebo-controlled, double-blind clinical trial. Arzneimittelforschung 57.1 (2007): 4–11.

Napryeyenko, O., et al. 2009. Efficacy and tolerability of *Ginkgo biloba* extract EGb 761 by type of dementia: analyses of a randomised controlled trial. J Neurol Sci, 283, 224–9.

Nathan P. Can the cognitive enhancing effects of ginkgo biloba be explained by its pharmacology? Med Hypotheses 55.6 (2000): 491–493.

Nicolai, S. P., Kruidenier, L. M., Bendermacher, B. L., et al. 2013. *Ginkgo biloba* for intermittent claudication. Cochrane Database Syst Rev, 6, CD006888.

Nishida S, Satoh H. Mechanisms for the vasodilations induced by *Ginkgo biloba* extract and its main constituent, bilobalide, in rat aorta. Life Sci 72.23 (2003): 2659–2667.

Oskouei, D.S., et al. 2013. The Effect of *Ginkgo biloba* on Functional Outcome of Patients with Acute Ischemic Stroke: A Double-blind, Placebo-controlled, Randomized Clinical Trial. Journal of Stroke and Cerebrovascular Diseases, 22, (8) e557–e563.

Ozgoli, G., et al. 2009. A randomized, placebo-controlled trial of *Ginkgo biloba* L. in treatment of premenstrual syndrome. J Altern Complement Med, 15, 845–51.

Ozturk G et al. The effect of Ginkgo extract EGb761 in cisplatin-induced peripheral neuropathy in mice. Toxicol Appl Pharmacol 196.1 (2004): 169–175.

Panda, V. S. & N, S. R. 2009. Evaluation of cardioprotective activity of *Ginkgo biloba* and *Ocimum sanctum* in rodents. Altern Med Rev, 14, 161–71.

Park, J. W., et al. 2011. Short-term effects of *Ginkgo biloba* extract on peripapillary retinal blood flow in normal tension glaucoma. Korean J Ophthalmol, 25, 323–8.

Park, Y. J., et al. 2013. Chemopreventive effects of *Ginkgo biloba* extract in estrogen-negative human breast cancer cells. Arch Pharm Res 36: 102–108.

Parsad D, et al. Effectiveness of oral *Ginkgo biloba* in treating limited, slowly spreading vitiligo. Clin Exp Dermatol 28.3 (2003): 285–287.

Peng H, et al. Effects of *Ginkgo biloba* extract on acute cerebral ischemia in rats analyzed by magnetic resonance spectroscopy. Acta Pharmacol Sin 24.5 (2003): 467–471.

Pierre, S. V., et al. 2008. The standardized *Ginkgo biloba* extract Egb-761 protects vascular endothelium exposed to oxidized low density lipoproteins. Cell Mol Biol (Noisy-le-grand), 54 Suppl, OL1032–42.

Pittler MH, Ernst E. *Ginkgo biloba* extract for the treatment of intermittent claudication: a meta-analysis of randomized trials. Am J Med 108.4 (2000): 276–281.

Pizzorno J, Murray M. Textbook of natural medicine. St Louis: Elsevier, 2006.

Puebla-Perez AM, et al. Effect of *Ginkgo biloba* extract, EGb 761, on the cellular immune response in a hypothalamic-pituitary-adrenal axis activation model in the rat. Int Immunopharmacol 3.1 (2003): 75–80.

Quaranta L et al. Effect of *Ginkgo biloba* extract on preexisting visual field damage in normal tension glaucoma. Ophthalmology 110.2 (2003): 359–362.

Ramassamy C et al. The *Ginkgo biloba* extract, EGb761, increases synaptosomal uptake of 5-hydroxytryptamine: in-vitro and ex-vivo studies. J Pharm Pharmacol 44.11 (1992): 943–945.

Reisser CH, Weidauer H. *Ginkgo biloba* extract EGb 761 or pentoxifylline for the treatment of sudden deafness: a randomized, reference-controlled, double-blind study. Acta Otolaryngol 121.5 (2001): 579–584.

Rejali D, et al. *Ginkgo biloba* does not benefit patients with tinnitus: a randomized placebo-controlled double-blind trial and meta-analysis of randomized trials. Clin Otolaryngol Allied Sci 29.3 (2004): 226–231.

Ribonnet, L., et al. 2011. Modulation of CYP1A1 activity by a *Ginkgo biloba* extract in the human intestinal Caco-2 cells. Toxicol Lett, 202, 193–202.

Rojas, P., et al. 2012. *Ginkgo biloba* extract (EGb 761) modulates the expression of dopamine-related genes in 1-methyl-4-phenyl-1,2,3,6-tetrahydropyridine-induced Parkinsonism in mice. Neuroscience, 223, 246–57.

Roland, P. D. & Nergard, C. S. 2012. [*Ginkgo biloba* — effect, adverse events and drug interaction.] Tidsskr Nor Laegeforen, 132, 956–9.

Roncin JP, et al. EGb 761 in control of acute mountain sickness and vascular reactivity to cold exposure. Aviat Space Environ Med 67.5 (1996): 445–452.

Russo, V., et al. 2009. Clinical efficacy of a *Ginkgo biloba* extract in the topical treatment of allergic conjunctivitis. Eur J Ophthalmol, 19, 331–6.

Ryu, K. H., et al. 2009. *Ginkgo biloba* extract enhances antiplatelet and antithrombotic effects of cilostazol without prolongation of bleeding time. Thromb Res, 124, 328–34.

Salehi, B., et al. 2010. *Ginkgo biloba* for attention-deficit/hyperactivity disorder in children and adolescents: a double blind, randomized controlled trial. Prog Neuropsychopharmacol Biol Psychiatry, 34, 76–80.

Sarris, J., et al. 2011. Complementary medicines (herbal and nutritional products) in the treatment of Attention Deficit Hyperactivity Disorder (ADHD): a systematic review of the evidence. Complement Ther Med, 19, 216–27.

Schneider R et al. Cardiac ischemia and reperfusion in spontaneously diabetic rats with and without application of EGb 761: I. Cardiomyocytes. Histol Histopathol 23.7 (2008): 807–817.

Schneider, R., et al. 2010. Cardiovascular autonomic neuropathy in spontaneously diabetic rats with and without application of EGb 761. Histol Histopathol, 25, 1581–90.

Scripnikov A, et al. Effects of *Ginkgo biloba* extract EGb 761 on neuropsychiatric symptoms of dementia: findings from a randomised controlled trial. Wien Med Wochenschr 157.13–14 (2007): 295–300.

Seupaul, R. A., et al. 2012. Pharmacologic prophylaxis for acute mountain sickness: a systematic shortcut review. Ann Emerg Med, 59, 307–317 e1.

Shevtsova EF, et al. [Mitochondria as the target for neuroprotectors.] Vestn Ross Akad Med Nauk 9 (2005): 13–117.

Shih JC et al. *Ginkgo biloba* abolishes aggression in mice lacking MAO A. Antioxid Redox Signal 2.3 (2000): 467–471.

Shim, S. H., et al. 2012. *Ginkgo biloba* extract and bilberry anthocyanins improve visual function in patients with normal tension glaucoma. J Med Food, 15, 818–23.

Singh B et al. Biology and chemistry of *Ginkgo biloba*. Fitoterapia 79.6 (2008): 401–418.

Singh, V., et al. 2010. Review and meta-analysis of usage of ginkgo as an adjunct therapy in chronic schizophrenia. Int J Neuropsychopharmacol, 13, 257–71.

Sloley BD et al. Identification of kaempferol as a monoamine oxidase inhibitor and potential Neuroprotectant in extracts of *Ginkgo biloba* leaves. J Pharm Pharmacol 52.4 (2000): 451–459.

Smith PF, et al. The neuroprotective properties of the *Ginkgo biloba* leaf: a review of the possible relationship to platelet-activating factor (PAF). J Ethnopharmacol 50.3 (1996): 131–139.

Smith JV et al. Anti-apoptotic properties of *Ginkgo biloba* extract EGb 761 in differentiated PC12 cells. Cell Mol Biol (Noisy-le-Grand) 48.6 (2002): 699–707.

Szczurko, O., et al. 2011. *Ginkgo biloba* for the treatment of vitilgo vulgaris: an open label pilot clinical trial. BMC Complement Altern Med, 11, 21.

Taavoni, S., et al. 2012. 160 Effect of *Ginkgo biloba* on menopausal women's sexual function: a randomized placebo controlled trial, Tehran, 2011. Maturitas, 71, Supplement 1, S65.

Taki, Y., et al. 2009. Time-dependent induction of hepatic cytochrome P450 enzyme activity and mRNA expression by bilobalide in rats. J Pharmacol Sci, 109, 459–62.

Tamborini A, Taurelle R. Value of standardized *Ginkgo biloba* extract (EGb 761) in the management of congestive symptoms of premenstrual syndrome. Rev Fr Gynecol Obstet 88.7–9 (1993): 447–457.

Tang J et al. Herb-drug interactions: effect of *Ginkgo biloba* extract on the pharmacokinetics of theophylline in rats. Food Chem Toxicol 45.12 (2007a): 2441–5.

Tang Y et al. The effect of *Ginkgo biloba* extract on the expression of PKCalpha in the inflammatory cells and the level of IL-5 in induced sputum of asthmatic patients. J Huazhong Univ Sci Technolog Med Sci 27.4 (2007b): 375–80.

Thanoon, I. A., et al. 2012. Oxidative Stress and C-Reactive Protein in Patients with Cerebrovascular Accident (Ischaemic Stroke): The role of *Ginkgo biloba* extract. Sultan Qaboos Univ Med J, 12, 197–205.

Tian YM et al. Effects of *Ginkgo biloba* extract (EGb 761) on hydroxyl radical-induced thymocyte apoptosis and on age-related thymic atrophy and peripheral immune dysfunctions in mice. Mech Ageing Dev 124.8–9 (2003): 977–983.

Tulsulkar, J. & Shah, Z. A. 2012. *Ginkgo biloba* prevents transient global ischemia-induced delayed hippocampal neuronal death through antioxidant and anti-inflammatory mechanism. Neurochem Int, 62, 189–197.

Usai, S., et al. 2011. Gingkolide B as migraine preventive treatment in young age: results at 1-year follow-up. Neurol Sci, 32 Suppl 1, S197–9.

Vale S. Subarachnoid haemorrhage associated with *Ginkgo biloba*. Lancet 352.9121 (1998): 36.

van Beek TA. Chemical analysis of *Ginkgo biloba* leaves and extracts. J Chromatogr A 967.1 (2002): 21–55.

Van Patot, M. C., et al. 2009. *Ginkgo biloba* for prevention of acute mountain sickness: does it work? High Alt Med Biol, 10, 33–43.

Vellas, B., et al. 2012. Long-term use of standardised *Ginkgo biloba* extract for the prevention of Alzheimer's disease (GuidAge): a randomised placebo-controlled trial. Lancet Neurol, 11, 851–9.

Villasenor-Garcia MM et al. Effect of *Ginkgo biloba* extract EGb 761 on the nonspecific and humoral immune responses in a hypothalamic-pituitary-adrenal axis activation model. Int Immunopharmacol 4.9 (2004): 1217–1222.

Von Boetticher, A. 2011. *Ginkgo biloba* extract in the treatment of tinnitus: a systematic review. Neuropsychiatr Dis Treat, 7, 441–7.

Wang J et al. Supervised exercise training combined with ginkgo biloba treatment for patients with peripheral arterial disease. Clin Rehabil 21.7 (2007): 579–586.

Wang, B. S., et al. 2010. Effectiveness of standardized ginkgo biloba extract on cognitive symptoms of dementia with a six-month treatment: a bivariate random effect meta-analysis. Pharmacopsychiatry, 43, 86–91.

Wang, W. W., et al. 2011. [The effect of extract of ginkgo biloba leaf during the formation of HBV-related hepatocellular carcinoma.] Zhonghua Shi Yan He Lin Chuang Bing Du Xue Za Zhi, 25, 325–7.

Wang, Z. Y., et al. 2012. [Ginkgolide B promotes axonal growth of retina ganglion cells by anti-apoptosis in vitro.] Sheng Li Xue Bao, 64, 417–24.

Watanabe CM et al. The in vivo neuromodulatory effects of the herbal medicine ginkgo biloba. Proc Natl Acad Sci U S A 98.12 (2001): 6577–6580.

Wei, J. M., et al. 2013. Ginkgo suppresses atherosclerosis through downregulating the expression of connexin 43 in rabbits. Arch Med Sci, 9, 340–6.

Weinmann, S., et al. 2010. Effects of *Ginkgo biloba* in dementia: systematic review and meta-analysis. BMC Geriatr, 10, 14.

Wettstein A. Cholinesterase inhibitors and Gingko extracts: are they comparable in the treatment of dementia? Comparison of published placebo-controlled efficacy studies of at least six months' duration. Phytomedicine 6.6 (2000): 393–401.

Wheatley D. Triple-blind, placebo-controlled trial of *Ginkgo biloba* in sexual dysfunction due to antidepressant drugs. Hum Psychopharmacol 19.8 (2004): 545–548.

Woelk H et al. *Ginkgo biloba* special extract EGb 761((R)) in generalized anxiety disorder and adjustment disorder with anxious mood: a randomized, double-blind, placebo-controlled trial. J Psychiatr Res (2007) 41: 472–480.

Wolf HR. Does *Ginkgo biloba* special extract EGb 761 provide additional effects on coagulation and bleeding when added to acetylsalicylic acid 500 mg daily? Drugs R D 7.3 (2006): 163–172.

Wu WR, Zhu XZ. Involvement of monoamine oxidase inhibition in neuroprotective and neurorestorative effects of *Ginkgo biloba* extract against MPTP-induced nigrostriatal dopaminergic toxicity in C57 mice. Life Sci 65.2 (1999): 157–164.

Wu, Y. Z., et al. 2008a. *Ginkgo biloba* extract improves coronary artery circulation in patients with coronary artery disease: contribution of plasma nitric oxide and endothelin-1. Phytother Res, 22, 734–9.

Wu, Z. M., et al. 2008b. *Ginkgo biloba* extract prevents against apoptosis induced by high glucose in human lens epithelial cells. Acta Pharmacol Sin, 29, 1042–50.

Wu YZ et al. *Ginkgo biloba* extract improves coronary artery circulation in patients with coronary artery disease: contribution of plasma nitric oxide and endothelin-1. Phytother Res 22.6 (2008c): 734–739.

Xie, Z. Q., et al. 2009. Molecular mechanisms underlying the cholesterol-lowering effect of *Ginkgo biloba* extract in hepatocytes: a comparative study with lovastatin. Acta Pharmacol Sin, 30, 1262–75.

Yancheva, S., et al. 2009. *Ginkgo biloba* extract EGb 761(R), donepezil or both combined in the treatment of Alzheimer's disease with neuropsychiatric features: a randomised, double-blind, exploratory trial. Aging Ment Health, 13, 183–90.

Yeh, K. Y., et al. 2008. *Ginkgo biloba* extract enhances male copulatory behavior and reduces serum prolactin levels in rats. Horm Behav, 53, 225–31.

Yeh, Y. C., et al. 2009. A standardized extract of *Ginkgo biloba* suppresses doxorubicin-induced oxidative stress and p53-mediated mitochondrial apoptosis in rat testes. Br J Pharmacol, 156, 48–61.

Yeung EY et al. Identification of *Ginkgo biloba* as a novel activator of pregnane X receptor. Drug Metab Dispos 36.11 (2008): 2270–2276.

Yoshitake, T., et al. 2010. The *Ginkgo biloba* extract EGb 761(R) and its main constituent flavonoids and ginkgolides increase extracellular dopamine levels in the rat prefrontal cortex. Br J Pharmacol, 159, 659–68.

Zadoyan, G., et al. 2012. Effect of *Ginkgo biloba* special extract EGb 761(R) on human cytochrome P450 activity: a cocktail interaction study in healthy volunteers. Eur J Clin Pharmacol, 68, 553–60.

Zeng X et al. *Ginkgo biloba* for acute ischaemic stroke. Cochrane Database Syst Rev 4 (2005): CD003691.

Zhang, S. J. & Xue, Z. Y. 2012. Effect of Western medicine therapy assisted by *Ginkgo biloba* tablet on vascular cognitive impairment of none dementia. Asian Pac J Trop Med, 5, 661–4.

Zhang, Y., et al. 2008. *Ginkgo biloba* Extract Kaempferol Inhibits Cell Proliferation and Induces Apoptosis in Pancreatic Cancer Cells. Journal of Surgical Research, 148, 17–23.

Zhang, W. F., et al. 2011. Extract of *Ginkgo biloba* treatment for tardive dyskinesia in schizophrenia: a randomized, double-blind, placebo-controlled trial. J Clin Psychiatry, 72, 615–21.
Zhang, X. Y., et al. 2012a. Brain-derived neurotrophic factor levels and its Val66Met gene polymorphism predict tardive dyskinesia treatment response to *Ginkgo biloba*. Biol Psychiatry, 72, 700–6.
Zhang, Z., et al. 2012b. Experimental evidence of *Ginkgo biloba* extract EGB as a neuroprotective agent in ischemia stroke rats. Brain Research Bulletin, 87, 193–198.
Zhao LZ et al. Induction of propranolol metabolism by *Ginkgo biloba* extract EGb 761 in rats. Curr Drug Metab 7.6 (2006): 577–587.
Zhao, M. X., et al. 2012. [Effects of *Ginkgo biloba* extract in improving episodic memory of patients with mild cognitive impairment: a randomized controlled trial.]. Zhong Xi Yi Jie He Xue Bao, 10, 628–34.
Zhou, Y. & Zeng, R. 2011. [Effects of *Ginkgo biloba* extract on anticoagulation and blood drug level of warfarin in healthy wolunteers]. Zhongguo Zhong Yao Za Zhi, 36, 2290–3.
Zhou, Z. Y., et al. 2010. Antioxidant and hepatoprotective effects of extract of ginkgo biloba in rats of non-alcoholic steatohepatitis. Saudi Med J, 31, 1114–8.
Zhou, L., et al. 2011. *Ginkgo biloba* extract enhances glucose tolerance in hyperinsulinism-induced hepatic cells. J Nat Med, 65, 50–6.
Zuo, X. C., et al. 2010. Effects of *Ginkgo biloba* extracts on diazepam metabolism: a pharmacokinetic study in healthy Chinese male subjects. Eur J Clin Pharmacol, 66, 503–9.

Glucosamine

OTHER NAMES

D-Glucosamine, amino monosaccharide, glucosamine sulfate, glucosamine hydrochloride, glucosamine hydroiodide, *N*-acetyl D-glucosamine, 2-amino-2-deoxy-beta-D-glucopyranose

BACKGROUND AND RELEVANT PHARMACOKINETICS

Glucosamine is a naturally occurring substance that is required for the production of proteoglycans, mucopolysaccharides and hyaluronic acid, which are substances that make up joint tissue, such as articular cartilage, tendons and synovial fluid. It is also a component of blood vessels, heart valves and mucus secretions (Kelly 1998).

Glucosamine sulfate is 90% absorbed after oral administration. The bioavailability is approximately 20% after first-pass metabolism (Aghazadeh-Habashi et al 2002). Unbound glucosamine is concentrated in the articular cartilage and the elimination half-life is 70 hours, with excretion as CO_2 in expired air, as well as by the kidneys and in faeces (Setnikar & Canali 1993). A study of the pharmacokinetics of glucosamine sulfate in humans found that it is rapidly absorbed after oral administration and its elimination half-life was tentatively estimated to average 15 hours, therefore supporting once-daily dosing (Persiani et al 2005). Twice-daily dosing with 500 mg of a time-release formula has also been shown to provide comparable serum levels after 24 hours as three divided doses of 500 mg (Basak et al 2004).

A further study suggests that glucosamine is bioavailable both systemically and at the joint, and that steady state concentrations in human plasma and synovial fluid were correlated and in line with levels deemed effective in in vitro studies (Persiani et al 2007). This is contrasted by the suggestion from a study of 18 people with osteoarthritis (OA) which found serum glucosamine levels were significantly less than those previously shown to have in vitro effects (Biggee et al 2006). Similar results were reported in an equine study that found levels attained in serum and synovial fluid were 500-fold lower than those reported to modify chondrocyte anabolic and catabolic activities in tissue and cell culture experiments (Laverty et al 2005).

It is interesting to note that co-adminstration of glucosamine and chondroitin has been observed to reduce plasma levels of glucosamine compared to administration of glucosamine alone (Jackson et al 2010). There is also some research being undertaken to improve the intestinal absorption of glucosamine, due to the large first pass effect. For example, one study found that glucosamine oral formulations containing chitosan (0.5% w/v) (QD-Glu solution and QD-Glu tablet) increased Cmax (2.8-fold) and AUC0-infinity (2.5-fold) of glucosamine (Qian et al 2013). Further pharmacokinetic studies in beagle dogs demonstrated that QD-Glu solution and QD-Glu tablets had higher relative bioavailabilities of 313% and 186%, compared to several other glucosamine products (Wellesse solution and Voltaflex tablet respectively).

CHEMICAL COMPONENTS

2-amino-2-deoxy-D-glucose

FOOD SOURCES

Glucosamine is present in chitin from the shells of prawns and other crustaceans. As a supplement, glucosamine is derived from marine exoskeletons or produced synthetically and is available in salt forms, including glucosamine sulfate, glucosamine hydrochloride, glucosamine hydroiodide and *N*-acetyl glucosamine. Glucosamine salts are likely to be completely ionised in the stomach, although clinical equivalence of the different salts has not been established. The purity and content of products has been questioned in the USA, where glucosamine is regarded as a food supplement and its quality was largely unregulated before GMP in 2010.

MAIN ACTIONS

Chondroprotective effect

Glucosamine is a primary substrate and stimulant of proteoglycan biosynthesis and inhibitor of proteoglycan degradation (Roman-Blas et al 2010). Glucosamine also stimulates synovial production of hyaluronic acid, a compound responsible for the lubricating and shock-absorbing properties of synovial fluid (McCarty 1998a, McCarty et al 2000) with the production of hyaluronic acid being higher in synovial cells than chondrocytes (Nagaoka et al 2012). Glucosamine also causes a statistically significant stimulation of proteoglycan production by chondrocytes from human osteoarthritic cartilage culture (Bassleer et al 1998) and modifies cultured OA chondrocyte metabolism by acting on protein kinase C, cellular phospholipase A_2, protein synthesis and possibly collagenase activation (Piperno et al 2000).

In animal models of OA, glucosamine has demonstrated limited site-specific, partial disease-modifying effects (Tiraloche et al 2005) which have been attributed to the inhibition of the cytokine intracellular signalling pathways and reversal of the proinflammatory and joint-degenerating effects of IL-1 (Roman-Blas et al 2010). In rabbits, *N*-acetyl glucosamine has been found to produce proliferation of matured cartilaginous tissues and matured cartilage substrate in experimentally produced cartilaginous injuries (Tamai et al 2003) and partially reverse structural effects of OA, restoring cartilage thickness to that of healthy joints and preventing superficial fibrillation (López et al 2013). In another animal model, co-administration with chondroitin was seen to prevent both biochemical and histological alterations and provide pain reduction (Silva et al 2009). Glucosamine is also reported to induce osteoblastic cell differentiation and suppress the osteoclastic cell differentiation, thereby increasing bone matrix deposition and decreasing bone resorption to modulate bone metabolism in OA (Nagaoka et al 2012).

An in vitro study using bovine chondrocytes suggested that the experimental effects of glucosamine were sensitive to the model, dose and length of treatment (de Mattei et al 2002). In another in vitro study, exogenous glucosamine was found not to stimulate chondroitin sulfate synthesis in human chondrocytes and the capacity to form glucosamine from glucose was estimated to be far in excess of the levels achievable through oral administration (Mroz & Silbert 2004). In human trials, glucosamine is suspected of reducing joint loading with decreased serum cartilage oligomeric matrix protein observed over a 12-week physical training period (Petersen et al 2010). Glucosamine, however, had no effect on type 2 collagen fragment levels in serum or urine in a 6-month RCT of 137 subjects with OA of the knee (Cibere et al 2005).

Part of the chondroprotective action of glucosamine sulfate is due to the provision of a source of additional inorganic sulfur, which is essential for glycosaminoglycan (GAG) synthesis as well as being a structural component of glutathione and other key enzymes, coenzymes and metabolites that play fundamental roles in cellular homeostasis and control of inflammation (Nimni & Cordoba 2006).

Anti-inflammatory

A number of in vitro and in vivo tests have identified anti-inflammatory activity for glucosamine (Nagaoka et al 2011). Anti-inflammatory and chondroprotective activities have been observed in human OA cartilage (Sumantran et al 2008). In vitro studies have found that glucosamine sulphate exerts anti-inflammatory effects by altering production of TNF-alpha, interleukins and prostaglandin E_2 in macrophage cells (Kim et al 2007), as well as suppression of mast cell activation (Sakai et al 2010).

Glucosamine restores proteoglycan synthesis and prevents the production of inflammatory mediators induced by the cytokine IL-1-beta in rat articular chondrocytes according to in vitro research (Gouze et al 2001). Glucosamine sulfate and *N*-acetyl glucosamine have also been found to inhibit IL-1-beta- and TNF-alpha-induced NO production in normal human articular chondrocytes (Shikhman et al 2001) and it is suggested that the anti-IL-1beta effect of glucosamine is accomplished by suppression of NF-κB activation. It is further suggested that glucosamine sulfate inhibits IL-1beta-stimulated gene expression of COX-2, inducible nitric oxide synthase, cytokines and metalloproteinases at concentrations found in human plasma and synovial fluid after administration of glucosamine sulfate standard oral doses (Roman-Blas 2010). It is further reported that glucosamine has epigenetic effects and can prevent cytokine-induced demethylation of a specific CpG site in the IL-1-beta promoter which is associated with decreased expression of IL-1-beta (Imagawa et al 2011).

Glucosamine demonstrates an ability to suppress PGE_2 production and partly suppress NO production in chondrocytes in vitro (Mello et al 2004, Nakamura et al 2004) and to suppress the production of matrix metalloproteases in normal chondrocytes and synoviocytes (Nakamura et al 2004). Glucosamine is further reported to exert an anti-inflammatory action through suppression of neutrophil function such as superoxide generation, phagocytosis, granule enzyme release and chemotaxis (Hua et al 2002).

Glucose metabolism

Exogenous glucosamine is actively taken up by cells. Its entry into cells is stimulated by insulin and involves the glucose transporter system (Pouwels et al 2001); however, the affinity of glucosamine for these transporters is substantially lower than that of glucose (Nelson et al 2000).

Early preliminary evidence suggested that glucosamine may cause changes in glucose metabolism and insulin secretion similar to those seen in type 2 diabetes in both rats (Balkan & Dunning 1994, Giaccari et al 1995, Lippiello et al 2000, Shankar et al 1998) and humans (Monauni et al 2000); however, these findings have been disputed (Echard et al 2001). In the 10 years following the original research, most clinical trial evidence has failed to find any significant effect on glucose metabolism in humans (Anderson et al 2005, Tannis et al 2004, Onigbinde et al 2011). It is suggested, however, that there could be some effect in people with impaired glucose tolerance or insulin resistance (Dostrovsky et al 2011).

Gastrointestinal protection

Glycoproteins are important in protecting the bowel mucosa from damage, and the breakdown of glycosaminoglycans is an important consequence of inflammation of mucosal surfaces (Salvatore et al 2000). Abnormalities in colonic glycoprotein synthesis have been implicated in the pathogenesis of ulcerative colitis and Crohn's disease (Burton & Anderson 1983, Winslet et al 1994).

OTHER ACTIONS

Glucosamine might have some activity against HIV. Preliminary evidence shows that it inhibits intracellular viral movement and blocks viral replication (Bagasra et al 1991). Other studies have found that glucosamine has immunosuppressive properties and can prolong graft survival in mice (Ma et al 2002). Oral, intraperitoneal and intravenously administered glucosamine significantly reduces CNS inflammation and demyelination in an animal model of multiple sclerosis (Zhang et al 2005).

CLINICAL USE

Osteoarthritis

There is very good evidence to suggest that glucosamine sulphate is effective in treating the symptoms of OA, in particular moderate severity OA, as well as slowing disease progression as per studies mainly investigating knee OA. This is further supported by studies with animal models that unequivocally confirm glucosamine has anti-inflammatory and disease modifying effects.

While there have been some inconsistencies in human studies, reviews of clinical trials generally confirm the efficacy of glucosamine sulphate in providing pain relief from OA whereas studies investigating glucosamine hydrochloride tend to produce inconsistent results (Black et al 2009, Bruyere & Reginster 2007, Chan and Ng 2011, Fox & Stephens 2009, Henrotin et al 2012, Kwoh et al 2013, Miller & Clegg 2011, Provenza et al 2014, Reginster et al 2007, 2012, Vangsness et al 2009, Wandel et al 2010, Wu et al 2013). Benefits appear most consistent when glucosamine sulfate is taken together with chondroitin sulfate long term.

Clinical note

In 2014, the European Society for Clinical and Economic Aspects of Osteoporosis and Osteoarthritis (ESCEO) gathered an international task force of 13 members to determine clinical management of patients with OA. They concluded that the first step for patients with OA and pain is to use either glucosamine sulfate +/− chondroitin sulphate or paracetamol on a regular basis, while NSAIDs should only be used as an advanced step, if response is not adequate. They recommended that the safer, more sensible approach is not to use paracetamol due to its side effects and questionable efficacy on pain with chronic use, but to recommend chronic symptomatic slow-acting drugs for osteoarthritis such as glucosamine sulphate (Bruyere et al 2014). Interestingly, they noted that US groups are reluctant to recommend dietary supplements due to quality issues, whereas there is less concern in Europe as pharmaceutical grade preparations are used.

One explanation for the inconsistent results could relate to dosing. Pharmacokinetic studies have shown that glucosamine is easily absorbed, but the current treatment doses (1500 mg/day) barely reach the required therapeutic concentration in plasma and tissue. Therefore, it is likely that many patients, in particular obese patients, are being under-dosed at the current tested concentrations (Aghazadeh-Habashi & Jamali 2011, Henrotin et al 2012). Other reasons for some of the inconsistent results include: inconsistency in the chemical potency of some products used as well as variable and erratic bioavailability indices. Some support for a higher dose was recently obtained via a 12-week randomised study that showed 3000 mg/day of glucosamine sulphate provided effective symptom relief in knee OA. All outcome measures (WOMAC and Lequesne algofunctional indices) were significantly improved (Coulson et al 2013).

Compared to standard treatments

Several clinical studies indicate that glucosamine is at least as effective as NSAIDs in treating the symptoms of OA however the effect takes longer to be established (approximately 2–6 weeks) (Herrero-Beaumont et al 2007, Muller-Fassbender et al 1994, Reichelt et al 1994, Rovati 1992, Ruane & Griffiths 2002). In addition, a double-blind, random controlled trial (RCT) involving 318 people with moderately severe knee OA showed that more people responded to daily glucosamine sulphate (1500 mg/day) than paracetamol (3 gm/day) or placebo over 6 months, as seen by improvements to the Lequesne score (Herrero-Beaumont et al 2007).

The first Cochrane systematic review was published in 2003 and analysed results from 16 RCTs testing glucosamine for OA. It concluded that 'there is good evidence that glucosamine is both effective and safe in treating OA' and that 'glucosamine therapy may indeed represent a significant breakthrough in the pharmacological management of OA' (Towheed et al 2003). The most recent Cochrane review (updated in 2008) looked at 20 studies involving a total of 2570 patients and found that the Rottapharm glucosamine sulfate preparation was superior to placebo in the treatment of pain and functional impairment, whereas studies using non-Rottapharm glucosamine hydrochloride preparations failed to show benefit in pain and function (Towheed et al 2006).

The first placebo-controlled clinical trials investigating glucosamine in OA were published in the early 1980s. Drovanti et al (1980) showed that a dose of 1500 mg glucosamine sulfate significantly reduced symptoms of OA, almost twice as effectively and twice as fast as placebo. Perhaps the most exciting results were found when electron microscopy analysis of cartilage showed that those people taking glucosamine sulfate had cartilage more similar to healthy joints than the placebo group. Based on this finding, researchers suggested that glucosamine sulfate had not only provided symptom relief but also had the potential to induce rebuilding of the damaged cartilage.

Since that time, multiple human clinical trials lasting from a few weeks (Coulson et al 2013, Crolle & D'Este 1980, Drovanti et al 1980, Lopes Vaz 1982, McAlindon 2001, Pujalte et al 1980, Qiu et al 1998) to 3 years (Pavelka et al 2002, Reginster et al 2001), as well as systematic reviews (Poolsup et al 2005, Towheed et al 2003, 2006) and meta-analyses (McAlindon et al 2000, Richy et al 2003) have shown that glucosamine sulfate (1500 mg/day) can significantly improve symptoms of pain and functionality measures in patients with OA of the knee, with side effects comparable to those of placebo. This is not to say that all studies have produced positive results for symptom relief in OA.

Probably the most well-known study showing 'apparent' negative results was published in 2005 after the National Institutes of Health (NIH) spent US$14 million on a Glucosamine hydrochloride and Chondroitin Arthritis Intervention Trial (GAIT). The 24-week, placebo-controlled, parallel, double-blind, five-arm trial involving 1583 patients aimed to answer the question as to whether glucosamine hydrochloride and/or chondroitin was more effective than placebo or the COX-2 inhibitor celecoxib for symptom relief (Clegg et al 2006, NIH 2002). The results of this study provide evidence that glucosamine hydrochloride and chondroitin are more effective when given in combination than when either substance is given alone and that combined treatment with glucosamine hydrochloride and chondroitin is more effective than celecoxib for treating moderate-to-severe, but not mild, arthritis. Furthermore, the combined treatment was significantly better than placebo for patients with either mild or moderate-to-severe disease when the internationally accepted Outcome Measures in Rheumatology-Osteoarthritis Research Society International (OMERACT-OARSI) response criteria for judging clinical trials of OA was used (Clegg et al 2006). A 2-year sub-study however, found no clinically important differences in symptoms or function with any treatments compared to placebo (Sawitzke et al 2010) and no reductions in joint space narrowing, although there was a trend for improvement in knees with Kellgren and Lawrence (K/L) grade 2 radiographic OA. The authors acknowledge that the statistical power of this 2-year follow-up study was diminished by the limited sample size, variance of joint space width measurements and a smaller than expected loss in joint space (Sawitzke et al 2008).

The design and overall inconclusive results of the GAIT trial have been strongly criticised for the fact that the trial included a large number of people with very mild disease at baseline who were more likely to be susceptible to placebo (as evidenced by the very high (60%) placebo response) and who were given ready access to rescue medication. Furthermore, the unusually high 50% drop-out rate at 2 years meant that the structural study was underpowered. The use of intention-to-treat rather than an according-to-protocol analysis further compromised the ability to detect any significant differences (Pelletier et al 2010).

Long-term use

A meta-analysis of six studies involving 1052 cases suggests that daily administration of glucosamine sulfate delays radiological progression of OA of the knee after 3 years (Lee et al 2010). A small to moderate protective effect on minimum joint space narrowing ($P < 0.001$) was observed after long-term use, but not yet apparent after the first 12 months. This was further confirmed in a more recent 2013 meta-analysis of 19 RCTs ($n = 3159$) which identified that long-term use (over 6 months) of glucosamine sulphate exerts disease-modifying effects in OA (Wu et al 2013).

The first of these long term structural studies was performed by Reginster et al (2000) and compared the effects of 1500 mg glucosamine sulfate with placebo daily over 3 years in 212 patients aged over 50 years with primary knee OA. This was heralded as a landmark study at the time because it not only detected modest symptom-relieving effects, but also was the first to identify significant joint-preserving activity with long-term use. Two years later, Pavelka et al confirmed these results in another randomised, double-blind study that involved 202 patients with knee OA (Pavelka et al 2002) and once again observed that long-term treatment with glucosamine sulfate retarded disease progression. A post hoc analysis of these studies found that the disease-modifying effect was evident in 319 postmenopausal women (Bruyere et al 2004) and another sub-analysis found that patients with less severe radiographic knee OA, who are likely to experience the most dramatic disease progression, may be particularly responsive to treatment with glucosamine (Bruyere et al 2003). A 1-year trial involving 104 subjects with OA of the hands, hip and knee also found that treatment with both glucosamine and chondroitin reduced pain and significantly slowed disease progression as measured by radiographs and measures of urinary C-terminal cross-linking telopeptides of type I collagen (Scarpellini et al 2008).

A recent 2-year double blind RCT with 605 participants that compared glucosamine sulfate (1500 mg/day) with or without chondroitin sulfate (1200 mg/day) to placebo, found that while those in the combination group experienced significant reduction in joint space narrowing after 2 years, and all groups experienced a reduction in pain, none of the treatment groups demonstrated significant symptomatic benefit above placebo (Fransen et al 2014).

Furthermore, results confirming a disease-modifying effect using cartilage volume assessment were also obtained in the National Institutes of Health Osteoarthritis Initiative (OAI) (a longitudinal observational cohort study) which analysed a sub-group of 600 people with knee osteoarthritis, who were followed over a 2-year period (Martel-Pelletier et al 2013). The cohort had complete radiographic and MRI data for the most symptomatic knee enabling close observation of disease progression. Importantly, this was the first study to use fully automated MRI analysis and not rely on manual or semi-automated techniques. The protective effect of glucosamine plus chondroitin appears to mainly target the medial subregions in subjects with less severe damage and in the more early stages of knee OA. This is highly relevant as the MRI parameter of medial compartment cartilage volume/thickness loss seems to be able to predict progression to total knee replacement, according to a recent report by the European Society for Clinical and Economic Aspects of Osteoporosis and Osteoarthritis (ESCEO). While this was not a controlled study, over 85% of subjects that reported using glucosamine plus chondroitin stated they did this nearly every day or every day; however, no details were obtained about the forms or doses used.

It is therefore interesting to note the results of a pharmacoeconomic study which suggests that treatment with glucosamine sulfate for at least 12 months results in significant reduction in health resource utilisation even after treatment is discontinued. This study, which involved 275 subjects previously involved in 12-month glucosamine intervention trials, followed subjects for up to 5 years after treatment was discontinued (making up a total of 2178 patient-years of observation). The study showed that total knee replacement had occurred in over twice as many patients from the placebo group (19/131 or 14.5%), than in those formerly receiving glucosamine sulphate (9/144 or 6.3%) (Bruyere et al 2008).

Clinical note: Theories to explain inconsistencies across studies

Although many forms of glucosamine are used in practice, there is significantly more evidence supporting the use of the glucosamine sulfate than glucosamine hydrochloride. It has been suggested the inconsistent results may be due to the type of preparation, inadequate allocation concealment and industry bias as most clinical trials of glucosamine sulfate have used a specific patented oral formulation from Rottapharm, Italy, which is available as a prescription medicine in Europe (Vlad et al 2007). The greater efficacy seen with the Rottapharm glucosamine sulfate formulation may be due to the fact it uses vacuum sealed sachets to protect the physiologically active and highly hygroscopic, crystalline glucosamine sulfate from degradation in air, while the less hygroscopic 'stabilised' glucosamine hydrochloride preparations have been found to crystallise out of solution and therefore may contain less than the optimal amount of the physiologically active ingredient (Sahoo et al 2012). Pharmacokinetic studies have also suggested that the current treatment doses (500 mg three times daily) barely reach the required therapeutic concentration in plasma and tissue and it is likely that many patients are being under-dosed at the current tested concentrations (Aghazadeh-Habashi & Jamali 2011, Henrotin et al 2012). This is most likely with obese patients who tend to require higher doses of many medications. Henrotin et al (2012) further suggest that inconsistent results are likely to be due to inconsistency in the chemical potency of some products used as well as variable and erratic bioavailability indices.

G

Combination therapy

With chondroitin sulfate (see Chondroitin monograph for more information)

Chondroitin sulfate and glucosamine are frequently marketed together in combination products and many studies suggest that this combination is effective in treating symptoms (Clegg et al 2006, Das & Hammad 2000, Leffler et al 1999, McAlindon et al 2000, Nguyen et al 2001, NIH 2002) and reducing joint space narrowing (Rai et al 2004). In a cluster-randomised, placebo-controlled trial in 251 patients, a combination of chondroitin sulfate and glucosamine hydrochloride but not glucosamine hydrochloride alone was found to be effective in alleviating symptoms and improving the dysfunction with Kashin-Beck disease (Yue et al 2012). This is supported by in vitro studies using horse cartilage, which report that a combination of glucosamine sulfate and chondroitin sulfate can partially mitigate the catabolic response to inflammatory stress and mechanical trauma (Harlan et al 2012) and that combination treatment is more effective than either product alone in preventing articular cartilage glycosaminoglycan degradation (Dechant et al 2005). Further support for combination therapy comes from an in vivo study of rats, which found that combined treatment with chondroitin and glucosamine sulfate prevented the development of cartilage damage and was associated with a reduction in IL-1-beta and matrix metalloprotease-9 synthesis (Chou et al 2005). While combination therapy with glucosamine and chondroitin is supported by clinical evidence, the mechanism of any synergistic action is unknown. Furthermore, research indicates that co-administration of chondroitin actually reduces the uptake of glucosamine sulphate resulting in reduced circulating plasma levels. Thus, it is suggested that any combined effect may be due to effects on the gut lining or liver rather than the joint space (Jackson et al 2010).

With omega-3 EFAs

Results from a recent study further suggest that glucosamine may be more effective in combination with omega-3 fatty acids. A recent RCT involving 177 patients with moderate to severe hip or knee osteoarthritis compared glucosamine sulfate (1500 mg/day) alone with glucosamine sulfate in combination with the omega-3 polyunsaturated fatty acids eicosapentaenoic acid (EPA) and docosahexaenoic acid (DHA). After 26 weeks the combination therapy group was significantly superior to glucosamine sulphate alone in reducing WOMAC by either 80% ($P = 0.044$) or 90% ($P = 0.015$) (Gruenwald et al 2009).

With MSM

In a 12-week, randomised, placebo-controlled trial of glucosamine and methylsulfonylmethane involving 118 patients, combined therapy was found to produce a greater and more rapid reduction in pain, swelling and loss of function than either agent alone (Usha & Naidu 2004).

Topical, with camphor

A topical preparation containing glucosamine along with chondroitin and camphor has been shown to reduce pain from OA of the knee in one randomised controlled trial (Cohen et al 2003).

With NSAIDs

Although glucosamine has not been shown to have direct analgesic activity, certain combinations with non-opioid analgesics have demonstrated synergistic (e.g. ibuprofen and ketoprofen), additive (e.g. diclofenac, indomethacin, naproxen and piroxicam) or sub-additive (e.g. aspirin and paracetamol) effects in animal pain models, suggesting that combinations of certain ratios of glucosamine and specific non-steroidal anti-inflammatory drugs (NSAIDs) might enhance pain relief or provide adequate pain relief with lower doses of NSAIDs (Tallarida et al 2003).

Comparisons with NSAIDs

There are many studies suggesting that glucosamine is at least as effective as NSAIDs in treating the symptoms of OA (Herrero-Beaumont et al 2007, Muller-Fassbender et al 1994, Reichelt et al 1994, Rovati 1992, Ruane & Griffiths 2002), although glucosamine has a slower onset of action, taking 2–6 weeks to establish an effect. The GAIT trial (see earlier) found that the combination of glucosamine hydrochloride and chondroitin was more effective than celecoxib in treating moderate to severe OA in the shorter term, whereas glucosamine alone was not (Clegg et al 2006).

Inflammatory bowel disease

In vitro and in vivo studies suggest that glucosamine may be useful in treating inflammatory bowel disease with in vitro studies demonstrating suppression of cytokine-induced activation of intestinal epithelial cells and in vivo studies finding that glucosamine improved clinical symptoms and suppressed colonic inflammation and tissue injury in a rat model of inflammatory bowel diseases (Yomogida et al 2008). The anti-inflammatory activity of glucosamine is partly mediated by an increased production of heparan sulfate proteoglycans by the vascular endothelium, thereby improving the endothelium's barrier function (McCarty 1998b). It is possible that the step in glycoprotein synthesis involving the amino sugar is relatively deficient in patients with inflammatory bowel disease and this could reduce the synthesis of the glycoprotein cover that protects the mucosa from damage by bowel contents (Burton & Anderson 1983, Winslet et al 1994). In a pilot study, *N*-acetyl glucosamine proved beneficial in children with chronic inflammatory bowel disease (Salvatore et al 2000).

Chronic lower back pain

A systematic review of 3 RCTs concluded that there was insufficient data to determine whether the use of glucosamine is useful for lower back pain (Sodha et al 2013). Wilkens et al (2012) conducted a double blind RCT over 6 months of 250 subjects with chronic lower back pain (>6 months) and MRI findings indicating degenerative lumbar disease, finding no significant pain relieving effects with glucosamine sulfate (1500 mg/day) (Wilkens et al 2012). Similarly, no pain relief was observed in a small double blind, placebo controlled, crossover study which tested a combination of glucosamine HCl (1500 mg/day), chondroitin sulfate (1200 mg/day) and manganese ascorbate (228 mg/day) over 16 weeks (Leffler et al 1999). In contrast, Tant et al (2005) conducted an open label, RCT of glucosamine taken over 12 weeks in combination with other ingredients such as MSM (methylsulfonylmethane) and found a clinically significant reduction in pain; however, the trial was an open study using a multiple ingredient combination treatment.

OTHER USES

There is the suggestion from one small RCT that glucosamine may provide symptomatic relief for people with rheumatoid arthritis (Nakamura et al 2007).

Veterinary use

Glucosamine demonstrates benefits in alleviating symptoms of degenerative joint disease in both horses (Forsyth et al 2006, Baccarin et al 2012) and dogs (McCarthy et al 2007).

Skincare use

It has been suggested that glucosamine may be a suitable cosmetic ingredient for use in skin care products. Because of its stimulation of hyaluronic acid synthesis, glucosamine has been shown to accelerate wound healing, improve skin hydration and decrease wrinkles. In addition, as an inhibitor of tyrosinase activation, it inhibits melanin production and is useful in treatment of disorders of hyperpigmentation (Bissett 2006). This is supported by an 8-week, double-blind, placebo-controlled trial, which found that hyperpigmentation was reduced with topical use of *N*-acetyl glucosamine with the effect being enhanced by niacinamide (Bissett et al 2007).

DOSAGE RANGE

- Typical dosing is 1500 mg glucosamine (either HCl or sulphate)/day (500 mg three times daily). This is based on preclinical animal models which used 20 mg/kg of body weight per day, which translates to 1500 mg/day for a 75 kg adult. Higher dosing may therefore be required in heavier individuals.
- A 2–3-month trial is generally used to determine whether it is effective for an individual patient. Use for 3+ years is required to slow down knee joint degeneration and potentially reduce the risk of knee replacement.
- Intramuscular glucosamine sulfate: 400 or 800 mg three times/week (Reichelt et al 1994) for 4–6 weeks or longer if required.
- Glucosamine sulfate, hydrochloride, hydroiodide and *N*-acetyl forms are available. Most research has been done on the sulfate forms. Topical, intravenous, intramuscular and intraarticular forms are also available in some countries.

ADVERSE REACTIONS

Glucosamine has been used safely in multiple clinical trials lasting from 4 weeks to 3 years with minimal or no adverse effects (Lopes Vaz 1982, Pavelka et al 2002, Pujalte et al 1980, Reginster et al 2001). A 2006 Cochrane systematic review concluded that glucosamine is as safe as placebo (Towheed et al 2006). Glucosamine has an observed safe level (OSL) of 2000 mg/day and while it is considered safe, some uncommon and minor adverse effects have been reported, including epigastric pain or tenderness (3.5%), heartburn (2.7%), diarrhoea (2.5%) and nausea (1%) (Sherman et al 2012).

Glucosamine sulphate has no significant effect on serum lipids (Albert et al 2007, Østergaard et al 2007). While it is unlikely that glucosamine has any significant effects on glucose tolerance, people with impaired glucose tolerance or insulin resistance should be monitored (Dostrovsky et al 2011).

There is one case report of asthma being exacerbated by glucosamine–chondroitin supplementation (Tallia & Cardone 2002).

Practice points/Patient counselling

- Glucosamine is a naturally occurring building block of joint tissue and cartilage.
- Glucosamine sulphate is an effective symptomatic treatment for pain and disability associated with OA, with most research conducted with knee OA. When used long term (more than 6 months) it slows the progression of the disease, and appears to work best long-term with chondroitin sulfate.
- It is considered extremely safe and may reduce the need for NSAIDs (which can have serious side effects).
- People who are overweight or obese may require higher doses than the usual dose of 1500 mg/day.
- People with severe shellfish allergy should be advised to use a form that is not derived from shellfish.
- Patients with diabetes should monitor their blood glucose levels while taking glucosamine, although no significant changes are anticipated.

Clinical note — Should people with diabetes avoid glucosamine?

Clinicians' concern about the safety of glucosamine in diabetes were probably first fuelled by an article published in *Lancet* in 1999 (Adams 1999). The article entitled 'Hype about glucosamine' by Adams stated that glucosamine increases glucose resistance in normal and in experimentally diabetic animals (McClain & Crook 1996) and intravenous glucosamine in doses as low as 0.1 mg/kg/minute result in a 50% reduction in the rate of glucose uptake in skeletal muscle (Baron et al 1995). Adams concluded by suggesting that perhaps all people, but especially those who are overweight or have diabetes, should be urged to have caution when using glucosamine. In 2005, a critical review of 33 clinical studies involving 3063 human subjects concluded that glucosamine does not affect glucose metabolism, and that there are no adverse effects of oral glucosamine administration on blood, urine or faecal parameters (Anderson et al 2005). A more recent systematic review of 11 studies, however, suggests that glucosamine may have some effect on glucose metabolism in people with impaired glucose tolerance or insulin resistance and that more studies are required before definitive conclusion can be made (Dostrovsky et al 2011).

SIGNIFICANT INTERACTIONS

Controlled studies are not available so interactions remain speculative and are based on evidence of pharmacological activity.

Non-steroidal anti-inflammatory drugs

Glucosamine reduces the requirements for NSAID use by people with knee OA according to a large French study (Bertin & Taieb 2013) — drug dosage may require modification after several weeks' glucosamine use — a potentially beneficial combination.

Warfarin

Case reports exist of glucosamine and glucosamine/chondroitin combinations increasing bruising, bleeding and INR amongst people taking warfarin (Knudsen & Sokol 2008). Until the interaction can be tested in a controlled study, caution is advised.

CONTRAINDICATIONS AND PRECAUTIONS

Diabetics using glucosamine should have their blood sugar levels checked regularly.

Glucosamine is made from shellfish and, although it is not extracted from the protein component and appears to pose no threat to shrimp-allergic individuals (Villacis et al 2006), it should be used with caution in patients with shellfish allergy.

Whether glucosamine poses a serious bleeding risk in major surgery is unclear. Multiple case reports suggesting an interaction between warfarin and glucosamine have been collected by the FDA and WHO however it is unknown whether the interaction is pharmacokinetic or pharmacodynamic (Knudsen & Sokol 2008). Of the 21 documented case reports indicating increased INR and held in the WHO adverse drug reaction database, 17 resolved when glucosamine was ceased. While this does not provide strong evidence that glucosamine used by itself will cause bleeding, caution is advised. Due to the fact that glucosamine is long term therapy, suspending use one week before major surgery and resuming use afterwards seems reasonable.

PREGNANCY USE

Insufficient reliable information is available to advise on safety in pregnancy. Some limited data suggest no increased risk for major malformations or other adverse fetal effects with glucosamine use during pregnancy (Sivojelezova et al 2007).

PATIENTS' FAQs

What will this supplement do for me?

Multiple scientific studies have shown that glucosamine sulfate reduces symptoms of OA and also slows progression of the condition when used long-term. The sulfate form is superior to the hydrochloride form for improving symptoms. Some people find that they do not require NSAIDs as often when taking it.

When will it start to work?

Symptom relief generally takes 2–6 weeks to establish, but joint protection effects occur only with long-term use of at least 6 months to several years.

Are there any safety issues?

Although considered very safe for the general population, it should be used with caution in people with severe shellfish allergies.

REFERENCES

Adams ME. Hype about glucosamine. Lancet 354.9176 (1999): 353–354.

Aghazadeh-Habashi A et al. Single dose pharmacokinetics and bioavailability of glucosamine in the rat. J Pharmacy Pharm Sci 5.2 (2002): 181–184.

Aghazadeh-Habashi A, Jamali F. The glucosamine controversy; a pharmacokinetic issue. J Pharm Pharm Sci 14.2 (2011): 264–273.

Albert SG et al. The effect of glucosamine on serum HDL cholesterol and apolipoprotein AI levels in people with diabetes. Diabetes Care 30.11 (2007): 2800–2803.

Anderson JW et al. Glucosamine effects in humans: a review of effects on glucose metabolism, side effects, safety considerations and efficacy. Food Chem Toxicol 43.2 (2005): 187–201.

Baccarin RYA et al. Urinary glycosaminoglycans in horse osteoarthritis. Effects of chondroitin sulfate and glucosamine. Research in Veterinary Science 93.1 (2012): 88–96.

Bagasra O et al. Anti-human immunodeficiency virus type 1 activity of sulfated monosaccharides: comparison with sulfated polysaccharides and other polyions. J Infect Dis 164.6 (1991): 1082–1090.

Balkan B, Dunning BE. Glucosamine inhibits glucokinase in vitro and produces a glucose-specific impairment of in vivo insulin secretion in rats. Diabetes 43.10 (1994): 1173–1179.

Baron AD et al. Glucosamine induces insulin resistance in vivo by affecting GLUT 4 translocation in skeletal muscle. Implications for glucose toxicity. J Clin Invest 96.6 (1995): 2792–2801.

Basak M et al. Comparative bioavailability of a novel timed release and powder-filled glucosamine sulfate formulation: a multi-dose, randomized, crossover study. Int J Clin Pharmacol Ther 42.11 (2004): 597–601.

Bassleer C, Rovati L, Franchimont P. Stimulation of proteoglycan production by glucosamine sulfate in chondrocytes isolated from human osteoarthritic articular cartilage in vitro. Osteoarthritis Cartilage 6.6 (1998): 427–434.

Bertin P, Taieb C. NSAID-sparing effect of glucosamine hydrochloride in patients with knee osteoarthritis: an analysis of data from a French database. Curr Med Res Opin (2013).

Biggee BA et al. Low levels of human serum glucosamine after ingestion of glucosamine sulphate relative to capability for peripheral effectiveness. Ann Rheum Dis 65.2 (2006): 222–226.

Bissett DL et al. Reduction in the appearance of facial hyperpigmentation by topical N-acetyl glucosamine. J Cosmet Dermatol 6.1 (2007): 20–26.

Bissett DL. Glucosamine: an ingredient with skin and other benefits. J Cosmet Dermatol 5.4 (2006): 309–15.

Black C et al. The clinical effectiveness of glucosamine and chondroitin supplements in slowing or arresting progression of osteoarthritis of the knee: a systematic review and economic evaluation. Health Technology Assessment 13(52) (2009).

Bruyere O et al. Correlation between radiographic severity of knee osteoarthritis and future disease progression: results from a 3-year prospective, placebo-controlled study evaluating the effect of glucosamine sulfate. Osteoarthritis Cartilage 11.1 (2003): 1–5.

Bruyere O et al. Glucosamine sulfate reduces osteoarthritis progression in postmenopausal women with knee osteoarthritis: evidence from two 3-year studies. Menopause 11.2 (2004): 138–143.

Bruyere O et al. Total joint replacement after glucosamine sulphate treatment in knee osteoarthritis: results of a mean 8-year observation of patients from two previous 3-year, randomised, placebo-controlled trials. Osteoarthritis Cartilage 16.2 (2008): 254–260.

Bruyere O, Reginster JY. Glucosamine and chondroitin sulfate as therapeutic agents for knee and hip osteoarthritis. Drugs Aging 24.7 (2007): 573–80.

Burton AF, Anderson FH. Decreased incorporation of 14C-glucosamine relative to 3H-N-acetyl glucosamine in the intestinal mucosa of patients with inflammatory bowel disease. Am J Gastroenterol 78.1 (1983): 19–22.

Chan KOW, Ng GYF. A review on the effects of glucosamine for knee osteoarthritis based on human and animal studies. Hong Kong Physiotherapy Journal 29.2 (2011): 42–52.

Chou MM et al. Effects of chondroitin and glucosamine sulfate in a dietary bar formulation on inflammation, interleukin-1-beta, matrix metalloprotease-9, and cartilage damage in arthritis. Exp Biol Med 230.4 (2005): 255–262.

Cibere J et al. Glucosamine sulfate and cartilage type II collagen degradation in patients with knee osteoarthritis: randomized discontinuation trial results employing biomarkers. J Rheumatol 32.5 (2005): 896–902.

Clegg DO et al. Glucosamine, chondroitin sulfate, and the two in combination for painful knee osteoarthritis. N Engl J Med 354.8 (2006): 795–808.

Cohen M et al. A randomized double blind, placebo controlled trial of a topical cream containing glucosamine sulfate, chondroitin sulfate, and camphor for osteoarthritis of the knee. J Rheumatol 30 (2003): 523–528.

Consumer Lab 2; Product review: glucosamine and chondroitin. Available at www.consumerlab.com (accessed January 2006).

Coulson S et al. Green-lipped mussel extract (Perna canaliculus) and glucosamine sulphate in patients with knee osteoarthritis: therapeutic efficacy and effects on gastrointestinal microbiota profiles. Inflammopharmacology 21.1 (2013): 79–90.

Crolle G, D'Este E. Glucosamine sulphate for the management of arthrosis: a controlled clinical investigation. Curr Med Res Opin 7.2 (1980): 104–109.

Das A Jr, Hammad TA. Efficacy of a combination of FCHG49 glucosamine hydrochloride, TRH122 low molecular weight sodium chondroitin sulfate and manganese ascorbate in the management of knee osteoarthritis. Osteoarthritis Cartilage 8.5 (2000): 343–350.
de Mattei M et al. High doses of glucosamine-HCl have detrimental effects on bovine articular cartilage explants cultured in vitro. Osteoarthritis Cartilage 10.10 (2002): 816–825.
Dechant JE et al. Effects of glucosamine hydrochloride and chondroitin sulphate, alone and in combination, on normal and interleukin-1 conditioned equine articular cartilage explant metabolism. Equine Vet J 37.3 (2005): 227–231.
Dostrovsky NR et al. The effect of glucosamine on glucose metabolism in humans: a systematic review of the literature. Osteoarthritis and Cartilage 19.4 (2011): 375–380.
Drovanti A, Bignamini AA, Rovati AL. Therapeutic activity of oral glucosamine sulfate in osteoarthrosis: a placebo-controlled double-blind investigation. Clin Ther 3.4 (1980): 260–272.
Echard BW et al. Effects of oral glucosamine and chondroitin sulfate alone and in combination on the metabolism of SHR and SD rats. Mol Cell Biochem 225 (2001): 85–91.
Forsyth RK et al. Double blind investigation of the effects of oral supplementation of combined glucosamine hydrochloride (GHCL) and chondroitin sulphate (CS) on stride characteristics of veteran horses. Equine Vet J 36 (Suppl) (2006): 622–625.
Fox BA, Stephens, MM. Glucosamine/chondroitin/primorine combination therapy for osteoarthritis. Drugs Today (Barc.) 45.1 (2009): 21–31.
Fransen M et al. Glucosamine and chondroitin for knee osteoarthritis: a double-blind randomised placebo-controlled clinical trial evaluating single and combination regimens. Annals of Rheumatic Diseases 0 (2014): 1–8.
Giaccari A et al. In vivo effects of glucosamine on insulin secretion and insulin sensitivity in the rat: possible relevance to the maladaptive responses to chronic hyperglycaemia. Diabetologia 38.5 (1995): 518–524.
Gouze JN et al. Interleukin-1beta down-regulates the expression of glucuronosyltransferase I, a key enzyme priming glycosaminoglycan biosynthesis: influence of glucosamine on interleukin-1beta-mediated effects in rat chondrocytes. Arthritis Rheum 44.2 (2001): 351–360.
Gruenwald J et al. Effect of glucosamine sulfate with or without omega-3 fatty acids in patients with osteoarthritis. Adv Ther 26.9 (2009): 858–871.
Harlan RS et al. The Effect of Glucosamine and Chondroitin on Stressed Equine Cartilage Explants. Journal of Equine Veterinary Science 32.1 (2012): 12–14.
Henrotin, Y et al. Is there any scientific evidence for the use of glucosamine in the management of human osteoarthritis? Arthritis Res Ther 14.1(2012): 201.
Herrero-Beaumont G et al. Glucosamine sulfate in the treatment of knee osteoarthritis symptoms: a randomized, double-blind, placebo-controlled study using acetaminophen as a side comparator. Arthritis Rheum 56.2 (2007): 555–67.
Hua J, Sakamoto K, Nagaoka I. Inhibitory actions of glucosamine, a therapeutic agent for osteoarthritis, on the functions of neutrophils. J Leukocyte Biol 71.4 (2002): 632–640.
Imagawa K et al. The epigenetic effect of glucosamine and a nuclear factor-kappa B (NF-kB) inhibitor on primary human chondrocytes — Implications for osteoarthritis. Biochemical and Biophysical Research Communications 405.3 (2011): 362–367.
Jackson CG et al. The human pharmacokinetics of oral ingestion of glucosamine and chondroitin sulfate taken separately or in combination. Osteoarthritis and Cartilage 18(3) (2010): 297–302.
Kelly GS. The role of glucosamine sulfate and chondroitin sulfates in the treatment of degenerative joint disease. Altern Med Rev 3.1 (1998): 27–39.
Kim MM et al. Glucosamine sulfate promotes osteoblastic differentiation of MG-63 cells via anti-inflammatory effect. Bioorg Med Chem Lett 17.7 (2007): 1938–1942.
Knudsen JF, Sokol GH. Potential glucosamine-warfarin interaction resulting in increased international normalized ratio: case report and review of the literature and MedWatch database. Pharmacotherapy, 28.4 (2008): 540–548.
Laverty S et al. Synovial fluid levels and serum pharmacokinetics in a large animal model following treatment with oral glucosamine at clinically relevant doses. Arthritis Rheum 52.1 (2005): 181–191.
Lee YH et al. Effect of glucosamine or chondroitin sulfate on the osteoarthritis progression: a meta-analysis. Rheumatology International 30 (2010): 357–363.
Leffler CT et al. Glucosamine, chondroitin, and manganese ascorbate for degenerative joint disease of the knee or low back: a randomized, double-blind, placebo-controlled pilot study. Mil Med 164.2 (1999): 85–91.
Lippiello L et al. In vivo chondroprotection and metabolic synergy of glucosamine and chondroitin sulfate. Clin Orthopaed Rel Res 381 (2000): 229–240.
Lopes Vaz A. Double-blind clinical evaluation of the relative efficacy of ibuprofen and glucosamine sulphate in the management of osteoarthrosis of the knee in out-patients. Curr Med Res Opin 8.3 (1982): 145–149.
López M et al. Effects of Glucosamine Sulphate, Chondroitin Sulphate and Hyaluronic Acid on Articular Cartilage. Journal of Comparative Pathology 148.1 (2013): 97.
Ma L et al. Immunosuppressive effects of glucosamine. J Biol Chem 277.42 (2002): 39343–39349.
Martel-Pelletier J et al. First-line analysis of the effects of treatment on progression of structural changes in knee osteoarthritis over 24 months: data from the osteoarthritis initiative progression cohort. Ann.Rheum.Dis. (2013).
McAlindon T. Glucosamine and chondroitin for osteoarthritis? Bull Rheum Dis 50.7 (2001): 1–4.
McAlindon TE et al. Glucosamine and chondroitin for treatment of osteoarthritis: a systematic quality assessment and meta-analysis [Comment]. JAMA 283.11 (2000): 1469–1475.
McCarthy G et al. Randomised double-blind, positive-controlled trial to assess the efficacy of glucosamine/chondroitin sulfate for the treatment of dogs with osteoarthritis. Vet J 174.1 (2007): 54–61.
McCarty MF, Russell AL, Seed MP. Sulfated glycosaminoglycans and glucosamine may synergize in promoting synovial hyaluronic acid synthesis. Med Hypotheses 54.5 (2000): 798–802.
McCarty MF. Enhanced synovial production of hyaluronic acid may explain rapid clinical response to high-dose glucosamine in osteoarthritis. Med Hypotheses 50.6 (1998a): 507–10.

McCarty MF. Vascular heparan sulfates may limit the ability of leukocytes to penetrate the endothelial barrier: implications for use of glucosamine in inflammatory disorders. Med Hypotheses 51.1 (1998b): 11–15.
McClain DA, Crook ED. Hexosamines and insulin resistance. Diabetes 45.8 (1996): 1003–1009.
Mello DM et al. Comparison of inhibitory effects of glucosamine and mannosamine on bovine articular cartilage degradation in vitro. Am J Vet Res 65.10 (2004): 1440–1445.
Miller KL, Clegg DO. Glucosamine and chondroitin sulfate. Rheum Dis Clin North Am 37.1 (2011): 103–118.
Monauni T et al. Effects of glucosamine infusion on insulin secretion and insulin action in humans. Diabetes 49.6 (2000): 926–935.
Mroz PJ, Silbert JE. Use of 3H-glucosamine and 35S-sulfate with cultured human chondrocytes to determine the effect of glucosamine concentration on formation of chondroitin sulfate. Arthritis Rheum 50.11 (2004): 3574–3579.
Muller-Fassbender H et al. Glucosamine sulfate compared to ibuprofen in osteoarthritis of the knee. Osteoarthritis Cartilage 2.1 (1994): 61–69.
Nagaoka I et al. Chapter 22 — Biological Activities of Glucosamine and Its Related Substances. Advances in Food and Nutrition Research. K. Se-Kwon, Academic Press 65 (2012): 337–352.
Nagaoka I et al. Recent aspects of the anti-inflammatory actions of glucosamine. Carbohydrate Polymers 84.2 (2011): 825–830.
Nakamura H et al. Effects of glucosamine administration on patients with rheumatoid arthritis. Rheumatol Int 27.3 (2007): 213–2118.
Nakamura H et al. Effects of glucosamine hydrochloride on the production of prostaglandin E2, nitric oxide and metalloproteases by chondrocytes and synoviocytes in osteoarthritis. Clin Exp Rheumatol 22.3 (2004): 293–299.
National Institutes of Health NIH; National Centre for Complementary and Alternative Medicine GAIT Study, 2002. www.nih.com (accessed January 2008).
Nelson BA, Robinson KA, Buse MG. High glucose and glucosamine induce insulin resistance via different mechanisms in 3T3-L1 adipocytes. Diabetes 49.6 (2000): 981–991.
Nguyen P et al. A randomized double-blind clinical trial of the effect of chondroitin sulfate and glucosamine hydrochloride on temporomandibular joint disorders: a pilot study. Cranio 19.2 (2001): 130–139.
Nimni ME, Cordoba F. Chondroitin sulfate and sulfur containing chondroprotective agents: Is there a basis for their pharmacological action? Curr Rheum Rev 2.2 (2006): 137–149.
Onigbinde AT et al. Acute effects of combination of glucosamine sulphate lontophoresis with exercise on fasting plasma glucose of participants with knee osteoarthritis. Hong Kong Physiotherapy Journal 29.2 (2011): 79–85.
Østergaard K et al. The effect of glucosamine sulphate on the blood levels of cholesterol or triglycerides — a clinical study. Ugeskr Laeger 169.5 (2007): 407–410.
Pavelka K et al. Glucosamine sulfate use and delay of progression of knee osteoarthritis: a 3-year, randomized, placebo-controlled, double-blind study. Arch Intern Med 162.18 (2002): 2113–2123.
Pelletier JP et al. Long term knee OA trial design: an ounce of prevention is worth a pound of cure. Annals of Rheumatic Diseases Letter to Editor (2010).
Persiani S et al. Glucosamine oral bioavailability and plasma pharmacokinetics after increasing doses of crystalline glucosamine sulfate in man. Osteoarthritis Cartilage 13.12 (2005): 1041–1049.
Persiani S et al. Synovial and plasma glucosamine concentrations in osteoarthritic patients following oral crystalline glucosamine sulphate at therapeutic dose. Osteoarthritis Cartilage 15.7 (2007): 764–772.
Petersen SG et al. Glucosamine but not ibuprofen alters cartilage turnover in osteoarthritis patients in response to physical training. Osteoarthritis and Cartilage 18.1 (2010): 34–40.
Piperno M et al. Glucosamine sulfate modulates dysregulated activities of human osteoarthritic chondrocytes in vitro. Osteoarthritis Cartilage 8.3 (2000): 207–212.
Poolsup N et al. Glucosamine long-term treatment and the progression of knee osteoarthritis: systematic review of randomized controlled trials. Ann Pharmacother 39.6 (2005): 1080–1087.
Pouwels MJ et al. Short-term glucosamine infusion does not affect insulin sensitivity in humans. J Clin Endocrinol Metab 86.5 (2001): 2099–2103.
Provenza JR et al. Combined glucosamine and chondroitin sulfate, once or three times daily, provides clinically relevant analgesia in knee osteoarthritis. Clin Rheumatol 2014 [Epub ahead of print].
Pujalte JM, Llavore EP, Ylescupidez FR. Double-blind clinical evaluation of oral glucosamine sulphate in the basic treatment of osteoarthrosis. Curr Med Res Opinion 7.2 (1980): 110–1114.
Qian, S et al. Bioavailability enhancement of glucosamine hydrochloride by chitosan. Int.J Pharm., 455.1–2 (2013): 365–373.
Qiu GX et al. Efficacy and safety of glucosamine sulfate versus ibuprofen in patients with knee osteoarthritis. Arzneimittelforschung 48.5 (1998): 469–474.
Rai J et al. Efficacy of chondroitin sulfate and glucosamine sulfate in the progression of symptomatic knee osteoarthritis: a randomized, placebo-controlled, double blind study. Bull Postgrad Inst Med Educ Res Chandigarh 38.1 (2004): 18–22.
Reginster JY et al. Evidence of nutriceutical effectiveness in the treatment of osteoarthritis. Curr Rheumatol Rep 2.6 (2000): 472–477.
Reginster JY et al. Long-term effects of glucosamine sulphate on osteoarthritis progression: a randomised, placebo-controlled clinical trial [Comment]. Lancet 357.9252 (2001): 251–256.
Reginster JY et al. Current role of glucosamine in the treatment of osteoarthritis. Rheumatology (Oxford) 46.5 (2007): 731–5.
Reginster J-YN et al. Role of glucosamine in the treatment for osteoarthritis. Rheumatology International 32 (2012): 2959–2967.
Reichelt A et al. Efficacy and safety of intramuscular glucosamine sulfate in osteoarthritis of the knee: a randomised, placebo-controlled, double-blind study. Arzneimittelforschung 44.1 (1994): 75–80.
Richy F et al. Structural and symptomatic efficacy of glucosamine and chondroitin in knee osteoarthritis: a comprehensive meta-analysis. Arch Intern Med 163.13 (2003): 1514–1522.

Roman-Blas J et al. Glucosamine sulfate for knee osteoarthritis: science and evidence-based use. Therapy 7.6 (2010): 591–604.
Rovati LC. Clinical research in osteoarthritis: design and results of short-term and long-term trials with disease-modifying drugs. Int J Tissue React 14.5 (1992): 243–251.
Ruane R, Griffiths P. Glucosamine therapy compared to ibuprofen for joint pain. Br J Community Nurs 7.3 (2002): 148–152.
Sahoo SC et al. Glucosamine Salts: Resolving Ambiguities over the Market-Based Compositions Crystal Growth and Design 12 (2012): 5148–5154.
Sakai S et al. Effect of glucosamine and related compounds on the degranulation of mast cells and ear swelling induced by dinitrofluorobenzene in mice. Life Sciences 86(9–10) (2010): 337–343.
Salvatore S et al. A pilot study of N-acetyl glucosamine, a nutritional substrate for glycosaminoglycan synthesis, in paediatric chronic inflammatory bowel disease. Aliment Pharmacol Ther 14.12 (2000): 1567–1579.
Sawitzke AD et al. The effect of glucosamine and/or chondroitin sulfate on the progression of knee osteoarthritis: a report from the glucosamine/chondroitin arthritis intervention trial. Arthritis Rheum 58.10 (2008): 3183–91.
Sawitzke AD et al Clinical efficacy and safety of glucosamine, chondroitin sulphate, their combination, celecoxib or placebo taken to treat osteoarthritis of the knee: 2-year results from GAIT. Annals of Rheumatic Diseases 69 (2010): 1459–1464.
Scarpellini M et al. Biomarkers, type II collagen, glucosamine and chondroitin sulfate in osteoarthritis follow-up: the Magenta osteoarthritis study. J Orthop Traumatol 9.2 (2008): 81–87.
Setnikar IP, Canali S. Pharmacokinetics of glucosamine in man. Arzneimittelforschung 43.10 (1993): 1109–1113.
Shankar RR et al. Glucosamine infusion in rats mimics the beta-cell dysfunction of non-insulin-dependent diabetes mellitus. Metabolism 47.5 (1998): 573–577.
Sherman AL et al Use of Glucosamine and Chondroitin in Persons With Osteoarthritis. PM&R 4(5, Supplement) (2012): S110–S116.
Shikhman AR et al. N-acetylglucosamine prevents IL-1 beta-mediated activation of human chondrocytes. J Immunol 166.8 (2001): 5155–5160.
Silva FS Jr et al. Combined glucosamine and chondroitin sulfate provides functional and structural benefit in the anterior cruciate ligament transection model. Clin Rheumatol 28.2 (2009): 109–117.
Sivojelezova A et al. Glucosamine use in pregnancy: an evaluation of pregnancy outcome. J Womens Health (Larchmt) 16.3 (2007): 345–348.
Sodha, R et al. The use of glucosamine for chronic low back pain: a systematic review of randomised control trials. BMJ Open 3.6 (2013).
Sumantran VN et al. The relationship between chondroprotective and antiinflammatory effects of Withania somnifera root and glucosamine sulphate on human osteoarthritic cartilage in vitro. Phytother Res 22.10 (2008): 1342–1348.
Tallarida RJ et al. Antinociceptive synergy, additivity, and subadditivity with combinations of oral glucosamine plus nonopioid analgesics in mice. J Pharmacol Exp Ther 307.2 (2003): 699–704.
Tallia AF, Cardone DA. Asthma exacerbation associated with glucosamine-chondroitin supplement. J Am Board Fam Pract 15.6 (2002): 481–484.
Tamai Y et al. Enhanced healing of cartilaginous injuries by N-acetyl-glucosamine and glucuronic acid. Carbohydr Polym 54.2 (2003): 251–262.
Tannis AJ et al. Effect of glucosamine supplementation on fasting and non-fasting plasma glucose and serum insulin concentrations in healthy individuals. Osteoarthritis Cartilage 2.6 (2004): 506–511.
Tant L et al. Open-label, randomized, controlled pilot study of the effects of a glucosamine complex on low back pain. Curr Ther Res 66 (2005): 511–21.
Tiraloche G et al. Effect of oral glucosamine on cartilage degradation in a rabbit model of osteoarthritis. Arthritis Rheum 52.4 (2005): 1118–1128.
Towheed TE et al. Glucosamine therapy for treating osteoarthritis. Cochrane Database Syst Rev 1 (2003).
Towheed TE et al. Glucosamine therapy for treating osteoarthritis. Cochrane Database Syst Rev 2 (2006).
Usha PR, Naidu MUR. Randomised, double-blind, parallel, placebo-controlled study of oral glucosamine, methylsulfonylmethane and their combination in osteoarthritis. Clin Drug Invest 24.6 (2004): 353–363.
Vangsness CT Jr et al. A review of evidence-based medicine for glucosamine and chondroitin sulfate use in knee osteoarthritis. Arthroscopy 25.1 (2009): 86–94.
Villacis J et al. Do shrimp-allergic individuals tolerate shrimp-derived glucosamine? Clin Exp Allergy 36.11 (2006): 1457–1461.
Vlad SC et al. Glucosamine for pain in osteoarthritis: why do trial results differ? Arthritis Rheum 56.7 (2007): 2267–2277.
Wandel S et al. Effects of glucosamine, chondroitin, or placebo in patients with osteoarthritis of hip or knee: network meta-analysis. BMJ 341 (2010): c4675.
Wilkens P et al. No effect of 6-month intake of glucosamine sulfate on Modic changes or high intensity zones in the lumbar spine: sub-group analysis of a randomized controlled trial. J Negat Results Biomed 11.13 (2012).
Winslet MC et al. Mucosal glucosamine synthetase activity in inflammatory bowel disease. Dig Dis Sci 39.3 (1994): 540–544.
Wu, D et al. Efficacies of different preparations of glucosamine for the treatment of osteoarthritis: a meta-analysis of randomised, double-blind, placebo-controlled trials. Int.J Clin Pract 67.6 (2013): 585–594.
Yomogida S et al. Glucosamine, a naturally occurring amino monosaccharide, suppresses dextran sulfate sodium-induced colitis in rats. Int J Mol Med 22.3 (2008): 317–323.
Yue J et al. Chondroitin sulfate and/or glucosamine hydrochloride for Kashin-Beck disease: a cluster-randomized, placebo-controlled study. Osteoarthritis and Cartilage 20.7 (2012): 622–629.
Zhang GX et al. Glucosamine abrogates the acute phase of experimental autoimmune encephalomyelitis by induction of Th2 response. J Immunol 175.11 (2005): 7202–7208.

Green tea

HISTORICAL NOTE Tea has been a popular beverage for thousands of years and was originally grown in China, dating back 5000 years, where it has been used as part of various ceremonies and to maintain alertness. Green tea and the partially fermented oolong tea have remained popular beverages in Asia since that time, whereas black tea is the preferred beverage in many English-speaking countries. Tea was introduced to the Western culture in the sixth century by Turkish traders (Ulbricht & Basch 2005). Second to water, tea is now considered to be the world's most popular beverage.

Clinical note — The difference between teas

Black, green and oolong tea are produced from the same plant (*Camellia sinensis*) but differ in polyphenol content according to the way the leaves are processed. Black tea is made from oxidised leaves, whereas oolong tea is made from partially oxidised leaves and green tea leaves are not oxidised at all. Because the oxidising process converts many polyphenolic compounds into others with less activity, green tea is considered to have the strongest therapeutic effects and the highest polyphenol content (Lin et al 2003). Caffeine concentrations also vary between the different teas: black tea > oolong tea > green tea > fresh tea leaf (Lin et al 2003). Variation in caffeine content is further influenced by growing conditions, manufacturing processes and size of the tea leaves (Astill et al 2001). The highest-quality leaves are the first spring leaf buds, called the 'first flush'. The next set of leaf buds produced is called the 'second flush' and considered to be of poorer quality. Tea varieties also reflect the area they are grown in (e.g. Darjeeling in India), the form produced (e.g. pekoe is cut, gunpowder is rolled) and processing method (black, oolong or green) (Ulbricht & Basch 2005).

COMMON NAME

Green tea

OTHER NAMES

Chinese tea, camellia tea, gruner tea, Matsu-cha, green Sencha tea, Japanese tea, Yame tea

BOTANICAL NAME/FAMILY

Camellia sinensis (family Theaceae)

PLANT PART USED

Leaf

CHEMICAL COMPONENTS

The composition of green tea varies according to the growing and harvesting methods, but the most abundant components are polyphenols, which are predominantly flavonoids (e.g. catechin, epicatechin, epicatechin gallate, epigallocatechin gallate, proanthocyanidins). Caffeine content in green tea varies but is estimated at about 3%, along with very small amounts of the other common methylxanthines, theobromine and theophylline (Graham 1992). It also contains many other constituents, such as tannin, diphenylamine, oxalic acid, trace elements and vitamins.

Epigallocatechin gallate is one of the most abundant polyphenols in tea and is regarded as the most important pharmacologically active component.

MAIN ACTIONS

It is suspected that the polyphenol content is chiefly responsible for the chemoprotective, antiproliferative, antimicrobial and antioxidant activity of green tea. The caffeine content is predominantly responsible for central nervous system (CNS) activity and an interaction between both appears necessary for increasing thermogenesis.

Antioxidant

Green tea has consistently demonstrated strong antioxidant activity. A recent systematic review of 31 controlled intervention studies concluded that green tea reduced lipid peroxidation and increased antioxidant capacity when the beverage was consumed regularly (0.6–1.5 litres a day) (Ellinger et al 2011). In a controlled human trial, 24 healthy women consumed two cups of green tea (250 mg catechins/day) for 42 days (Erba et al 2005). The results showed a significant increase in plasma antioxidant status, reduced plasma peroxides and reduced low-density lipoprotein (LDL) cholesterol when compared with controls. Several other in vitro animal and human studies have also demonstrated that green tea inhibits lipid peroxidation and scavenges hydroxyl and superoxide radicals (Leenen et al 2000, Rietveld & Wiseman 2003, Sung et al 2000).

Antibacterial activity

Green tea extract has moderate and wide-spectrum inhibitory effects on the growth of many types of pathogenic bacteria, according to in vitro tests, including seven strains of *Staphylococcus* spp., seven strains of *Streptococcus* spp., 26 strains of *Salmonella*, 19 strains of *Escherichia coli* spp. and one strain of *Corynebacterium suis* (Ishihara et al 2001). In one in vitro study green tea was effective against most of the 111 bacteria tested, including two genera of Gram-positive and seven genera of Gram-negative bacteria. It was also confirmed that in vivo it could protect against *Salmonella typhimurium* (Bandyopadhyay et al 2005).

Recent in vitro research is looking at a possible role for (–)(–)-epigallocatechin-3-gallate (EGCG) in fighting antibiotic-resistant bacteria. It has been shown to be effective against 21 clinical isolates of *Acinetobacter baumannii*, a common cause of infection in intensive-care units, and against the antibiotic resistant *Stenotrophomonas maltophilia* (Gordon & Wareham 2010, Osterburg et al 2009).

Green tea has also been found to inhibit *Helicobacter pylori* in animal models (Matsubara et al 2003, Stoicov et al 2009). According to one study, which compared the antibacterial activity of black, green and oolong tea, it seems that fermentation adversely affects antibacterial activity, as green tea exhibited the strongest effects, and black tea the weakest (Chou et al 1999). An in vitro study has demonstrated that green tea can significantly lower bacterial endotoxin-induced cytokine release and therefore may reduce mortality from sepsis. Part of the antibacterial activity may be a selective antiadhesive effect, with green tea inhibiting pathogen adhesion to cells (Lee et al 2009).

Oral pathogens

In a recent randomised controlled trial (RCT), 66 healthy subjects rinsed with a green tea extract for 1 minute three times a week, and at the end of 4 and 7 days there was a significant reduction in *Streptococcus mutans* and lactobacilli in the green tea group (Ferrazzano et al 2011). Both in vitro and in vivo tests have identified strong antibacterial activity against a range of oral pathogens, such as *Streptococcus mutans*, *S. salivarius* and *E. coli* (Otake et al 1991, Rasheed & Haider 1998). The mechanism of action appears to involve antiadhesion effects, with the strongest activity associated with epigallocatechin gallate and epicatechin gallate. Green tea catechins (GTCs) have also showed an antibacterial effect against *Porphyromonas gingivalis* and *Prevotella* spp. in vitro (Araghizadeh et al 2013, Hirasawa et al 2002). Furthermore, green tea polyphenols, especially epigallocatechin gallate, have been found to completely inhibit the growth and adherence of *Porphyromonas gingivalis* on buccal epithelial cells (Sakanaka et al 1996).

Antiviral activity

A number of in vitro studies have shown that epigallocatechin gallate strongly inhibits HIV replication (Chang et al 1994, Fassina et al 2002, Liu et al 2005, Tao 1992, Williamson et al 2006) and inhibits attachment of HIV virus to T cells (Nance et al 2009). The theaflavins from black tea have shown even stronger anti-HIV activity than catechins in vitro by inhibiting viral entry into target cells (Liu et al 2005). Antiviral activity has also been identified against Epstein–Barr virus, herpes simplex virus 1, influenza A and B, rotavirus and enterovirus (Chang et al 2003, de Oliveira et al 2013, Imanishi et al 2002, Isaacs et al 2008, Mukoyama et al 1991, Tao 1992, Weber et al 2003). EGCG and epicatechin gallate show antiviral activity inhibiting influenza virus replication in vitro with differences in the strength of the antiviral activity depending on the strain of influenza (Song et al 2005). In vitro research shows green tea extract and EGCG inhibit human papillomavirus in human cervical cancer cells (Tang et al 2008). Antiviral activity seems to be attributable to interference with virus adsorption (Mukoyama et al 1991).

Antimalarial

Antimalarial properties have been shown in vitro, with crude extract of green tea, EGCG and epicatechin gallate strongly inhibiting *Plasmodium falciparum* growth (Sannella et al 2007).

Anticarcinogenic

Several in vitro studies have shown a dose-dependent decreased proliferation and/or increased apoptosis in a variety of cancer cell lines (lung, prostate, colon, stomach, pancreatic, bladder, oral, leukaemia, breast, cervical and bone) (Garcia et al 2006, Gupta et al 2003, Han et al 2009, Honicke et al 2012, Kavanagh et al 2001, Khan et al 2009a, Kinjo et al 2002, Qanungo et al 2005, Qin et al 2007, Sen & Chatterjee 2011, Shimizu et al 2005, Siddiqui et al 2011, Srinivasan et al 2008, Valcic et al 1996, Wang & Bachrach 2002, Yamauchi et al 2009, Yoo et al 2002, Zhang et al 2002, Zou et al 2010). Additionally, photochemopreventive effects for green tea and epigallocatechin gallate have been demonstrated in vitro, in vivo and on human skin for the prevention of skin cancer (Afaq et al 2003, Katiyar 2011) and apoptosis of skin tumour cells (Mantena et al 2005).

The mechanism of action by which tea polyphenols exert antimutagenic and antitumorigenic effects is still largely speculative. A review of research suggests there is increasing experimental evidence of multiple signalling pathways and reducing cancer metastasis (Khan & Mukhtar 2010, Thakur et al 2012). A systematic review of in vitro and in vivo studies on epithelial ovarian cancer cells concluded green tea components had an impact on cell signalling, cell motility, angiogenesis, apoptosis and inflammation (Trudel et al 2012). The following has been observed: inhibition of the large multicatalytic protease and metalloproteinases, which are involved in tumour survival and metastasis, respectively, and inhibition of many tumour-associated protein kinases, while not affecting kinase activity in normal cells (Kazi et al 2002, Wang & Bachrach 2002). Tea polyphenols have also been found to inhibit some cancer-related proteins that regulate DNA replication and transformation. There is increasing evidence that catechins possess antiangiogenic properties (Sachinidis & Hescheler 2002). Inhibition of angiogenic factors and antitumour immune reactivity, including an increase in cytotoxic T-lymphocyte cells, was found to be the mechanism of action in preventing photocarcinogenesis (Mantena et al 2005). Recent work suggests tea polyphenols may inhibit microsomal aromatase and 5 alpha-reductase, so suppressing prostate carcinogenesis. Tea catechins may work to suppress proteasomal activities, thereby inhibiting breast cancer cell proliferation (Ho et al 2009). Modification of oestrogen metabolism was found with both premenopausal and menopausal women, which may modify the risk of breast cancer (Fuhrman et al 2013).

G

Adjunct in cancer treatment

There has been some exploratory in vitro research to study the combination of green tea and anticancer drugs, with findings suggesting that EGCG with cyclooxygenase-2 inhibitors increased apoptosis mediated through the MAPK signalling pathway and the combination of EGCG and tamoxifen increased the effectiveness in apoptosis more than tamoxifen alone (Suganuma et al 2011). In this cell culture research the issue of ovarian cancer cells developing resistance to chemotherapy was explored. They found EGCG and sulforaphane from cruciferous vegetables may offer a novel treatment in ovarian cancer. The combination of EGCG and sulforaphane increased apoptosis significantly after 6 days of treatment in cells that were resistant to paclitaxel and it may offer a solution for overcoming paclitaxel resistance in this disease (Chen et al 2013). This initial in vitro work may point the way to future research.

Antihypertensive

Recent human studies have found antihypertensive benefit, with a small RCT reporting significant reduction in both systolic and diastolic blood pressure in obese patients with hypertension (Bogdanski et al 2012) and other studies reporting blood pressure-lowering effects (Brown et al 2009, Nantz et al 2009). In vitro experiments using green tea extracts have identified angiotensin-converting enzyme inhibition (Persson et al 2006). Animal experiments have also shown that a green tea extract protected against arterial hypertension induced by angiotensin II (Antonello et al 2007).

Cardioprotective

Studies on animals and humans find that green tea has multiple mechanisms that have an impact on the cardiovascular system, including lipid lowering, hypocholesterolaemic, anti-inflammatory, antithrombogenic, antioxidant, antihypertensive and antiatherosclerotic (Babu & Liu 2008, Neves et al 2008) and shows a beneficial effect on endothelial function in healthy volunteers (Alexopoulos et al 2008). The catechins in the green tea also have the ability to prevent atherosclerosis, as well as inhibiting thrombogenesis through a platelet aggregation action (Bhardwaj & Khanna 2013).

Neuroprotective/neurorescue

Neuroprotective activity refers to the use of an agent before exposure to a neurotoxin which prevents toxicity. Neurorescue is a different term which refers to the use of an agent after exposure to a neurotoxin, which is able to reverse toxicity effects. In vitro and animal research indicates that EGCG found in green tea has the ability to act as both a neuroprotective and a neurorescue agent (Guo et al 2007, Hou et al 2008, Jeong et al 2007). In vitro tests reveal that EGCG reduces apoptosis of human neuroblastoma cells (Avramovich-Tirosh et al 2007). Additionally, in vivo studies have found a neuroprotective effect for EGCG on dopamine neurons, which is being further investigated as a potential preventive treatment in Parkinson's disease (Guo et al 2007, Jeong et al 2007). Animal research has found a number of neuroprotective benefits, such as reducing neuronal cell death, of EGCG in multiple sclerosis (Herges et al 2011), following a traumatic brain injury (Itoh et al 2011) and protecting the retina against neurodegeneration in a rat diabetic retinopathy model (Silva et al 2013). In vitro epicatechin and EGCG have been shown to have a neuroprotective effect which may be suitable for the neurological complications associated with HIV infection (Nath et al 2012).

Two animal studies found that EGCG reduced beta-amyloid deposition — one study reported 60% reduction in the frontal cortex and 52% in the hippocampus over the 3 months of the study (Li et al 2006, Rezai-Zadeh et al 2008). This may have implications in the development and progression of Alzheimer's dementia and is being further investigated in other models. Beta-amyloid deposition impacts on mitochondrial function and recent in vitro and in vivo research suggests EGCG can restore and protect brain mitochondrial function and integrity (Dragicevic et al 2011).

Numerous in vitro and animal models suggest several different mechanisms of action appear to be responsible for neuroprotective and neurorescue activity, including antioxidant, iron chelating, anti-inflammatory, cell apoptosis, signal transduction, gene regulation and an effect on amyloid precursor protein (Assuncao et al 2010, Biasibetti et al 2013, Mandel et al 2006, Ostrowska et al 2007). These actions taken together make green tea polyphenols a promising agent in reversing age-related neuronal decline (Andrade & Assuncao 2012). A rat model found improvement in spatial learning and memory over long-term treatment, with green tea protecting against oxidative damage in the rat hippocampal region (Assuncao et al 2011). In an aged rat model improved cognitive function after EGCG might be due to its impact on neurotransmitters, with a positive effect found for dopamine, acetylcholine and serotonin (Srividhya et al 2012).

Iron chelation

EGCG has been shown to chelate metals such as iron, zinc and copper (Guo et al 1996, Kumamoto et al 2001). Since the accumulation of iron has been implicated in the aetiology of both Alzheimer's dementia and Parkinson's disease and in vivo research shows EGCG's iron-chelating effect penetrates the brain barrier, it may offer neuroprotective and neurorescue effects in these diseases. EGCG has further been shown to reduce amyloid precursor protein and beta-amyloid peptide, most likely due to its iron-chelating activity (Reznichenko et al 2006). It is possible that iron chelation effects enabling iron to be removed from the brain may provide a novel therapy to prevent progression in neurodegenerative diseases (Mandel et al 2007).

Thermogenic activity

Although the thermogenic activity of green tea is often attributed to its caffeine content, an in vivo study has shown that stimulation of brown adipose tissue thermogenesis occurs to a greater extent than would be expected from the caffeine content alone (Dulloo et al 2000). The interaction between catechin polyphenols and caffeine on stimulating noradrenaline release and reducing noradrenaline catabolism may be responsible. Clinical investigation has produced similar results, with green tea consumption significantly increasing 24-hour energy expenditure and urinary noradrenaline excretion, whereas an equivalent concentration of caffeine had no effect on these measures (Dulloo et al 2000).

OTHER ACTIONS

Green tea exhibits a variety of other pharmacological actions, such as anti-inflammatory activity, CNS stimulation, inhibition of platelet aggregation, stimulation of gastric acid secretion and diuresis, increased mental alertness, relaxation of extracerebral vascular and bronchial smooth muscle, and reduced cholesterol, triglyceride and leptin levels (Fassina et al 2002, Sayama et al 2000). Recent in vitro and animal models suggest potential as a therapeutic agent for T-cell-mediated autoimmune conditions (Pae & Wu 2013). A significant genoprotective effect was found with an in vitro study and a small human trial using a biomarker of oxidative stress (Han et al 2011).

Some animal studies suggest that EGCG activates gamma-aminobutyric acid (GABA)-A receptors, causing sedative and hypnotic effects (Adachi et al 2006, Vignes et al 2006). A number of rat experiments have shown memory improvement in older animals. Improved spatial cognition learning ability in rats was demonstrated after the administration of long-term GTCs (Haque et al 2006). Significant improvement in memory and learning was found in older rats administered with green tea extract over 8 weeks (Kaur et al 2008).

Hepatoprotective

Preliminary evidence from in vitro experiments demonstrates hepatoprotective activity with GTCs improving insulin sensitivity, decreasing lipids and through their antioxidant and anti-inflammatory actions (Masterjohn & Bruno 2012, Ueno et al 2009).

Antithyroid

In vitro research and a recent rat model has found catechins have an antithyroid action, decreasing the activities of thyroid peroxidase and the synthesis of thyroid hormone (Chandra & De 2013). An action preventing autoimmune inflammation in an animal model suggests EGCG may delay or manage autoimmune disorders such as Sjögren's syndrome (Gillespie et al 2008). Another recent animal model of multiple sclerosis reported a protection against autoimmune expression by inhibiting immune cell infiltration and modulating proautoimmune cells and antiautoimmune cells (Meydani 2011). In vitro and in vivo studies and some preclinical research suggests an antiarthritic and antirheumatic activity for EGCG (Ahmed 2010).

CLINICAL USE

Evidence is largely based on epidemiological studies, with few clinical studies available.

Cancer prevention

It is still unclear whether green tea consumption reduces the incidence of all cancers or has any effect on mortality; however, studies of individual cancers show some protective effects. Supportive evidence is most consistent for breast, ovarian, endometrial and prostate cancers, with some supportive evidence for colerectal, pancreatic cancers and leukaemia and less consistent evidence for lung, liver, bladder, oesophageal and gastric cancers.

All cancers

A Cochrane review concluded that there was conflicting evidence regarding an inverse association between green tea drinking and cancer risk and suggests it remains unproven as a cancer intervention (Boehm et al 2009). Other systematic reviews and meta-analyses have suggested a trend towards protection in breast and prostate cancers and improved survival rates in epithelial ovarian cancer (Clement 2009, Johnson et al 2012). Another review concluded that green tea was associated with a reduced risk of upper gastrointestinal tract cancers and had a beneficial role in breast cancer. However they suggested results on overall cancer prevention were inconclusive (Yuan et al 2011). A 2003 study using 13-year follow-up data found increased green tea consumption was associated with an apparent delay of cancer onset and death, and all-cause deaths (Nakachi et al 2003).

The conflicting results from different studies and reviewers may be due to confounding factors in different populations, dosages and differences in the EGCG content of green teas.

Breast cancer

There appears to be a benefit of green tea drinking of three or more cups daily with reduction in the risk of breast cancer. Some recent studies are suggesting the aromatase-inhibiting action may be more effective for women drinking green tea premenopause, which may delay onset of breast cancer later in life. A meta-analysis of three cohort studies from Japan and one population case-control study from the United States concluded that green tea consumption reduced the risk of breast cancer (Sun et al 2006). Similar protective effects were observed in a case–control study in China, which found that regular drinking of green tea reduced breast cancer risk (Zhang et al 2007a). In a meta-analysis of nine studies — seven studies on the incidence and two on the recurrence of breast cancer — consumption of three or more cups of green tea daily was associated with reduced recurrence (pooled relative risk [RR] = 0.73, 95% confidence interval [CI]: 0.56–0.96). No association was found in the cohort studies for reduced incidence of breast cancer; however the case-control studies did find an inverse association with incidence (pooled RR 0.81, 95% CI: 0.75–0.88) (Ogunleye et al 2010). In this review it is suggested that the difference in numbers of pre- or postmenopausal women in the case-controlled or cohort studies may explain the conflicting results. One review examining data from the Shanghai Women's Health Study (n = 74,942 Chinese women) considered the hypothesis that, because of the difference in oestrogens pre- and postmenopause, and green tea's aromatase-inhibiting action, tea-drinking protection might depend on menopausal status. Their analysis found that regularly drinking green tea from 25 years of age may delay the onset of breast cancer, suggesting a largely beneficial effect in premenopausal women (Dai et al 2010). This hypothesis may explain in part some of the conflicting evidence from studies, but larger studies and RCTs are required to confirm findings.

Ovarian cancer

A recent meta-analysis included six case-control and cohort studies with a total of 9113 subjects (3842 cases and 5271 controls) reporting that green tea drinking can significantly decrease the risk of ovarian cancer (odds ratio [OR] 0.81; 95% CI: 0.73–0.89; $P < 0.0001$). More research is suggested to assess different teas and dosages, and how different subgroups are affected (Gao et al 2013). The case-control Australian Ovarian Cancer Study conducted over 3.5 years (1368 patients and 1416 controls) reported a significant inverse association between green tea drinking (four or more cups) and ovarian cancer. They found no difference between green and black tea consumption and there was no dose-response effect. The same authors conducted a meta-analysis (which included 17 studies) and found a trend towards green tea drinking and ovarian cancer prevention (Nagle et al 2010). A 2011 review of the literature found only four case-control studies (Goodman 2003, Nagle et al 2010, Song et al 2008, Zhang et al 2002) of green tea and ovarian cancer and a meta-analysis of these studies found evidence of a combined inverse association (OR 0.66; 95% CI: 0.54–0.80) between green tea drinking and ovarian cancer, with a 32% reduction in risk for green tea drinkers. Both prospective and retrospective observational analysis found an inverse association; however the authors suggested caution in interpretation of the results, with very different levels of tea drunk in the studies and lack of prospective cohort results (Butler & Wu 2011). A systematic review of in vitro, in vivo and epidemiological studies on epithelial ovarian cancer included four case-control studies and concluded that it was difficult to extrapolate data as the catechins in the green tea varied, there were different cup sizes and various definitions of high tea intake. Despite these factors it did appear that green tea consumption was associated with a decreased ovarian cancer risk and better prognosis of the disease (Trudel et al 2012).

Endometrial cancer

Green tea drinking was found to be mildly protective against endometrial cancer risk in a population-based case–control study in China where 995 cases were interviewed. This protective effect might be limited to premenopausal women (Gao et al 2005). A total of two cohort and five case-control studies were included in a meta-analysis that reported a significant reduction in risk of endometrial cancer for green tea drinkers, with an increase of two cups a day associated with a reduction in risk of endometrial cancer by 25% (Tang et al 2009b). A more recent review and meta-analysis of six observational studies confirmed a dose-dependent protective role of green tea drinking and endometrial cancer risk, suggesting a 23% reduction in risk for regular green tea drinkers (OR 0.78; 95% CI: 0.62–0.98). However the authors suggest caution in interpreting the results because of the differences in green teas and the amount of tea consumed (Butler & Wu 2011).

Prostate cancer

Although evidence is inconclusive, there is a mounting body of research showing a preventive role for reducing the risk of prostate cancer with a therapeutic dose of five or more cups of green tea a day. A Cochrane review included five studies and reported that in the higher-quality observational studies and in the only RCT there was a decreased risk of prostate cancer with high consumption of green tea (Boehm et al 2009). A case-control study in China with 130 prostate cancer patients found that green tea was protective against prostate cancer, with lower risk associated with an increase in the frequency, duration and quantity of green tea consumed (Jian et al 2004). Drinking green tea was also associated with a reduction in the risk of advanced prostate cancer in 49,920 men aged 40–69 years who completed questionnaires over a 10-year period in the Japan Public Health Center-based Prospective Study. The effect was dose-dependent and strongest for men drinking five or more cups/day compared with less than 1 cup/day (Kurahashi et al 2008). The more recent evidence appears to be inconclusive, with mixed results from a number of clinical trials and population studies (Henning et al 2011, Khan et al 2009a, Lee & Pasalich 2013). A meta-analysis of observational studies included seven studies with green tea and reported a borderline significant decrease (38%) in prostate cancer risk for Asian populations with high green tea consumption (Zheng et al 2011a). One of the plausible reasons for the conflicting evidence is that some studies include low tea consumption, which may skew the results, as it appears that dosage is important in cancer protection.

Colorectal cancer

A recent meta-analysis of 13 case-control studies found a weak, non-statistically-significant reduction in colorectal cancer risk for those drinking high doses of green tea (Wang et al 2012c). This benefit did not seem to extend to US and European populations. More research would be required to confirm these findings. A meta-analysis of six prospective cohort studies (including 1675 cases of colorectal cancer) reported that in Shanghai populations there was an inverse risk between green tea consumption and the incidence of colon and colorectal cancers. The results overall were insufficient to suggest green tea may protect against colorectal cancer (Wang et al 2012e).

Pancreatic cancer

A recent Chinese population-based case-control study (908 patients with pancreatic cancer and 1067 healthy controls) found that women had a 32% less risk of pancreatic cancer with regular low-temperature green tea consumption, especially drinking higher amounts and with long-term use. Drinking more than 150 g of dry tea leaves per month (also lower-temperature tea) resulted in a reduction in risk by 43% (OR 0.56, 95% CI 0.32–0.98) for women compared with non-tea drinkers. With men there was only an association between pancreatic cancer risk and tea for regular tea drinkers consuming lukewarm and cool tea compared to hot tea (Wang et al 2012b).

Leukaemia

Leukaemia risk may be reduced with drinking sufficient amounts of green tea. The protective effect was significant in the 16–29-year age range with higher amounts of green tea consumption; there was no significant relationship to green tea drinking and leukaemia risk in younger people in the 0–15-year age range. These findings were from a population-based study in Taiwan (Kuo et al 2009). A hospital-based case-control study (107 patients) in China found that there was a reduction of risk in adult leukaemia with high green tea consumption (Zhang et al 2007b).

Lung cancer

A systematic review of epidemiological studies on the risk of lung cancer and tea drinking found a significant reduction in risk for the high-level tea drinkers in only four out of 20 studies. Overall the review found a small benefit for green tea drinking in reducing the risk of lung cancer, which was especially noticeable in those who had never smoked (Arts 2008). A meta-analysis including 22 studies (12 studies on green tea only) also reported a borderline significant association with a 22% reduction in the risk of developing lung cancer for the highest green tea drinkers. Increasing green tea by two cups a day was shown to reduce lung cancer risk by 18% (Tang et al 2009a). This was confirmed in a dose–response analysis of six studies where a significant non-linear relationship between green tea and risk of lung cancer was reported. This beneficial effect was especially strong in those drinking more than seven cups a day (Wang et al 2012d). It appears that green tea may have a small beneficial effect in reducing lung cancer risk but, as a recent systematic review suggests, more well-designed studies are needed (Fritz et al 2013).

Liver cancer

The protective effect of green tea drinking to reduce liver cancer risk appears to be stronger for high-risk patients with hepatitis B or C and also for long-term green tea drinkers. A recent meta-analysis included 13 epidemiological studies (six case-control and seven prospective cohort studies) and reported borderline significance showing green tea was preventive (for both men and women) in reducing the risk of developing primary liver cancer (Fon Sing et al 2011). Evidence is conflicting and one analysis of data from a Japanese Public Health Cohort study with 18,815 subjects found no association with green tea drinking and liver cancer risk (Inoue et al 2009a). However another larger Japanese cohort study (Ohsaki Cohort Study, following 41,761 subjects over 9 years) found a significant reduction in risk for liver cancer and green tea for men and women drinking five or more cups of green tea a day (Ui et al 2009). The differences in reporting data may be linked to quantity of tea drunk, number of years of green tea drinking and also whether the group had a high- or low-risk cohort. A recent case-control study of 204 hepatocellular carcinoma (HCC) patients and 415 healthy controls found that drinking high amounts of green tea for longer periods of time resulted in a protective effect, with those drinking green tea for over 30 years having the lowest risk. In the subgroup of patients with chronic hepatitis infection, the risk of HCC in non-green tea drinkers was twice that of those consuming green tea. Further research in this subgroup of people with a higher HCC risk may be warranted (Li et al 2011). According to a placebo-controlled, randomised study, green tea polyphenols may reduce the incidence of HCC in high-risk patients (Yu et al 2006). The study involved 1209 males, who tested positive for hepatitis B virus and then were allocated to the control group or active treatment with green tea polyphenols (two capsules daily of 500 mg). The trial lasted 3 years, with a further 2-year follow-up period. Ten cases of HCC were reported in the green tea group and 18 cases in the placebo group.

Bladder/kidney cancer

A recent meta-analysis included five case-control or cohort studies specifically for green tea and bladder cancer and no association was found between bladder cancer risk and green tea consumption (Wu et al 2013), although a meta-analysis in the same year suggested that Asian people drinking green tea may benefit and a protective effect on bladder cancer was found in this subgroup (Wang et al 2013). More research is indicated to confirm this finding and to discover why the benefit may be only for Asian populations, but the type of green tea may be a possible reason.

A hospital-based case-control study was undertaken in China, in which 250 patients diagnosed with clear cell renal cell carcinoma were compared with healthy controls. The research found green tea consumption of 500 mL or more a day was inversely associated with clear cell renal cell carcinoma risk (Wang et al 2012a).

Oesophageal cancer

Ten epidemiological studies (eight case-control and two cohort studies; n = 33,731) were included in a meta-analysis of green tea consumption and oesophageal cancer risk. There was no association with low or high green tea consumption and oesophageal cancer, except in a subgroup analysis, where the authors reported a protective effect of any level of green tea drinking and oesophageal cancer for women (high green tea consumption: RR/OR = 0.32, 95% CI: 0.10–0.54; medium consumption: RR/OR = 0.43, 95% CI: 0.21–0.66; low consumption: RR/OR = 0.45, 95% CI: 0.10–0.79) (Zheng et al 2012). Another systematic review and meta-analysis of green tea, black tea and coffee and oesophageal cancer risk included 13 green tea studies (one cohort and the 12 case-controls) and the authors reported a significant association for the highest green tea drinkers in the case-control studies (OR = 0.70; 95% CI: 0.51–0.96, $P <$ 0.001) and for the Chinese studies (OR = 0.64; 95% CI: 0.44–0.95, $P < 0.001$) and a more pronounced inverse association for women (Zheng et al 2013a). It is recommended that further studies with control of dose and the temperature of the tea be undertaken.

Gastric cancer

There is conflicting research on the benefit of green tea in reducing gastric cancer risk according to a Cochrane review on green tea and cancer (Boehm et al 2009). However, there may be a trend towards significance for higher green tea consumption (five or more cups per day) and this is especially noted in women and in Chinese populations. A recent review of epidemiological evidence included 17 Japanese and Chinese studies (10 case-control and seven cohort studies). This review concluded that the evidence was insufficient to suggest that green tea reduces the risk of gastric cancer. They found seven studies with no association, eight with an inverse association and one study showing a positive association; however, they do suggest that *Helicobacter pylori* infection may be a confounding factor and that future research should include this subgroup (Hou et al 2013). A pooled analysis of six Japanese cohort studies (total of 219,080 individuals) reported no significant association of green tea drinking and reduction in gastric cancer risk for men; however, women drinking five or more cups a day had a significant reduction in risk of distal gastric cancer (with no significant effect seen on proximal gastric cancer) (Inoue et al 2009b). A later systematic review of epidemiological studies in Japan agreed with this finding, reporting a protective effect for women reducing gastric cancer risk. They included eight cohort studies and three case-control studies and, when analysing only the case-control studies, they found a weak association with gastric cancer reduction and green tea but not in the cohort studies (Sasazuki et al 2012). This difference in results reported from case-control and cohort studies was also found in an earlier meta-analysis (Myung et al 2009). One meta-analysis (seven cohort, 10 case-control and one population-based nested case-control study) reported a statistically significant 14% reduced risk of stomach cancer for people drinking five or more cups of green tea. The five Chinese studies showed a stronger stomach cancer risk reduction than the Japanese studies. The authors recommend further research confined to higher green tea drinkers to confirm the findings (Kang et al 2010). A note of caution from a population-based case-control study ($n = 200$) found that drinking tea at a very hot temperature might be associated with an increased risk of gastric cancer (Mao et al 2011).

Cancer treatment

Studies have been conducted with various doses of green tea and GTCs in different cancers, producing mixed results.

Overall, the current evidence does not support the use of green tea as a cancer treatment; however, there are some exceptions, which suggest an adjunctive role.

Epithelial ovarian cancer

Green tea increased the survival rate of patients with epithelial ovarian cancer in a cohort of 309 Chinese women (Zhang et al 2004). Most (77.9%) of the women in the treatment group were alive at the 3-year follow-up, as compared with 47.9% of the control group.

Cervical cancer

In an RCT, 90 patients with cervical lesions infected with human papillomavirus were given either a capsule containing 200 mg EGCG and/or an ointment containing 200 mg Polyphenon E, to be applied daily (Ahn et al 2003). There was a 69% response rate (35 out of 51 patients) for those on treatment when compared with a 10% response rate for controls ($P < 0.05$), with the ointment showing the best effects.

Colorectal cancer

A pilot study was undertaken with 136 patients with colorectal adenomas, which are considered to be a precursor to colorectal cancers. This randomised trial in Japan increased green tea intake from an average of six cups a day to the equivalent of 10 cups a day by supplementing with green tea extract tablets. This involved supplementing the treatment group with 1.5 g of green tea extract per day for 12 months while both placebo and treatment group continued their green tea drinking. At the end of the intervention metachronous adenomas were evident in 31% (20 of 65) of the control and 15% (9 of 60) of the green tea extract group (RR 0.49; 95% CI, 0.24–0.99; $P < 0.05$) and the size of the relapsed adenomas was smaller in the treated group, illustrating a potential chemopreventive role for green tea extract (Shimizu et al 2008).

Oral premalignant lesions

A phase II RCT with 39 patients with oral premalignant lesions gave the treatment group of patients 500, 750 or 1000 mg of green tea extract three times a day for 12 weeks. On biopsy the green tea extract group had improved histology, especially at the two higher doses, although this was not statistically significant. During the follow-up (median time of 27.5 months) 15 of the patients developed oral cancer and there was no difference between oral cancer-free survival between the placebo and green tea extract groups. It is thought that the green tea extract may act through stromal vascular endothelial growth factor and the research suggests that longer-term trials are needed (Tsao et al 2009).

Prostate cancer

Several studies have been conducted in men with established prostate cancer. GTCs may have a role in arresting disease development in prostate cancer according to a double-blind, placebo-controlled study (Bettuzzi et al 2008). Sixty volunteers with high-grade prostate intraepithelial neoplasis and therefore at high risk of prostate cancer were treated with GTCs (three capsules of 200 mg/day) or placebo over 12 months. Of the 30 men in the GTC group, only one tumour was diagnosed, as opposed to nine cases in the placebo group. The GTC group also scored higher on the quality-of-life scores and had reduced lower urinary tract symptoms and no side effects were detected (Bettuzzi et al 2006). An update for this trial was undertaken 2 years later to see if the prostate cancer was merely delayed rather than prevented in the green tea group. Half the original subjects (equal numbers from placebo and green tea cohorts) agreed to further investigations, which detected one more tumour in the GTC group and two more in the placebo group. These results suggest that GTC given for a year may offer long-term protection within this at-risk group and might be useful as first-line preventive therapy. More recently, a small open-label study of 26 men (aged 41–68 years) with a recent diagnosis of prostate cancer (stage I, II or III) were given 800 mg EGCG (Polyphenon E) daily in the time between biopsy and radical prostatectomy and serum levels of prostate-specific antigen, hepatocyte growth factor, insulin-like growth factor-1 and vascular endothelial growth factor all decreased significantly with the median dosing period of 34.5 days. The authors also noted that there were no adverse effects on the liver observed during the study (McLarty et al 2009). This same trend was found in a RCT of 50 diagnosed prostate cancer patients given Polyphenon E or placebo for 3–6 weeks prior to surgery. Although not significant, biomarkers did show some chemopreventive potential with decreased prostate-specific antigen and insulin-like growth factors. However, it was found that apoptosis and angiogenesis did not differ in either group and the bioavailability of the polyphenols in the prostate tissue was low (Nguyen et al 2012). The authors suggested that longer term and larger controlled trials would be useful to verify findings.

In contrast, a small study testing green tea (6 g/day) in patients with pre-existing androgen-independent prostate cancer found little effect on PSA levels (Jatoi et al 2003). Similar results were obtained in a small study of 19 patients with hormone-refractory prostate cancer given a lower dose of 250 mg capsules of green tea twice a day (Choan et al 2005). It is likely that both these studies did not use a green tea treatment with sufficient concentrations of catechins or a high enough dose.

Leukaemia

A clinical trial with 42 patients with Rai stage 0–II early stage of chronic lymphocytic leukaemia, who were asymptomatic and not eligible to begin chemotherapy, were given Polyphenon E (2000 mg twice daily) for up to 6 months and found declines in the absolute lymphocyte count and lymphadenopathy in the majority of patients (Shanafelt et al 2013). This is a possible novel use as a low-toxicity early intervention, but randomised trials are needed to affirm these findings.

Adjunct in breast cancer treatment

Ten radiotherapy patients with non-inflammatory breast cancer (locally advanced) in a small 8-week study were randomly assigned to radiotherapy plus EGCG (400 mg three times daily) or radiotherapy plus placebo. The green tea treatment group showed serum changes, including suppression of cell proliferation and invasion, a reduction in metalloproteinase-9 and metalloproteinase-2 expression and lower serum vascular endothelial growth factor. This additive apoptotic effect with the radiation treatment suggests that green tea polyphenols have potential as an adjunctive treatment in breast cancer (Zhang et al 2012a).

Reducing cancer drug side effects

An animal study has suggested a possible novel use of green tea to protect against nephrotoxicity caused by the use of cisplatin, a chemotherapy drug used to treat a variety of cancers (Khan et al 2009b).

Some recent research has experimented with nanochemoprevention with encapsulated EGCG which enhanced the bioavailability of the EGCG by 10-fold. In the future this nanoparticle-mediated delivery could be used to reduce toxicity side effects of chemotherapy drugs (Siddiqui et al 2009).

Cardiovascular protection

Epidemiological studies suggest that green tea consumption is associated with a reduced risk of cardiovascular disease (CVD) (Kuriyama 2008, Maeda et al 2003). Its antioxidant effects may explain some of the CVD benefits and a recent systematic review of 31 RCTs found 0.6–1.5 L/day of green tea increased antioxidant capacity and reduced lipid peroxidation (Ellinger et al 2011). A systematic review of literature reported that observational studies indicated protection against stroke, atherosclerosis and hypertension for green tea drinkers (Clement 2009) and a recent review included four systematic reviews (Hooper et al 2008, Kim et al 2011, Wang et al 2011, Zheng et al 2011b) and meta-analysis, suggesting that, although evidence is not robust for a reduction in coronary artery disease (CAD), some RCTs do indicate that green tea may be effective in reducing LDLs and total cholesterol (Johnson et al 2012). This is confirmed by a recent Cochrane review reporting on 11 RCTs (n = 821), with seven of these trials on green tea alone (five on green tea tablets or capsules and two with tea drinking). The authors concluded that total cholesterol, LDL-cholesterol and blood pressure were significantly reduced with green tea consumption. They recommend caution in interpreting these results, as there were only a small number of studies in this analysis (Hartley et al 2013).

G

A 2000 prospective cohort study of 8552 people in Japan found that those consuming more than 10 cups a day, compared with those consuming fewer than three cups, had a decreased relative risk of death from CVD (Nakachi et al 2000). The Ohsaki National Health Insurance Cohort Study was a population-based study in Japan, spanning 11 years (1995–2005) with 40,530 Japanese adults aged 40–79 years. At baseline, no participants had cancer or coronary heart disease. The study identified an inverse association between green tea consumption and mortality due to CVD (especially mortality due to stroke) as well as all other causes. A significant protective effect was shown at a dose of five cups or more daily for men and three or more cups daily for women. Overall, the protective effects were greatest for women compared to men (Kuriyama et al 2006b). The investigators suggested higher smoking levels in men may have reduced potential benefits in this group (Cheng 2007).

Some 76,979 subjects from another Japanese study (Japan Collaborative Cohort Study for Evaluation of Cancer Risk) were included in a prospective study assessing tea drinking and mortality from CVD. The individuals did not have coronary heart disease nor had they had a stroke at the onset of the study. There were 1362 deaths from strokes and 650 deaths from CVD over the 13.1-year follow-up. The analysis found that a moderate intake of green tea was associated with lower CVD mortality. For coronary heart disease this benefit was more for women, who drank six or more cups of green tea a day (a 38% lower risk of mortality) (Mineharu et al 2011). Similarly, analysis from the Japan Public Health Center-Based Study, with a slightly larger cohort of 82,369, found that higher green tea drinkers had an inverse association with strokes (especially intracerebral haemorrhage) and CVD in the general population. The participants completed self-administered food frequency questionnaires over a 13-year period (Kokubo et al 2013).

Elderly people in a Japanese population-based study of 14,001 were followed for 6 years and drinking seven or more cups a day exerted a reduced risk of cardiovascular mortality (Suzuki et al 2009). A meta-analysis that included data from nine epidemiological studies with 4378 stroke incidences found a 21% lower risk of stroke among green or black tea drinkers if they consumed three or more cups a day (Arab et al 2009). These benefits of green tea drinking were not confirmed in a Dutch population study using a validated food frequency questionnaire (n = 37,514) over 13 years, where they found no correlation with tea drinking and stroke. The difference in findings with other population studies may be because most of the tea was black and not green tea (de Koning Gans et al 2010). Well-designed RCTs would be helpful to establish a benefit in reducing risk of stroke. However, this same large Dutch cohort of healthy men and women did appear to benefit from a reduction in coronary heart disease mortality by drinking three to six cups of tea a day (some green tea but mainly black tea). Relatively few people died from either stroke or coronary heart disease during the study, making associations with tea drinking difficult to evaluate (de Koning Gans et al 2010). In a later meta-analysis (13 studies on black tea and five studies with green tea), green but not black tea showed a significant association with reducing risk for the highest green tea drinkers. Including an additional cup of green tea per day was associated with a 10% decrease in CAD risk. This inverse association between green tea and CAD was found in the case-control studies, which may not be strong evidence given problems with recall or selection bias in retrospective studies. Thus the authors suggest the protective role of green tea is tentative and large prospective cohort studies are needed (Wang et al 2011). It may be that the catechins in green tea provide protection in CAD, whereas black tea benefits are more associated with heart disease (Di Castelnuovo et al 2012).

Lipid lowering

An increasing body of research suggests that green tea given to patients with hypercholesterolaemia may lower total and LDL-cholesterol levels but there is less robust evidence that triglycerides or high-density lipoproteins (HDLs) are impacted.

A recent Cochrane review included evidence from seven RCTs on green tea with varied doses (five studies with 375–600 mg daily of green tea extract and two studies on green tea beverages). The review reported a statistically significant reduction in total cholesterol (MD –0.62 mmol/L, 95% CI –0.77 to –0.46) and LDL-cholesterol (MD –0.64 mmol/L, 95% CI –0.77 to –0.52) compared to placebo, with a trend towards a reduction in triglycerides (Hartley et al 2013). A meta-analysis including 20 trials found that total and LDL-cholesterol levels were lowered with green tea but no effect was found on HDL-cholesterol or triglycerides. Subgroup analysis suggested that people with normal cholesterol levels found no benefit and there appeared to be no significant effect with green tea capsules. The heterogeneity of the studies limits the meta-analysis. It appears that higher-dose catechins may be more effective and further studies on dose and duration of green tea drinking are needed (Kim et al 2011). Another meta-analysis in the same year included 14 RCTs (n = 1136) and confirmed that green tea reduced both total and LDL-cholesterol but exerted no effect on HDLs, although these researchers found both green tea drinking and extracts were beneficial (Zheng et al 2011b).

A significant reduction in LDL-cholesterol and triglycerides and marked increase in HDL-cholesterol was also found for green tea consumption (400 mg given three times daily) in a double-blind, placebo, RCT of 78 obese women conducted over 12 weeks (Hsu et al 2008). Similar results were obtained in an early cross-sectional study involving 1371 men aged over 40 years (Imai & Nakachi 1995). The study showed that increased green tea consumption was associated with decreased serum concentrations of total cholesterol and triglyceride and an increase in HDL, together with a decrease in LDL and very-low-density lipoprotein cholesterols. Fifty-six obese hypertensive patients entered a randomised, double-blind, placebo-controlled trial and green tea supplementation did increase HDL-cholesterol as well as lower total and LDL-cholesterol. The treated group were given a green tea extract capsule (379 mg) daily for 3 months (Bogdanski et al 2012). Other studies have found no significant HDL effect which may be limited to patient subgroups.

In contrast, the inclusion of 3 g/day (145 mg of EGCG in 500 mL water daily) of green tea to a cholesterol-lowering diet provided no further lipid-lowering effects according to a study of 100 hypercholesterolaemic patients (Bertipaglia de Santana et al 2008). While green tea increased antioxidant potential, there was no significant reduction in any cholesterol parameters. This result may be explained by the low dose compared to other studies.

Hypertension

Research is now beginning to find antihypertensive benefits for green tea and large, longer-term, well-designed studies are needed. A recent Cochrane review included three trials which measured blood pressure (Bogdanski et al 2012, Nantz et al 2009) and on analysis found a statistically significant reduction in both systolic (MD −3.18 mmHg, 95% CI −5.25 to −1.11) and diastolic blood pressure (MD −3.42, 95% CI −4.54 to −2.30) (Hartley et al 2013). Blood pressure was significantly reduced in an RCT of 56 obese, hypertensive patients taking one capsule a day of 379 mg of a green tea extract (with 208 mg of EGCG from Olimp Labs, Debica, Poland) for over 3 months. At the end of the trial both systolic and diastolic blood pressure had reduced significantly, tumour necrosis factor-α and C-reactive protein were significantly reduced, fasting glucose and insulin levels had lowered, along with a reduction in LDL and total cholesterol and an increase in HDL-cholesterol. This small study shows promise for a multifaceted benefit for obese patients with hypertension (Bogdanski et al 2012). Another small trial with 46 obese male patients found a reduction in diastolic blood pressure (by a modest 2.5 mmHg) but no other metabolic effects were observed. The intervention was a 400 mg capsule twice a day for 8 weeks (Teavigo with 97% pure EGCG) (Brown et al 2009). In a randomised, double-blind placebo study of 111 healthy volunteers a green tea extract (200 mg decaffeinated catechin green tea extract Cardio Guard) was given twice daily. There was a reduction in systolic (5 mmHg) and diastolic (4 mmHg) blood pressure after only 3 weeks and after 3 months systolic blood pressure remained significantly lower. Other cardiovascular markers, including total and LDL-cholesterol-lowering effects, were also noted and there was a 42% reduction in serum amyloid-α (a marker of chronic inflammation) (Nantz et al 2009).

Weight loss

Animal studies have found that green tea consumption reduces food intake, decreases leptin levels and body weight and increases thermogenesis.

Clinical studies investigating the effects of green tea on weight loss have produced mixed results; however green tea in some studies suggests moderate weight loss, reduction in waist circumference and improvement in metabolic parameters and may be helpful when combined with an exercise program. The wide disparity in green teas, green tea extracts and dosage protocols hampers the pooling of results, in meta-analyses, in a meaningful way.

A recent Cochrane review included RCTs of overweight adults with trials of at least 12 weeks. They included six studies outside Japan; a small, non-significant reduction in weight, waist circumference and body mass index (BMI) was found which was unlikely to be clinically relevant. The data from the eight Japanese studies could not be pooled and again some small non-significant improvements in weight loss were seen in some studies. There was no significant benefit on weight maintenance (Jurgens et al 2012). A meta-analysis including 11 studies suggests that green tea has a small beneficial effect on weight loss and weight maintenance (Hursel et al 2009). A systematic review and meta-analysis comparing GTC benefits with and without caffeine found, of the 15 studies included, that the GTCs alone did not show anthropometric benefit; however GTCs with caffeine showed modest benefit with reduced weight, BMI and waist circumference compared with caffeine alone (Phung et al 2010).

One open study found that a green tea extract AR25 (80% ethanolic dry extract standardised at 25% catechins) taken by moderately obese patients resulted in a 4.6% decrease in body weight and 4.5% decrease in waist circumference after 3 months' treatment (Chantre & Lairon 2002). Both groups lost the same amount of weight and displayed similar metabolic parameters at the end of the study period. An RCT study in Thailand was undertaken over 12 weeks with 60 obese individuals all given a similar diet of three meals a day with 65% carbohydrates, 15% protein and 20% fat. There was no significant difference in weight loss at week 4 but at weeks 8 and 12 weight reduction was significantly greater in the green tea group than the placebo group. The difference in weight loss between the groups was 2.70 kg at 4 weeks, 5.10 kg at 8 weeks and 3.3 kg at 12 weeks. Researchers suggested the effects were due to changes in resting energy expenditure and fat oxidation (Auvichayapat et al 2008). However, two other studies produced negative findings. One double-blind, placebo-controlled parallel trial, with 46 women attempting a weight-loss program over 87 days, showed no difference between the green tea group and the placebo group (Diepvens et al 2005). Another double-blind, placebo RCT, with 78 obese women, also showed no significant difference in body weight, BMI or waist circumference after taking a green tea extract capsule of 400 mg three times a day for 12 weeks (Hsu et al 2008). An RCT (n = 104) of Chinese participants with high levels of visceral fat found a significant reduction in abdominal visceral fat and body weight by drinking a catechin-enriched green tea (609.3 mg catechins and 68.7 mg caffeine) daily for 12 weeks (Zhang et al 2012b).

A randomised clinical trial using a highly bioavailable form of green tea (Monoselect Camellia containing GreenSelect Phytosome) was used in a study with 100 overweight participants who were all assigned low-calorie diets and half of them given the green tea extract. After 90 days the diet-only group lost 5 kg in weight while the diet plus green tea group lost 14 kg. Males in the study also experienced a significant reduction in waistline measurement by 14% compared to 7% in the diet-only group. Other metabolic parameters were improved in both groups, including LDL, HDL-cholesterol, triglycerides, growth hormone, insulin and cortisol. This particular green tea extract appears to potentiate weight loss in combination with a calorie-controlled diet (Di Pierro et al 2009). More research is needed to confirm the findings of this bioavailable form of green tea.

There is some emerging research on benefit for obese patients with metabolic syndrome due to the effect green tea has on weight loss, lowering of lipids, improving blood glucose regulation and cardiovascular health (Thielecke & Boschmann 2009). A randomised, controlled prospective trial with 35 participants with obesity and metabolic syndrome were assigned placebo, four cups of green tea (equivalent of 440 mg EGCG) or green tea extract (two capsules a day totalling 460 mg EGCG). After 8 weeks a significant reduction in body weight and BMI was reported in both the green tea groups. Biomarkers of oxidative stress and lipid peroxidation including LDL-cholesterol also had a modest reduction. In this subgroup green tea may have potential, and further research would be recommended to confirm the findings (Basu et al 2010).

A small intervention study of elderly patients with metabolic syndrome found that drinking three cups of green tea a day for 60 days significantly reduced weight, waist circumference and BMI compared to placebo. There were no changes in biochemical parameters (Vieira Senger et al 2012). In a recent RCT with 46 obese participants given green tea extract (379 mg a day) or placebo over

3 months, the supplemented group had a reduction in BMI, waist circumference, total and LDL-cholesterol, triglycerides and glucose. The green tea extract group also saw an increase in antioxidant levels and zinc, HDL-cholesterol and magnesium, although iron levels were lower than the placebo group. This study shows potential for multieffect benefits for obese patients taking green tea extract (Suliburska et al 2012).

Combination of green tea with exercise for weight loss

Some small trials have shown additional benefits when dietary changes and exercise have been included in the studies. A recent double-blind, placebo-controlled trial with 36 overweight or obese women included dietary changes and resistance training over a 4-week period. They reported significant increases in resting metabolic rate, lean body mass and strength and significant reduction in waist circumference, body fat and triglycerides when combining green tea with resistance training compared with placebo and resistance training only (Cardoso et al 2013). Another study (n = 107) of overweight or obese participants over 12 weeks randomly assigned a green tea drink (625 mg catechins and 39 mg caffeine) or control drink (39 mg caffeine) and all participants were asked to do 180 minutes of moderate-intensity exercise each week. The trend (non-significant) was towards a reduction in weight, subcutaneous abdominal fat and triglycerides in the catechin group (Maki et al 2009). Further research is needed to see if green tea enhances the weight loss benefits of an exercise training program.

Diabetes

Animal studies have identified that green tea polyphenols reduce serum glucose levels and improve kidney function in diabetes (Rhee et al 2002, Sabu et al 2002) and may be helpful in preventing diabetic nephropathy (Kang et al 2012). Evidence from human trials has been contradictory and it may be that green tea is beneficial for some subgroups. A recent meta-analysis of 17 trials (including seven high-quality trials with the remainder low-quality) reported significant lowering of fasting glucose concentrations (−0.09 mmol/L; 95% CI: −015 to −0.03 mmol/L; $P < 0.01$) compared with controls and with HbA_{1C} (−0.30%; 95% CI: −0.37, −0.22%; $P \leq 0.01$). There was no significant change in fasting insulin or homeostatic model assessment of insulin resistance (HOMA-IR) values. Interestingly, subgroup analysis found that green tea lowered fasting glucose in those at risk of metabolic syndrome but not in healthy subjects and a high dose of catechins was more effective. In further analysis the higher-quality trials also showed green tea significantly reduced fasting insulin (Liu et al 2013). Another meta-analysis in the same year included 22 RCTs with 1584 participants and found a significant decrease in fasting blood glucose with GTCs (with or without caffeine) (−1.48 mg/dL; 95% CI: −2.57, −0.40 mg/dL) over a 12-week time period, but not in the shorter treatment protocols under 12 weeks. No significant effect was found with fasting blood insulin, HbA_{1C} or insulin resistance (HOMA-IR), but this could be because only a small number of the trials actually reported on these parameters. The trials included in this meta-analysis were pooled studies with diabetic, obese, metabolic syndrome and healthy patients; therefore outcome for diabetic patients alone may differ. The authors report conflicting results on dose of green tea consumption for the glucose metabolism effect and suggest further research is needed on the dose-response relationship and also to understand more about postprandial glycaemic variables (Zheng et al 2013b). One double-blind RCT with 49 individuals with type 2 diabetes mellitus found no significant hypoglycaemic effects for green tea given at 375 mg or

750 mg/day (MacKenzie et al 2007). Another RCT of 66 diabetic patients found 500 mg/day of green tea polyphenols had no clear effect on blood glucose or insulin resistance markers (Fukino et al 2005). A more recent randomised, double-blind and placebo-controlled trial with 68 obese type 2 diabetics found no significant difference in diabetic markers over 16 weeks with a decaffeinated green tea extract (500 mg three times daily 30 minutes after meals). However, some within-group comparisons did find significant reduction in HbA_{1C}, waist circumference, HOMA-IR index and insulin levels and increase in the appetite-regulating hormone ghrelin (Hsu et al 2011). A cross-over RCT with 60 borderline diabetic patients reported a significant reduction in HbA_{1C} levels and a borderline significant reduction in diastolic blood pressure after 2 months of green tea extract powder (456 mg catechins) daily. No changes were noted for weight, BMI, systolic blood pressure, lipids or fasting serum glucose levels (Fukino et al 2008). The bioavailability of some green tea extracts may vary and in some studies serum EGCG was detected in only half the subjects after early-morning testing, which could explain why some researchers report significant changes to diabetic markers and others non-significant changes. It appears that taking the green tea extract for at least 12 weeks is more beneficial and in most studies some of the diabetic markers are positively impacted, even if modestly so.

An epidemiological study of 542 men and women, aged over 65 years, from the Mediterranean islands found that tea consumption (green and black) was associated with reduced levels of fasting glucose but this was only in the non-obese subjects (Polychronopoulos et al 2008). The same MEDIS study in the Mediterranean islands evaluated 300 elderly men and women and found that long-term tea drinking (green and black) was associated with a reduction of risk of type 2 diabetes (Panagiotakos et al 2009).

Dental caries and gingivitis

Green tea extract tablets, gels, mouthwash and chewable oral preparations have been investigated for effects on dental plaque formation and gingival health under RCT conditions, overall producing favourable results (Liu & Chi 2000). Recent research also suggests potential for preventing caries.

A double-blind study investigated the effects of GTCs and polyphenols on the gingiva when used in the form of chewable oral sweets (Krahwinkel & Willershausen 2000). Compared with placebo, the green tea product chewed eight times a day significantly decreased gingival inflammation and improved periodontal structures before the 21-day test period was complete.

Another study investigated Chinese green tea polyphenol tablets for effects on plaque formation in 150 volunteers (Liu & Chi 2000). The randomised, controlled crossover study showed that green tea polyphenol tablets used for 2 weeks were able to reduce the plaque index compared with placebo treatment. Thirty chronic periodontitis patients were included in an RCT, with the treated group using a thermo-reversible sustained-release green tea gel. At the end of the 4-week trial the green tea group had a significant reduction in oral pocket depth and gingival index, showing a benefit and reduction in inflammation in these periodontitis patients (Chava & Vedula 2013).

A recent pilot study in a dental clinic concluded that rinsing with a green tea solution strongly inhibited *Streptococcus mutans* growth in saliva and plaque and reduced the gingival bleeding index score. The authors suggested further research to find out if a green tea mouthwash can reduce the prevalence of dental caries (Awadalla et al 2011). Another single-blinded RCT gave 25 high school female students, with gingivitis, a green tea mouthwash twice a day. They reported improvements on all periodontal indices over the 5-week study, although these improvements were not statistically significant (Jenabian et al 2012). In an RCT with 60 children a green tea mouthwash was as effective as sodium fluoride in reducing oral *S. mutans* and lactobacillus indicating a potential use for reduction in caries (Tehrani et al 2011).

Green tea drinking, in a study with 940 Japanese men, has also been found to have a small inverse association with periodontal disease (Kushiyama et al 2009).

Genital warts

A number of recent trials have shown good effectivity for a topical treatment (Polyphenon E, Medigene EU) containing a fixed amount of GTCs in the treatment of genital warts. The product is marketed as Veregen in the United States. It is thought the mechanism of action is a combination of immune enhancement, cell apoptosis and inhibition of human papillomavirus (Stockfleth & Meyer 2012).

A systematic review and meta-analysis included three RCTs of Polyphenon E (Gross 2008, Stockfleth et al 2008, Tatti et al 2008) with a total of 660 men and 587 women. It reported a significantly higher chance of complete clearance with the green tea product and very low recurrence rates with both the 10% ointment cream and 15% ointment. There was good tolerability, although some side effects were noted of erythema and localised skin itching (Tzellos et al 2011). Healing of genital warts occurred in 54.9% of patients using Polyphenon E ointment compared with 35.4% of patients receiving placebo in three placebo-controlled clinical studies (n = 1400) (Gross 2008). Another trial with the same Polyphenon E topical treatment evaluated 503 patients, with external genital and perianal warts, who were randomised to be treated with a 15% or 10% ointment or placebo. Treatment was applied three times a day for up to 16 weeks. After follow-up, 12 weeks later, 53% of patients with the 15% strength ointment had complete clearance, 51% for the 10% ointment and 37% for the control vehicle. A greater number of women experienced total clearance of all warts (with the Polyphenon E treatment compared to men, 60% compared to 45%: Stockfleth et al 2008). Another double-blind, placebo-controlled RCT of 502 patients with genital and perianal warts used a topical treatment of sinecatechins (a defined green tea extract), which was found to be effective and well tolerated. The findings were significant at weeks 4 and 6 and at subsequent visits over the 16-week trial. Complete clearance of warts was obtained in 57% of patients compared with only 33% with the control group (Tatti et al 2008).

Infections

Influenza

A potential novel use of green tea has been studied preventing influenza infection. A randomised, double-blind, placebo-controlled trial found the green tea group had significantly lower incidence of flu, a lower incidence of viral antigen measured in the laboratory and a significantly longer time free from the influenza infection from the start of the green tea intervention. This 5-month RCT with 200 health workers during the flu season administered six capsules of green tea extract a day (total catechins 378 mg/day and theanine 210 mg/day) or placebo. Larger trials are needed but this study may demonstrate a potential use as a prophylactic agent for influenza (Matsumoto et al 2011).

An observational study of 2663 schoolchildren in Japan gained information from questionnaires during the flu season and found an inverse association between drinking 1–5 cups a day of green tea and influenza infection (Park et al 2011).

Pneumonia

The Ohsaki cohort study in Japan followed up 19,079 men and 21,493 women (aged 40–79 years) and found 406 reported deaths from pneumonia and, although no significant association was found for men drinking green tea, it was found that green tea consumption for women did reduce the risk of dying from pneumonia (Watanabe et al 2009).

Tuberculosis

A study of 200 newly diagnosed patients with acid-fast bacilli-positive pulmonary tuberculosis were randomly assigned to receive catechin (500 mcg) or placebo. Patients were undergoing conventional treatment and after 1 and 4 months the patients with the green tea extract had a reduction in oxidative stress (Agarwal et al 2010). With further studies there may be a role for green tea extract as an adjuvant therapy in tuberculosis patients.

Sunburn protection and skin ageing

More than 150 in vitro and in vivo studies have reported the benefits of green tea for the skin (Hsu 2005). Many mechanisms appear to be responsible: green tea protects against ultraviolet and psoralen + ultraviolet A-induced carcinogenesis and DNA damage and is a potent antioxidant, anti-inflammatory, anticarcinogenic and vulnerary (Hsu 2005). Research with human volunteers has found that topical application of green tea to skin half an hour before ultraviolet exposure protects against the development of sunburn and epidermal damage (Elmets et al 2001). The effect is dose-dependent and strongest for the EGCG and epicatechin gallate polyphenols.

A 2-year, double-blind randomised placebo-controlled trial of oral supplementation of green tea reported significant improvement at 6 months in solar damage and improvement at 12 months in erythema and telangiectasias, although these improvements were not sustained to the 2-year end of the trial. At the end of 2 years there was no significant improvement in photoageing of the skin. The trial included 56 women who were randomised to take 250 mg of green tea polyphenols twice a day or placebo. This was a low dose of green tea extract and further research may be useful to confirm findings (Janjua et al 2009).

Liver disease

A recent meta-analysis reported borderline significance showing green tea was preventive (for both men and women) in reducing the risk of developing primary liver cancer (Fon Sing et al 2011). A systematic review of 10 studies showed that increased green tea consumption is associated with a reduced risk of liver disease. The studies were published between the years 1995 and 2005, with numbers of subjects ranging from 52 to 29,090. Of the 10 studies, four were RCTs, two cohort, one case–control and three cross-sectional studies. Among them, eight studies were conducted in China, one in Japan and the other in the United States. Most of the studies used adjustments such as age, sex, smoking and drinking to control potential confounders and the study periods varied from less than 6 months to more than 6 years. Eight studies yielded statistically significant results, showing a protective role of green tea against liver disease, whereas two studies only showed a partial tendency. Also, four studies showed a positive association between green tea intake and attenuation of liver disease. When considering the protective effects of green tea against subgroups of liver diseases, it seems that they are more effective in fatty liver disease and liver disorders (Jin et al 2008); The protective effect of green tea drinking to reduce liver cancer risk appears to be stronger for high-risk patients with hepatitis B or C and also for long-term green tea drinkers. Despite these promising results, more rigorous double-blind studies are still required to confirm the results as the studies used in the review were heterogeneous and differed in the design, outcome, tea dosage and other aspects.

OTHER USES

Green tea has many other uses, based on results of animal or in vitro tests or on the known pharmacological activity of constituents such as tannin and caffeine. Some of these other uses are treatment of diarrhoea, Crohn's disease, dyspepsia and other digestive symptoms, promoting alertness and cognitive performance, reducing symptoms of headache and promoting diuresis.

Allergic rhinitis

A novel study suggests drinking tea may provide benefits for seasonal allergic rhinitis. The trial was an open-label, single-dose, randomised study of 38 subjects in Japan. Half the participants drank the benifuuki green tea (34 mg *O*-methylated catechin) daily for 1.5 months before the cedar pollen season while the other group commenced at the start of the pollen season. The symptoms of throat pain, nose blowing and disturbance in daily life were significantly lower in the group taking the tea for the longer period pre-pollen season. This same group of researchers had previously reported that benifuuki green tea containing *O*-methylated catechin had reduced perennial or seasonal rhinitis whereas the placebo green tea did not. It may be the *O*-methylated catechins are required for this effect and more studies are warranted (Maeda-Yamamoto et al 2009).

Ulcerative colitis

Animal studies have shown anti-inflammatory activity in colitis (Varilek et al 2001, Westphal et al 2008). A double-blinded pilot study of 20 patients with mild to moderate ulcerative colitis achieved a 53% remission rate compared with 0% for placebo after daily doses of Polyphenon E (400 mg or 800 mg of EGCG daily) for 56 days. The remission results were based on the ulcerative colitis disease activity index and the inflammatory bowel disease questionnaire and 10 of the 15 patients in the Polyphenon E group responded to treatment. The authors suggest Polyphenon E may offer a novel therapy for mild to moderate ulcerative colitis (Dryden et al 2013).

Dementia/cognitive impairment

Several in vivo studies have demonstrated memory improvement in older animals for green tea extract and improvements in spatial cognition learning ability after long-term administration of GTCs (Haque et al 2006, Kaur et al 2008). In healthy adults a small RCT with 27 participants found a significant improvement in cerebral blood flow with the lower dose of 135 mg of EGCG (and not with the higher dose of 270 mg). These doses were given on two separate days and no significant improvement was found with mood or cognitive performance (Wightman et al 2012). A community-based self-administered questionnaire of 1003 Japanese geriatric people found that greater ingestion of green tea was associated with lower cognitive impairment (Kuriyama et al 2006a). Green tea intake was significantly associated with better cognitive performance in a 2-year follow-up study of Japanese elderly (Hasegawa et al 2005).

Depression

Novel research in Japan with 537 men and women in a cross-sectional study, using a validated dietary questionnaire, found a 51% lower prevalence of depression in those drinking four or more cups of green tea a day compared to one cup (Pham et al 2013).

Beta-thalassaemia

In vitro research shows green tea (tannins) chelates iron, which could prove useful in patients with conditions such as beta-thalassaemia (Srichairatanakool et al 2006). Beta-thalassaemic mice (with iron overload due to transfusions) were fed green tea extract and a reduction in liver iron content resulted. This may prove to be a novel therapy to chelate liver iron overload in beta-thalassaemia patients (Saewong et al 2010).

Amyloid light-chain amyloidosis

This rare disease, causing amyloid deposits in different organs, can affect the heart. Green tea's cardiac benefits may be useful in this condition when there is cardiac involvement. In a small longitudinal observational study of 59 patients with amyloid light-chain amyloidosis with cardiac involvement it was found that green tea polyphenol EGCG produced a significant reduction in left ventricular wall thickness. A reduction of 2 mm of wall thickness occurred in 11 patients; heart functionality was also improved, as was left ventricular ejection fraction. The patients either drank 1.5–2 L of green tea daily or consumed green tea extracts of 600–800 mg EGCG over a 6-month time period (Mereles et al 2010). This novel study requires more research to confirm findings.

Renal failure

Green tea extract blocks the development of cardiac hypertrophy in experimental renal failure and reduces oxidative stress, according to the results of investigation with animal models (Priyadarshi et al 2003, Yokozawa et al 1996).

Urinary stones

Two in vivo and in vitro studies have shown that green tea's antioxidant action may inhibit kidney stone formation (Itoh et al 2005, Jeong et al 2006).

Osteoporosis

There are several in vitro and animal studies as well as emerging human epidemiological research showing promise for green tea in improving bone health. Its mechanism of action is thought to be enhancing osteoblast activity, reducing osteoclasts plus osteoprotection through anti-inflammatory and antioxidant action, leading to a reduction in bone loss (Shen et al 2009, 2011, Tokuda et al 2008). Clinical studies are needed to confirm these findings and to assess if green tea results in fracture reduction. In a study, 150 postmenopausal women with osteopenia were randomised to have green tea supplement (500 mg daily) and/or tai chi exercise over 6 months. Muscle strength and bone formation biomarkers were improved by both green tea and tai chi exercise (Shen et al 2012).

DOSAGE RANGE

The dose varies depending on the indication it is being used for. Some research suggests 8–10 cups of green tea/day are required for effects whereas others indicate only 3–5 cups of green tea/day are required. It is likely that the dose also depends on the quality of the green tea and the concentration of GTCs in the preparation When used as a green tea extract in capsule form in high doses for long periods, green tea may have the potential to have adverse effects (Schonthal 2011).

- For external genital and perianal warts: Polyphenon E 10–15% strength ointment applied three times daily.
- For reduced risk of cancers: five or more cups daily.
- For CVD protection: 3–10 cups daily.
- For treatment for periodontal disease: use of gel, chewable tablets or mouthwash twice daily for 2–4 weeks.

ADVERSE REACTIONS

Due to the caffeine content of the herb, CNS stimulation and diuresis are possible when consumed in large amounts. Teeth staining is also possible due to the tannin content of the herb.

One clinical study found an absence of any severe adverse effects when 15 green tea tablets were taken daily (2.25 g green tea extracts, 337.5 mg EGCG and 135 mg caffeine) for 6 months (Fujiki et al 1999). One trial with high-dose green tea (600 mg/day) reported adverse effects in 69% of the patients with a range of adverse effects, including insomnia, fatigue, nausea, vomiting, diarrhoea, abdominal pain and confusion (Jatoi et al 2003).

There are rare, idiosyncratic reports of altered liver function with the consumption of green tea. A review of green tea and hepatic reactions found 34 cases of hepatitis with a positive rechallenge in 29 cases. There was one reported death (where there were other confounding factors, such as drugs and alcohol) and a positive rechallenge in seven cases. The authors suggest a causal association between green tea and liver damage which could be related to particular conditions and concomitant medications may be part of the picture (Mazzanti et al 2009). Frequently the green tea products were not fully analysed and others contained a herbal combination, making it difficult to definitively establish a causal relationship between green tea extracts and hepatotoxicity (Schonthal 2011). The US pharmacopeia similarly reports 27 cases where green tea is a possible causality and seven cases as a probable causality of liver damage. They reported that liver issues may be worse if the extract is taken under fasting conditions or on an empty stomach. This committee concluded that, when dietary supplements are formulated and manufactured appropriately, there are no significant safety issues with green tea but there should be caution with use (Sarma et al 2008). Another case report of acute hepatitis occurred in 2009 after consuming a green tea supplement; other causes were excluded and there was a rapid recovery after cessation of the supplement. However other studies have demonstrated no hepatotoxic effects, such as the placebo-controlled parallel study with healthy men taking six capsules of green tea extract daily (714 mg/day green tea polyphenols) for 3 weeks, where no significant changes in biomarkers of liver function or cardiovascular risk markers were found (Frank et al 2009). This was only a small study of 17 and so had no statistical power. Other studies have shown green tea to be effective in reducing liver disease (Jin et al 2008) and liver cancer (Ui et al 2009) and one trial using 1.3 g daily of GTCs reported no abnormalities in liver function tests when used for the duration of around 34 days (McLarty et al 2009).

There is one case report of thrombotic thrombocytopenic purpura after a 38-year-old woman consumed a weight loss product containing green tea extract (200 mg) for 2 months. After being hospitalised for 20 days and treated, her neurological symptoms reduced and platelet count and haematocrit levels normalised. The green tea preparation has been classed as a 'possible' cause of this condition developing in this woman and, as there are no other reported cases, it has been suggested that this could be an idiosyncratic drug reaction. The authors suggest that doctors be aware of this rare condition developing after ingesting green tea (Liatsos et al 2010).

When used over a 16-week period for genital warts, erythema and localised skin itching may occur (Tzellos et al 2011).

SIGNIFICANT INTERACTIONS

Few controlled studies are available for green tea, so interactions are speculative and based on evidence of pharmacological activity or known actions of key constituents such as caffeine and tannins.

Anticoagulants

Antagonistic interaction — a case of excessive consumption (2.25–4.5 L of green tea/day) was reported to inhibit warfarin activity and decrease the international normalised ratio (Taylor & Wilt 1999). Whether this is an exceptional case or representative of an expected interaction remains to be determined.

Hypoglycaemic agents

Caffeine-containing beverages can increase blood sugar levels when used in sufficient quantity (200 mg of caffeine); however, hypoglycaemic activity has been reported for green tea, which could theoretically negate this effect (Ulbricht & Basch 2005) — the outcome of this combination is uncertain, therefore observe the patient.

Iron

Tannins found in herbs such as *Camellia sinensis* can bind to iron and reduce its absorption — separate doses by at least 2 hours. Protein and iron have also been found to interact with tea polyphenols and decrease their antioxidant effects in vitro (Alexandropoulou et al 2006). The clinical significance of this is as yet unknown.

CNS stimulants

Based on the caffeine content of the herb, high intakes of green tea can theoretically increase the CNS stimulation effects of drugs such as nicotine and beta-adrenergic agonists (e.g. salbutamol); however, the clinical significance of this is unknown — observe patient.

CNS depressants

Based on the caffeine content of the herb, high intakes of green tea can theoretically decrease the CNS-depressant effects of drugs such as benzodiazepines; however, the clinical significance of this is unknown — observe patient.

Antidepressants

Based on theoretical considerations, caution is advised when using highly concentrated supplements with monoamine oxidase inhibitors or dopamimetic drugs because catechins are metabolised by catechol-*O*-methyltransferase (Shord et al 2009).

Bortezomib (BZM) and other boronic acid-based proteasome inhibitors

EGCG was tested in vitro and in vivo to investigate whether combining it with the proteasome inhibitor BZM, commonly used in the treatment of multiple myeloma, would result in an increase in the drug's antitumour activity (Golden et al 2009). Green tea extract almost completely blocked the effects of BZM both in vitro and in vivo — avoid.

Diuretics

Based on the caffeine content of the herb, high intakes of green tea can theoretically increase the diuretic effects of drugs such as frusemide; however, the clinical significance of this is unknown — observe patient.

Drugs metabolised by cytochrome P450 system

The inhibitory effect of caffeine on CYP1A2 may cause other interactions, but this is speculative for green tea. In vitro and animal research has shown that green tea inhibits CYP3A4 metabolism and a probable inhibition of intestinal CYP3A4, but clinical relevance is unknown (Engdal & Nilsen 2009, Fukuda et al 2009). A small trial with 42 volunteers giving 800 mg of green tea a day suggested that drugs metabolised by the CYP enzymes were unlikely to be significantly affected (Chow et al 2006).

CONTRAINDICATIONS AND PRECAUTIONS

Excessive intake will increase the likelihood of adverse effects due to the caffeine content and therefore is not recommended for people with hypertension, cardiac arrhythmias, severe liver disease, anxiety or psychiatric disorders or insomnia. It is considered safe when consumed as a tea in moderate amounts but should not be consumed to excess and is generally better on a full rather than empty stomach. However, if taken too close to meals, the tannin content of green tea will inhibit iron absorption.

PREGNANCY USE

Usual dietary intakes appear safe; however, excessive use is not recommended due to the caffeine content of green tea. It may also be prudent to avoid or drink small quantities of green tea in pregnancy due to its potential to chelate iron and a recent study linking high green tea intake with lower levels of folate in pregnant women (Shiraishi et al 2010).

PATIENTS' FAQs

What will this herb do for me?

Green tea has strong antioxidant effects and some population studies suggest that regular consumption may reduce the risk of cancer and CVD. Early research has found it may be useful for sunburn protection, reducing dental plaque formation, colitis, diabetes, flu prevention, renal disease, improving memory and cognition and as an antiseptic. However, further research is required.

When will it start to work?

This will depend on the reason it is being used. Preventive health benefits are likely to take several years of regular daily tea consumption. Effects on oral health care appear to develop more quickly, within 2 weeks.

Are there any safety issues?

Research suggests that green tea is a safe substance when used in usual dietary doses, but excessive consumption may produce side effects, chiefly because of the caffeine content.

Practice points/Patient counselling

- Green tea is made from the same plant as black tea, but it contains greater amounts of polyphenols and generally less caffeine.
- Green tea has been found to have significant antioxidant activity and protects against sunburn when applied topically.
- It has antibacterial activity and is used in oral preparations to reduce plaque and improve gingival health.
- Several in vitro and animal studies have shown anticarcinogenic activity for a range of cancers and some epidemiological evidence further suggests cancer-protective effects may occur, especially for reducing the risk of breast, prostate, endometrial, ovarian, colerectal and pancreatic cancers and leukaemia; however, further research is required. Patients with a high risk of prostate or liver cancer (due to hepatitis B) may benefit from regular green tea drinking.
- Epidemiological evidence suggests green tea may reduce CVD, especially stroke risk. Some clinical trials have demonstrated a reduction in LDL-cholesterol and antihypertensive effect.
- Preliminary evidence from animal studies has shown that it increases thermogenesis, decreases appetite, reduces inflammation in colitis, reduces glucose levels in diabetes, may be useful in renal failure and has the potential to improve cognitive function in the elderly and be used in Alzheimer's and Parkinson's diseases. Early clinical trials have shown specific green teas (benifuuki tea) may be preventive for allergic rhinitis and green tea drinking may reduce depression.
- Some clinical studies show inconsistent, but possibly modest, benefits in diabetes treatment.
- It is not known whether the use will promote weight loss in humans as research results are inconsistent; however, it may assist with modest weight reduction, especially when combined with exercise.
- A proprietary ointment made from a fixed concentration of GTCs is effective in the treatment of genital warts.

REFERENCES

Adachi N et al. (–)-Epigallocatechin gallate attenuates acute stress responses through GABAergic system in the brain. Eur J Pharmacol 531.1–3 (2006): 171–175.

Afaq F et al. Inhibition of ultraviolet B-mediated activation of nuclear factor kappaB in normal human epidermal keratinocytes by green tea constituent (–)-epigallocatechin-3-gallate. Oncogene 22.7 (2003): 1035–1044.

Agarwal, A., et al. 2010. Effect of green tea extract (catechins) in reducing oxidative stress seen in patients of pulmonary tuberculosis on DOTS Cat I regimen. Phytomedicine, 17, 23–7.

Ahmed, S. 2010. Green tea polyphenol epigallocatechin 3-gallate in arthritis: progress and promise. Arthritis Res Ther, 12, 208.

Ahn WS et al. Protective effects of green tea extracts (polyphenon E and EGCG) on human cervical lesions. Eur J Cancer Prev 12.5 (2003): 383–390.

Alexandropoulou I, et al. Effects of iron, ascorbate, meat and casein on the antioxidant capacity of green tea under conditions of in vitro digestion. Food Chem 94 (2006): 359–365.

Alexopoulos, N., et al. 2008. The acute effect of green tea consumption on endothelial function in healthy individuals. Eur J Cardiovasc Prev Rehabil, 15, 300–5.

Andrade, J. P. & Assuncao, M. 2012. Protective effects of chronic green tea consumption on age-related neurodegeneration. Curr Pharm Des, 18, 4–14.

Antonello M et al. Prevention of hypertension, cardiovascular damage and endothelial dysfunction with green tea extracts. Am J Hypertens 20.12 (2007): 1321–1328.

Arab, L., et al. 2009. Green and black tea consumption and risk of stroke: a meta-analysis. Stroke, 40, 1786–92.

Araghizadeh, A., et al. 2013. Inhibitory Activity of Green Tea (*Camellia sinensis*) Extract on Some Clinically Isolated Cariogenic and Periodontopathic Bacteria. Med Princ Pract 22: 368–372.

Arts, I. C. 2008. A review of the epidemiological evidence on tea, flavonoids, and lung cancer. J Nutr, 138, 1561S-1566S.

Assuncao, M., et al. 2010. Green tea averts age-dependent decline of hippocampal signaling systems related to antioxidant defenses and survival. Free Radic Biol Med, 48, 831–8.

Assuncao, M., et al. 2011. Chronic green tea consumption prevents age-related changes in rat hippocampal formation. Neurobiol Aging, 32, 707–17.

Astill C et al. Factors affecting the caffeine and polyphenol contents of black and green tea infusions. J Agric Food Chem 49.11 (2001): 5340–5347.

Auvichayapat P et al. Effectiveness of green tea on weight reduction in obese Thais: a randomized, controlled trial. Physiol Behav 93.3 (2008): 486–491.

Avramovich-Tirosh Y et al. Neurorescue activity, APP regulation and amyloid-beta peptide reduction by novel multi-functional brain permeable iron-chelating antioxidants, M-30 and green tea polyphenol, EGCG. Curr Alzheimer Res 4.4 (2007): 403–411.

Awadalla, H. I., et al. 2011. A pilot study of the role of green tea use on oral health. Int J Dent Hyg, 9, 110–6.

Babu PV, Liu D. Green tea catechins and cardiovascular health: an update. Curr Med Chem 15.18 (2008): 1840–1850.

Bandyopadhyay D et al. In vitro and in vivo antimicrobial action of tea: the commonest beverage of Asia. Biol Pharm Bull 28.11 (2005): 2125–2127.

Basu, A., et al. 2010. Green tea supplementation affects body weight, lipids, and lipid peroxidation in obese subjects with metabolic syndrome. J Am Coll Nutr, 29, 31–40.

Bertipaglia de Santana M et al. Association between soy and green tea (*Camellia sinensis*) diminishes hypercholesterolemia and increases total plasma antioxidant potential in dyslipidemic subjects. Nutrition 24.6 (2008): 562–568.

Bettuzzi S et al. Chemoprevention of human prostate cancer by oral administration of green tea catechins in volunteers with high-grade prostate intraepithelial neoplasia: a preliminary report from a one-year proof-of-principle study. Cancer Res 66.2 (2006): 1234–1240.

Bettuzzi S et al. Inhibition of human prostate cancer progression by administration of green tea catechins: a two years later follow-up update. Eur Urol Supplements 7.3 (2008): 279.

Bhardwaj, P. & Khanna, D. 2013. Green tea catechins: defensive role in cardiovascular disorders. Chin J Nat Med, 11, 345–53.

Biasibetti, R., et al. 2013. Green tea (–)epigallocatechin-3-gallate reverses oxidative stress and reduces acetylcholinesterase activity in a streptozotocin-induced model of dementia. Behav Brain Res, 236, 186–93.

Boehm, K., et al. 2009. Green tea (*Camellia sinensis*) for the prevention of cancer. Cochrane Database Syst Rev, CD005004.

Bogdanski, P., et al. 2012. Green tea extract reduces blood pressure, inflammatory biomarkers, and oxidative stress and improves parameters associated with insulin resistance in obese, hypertensive patients. Nutr Res, 32, 421–7.

Brown, A. L., et al. 2009. Effects of dietary supplementation with the green tea polyphenol epigallocatechin-3-gallate on insulin resistance and associated metabolic risk factors: randomized controlled trial. Br J Nutr, 101, 886–94.

Butler, L. M. & Wu, A. H. 2011. Green and black tea in relation to gynecologic cancers. Mol Nutr Food Res, 55, 931–40.

Cardoso, G. A., et al. 2013. The effects of green tea consumption and resistance training on body composition and resting metabolic rate in overweight or obese women. J Med Food, 16, 120–7.

Chandra, A. K. & De, N. 2013. Catechin induced modulation in the activities of thyroid hormone synthesizing enzymes leading to hypothyroidism. Mol Cell Biochem, 374, 37–48.

Chang CW, et al. Inhibitory effects of polyphenolic catechins from Chinese green tea on HIV reverse transcriptase activity. J Biomed Sci 1.3 (1994): 163–166.

Chang LK et al. Inhibition of Epstein–Barr virus lytic cycle by (–)-epigallocatechin gallate. Biochem Biophys Res Commun 301.4 (2003): 1062–1068.

Chantre P, Lairon D. Recent findings of green tea extract AR25 (Exolise) and its activity for the treatment of obesity. Phytomedicine 9.1 (2002): 3–8.

Chava, V. K. & Vedula, B. D. 2013. Thermo reversible green tea catechin gel for local application in chronic periodontitis- a 4 week clinical trial. J Periodontol 84: 1290.

Chen, H., et al. 2013. Epigallocatechin gallate and sulforaphane combination treatment induce apoptosis in paclitaxel-resistant ovarian cancer cells through hTERT and Bcl-2 down-regulation. Exp Cell Res, 319, 697–706.

Cheng TO. Why is green tea more cardioprotective in women than in men? Int J Cardiol 122.3 (2007): 244.

Choan E et al. A prospective clinical trial of green tea for hormone refractory prostate cancer: An evaluation of the complementary/alternative therapy approach. Urol Oncol 23.2 (2005): 108–113.

Chou CC, et al. Antimicrobial activity of tea as affected by the degree of fermentation and manufacturing season. Int J Food Microbiol 48.2 (1999): 125–130.

Chow HH et al. Effects of repeated green tea catechin administration on human cytochrome P450 activity. Cancer Epidemiol Biomarkers Prev 15.12 (2006): 2473–2476.

Clement, Y. 2009. Can green tea do that? A literature review of the clinical evidence. Prev Med, 49, 83–7.

Dai, Q., et al. 2010. Is green tea drinking associated with a later onset of breast cancer? Ann Epidemiol, 20, 74–81.

De Koning Gans, J. M., et al. 2010. Tea and coffee consumption and cardiovascular morbidity and mortality. Arterioscler Thromb Vasc Biol, 30, 1665–71.

De Oliveira, A., et al. 2013. Inhibition of herpes simplex virus type 1 with the modified green tea polyphenol palmitoyl-epigallocatechin gallate. Food Chem Toxicol, 52, 207–15.

Di Castelnuovo, A., et al. 2012. Consumption of cocoa, tea and coffee and risk of cardiovascular disease. Eur J Intern Med, 23, 15–25.

Diepvens K et al. Effect of green tea on resting energy expenditure and substrate oxidation during weight loss in overweight females. Br J Nutr 94.6 (2005): 1026–1034.

Di Pierro, F., et al. 2009. Greenselect Phytosome as an adjunct to a low-calorie diet for treatment of obesity: a clinical trial. Altern Med Rev, 14, 154–60.

G

Dragicevic, N., et al. 2011. Green Tea Epigallocatechin-3-Gallate (EGCG) and Other Flavonoids Reduce Alzheimer's Amyloid-Induced Mitochondrial Dysfunction. Journal of Alzheimer's Disease, 26, 507–521.

Dryden, G. W., et al. 2013. A pilot study to evaluate the safety and efficacy of an oral dose of (–)-epigallocatechin-3-gallate-rich polyphenon e in patients with mild to moderate ulcerative colitis. Inflamm Bowel Dis, 19, 1904–12.

Dulloo AG et al. Green tea and thermogenesis: interactions between catechin-polyphenols, caffeine and sympathetic activity. Int J Obes Relat Metab Disord 24.2 (2000): 252–258.

Ellinger, S., et al. 2011. Consumption of green tea or green tea products: is there an evidence for antioxidant effects from controlled interventional studies? Phytomedicine, 18, 903–15.

Elmets CA et al. Cutaneous photoprotection from ultraviolet injury by green tea polyphenols. J Am Acad Dermatol 44.3 (2001): 425–432.

Engdal, S. & Nilsen, O. G. 2009. In vitro inhibition of CYP3A4 by herbal remedies frequently used by cancer patients. Phytother Res, 23, 906–12.

Erba D et al. Effectiveness of moderate green tea consumption on antioxidative status and plasma lipid profile in humans. J Nutr Biochem 16.3 (2005): 144–149.

Fassina G et al. Polyphenolic antioxidant (–)-epigallocatechin-3-gallate from green tea as a candidate anti-HIV agent. AIDS 16.6 (2002): 939–941.

Ferrazzano, G. F., et al. 2011. Antimicrobial properties of green tea extract against cariogenic microflora: an in vivo study. J Med Food, 14, 907–11.

Fon Sing, M., et al. 2011. Epidemiological studies of the association between tea drinking and primary liver cancer: a meta-analysis. Eur J Cancer Prev, 20, 157–65.

Frank, J., et al. 2009. Daily consumption of an aqueous green tea extract supplement does not impair liver function or alter cardiovascular disease risk biomarkers in healthy men. J Nutr, 139, 58–62.

Fritz, H., et al. 2013. Green tea and lung cancer: a systematic review. Integr Cancer Ther, 12, 7–24.

Fuhrman, B. J., et al. 2013. Green tea intake is associated with urinary estrogen profiles in Japanese-American women. Nutr J 12: 25.

Fujiki H et al. Mechanistic findings of green tea as cancer preventive for humans. Proc Soc Exp Biol Med 220.4 (1999): 225–228.

Fukino Y et al. Randomized controlled trial for an effect of green tea consumption on insulin resistance and inflammation markers. J Nutr Sci Vitaminol (Tokyo) 51.5 (2005): 335–42.

Fukino, Y., et al. 2008. Randomized controlled trial for an effect of green tea-extract powder supplementation on glucose abnormalities. Eur J Clin Nutr, 62, 953–60.

Fukuda, I., et al. 2009. Suppression of cytochrome P450 1A1 expression induced by 2,3,7,8-tetrachlorodibenzo-p-dioxin in mouse hepatoma hepa-1c1c7 cells treated with serum of (–)-epigallocatechin-3-gallate- and green tea extract-administered rats. Biosci Biotechnol Biochem, 73, 1206–8.

Gao J et al. [Green tea consumption and the risk of endometrial cancer: a population-based case-control study in urban Shanghai]. Zhonghua Liu Xing Bing Xue Za Zhi 26.5 (2005): 323–327.

Gao, M., et al. 2013. Meta-analysis of Green Tea Drinking and the Prevalence of Gynecological Tumors in Women. Asia Pac J Public Health.

Garcia F et al. Apoptosis induction by green tea compounds in cervical cancer cells. Eur J Cancer Supplements 4.1 (2006): 58.

Gillespie, K., et al. 2008. Effects of oral consumption of the green tea polyphenol EGCG in a murine model for human Sjogren's syndrome, an autoimmune disease. Life Sci, 83, 581–8.

Golden EB et al. Green tea polyphenols block the anticancer effects of bortezomib and other boronic acid-based proteasome inhibitors. Blood 113.23 (2009): 5927–37.

Gordon, N. C. & Wareham, D. W. 2010. Antimicrobial activity of the green tea polyphenol (–)-epigallocatechin-3-gallate (EGCG) against clinical isolates of *Stenotrophomonas maltophilia.* Int J Antimicrob Agents, 36, 129–31.

Graham HN. Green tea composition, consumption, and polyphenol chemistry. Prev Med 21.3 (1992): 334–350.

Gross G. [Polyphenon E. A new topical therapy for condylomata acuminata.] Hautarzt 59.1 (2008): 31–35.

Guo Q et al. Studies on protective mechanisms of four components of green tea polyphenols against lipid peroxidation in synaptosomes. Biochim Biophys Acta 1304.3 (1996): 210–222.

Guo S et al. Protective effects of green tea polyphenols in the 6-OHDA rat model of Parkinson's disease through inhibition of ROS-NO pathway. Biol Psychiatry 62.12 (2007): 1353–1362.

Gupta S, et al. Molecular pathway for (–)-epigallocatechin-3-gallate-induced cell cycle arrest and apoptosis of human prostate carcinoma cells. Arch Biochem Biophys 410.1 (2003): 177–185.

Han, D. H., et al. 2009. Anti-proliferative and apoptosis induction activity of green tea polyphenols on human promyelocytic leukemia HL-60 cells. Anticancer Res, 29, 1417–21.

Han, K. C., et al. 2011. Genoprotective effects of green tea (*Camellia sinensis*) in human subjects: results of a controlled supplementation trial. Br J Nutr, 105, 171–9.

Haque AM et al. Long-term administration of green tea catechins improves spatial cognition learning ability in rats. J Nutr 136.4 (2006): 1043–1047.

Hartley, L., et al. 2013. Green and black tea for the primary prevention of cardiovascular disease. Cochrane Database Syst Rev, 6, CD009934.

Hasegawa T et al. Protective effect of Japanese green tea against cognitive impairment in the elderly, a two-years follow-up observation. Alzheimers Dement 1.1 (Suppl 1) (2005): S100.

Henning, S. M., et al. 2011. Chemopreventive effects of tea in prostate cancer: green tea versus black tea. Mol Nutr Food Res, 55, 905–20.

Herges, K., et al. 2011. Neuroprotective effect of combination therapy of glatiramer acetate and epigallocatechin-3-gallate in neuroinflammation. PLoS One, 6, e25456.

Hirasawa M et al. Improvement of periodontal status by green tea catechin using a local delivery system: a clinical pilot study. J Periodontal Res 37.6 (2002): 433–8.

Ho C -T et al. Tea & tea products: chemistry & health promoting properties. CRC Press, Boka Raton, (2009).

Honicke, A. S., et al. 2012. Combined administration of EGCG and IL-1 receptor antagonist efficiently downregulates IL-1-induced tumorigenic factors in U-2 OS human osteosarcoma cells. Int J Oncol, 41, 753–8.

Hooper L et al. Flavonoids, fl avonoid-rich foods, and cardiovascular risk: a meta-analysis of randomized controlled trials. Am J Clin Nutr 88.1 (2008): 38–50.

Hou R-R et al. Neuroprotective effects of (-)-epigallocatechin-3-gallate (EGCG) on paraquat-induced apoptosis in PC12 cells. Cell Biol Int 32.1 (2008): 22–30.

Hou, I. C., et al. 2013. Green tea and the risk of gastric cancer: Epidemiological evidence. World J Gastroenterol, 19, 3713–22.

Hsu S. Green tea and the skin. J Am Acad Dermatol 52.6 (2005): 1049–59.

Hsu C -H et al. Effect of green tea extract on obese women: a randomized, double-blind, placebo-controlled clinical trial. Clin Nutr 27.3 (2008) : 363–70.

Hsu, C. H., et al. 2011. Does supplementation with green tea extract improve insulin resistance in obese type 2 diabetics? A randomized, double-blind, and placebo-controlled clinical trial. Altern Med Rev, 16, 157–63.

Hursel, R., et al. 2009. The effects of green tea on weight loss and weight maintenance: a meta-analysis. Int J Obes (Lond), 33, 956–61.

Imai K, Nakachi K. Cross sectional study of effects of drinking green tea on cardiovascular and liver diseases. BMJ 310.6981 (1995): 693–6.

Imanishi N et al. Additional inhibitory effect of tea extract on the growth of infl uenza A and B viruses in MDCK cells. Microbiol Immunol 46.7 (2002): 491–4.

Inoue, M., et al. 2009a. Effect of coffee and green tea consumption on the risk of liver cancer: cohort analysis by hepatitis virus infection status. Cancer Epidemiol Biomarkers Prev, 18, 1746–53.

Inoue, M., et al. 2009b. Green tea consumption and gastric cancer in Japanese: a pooled analysis of six cohort studies. Gut, 58, 1323–32.

Isaacs C E et al. Epigallocatechin gallate inactivates clinical isolates of herpes simplex virus. Antimicrob Agents Chemother 52.3 (2008): 962–70.

Ishihara N et al. Improvement of intestinal microfl ora balance and prevention of digestive and respiratory organ diseases in calves by green tea extracts. Livest Prod Sci 68.2–3 (2001): 217–29.

Itoh Y et al. Preventive effects of green tea on renal stone formation and the role of oxidative stress in nephrolithiasis. J Urol 173.1 (2005): 271–5.

Itoh, T., et al. 2011. (–)-Epigallocatechin-3-gallate protects against neuronal cell death and improves cerebral function after traumatic brain injury in rats. Neuromolecular Med, 13, 300–9.

Janjua, R., et al. 2009. A two-year, double-blind, randomized placebo-controlled trial of oral green tea polyphenols on the long-term clinical and histologic appearance of photoaging skin. Dermatol Surg, 35, 1057–65.

Jatoi A et al. A phase II trial of green tea in the treatment of patients with androgen independent metastatic prostate carcinoma. Cancer 97.6 (2003): 1442–6.

Jenabian, N., et al. 2012. The effect of *Camellia sinensis* (green tea) mouthwash on plaque-induced gingivitis: a single-blinded randomized controlled clinical trial. Daru, 20, 39.

Jeong BC et al. Effects of green tea on urinary stone formation: an in vivo and in vitro study. J Endourol 20.5 (2006): 356–361.

Jeong H-S et al. Effects of (–) epigallocatechin-3-gallate on the activity of substantia nigra dopaminergic neurons. Brain Res 1130 (2007): 114–1118.

Jian L et al. Protective effect of green tea against prostate cancer: a case-control study in southeast China. Int J Cancer 108.1 (2004): 130–135.

Jin X, et al. Green tea consumption and liver disease: a systematic review. Liver Int 28.7 (2008): 990–996.

Johnson, R., et al. 2012. Green tea and green tea catechin extracts: an overview of the clinical evidence. Maturitas, 73, 280–7.

Jurgens, T. M., et al. 2012. Green tea for weight loss and weight maintenance in overweight or obese adults. Cochrane Database Syst Rev, 12, CD008650.

Kang, H., et al. 2010. Green tea consumption and stomach cancer risk: a meta-analysis. Epidemiol Health, 32, e2010001.

Kang, M. Y., et al. 2012. Preventive effects of green tea (*Camellia sinensis* var. assamica) on diabetic nephropathy. Yonsei Med J, 53, 138–44.

Katiyar, S. K. 2011. Green tea prevents non-melanoma skin cancer by enhancing DNA repair. Arch Biochem Biophys, 508, 152–8.

Kaur T et al. Effects of green tea extract on learning, memory, behavior and acetylcholinesterase activity in young and old male rats. Brain Cogn 67.1 (2008): 25–30.

Kavanagh KT et al. Green tea extracts decrease carcinogen-induced mammary tumor burden in rats and rate of breast cancer cell proliferation in culture. J Cell Biochem 82.3 (2001): 387–398.

Kazi A et al. Potential molecular targets of tea polyphenols in human tumor cells: significance in cancer prevention. In Vivo 16.6 (2002): 397–403.

Khan, N. & Mukhtar, H. 2010. Cancer and metastasis: prevention and treatment by green tea. Cancer Metastasis Rev, 29, 435–45.

Khan, N., et al. 2009a. Review: green tea polyphenols in chemoprevention of prostate cancer: preclinical and clinical studies. Nutr Cancer, 61, 836–41.

Khan, S. A., et al. 2009b. Studies on the protective effect of green tea against cisplatin induced nephrotoxicity. Pharmacological Research, 60, 382–391.

Kim, A., et al. 2011. Green tea catechins decrease total and low-density lipoprotein cholesterol: a systematic review and meta-analysis. J Am Diet Assoc, 111, 1720–9.

Kinjo J et al. Activity-guided fractionation of green tea extract with antiproliferative activity against human stomach cancer cells. Biol Pharm Bull 25.9 (2002): 1238–1240.

Kokubo, Y., et al. 2013. The impact of green tea and coffee consumption on the reduced risk of stroke incidence in Japanese population: the Japan Public Health Center-Based Study Cohort. Stroke 44: 1369–1374.

Krahwinkel T, Willershausen B. The effect of sugar-free green tea chew candies on the degree of inflammation of the gingiva. Eur J Med Res 5.11 (2000): 463–467.

Kumamoto M et al. Effects of pH and metal ions on antioxidative activities of catechins. Biosci Biotechnol Biochem 65.1 (2001): 126–132.

Kuo YC et al. A population-based, case-control study of green tea consumption and leukemia risk in southwestern Taiwan. Cancer Causes Control 20.1 (2009): 57–765.

Kurahashi N et al. Green tea consumption and prostate cancer risk in Japanese men: a prospective study. Am J Epidemiol 167.1 (2008): 71–77.

Kuriyama, S. 2008. The relation between green tea consumption and cardiovascular disease as evidenced by epidemiological studies. J Nutr, 138, 1548S-1553S.

Kuriyama S et al. Green tea consumption and cognitive function: a cross-sectional study from the Tsurugaya Project 1. Am J Clin Nutr 83.2 (2006a): 355–361.

Kuriyama S et al. Green tea consumption and mortality due to cardiovascular disease, cancer, and all causes in Japan: the Ohsaki study. JAMA 296.10 (2006b): 1255–1265.

Kushiyama, M., et al. 2009. Relationship between intake of green tea and periodontal disease. J Periodontol, 80, 372–7.

Lee, A. H. & Pasalich, M. 2013. Chapter 64 — Protective Aspects of Tea and Prostate Cancer: Emerging Evidence. Tea in Health and Disease Prevention. Amsterdam: Academic Press.

Lee, J. H., et al. 2009. In vitro anti-adhesive activity of green tea extract against pathogen adhesion. Phytother Res, 23, 460–6.

Leenen R et al. A single dose of tea with or without milk increases plasma antioxidant activity in humans. Eur J Clin Nutr 54.1 (2000): 87–92.

Li Q et al. Oral administration of green tea epigallocatechin-3-gallate (EGCG) reduces amyloid beta deposition in transgenic mouse model of Alzheimer's disease. Exp Neurol 198.2 (2006): 576.

Li, Y., et al. 2011. Green tea consumption, inflammation and the risk of primary hepatocellular carcinoma in a Chinese population. Cancer Epidemiol, 35, 362–8.

Liatsos, G. D., et al. 2010. Possible green tea-induced thrombotic thrombocytopenic purpura. Am J Health Syst Pharm, 67, 531–4.

Lin YS et al. Factors affecting the levels of tea polyphenols and caffeine in tea leaves. J Agric Food Chem 51.7 (2003): 1864–1873.

Liu T, Chi Y. Experimental study on polyphenol anti plaque effect in humans. Zhonghua Kou Qiang Yi Xue Za Zhi 35.5 (2000): 383–384.

Liu S et al. Theaflavin derivatives in black tea and catechin derivatives in green tea inhibit HIV-1 entry by targeting gp41. Biochim Biophys Acta 1723.1–3 (2005): 270–281.

Liu, K., et al. 2013. Effect of green tea on glucose control and insulin sensitivity: a meta-analysis of 17 randomized controlled trials. Am J Clin Nutr 98: 340–348.

MacKenzie T, et al. The effect of an extract of green and black tea on glucose control in adults with type 2 diabetes mellitus: double-blind randomized study. Metabolism 56.10 (2007): 1340–13444.

Maeda K et al. Green tea catechins inhibit the cultured smooth muscle cell invasion through the basement barrier. Atherosclerosis 166.1 (2003): 23–30.

Maeda-Yamamoto, M., et al. 2009. The efficacy of early treatment of seasonal allergic rhinitis with benifuuki green tea containing O-methylated catechin before pollen exposure: an open randomized study. Allergol Int, 58, 437–44.

Maki, K. C., et al. 2009. Green tea catechin consumption enhances exercise-induced abdominal fat loss in overweight and obese adults. J Nutr, 139, 264–70.

Mandel S et al. Green tea catechins as brain-permeable, natural iron chelators-antioxidants for the treatment of neurodegenerative disorders. Mol Nutr Food Res 50.2 (2006): 229–234.

Mandel S et al. Iron dysregulation in Alzheimer's disease: multimodal brain permeable iron chelating drugs, possessing neuroprotective-neurorescue and amyloid precursor protein-processing regulatory activities as therapeutic agents. Prog Neurobiol 82.6 (2007): 348–360.

Mantena SK, et al. Epigallocatechin-3-gallate inhibits photocarcinogenesis through inhibition of angiogenic factors and activation of CD8 + T cells in tumors. Photochem Photobiol 81.5 (2005): 1174–1179.

Mao, X. Q., et al. 2011. Green tea drinking habits and gastric cancer in southwest China. Asian Pac J Cancer Prev, 12, 2179–82.

Masterjohn, C. & Bruno, R. S. 2012. Therapeutic potential of green tea in nonalcoholic fatty liver disease. Nutr Rev, 70, 41–56.

Matsubara S et al. Suppression of *Helicobacter pylori*-induced gastritis by green tea extract in Mongolian gerbils. Biochem Biophys Res Commun 310.3 (2003): 715–7119.

Matsumoto, K., et al. 2011. Effects of green tea catechins and theanine on preventing influenza infection among healthcare workers: a randomized controlled trial. BMC Complement Altern Med, 11, 15.

Mazzanti, G., et al. 2009. Hepatotoxicity from green tea: a review of the literature and two unpublished cases. Eur J Clin Pharmacol, 65, 331–41.

McLarty, J., et al. 2009. Tea polyphenols decrease serum levels of prostate-specific antigen, hepatocyte growth factor, and vascular endothelial growth factor in prostate cancer patients and inhibit production of hepatocyte growth factor and vascular endothelial growth factor in vitro. Cancer Prev Res (Phila), 2, 673–82.

Mereles, D., et al. 2010. Effects of the main green tea polyphenol epigallocatechin-3-gallate on cardiac involvement in patients with AL amyloidosis. Clin Res Cardiol, 99, 483–90.

Meydani, S. N. 2011. Green tea and autoimmune disorders: Impact on pathogenesis and the underlying mechanisms. Clinical Biochemistry, 44, S19-S20.

Mineharu, Y., et al. 2011. Coffee, green tea, black tea and oolong tea consumption and risk of mortality from cardiovascular disease in Japanese men and women. J Epidemiol Community Health, 65, 230–40.
Mukoyama A et al. Inhibition of rotavirus and enterovirus infections by tea extracts. Jpn J Med Sci Biol 44.4 (1991): 181–186.
Myung, S. K., et al. 2009. Green tea consumption and risk of stomach cancer: a meta-analysis of epidemiologic studies. Int J Cancer, 124, 670–7.
Nagle, C. M., et al. 2010. Tea consumption and risk of ovarian cancer. Cancer Causes Control, 21, 1485–91.
Nakachi K et al. Preventive effects of drinking green tea on cancer and cardiovascular disease: epidemiological evidence for multiple targeting prevention. Biofactors 13.1–4 (2000): 49–54.
Nakachi K, et al. Can teatime increase one's lifetime? Ageing Res Rev 2.1 (2003): 1–110.
Nance, C. L., et al. 2009. Preclinical development of the green tea catechin, epigallocatechin gallate, as an HIV-1 therapy. J Allergy Clin Immunol, 123, 459–65.
Nantz, M. P., et al. 2009. Standardized capsule of *Camellia sinensis* lowers cardiovascular risk factors in a randomized, double-blind, placebo-controlled study. Nutrition, 25, 147–54.
Nath, S., et al. 2012. Catechins protect neurons against mitochondrial toxins and HIV proteins via activation of the BDNF pathway. J Neurovirol, 18, 445–55.
Neves, D., et al. 2008. Does regular consumption of green tea influence expression of vascular endothelial growth factor and its receptor in aged rat erectile tissue? Possible implications for vasculogenic erectile dysfunction progression. Age (Dordr), 30, 217–28.
Nguyen, M. M., et al. 2012. Randomized, double-blind, placebo-controlled trial of polyphenon E in prostate cancer patients before prostatectomy: evaluation of potential chemopreventive activities. Cancer Prev Res (Phila), 5, 290–8.
Ogunleye, A. A., et al. 2010. Green tea consumption and breast cancer risk or recurrence: a meta-analysis. Breast Cancer Res Treat, 119, 477–84.
Osterburg, A., et al. 2009. Highly antibiotic-resistant *Acinetobacter baumannii* clinical isolates are killed by the green tea polyphenol (–)-epigallocatechin-3-gallate (EGCG). Clin Microbiol Infect, 15, 341–6.
Ostrowska J et al. Green and black tea in brain protection. Oxidative Stress and Neurodegenerative Disorders. Amsterdam, Elsevier Science B.V. (2007), pp 581–605.
Otake S et al. Anticaries effects of polyphenolic compounds from Japanese green tea. Caries Res 25.6 (1991): 438–443.
Pae, M. & Wu, D. 2013. Immunomodulating effects of epigallocatechin-3-gallate from green tea: mechanisms and applications. Food Funct 4: 1287–1303.
Panagiotakos, D. B., et al. 2009. Long-term tea intake is associated with reduced prevalence of (type 2) diabetes mellitus among elderly people from Mediterranean islands: MEDIS epidemiological study. Yonsei Med J, 50, 31–8.
Park, M., et al. 2011. Green tea consumption is inversely associated with the incidence of influenza infection among schoolchildren in a tea plantation area of Japan. J Nutr, 141, 1862–70.
Persson IA et al. Tea flavanols inhibit angiotensin-converting enzyme activity and increase nitric oxide production in human endothelial cells. J Pharm Pharmacol 58.8 (2006): 1139–1144.
Pham, N. M., et al. 2013. Green tea and coffee consumption is inversely associated with depressive symptoms in a Japanese working population. Public Health Nutr, 1–9.
Phung, O. J., et al. 2010. Effect of green tea catechins with or without caffeine on anthropometric measures: a systematic review and meta-analysis. Am J Clin Nutr, 91, 73–81.
Polychronopoulos E et al. Effects of black and green tea consumption on blood glucose levels in non-obese elderly men and women from Mediterranean Islands (MEDIS epidemiological study). Eur J Nutr 47.1 (2008): 10–116.
Priyadarshi S et al. Effect of green tea extract on cardiac hypertrophy following 5/6 nephrectomy in the rat. Kidney Int 63.5 (2003): 1785–1790.
Qanungo S et al. Epigallocatechin-3-gallate induces mitochondrial membrane depolarization and caspase-dependent apoptosis in pancreatic cancer cells. Carcinogenesis 26.5 (2005): 958–967.
Qin J et al. A component of green tea, (–)-epigallocatechin-3-gallate, promotes apoptosis in T24 human bladder cancer cells via modulation of the PI3K/Akt pathway and Bcl-2 family proteins. Biochem Biophys Res Commun 354.4 (2007): 852–857.
Rasheed A, Haider M. Antibacterial activity of *Camellia sinensis* extracts against dental caries. Arch Pharm Res 21.3 (1998): 348–352.
Rezai-Zadeh K et al. Green tea epigallocatechin-3-gallate (EGCG) reduces [beta]-amyloid mediated cognitive impairment and modulates tau pathology in Alzheimer transgenic mice. Brain Res 1214 (2008): 177–187.
Reznichenko L et al. Reduction of iron-regulated amyloid precursor protein and beta-amyloid peptide by (–)-epigallocatechin-3-gallate in cell cultures: implications for iron chelation in Alzheimer's disease. J Neurochem 97.2 (2006): 527–536.
Rhee SJ, et al. Effects of green tea catechin on prostaglandin synthesis of renal glomerular and renal dysfunction in streptozotocin-induced diabetic rats. Asia Pac J Clin Nutr 11.3 (2002): 232–236.
Rietveld A, Wiseman S. Antioxidant effects of tea: evidence from human clinical trials. J Nutr 133.10 (2003): 3285–92S.
Sabu MC, et al. Anti-diabetic activity of green tea polyphenols and their role in reducing oxidative stress in experimental diabetes. J Ethnopharmacol 83.1–2 (2002): 109–116.
Sachinidis A, Hescheler J. Are catechins natural tyrosine kinase inhibitors? Drug News Perspect 15.7 (2002): 432–438.
Saewong, T., et al. 2010. Effects of green tea on iron accumulation and oxidative stress in livers of iron-challenged thalassemic mice. Med Chem, 6, 57–64.
Sakanaka S et al. Inhibitory effects of green tea polyphenols on growth and cellular adherence of an oral bacterium, *Porphyromonas gingivalis*. Biosci Biotechnol Biochem 60.5 (1996): 745–749.

Sannella AR et al. Antimalarial properties of green tea. Biochemical and Biochem Biophys Res Commun 353.1 (2007): 177–181.

Sarma, D. N., et al. 2008. Safety of Green Tea Extracts : A Systematic Review by the US Pharmacopeia. Drug Safety, 31, 469–484.

Sasazuki, S., et al. 2012. Green tea consumption and gastric cancer risk: an evaluation based on a systematic review of epidemiologic evidence among the Japanese population. Jpn J Clin Oncol, 42, 335–46.

Sayama K et al. Effects of green tea on growth, food utilization and lipid metabolism in mice. In Vivo 14.4 (2000): 481–484.

Schonthal, A. H. 2011. Adverse effects of concentrated green tea extracts. Mol Nutr Food Res, 55, 874–85.

Sen, T. & Chatterjee, A. 2011. Epigallocatechin-3-gallate (EGCG) downregulates EGF-induced MMP-9 in breast cancer cells: involvement of integrin receptor alpha5beta1 in the process. Eur J Nutr, 50, 465–78.

Shanafelt, T. D., et al. 2013. Phase 2 trial of daily, oral Polyphenon E in patients with asymptomatic, Rai stage 0 to II chronic lymphocytic leukemia. Cancer, 119, 363–70.

Shen, C. L., et al. 2009. Green tea and bone metabolism. Nutr Res, 29, 437–56.

Shen, C. L., et al. 2011. Green tea and bone health: Evidence from laboratory studies. Pharmacol Res, 64, 155–61.

Shen, C. L., et al. 2012. Effect of green tea and Tai Chi on bone health in postmenopausal osteopenic women: a 6-month randomized placebo-controlled trial. Osteoporos Int, 23, 1541–52.

Shimizu M et al. EGCG inhibits activation of the insulin-like growth factor-1 receptor in human colon cancer cells. Biochem Biophys Res Commun 334.3 (2005): 947–953.

Shimizu, M., et al. 2008. Green tea extracts for the prevention of metachronous colorectal adenomas: a pilot study. Cancer Epidemiol Biomarkers Prev, 17, 3020–5.

Shiraishi, M., et al. 2010. Association between the serum folate levels and tea consumption during pregnancy. Biosci Trends, 4, 225–30.

Shord, S. S., et al. 2009. Drug-botanical interactions: a review of the laboratory, animal, and human data for 8 common botanicals. Integr Cancer Ther, 8, 208–27.

Siddiqui, I. A., et al. 2009. Introducing nanochemoprevention as a novel approach for cancer control: proof of principle with green tea polyphenol epigallocatechin-3-gallate. Cancer Res, 69, 1712–6.

Siddiqui, I. A., et al. 2011. Green tea polyphenol EGCG blunts androgen receptor function in prostate cancer. FASEB J, 25, 1198–207.

Silva, K. C., et al. 2013. Green tea is neuroprotective in diabetic retinopathy. Invest Ophthalmol Vis Sci, 54, 1325–36.

Song J-M, et al. Antiviral effect of catechins in green tea on influenza virus. Antiviral Res 68.2 (2005): 66–74.

Song L et al. P345 Effects of green tea on lipids blood pressure and vasorelaxation in rats with hypercholesterolaemia-induced hypertension. Int J Cardiol 125 (Suppl 1) (2008): S64.

Srichairatanakool S et al. Iron-chelating and free-radical scavenging activities of microwave-processed green tea in iron overload. Hemoglobin 30.2 (2006): 311–327.

Srinivasan P et al. Chemopreventive and therapeutic modulation of green tea polyphenols on drug metabolizing enzymes in 4-Nitroquinoline 1-oxide induced oral cancer. Chem Biol Interact 172.3 (2008): 224–234.

Srividhya, R., et al. 2012. Impact of epigallo catechin-3-gallate on acetylcholine-acetylcholine esterase cycle in aged rat brain. Neurochem Int, 60, 517–22.

Stockfleth, E. & Meyer, T. 2012. The use of sinecatechins (polyphenon E) ointment for treatment of external genital warts. Expert Opin Biol Ther, 12, 783–93.

Stockfleth E et al. Topical Polyphenon E in the treatment of external genital and perianal warts: a randomized controlled trial. Br J Dermatol 158.6 (2008): 1329–1338.

Stoicov, C., et al. 2009. Green tea inhibits *Helicobacter* growth in vivo and in vitro. Int J Antimicrob Agents, 33, 473–8.

Suganuma, M., et al. 2011. New cancer treatment strategy using combination of green tea catechins and anticancer drugs. Cancer Sci, 102, 317–23.

Suliburska, J., et al. 2012. Effects of green tea supplementation on elements, total antioxidants, lipids, and glucose values in the serum of obese patients. Biol Trace Elem Res, 149, 315–22.

Sun CL et al. Green tea, black tea and breast cancer risk: a meta-analysis of epidemiological studies. Carcinogenesis 27.7 (2006): 1310–13115.

Sung H et al. In vivo antioxidant effect of green tea. Eur J Clin Nutr 54.7 (2000): 527–529.

Suzuki, E., et al. 2009. Green Tea Consumption and Mortality among Japanese Elderly People: The Prospective Shizuoka Elderly Cohort. Ann Epidemiol, 19, 732–739.

Tang, X. D., et al. 2008. [Effects of green tea extract on expression of human papillomavirus type 16 oncoproteins-induced hypoxia-inducible factor-1alpha and vascular endothelial growth factor in human cervical carcinoma cells.] Zhonghua Yi Xue Za Zhi, 88, 2872–7.

Tang, N., et al. 2009a. Green tea, black tea consumption and risk of lung cancer: a meta-analysis. Lung Cancer, 65, 274–83.

Tang, N. P., et al. 2009b. Tea consumption and risk of endometrial cancer: a metaanalysis. Am J Obstet Gynecol, 201, 605 e1–8.

Tao P. The inhibitory effects of catechin derivatives on the activities of human immunodeficiency virus reverse transcriptase and DNA polymerases. Zhongguo Yi Xue Ke Xue Yuan Xue Bao 14.5 (1992): 334–338.

Tatti S et al. Sinecatechins, a defined green tea extract, in the treatment of external anogenital warts: a randomized controlled trial. Obstet Gynecol 111.6 (2008): 1371–1379.

Taylor JR, Wilt VM. Probable antagonism of warfarin by green tea. Ann Pharmacother 33.4 (1999): 426–428.

Tehrani, M. H., et al. 2011. Comparing *Streptococcus mutans* and *Lactobacillus* colony count changes following green tea mouth rinse or sodium fluoride mouth rinse use in children (Randomized double-blind controlled clinical trial). Dent Res J (Isfahan), 8, S58–63.

Thakur, V. S., et al. 2012. The chemopreventive and chemotherapeutic potentials of tea polyphenols. Curr Pharm Biotechnol, 13, 191–9.

Thielecke, F. & Boschmann, M. 2009. The potential role of green tea catechins in the prevention of the metabolic syndrome - a review. Phytochemistry, 70, 11–24.

Tokuda, H., et al. 2008. (–)-Epigallocatechin gallate inhibits basic fibroblast growth factor-stimulated interleukin-6 synthesis in osteoblasts. Horm Metab Res, 40, 674–8.

Trudel, D., et al. 2012. Green tea for ovarian cancer prevention and treatment: a systematic review of the in vitro, in vivo and epidemiological studies. Gynecol Oncol, 126, 491–8.

Tsao, A. S., et al. 2009. Phase II randomized, placebo-controlled trial of green tea extract in patients with high-risk oral premalignant lesions. Cancer Prev Res (Phila), 2, 931–41.

Tzellos, T. G., et al. 2011. Efficacy, safety and tolerability of green tea catechins in the treatment of external anogenital warts: a systematic review and meta-analysis. J Eur Acad Dermatol Venereol, 25, 345–53.

Ueno, T., et al. 2009. Epigallocatechin-3-gallate improves nonalcoholic steatohepatitis model mice expressing nuclear sterol regulatory element binding protein-1c in adipose tissue. Int J Mol Med, 24, 17–22.

Ui, A., et al. 2009. Green tea consumption and the risk of liver cancer in Japan: the Ohsaki Cohort study. Cancer Causes Control, 20, 1939–45.

Ulbricht CE, Basch EM. Natural standard herb and supplement reference. St Louis: Mosby, 2005.

Valcic S et al. Inhibitory effect of six green tea catechins and caffeine on the growth of four selected human tumor cell lines. Anticancer Drugs 7.4 (1996): 461–468.

Varilek GW et al. Green tea polyphenol extract attenuates inflammation in interleukin-2-deficient mice, a model of autoimmunity. J Nutr 131.7 (2001): 2034–2039.

Vieira Senger, A. E., et al. 2012. Effect of green tea (*Camellia sinensis*) consumption on the components of metabolic syndrome in elderly. J Nutr Health Aging, 16, 738–42.

Vignes M et al. Anxiolytic properties of green tea polyphenol (–)-epigallocatechin gallate (EGCG). Brain Res 1110.1 (2006): 102–115.

Wang YC, Bachrach U. The specific anti-cancer activity of green tea (–)-epigallocatechin-3-gallate (EGCG). Amino Acids 22.2 (2002): 131–143.

Wang, Z. M., et al. 2011. Black and green tea consumption and the risk of coronary artery disease: a meta-analysis. Am J Clin Nutr, 93, 506–15.

Wang, G., et al. 2012a. Risk factor for clear cell renal cell carcinoma in Chinese population: a case-control study. Cancer Epidemiol, 36, 177–82.

Wang, J., et al. 2012b. Green tea drinking and risk of pancreatic cancer: A large-scale, population-based case–control study in urban Shanghai. Cancer Epidemiol, 36, e354-e358.

Wang, X. J., et al. 2012c. Association between green tea and colorectal cancer risk: a meta-analysis of 13 case-control studies. Asian Pac J Cancer Prev, 13, 3123–7.

Wang, Y., et al. 2012d. Coffee and tea consumption and risk of lung cancer: a dose-response analysis of observational studies. Lung Cancer, 78, 169–70.

Wang, Z. H., et al. 2012e. Green tea and incidence of colorectal cancer: evidence from prospective cohort studies. Nutr Cancer, 64, 1143–52.

Wang, X., et al. 2013. A meta-analysis of tea consumption and the risk of bladder cancer. Urol Int, 90, 10–6.

Watanabe, I., et al. 2009. Green tea and death from pneumonia in Japan: the Ohsaki cohort study. Am J Clin Nutr, 90, 672–9.

Weber JM et al. Inhibition of adenovirus infection and adenain by green tea catechins. Antiviral Res 58.2 (2003): 167–173.

Westphal S et al. S1753 EGCG, a Major Component of Green Tea Catechins Attenuates Inflammatory Responses in Two Different Mouse Colitis Models. Gastroenterology 134 (4 Suppl 1) (2008): A–263.

Wightman, E. L., et al. 2012. Epigallocatechin gallate, cerebral blood flow parameters, cognitive performance and mood in healthy humans: a double-blind, placebo-controlled, crossover investigation. Hum Psychopharmacol, 27, 177–86.

Williamson MP et al. Epigallocatechin gallate, the main polyphenol in green tea, binds to the T-cell receptor, CD4: Potential for HIV-1 therapy. J Allergy Clin Immunol 118.6 (2006): 1369–1374.

Wu, S., et al. 2013. The association of tea consumption with bladder cancer risk: a meta-analysis. Asia Pac J Clin Nutr, 22, 128–37.

Yamauchi, R., et al. 2009. Identification of epigallocatechin-3-gallate in green tea polyphenols as a potent inducer of p53-dependent apoptosis in the human lung cancer cell line A549. Toxicol In Vitro, 23, 834–9.

Yokozawa T et al. Effectiveness of green tea tannin on rats with chronic renal failure. Biosci Biotechnol Biochem 60.6 (1996): 1000–1005.

Yoo HG et al. Induction of apoptosis by the green tea flavonol (–)-epigallocatechin-3-gallate in human endothelial ECV 304 cells. Anticancer Res 22.6A (2002): 3373–3378.

Yu J et al. Chemoprevention trial of green tea polyphenols in high-risk population of liver cancer in southern Guangxi, China. AACR Meeting Abstracts 2006 (1) (2006): 1148–a.

Yuan, J. M., et al. 2011. Tea and cancer prevention: epidemiological studies. Pharmacol Res, 64, 123–35.

Zhang H et al. Modification of lung cancer susceptibility by green tea extract as measured by the comet assay. Cancer Detect Prev 26.6 (2002): 411–4118.

Zhang M et al. Green tea consumption enhances survival of epithelial ovarian cancer. Int J Cancer 112.3 (2004): 465–469.

Zhang M et al. Green tea and the prevention of breast cancer: a case-control study in Southeast China. Carcinogenesis 28.5 (2007a): 1074–1078.

Zhang, M., et al. 2007b. Possible protective effect of green tea intake on risk of adult leukaemia. Br J Cancer, 98, 168–170.

Zhang, G., et al. 2012a. Anti-cancer activities of tea epigallocatechin-3-gallate in breast cancer patients under radiotherapy. Curr Mol Med, 12, 163–76.

Zhang, Y., et al. 2012b. Effects of catechin-enriched green tea beverage on visceral fat loss in adults with a high proportion of visceral fat: A double-blind, placebo-controlled, randomized trial. Journal of Functional Foods, 4, 315–322.
Zheng, J., et al. 2011a. Green tea and black tea consumption and prostate cancer risk: an exploratory meta-analysis of observational studies. Nutr Cancer, 63, 663–72.
Zheng, X. X., et al. 2011b. Green tea intake lowers fasting serum total and LDL cholesterol in adults: a meta-analysis of 14 randomized controlled trials. Am J Clin Nutr, 94, 601–10.
Zheng, P., et al. 2012. Green tea consumption and risk of esophageal cancer: a meta-analysis of epidemiologic studies. BMC Gastroenterol, 12, 165.
Zheng, J. S., et al. 2013a. Effects of green tea, black tea, and coffee consumption on the risk of esophageal cancer: a systematic review and meta-analysis of observational studies. Nutr Cancer, 65, 1–16.
Zheng, X. X., et al. 2013b. Effects of green tea catechins with or without caffeine on glycemic control in adults: a meta-analysis of randomized controlled trials. Am J Clin Nutr 97: 750–762.
Zou, C., et al. 2010. Green tea compound in chemoprevention of cervical cancer. Int J Gynecol Cancer, 20, 617–24.

Iodine

BACKGROUND AND RELEVANT PHARMACOKINETICS

Iodine is an essential trace element required for proper functioning of the thyroid gland. It is mainly consumed as iodide salts obtained from sea salt, shellfish and seawater fish and vegetables, which are more bioavailable than the organic forms. The iodine content of soil is considered to be one of the most variable of all minerals, influenced by local geography and the type and quantity of fertiliser used in agriculture (Groff et al 2009). There is evidence of iodine-deficient soils in many regions of Australia. Dietary iodine content is also significantly influenced by agricultural iodine-containing compounds, used in irrigation products, fertiliser and livestock feeds (Zimmermann et al 2008).

Iodide is rapidly absorbed from the stomach to the small intestine and distributed via the blood to a range of tissues, most notably the thyroid, which traps iodide through an ATP-dependent iodide pump called the sodium iodide symporter. The thyroid contains 80% of the body's iodine pool, which is approximately 15 mg in adults. Also found in high concentrations in the salivary, gastric and mammary glands (exclusively during pregnancy and lactation in the latter), iodine's uptake is regulated by thyroid-stimulating hormone (TSH) (Groff et al 2009, Kohlmeier 2003).

Excess iodine is excreted via the kidneys when the needs of the thyroid have been met (Kohlmeier 2003), therefore urine concentrations are used as a means of assessing iodine status. Interestingly, there is no renal conservation mechanism for this mineral and the only evidence of iodine preservation comes from the scavenging and recycling of thyroid hormones by the selenium-dependent deiodinase DII (Kohlmeier 2003). Of the total amount excreted, 20% occurs via faeces and additional losses can occur through sweat, which, although a minor eliminatory pathway under normal circumstances, can be a significant contributor for people living in hot climates with low dietary consumption (Groff et al 2009).

FOOD SOURCES

Iodine can occur in foods as either an inorganic or organic salt, or as thyroxine in animal sources. Unlike many other essential nutrients, the organic form of iodine found in animal products has poor bioavailability, whereas the iodide salts found in the sea are almost completely absorbed (Jones 2002).

However, irrespective of whether it is animal or plant derived, food from the land has enormous variability in terms of iodine content, from 1 to 10 microgram/kg (Geissler & Powers 2005), due to iodine's high solubility and therefore susceptibility to leaching (Wahlqvist 2002).

Additionally, chemicals known as goitrogens are naturally found in some foods (e.g. brassica [cabbage] family), and these interfere with iodine utilisation and thyroid hormone production.

Best sources

Due to the high saltwater levels of bioavailable iodide, all sea-dwelling creatures, animal or plant, are considered as superior dietary sources.

- Seawater fish
- Shellfish
- Sea vegetables such as seaweeds
- Iodised salt (fortified form of table salt) — providing 20–40 microgram/g
- Recommended for use in Australia by the Foods Standard Australia New Zealand
- Commercially manufactured breads due to the iodate dough oxidisers
- Dairy milk (variable)

In Australia, milk no longer supplies a significant amount of iodine, whereas in the United Kingdom it is still an important dietary source because of the use of both supplemented feeds and iodine-based antiseptics in the dairy industry (Geissler & Powers 2005).

DEFICIENCY SIGNS AND SYMPTOMS

Primary deficiency

Iodine status is considered optimal in a population if the median urinary iodine concentration (MUIC) lies between 100 and 200 micrograms/L. An MUIC of between 50 and 100 micrograms/L is defined as a mild iodine deficiency; 29–49 micrograms/L as moderate deficiency and <20 micrograms/L as severe iodine deficiency. Intervention, such as fortification of salt, is recommended where a population MUIC is <100 micrograms/L. Urinary iodine concentration alone is not however considered an accurate measure of individual iodine status due to high intra-individual variability (Australian Population Health Development Principal Committee [APHDPC] 2007).

Inadequate intake of iodine leads to a decreased thyroid function which results in a collection of physical and mental disorders referred to as 'iodine deficiency disorders' (IDD). These disorders range from being mild to life-threatening (Groff et al 2009, Eastman 2012). A normal adult thyroid contains up to 20 mg of iodine, but this may drop as low as 20 micrograms in cases of chronic iodine deficiency (Zimmerman 2011).

In situations of moderate iodine deficiency, TSH induces thyroid hypertrophy in order to concentrate iodide, resulting in goitre. Most of these cases remain euthyroid, but in cases of severe iodine deficiency, myxoedema may result in adults and cretinism in infants, both of which are serious conditions.

Myxoedema is characterised by swelling of the hands, face, feet and peri-orbital tissues and can lead to coma and death if sufficiently severe and left untreated. Endemic cretinism is divided into two forms, neurological or myxoedematous, depending on the interplay of genetics and iodine deficiency. Usually, children with neurological cretinism are mentally deficient and often deaf–mute, but of normal height and strength and may have goitre. Myxoedematous cretinism is characterised by dwarfism, mental deficiency, dry skin, large tongue, umbilical hernia, muscular incoordination and puffy facial features. Concomitant selenium deficiency may be a contributing factor in myxoedematous cretinism. Early treatment with thyroid hormone supplementation can promote normal physical growth; however, intellectual disability may not be prevented and in very severe cases death may ensue.

Although severe iodine deficiency is rare in Australia and New Zealand, the Australian Population Health Development Principal Committee reports a high incidence of mild to moderate iodine deficiency in primary-school-aged children in Australia and New Zealand (APHDPC 2007). Many parts of the world have notoriously low iodine levels, which is attributed to factors such as depletion in soils, low intake of iodised salt and fish farming practices (Kotsirilos et al 2011). Countries where iodine deficiency is a primary concern include China, Latin America, Southeast Asia and the eastern Mediterranean (Wahlqvist 2002). A report conducted by the World Health Organization in 2007 found that while many countries had succeeded in reaching optimal iodine nutrition through enhanced monitoring and fortification programs over the past decade, worldwide, an estimated almost 2 billion people still have insufficient iodine intakes, including one-third of all school-going children (Zimmerman 2011). Iodine deficiency is considered the single most important cause of preventable mental retardation and brain damage worldwide (APHDPC 2007).

Fetal deficiency

The fetus depends solely on maternal thyroid hormones during the first trimester of pregnancy (Soldin et al 2002) and iodine deficiency uncorrected prior to mid-gestation results in irreversible brain damage (de Escobar et al 2007). To accommodate for this, increasing plasma volume, renal clearance and the increased thyroid hormone degradation secondary to hyperactivity of the uterine–placental deiodinases, healthy pregnant women exhibit a surge in T_4 production, partly under the stimulation of human chorionic gonadotrophin (HCG). From week 11 of gestation, fetal thyroid hormone synthesis usually begins, still dependent on maternal provision of iodine and at term a residual 20–40% of T_4 found in cord blood is of maternal origin (de Escobar et al 2008, Delange 2007, Glinoer 2007, Zimmermann 2008). These demands necessitate an approximately 100% increase (e.g. 250–300 microgram/day) (de Escobar et al 2008, Delange 2007) in maternal iodine intake from conception and throughout the pregnancy. Should such needs go unmet, the mother will adapt by preferentially producing T_3 to stave off both clinical and biochemical hypothyroidism. The fetus, however, yet to develop rapid adaptations to circulating iodine levels, will exhibit reductions of all thyroid hormones and develop hypothyroidism in spite of the mother's euthyroid state (de Escobar et al 2008).

Adequate iodine and healthy functioning of both the maternal and the fetal thyroid glands play a critical role in fetal neuropsycho-intellectual development, due to its role in neuronal migration and myelination, with brain damage risk secondary to a deficiency, peaking in the second trimester and the early neonatal period. Studies have also confirmed that 'mild but measurable' psychomotor deficits in early childhood can result from subclinical hypothyroidism and hypothyroxaemia caused by mild-to-moderate iodine deficiency in pregnancy (Glinoer 2007, Soldin et al 2002). Finally, severe iodine deficiency during pregnancy also increases risk of stillbirths, miscarriage, perinatal mortality and congenital abnormalities (Zimmermann 2008).

Because of the severe neurological consequences of untreated congenital hypothyroidism, neonatal screening programs have been established in some developed countries; however, early or pre-pregnancy detection of subclinical iodine deficiency would be most effective (Ares et al 2008).

Premature infant deficiency

Premature infants face a significantly elevated risk of iodine deficiency secondary to a collusion of factors: interruption of maternal supply (small amounts of breast milk provide substantially smaller quantities of iodine than placental transfer), immaturity of the hypothalamic pituitary thyroid axis and the deiodinase systems, maternal antibodies and postnatal exposure to drugs (e.g. dopamine, heparin, corticosteroids) (Ares et al 2008). Research suggests that 75% of premature neonates demonstrate a negative iodine balance at 5 days post-partum prior to intentional repletion.

Secondary deficiency

High consumption of goitrogens can induce a secondary deficiency state. Goitrogens are substances that inhibit iodine metabolism and include thiocyanates found in the cabbage family (e.g. cabbage, kale, cauliflower, broccoli, turnips and Brussels sprouts) and in linseed, cassava, millet, soybean and competing entities, such as other members of the halogen family (e.g. bromine, fluorine and lithium, as well as arsenic) (Groff et al 2009). Most researchers agree, however, that moderate intake of goitrogens in the diet is not an issue, except when accompanied by low iodine consumption (Groff et al 2009, Kohlmeier 2003). A very rare cause of secondary iodine deficiency and hypothyroidism is TSH deficiency.

Low selenium intake

Low dietary intake of selenium is a factor that exacerbates the effects of iodine deficiency. Selenium is found in the thyroid gland in high concentrations, and while iodine is required for thyroid hormone synthesis, selenium-dependent enzymes are required for the peripheral conversion of thyroxine (T_4) to its biologically active form triiodothyronine (T_3) (Higdon 2003), as well as the general recycling of iodine. Selenium deficiency results in decreased T_4 catabolism, which leads to increased production of peroxide and thyroid cell destruction, fibrosis and functional failure.

SIGNS AND SYMPTOMS

Overall, in addition to highly visible goitre, moderate-to-severe iodine deficiency produces subtle but widespread effects secondary to hypothyroidism, including reduced educability, apathy and impaired productivity, culminating ultimately in poor social and economic development (Zimmermann 2008).

Mild hypothyroidism

This refers to biochemical evidence of thyroid hormone deficiency in patients who have few or no apparent clinical features of hypothyroidism. Current literature does not adequately describe the health consequences of a mild iodine deficiency, although there is reasonable evidence of an association between a mild iodine deficiency and suboptimal neurological development in children such as a reduced IQ.

Congenital hypothyroidism

The majority of infants appear normal at birth and <10% are diagnosed with hypothyroidism based on the following clinical features:

- prolonged jaundice
- feeding problems
- hypotonia

- enlarged tongue
- delayed bone maturation
- umbilical hernia.

Importantly, permanent neurological damage results if treatment is delayed.

Adult hypothyroidism

According to Beers (2005), the clinical signs of hypothyroidism in adults are as follows:

- weakness, tiredness and sleepiness
- dry skin
- cold intolerance
- hair loss and diffuse alopecia
- poor memory and difficulty concentrating
- constipation
- reduced appetite and weight gain
- dyspnoea
- hoarse voice
- increased susceptibility to infectious diseases
- increased susceptibility to cardiovascular diseases
- paraesthesia
- puffy hands, feet and face and peripheral oedema
- impaired hearing
- menorrhagia (later amenorrhoea)
- carpal tunnel and other entrapment syndromes are common, as is impairment of muscle function with stiffness, cramps and pain
- reduced myocardial contractility and pulse rate, leading to a reduced stroke volume and bradycardia.

In adults, mild–moderate iodine deficiency also results in higher rates of more aggressive subtypes of thyroid cancer and an increased risk of (non) toxic goitre (Zimmermann 2008).

MAIN ACTIONS

Thyroid hormone production

Iodine is essential for the manufacture of T_4 and T_3, which are hormones that influence growth, maturation, thermogenesis, oxidation, myelination of the CNS and the metabolism of all tissues (Jones 2002). The thyroid hormones, especially T_3, exert their effects by binding to nuclear receptors on cell surfaces, which in turn trigger binding of the zinc fingers of the receptor protein to the DNA (Groff et al 2009).

OTHER ACTIONS

Due to the concentration of appreciable iodine levels in a range of other tissues, including salivary, gastric and lactating mammary glands, and the ovaries, questions remain about potential additional actions of iodine. One hypothesis postulates iodine as an indirect antioxidant, via its capacity to reduce elevated TSH, a trigger of increased peroxide levels in the body (Smyth 2003).

CLINICAL USE

Increased iodine intake can be achieved through dietary modification and supplementation with tablets. Dietary modification usually refers to increased intake of iodised salt, but may also refer to use of iodised water, iodised vegetable oil or seafood or the use of iodised salt in bread manufacture.

Treatment and prevention of deficiency

Iodine deficiency is accepted as the most common cause of brain damage worldwide, with IDD affecting 740 million people (Higdon 2003). Although it is well accepted that severe deficiency is responsible, evidence is now emerging that mild deficiency during pregnancy is also important and can have subtle effects on brain development, lowering intellectual functioning and inducing psychomotor deficits in early childhood (Glinoer 2007). Preliminary data are also emerging to suggest an association between iodine deficiency hypothyroidism of pregnancy and the incidence of attention-deficit/hyperactivity disorder (ADHD) in the offspring; however, this still requires confirmation in larger studies (Soldin et al 2002, Vermiglio et al 2004).

Pregnancy

Severe iodine deficiency is uncommon in Western countries, such as Australia and New Zealand, but several local surveys have identified that mild-to-moderate deficiency is more prevalent than once thought. The published studies on iodine status in pregnant Australians are limited to New South Wales, Victoria and Tasmania; however, the results are of concern as they consistently suggest that iodine intake is inadequate, with median urinary iodine concentrations (MUIC) ranging from 47–104 micrograms/L, well below the adequate range of 150–249 micrograms/L as defined by WHO for pregnant women (APHPDC 2007).

A research group at Monash Medical Centre in Melbourne screened 802 pregnant women and found that 48.4% of Caucasian women had urinary iodine concentration (UIC) below 50 microgram/L compared to 38.4% of Vietnamese women and 40.8% of Indian/Sri Lankan women (Hamrosi et al 2005). A study conducted at a Sydney hospital involving 81 women attending a 'high' risk clinic found moderate-to-severe iodine deficiency in 18.8% of subjects and mild iodine deficiency in another 29.6% (Gunton et al 1999), the former clearly too close to the WHO maximum acceptable level of 20%. This study also revealed that almost 5% of the sample had MUIC < 25 microgram/L.

Aside from fortification programs in populations affected by severe iodine deficiency, there have been several RCTs of iodine supplementation in mild-to-moderately deficient pregnant women (Zimmermann 2008). While treatment effects include reductions in maternal and newborn thyroid size and, in some, reduced maternal TSH, none of the studies have demonstrated a positive effect on T_4 and T_3 of mother or child, or measured longer term clinical outcomes. Future research needs to address these issues.

Infants

An investigation of infant TSH levels within 72 hours of birth at the Royal North Shore Hospital in Sydney suggests that endemic IDD may be emerging (McElduff et al 2002). Currently, the WHO recommends that less than 3% of newborns should have TSH levels greater than 5 mIU/L and of the 1773 infants enrolled in the study, 5–10% had a TSH reading > 5 mIU/L.

Children and adolescents

Evidence of iodine deficiency has also been demonstrated in Australian schoolchildren (Li et al 2006). Iodine status in schoolchildren is based on median UIC values and is categorised as normal (UIE ≥ 100 microgram/L), or as mild (UIE 50–99 microgram/L), moderate (UIE 20–49 microgram/L) or severe deficiency (UIE < 20 microgram/L). The UIC is considered in combination with the child's sex, year of school and presence of goitre.

I

A study of Melbourne schoolchildren aged 11–18 years found that 76% (439/577) had abnormal UIC values, with 27% (156/577) possessing values consistent with moderate-to-severe iodine deficiency (McDonnell et al 2003). The median UIC value in girls was lower than that in boys (64 microgram/L vs 82 microgram/L), and girls had significantly lower UIC values overall ($P < 0.002$). A study of 324 schoolchildren aged 5–13 years from the Central Coast of New South Wales produced similar results; there was a median UIC concentration of 82 microgram/L, with 14% of children having levels below 50 microgram/L (Guttikonda et al 2003).

These findings were confirmed in the Australian National Iodine Nutrition Study, which identified inadequate iodine intake in the Australian population and called for the urgent implementation of mandatory iodisation of all edible salt in Australia (Li et al 2006). The study consisted of a survey of 1709 schoolchildren aged 8–10 years in the five mainland Australian States and was conducted between July 2003 and December 2004. It found that, overall, children in mainland Australia are borderline iodine deficient, with a national median UIC of 104 microgram/L. On a state basis, children in Victoria and New South Wales are mildly iodine deficient, with median UIC levels of 89 microgram/L and 73.5 microgram/L, respectively; South Australian children are borderline iodine deficient, with a median UIC of 101 microgram/L, whereas both Queensland and Western Australian children are iodine sufficient, with median UIC levels of 136.5 microgram/L and 142.5 microgram/L, respectively. Researchers attributed the decline in iodine intake to changes within the dairy industry, with chlorine-containing sanitisers now replacing iodine-containing sanitisers and a decreased intake of iodised salt.

In 2001, an iodine supplementation program was initiated in Tasmania because it was identified as an area of endemic goitre by the Department of Health Services. The program involves the use of iodised salt in 80% of Tasmania's bread production and aims to reduce the incidence of iodine deficiency. Despite encouraging preliminary data (Doyle & Seal 2003), iodine levels are still inadequate according to the WHO standards. There have been conflicting opinions about the success of this program, with the largest study demonstrating evidence of ongoing iodine deficiency (Guttikonda et al 2002, Seal et al 2003).

Iodine deficiency in children and adolescents is associated with poorer school performance, reduced achievement motivation and a higher incidence of learning disabilities (Tiwari et al 1996, Zimmermann 2008). A meta-analysis of 18 studies from eight countries of people aged between 2 and 30 years showed that iodine deficiency alone reduced mean IQ scores by 13.5 points in children (Bleichrodt et al 1996). Iodine repletion studies in children have yielded improved somatic growth, partial reversal of cognitive impairment and normalisation of age of onset of puberty; however, the strength of the evidence is hampered by methodological issues (Markou et al 2008, Zimmermann et al 2006, Zimmermann 2008).

Clinical note — Why is iodine deficiency on the rise?

In spite of increased rates of household iodised salt use globally since 1990, iodine intakes in Australia are falling (Zimmermann 2008). The emergence or re-emergence of iodine deficiency, however, is not limited to Australia; median urinary iodine concentration had declined by more than 50% between 1971 and 1994 in the United States (Gunton et al 1999, Zimmerman 2008).

Several reasons have been proposed to explain the emergence of iodine deficiency in developed countries. Firstly, from the 1960s, milk had become an unplanned major dietary source of iodine due to residues left from sanitising agents used in the dairy industry. However, from the 1990s, the use of iodine-containing sanitisers were gradually replaced with chlorine-containing substitutes and better practice standards, resulting in significantly reduced iodine concentrations in milk. The significance of this change within the dairy industry was recently shown by Li et al (2006), who compared the iodine content of Australian milk products from 1975 and 2004. The researchers identified mean iodine concentrations of 593.5 microgram/L and 583 microgram/L from samples taken from Victoria and New South Wales (NSW), respectively in 1975 compared to a median concentration of 195 microgram/L in 2004 (250 mL providing 50–60 microgram iodine). Interestingly, the same researchers demonstrated that dairy products and water in northern and central Queensland contained higher iodine levels, which may explain the lower incidence of iodine deficiency in these areas (Li et al 2006). In spite of this, a survey of dietary habits of Tasmanian schoolchildren has revealed that consumption of dairy products is associated with improved iodine status (Hynes et al 2004), a case of some being better than none.

A second reason may relate to public health campaigns that have resulted in increased awareness of the potential adverse effects of salt and reduced its consumption, but failed to highlight the potential benefits of a moderate intake of iodised salt. The last decade has also seen the use of non-iodised rock salt in salt-grinders becoming more fashionable than the use of traditional iodised salt, although in recent years, iodised rock salt has become available. In addition, few food manufacturers use iodised salt in their products, further reducing exposure to iodine (Gunton et al 1999).The trend towards an increased consumption of processed foods has also impacted on iodine status, as only 0.5% of salt used in commercial manufacture is iodised.

Lastly, the mineral depletion of soils is another possible contributing factor, in particular, the depletion of selenium. Due to its role in iodine utilisation, a selenium deficiency would potentiate the effects of an iodine deficiency. Flooding, erosion and glaciation have also contributed to leaching of iodine from soil.

Other theoretical considerations include increased environmental exposure to halogens, such as fluorine and chlorine, and increased consumption of goitrogens, such as soy, in the diet.

Although identifying the key factors responsible for the increased incidence of iodine deficiency is important (Thomson 2004), many authors argue that implementation of national iodine monitoring and surveillance of the iodine content in foods are the most immediate concern (Li et al 2006, McDonnell et al 2003). Lessons learnt from Tasmania's iodine supplementation program, where statewide bread fortification failed to reduce the prevalence of iodine deficiency in children, indicate that greater efforts are required to create significant improvements in iodine status.

Adults

A study of non-pregnant adults in 1999 demonstrated iodine deficiency in 26.3% of 'healthy' subjects and 34.1% of diabetic subjects (Gunton et al 1999).

Non-toxic goitre thyroidectomy

One 12-month study involving 139 patients who had undergone thyroidectomy for non-toxic goitre identified that supplementing L-thyroxine therapy with iodised salt produced significant improvements in thyroid function compared with stand-alone L-thyroxine therapy (Carella et al 2002).

Antiseptic

Iodine solution has been used as a topical antiseptic in the treatment of superficial wounds for more than a century and is still widely used for this indication. It is a highly effective method of decontaminating intact skin and minor wounds and has a low toxicity profile. Povidone–iodine preparations have replaced older iodine solutions and are now the most commonly used form. Results from a systematic review of 27 randomised clinical trials on chronic and acute wound care demonstrated that iodine shows either equivalent or superior benefits to both non-antiseptic wound dressings (paraffin dressings, dextranomer or zinc paste) and other antiseptic agents (silver sulfadiazine cream or chlorhexidine dressings). The review also noted that use of topical iodine did not adversely affect thyroid function, cause significant allergic responses or reduce the speed of wound healing (Vermeulen et al 2010). Povidone–iodine has also been shown to be an effective disinfectant in ocular surgery as well as being an oral antibacterial agent.

Although the treatment is considered safe, a number of reports of iodine toxicity in newborns receiving ongoing treatment with topical iodine-based solutions suggest that it should be used with caution as an ongoing treatment in this group and TSH monitoring considered where appropriate.

Water purification

Iodine-releasing tablets and iodine tincture have been used for many years to decontaminate water and have been used by the United States Army since World War II. A weak aqueous solution of 3–5 ppm of elemental iodine can destroy a wide range of enteroviruses, amoebae and their cysts, bacteria and algae. Under temperate conditions of 25°C, the disinfection process takes 15 minutes, and longer in colder conditions. Adding to the versatility of iodine as a water decontamination agent is its ability to act over a wide range of pH and still be effective in the presence of ammonia and amino ions from nitrogenous wastes that may be also present in the water (Kahn & Visscher 1975). Heiner et al (2010) reported that a 10% povidone–iodine (PVI) solution at a concentration of at least 1 : 1000 in water is an effective bactericidal agent against *Escherichia coli* (*E. coli*), which is the most common cause of traveller's diarrhoea. Disinfection of the water occurred after 15 minutes of contact time with the iodine.

OTHER USES

Fibrocystic breast disease and cyclic mastalgia

A 1993 review that focused on three clinical studies suggested that iodine supplementation may improve objective and subjective outcomes, including pain and fibrosis, for women with fibrocystic breast disease and cyclic mastalgia (Ghent et al 1993). Together the trials involved 1000 women and used a variety of different forms, the most successful being molecular iodine at a dose of 0.08 mg/kg (approximately equivalent to 500 microgram/day in a 60 kg woman) (Ghent et al 1993).

Recently, a placebo-controlled trial conducted with 11 euthyroid women with cyclic mastalgia tested different doses of molecular iodine ranging from 1.5 to 6 mg/day and showed that after 3 months of treatment, 50% of patients consuming 3 or 6 mg/day experienced a significant decrease in pain (Kessler 2004). Although no dose-related adverse events were detected, further investigation is required to confirm both efficacy and safety.

Breast cancer

There is suggestive evidence of a preventive role for iodine in breast cancer. As far back as 1896, research suggested a link between iodine deficiency, thyroid disease and breast cancer (Gago-Dominguez & Castelao 2008, Smyth 2003, Stoddard et al 2008). Epidemiological data have demonstrated a correlation between increased incidence of breast cancer and a range of thyroid conditions, most notably hypothyroidism, with both conditions demonstrating peak incidence in postmenopausal women (Gago-Dominguez & Castelao 2008, Smyth 2003). A prospective study of peri- and postmenopausal women revealed that low free T_4 was an independent risk for the development of breast cancer (OR 2.3). Another study found that the premenopausal women treated for differentiated thyroid cancer with radioactive iodine were at an increased risk of developing breast cancer over the following 5–20 years (Gago-Dominguez & Castelao 2008). In addition, the observed low rates of breast cancer in Japanese women consuming a traditional diet are speculated to be partly due to a high dietary iodine intake, further suggesting a protective effect (Patrick 2008). Notably, this protection disappears when Japanese women consume a 'Western diet'.

It is noteworthy that both the thyroid and the breast share the capacity to concentrate iodide, which exerts both an oxidant effect, triggering and facilitating apoptosis, and antioxidant effect, protecting cells from peroxidative damage (Gago-Dominguez & Castelao 2008, Venturi 2001) and converting it to iodine. The thyroid retains this capacity throughout life, whereas the healthy breast can only concentrate iodide during pregnancy and lactation; states associated with a reduced risk of breast cancer. Curiously, approximately 80% of breast cancers also demonstrate iodide uptake (Stoddard et al 2008). It has been theorised that with iodine insufficiency during pregnancy and lactation, the protective effect of iodide may be compromised, concomitant with diminished oxidant and antioxidant activities. Researchers speculate that this scenario may be compounded by co-existing selenium deficiency (Turken et al 2003).

Besides the diminished antioxidant effect, studies with animal models show that iodine deficiency results in changes in the mammary gland that make it more sensitive to the effects of oestradiol (Stoddard et al 2008, Strum 1979). Iodine has been implicated in the synthesis of alpha-oestrogen receptors, down-regulation of several oestrogen-responsive genes and increased expression of the cytochrome P450 genes responsible for its phase I detoxification (Stoddard et al 2008). Together with other sources of evidence, it is clear that the potential protective effect of iodine against breast cancer is independent of its thyroid role (Stoddard et al 2008).

At present, the only interventional evidence comes from rat studies, demonstrating that administration of Lugol's iodine or iodine-rich Wakame seaweed suppressed the development of induced mammary tumours (Funahashi et al 2001) and in vitro evidence confirming that molecular iodine induces apoptosis in breast cancer cell lines (Shrivastava et al 2006). In light of ongoing evidence of a superior effect of molecular iodine rather than iodide in relation to breast pathology in both animals and humans, rigorous human studies using this form are required (Patrick 2008, Stoddard et al 2008).

Prevention of attention-deficit hyperactivity disorder

Emerging data from research conducted over the past 15 years suggest a possible link between low maternal iodine status and increased risk of ADHD in the offspring. According to a report published in 2004, 11 of 16 children born to women living in a moderately iodine-deficient region in Italy developed ADHD compared to no offspring from the 11 control mothers living in a marginally iodine-deficient region (Vermiglio et al 2004).

On the other hand, another group of researchers investigated whether T_4 levels at birth could represent a biomarker for later development of ADHD and found that all newborns in the sample had T_4 within the normal range and no correlation between values and risk could be demonstrated (Soldin et al 2002, Soldin et al 2003). This evidence invalidated TSH levels as a biomarker of risk, but does not disprove a link between iodine and ADHD, as earlier studies found that those newborns who later developed ADHD were all euthyroid at birth (Vermiglio et al 2004).

Although further investigation is required to clarify these observations, they have provided a new avenue for ADHD research.

DOSAGE RANGE

Australia and New Zealand recommended daily intake (RDI)

- Infants
  - 0–6 months: 90 microgram/day.
  - 7–12 months: 110 microgram/day.
- Children
  - 1–3 years: 90 microgram/day.
  - 4–8 years: 90 microgram/day.
  - 9–14 years: 120 microgram/day.
  - >14 years: 150 microgram/day.
- Adults: 150 microgram/day.
- Pregnancy: 220 microgram/day.
- Lactation: 270 microgram/day.
- Upper level of intake
  - 1–3 years: 200 microgram/day.
  - 4–8 years: 300 microgram/day.
  - 9–13 years: 600 microgram/day.
  - 14–18 years (including pregnancy, lactation): 900 microgram/day.
  - Adults >18 years (including pregnancy, lactation): 1100 microgram/day.

These are the revised Australian RDIs (2006), which are more closely aligned with the WHO recommendations than previously.

According to clinical studies

- ADHD prevention: adequate intake to prevent maternal deficiency (approximately 250 microgram/day)
- Topical antimicrobial: Various concentrations have been used depending on site, type and severity of the wound, with a range of 2–10% povidone-iodine being the most commonly used.
- Fibrocystic breast disease and cyclic mastalgia: 1.5–6 mg iodine/day for 6–18 months.
- Breast cancer prevention: dose is unknown; however, it is suggested that women meet RDI to prevent deficiency.
- Water disinfectant: Widely used practice suggests 3–10 drops iodine tincture per litre of water provides an antibacterial effect after 15 minutes.

TOXICITY

Chronic iodine toxicity results when iodide intake is approximately 2 mg daily or greater (Beers 2005). Overconsumption of iodine can cause gastrointestinal irritation, abdominal pain, nausea, vomiting and diarrhoea, cardiovascular symptoms and can induce both hypo- and hyperthyroidism, depending on the patient's preexisting susceptibility (Wahlqvist 2002, Zimmermann 2008). Excess iodine during pregnancy has also been associated with increased risk of postpartum thyroiditis (Guan et al 2005). Alternatively, there are many cases in which excesses have been tolerated without any overt consequences, particularly in individuals with healthy thyroid function (Geissler & Powers 2005, Groff et al 2009, Zimmermann 2008). Chronic ingestion of ≥500 microgram/day by children has resulted in increased thyroid size (Zimmermann 2008). Intake of very high doses can lead to a brassy taste in the mouth, increased salivation, gastric irritation and acneiform skin lesions.

SIGNIFICANT INTERACTIONS

Goitrogens

These are substances that interfere with iodine utilisation, uptake into the thyroid or thyroid hormone production. These include thiocyanates found in the cabbage family (e.g. cabbage, kale, cauliflower, broccoli, turnips and Brussels sprouts) and in linseed, cassava, millet and soybean — separate intake of iodine and goitrogens where possible. Smoking has also been shown to increase thiocyanate levels and reduce iodine content in the breastmilk of smoking mothers (Zimmermann et al 2008). Other chemical goitrogens include perchlorate and disulphides, the latter from coal processes and there is accumulating evidence of thyroid endocrine disruptors in the form of ingredients used in cosmetics, as pesticides or plasticisers. Major targets are the sodium–iodide symporter (NIS), the haemoprotein thyroperoxidase (TPO), the T_4 distributor protein transthyretin (TTR) and the deiodinases (Köhrle 2008).

Soy

The actions of this particular goitrogen are two-fold: ingestion of soy appears to inhibit iodine absorption to some extent (particularly when presented in its thyroxine form in the gut) and also high levels of the isoflavones, genistein and daidzein, can inhibit T_3 and T_4 production — separate intake of iodine and goitrogens where possible. Particular attention should be paid to minimising soy consumption in individuals taking thyroid hormone supplementation, as it has been shown that soy consumption can increase dosage requirements.

Selenium

Selenium is intrinsic to the metabolism and activity of the thyroid hormones, facilitating the conversion of T_4 to T_3 and is also responsible for the only iodine recycling pathway of the body through the action of the deiodinases on excess or unnecessary thyroid hormones to release the iodine — beneficial interaction.

CONTRAINDICATIONS AND PRECAUTIONS

Thyroid conditions

Due to the complex and diverse causes of thyroid conditions, it is advised that iodine supplementation should be avoided unless under the supervision of a medical practitioner.

Practice points/Patient counselling

- Iodine is an essential trace element required for healthy functioning of the thyroid gland and for normal growth and development.
- It is mainly consumed as iodide salts from sea salt, shellfish, seawater fish and vegetables.
- Iodine is essential for the manufacture of thyroxine (T_4) and liothyronine (T_3), which are hormones that influence growth, maturation, thermogenesis, oxidation, myelination of the CNS and the metabolism of all tissues (Jones 2002).
- Iodine supplementation is commonly used to prevent and treat deficiency. There is also some evidence that it may reduce pain in fibrocystic breast disease and cyclic mastalgia and suggestive evidence of a protective role against breast cancer; however, rigorous research is required to confirm these observations.
- Current evidence points to widespread mild-to-moderate iodine deficiency in Australia, suggesting that dietary intake is inadequate and supplementation or fortification of foods with additional iodine may be required. Use of iodised salt is recommended.

PREGNANCY USE

Up until 2006, the Australian recommended daily intake of iodine was 150 micrograms for pregnant women and 170 micrograms for lactating women; however, reflecting new research, the Australian RDI levels for pregnancy and lactation have been revised and increased to 220 micrograms and 270 micrograms respectively. Care should be taken to avoid ingestion of excessive amounts during pregnancy due to suspected links with increased rates of postpartum thyroiditis and other disorders of thyroid function (Guan et al 2005).

PATIENTS' FAQs

What will this supplement do for me?

Adequate intake of iodine is critical for healthy thyroid function and normal growth and development. Ensuring adequate intake becomes critical during pregnancy and breastfeeding when the infant is solely dependent on the mother's intake for normal growth and brain development. Currently, there is some suggestive evidence that adequate iodine particularly during the female reproductive years may be protective against breast cancer and supplementation may relieve symptoms of breast pain in fibrocystic breast disease and cyclic mastalgia.

When will it start to work?

The time frames depend on the indication it is being used to treat and the level of deficiency. In the case of breast pain, studies suggest that 3 months of treatment are required to attain significant symptom relief.

Are there any safety issues?

People with preexisting thyroid conditions should only increase iodine intake under professional supervision. Doses in excess of the RDI should be avoided unless under the supervision of a medical practitioner.

REFERENCES

APHDPC. The prevalence and severity of iodine deficiency in Australia. Prepared for the Australian Population Health Development Principal Committee (APHDPC) (2007). Available online www.foodstandards.gov.au (accessed 24/01/2013)

Ares S, Quero J, de Escobar GM. Iodine balance, iatrogenic excess, and thyroid dysfunction in premature newborns. Semin Perinatol 32.6 (2008): 407–412.

Beers MH. Merck manual home edition. Whitehouse, NJ: Merck, 2005. www.merck.com (accessed 04-04-2006).

Bleichrodt N et al. The benefits of adequate iodine intake. Nutr Rev 54.4 (1996): S72–S78.

Carella C et al. Iodized salt improves the effectiveness of L-thyroxine therapy after surgery for nontoxic goitre: a prospective and randomized study. Clin Endocrinol (Oxf) 57.4 (2002): 507–513.

de Escobar GM et al. The changing role of national thyroid hormones in fetal brain development. Seminars in Perinatology 32.6 (2008): 407–412.

de Escobar GM, Obregon MJ, del Rey FE. Iodine deficiency and brain development in the first half of pregnancy. Public Health Nutr 10.12A (2007): 1554–1570.

Delange F. Iodine requirements during pregnancy, lactation and the neonatal period and indicators of optimal iodine nutrition. Public Health Nutr 10.12A (2007): 1581–1583.

Doyle Z, Seal J. The Tasmanian iodine monitoring program in schools. Asia Pacific J Clin Nutr 12 (Suppl) (2003): S14.

Eastman CJ. Screening for thyroid disease and iodine deficiency. Pathology 442. 2 (2012): 153–159.

Funahashi H et al. Seaweed prevents breast cancer? Jpn J Cancer Res 92.5 (2001): 483–487.

Gago-Dominguez M, Castelao JE. Role of lipid peroxidation and oxidative stress in the association between thyroid diseases and breast cancer. Crit Rev Oncol Hematol 68.2 (2008): 107–114.

Geissler C, Powers H (eds), Human nutrition, 11th edn. London: Elsevier, 2005.

Ghent WR et al. Iodine replacement in fibrocystic disease of the breast. Can J Surg 36.5 (1993): 453–460.

Glinoer D. The importancec of iodine nutrition during pregnancy. Public Health Nutr 10.12A (2007): 1542–1546.

Groff S et al. Advanced nutrition and human metabolism, 4th edn. Belmont, CA: Wadsworth Thomson Learning, 2009.

Guan H et al. High iodine intake is a risk factor of post-partum thyroiditis: result of a survey from Shenyang, China. J Endocrinol Invest 28.10 (2005): 876–881.

Gunton JE et al. Iodine deficiency in ambulatory participants at a Sydney teaching hospital: is Australia truly iodine replete? Med J Aust 171.9 (1999): 467–470.

Guttikonda K et al. Iodine deficiency in urban primary school children: a cross-sectional analysis. Med J Aust 179.7 (2003): 346–348.

Guttikonda K et al. Recurrent iodine deficiency in Tasmania, Australia: a salutary lesson in sustainable iodine prophylaxis and its monitoring. J Clin Endocrinol Metab 87.6 (2002): 2809–2815.

Hamrosi MA, Wallace EM, Riley MD. Iodine status in pregnant women living in Melbourne differs by ethnic group. Asia Pac J Clin Nutr 14.1 (2005): 27–31.

Heiner JD et al. 10% Povidine–iodine may be a practical field water disinfectant. Wilderness & Environmental Medicine 21 (2010): 332–336.

Higdon J. An evidence-based approach to vitamins and minerals. In: Iodine. New York: Thieme, 2003, pp 130–137.

Hynes KL et al. Persistent iodine deficiency in a cohort of Tasmanian school children: associations with socio-economic status, geographical location and dietary factors. Aust NZ J Public Health 28.5 (2004): 476–481.

Jones GP. Minerals. in: Wahlqvist M (ed). Food and nutrition, 2nd edn. Sydney: Allen & Unwin, 2002, pp 275–276.

Kahn FH, Visscher BR. Water disinfection in the wilderness: a simple, effective method of iodination. West J Med 122.5 (1975): 450–453.

Kessler JH. The effect of supraphysiologic levels of iodine on patients with cyclic mastalgia. Breast J 10.4 (2004): 328–336.

Kohlmeier M. Nutrient metabolism. London: Elsevier, 2003.

Köhrle J. Environment and endocrinology: the case of thyroidology. Ann Endocrinol (Paris) 69.2 (2008): 116–122.

Kotsirilos V et al. A guide to evidence-based integrative and complementary medicine. Chatsworth, NSW, Churchill Livingstone Elsevier (2011).

Li M et al. Are Australian children iodine deficient? Results of the Australian National Iodine Nutrition Study. Med J Aust 184.4 (2006): 165–169.

Markou K et al. Treating iodine deficiency: long-term effects of iodine repletion on growth and pubertal development in school-age children. Thyroid 18.4 (2008): 449–454.

McDonnell CM, Harris M, Zacharin MR. Iodine deficiency and goitre in schoolchildren in Melbourne, 2001. Med J Aust 178.4 (2003): 159–162.

McElduff A et al. Neonatal thyroid-stimulating hormone concentrations in northern Sydney: further indications of mild iodine deficiency? Med J Aust 176.7 (2002): 317–320.

Patrick L. Iodine: deficiency and therapeutic considerations. Altern Med Rev 13.2 (2008): 116–127.

Seal JA et al. Tasmania: doing its wee bit for iodine nutrition [Letter]. Med J Aust 179.8 (2003): 451–452.

Shrivastava A et al. Molecular iodine induces caspase-independent apoptosis in human breast carcinoma cells involving the mitochondria-mediated pathway. J Biol Chem 281.28 (2006): 19762–19771.

Smyth PP. The thyroid, iodine and breast cancer. Breast Cancer Res 5.5 (2003): 235–238 [Epub ahead of print].

Soldin OP et al. Lack of a relation between human neonatal thyroxine and pediatric neurobehavioral disorders. Thyroid 13.2 (2003): 193–198.

Soldin OP et al. Newborn thyroxine levels and childhood ADHD. Clin Biochem 35.2 (2002): 131–136.

Stoddard FR et al. Iodine alters gene expression in the MCF7 breast cancer cell line: evidence for an anti-estrogen effect of iodine. Int J Med Sci 5.4 (2008): 189–196.

Strum JM. Effect of iodide-deficiency on rat mammary gland. Virchows Arch B Cell Pathol Incl Mol Pathol 30.2 (1979): 209–220.
Thomson CD. Selenium and iodine intakes and status in New Zealand and Australia. Br J Nutr 91.5 (2004): 661–672.
Tiwari BD et al. Learning disabilities and poor motivation to achieve due to prolonged iodine deficiency. Am J Clin Nutr 63.5 (1996): 782–7816.
Turken O et al. Breast cancer in association with thyroid disorders. Breast Cancer Res 5.5 (2003): R110–R1113.
Venturi S. Is there a role for iodine in breast diseases? Breast 10.5 (2001): 379–382.
Vermeulen H et al. Benefit and harm of iodine in wound care: a systematic review. Journal of Hospital Infection 76 (2010): 191–199.
Vermiglio F et al. Attention deficit and hyperactivity disorders in the offspring of mothers exposed to mild-moderate iodine deficiency: a possible novel iodine deficiency disorder in developed countries. J Clin Endocrinol Metab 89.12 (2004): 6054–6060.
Wahlqvist M (ed). Food and nutrition, 2nd edn. Sydney: Allen & Unwin, 2002.
Zimmerman MB. The role of iodine in human growth and development. Seminars in Cell Development Biology 22 (2011): 645–652.
Zimmermann MB et al. Iodine supplementation improves cognition in iodine-deficient schoolchildren in Albania: a randomized, controlled, double-blind study. Am J Clin Nutr 83.1 (2006): 108–114.
Zimmermann MB, Jooste PL, Pandav CS. Iodine-deficiency disorders. Lancet 372.9645 (2008): 1251–1262.
Zimmermann MB. Iodine requirements and the risks and benefits of correcting iodine deficiency in populations. J Trace Elem Med Biol 22.2 (2008): 81–92.

Iron

BACKGROUND AND RELEVANT PHARMACOKINETICS

Iron is an essential mineral, vital to human health. The average human body contains 2–4 g of iron. Iron is found in the body in: haemoglobin (65%); myoglobin (10%); enzymes (1–5%); with the remaining approximately 20% of body iron being found in storage or in the blood (Gropper & Smith 2013).

Although the metal exists in several oxidation states in nature, only the ferrous (Fe^{2+}) and ferric (Fe^{3+}) forms are stable in the aqueous environment of the body (Gropper & Smith 2013).

Iron is found in the haem form, which comes from animal sources, and the non-haem form, derived from plants and dairy products.

The haem form of iron is more soluble than the non-haem form and is absorbed 2–3 times more readily. Absorption of haem iron occurs across the brush border of the small intestine, especially in the proximal region, and is facilitated by haem carrier protein 1 (hcp1). Non-haem iron is bound to other substances in food when ingested, and must first be enzymatically released by gastric secretions such as hydrochloric acid and pepsin before absorption can occur. Non-haem iron in the ferrous form (Fe^{2+}) is absorbed more readily than iron in the ferric (Fe^{3+}) form, and occurs primarily in the duodenum with the aid of divalent mineral transporter 1. Iron in the ferric form (Fe^{3+}) is susceptible to aggregation and precipitation in the alkaline environment of the small intestine which impairs absorption (Gropper & Smith 2013). Intestinal absorption of non-haem iron is influenced by a number of factors, as summarised below.

Solubility enhancers of non-haem iron

- Acids (including ascorbic acid) aid solubility of non-haem iron, thus improving absorption; the addition of 20 mg ascorbic acid has been shown to increase non-haem iron absorption by 39% (Hallberg et al 2003)

- Sugars (e.g. fructose and sorbitol) aid absorption
- Mucin
- Meat stimulates digestive secretions, and breakdown products such as cysteine-containing peptides aid absorption (Hurrell et al 1988). The addition of red meat increases non-haem iron absorption by 85% (Hallberg et al 2003). This appears to be dose-dependent, as a study found that the addition of 60 g Danish pork meat three times daily improved the absorption of non-haem iron from 5.3% to 7.9% (Bach-Kristensen et al 2005), although the addition of smaller amounts was not as effective (Baech et al 2003)
- The addition of fish to a high-phytate bean meal has also been shown to increase iron absorption (Navas-Carretero et al 2008)
- Alcohol improves iron uptake. The consumption of up to two alcoholic drinks per day is associated with reduced risk of iron deficiency and more than two can increase the risk of iron overload (Ioannou et al 2004).

Solubility inhibitors of non-haem iron

- Polyphenols, including tannin derivatives of gallic acid. A number of studies have shown that tea catechins can inhibit intestinal non-haem iron absorption (Ullmann et al 2005); however, polyphenols do not have chelating effects on cooked haem iron (Breet et al 2005). Overall, tea consumption has been reported to reduce non-haem iron absorption by 60% (Kaltwasser et al 1998) and coffee consumption by 40% when taken with or shortly after a meal (Gropper & Smith 2013).

Recent studies suggest that impaired absorption is unlikely to be significant in people with normal iron stores (Breet et al 2005, Ullmann et al 2005). The addition of milk to tea may reduce the chelating effects.

- Phytic acid or phytates (whole grains, legumes, maize) (Gropper & Smith 2013)
- Oxalic acid (spinach, chard, chocolate, berries, tea) (Gropper & Smith 2013)
- Phosvitin, a protein found in egg yolks (Gropper & Smith 2013)
- Calcium — a transient inhibitory effect has been observed which does not occur with long-term high-dose calcium intake (Lonnerdal 2010). This includes calcium found in dairy foods, and other forms such as calcium phosphate, calcium citrate, calcium carbonate and calcium chloride; when consumed in amounts of 300–600 mg, it significantly impairs iron absorption (ferrous sulfate and dietary iron) (Gropper & Smith 2013)
- Zinc competes with iron for absorption (Gropper & Smith 2013) — inorganic zinc supplements may reduce iron absorption by 66–80% (Crofton et al 1989), and supplements containing both iron and zinc may not be as efficacious as the same doses given in isolation (Fischer Walker et al 2005, Lind et al 2003). Nutrients consumed in a meal may not be as affected (Whittaker 1998)
- Manganese may reduce absorption by 22–40% (Rossander-Hulten et al 1991)
- Rapid intestinal transit time (Gropper & Smith 2013)
- Malabsorption syndromes (Gropper & Smith 2013)
- *Helicobacter pylori* infection (Ciacci et al 2004, Duque et al 2010)
- Gastrointestinal blood loss (Higgins & Rockey 2003)
- Insufficient digestive secretions (including achlorhydria), or raised gastric pH due to age-related decrease in gastric acid production
- Antacids, H_2 antagonists and proton pump inhibitor drugs due to raising pH within the gastrointestinal tract.

Systemic and local mechanisms have also been identified which regulate iron absorption and play a role in iron homeostasis. Hepcidin, a 25-amino-acid peptide, is the regulatory protein for systemic iron absorption from intestinal enterocytes as well as for the efflux of iron from macrophages. Factors that alter hepcidin levels, such as inflammation, infection and hypoxia, will in turn have an effect on iron levels, although exact mechanisms are yet to be fully elucidated. Local regulatory mechanisms involve an iron-responsive element/iron-regulatory protein system, which affects the regulation of proteins involved in iron metabolism. Disturbances in these local or systemic iron absorption regulatory mechanisms are implicated in both iron-loading and iron-deficiency disorders (Fuqua et al 2012).

Clinical note — Factors affecting the absorption of iron
If the dietary intake of iron is adequate, it is often assumed that a patient's iron levels will be within the normal range. In practice, this is not always the case as absorption is significantly affected by a number of factors, thereby increasing or decreasing the amount of ingested dietary iron that reaches the systemic circulation.

CHEMICAL COMPONENTS

Ferrous sulfate is the most widely studied form and is generally considered the treatment of choice based on proven efficacy, cost and tolerability, especially when administered as oral sustained-release preparations (Santiago 2012). Other ferrous forms include ascorbate, carbonate, citrate, fumarate, gluconate, lactate, succinate and tartrate (non-haem iron). Iron from ferrous sulfate has a significantly greater bioavailability than ferrous glycine chelate or ferric ethylenediamine tetraacetic acid (EDTA) (Ferreira da Silva et al 2004). Other ferric forms include ammonium citrate, chloride, citrate, pyrophosphate and sulfate. Amino acid chelates, such as iron glycine, are also available. Dietary ferritin is as equally well absorbed as ferrous sulfate and therefore food sources are likely to be effective (Davila-Hicks et al 2004). Cooking in iron pots may also improve iron status (Geerligs et al 2003).

FOOD SOURCES

The average Western diet is estimated to contain 5–7 mg iron/1000 kcal.

Haem iron

About 50–60% of the iron in animal sources is in the haem form. Sources include liver, lean red meat, poultry, fish, oysters, clams, shellfish, kidney and heart.

Non-haem iron

This is found in plant and dairy products in the form of iron salts and makes up about 85% of the average intake. Sources include egg yolks, nuts, legumes, fruit, dried fruit, raisins, dark molasses, vegetables, including beetroot, grains and tofu. Dairy is a relatively poor source of iron.

A number of iron-fortified foods are also available and include wholegrain and enriched bread, pasta, cereal, soy sauce, Thai fish sauce, milk, orange juice and wines.

Considering that minerals such as calcium may reduce iron absorption, fortification of some foods may be relatively ineffectual unless absorption enhancers such as vitamin C are also included (Davidsson et al 1998).

DEFICIENCY SIGNS AND SYMPTOMS

Iron deficiency is the most common and widespread nutritional disorder in the world, affecting approximately 1.6 billion people according to World Health Organization reports (de Benoist et al 2008). Iron deficiency may occur with or without anaemia (Gillespie et al 1991); however an estimated 50% of all anaemias worldwide are attributed to a deficiency in iron (Stoltzfus 2003).

The term iron deficiency is used when there are no iron stores that can be mobilised and there are signs of a compromised supply of iron to tissues; however this has not yet led to a low haemoglobin level and thus a classification of 'anaemia' (Rattehalli et al 2013). A mild deficiency, without anaemia, will still result in symptoms such as mood changes, poor concentration, fatigue and reduced physical performance and may still warrant iron replenishment, especially in vulnerable patient groups (Rattehalli et al 2013).

Iron-deficiency anaemia results when an ongoing iron deficiency results in reduced erthyropoiesis and a drop in haemoglobin levels, which leads to a decrease in red blood cell count and mean corpuscle volume. The World Health Organization defines anaemia in terms of a haemoglobin concentration <13 g/dL for men and <12 g/dL for non-pregnant women. Iron-deficiency anaemia is associated with an increased risk of maternal and child mortality, especially in developing countries, and results in reduced work capacity and physical performance in adults, and in children leads to a reduced ability to learn and develop physically.

Signs and symptoms include:

- Fatigue and lethargy
- Decreased resistance to infection
- Cardiovascular and respiratory changes, which can progress to cardiac failure if left untreated
- Increased lead absorption, which in turn inhibits haem synthesis
- Decreased selenium and glutathione peroxidase levels
- Pale inside lower eyelid or mouth
- Pale-coloured nail bed
- Pale lines on stretched palm (palmar creases)
- Ridged, spoon-shaped, thin flat nails
- Brittle hair
- Impaired cognitive and motor function
- Adverse pregnancy outcomes and increased perinatal maternal mortality (NMCD 2005)
- Reduced thyroid function and ability to make thyroid hormones (Beard et al 1990)
- Difficulty maintaining body temperature in a cold environment.

Risk groups for iron deficiency

The four main population groups that are most at risk of developing iron deficiency are:

1. Young children (6 months–4 years), due to factors such as inadequate dietary intake, inadequate reserves to meet physiological requirements, rapid growth phases, low iron content in milk
2. Adolescents, due to pubertal growth spurts and increased need to match expansion in mass of red blood cells
3. Women during child-bearing years, due to menstrual blood loss
4. Pregnant women, due to increased fetal demands, expanding blood volume and blood loss associated with childbirth (Gropper & Smith 2013).

Primary deficiency

Primary deficiency is most common in vegetarians, the elderly, those with protein-calorie malnutrition, and during periods of increased iron requirement due to expanded blood volume in infancy, adolescence and pregnancy.

Secondary deficiency

Underlying causes of iron-deficiency anaemia include blood loss, inefficient absorption due to gastrointestinal disturbances and increased destruction of red blood cells.

- Blood loss (menstruation, menorrhagia, bleeding haemorrhoids, parasites, bleeding peptic ulcer, malignancy, *Helicobacter pylori* infection, gastrointestinal bleeding due to medication such as non-steroidal anti-inflammatory drugs)
- Inefficient absorption (chronic gastrointestinal disturbances, malabsorption syndromes, coeliac disease) (Annibale et al 2001)
- Increased destruction of red blood cells (malaria, high-intensity exercise).

Note: The majority of iron utilised in erythropoiesis is provided by recovered iron from old erythrocytes (Handelman & Levin 2008), thus a failure in this system will also impact on iron status.

> ***Clinical note — Testing for iron deficiency***
>
> In iron-deficiency anaemia, storage iron declines until the delivery of iron to bone marrow is insufficient for erythropoiesis to occur. In the early stages, blood tests will reveal low plasma ferritin, followed by decreased plasma iron and transferrin saturation, and ultimately low haemoglobin in red blood cells (Handelman & Levin 2008). As isolated haemoglobin has both low specificity and low sensitivity for determining iron status, the optimal diagnostic approach is to measure the serum ferritin as an index of iron stores and the serum transferrin receptor as an index of tissue iron deficiency (Cook 2005, Flesland et al 2004, Mei et al 2005). Iron deficiency is associated with a plasma ferritin concentration of <12 ng/mL. In the presence of infection or inflammation, however, plasma ferritin levels are a less reliable indicator of iron status. Inflammation or infection lead to a rise in plasma ferritin concentration and it may therefore still appear within normal range or high, even though iron levels are depleted (Gropper & Smith 2013).

MAIN ACTIONS

Iron plays a central role in many biochemical processes in the body.

Oxygen transport and storage

The key function of iron is to facilitate oxygen transport by haemoglobin, the oxygen-carrying pigment of erythrocytes. It is also involved in oxygen storage by myoglobin, an iron-containing protein that transports and stores oxygen within muscle and releases it to meet increased metabolic demands during muscle contraction.

Immunity

Iron is vital for the proliferation of all cells, including those of the immune system. In vitro and in vivo studies have indicated a link between iron deficiency and impaired T-lymphocyte proliferation. In anaemic children in Bolivia who received iron treatment for 3 months, the proportion of circulating immature T lymphocytes decreased from 18.3% to 9.2% (Sejas et al 2008).

Iron deficiency causes several defects in both humoral and cellular immunity (Bowlus 2003), including a reduction in peripheral T cells secondary to atrophy of the thymus and inhibition of thymocyte proliferation (Bowlus 2003) and a reduction in interleukin-2 (IL-2) production (Bergman et al 2004). Reduced IL-2 production may partly explain the increased susceptibility to infections and cancer in patients with iron-deficiency anaemia (Bergman et al 2004). Supplementation of ferrous sulfate (60 mg Fe) once daily for 8 weeks has been shown to reduce the incidence and duration of upper respiratory tract infections in children (De-Silva et al 2003).

However, there is also preliminary evidence that iron may be implicated in the pathogenesis of autoimmune disorders, including systemic lupus erythematosus, scleroderma, type 1 diabetes, Goodpasture's syndrome, multiple sclerosis and rheumatoid arthritis (Bowlus 2003). A review conducted by Recalcati et al (2012) highlights the importance of macrophages in autoimmune diseases, and the potential role that iron retention may play in promoting the proinflammatory, pathogenic activity of M1 macrophages, rather than allowing for modulation by the anti-inflammatory action of M2 macrophages. In this way, iron accumulation in macrophages may potentially exacerbate autoimmune disease (Recalcati et al 2012).

Protein and enzyme systems

Iron forms a part of several proteins and is a cofactor for many different enzymes. Processes in which iron plays a role include:

- Production of adenosine triphosphate and cellular respiration
- Amino acid metabolism (e.g. arginine, phenylalanine, tryptophan, tyrosine)
- Carbohydrate metabolism
- As a component of enzymes, including catalase, myeloperoxidase, thyroperoxidase and oxidoreductase, providing protection against free radical damage
- Synthesis of carnitine and niacin
- Synthesis of nitric oxide, which plays a role in blood pressure regulation, intestinal motility, macrophage function and inhibition of platelet aggregation
- Synthesis and function of hormones (e.g. thyroid hormone) and neurotransmitters (serotonin, dopamine and noradrenaline)
- Synthesis of procollagen and elastin.

CLINICAL USE

Iron supplementation is used to prevent deficiency in at-risk populations and also to rectify deficiency states. The best form of iron to use, administration form and dosage regimen are yet to be determined and likely to vary depending on the individual presentation. This review will mainly focus on oral supplementation as this is the most commonly used form. Oral ferrous iron supplements are a popular commercial form which is available in complexes as ferrous sulfate or ferrous fumarate, but may also be found in complexes with succinate, citrate, tartrate, lactate and gluconate. Amino acid-iron chelates such as iron glycine are also available. Administration in the chelate form has not been shown to provide better absorption than administration of iron as ferrous sulfate (Gropper & Smith 2013).

Iron deficiency and iron-deficiency anaemia

Ferrous sulfate is the most commonly used oral treatment for iron deficiency and iron-deficiency anaemia. Daily iron therapy has been shown to be the most effective treatment, but is associated with a higher incidence of adverse effects, such as nausea, constipation and dental discolouration, as well as poor compliance, and may not be feasible in all population groups (Fernandez-Gaxiola & De-Regil 2011). In practice, it is often prescribed in divided doses rather than a single, larger daily dose in an attempt to reduce the incidence and severity of these side effects.

Intermittent iron therapy is less effective than daily iron therapy in the prevention and treatment of iron-deficiency anaemia, but still a successful alternative strategy where daily supplementation is not possible, according to a recent Cochrane review of 21 trials involving 10,258 women in their menstrual years (Fernandez-Gaxiola & De-Regil 2011).

Previous evidence also suggested that weekly administration of iron was an effective strategy for the treatment and prevention of iron deficiency and iron-deficiency anaemia in most population groups, including pregnant women and children (Agarwal et al 2003, Mukhopadhyay et al 2004, Siddiqui et al 2004, Sungthong et al 2004, Yang et al 2004). Although this is associated with lower cost, fewer side effects and improved compliance (Haidar et al 2003), this notion has been challenged when twice-weekly doses of iron (ferrous dextran containing 60 mg elemental iron) for 12 months failed to improve haemoglobin or serum ferritin (iron stores) in children or adults (Olsen et al 2006). The results from some studies suggest that weekly doses may assist in maintenance but may not improve iron status (Wijaya-Erhardt et al 2007). To achieve a better result, it may be necessary to use higher weekly doses and also address concomitant nutritional deficiencies and other factors affecting iron absorption.

Children

According to a 2013 meta-analysis by Thompson et al, iron supplementation in children aged 2–5 years increases both haemoglobin and ferritin levels and may also lead to a small improvement in cognitive, but not physical, development in this age group (Thompson et al 2013). Benefits for growth appear most likely if iron is given together with a combination of micronutrients according to systematic reviews and meta-analyses (Allen et al 2009, Ramakrishnan et al 2004, 2009, Sachdev et al 2005).

Daily iron supplementation is more effective than intermittent supplementation in children under 12 years, according to a 2011 Cochrane systematic review (De-Regil et al 2011). Despite this, intermittent supplementation is still better than placebo and presents an effective solution should daily supplementation not be possible. It may also be associated with fewer side effects, according to a 2004 study of 60 children (age 5–10 years) with iron-deficiency anaemia given ferrous sulfate (200 mg) weekly for 2 months and compared to daily treatment with the same dose (Siddiqui et al 2004). Another study found that children receiving weekly doses of ferrous sulfate (300 mg) had similar improvements in haemoglobin, but a significantly higher increase in IQ, compared to those taking the same dose of iron 5 days per week (Sungthong et al 2004).

Preliminary data suggests that low iron status and low serum ferritin concentration should be investigated in children presenting with febrile seizures as these may be risk factors for the development of this condition (Zareifar et al 2012).

Elderly

The prevalence of iron-deficiency anaemia increases with age. This is mainly due to a combination of factors, including poor dietary intake together with decreased digestive function, use of medications affecting uptake and disease states associated with chronic inflammation, gastrointestinal bleeding and malabsorption, renal failure, portal hypertension, colorectal cancer and angiodysplasia (Andres et al 2008).

Elderly patients are particularly vulnerable to the dose-dependent adverse effects of iron supplementation, and should be given the lowest effective dose. A randomised controlled trial (RCT) of 90 hospitalised elderly patients demonstrated that 15 mg of liquid ferrous gluconate produced similar improvements in haemoglobin and ferritin over 60 days to 150 mg of ferrous calcium citrate tablets without the negative side effects (Rimon et al 2005). Iron supplementation appears to be effective and safe for the treatment of comorbid anaemia in elderly patients undergoing knee or hip surgery, according to recent meta-analysis (Yang et al 2011).

In all cases the lowest safe and effective dose at the lowest frequency of dosing should be used to correct iron deficiency with or without anaemia.

It is becoming clearer that long-term iron deficiency is also associated with an increased risk for cardiovascular disease and all-cause mortality in the elderly (Hsu et al 2013) and has implications in congestive heart failure (CHF). Anaemia is reported in over 50% of patients with CHF, and is associated with an increased risk of death compared to non-anaemic CHF patients (Avni et al 2012). Iron deficiency has also been highlighted as a potential problem in CHF patients, decreasing aerobic performance and exercise tolerance, and may be a predictor of disease severity and mortality (Klip et al 2012). A recent review reported that intravenous iron supplementation (1000–2000 mg total dose) may improve exercise capacity and quality of life and reduce the need for hospitalisation in CHF patients. Benefits were also reported in non-anaemic patients, suggesting that anaemia is not the only reason for improvement in symptoms of CHF with use of iron supplementation (Avni et al 2012).

Pregnancy

Women taking iron supplementation during pregnancy are at less risk of giving birth to babies of low birth weight (<2500 g) and more likely to have a baby with a higher mean birth weight than women not taking iron supplements, according to a recent Cochrane review of 43 trials (*n* = 27,400) (Pena-Rosas et al 2012). Prophylactic use of iron supplementation reduced the risk of iron deficiency at term by 57% and/or iron-deficiency anaemia by 70%. In the review, iron supplementation was also associated with a marginally higher risk of maternal adverse effects and raised haemoglobin levels, suggesting a need for updating recommendations on dosing and iron supplementation regimens. Improved birth weight with iron supplementation was also reported in a 2013 review of 48 RCTs (*n* = 17,793 women) and 44 cohort studies, involving almost 2 million women (Haider et al 2013). It was found to significantly decrease the risk of iron-deficiency anaemia in pregnancy and substantially improved birth weight in a linear dose–response manner.

Due to the possibility of uncontrolled lipid peroxidation, predictive of adverse effects for mother and fetus, iron supplementation should be prescribed on the basis of biological criteria, not on the assumption of anaemia alone (Lachili et al 2001) and the minimum dose possible should be used. Low-dose iron supplements (20 mg elemental iron) have demonstrated efficacy in treating anaemia in pregnancy with fewer gastrointestinal side effects (Zhou et al 2009).

According to trials, a supplement of 40 mg ferrous iron/day from 18 weeks' gestation appears adequate to prevent iron deficiency in 90% of women and iron-deficiency anaemia in at least 95% of women during pregnancy and postpartum (Milman et al 2004). A single weekly dose of 200 mg elemental iron, however, may be sufficient, as this has been shown to be comparable with 100 mg elemental iron daily on erythrocyte indices (Mukhopadhyay et al 2004). Other trials have found that low doses of sodium feredetate (33 mg and 66 mg of elemental iron given twice daily) produced comparable results to ferrous fumarate (100 mg elemental iron given twice daily), with no reports of adverse effects (Sarkate et al 2007).

Although iron supplementation is often used as stand-alone treatment in pregnant iron-deficient women, one RCT indicated that a combination of iron and folate therapy (80 mg iron protein succinylate, with 0.370 mg folinic acid daily) for 60 days produces a better therapeutic response than iron-only supplementation (Juarez-Vazquez et al 2002).

Postpartum anaemia

Postpartum anaemia is associated with breathlessness, tiredness, palpitations, maternal infections and impaired mood and cognition. A 2004 Cochrane review suggested that further high-quality trials were required before the benefits of iron supplementation or iron-rich diets in the treatment of postpartum anaemia could be established (Dodd et al 2004). Since then a randomised placebo-controlled study of iron sulfate (80 mg daily) for 12 weeks starting 24–48 hours after delivery demonstrated an improvement in haemoglobin levels and iron stores (Krafft et al 2005) and supplementation of ferrous sulfate (125 mg) with folate (10 mcg) and vitamin C (25 mg) demonstrated improvements in cognitive function, as well as depression and stress compared with folate and vitamin C alone (Beard et al 2005). However, further studies are still warranted.

Restless-leg syndrome

Low serum iron levels are frequently seen in patients with restless-leg syndrome. Whether this is a cause or consequence of the syndrome remains unclear. A Cochrane review of six RCTs (n = 192) concluded that currently there is insufficient evidence to determine whether iron supplementation would be of benefit in the treatment of restless-leg syndrome (Trotti et al 2012). The trials included patients with and without iron deficiency.

Unexplained fatigue without anaemia

Iron supplementation may be considered as a treatment in non-anaemic menstruating women with haemoglobin levels within normal range (>120 g/L) who complain of unexplained fatigue without identifiable secondary causes.

A recent multicentre RCT involving 198 women aged 18–53 years assessed the effect of oral iron therapy for 12 weeks in women with considerable fatigue without obvious clinical cause. Eligibility criteria included ferritin levels of <50 mcg/L and haemoglobin levels >12 g/dL (120 g/L). Iron supplementation (80 mg elemental iron/day as ferrous sulfate for 12 weeks) was shown to decrease fatigue by 47.7% in the treatment group compared to 28.8% in the placebo group ($P = 0.02$). No significant effects on anxiety or quality of life unrelated to fatigue were observed (Vaucher et al 2012). These findings support earlier research by Verdon and colleagues (2003), who conducted a double-blind, randomised placebo-controlled trial designed to determine the subjective response to iron therapy in non-anaemic women (haemoglobin > 117 g/L) with unexplained fatigue. This study found that supplementation with oral ferrous sulfate (80 mg/day elemental iron) for 4 weeks reduced the level of fatigue in the iron group by 29% compared with 13% in the placebo group. Subgroup analysis showed that only women with ferritin concentrations <50 mcg/L improved with oral supplementation. This was common in 85% of subjects and 51% of subjects had ferritin concentrations <20 mcg/L (Verdon et al 2003). It has been suggested that the current reference levels for women may need to be revised.

Improving athletic performance

Sports anaemia is a common finding among professional and non-professional athletes engaging in strenuous physical activity. Optimal iron balance is important to maintain athletic performance, yet elite athletes appear to be at greater risk of developing iron deficiency (Reinke et al 2012).

Possible mechanisms include: increased iron loss due to factors such as sweating, gastrointestinal bleeding and inflammation (McClung 2012). Proinflammatory cytokines such as IL-6 stimulate expression of hepcidin, a hormone that reduces absorption of iron in the enterocyte, while promoting the sequestering of iron in macrophages (McClung & Karl 2009). Some athletes may also consume carefully controlled diets which are low in meat and other sources of haem iron, yet high in grains and vegetable products that inhibit iron absorption (McClung 2012). Another possibility is dilutional pseudoanaemia, which is caused by plasma volume expansion greater than that of the red blood cell mass, but does not reflect actual blood loss and will generally normalise within 3–5 days of ceasing training; intravascular haemolysis due to mechanical trauma such as 'foot strike haemolysis', which can result in urinary loss of iron; or transient ischaemia resulting from vasoconstriction of the splanchnic and renal vessels, which can also result in blood loss from the gastrointestinal and urinary tracts (Merkel et al 2005).

In a placebo-controlled trial, iron supplementation (50 mg ferrous sulfate twice daily) for 6 weeks significantly improved iron status and maximal oxygen uptake (VO_{2max}) after 4 weeks' concurrent aerobic training in previously marginally deficient and untrained women (Brownlie et al 2002). In a later randomised double-blind placebo-controlled study of 41 untrained iron-deficient women without anaemia, ferrous sulfate (100 mg) for 6 weeks improved endurance capacity after aerobic training (Brownlie et al 2004). However, a review concluded that the current evidence does not justify the use of supplementation solely for the purpose of performance enhancement (Rodenberg & Gustafson 2007).

Due to the potential side effects of inappropriate iron supplementation and the possibility of masking more serious underlying complaints, athletes should only be supplemented if iron deficiency is established on the basis of biological criteria (Zoller & Vogel 2004). Short recuperation periods between intense athletic training may also allow for some recovery of iron storage; however, it may not be sufficient to fully normalise decreased iron levels and iron deficiency in athletes. Monitoring of iron status in elite athletes is recommended (Reinke et al 2012).

Anaemia of inflammation/chronic disease

In this form of anaemia storage iron is often abundant but not available for erythropoiesis. Thus, elevated markers of inflammation should be used for diagnosis. Treatment is difficult but often involves intravenous iron and erythropoietin (EPO) supplements (Handelman & Levin 2008). Emerging future therapies for anaemia associated with chronic inflammation and autoimmune disease may include iron chelation anticytokine administration, modulation of EPO receptors, use of erythropoietin-stimulating agents and agonists/antagonists to modulate the levels of the proteins hepcidin and ferroportin, which are involved with iron homeostasis (Recalcati et al 2012).

Cognitive function

Iron deficiency and iron-deficiency anaemia are associated with impaired cognitive function, which suggests that iron supplementation may have a potential role in improving cognitive function. Iron deficiency has been associated with delayed achievement of developmental motor milestones in a study of infants aged 9–10 months (Shafir et al 2008) and poor cognitive and motor development with behavioural problems (Otero et al 2004).

A systematic review and meta-analysis of 14 RCTs reported that iron supplementation results in a slight improvement (2.5 points) in IQ in anaemic participants ($P = 0.0002$), but not in non-anaemic ones (Falkingham et al 2010). Most of the studies included in the review were conducted on children or adolescents, but some studies in women were also included. Interestingly, iron supplementation may also improve attention and concentration in adolescents and women, irrespective of baseline iron status, although it was not found to have a significant effect on memory, psychomotor function or scholastic achievement (Falkingham et al 2010).

Modest improvements in mental development scores were found for iron supplementation according to a systematic review; however benefits were more prevalent in those who were initially anaemic or iron deficient (Sachdev et al 2005). Two-month supplementation of 15 mg iron (and multivitamin) was better than a multivitamin alone in preschoolers with iron-deficiency anaemia as it resulted in improvements to discrimination (specifically selective attention), accuracy and efficiency (Metallinos-Katsaras et al 2004). Another study found that iron deficiency was associated with compromised working memory in children between the ages of 8 and 10, with iron supplementation being able to restore attention and cognitive capabilities in this group (Otero et al 2008).

An increased incidence of iron deficiency and iron-deficiency anaemia has been reported in children with autistic spectrum disorders; this appears to be mainly due to low iron intake relating to feeding difficulties and food selectivity. These low iron levels may exacerbate the severity of psychomotor and behavioural problems in these children (Bilgic et al 2010).

In adults, iron deficiency in the absence of anaemia has been reported to impair cognitive function in a small study conducted on premenopausal women (Blanton et al 2011). Another study found that iron supplementation improved cognitive function and depression in postpartum anaemic women (Beard et al 2005).

Attention-deficit hyperactivity disorder (ADHD) in children

Whether iron supplementation has benefits in ADHD is difficult to determine at this stage due to a lack of RCTs; however, preliminary research suggests it may be of use in improving some aspects of ADHD. In particular, it appears that iron deficiency may contribute to behavioural problems, including ADHD (as well as restless-leg syndrome and Tourette's) due to an influence on the metabolism of dopamine and other catecholamines (Cortese et al 2008). As a result, children with ADHD and a positive family history of restless-leg syndrome appear to be at increased risk for severe ADHD symptoms (Konofal et al 2007). Iron supplementation (80 mg/day) for 12 weeks significantly improved ADHD symptoms in children with low serum ferritin levels but without anaemia. The mean Clinical Global Impression-Severity ($P < 0.01$) and ADHD Rating Scale ($P < 0.008$) were improved in a manner comparable to pharmaceutical stimulants (Konofal et al 2008).

Perioperative care

Iron is sometimes given before surgery to reduce postoperative decreases in haemoglobin (Andrews et al 1997). However, this use is contentious and numerous studies have failed to report benefits for preoperative autologous blood collection (Cid et al 2005) or for correcting anaemia associated with cardiac surgery (Madi-Jebara et al 2004) or orthopaedic surgery, such as hip or knee arthroplasty (Mundy et al 2005, Weatherall & Maling 2004). In a more recent randomised placebo-controlled trial in patients undergoing colorectal surgery, oral ferrous sulfate (200 mg TDS) for 2 weeks preoperatively resulted in increased mean haemoglobin and ferritin concentrations, and reduced the need for operative blood transfusion (mean 0 units transfused [range, 0–4 units] versus 2 units transfused [range, 0–11 units]; $P = 0.031$; 95% confidence interval 0.13–2.59) (Lidder et al 2007).

Gastric bypass patients

Iron deficiency may develop after gastric bypass due to red meat intolerance, diminished gastric acid secretion and exclusion of the duodenum from the gastrointestinal tract. Patients require lifelong follow-up of haematological and iron parameters since iron deficiency and anaemia may develop years after surgery and, once developed, may prove refractory to oral treatment, resulting in the need for parenteral iron, blood transfusions or surgical interventions (Love & Billett 2008).

Blood donors

Iron supplementation (150 mg ferrous sulfate three times daily) for 1 week following blood donation reduced the decline in haemoglobin concentration and maintained haematocrit, serum iron, serum ferritin and percentage saturation (Maghsudlu et al 2008). Normalisation of low haemoglobin, and thus blood donor retention, may be further enhanced by a standardised protocol offering iron supplementation and simple oral and written advice based on plasma ferritin measurements (Magnussen et al 2008).

OTHER USES

Breath-holding spells

According to one RCT in iron-deficient children, iron supplementation significantly reduced the incidence of breath-holding spells (Daoud et al 1997). No further research on this indication for iron supplements appears to have been conducted, according to a Cochrane review (Zehetner et al 2010).

Haemodialysis

Intravenous iron is frequently, but contentiously, prescribed for the aggressive management of anaemia associated with dialysis (Agarwal et al 2004, Gillespie & Wolf 2004, Ruiz-Jaramillo et al 2004). CYP3A4 activity is reduced in haemodialysis patients, which may be related to functional iron deficiency. However, with the exception of a subset of haemodialysis patients with low baseline CYP3A4 activity, intravenous iron does not appear to have a significant effect on hepatic CYP3A4 (Pai et al 2007). It has been suggested that strategies to improve vitamin C status and to decrease inflammation would lead to better utilisation of iron in these patients (Handelman 2007).

Hypothyroidism

Adjunct therapy in thyroid disorders

Iron supplementation as adjunct therapy to iodine supplementation results in greater improved thyroid function than giving iodine alone in populations that are deficient in both nutrients (Hess 2010). For patients with comorbid iron-deficiency anaemia and subclinical hypothyroidism, but raised thyroid-stimulating hormone levels, the addition of levothyroxine (50 mcg/day) to iron supplementation (ferrous sulfate 65 mg/day) resulted in better outcomes of both conditions than monotherapy with either iron or levothyroxine, according to one small study of 60 patients (Ravanbod et al 2013). The authors suggest that all patients with iron-deficiency anaemia of unknown aetiology should also be investigated for subclinical hypothyroidism.

DOSAGE RANGE

- Therapeutic dose: Generally 2–5 mg/kg/day; depending on the condition being treated. In many cases the equivalent of this dose may be given as a weekly

TABLE 1 AUSTRALIAN RECOMMENDED DAILY INTAKE (RDI) BY AGE AND SEX

Age	Australian RDI (mg/day)
Infants (0–6 months; breastfed)	0.2
Infants (7–12 months)	11
Children (1–8 years)	9–10
Girls (9–13 years)	8
Girls (14–18 years)	15
Boys (9–13 years)	8
Boys (14–18 years)	11
Men (>18 years)	8
Women (18 to menopause)	18
After menopause	8
Pregnancy	27
Lactation	9

dose rather than a daily dose. The duration of therapy may need to be individualised until iron stores are replenished.

- In cases of deficiency, initial effects on haemoglobin and erythrocyte concentrations take about 2 weeks but it may take 6–12 months to build iron stores (Gropper & Smith 2013).
- The Australian Iron Status Advisory Panel advocates dietary intervention as the first treatment option for mild iron deficiency (serum ferritin 10–15 mcg/L) (Patterson et al 2001). Trials have shown a significant increase in serum ferritin levels (26%) using dietary intervention alone (Heath et al 2001).

In Table 1, the RDI of iron is expressed as a range to allow for differences in bioavailability of iron from different Australian foods.

Studies have shown that there can be a significant sex difference in haemoglobin and other indicators of iron status during infancy. Some of these may be genetically determined, whereas others seem to reflect an increased incidence of true iron deficiency in boys (Domellof et al 2002).

TOXICITY

Iron toxicity causes severe organ damage and eventually death. The most pronounced effects are haemorrhagic necrosis of the gastrointestinal tract, which manifests as vomiting, bloody diarrhoea and hepatotoxicity. Acute overdose or iron accumulation may progress to shock and/or impaired consciousness (Singhi & Baranwal 2003). Iron overdose in pregnant women has been associated with spontaneous abortion, preterm delivery and maternal death (Tran et al 2000). Excess iron accumulation is being investigated as a potential contributing factor for the development of diseases such as Parkinson's and Alzheimer's disease

(Dwyer et al 2009, Rhodes & Ritz 2008, Sian-Hulsmann et al 2011). Some studies suggests that chronic iron overload may contribute to the development of type 2 diabetes and coronary heart disease; however, further research is required to confirm these associations (Mojiminiyi et al 2008).

Conditions that increase risk of toxicity include:

- Haemochromatosis (iron overload) — excess absorption and accumulation of iron in the body, which can cause organ and tissue damage (especially liver, heart and pancreas) and an increased risk for hepatic carcinoma. The most important causes are a genetic disorder (hereditary haemochromatosis), which leads to abnormal iron absorption, or as a secondary consequence of a transfusion, or repeated transfusions.
- Haemosiderosis — iron overload without tissue damage.
- Iron-loading anaemias — thalassaemia and sideroblastic anaemia.

ADVERSE REACTIONS

Oral supplements may cause gastrointestinal disturbances such as nausea, diarrhoea, constipation, heartburn and upper gastric discomfort, and may cause stools to blacken.

Taking supplements with food appears to reduce the possibility of gastrointestinal side effects. Liquid iron preparations can discolour teeth — brush teeth after use.

Intermittent dosing on a weekly basis rather than a daily basis may also reduce side effects.

In the absence of appropriate storage or chelation, excess free iron can readily participate in the formation of toxic free radicals, inducing oxidative stress and apoptosis (Whitnall & Richardson 2006). Iron depletion leads to decreased availability of redox-active iron in vivo and appears to reduce atherosclerotic lesion size and increase plaque stability (Sullivan & Mascitelli 2007). Iron toxicity and subsequent organ damage can develop from long-term excessive intake.

There is preliminary evidence that iron may be implicated in the pathogenesis of autoimmune disorders (Bowlus 2003) and neurodegenerative diseases (Whitnall & Richardson 2006) and that moderately elevated iron stores may be associated with an overall increased risk for cancer, especially colorectal cancer (McCarty 2003). In younger people iron depletion is associated with a reduced risk of all-cause mortality (Sullivan & Mascitelli 2007), although numerous confounding factors cannot be ignored. While haem iron intake from red meat may present a risk for increased blood pressure, non-haem dietary intake may slightly reduce systolic blood pressure (Tzoulaki et al 2008). For the time being, supplementation without demonstrated biological need cannot be justified as the potential risks may outweigh any short-term benefits.

SIGNIFICANT INTERACTIONS

Iron interacts with a variety of foods, herbs and drugs through several different mechanisms. Most commonly, the formation of insoluble complexes occurs whereby both iron and drug absorption is hindered. Separation of doses by several hours will often reduce the severity of this type of interaction. Additionally, substances that alter gastric pH have the theoretical ability to reduce iron absorption. A summary of interactions is presented in Table 2 for easy reference.

TABLE 2 SUMMARY OF IRON INTERACTIONS

Drug/ therapeutic substance	Mechanism	Possible outcome	Action required
Angiotensin-converting enzyme (ACE) inhibitors	Oral iron supplementation with ferrous sulfate 200 mg may suppress cough induced by ACE inhibitors through an effect on nitric oxide generation (Bhalla et al 2011, Lee et al 2001)	Reduced drug adverse effect	Beneficial interaction possible
Antacids and products containing aluminium, calcium or magnesium	Reduces iron absorption (O'Neil-Cutting & Crosby 1986)	Reduced effect of iron	Separate doses by at least 2 h
Ascorbic acid	Increases iron absorption	Increased effects of iron	Beneficial interaction is possible — caution in haemochromatosis
Cholestyramine and colestipol	In vitro investigations have shown that cholestyramine and colestipol both bind iron citrate (Leonard et al 1979)	Reduced drug and iron effect	Monitor for iron efficacy if cholestyramine is being used concurrently. Separate doses by 4 h. Increased iron intake may be required with long-term therapy
Cimetidine	Iron can bind cimetidine in the gastrointestinal tract and reduce its absorption (Campbell et al 1993)	Reduced drug and iron effect	Separate doses by at least 2 h
Dairy products and eggs	May reduce iron absorption	Reduced effect of iron	Monitor for iron efficacy
Erythropoietin	Pharmacodynamic interaction (Carnielli et al 1998). In patients with chemotherapy-related anaemia without iron deficiency, the addition of intravenous iron supplementation may improve the success of darbepoetin (92.5% versus 70% for darbepoetin alone; $P = 0.0033$) without increasing toxicity (Pedrazzoli et al 2008)	Additive pharmacological effect possible	Beneficial interaction is possible

TABLE 2 SUMMARY OF IRON INTERACTIONS *(continued)*			
Drug/ therapeutic substance	**Mechanism**	**Possible outcome**	**Action required**
H_2-receptor antagonists (antiulcer drugs)	Iron absorption is dependent upon gastric pH; therefore, medications that affect gastric pH may interfere with absorption of iron (Aymard et al 1988)	Reduced effect of iron	Monitor for iron efficacy if these drugs are being used concurrently
Haloperidol	May cause decreased blood levels of iron (Leenders et al 1994, Threlkeld 1999)	Reduced effect of iron	Monitor for iron efficacy if these drugs are being used concurrently. Increased iron intake may be required with long-term therapy
L-Dopa and carbidopa	May reduce bioavailability of carbidopa and L-dopa (van Woert et al 1977)	Reduced drug effect	Separate doses by 2 h
Omeprazole and other proton pump inhibitors	Reduced iron absorption due to changes in gastric pH	Reduced effect of iron	Monitor for iron efficacy if omeprazole is being used concurrently
Penicillamine	Reduced drug and iron absorption	Reduced drug and iron effect	Separate doses by at least 2 h. Sudden withdrawal of iron during penicillamine use has been associated with penicillamine toxicity and kidney damage (Harkness & Blake 1982) — caution
Quinolone antibiotics (e.g. norfloxacin)	Reduced drug absorption (Brouwers 1992)	Reduced drug effect	Take drug 2 h before or 4–6 h after iron dosing. Monitor patient for continued antibiotic efficacy
Sulfasalazine	May bind together, decreasing the absorption of both (Dukes & Duncan 1995)	Reduced drug and iron effect	Separate doses by at least 2 h
Tannins — herbs with significant tannin content (e.g. green tea, bilberry, raspberry leaf)	Tannin can bind to iron and reduce its absorption	Reduced effect of iron	Monitor for iron efficacy if these herbs are being used concurrently. Separate doses by 2 h

Continued

TABLE 2 SUMMARY OF IRON INTERACTIONS *(continued)*

Drug/ therapeutic substance	Mechanism	Possible outcome	Action required
Tetracycline antibiotics (e.g. minocycline, doxycycline)	While early studies suggested reduced drug and iron absorption (Neuvonen 1976), more recent human data found no effect on erythrocyte iron uptake when in patients taking 100 mg iron orally and oral tetracycline (Potgieter et al 2007)	Reduced drug effect	Monitor for iron efficacy if tetracyclines are being used long-term. Separate doses by 4 h
L-Thyroxine	Decreased drug absorption possible. Iron supplements may decrease absorption of thyroid medication; however, iron deficiency may impair the body's ability to make thyroid hormones	Reduced drug effect	Thyroid function should be monitored and L-thyroxine dose may need alteration during treatment with iron. Separate doses by at least 2–4 h (Shakir et al 1997)
Vitamin A	Iron supplementation may cause a redistribution of retinol, inducing vitamin A deficiency in infants with marginal vitamin A status (Wieringa et al 2003)	Redistribution of retinol	Iron supplementation in infants should be accompanied by measures to improve vitamin A status

Practice points/Patient counselling

- Iron is an essential mineral that facilitates oxygen transport and storage in the body and is part of many enzyme systems.
- Haem iron, found in animal products, is absorbed two- to threefold better than non-haem forms found in vegetable sources. However, iron absorption is influenced by many factors, such as other foods ingested, medicines and gastric activity.
- Iron deficiency is the most common nutritional deficiency in the world and may occur with or without anaemia. Excessive blood loss during menstruation is the most common cause.
- Supplements are generally used to treat or prevent deficiency. Excess iron can be dangerous and can lead to organ damage and death.
- As inappropriate iron supplementation can inhibit growth in non-deficient children and adversely affect pregnancy outcomes, iron status should be tested before administration.
- Correction of iron deficiency with or without anaemia may be achieved with lower doses than those recommended in some trials. In many cases, once-weekly dosing of iron is as effective as daily dosing and improves compliance, while reducing side effects and cost.
- Oral liquid iron supplements should be diluted with water and drunk through a straw to prevent discolouration of teeth, especially if used long-term.

CONTRAINDICATIONS AND PRECAUTIONS

Iron poisoning can occur due to accidental ingestion of excess iron supplements. As such, iron supplements should be kept in childproof bottles and out of the reach of children.

Caution should be exercised when supplementing iron to infants or children with apparently normal growth when the iron status of the child is unknown. A double-blind placebo-controlled trial showed that, while iron therapy produced a significant improvement of mean monthly weight gain and linear growth in iron-deficient children, it significantly decreased the weight gain and linear growth of iron-replete children (Majumdar et al 2003). This study confirms the results of earlier studies (Dewey et al 2002).

Iron supplements should not be used in haemochromatosis, haemosiderosis or iron-loading anaemias (thalassaemia, sideroblastic anaemia).

Daily oral iron supplementation providing 50 mg elemental iron for 8 weeks did not result in increased oxidative damage in the plasma of college-aged women (Gropper et al 2003). However, more recently 100 mg doses of iron daily for 8 weeks were shown to increase lipid peroxidation. As iron status and duration of supplementation increased, so too did indicators of lipid peroxidation (King et al 2008). As the use of iron supplements may potentially result in oxidative damage, risk should always be assessed against benefit before prescribing iron supplements.

Elevated levels of serum ferritin have been implicated in the pathogenesis of vascular (and other) diseases, although this remains controversial (McCarty 2003, Zacharski et al 2004).

Haem-rich flesh foods may need to be limited in people with insulin resistance due to a possible link with increased cancer risk mediated by iron excess in such populations (McCarty 2003).

Iron supplementation should be prescribed on the basis of biological criteria, not on the assumption of anaemia alone, as unnecessary iron supplementation can result in adverse effects. The lowest safe and effective dose and frequency of dose should be recommended.

PREGNANCY USE

Oral iron preparations are considered safe in pregnancy; while adequate iron in pregnancy is important, unnecessary iron supplementation can result in uncontrolled lipid peroxidation (Lachili et al 2001), lowered serum levels of copper and zinc (Ziaei et al 2008), low birth weight and maternal hypertension disorder (Ziaei et al 2007). As a result, iron supplementation should be prescribed on the basis of biological criteria, and the woman's iron status should be assessed first, rather than basing it on the assumption of anaemia alone.

PATIENTS' FAQs

What will this supplement do for me?

Iron is necessary for health and wellbeing. It facilitates oxygen transport and storage in the body and is part of many enzyme systems. Iron deficiency is the most common nutrient deficiency in the world.

When will it start to work?

Iron deficiency responds to supplementation within 2 weeks; however, 6–12 months may be required to build up the body's iron stores.

Are there any safety issues?

Excess iron can be dangerous and ultimately can lead to severe organ damage and death.

REFERENCES

Agarwal KN et al. Anemia prophylaxis in adolescent school girls by weekly or daily iron-folate supplementation. Indian Pediatr 40.4 (2003): 296–301.

Agarwal R et al. Oxidative stress and renal injury with intravenous iron in patients with chronic kidney disease. Kidney Int 65.6 (2004): 2279–2289.

Allen LH, et al. Provision of multiple rather than two or few micronutrients more effectively improves growth and other outcomes in micronutrient-deficient children and adults. J Nutri 139.5 (2009): 1022–30

Andres E et al. Update of nutrient-deficiency anemia in the elderly. European Journal of Internal Medicine. 19 (2008): 488–493

Andrews CM, et al. Iron pre-load for major joint replacement. Transfus Med 7.4 (1997): 281–286.

Annibale B et al. Efficacy of gluten-free diet alone on recovery from iron deficiency anemia in adult celiac patients. Am J Gastroenterol 96.1 (2001): 132–137.

Avni T, et al. Iron supplementation for the treatment of chronic heart failure and iron deficiency: systematic review and meta-analysis. European Journal of Heart Failure 14 (2012):423–429

Aymard JP et al. Haematological adverse effects of histamine H2-receptor antagonists. Med Toxicol Adverse Drug Exp 3 (1988): 430–448.

Bach-Kristensen M et al. Pork meat increases iron absorption from a 5-day fully controlled diet when compared to a vegetarian diet with similar vitamin C and phytic acid content. Br J Nutr 94.1 (2005): 78–83.

Baech SB et al. Nonheme-iron absorption from a phytate-rich meal is increased by the addition of small amounts of pork meat. Am J Clin Nutr 77.1 (2003): 173–179.

Beard JL, et al. Impaired thermoregulation and thyroid function in iron-deficiency anaemia. Am J Clin Nutr 52 (1990): 813–8119.

Beard JL et al. Maternal iron deficiency anemia affects postpartum emotions and cognition. J Nutrition 135.2 (2005): 267–272.

Bergman M et al. In vitro cytokine production in patients with iron deficiency anemia. Clin Immunol 113.3 (2004): 340–344.

Bhalla P, et al. Attenuation of angiotensin converting enzyme inhibitor induced cough by iron supplementation: role of nitric oxide. J Renin Angiotensin Aldosterone Syst. 12.4 (2011):491–7

Bilgic A et al. Iron deficiency in preschool children with autistic spectrum disorders. Research in Autism Spectrum Disorders 4 (2010):639–644

Blanton CA, et al. Iron deficiency without anaemia impairs cognitive function in premenopausal women. Appetite 57 (2011): 553–569

Bowlus CL. The role of iron in T cell development and autoimmunity.Autoimmun Rev 2.2 (2003): 73–78.

Breet P et al. Actions of black tea and Rooibos on iron status of primary school children. Nutr Res 25.11 (2005): 983–994.

Brouwers J. Drug interactions with quinolone antibacterials. Drug Safety 7.4 (1992): 268–281.

Brownlie T et al. Marginal iron deficiency without anemia impairs aerobic adaptation among previously untrained women. Am J Clin Nutr 75.4 (2002): 734–742.

Brownlie T et al. Tissue iron deficiency without anemia impairs adaptation in endurance capacity after aerobic training in previously untrained women. Am J Clin Nutr 79.3 (2004): 437–443.

Campbell NR et al. Ferrous sulfate reduces cimetidine absorption. Dig Dis Sci 38.5 (1993): 950–954.

Carnielli VP, et al. Iron supplementation enhances responses to high doses of recombinant human erythropoietin in preterm infants.Arch Dis Child Fetal Neonatal Ed 79.1 (1998): F44–F48.

Ciacci C et al. *Helicobacter pylori* impairs iron absorption in infected individuals. Dig Liver Dis 36.7 (2004): 455–460.

Cid J et al. [Oral iron and folic acid supplements in a preoperative autologous blood collection program: a randomized study.] Med Clin (Barc) 124.18 (2005): 690–691.

Cook JD. Diagnosis and management of iron-deficiency anaemia. Best Pract Res Clin Haematol 18.2 (2005): 319–332.

Cortese S et al. Attention-deficit/hyperactivity disorder, Tourette's syndrome, and restless legs syndrome: the iron hypothesis. Med Hypotheses 70.6 (2008): 1128–1132.

Crofton R et al. Inorganic zinc and the absorption of ferrous iron. Am J Clin Nutr 50 (1989): 141–144.

Daoud AS et al. Effectiveness of iron therapy on breath-holding spells. J Pediatr 130.4 (1997): 547–550.

Davidsson L et al. Influence of ascorbic acid on iron absorption from an iron-fortified, chocolate-flavored milk drink in Jamaican children. Am J Clin Nutr May 67.5 (1998): 873–877.

Davila-Hicks P, et al. Iron in ferritin or in salts (ferrous sulfate) is equally bioavailable in nonanemic women. Am J Clin Nutr 80.4 (2004): 936–940.

de Benoist B, et al. (2008) Worldwide prevalence of anaemia 1993–2005. WHO global database on anaemia. Accessed March 2013. Available at URL: http://www.who.int/vmnis/publications/anaemia_prevalence/en/index.html

De-Regil LM et al. Intermittent iron supplementation for improving nutrition and development in children under 12 years of age. Cochrane Database of Syst Rev (2011) CD009085.

De-Silva A et al. Iron supplementation improves iron status and reduces morbidity in children with or without upper respiratory tract infections: a randomized controlled study in Colombo, Sri Lanka. Am J Clin Nutr 77.1 (2003): 234–241.

Dewey KG et al. Iron supplementation affects growth and morbidity of breast-fed infants: results of a randomized trial in Sweden and Honduras. J Nutr 132.11 (2002): 3249–3255.

Dodd J, et al. Treatment for women with postpartum iron deficiency anaemia. Cochrane Database Syst Rev 4 (2004): CD004222.

Domellof M et al. Sex differences in iron status during infancy. Pediatrics 110.3 (2002): 545–552.

Dukes DE Jr, Duncan BS. Applied Therapeutics: The clinical use of drugs, 6th edn. Philadelphia: Lippincott Williams & Wilkins, 1995, pp 24–7.

Duque X et al. Effect of eradication of *Helicobacter pylori* and iron supplementation on the iron status of children with iron deficiency. Archives of Medical Research 40 (2010): 38–45

Dwyer BE et al. Getting the iron out: phlebotomy for Alzheimer's disease?. Med Hypothesis 75.5 (2009): 504–9

Falkingham M et al. The effects of oral iron supplementation on cognition in older children and adults: a systematic review and meta-analysis. Nutrition Journal 9.4 (2010).

Fernandez-Gaxiola AC, De-Regil LM. Intermittent iron supplementation for reducing anaemia and its associated impairments in menstruating women. Cochrane Database of Syst Rev 12 (2011) CD009218

Ferreira da Silva L, et al. Serum iron analysis of adults receiving three different iron compounds. Nutr Res 24.8 (2004): 603–611.

Fischer Walker C et al. Interactive effects of iron and zinc on biochemical and functional outcomes in supplementation trials. Am J Clin Nutri 82 (2005):5–12

Flesland O et al. Transferring receptor in serum. A new tool in the diagnosis and prevention of iron deficiency in blood donors. Transf Aph Sci 31.1 (2004): 11–16.

Fuqua BK, et al. Intestinal iron absorption. Journal of Trace Elements in Medicine and Biology. 26 (2012):115–119

Geerligs PP et al. The effect on haemoglobin of the use of iron cooking pots in rural Malawian households in an area with high malaria prevalence: a randomized trial. Trop Med Int Health 8.4 (2003): 310–3115.

Gillespie RS, Wolf FM. Intravenous iron therapy in pediatric hemodialysis patients: a meta-analysis. Pediatr Nephrol 19.6 (2004): 662–666.

Gillespie S, et al (eds). Controlling iron deficiency. Geneva, Switzerland: United Nations Administrative Committee on Coordination/Subcommittee on Nutrition. State-of-the-Art Series: Nutrition Policy, Discussion Paper No. 9, 1991.

Gropper SS, Smith JL, Advanced Nutrition and Human Metabolism, 6th edition. Belmont, CA: Wadsworth (2013): 481–500

Gropper SS, et al. Non-anemic iron deficiency, oral iron supplementation, and oxidative damage in college-aged females. J Nutr Biochem 14.7 (2003): 409–415.

Haidar J et al. Daily versus weekly iron supplementation and prevention of iron deficiency anaemia in lactating women. East Afr Med J 80.1 (2003): 11–116.

Haider BA et al. Anaemia, prenatal iron use, and risk of adverse pregnancy outcomes: systematic review and meta-analysis. BMJ. 346 (2013):f3443

Hallberg L et al. The role of meat to improve the critical iron balance during weaning. Pediatrics 111.4 Pt. 1 (2003): 864–870.

Handelman GJ. Newer strategies for anemia prevention in hemodialysis. Int J Artif Organs 30.11 (2007): 1014–10119.

Handelman GJ, Levin NW. Iron and anemia in human biology: a review of mechanisms. Heart Fail Rev 13.4 (2008): 393–404.

Harkness JAL, Blake DR. Penicillamine nephropathy and iron. Lancet 2 (1982): 1368–1369.

Heath AL et al. Can dietary treatment of non-anemic iron deficiency improve iron status? J Am Coll Nutr 20.5 (2001): 477–484.

Hess SY. The impact of common micronutrient deficiencies on iodine and thyroid metabolism: the evidence from human studies. Best Practice & Research Clinical Endocrinology & Metabolism. 24. 1 (2010):117–32

Higgins PDR, Rockey DC. Iron-deficiency anemia. Tech Gastrointest Endosc 5.3 (2003): 134–141.

Hsu HS et al. Iron deficiency with increased risk of cardiovascular disease an all-cause mortality in the elderly living in long-term care facilities. Nutrition (2013):29: 737–743.

Hurrell R et al. Iron absorption in humans: bovine serum albumin compared with beef muscle and egg white. Am J Clin Nutr 47 (1988): 102–107.

Ioannou GN et al. The effect of alcohol consumption on the prevalence of iron overload, iron deficiency, and iron deficiency anemia. Gastroenterology 126.5 (2004): 1293–1301.

Juarez-Vazquez J, et al. Iron plus folate is more effective than iron alone in the treatment of iron deficiency anaemia in pregnancy: a randomised, double blind clinical trial. Br J Obstet Gynaecol 109.9 (2002): 1009–1014.

Kaltwasser JP et al. Clinical trial on the effect of regular tea drinking on iron accumulation in genetic haemochromatosis. Gut 43.5 (1998): 699–704.

King SM et al. Daily supplementation with iron increases lipid peroxidation in young women with low iron stores. Exp Biol Med (Maywood) 233.6 (2008): 701–707.

Klip IT et al. Prevalence, predictors and prognosis of iron deficiency in patients with chronic heart failure: an international pooled analysis of 1,506 patients. Journal of American College of Cardiology. 59.13 (2012):E1045

Konofal E et al. Impact of restless legs syndrome and iron deficiency on attention-deficit/hyperactivity disorder in children. Sleep Med 8.7–8 (2007): 711–715.

Konofal E et al. Effects of iron supplementation on attention deficit hyperactivity disorder in children. Pediatr Neurol 38.1 (2008): 20–226.

Krafft A, et al. Effect of postpartum iron supplementation on red cell and iron parameters in non-anaemic iron-deficient women: a randomised placebo-controlled study. Br J Obstet Gynaecol 112.4 (2005): 445–450.

Lachili B et al. Increased lipid peroxidation in pregnant women after iron and vitamin C supplementation. Biol Trace Elem Res 83.2 (2001): 103–110.
Lee SC, et al. Iron supplementation inhibits cough associated with ACE Inhibitors. Hypertension 38 (2001): 166–170.
Leenders KL et al. Blood to brain iron uptake in one rhesus monkey using [Fe-52]-citrate and positron emission tomography (PET): influence of haloperidol. J Neural Transm 43 (Suppl) (1994): 123–132.
Leonard JP et al. In vitro binding of various biological substances by two hypocholesterolaemic resins: Cholestyramine and colestipol. Arzneim Forsch/Drug Res 29 (1979): 979–981.
Lidder PG et al. Pre-operative oral iron supplementation reduces blood transfusion in colorectal surgery — a prospective, randomised, controlled trial. Ann R Coll Surg Engl 89.4 (2007): 418–421.
Lind T et al. A community-based randomized controlled trial of iron and zinc supplementation in Indonesian infants: interactions between iron and zinc. Am J Clin Nutr 77.4 (2003): 883–890.
Lonnerdal B. Calcium and iron absorption-mechanisms and public relevance. International Journal for Vitamin & Nutrition Research 80 (2010):293–299
Love AL, Billett HH. Obesity, bariatric surgery, and iron deficiency: true, true, true and related. Am J Hematol 83.5 (2008): 403–409.
Madi-Jebara SN et al. Postoperative intravenous iron used alone or in combination with low-dose erythropoietin is not effective for correction of anemia after cardiac surgery. J Cardiothorac Vasc Anesth 18.1 (2004): 59–63.
Maghsudlu M et al. Short-term ferrous sulfate supplementation in female blood donors. Transfusion 48.6 (2008): 1192–1197.
Magnussen K, et al. The effect of a standardized protocol for iron supplementation to blood donors low in hemoglobin concentration. Transfusion 48.4 (2008): 749–754.
Majumdar I et al. The effect of iron therapy on the growth of iron-replete and iron-deplete children. J Trop Pediatr 49.2 (2003): 84–88.
McCarty MF. Hyperinsulinemia may boost both hematocrit and iron absorption by up-regulating activity of hypoxia-inducible factor-1[alpha]. Med Hypoth 61.5–6 (2003): 567–573.
McClung JP. Iron status and the female athlete. Journal of Trace Elements in Medicine and Biology. 26 (2012):124–126
McClung JP, Karl JP. Iron deficiency and obesity: the contribution of inflammation and diminished iron absorption. Nutri Rev 67 (2009):100–4
Mei Z et al. Hemoglobin and ferritin are currently the most efficient indicators of population response to iron interventions: an analysis of nine randomized controlled trials. J Nutr 135.8 (2005): 1974–1980.
Merkel D et al. Prevalence of iron deficiency and anemia among strenuously trained adolescents. J Adolesc Health 37.3 (2005): 220–223.
Metallinos-Katsaras E et al. Effect of iron supplementation on cognition in Greek preschoolers. Eur J Clin Nutr 58.11 (2004): 1532–1542.
Milman N et al. Iron prophylaxis during pregnancy: how much iron is needed? A randomized dose-response study of 20–80 mg ferrous iron daily in pregnant women. Acta Obstet Gynecol Scand 84.3 (2004): 238–247.
Mojiminiyi OA, et al. Body iron stores in relation to the metabolic syndrome, glycemic control and complications in female patients with type 2 diabetes. Nutrition, Metabolism & cardiovascular Diseases 18 (2008):559–566
Mukhopadhyay A et al. Erythrocyte indices in pregnancy: effect of intermittent iron supplementation. Natl Med J India 17.3 (2004): 135–137.
Mundy GM, et al. The effect of iron supplementation on the level of haemoglobin after lower limb arthroplasty. J Bone Joint Surg Br 87.2 (2005): 213–2117.
Navas-Carretero S et al. Oily fish increases iron bioavailability of a phytate rich meal in young iron deficient women. J Am CollNutr 27.1 (2008): 96–101.
Neuvonen PJ. Interactions with the absorption of tetracyclines. Drugs 11.1 (1976): 45–54.
NMCD (Natural Medicines Comprehensive Database) Iron. Available online: http://www.naturaldatabase.com 10 November 2005.
Olsen A et al. Failure of twice-weekly iron supplementation to increase blood haemoglobin and serum ferritin concentrations: results of a randomized controlled trial. Ann Trop Med Parasitol 100.3 (2006): 251–263.
O'Neil-Cutting MA, Crosby WH. The effect of antacids on the absorption of simultaneously ingested iron. JAMA 255 (1986): 1468–1470.
Otero GA et al. Iron supplementation brings up a lacking P300 in iron deficient children. Clin Neurophysiol 115.10 (2004): 2259–2266.
Otero GA et al. Working memory impairment and recovery in iron deficient children. Clinical Neurophysiology 119 (2008): 1739–1746
Pai AB et al. Effect of intravenous iron supplementation on hepatic cytochrome P450 3A4 activity in hemodialysis patients: a prospective, open-label study. Clin Ther 29.12 (2007): 2699–2705.
Patterson AJ et al. Dietary treatment of iron deficiency in women of childbearing age. Am J Clin Nutr 74.5 (2001): 650–656.
Pedrazzoli P et al. Randomized trial of intravenous iron supplementation in patients with chemotherapy-related anemia without iron deficiency treated with darbepoetin alpha. J Clin Oncol 26.10 (2008): 1619–1625.
Pena-Rosas JP et al. Daily oral iron supplementation during pregnancy. Cochrane Database Syst Rev (2012) doi:10/1002/14651858.CD004736.pub4
Potgieter MA et al. Effect of oral tetracycline on iron absorption from iron(III)-hydroxide polymaltose complex in patients with iron deficiency anemia /a single-centre randomized controlled isotope study. Arzneimittelforschung 57.6A (2007): 376–384.
Ramakrishnan U et al. Multimicronutrient interventions but not vitamin a or iron interventions alone improve child growth: results of 3 meta-analyses. J Nutr 134.10(2004): 2592–602
Ramakrishnan U, et al. Effects of micronutrients on growth of children under 5 y of age: meta-analyses of single and multiple nutrient interventions. Am J Clin Nutr 89.1 (2009): 191–203

Rattehalli D et al. Iron deficiency without anaemia: do not wait for the haemoglobin to drop? Health Policy and Technology 2 (2013):45–5

Ravanbod M et al. Treatment of iron-deficiency anaemia in patients with subclinical hypothyroidism. American Journal of Medicine 126 (2013): 420–424.

Recalcati S et al. Iron levels in polarized macrophages: regulation of immunity and autoimmunity. Autoimmun Rev 11.12 (2012): 883–889.

Reinke S et al. Absolute and functional iron deficiency in professional athletes during training and recovery. International Journal of cardiology 156 (2012):186–191

Rhodes SL, Ritz B. Genetics of iron regulation and the possible role of iron in Parkinson's disease. Neurobiology of Disease 32 (2008):183–195

Rimon E et al. Are we giving too much iron? Low-dose iron therapy is effective in octogenarians. Am J Med 118.10 (2005): 1142–1147.

Rodenberg RE, Gustafson S. Iron as an ergogenic aid: ironclad evidence? Curr Sports Med Rep 6.4 (2007): 258–264.

Rossander-Hulten L et al. Competitive inhibition of iron absorption by manganese and zinc. Am J Clin Nutr 54 (1991): 152–156.

Ruiz-Jaramillo M-L et al. Intermittent versus maintenance iron therapy in children on hemodialysis: a randomized study. Pediatr Nephrol 19.1 (2004): 77–81.

Sachdev H, et al. Effect of iron supplementation on mental and motor development in children: systematic review of randomised controlled trials. Public Health Nutr 8.2 (2005): 117–132.

Santiago P. Ferrous versus ferric oral iron formulations for the treatment of iron deficiency: A clinical overview. Scientific World Journal (2012) 2012: 846824.

Sarkate P et al. A randomised double-blind study comparing sodium feredetate with ferrous fumarate in anaemia in pregnancy. J Indian Med Assoc 105.5 (2007): 278, 280–281, 284.

Sejas E et al. Iron supplementation in previously anemic Bolivian children normalized hematologic parameters, but not immunologic parameters. J Trop Pediatr 54.3 (2008): 164–168.

Shafir T et al. Iron deficiency and infant motor development. Early Human Development 84 (2008):479–485

Shakir KM et al. Ferrous sulfate-induced increase in requirement for thyroxine in a patient with primary hypothyroidism. South Med J 90.6 (1997): 637–639.

Sian-Hulsmann J et al. The relevance of iron in the pathogenesis of Parkinson's disease. J Neurochem 118.6 (2011):939–57

Siddiqui IA, et al. Efficacy of daily vs. weekly supplementation of iron in schoolchildren with low iron status. J Trop Pediatr 50.5 (2004): 276–278.

Singhi S, Baranwal AK. Acute iron poisoning: clinical picture, intensive care needs and outcome. Indian Pediatr 40.12 (2003): 1177–82

Stoltzfus R. Iron deficiency: global prevalence and consequences. Food Nutr Bull 24.4 (2003):S99–103

Sullivan JL, Mascitelli L. [Current status of the iron hypothesis of cardiovascular diseases.] Recent Prog Med 98.7–8 (2007): 373–377.

Sungthong R et al. Once-weekly and 5-days a week iron supplementation differentially affect cognitive function but not school performance in Thai children. J Nutr 134.9 (2004): 2349–2354.

Thompson J, et al. Effects of daily iron supplementation in 2-to-5-year old children: systematic review and meta-analysis. Pediatrics 131.4 (2013):739–53

Threlkeld DS (ed.). Central nervous system drugs, antipsychotic agents. In: Facts and comparisons drug information. St Louis, MO: Wolter Kluwer Health, 1998, pp 266k–266m. Cited in: Lininger SW et al (eds). A–Z Guide to drug–herb–vitamin interactions. Roseville, CA: Healthnotes, 1999.

Tran T et al. Intentional iron overdose in pregnancy-management and outcome. J Emerg Med 18. 2 (2000): 225–8

Trotti LM, et al. Iron for restless leg syndrome (review). Cochrane Database Syst Rev 5 (2012): CD007834.

Tzoulaki I et al. Relation of iron and red meat intake to blood pressure: cross sectional epidemiological study. BMJ 337 (2008): a258.

Ullmann U et al. Epigallocatechingallate (EGCG) (TEAVIGO) does not impair nonhaem-iron absorption in man. Phytomedicine 12.6–7 (2005): 410–4115.

Van Woert MH et al. Long-term therapy of monoclonus and other neurological disorders with L-5-hydroxytryptophan and carbidopa. N Engl J Med 296 (1977): 70–75.

Vaucher P et al. Effect of iron supplementation on fatigue in anaemic menstruating women with low ferritin: a randomized controlled trial. CMAJ 184.11 (2012):1247–1254

Verdon F et al. Iron supplementation for unexplained fatigue in non-anaemic women: double blind randomised placebo controlled trial (Primary care). BMJ 326.7399 (2003): 1124.

Weatherall M, Maling TJ. Oral iron therapy for anaemia after orthopaedic surgery: randomized clinical trial. Aust NZ J Surg 74.12 (2004): 1049–1051.

Whitnall M, Richardson DR. Iron: a new target for pharmacological intervention in neurodegenerative diseases. Semin Pediatr Neurol 13.3 (2006): 186–197.

Whittaker P. Iron and zinc interactions in humans. Am J Clin Nutr 68 (1998): 442–6S.

Wieringa FT et al. Redistribution of vitamin A after iron supplementation in Indonesian infants. Am J Clin Nutr 77.3 (2003): 651–657.

Wijaya-Erhardt M et al. Effect of daily or weekly multiple-micronutrient and iron foodlike tablets on body iron stores of Indonesian infants aged 6–12 mo: a double-blind, randomized, placebo-controlled trial. Am J Clin Nutr 86.6 (2007): 1680–1686.

Yang Q, et al. Effect of daily or once weekly iron supplementation on growth and iron status of preschool children. Wei Sheng Yan Jiu 33.2 (2004): 205–207.

Yang Y et al. Efficacy and safety of iron supplementation for the elderly patients undergoing hip or knee surgery: A meta-analysis of randomized controlled trials. Journal of Surgical Research 171.2 (2011) e201-e207

Zacharski LR et al. Implementation of an iron reduction protocol in patients with peripheral vascular disease: VA cooperative study no. 410: The Iron (FE) and Atherosclerosis Study (FEAST). Am Heart J 148.3 (2004): 386–392.
Zareifar S et al. Association between iron status and febrile seizures in children. Seizure 21.8 (2012): 603–605.
Zehetner AA et al. Iron supplementation for breath-holding attacks in children. Cochrane Database Syst Rev 12.5 (2010): CD008132.
Zhou SJ et al. Should we lower the dose of iron when treating anaemia in pregnancy? A randomized dose-response trial. Eur J Clin Nutr (2009): 63: 183–190.
Ziaei S et al. A randomised placebo-controlled trial to determine the effect of iron supplementation on pregnancy outcome in pregnant women with haemoglobin> or = 13.2 g/dl. BJOG 114.6 (2007): 684–688.
Ziaei S et al. The effects of iron supplementation on serum copper and zinc levels in pregnant women with high-normal hemoglobin. Int J Gynaecol Obstet 100.2 (2008): 133–135.
Zoller H, Vogel W. Iron supplementation in athletes: first do no harm. Nutrition 20.7–8 (2004): 615–6119.

L-Glutamine

HISTORICAL NOTE Glutamine and glutamate were originally described in the mid 19th century and their functions began to be examined in the early 20th century. The role of glutamine in the immune system and gastrointestinal tract has been investigated since the 1980s.

BACKGROUND AND RELEVANT PHARMACOKINETICS

L-Glutamine is a conditionally essential amino acid found in all life forms and the most abundant amino acid in the human body. During conditions of metabolic stress characterised by catabolism and negative nitrogen balance, such as trauma (including surgical trauma), prolonged stress, glucocorticoid use, excessive exercise, starvation, infection, sepsis, cancer and severe burns, the body is unable to synthesise L-glutamine in sufficient quantities to meet biological needs and it becomes essential to have an exogenous intake (Miller 1999, PDRHealth 2006a).

L-Glutamine is absorbed from the lumen of the small intestine by active transport (Meng et al 2003) and is then transported to the liver via the portal circulation and enters the systemic circulation, where it is distributed to various tissues and transported into cells via an active process. Elimination occurs via glomerular filtration and it is almost completely reabsorbed by the renal tubules. Some metabolism of L-glutamine takes place in the enterocytes and hepatocytes and it is involved in various metabolic activities, including the synthesis of L-glutamate (catalysed by glutaminase), proteins, glutathione, pyrimidine and purine nucleotides and amino sugars. L-glutamate is converted to L-glutamine by glutamine synthase in the presence of ammonia, adenosine triphosphate (ATP) and magnesium or manganese.

L-Glutamine is synthesised endogenously from other amino acids, predominantly branched-chain amino acids and glutamate, and stored in skeletal muscles, where it comprises around 60% of the free amino acids and makes up 4–5% of muscle protein. In times of metabolic stress, glutamine is released into the circulation and transported to tissues in need (Kohlmeier 2003, Miller 1999, PDRHealth 2006a).

L-Glutamine is not very soluble or stable in solution, especially upon heating for sterilisation, and as a result, until recently, was not included in total parenteral nutrition (TPN). The more soluble and stable glutamine dipeptides are now commonly used as the delivery forms in TPN solutions and some nutritional supplements (Kohlmeier 2003, PDRHealth 2006b).

Common forms available

The terms L-glutamine and glutamine are often used interchangeably. L-glutamine is the amide form of L-glutamic acid and contains 15.7% nitrogen (Kohlmeier 2003). It is also known as 2-aminoglutaramic acid, levoglutamide, (S)-2,5-diamino-5-oxopentaenoic acid and glutamic acid 5-amide. Glutamic acid is a non-essential amino acid and glutamine is the aminated form of glutamic acid. Glutamic acid is found in many foods, such as grain cereals (barley, wheat, flax, sorghum, rye), nuts and seeds, dairy foods and meat. L-glutamic acid is commonly used as a supplement in sports nutrition. Salts and carboxylate anions of glutamic acid are known as glutamates (such as sodium glutamate, potassium glutamate). Glutamate is involved in cellular metabolism and it is an abundant neurotransmitter.

Two synthetic glutamine dipeptides that may be used in TPN are L-alanyl-L-glutamine and glycyl-L-glutamine. D-Glutamine, the stereoisomer of L-glutamine, has no known biological activity (Kohlmeier 2003, PDRHealth 2006b).

Since the late 1960s, L-glutamine has been manufactured for pharmaceutical use using a fermentation broth. The manufacture of high-quality, low-cost L-glutamine requires a strain of microorganism with good production efficiency and minimum byproducts. Impurities can then be removed from the broth using a nanofiltration membrane to obtain a fine crystalline powder (Kusumoto 2001, Li et al 2003).

FOOD SOURCES

Typical dietary intake of L-glutamine is 5–10 g/day (Miller 1999). Sources include animal and plant proteins, vegetable juices (especially cabbage), eggs, wheat, soybeans and fermented foods, such as miso and yoghurt (Kohlmeier 2003, PDRHealth 2006a).

DEFICIENCY SIGNS AND SYMPTOMS

Although traditionally considered a non-essential amino acid, L-glutamine is now considered 'conditionally essential' during periods of metabolic stress characterised by catabolism and negative nitrogen balance.

Critical illness, stress and injury can lead to a significant decrease in plasma levels of L-glutamine which, if severe, can increase the risk of mortality (Boelens et al 2001, Wischmeyer 2003).

Prolonged protein malnutrition may cause growth inhibition, muscle wasting and organ damage (Kohlmeier 2003). In the absence of sufficient plasma glutamine, the body will break down skeletal muscle stores, and gut integrity (gut mucosal barrier function) and immunity will be compromised. Because L-glutamine is utilised during exercise, a more recent phenomenon of deficiency has been explored and glutamine depletion has been linked with 'overtraining syndrome'.

MAIN ACTIONS

L-Glutamine has many important biological functions within the human body. It is an important fuel for the intestinal mucosal cells, hepatocytes and rapidly proliferating cells of the immune system, particularly lymphocytes and monocytes, assists in the regulation of acid balance, thus preventing acidosis, acts as a nitrogen shuttle protecting the body from high levels of ammonia, and is involved in the synthesis of amino acids (including L-glutamate), gamma-aminobutyric acid

(GABA), glutathione (an important antioxidant), purine and pyramidine nucleotides, amino acid sugars in glycoproteins and glycans, and nicotinamide adenosine dinucleotide (NAD). It is also involved in protein synthesis and energy production (Boelens et al 2001, Kohlmeier 2003, Miller 1999, Niihara et al 2005, Patel et al 2001, PDRHealth 2006a).

Gastrointestinal protection/repair

According to in vitro and in vivo research, L-glutamine aids in the proliferation and repair of intestinal cells (Chun et al 1997, Rhoads et al 1997, Scheppach et al 1996) and is the preferred respiratory fuel for enterocytes (and also utilised by colonocytes) (Miller 1999). It is thus vital for maintaining the integrity of the intestinal lining and preventing the translocation of microbes and endotoxins into the body. In addition, L-glutamine helps to maintain secretory immunoglobulin A (IgA), which functions primarily by preventing the attachment of bacteria to mucosal cells (PDRHealth 2006a, Yu et al 1996).

According to evidence from animal studies, it may also assist in preventing atrophy following colostomy (Paulo 2002) and irradiation (Diestel et al 2005), and intestinal injury by inhibiting intestinal cytokine release (Akisu et al 2003). L-glutamine depletion induces apoptosis by triggering intercellular events that lead to cell death (Paquette et al 2005), resulting in altered epithelial barrier competence (increased intestinal permeability), bacterial translocation and increased mortality. Under experimental conditions, L-glutamine may assist in maintaining intestinal barrier function by increasing epithelial resistance to apoptotic injury, reducing oxidative damage, attenuating programmed cell death and promoting re-epithelialisation (Masuko 2002, Ropeleski et al 2005, Scheppach et al 1996) and may thus reduce bacterial and endotoxin translocation (Chun et al 1997).

Immunomodulation

L-Glutamine has demonstrated immunomodulatory activity in animal models of infection and trauma, as well as trauma in humans. L-Glutamine acts as the preferred respiratory fuel for lymphocytes, is essential for cell proliferation, and can enhance the function of stimulated immune cells.

Extracellular glutamine concentration affects lymphocyte, interleukin-2 and interferon-gamma proliferation, cytokine production, phagocytic and secretory macrophage activities and neutrophil bacterial killing (Miller 1999, Newsholme 2001, PDRHealth 2006a). In humans, L-glutamine may enhance both phagocytosis and reactive oxygen intermediate production by neutrophils (Furukawa et al 2000) and support the restoration of type-1T lymphocyte responsiveness following trauma (Boelens et al 2004). In a randomised trial, there was a reduced frequency of pneumonia, sepsis and bacteraemia in patients with multiple traumas who received glutamine-supplemented enteral nutrition (Houdijk et al 1998).

In addition, effects on the gastrointestinal tract may contribute significantly to immune defence by maintaining gut-associated lymphoid tissue and secretory IgA (preventing the attachment of bacteria to the gut mucosa) and maintaining gut integrity (thus preventing the translocation of microbes and their toxins, especially Gram-negative bacteria from the large intestine) (Miller 1999, Yu et al 1996).

Antioxidant

As a precursor to glutathione (together with cysteine and glycine), L-glutamine can assist in ameliorating the oxidation that occurs during metabolic stress. Glutathione protects epithelial cell membranes from damage, and its depletion can negatively affect gut barrier function and result in severe degeneration of colonic and jejunal epithelial cells (Iantomasi 1994, Ziegler et al 1999). In animal studies, it has also been shown to inhibit fatty acid oxidation, resulting in a reduction in body weight and alleviation of hyperglycaemia and hyperinsulinaemia in mice fed a high-fat diet (Opara et al 1996).

Anabolic/anticatabolic

As L-glutamine is stored primarily in skeletal muscles and becomes conditionally essential under conditions of metabolic stress, the anticatabolic/anabolic properties of supplemented L-glutamine are likely due to a sparing effect on skeletal muscle stores.

Following strenuous exercise, glutamine levels are depleted by approximately 20%, resulting in immunodepression (Castell 2003, Castell & Newsholme 1997, Rogero et al 2002). As a result supplemental L-glutamine may be of benefit in athletes to prevent the deleterious effects of glutamine depletion associated with 'overtraining syndrome'. Evidence supporting a direct ergogenic effect is currently lacking.

Cardioprotective

In vitro, L-glutamine has been shown to assist in the maintenance of myocardial glutamate, ATP and phosphocreatine, and in the prevention of lactate accumulation (Khogali et al 1998). In addition to its antioxidant properties and effects on hyperglycaemia and hyperinsulinaemia (Opara et al 1996), this may suggest a possible role as a cardioprotective agent.

L

A recent randomised, double-blind, placebo-controlled study by Lomivorotov et al (2013) reported no cardioprotective benefit of perioperative use of N_2-L-alanyl-L-glutamine (0.4 g/kg/day of 20% solution of N_2-L-alanyl-L-glutamine [Dipeptiven, Fresenius Kabi, Germany]) in 32 patients with type 2 diabetes who underwent cardiopulmonary bypass surgery compared to the control group of 32 patients who received 0.9% NaCl.

However glutamine supplementation was reported to be cardioprotective in the first 24 hours postoperatively, as assessed by dynamics of troponin I in a study of patients with ischaemic heart disease who underwent cardiopulmonary bypass surgery. The perioperative glutamine-supplemented group of 25 patients (0.4 g/kg glutamine [Dipeptiven, 20% solution] per day) was compared to 25 patients in the control group who were administered a placebo (0.9% NaCl) (Lomivorotov et al 2011) and the dynamics of troponin I were assessed at 30 minutes, and at 6, 24 and 48 hours after surgery.

In a small, randomised double-blind study, 14 patients who required cardiopulmonary bypass surgery were placed in two groups. One group of 7 patients received oral alanyl-glutamine (25 g twice daily) for 3 days prior to surgery and the other group served as a control and received maltodextrin. The glutamine-supplemented group was reported to have significantly reduced myocardial injury and clinical complications (Sufit et al 2012).

Clinical note — Total parenteral nutrition

L-Glutamine is not very soluble or stable in solution, especially upon heating for sterilisation. As a result, until recently it was not included in TPN, resulting in compromised glutamine status in patients for whom reduced immune status and increased intestinal permeability could potentially increase the risk of morbid infection and mortality. The more soluble and stable synthetic glutamine dipeptides (L-alanyl-L-glutamine and glycyl-L-glutamine) have now been developed as delivery forms of L-glutamine for use in TPN. The dipeptide forms can also be used orally and have demonstrated a potential for greater bioavailability than glutamine alone (Macedo Rogero et al 2004).

Numerous studies have now been conducted using glutamine dipeptides in TPN and have shown benefit in preventing deterioration of gut permeability and preserving mucosal structure (Hall et al 1996, Jiang et al 1999, PDRHealth 2006a, van der Hulst et al 1993). In addition, animal studies suggest that glutamine-enriched TPN may attenuate the suppression of CYP3A and CYP2C usually associated with TPN (Shaw et al 2002). The addition of glutamine to TPN in preterm infants also appears to hasten improvements in hepatic function (Wang et al 2013).

In a meta-analysis of European and Asian randomised controlled trials (RCTs) in elective surgery patients, 13 studies (pooled $n = 355$) met inclusion criteria and demonstrated a significant reduction in infectious complication and length of hospital stay (weighted mean difference [WMD] of 3.86 days) (Jiang et al 2004). Conversely, a small study using glutamine (10 g) as part of home parenteral nutrition for 6 months did not reveal any significant effects compared to placebo for infective complications (36% vs 55%; $P = 0.67$), nutritional status, intestinal permeability or quality of life. It should be noted that plasma glutamine concentrations were also not affected in this study (Culkin et al 2008).

Neurotransmission

Disturbances of glutamine metabolism and/or transport may contribute to changes in glutamatergic or GABAergic transmission associated with different pathological conditions of the brain, such as epilepsy, hepatic encephalopathy and manganese encephalopathy. Glutamine appears to affect neurotransmission by interacting with the *N*-methyl-D-aspartate class of glutamine receptors (Albrecht et al 2010).

CLINICAL USE

Deficiency: prevention and treatment

During periods of increased need, L-glutamine is considered conditionally essential. Glutamine depletion can result in increased intestinal permeability, microbial translocation across the gut barrier, impaired wound healing, sepsis and multiple organ failure (Miller 1999). Experimental studies have proposed a number of benefits for patients with conditions that increase glutamine requirements. The suggested mechanisms include effects on proinflammatory cytokine expression, gut integrity, enhanced ability to mount a stress response and improved immune cell function, and studies have shown potential benefit with regard to mortality, length of hospital stay and infection.

To date, the results of studies using glutamine dipeptides in TPN have proven to be very promising in treating patients for whom enteral feeding is impossible. Benefits from studies of enteral glutamine supplementation have tended to be less pronounced, but preliminary trials have demonstrated benefits in some conditions, especially at high doses (e.g. 30 g/day enterally) (Wischmeyer 2003).

Critical care settings

A systematic review found trends to suggest that parenteral and enteral glutamine supplementation may reduce mortality, the development of infection and organ failure in critical illness; however, poor study design and possible publication bias limit what conclusions can be drawn from the current data (Avenell 2006).

A recent meta-analysis of 14 RCTs ($n = 587$) found that people given parenteral nutrition supplemented with glutamine dipeptide had a shorter length of hospital stay and a significant decrease in infectious complications (relative risk [RR] = 0.69; $P = 0.02$) compared to the group receiving standard parenteral nutrition (Wang et al 2010).

Similarly, in a recent meta-analysis by Bollhalder et al (2013) that included 40 RCTs, parenteral glutamine supplementation was associated with a significant reduction in infections (RR = 0.83) and a non-significant reduction in short-term mortality (RR = 0.89) and length of stay, although a significant reduction in mortality was not verified, in contrast to previous meta-analyses.

Likewise, a more recent meta-analysis by Chen et al (2014) that included 15 studies of 2862 critically ill patients in a number of settings, including surgical intensive care unit (ICU) subgroup and parenteral nutrition subgroup, reported that, compared to control groups, glutamine supplementation significantly reduced the incidence of hospital-acquired infections (RR 0.85; 95% confidence interval [CI] 0.74–0.97; $P = 0.02$). However, in 14 studies with 2777 patients, there was no benefit in overall mortality or length of hospital stay, although the mortality rate was significantly higher (RR 1.18; 95% CI 1.02–1.38; $P = 0.03$) in high glutamine dosage subgroup (above 0.5 g/kg/day).

Abdominal surgery and trauma

Parenteral supplementation of glutamine in critically ill patients has been shown to improve survival rate and minimise infectious complications, costs and length of hospital stay; however, the role of enteral glutamine supplementation remains controversial (Al Balushi et al 2013).

A meta-analysis of nine RCTs involving 373 patients was performed to assess the clinical and economical validity of glutamine dipeptide supplementation to parenteral nutrition in patients undergoing abdominal surgery. The review concluded that glutamine dipeptide has a positive effect in decreasing postoperative infectious morbidity (odds ratio [OR] = 0.24, $P = 0.04$), shortening the length of hospital stay (WMD = −3.55, 95% $P < 0.00001$) and improving postoperative cumulative nitrogen balance (WMD = 8.35, $P = 0.002$). No serious adverse effects were identified (Zheng 2006).

Enteral supplementation has not been shown to be as effective in abdominal trauma. In one trial, 120 patients with peritonitis or abdominal trauma were randomised to receive either enteral glutamine (45 g/day for 5 days) in addition to standard care ($n = 63$) or standard care alone ($n = 57$). No statistically significant benefits were noted in the treatment group for serum malondialdehyde or glutathione levels, infectious complications, survival rate or duration of hospital stay (Kumar et al 2007).

Trauma

Enteral glutamine has been shown to be protective to the gut in experimental models of shock and thus improve clinical outcomes. In a pilot study, enteral glutamine was administered during active shock resuscitation (0.5 g/kg/day during the first 24 hours) and continued for 10 days through the early postinjury period. The treatment was found to be safe and improved gastrointestinal tolerance (vomiting, nasogastric output, diarrhoea and distension). ICU and hospital length of stay were comparable (McQuiggan et al 2008). In a randomised trial using glutamine-enriched enteral nutrition in patients with multiple traumas, there was a reduction in the incidence of pneumonia, sepsis and bacteraemia (Houdijk et al 1998). Parenteral supplementation of alanyl-glutamine dipeptide may also result in better insulin sensitivity in multiple-trauma patients (Bakalar et al 2006).

Burns

Acute burn injury results in depletion of plasma and muscle glutamine, which contributes to muscle wasting, weight loss and infection. In critical illness, supplementation has been shown to minimise these effects and reduce the rate of mortality and length of stay (Windle 2006). In a double-blind controlled trial, 48 severely burned patients (total burn surface area 30–75%, full-thickness burn area 20–58%) were randomised into treatment (n = 25; 0.5 g/kg/day glutamine granules for 14 days with oral or tube feeding) or control group (n = 23; glycine placebo). The results indicated that significantly reduced plasma glutamine and damaged immunological function occurred and supplementation with glutamine granules increased plasma glutamine concentration and reduced the degree of immunosuppression. Glutamine improved immunological function (especially cellular immunity), wound healing and length of hospital stay (46.59 ± 12.98 days vs 55.68 ± 17.36 days, $P < 0.05$) (Peng et al 2006).

According to animal studies, oral glutamine supplementation may reduce bacterial and endotoxin translocation after burns by maintaining secretory IgA in the intestinal mucosa (Yu et al 1996). Systematic reviews and practice guidelines generally support glutamine supplementation in critical illness; however, in large or severe burns or inhalation injury there may be a prolonged critical illness phase (>4 weeks). Further research focusing on enteral and parenteral glutamine supplementation and long-term use is required (Windle 2006).

A recent meta-analysis of glutamine supplementation in critically ill patients with burns reported a reduction in mortality in hospital and complications due to Gram-negative bacteraemia (Lin et al 2013). The meta-analysis included four RCTs which involved 155 patients. The total burn surface area ($P = 0.34$) was similar in both glutamine and control groups at baseline; however, treatment with glutamine induced a significant decrease in the number of patients with Gram-negative bacteraemia (OR 0.27; $P = 0.04$) and hospital mortality (OR = 0.13; $P = 0.004$), and there was no statistical difference for the length of hospital stay.

Infants

Enteral and parenteral glutamine supplementation in preterm infants has been shown to have some beneficial effects on neonatal morbidity and mortality; however, these results are controversial (Korkmaz et al 2007).

In a short-term study of preterm infants (birth weight ≤ 1500 g) who received either enteral glutamine supplementation (n = 36; 300 mg/kg/day adjusted over time according to the current weight) or placebo (n = 33) between 8 and 120 days of life, the glutamine-supplemented group had significantly higher mean weight, length, head circumference, left upper mid-arm circumference and left mid-thigh circumference than the control group at the end of the fourth month. The effects appeared to occur in a time-dependent pattern (Korkmaz et al 2007). Another study reported that oral supplementation (0.25 mg/kg body weight) with glutamine did not improve growth or intestinal permeability (lactulose : mannitol ratio: 0.29 [95% CI 0.23–0.35] and 0.26 [95% CI: 0.21–0.32]) in malnourished Gambian infants (Williams et al 2007). It should be noted, however, that this dose is exceptionally low compared to other trials. The dose, route of administration and length of supplementation require further elucidation in larger-scale trials before full assessment can be made.

Experimental data have suggested that, by stimulating the rate of recovery of the villi and lipid-synthesising enzymes, L-glutamine treatments could improve the efficacy of enteral feeding in infants recovering from bowel damage (Ahdieh et al 1998). However, a recent Cochrane review concluded insufficient data were available from RCTs to determine whether glutamine supplementation confers clinically significant benefits for infants with severe gastrointestinal disease (Wagner et al 2012).

Some authors have suggested that early glutamine supplementation may also provide longer-term benefits. Enteral glutamine supplementation (300 mg/kg/day) between 3 and 30 days of life has been shown to lower the incidence of atopic dermatitis (OR 0.13; 95% CI 0.02–0.97) but not the incidence of bronchial hyperreactivity and infectious diseases (upper respiratory, lower respiratory and gastrointestinal) during the first year of life (van den Berg et al 2007). Follow-up of 52 very preterm babies who received glutamine supplementation in their first month of life revealed that there was an increase in white matter, hippocampus and brainstem volumes at school age, and this was mediated by a decrease in serious neonatal infections (de Kieviet et al 2012).

Despite the many encouraging results, a recent Cochrane review of 11 RCTs (five trials of enteral glutamine supplementation and six trials of parenteral glutamine supplementation) that included 2771 preterm infants reported that glutamine supplementation did not have a significant effect on mortality or major neonatal morbidities, including the incidence of invasive infection and necrotising enterocolitis (Moe-Byrne et al 2012).

Strenuous exercise

Following strenuous exercise, glutamine levels are depleted approximately 20%, resulting in immunodepression (Castell 2003, Castell & Newsholme 1997, Rogero et al 2002). However the role of glutamine supplementation in preventing postexercise effects on immune function is controversial (Gleeson 2008). The type of training is important to note, as although previous reports suggest decreased glutamine concentrations in overtrained athletes, progressive endurance training may lead to steady increases in plasma glutamine levels (Kargotich et al 2007).

L

The provision of glutamine after exercise has been shown to improve immune status (Castell & Newsholme 1997). In a study of 200 elite runners and rowers given a glutamine or placebo drink immediately after and again 2 hours after strenuous exercise, 151 participants returned questionnaires reporting the incidence of infection over the subsequent 7 days. The percentage of athletes reporting no infections was considerably higher in the glutamine group (81%, $n = 72$) compared to the placebo group (49%, $n = 79$, $P < 0.001$) (Castell et al 1996).

During recovery from strenuous exercise, rates of lymphocyte apoptosis, hyperammonaemia and whole-body proteolysis may be affected by glutamine supplementation. In a small study of nine triathletes, glutamine supplementation (four tablets of 700 mg of hydrolysed whey protein enriched with 175 mg of glutamine dipeptide dissolved in 250 mL water) partially prevented lymphocyte apoptosis induced by exhaustive exercise, possibly by a protective effect on mitochondrial function (Cury-Boaventura et al 2008). Both intermittent and continuous-intensity exercises increase ammonia, urate, urea and creatinine in the blood stream. Chronic glutamine supplementation (100 mg/kg body weight) given immediately before exercise may partially protect against elevated ammonia but not urate, urea or creatinine (Bassini-Cameron et al 2008). The addition of glutamine (300 mg/kg body weight) to an oral carbohydrate (1 g/kg/h) and essential amino acid (9.25 g) solution had no effect on postexercise muscle glycogen resynthesis or muscle protein synthesis, but may suppress a rise in whole-body proteolysis during the later stages of recovery (Wilkinson et al 2006).

Conversely, a trial assessing the possible ergogenic effects of glutamine supplementation (300 mg/kg body weight) to improve high-intensity exercise performance in trained males was unable to determine a beneficial effect (Haub et al 1998). Currently, the use of glutamine to enhance exercise performance is speculative at best and the cost of the high doses indicated must be considered. Further large-scale research is required to elucidate any potentially beneficial effects.

Care should be taken in people with diabetes as a small study revealed an increase in postexercise overnight hypoglycaemia in adolescents with type 1 diabetes who received a glutamine drink (0.25 g/kg/dose) pre-exercise and at bedtime (Mauras et al 2010).

Gut repair

Preliminary research on enteral (as well as parenteral) glutamine supplementation suggested promise for the use of glutamine in gut repair by: (1) protecting the intestinal mucosa from damage and promoting repair, thus improving intestinal permeability and reducing subsequent microbial and endotoxin translocation, promoting glutathione and secretory IgA; and (2) improving gut immunity. However, while there is some evidence for the use of glutamine in TPN (Hall et al 1996), clinical evidence using oral supplementation is less convincing. As in vitro data suggest that the colonic mucosa receives its nutrients preferentially from the luminal (not vascular) side (Roediger 1986), it has been suggested that glutamine should be more effective when delivered by the enteral route (Kouznetsova et al 1999). This has yet to be determined in clinical trials.

L-Glutamine enemas, twice daily for 7 days, have been shown to reduce mucosal damage and inflammation in experimental models of colitis in rats (Kaya et al 1999); however, preliminary trials in humans using parenteral glutamine (da Gama Torres et al 2008) and oral supplementation in malnourished preterm infants (Williams et al 2007) have not confirmed benefits for intestinal permeability.

Postoperative administration of TPN supplemented with a combination of glutamine and recombinant human growth hormone in patients following portal hypertension surgery prevented intestinal mucous membrane atrophy and preserved intestinal integrity, although the role of glutamine is unclear (Tang et al 2007). In a 1998 randomised, double-blind, placebo-controlled, 4-week trial of 24 HIV patients with abnormal intestinal permeability using 0, 4 or 8 g/day of glutamine, the authors reported a dose-dependent trend towards improved intestinal permeability and enhanced intestinal absorption with glutamine supplementation and recommended further studies to be carried out with higher doses (e.g. 20 g/day) over a longer study period (Noyer et al 1998). It is difficult to extrapolate the findings of this study to the wider community for the purpose of gut repair as there are factors involved in HIV/AIDS that may increase the biological demand for glutamine. Longer-term studies may provide more convincing results; however, it is possible that glutamine only stabilises gut barrier function under certain conditions and more research is required to elucidate these.

Crohn's disease

In a controlled trial, consecutive patients in remission from Crohn's disease with an abnormal intestinal permeability were randomised to receive oral glutamine or whey protein (0.5 g/kg ideal body weight/day). After 2 months intestinal permeability and morphology had improved significantly in both the glutamine and whey groups (Benjamin et al 2012). Previously a 4-week study on 18 children with active Crohn's disease fed a glutamine-enriched polymeric diet (Akobeng et al 2000) was unable to demonstrate benefits.

HIV

L-Glutamine has been shown to improve glutathione levels and significantly increase lean body mass in HIV patients (Patrick 2000); however, not all studies confirm this latter effect (Huffman & Walgren 2003). A recent study of 12 treated patients (six men and six women, 22–45 years old) and 20 healthy controls (10 men and 10 women, 20–59 years old) who were randomly assigned to 7-day dietary supplements containing *N*-acetylcysteine (1 g/day) or glutamine (20 g/day), with a 7-day washout period ingesting their usual diet, reported an increase in total glutathione by glutamine supplementation (Borges-Santos et al 2012). Improvements in intestinal absorption have also been reported in HIV patients receiving isonitrogenous doses of alanyl-glutamine (24 g/day for 10 days) (Leite et al 2013). Combined therapy with arginine and the leucine metabolite beta-hydroxy-beta-methylbutyrate has been shown to reverse lean tissue loss in HIV and cancer patients (Rathmacher et al 2004).

During initial HIV infection, the rapid turnover and proliferation of immune cells increase glutamine requirements and later the repeated episodes of infection, fever and diarrhoea may lead to further depletion. As a result, the doses used in the trial mentioned above (4 g and 8 g) may have been insufficient to meet the increased requirement in such patients (Noyer et al 1998).

Highly active antiretroviral therapy may be associated with diarrhoea and other gastrointestinal side effects. In a prospective, randomised, double-blind crossover study, HIV-infected patients with nelfinavir-associated diarrhoea (for >1 month) received L-glutamine (30 g/day) or placebo for 10 days. Glutamine supplementation resulted in a significant reduction in the severity of nelfinavir-associated diarrhoea (Huffman & Walgren 2003). A prospective 12-week trial of 35 HIV-positive men experiencing diarrhoea as a result of nelfinavir or lopinavir/ritonavir therapy was also conducted using probiotics and soluble fibre. When glutamine (30 g/day) was added to the regimen of non-responders at week 4, the response rate improved (Heiser et al 2004).

Cancer prevention

In addition to being the major fuel source for rapidly proliferating intestinal and immune cells, L-glutamine is the main fuel source for many rapidly growing tumours and, as a result, tumour growth is associated with a depletion in glutamine and glutathione stores and a depression of natural killer (NK) cell activity (Fahr et al 1994, Miller 1999). The increased intestinal permeability, immune suppression and oxidative damage that may result may further compromise the body's ability to deal with the tumour. While concerns exist, and are supported by in vitro evidence, that glutamine supplementation may feed the tumour, animal studies suggest that glutamine supplementation may assist in decreasing tumour growth by enhancing NK cell activity (Fahr et al 1994, Miller 1999). Animal studies have demonstrated that glutamine supplementation prevents the promotion of tumour cells in an implantable breast cancer model (Kaufmann et al 2003). The exact effects in different human tumour cell lines require further elucidation.

Clinical note — Cancer therapy

Side effects of chemotherapy and radiation therapy can significantly affect the quality of life of patients undergoing treatment for cancer. A number of trials have demonstrated the benefits of glutamine supplementation for improving side effects such as oral pain and inflammation, increased gut permeability and reduced lymphocyte count.

The provision of 15 g of oral glutamine three times daily appears to significantly reduce the incidence of severe radiation-induced diarrhoea (Kucuktulu et al 2013). Similarly, in a retrospective randomised experimental study of 46 patients with lung cancer who were treated with thoracic radiotherapy, the severity of acute radiotherapy-induced oesophagitis was significantly reduced ($P < 0.0001$) in those who were given 30 g prophylactic oral glutamine powder daily (Tutanc et al 2013).

Gastrointestinal effects

A number of studies have reported that adding glutamine to chemotherapy appears to reduce the incidence and severity of oral mucositis, a frequent complication of mucotoxic cancer therapy, which causes significant oral pain, increased infection risk and impaired functioning (Peterson et al 2007). For instance, oral glutamine (30 g/day) appears to reduce the incidence of fluorouracil/leucovorin-induced mucositis/stomatitis (9% vs 38% in the control group; $P < 0.001$) (Choi et al 2007). Reduced oral pain and inflammation have also been observed in patients receiving radiation and chemotherapy during bone marrow transplantation taking oral glutamine (1 g four times daily) (Miller 1999). In a retrospective study involving 41 patients with stage III lung carcinoma treated with thoracic irradiation, prophylactic supplementation with powdered glutamine (10 g/8 h) was found to be associated with a 27% lower incidence of grade 2 or 3 acute radiation-induced oesophagitis (ARIE), a 6-day delay in ARIE (22 days vs 16 days) and weight gain during radiotherapy (Topkan et al 2009).

In another study, L-glutamine (4 g twice daily, swish and swallow) was given to 12 patients receiving doxorubicin, one receiving etoposide, and one receiving ifosfamide, etoposide and carboplatinum from day 1 of chemotherapy for 28 days or for 4 days past the resolution of any postchemotherapy mucositis. Oral supplementation with glutamine significantly decreased the severity of chemotherapy-induced stomatitis (Skubitz & Anderson 1996). In a small study, parenteral glutamine supplementation was shown to protect the gastrointestinal mucosa against fluorouracil/calcium-folinate chemotherapy-induced damage (Decker-Baumann et al 1999). Yoshida et al (1998, 2001) have also shown that 30 g/day L-glutamine for 28 days attenuates the increased gut permeability and reduced lymphocyte count observed in patients undergoing cisplatin and fluorouracil therapy for oesophageal cancer.

In a small phase I trial ($n = 15$), glutamine was co-administered in an attempt to escalate the dose of a chemoradiotherapy regimen (weekly paclitaxel and carboplatin with concurrent radiation therapy). The addition was deemed unsuccessful due to multiple severe toxicities, including haematological toxicities and oesophagitis (Jazieh et al 2007). The role of glutamine in reducing taxane-associated dysgeusia (taste alteration) appears limited (Strasser et al 2008).

In a double-blind, placebo-controlled, randomised trial, oral glutamine (18 g/day) or placebo was given to 70 chemotherapy-naive patients with colorectal cancer 5 days prior to their first cycle of fluorouracil (450 mg/m^2) in association with folinic acid (100 mg/m^2), which was administered intravenously for 5 days. Glutamine treatment was continued for 15 days and was shown to reduce the negative effects on intestinal absorption and permeability induced by the chemotherapy and to potentially reduce diarrhoea (Daniele et al 2001). L-Glutamine may also reverse the decrease in goblet cells induced by fluorouracil (Tanaka & Takeuchi 2002).

More recent studies have further investigated the utility of glutamine supplementation in different patient groups receiving various modes of nutrition support and a variety of glutamine dosages.

A randomised study of 70 patients (Chattopadhyay et al 2014) reported that oral glutamine (10 g in 1 L of water 2 hours before radiotherapy treatment for 5 days/week on treatment days only; n = 35) reduced the severity and duration of oral mucositis in head and neck cancer patients receiving primary or adjuvant radiation therapy compared to patients in the control group (n = 35) who did not receive the glutamine.

A recent systematic review of 131 studies that included 10,514 participants evaluated the effectiveness of a range of prophylactic agents, including glutamine supplementation for oral mucositis in patients with cancer receiving treatment, compared with other potentially active interventions, placebo or no treatment, and reported that there was some benefit with intravenous glutamine (Worthington et al 2011).

However a more recent systematic review investigating natural agents in the management of oral mucositis has made a recommendation against the use of intravenous glutamine in patients receiving high-dose chemotherapy prior to haematopoietic stem cell transplant (level II evidence) (Yarom et al 2013).

In particular an earlier study by Pytlík et al (2002) had reported that intravenous glutamine made mucositis worse and was significantly associated with more relapses (P = 0.02) and higher mortality (P = 0.05).

In contrast, Gibson et al (2013) reported in their systematic review that new research did not support earlier observations of toxicity associated with glutamine supplementation and therefore they were unable to make a clinical guideline regarding glutamine supplementation for gastrointestinal mucositis, whereas the previous guideline was not to use systemic glutamine.

In regard to use in children, the evidence is less clear. A recent systematic review by Qutob et al (2013) investigated the evidence for the use of agents regarding the prevention of oral mucositis in children and concluded that, due to conflicting results, certain agents such as oral or enteral glutamine should be avoided until their efficacy is confirmed by further research.

Chemotherapy-induced diarrhoea

Chemotherapy-induced diarrhoea is a significant adverse effect during treatment with chemotherapy. A recent meta-analysis of eight RCTs (five studies with glutamine administered intravenously and three studies where glutamine was taken orally) included 298 patients (147 patients who received glutamine supplementation [16–40 g/day] and 151 patients who received a placebo), and reported a statistically significant reduction in the duration of diarrhoea in the glutamine-supplemented group, although there was no significant difference in the severity of diarrhoea between the groups (Sun et al 2012).

In a small randomised double-blind, placebo-controlled pilot study of 33 patients with rectal cancer, 30 g of glutamine was given in three doses per day for 5 weeks during preoperative radiochemotherapy and the placebo was given as 30 g of maltodextrin. There was no difference between groups in the frequency and severity of diarrhoea during radiochemotherapy (P = 0.5 and P = 0.39 respectively) (Rotovnik Kozjek et al 2011).

Chemotherapy-induced peripheral neuropathy

Chemotherapy-induced peripheral neuropathy is a significant adverse effect associated with neurotoxic chemotherapy (especially taxanes, platinum compounds and vinca alkaloids). In a review, two studies were identified that suggested beneficial effects. In one study, oral glutamine was found to be effective in reducing peripheral neuropathy associated with high-dose paclitaxel, resulting in a reduction in numbness, dysaesthesias and motor weakness, as well as a smaller loss of vibratory sensation (Amara 2008). Another study found that the addition of oral glutamine (15 g twice daily for 7 consecutive days every 2 weeks, starting on the day of oxaliplatin infusion) resulted in a significant reduction in the incidence and severity of peripheral neuropathy, less interference with activities of daily living (16.7% versus 40.9%) and less need for oxaliplatin dose reduction due to adverse effects (7.1% vs 27.3%). The addition of glutamine did not affect response to chemotherapy or survival (Wang et al 2007).

Other benefits

In one report, L-glutamine (10 g three times daily), given 24 hours after receiving paclitaxel, appeared to prevent the development of myalgia and arthralgia associated with treatment (PDRHealth 2006a). In children with solid tumours receiving chemotherapy, oral glutamine supplementation (4 $g/m^2/day$) may improve nutritional and immunological parameters and reduce requirements for antibiotics (Okur et al 2006). Glutamine may also increase tumour methotrexate concentration and tumouricidal activity and reduce side effects and mortality rates (Miller 1999, PDRHealth 2006a).

OTHER USES

Growth and development

In a prospective randomised, double-blind, placebo-controlled 1-year study of 120 young Brazilian shantytown children aged from 2 months to 9 years who were given glutamine alone (16 g daily for 10 days at start of the study) or a combination of glutamine + zinc + vitamin, improved intestinal barrier function was seen, as measured by the percentage of lactulose urinary excretion and the lactulose : mannitol absorption ratio. Glutamine treatment significantly improved weight-for-height z-scores compared to the placebo-glycine control group (Lima et al 2014).

Radiation injury

In a recent double-blind study the beneficial effects of oral glutamine supplementation on radiation injury were investigated in women undergoing radiation therapy for breast cancer. In the 8-week study, 17 patients were randomised to receive either the supplementary glutamine (0.5 g/kg/day; $n = 9$) or a placebo (dextrose, 25 g/day; $n = 8$) three times daily during 6 weeks of radiation therapy. The patients were followed for 2 years for assessment of radiation injury using the Radiation Therapy Oncology Group scales. The study reported reduced acute radiation morbidity and pain in the glutamine-supplemented group (Rubio et al 2013).

Alcoholism

Preliminary studies suggested a potential for glutamine to reduce alcohol cravings; however, these effects have not yet been studied in controlled trials on humans (PDRHealth 2006a). More recently, in vitro research has suggested that glutamine supplementation may inhibit the deleterious effects of alcohol on the tight junctions of the gut mucosa and in turn reduce the increased risk for gastrointestinal cancers in alcoholics (Basuroy et al 2005, Seth et al 2004).

Acute pancreatitis

The enteral administration of L-glutamine (15 mg/kg/day) to rats with acute pancreatitis resulted in a reduction in necrosis and infectious complications by decreasing the bacterial translocation rate (Avsar et al 2001).

Sickle cell disease

Orally administered L-glutamine improves the NAD redox potential of sickle red blood cells. Investigations of blood samples taken from five adult patients with sickle cell anaemia who had been on L-glutamine (30 g/day) therapy for at least 4 weeks consistently resulted in improvement of sickle red blood cell adhesion to human umbilical vein endothelial cells compared to the control group. The authors conclude that these results suggest positive physiological effects for L-glutamine in sickle cell disease (Niihara et al 2005).

Other conditions

Glutamine is a popular supplement in naturopathic practice and sometimes used for conditions that may be associated with compromised intestinal permeability, such as food allergies, leaky gut syndrome and malabsorption syndromes, including diarrhoea. It may also be used for conditions such as dermatitis and general fatigue, based on the theory that compromised intestinal permeability provides the opportunity for undigested food particles (especially proteins) to enter the systemic circulation and gives rise to an unwanted immune response that manifests as a skin reaction or as lethargy.

L

DOSAGE RANGE

Naturally-occurring food proteins contain 4–8% of their amino acid residues as glutamine and so the daily consumption is usually less than 10 g/day (Hall et al 1996).

Supplemental L-glutamine is available for oral and enteral use (in capsules, tablets and powder form) and in a dipeptide form for parenteral use.

While solubility and stability are primarily factors for TPN solutions, several factors should also be considered when using oral supplements, as powder forms are often mixed into a solution to enable easy administration of higher doses: 1 g of L-glutamine dissolves in 20.8 mL of water at 30°C (PDRHealth 2006a) and is stable for up to 22 days if stored at 4°C (Hornsby-Lewis et al 1994). Ideally, powdered formulas should be consumed immediately after mixing.

- Gut repair: 7–21 g taken orally as a single dose or in divided doses.
- Cancer therapy: 2–4 g twice daily swished in the mouth and swallowed (up to 45 g has been used in trials and given orally in divided doses).
- Critical illness: 5 g/500 mL of enteral feeding solution.
- HIV: 30 g/day taken orally as a single dose or in divided doses.
- Infection: 12–30.5 g in an enteral feeding solution.
- Infants: 300 mg/kg/day added to breast milk or to preterm formula.

ADVERSE REACTIONS

Toxicity studies in rats fed up to 5% of their diet in L-glutamine showed no toxic events (Tsubuku et al 2004) and glutamine dose–response studies have demonstrated 'good tolerance without untoward clinical or biochemical effects' (Ziegler et al 1999). Based on the available published human clinical trial data, glutamine intakes up to 14 g/day appear to be safe in normal healthy adults. Higher levels have been tested without adverse effects and may be safe; however, the data for intakes above 14 g are not sufficient for a confident conclusion of long-term safety (Shao & Hathcock 2008).

Most adverse reactions are mild and uncommon; they include gastrointestinal complaints such as constipation and bloating (PDRHealth 2006a). No evidence of harm has been observed in the studies conducted to date (Wischmeyer 2003).

A report exists of mania in two hypomanic patients after self-medication with up to 4 g/day glutamine (Membane 1984). As glutamine is a precursor of GABA, this may provide a possible explanation.

Two cases of a transient increase in liver enzyme levels have also been reported (Hornsby-Lewis et al 1994).

SIGNIFICANT INTERACTIONS

Radiation and chemotherapy

Benefits have been observed for the use of L-glutamine during radiation and chemotherapy (see 'Clinical note — Cancer therapy', above).

Indomethacin/NSAIDs

Concomitant use of L-glutamine (7 g three times daily) and indomethacin may ameliorate the increased intestinal permeability caused by indomethacin. The inclusion of misoprostol may also have a synergistic effect with this combination (Hond et al 1999, PDRHealth 2006a, Tanaka & Takeuchi 2002) — beneficial interaction possible.

Human growth hormone

In patients with severe short-bowel syndrome, concomitant use of L-glutamine and human growth hormone may enhance nutrient absorption (PDRHealth 2006a).

CONTRAINDICATIONS AND PRECAUTIONS

It is contraindicated in patients with hypersensitivity to glutamine or hepatic disease or any condition where there is a risk of accumulation of nitrogenous wastes in the blood, thus increasing the risk of ammonia-induced encephalopathy and coma.

It should only be used in people with chronic renal failure under professional supervision.

PREGNANCY USE

Safety in pregnancy has not been established; however, doses in line with normal dietary intake (approximately 10 g/day) are unlikely to be cause for concern.

PATIENTS' FAQs

What will this supplement do for me?

L-Glutamine is an amino acid that is used by the immune systems and intestinal cells as a fuel source. People with critical illnesses, stress, burns, injury or having undergone surgery or undertaking strenuous physical exercise require an increased intake to restore glutamine levels to normal and avoid loss of muscle mass and compromised immune function. It also promotes gastrointestinal repair and may improve tolerance to some anticancer treatments.

When will it start to work?

This will depend on the indication for which it is being used.

Are there any safety issues?

Glutamine appears to be a safe supplement; however, it should not be used by people who are hypersensitive to this compound, those with liver disease or any condition where there is a risk of accumulation of nitrogenous wastes in the blood (e.g. Reye's syndrome).

It should be used only by people with chronic renal failure under professional supervision.

REFERENCES

Ahdieh N et al. L-glutamine and transforming growth factor-alpha enhance recovery of monoacylglycerol acyltransferase and diacylglycerol acyltransferase activity in porcine postischemic ileum. Pediatr Res 43.2 (X) (1998): 227–233.

Akisu M et al. The role of dietary supplementation with L-glutamine in inflammatory mediator release and intestinal injury in hypoxia/reoxygenation-induced experimental necrotizing enterocolitis. Ann Nutr Metab 47.6 (2003): 262–266.

Akobeng A et al. Double-blind randomized controlled trial of glutamine-enriched polymeric diet in the treatment of active Crohn's disease. J Pediatr Gastroenterol Nutr 30.1 (2000): 78–84.

Al Balushi, R.M., et al. (2013). The clinical role of glutamine supplementation in patients with multiple trauma: A narrative review. Anaesth Intensive Care, 41(1), 24–34.

Albrecht, J., et al. (2010). Roles of glutamine in neurotransmission. Neuron Glia Biol, 6(4), 263–276.

Amara S. Oral glutamine for the prevention of chemotherapy-induced peripheral neuropathy. Ann Pharmacother 42.10 (2008): 1481–1485.

Avenell A. Glutamine in critical care: current evidence from systematic reviews. Proc Nutr Soc 65.3 (2006): 236–241.

Avsar F et al. Effects of oral L-glutamine, insulin and laxative on bacterial translocation in acute pancreatitis. Turk J Med Sci 31.4 (2001): 297–301.

Bakalar B et al. Parenterally administered dipeptide alanyl-glutamine prevents worsening of insulin sensitivity in multiple-trauma patients. Crit Care Med 34.2 (2006): 381–386.

Bassini-Cameron A et al. Glutamine protects against increases in blood ammonia in football players in an exercise intensity-dependent way. Br J Sports Med 42.4 (2008): 260–266.

Basuroy S et al. Acetaldehyde disrupts tight junctions and adherens junctions in human colonic mucosa: protection by EGF and l-glutamine. Am J Physiol Gastrointest Liver Physiol 289.2 (2005): G367–G375.

Benjamin, J., et al. (2012). Glutamine and whey protein improve intestinal permeability and morphology in patients with Crohn's disease: A randomized controlled trial. Dig Dis Sci, 57(4), 1000–1012.

Boelens PG et al. Glutamine alimentation in catabolic state. J Nutr 131 (9 Suppl) (2001): 2569–77S; discussion 2590S.

Boelens PG et al. Glutamine-enriched enteral nutrition increases in vitro interferon-gamma production but does not influence the in vivo specific antibody response to KLH after severe trauma: A prospective, double blind, randomized clinical study. Clin Nutr 23.3 (2004): 391–400.

Bollhalder L, et al. A systematic literature review and meta-analysis of randomized clinical trials of parenteral glutamine supplementation. Clin Nutr.;32(2) (2013):213–23.

Borges-Santos MD, et al. Plasma glutathione of HIV$^+$ patients responded positively and differently to dietary supplementation with cysteine or glutamine. Nutrition.28(7–8) (2012):753–6.

Castell L. Glutamine supplementation in vitro and in vivo, in exercise and in immunodepression. Sports Med 33.5 (2003): 323–345.

Castell LM, Newsholme EA. The effects of oral glutamine supplementation on athletes after prolonged, exhaustive exercise. Nutrition 13.7–8 (1997): 738–742.

Castell LM, et al. Does glutamine have a role in reducing infections in athletes?. Eur J Appl Physiol Occup Physiol 73.5 (1996): 488–490.

Chattopadhyay S, Saha A, Azam M, Mukherjee A, Sur PK. Role of oral glutamine in alleviation and prevention of radiation-induced oral mucositis: A prospective randomized study. South Asian J Cancer. 2014 Jan;3(1):8–12.

Chen QH, et al. The effect of glutamine therapy on outcomes in critically ill patients: a meta-analysis of randomized controlled trials. Crit Care. 2014 Jan 9;18(1):R8.

Choi K et al. The effect of oral glutamine on 5-fluorouracil/leucovorin-induced mucositis/stomatitis assessed by intestinal permeability test. Clin Nutr 26.1 (2007): 57–62.

Chun H et al. Effect of enteral glutamine on intestinal permeability and bacterial translocation after abdominal radiation injury in rats. J Gastroenterol 32 (1997): 189–195.

Culkin A et al. A double-blind, randomized, controlled crossover trial of glutamine supplementation in home parenteral nutrition. Eur J Clin Nutr 62.5 (2008): 575–583.

Cury-Boaventura MF et al. Effects of exercise on leukocyte death: prevention by hydrolyzed whey protein enriched with glutamine dipeptide. Eur J Appl Physiol 103.3 (2008): 289–294.

da Gama Torres HO et al. Efficacy of glutamine-supplemented parenteral nutrition on short-term survival following allo-SCT: a randomized study. Bone Marrow Transplant 41.12 (2008): 1021–1027.

Daniele B et al. Oral glutamine in the prevention of fluorouracil induced intestinal toxicity: a double blind, placebo controlled, randomised trial. Gut 48.1 (2001): 28–33.

Decker-Baumann C et al. Reduction of chemotherapy-induced side-effects by parenteral glutamine supplementation in patients with metastatic colorectal cancer. Eur J Cancer 35.2 (1999): 202–207.

de Kieviet, J.F., et al. (2012). Effects of glutamine on brain development in very preterm children at school age. Pediatrics, 130(5), e1121–1127.

Diestel CF et al. [Effect of oral supplement of L-glutamine in colonic wall of rats subjected to abdominal irradiation.] Acta Cir Bras 20 (Suppl 1) (2005): 94–100.

Fahr MJ, et al. Vars Research Award. Glutamine enhances immunoregulation of tumor growth. J Parenter Enteral Nutr 18.6 (1994): 471–476.

Furukawa S et al. Supplemental glutamine augments phagocytosis and reactive oxygen intermediate production by neutrophils and monocytes from postoperative patients in vitro. Nutrition 16.5 (2000): 323–329.

Gibson RJ, et al. Systematic review of agents for the management of gastrointestinal mucositis in cancer patients. Support Care Cancer. 2013 Jan;21(1):313–26.

Gleeson, M. (2008). Dosing and efficacy of glutamine supplementation in human exercise and sport training. J Nutr, 138(10), 2045S–2049S.

Hall J et al. Glutamine. Br J Surg 83 (1996): 305–312.

Haub MD et al. Acute l-glutamine ingestion does not improve maximal effort exercise. J Sports Med Phys Fitness 38.3 (1998): 240–244.

Heiser CR et al. Probiotics, soluble fiber, and l-Glutamine (GLN) reduce nelfinavir (NFV)- or lopinavir/ritonavir (LPV/r)-related diarrhea. J Int Assoc Physicians AIDS Care (Chic Ill) 3.4 (2004): 121–129.

Hond ED et al. Effect of glutamine on the intestinal permeability changes induced by indomethacin in humans. Aliment Pharmacol Ther 13.5 (1999): 679–685.

Hornsby-Lewis L et al. L-glutamine supplementation in home total parenteral nutrition patients: stability, safety and affects on intestinal absorption. J Parenter Enteral Nutr 18 (1994): 268–273.

Houdijk AP et al. Randomised trial of glutamine-enriched enteral nutrition on infectious morbidity in patients with multiple trauma. Lancet 352.9130 (1998): 772–776.

Huffman FG, Walgren ME. l-glutamine supplementation improves nelfinavir-associated diarrhea in HIV-infected individuals. HIV Clin Trials 4.5 (2003): 324–329.

Iantomasi T. Glutathione metabolism in Crohn's disease. Biochem Med Metab Biol 53 (1994): 87–91.

Jazieh AR et al. Phase I clinical trial of concurrent paclitaxel, carboplatin, and external beam chest irradiation with glutamine in patients with locally advanced non-small cell lung cancer. Cancer Invest 25.5 (2007): 294–298.

Jiang ZM et al. The impact of alanyl-glutamine on clinical safety, nitrogen balance, intestinal permeability, and clinical outcome in postoperative patients: a randomised, double blind, controlled study of 120 patients. J Parenter Enteral Nutr 23 (1999): S62–S66.

Jiang ZM et al. The impact of glutamine dipeptides on outcome of surgical patients: systematic review of randomized controlled trials from Europe and Asia. Clin Nutr Suppl 1.1 (2004): 17–23.

Kargotich S et al. Monitoring 6 weeks of progressive endurance training with plasma glutamine. Int J Sports Med 28.3 (2007): 211–216.

Kaufmann Y et al. Effect of glutamine on the initiation and promotion phases of DMBA-induced mammary tumor development. J Parenter Enteral Nutr 27.6 (2003): 411–4118.

Kaya E et al. L-glutamine enemas attenuate mucosal injury in experimental colitis. Dis Colon Rectum 42.9 (1999): 1209–1215.

Khogali SE et al. Effects of L-glutamine on post-ischaemic cardiac function: protection and rescue. J Mol Cell Cardiol 30.4 (1998): 819–827.

Kohlmeier M. Glutamine. In: Nutrient metabolism. St Louis: Elsevier, 2003, pp. 280–288.

Korkmaz A et al. Long-term enteral glutamine supplementation in very low birth weight infants: effects on growth parameters. Turk J Pediatr 49.1 (2007): 37–44.

Kouznetsova L et al. Glutamine reduces phorbol-12,13-dibutyrate-induced macromolecular hyperpermeability in HT-29Cl.19A intestinal cells. J Parenter Enteral Nutr 23.3 (1999): 136–139.

Kucuktulu, E., et al. (2013). The protective effects of glutamine on radiation-induced diarrhea. Support Care Cancer, 21(4), 1071–1075.

Kumar S et al. Effect of oral glutamine administration on oxidative stress, morbidity and mortality in critically ill surgical patients. Indian J Gastroenterol 26.2 (2007): 70–73.

Kusumoto I. Industrial production of L-glutamine. J Nutr 131 (9 Suppl) (2001): 2552–5S.

Li S et al. Separation of L-glutamine from fermentation broth by nanofiltration. J Membr Sci 222.1–2 (2003): 191–201.

Lima AA, et al. Effects of glutamine alone or in combination with zinc and vitamin A on growth, intestinal barrier function, stress and satiety-related hormones in Brazilian shantytown children. Clinics (Sao Paulo). 2014 Apr;69(4):225–33.

Lin JJ, et al. A meta-analysis of trials using the intention to treat principle for glutamine supplementation in critically ill patients with burn. Burns. 2013; 39: 565–570.

Lomivorotov VV et al Glutamine is cardioprotective in patients with ischemic heart disease following cardiopulmonary bypass. Heart Surg Forum. 2011 Dec;14(6):E384–8.

Lomivorotov VV, et al. Does glutamine promote benefits for patients with diabetes mellitus scheduled for cardiac surgery? Heart Lung Circ. 2013 May;22(5):360–5.

Macedo Rogero M et al. Plasma and tissue glutamine response to acute and chronic supplementation with L-glutamine and L-alanyl-L-glutamine in rats. Nutr Res 24.4 (2004): 261–270.

Masuko Y. Impact of stress response genes induced by L-glutamine on warm ischemia and reperfusion injury in the rat small intestine. Hokkaido Igaku Zasshi 77.2 (2002): 169–183.

Mauras, N., et al. (2010). Effects of glutamine on glycemic control during and after exercise in adolescents with type 1 diabetes: A pilot study. Diabetes Care, 33(9), 1951–1953.

McQuiggan M et al. Enteral glutamine during active shock resuscitation is safe and enhances tolerance of enteral feeding. J Parenter Enteral Nutr 32.1 (2008): 28–35.
Membane A. L-Glutamine and mania (letter). Am J Psychiatry 141 (1984): 1302–1303.
Meng Q et al. Regulation of intestinal glutamine absorption by transforming growth factor-beta. J Surg Res 114.2 (2003): 257–258.
Miller AL. Therapeutic considerations of L-glutamine: a review of the literature. Altern Med Rev 4.4 (1999): 239–247.
Moe-Byrne T, et al. Glutamine supplementation to prevent morbidity and mortality in preterm infants. Cochrane Database Syst Rev. 2012 Mar 14;3:CD001457.
Newsholme P. Why is L-glutamine metabolism important to cells of the immune system in health, postinjury, surgery or infection? J Nutr 131 (9 Suppl) (2001): 2515–222S: discussion 2523–4S.
Niihara Y et al. L-Glutamine therapy reduces endothelial adhesion of sickle red blood cells to human umbilical vein endothelial cells. BMC Blood Disord 5.4 (2005).
Noyer CM et al. A double-blind placebo-controlled pilot study of glutamine therapy for abnormal intestinal permeability in patients with AIDS. Am J Gastroenterol 93.6 (1998): 972–975.
Okur A et al. Effects of oral glutamine supplementation on children with solid tumors receiving chemotherapy. Pediatr Hematol Oncol 23.4 (2006): 277–285.
Opara EC et al. l-Glutamine supplementation of a high fat diet reduces body weight and attenuates hyperglycemia and hyperinsulinemia in C57BL/6J mice. J Nutr 126.1 (1996): 273–279.
Paquette JC, et al. Rapid induction of the intrinsic apoptotic pathway by L-glutamine starvation. J Cell Physiol 202.3 (2005): 912–921.
Patel AB et al. Glutamine is the major precursor for GABA synthesis in rat neocortex in vivo following acute GABA-transaminase inhibition. Brain Res 919.2 (2001): 207–220.
Patrick L. Nutrients and HIV. part three: N-acetylcysteine, alpha-lipoic acid, L-glutamine, and L-carnitine. Altern Med Rev 5.4 (2000): 290–305.
Paulo FL. Effects of oral supplement of L-glutamine on diverted colon wall. J Cell Mol Med 6.3 (2002): 377–382.
PDRHealth. L-Glutamine. PDRHealth [online]. Thomson Healthcare. www.pdrhealth (accessed 03–06), 2006a.
PDRHealth. Glutamine peptides. PDRHealth [online]. Thomson Healthcare. www.pdrhealth (accessed 03–06), 2006b.
Peng X et al. Glutamine granule-supplemented enteral nutrition maintains immunological function in severely burned patients. Burns 32.5 (2006): 589–593.
Peterson DE, et al. Randomized, placebo-controlled trial of Saforis for prevention and treatment of oral mucositis in breast cancer patients receiving anthracycline-based chemotherapy. Cancer 109.2 (2007): 322–331.
Pytlík R, et al (2002) Standardized parenteral alanyl-glutamine dipeptide supplementation is not beneficial in autologous transplant patients: a randomized, double-blind, placebo controlled study. Bone Marrow Transplant 30:953–961.
Qutob AF, et al. Prevention of oral mucositis in children receiving cancer therapy: a systematic review and evidence-based analysis. Oral Oncol.49(2) (2013):102–7.
Rathmacher JA et al. Supplementation with a combination of beta-hydroxy-beta-methylbutyrate (HMB), arginine, and glutamine is safe and could improve hematological parameters. J Parenter Enteral Nutr 28.2 (2004): 65–75.
Rhoads JM et al. L-glutamine stimulates intestinal cell proliferation and activates mitogen-activated protein kinases. Am J Physiol 272.5 (Pt 1) (1997): G943–G953.
Roediger WE. Metabolic basis of starvation diarrhoea: implications for treatment. Lancet 1.8489 (1986): 1082–1084.
Rogero M et al. Effect of L-glutamine and L-alanyl-L-glutamine supplementation on the response to delayed-type hypersensitivity test (DTH) in rats submitted to intense training. Rev Bras Cienc Farm 38.4 (2002): 487–497.
Ropeleski MJ et al. Anti-apoptotic effects of L-glutamine-mediated transcriptional modulation of the heat shock protein 72 during heat shock. Gastroenterology 129.1 (2005): 170–184.
Rotovnik Kozjek N, et al. Oral glutamine supplementation during preoperative radiochemotherapy in patients with rectal cancer: a randomised double blinded, placebo controlled pilot study. Clin Nutr.30(5) (2011):567–70.
Rubio I, et al. Oral glutamine reduces radiation morbidity in breast conservation surgery. JPEN J Parenter Enteral Nutr. 2013 Sep;37(5):623–30.
Scheppach W et al. Effect of L-glutamine and n-butyrate on the restitution of rat colonic mucosa after acid induced injury. Gut 38.6 (1996): 878–885.
Seth A et al. L-Glutamine ameliorates acetaldehyde-induced increase in paracellular permeability in Caco-2 cell monolayer. Am J Physiol Gastrointest Liver Physiol 287.3 (2004): G510–G517.
Shao A, Hathcock JN. Risk assessment for the amino acids taurine, L-glutamine and L-arginine. Regul Toxicol Pharmacol 50.3 (2008): 376–399.
Shaw AA et al. The influence of L-glutamine on the depression of hepatic cytochrome P450 activity in male rats caused by total parenteral nutrition. Drug Metab Dispos 30.2 (2002): 177–182.
Skubitz KM, Anderson PM. Oral glutamine to prevent chemotherapy induced stomatitis: A pilot study. J Lab Clin Med 127.2 (1996): 223–228.
Strasser F et al. Prevention of docetaxel- or paclitaxel-associated taste alterations in cancer patients with oral glutamine: a randomized, placebo-controlled, double-blind study. Oncologist 13.3 (2008): 337–346.
Sufit A, et al. Pharmacologically dosed oral glutamine reduces myocardial injury in patients undergoing cardiac surgery: a randomized pilot feasibility trial. JPEN J Parenter Enteral Nutr. 2012 Sep;36(5):556–61. 2012
Sun J, et al. Glutamine for chemotherapy induced diarrhea: a meta-analysis. Asia Pac J Clin Nutr. 21(3) (2012):380–5.
Tanaka A, Takeuchi K. Prophylactic effect of L-glutamine against intestinal derangement induced 5-fluorouracil or indomethacin in rats. Jpn Pharmacol Ther 30.6 (2002): 455–462.
Tang ZF et al. Glutamine and recombinant human growth hormone protect intestinal barrier function following portal hypertension surgery. World J Gastroenterol 13.15 (2007): 2223–2228.

Topkan E et al. Prevention of acute radiation-induced esophagitis with glutamine in non-small cell lung cancer patients treated with radiotherapy: evaluation of clinical and dosimetric parameters. Lung Cancer 2009, 63(3):393–399.
Tutanc, O.D., et al. (2013). The efficacy of oral glutamine in prevention of acute radiotherapy-induced esophagitis in patients with lung cancer. Contemp Oncol (Pozn), 17(6), 520–524.
Tsubuku S et al. Thirteen-week oral toxicity study of L-glutamine in rats. Int J Toxicol 23.2 (2004): 107–112.
van den Berg A et al. Glutamine-enriched enteral nutrition in very low-birth-weight infants: effect on the incidence of allergic and infectious diseases in the first year of life. Arch Pediatr Adolesc Med 161.11 (2007): 1095–1101.
van der Hulst RRWJ et al. Glutamine and the preservation of gut integrity. Lancet 341.8857 (1993): 1363–1365.
Wagner JV, et al. Glutamine supplementation for young infants with severe gastrointestinal disease. Cochrane Database Syst Rev. 2012 Jul 11;7:CD005947.
Wang WS et al. Oral glutamine is effective for preventing oxaliplatin-induced neuropathy in colorectal cancer patients. Oncologist 12.3 (2007): 312–319.
Wang Y, et al. The impact of glutamine dipeptide-supplemented parenteral nutrition on outcomes of surgical patients: a meta-analysis of randomized clinical trials. JPEN J Parenter Enteral Nutr. 34(5) (2010):521–9.
Wang, Y.,et al. (2013). Glutamine supplementation in preterm infants receiving parenteral nutrition leads to an early improvement in liver function. Asia Pac J Clin Nutr, 22(4), 530–536.
Wilkinson SB et al. Addition of glutamine to essential amino acids and carbohydrate does not enhance anabolism in young human males following exercise. Appl Physiol Nutr Metab 31.5 (2006): 518–529.
Williams EA, et al. A double-blind, placebo-controlled, glutamine-supplementation trial in growth-faltering Gambian infants. Am J Clin Nutr 86.2 (2007): 421–427.
Windle EM. Glutamine supplementation in critical illness: evidence, recommendations, and implications for clinical practice in burn care. J Burn Care Res 27.6 (2006): 764–772.
Wischmeyer PE. Clinical applications of L-glutamine: past, present, and future. Nutr Clin Pract 18.5 (2003): 377–385.
Worthington HV, et al. Interventions for preventing oral mucositis for patients with cancer receiving treatment. Cochrane Database Syst Rev. 2011 Apr 13;(4):CD000978.
Yarom N, et al. Systematic review of natural agents for the management of oral mucositis in cancer patients. study, 2013 Nov;21(11):3209–21.
Yoshida S et al. Effects of glutamine supplements and radiochemotherapy on systemic immune and gut barrier function in patients with advanced esophageal cancer. Ann Surg 227.4 (1998): 485–491.
Yoshida S et al. Glutamine supplementation in cancer patients. Nutrition 17.9 (2001): 766–768.
Yu B, et al. Enhancement of gut immune function by early enteral feeding enriched with L-glutamine in severe burned miniswine. Zhonghua Zheng Xing Shao Shang Wai Ke Za Zhi 12.2 (1996): 98–100.
Zheng YM. Glutamine dipeptide for parenteral nutrition in abdominal surgery: a meta-analysis of randomized controlled trials. World J Gastroenterol 12.46 (2006): 7537–7541.
Ziegler T et al. Interactions between nutrients and peptide growth factors in intestinal growth, repair and function. J Parenter Enteral Nutr 23 (1999): S174–S183.

L-Lysine

BACKGROUND

L-Lysine is an amino acid which is absorbed from the small intestine and then transported to the liver via the portal circulation where it is involved in protein biosynthesis and is partly metabolised.

CHEMICAL COMPONENTS

L-Lysine is the biologically active stereoisomer of lysine.

MAIN ACTIONS

Essential amino acid

The human body cannot synthesise L-lysine so it must be taken through the diet. The richest sources of L-lysine are animal proteins such as meat and poultry. It is also found to lesser extents in eggs, beans and dairy products (Bratman & Kroll 2000).

Antiviral

L-Lysine has an inhibitory effect on the multiplication of herpes simplex virus (HSV) in cell cultures (Griffith et al 1981, Milman et al 1980). It appears to act as an antimetabolite and competes with arginine for inclusion into viral replicative processes (Griffith et al 1981). As such, lysine retards the viral growth-promoting action of arginine.

Calcium regulation

L-Lysine may be involved in the cellular absorption, regulation and use of calcium (Civitelli et al 1992). In vitro tests with human osteoblasts indicate that lysine has a positive effect on osteoblast proliferation, activation and differentiation (Torricelli et al 2003).

Inhibition of protein glycation and advanced glycation end products

L-Lysine inhibits protein glycation and the role of supplementary lysine has been investigated for the prevention of protein glycation and inhibition of the formation of advanced glycation end products. Under hyperglycaemic conditions, production of fibrin is increased by glycated fibrinogen and human studies report that lysine supplementation significantly reduces fibrinogen activity in diabetic patients ($P < 0.05$). As an inhibitor of glycation, lysine may therefore reduce fibrinogen's non-enzymatic glycation and rectify its structure and function (Mirmiranpour et al 2012).

L

OTHER ACTIONS

L-Lysine is required for biosynthesis of collagen, elastin and carnitine. Studies in animal models have reported that lysine deficiency can have a negative impact on carnitine synthesis which results in a reduction in carnitine levels and an increase in lipid levels. The addition of lysine in a lysine-deficient diet improves both triglyceride and carnitine levels (Khan & Bamji 1979). However in human studies supplementation of 1 g lysine daily for 12 weeks has failed to demonstrate benefits for lipid profiles (Hlais et al 2012).

CLINICAL USE

Herpes simplex — prevention and treatment

The most common use for oral lysine supplements in practice is to prevent and treat outbreaks of herpes simplex labialis. Most clinical research was conducted in the 1980s, generally producing positive results for reducing recurrences when used in high doses, long-term and possibly also reducing severity and improving healing time, but this is less consistent (Digiovanna & Blank 1984, Griffith et al 1978, 1987, McCune et al 1984, Milman et al 1978, 1980, Simon et al 1985, Thein & Hurt 1984, Walsh et al 1983, Wright 1994).

Preventing an outbreak

The majority of double-blind, placebo-controlled randomised controlled trials have shown oral L-lysine supplementation to be effective for decreasing the frequency of outbreaks.

One randomised, double-blind crossover study found that supplementation with 1000 mg/day of L-lysine together with a low arginine diet over 24 weeks decreased the recurrence rate of HSV attacks in non-immunocompromised subjects (McCune et al 1984). A group taking a lower dose of 500 mg daily experienced similar results to placebo. Another double-blind trial compared the effects of 1000 mg L-lysine three times daily for 6 months with placebo treatment in 52 subjects. Once again, oral L-lysine was found to decrease recurrence rates (Griffith et al 1987). An open study of 45 patients with recurring HSV infection found that L-lysine supplementation reduced recurrence when taken at concentrations between 312 and 1200 mg/day in single or multiple doses (Griffith et al 1978). Thein and Hurt (1984) conducted a 12-month, double-blind crossover trial involving 26 subjects with recurring herpes lesions and found that a dose of 1000 mg/day L-lysine in combination with dietary arginine restriction had protective effects against lesion formation. Furthermore, once supplementation ceased, an increase in lesion frequency occurred. This study went further than others, identifying that serum lysine levels need to exceed 165 nmol/mL in order for clinical effects to become significant.

An observational study of 1534 volunteers asking about the perceived effectiveness of lysine supplements to treat cold sores, canker sores or genital herpes over a 6-month trial period indicated positive results (Walsh et al 1983). Of those people with cold sores or fever blisters, 92% claimed lysine supplements were 'very effective' or 'an effective form' of treatment and 81% of those with genital herpes and who had tried other forms of treatment also claimed positive results.

A crossover study by Milman et al (1980) found that significantly more patients receiving treatment with L-lysine 500 mg twice daily for 12 weeks experienced a reduction in infection occurrence compared to placebo (27.7% versus 12.3%; $P < 0.05$). However, the total number of recurrences was 12.5% lower in the active treatment group compared to the placebo group, but not statistically significant.

In contrast, a small double-blind study of 21 participants found oral lysine hydrochloride therapy (400 mg three times a day) did not reduce the frequency, duration or severity of herpes simplex infections (Digiovanna & Blank 1984). A later study by Simon et al (1985) suggests that there is a dose response. In their study, 31 people with diagnosed herpes labialis or genitalis took two capsules twice a day for 3 months (1000 mg/day), then 18 patients took 750 mg/day for 3 more months (Simon et al 1985). The group taking the higher dose had fewer recurrences than predicted while taking 1000 mg/day (17 recurrences versus 42.6 predicted) but during the second 3-month period (750 mg/day or placebo) there was no significant difference between actual and predicted recurrences (17 recurrences versus 16.8 predicted in the treatment group and 16 recurrences versus 21.8 predicted in the placebo group).

Reducing severity and/or healing time

Griffith et al (1987) found that a higher dose of 1000 mg three times daily significantly reduced symptom severity and healing time. More specifically, healing time was reduced by a mean ± SD of 2.3 ± 0.7 days in the lysine group, versus 0.2 ± 0.6 day with placebo ($P < 0.1$). More patients in the lysine group than the placebo group reported their symptoms to be 'milder' (74% versus 28%; $P < 0.01$). The treatment group had been taking L-lysine long-term as a means of reducing outbreak frequency.

Previously, Griffith et al (1978) showed that L-lysine taken at doses between 312 mg/day and 1200 mg/day accelerated recovery time during an outbreak, whereas a double-blind, placebo-controlled study by Milman et al (1978) showed that the lower dose of L-lysine 1000 mg taken at the first sign of an outbreak was no better than placebo for reducing severity or enhancing healing rate. McCune et al (1984) also did not find that a daily dose of 1000 mg/day reduced healing time during an outbreak in non-immunocompromised volunteers.

The effect of lysine on herpes may depend on variables such as the overall dietary ratio of lysine to arginine and the additional dose of supplemental lysine.

In practice, doses of >3000 mg/day are used as treatment during an acute episode, based on the positive findings of the Griffith study. This is combined with a diet low in arginine-rich foods, such as chocolate, peas, nuts and beer, and high in lysine-rich foods, such as baked beans and eggs.

A small pilot study examined the use of a topical preparation SuperLysine Plus+ cream containing lysine plus other nutrients (zinc oxide, vitamins A, D and E and lithium carbonate 3X) and botanicals (extracts of propolis, calendula, echinacea and goldenseal) in relieving the symptoms of herpes simplex. Patients with signs and symptoms of an active cold sore of less than 24 hours duration applied the ointment to the lesions 2-hourly during waking hours. Symptoms, including severity of tingling, burning and tenderness, showed significant improvement by day 3 except oozing, and 40% of patients had full resolution; 87% of patients had full resolution after day 6 (Singh et al 2005).

OTHER USES

Diabetes/hyperlipidaemia

Mirmiranpour et al (2012) investigated changes in fibrinogen activity in 50 subjects with type 2 diabetes mellitus (aged ≥40 years). The subjects were randomised to receive either 3 g of L-Lysine monohydrochloride or placebo daily for 3 months. Patients also received the antidiabetic drugs metformin and glibenclamide.The authors reported that fibrinogen activity in the diabetic patients was significantly reduced ($P < 0.05$) in the lysine-supplemented group compared to the placebo group, although there were no changes in the prothrombin time and partial thromboplastin time.

Body composition

A high-lysine diet (80 mg/kg/day) for 8 weeks in well and undernourished healthy males resulted in a small positive effect (~+7.5%) on muscle strength compared to those on low-lysine diets (Unni et al 2012). However most of the studies investigating lysine on body composition have used mixed formulations of amino acids.

Lysine has been reported to stimulate muscle protein anabolism; arginine stimulates whole-body protein synthesis and beta-hydroxy-beta-methylbutyrate has been shown to prevent excessive muscle proteolysis. A double-blind, randomised study (Flakoll et al 2004) investigated the effect of daily supplementation with lysine (1.5 g), arginine (5 g) and beta-hydroxy-beta-methylbutyrate (2 g) on strength, functionality, body composition and protein metabolism in 50 elderly women (mean age 76.7 years). The control group received an isocaloric isonitrogenous mixture (1.8 g of nitrogen) that contained non-essential amino acids (5.6 g of alanine, 0.9 g of glutamic acid, 3.1 g of glycine and 2.2 g of serine). The treatment group had increased measurements of functionality, lean tissue and protein synthesis ($P < 0.05$) after 12 weeks. Similarly, a subsequent double-blind randomised 1-year-long study (Baier et al 2009) investigated the effects of daily consumption of the same supplement in elderly men and women (76 ± 1.6 years) over 1 year. Compared to the control group ($n = 37$), there was a significant increase in protein turnover and fat-free mass ($P = 0.05$) in the treatment group ($n = 40$). Recently post hoc analysis of muscle strength based on the participants' vitamin D status was conducted because of the association of increased serum vitamin D levels with an increase in muscle function. The analysis revealed that vitamin D status did not affect fat-free mass, although muscle strength was increased significantly in the supplement group ($P < 0.01$) but only in those with adequate (≥30 ng 25OH-vitamin D_3/mL) vitamin D levels (Fuller et al 2011). The role that lysine plays in this combination is unclear.

L

Osteoporosis prevention

Two studies have investigated the effects of oral L-lysine supplementation on calcium use to determine whether L-lysine has a role in the prevention of osteoporosis. In these tests, oral L-lysine was shown to significantly increase intestinal absorption of calcium and decrease renal excretion in both healthy women and those with osteoporosis (Civitelli et al 1992).

Anxiety and mood disturbances

A systematic review of nutritional and herbal supplements for anxiety and anxiety-related disorder reported that there is evidence for the use of supplemental L-lysine in combination with L-arginine (Lakhan & Vieira 2010). According to a randomised, double-blind trial, fortification of lysine in a wheat-based (L-lysine-deficient) diet significantly reduced anxiety score in males, but not females with high baseline anxiety. It is suspected that L-lysine's action as a 5-HT_4 receptor antagonist and benzodiazepine receptor agonist is responsible for the observed effect (Smriga et al 2004). In a double-blind, randomised placebo-controlled study, Smriga et al (2007) evaluated the efficacy of combined lysine and arginine supplementation on reducing anxiety and stress response hormonal levels. Patients were given 1.32 g each of L-lysine and L-arginine twice daily for 1 week, estimated to be a 50% increase in total intake. Compared to placebo, long-term and stress-induced anxiety levels were reduced in both genders in the treatment group, and basal levels of salivary cortisol and chromogranin-A (a measure of sympathetic stress response) were significantly reduced in males (Smriga et al 2007). In contrast, a prospective study of 29,133 men (aged 50–69 years) found no association between L-lysine intake and depressed mood (Hakkarainen et al 2003).

It is believed that the brain's nitric oxide signalling system may be involved in the pathophysiology of schizophrenia. In a small, randomised single-blinded cross-over study, 10 patients with schizophrenia received L-lysine (6 g/day) or placebo in addition to their conventional antipsychotic medication for 4 weeks before being crossed over to the alternative phase of the study. During the lysine phase participants showed a significant decrease in positive symptoms, as assessed by the Positive and Negative Syndrome Scale. These encouraging results deserve further investigation in larger studies in future (Wass et al 2011).

Cancer treatment (in combination)

Preliminary research has been conducted into the possible protective or treatment effects of lysine in combination with other nutritional components.

A formulation of lysine combined with other compounds (proline, arginine, vitamin C and green tea extract) has been used in several in vitro and in vivo studies, suggesting it may be beneficial in cancer treatment by inhibiting the growth, invasion and metastasis of tumour cells via inhibiting metalloproteinases which trigger excellular matrix degradation (Roomi et al 2004, 2005a–e, 2006a–e, Roomi 2006). In contrast to this, however, an in vivo study conducted on mice found L-lysine and vitamin C Lysin C Drink, alone or in combination with epigallocatechin-gallate and amino acids Epican forte, was not effective as a prophylactic or treatment in reducing primary tumour growth (neuroblastoma model) or in preventing metastases (Lode et al 2008).

Lysinuric protein intolerance

Lysinuric protein intolerance is an autosomal recessive transport disorder of the cationic amino acids which leads to decreased intestinal absorption and excessive renal loss of lysine, arginine and ornithine. Usual treatment involves restriction of protein and citrulline supplementation, which corrects many side effects except those related to lysine deficiency. Long-term low-dose lysine supplementation improves plasma lysine concentration in patients and may help correct chronic lysine deficiency without causing side effects such as hyperammonaemia (Tanner et al 2007).

DOSAGE RANGE

Herpes simplex infections

- Prevention: 1000–3000 mg/day taken long-term (at least 6 months) together with a low-arginine diet.
- Acute treatment: minimum 3000 mg/day in divided doses taken between meals until lesions have healed.

Osteoporosis prevention

- 400–800 mg L-lysine taken together with calcium supplementation.

TOXICITY

Not known.

ADVERSE REACTIONS

Doses greater than 10–15 g/day may cause gastrointestinal discomfort with symptoms of nausea, vomiting and diarrhoea.

SIGNIFICANT INTERACTIONS

L

Calcium

Clinical tests have found L-lysine enhances intestinal absorption and decreases renal excretion of calcium (Civitelli et al 1992) — potentially beneficial interaction.

Practice points/Patient counselling

- L-Lysine is an essential amino acid found in foods such as animal proteins, eggs and milk.
- It has been shown to inhibit HSV multiplication in vitro.
- Supplemental L-lysine is popular as a prophylactic and treatment for HSV.
- Studies have yielded inconsistent results suggesting that there may be individual variation in responses. Due to its safety, a trial is worthwhile to determine individual response.
- Doses used as prophylaxis range from 1000 to 3000 mg/day, with treatment doses generally above 3000 mg/day.
- L-Lysine may also enhance intestinal absorption of calcium and reduces its renal excretion.

CONTRAINDICATIONS AND PRECAUTIONS

Contraindicated in people with the rare genetic disorder hyperlysinaemia/hyperlysinuria (Hendler & Rorvik 2001). High-dose lysine supplements should be used with caution in hypercalcaemic states, and by people with kidney or liver disease.

In children with pyridoxine-dependent epilepsy caused by antiquitin deficiency, a lysine-restricted diet as an adjunct to pyridoxine therapy appears to potentially decrease neurotoxic biomarkers and improve developmental outcomes (van Karnebeek et al 2012). As such lysine supplementation may not be suitable in such patients until more is known.

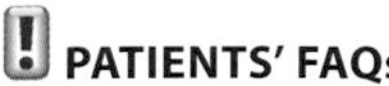

Safety is unknown for high-dose supplements; however, dietary intake levels are safe.

PATIENTS' FAQs

What will this supplement do for me?

L-Lysine supplements taken long-term appear to reduce the frequency of herpes simplex outbreaks and possibly reduce the severity and enhance healing. It may also improve the way the body absorbs and retains calcium.

When will it start to work?

Studies suggest that several months' treatment may be required, with a long-term approach recommended for prophylaxis against herpes simplex outbreaks.

Are there any safety issues?

L-Lysine appears to be a very safe supplement, although safety has not been established in pregnancy and lactation for high-dose supplements.

REFERENCES

Baier S, et al. Year-long changes in protein metabolism in elderly men and women supplemented with a nutrition cocktail of beta-hydroxy-beta-methylbutyrate (HMB), L-arginine, and L-lysine. JPEN J Parenter Enteral Nutr. 33(1) (2009):71–82.

Bratman S, Kroll D. Natural health bible. Rocklin, CA: Prima Health, 2000.

Civitelli R et al. Dietary L-lysine and calcium metabolism in humans. Nutrition 8.6 (1992): 400–405.

Digiovanna JJ, Blank H. Failure of lysine in frequently recurrent herpes simplex infection: Treatment and prophylaxis. Arch Dermatol 120.1 (1984): 48–51.

Flakoll P, et al. Effect of beta-hydroxy-beta-methylbutyrate, arginine, and lysine supplementation on strength, functionality, body composition, and protein metabolism in elderly women. Nutrition 20 (2004):445–451.

Fuller JC Jr, et al. Vitamin D status affects strength gains in older adults supplemented with a combination of β-hydroxy-β-methylbutyrate, arginine, and lysine: a cohort study. JPEN J Parenter Enteral Nutr. 35(6) (2011):757–62.

Griffith RS, et al. A multicentered study of lysine therapy in herpes simplex infection. Dermatologica 156.5 (1978): 257–267.

Griffith RS, et al. Relation of arginine-lysine antagonism to herpes simplex growth in tissue culture. Chemotherapy 27.3 (1981): 209–213.

Griffith RS et al. Success of L-lysine therapy in frequently recurrent herpes simplex infection. Treatment and prophylaxis. Dermatologica 175.4 (1987): 183–190.

Hakkarainen R et al. Association of dietary amino acids with low mood. Depression Anxiety 18.2 (2003): 89–94.

Hendler SS, Rorvik D (eds). PDR for Nutritional Supplements. Montvale, NJ: Medical Economics Co., 2001.

Hlais S, et al. Effect of lysine, vitamin B(6), and carnitine supplementation on the lipid profile of male patients with hypertriglyceridemia: a 12-week, open-label, randomized, placebo-controlled trial. Clin Ther. 34(8) (2012):1674–82.

Khan L, Bamji MS. Tissue carnitine deficiency due to dietary lysine deficiency: triglyceride accumulation and concomitant impairment in fatty acid oxidation. J Nutr. 109 (1979):24–31.

Lakhan SE, Vieira KF. Nutritional and herbal supplements for anxiety and anxiety-related disorders: a systematic review. Nutrition Journal. 9 (2010): 42–55.

Lode HN et al. Nutrient mixture including vitamin C, L-lysine, L-proline, and epigallocatechin is ineffective against tumor growth and metastasis in a syngeneic neuroblastoma model. Pediatr Blood Cancer 50.2 (2008): 284–288.

McCune MA et al. Treatment of recurrent herpes simplex infections with L-lysine monohydrochloride. Cutis 34.4 (1984): 366–373.

Milman N, et al. Failure of lysine treatment in recurrent herpes simplex labialis. Lancet 2.8096 (1978): 942.

Milman N, et al. Lysine prophylaxis in recurrent herpes simplex labialis: a double-blind, controlled crossover study. Acta Derm Venereol 60.1 (1980): 85–87.

Mirmiranpour H, et al. Investigation of the mechanism(s) involved in decreasing increased fibrinogen activity in hyperglycemic conditions using L-lysine supplementation. Thromb Res. 130(3) (2012):e13–9.

Roomi MW. Antitumor effect of ascorbic acid, lysine, proline, arginine, and green tea extract on bladder cancer cell line T-24. Int J Urol 13.4 (2006): 415–19.

Roomi MW, et al. Anti-tumor effect of ascorbic acid, lysine, proline, arginine, and epigallocatechin gallate on prostate cancer cell lines PC-3, LNCaP, and DU145. Res Commun Mol Pathol Pharmacol 115–116 (2004): 251–264.

Roomi MW et al. Antitumor effect of a combination of lysine, proline, arginine, ascorbic acid, and green tea extract on pancreatic cancer cell line MIA PaCa-2. Int J Gastrointest Cancer 35.2 (2005a): 97–102.

Roomi MW et al. In vitro and in vivo antitumorigenic activity of a mixture of lysine, proline, ascorbic acid, and green tea extract on human breast cancer lines MDA-MB-231 and MCF-7. Med Oncol 22.2 (2005b): 129–38.

Roomi MW et al. In vivo antitumor effect of ascorbic acid, lysine, proline and green tea extract on human colon cancer cell HCT 116 xenografts in nude mice: evaluation of tumor growth and immunohistochemistry. Oncol Rep 13.3 (2005c): 421–5.

Roomi MW et al. In vivo antitumor effect of ascorbic acid, lysine, proline and green tea extract on human prostate cancer PC-3 xenografts in nude mice: evaluation of tumor growth and immunohistochemistry. In Vivo 19.1 (2005d): 179–83.

Roomi MW et al. Inhibitory effect of a mixture containing ascorbic acid, lysine, proline and green tea extract on critical parameters in angiogenesis. Oncol Rep 14.4 (2005e): 807–815.

Roomi MW et al. In vivo and in vitro antitumor effect of ascorbic acid, lysine, proline, arginine, and green tea extract on human fibrosarcoma cells HT-1080. Med Oncol 23.1 (2006a): 105–11.

Roomi MW et al. Inhibition of matrix metalloproteinase-2 secretion and invasion by human ovarian cancer cell line SK-OV-3 with lysine, proline, arginine, ascorbic acid and green tea extract. J Obstet Gynaecol Res 32.2 (2006b): 148–54.

Roomi MW et al. Inhibition of pulmonary metastasis of melanoma b16fo cells in C57BL/6 mice by a nutrient mixture consisting of ascorbic acid, lysine, proline, arginine, and green tea extract. Exp Lung Res 32.10 (2006c): 517–530.

Roomi MW et al. Suppression of human cervical cancer cell lines Hela and DoTc2 4510 by a mixture of lysine, proline, ascorbic acid, and green tea extract. Int J Gynecol Cancer 16 3 (2006d): 1241–47.

Roomi MW et al. In vivo and in vitro antitumor effect of ascorbic acid, lysine, proline and green tea extract on human melanoma cell line A2058. In Vivo 20.1 (2006e): 25–32.

Simon, C.A., et al. 1985. Failure of lysine in frequently recurrent herpes simplex infection. Arch.Dermatol., 121, (2) 167–168.

Singh BB et al. Safety and effectiveness of an L-lysine, zinc, and herbal-based product on the treatment of facial and circumoral herpes. Altern Med Rev 10.2 (2005): 123–127.

Smriga M et al. Lysine fortification reduces anxiety and lessens stress in family member in economically weak communities in Northwest Syria. Proc Natl Acad Sci USA 101.22 (2004): 8285–8288.

Smriga M et al. Oral treatment with L-lysine and L-arginine reduces anxiety and basal cortisol levels in healthy humans. Biomed Res 28.2 (2007): 85–90.

Tanner LM et al. Long-term oral lysine supplementation in lysinuric protein intolerance. Metabolism 56.2 (2007): 185–189.

Thein DJ, Hurt WC. Lysine as a prophylactic agent in the treatment of recurrent herpes simplex labialis. Oral Surg Oral Med Oral Pathol 58.6 (1984): 659–666.

Torricelli P et al. Human osteopenic bone-derived osteoblasts: essential amino acids treatment effects. Artif Cells Blood Substit Immobil Biotechnol 31.1 (2003): 35–46.

Unni, U.S., et al. (2012). The effect of a controlled 8-week metabolic ward based lysine supplementation on muscle function, insulin sensitivity and leucine kinetics in young men. Clin Nutr, 31(6), 903–910.

van Karnebeek, C.D., et al. (2012). Lysine restricted diet for pyridoxine-dependent epilepsy: First evidence and future trials. Mol Genet Metab, 107(3), 335–344.

Walsh DE, et al. Subjective response to lysine in the therapy of herpes simplex. J Antimicrob Chemother 12 (1983): 489–496.

Wass, C., et al. (2011). L-lysine as adjunctive treatment in patients with schizophrenia: A single-blinded, randomized, cross-over pilot study. BMC Med, 9, 40.

Wright EF. Clinical effectiveness of lysine in treating recurrent aphthous ulcers and herpes labialis. Gen Dent 42.1 (1994): 40–42.

L

Lutein and zeaxanthin

BACKGROUND AND RELEVANT PHARMACOKINETICS

Lutein and its isomer, zeaxanthin, are yellow-coloured, xanthophyll carotenoids that are not converted into vitamin A. The bioavailability of lutein and zeaxanthin from food sources is influenced by the food matrix and by the type and extent of food processing, but most notably by the presence of fat in the diet (Castenmiller et al 1999), with dietary fat intake being inversely related to serum levels (Nolan et al 2004). Cooking may increase their bioavailability by disrupting the cellular matrix and protein complexes, and supplemental sources may be significantly more bioavailable than food sources (Castenmiller et al 1999). It has also been observed that plasma responses to cholesterol and carotenoids are related (Clark et al 2006, Karppi et al 2010) and that the bioavailability of zeaxanthin from freeze-dried wolfberries is enhanced threefold when consumed in hot skimmed milk compared to hot water or warm milk (Benzie et al 2006). One clinical study found that plasma lutein was higher when lutein was consumed with a high-fat spread (207% increase) than with a low-fat spread (88% increase) (Roodenburg et al 2000). This was supported by a small in vitro study showing that dietary lutein is absorbed more efficiently with 24 g of avocado oil or 150 g of avocado fruit (Unlu et al 2005). For each 10% increase in dietary lutein and zeaxanthin, serum levels are seen to increase by 1% (Gruber et al 2004).

When ingested, lutein and zeaxanthin are transported from the intestine to the liver via chylomicrons. They are then transported via low-density lipoproteins (LDL) and high-density lipoproteins (HDL) to various parts of the body (Yeum & Russell 2002). Lutein and zeaxanthin are present in the eye, blood serum, skin, cervix, brain, breast and adipose tissue. In the eye, lutein is more prominent at the edges of the retina and in the rods (Bernstein et al 2001, Bone et al 1997). Lutein appears to undergo some metabolism in the retina to *meso*-zeaxanthin in most, but not all people. This accounts for lower retinal levels of lutein and higher relative levels of meso-zeaxanthin in the central macular and visa versa in the peripheral macular (Bone et al 1993). As such, meso-zeaxanthin and zeaxanthin are the predominant carotenoids in the foveal region, whereas lutein predominates in the parafoveal region (Bone et al 1988, Snodderly et al 1991). In particular, zeaxanthin is primarily concentrated in the centre of the retina and the cones, where it is present in concentrations nearly 1000-fold of those found in other tissues, thus giving the macula lutea or yellow spot of the retina its characteristic colour (Krinsky et al 2003). It is suggested, however, that during supplementation with xanthophylls, lutein is predominantly deposited in the fovea, while zeaxanthin deposition appears to cover a wider retinal area (Schalch et al 2007).

Lower serum concentrations of zeaxanthin have been associated with male gender, smoking, younger age, lower non-HDL cholesterol, greater ethanol consumption and higher body mass index (Brady et al 1996). Lutein and zeaxanthin, together with other carotenoids, have also been found to be lower in people with chronic cholestatic liver disease, which can be attributed to malabsorption of fat soluble vitamins, as well as other mechanisms of hepatic release (Floreani et al 2000). In an epidemiological study involving 7059 participants, lower serum lutein and zeaxanthin levels were significantly associated with smoking, heavy drinking, being white, female, not physically active, having lower dietary lutein and zeaxanthin, a higher percentage of fat mass, a higher waist–hip ratio, lower serum cholesterol, a higher white blood cell count and high levels of C-reactive protein (Gruber et al 2004).

In a pharmacokinetic study involving 20 healthy volunteers, serum zeaxanthin levels were found to have an effective half-life for accumulation of 5 days and a terminal elimination half-life of around 12 days (Hartmann et al 2004). This was confirmed by another study that also found that lutein did not affect the concentrations of other carotenoids in healthy volunteers (Thurmann et al 2005). Similarly, high doses (50 mg) of beta-carotene over 5 years were not found to influence serum levels of lutein and zeaxanthin (Mayne et al 1998). It has been suggested that the associations between macula pigment density and serum lutein, serum zeaxanthin and adipose lutein concentrations are stronger in men (Broekmans et al 2002, Johnson et al 2000) and that the processes governing accumulation and/or stabilisation of zeaxanthin in fat tissue are different for males and females (Nolan et al 2004). This is supported by the finding that serum lutein and zeaxanthin concentrations vary with the menstrual cycle, with levels being higher in the late follicular than in the luteal phase (Forman et al 1998).

CHEMICAL COMPONENTS

Lutein and zeaxanthin are isomers and have identical chemical formulas, differing only in the location of a double bond in one of the hydroxyl groups. Lutein is known as beta, epsilon-carotene-3,3′-diol, whereas zeaxanthin is known as all-*trans* beta-carotene-3,3′-diol.

FOOD SOURCES

Foods differ in their relative amounts of lutein and zeaxanthin, with lutein generally being more abundant. Lutein is found in dark green leafy vegetables such as spinach and kale, as well as in sweetcorn and egg yolks, whereas zeaxanthin is found in sweetcorn, egg yolk, orange peppers (capsicums), persimmons, tangerines, mandarins and oranges. Goji berries are a very rich source of zeaxanthin.

Lutein, zeaxanthin and *meso*-zeaxanthin are primarily extracted from marigold flowers (*Tagetes erecta*) for use in supplements and are available in either free or esterified form. The esters typically contain two fatty acid groups that must be cleaved by pancreatic esterases and their absorption requires higher levels of dietary fat (Roodenburg et al 2000); however, addition of omega-long-chain polyunsaturated fatty acids to oral supplementation of lutein/zeaxanthin has not been found to change serum levels of lutein and zeaxanthin (Huang et al 2008).

DEFICIENCY SIGNS AND SYMPTOMS

L

Zeaxanthin and lutein can be considered conditionally essential nutrients because low serum levels or low dietary intakes are associated with low macular pigment density (Mares et al 2006) and increased risk of age-related macular degeneration (ARMD) (Semba & Dagnelie 2003).

Epidemiological studies have also found an association between low serum carotenoid levels, including lutein and zeaxanthin levels, with all-cause mortality (De Waart et al 2001), the risk of inflammatory polyarthritis (Pattison et al 2005), breast cancer (Tamimi et al 2005), prostate cancer (Jian et al 2005), colon cancer (Nkondjock & Ghadirian 2004), cervical cancer (Garcia-Closas et al 2005, Kim et al 2004), human papillomavirus persistence (Garcia-Closas et al 2005), type 2 diabetes and impaired glucose metabolism (Coyne et al 2005), chronic cholestatic liver diseases (Floreani et al 2000), Alzheimer's disease and vascular dementia (Polidori et al 2004) and low fruit and vegetable consumption (Al-Delaimy et al 2005).

Carotenoids have also emerged as an excellent tissue marker for a diet rich in fruit and vegetables, and measurement of plasma and tissue carotenoids is considered to have an important role in defining optimal diets (Al-Delaimy et al 2005, Brevik et al 2004, Handelman 2001).

MAIN ACTIONS

Antioxidant

Lutein and zeaxanthin are both powerful antioxidants, with activity having been demonstrated in a number of in vitro and in vivo tests (Higashi-Okai et al 2001, Iannone et al 1998, Muriach et al 2008, Naguib 2000). In vitro studies of human lens epithelial cells also indicate that their antioxidant activity may protect the lens from ultraviolet (UV) B radiation (Chitchumroonchokchai et al 2004). According to animal studies, lutein increases glutathione levels and reduces retinal apoptosis following ischaemic reperfusion (Dilsiz et al 2005). Lutein was also found to significantly protect against injury associated with oxidative stress in rat intestinal tissues following ischaemia-reperfusion (Sato et al 2011).

Lutein supplementation of 20 mg daily over 12 weeks was shown to significantly reduce C-reactive protein levels and lipid peroxidation, as well as increase total antioxidant capacity, in a randomised placebo-controlled trial of healthy volunteers (n = 117; Wang et al 2013). In contrast, a smaller study of 20 well-nourished adults aged 50–70 years found that supplementation of lutein (12 mg daily) for 112 days resulted in increased plasma antioxidant concentration but no significant changes in antioxidant activity or lipid peroxidation (Li et al 2010).

Blue light filter

The yellow colour of lutein and zeaxanthin is due to their ability to absorb blue light, which is believed to contribute to their protective function because blue light is at the high-energy, and therefore the most damaging, end of the visible spectrum (Krinsky et al 2003). Lutein and zeaxanthin thus serve as 'natural sunglasses' (Rehak et al 2008) that act as an optical filter for blue light, reducing chromatic aberration and preventing damage to the photoreceptor cell layer (Krinsky et al 2003). An in vivo study confirmed that lutein afforded protection against light-induced retinal damage in mice, which was associated with reduced markers of DNA damage in photoreceptor cells, and upregulation of the prosurvival gene 'eyes absent' (Sasaki et al 2012). The reduction of light-induced oxidative stress was thought to contribute to protection against DNA strand damage.

Macular pigment development

Lutein and zeaxanthin are entirely of dietary origin and are initially absent in newborns but gradually accumulate over time (Nussbaum et al 1981). It has been generally accepted that macular pigment density decreases with age; however, there are conflicting results. In one prospective, observational study involving 390 patients, macular pigment density was not found to change significantly with age, even when elderly subjects with cataracts and ARMD were considered (Ciulla & Hammond 2004). Other studies, however, have found that macular pigment does indeed decline with age in both normal eyes (Beatty et al 2001, Bernstein et al 2002) and those with ARMD (Bernstein et al 2002) and Stargardt macular dystrophy (Zhao et al 2003), but not in retinitis pigmentosa or choroideraemia (Zhao et al 2003).

Although lutein and zeaxanthin levels in the serum, diet and retina correlate, the nature of the relationships between lutein and zeaxanthin in foodstuffs, blood and the macula is confounded by many variables, including processes that influence digestion, absorption and transport and accumulation and stabilisation of the carotenoids in the tissues (Beatty et al 2004). It is suggested, however, that lutein and zeaxanthin are transported into an individual's retina in the same proportions found in his or her blood (Bone et al 1997). An in vitro study using retinal pigment epithelial cells found that both lutein and zeaxanthin modulate inflammatory responses to photo-oxidation, providing a possible mechanism for these compounds' effects in ARMD (Bain et al 2012).

Immunomodulation

Lutein modulates cellular and humoral-mediated immune responses, according to animal studies (Kim et al 2000a, 2000b). In particular, high levels of C-reactive protein and a high white blood cell count have been identified in individuals with low serum levels of lutein (Gruber et al 2004). In a case-controlled study, serum lutein and zeaxanthin, together with other carotenoids, were also found to be lower in children with acute-phase infections compared to healthy controls (Cser et al 2004).

Anti-inflammatory

Lutein supplementation (20 mg daily) in early atherosclerosis patients ($n = 65$) was found to significantly reduce serum cytokines interleukin-6 and monocyte chemotactic protein-1 after 3 months compared to placebo (Xu et al 2013). This also correlated with reduced serum LDL and triglyceride levels in patients receiving lutein, though this study may be insufficiently powered to draw meaningful conclusions. Further studies are recommended to clarify lutein's anti-inflammatory effects.

Photoprotection

According to animal studies, lutein reduces the risk of sunburn, as well as local UVB radiation-induced immune suppression and reactive oxygen species generation (Lee et al 2004), and directly protects against photoageing and photocarcinogenesis (Astner et al 2007). A protective effect on skin cancer, however, has not been observed in human cohort studies. One prospective cohort study involving 43,867 men and 85,944 women found no significant inverse association between intake of lutein and squamous cell carcinoma (Fung et al 2003), while an increased risk of squamous cell carcinoma was observed for people with multiple prior non-melanoma skin cancers and high serum levels of lutein and zeaxanthin (Dorgan et al 2004).

While a protective effect against skin cancer is uncertain, there is evidence to suggest that supplementation with lutein and zeaxanthin may improve general skin health and simultaneously help to minimise signs of premature ageing (Maci 2007). A double-blind, placebo-controlled study that examined surface lipids, hydration, photoprotective activity, skin elasticity and skin lipid peroxidation found that oral and/or topical administration of either lutein or zeaxanthin provided antioxidant protection, with the greatest protection being seen with combined administration of lutein and zeaxanthin (Palombo et al 2007). The clinical significance of these findings is uncertain.

L

CLINICAL USE

Lutein and zeaxanthin supplementation is most often used for preventing and/or treating various ocular conditions.

Age-related macular degeneration

ARMD is the leading cause of irreversible visual dysfunction in individuals over 65 years in Western society. People with ARMD are classified as having early-stage disease (early ARMD), in which visual function is affected, or late ARMD (generally characterised as either 'wet' neovascular ARMD or 'dry' atrophic ARMD, or both) in which central vision is severely compromised or lost (Bowes et al 2013). Atrophic ARMD accounts for 90% of all ARMD cases (Richer et al 2004).

The evidence that lifetime oxidative stress plays an important role in the development of ARMD is now compelling (Hogg & Chakravarthy 2004). ARMD is thought to be the result of free radical damage to photoreceptors within the macula, and therefore it is suspected that inefficient macular antioxidant systems play a role in disease development. After ageing, smoking is the next significant risk factor, most likely due to antioxidant depletion and increased oxidative stress. Smoking is also associated with lower levels of macular xanthophyll pigments such as lutein. Diets low in fruit and vegetables, excessive exposure to sunlight and blue light and use of photosensitising medicines are other factors known to increase the risk of developing ARMD (Richer et al 2004).

Epidemiological and autopsy studies have found an inverse relationship between lutein and zeaxanthin intake and macular pigment density (Bone et al 2001,

Curran-Celentano et al 2001). The presence of unusually high levels of macular carotenoids in older donors who were regularly consuming high-dose lutein supplements further supports the hypothesis that long-term high intake of lutein can raise levels of macular pigment (Bhosale et al 2007). Similarly, clinical studies have also confirmed the association between macular pigmentation, dietary lutein intake and serum lutein levels (Burke et al 2005, Mares et al 2006, Yao et al 2013).

Lutein supplementation can also effectively increase plasma lutein and macular pigment density in most people with established ARMD (Bernstein et al 2002, Richer et al 2004, 2011, Wang et al 2007) and also in healthy controls (Koh et al 2004), demonstrating that both a diseased and a healthy macula can accumulate and stabilise lutein and/or zeaxanthin (Koh et al 2004). An increase in macular pigment density develops within 4 weeks of increasing lutein, according to clinical studies (Berendschot et al 2000, Hammond et al 1997). Interestingly, it was recently discovered that the variability in retinal macular pigment response to increased lutein intake is due to underlying genetic variants (Yonova-Doing et al 2013). Clinical research further indicates that people with lower starting lutein levels experience greater protective effects when increasing lutein consumption in regard to age-related maculopathy (which precedes ARMD) (Cho et al 2004). There is also evidence from the Lutein Antioxidant Supplementation Trial (LAST) II that people with established atrophic ARMD starting with the lowest macular pigment optical density (MPOD) experience the greatest increases in MPOD when taking lutein or lutein + antioxidant supplements over 12 months (Richer et al 2007). These combined results are helping to clarify who is most likely to experience benefits from increased lutein intake and the variability in clinical trial results to date.

At least 16 epidemiological studies have reported a link between lutein and zeaxanthin and ARMD risk, supporting the theory that higher intakes and/or plasma levels of these macular pigments may be protective (Elliott & Williams 2012). A 2012 systematic review and meta-analysis concluded that, while dietary intake of lutein and zeaxanthin was not significantly associated with reduced risk of early ARMD onset, it was associated with protection in late ARMD (relative risk 0.74; Ma et al 2012). Joachim et al (2014) reported that dietary lutein-zeaxanthin intake was associated with decreased likelihood of progression from reticular drusen to late ARMD (adjusted odds ratio 0.5; 95% confidence interval 0.3–1.0), as based on the most recent results from the Blue Mountains Eye Study (n = 3654), which involves 5-year, 10-year and 15-year follow-up examinations. Using data from the same study cohort together with data from the Rotterdam Study, Wang et al (2014) reported that people with a high ARMD genetic risk and the highest intake of lutein/zeaxanthin had a >20% reduced risk of early ARMD compared to people with a low genetic risk having a high intake of lutein/zeaxanthin.

For people with established ARMD, several important benefits have been reported with increased lutein intake, often when combined with other antioxidant nutrients. Improvements of up to 92% in visual acuity tests were observed when subjects with atrophic ARMD consumed a diet designed to contain approximately 150 g of spinach 4–7 times a week, according to an early pilot study (Richer 1999). A small pilot study by Falsini et al (2003) involving 30 patients with early ARMD and visual acuity of 6/9 or better experienced improved macular function with the use of daily lutein (15 mg) + vitamin E (20 mg) and nicotinamide (18 mg) for 180 days; this improvement was lost when supplementation was stopped (Falsini et al 2003).

Richer et al (2004) subsequently conducted a much larger study which found that lutein supplements (10 mg/day) improved some symptoms of atrophic ARMD after 12 months, such as contrast sensitivity, glare recovery and near vision acuity, while also increasing macular pigment density. The groups receiving lutein + antioxidants (including zinc) demonstrated even broader effects compared to lutein alone or placebo. LAST, conducted by Richer et al (2004), was a double-blind, randomised, placebo-controlled study involving 90 subjects. In addition to improving most measures of quality of vision, both the lutein (FloraGloB, Kemin Foods International, USA) and lutein plus antioxidant (OcuPower, Nutraceutical Sciences Institute (NSI), USA) groups achieved an increase of 36% and 43%, respectively, in macular pigment density, whereas the placebo group experienced a slight decrease (Richer et al 2004). In other studies, lutein supplementation has been shown to increase macular pigment optical density and contrast and glare sensitivity compared to placebo (Yao et al 2013), and was seen to improve visual performance at low illumination, yet this was not correlated with macular pigment density (Kvansakul et al 2006).

More recently, a double-blind, placebo-controlled trial reported that macular pigment optical density and best-corrected visual acuity were significantly improved in patients with non-exudative ARMD (n = 172) after taking a combination of lutein (10–20 mg) + zeaxanthin (1–2 mg) + omega-3 fatty acids (100–200 mg docosahexaenoic acid and 30–60 mg eicosapentaenoic acid) + antioxidants over 12 months (Dawczynski et al 2013). Two doses were used and both were as effective as each other but better than placebo, suggesting the lower dose saturated retinal levels and no further benefits could be achieved with a higher dose. A low dose of 6 mg daily of lutein is not effective according to a small double-blind, randomised controlled trial conducted over 60 weeks involving people with ARMD (Bartlett & Eperjesi 2007).

In regard to delaying the progression of ARMD, the AREDS2 study found that general antioxidant supplementation (original AREDS formula) was not enhanced by the addition of lutein (10 mg) and zeaxanthin (2 mg) (The AREDS2 Research Group 2013b). More recently, combinations of lutein and zeaxanthin combined with meso-xanthin have been tested in AMD. The Central Retinal Enrichment Supplementation Trials (CREST) are underway and will investigate the potential impact of macular pigment (MP) enrichment, following supplementation with a formulation containing 10 mg lutein (L), 2 mg zeaxanthin (Z) and 10 mg meso-zeaxanthin (MZ), on visual function in normal subjects and in subjects with early age-related macular degeneration (Akuffo et al 2014).

L

Cataracts

Lens density has been found to inversely correlate with macular lutein and zeaxanthin levels (Hammond et al 1997) and numerous observational studies have found that increased consumption of foods high in lutein and zeaxanthin is associated with a decreased risk for cataracts (Brown et al 1999, Delcourt et al 2006, Tavani et al 1996). In one study involving 77,466 female nurses from the Nurses' Health Study, those with the highest quintile for consumption of zeaxanthin and lutein were found to have a 22% reduction in the risk of cataract extraction (Chasan-Taber et al 1999). Similarly, a study of 1802 women aged 50–79 years found that women in the highest quintile category of diet or serum levels of lutein and zeaxanthin were 32% less likely to have nuclear cataract as compared with those in the lowest quintile category (Moeller et al 2008). A further epidemiological study of 3271 Melbourne residents found that, while cortical and posterior subcapsular cataracts were not significantly associated with lutein or zeaxanthin intake, high dietary lutein and zeaxanthin intake was inversely associated with the prevalence of nuclear cataract (Vu et al 2006). The link between lutein and cataracts is further supported by a small randomised, placebo-controlled trial of 17 patients with clinically diagnosed age-related cataracts that found that supplementation with lutein 15 mg three times weekly for up to 2 years resulted in improved visual performance (visual acuity and glare sensitivity) compared with placebo (Olmedilla et al 2003).

These results contrast with those from a cohort study of 478 women without previously diagnosed cataracts, which failed to detect a significant inverse relationship between lutein intake and lens opacities over a 13–15-year follow-up period (Jacques et al 2001). The AREDS2 randomised clinical trial also determined that daily supplementation with lutein (10 mg) and zeaxanthin (2 mg) had no statistically significant effects on rates of cataract surgery or vision loss in adults aged 50–85 years at risk for progression to advanced ARMD (The AREDS2 Research Group 2013a).

Retinitis pigmentosa

In a double-blind, randomised, placebo-controlled crossover trial, supplementation with lutein (10 mg/day) for 12 weeks followed by 30 mg/day for 12 weeks was found to improve visual field and possibly visual acuity in 34 patients with retinitis pigmentosa (Bahrami et al 2006). A further study found that daily supplementation with 40 mg of lutein over 9 weeks followed by 20 mg for a further 16 weeks significantly improved visual acuity in 16 subjects with retinitis pigmentosa, many of whom were also taking other supplements (Dagnelie et al 2000).

Clinical note

The macula (central retina) contains a yellow pigment comprising the dietary carotenoids lutein (L), zeaxanthin (Z), and meso-zeaxanthin, known as macular pigment (MP). The concentrations of MP's constituent carotenoids in retina and brain tissue correlate, and there is a biologically plausible rationale, supported by emerging evidence, that MP's constituent carotenoids are also important for cognitive function (Nolan et al 2014).

Retinopathy of prematurity

Supplementation of lutein and zeaxanthin in preterm infants did not prevent the occurrence of retinopathy of prematurity or outcome at hospital discharge compared to placebo in a randomised controlled trial of 114 infants of ≤32 weeks' gestation (Dani et al 2012).

Cancer prevention

High dietary intake of lutein has been associated with reduced risk of some cancers, most notably endometrial and ovarian cancer, but not all cancers, according to epidemiological evidence (Freudenheim et al 1996, Fung et al 2003, Gann et al 1999, Giovannucci et al 1995, Huang et al 2003, Ito et al 2003, Lu et al 2001, McCann et al 2000, Michaud et al 2000, Nomura et al 1997, Schuurman et al 2002, Terry et al 2002).

Lung cancer

Three large population studies of diet and lung cancer have revealed a non-significant association between high lutein intake and lower risk of lung cancer (Ito et al 2003, Michaud et al 2000, Ziegler et al 1996), and a significant trend was observed in another population-based case–control study (Le Marchand et al 1993). A nested case–control study also found that serum lutein and zeaxanthin were lower in those with lung cancer than in controls (Comstock et al 1997). These results are contrasted with those from a case–control study of 108 cases of lung cancer in a Chinese occupational cohort that found that higher serum carotenoid levels, including lutein and zeaxanthin, were significantly associated with increased lung cancer risk among alcohol drinkers, while having a possible protective association among non-drinkers (Ratnasinghe et al 2000).

Cervical cancer

A 2005 systematic review suggests that lutein/zeaxanthin is likely to have a protective effect for cervical neoplasia and possibly for human papillomavirus persistence (Garcia-Closas et al 2005).

Endometrial cancer

An epidemiological study involving 232 patients with endometrial cancer and 639 controls found that an intake of more than 7.3 mg/day of lutein was associated with a 70% reduced risk of endometrial cancer (McCann et al 2000).

Ovarian cancer

A case–control study found that weekly intake of lutein of more than 24 mg was associated with a 40% reduction in the risk for developing ovarian cancer compared with weekly consumption of less than 3.8 mcg (Bertone et al 2001).

Breast cancer

High lutein and zeaxanthin intake has been related to reduced risk of breast cancer (Dorgan et al 1998, Toniolo et al 2001). High lutein intake (>7 mg/day) was associated with a 53% reduction in the risk of developing breast cancer compared with low consumption (<3.7 mg/day) in a population-based case-control study of 608 premenopausal women over age 40 (Freudenheim et al 1996). Similar risk reductions were found in a nested case-control study of 540 New York women (Toniolo et al 2001) and another nested case–control study of 969 cases of breast cancer and matched controls from the Nurses' Health Study found that the risk of breast cancer was 25–35% less for women with the highest quintile compared with that for women with the lowest quintile of lutein/zeaxanthin and total carotenoid intake (Tamimi et al 2005). Although this association is encouraging, another study of 4697 women followed over 25 years found no significant relationships between lutein intake and breast cancer risk (Jarvinen et al 1997).

Gastric cancer

High serum lutein levels have been associated with a higher incidence of gastric carcinoma, according to a cohort study of 29,584 patients with oesophageal and stomach cancer (Abnet et al 2003); however, this association requires further investigation.

Bowel cancer

The relationship between lutein and zeaxanthin intake and colon cancer is uncertain. A case-control study involving 1993 cases of colon cancer and 2410 controls found that lutein intake, as measured by a food frequency score, was inversely associated with colon cancer and another case–control study of 223 subjects with histologically confirmed colon or rectal cancer identified a non-significant inverse association with lutein (Levi et al 2000). A cohort analysis of 5629 women, however, found no such association (Terry et al 2002). A case-controlled study found that women with high intakes of long-chain polyunsaturated fatty acids had an inverse association between lutein and zeaxanthin intake and the risk of colon cancer (Nkondjock & Ghadirian 2004). Further investigation is required to clarify these findings because animal studies suggest low doses of lutein inhibit aberrant crypt foci formation, whereas high doses may increase the risk by 9–59% (Raju et al 2005).

Prostate cancer

Overall, epidemiological evidence suggests that lutein and zeaxanthin intake has no influence over the risk of prostate cancer (Bosetti et al 2004, Gann et al 1999, Giovannucci et al 1995, Huang et al 2003, Lu et al 2001, Nomura et al 1997, Schuurman et al 2002). However, when lutein was included as part of a mixed carotenoid and tocopherol extract, the combination was effective in an in vitro study of prostate cancer cell lines (Lu et al 2005). A case-controlled study of 130 patients with adenocarcinoma of the prostate found that prostate cancer risk was seen to decline with increasing consumption of carotenoids, including lycopene, alpha-carotene, beta-carotene, beta-cryptoxanthin, lutein and zeaxanthin (Jian et al 2005).

Laryngeal cancer

A case–control study involving 537 subjects identified an inverse relationship between dietary lutein and zeaxanthin intake, together with the intake of other carotenoids, and the risk of laryngeal cancer (Bidoli et al 2003).

OTHER USES

Lutein and zeaxanthin may be used as part of a general antioxidant supplement, often taken in conjunction with other carotenoids in cases where there is known or suspected increased oxidative load.

Sleep duration

Reduced lutein and zeaxanthin intake may be associated with reduced sleep duration; however more studies are needed to confirm this preliminary finding (Grandner 2013).

Cognitive impairment

Dementia has been found to be associated with increased protein oxidative modification and the depletion of a large spectrum of antioxidant micronutrients, including lutein and zeaxanthin (Polidori et al 2004). In a clinical study of 25 subjects with mild cognitive impairment, 63 subjects with Alzheimer's disease and 56 healthy individuals found that serum lutein levels were lowest in the first two groups, particularly those with Alzheimer's disease (Rinaldi et al 2003), while a double-blind trial of 49 women aged 60–80 years found improved cognitive function after supplementation with a combination of docosahexaenoic acid and lutein (Johnson et al 2008).

A large, population-based study of adults aged over 50 years identified that low macular pigment density was associated with lower cognitive performance (Feeney et al 2013). This, however, was not an intervention-based study and therefore was not able to determine the effect of exogenous lutein supplementation in acutely improving cognitive parameters.

Atherosclerosis

The relationship between lutein and zeaxanthin status and atherosclerosis is being investigated but remains unclear. Plasma levels of lutein, beta-cryptoxanthin and zeaxanthin were correlated to carotid intima media thickness in a 3-year case-controlled study of 231 subjects (Iribarren et al 1997), as well as in an 18-month epidemiological study of 573 subjects, suggesting that these carotenoids may be protective against early atherosclerosis (Dwyer et al 2004). Lutein intake has also been found to be inversely associated with the risk of ischaemic stroke in an observational study involving 43,738 males (Ascherio et al 1999), as well as being inversely associated with the risk of subarachnoid haemorrhage in a cohort study of 26,593 male smokers (Hirvonen et al 2000). Serum levels of lutein and zeaxanthin, however, were not associated with atherosclerosis risk in a case–control study involving 108 cases of aortic atherosclerosis in an elderly population (Klipstein-Grobusch et al 2000).

The foregoing findings contrast with those from two case-controlled studies that found a positive correlation between lutein and zeaxanthin levels and cardiovascular risk. A nested, case-control study of 499 cases of cardiovascular disease with matched controls taken from the Physicians' Health Study found that concentrations of plasma lutein, zeaxanthin and retinol corresponded to a moderate increase in cardiovascular disease (Sesso et al 2005). Similarly, myocardial infarction risk was positively associated with lutein and zeaxanthin levels in adipose tissue and diet in a case-controlled study of 1456 cases of first acute myocardial infarction and matched controls (Kabagambe et al 2005). The clinical significance of these findings is unclear and requires further investigation.

DOSAGE RANGE

According to clinical studies

- Macular protection: lutein 6–20 mg/day; zeaxanthin 2–5 mg/day.
- The original AREDS formulation contained vitamin C, vitamin E, beta-carotene, zinc and copper.
- The successful AREDS2 formulation contained lutein and zeaxanthin instead of beta-carotene.
- Atrophic ARMD: improving visual quality — 10 mg lutein daily, ideally in combination with other antioxidants and possibly omega-3 essential fatty acids for better effects.
- Cataracts — improving visual performance: lutein 15 mg three times weekly.

TOXICITY

Dietary amounts and those used in clinical studies are considered safe.

ADVERSE REACTIONS

Lutein and zeaxanthin supplements are well tolerated.

SIGNIFICANT INTERACTIONS

Vitamin C

Lutein showed increased antioxidant efficacy with vitamin C in an animal study (Blakely et al 2003). Further to this, a small in vivo study showed that 2000 mg of vitamin C enhanced the absorption of lutein (Tanumihardjo et al 2005).

Vitamin E

Vitamin E showed increased antioxidant efficacy with lutein according to an animal study (Blakely et al 2003).

Phytosterols

High dietary intake of phytosterol esters (6.6 g/day) reduced plasma levels of lutein by 14% in a small clinical trial; however, this was reversed by increasing fruit and vegetable intake (Clifton et al 2004).

Orlistat

Theoretically, long-term use of orlistat leads to reduced plasma levels of lutein due to reduced gastric absorption (Australian Medicines Handbook) — increased dietary intake of lutein should be considered.

Olestra

Lutein and zeaxanthin levels have been found to decrease with long-term use of olestra (Tulley et al 2005) — increased dietary intake of lutein should be considered.

> ***CONTRAINDICATIONS AND PRECAUTIONS***
>
> Lutein and zeaxanthin are contraindicated in people with a hypersensitivity to these carotenoids or their food sources.

> ***PREGNANCY USE***
>
> Eating dietary amounts of foods rich in lutein and zeaxanthin is likely to be safe. Women at risk of premature rupture of the membranes are cautioned against very high intake because one study observed a fourfold greater risk of membrane rupture with high serum lutein levels (Mathews & Neil 2005).

Practice points/Patient counselling

- Lutein and zeaxanthin are antioxidant carotenoids found in spinach, corn, egg yolk, squash and greens. Goji berries are a particularly rich source of zeaxanthin.
- Lutein and zeaxanthin are essential for the development of macular pigment, which protects photoreceptor cells in the retina from free radical damage.
- Epidemiological studies have generally found an inverse relationship between lutein and zeaxanthin intake and macular degeneration; increased intakes will reduce the incidence of ARMD in some populations, but not all.
- People with established 'dry' macular degeneration may experience improved visual quality with lutein supplementation.
- Long-term use of lutein supplements may increase visual performance in people with pre-existing cataracts.
- High dietary intake of lutein has been associated with reduced risk of some cancers, most notably endometrial and ovarian cancer, but not all cancers, according to epidemiological evidence.
- Supplements containing lutein and zeaxanthin should be taken with food as dietary fat improves their absorption.

PATIENTS' FAQs

What will this supplement do for me?

Lutein and zeaxanthin are important for eye health. They improve visual quality in people with established 'dry' ARMD and may reduce the risk of progressing to ARMD in some at-risk people. There may also be some protection against developing certain cancers when consumed over time.

When will it start to work?

Increased intake of lutein can improve macular health within 4 weeks; however, clinical effects develop slowly and may not be detected for 6 months. In regard to improving visual performance in people with pre-existing cataracts, effects take even longer (≈2 years).

Are there any safety issues?

Lutein and zeaxanthin are generally considered safe.

REFERENCES

Abnet CC et al. Prospective study of serum retinol, beta-carotene, beta-cryptoxanthin, and lutein/zeaxanthin and esophageal and gastric cancers in China. Cancer Causes Control 14.7 (2003): 645–655.

Al-Delaimy WK et al. Plasma carotenoids as biomarkers of intake of fruits and vegetables: ecological-level correlations in the European Prospective Investigation into Cancer and Nutrition (EPIC). Eur J Clin Nutr 59.12 (2005): 1397–1408.

Akuffo KO et al. Central Retinal Enrichment Supplementation Trials (CREST): design and methodology of the CREST randomized controlled trials. Ophthalmic Epidemiol 21.2 (2014): 111-123.

Ascherio A et al. Relation of consumption of vitamin E, vitamin C, and carotenoids to risk for stroke among men in the United States. Ann Intern Med 130.12 (1999): 963–970.

Astner S et al. Dietary lutein/zeaxanthin partially reduces photoaging and photocarcinogenesis in chronically UVB-irradiated Skh-1 hairless mice. Skin Pharmacol Physiol 20.6 (2007): 283–291.

Australian Medicines Handbook. Royal Australian College of General Practitioners, the Pharmaceutical Society of Australia and the Australasian Society of Clinical and Experimental Pharmacologists and Toxicologists. www.amh.hcn.net.au (accessed 06-12-05).

Bahrami H, et al. Lutein supplementation in retinitis pigmentosa: PC-based vision assessment in a randomized double-masked placebo-controlled clinical trial [NCT00029289]. BMC Ophthalmol 6 (2006): 23.

Bain Q et al. Lutein and zeaxanthin supplementation reduces photooxidative damage and modulates the expression of inflammation-related genes in retinal pigment epithelial cells. Free Radic Biol Med 53.6 (2012): 1298–1307.

Bartlett HE, Eperjesi F. Effect of lutein and antioxidant dietary supplementation on contrast sensitivity in age-related macular disease: a randomized controlled trial. Eur J Clin Nutr 61.9 (2007): 1121–1127.

Beatty S et al. Macular pigment and risk for age-related macular degeneration in subjects from a Northern European population. Invest Ophthalmol Vis Sci 42.2 (2001): 439–446.

Beatty S et al. Macular pigment optical density and its relationship with serum and dietary levels of lutein and zeaxanthin. Arch Biochem Biophys 430.1 (2004): 70–76.

Benzie IF et al. Enhanced bioavailability of zeaxanthin in a milk-based formulation of wolfberry (Gou Qi Zi; *Fructus barbarum* L.). Br J Nutr 96.1 (2006): 154–160.

Berendschot TT et al. Influence of lutein supplementation on macular pigment, assessed with two objective techniques. Invest Ophthalmol Vis Sci 41.11 (2000): 3322–3326.

Bernstein PS et al. Identification and quantification of carotenoids and their metabolites in the tissues of the human eye. Exp Eye Res 72.3 (2001): 215–223.

Bernstein PS et al. Resonance Raman measurement of macular carotenoids in normal subjects and in age-related macular degeneration patients. Ophthalmology 109.10 (2002): 1780–1787.

Bertone ER et al. A population-based case-control study of carotenoid and vitamin A intake and ovarian cancer (United States). Cancer Causes Control 12.1 (2001): 83–90.

Bhosale P, et al. HPLC measurement of ocular carotenoid levels in human donor eyes in the lutein supplementation era. Investigative Ophthalmology and Visual Science 48.2 (2007): 543–54549.

Bidoli E et al. Micronutrients and laryngeal cancer risk in Italy and Switzerland: a case control study. Cancer Causes Control 14.5 (2003): 477–484.

Blakely S et al. Lutein interacts with ascorbic acid more frequently than with (alpha)-tocopherol to alter biomarkers of oxidative stress in female Zucker obese rats. J Nutr 133.9 (2003): 2838–2844.

Bone R et al. Distribution of lutein and zeaxanthin stereoisomers in the human retina. Exp Eye Res 64.2 (1997): 211–2118.

Bone R et al. Macular pigment in donor eyes with and without AMD: a case-control study. Invest Ophthalmol Vis Sci 42.1 (2001): 235–240.

Bosetti C et al. Retinol, carotenoids and the risk of prostate cancer: a case-control study from Italy. Int J Cancer 112.4 (2004): 689–692.

Bowes, R.C., et al. 2013. Dry age-related macular degeneration: mechanisms, therapeutic targets, and imaging. Invest Ophthalmol.Vis.Sci., 54, (14) ORSF68–ORSF80.

Brady WE et al. Human serum carotenoid concentrations are related to physiologic and lifestyle factors. J Nutr 126.1 (1996): 129–137.

Brevik A et al. Six carotenoids in plasma used to assess recommended intake of fruits and vegetables in a controlled feeding study. Eur J Clin Nutr 58.8 (2004): 1166–1173.

Broekmans WM et al. Macular pigment density in relation to serum and adipose tissue concentrations of lutein and serum concentrations of zeaxanthin. Am J Clin Nutr 76.3 (2002): 595–603.

Brown L et al. A prospective study of carotenoid intake and risk of cataract extraction in US men. Am J Clin Nutr 70.4 (1999): 517–524.

Burke JD, et al. Diet and serum carotenoid concentrations affect macular pigment optical density in adults 45 years and older. J Nutr 135.5 (2005): 1208–1215.

Castenmiller JJ et al. The food matrix of spinach is a limiting factor in determining the bioavailability of beta-carotene and to a lesser extent of lutein in humans. J Nutr 129.2 (1999): 349–355.

L

Chasan-Taber L et al. A prospective study of vitamin supplement intake and cataract extraction among U.S. women. Epidemiology 10.6 (1999): 679–684.

Chitchumroonchokchai C et al. Xanthophylls and [alpha]-tocopherol decrease UVB-induced lipid peroxidation and stress signaling in human lens epithelial cells. J Nutr 134.12 (2004): 3225–3232.

Cho E, et al. Prospective study of intake of fruits, vegetables, vitamins, and carotenoids and risk of age-related maculopathy. Arch Ophthalmol 2004;122:883–92.

Ciulla TA, Hammond BR Jr. Macular pigment density and aging, assessed in the normal elderly and those with cataracts and age-related macular degeneration. Am J Ophthalmol 138.4 (2004): 582–587.

Clark RM et al. Hypo- and hyperresponse to egg cholesterol predicts plasma lutein and beta-carotene concentrations in men and women. J Nutr 136.3 (2006): 601–607.

Clifton PM et al. High dietary intake of phytosterol esters decreases carotenoids and increases plasma plant sterol levels with no additional cholesterol lowering. J Lipid Res 45.8 (2004): 1493–1499.

Comstock GW et al. The risk of developing lung cancer associated with antioxidants in the blood: ascorbic acid, carotenoids, alpha-tocopherol, selenium, and total peroxyl radical absorbing capacity. Cancer Epidemiol Biomarkers Prev 6.11 (1997): 907–916.

Coyne T et al. Diabetes mellitus and serum carotenoids: findings of a population-based study in Queensland. Australia. Am J Clin Nutr 82.3 (2005): 685–693.

Cser MA et al. Serum carotenoid and retinol levels during childhood infections. Ann Nutr Metab 48.3 (2004): 156.

Curran-Celentano J et al. Relation between dietary intake, serum concentrations, and retinal concentrations of lutein and zeaxanthin in adults in a Midwest population. Am J Clin Nutr 74.6 (2001): 796–802.

Dagnelie G, et al. Lutein improves visual function in some patients with retinal degeneration: a pilot study via the Internet. Optometry 71 (2000): 147–164.

Dani C et al. Lutein and zeaxanthin supplementation in preterm infants to prevent retinopathy of prematurity: a randomized controlled study. J Matern Fetal Neonatal Med 25.5 (2012): 523–527

Dawczynski J et al. Long term effects of lutein, zeaxanthin and omega-3-LCPUFAs supplementation on optical density of macular pigment in AMD patients: the LUTEGA study. Graefes Arch Clin Exp Ophthalmol 251.12 (2013): 2711–2723

Delcourt C et al. Plasma lutein and zeaxanthin and other carotenoids as modifiable risk factors for age-related maculopathy and cataract: The POLA study. Investigative Ophthalmology and Visual Science 47.6 (2006): 2329–2335.

De Waart FG et al. Serum carotenoids, [alpha]-tocopherol and mortality risk in a prospective study among Dutch elderly. Int J Epidemiol 30.1 (2001): 136–143.

Dilsiz N et al. Protective effects of various antioxidants during ischemia-reperfusion in the rat retina. Graefe's Arch Clin Exp Ophthalmol (2005): 1–7.

Dorgan JF et al. Relationships of serum carotenoids, retinol, [alpha]-tocopherol, and selenium with breast cancer risk: results from a prospective study in Columbia, Missouri (United States). Cancer Causes Control 9.1 (1998): 89–97.

Dorgan JF et al. Serum carotenoids and (alpha)-tocopherol and risk of nonmelanoma skin cancer. Cancer Epidemiol Biomarkers Prev 13.8 (2004): 1276–1282.

Dwyer JH et al. Progression of carotid intima-media thickness and plasma antioxidants: the Los Angeles Atherosclerosis Study. Arterioscler Thromb Vasc Biol 24.2 (2004): 313–3119.

Elliott, J.G. & Williams, N.S. 2012. Nutrients in the battle against age-related eye diseases. Optometry., 83, (1) 47–55.

Falsini B et al. Influence of short-term antioxidant supplementation on macular function in age-related maculopathy: a pilot study including electrophysiologic assessment. Ophthalmology 110.1 (2003): 51–60.

Feeney J et al. Low macular pigment opticl density is associated with lower cognitive performance in a large, population-based sample of older adults. Neurobiol Aging 34.11 (2013): 2449–2456

Floreani A et al. Plasma antioxidant levels in chronic cholestatic liver diseases. Aliment Pharmacol Ther 14.3 (2000): 353–358.

Forman MR et al. Effect of menstrual cycle phase on the concentration of individual carotenoids in lipoproteins of premenopausal women: a controlled dietary study. Am J Clin Nutr 67.1 (1998): 81–87.

Freudenheim JL et al. Premenopausal breast cancer risk and intake of vegetables, fruits, and related nutrients. J Natl Cancer Inst 88.6 (1996): 340–348.

Fung TT et al. Vitamin and carotenoid intake and risk of squamous cell carcinoma of the skin. Int J Cancer 103.1 (2003): 110–1115.

Gann PH et al. Lower prostate cancer risk in men with elevated plasma lycopene levels: results of a prospective analysis. Cancer Res 59.6 (1999): 1225–1230.

Garcia-Closas R et al. The role of diet and nutrition in cervical carcinogenesis: a review of recent evidence. Int J Cancer 117.4 (2005): 629–637.

Giovannucci E et al. Intake of carotenoids and retinol in relation to risk of prostate cancer. J Natl Cancer Inst 87.23 (1995): 1767–1776.

Grandner MA. Dietary nutrients associated with short and long sleep duration. Data from a nationally representation sample. Appetite 64 (2013): 71–80

Gruber M et al. Correlates of serum lutein + zeaxanthin: findings from the Third National Health and Nutr Examination Survey. J Nutr 134.9 (2004): 2387–2394.

Hammond BR Jr et al. Dietary modification of human macular pigment density. Invest Ophthalmol Vis Sci 38.9 (1997): 1795–1801.

Handelman GJ. The evolving role of carotenoids in human biochemistry. Nutrition 17.10 (2001): 818–822.

Hartmann D et al. Plasma kinetics of zeaxanthin and 3′-dehydro-lutein after multiple oral doses of synthetic zeaxanthin. Am J Clin Nutr 79.3 (2004): 410–417.

Higashi-Okai K et al. Identification and antioxidant activity of several pigments from the residual green tea (*Camellia sinensis*) after hot water extraction. J Univ Occup Environ Health 23.4 (2001): 335–344.

Hirvonen T et al. Intake of flavonoids, carotenoids, vitamins C and E, and risk of stroke in male smokers. Stroke 31.10 (2000): 2301–2306.

Hogg R, Chakravarthy U. AMD and micronutrient antioxidants. Current Eye Res 29.6 (2004): 387–401.

Huang HY et al. Prospective study of antioxidant micronutrients in the blood and the risk of developing prostate cancer. Am J Epidemiol 157.4 (2003): 335–344.

Huang LL et al. Oral supplementation of lutein/zeaxanthin and omega-3 long chain polyunsaturated fatty acids in persons aged 60 years or older, with or without AMD. Invest Ophthalmol & Vis Sci 49.9 (2008): 3864–3869.

Iannone A et al. Antioxidant activity of carotenoids: an electron-spin resonance study on beta-carotene and lutein interaction with free radicals generated in a chemical system. J Biochem Mol Toxicol 12.5 (1998): 299–304.

Iribarren C et al. Association of serum vitamin levels, LDL susceptibility to oxidation, and autoantibodies against MDA-LDL with carotid atherosclerosis: a case-control study: the ARIC Study Investigators (Atherosclerosis Risk in Communities). Arterioscler Thromb Vasc Biol 17.6 (1997): 1171–1177.

Ito Y et al. Serum carotenoids and mortality from lung cancer: a case-control study nested in the Japan Collaborative Cohort (JACC) study. Cancer Sci 94.1 (2003): 57–63.

Jacques PF et al. Long-term nutrient intake and early age-related nuclear lens opacities. Arch Ophthalmol 119.7 (2001): 1009–1019.

Jarvinen R et al. Diet and breast cancer risk in a cohort of Finnish women. Cancer Lett 114.1–2 (1997): 251–253.

Jian L et al. Do dietary lycopene and other carotenoids protect against prostate cancer? Int J Cancer 113.6 (2005): 1010–10114.

Joachim, N., et al. 2014. Incidence and progression of reticular drusen in age-related macular degeneration: findings from an older Australian cohort. Ophthalmology 121: 917–925.

Johnson E et al. Relation among serum and tissue concentrations of lutein and zeaxanthin and macular pigment density. Am J Clin Nutr 71.6 (2000): 1555–1562.

Johnson EJ et al. Cognitive findings of an exploratory trial of docosahexaenoic acid and lutein supplementation in older women. Nutr Neurosci 11.2 (2008): 75–83.

Kabagambe EK et al. Some dietary and adipose tissue carotenoids are associated with the risk of nonfatal acute myocardial infarction in Costa Rica. J Nutr 135.7 (2005): 1763–1769.

Karppi J et al. Lycopene, lutein and β-carotene as determinants of LDL conjugated dienes in serum. Atherosclerosis 209.2 (2010): 565–572

Kim HW et al. Dietary lutein stimulates immune response in the canine. Vet Immunol Immunopathol 74.3–4 (2000a): 315–27.

Kim HW et al. Modulation of humoral and cell-mediated immune responses by dietary lutein in cats. Vet Immunol Immunopathol 73.3–4 (2000b): 331–41.

Kim YT et al. Relation between deranged antioxidant system and cervical neoplasia. Int J Gynecol Cancer 14.5 (2004): 889–895.

Klipstein-Grobusch K et al. Serum carotenoids and atherosclerosis: the Rotterdam Study. Atherosclerosis 148.1 (2000): 49–56.

Koh HH et al. Plasma and macular responses to lutein supplement in subjects with and without age-related maculopathy: a pilot study. Exp Eye Res 79.1 (2004): 21–27.

Krinsky NI, et al. Biologic mechanisms of the protective role of lutein and zeaxanthin in the eye. Annu Rev Nutr 23 (2003): 171–201.

Kvansakul J et al. Supplementation with the carotenoids lutein or zeaxanthin improves human visual performance. Ophthalmic and Physiological Optics 26.4 (2006): 362–371.

Lee EH et al. Dietary lutein reduces ultraviolet radiation-induced inflammation and immunosuppression. J Invest Dermatol 122.2 (2004): 510–5117.

Le Marchand L et al. Intake of specific carotenoids and lung cancer risk. Cancer Epidemiol Biomarkers Prev 2.3 (1993): 183–187.

Levi F et al. Selected micronutrients and colorectal cancer. a case-control study from the canton of Vaud. Switzerland. Eur J Cancer 36.16 (2000): 2115–21119.

Li L et al. Supplementation with lutein or lutein plus green tea extracts does not change oxidative stress in adequately nourished older adults. J Nutr Biochem 21.6 (2010): 544–549

Lu QY et al. Inverse associations between plasma lycopene and other carotenoids and prostate cancer. Cancer Epidemiol Biomarkers Prev 10.7 (2001): 749–756.

Lu QY et al. Inhibition of prostate cancer cell growth by an avocado extract: role of lipid-soluble bioactive substances. J Nutr Biochem 16.1 (2005): 23–30.

Ma L et al. Lutein and zeaxanthin intake and the risk of age-related macular degeneration: a systematic review and meta-analysis. Br J Nutr 107.3 (2012): 350–359

Maci S. Nutritional support against skin ageing: New scientific evidence for the role of lutein. Agro Food Industry Hi-Tech 18.5 (2007): 42–44.

Mares J et al. Predictors of optical density of lutein and zeaxanthin in retinas of older women in the Carotenoids in Age-Related Eye Disease Study, an ancillary study of the Women's Health Initiative. Am J Clin Nutr 84.5 (2006): 1107–1122.

Mathews F, Neil A. Antioxidants and preterm prelabour rupture of the membranes. Br J Obstet Gynaecol 112.5 (2005): 588–594.

Mayne ST et al. Effect of supplemental [beta]-carotene on plasma concentrations of carotenoids, retinol, and [alpha]-tocopherol in humans. Am J Clin Nutr 68.3 (1998): 642–647.

McCann SE et al. Diet in the epidemiology of endometrial cancer in western New York (United States). Cancer Causes Control 11.10 (2000): 965–974.

Michaud DS et al. Intake of specific carotenoids and risk of lung cancer in 2 prospective US cohorts. Am J Clin Nutr 72.4 (2000): 990–997.

Moeller SM et al. Associations between age-related nuclear cataract and lutein and zeaxanthin in the diet and serum in the carotenoids in the age-related eye disease study (CAREDS), an ancillary study of the Women's Health Initiative. Arch Ophthalmol 126.3 (2008): 354–364.

Muriach M et al. Lutein prevents the effect of high glucose levels on immune system cells in vivo and in vitro. J Physiol Biochem 64.2 (2008): 149–158.

Naguib YM. Antioxidant activities of astaxanthin and related carotenoids. J Agric Food Chem 48.4 (2000): 1150–1154.

Nkondjock A, Ghadirian P. Dietary carotenoids and risk of colon cancer: Case-control study. Int J Cancer 110.1 (2004): 110–1116.

Nolan JM et al. Macular pigment, visual function, and macular disease among subjects with Alzheimer's disease: An exploratory study. J Alzheimers Dis 2014. [Epub ahead of print]

Nolan J et al. Macular pigment and percentage of body fat. Invest Ophthalmol Vis Sci 45.11 (2004): 3940–3950.

Nomura AM et al. Serum micronutrients and prostate cancer in Japanese Americans in Hawaii. Cancer Epidemiol Biomarkers Prev 6.7 (1997): 487–491.

Nussbaum JJ, et al. Historic perspectives: Macular yellow pigment: the first 200 years. Retina 1.4 (1981): 296–310.

Olmedilla B et al. Lutein, but not alpha-tocopherol, supplementation improves visual function in patients with age-related cataracts: a 2-y double-blind, placebo-controlled pilot study. Nutr 19.1 (2003): 21–24.

Palombo P et al. Beneficial long-term effects of combined oral/topical antioxidant treatment with the carotenoids lutein and zeaxanthin on human skin: A double-blind, placebo-controlled study. Skin Pharmacol Physiol 20.4 (2007): 199–210.

Pattison DJ et al. Dietary beta-cryptoxanthin and inflammatory polyarthritis: results from a population-based prospective study. Am J Clin Nutr 82.2 (2005): 451–455.

Polidori MC et al. Plasma antioxidant status, immunoglobulin G oxidation and lipid peroxidation in demented patients: Relevance to Alzheimer disease and vascular dementia. Dementia Geriatr Cognitive Disord 18.3–4 (2004): 265–270.

Raju J et al. Low doses of beta-carotene and lutein inhibit AOM-induced rat colonic ACF formation but high doses augment ACF incidence. Int J Cancer 113.5 (2005): 798–802.

Ratnasinghe DM et al. Serum carotenoids are associated with increased lung cancer risk among alcohol drinkers, but not among non-drinkers in a cohort of tin miners. Alcohol Alcoholism 35.4 (2000): 355–360.

Rehak M, et al. Lutein and antioxidants in the prevention of age-related macular degeneration. Lutein und Antioxidantien zur Pravention der AMD 105.1 (2008): 37–45.

Richer S. ARMD-pilot (case series) environmental intervention data. J Am Optom Assoc 70 (1999): 24–36.

Richer S et al. Double-masked, placebo-controlled, randomized trial of lutein and antioxidant supplementation in the intervention of atrophic age-related macular degeneration: the Veterans LAST study (Lutein Antioxidant Supplementation Trial). Optometry 75 (2004): 216–230.

Richer, S., et al. 2007. LAST II: Differential temporal responses of macular pigment optical density in patients with atrophic age-related macular degeneration to dietary supplementation with xanthophylls. Optometry., 78, (5) 213–219.

Richer SP et al. Randomised, double-blind, placebo-controlled study of zeaxanthin and visual function in patients with atrophic age-related macular degeneration: The Zeaxanthin and Visual Function Study (ZVF) FDA IND #78, 973. J Am Optom Assoc 82.11 (2011): 667–680

Rinaldi P et al. Plasma antioxidants are similarly depleted in mild cognitive impairment and in Alzheimer's disease. Neurobiol Aging 24.7 (2003): 915–9119

Roodenburg AJ et al. Amount of fat in the diet affects bioavailability of lutein esters but not of alpha-carotene, beta-carotene, and vitamin E in humans. Am J Clin Nutr 71.5 (2000): 1187–1193.

Sasaki M et al. Biological role of lutein in the light-induced retinal degeneration. J Nutr Biochem 23.5 (2012): 423–429

Sato Y et al. Protective effect of lutein after ischemia-reperfusion in the small intestine. Food Chem 127.3 (2011): 893–898

Schalch W et al. Xanthophyll accumulation in the human retina during supplementation with lutein or zeaxanthin — the LUXEA (LUtein Xanthophyll Eye Accumulation) study. Arch Biochem Biophys 458.2 (2007): 128–135.

Schuurman AG et al. A prospective cohort study on intake of retinol, vitamins C and E, and carotenoids and prostate cancer risk (Netherlands). Cancer Causes Control 13.6 (2002): 573–582.

Semba RD, Dagnelie G. Are lutein and zeaxanthin conditionally essential nutrients for eye health? Med Hypotheses 61.4 (2003): 465–472.

Sesso HD et al. Plasma lycopene, other carotenoids, and retinol and the risk of cardiovascular disease in men. Am J Clin Nutr 81.5 (2005): 990–997.

Tamimi RM et al. Plasma carotenoids, retinol, and tocopherols and risk of breast cancer. Am J Epidemiol 161.2 (2005): 153.

Tanumihardjo SA, et al. Lutein absorption is facilitated with cosupplementation of ascorbic acid in young adults. J Am Dietetic Assoc 105.1 (2005): 114–1118.

Tavani A, et al. Food and nutrient intake and risk of cataract. Ann Epidemiol 6 (1996): 41–46.

Terry P et al. Dietary carotenoid intake and colorectal cancer risk. Nutr Cancer 42.2 (2002): 167–172.

The AREDS2 Research Group. Lutein / zeaxanthin for the treatment of age-related cataract: AREDS2 randomised trial report no. 4. JAMA Ophthalmol 131.7 (2013a): 843–850.

The AREDS2 Research Group. Lutein + zeaxanthin and omega-3 fatty acids for age-related macular degeneration: the Age-Related Eye Disease Study 2 (AREDS2) randomized clinical trial. JAMA 309.19 (2013b): 2005–2015

Thurmann PA et al. Plasma kinetics of lutein, zeaxanthin, and 3-dehydro-lutein after multiple oral doses of a lutein supplement. Am J Clin Nutr 82.1 (2005): 88–97.

Toniolo P et al. Serum carotenoids and breast cancer. Am J Epidemiol 153.12 (2001): 1142–1147.

Tulley RT et al. Daily intake of multivitamins during long-term intake of olestra in men prevents declines in serum vitamins A and E but not carotenoids. J Nutr 135.6 (2005): 1456–1461.

Unlu NZ et al. Carotenoid absorption from salad and salsa by humans is enhanced by the addition of avocado or avocado oil. J Nutr 135.3 (2005): 431.
Vu HT et al. Lutein and zeaxanthin and the risk of cataract: the Melbourne Visual Impairment Project. Invest Ophthalmol Vis Sci 47.9 (2006): 3783–3786.
Wang W et al. Effect of dietary lutein and zeaxanthin on plasma carotenoids and their transport in lipoproteins in age-related macular degeneration. Am J Clin Nutr 85.3 (2007): 762–769.
Wang MX et al. Lutein supplementation reduces plasma lipid peroxidation and C-reactive protein in healthy nonsmokers. Atherosclerosis 227.2 (2013): 380–385
Wang, J.J., et al. 2014. Genetic susceptibility, dietary antioxidants, and long-term incidence of age-related macular degeneration in two populations. Ophthalmology 121: 667–675.
Xu XR et al. Effects of lutein supplement on serum inflammatory cytokines, ApoE and lipid profiles in early atherosclerosis population. J Atheroscler Thromb 20.2 (2013): 170–177
Yao Y et al. Lutein supplementation improves visual performance in Chinese drivers: 1 year randomised, double-blind, placebo-controlled study. Nutrition 29.7–8 (2013): 958–964.
Yeum KJ, Russell RM. Carotenoid bioavailability and bioconversion. Ann Rev Nutr 22 (2002): 483–504.
Yonova-Doing, E., et al. 2013. Candidate gene study of macular response to supplemental lutein and zeaxanthin. Exp.Eye Res., 115, 172–177
Zhao D-Y et al. Resonance Raman measurement of macular carotenoids in retinal, choroidal, and macular dystrophies. Arch Ophthalmol 121.7 (2003): 967–972.
Ziegler RG et al. Importance of alpha-carotene, beta-carotene, and other phytochemicals in the etiology of lung cancer. J Natl Cancer Inst 88.9 (1996): 612–6115.

Magnesium

M

HISTORICAL NOTE 'Magnesium' comes from the name of the ancient Greek city Magnesia, where large deposits of magnesium were found. In the form of Epsom salts, magnesium has long been used therapeutically as a laxative although it is also used in many other ways, such as a foot soak to soften rough spots and absorb foot odour and as a bath additive to ease muscle aches and pains. Supplemental magnesium in recent years is commonly ingested to alleviate musculoskeletal pains and cramping.

BACKGROUND AND RELEVANT PHARMACOKINETICS

Magnesium is an essential mineral and critical cofactor for over 300 biochemical processes, such as adenosine triphosphate (ATP) manufacture, critical to phosphorylation reactions. It is also necessary for DNA, RNA protein synthesis, carbohydrate metabolism, bone formation and cellular signal transduction (Allen 2013, Hartwig 2001, Rude et al 2009). Magnesium may also serve as an immunomodulator regulating NF-κB activation and cytokine production. In this role it may limit systemic inflammation and corresponding general markers such as C-reactive protein (Chacko et al 2010, Song et al 2007). It is the fourth most abundant cation in the body, with 50–60% sequestered in the bone, the remainder distributed equally between muscle and non-muscular soft tissue. Only about 1% of total body magnesium is found in the extracellular fluid. Dietary intake, renal and intestinal function finely balance and maintain plasma magnesium concentrations.

Absorption of dietary magnesium starts within 1 hour of ingestion, and occurs along the entire length of the bowel, with salts of high solubility having the most complete absorption (e.g. magnesium citrate). Normal magnesium absorption occurs passively at a rate of approximately 90% through the paracellular pathway. Active transport may occur only where extremely low dietary magnesium magnesium intake is observed, i.e. it is thought that magnesium absorption may be enhanced in bowel disorders, which must be considered when suggesting magnesium supplementation for these conditions (Allen 2013, Swaminathan 2003, Topf & Murray 2003). Magnesium absorption requires selenium, parathyroid hormone (PTH) and vitamins B_6 and D and is hindered by phytate, fibre, alcohol, excess saturated fat and the presence of unabsorbed fatty acids, high phosphorus or calcium intake (Johnson 2001, Saris et al 2000). However, calcium is no longer perceived to be as antagonistic to magnesium uptake as previously thought, while research using test meals may show negative interaction — in contrast to long-term balance studies (Andon et al 1996, Fine et al 1991, Gropper et al 2009, Lewis et al 1989). Some authors suggest that such nutrient interactions only become significant in situations of low magnesium intake (Gropper et al 2009, Lewis et al 1989). Healthy people absorb 30–50% of ingested magnesium; increasing to 70% bioavailability in cases of low intake or deficiency (Allen 2013, Braunwald et al 2003). Other research suggests that fructo-oligosaccharides may improve magnesium absorption, particularly in adolescent girls (Ellen 2009).

Although currently it is undisputed that magnesium metabolism is regulated, the identity of such regulators remains largely obscured (Gropper et al 2009). While a number of hormones affect magnesium homeostasis they fail to explain every facet. What is understood to date is that magnesium homeostasis is regulated via a filtration–reabsorption process in the kidneys. Magnesium conservation is facilitated when magnesium is deficit, and excreted when surfeit (Quamme 2008). Reabsorption occurs in the ascending loop of Henle mediated by mechanisms involving paracellin-1, where sodium-assisted potential is generated to enhance transepithelial transport. Therefore medications that impact sodium resorption, such as loop diuretics, osmotic diuretics and changes in extracellular fluid volume expansion, may enhance the excretion of magnesium (Allen 2013).

While hormones central to calcium homeostasis, e.g. PTH, play a role in magnesium metabolism, this is a greatly diminished one compared to calcium (Shils & Rude 1996). Additional regulators include adrenergic signalling pathways, insulin, oestrogen and growth hormone (Rude & Shils 2006). Some researchers suggest that the real locus of control over magnesium homeostasis may be independent of hormones; instead there may be a combination of fractional absorption, renal excretion and transmembranous cation flux (Gropper et al 2009).

Once absorbed, magnesium travels to the liver, enters the systemic circulation and is transported around the body, to be ultimately excreted via the kidneys, with urine representing the major excretory pathway. Consequently, the kidney is pivotal in homeostatic control, rapidly adjusting to changing dietary intake (Rude & Shils 2006). Renal handling of magnesium is subject to additional negative influences. For example, increased calcium (≈ 2600 mg/day) (NHMRC 2005), sodium, protein, caffeine and alcohol consumption (Allen 2013, Gropper et al 2009, Rude 2010, Rude & Shils 2006), B_6 depletion (Turnlund et al 1992), glycosuria, stress (Allen 2013, Khan et al 1999, Rude & Shils 2006, Turnlund et al 1992, Walti et al 2003), elevated thyroid hormones (Wester 1987), protein intakes either above or below recommended levels (Wester 1987) and increases in net endogenous acid production (Rylander et al 2006) all impair the kidney's capacity to reabsorb magnesium. Additional minor losses occur through sweat and faeces (Gropper et al 2009, Rude & Shils 2006).

Magnesium assessment

In spite of intense ongoing research, there is still no simple, rapid and accurate laboratory test to determine total body magnesium status in humans (Arnaud

2008, Feillet-Coudray et al 2000). In particular, as with many of the minerals, there is an urgent need to identify a functional or biological marker of magnesium status, similar to the role of ferritin in iron assessment (Arnaud 2008). While serum testing is still frequently performed, it is only indicative of severe depletion, as evidenced by values <0.75 mmol/L and while some studies demonstrate a correlation between these values and the magnesium content of other tissues, many do not (Arnaud 2008). Some researchers suggest that serum values 0.75–0.85 mmol/L warrant further investigation with more sensitive tests.

Erythrocytes naturally contain large amounts of magnesium and experimental depletion is reflected by declining red blood cell (RBC) concentrations within weeks. A criticism of this method relates to repletion studies which found greater increases in serum magnesium following supplementation than reflected in the RBC; however, one could argue that the diminished response is a more accurate reflection of delayed intracellular recovery. Both animal and human studies have shown magnesium concentrations in white blood cells, e.g. lymphocytes, to be a particularly accurate indicator of magnesium content of both skeletal and cardiac tissues, which, given their functional significance, represents an attractive option. Actual muscle biopsies are believed to be an excellent indicator of body status; however, due to their invasive nature, they are rarely used (Arnaud 2008).

Increasingly, however, magnesium loading tests are probably the best assessment (Allen 2013, Arnaud 2008). The procedure involves either oral or intravenous (IV) loading with magnesium (e.g. 500–700 mg) followed by collection of 24-hour urine. Generally, excretion of <70% is considered indicative of magnesium deficiency. One of the significant disadvantages of this method is the lack of standardisation, e.g. form and dose of magnesium administered, which is critical for ensuring its sensitivity and reproducibility. Additionally, this test should only be used in individuals with healthy renal function generally and absorptive capacity specifically in oral loading. Exchangeable magnesium pool tests requiring magnesium stable isotopes is a novel approach to magnesium assessment; more studies and human trials are needed (Allen 2013).

FOOD SOURCES

Good dietary sources of magnesium include, in descending order, dark green leafy vegetables, legumes, wholegrain cereals, nuts, fruit, fish, most meat, whole full-fat milk, cheese, eggs, cocoa, soy flour, mineral water and hard water (Allen 2013). In some communities, 'hard tap water' contains significant amounts of magnesium. Food processing and refining remove a substantial amount of naturally occurring magnesium from the food chain — up to 80% in refined grains (Insel et al 2013). High-fibre foods can limit the amount of magnesium absorbed from food but those containing fermentable carbohydrates (e.g. oligosaccharides, pectin) can improve magnesium absorption.

DEFICIENCY SIGNS AND SYMPTOMS

When reduced intakes or increased losses of magnesium, potassium or phosphorus occur (the three major intracellular elements), losses of the others generally follow. As such, many deficiency symptoms are also due to alterations in potassium and/or phosphorus status and manifest as neurological or neuromuscular symptoms.

Symptoms of deficiency include:

- anorexia and weight loss
- nausea and vomiting

- muscular weakness and spasms
- numbness, tingling, cramps
- spontaneous carpal–pedal spasm
- vertigo, ataxia, athetoid, choreiform movements
- lethargy
- difficulty remembering things
- apathy and melancholy
- confusion
- dysregulation of biorhythms (some sleep and mental health disorders, including insomnia)
- depression
- mental confusion, decreased attention span and poor concentration
- personality changes
- hyperirritability and excitability
- vertigo
- cardiac arrhythmia, tetany and ultimately convulsions can develop if deficiency is prolonged.

Although magnesium deficiency is a common clinical problem, serum levels are often overlooked or not measured in patients at risk for the disorder. About 10% of patients admitted to hospitals and up to 65% of patients in intensive care units may be magnesium-deficient (Braunwald et al 2003).

Low magnesium states are associated with several serious diseases such as congestive heart failure, ischaemic heart disease, atherogenesis, atherosclerosis, cardiac arrhythmias, hypertension, mitral valve prolapse, metabolic syndrome, diabetes mellitus, hyperlipidaemia, pre-eclampsia (PE) and eclampsia and osteoporosis, although the latter demonstrates conflicting evidence (Allen 2013, Fox et al 2001, Guerrero-Romero & Rodriguez-Moran 2002, Rude & Shils 2006). Epidemiological evidence suggests that a low dietary intake of magnesium is also associated with impaired lung function, bronchial hyperreactivity and wheezing, and risk of stroke (Ascherio et al 1998, Hill et al 1997). Magnesium deficiency may also play a role in the pathophysiology of Tourette's syndrome (Grimaldi 2002).

Primary deficiency

A primary deficiency is rare in healthy people as the kidneys are extremely efficient at maintaining magnesium homeostasis. Studies of experimental magnesium depletion demonstrate that it takes months of intentional magnesium deprivation to induce a deficiency and even then, its presentation is 'vague' and idiosyncratic (Shils & Rude 1996, Wester 1987).

Marginal deficiencies are far more common and very often undiagnosed. There is evidence that daily magnesium intake has declined substantially since the beginning of the last century, with dietary surveys showing the average intake in Western countries is often below the recommended dietary intake (RDI) (Ford & Mokdad 2003, Lukaski 2000, Rude & Shils 2006, Saris et al 2000). Those particularly susceptible to inadequate dietary intakes are institutionalised elderly and the elderly in general (McKeown et al 2008, Woods et al 2009).

Secondary deficiency

In contrast to the low rates of reported primary magnesium deficiency, secondary deficiency is far more common and seen in both the acutely and the chronically ill (Gropper et al 2009, Shils 1964). Most magnesium deficiencies occur due to a combination of insufficient dietary intake and/or intestinal malabsorption and increased magnesium depletion or excretion. There are many factors that predispose to deficiency and the most common are listed in Table 1.

TABLE 1 RISK FACTORS FOR MAGNESIUM DEPLETION AND DEFICIENCY	
Dietary	Excessive intake of ethanol, salt, phosphoric acid (soft drinks), caffeine Sodium deficit (via drug administration) Protein-energy malnutrition. There is evidence that magnesium balance remains positive despite reduced recommended dietary intake as long as protein >30 g/day Chronic excessive magnesium intake
Endocrine disorders	Hyperaldosteronism Hyperparathyroidism with hypercalcaemia Hyperthyroidism Diabetes mellitus and glycosuria
Lifestyle	Profuse sweating Intense, prolonged stress Alcohol ingestion
Gastrointestinal disorders (gastrointestinal tract [GIT] absorptive surface pathology or reduced transit time or increased upper GIT loss)	Coeliac disease Infections Inflammatory bowel disease Malabsorption syndromes Biliary and intestinal fistula Pancreatitis Partial bowel obstruction Vomiting/diarrhoea
Elevated cortisol levels	Chronic stress Sleep deprivation Athletes and high-frequency exercise
Pharmaceutical drugs	Aminoglycoside antibiotics Amphotericin B Antivirals (ribavirin, foscavir) Carboplatin, cisplatin Cetuximab, panitumumab Corticosteroids Cyclosporin Digoxin Loop diuretics Oestrogens Osmotic diuretics Penicillamine Pentamidine Proton pump inhibitors Tacrolimus Tetracycline antibiotics
Renal	Metabolic disorders Renal failure Acidosis Nephrotoxic drugs (e.g. cisplatin, cyclosporin)

Continued

M

TABLE 1 RISK FACTORS FOR MAGNESIUM DEPLETION AND DEFICIENCY *(continued)*	
Other	Hyperthermia Hypercatabolic states such as burns Phosphate depletion Potassium depletion Pregnancy Lactation (prolonged (>12 months) or excessive lactation) Excessive menstruation Long-term parenteral nutrition combined with loss of body fluids (e.g. diarrhoea) Parasitic infection (e.g. pinworms)

Source: Allen (2013), Braunwald et al (2003), Johnson (2001), McDermott et al (1991), Sanders et al (1999), Shils et al (1999).

Medicines increasing risk of deficiency

Many pharmaceutical drugs have the potential to cause hypomagnesaemia.

MAIN ACTIONS

Magnesium plays an essential role in a wide range of fundamental biological reactions in the body. It is involved in over 300 essential enzymatic reactions and is necessary for every major biological process. It is especially important for those enzymes that use nucleotides as cofactors or substrates and plays a role in many processes that are of central importance in the biochemistry of each cell, particularly in energy metabolism. It is also required for many other important biological functions, such as:

- nerve conduction
- regulation of vascular tone
- muscle activity
- amino acid and protein synthesis
- DNA synthesis and degradation
- immune function
- ATP production
- blood clotting
- natural calcium antagonist.

Interaction with other nutrients

Magnesium is extremely important for the metabolism of calcium, potassium, phosphorus, zinc, copper, iron, sodium, lead and cadmium and the intracellular homeostasis and activation of thiamine (Johnson 2001). It acts as a calcium antagonist and positively interacts with nutrients such as potassium, phosphorus, vitamin B_6 and boron.

OTHER ACTIONS

In its macro form, oral inorganic magnesium salts have a laxative and antacid activity and are practically insoluble in water.

CLINICAL USE

In practice, magnesium is administered by various routes, such as intramuscular injection and intravenous infusion. This review will focus only on oral magnesium, as this is the form most commonly used by healthcare professionals and the general public, outside the hospital setting.

Deficiency: treatment and prevention

Magnesium supplementation is used to prevent and/or treat magnesium deficiency. This is achieved using either oral or parenteral administration forms. Ideally, forms of magnesium less likely to induce diarrhoea are recommended for long-term use. Table 1 lists the diet, lifestyle, comorbidities and pharmaceutical medications which can increase the risk of hypomagnesaemia. Sometimes, sub-optimal magnesium states are associated with other electrolyte imbalances, such as calcium and potassium.

Healthy representation of total plasma magnesium levels are 0.86 mmol/L, between a reference value of 0.75–0.96 mmol/L. Low total plasma magnesium levels <0.7 mmol/L (1.8 mg/dL, 1.5 mEq/L) are indicative of magnesium deficiency, although symptoms occur when total plasma magnesium is <0.5 mmol/L (1.2 mg/dL, 1.0 mEq/L). It should be noted that total plasma magnesium may not be a good indicator of magnesium status, as low plasma levels may exist with low intracellular magnesium. Further investigation is needed to ascertain accurate measurement of magnesium status (Allen 2013, Braunwald et al 2003).

Constipation

In high doses magnesium exerts a laxative effect, which is used in practice for the short-term treatment of constipation and in order to get the bowel ready for surgical or diagnostic procedures. It is often used in the form of magnesium hydroxide (milk of magnesia) or magnesium sulfate (Epsom salts) (Guerrera et al 2009).

Dyspepsia

As magnesium hydroxide (milk of magnesia), oral magnesium is used to reduce symptoms of dyspepsia and gastric acidity and acts as an antacid by forming magnesium chloride in the stomach. Magnesium oxide is also used for its antacid properties, which are greater than magnesium carbonate and sodium bicarbonate (Coffin et al 2011, Reynolds et al 1982). Magnesium trisilicate is the form used when a prolonged antacid activity is required.

Clinical note — Magnesium citrate and orotate: superior supplements?

Magnesium supplements come in a variety of salts (e.g. citrate, oxide, gluconate, acetate, orotate); however their bioavailability varies. Current evidence, although not clearly demonstrating superiority of one preparation over another, supports the use in general of organic over inorganic forms (Coudray et al 2005, Firoz & Graber 2001, Lindberg et al 1990, Walker et al 2003). In particular, investigations of magnesium orotate (Lindberg et al 1990), citrate (Walker et al 2003) and gluconate (Coudray et al 2005) demonstrate high solubility and bioavailability. Magnesium orotate has attracted further attention regarding its potential synergism with magnesium in terms of repair of damaged myocardium (Classen 2004, Zeana 1999).

According to one randomised, double-blind, placebo-controlled study, magnesium amino chelate and magnesium citrate are better absorbed than magnesium oxide in healthy individuals (Walker et al 2003). Of the three, magnesium citrate led to the greatest increase in mean serum magnesium, a result evident after acute dosing (24 hours) and chronic dosing (60 days). Furthermore, although mean erythrocyte magnesium concentration showed no differences among groups, chronic magnesium citrate supplementation resulted in the greatest mean salivary magnesium concentration compared with all other treatments.

Cardiovascular disease (CVD)

Whether adequate magnesium intake has a protective effect against the development of CVD appears likely, based on the balance of evidence; however some studies remain inconclusive. This is largely based on epidemiological evidence which continues to strongly link magnesium deficiency to numerous CVD presentations, including congestive heart failure, ischaemic heart disease, cardiac arrhythmias, hypertension, mitral valve prolapse, stroke, non-occlusive myocardial infarction and hyperlipidaemia (Alon et al 2006, Flight & Clifton 2006, Fox et al 2001, Frishman et al 2005, Gropper et al 2009, Guerrero-Romero & Rodriguez-Moran 2002, Haenni et al 1998, Klevay & Milne 2002, Ma et al 1995, Rasmussen et al 1988, Rude & Shils 2006, Saris et al 2000, Song et al 2006, Xu et al 2012, Zhang et al 2012).

Xu et al (2012), in their meta-analysis of >210,000 people with cardiovascular history and CVD incidence and mortality, suggest that the evidence is weighted more towards protective factors in women than men. The Japan Collaborative Cohort study produced similar findings; however the authors state that this may be due to confounders such as a propensity of men to more risky lifestyle factors such as high-energy drinks, smoking and alcohol consumption (Zhang et al 2012).

A protective effect from hard water consumption, and in particular magnesium intake from this source, against CVD has been hypothesised for many years, culminating in a meta-analysis which determined a pooled odds ratio of 0.75 for cardiovascular mortality (Catling et al 2008).

Although the pathophysiology of each condition is multifactorial, the multiple biological effects of magnesium in the cardiovascular system suggest an important cardioprotective role. In the heart, magnesium acts as a calcium-channel blocker and promotes resting polarisation of the cell membrane, thereby reducing arrhythmias (Shattock et al 1987). It also helps to prevent serum coagulation (Frishman et al 2005). Low magnesium selectively impairs the release of nitric oxide from the coronary endothelium, resulting in vasoconstriction and possibly coronary embolism. Magnesium plays a role in blood lipid levels with detrimental changes, e.g. increased oxidation of low-density lipoproteins (LDLs), as well as generally increased oxidation, evident in hypomagnesaemia (Rude & Shils 2006). In experimental animals, dietary magnesium deficiency exacerbates atherosclerosis and vascular damage because it has a modulatory role in controlling lipid metabolism in the arterial wall.

Mitral valve prolapse

It has been suggested that hypomagnesaemia is common in patients with mitral valve prolapse and therefore supplementation to correct this deficiency could exert beneficial clinical effects (Kitlinski et al 2004). In 1997, one study of 141 subjects with symptomatic mitral valve prolapse confirmed this suspicion by identifying hypomagnesaemia in 60% of patients (Lichodziejewska et al 1997). A randomised, double-blind, crossover study followed those magnesium-deficient people and found that 5 weeks' magnesium supplementation significantly alleviated symptoms of weakness, chest pain, dyspnoea, palpitation and anxiety (Lichodziejewska et al 1997). The dose regimen used was three tablets of magnesium carbonate 600 mg (7 mmol elementary magnesium) daily for the first week followed by two tablets daily until the fifth week. New research in this area is sadly lacking; the most recent article was presented in a paediatric study of the prevalence of hypomagnesaemia in mitral valve prolapse syndrome. A small percentage of the patients had serum magnesium levels <1.5 mg/dL after therapy symptoms of chest pain decreased (Amoozagar et al 2012).

Symptoms of coronary artery disease (CAD)

In 2003, the results from a multicentre, double-blind randomised controlled trial (RCT) showed that 6 months' oral magnesium supplementation in patients with CAD resulted in a significant improvement in exercise tolerance, exercise-induced chest pain and quality of life compared to placebo (Shechter et al 2003). The study used oral magnesium citrate (15 mmol twice daily) as Magnosolv-Granulat (total magnesium 365 mg). Previously, randomised placebo-controlled studies have shown that oral magnesium supplementation in CAD patients is associated with significant improvement in brachial artery endothelial function and inhibits platelet-dependent thrombosis, providing several potential mechanisms by which magnesium could beneficially alter outcomes in these patients. Additionally, Shechter (2010) suggests magnesium supplementation has theoretical benefits in hospitalised and elderly patients as cardioprotective therapy in CAD (Shechter et al 1999, 2000, 2010).

Hypertension

Epidemiological evidence suggests an inverse relationship between blood pressure and serum magnesium, while large well-designed prospective studies report that magnesium-rich diets may lower blood pressure, particularly in older individuals (Sontia & Touryz 2007). Magnesium modulates vascular tone and reactivity both directly, e.g. calcium-channel blocker, and indirectly, e.g. prostacyclin, and alters vascular responsivity to vasoactive agonists. However, magnesium deficiency does not appear universal amongst hypertensive patients and several subgroups have been identified as characteristically demonstrating both pathologies. These include individuals of African descent, obese patients, patients with severe or malignant presentations and those also diagnosed with metabolic syndrome.

M

This may partly explain the mixed findings produced from magnesium supplementation studies, as well as additional heterogeneities in study designs, such as the salts used, dose administered, sample size and trial duration (Sontia & Touryz 2007). Modest but significant success (≈ −2 to −5 mmHg), however, has been achieved, particularly in those patients deficient at baseline, African American individuals and those patients with diuretic-associated hypertension (Rude & Shils 2006, Sontia & Touryz 2007, Witteman et al 1994). Patients who are considered metabolically obese normal-weight people (also deficient at baseline) demonstrate lowered mean systolic (−2.1 vs 3.9% mmHg, $P < 0.05$) and diastolic (−3.8 vs 7.5% mmHg, $P < 0.05$) benefit from IV magnesium supplementation (equivalent: 382 mg magnesium) when compared to controls (Rodriguez-Moran & Guerrero-Romero 2014).

Stroke protection

A prospective study of 43,738 men (Health Professional Follow-up Study) conducted over 8 years showed an inverse association between dietary magnesium intake and the risk of total stroke (Ascherio et al 1998). This association was stronger in hypertensive than normotensive men and was not materially altered by adjustments for blood pressure levels. This association was confirmed in a later study of male smokers (Larsson et al 2008). Following adjustment for age and other cardiovascular risks, high magnesium intake was associated with a statistically significant reduced risk of cerebral infarct, with a relative risk of 0.85 across men of all ages or 0.76 in those men aged <60 years, while the dietary intake of other minerals did not appear to convey any protection. It is also interesting to note that low concentrations of magnesium in the serum or cerebrospinal fluid in acute ischaemic stroke patients at admission or within 48 hours of onset of the stroke predict both greater neurological deficits, e.g. paresis, and higher

1-week mortality (Bayir et al 2009, Cojocaru et al 2007). In a meta-analysis of eight cohort studies — 8367 stroke cases amongst 304,551 people — a significant inverse association between high magnesium intake (range 228–471 mg magnesium day) and risk of stroke was found. More specifically, the people with the highest magnesium intake experienced an 11% reduction in the relative risk of stroke (Nie et al 2012). Findings were confirmed by the National Institutes of Health Stroke Scale, appearing as a dose–response relationship between magnesium serum levels and risk of death, in an epidemiological study in China (Feng et al 2012).

Dyslipidaemia

Oral magnesium supplementation (magnesium oxide 12 mmol/day) taken over 3 months effectively reduced plasma lipids compared with placebo in people with ischaemic heart disease (Rasmussen et al 1989). The double-blind study showed that magnesium produced a statistically significant 13% increase in molar ratio of apolipoprotein A1:apolipoprotein B, compared with a 2% increase in the placebo group. This was caused by a decrease in apolipoprotein B concentrations, which were reduced by 15% in the magnesium group as compared with a slight increase in the placebo group. Additionally, triglyceride levels decreased by 27% after magnesium treatment.

In a later study measuring serum lipids and insulin sensitivity (IS) in 48 patients with mild uncomplicated hypertension, oral magnesium (600 mg pidolate) was administered with concurrent lifestyle recommendations. In the control group there were no changes to oral glucose tolerance test-derived IS indices, nor serum lipids, whereas the active treatment group experienced increased IS indices and decreased triglycerides, LDL and total cholesterol, with elevated high-density lipoprotein (HDL) levels (Hadjistavri et al 2010).

A study of 50 healthy volunteers by Marken et al (1989) found no change in lipid profile in a double-blind, crossover RCT using magnesium oxide (400 mg twice daily) for 60 days. This may be due to the fact that participants had lipid levels within the normal range at baseline.

Arrhythmia prevention

In congestive heart failure

Although magnesium is usually administered intravenously when indicated in this condition, one controlled study using oral magnesium showed that it significantly reduced the incidence of arrhythmias in patients with stable congestive heart failure (Bashir et al 1993). The double-blind crossover study used magnesium chloride (3204 mg/day in divided doses). Its role in sudden cardiac death as a result of fatal ventricular arrhythmia was observed in a prospective women's cohort, where higher plasma magnesium from dietary intake was associated with lower risk of sudden cardiac death (Chiuve et al 2011).

Postoperative recovery from cardiac surgery

An interesting Australian study employed a range of preoperative treatments addressing mental, physical and metabolic components, including magnesium. The results of this RCT, using 1200 mg magnesium orotate, together with 300 mg CoQ10, 300 mg alpha-lipoic acid and 3 g omega-3 essential fatty acids administered daily 1 month prior to surgery, suggest an enhanced postoperative recovery and improved quality of life (Hadj et al 2006). IV administration of magnesium sulfate is also used to reduce the risk of atrial fibrillation postsurgery (Burgess et al 2006).

Postsurgical pain

Systemic magnesium has been used with some scepticism in the management of postoperative pain management. Magnesium was examined in both intraoperative and postoperative patient observations in a vast variety of surgical procedures. The perioperative meta-analysis of 20 RCTs suggests a use for magnesium to reduce opioid consumption and mitigate postoperative pain. In the cardiac patients (three studies) no adverse effects were noted (De Oliveira et al 2013).

Migraine headaches: prevention

People who suffer with recurrent migraines appear to have lower intracellular magnesium levels (demonstrated in both red and white blood cells) than those who do not experience migraines. (See Feverfew monograph for more information about migraine aetiology.) The low magnesium level is believed to result in cerebral artery spasm and increased release of substance P and other pain mediators (Woolhouse 2005).

Two randomised, double-blind studies using high-dose oral magnesium have found it to be useful in migraine sufferers, reducing frequency and/or number of days with migraine headache (Peikert et al 1996, Taubert 1994). One placebo-controlled study using a lower dose found no benefit in reducing the frequency of migraine headaches (Pfaffenrath et al 1996).

A dose of 24 mmol/L magnesium (600 mg trimagnesium dicitrate) taken daily over 12 weeks produced a 42% reduction in frequency of attack compared with 16% with placebo in one study of 81 patients, with a mean attack frequency of 3.6 migraine headaches each month (Peikert et al 1996). Effects were observed after week 9 and treatment also significantly decreased the duration of each migraine. Significant decreases in migraine frequency were also observed in a crossover study that used the same dose and form of oral magnesium (Taubert 1994). In a recent study, 300 mg magnesium, in combination with other B vitamins and a standardised extract of feverfew magnesium, was stated as probably prophylactic for migraine treatment (Holland et al 2012). However research on the use of single magnesium supplementation in the reduction of migraine headaches is limited.

M

Clinical note — What is the link between magnesium and migraine?

Magnesium seems to play a significant role in the pathogenesis of migraine, with low brain levels and impaired magnesium metabolism reported in migraine sufferers (Thomas et al 2000). Magnesium has an effect on serotonin receptors, nitric oxide synthesis and release and a variety of other migraine-related receptors and neurotransmitters. It is also essential for mitochondrial function within the cell. The available evidence suggests that up to 50% of patients during an acute migraine attack have lowered levels of ionised magnesium (Mauskop & Altura 1998). Pilot studies of migraine patients have suggested that disordered energy metabolism or magnesium deficiencies may be responsible for hyperexcitability of neuronal tissue in migraine patients (Boska et al 2002). As such, factors that decrease neuronal excitability, such as magnesium, may alter the threshold for triggering attacks (Boska et al 2002). The efficacy of magnesium is stated as probably effective for migraine prevention (Holland et al 2012).

Menstrual migraine headache

Oral magnesium supplementation decreases pain, premenstrual symptoms and the number of days with migraine headache, according to two double-blind, placebo-controlled studies (Facchinetti et al 1991a, Peikert et al 1996). In the earlier study, treatment consisted of 360 mg/day of magnesium (pyrrolidone carboxylic acid) starting on day 15 of the menstrual cycle and continuing until the onset of menses. In the second study 600 mg of trimagnesium dicitrate was administered every morning. Both studies suggest a benefit in the reduction of symptoms (Mauskop & Varughese 2012).

Migraine prophylaxis in children

Oral magnesium oxide (9 mg/kg/day) given in three divided doses with food may decrease headache frequency and severity, according to a multicentre, randomised, double-blind, placebo-controlled trial (Wang et al 2003). The 16-week study involved children aged 3–17 years who reported a 4-week history of at least weekly moderate to severe headache with a throbbing or pulsatile quality, associated anorexia/nausea, vomiting, photophobia, sonophobia or relief with sleep, but no fever or evidence of infection. Of note, 27% of subjects (n = 42 magnesium oxide; n = 44 placebo) failed to complete the study, thereby hindering interpretation of the results. While promising, there has been little further investigation so the evidence to date can be described as limited, with further research required (Orr & Venkateswaran 2014).

Attention-deficit hyperactivity disorder (ADHD)

The role of magnesium status and supplementation in ADHD remains unclear.

Several studies have demonstrated a positive correlation between magnesium status and ADHD pathology. Reported prevalence of hypomagnesaemia varies between 50% and 95% (Kozielec & Starobrat-Hermelin 1997, Mousain-Bosc et al 2004). It has been hypothesised that a genetic mutation involving the TRPM6 gene, which is crucial for magnesium transport and homeostasis, may be implicated, therefore making deficiency possible irrespective of adequate dietary intake (Mousain-Bosc et al 2004). There have been three magnesium supplementation studies in combination with vitamin B_6 (6 mg/kg/day magnesium ± 0.6–0.8 mg/kg/day vitamin B_6), producing significant behavioural improvement (Mousain-Bosc et al 2004). Magnesium–B_6 treatment led to a rise in erythrocyte magnesium levels; when treatment ceased, behavioural symptoms reappeared within a few weeks, concurrent with lowered erythrocyte magnesium levels (Mousain-Bosc et al 2006).

More recently, a systematic review of magnesium monotherapy in ADHD by Ghanizadeh (2013) concluded there are no well-controlled trials available to support the efficacy of magnesium in ADHD, even though preliminary reports are promising. Part of the difficulties arise from the fact that some pharmaceutical stimulants affect magnesium plasma levels, baseline levels of children with ADHD in the studies are unknown and confounders such as B_6 deficiency (which negatively affects magnesium balance), dietary intake and kidney/liver function are not usually taken into account.

Autism spectrum disorders (ASD)

Research suggests that people with ASD generally demonstrate RBC magnesium depletion (Mousain-Bosc et al 2006, Priya 2011, Strambi et al 2006). In spite of two negative reviews published 10 years apart (Nye & Brice 2005, Pfeiffer et al 1995), enthusiasm regarding the use of magnesium as an adjunct to high-dose vitamin B_6 therapy (6 mg/kg/day with 0.6–0.8 mg/kg/day vitamin B_6) in ASD continues (Kidd 2002, Mousain-Bosc et al 2006). Whether magnesium ultimately proves to be a successful adjunctive treatment remains unclear as currently there are limited trials and poor methodological rigour (Ghanizadeh 2103, Kidd 2002, Nye & Brice 2005, Pfeiffer et al 1995).

It has been proposed by Yasuda and Tsutsui (2013) that the pathogenesis of autism may somehow relate to low zinc and magnesium levels coupled with high aluminium, cadmium, lead, mercury and arsenic. This complex interplay of nutritional factors needs further exploration to be confirmed.

Kidney stone prevention

Magnesium deficiency is one of many risk factors for the development of kidney stones (Anderson 2002, Seiner 2005). Others include nutritional deficiencies of water, calcium, potassium and vitamin B_6, excessive intakes of animal protein, fat, sugar, oxalates, colas, alcohol, caffeine, salt and vitamin D, lifestyle factors and a positive family history.

A prospective double-blind study of 64 patients who were randomly assigned to receive placebo or potassium–magnesium citrate (42 mEq potassium, 21 mEq magnesium and 63 mEq citrate) daily for up to 3 years showed that the combination supplement reduced the risk of developing recurrent calcium oxalate kidney stones by 85% (Ettinger et al 1997). In a recent epidemiological study (European Prospective Investigation into Cancer and Nutrition: EPIC), participants with higher levels of fresh fruit, wholegrain fibre and dietary magnesium (low range 282, higher range 481 mg/day) were found to have a lower risk of kidney stone formation (Turney et al 2014).

M

Premenstrual syndrome (PMS)

Three early double-blind studies using oral magnesium supplements in women with PMS produced positive results for decreasing symptoms such as fluid retention and mood swings (Facchinetti et al 1991b, Rosenstein et al 1994, Walker et al 1998). According to these, clinical effects develop slowly, starting during the second menstrual cycle. More recently, an open-label study of magnesium (250 mg) in PMS showed a 35% reduction in symptoms as assessed by investigators and 33.5% improvement as assessed by participants (Quaranta et al 2007). The study of 41 women with PMS used a modified-release magnesium tablet taken at intermittent times over three menstrual cycles, beginning 20 days after the start of their last menstrual period and continuing until the start of their next menstrual period.

Although it is not clear what mechanism of action is responsible, some, but not all, studies have identified decreased magnesium concentrations in both RBC and mononuclear blood cells of women with PMS (Khine et al 2006, Rosenstein et al 1994).

To date, the evidence overall remains promising for magnesium supplementation for some women with PMS; however further studies are required for a definitive conclusion to be made (Whelan et al 2009).

Dysmenorrhoea

A Cochrane review of seven RCTs investigating the effects of various treatments for dysmenorrhoea included three trials comparing magnesium with placebo. Overall, magnesium was found to be more effective than placebo for pain relief and resulted in less extra medication being required (Doty & Attaran 2009, Wilson & Murphy 2001). It appears that decreased serum magnesium is associated with dysmenorrhoea in young female adults; however evaluation of effective dosing is not available (Kibirian 2011, Yakubova 2012).

Osteoporosis prevention

Magnesium comprises about 1% of bone mineral and is involved in a number of activities supporting bone strength, preservation and remodelling. Epidemiological studies have linked increased magnesium consumption, as part of an alkaline diet, with improved bone mineral density (BMD) (Tucker et al 1999). Chronic magnesium deficiency compromises bone health by increasing the size and brittleness of the bone crystals, inducing hypocalcaemia and possibly increasing inflammatory cytokines (Rude & Shils 2006). Therefore, low magnesium states increase the risk of osteoporosis. Several studies have investigated the effects of supplemental magnesium on bone density, generally yielding positive effects in both men and women (Tucker 2009).

One long-term study has reported an increase in bone density for magnesium hydroxide supplementation in a group of menopausal women (Sojka & Weaver 1995). After the 2-year test period, fracture incidence was also reduced. Another 2-year study showed that magnesium supplementation in postmenopausal women with osteoporosis results in increased bone mass at the wrist after 1 year, with no further increase after 2 years of supplementation (Stendig-Lindberg et al 1993). The regimen used here was oral magnesium 750 mg/day for the first 6 months, followed by 250 mg/day thereafter. In the Women's Health Initiative Observational Study, observing risk factors for osteoporotic fractures and altered BMD, low magnesium intake was associated with lower-bone (whole body, including hip) mineral density, but this did not translate to increased risk of fracture. In women who consumed magnesium via food and supplementation, baseline hip BMD and whole-body BMD was 2–3% higher than controls (Orchard et al 2014).

Clinical note — Peak bone mass

The best opportunity to influence bone mass occurs early in life. It has been estimated that approximately 40% of peak bone mass is accumulated during adolescence, with peak bone mass in the hip achieved by age 16–18 years (Weaver 2000). The spinal vertebrae are still able to increase in mass until the third decade of life, when total peak bone mass reaches 99% by age 26.6 years (± 3.7 years). As such, ensuring an adequate intake of calcium and magnesium early in life is essential for attaining optimal bone mass.

Fibromyalgia

A study of 60 premenopasual women diagnosed with fibromyalgia according to the American College of Radiology criteria and 20 healthy women matched for age and weight found that oral magnesium citrate (300 mg/day) significantly reduced the number of tender points, tender point index and Beck depression scores by the end of the 8-week treatment period (Bagis et al 2013). Interestingly, the serum and erythrocyte magnesium levels were significantly lower in patients with fibromyalgia than in the controls and there was a negative correlation between the magnesium levels and fibromyalgia symptoms.

Asthma

There is some evidence that asthmatics have low intracellular (both red and white blood cells) magnesium (Dominguez et al 1998, Mircetic et al 2001, Sedighi et al 2006). This has relevance in asthma because healthy magnesium concentrations inhibit calcium entering smooth muscles such as those in the airways and therefore potentially reduce bronchospasm (Dominguez et al 1998, Gropper et al 2009). In addition, magnesium influences pulmonary vascular muscle contractility, mast cell granulation and neurohumoral mediator release (Mathew & Altura 1988).

Results of two randomised, double-blind studies suggest that oral supplements may also significantly alleviate asthma symptoms (Bede et al 2003, Hill et al 1997). Hill et al found that treatment improved symptoms, although it failed to change objective measures of air flow or airway reactivity, and Bede et al found a significant decrease in bronchodilator use after 8 weeks compared with placebo. This was a 12-week study using oral magnesium citrate in 89 children (4–16 years) with mild or moderate persistent bronchial asthma. The dose used was 200 mg daily for children aged 7 years and 290 mg for those older than 7 years. Adding to this, a randomised double-blind trial of magnesium glycine (300 mg/day) in 37 subjects aged 7–19 years over 2 months resulted in a statistically significant reduction in bronchial reactivity, skin responses to recognised antigens and salbutamol use in the treatment group compared to placebo (Gontijo-Amaral et al 2007). Kasaks (2013) suggests magnesium supplementation may be a useful adjunct to medical management to reduce airway hyperresponsiveness and improve perceived quality of life and asthma control.

Pregnancy

Six studies suggest magnesium intake in pregnant women is less than the recommended values and gene expression at week 37 of TRPM6 denotes higher urinary excretion of magnesium, indicating an increased demand in pregnant women (Rylander 2014).

Pregnancy-induced hypertension

A double-blind RCT of pregnant primagravida women given an oral supply of 300 mg magnesium citrate from pregnancy week 25 found that the average diastolic blood pressure at week 37 was significantly lower than in the placebo group ($P = 0.031$) and the number of women with an increase in diastolic blood pressure of ≥15 mmHg was also significantly lower than with placebo ($P = 0.011$) (Bullarbo et al 2013).

Pregnancy-induced leg cramps

A 2002 Cochrane review of five RCTs of treatments for leg cramps in pregnancy concluded that the best evidence is for magnesium lactate or citrate taken as 5 mmol in the morning and 10 mmol in the evening (Young & Jewell 2002). According to a more recent double-blind RCT involving 45 women, short-term use of magnesium supplementation (120 mg magnesium citrate and magnesium lactate 360 mg daily) over 2 weeks was insufficient to modify the intensity or frequency of leg cramps compared to placebo (Nygaard et al 2008). Possibly another dose or longer-term use would be more beneficial; however this remains to be tested.

Preterm birth and low birth weight

A 2001 Cochrane review of seven studies involving 2689 women concluded that, although not all trials were positive, oral magnesium taken before the 25th week of gestation was associated with a lower frequency of preterm birth, a lower frequency of low birth weight and fewer small-for-gestational-age infants. Additionally, fewer hospitalisations during pregnancy and fewer cases of antepartum haemorrhage were associated with magnesium use (Makrides & Crowther 2014).

Pre-eclampsia and eclampsia

Parenteral magnesium is used for preventing and managing PE and eclampsia. In particular, magnesium sulfate administered intravenously or intramuscularly is used.

M

An interesting longitudinal study revealed that, while serum magnesium levels decline in both healthy and pre-eclamptic pregnant women, such a decrease occurs earlier in those women who later develop PE (Sontia & Touryz 2007). Lower measures of erythrocyte, brain and muscle magnesium have recently been observed in PE women compared to those with normal pregnancies. In addition, there was a lower risk of hypertension in PE women with higher magnesium intake. More specifically, the study of 50 patients with PE and 50 controls demonstrated severe PE with erythrocyte magnesium levels 0.62 mmol/L, mild PE with erythrocyte magnesium of 0.67 mmol/L, and normal with 0.79 mmol/L (Rylander 2014).

Diabetes mellitus

A strong association between magnesium, diabetes and hypertension has been established (Ascherio et al 1998, Dasgupta et al 2012, Sontia & Touryz 2007). Deficiency aggravates insulin resistance and contributes to an increased risk of CVD in people with diabetes.

Type 1 diabetes mellitus (T1DM)

Hypomagnesaemia is present in 25–38% of all diabetic patients secondary to glycosuria and magnesium redistribution (Paolisso et al 1992). Such depletion may occur early in the pathology, with T1DM children demonstrating progressive deterioration of serum levels within 2 years of diagnosis in some (Tuvemo et al 1997), but not all, studies. Magnesium depletion in T1DM has also been linked to earlier atherosclerotic development (Atabek et al 2006, Djurhuus et al 1999), polyneuropathy (De Leeuw et al 2004), advanced retinopathy (de Valk et al 1999) and immunosuppression (Cojocaru et al 2006). Supplementation studies have produced mixed results (Eibl et al 1998); however, magnesium supplementation may reduce risks of secondary pathology.

Consistent with these findings, some researchers suggest T1DM patients receive a high dose in the first month of treatment to normalise RBC and serum magnesium and then remain on continuous lower-dose supplementation (e.g. 300 mg/day) in order to avoid a return to hypomagnesaemia (Eibl et al 1998). Lower serum magnesium levels are found in young patients with poor glycaemic control (0.79 ± 0.09 vs 0.82 ± 0.09 mmol/L, respectively; $P = 0.002$). In youths with T1DM, low magnesium levels provide inadequate glycaemic control ($HbA_{1C} > 7.5\%$). Higher levels of magnesium concentration present a decrease of 1.7% in HbA_{1C} (Galli-Tsinopoulou et al 2014).

Type 2 diabetes mellitus (T2DM)

Epidemiological studies have drawn a link between poor dietary and/or serum magnesium and an increased risk of T2DM (Chambers et al 2006, Dasgupta et al 2012, He et al 2006, van Dam et al 2006). In one large study those in the lowest tertile of magnesium and fibre intakes exhibited a three to four times greater risk (Bo et al 2006). Serum magnesium depletion is also evident in ≈ 25–38% patients. Hypomagnesaemia in diabetic patients appears to exacerbate impaired insulin resistance, elevated fasting blood glucose and HbA_{1C} concentrations (He et al 2006, Walti et al 2003). Oral magnesium (magnesium chloride 2.5 g/day for 4 months) adjunctive to hypoglycaemic medication has produced reductions of fasting glucose (−37.5%), HbA_{1C} (−30.4%), homeostasis model assessment-insulin resistance index (−9.5%) and insulin (Rodriguez-Moran & Guerrero-Romero 2003), while other studies demonstrate increased insulin levels with improved action (Paolisso et al 1992). In another study, a combination of magnesium (200 mg/day), zinc (30 mg/day) and vitamins (C 200 mg/day and E 150 mg/day) over 3 months significantly increased levels of HDL and apo-A1 24% and 8.8%, respectively (Farvid et al 2004).

Several RCTs and a meta-analysis of prospective cohort studies investigating oral magnesium supplementation have shown improvements in diabetic control (Dong et al 2011, Paolisso et al 1992, Rodriguez-Moran & Guerrero-Romero 2003). A double-blind trial that involved 63 patients with T2DM and reduced serum magnesium levels (treated with glibenclamide) demonstrated that the addition of oral magnesium over 16 weeks significantly improves IS and metabolic control (Rodriguez-Moran & Guerrero-Romero 2003). In a meta-analysis of prospective cohort studies involving 536,318 participants, a dose-responsive relative risk for type 2 diabetes for 100 mg/day increment in magnesium intake was 0.86 (95% confidence interval 0.82–0.89) (Dong et al 2011).

Chronic leg cramps

Two randomised, double-blind studies have investigated the use of oral magnesium supplements in people with leg cramps. Frusso et al (1999) conducted a crossover trial involving 45 individuals who had experienced at least six cramps during the previous month. Subjects were given 1 month of oral magnesium citrate (900 mg twice daily) followed by a matching placebo for 1 month, or vice versa. This treatment regimen failed to reduce the severity, duration or number of nocturnal leg cramps. In contrast, Roffe et al (2002) tested magnesium citrate equivalent to 300 mg magnesium in subjects suffering regular leg cramps and identified a trend towards fewer cramps with active treatment ($P = 0.07$). Significantly more subjects thought that the treatment had helped after magnesium than after placebo — 36 (78%) and 25 (54%) respectively. Interestingly, in both studies patients improved over time regardless of the treatment they received.

Although two additional studies in athletes found no correlation between cramping incidence and serum magnesium, the authors suggest that the cramping was caused by increased neuromuscular excitability (Schwellnus et al 2004, Sulzer et al 2005), which is a classic feature of magnesium deficiency (Rude & Shils 2006). As is the case with much magnesium research, more accurate and validated assessment methods may be required to elicit the true relationship between magnesium status and this presentation.

Cancer

Colorectal cancer (CRC)

A meta-analysis of prospective studies suggests that higher magnesium intake is inversely related to the risk of CRC. In dose–response analyses, summary relative risks for incremental magnesium intake of 50 mg/day in colorectal, colon and rectal cancer were 0.95, 0.93 and 0.93 respectively. In a case–control study on colorectal adenomas (three) and carcinomas (six prospective cohort studies) meta-analysis, for every 100-mg/day elevation in magnesium intake, there was an associated 13% lower risk of colorectal adenomas and 12% lower risk of CRC (Chen et al 2012, Wark et al 2012).

Lung cancer

There is limited evidence to suggest an association between risk of lung cancer and lower calcium and magnesium levels (Cheng et al 2012).

Prostate cancer

There is a possible relationship between low blood magnesium levels and high calcium-to-magnesium ratio and high-grade prostate cancer. More studies are needed (Dai et al 2011).

M

OTHER POSSIBLE USES

Oral magnesium supplements are used in a variety of different conditions, most notably those involving muscle spasm or tension, pain and/or psychological and physical symptoms of stress and hyperexcitability. This includes irritable bowel syndrome, restless legs syndrome, chronic fatigue syndrome, anxiety states, tension headaches and insomnia. Preliminary evidence suggests that it may be beneficial for women with detrusor muscle instability (incontinence) or sensory urgency.

DOSAGE RANGE

Australian RDI for adults

Men

- 19–30 years: 400 mg/day.
- >30 years: 420 mg/day.

Women

- 19–30 years: 310 mg/day.
- >30 years: 320 mg/day.

Pregnancy

- ≤18 years: 400 mg/day.
- >19–30 years: 350 mg/day.
- >31–50 years: 360 mg/day.

Lactation

- ≤18 years: 360 mg/day.
- >18–30 years: 310 mg/day.
- >31–50 years: 320 mg/day.

According to clinical studies

- ADHD: 6 mg/kg/day ± 0.6–0.8 mg/kg/day vitamin B_6.
- Arrhythmia prevention in congestive heart failure: magnesium chloride 3204 mg/day in divided doses.
- ASD: 6 mg/kg/day ± 0.6–0.8 mg/kg/day vitamin B_6.
- CAD symptoms: oral magnesium citrate (15 mmol twice daily as Magnosolv-Granulat, total magnesium 365 mg).
- Cancer risk reduction CRC: >100 mg/day.
- Dyslipidaemia: 600 mg/day magnesium pidolate.
- Fibromylagia: 300 mg/day.
- Hypertension: 360–600 mg/day.
- Kidney stone prevention: magnesium hydroxide 400–500 mg/day.
- Migraine: 600 mg trimagnesium dicitrate daily.
- Migraine prophylaxis in children: magnesium oxide (9 mg/kg/day).
- Mitral valve prolapse: three tablets magnesium carbonate 600 mg (7 mmol of elementary magnesium) daily for the first week followed by two tablets daily.
- Nocturnal leg cramps: magnesium citrate equivalent to 300 mg magnesium daily.
- Osteoporosis prevention: taken on an empty stomach, 250 mg three times daily for 6 months, followed by 250 mg/day for 18 months.
- Paediatric asthma: magnesium citrate 200–300 mg daily.
- PMS general symptoms: 260 mg/day.
- PMS fluid retention symptoms: 200 mg magnesium (as magnesium oxide) daily.

- PMS mood swings: magnesium pyrrolidone carboxylic acid (360 mg) taken three times daily, from day 15 of the menstrual cycle to the onset of menstrual flow.
- Postoperative recovery from cardiac surgery: 1200 mg magnesium orotate in combination with 300 mg CoQ10, 300 mg alpha-lipoic acid and 3 g omega-3 oils taken daily 1 month prior to surgery.
- Stroke prevention 228–471 mg/day.
- T1DM: initial high dose to normalise serum levels and then continuous 300 mg daily.
- T2DM: 2.5 g magnesium dichloride daily or 300 mg elemental magnesium in combination with 30 mg zinc, 250 mg vitamin C and 150 mg vitamin E daily.

ADVERSE REACTIONS

The most common adverse effects of oral supplements are diarrhoea (18.6%) and gastric irritation (4.7%) (Peikert et al 1996). It can be found as a primary ingredient in some laxatives (magnesium hydroxide) providing 500 mg of elemental magnesium (Guerrera et al 2009). Typically, doses of inorganic preparations supplying above 350 mg/day (elemental) may be associated with adverse effects. Dividing total daily supplemental amounts over two to three separate doses may help to reduce this risk and maximise bioavailability.

TOXICITY

The possibility of hypermagnesaemia is rare, and is seen mostly in the elderly, people with renal insufficiency, dialysis or with serious bowel disorders.

Mild hypermagnesaemia signs and symptoms are subtle, such as light-headedness, headache, nausea, flushing and warmth.

At levels between 6 and 12 mg/dL (5–10 mEq/L), electrocardiographic changes occur with prolonged reportedly similar changes to hyperkalaemia. Concentrations of 9–12 mg/dL may increase hypotension, loss of deep tendon reflex and somnolence. Levels >12 mg/dL (10 mEq/L) may initiate muscle paralysis, arrhythmias, hypoventilations, stupor, sinoatrial and atrioventricular block and ventricular arrhythmias. Levels exceeding 15.6 mg/dL (13 mEq/L) may result in coma, respiratory arrest and cardiac asystole (Jhang et al 2013).

SIGNIFICANT INTERACTIONS

The interactions included in this section are relevant for oral supplementation and do not refer to other administration routes, although there may be an overlap.

Alcohol

Alcohol consumption results in increased urinary losses of magnesium and therefore with higher chronic ingestion additional magnesium replacement may be necessary.

Aminoglycosides (e.g. gentamicin)

Drug may reduce absorption of magnesium — monitor for signs and symptoms of magnesium deficiency, as increased magnesium intake may be required with long-term therapy.

Calcium

Magnesium and calcium deficiencies usually coexist due to magnesium's key role in active PTH and vitamin D production (Gropper et al 2009, Rude & Shils 2006, Wester 1987). Conversely, if magnesium intakes are excessive, calcium levels decline due to inhibition of PTH release and increased renal excretion. There is additional redistribution with impaired calcium influx and release from intracellular stores. Magnesium can also bind calcium-binding sites and mimic its actions (Gropper et al 2009, Rude & Shils 2006).

Calcium-channel blockers

Magnesium may enhance the hypotensive effect of calcium-channel blockers: monitor patients and their drug requirements — possible beneficial interaction under supervision.

Fluoroquinolones

Magnesium may decrease absorption of fluoroquinolone antibiotics — separate doses by at least 2 hours before or 4 hours after oral magnesium.

Loop diuretics and thiazide diuretics

Increased magnesium intake may be required with long-term therapy because of increased urinary excretion — monitor magnesium efficacy and status with long-term drug use.

Potassium

Hypomagnesaemia results in hypokalaemia due to increased potassium efflux from cells and renal excretion (Gropper et al 2009, Rude & Shils 2006).

Potassium-sparing diuretics

May increase the effects of supplemental magnesium — observe patients taking this combination.

Tetracycline antibiotics

Tetracyclines form insoluble complexes with magnesium, thereby reducing absorption of both — separate doses by at least 2 hours.

Dasatinib

May increase magnesium blood levels — observe (Vest & Cho 2012).

Neuromuscular blockers

May potentiate effects of neuroblockers — observe (Amgen Inc 2012, Kim et al 2012).

L-thyroxine

Case studies suggest reduced effectiveness of levothyroxine with magnesium-containing antacids and laxatives (Pinard et al 2003) — observe.

CONTRAINDICATIONS AND PRECAUTIONS

- Magnesium supplementation should be done cautiously in people with compromised renal function and is contraindicated in renal failure and heart block (unless a pacemaker is present).
- Hypermagnesaemia can develop in patients with renal failure and receiving magnesium-containing antacids or laxatives and with accidental Epsom salt ingestion.
- Overuse of magnesium hydroxide or magnesium sulfate may cause deficiencies of other minerals or lead to toxicity.

PREGNANCY USE

Pregnant women and nursing mothers are advised to consume sufficient magnesium (see Australian RDI under Dosage range, above).

PATIENTS' FAQs

What will this supplement do for me?

Magnesium is essential for health and wellbeing. Although used to prevent or treat deficiency states, it is also used to alleviate many conditions, such as CVD and PMS, and prevent migraine and muscular spasms.

When will it start to work?

This will depend on the indication it is being used to treat.

Are there any safety issues?

In high doses, some magnesium supplements can cause diarrhoea. High-dose supplements should not be used by people with severe kidney disease or heart block.

Practice points/Patient counselling

- Magnesium is an essential mineral in human nutrition with a wide range of biological functions.
- Low magnesium states are associated with several serious diseases, such as congestive heart failure, ischaemic heart disease, cardiac arrhythmias, hypertension, mitral valve prolapse, metabolic syndrome, stroke, diabetes mellitus, hyperlipidaemia, pre-eclampsia and eclampsia.
- Although supplementation is traditionally used to correct or avoid deficiency states, research has also shown a role in the management of numerous disease states, e.g. asthma, CVD, PMS, dysmenorrhoea, migraine prevention, diabetes, kidney stone prevention, osteoporosis prevention, dyspepsia and constipation. Preliminary research also suggests a possible benefit in ADHD, autism, women with detrusor muscle instability (incontinence) and pregnancy-induced leg cramps.
- Oral magnesium supplements are also used in a variety of different conditions, most notably those involving muscle spasm or tension, pain and/or psychological and physical symptoms of stress and hyperexcitability.
- Numerous drug interactions exist, so care should be taken to ensure safe use.

M

REFERENCES

Allen LH Magnesium. Encyclopedia of Human Nutrition (3rd edn) 2013;131–135.

Alon I et al. Intracellular magnesium in elderly patients with heart failure: effects of diabetes and renal dysfunction. J Trace Elem Med Biol 20.4 (2006): 221–226.

Amgen Inc. Vectibix (panitumumab) prescribing information (revised 08/2012). Available at http://pi.amgen.com/united_states/vectibix/vectibix_pi.pdf. Accessed October 3, 2012.

Amoozagar H, et al. The prevalence of hypomagnesaemia in pediatric patients with mitral valve prolapse syndrome and the effect of Mg therapy, 2012. Int Cardiovasc Res J 6:3;92–5.

Anderson RA. A complementary approach to urolithiasis prevention. World J Urol 20.5 (2002): 294–301.

Andon M et al. Magnesium balance in adolescent females consuming a low- or high-calcium diet. AJCN 63 (1996): 950–953.

Arnaud MJ. Update on the assessment of magnesium status. Br J Nutr 99 (Suppl 3) (2008): S24–S36.

Ascherio A et al. Intake of potassium, magnesium, calcium, and fiber and risk of stroke among US men. Circulation 98.12 (1998): 1198–1204.

Atabek M et al. Serum magnesium concentrations in type 1 diabetic patients: relation to early atherosclerosis (abstract). Diabetes Res Clin Pract 72.1 (2006): 42–47.

Bagis, S., et al. 2013. Is magnesium citrate treatment effective on pain, clinical parameters and functional status in patients with fibromyalgia? Rheumatol.Int., 33, (1) 167–172.

Bashir Y et al. Effects of long-term oral magnesium chloride replacement in congestive heart failure secondary to coronary artery disease. Am J Cardiol 72.15 (1993): 1156–1162.

Bayir A et al. Serum and cerebrospinal fluid magnesium levels, Glasgow coma scores, and in-hospital mortality in patients with acute stroke. Biol Trace Elem Res (2009 Jan 23): Epub ahead of print.

Bede O et al. Urinary magnesium excretion in asthmatic children receiving magnesium supplementation: a randomized, placebo-controlled, double-blind study. Magnes Res 16.4 (2003): 262–270.

Bo S et al. Dietary magnesium and fiber intakes and inflammatory and metabolic indicators in middle-aged subjects from a population-based cohort. AJCN 84.5 (2006): 1062–1069.

Boska MD et al. Contrasts in cortical magnesium, phospholipid and energy metabolism between migraine syndromes. Neurology 58.8 (2002): 1227–1233.

Braunwald E et al. Harrison's principles of internal medicine. New York: McGraw Hill, 2003.

Bullarbo, M., et al. 2013. Magnesium supplementation to prevent high blood pressure in pregnancy: a randomised placebo control trial. Arch.Gynecol.Obstet., 288, (6) 1269–1274.

Burgess DC, et al. Interventions for prevention of post-operative atrial fibrillation and its complications after cardiac surgery: a meta-analysis. Eur Heart J 27.23 (2006): 2846–2857.

Catling LA et al. A systematic review of analytical observational studies investigating the association between cardiovascular disease and drinking water hardness. J Water Health 6.4 (2008): 433–42.

Chacko SA, et al. Relations of dietary magnesium intake to biomarkers of inflammation and endothelial dysfunction in an ethnically diverse cohort of postmenopausal women. Diabetes Care 2010;33(2):304–310.

Chambers E et al. Serum magnesium and type-2 diabetes in African Americans and Hispanics: a New York Cohort. J Am Coll Nutr 25.6 (2006): 509–513.

Chen, G. C., et al. Magnesium intake and risk of colorectal cancer: a meta-analysis of prospective studies. Eur J Clin Nutr. 2012. 66(11):1182–6.

Cheng, M. H., et al. Calcium and magnesium in drinking-water and risk of death from lung cancer in women. Magnesium Research. 25(3):112–119, 2012.

Chiuve, S. E., et al. Plasma and dietary magnesium and risk of sudden cardiac death in women. American Journal of Clinical Nutrition. 93(2):253–260, 2011.

Classen H. Magnesium orotate — experimental and clinical evidence. Rom J Intern Med 42.3 (2004): 491–501.

Coffin B, et al. Efficacy of a simethicone, activated charcoal and magnesium oxide combination (Carbosymag ®) in functional dyspepsia: Results of a general practice-based randomized trial. Clinics and Research in Hepatology and Gastroenterology 2011: 35;6–7;494–499.

Cojocaru M et al. The effect of magnesium deficit on serum immunoglobulin concentrations in type 1 diabetes mellitus. Rom J Intern Med 44.1 (2006): 61–67.

Cojocaru IM et al. Serum magnesium in patients with acute ischemic stroke. Rom J Intern Med 45.3 (2007): 269–273.

Coudray C et al. Study of magnesium bioavailability from the organic and inorganic Mg salts in Mg-depleted rats using a stable isotope approach. Magnes Res 18.4 (2005): 215–223.

Dai, Q., et al. Blood magnesium, and the interaction with calcium, on the risk of high-grade prostate cancer. PLoS One. 6(4):e18237, 2011.

Dasgupta A, et al. Hypomagnesemia in type 2 diabetes mellitus. Indian J Endocrin Metab. 2012; 16:6; 1000–1003.

Djurhuus MS et al. Effect of moderate improve- ment in metabolic control on magnesium and lipid concentrations in patients with type 1 diabetes. Diabetes Care 22.4 (1999): 546–554.

De Leeuw I et al. Long term magnesium supplementation influences favourably the natural evolution of neuropathy in Mg-depleted type 1 diabetic patients (1DM). (abstract). Magnes Res 17.2 (2004): 109–114.

de Valk H et al. Plasma magnesium concentration and progression of retinopathy. Diabetes Care 22.5 (1999): 864–865.

Dominguez L et al. Bronchial reactivity and intracellular magnesium: a possible mechanism for the bronchodilating effects of magnesium in asthma (abstract). Clin Sci (Lond) 95.2 (1998): 137–142.

Dong Jy, et al. Magnesium intake and risk of type 2 diabetes:meta-analysis of prospective cohort studies. Diabetes Care 2011. 34:9;2116–22.

Doty E. & Attaran C. (2009). Managing primary dysmenorrhea. Journal of Pediatric and Adolescent Gynecology 19 (5): 341–344.

Eibl N, et al. Magnesium supplementation in type 2 diabetes (Letter). Diabetes Care 21 (1998): 2031–2032.

Ellen GHM. Short-chain fructo-oligosaccharides improve magnesium absorption in adolescent girls with a low calcium intake. Nutr Res 29.4 (2009): 229–237.

Ettinger B et al. Potassium-magnesium citrate is an effective prophylaxis against recurrent calcium oxalate nephrolithiasis. J Urol 158.6 (1997): 2069–2073.

Facchinetti F et al. Magnesium prophylaxis of menstrual migraine: effects on intracellular magnesium. Headache 31.5 (1991a): 298–301.

Facchinetti F et al. Oral magnesium successfully relieves premenstrual mood changes. Obstet Gynecol 78.2 (1991b): 177–81.

Farvid MS et al. The impact of vitamins and/or mineral supplementation on blood pressure in type 2 diabetes. J Am Coll Nutr 23.3 (2004): 272–9.

Feillet-Coudray C et al. Exchangeable magnesium pool masses reflect the magnesium status of rats. J Nutr 130.9 (2000): 2306–2311.

Feng, P., et al. Association between concentrations of serum magnesium and the short-term outcome of patients with acute ischemic stroke. Department of Epidemiology, School Of Public Health of medical College, China 2012. 33(11):1171–1175.

Fine K et al. Intestinal absorption of magnesium from food and supplements. J Clin Invest 88 (1991): 396–402.
Firoz M, Graber M. Bioavailability of US commercial magnesium preparations. Magnes Res 14.4 (2001): 257–262.
Flight I, Clifton P. Cereal grains and legumes in the prevention of coronary heart disease and stroke: a review of the literature. Eur J Clin Nutr 60.10 (2006): 1145–1159.
Ford E, Mokdad A. Dietary magnesium intake in a national sample of U.S. adults. J.Nutr 133 (2003): 2879–2882.
Fox C, et al. Magnesium: its proven and potential clinical significance. South Med J 94.12 (2001): 1195–1201.
Frishman WH, et al. Alternative and complementary medical approaches in the prevention and treatment of cardiovascular disease. Current Prob Cardiol 30.8 (2005): 383–459.
Frusso R et al. Magnesium for the treatment of nocturnal leg cramps: a crossover randomized trial. J Fam Pract 48.11 (1999): 868–871.
Galli-Tsinopoulou A et al., Association between magnesium concentration and HbA1c in children and adolescents with type 1 diabetes mellitus. Journal of Diabetes 2014 ;6;4; 369–377.
Ghanizadeh A. A systematic review of magnesium therapy for treating ADHD. Archives of Iranian Medicine 2013 16:7; 412–417.
Gontijo-Amaral C et al. Oral magnesium supplementation in asthmatic children: a double-blind randomized placebo-controlled trial. Eur J Clin Nutr 61.1 (2007): 54–60.
Grimaldi BL. The central role of magnesium deficiency in Tourette's syndrome: causal relationships between magnesium deficiency, altered biochemical pathways and symptoms relating to Tourette's syndrome and several reported comorbid conditions. Med Hypotheses 58.1 (2002): 47–60.
Gropper S, et al. Advanced nutrition and human metabolism, 5th edn. Belmont: Thomson Wadsworth, 2009.
Guerrera MP, et al. Therapeutic uses of magnesium. Am Fam Physician 2009;80:157–62.
Guerrero-Romero F, Rodriguez-Moran M. Low serum magnesium levels and metabolic syndrome. Acta Diabetol 39.4 (2002): 209–213.
Hadj A et al. Pre-operative preparation for cardiac surgey utilising a combination of metabolic, physical and mental therapy. Heart Lung Circ 15.3 (2006): 172–181.
Hadjistavri, L. S., et al. Beneficial effects of oral magnesium supplementation on insulin sensitivity and serum lipid profile. Med Sci Monit. 16(6):13–18, 2010.
Haenni A, et al. Atherogenic lipid fractions are related to ionized magnesium status. AJCN 67 (1998): 202–207.
Hartwig A. Role of magnesium in genomic stability. Mutat Res. 2001;475(1–2):113–121.
He K et al. Magnesium intake and incidence of metabolic syndrome among young adults. Circulation 113 (2006): 1675–1682.
Hill J et al. Investigation of the effect of short-term change in dietary magnesium intake in asthma. Eur Respir J 10.10 (1997): 2225–2229.
Holland S, et al. Evidence-based guideline update: NSAIDs and other complementary treatments for episodic migraine prevention in adults. Neurology 2012;78:1346–53.
Jhang WK, et al. Severe hypermagnesemia presenting with abnormal electrocardiographic findings similar to those of hyperkalemia in a child undergoing peritoneal dialysis. Korean J Pediatr. 2013:56;7:308–311.
Johnson S. The multifaceted and widespread pathology of magnesium deficiency. Med Hypotheses 56.2 (2001): 163–170.
Khan L et al. Serum and urinary magnesium in young diabetic subjects in Bangladesh. AJCN 69 (1999): 70–73.
Khine K et al. Magnesium (Mg) retention and mood effects after intravenous Mg infusion in premenstrual dysphoric disorder. Biol Psychiatry 59.4 (2006): 327–333.
Kidd P. Autism, an extreme challenge to integrative medicine. Part II: Medical management. Alt Med Rev 7.6 (2002): 472–499.
Kim MH, et al. A randomised controlled trial comparing rocuronium priming, magnesium pre-treatment and a combination of the two methods. Anaesthesia. 2012;67(7):748–754.
Kitlinski M et al. Is magnesium deficit in lymphocytes a part of the mitral valve prolapse syndrome? Magnes Res 17.1 (2004): 39–45.
Klevay L, Milne D. Low dietary magnesium increases supraventricular ectopy. AJCN 75 (2002): 550–554.
Kozielec T, Starobrat-Hermelin B. Assessment of magnesium levels in children with attention deficit hyperactivity disorder (ADHD). Magnes Res 10.2 (1997): 143–148.
Larsson SC et al. Magnesium, calcium, potassium, and sodium intakes and risk of stroke in male smokers. Arch Intern Med 168.5 (2008): 459–465.
Lewis N et al. Calcium supplements and milk: effects on acid-base balance and on retention of calcium magnesium, phosphorus. AJCN 49 (1989): 527–533.
Lichodziejewska B et al. Clinical symptoms of mitral valve prolapse are related to hypomagnesemia and attenuated by magnesium supplementation. Am J Cardiol 79.6 (1997): 768–772.
Lindberg J et al. Magnesium bioavailability from magnesium citrate and magnesium oxide. J Am Coll Nutr 9.1 (1990): 48–55.
Lukaski H. Magnesium, zinc, and chromium nutriture and physical activity. AJCN 72 (Suppl) (2000): 585S–593S.
Ma J et al. Associations of serum and dietary magnesium with cardiovascular disease, hypertension, diabetes, insulin, and carotid arterial wall thickness: the ARIC study. (Atherosclerosis Risk in Communities Study). J Clin Epidemiol 48.7 (1995): 927–940.
Makrides M., Crowther CA. Magnesium supplementation in pregnancy. Cochrane Database Syst Rev. 2014;4:CD000937.
Marken PA et al. Effects of magnesium oxide on the lipid profile of healthy volunteers. Atherosclerosis 77 (1989): 37–42.
Mathew R, Altura BM. Magnesium and the lungs. Magnesium 7.4 (1988): 173–187.
Mauskop A, Altura BM. Role of magnesium in the pathogenesis and treatment of migraines. Clin Neurosci 5.1 (1998): 24–27.

Mauskop A, Varughese J. Why all migraine patients should be treated with magnesium. Journal of Neural Transmission 2012; 119:5:575–9.

McDermott KC, et al. The diagnosis and management of hypomagnesemia: a unique treatment approach and case report. Oncol Nurs Forum 18.7 (1991): 1145–1152.

McKeown NM, et al. Dietary magnesium intake is related to metabolic syndrome in older Americans. Eur J Nutr. Jun 2008;47(4):210–216.

Mircetic R et al. Magnesium concentration in plasma, leukocytes and urine of children with intermittent asthma (abstract). Clin Chim Acta 312.1–2 (2001): 197–203.

Mousain-Bosc M et al. Magnesium VitB6 Intake reduces central nervous system hyperexcitability in children. J Am Coll Nutr 23.5 (2004): 545S–548S.

Mousain-Bosc M et al. Improvement of neurobehavioural disorders in children supplemented with magnesium-vitamin B6. II. Pervasive developmental disorder (abstract). Magnes Res 19.1 (2006a): 53–62.

Mousain-Bosc, M., et al. Improvement of neurobehavioral disorders in children supplemented with magnesium-vitamin B6. I. Attention deficit hyperactivity disorders. Magnesium Research. 19(1):46–52, 2006b.

NHMRC. Nutrient reference values for Australia and New Zealand including recommended dietary intakes: Australian Government Department of Health and Ageing, Canberra, 2005.

Nie ZL, et al. Magnesium intake and incidence of stroke: Meta analysis of cohort studies. Nutrition, Metabolism and Cardiovascular Diseases 2013. 23:3; 169–176.

Nye C, Brice A. Combined vitamin B6-magnesium treatment in autism spectrum disorder. Cochrane Database Syst Rev 19.4 (2005): CD003497.

Nygaard IH, et al. Does oral magnesium substitution relieve pregnancy-induced leg cramps? European Journal of Obstetrics & Gynecology and Reproductive Biology 2008:141;1;23–26.

Orchard TS et al. Magnesium intake, bone mineral density, and fractures: results from the Women's Health Initiative Observational Study. Am J Clin Nutr 2014: 99;4;926–933.

Orr SL, Venkateswaran S. Nutraceuticals in the prophylaxis of pediatric migraine: Evidence-based review and recommendations. 2014 Cephalalgia. abstract available online http://www.ncbi.nlm.nih.gov/pubmed/24443395 ?dopt=Abstract accessed 14 th June 2014.

Paolisso G et al. Daily magnesium supplements improve glucose handling in elderly subjects. Am J Clin Nutr 55.6 (1992): 1161–1167.

Peikert A, et al. Prophylaxis of migraine with oral magnesium: results from a prospective, multi-center, placebo-controlled and double-blind randomized study. Cephalalgia 16.4 (1996): 257–263.

Pfaffenrath V et al. Magnesium in the prophylaxis of migraine: a double-blind placebo-controlled study. Cephalalgia 16.6 (1996): 436–440.

Pfeiffer S et al. Efficacy of vitamin B6 and magnesium in the treatment of autism: a methodology review and summary of outcomes. J Autism Dev Disord 25.5 (1995): 481–493.

Pinard AM, et al. Magnesium potentiates neuromuscular blockade with cisatracurium during cardiac surgery. Can J Anaesth. Feb 2003;50(2):172–178.

Quamme GA. Recent developments in intestinal magnesium absorption. Curr Opin Gastroenterol. Mar 2008;24(2):230–235.

Quaranta S et al. Pilot study of the efficacy and safety of a modified-release magnesium 250 mg tablet (Sincromag) for the treatment of premenstrual syndrome. Clin Drug Investig 27.1 (2007): 51–58.

Rasmussen HS et al. Magnesium deficiency in patients with ischemic heart disease with and without acute myocardial infarction uncovered by an intravenous loading test. Arch Intern Med 148.2 (1988): 329–332.

Rasmussen HS et al. Influence of magnesium substitution therapy on blood lipid composition in patients with ischemic heart disease: a double-blind, placebo controlled study. Arch Intern Med 149.5 (1989): 1050–1053.

Reynolds JEF et al. Martindale extra pharmacopoeia, 28th edn. London: The Pharmaceutical Press, 1982.

Rodriguez-Moran M, Guerrero-Romero F. Oral magnesium supplementation improves insulin sensitivity and metabolic control in type 2 diabetic subjects: a randomized double-blind controlled trial. Diabetes Care 26.4 (2003): 1147–1152.

Rodriguez-Moran M, Guerrero-Romero F. Oral magnesium supplementation improves the metabolic profile of metabolically obese, normal weight individuals: A randomized double blind, placebo-controlled trial. Archives of Medical Research 2014. Online http://www.sciencedirect.com/science/article/pii/S0188440914000782 accessed 12th June 2014.

Roffe C et al. Randomised, cross-over, placebo controlled trial of magnesium citrate in the treatment of chronic persistent leg cramps. Med Sci Monit 8.5 (2002): CR326–CR330.

Rosenstein DL et al. Magnesium measures across the menstrual cycle in premenstrual syndrome. Biol Psychiatry 35.8 (1994): 557–561.

Rude RK. Magnesium. In: Coates PM et al. eds. Encyclopedia of dietary supplements, 2nd edn. New York, NY: Informa Healthcare; 2010:527–37.

Rude R, Shils M. Magnesium. In: Shils M (ed), Modern nutrition in health and disease, 10th edn. Baltimore: Lippincott, Williams & Wilkins, 2006, pp 223–47.

Rude RK, et al. Skeletal and hormonal effects of magnesium deficiency. J Am Coll Nutr 2009;28(2):131–141.

Rylander R, Magnesium in pregnancy blood pressure and pre-eclampsia — A review. Pregnancy Hypertension 4, (2), 2014, 146–149.

Rylander R et al. Acid-base status affects renal magnesium losses in healthy, elderly persons. J.Nutr 136.9 (2006): 2374–2377.

Sanders GT, et al Magnesium in disease: a review with special emphasis on the serum ionized magnesium. Clin Chem Lab Med 37.11–12 (1999): 1011–1033.

Saris NE et al. Magnesium: an update on physiological, clinical and analytical aspects. Clin Chim Acta 294.1–2 (2000): 1–26.

Schwellnus M et al. Serum electrolyte concentrations and hydration status are not associated with exercise associated muscle cramping (EAMC) in distance runners. Br J Sports Med 38.4 (2004): 488.

Sedighi M et al. Low magnesium concentration in erythrocytes of children with acute asthma (abstract). Iran J Allergy Asthma Immunol 5.4 (2006): 183–186.

Shattock MJ, et al. The ionic basis of the anti-ischemic and anti-arrhythmic properties of magnesium in the heart. J Am Coll Nutr 6.1 (1987): 27–33.

Shechter M, Magnesium and cardiovascular system. Magnesium Research 2010, 23:2;60–72.

Shechter M et al. Oral magnesium supplementation inhibits platelet-dependent thrombosis in patients with coronary artery disease. Am J Cardiol 84.2 (1999): 152–156.

Shechter M et al. Oral magnesium therapy improves endothelial function in patients with coronary artery disease. Circulation 102.19 (2000): 2353–2358.

Shechter M et al. Effects of oral magnesium therapy on exercise tolerance, exercise-induced chest pain, and quality of life in patients with coronary artery disease. Am J Cardiol 91.5 (2003): 517–521.

Shils M. Experimental human magnesium depletion. AJCN 15 (1964): 133–143.

Shils M, Rude R. Deliberations and evaluations of the approaches endpoints and paradigms for magnesium dietary recommendations. J Nutr 126 (1996): 2398S–2403S.

Shils ME et al. Magnesium. In: Modern nutrition in health and disease, 9th edn. Baltimore: Williams and Wilkins, 1999; Ch 9.

Sojka JE, Weaver CM. Magnesium supplementation and osteoporosis. Nutr Rev 53.3 (1995): 71–74.

Song Y et al. Dietary magnesium intake and risk of incident hypertension among middle-aged and older US women in a 10-year follow-up study. Am J Cardiol 98.12 (2006): 1616–1621.

Song Y, et al. Magnesium intake and plasma concentrations of markers of systemic inflammation and endothelial dysfunction in women. Am J Clin Nutr 2007;85(4):1068–1074.

Sontia B, Touryz RM. Role of magnesium in hypertension. Arch Biochem Biophys 458.1 (2007): 33–39.

Stendig-Lindberg G, et al. Trabecular bone density in a two year controlled trial of perioral magnesium in osteoporosis. Magnes Res 6.2 (1993): 155–163.

Strambi M et al. Magnesium profile in autism. Biol Trace Elem Res 109.2 (2006): 97–104.

Sulzer N, et al. Serum electrolytes in Ironman triathletes with exercise-associated muscle cramping (abstract). Med Sci Sports Exerc 37.7 (2005): 1081–1085.

Swaminathan R. Magnesium metabolism and its disorders. Clin Biochem Rev 2003;24(2):47–66.

Taubert K. Magnesium in migraine: results of a multicenter pilot study. Fortschr Med 112.24 (1994): 328–330.

Thomas J et al. Free and total magnesium in lymphocytes of migraine patients: effect of magnesium-rich mineral water intake. Clin Chim Acta 295.1–2 (2000): 63–75.

Topf JM, Murray PT. Hypomagnesemia and hypermagnesemia. Rev Endocr Metab Disord. May 2003;4(2):195–206.

Tucker KL. Osteoporosis prevention and nutrition. Curr Osteoporos Rep 2009; 7:111–7.

Tucker K et al. Potassium magnesium, and fruit and vegetable intakes are associated with greater bone mineral density in elderly men and women. AJCN 69 (1999): 727–736.

Turney BW et al. Diet and risk of kidney stones in the Oxford cohort of the European Prospective Investigation into Cancer and Nutrition (EPIC). Eur J Epidemiol 2014, 29: 363–369.

Turnlund J et al. Vitamin B-6 depletion followed by repletion with animal- or plant-source diets and calcium and magnesium metabolism in young women. AJCN 56 (1992): 905–910.

Tuvemo T et al. Serum magnesium and protein concentrations during the first five years of insulin-dependent diabetes in children. Acta Paediatr 418 (Suppl) (1997): 7–10.

van Dam R et al. Dietary calcium and magnesium, major food sources, and risk of type 2 diabetes in U.S. black women. Diabetes Care 29 (2006): 2238–2243.

Vest AR, Cho LS. Hypertension in pregnancy. Cardiol Clin 2012;30(3):407–423.

Walker AF et al. Magnesium supplementation alleviates premenstrual symptoms of fluid retention. J Womens Health 7.9 (1998): 1157–1165.

Walker AF et al. Mg citrate found more bioavailable than other Mg preparations in a randomised, double-blind study. Magnes Res 16.3 (2003): 183–191.

Walti M et al. Measurement of magnesium absorption and retention in type 2 diabetic patients with the use of stable isotopes. AJCN 78 (2003): 448–453.

Wang F et al. Oral magnesium oxide prophylaxis of frequent migrainous headache in children: a randomized, double-blind, placebo-controlled trial. Headache 43.6 (2003): 601–610.

Wark, P. A., et al. Magnesium intake and colorectal tumor risk: a case-control study and meta-analysis. American Journal of Clinical Nutrition. 96(3):622–631, 2012.

Weaver CM. Calcium and magnesium requirements of children and adolescents and peak bone mass. Nutrition 16.7–8 (2000): 514–5116.

Wester P. Magnesium. AJCN 45 (1987): 1305–1312.

Whelan AM, et al. Herbs, vitamins and minerals in the treatment of premenstrual syndrome: a systematic review. Canadian Journal of Clinical Pharmacology 2009; 16;3;e 407–429.

Wilson ML, Murphy PA. Herbal and dietary therapies for primary and secondary dysmenorrhoea. Cochrane Database Syst Rev 3 (2001): CD002124.

Witteman J et al. Reduction of blood pressure with oral magnesium supplementation in women with mild to moderate hypertension. AJCN 60 (1994): 129–135.

Woods JL, et al. Malnutrition on the menu: Nutritional status of institutionalized elderly Australians in low level care. 2009 JNHA: Geriatric Science 13:8 p 693.

Woolhouse M. Migraine and tension headache — a complementary and alternative approach. Aust Fam Physician 34.8 (2005): 647–651.

Xu T, et al. Magnesium intake and cardiovascular disease mortality: A meta-analysis of prospective cohort studies. International Journal of Cardiology, 2012. 167:6:3044–3047.

Yakubova O. Relationship of connective tissue dysplasia and hypomagnesemia in genesis of juvenile dysmenorrhea. European Medical, Health and Pharmaceutical Journal 2012;3;5–6.

Yasuda H, and Tsutsui T. Assessment of infantile mineral imbalances in austism spectrum disorders (ASDs). Int J Environ Res Public Health 2013:10: 6027–6043.
Young GL, Jewell D. Interventions for leg cramps in pregnancy. Cochrane Database Syst Rev 1 (2002): CD000121.
Zeana C. Magnesium orotate in myocardial and neuronal protection. Rom J Intern Med 37.1 (1999): 91–97.
Zhang W, et al. Associations of dietary magnesium intake with mortality from cardiovascular disease: The JACC study 2012. Atherosclerosis 221;2; 587–695.

New Zealand green-lipped mussel

HISTORICAL NOTE The Mytilidae are a family of bivalve molluscs that first appeared approximately 400 million years ago (Scotti et al 2001). In New Zealand, they include the green-lipped mussel, which is also known as *Perna canaliculus* and has the Māori name kuku. Green-lipped mussel forms an important component of the traditional diet of coastal Māori people in New Zealand. Interest in the potential therapeutic use of green-lipped mussel as a natural anti-inflammatory began about four decades ago when it was observed that coastal Māoris had a lower incidence of arthritis than those living inland.

BACKGROUND AND RELEVANT PHARMACOKINETICS

There is insufficient reliable information available.

CHEMICAL COMPONENTS

Green-lipped mussel contains a number of constituents, of which the protein (61%) and lipid content (5%) are considered the most important for pharmacological activity. Virtually all of the protein content is comprised of pernin, a self-aggregating glycoprotein rich in histidine and aspartic acid, while the lipid content is comprised of polyunsaturated fatty acids including omega-3 EFAs, free fatty acids, furan fatty acid, sterols, sterol esters and triglycerides. Other constituents include carbohydrates (13%), glucosaminoglycans (12%), minerals (5%) and water (4%) (Scotti et al 2001, Wakimoto et al 2011).

The green-lipped mussel also contain toxins, including BTXB4, a B4 analogue of brevetoxin, yessotoxins, pectenotoxin and okadaic acid (Mackenzie et al 2002, Morohashi et al 1999). BTXB4 has been associated with neurotoxic shellfish poisoning and has been identified as the most significant toxin in green-lipped mussel (Morohashi et al 1999).

MAIN ACTIONS

Most investigation has been conducted with the commercial preparations: Seatone and Lyprinol.

Anti-Inflammatory

Significant anti-inflammatory activity has been observed with the New Zealand green-lipped mussel, which forms the basis of much of its clinical use (Halpern 2000, McPhee et al 2007, Miller & Ormrod 1980, Miller et al 1993). Multiple mechanisms of action have been demonstrated in preclinical tests and include inhibition of the 5-lipoxygenase pathway and synthesis of leukotriene B_4, as well as inhibition of PGE_2 production by activated macrophages and prostaglandin inhibitor actions (Miller & Wu 1984, Miller et al 1993), and potent inhibition of the cyclo-oxygenase COX-1 and COX-2 enzyme pathways (Lawson et al 2007, Mani & Lawson 2006, McPhee et al 2007), with some findings suggesting preferential blockade of COX-2 enzyme activity over COX-1 activity (Efthimiou & Kukar 2010).

Inhibition of IgG, TNF-α, IL-1, IL-2 and IL-6 by green-lipped mussel extract has been demonstrated in an in vitro study by Mani and Lawson (2006) and in vivo research indicates that green-lipped mussel decreases anti-collagen antibody levels, inhibiting production of pro-inflammatory cytokines (TNF-α, IL-12p40) and reduces superoxide release (Lawson et al 2007).

The most important constituents responsible for these mechanisms of action are the various fatty acids found in green-lipped mussel.

The omega-3 fatty acids EPA and DHA have been isolated in green-lipped mussel (Murphy et al 2003), in addition to a unique series of other omega-3 polyunsaturated fatty acids (C18:4, C19:4, C20:4, C21:5) which may confer a more potent anti-inflammatory action than DHA and EPA, via competitive inhibition of arachidonic acid metabolism, reducing both leukotriene and prostaglandin synthesis (Treschow et al 2007). Furan fatty acids (F-acids), compounds found only in algae and in a limited number of marine animals, are thought to be other key therapeutic components of green-lipped mussel, which exhibits more potent anti-inflammatory activity than the omega-3 fatty acid, EPA (Wakimoto et al 2011). These unstable fatty acids also have potent free-radical-scavenging activity, especially reducing lipid peroxidation.

OTHER ACTIONS

N

In addition to anti-inflammatory and antioxidant activity, green-lipped mussel has demonstrated antihistamine activity and immunomodulatory properties, as well as endocrine actions and uterine effects (Ulbricht et al 2009). The protein, polysaccharide and lipid fractions are reportedly the bioactive components responsible for these actions (McPhee et al 2007).

CLINICAL USE

In clinical practice, green-lipped mussel is chiefly used for indications characterised by inflammation.

Osteoarthritis

The clinical evidence to support the use of green-lipped mussel (GLM) in osteoarthritis is promising and supported by mechanistic studies demonstrating an effect on inflammatory pathways.

In 2013, a non-blinded randomised clinical trial (RCT) was conducted with 38 subjects diagnosed with knee osteoarthritis (OA) (Coulson et al 2013). Each volunteer received either 3000 mg/day of a whole GLM extract or 3000 mg/day of glucosamine sulphate (GS) orally for 12 weeks. A significant improvement was seen with GLM treatment using the Western Ontario McMaster Universities Arthritis Index (WOMAC) and the Lequesne algofunctional indices ($P < 0.05$) after the test period.

Previously, an open study of 21 subjects with knee OA found that treatment with 3000 mg/day of green-lipped mussel extract for 8 weeks provided a significant improvement for the Lequesne and WOMAC ($P < 0.001$), thereby demonstrating improvements in knee joint pain, stiffness and mobility. The doses used by Coulson and colleagues exceeded those previously tested (maximum 1150 mg/day), which may have contributed to the positive findings.

A 2008 systematic review by Brien et al identified four RCTs where green-lipped mussel was used as an adjunct to standard therapy in mild to moderate osteoarthritis. In three studies, GLM was compared to placebo and in the fourth, a GLM lipid extract was compared to a stabilised powder extract. Results from the two studies considered to be of higher quality suggested that GLM may be superior to placebo for the treatment of mild to moderate OA (Brien et al 2008).

Rheumatoid arthritis (RA)

In contrast, evidence is less supportive of the use of GLM in RA as clinical studies with Seatone have produced inconsistent results. Whether the negative results are due to insufficient dosage or lack of any real effect remains to be tested further.

The first clinical trials testing Seatone in RA were conducted in the 1980s. Huskisson et al (1981) conducted a 4-week study of Seatone 300 mg three times a day as an adjunct to standard therapy in RA (n = 26). It failed to show a significant benefit compared to placebo (Huskisson et al 1981). Another RCT using Seatone in 35 patients with RA found no significant difference in chemical or clinical parameters compared with placebo, after 6 months' use (Larkin et al 1985). A more recent RCT of 28 patients using Seatone over 3 months, with a follow-up phase of another 3 months, reported that active treatment was effective in reducing symptoms of RA in 68% of the treatment group (Gibson & Gibson 1998). This study was subsequently criticised as the subjects served as their own controls in the second phase of the study, and because treatment group were further subdivided into responders and non-responders making interpretation of the results difficult (Cobb & Ernst 2006).

Asthma

To date, two studies have investigated GLM in asthma, producing promising results. A 2002 study of 46 patients with asthma compared Lyprinol (2 capsules twice daily) to placebo twice daily over 8 weeks under double-blind randomised test conditions (Emelyanov et al 2002). Active treatment resulted in a significant improvement on several parameters, such as daytime wheeze, reduced concentration of exhaled H_2O_2 (marker of airway inflammation) and an increase in morning peak expiratory flow (PEF), compared with placebo, but it did not improve night awakenings or reduce the use of beta-agonist bronchodilators or forced expiratory volume in 1-sec (FEV_1).The Lyprinol product contains GLM oil as 50 mg per capsule.

More recently in 2013, treatment with a GLM product (Lyprinol/Omega XL) was tested for effects on airway inflammation and the bronchoconstrictor response to eucapnic voluntary hyperpnoea (EVH) in asthmatics (Mickleborough et al 2013). The placebo controlled double-blind randomised crossover trial involved 23 asthmatic volunteers with clinically treated mild to moderate persistent asthma and a resting forced expiratory volume in 1-sec (FEV_1) of >65% predicted, and EIB as demonstrated by a greater than 10% drop in FEV_1 following a eucapnic voluntary hyperventilation (EVH) challenge. All subjects had a history of shortness of breath, chest tightness and intermittent wheezing following exercise, which was relieved by bronchodilator therapy and none were taking any maintenance medications (e.g. corticosteroids and leukotriene modifiers) at the time of the study.

Treatment consisted of 3 weeks of Lyprinol/Omega XL (8 capsules daily) or placebo followed by a 2-week washout period, before crossing over to the alternative arm. Additionally, all subjects were reviewed to ensure dietary intake was unchanged during the test period, in particular omega-3 EFA intake. Active treatment was found to significantly improve asthma symptom scores ($P < 0.05$), reduce bronchodilator use ($P < 0.05$) and reduce the maximum fall in post-EVH FEV_1 compared to usual and placebo ($P < 0.05$). It appears that effects are slow-acting as a reduction in bronchodilator use was only evident after 1 week of treatment.

OTHER USES

Veterinary use for osteoarthritis

New Zealand GLM shows promise as a treatment option for dogs, cats and horses with joint disease. In dogs, the most common form of joint disease is OA, which has been successfully treated by green-lipped mussel powder in one double-blind RCT (Bierer & Bui 2002). Active treatment was shown to significantly improve total arthritic score, and alleviate joint pain and swelling at the end of week six compared with controls. More specifically, 83% of dogs in the active treatment group experienced a 30% or greater reduction in total arthritic scores and of these, 18% showed a 70% or greater improvement. Only 7% of controls showed a 30% or greater improvement, with no dogs showing a 50% or greater improvement. The doses of GLM powder ranged from 450 mg to 1000 mg/day, depending on body weight. Another randomised double-blind study of 45 dogs with OA reported that the dogs treated with green-lipped mussel showed significant improvements according to veterinary pain and mobility scales compared to placebo. However, these benefits were not as great as those observed in the dogs treated with carprofen, a non-steroidal anti-inflammatory drug (Hielm-Bjorkman et al 2009). A further study was conducted including 81 dogs with a diagnosis of mild-moderate degenerative joint disease. Daily oral consumption of an extract of green lipped mussel appeared to reduce clinical signs of disease (Pollard et al 2006).

GLM extract has also been evaluated in cats diagnosed with degenerative joint disease. In one study of 45 cats, the animals in the treatment group were given a diet high in EPA/DHA, green-lipped mussel extract and supplemental glucosamine/chondroitin. Although improvements in mobility were reported, it is unclear how much of this benefit can be attributed to green-lipped mussel (Lascelles et al 2010).

Lyophilised products from green-lipped mussel (*Perna canaliculus* [LPPC]) are also used in horses to treat OA. A double-blind, multi-centre RCT evaluating horses with primary fetlock lameness found treatment with oral LPPC 25 mg/kg bwt/day for 56 days produced a significant reduction in severity of lameness ($P < 0.001$), improved response to the joint flexion test ($P < 0.001$) and reduced joint pain ($P = 0.014$) when compared with horses treated with placebo (Cayzer et al 2012).

Inflammatory bowel disease

Findings from a preliminary animal study suggest green-lipped mussel may be of potential benefit in inflammatory bowel disease (IBD). A study compared the anti-inflammatory effects of green-lipped mussel (Lyprinol containing <1 mg omega-3 fatty acids/day) to that of fish oils (given at a dose 55 mg omega-3 fatty acids/day) in mice with experimentally induced IBD. The mice treated with Lyprinol showed significantly less weight loss, disease activity index scores and colonic damage than those treated with omega-3 fatty acids ($P < 0.05$) after 13 days (Tenikoff et al 2005). Based on these results, the researchers proposed that GLM has a potential therapeutic benefit in IBD due to a mechanism or constituent unrelated to omega-3 fatty acids content (Tenikoff et al 2005). Human trials are now required to determine whether the effect is clinically significant.

Muscle damage and soreness in athletes — no effect

A double-blind RCT found GLM was ineffective in reducing delayed onset muscle soreness, inflammatory markers or muscle damage after exercise. Twenty well-trained male athletes from various sports disciplines were randomly assigned to either Lyprinol 200 mg/day or placebo, taken for 8 weeks prior to an intense exercise intervention (Pumpa et al 2011).

Cancer — no effect

Some research has been conducted with New Zealand GLM in the management of certain cancers as in vivo and in vitro studies suggest that inhibition of lipo-oxygenase pathways may arrest tumour growth in some cancers, especially prostate cancer and green-lipped mussel is a potent natural lipo-oxygenase inhibitor (Sukumaran et al 2010). An open-labelled clinical study involving 19 subjects found that GLM (Lyprinol) produced no clinical benefits in the management of advanced, treatment-refractory, prostate or breast cancer (Sukumaran et al 2010).

DOSAGE RANGE

Doses provided are based on the available clinical research. In addition, there is no well-known standardisation for green lipped mussel and efficacy may vary between manufacturers and between different batches (Ulbricht et al 2009).

- Asthma — Lyprinol/Omega XL taken as 8 capsules daily or Lyprinol taken as 4 capsules daily.
- Osteoarthritis — two studies showed significant symptomatic improvement at a dose of 3000 mg/day.

TOXICITY

GLM contain the toxin brevetoxin B4 (BTXB4), which has been associated with neurotoxic shellfish poisoning (Morohashi et al 1999). Regular ingestion of New Zealand green-lipped mussels does not appear to lead to heavy metal toxicity according to traditional dietary use by Māori people, nor according to a preliminary laboratory investigation (Whyte et al 2009). Insufficient reliable information is available to determine toxicity of supplemental green-lipped mussel.

ADVERSE REACTIONS

Gastrointestinal discomfort, nausea, gout and skin rashes have been reported (Ahern et al 1980, Brooks 1980). There have been three case reports in the literature suggesting that green-lipped mussel may be associated with rare incidences of liver dysfunction, however causality is difficult to ascertain (Abdulazim et al 2012). Raised liver enzymes were reported in two cancer patients participating in a small study (n = 17) on the safety and tolerability of green-lipped mussel as adjunct therapy. One of the two patients had significant metastatic liver involvement and this was reported as the most likely reason for raised liver enzymes. The other patient had normal liver function at baseline and no liver cancer involvement. The dose of green-lipped mussel at which liver abnormalities were reported was not specified, nor were any other medications taken by the patients described (Sukumaran et al 2010).

SIGNIFICANT INTERACTIONS

Insufficient reliable information exists regarding clinical interactions with green lipped mussel; however, in vivo studies suggest possible interactions with some medications.

Anti-inflammatory agents

Due to the anti-inflammatory activity of GLM, concomitant use with these medications can theoretically result in enhanced anti-inflammatory effects or a reduction in drug dosage — beneficial.

CONTRAINDICATIONS AND PRECAUTIONS

Contraindicated in people with allergies to shellfish. Rash, swelling of extremities and mouth, tingling, chest tightness and breathing difficulties have been reported (Ulbricht et al 2009). Lung dysfunction and a range of respiratory symptoms were reported in 32.3% of workers employed as New Zealand mussels openers, according to one study of 224 employees (Glass et al 1998). Whether the same effect is seen with manufactured GLM extracts taken orally remains to be seen.

Use with caution in people with hypertension, as the sodium content could theoretically raise blood pressure.

PREGNANCY USE

Insufficient reliable information is available to assess safety.

Practice points/Patient counselling

- New Zealand green-lipped mussel has been used to treat arthritis by the New Zealand Māoris for many years.
- Significant anti-inflammatory activity has been observed in both animals and humans.
- Several clinical trials have produced promising results for GLM in the symptomatic treatment of OA.
- Two clinical trials also suggest a possible role in asthma management.
- Significant symptom relief has been observed for GLM in dogs with osteoarthritis and cats and horses with joint disease.
- The most common side effects associated with GLM are gastrointestinal discomfort, nausea, gout and skin rashes.

PATIENTS' FAQs

What will this supplement do for me?

Some studies have shown that NZ green-lipped mussel exerts significant anti-inflammatory activity and is likely to relieve symptoms of OA when taken for several weeks, Two studies also suggest a possible role in the treatment of asthma.

When will it start to work?

Effects in osteoarthritis are likely to be seen within 8 weeks of use. Effects with a combination of GLM and omega-3 EFAS developed within 3 weeks in the management of mild-to-moderate asthma.

Are there any safety issues?

GLM should not be taken by people with allergies to shellfish and should be used with caution by people with high blood pressure due to the sodium content.

REFERENCES

Abdulazim A et al. Acute hepatitis induced by Lyprinol, the lipid extract of the green-lipped mussel (Pernacanaliculus), in a patient with polyarthrosis. Case Reports in Hepatology. Article 135146 (2012). doi:10.1155/2012/135146

Ahern MJ et al. Granulomatous hepatitis and Seatone. Med J Aust 2.3 (1980): 151–152.

Bierer TL, Bui LM. Improvement of arthritic signs in dogs fed green-lipped mussel (Pernacanaliculus). J Nutr 132.6 Suppl 2 (2002): 1634–1636S.

Brien S et al. Systematic review of the nutritional supplement Pernacanaliculus (green-lipped mussel) in the treatment of osteoarthritis. Q J Med 101 (2008):167–179. doi:10.1093/qjmed/hcm108.

Brooks PM. Side effects from Seatone. Med J Aust 2.3 (1980): 158.

Cayzer J et al. A randomised, double-blinded, placebo-controlled study on the efficacy of a unique extract of green-lipped mussel (Perna canaliculus) in horses with chronic fetlock lameness attributed to osteoarthritis. Equine Vet J 44.4 (2012) 393–398.

Cobb CS, Ernst E. Systematic review of a marine nutriceitical supplement in clinical trials for arthritis: the effectiveness of the New Zealndgree-lipped mussel Pernacanaliculus. Clinical Rheumatology 25 (2006): 275–284.

Coulson S et al. Green-lipped mussel extract (Perna canaliculus) and glucosamine sulphate in patients with knee osteoarthritis: therapeutic efficacy and effects on gastrointestinal microbiota profiles. Inflammopharmacology 21.1 (2013): 79–90.

Efthimiou P, Kukar M. Complementary and alternative medicine use in rheumatoid arthritis: prosed mechanism of action and efficacy of commonly used modalities. RheumatolInt 30.(2010): 571–586.

Emelyanov A et al. Treatment of asthma with lipid extract of New Zealand green-lipped mussel: a randomised clinical trial. EurRespir J 20.3 (2002): 596–600.

Gibson SLM, Gibson RG. The treatment of arthritis with a lipid extract of Perna canaliculis: a randomised trial. Comp Ther Med 6 (1998):122–126.

Glass WI et al. Work-related respiratory symptoms and lung function in New Zealand mussel openers. Am J Ind Med. 34.2 (1998):163–168.

Halpern GM. Anti-inflammatory effects of a stabilized lipid extract of Pernacanaliculus (Lyprinol). AllergImmunol (Paris) 32.7 (2000): 272–278.

Hielm-Bjorkman A et al. Evaluating complementary therapies for canine osteoarthritis Part 1: green-lipped mussel (Pernacanaliculus). eCam 6.3 (2009): 365–373.

Huskisson EC et al. Seatone is ineffective in rheumatoid arthritis. Br Med J (Clin Res Ed) 4.25 (1981): 1358–1359.

Larkin JG, Capell HA, Sturrock RD. Seatone in rheumatoid arthritis: a six-month placebo-controlled study. Ann Rheum Dis 44.3 (1985): 199–201.

Lascelles BDX et al. Evaluation of a therapeutic diet for feline degenerative joint disease. J Vet Intern Med 24 (2010): 487–495.

Lawson BR et al. Immunomodulation of murine collagen-induced arthritis by N,N-dimethylglycine and a preparation of Pernacanaliculus. BMC Complementary and Alternative Medicine 7.20 (2007).

Mackenzie L et al. Complex toxin profiles in phytoplankton and greenshell mussels (Pernacanaliculus) revealed by LC-MS/MS analysis. Toxicon. 40.9 (2002): 1321–1330.

Mani S, Lawson JW. In vitro modulation of inflammatory cytokine and IgG levels by extracts of Pernacanaliculus. BMC Complemen Alt Med 6.1 (2006).

McPhee S et al. Anti-cyclooxygenase effects of lipid extarcts from the New Zealand green-lipped mussel, Pernacanaliculus. Comparative Biochemistry and Physiology, part B 146 (2007): 346–356.

Mickleborough TD et al. Marine lipid fraction PCSO-524 (lyprinol/omega XL) of the New Zealand green lipped mussel attenuates hyperpnea-induced bronchoconstriction in asthma. Respir Med, 107.8 (2013): 1152–1163.

Miller T, Wu H. In vivo evidence for prostaglandin inhibitory activity in New Zealand green-lipped mussel extract. NZ Med J 97.757 (1984): 355–357.

Miller TE et al. Anti-inflammatory activity of glycogen extracted from Pernacanaliculus (NZ green-lipped mussel). Agents Actions 38 (1993): C139–42.

Miller TE, Ormrod D. The anti-inflammatory activity of Pernacanaliculus (NZ green lipped mussel). NZ Med J 92.667 (1980): 187–193.

Morohashi A et al. Brevetoxin B4 isolated from greenshell mussels Pernacanaliculus, the major toxin involved in neurotoxic shellfish poisoning in New Zealand. Natural Toxins 7.2 (1999): 45–48.

Murphy KJ et al. Fatty acid and sterol composition of frozen and freeze-dried Mew Zealand green lipped mussel (Pernacanaliculus) from three sites in New Zealand. Asia Pac. J. Clin. Nutr. 12 (2003): 50–60.

Pollard B et al. Clinival efficacy and tolerance of an extract of green-lipped mussel (Pernacanaliculus) in dogs presumptively diagnosed with degenerative joint disease. New Zealand Veterinary Journal 54.3 (2006): 114–118.

Pumpa KL et al. The effects of Lyprinol® on delayed onset musclesoreness and muscle damage in well trainedathletes: A double-blind randomised controlled trial. Complemen Ther Med 19 (2011): 311–318.

Scotti PD et al. Pernin: a novel, self-aggregating haemolymph protein from the New Zealand green-lipped mussel, Pernacanaliculus (Bivalvia: Mytilidae). Comp Biochem Physiol B Biochem Mol Biol 128.4 (2001): 767–779.

Sukumaran S et al. A phase 1 study to determine the safety, tolerability and maximum tolerated dose of green-lipped mussel (Pernacanaliculus) lipid extract in patients with advanced prostate and breast cancer. Annals Oncol 21.5 (2010): 1089–1093.

Tenikoff D et al. Lyprinol (stabilized lipid extract of New Zealand green-lipped mussel): a potential preventative treatment modality for inflammatory bowel disease. J Gastroenterol 40.4 (2005): 361–365.

Treschow AP et al. Novel anti-inflammatory ω-3 PUFA's from the New Zealand green-lipped mussel, Pernacanaliculus. Comparative Biochemistry and Physiology, part B 147 (2007): 645–656.
Ulbricht C et al. An Evidence-based systematic review of green-lipped mussel (Pernacanaliculus) by the Natural Standard Research Collaboration. J Diet Supplements 6.1 (2009): 54–90.
Wakimoto T et al. Furan fatty acid as an anti-inflammatory component from the green-lipped mussel Pernacanaliculus. PNAS 108.42 (2011).
Whyte ALH et al. Human dietary exposure to heavy metals via the consumption of greenshell mussels (PernacanaliculusGmelin 1791) from the Bay of Islands, Northern New Zealand. Science of the Total Environment 407 (2009): 4348–4355.

Passionflower

HISTORICAL NOTE Legend has it that this herb received its name because the corona resembles the crown of thorns worn by Christ during the crucifixion. A popular sedative medicine in the early 20th century, it was listed in the US National Formulary until 1936.

COMMON NAME

Passionflower

OTHER NAMES

Apricot vine, granadilla, Jamaican honeysuckle, Maypop passion flower, maracuja, passion vine, water lemon

BOTANICAL NAME/FAMILY

Passiflora incarnata (family Passifloraceae)

PLANT PARTS USED

Aerial parts, particularly leaves

CHEMICAL COMPONENTS

Flavonoids and related compounds (including apigenin, quercetin, kaempferol and chrysin), maltol, coumarin derivatives, indole alkaloids (mainly harman, harmaline, harmine), phytosterols (stigmasterol), sugars and small amounts of essential oil.

Note: Some research trials use other species of *Passiflora*, notably *P. edulis*, *P. alata* or *P. caerulea*. Each species contains similar, but not equivalent, constituents and may have different pharmacological properties and effects.

Harmine

Research has been conducted with several key constituents found in passionflower, in particular harmine and harman. Harmine is a β-carboline alkaloid, a compound class known to be strong inhibitors of monoamine oxidase which metabolises catecholamine neurotransmitters. Harmine exhibits various pharmacological effects both in vitro and in vivo, such as improvement of insulin sensitivity, a vasorelaxant effect and an antidepressant effect. In vitro and ex vivo models also show that harmine inhibits osteoclast differentiation and suppresses bone loss. In vivo studies on mice have demonstrated that harmine was able to prevent bone loss in osteoporosis models (Yonezawa et al 2011).

Harman

Numerous in vitro and in vivo trials have been conducted on the constituent known as harman suggesting mild monoamine oxidase A inhibitory activity (Adell et al 1996), inhibition of HIV replication (Ishida et al 2001), vasorelaxant activity (Shi et al 2000) and effects on gamma-aminobutyric acid (GABA) release (Dolzhenko & Komissarov 1984).

However, harman is not considered to be one of the main active constituents in the herb and is not present in biologically active concentrations in the dosage range used for passionflower. As such, results obtained using isolated harman in vitro and in vivo cannot necessarily be extrapolated to the use of passionflower in humans.

Harman has also been identified in beer, and to a lesser extent in wine, both of which contain levels far in excess of those found in passionflower at therapeutic doses.

MAIN ACTIONS

Anxiolytic and sedative activity

Several in vivo studies have demonstrated the anxiolytic effects of *Passiflora* extract (Della Loggia et al 1981, Dhawan et al 2001, Soulimani et al 1997). Behavioural tests in mice have also demonstrated that high doses have a sedative effect (Soulimani et al 1997).

The mechanism of action has been unclear until recently, as some research suggested stimulation of GABA release or an interaction with GABA receptors, and other research observed no interaction with GABA benzodiazepine receptors (Zanoli et al 2000). This may be due to different *Passiflora* species being used in research, as well as different routes of administration.

In 1999, an in vitro study showed inhibition of GABA-A binding with *Passiflora* extract (Simmen et al 1999). A more recent study has determined that, indeed, the anxiolytic effects of *P. incarnata* are mediated via the GABAergic system (Grundman et al 2008). This was confirmed yet again in 2011, whereby numerous pharmacological effects of *Passiflora incarnata* were shown to be mediated via modulation of the GABA system including affinity to GABA-A and GABA-B receptors, and effects on GABA uptake in vitro (Appel et al 2011).

Anticonvulsant

A hydroalcoholic extract of *Passiflora* (Pasipay 0.4 mg/kg) has demonstrated anticonvulsant activity in vivo (Nassiri-Asl et al 2007). The extract was shown to delay onset and decrease the duration of seizures compared to placebo. It appeared to work through GABAergic and opioid pathways; however more research is needed to confirm the mechanism.

OTHER ACTIONS

Recent in vitro and rat studies demonstrated that *Passiflora* enhances the potency of St John's wort's antidepressant action (Fiebich et al 2011).

Antiepileptic

Passiflora significantly reduced the severity of seizures in vivo, and ameliorated postictal (the period immediately after a seizure) depression, possibly due to its ability to retain serotonin and noradrenaline levels of the brain. This is worthy of further consideration as the standard anticonvulsive therapies such as diazepam tend to worsen postictal depression (Singh et al 2012).

Aphrodisiac

Tests in mice have identified significant aphrodisiac properties associated with high doses of *Passiflora* extract (Dhawan et al 2003a). A benzoflavone moiety may be chiefly responsible, as tests with this isolated compound were found to increase libido and fertility of male rats after 30 days' treatment (Dhawan et al 2002a).

Antitussive and antiasthmatic activity

P. incarnata was as effective as codeine phosphate in suppressing a sulfur dioxide-induced cough in mice (Dhawan & Sharma 2002). Passionflower (100 mg/kg) was also able to prevent dyspnoea-related convulsions in guinea pigs with acetylcholine-induced bronchospasm (Dhawan et al 2003b).

Antidiabetic

In the Ayurvedic system, the leaves of *P. incarnata* are used for their antidiabetic properties. Recent tests using mice confirm hypoglycaemic and hypolipidaemic effects, with improvement in glucose tolerance and lipid profile as well as regeneration of pancreatic islets of Langerhans (Gupta et al 2012).

Nicotine withdrawal

Promising new in vivo research suggests that passionflower extract has the potential to ameliorate the signs of nicotine sensitisation (Breivogel & Jamerson 2012). This builds on previous research which identified a benzoflavone moiety in *Passiflora* which, when given acutely to test animals as a single 20 mg/kg dose, prevented some of the nicotine withdrawal effects (Dhawan et al 2002c).

CLINICAL USE

Preclinical research and traditional evidence suggest *Passiflora* can play a role in the symptomatic relief of anxiety. The clinical evidence currently available supports this and shows benefits for anxiety and possibly insomnia and opiate withdrawal. However, evidence comes from only a handful of randomised controlled trials, so ideally, larger controlled trials are required to further clarify its role in practice.

Anxiety and nervous restlessness

Passiflora extract is a popular herb for nervousness and anxiety and is most often prescribed in combination with other herbs such as valerian and St John's wort.

At least three clinical trials have confirmed the efficacy of passionflower treatment for symptoms of anxiety. Two trials found that treatment with passiflora before surgery relieved anxiety and one trial investigated its use in generalised anxiety disorder (GAD), finding positive results (Lakhan & Vieira 2010).

Treatment with passionflower extract (45 drops/day) was compared to oxazepam (30 mg/day) in a double-blind study involving 36 volunteers with GAD and found both treatments were equally effective anxiolytics in this population. Both treatments were used for 4 weeks. Passionflower treatment had a slower onset of action compared to oxazepam; however, the herbal group also reported less job impairment (Akhondzadeh et al 2001a).

Commission E approved passionflower for this indication (Blumenthal et al 2000).

Presurgery use

Two studies have investigated the use of passiflora to relieve anxiety before surgery. In the first study, 60 patients were randomised to two groups and given passionflower (500 mg; Passipy Iran Darouk) or placebo 90 minutes before surgery (Movafegh et al 2008). Anxiety scores were significantly lower in the active treatment group compared to the placebo group, while other parameters such as psychological and physiological recovery were the same for both groups.

Anxiolytic activity was confirmed in a more recent randomised, double-blind, placebo-controlled study involving 60 patients about to undergo spinal anaesthesia. Thirty minutes before the procedure, patients were randomly assigned to receive either oral *Passiflora incarnata* extract or placebo. The passiflora extract was found to reduce the increase in anxiety before spinal anaesthesia without changing psychomotor function test results, sedation level or haemodynamics (Aslanargun et al 2012).

IN COMBINATION

A formulated extract containing passionflower, St John's wort and valerian was tested on 16 healthy adults in a randomised, placebo-controlled crossover study. Electroencephalogram (EEG) recordings were performed 0.5, 1.5, 3 and 4 hours after administration of the preparation and analysis revealed a difference to placebo 3 and 4 hours after intake. Analysis of the neurophysiological changes following the intake of the preparation showed a similarity of brain frequency changes on the EEG to those of calming and antidepressive drugs without impairment of cognition (Dimpfel et al 2011).

Previously, an anxiolytic effect was observed in a randomised, placebo-controlled study of 182 people diagnosed with adjustment disorder and anxious mood who were treated with a combination of *Crataegus oxyacantha, Ballota foetida, Valeriana officinalis, Cola nitida* and *Paullinia cupana* in a commercial product known as Euphytose, taken as two tablets three times daily for 28 days (Bourin et al 1997).

Opiate withdrawal

A randomised double-blind study involving 65 subjects with opiate addiction compared the effects of clonidine and placebo with clonidine and passiflora extract over a 14-day period. The fixed daily dose was 60 drops of passiflora extract and a maximum daily dose of 0.8 mg of clonidine administered in three divided doses.

The combination treatment of clonidine and passiflora extract was significantly better at alleviating the psychological symptoms associated with withdrawal; however, no differences in physical symptoms were seen between the groups (Akhondzadeh et al 2001b).

Insomnia

Currently, in vivo evidence supports the sedative activity of passiflora when used in high doses. There has been only one small randomised controlled trial (n = 41) that compared 2 g of passionflower tea to placebo before sleep and demonstrated an improvement for subjective sleep quality but no other significant findings on other sleep outcomes (Ngan & Conduit 2011). Preclinical research suggests it should have potential for this indication.

IN COMBINATION

A herbal combination consisting of standardised extracts of *Valeriana officinalis* (300 mg; standardised to 0.8% total valerinic acid), *Passiflora incarnata* (80 mg; standardised to 4% isovitexin) and *Humulus lupulus* (30 mg; standardised to 0.35% rutin) may be a suitable alternative to zolpidem as a treatment for primary insomnia, according to a recent randomised, double-blind study (Maroo et al 2013). The study of 91 people with primary insomnia identified that the herbal combination was as effective as zolpidem in significantly improving total sleep time, sleep latency, number of nightly awakenings and insomnia severity index scores. Interestingly, the Epworth sleepiness scores did not change significantly over the study period for either group.

In regard to safety, 12 people in the herbal group and 16 treated with zolpidem reported side effects, with drowsiness the most common. Most were mild and not serious.

OTHER USES

Traditional uses

Traditionally, passionflower has been used to treat neuralgia, generalised seizures, hysteria and insomnia. It has also been used to treat diarrhoea, dysentery and dysmenorrhoea by acting on the nervous system.

DOSAGE RANGE

- Dried herb: 2 g three to four times daily.
- Infusion of dried herb: 0.25–2 g three to four times daily.
- Fluid extract (1:1) (g/mL): 2 mL three to four times daily in 150 mL of water.
- Tincture (1:5) (g/mL): 10 mL three to four times daily.

TOXICITY

Not known.

ADVERSE REACTIONS

Drowsiness is the most common side effect according to the available clinical research.

One human study found that *Passiflora* extract has a significantly lower incidence of impairment of job performance compared with oxazepam (Akhondzadeh et al 2001b). One case reports a 34-year-old woman who developed severe nausea, vomiting, drowsiness and episodes of non-sustained ventricular tachycardia following administration of passionflower at therapeutic doses (Fisher et al 2000).

SIGNIFICANT INTERACTIONS

Controlled studies are not available; therefore, interactions are based on evidence of pharmacological activity and are theoretical.

Benzodiazepines

Additive effects are theoretically possible at high doses. There has been one case report of a patient taking passiflora and valerian while also taking lorazepam and developing shaking hands, dizziness, throbbing and muscular fatigue (Carrasco et al 2009). It is not known if the treatment was tested for authenticity or contamination, so causality is difficult to ascertain.

Use with caution and monitor drug dosage — possible beneficial interaction under medical supervision.

Note: *Passiflora* may be a useful support during benzodiazepine withdrawal.

Barbiturates

Additive central nervous system sedation is theoretically possible. Use with caution and monitor drug dosage — possible beneficial interaction under medical supervision.

Practice points/Patient counselling

- Both human and animal studies confirm passionflower has significant anxiolytic activity and reduces the symptoms of anxiety.
- When used 30 minutes before surgery, it appears to reduce nervousness.
- One randomised study found that it has significantly less negative effects on performance than 30 mg oxazepam, yet is as effective for GAD.
- Maximal effects may require several days of regular intake.
- It is not known whether physical tolerance develops.
- One study has shown it improves psychological symptoms during opiate withdrawal when used together with clonidine.
- In practice, it is often prescribed with other herbs for stronger effects in anxiety and insomnia.

CONTRAINDICATIONS AND PRECAUTIONS

Whether concomitant use of high doses of passiflora adversely affects people's ability to drive a car or operate heavy machinery should be evaluated on an individual case-by-case basis.

PREGNANCY USE

Passionflower has demonstrated the ability to increase uterine contractions in an isolated rat uterus model when compared to control tissue (Sadraei et al 2003). Whether this has any adverse effects in pregnancy remains unknown. Caution is advised until safety is better established.

PATIENTS' FAQs

What will this herb do for me?

Passionflower has anxiolytic effects that help reduce symptoms of anxiety. It might also be useful for insomnia, especially when used as part of a herbal combination. There is some research suggesting it may help ease the symptoms of opiate withdrawal.

When will it start to work?

When being used for anxiety, it may take 3–4 weeks before significant effects are seen.

Are there any safety issues?

Overall, passionflower does not appear to impair job performance but some people have reported drowsiness. However, it may theoretically interact with other sedative medicines when used in high doses. Other interactions are theoretically possible, so use should be monitored by a healthcare professional.

REFERENCES

Adell A, et al. Action of harman (1-methyl-beta-carboline) on the brain: body temperature and in vivo efflux of 5-HT from hippocampus of the rat. Neuropharmacology 35.8 (1996): 1101–1107.

Akhondzadeh S et al. Passionflower in the treatment of opiates withdrawal: a double-blind randomized controlled trial. J Clin Pharm Ther 26.5 (2001a): 369–73.

Akhondzadeh S et al. Passionflower in the treatment of generalized anxiety: a pilot double-blind randomized controlled trial with oxazepam. J Clin Pharm Ther 26.5 (2001b): 363–7.

Appel, K., et al. 2011. Modulation of the gamma-aminobutyric acid (GABA) system by *Passiflora incarnata* L. Phytother.Res., 25, (6) 838–843.

Aslanargun, P., et al. (2012). *Passiflora incarnata* Linneaus as an anxiolytic before spinal anesthesia. J Anesth., 26(1), 39–44.

Blumenthal M, et al (eds). Herbal medicine: expanded Commission E monographs. Austin, TX: Integrative Medicine Communications, 2000.

Bourin, M., et al. 1997. A combination of plant extracts in the treatment of outpatients with adjustment disorder with anxious mood: controlled study versus placebo. Fundam.Clin. Pharmacol., 11, (2) 127–132.

Breivogel, C., & Jamerson, B. (2012). Passion flower extract antagonizes the expression of nicotine locomotor sensitization in rats. Pharm Biol., 50(10), 1310–1316.

Carrasco, M. C., et al. (2009). Interactions of *Valeriana officinalis* L. and *Passiflora incarnata* L. in a patient treated with lorazepam. Phytother. Res., 23, 1795–1796.

Della Loggia R, et al. Evaluation of the activity on the mouse CNS of several plant extracts and a combination of them. Riv Neurol 51.5 (1981): 297–310.

Dhawan K, Sharma A. Antitussive activity of the methanol extract of *Passiflora incarnata* leaves. Fitoterapia 73.5 (2002): 397–399.

Dhawan K, et al. Anxiolytic activity of aerial and underground parts of *Passiflora incarnata.* Fitoterapia 72.8 (2001): 922–926.

Dhawan K, et al. Beneficial effects of chrysin and benzoflavone on virility in 2-year-old male rats. J Med Food 5.1 (2002a): 43–8.

Dhawan K, et al. Suppression of alcohol-cessation-oriented hyper-anxiety by the benzoflavone moiety of *Passiflora incarnata* Linneaus in mice. J Ethnopharmacol 81.2 (2002c): 239–44.

Dhawan K, et al. Aphrodisiac activity of methanol extract of leaves of *Passiflora incarnata* Linn. in mice. Phytother Res 17.4 (2003a): 401–3.

Dhawan K, et al. Antiasthmatic activity of the methanol extract of leaves of Passiflora incarnata. Phytother Res 17.7 (2003b): 821–2.

Dimpfel, W., et al. (2011). Early effect of NEURAPAS® balance on current source density (CSD) of human EEG. Links Export Central Citation BMC psychiatry, 11, 123.

Dolzhenko AT, Komissarov IV. GABA-ergic effects of harman independent of its influence on benzodiazepine receptors. Bull Eksp Biol Med 98.10 (1984): 446–448.

Fiebich, B., et al. (2011). Pharmacological studies in an herbal drug combination of St. John's Wort (*Hypericum perforatum*) and passion flower (*Passiflora incarnata*): In vitro and in vivo evidence of synergy between *Hypericum* and *Passiflora* in antidepressant pharmacological models. Fitoterapia, 82(3), 474–480.

Fisher AA, et al. Toxicity of *Passiflora incarnata* L. J Toxicol Clin Toxicol 38.1 (2000): 63–66.

Grundman, O., et al. (2008). Anxiolytic activity of a phytochemically characterized *Passiflora incarnata* extract is mediated via the GABAergic system. Planta medica, 74(15).

Gupta, K., et al. (2012). Antidiabetic activity of *Passiflora incarnata* Linn. in streptozotocin-induced diabetes in mice. Journal of Ethnopharmacology, 139, 801–806.

Ishida J et al. Anti-AIDS agents. 46: Anti-HIV activity of harman, an anti-HIV principle from *Symplocos setchuensis*, and its derivatives. Nat Prod 64.7 (2001): 958–960.

Lakhan, S.E. & Vieira, K.F. 2010. Nutritional and herbal supplements for anxiety and anxiety-related disorders: systematic review. Nutr.J, 9, 42.

Maroo, N., et al. 2013. Efficacy and safety of a polyherbal sedative-hypnotic formulation NSF-3 in primary insomnia in comparison to zolpidem: a randomized controlled trial. Indian J Pharmacol., 45, (1) 34–39.

Movafegh A et al. Preoperative oral *Passiflora incarnata* reduces anxiety in ambulatory surgery patients: a double-blind, placebo-controlled study. Anesth Analg 106.6 (2008): 1728–1732.

Nassiri-Asl M, et al. Anticonvulsant effects of aerial parts of *Passiflora incarnata* extract in mice: involvement of benzodiazepine and opioid receptors. BMC Complement Altern Med 7 (2007): 26.

Ngan, A., & Conduit, R. (2011). A double-blind placebo-controlled investigation of the effects of *Passiflora incarnata* (passionflower) herbal tea on subjective sleep quality. Phtyotherapy Research. 25: 1153–1159.

Sadraei H, et al. Extract of *Zataria multiflora* and *Carum carvi* essential oils and hydroalcoholic extracts of *Passiflora incarnata, Berberis intejerrimat* and *Crocus sativus* on rat isolated uterus contractions. Int J Aromather 13.2–3 (2003): 121–127.

Shi CC et al. Vasorelaxant effect of harman. Eur J Pharmacol 390.3 (2000): 319–325.

Simmen U et al. Extracts and constituents of *Hypericum perforatum* inhibit the binding of various ligands to recombinant receptors expressed with the Semliki Forest virus system. J Recept Signal Transduct Res 19.1–4 (1999): 59–74.

Singh, B., et al. (2012). Dual protective effect of *Passiflora incarnata* in epilepsy and associated post-ictal depression. Journal of Ethnopharmacology, 139(1), 273–279.

Soulimani R et al. Behavioural effects of *Passiflora incarnata* L. and its indole alkaloid and flavonoid derivatives and maltol in the mouse. J Ethnopharmacol 57.1 (1997): 11–20.

Yonezawa, T., et al. (2011). Harmine, a β-carboline alkaloid, inhibits osteoclast differentiation and bone resorption in vitro and in vivo. European Journal of Pharmacology, 650, 511–518.

Zanoli P, Avallone R, Baraldi M. Behavioral characterisation of the flavonoids apigenin and chrysin. Fitoterapia 71 (Suppl 1) (2000): S117–S123.

P

Pelargonium

HISTORICAL NOTE *Pelargonium sidoides* DC. (Geraniaceae) is an important traditional medicine in South Africa where it has been used to treat diarrhoea, dysentery, coughs and colds, tuberculosis and gastrointestinal conditions. This and other South African traditional medicines were often referred to by their original Khoi-Khoi name *rabas*, and were amongst the first to be recorded by early explorers such as van der Stel (1685) and Thunberg (1773). The most detailed account of the value and uses of *P. sidoides* is that of Smith (1895), who listed *P. reniforme/P. sidoides* as the first of five species used in the treatment of dysentery (Brendler & van Wyk 2008). The herb was introduced to Europe by the Englishman Charles Henry Stevens and is now a popular, commercially produced herbal medicine, listed in the European Pharmacopoeia (Brendler & van Wyk 2008).

***Clinical note — Is it* P. sidoides *or* P. reniforme?**
P. sidoides is predominantly found over large parts of the interior of southern Africa, but also occurs in coastal mountain ranges. The product may be adulterated with the very similar-looking *P. reniforme* and the two species often grow side by side. The phytochemical composition of the roots of *P. sidoides* is similar to *P. reniforme*, reflecting the close botanical relationship between the two species (Brendler & van Wyk 2008, Kolodziej 2007). Morphological distinction of the dried product is extremely difficult and chemical analysis is the only reliable method of telling them apart.

COMMON NAME

South African geranium

OTHER NAMES

Geranium, EPs 7630, Geranien, geranium root, Ikhubalo, Icwayiba, i-Yeza lezi-kali, Kaloba, Kalwerbossie, Pelargonien, pelargonium root, Rabas, Rabassam, silverleaf geranium, Umckaloabo, Uvendle

BOTANICAL NAME/FAMILY

Pelargonium sidoides (family: Geraniaceae)

PLANT PARTS USED

Root

CHEMICAL COMPONENTS

Oligomeric and polymeric proanthocyanidins are present in significant amounts: the putative precursors afzelechin, catechin and gallocatechin have been isolated; and highly oxygenated coumarins. Gallic acid is consistently found in high concentrations in the plant material and the minerals calcium and silica (Kolodziej 2007, Kolodziej et al 2003).

Coumarins and phenolic compounds, including simple phenolic acids and proanthocyanidins, are the principal compounds found in the special extract, EPs 7630 (Kolodziej 2007). Gallic acid occurs in low amounts in EPs 7630 (Kolodziej 2007).

MAIN ACTIONS

Antibacterial activity

Different in vitro evaluations of the herbal preparation from the roots of *P. sidoides* and its isolated constituents demonstrated pharmacological activities, including moderate, direct antibacterial effects against a panel of pathogenic bacteria that are responsible for numerous respiratory tract infections (RTIs), several multi-resistant strains of *Staphylococcus aureus*, also *Streptococcus pneumoniae*, *Haemophilus influenzae*, *Moraxella catarrhalis* and *Mycobacterium tuberculosis* (Kolodziej et al 2003, Lizogub et al 2007, Mativandlela et al 2006).

Antiadhesion properties

Antiadhesive properties of pelargonium have been demonstrated for several bacteria, including *Helicobacter pylori,* and is thought to be one of the mechanisms responsible for its antimicrobial activity (Beil & Kilian 2007, Wittschier et al 2007).

Immune enhancement

The root extract also exhibits notable immune modulatory capabilities. The immune modulatory activities are mediated mainly by the release of tumour necrosis factor-alpha and nitric oxides, the stimulation of interferon-beta, the increase of natural killer cell activity and interferon-like activity (Kolodziej et al 2003, Lizogub et al 2007). Improved phagocytosis has also been demonstrated in vitro.

Antiviral activity

Direct antiviral activity against herpesvirus 1 and 2 has been demonstrated (Schnitzler et al 2008). *P. sidoides* extract affects the virus before penetration into the host cell and reveals a different mode of action when compared to aciclovir; it might be suitable for topical therapeutic use as antiviral drug in both labial and genital herpes infection. Through induction of the interferon system and upregulation of cytokines, important in protecting host cells from viral infection, the herb can be expected to exhibit antiviral activity in vivo (Engler et al 2009).

OTHER ACTIONS

A variety of mechanisms account for its symptom-relieving effects in RTIs.

The liquid extract acts as an expectorant and reduces sputum production, allowing the body to expel mucus, thereby making conditions less suitable for the multiplication of the bacteria and viruses. It has also been shown to increase cilia beat frequency in nasal epithelia.

CLINICAL USE

Most research has been conducted with a standardised liquid herbal extract of the roots of *P. sidoides* (1 : 8–10), extraction solvent: ethanol 11% (wt/wt) produced by Willmar Schwabe Pharmaceuticals, Karlsruhe, Germany, also known as EPs 7630 (Umckaloabo, marketed by Spitzner Arzneimittel, Ettlingen, Germany). It has been approved for use in over 30 countries, including Australia.

Clinical note — The difficult and winding road to successful commercialisation

It is believed that the medicinal properties of *Pelargonium sidoides* were first recognised and applied by traditional tribal healers in South Africa many centuries ago. It first came to the attention of Europeans in the early 1900s, as a result of a serendipitous meeting between an Englishman, Charles Henry Stevens, and a traditional Zulu healer. In 1897, Stevens was sent to South Africa by his doctor to recover from pulmonary tuberculosis. While there, he was treated by a traditional Zulu healer with a root concoction that successfully cured his condition (Bladt & Wagner 2007). Seeing the need for such a medicine back home and no doubt the commercial opportunity, Stevens called the tuberculosis treatment 'Umckaloabo', which he commercially manufactured once back in England. The treatment also became known as the 'Stevens' cure' and caused controversy amongst the medical establishment, which sought to discredit him by labelling Stevens a 'quack'. After his death in 1942, Stevens' son sold the business to a drug manufacturer in Germany. The exact herbal ingredient in the remedy and its source were kept secret and shrouded in mystery until well into the 1970s, when the plant ingredient was finally identified as *P. sidoides* by S. Bladt, while undertaking research for her thesis in Germany (Bladt & Wagner 2007). After the conduct of scientific and clinical trials, the herb was once again commercially manufactured in Europe with great success, with an annual turnover in Germany of 80 million Deutschmark in 2006 (Brendler & van Wyk 2008).

Respiratory tract infections — bronchitis, common cold, sinusitis

In the light of inappropriate antibiotic use and increasing drug resistance rates worldwide, the need for an alternative, effective remedy for respiratory tract conditions is crucial. *P. sidoides* has been investigated as one such medicine and represents a promising treatment for the management of RTIs. It has achieved widespread popularity in Germany over the last 50 years, where it is approved for the treatment of acute bronchitis, acute tonsillopharyngitis and acute sinusitis. The standardised, liquid extract is now a registered medicine on the Australian Register of Therapeutic Goods and has been given an AUST R number, signifying claims have been evaluated by the Therapeutic Goods Administration for which there is good supportive scientific evidence.

Overall, the available evidence indicates that pelargonium is likely to be beneficial in the treatment of acute, mild to moderate bronchitis, acute rhinosinusitis and the common cold in adults. Paediatric trials suggest a potential benefit in acute bronchitis and in alleviating several common RTI symptoms, in particular, nasal congestion.

The scientific investigation of *P. sidoides* in the treatment of various RTIs really began in earnest in the 1990s (Brendler & van Wyk 2008). The earliest trials were mainly observational studies, whereas more recent studies tend to be placebo-controlled randomised trials and focus on acute bronchitis, although observational studies are still performed. The results of the individual research reports are compelling, particularly as there are no good treatment options for viral RTIs and bacterial RTIs are becoming increasingly difficult to treat.

One of the largest adult studies published to date was a randomised, double-blind, placebo-controlled, multicentre study of 406 adults with acute bronchitis published in 2010 (Matthys et al 2010). Patients were randomly assigned to one of four parallel treatment groups to receive different doses of EPs 7630 tablets

(10 mg EPs 7630 tablets three times a day (30 mg group), 20 mg EPs 7630 tablets three times a day (60 mg group), 30 mg EPs 7630 tablets three times a day (90 mg group)) or placebo three times a day for a treatment period of 7 days. Bronchitis-specific symptoms were measured from baseline to day 7 and the groups were compared. Overall, the participants receiving EPs 7630 tablets had a statistically significant improvement in symptoms compared to the placebo group. The best results were obtained for the two higher-dosage regimens. When the incidence of side effects was considered, the optimal dose was 20 mg tablets of EPs 7630 taken three times daily.

Two new paediatric studies have been published since 2009, both in 2012. They continue to build the supportive evidence base for *Pelargonium sidoides* as a medicine for the treatment of common symptoms associated with RTIs, in particular, nasal congestion.

A randomised, placebo-controlled study by Patiroglu et al (2012) involved 28 children aged between 1 and 5 years with transient hypogammaglobulinaemia of infancy, one of the more common immune deficiencies of childhood. In this study, 14 participants were treated with *Pelargonium sidoides* for 1 week (10 drops three times a day), while 14 were given placebo during an episode of upper RTI. Active treatment with *P. sidoides* resulted in significantly improved appetite by day 5, a good representative factor in terms of indicating the general state of health of children. A highly relevant improvement was observed for nasal congestion in the *P. sidoides* extract group, compared to no improvement in the placebo group. On day 7, 71.4% of children taking active treatment had no nasal congestion compared with 21.5% in the placebo group. In contrast, no improvements were detected between the *P. sidoides* extract group and the placebo group for daily and nocturnal cough, fever or pain.

The prevention of an asthma attack during an upper RTI by 5 days of pelargonium treatment was tested in a randomised study of 61 children (Tahan et al 2012). This is based on the fact that viral infections have been implicated in most (>80%) asthma exacerbations in children. When the active treatment and placebo groups were compared, those receiving liquid *P. sidoides* had a significant decrease in cough frequency and nasal congestion and a statistically significant reduced frequency of developing an asthma attack. No significant changes were reported for fever or muscle aches and pains. The dosage schedule used was: for 1–5 years, 10 drops three times a day; for 6–12 years, 20 drops three times a day; for 12 years and above, 30 drops three times a day.

Previously, in 2008 a Cochrane systematic review was published in which authors evaluated data from eight randomised control trials (RCTs) and concluded that *P. sidoides* may be effective in alleviating symptoms of acute bronchitis, rhinosinusitis and the common cold in adults, but the findings were not yet definitive (Timmer et al 2008). The authors identified two RCTs that showed *P. sidoides* was effective in relieving all symptoms, and in particular cough and sputum production in adults with acute bronchitis, although a third study showed that the preparation was only effective for treating sputum reduction. Similarly, *P. sidoides* was effective in resolving symptoms of acute bronchitis in two out of three paediatric studies. One RCT of 104 adults was included in the review, showing significant treatment effects in acute rhinosinusitis for the resolution of all symptoms as well as the key symptoms of nasal discharge and headache resolution.

The results obtained by studies using tablet preparations included in this review were different from those using the liquid preparation. Based on this, the authors stated that the liquid preparation (alcoholic solution) may be associated with improvement in some symptoms of acute bronchitis in both children and adults

— in particular sputum production and cough — but tablet preparations produced fewer or no potential beneficial effects in both children and adults. The cause of this difference is unknown and may be due to chance or differences in constituent bioavailability or in the product's phytochemical constituents. Another caution expressed by the review authors was of the use of non-validated symptom scales as a primary end point and the subjective nature of the results.

The same year, a review was published in *Phytomedicine* that analysed six RCTs, of which four were suitable for statistical pooling (Agbabiaka et al 2008). One study compared EPs 7630 against conventional non-antibiotic treatment (acetyl-cysteine); the other five studies tested EPs 7630 against placebo. All RCTs reported findings suggesting the effectiveness of EPs 7630 in treating acute bronchitis. When a meta-analysis of the four placebo-controlled RCTs was conducted, the results confirmed that EPs 7630 significantly reduced bronchitis symptom scores in patients with acute bronchitis by day 7.

Common cold

A multicentre, randomised, double-blind trial by Lizogub et al (2007) involved 107 participants with cold symptoms present for between 24 and 48 hours. It demonstrated that treatment with liquid extract of *P. sidoides* significantly hastened recovery from the common cold, and markedly improved individual symptoms, most notably nasal congestion and drainage, sneezing, sore throat, hoarseness and headache. The group receiving active treatment also experienced significantly higher remission and improvement in rates of other cold-related symptoms compared to placebo, such as limb pain (95.5% vs 74%), general weakness (79% vs 35%), exhaustion (85% vs 43%) and fatigue (89% vs 60.5%) (Lizogub et al 2007). The study compared 30 drops (1.5 mL) of liquid herbal pelargonium three times daily to placebo for a maximum of 10 days. After 10 days, substantially more people receiving the herbal treatment were considered clinically cured than the placebo group (78.8% vs 31.4%; $P < 0.0001$). All (100%) of patients receiving pelargonium judged tolerability of treatment as good or very good.

Immune modulation in athletes

Exhaustive physical exercise is associated with increased frequency of upper RTIs, probably due to a compromised immune response. A double-blind, placebo-controlled study involving male marathon runners found that treatment with *P. sidoides* extract modulated the production of secretory immunoglobulin A in saliva, both interleukin-15 (IL-15) and IL-6 in serum, and IL-15 in the nasal mucosa after an intense running session. Secretory immunoglobulin A levels were increased, while levels of IL-15 and IL-6 were decreased, thereby indicating a strong modulating influence on the immune response (Luna et al 2011). The treatment schedule consisted of umckaloabo or placebo (3 × 30 drops/day) for 28 consecutive days before training and testing.

OTHER USES

The traditional uses of tuberous *Pelargonium* species mainly involve ailments of the gastrointestinal tract (diarrhoea and dysentery) and respiratory tract, although Smith (1895) made a case for it being used as a general tonic.

It is also used as a gripe water for infants ('upset stomach', 'air in the intestine'). The crushed root is mixed with water and a teaspoonful of the red infusion is taken orally (Brendler & van Wyk 2008).

The aerial parts have also been used traditionally as a wound-healing agent. This may be due to their high tannin content that would contribute to its astringent effect (Kolodziej 2007).

Practice points/Patient counselling

- *P. sidoides* is a traditional herbal medicine originating from South Africa and now extremely popular in Europe, particularly Germany, and available in Australia.
- The herb demonstrates antibacterial and antiviral activity and enhances non-specific immune function; it also has activity against herpesvirus 1 and 2.
- Observational and randomised studies indicate *Pelargonium sidoides* liquid extract EPs 7630 may provide benefits in the treatment in acute, mild to moderate bronchitis, acute rhinosinusitis and possibly the common cold in adults, acute bronchitis in children and in alleviating several common RTI symptoms, in particular, nasal congestion.
- It appears to hasten recovery from the common cold, reduce symptoms and improve associated fatigue and weakness and may have a role in the acute treatment of other, uncomplicated respiratory infections.
- It is generally well tolerated; however, gastrointestinal side effects and allergic skin reactions have been reported with use.

DOSAGE RANGE

Dried herb: 0.4 g/day

According to clinical studies

Treatment of acute bronchitis

General dosage: Adults and children over 12 years: 30 drops (1.5 mL) of liquid extract herbal pelargonium three times daily before meals for up to 10 days.

Adults — for acute bronchitis symptoms: 20 mg tablets of EPs 7630 taken three times daily.

Children aged 6–12 years: 20 drops (1.0 mL) three times per day.

Children aged 2–5 years: 10 drops three times a day.

Treatment for the common cold

Adults: 30 drops (1.5 mL) of liquid herbal pelargonium three times daily.

Acute sinusitis treatment

Adults: 60 drops three times a day.

Reducing the frequency of an asthma attack during respiratory tract infection in children with mild asthma

1–5 years: 10 drops three times a day.

6–12 years: 20 drops three times a day.

Over 12 years of age: 30 drops three times a day.

TOXICITY

Not known.

ADVERSE REACTIONS

Evidence from clinical trials and postmarket surveillance studies indicates few serious adverse events, all found to be unrelated to the medicine, and only mild side effects, which tended to be limited to gastrointestinal symptoms such as nausea, vomiting, diarrhoea or heartburn, and rashes. Allergic skin reactions with pruritus and urticaria have been reported in trials.

SIGNIFICANT INTERACTIONS

Controlled clinical studies are not available; therefore, interactions are based on evidence of activity and are largely theoretical and speculative.

Immunosuppressant drugs

Theoretically, use of this herb may reduce the effectiveness of immunosuppressant medication — avoid until safety can be established.

CONTRAINDICATIONS AND PRECAUTIONS

People with an allergy to the geranium family of plants should avoid this herb.

PREGNANCY USE

It appears safe in pregnancy based on studies using animal models of reproduction and development whereby no effects on fertility or development were detected at up to 2700 mg/kg body weight/day EPs 7630.

PATIENTS' FAQs

What will this herb do for me?
Pelargonium sidoides has antibacterial and antiviral actions and will enhance immune function. It may provide benefits in the treatment in acute, mild to moderate bronchitis, acute rhinosinusitis and possibly the common cold in adults, acute bronchitis in children and in alleviating several common RTI symptoms, in particular, nasal congestion.

When will it start to work?
It should be started at the first sign of infection and a course of treatment is 6–10 days. When used as acute treatment for the common cold, symptom relief may be noticeable within 3 days and significant after 5 days. Symptom relief may take longer to fully establish in cases of acute bronchitis and rhinosinusitis.

Are there any safety issues?
It is generally well tolerated; however; gastrointestinal side effects and allergic skin reactions have been reported with use.

REFERENCES

Agbabiaka TB, et al. *Pelargonium sidoides* for acute bronchitis: a systematic review and meta-analysis. Phytomedicine 15.5 (2008): 378–385.

Beil, W. & Kilian, P. 2007. EPs 7630, an extract from *Pelargonium sidoides* roots inhibits adherence of *Helicobacter pylori* to gastric epithelial cells. Phytomedicine, 14 (Suppl 6), 5–8.

Bladt S, Wagner H. From the Zulu medicine to the European phytomedicine Umckaloabo. Phytomedicine 14 (Suppl 6) (2007): 2–4.

Brendler T, van Wyk BE. A historical, scientific and commercial perspective on the medicinal use of *Pelargonium sidoides* (Geraniaceae). J Ethnopharmacol 119.3 (2008): 420–433.

Engler RJM et al. Complementary and alternative medicine for the allergist-immunologist: where do I start? J Allergy Clin Immunol 123.2 (2009): 309–316.

Kolodziej H et al. Pharmacological profile of extracts of *Pelargonium sidoides* and their constituents. Phytomedicine 10 Suppl 4 (2003): 18–24.

Kolodziej H. Fascinating metabolic pools of *Pelargonium sidoides* and *Pelargonium reniforme*, traditional and phytomedicinal sources of the herbal medicine Umckaloabo. Phytomedicine 14.Suppl 6 (2007): 9–17.

Lizogub VG, et al. Efficacy of a *Pelargonium sidoides* preparation in patients with the common cold: a randomized, double blind, placebo-controlled clinical trial. NY: Explore 3.6 (2007): 573–84.
Luna, L.A., Jr., et al. 2011. Immune responses induced by *Pelargonium sidoides* extract in serum and nasal mucosa of athletes after exhaustive exercise: modulation of secretory IgA, IL-6 and IL-15. Phytomedicine, 18, (4) 303–308.
Mativandlela SPN, et al. Antibacterial, antifungal and antitubercular activity of (the roots of) *Pelargonium reniforme* (CURT) and *Pelargonium sidoides* (DC) (Geraniaceae) root extracts. S Afr J Bot 72.2 (2006): 232–237.
Matthys H, et al. [*Pelargonium sidoides* in acute bronchitis — Health related quality of life and patient-reported outcome in adults receiving EPs 7630 treatment.] Wien Med Wochenschr 2010;160(21–22):564–570.
Patiroglu T, et al. The efficacy of *Pelargonium sidoides* in the treatment of upper respiratory tract infections in children with transient hypogammaglobulinemia of infancy. Phytomedicine 2012;19(11):958–961.
Schnitzler P et al. Efficacy of an aqueous *Pelargonium sidoides* extract against herpesvirus. Phytomedicine 15.12 (2008): 1108–1116.
Tahan F, Yaman M. Can the *Pelargonium sidoides* root extract EPs((R)) 7630 prevent asthma attacks during viral infections of the upper respiratory tract in children? Phytomedicine 2012; 20: 148–150.
Timmer A et al. *Pelargonium sidoides* extract for acute respiratory tract infections. Cochrane Database Syst Rev 3 (2008): CD006323.
Wittschier, N., et al. 2007. An extract of *Pelargonium sidoides* (EPs 7630) inhibits in situ adhesion of *Helicobacter pylori* to human stomach. Phytomedicine, 14, (4) 285–288.

Prebiotics

HISTORICAL NOTE Gibson & Roberfroid (1995) introduced the concept of prebiotic as 'a non-digestible food ingredient that beneficially affects the host by selectively stimulating the growth and/or activity of one or a limited number of bacteria in the colon and thus improves health'. This concept has been further developed to define prebiotics as 'selectively fermented ingredients that allow specific changes, both in the composition and/or activity of the gastrointestinal microflora that confer benefits upon host wellbeing and health' (Roberfroid 2007b).

P

BACKGROUND AND RELEVANT PHARMACOKINETICS

Numerous components appear to have prebiotic characteristics, but some will not be classified as prebiotics because they may not meet all the criteria, i.e. not metabolised (hydrolysed or absorbed) in the upper gastrointestinal tract (GIT), demonstrate selective fermentation by one or a limited number of potentially beneficial intestinal bacteria and change the colonic microflora to a healthier composition (Gibson & Roberfroid 1995, Roberfroid 2007b). To date, the most well-researched prebiotics are inulin, lactulose, fructooligosaccharides (FOS) and galactooligosaccharides (GOS) (Roberfroid 2007a).

One of the key characteristics of prebiotics is to stimulate the selective growth of intestinal microorganisms and, in particular, the growth of lactobacilli and bifidobacteria.

Studies have demonstrated that the intestinal microflora of breastfed infants is characterised by high levels of bifidobacteria and lactic acid bacteria because oligosaccharides occur naturally in breastmilk. Formula-fed infants were found to have more *Bacteroides*, clostridia and Enterobacteriaceae and lower levels of the beneficial microorganisms (Coppa et al 2006).

Bifidobacteria are well-known defences against pathogenic bacteria and are significant for promoting gut health (Brunser et al 2006, Cummings & Macfarlane 2002, Gibson 1998, Gibson & Roberfroid 1995). In addition to stabilising the gut microflora, prebiotics may have a role in allergy: reports indicate that infants with allergy had lower levels of lactobacilli and bifidobacteria (Bjorksten et al 2001) and feeding prebiotics was able to rectify this. Increasingly, prebiotics have been added to infant milk formulas in order to simulate the composition of human breastmilk prebiotic oligosaccharides.

In recent years, there has been a focus on using multiple prebiotics together rather than a single component; combinations of long-chain FOS and short-chain GOS have been utilised mainly because different gastrointestinal microorganisms may require different substrates for optimal growth.

In both adults and the young, prebiotics are reported to have other health-promoting properties and they may have a role in the management of a number of diseases and conditions. Altered gastrointestinal microflora and abnormal colonic fermentation are also noted in some conditions, such as inflammatory bowel disease (IBD) and irritable bowel syndrome (IBS) (King et al 1998); treatment with prebiotics or synbiotics may normalise the altered microflora.

Prebiotics as indigestible components are known to have laxative properties and are used as bulking agents for gastrointestinal health. The end products of the prebiotic fermentation in the colon are short-chain fatty acids (SCFAs), while have direct effects on the intestinal cells and stimulate intestinal peristalsis (Gibson 1998, 1999, Gibson & Roberfroid 1995, Gibson et al 1995).

Both lactobacilli and bifidobacteria species in the colon have important roles in immune stimulation and prevention of infection and diarrhoea (Gorbach et al 1987, Macfarlane et al 2006, Saavedra et al 1994). Some bifidobacteria and lactobacilli strains may have antimutagenic and antitumour properties; prebiotics such as inulin appear to inhibit colonic cancer cell growth (Pool-Zobel & Sauer 2007).

Prebiotics also demonstrate anti-inflammatory activity in the GIT, with lactulose, inulin and FOS all demonstrating GIT anti-inflammatory activity in animal models and/or human research (Cherbut et al 2003, Koleva et al 2012, Lara-Villoslada et al 2006, Looijer–Van Langen & Dieleman 2009, Yasuda et al 2012).

CHEMICAL COMPONENTS

Prebiotics are principally oligosaccharides or disaccharides, of which there are various types: oligofructose, inulins, isomaltooligosaccharides, lactosucrose, GOS, lactulose, pyrodextrins and xylooligosaccharides. Potential prebiotics, their food sources and their targeted microorganisms are highlighted in Table 1.

Inulins are multiple fructose units and inulin degradation results in oligofructose. GOS occur naturally in breastmilk. Fructans are linear or branched fructose polymers and the GOS are synthesised from lactose by the action of beta-galactosidase. FOS are the inulin-type fructans that can be readily obtained from plant sources. Both GOS and FOS are widely used in the food industry (Yang & Silva 1995).

Clinical note — The hygiene hypothesis

The intestinal microflora is crucial for the development of the immune system (Ouwehand et al 2002) and the 'hygiene theory' suggests that exposure to microorganisms is required for this. The consumption of foods containing microorganisms for health-promoting properties has a long history. Probiotics are microorganisms that can 'beneficially affect the host physiology by modulating mucosal and systemic immunity, as well as improving nutritional and microbial balance of the intestinal tract' (Gibson & Roberfroid 1995, Salminen et al 1998).

TABLE 1 PREBIOTIC SUBSTANCES AND THE ORGANISMS WHOSE GROWTH THEY PROMOTE (HUDSON & MARSH 1995, TERAMOTO ET AL 1996, TEURI & KORPELA 1998, VAN LOO ET AL 1995, 1998)

Prebiotic compound	Food sources	Targeted microorganisms
β-glucooligomers	Oats	*Lactobacillus* spp.
Fructooligosaccharides and inulin	Jerusalem artichokes, garlic, onions, chicory roots, asparagus, wheat	*Bifidobacterium* spp.
Galactooligosaccharides	Cow's milk, yoghurt, human milk	*Bifidobacterium* spp.
Galactosyl lactose	Human milk	*Bifidobacterium* spp.
Lactitol	None known	*Lactobacillus* spp.; *Bifidobacterium* spp.
Lactosucrose	None	*Bifidobacterium* spp.
Lactulose	UHT milk	*Lactobacillus* spp.; *Bifidobacterium* spp.
Polydextrose	None known	*Lactobacillus* spp.; *Bifidobacterium* spp.
Raffinose	Legumes, beets	*Lactobacillus* spp.; *Bifidobacterium* spp.
Xylooligosaccharides	Oats	*Bifidobacterium* spp.

P

Clinical note — Synbiotics

Synbiotics are products that contain both probiotic and prebiotic agents (Schrezenmeir & de Vrese 2001). The combination is supposed to enhance the survival of the probiotic bacteria through the upper GIT, improve implantation of the probiotic in the colon and have a stimulating effect on the growth and/or activities of both the exogenously-provided probiotic strain(s) and the endogenous inhabitants of the bowel (Casiraghi et al 2007). In recent years, there has been a trend to increasingly use synbiotics for a synergistic health-promoting effect, but this also makes it difficult to evaluate the individual effects of each component.

FOOD SOURCES

Low levels of prebiotic compounds can be found in artichokes, asparagus, bananas, chicory root, garlic, leek, onions and wheat. Inulin and oligofructose occur naturally in these foods. Commercially produced prebiotics are extracted from chicory roots or Jerusalem artichokes or synthesised from sucrose and are used widely in the food industry. Dietary intake of prebiotics is variable, with the intake for Americans being in the range 1–4 g/day and on average a higher intake among Europeans, who consume 3–10 g/day (Delzenne 2003).

DEFICIENCY SIGNS AND SYMPTOMS

Clear deficiency signs are difficult to establish because the symptoms may vary enormously. Local signs and symptoms of disruption of the intestinal microflora leading to an imbalance (intestinal dysbiosis) include bloating, flatulence, abdominal pain, diarrhoea and/or constipation and fungal overgrowth (such as *Candida*). An imbalance in the gastrointestinal microflora can be caused by the use of antibiotics, GIT infections, stress and dietary factors (Hawrelak & Myers 2004). Administration of prebiotics, probiotics or synbiotics is used as a means of restoring this microflora imbalance.

MAIN ACTIONS

The health benefits claimed for prebiotics mainly stem from their ability to increase numbers of beneficial organisms in the colon, modulate the immune response, reduce numbers of potentially pathogenic microorganisms (PPMs) in the GIT and stimulate SCFA production.

Stimulation of beneficial bacteria and prevention of GIT infections

Many animal and human studies have demonstrated that prebiotics modulate the gut microflora by increasing bifidobacteria and lactobacilli levels (Bouhnik et al 1997, Gibson & Wang 1994, Langlands et al 2004).

Prebiotics are fermented by the microflora in the proximal colon, resulting in the production of SCFAs (acetic, propionic and butyrate acids) and gas (CO_2 and H_2). Consequently, the lower intraluminal pH inhibits the growth of PPMs while simultaneously creating an atmosphere more conducive to the growth of lactobacilli and bifidobacteria (Walker et al 2005). As a result of prebiotics stimulating the growth of beneficial bacteria, these microorganisms secrete antimicrobial compounds and can inhibit colonisation of the pathogenic bacteria and prevent their adherence to the intestinal epithelium (Shoaf-Sweeney & Hutkins 2009). Adherence can also be limited as a result of the oligosaccharide's terminal sugars interfering with the receptors on the pathogenic bacteria (Hopkins & Macfarlane 2003, Zopf & Roth 1996): reduced adherence of enteropathogenic *Escherichia coli* in HeP and Caco-2 cells has been noted with GOS, for example (Shoaf et al 2006). GOS have also been shown to inhibit binding of *Vibrio cholerae* toxin to its receptor in the human GIT (Sinclair et al 2009) and reduce colonisation and pathology associated with *Salmonella typhimurium* infection in a murine model (Searle et al 2009).

Immunomodulation and enhanced mucin production

The mechanisms whereby prebiotics have immunomodulatory effects (modulate cytokine and antibody production) are largely unknown and the proposed mechanisms include beneficial changes in the intestinal microflora and increased production of both mucin and SCFAs. There may also be changes in the gut-associated lymphoid tissues (GALT) as a result of prebiotic fermentation in the colon (Forchielli & Walker 2005). The SCFAs are beneficial to the host as an energy source and enhance mucosal integrity with increased production of mucin, binding to receptors on immune cells within GALT and limiting translocation. Mucin may limit bacterial translocation and acts as a barrier against luminal contents by protectively covering the intestinal epithelial cells. There is little information about the effects of prebiotics on mucin production, but both animal and human research has noted increased mucin production associated with inulin and FOS supplementation (Fontaine et al 1996, Ten Bruggencate et al 2006). This increase appears to be mediated via increases in mucin 3 gene expression, as well as increases in colon crypt depth with more mucin-secreting goblet cells per crypt (Paturi et al 2012).

Both prebiotics and probiotics are reported to have beneficial effects in reducing the effects of colitis by altering the gastrointestinal microflora due to stimulating growth of the protective bacteria and reducing colonisation with potentially hazardous bacteria (Sartor 2004). Prebiotics (mainly inulin and FOS) may also ameliorate inflammation as a result of reducing the activity of proinflammatory transcription factors (e.g. NF-κB), and by the increased production of SCFAs (Cavin et al 2005, Holma et al 2002, Kinoshita et al 2002, Millard et al 2002). Animal studies show conflicting findings, with the majority reporting a reduction in inflammation with prebiotic supplementation (Cherbut et al 2003) and others reporting that there is no protection from FOS or GOS in rat models of colitis (Looijer-Van Langen & Dieleman 2009). In recent years, some human studies have been undertaken and mixed results are reported. Butyrate is a major source of energy for colonocytes, and in vitro studies indicate that butyrate has anti-inflammatory effects (Saemann et al 2000, Segain et al 2000); butyrate and acetate also enhance mucin secretion.

Cancer prevention

Various in vitro and animal studies have been conducted to investigate the role of prebiotics and synbiotics for their anticancer effects, but there are only a limited number of studies in humans (Pool-Zobel & Sauer 2007). Animal studies have shown that prebiotic treatment is beneficial in reducing precancerous aberrant crypt foci and the effects may be more pronounced with synbiotics. Rowland et al (1998) reported that the effect is enhanced with synbiotics such as inulin plus *Bifidobacterium longum* in their study of azoxymethane-induced aberrant crypt foci in rats. Oligofructose-enriched inulin plus *Lactobacillus rhamnosus* and *B. lactis* treatment prevented azoxymethane-induced suppression of natural killer (NK) cell activity in Peyer's patches (Roller et al 2004) and, similarly, a study (Le Leu et al 2005) demonstrated increased apoptotic response with resistant starch plus *B. lactis* treatment.

OTHER ACTIONS

P

Mineral metabolism

Animal studies have indicated that prebiotics such as inulin and oligofructose can affect calcium bioavailability and increase calcium absorption. A number of mechanisms have been proposed for this action, including the increased production of SCFAs, which increase the solubility of minerals and also facilitate the colonic absorption of calcium and magnesium (Demigne et al 2008).

Improved bioavailability of phyto-oestrogens

An interesting animal (rat) study has found that concurrent consumption of FOS and the soy isoflavones, genistein and daidzein, significantly improved the bioavailability of these compounds. The relative absorption of genistein was ~20% higher in FOS-fed rats than in controls. In addition, the presence of both phyto-oestrogens in serum was maintained for longer in FOS-fed rats than in controls, suggesting that FOS enhanced colonic absorption of these compounds (Uehara et al 2001).

This result may be especially relevant to women postantibiotic therapy, where the metabolism and subsequent absorption of phyto-oestrogens appear to be impaired (Kilkkinen et al 2002). Bifidobacteria have been shown to possess β-glucosidase activity, and FOS administration has resulted in enhanced β-glucosidase activity in animal models (Rowland et al 1998) as well as improved phyto-oestrogen bioavailability (Ohta et al 2002). FOS consumption not only aids in the re-establishment of a healthy GIT microflora, but its consumption also increases colonic β-glucosidase activity, resulting in enhanced deglycosylation and thus increased colonic concentrations of the medicinally active aglycones.

The synergistic effect of FOS supplementation with soy isoflavones on bone health has been observed in an osteopenic rat model, where coadministration of the two agents was found to exert the strongest effect in inhibiting bone loss in rats. This was due, at least in part, to FOS-induced increases in calcium absorption and equol production (Kimira et al 2012). Another study utilising an ovariectomised rat model of osteoporosis also found a strong synergistic effect between soy isoflavones and FOS supplementation in preventing bone loss (Hooshmand et al 2010).

CLINICAL USE

Irritable bowel syndrome

A multicentre, double-blind randomised controlled trial (RCT) by Olesen and Gudmand-Hoyer (2000) did not find benefits for the use of FOS in the treatment of IBS, similar to the findings of Hunter et al (1999), who utilised oligofructose in their double crossover study investigating IBS.

Conversely, in a randomised, single-blind, placebo-controlled, crossover trial, supplementation of 3.5 g/day of GOS to subjects with IBS significantly improved stool consistency, flatulence scores, bloating scores and overall IBS symptom scores compared to placebo (all $P < 0.05$) over a 4-week treatment period. Supplementation of 7 g/day resulted in significant improvements in overall IBS symptom scores and a reduction in anxiety levels compared to placebo (both $P < 0.05$). However, there was also a significant increase in bloating scores relative to baseline when subjects were taking the higher dosage ($P < 0.05$) (Silk et al 2009).

Inflammatory bowel disease

In a study of patients with active IBD, 14 patients presenting with ulcerative colitis (UC) and 17 patients presenting with Crohn's disease (CD) received either standard medication treatment or the medications with an additional 10 g/day lactulose dose for 4 months. At the end of the study there were no differences in the clinical or endoscopic score, although the UC group receiving the lactulose treatment reported an improved quality of life compared to the control group ($P = 0.04$) (Hafer et al 2007).

Crohn's disease

At present, the role of prebiotics in the management of CD remains unknown due to a limited number of studies.

A small open-label study of 10 patients with active ileocolonic CD who were treated with FOS (15 g/day for 3 weeks) reported a significant reduction in disease activity scores (30% reduction; $P < 0.01$) and inflammation, with an increase in interleukin-10 (IL-10)-positive dendritic cells and Toll-like receptor 2 and Toll-like receptor 4 expression. It is noteworthy that patients entering remission had increased mucosal-associated bifidobacteria (Lindsay et al 2006).

This positive, but small, open-label trial was followed up with a double-blind, placebo-controlled RCT. One hundred and three subjects with active CD were supplemented with 15 g/day FOS or placebo for 4 weeks in conjunction with standard medications. While there was an increased percentage of IL-10-positive dendritic cells ($P = 0.035$), there was no significant difference in response rate or rate of remission. Surprisingly, there were no changes in faecal bifidobacterial concentrations in the FOS-treated group. It is also worth noting that 19% of the FOS-treated group withdrew from the trial due to adverse gastrointestinal effects (flatulence, borborygmi and abdominal pain) (Benjamin et al 2011).

In a small, randomised, open-label trial, Hafer et al (2007) investigated the efficacy of lactulose therapy (10 g/day for 4 months) compared to standard care in patients with CD (n = 17). No significant improvements in clinical activity index, endoscopic score or immunohistochemical parameters were observed in CD patients receiving lactulose, in comparison to controls (Hafer et al 2007).

A RCT of 30 patients with CD postoperative ileocaecal resection, who were treated with Synbiotic 2000, a combination of four prebiotic components plus a probiotic mixture of four lactic acid strains (*Pediococcus pentosaceus*, *Lactobacillus raffinolactis*, *Lactobacillus paracasei* subsp. *paracasei* F19, *Lactobacillus plantarum*, 2.5 g beta-glucans, 2.5 g inulin, 2.5 g pectin, 2.5 g resistant starch), did not show prevention of relapse 24 months later (Chermesh et al 2007). In another study (duration: 13.0 ± 4.5 months) (Fujimori et al 2007), 10 non-hospitalised patients with active CD were treated with high-dose synbiotic therapy consisting of bifidobacterium and lactobacillus (75 billion colony-forming units (CFU)/day) plus psyllium (9.9 g/day); only three patients did not experience any benefit.

These differing results may be due to the variation in fibres used in the trials, as well as differences in the probiotic strains utilised.

Ulcerative colitis

The results from a number of animal studies have indicated that prebiotics may be of therapeutic value in UC and preliminary human studies appear to show similar results. A small randomised, double-blind, placebo-controlled trial evaluated 19 patients with active UC (mild/moderate). Subjects received prebiotic treatment (12 g/day of oligofructose-enriched inulin, ratio 1 : 1) or placebo plus 3 g/day of mesalazine for 2 weeks. Subjects in the prebiotic group experienced significantly fewer dyspeptic symptoms and a reduction of intestinal inflammation, as determined by faecal calprotectin levels, which decreased after 1 week of treatment (from 4377 to 1033; $P < 0.05$). However, there was no change in prostaglandin E_2 secretion and IL-8 production (Casellas et al 2007).

The effectiveness of lactulose therapy in UC was evaluated in a small, randomised, open-label trial. Seven subjects consumed 10 g/day of lactulose in conjunction with their standard medications for 4 months, while another seven received standard care only. There was a significant improvement seen in the clinical activity index in the lactulose-treated group (54% reduction; $P = 0.047$ compared to baseline). The decrease in the clinical activity index was not significant when compared to controls, however ($P = 0.09$). Four patients in the lactulose group achieved remission versus none in the control group. Quality-of-life scores significantly improved in the lactulose group compared to controls ($P = 0.037$) and there was also a trend for a reduction in steroid dose ($P = 0.063$) in this group (Hafer et al 2007).

In a double-blind RCT of 18 patients with active UC, synbiotic treatment with 12 g oligofructose-enriched inulin (1 : 1) plus *Bifidobacterium longum* for 4 weeks resulted in reduced colonic inflammation, decreased human beta-defensin mRNA, tumour necrosis factor-alpha and IL-1alpha, and improved sigmoidoscopy scores, although there was no difference in clinical measures (Furrie et al 2005).

In another RCT, the efficacy of synbiotic therapy was compared to either prebiotics or probiotics and involved 120 outpatients with UC in remission (Fujimori et al 2009). Each group of patients enrolled in the study were treated with either one capsule per day consisting of *B. longum* 2×10^9 CFU (probiotic

P

group) or 2 × 4 g doses of psyllium (prebiotic group) or both the probiotic plus prebiotic (synbiotic group) for 4 weeks. At the end of the study, C-reactive protein decreased significantly (P = 0.04) and the quality-of-life scores in the Inflammatory Bowel Disease Questionnaires were also significantly improved for the synbiotic treated group; the score for bowel function was significant in the prebiotic group (P = 0.04).

Pouchitis

There are only a limited number of studies that have investigated the role of prebiotics or synbotics in pouchitis.

A small open-label study of 10 patients with pouchitis (antibiotic-refractory or antibiotic-dependent) treated with a synbiotic mixture of FOS plus *Lactobacillus rhamnosus* GG reported complete remission as determined by clinical and endoscopic criteria (Friedman & George 2000). In a crossover study of 20 patients with ileal pouch–anal anastomosis, daily treatment with 24 g of inulin or placebo for 3 weeks did not change the clinical activity scores, although there was a reduction in inflammation (P = 0.01) and increased faecal butyrate concentrations. Lactobacilli and bifidobacteria levels were not affected, although a significant reduction in faecal levels of *Bacteroides fragilis* was reported (Welters et al 2002).

Constipation

The use of lactulose has a long history and it has been used successfully as an osmotic laxative to treat constipation (de Schryver et al 2005, Petticrew et al 1997). Likewise, FOS and GOS also have laxative effects: Gibson et al (1995) demonstrated that feeding 15 g of FOS or 15 g inulin per day could significantly increase stool output. Utilising 9 g GOS/day, one study found an increase in defecation frequency (from 5.9 to 7.1 movements/week) in elderly subjects over a 2-week treatment period. There was also a trend for easier defecation (P = 0.07) during the GOS phase of the trial (Teuri & Korpela 1998).

Two RCTs evaluated the laxative effects of GOS in healthy adult subjects with a tendency to constipation. At a daily dose of 5 and 10 g there were significant improvements in defecation frequency — from 0.92 to 1.07 movements daily ($P < 0.05$) and from 0.85 to 0.97 times per day ($P < 0.05$), respectively (Niittyen et al 2007).

Diarrhoea

Various prebiotic components have been utilised in clinical trials to evaluate their efficacy in diarrhoea of different origins.

Traveller's diarrhoea

A double-blind RCT of 244 people travelling to medium–high-risk destinations and at risk of traveller's diarrhoea reported that those subjects who were treated with FOS (10 g) experienced increased wellbeing and less severe diarrhoea, although there was no significant difference in the incidence of diarrhoea (Cummings et al 2001).

A more recent double-blind RCT evaluated the potential of GOS administration to prevent traveller's diarrhoea. Subjects ingested 2.6 g GOS once daily starting 7 days before reaching their holiday destination and continued taking it daily throughout their holiday. Compared to the placebo group, subjects in the GOS group experienced a 40% decrease in the incidence ($P < 0.05$) and a 48% reduction in duration of traveller's diarrhoea ($P < 0.05$). Additionally, they suffered less abdominal pain ($P < 0.05$) and experienced improved quality of life ($P < 0.05$) (Drakoularakou et al 2009).

Clostridium difficile-associated diarrhoea (CDAD)

In a double-blind RCT, 142 patients with CDAD in hospital were randomised to receive oligofructose or placebo as well as the standard antibiotic treatment for 30 days and followed up 30 days later. It was found that the prebiotic-treated patients had increased bifidobacteria levels and reduction in the rate of relapse and experienced significantly less diarrhoea compared to placebo (8% vs 34%, $P < 0.001$) (Lewis et al 2005a).

In another double-blind RCT of 435 hospitalised patients who were receiving antibiotics, treatment with oligofructose for 7 days was compared to placebo. After a 7-day follow-up period, there was a significant increase in bifidobacteria concentrations in the prebiotic group, although there was no difference in the incidence of *Clostridium difficile* (Lewis et al 2005b).

Allergic disease and food hypersensitivity

Clinical trials confirm that prebiotic-enhanced infant formula ingested during the first 6 months of life reduces the risk of atopic disease. The effect is not limited to the 6-month treatment period but seems to provide longer-term protection.

In a double-blind RCT, Moro et al (2006) evaluated the effects of a prebiotic-enhanced infant formula (FOS and GOS combination) on the incidence of atopic dermatitis during the first 6 months of life in formula-fed infants at high risk of atopy development. Atopic dermatitis developed in 23% of infants in the control group compared to 10% in the prebiotic group ($P = 0.014$) over the 6-month intervention period. Subjects in the prebiotic group were also found to have significantly reduced plasma levels of total IgE ($P = 0.007$), IgG_2 ($P = 0.029$) and IgG_3 ($P = 0.0343$), as well as cow's milk protein-specific IgG_1 ($P = 0.015$), suggesting that FOS and GOS supplementation induces an antiallergic antibody profile (Nauta et al 2008).

These same infants were followed up over the next 18 months. Those infants who received the prebiotic-enhanced formula for the first 6 months of life were at reduced risk of developing atopic disease over the follow-up period. Infants in the control group experienced a significantly higher rate of atopic disease, such as atopic dermatitis (27.9% vs 13.6%), recurrent wheezing (20.6% vs 7.6%) and allergic urticaria (10.3% vs 1.5%) compared to infants in the prebiotic group (all $P < 0.05$) (Arslanoglu et al 2010).

A Cochrane systematic review (Osborn & Sinn 2013) investigated the effectiveness of prebiotics for the prevention of allergic disease or food hypersensitivity in infants. Four studies including 1428 infants were eligible for inclusion. Meta-analysis of two studies (226 infants) found no significant difference in rates of infant asthma, although significant heterogeneity was observed between the two studies. Meta-analysis of four studies found a significant reduction in eczema incidence in the prebiotic-treated groups (1218 infants, typical risk ratio 0.68; $P = 0.03$), with no statistically significant heterogeneity found between studies.

Improved immune response

Prebiotics, like FOS, have long been suggested to have immune-enhancing effects (Bornet & Brouns 2002, Watz et al 2005). It is, however, only recently that human trials with hard end points have been completed, in both children and adults.

Use in children

Various studies have evaluated whether long-term prebiotic use reduces the incidence of various infections and reduces the use of antibiotic medication, overall producing positive results.

One of the first of these trials investigated the effects of a prebiotic mixture (containing a combination of FOS and GOS) in protecting against infection during the first 6 months of life in formula-fed infants. In this randomised, double-blind, placebo-controlled trial, infants allocated to the prebiotic group experienced significantly fewer episodes of all types of infections combined ($P = 0.01$) compared to those in the placebo group. There was also a trend for fewer episodes of upper respiratory tract infection ($P = 0.07$) and fewer infections requiring antibiotic treatment ($P = 0.10$) in the prebiotic group. Additionally, the cumulative incidence of recurring infection and recurring respiratory tract infection was 3.9% and 2.9% in the prebiotic group versus 13.5% and 9.6% in the placebo group, respectively ($P < 0.05$) (Arslanoglu et al 2008).

This same infant cohort was followed up over the next 1.5 years. Those infants who received the prebiotic-enhanced formula for the first 6 months of life experienced significantly fewer episodes of medically-diagnosed respiratory tract infections ($P < 0.01$), fever episodes ($P < 0.00001$) and fewer antibiotic prescriptions ($P < 0.05$) compared to those in the placebo group (Arslanoglu et al 2010).

In an open-label, placebo-controlled, randomised study, Bruzzese et al (2009) also investigated the efficacy of a prebiotic-enhanced infant formula (a combination of GOS and FOS) on infection incidence in infants. The prebiotic-enhanced formula or a standard infant formula was consumed over the initial 12 months of life. During this period, the incidence of gastroenteritis was 59% lower in the prebiotic group ($P = 0.015$). Additionally, the number of children suffering from recurrent upper respiratory tract infections tended to be lower in the prebiotic group (28% vs 45%; $P = 0.06$) and the number of children prescribed multiple antibiotic courses per year was also lower (40% vs 66%; $P = 0.004$)

A shorter double-blind RCT was conducted involving children (aged 7–19 months) attending day-care centres. The authors found that 21 days of treatment with FOS significantly reduced the number of infectious diseases requiring antibiotic treatment ($P < 0.001$), episodes of diarrhoea and vomiting ($P < 0.001$) and episodes of fever ($P < 0.05$) compared to controls (Waligora-Dupriet et al 2007). In another RCT investigating the effects of FOS in toddlers (4–24-month-olds) attending day care, FOS administration was found to significantly reduce antibiotic use (32% reduction; $P = 0.001$) and day-care absenteeism (61% decrease; $P = 0.025$) compared to those in the control group. There was also a 34% reduction in episodes of fever in combination with any cold symptoms ($P = 0.001$) and a 61% decrease in episodes of fever in association with diarrhoea ($P < 0.05$) in the FOS-supplemented group (Saavedra & Tschernia 2002).

Use in adults

Treatment with GOS for 8 weeks around exam time had multiple beneficial effects according to a double-blind RCT involving 427 academically stressed undergraduate students. Students received placebo, 2.5 or 5.0 g GOS daily for 8 weeks. Active treatment resulted in a significant reduction in stress-induced gastrointestinal symptoms such as diarrhoea ($P = 0.0298$) and constipation ($P = 0.0003$). Additionally, the lower dose of GOS was associated with lower cold and flu symptom intensity. The higher dose was found to reduce the probability of having a sick day by 40% in normal-weight individuals ($P = 0.0002$). However, this protective effect was not observed in overweight or obese patients. The authors theorised that the lack of efficacy in overweight patients was due to differences in the baseline microbiota (e.g. fewer bifidobacteria) (Hughes et al 2011).

In another randomised, double-blind, placebo-controlled, crossover trial, the impact of GOS supplementation (2.75 g/day) on immune parameters in healthy elderly subjects was assessed. Forty-four subjects took part in this 24-week trial (2 × 10-week treatment periods with a 4-week washout in between). Ten weeks of GOS supplementation was found to not only significantly increase faecal populations of bifidobacteria and decrease the quantity of less beneficial bacteria (*E. coli*, *Bacteroides* spp., *Clostridium* spp. and *Desulfovibrio* spp.) compared to the control period, but also significantly increase NK cell activity, phagocytic activity of leucocytes and the production of the anti-inflammatory cytokine IL-10. GOS supplementation also resulted in a significant reduction in the production of proinflammatory cytokines (IL-6, IL-1beta and tumour necrosis factor-alpha) (Vulevic et al 2008).

Prebiotic supplementation has also been tested in an HIV-positive population, showing benefits. In a double-blind RCT, 57 highly active antiretroviral therapy (HAART)-naive HIV-1-infected adults received either a unique prebiotic mixture (GOS, long-chain FOS and pectin hydrolysate-derived acidic oligosaccharides) or placebo for 12 weeks. Subjects in the prebiotic group demonstrated significant improvements in the gut microbiota composition, a reduction of soluble CD14 and $CD4^+$ T-cell activation and increased NK cell activity compared to controls (Gori et al 2011).

Cancer of the colon

Administration of lactulose or oligofructose-enriched inulin to healthy volunteers resulted in a significant decrease in colonic beta-glucuronidase activity, which is considered protective against colon cancer development (De Preter et al 2008). A randomised, double-blind, placebo-controlled study investigated the effects of a synbiotic mixture on immune modulation in patients with colon cancer (n = 34) post 'curative resection' and polypectomised patients (n = 40). The synbiotic-treated group received encapsulated *Lactobacillus rhamnosus* GG 1 × 10^{10} CFU + *Bifidobacterium lactis* Bb12 1 × 10^{10} CFU plus 10 g of inulin enriched with oligofructose on a daily basis for 12 weeks. Overall, both groups receiving the synbiotic treatment demonstrated minor effects on some of the immune markers (Roller et al 2007). Likewise, in another randomised, double-blind, placebo-controlled study of 80 patients (37 colon cancer and 43 polypectomised) by this group, a number of colorectal cancer biomarkers were positively affected by 12 weeks' synbiotic treatment (Rafter et al 2007).

A randomised clinical trial conducted by Roncucci et al (1993) demonstrated the ability of lactulose to prevent the growth of resected colorectal polyps. Lactulose administration (20 g/day) reduced the recurrence rates of colonic polyps by 66% ($P < 0.02$) as compared to controls.

Prevention of urinary tract infections

Two human studies have demonstrated the efficacy of lactulose therapy in the prevention of urinary tract infections. McCutcheon and Fulton (1989) conducted a retrospective study using 45 elderly, long-term hospital patients as subjects. The study found that daily lactulose therapy for 6 months (30 mL lactulose syrup/day) resulted in a significant reduction in urinary tract infections compared to controls ($P < 0.025$). Sixteen of the 17 lactulose-treated patients (94%) remained infection-free over the 6 months, compared to 16 of the 28 control patients (57%) ($P < 0.005$). In addition, there was a significant reduction in the number of antibiotic prescriptions ($P < 0.05$) and in the number of patients receiving antibiotics ($P < 0.005$) in the lactulose group.

In the second study, Mack et al (cited in Conn 1997) enrolled 75 elderly, hospitalised patients in a randomised, placebo-controlled trial. Thirty-eight patients received the placebo and 58 received lactulose therapy. Twelve per cent of the lactulose group developed urinary tract infections during the period of follow-up, compared to 32% in the control group ($P < 0.01$).

Bone health

Calcium absorption was significantly increased ($P = 0.04$) in women ingesting a yoghurt drink (2 × 200 mL/day) rich in GOS (20 g/day) according to a double-blind, crossover RCT. The study used a 9-day intervention period and involved 12 menopausal women (van den Heuvel et al 2000).

Griffin et al (2002) conducted a larger, randomised, crossover study of 59 young girls to investigate the effect of either inulin or inulin plus oligofructose (8 g/day) taken for 3 weeks in addition to 1500 mg/day calcium (two glasses of calcium-fortified orange juice); at the end of the study, the inulin plus oligofructose-treated group was reported to have significantly higher calcium absorption. Research by Abrams et al (2005) has supported these findings.

Promotion of satiety

FOS supplementation affects satiety and hunger, according to a single-blind, crossover, placebo-controlled trial (Cani et al 2006). Subjects who ingested 8 g of FOS twice daily (with breakfast and dinner) experienced a significant increase in satiety at both meals (both $P = 0.04$), but not at lunch. At dinner, FOS supplementation was also found to reduce hunger ($P = 0.04$) and prospective food consumption ($P = 0.05$). Energy intake at breakfast ($P = 0.01$) and lunch ($P = 0.03$) was also found to be significantly reduced after FOS supplementation, resulting in a 5% decrease in total energy intake per day.

A later double-blind RCT investigated the effects of a higher dose (21 g/day) of FOS over a 12-week period and found that active treatment resulted in a mean reduction of 1.03 kg bodyweight compared to a 0.45 kg increase in weight in the placebo group ($P = 0.01$). FOS consumption was also associated with a lower area under the curve (AUC) for ghrelin ($P = 0.004$) and a higher AUC for peptide YY ($P = 0.03$), suggesting an upregulation of satiety hormone secretion. These changes coincided with a reduction in self-reported caloric intake ($P < 0.05$). Serum glucose concentrations and insulin levels also significantly improved in the FOS group compared to baseline measures (both $P < 0.05$) (Parnell & Reimer 2009).

Metabolic syndrome

Treatment with GOS (2.75 g/day) for 12 weeks resulted in significant decreases in levels of plasma C-reactive protein ($P < 0.0012$), insulin ($P < 0.005$), total cholesterol ($P < 0.001$) and triglycerides ($P < 0.0005$) compared to placebo in a double-blind, crossover RCT involving 45 overweight adults with three or more risk factors associated with metabolic syndrome. The decreases in total cholesterol and triglycerides, while statistically significant, was not of a magnitude considered clinically significant (Vulevic et al 2013).

OTHER USES

Liver disease — hepatic encephalopathy

Lactulose has been used routinely as part of the treatment for hepatic encephalopathy, although the exact mechanism of its action is still undetermined. Lactulose treatment results in normalising of the intestinal microflora, lowering faecal pH, decreasing colonic ammonia production and increasing nitrogen excretion (Ballongue et al 1997, Elkington et al 1969). A meta-analysis of prebiotics in the treatment of minimal hepatic encephalopathy found lactulose treatment (five studies) to be associated with significant improvement in the condition (Shukla et al 2011). Lactulose therapy has also recently found in RCTs to effectively prevent the development of hepatic encephalopathy in patients with liver cirrhosis (Sharma et al 2012, Wen et al 2013).

Pancreatitis

Some studies have found that synbiotic supplementation was more beneficial than prebiotics alone for improved systemic inflammatory response in patients with acute pancreatitis (Olah et al 2005).

DOSAGE RANGE

Lactulose, FOS and GOS have all demonstrated dose-dependent responses in terms of altering the GIT microbiota, with larger doses inducing greater beneficial changes in the ecosystem. However, prebiotics are known to induce gastrointestinal side effects, such as abdominal pain, bloating, borborygmi and excessive flatulence when used in high doses; these symptoms tend to diminish over time or with dose reduction. Hence, the initial dose should be small and increased gradually dependent on gastrointestinal tolerance. Therapeutic dosage ranges are as follows: GOS: 2.5–20 g/day; FOS: 4–40 g/day; lactulose: 3–40 g/day.

TOXICITY

Overall, prebiotics have a good profile but their consumption can result in some adverse gastrointestinal side effects. (See Adverse reactions, below.)

ADVERSE REACTIONS

There are many reports of transient gastrointestinal side effects of prebiotic treatment; symptoms such as abdominal pain, bloating, diarrhoea and increased flatulence are commonly reported. The severity of the symptoms is dose-dependent.

A potentially more troubling aspect of prebiotic prescription is their possible enhancement of bacterial translocation, although the research results have been mixed, with some research finding a protective effect and other research finding the opposite, and others no effect. Studies in rats have shown that both inulin and FOS supplementation not only increased intestinal lactobacilli and bifidobacteria colonisation, but also enhanced translocation of *Salmonella enterica* serovar *enteritidis* and the caecal contents also contained *Salmonella*, although concurrent calcium intake was noted to resolve this problem (Bovee-Oudenhoven et al 2003, Ten Bruggencate et al 2004). On the other hand, reduced bacterial translocation to the liver has been reported in rats with dextran sulfate sodium-induced colitis when fed FOS (Osman et al 2006) and feeding mice a combination of FOS and inulin was found to protect against *Klebsiella pneumoniae* translocation (Silva et al 2009). In piglets, the addition of GOS or polydextrose to their diet had no impact on rates of bacterial translocation (Monaco et al 2011). In a human study of 72 elective surgery patients, synbiotic feeding (FOS in combination with four strains of probiotic bacteria) did not result in increased bacterial translocation (Anderson et al 2004).

A published case study has described an instance of anaphylaxis attributed to inulin found in vegetables and processed foods. This was later confirmed with skinprick testing and blinded food provocation testing (Gay-Crosier et al 2000). This allergy appears to be extremely rare considering the widespread consumption of FOS-containing foods. There is also one report describing an allergic reaction to lactulose ingestion in a child with severe milk allergy, presumably due to contamination of trace amounts of cow's milk protein in the preparation used (Maiello et al 2011).

P

SIGNIFICANT INTERACTIONS

Controlled studies are not available and at present there are no known drug interactions with prebiotics.

CONTRAINDICATIONS AND PRECAUTIONS

Prebiotics/synbiotics are contraindicated in those people who are hypersensitive to any component of the prebiotics/synbiotics-containing product. People with IBS who may have increased gas production should avoid high intakes of prebiotics (Serra et al 2001); low doses of GOS have, however, been found to decrease gas-related symptoms in IBS patients (Silk et al 2009). People with lactose intolerance should use lactulose with caution, as its use may cause more gastrointestinal adverse events than in lactose digesters (Teuri et al 1999). On the other hand, long-term ingestion of lactulose in lactose maldigesters has been found to increase their tolerance to lactose (Szilagyi et al 2001). Patients with fructose intolerance may also be more sensitive to the gastrointestinal adverse effects of FOS (Shepherd et al 2008).

One research group has found FOS intake to promote bacterial translocation and increase mucosal irritation in an animal model of *Salmonella* infection (Bovee-Oudenhoven et al 2003, Ten Bruggencate et al 2005). Hence, FOS supplementation may be contraindicated in patients with *Salmonella* enteritis.

PREGNANCY USE

Prebiotics found in the food chain (FOS, inulin and GOS) are considered safe to consume in pregnancy. Lactulose in laxative doses (10–20+ g in a single dose) carries a category B classification (Prather 2004).

Practice points/Patient counselling

- Prebiotics can be obtained from foods such as artichoke, Jerusalem artichokes, asparagus, bananas, chicory root, garlic, leek, onions and wheat, although not necessarily in clinically relevant amounts.
- Prebiotics may be combined with probiotics to produce synbiotics that will enable the two components to work together in synergy.
- Although prebiotics may improve the long-term bowel flora, prebiotic supplementation has many other benefits not associated with improvement in the ecosystem of the GIT.
- There is some evidence that prebiotics support both the development and the maintenance of a healthy immune system.
- Prebiotics have been used in the management of diarrhoea, constipation, other gastrointestinal disorders, bone health, allergic disease and food sensitivity.
- Continuous intake of prebiotics is required in order to maintain their health benefits.
- Some individuals may experience greater gastrointestinal discomfort with use, although some symptoms may subside over time and dose reduction can improve tolerance.

PATIENTS' FAQs

What will this supplement do for me?

Studies have shown that prebiotics are beneficial in the treatment of digestive disorders such as diarrhoea, constipation and some IBDs, such as ulcerative colitis, and also other conditions, such as IBS, food allergies and eczema. There is some evidence that prebiotics may be useful for bone health.

When will it start to work?

Usually prebiotics can exert beneficial effects for digestive disorders such as constipation and diarrhoea within 1–2 weeks, although continuous use for several weeks/months may produce long-term benefits and be necessary in the treatment of other disorders.

Are there any safety issues?

Generally, prebiotics have a good safety profile; however, high-dose supplementation can cause a number of gastrointestinal adverse effects, such as bloating, distension and increased flatulence. These effects are most often noted at the beginning of prebiotic therapy and are generally dose-related. Hence, in some patients it is advisable to commence prebiotic supplementation at a low dose and slowly increase to achieve the optimal dose over several weeks.

REFERENCES

Abrams SA et al. A combination of prebiotic short- and long-chain inulin-type fructans enhances calcium absorption and bone mineralization in young adolescents. Am J Clin Nutr 82.2 (2005): 471–476.

Anderson AD et al. Randomised clinical trial of synbiotic therapy in elective surgical patients. Gut 53 (2004): 241–245.

Arslanoglu S et al. Early dietary intervention with a mixture of prebiotic oligosaccharides reduces the incidence of allergic manifestations and infections during the first two years of life. J Nutr 138 (2008): 1091–1095.

Arslanoglu, S., et al. 2010. Early dietary intervention with a mixture of prebiotic oligosaccharides reduces the incidence of allergic manifestations and infections during the first two years of life. J Nutr, 138, 1091–1095.

Ballongue et al. Effects of lactulose and lactitol on colonic microflora and enzymatic activity. Scand J Gastroenterol 32.222 (1997): 41–44.

Benjamin, J. L., et al. 2011. Randomised, double-blind, placebo-controlled trial of fructo-oligosaccharides in active Crohn's disease. Gut, 60, 923–929.

Bjorksten B et al. Allergy development and the intestinal microflora during the first year of life. J Allergy Clin Immunol 108 (2001): 516–520.

Bornet, F. R. & Brouns, F. 2002. Immune-stimulating and gut health-promoting properties of short-chain fructo-oligosaccharides. Nutrition Reviews, 60, 326–334.

Bouhnik Y et al. Administration of transgalacto-oligosaccharides increases fecal bifidobacteria and modifies colonic fermentation metabolism in healthy humans. J Nutr 127 (1997): 444–448.

Bovee-Oudenhoven IM et al. Dietary fructo-oligosaccharides and lactulose inhibit intestinal colonisation but stimulate translocation of salmonella in rats. Gut 52 (2003): 1572–1578.

Brunser O et al. Effects of probiotic or prebiotic supplemented milk formulas on fecal microbiota composition of infants. Asia Pac J Clin Nutr 15 (2006): 368–376.

Bruzzese, E., et al. 2009. A formula containing galacto- and fructo-oligosaccharides prevents intestinal and extra-intestinal infections: An observational study. Clin Nutr, 28, 156–161.

Cani, P. D., et al. 2006. Oligofructose promotes satiety in healthy human: a pilot study. European Journal of Clinical Nutrition, 60, 567–572.

Casellas F et al. Oral oligofructose-enriched inulin supplementation in acute ulcerative colitis is well tolerated and associated with lowered faecal calprotectin. Aliment Pharmacol Ther 25 (2007): 1061–1067.

Casiraghi, M. C., et al. 2007. Effects of a synbiotic milk product on human intestinal ecosystem. Journal of Applied Microbiology, 103, 499–506.

Cavin C et al. Inhibition of the expression and activity of cyclooxygenase-2 by chicory extract. Biochem Biophys Res Commun 327 (2005): 742–749.

Cherbut C, et al. The prebiotic characteristics of fructooligosaccharides are necessary for reduction of TNBS-induced colitis in rats. J Nutr 133 (2003): 21–27.

Chermesh I et al. Failure of synbiotic 2000 to prevent postoperative recurrence of Crohn's disease. Dig Dis Sci 52 (2007): 385–389.

Coppa GV et al. Prebiotics in human milk: a review. Dig Liver Dis 38 (Suppl 2) (2006): S291–S294.

Cummings JH, Macfarlane GT. Gastrointestinal effects of prebiotics. Br J Nutr 87 (Suppl 2) (2002): S145–S151.

Cummings JH, et al. A study of fructo-oligosaccharides in the prevention of traveller's diarrhoea. Aliment Pharmacol Ther 15 (2001): 1139–1145.

Delzenne NM. Oligosaccharides: state of the art. Proc Nutr Soc 62 (2003): 177–182.

Demigne C et al. Comparison of native or reformulated chicory fructans, or non-purified chicory, on rat cecal fermentation and mineral metabolism. Eur J Nutr 47 (2008): 366–374.

de Preter, V., et al 2008. Effect of dietary intervention with different pre- and probiotics on intestinal bacterial enzyme activities. Eur J Clin Nutr, 62, 225–31.

de Schryver AM et al. Effects of regular physical activity on defecation pattern in middle-aged patients complaining of chronic constipation. Scand J Gastroenterol 40 (2005): 422–429.

Drakoularakou, A., et al. 2009. A double-blind, placebo-controlled, randomized human study assessing the capacity of a novelgalacto-oligosaccharide mixture in reducing travellers' diarrhoea. European Journal of Clinical Nutrition, 64, 146–152.

Elkington SG, et al. Lactulose in the treatment of chronic portal-systemic encephalopathy. N Engl J Med 281 (1969): 408–411.

Fontaine N et al. Intestinal mucin distribution in the germ-free rat and in the heteroxenic rat harbouring a human bacterial flora: effect of inulin in the diet. Br J Nutr 75.6 (1996): 881–892.

Forchielli ML, Walker WA. The role of gut-associated lymphoid tissues and mucosal defence. Br J Nutr 93 (Suppl 1) (2005): S41–S48.

Friedman G, George J. Treatment of refractory 'pouchitis' with prebiotic and probiotic therapy. Gastroenterology 118 (2000) G4167.

Fujimori S et al. High dose probiotic and prebiotic cotherapy for remission induction of active Crohn's disease. J Gastroenterol Hepatol 22.8 (2007): 1199–1204.

Fujimori S et al. A randomised controlled trial on the efficacy of synbiotic versus probiotic or prebiotic treatment to improve the quality of life in patients with ulcerative colitis. Nutrition 25.5 (2009): 520–5.

Furrie E et al. Synbiotic therapy (*Bifidobacterium longum*/Synergy 1) initiates resolution of inflammation in patients with active ulcerative colitis: a randomised controlled pilot trial. Gut 54 (2005): 242–249.

Gay-Crosier, F., et al. 2000. Anaphylaxis from inulin in vegetables and processed food [Letter]. New England Journal of Medicine, 342, 1372.

Gibson GR. Dietary modulation of the human gut microflora using prebiotics. Br J Nutr 80 (1998): S209–S212.

Gibson GR. Dietary modulation of the human gut microflora using the prebiotics oligofructose and inulin. J Nutr 129 (1999): 1438S–41S.

Gibson GR, Roberfroid MB. Dietary modulation of the human colonic microbiota: introducing the concept of prebiotics. J Nutr 125 (1995): 1401–1412.

Gibson GR, Wang X. Regulatory effects of bifidobacteria on the growth of other colonic bacteria. J Appl Bacteriol 77 (1994): 412–420.

Gibson GR et al. Selective stimulation of bifidobacteria in the human colon by oligofructose and inulin. Gastroenterology 108 (1995): 975–982.

Gorbach SL, Chang TW, Goldin B. Successful treatment of relapsing *Clostridium difficile* colitis with Lactobacillus GG. Lancet 262.8574 (1987): 1519.

Gori, A., et al. 2011. Specific prebiotics modulate gut microbiota and immune activation in HAART-naive HIV-infected adults: results of the "COPA" pilot randomized trial. Mucosal Immunol, 4, 554–63.

Griffin IJ, et al. Non-digestible oligosaccharides and calcium absorption in girls with adequate calcium intakes. Br J Nutr 87 (Suppl 2) (2002): S187–S191.

Hafer A et al. Effect of oral lactulose on clinical and immunohistochemical parameters in patients with inflammatory bowel disease: a pilot study. BMC Gastroenterol 7 (2007): 36.

Hawrelak, J. A. & Myers, S. P. 2004. Intestinal dysbiosis: A review of the literature. Alternative Medicine Review, 9, 180–197.

Holma R et al. Galacto-oligosaccharides stimulate the growth of bifidobacteria but fail to attenuate inflammation in experimental colitis in rats. Scand J Gastroenterol 37 (2002): 1042–1047.

Hooshmand, S., et al. 2010. Combination of genistin and fructooligosaccharides prevents bone loss in ovarian hormone deficiency. J Med Food, 13, 320–5.

Hopkins MJ, Macfarlane GT. Nondigestible oligosaccharides enhance bacterial colonisation resistance against *Clostridium difficile* in vitro. Appl Environ Microbiol 69 (2003): 1920–1927.

Hudson, M. J. & Marsh, P. D. 1995. Carbohydrate metabolism in the colon. In: Gibson, G. R. & Macfarlane, G. T. (eds.) Human Colonic Bacteria: Role in Nutrition, Physiology, and Pathology. Boca Raton: CRC Press.

Hughes, C., et al. 2011. Galactooligosaccharide supplementation reduces stress-induced gastrointestinal dysfunction and days of cold or flu: a randomized, double-blind, controlled trial in healthy university students. Am J Clin Nutr, 93, 1305–11.

Hunter JO, et al. Controlled trial of oligofructose in the management of irritable bowel syndrome. J Nutr 129 (7 Suppl) (1999): 1451S–3S.

Kilkkinen, A., et al. 2002. Use of oral antimicrobials decreases serum enterolactone concentration. American Journal of Epidemiology, 155, 472–477.

Kimira, Y., et al. 2012. Synergistic effect of isoflavone glycosides and fructooligosaccharides on postgastrectomy osteopenia in rats. J Clin Biochem Nutr, 51, 156–60.

King TS, et al. Abnormal colonic fermentation in irritable bowel syndrome. Lancet 352 (1998): 1187–1189.

Kinoshita M, et al. Butyrate reduces colonic paracellular permeability by enhancing PPARgamma activation. Biochem Biophys Res Commun 293 (2002): 827–831.

Koleva, P. T., et al. 2012. Inulin and fructo-oligosaccharides have divergent effects on colitis and commensal microbiota in HLA-B27 transgenic rats. Br J Nutr, 108, 1633–43.

Langlands SJ et al. Prebiotic carbohydrates modify the mucosa associated microflora of the human large bowel. Gut 53 (2004): 1610–1616.

Lara-Villoslada, F., et al. 2006. Short-chain fructooligosaccharides, in spite of being fermented in the upper part of the large intestine, have anti-inflammatory activity in the TNBS model of colitis. Eur J Nutr, 45, 418–25.

Le Leu RK et al. A synbiotic combination of resistant starch and *Bifidobacterium lactis* facilitates apoptotic deletion of carcinogen-damaged cells in rat colon. J Nutr 135 (2005): 996–1001.

Lewis S, et al. Effect of the prebiotic oligofructose on relapse of *Clostridium difficile*-associated diarrhoea: a randomised controlled study. Clin Gastroenterol Hepatol 3 (2005a): 442–8.

Lewis S et al. Failure of dietary oligofructose to prevent antibiotic-associated diarrhoea. Aliment Pharmacol Ther 21 (2005b): 469–77.

Lindsay JO et al. Clinical, microbiological, and immunological effects of fructo-oligosaccharide in patients with Crohn's disease. Gut 55 (2006): 348–355.

Looijer–Van Langen, M. A. C. & Dieleman, L. A. 2009. Prebiotics in chronic intestinal inflammation. Inflammatory Bowel Diseases, 15, 454–462.

Macfarlane S, et al. Review article: prebiotics in the gastrointestinal tract. Aliment Pharmacol Ther 24.5 (2006): 701–714.

Maiello, N., et al. 2011. Severe allergic reaction to lactulose in a child with milk allergy. Annals of Allergy, Asthma & Immunology, 107, 85.

McCutcheon, J. & Fulton, J. D. 1989. Lowered prevalence of infection with lactulose therapy in patients in long-term hospital care. Journal of Hospital Infection, 13, 81–86.

Millard AL et al. Butyrate affects differentiation, maturation and function of human monocyte-derived dendritic cells and macrophages. Clin Exp Immunol 130 (2002): 245–255.

Monaco, M. H., et al. 2011. Addition of polydextrose and galactooligosaccharide to formula does not affect bacterial translocation in the neonatal piglet. J Pediatr Gastroenterol Nutr, 52, 210–6.

Moro G et al. A mixture of prebiotic oligosaccharides reduces the incidence of atopic dermatitis during the first six months of age. Arch Dis Child 91 (2006): 814–819.

Nauta, A. J., et al. 2008. A specific mixture of short-chain galacto-oligosaccharides and long-chain fructo-oligosaccharides induced an anti-allergic Ig profile in infants at risk for allergy. Proceedings of the Nutrition Society, 67, E82.

Niittyen, L., et al. 2007. Galacto-oligosaccharides and bowel function. Scandinavian Journal of Food and Nutrition, 51, 62–66.

Ohta, A., et al. 2002. A combination of dietary fructooligosaccharides and isoflavone conjugates increases femoral bone mineral density and equol production in ovariectomized mice. Journal of Nutrition, 132, 2048–2054.

Olah A et al. Combination of early nasojejunal feeding with modern synbiotic therapy in the treatment of severe acute pancreatitis (prospective, randomised, double-blind study). Magy Seb 58 (2005): 173–178.

Olesen M, Gudmand-Hoyer E. Efficacy, safety, and tolerability of fructooligosaccharides in the treatment of irritable bowel syndrome. Am J Clin Nutr 72.6 (2000): 1570–1575.

Osborn DA, Sinn JK. Prebiotics in infants for prevention of allergic disease and food sensitivity. Cochrane Database Syst Rev Oct 17.4 (2013): CD006474.

Osman N et al. Bifidobacterium infantis strains with and without a combination of oligofructose and inulin (OFI) attenuate inflammation in DSS-induced colitis in rats. BMC Gastroenterol 6 (2006): 31.

Ouwehand A, et al. The role of the intestinal microflora for the development of the immune system in early childhood. Eur J Nutr 41 (Suppl 1) (2002): 132–137.

Parnell, J. A. & Reimer, R. A. 2009. Weight loss during oligofructose supplementation is associated with decreased ghrelin and increased peptide YY in overweight and obese adults. Am J Clin Nutr, 89, 1751–1759.

Paturi, G., et al. 2012. Effects of early dietary intervention with a fermentable fibre on colonic microbiota activity and mucin gene expression in newly weaned rats. Journal of Functional Foods, 4, 520–530.

Petticrew M, et al. Systematic review of the effectiveness of laxatives in the elderly. Health Technol Assess 1 (1997): 1–52.

Pool-Zobel BL, Sauer J. Overview of experimental data on reduction of colorectal cancer risk by inulin-type fructans. J Nutr 137 (2007): 2580S–4S.

Prather, C. 2004. Pregnancy-related constipation. Current Gastroenterology Reports, 6, 402–404.

Rafter J et al. Dietary synbiotics reduce cancer risk factors in polypectomized and colon cancer patients. Am J Clin Nutr 85.2 (2007): 488–496.

Roberfroid MB. Inulin-type fructans: functional food ingredients. J Nutr 137.11 (2007a): 2493S–502S.

Roberfroid, M. 2007b. Prebiotics: the concept revisited. J Nutr, 137, 830S-7S.

Roller M et al. Intestinal immunity of rats with colon cancer is modulated by oligofructose-enriched inulin combined with *Lactobacillus rhamnosus* and *Bifidobacterium lactis*. Br J Nutr 92 (2004): 931.

Roller M et al. Consumption of prebiotic inulin enriched with oligofructose in combination with the probiotics *Lactobacillus rhamnosus* and *Bifidobacterium lactis* has minor effects on selected immune parameters in polypectomised and colon cancer patients. Br J Nutr 97.4 (2007): 676–684.

Roncucci, L., et al. 1993. Antioxidant vitamins or lactulose for the prevention of the recurrence of colorectal polyps. Diseases of the Colon and Rectum, 67, 227–234.

Rowland IR et al. Effect of *Bifidobacterium longum* and inulin on gut bacterial metabolism and carcinogen-induced aberrant crypt foci in rats. Carcinogenesis 19 (1998): 281–285.

Saavedra, J. M. & Tschernia, A. 2002. Human studies with probiotics and prebiotics: clinical implications. Br J Nutr, 87 (suppl 2), S241–S246.

Saavedra JM et al. Feeding of *Bifidobacterium bifidum* and *Streptococcus thermophilus* to infants in hospital for prevention of diarrhea and shedding of rotavirus. Lancet 344 (1994): 1046–1049.

Saemann MD et al. Anti-inflammatory effects of sodium butyrate on human monocytes: potent inhibition of IL-12 and up-regulation of IL-10 production. FASEB J 14 (2000): 2380–2382.

Salminen S et al. Demonstration of safety of probiotics: a review. Int J Food Microbiol 44.1–2 (1998): 93–106.

Sartor RB. Therapeutic manipulation of the enteric microflora in inflammatory bowel diseases: antibiotics, probiotics, and prebiotics. Gastroenterology 126 (2004): 1620–1633.

Schrezenmeir, J. & de Vrese, M. 2001. Probiotics, prebiotics, and synbiotics-approaching a definition. American Journal of Clinical Nutrition, 73, 361–364.

Searle, L. E., et al. 2009. A mixture containing galactooligosaccharide, produced by the enzymic activity of *Bifidobacterium bifidum*, reduces *Salmonella enterica* serovar *Typhimurium* infection in mice. Journal of Medical Microbiology, 58, 37–48.

Segain JP et al. Butyrate inhibits inflammatory responses through NFkappaB inhibition: implications for Crohn's disease. Gut 47 (2000): 397–403.

Serra J, et al. Impaired transit and tolerance of intestinal gas in the irritable bowel syndrome. Gut 48 (2001): 14–19.

Sharma, P., et al. 2012. Primary prophylaxis of overt hepatic encephalopathy in patients with cirrhosis: an open labeled randomized controlled trial of lactulose versus no lactulose. J Gastroenterol Hepatol, 27, 1329–35.

Shepherd, S. J., et al. 2008. Dietary Triggers of Abdominal Symptoms in Patients With Irritable Bowel Syndrome: Randomized Placebo-Controlled Evidence. Clinical Gastroenterology and Hepatology, 6, 765–771.

Shoaf K et al. Prebiotic galactooligosaccharides reduce adherence of enteropathogenic *Escherichia coli* to tissue culture cells. Infect Immun 74 (2006): 6920–6928.

Shoaf-Sweeney KD, Hutkins RW. Adherence, anti-adherence, and oligosaccharides preventing pathogens from sticking to the host. Adv Food Nutr Res 55 (2009): 101–161.

Shukla, S., et al. 2011. Meta-analysis: the effects of gut flora modulation using prebiotics, probiotics and synbiotics on minimal hepatic encephalopathy. Aliment Pharmacol Ther, 33, 662–71.

Silk, D. B., et al. 2009. Clinical trial: the effects of a trans-galactooligosaccharide prebiotic on faecal microbiota and symptoms in irritable bowel syndrome. Alimentary Pharmacology & Therapeutics, 29, 508–518.

Silva, D. F. D., et al. 2009. Translocation of *Klebsiella* sp. in mice fed an enteral diet containing prebiotics. Revista de Nutrição, 22, 229–235.

Sinclair, H. R., et al. 2009. Galactooligosaccharides (GOS) inhibit *Vibrio cholerae* toxin binding to its GM1 receptor. J Agric Food Chem, 57, 3113–3119.

Szilagyi, A., et al. 2001. Improved parameters of lactose maldigestion using lactulose. Dig Dis Sci, 46, 1509–19.

Ten Bruggencate SJ et al. Dietary fructo-oligosaccharides and inulin decrease resistance of rats to salmonella: protective role of calcium. Gut 53 (2004): 530–535.

Ten Bruggencate, S. J. M., et al. 2005. Dietary Fructooligosaccharides Increase Intestinal Permeability in Rats. The Journal of Nutrition, 135, 837–842.

Ten Bruggencate, S. J. M., et al. 2006. Dietary Fructooligosaccharides Affect Intestinal Barrier Function in Healthy Men. The Journal of Nutrition, 136, 70–74.

Teramoto, F., et al. 1996. Effect of 4- B -D-galactosylsucrose (lactosucrose) on fecal microflora in patients with chronic inflammatory bowel disease. Journal of Gastroenterology, 31, 33–39.

Teuri, U. & Korpela, R. 1998. Galacto-oligosaccharides relieve constipation in elderly people. Annals of Nutrition and Metabolism, 42, 319–327.

Teuri, U., et al. 1999. Fructooligosaccharides and lactulose cause more symptoms in lactose maldigesters and subjects with pseudohypolactasia than in control lactose digesters. The American Journal of Clinical Nutrition, 69, 973–979.

Uehara, M., et al. 2001. Dietary fructooligosaccharides modify intestinal bioavailability of a single dose of genistein and daidzein and affect their urinary excretion and kinetics in blood of rats. Journal of Nutrition, 131, 787–795.

Van den Heuvel EG, et al. Transgalactooligosaccharides stimulate calcium absorption in postmenopausal women. J Nutr 130.12 (2000): 2938–2942.

Van Loo, J., et al. 1995. On the presence of inulin and oligofructose as natural ingredients in the Western diet. Critical Reviews in Food Science and Nutrition, 35, 525–552.

Van Loo, J., et al. 1998. Functional food properties of non-digestible oligosaccharides: a consensus report from the ENDO project (DGXII AIRII-CT94-1095). British Journal of Nutrition, 81, 121–132.

Vulevic, J., et al. 2008. Modulation of the fecal microflora profile and immune function by a novel trans-galactooligosaccharide mixture (B-GOS) in healthy elderly volunteers. Am J Clin Nutr, 88, 1438–46.

Vulevic, J., et al. 2013. A Mixture of trans-Galactooligosaccharides Reduces Markers of Metabolic Syndrome and Modulates the Fecal Microbiota and Immune Function of Overweight Adults. J Nutr, 143, 324–31.

Waligora-Dupriet, A. J., et al. 2007. Effect of oligofructose supplementation on gut microflora and well-being in young children attending a day care centre. Int J Food Microbiol, 113, 108–113.

Walker AW et al. pH and peptide supply can radically alter bacterial populations and short-chain fatty acid ratios within microbial communities from the human colon. Appl Environ Microbiol 71 (2005): 3692–3700.

Watz, B., et al. 2005. Inulin, oligofructose and immunomodulation. Br J Nutr, 93, S49–S55.

Welters CF et al. Effect of dietary inulin supplementation on inflammation of pouch mucosa in patients with an ileal pouch-anal anastomosis. Dis Colon Rectum 45 (2002): 621–627.

Wen, J., et al. 2013. Lactulose is highly potential in prophylaxis of hepatic encephalopathy in patients with cirrhosis and upper gastrointestinal bleeding: results of a controlled randomized trial. Digestion, 87, 132–8.

Yang ST, Silva EM. Novel products and new technologies for use of a familiar carbohydrate, milk lactose. J Dairy Sci 78 (1995): 2541–2562.

Yasuda, A., et al. 2012. Dietary supplementation with fructooligosaccharides attenuates allergic peritonitis in mice. Biochemical and Biophysical Research Communications, 422, 546–550.

Zopf D, Roth S. Oligosaccharide anti-infective agents. Lancet 347 (1996): 1017–1021.

Probiotics

HISTORICAL NOTE There is a long history of consuming fermented foods and beverages containing microorganisms to improve health. The term 'probiotic' is derived from Greek and means 'for life'. As far back as 1907, Metchnikoff, the Nobel laureate, popularised the idea that fermented milk products could beneficially alter the microflora of the gastrointestinal tract (GIT). He believed that many diseases, and even ageing itself, were caused by putrefaction of protein in the bowel by intestinal bacteria. Lactic acid-producing bacteria were thought to be able to inhibit the growth of putrefactive bacteria in the intestines and, thus, yoghurt consumption was recommended to correct this 'autointoxication' and improve the composition of the microflora (Metchnikoff 1907). The term 'probiotics' was first coined in 1965 and has since been applied to those live microorganisms that are able to promote health when consumed in sufficient quantities (FAO/WHO 2001). This definition includes fermented foods, as well as specific supplements containing freeze-dried bacteria. Although it has taken more than a century for scientists to investigate their health benefits, there are now several thousand studies published on probiotics, the majority published since 2000.

BACKGROUND AND RELEVANT PHARMACOKINETICS

Prior to birth, the GIT of the neonate is generally considered completely sterile, although new research findings suggest that there may be some degree of transfer from the mother's microbiota in utero. During delivery, the newborn is inoculated with microorganisms from the birth canal (ideally) and the mother's faecal flora, as well as from organisms in the environment (Matamoros et al 2013). Subsequently, growth of normal gut flora is influenced by factors such as composition of the maternal GIT microbiota, diet (breast milk vs formula), degree of hygiene, use of antibiotics or other medication, the environment and possibly genetic aspects. These microorganisms confer many health benefits by preventing the colonisation of the GIT with pathogenic microorganisms and by carrying out a number of biochemical functions, such as deconjugation and dehydroxylation of bile acids, the conversion of bilirubin to urobilinogen, generation of short-chain fatty acids (SCFA) and the metabolism of cholesterol to coprostanol (Bengmark 1998, Hill 1997). Additionally the microbiota modulates immune function, enhances GIT motility and gut barrier function, induces mucin production, improves digestion and nutrient absorption, metabolises xenobiotics (e.g. phytooestrogens), and produces vitamins K, B_1, B_2, B_6 and B_{12} (Fotiadis et al 2008, Hawrelak & Myers 2004, Isolauri 2012).

The gastrointestinal microbiota is reasonably resilient to change and remains fairly constant in adults, although research has shown that components such as pre- and probiotics can beneficially modulate the gut microflora, while antibiotics, chemotherapy, stress and a Western diet can negatively impact the ecosystem (Hawrelak & Myers 2004). It has been estimated that the intestines are host to 10^{14} microbes representing over 1000 different species (Rajilic-Stojanovic et al 2007), which includes yeasts, mostly *Candida albicans* (<0.1% of the microbiota) (Vandenplas et al 2007).

Probiotics can be obtained from the consumption of fermented foods as well as supplements. It is important to note, however, that probiotic organisms require

TABLE 1 THE DESIRABLE CHARACTERISTICS OF EFFECTIVE PROBIOTIC STRAINS

Characteristics	Functional benefit
Gastric acid and bile salt stability	Survival through stomach and small intestine
Adherence to intestinal mucosa	Believed to be essential for immune cell modulation and competitive inhibition of pathogens
Colonisation of intestinal tract	Multiplication in the intestines suggests that daily ingestion may not be needed; immune cell modulation
Human origin	Human origin should translate to the ability to survive conditions in the human gastrointestinal tract, as well as the possibility of species-specific health effects
Safety in food and documented clinical safety	Adverse effects absent or minimal; accurate identification (genus, species, strain)
Production of antimicrobial compounds	Normalisation of gastrointestinal tract flora; suppressed growth of pathogens
Antagonism against pathogenic organisms	Prevention of adhesion and toxin production by pathogens
Clinically documented and validated health effects	Clinicians can be confident of therapeutic effects; dose-response data for minimum effective dosage in different formulations are known
Increased shelf-life and stability during processing	All of the above properties should be maintained during storage and processing

Adapted from Mattila-Sandholm & Salminen (1998).

certain characteristics to enable them to exert maximum therapeutic effects. These qualities are summarised in Table 1.

Out of these characteristics, there are some that are considered most important for a probiotic to have therapeutic effects. These are: (1) gastric acid and bile salt stability; (2) an ability to adhere to the intestinal mucosa; and (3) an ability to colonise the intestinal tract (Dunne et al 2001). Some commercially available probiotic supplements and yoghurts contain strains that do not exhibit these vital characteristics. If a probiotic strain does not exhibit these characteristics, then it will be less effective than strains that do.

Recently, the concept that probiotics should be viable/live has been re-evaluated. Studies have shown that bacterial DNA sequences may have similar effects as the live bacteria in some situations, and therefore colonisation of the intestinal tract may not be a prerequisite for the action of probiotics (Jijon et al 2004, Rachmilewitz et al 2002). In addition, the mucosal immune system may not require direct contact with probiotics for beneficial effects as other routes of administration (such as the parenteral route) are also effective (Rachmilewitz et al 2004, Sheil et al 2004). However, there are significant species and strain differences between the probiotic microorganisms, and therefore, they do not all share the same characteristics.

At present, there are numerous uses of probiotics, and reports of their beneficial effects cover a wide range of diseases and conditions.

Clinical note — Prebiotics and synbiotics
Prebiotics are components that modify the environment of the GIT to selectively favour proliferation of the beneficial intestinal microflora, lactobacilli and bifidobacteria (Gibson & Roberfroid 1995). Prebiotics include oligofructose (fructooligosaccharides), inulin, lactulose and galactooligosaccharides. (See Prebiotics monograph.) Synbiotics contain both pre- and probiotics.

CHEMICAL COMPONENTS

There are many different microorganisms currently used as probiotics in supplement and functional food form. Table 2 provides examples of commonly used probiotic species.

Common probiotic microorganisms

To better understand how bacteria are named and classified, the following discussion may be helpful. Genus is the first name of a bacterium (e.g. *Lactobacillus*). It is somewhat general and refers to a grouping of organisms based on similarity of qualities, such as physical characteristics, metabolic needs and metabolic end products. Species is a bacterium's second name (e.g. *acidophilus*). It is a much more narrow classification based on shared common characteristics that distinguish them from other species. Strain is an even more specific classification that divides members of the same species into subgroups based on several properties that a bacterial strain has that are distinct from other members of that species (e.g. strain LA5) (McKane & Kandel 1986).

TABLE 2 SOME ORGANISMS THAT ARE CURRENTLY USED AS PROBIOTICS (LISTED BY GENUS AND SPECIES) (GOLDIN 1998, MACFARLANE & CUMMINGS 1999, MATTILA-SANDHOLM & SALMINEN 1998)

Lactobacillus spp.	*Bifidobacterium* spp.	*Bacillus* spp.	*Streptococcus* spp.	*Enterococcus* spp.	*Saccharomyces* spp.
acidophilus	*breve*	*coagulans*	*thermophilus*	*faecium*	*cerevisiae*
plantarum	*infantis*				
rhamnosus	*longum*				
paracasei	*bifidum*				
fermentum	*thermophilum*				
reuteri	*adolescentis*				
johnsonii	*animalis*				
brevis	*lactis*				
casei					
lactis					
delbrueckii					
gasseri					

P

Strain selectivity of action

Within each species of bacteria there is a multitude of strains. Some probiotic strains are resilient and strong, with a demonstrated capacity to survive passage through the upper GIT and inhibit pathogenic bacteria, whereas others are weak and cannot even survive transit through the stomach. It is vital to note that, just because one strain of bacteria in a given species has a proven action or characteristic, it does not always mean that another strain will too, even if they are closely related. Strains of bacteria within the same species can have significantly different actions, properties and characteristics, as these are all essentially strain-specific qualities (Guarner et al 2011, Marteau 2011). For example, *Lactobacillus plantarum* strain 299v has been shown to effectively reduce irritable bowel syndrome (IBS) symptoms (Ducrotte et al 2012), whereas administration of *L. plantarum* strain MF1298 may actually worsens IBS symptoms (Ligaarden et al 2010). Thus, to achieve the desired therapeutic result, it is imperative to prescribe the precise probiotic strains that have demonstrated therapeutic and clinical efficacy in the condition in question. Additionally, strains that work in one condition will not necessarily be as effective in other conditions. For example, *Lactobacillus rhamnosus* GG (LGG) appears to be effective in the prevention of antibiotic-associated side effects (Arvola et al 1999) but not of any demonstrable benefit in urinary tract infections (Kontiokari et al 2001). When reviewing the Clinical Use section below, it is important to take note of the strains that were used in the summarised trials, not just the species.

FOOD SOURCES

Traditional fermented foods, such as sauerkraut (Dedicatoria et al 1981), kim chi (Cheigh et al 1994), ogi (Oyewole 1997) and kefir (Garrote et al 2001), are rich sources of probiotic organisms. The most commonly consumed probiotic food in Australia and New Zealand is yoghurt. As research has suggested that the main yoghurt-producing bacteria (*Lactobacillus delbrueckii* ssp. *bulgaricus* and *Streptococcus thermophilus*) have limited therapeutic potential, human GIT-derived probiotic strains are now commonly added to yoghurt in an attempt to increase its therapeutic potential (e.g. strains of *Lactobacillus acidophilus* and *Bifidobacterium* spp.) (Molin 2001).

DEFICIENCY SIGNS AND SYMPTOMS

Clear deficiency signs are difficult to establish because the symptoms may vary enormously. Local signs and symptoms of disruption of the intestinal microflora leading to an imbalance (intestinal dysbiosis) include bloating, flatulence, abdominal pain, diarrhoea and/or constipation and fungal overgrowth (such as *Candida*). An imbalance in the gastrointestinal microflora can be caused by the use of antibiotics, GIT infections, stress and dietary factors (Hawrelak & Myers 2004). Administration of probiotics is often used as a means of restoring this microflora imbalance (Bengmark 1998, Hedin et al 2007, Hoveyda et al 2009, Kajander et al 2008, McFarland 2006, 2007, McFarland & Dublin 2008).

MAIN ACTIONS

The exact mechanisms by which probiotics accomplish their myriad of beneficial actions have become clearer over the past decade and we now know of several mechanisms that explain many of their favourable effects.

Immune modulation

A growing body of evidence indicates that some probiotic strains are capable of modulating the immune system at both the systemic and the mucosal level, affecting many cell types (e.g. epithelial cells, dendritic cells, natural killer cells). This immune response may take the form of increased secretion of immunoglobulin A (IgA) via interaction with mesenteric lymph nodes (Link-Amster et al 1994, Walker 2008), elevated numbers of natural killer cells or enhanced phagocytic activity of macrophages (Schiffrin et al 1997). Recent research has demonstrated that dendritic cells in the lamina propria can extend their appendices between epithelial cells, and, via Toll-like receptors on their surface, sample probiotic-bacterial molecular patterns. This interaction leads to the maturation of the dendritic cells and to the release of cytokines, which orchestrate the conversion of naive T-helper cells (Th0) into a mature, balanced response of T-helper cells (Th1, Th2 and Th3/Tr1) (Walker 2008).

Anti-inflammatory activity

Probiotic strains have been shown to have anti-inflammatory effects via a number of different mechanisms. They can secrete metabolites with anti-inflammatory properties (anti-tumour necrosis factor-α [TNF-α] effects) (Ménard et al 2004), they can interact with Toll-like receptors (Rachmilewitz et al 2004), downregulate the transcription of a number of genes encoding proinflammatory effectors (Tien et al 2006) and upregulate the production of anti-inflammatory cytokines (Imaoka et al 2008).

GIT transit time modification

Some probiotic strains can modify GIT transit. Two strains of bifidobacteria have been found to significantly speed colonic transit time (Meance et al 2001, Waller et al 2011), while a strain of propionibacteria has been shown to slow descending colon transit (Bougle et al 1999). The mechanisms by which probiotics alter GIT transit time have not yet been fully elucidated; however, it is postulated that a bacterial metabolite may impact sigmoid tone and alter colonic motility (Marteau et al 2002).

Induction of oral tolerance

The GIT microflora has been shown to play a crucial role in generating an adequate population of Th2 cells that are capable of oral tolerance induction (Sudo et al 1997). In the presence of intestinal dysbiosis, some probiotic strains can also help induce oral tolerance and help protect against the development of food allergies (Prioult et al 2003).

Decrease visceral hypersensitivity

Animal research has suggested that some probiotic strains are capable of decreasing visceral hypersensitivity, believed to be one of the main contributing factors in IBS and other functional gastrointestinal disorders (Ait-Belgnaoui et al 2006, Johnson et al 2011, McKernan et al 2010). The exact mechanisms are unknown, but another lactobacilli strain has been shown to decrease visceral hypersensitivity by inducing cannabinoid and opioid receptor expression in the colonic epithelium (Rousseaux et al 2007).

Competition for gastrointestinal adhesion sites

Many pathogenic organisms must associate with the GIT epithelium in order to colonise effectively. However some strains of bifidobacteria and lactobacilli can adhere to the epithelium and act as 'colonisation barriers' by preventing pathogens from adhering to the mucosa (Fuller & Gibson 1997). This effect has been demonstrated with LGG and *L. plantarum* 299v. Both of these organisms have shown the ability to inhibit attachment of *Escherichia coli* to human colon cells (Mack et al 1999).

Antagonism against potentially pathogenic microorganisms and viruses

One of the mechanisms by which probiotics exert their beneficial effects is via inducing changes to the GIT microflora; specifically by inhibiting the growth of potentially pathogenic organisms. Some probiotic strains are capable of producing inhibitory substances such as bacteriocins, lactic acid and toxic oxygen metabolites. Of the toxic oxygen metabolites, hydrogen peroxide is of major importance as it exerts a bactericidal effect on many pathogens (Kaur et al 2002). The ability to produce bacteriocins, hydrogen peroxide and other antimicrobial compounds is strain-dependent. Probiotics have demonstrated in vitro inhibitory activity against a range of potentially pathogenic microorganisms, such as *Helicobacter pylori, Clostridium difficile, Escherichia coli, Candida albicans, Salmonella enterica, Shigella sonnei* and *Vibrio cholerae* (Hasslof et al 2010, Naaber et al 2004, Sgouras et al 2004, Spinler et al 2008). Some probiotic strains (LGG and *Bifidobacterium lactis* Bb12) can also bind to viruses, such as rotaviruses, helping to prevent mucosa-associated viral infections (Salminen et al 2010). Several probiotic strains have also demonstrated the ability to bind or remove toxins, such as aflatoxins and cyanotoxins (Salminen et al 2010), as well as inhibit the effects of bacterial toxins, such as *Clostridium difficile* toxins A and B (Castagliuolo et al 1999). Specific strains have also been found to reduce the expression of virulence factors via inhibition of pathogen gene encoding (Corr et al 2009).

Selective gastrointestinal antimicrobial activity

Ingestion of selected probiotic strains has been found to significantly increase gastrointestinal populations of beneficial bacteria (i.e. lactobacilli or bifidobacteria), while simultaneously decreasing populations of less health-promoting genera (Ahmed et al 2007, Benno et al 1996, Mohan et al 2006).

Production of beneficial compounds

The production of SCFAs as metabolic byproducts is a characteristic which almost all probiotic strains share. These SCFAs help create a healthier colonic milieu by decreasing the luminal pH and some (e.g. butyrate) are used as energy sources by colonocytes (D'Argenio & Mazzacca 1999, Ng et al 2009). Other probiotic strains can help restore normal small intestinal architecture and upregulate intestinal brush border enzyme expression via the luminal release of polyamines (Buts et al 1986, 1994, Guillot et al 1995). These strains will have clinical utility in situations of small intestinal damage and decreased brush border enzyme activity, such as coeliac disease, Crohn's disease, or after small intestinal infections.

Strengthen the intestinal barrier

A number of probiotic strains have been found to increase mucin production in the gut via increases in mucin gene expression, which provides a protective coating between the lumen and intestinal epithelial cells (Caballero-Franco et al 2007, Mack et al 2003). Probiotics are also capable of directly strengthening the intestinal barrier. A strain of *Lactobacillus plantarum* (WCSF1) has been found to decrease paracellular intestinal permeability by increasing the relocation of occludin and zonulin into the tight junction between duodenal epithelial cells (Ahrne & Hagslatt 2011). Other strains appear to enhance barrier function via the preservation of enterocyte cytoskeleton architecture and enhancement of tight junctional protein structures (Ng et al 2009). Such strains should prove useful in the treatment and prevention of intestinal permeability.

Chemopreventive effects

Select probiotics may have anticancer properties. Different strains of *Lactobacillus acidophilus* and bifidobacteria have been studied to investigate their antimutagenic activity against chemical mutagens (Lankaputhra & Shah 1998).

Antimutagenic activity against chemical mutagens and promutagens has been demonstrated for different strains of *Lactobacillus acidophilus*, bifidobacteria and the organic acids usually produced by these probiotics, with live cells producing the most positive results (Lankaputhra & Shah 1998). Some probiotics also reduce faecal enzymes implicated in cancer initiation, while others produce butyric acid, which affects the turnover of colonocytes and neutralises the activity of dietary carcinogens, such as nitrosamines. Additionally, enhancing host immunity and qualitative and quantitative changes to the intestinal microflora and physicochemical conditions are important contributing factors (Hirayama & Rafter 1999).

OTHER ACTIONS

Several clinical studies have investigated lipid-lowering activity of probiotics (see section on Clinical Use, below).

> ***How to choose an effective probiotic supplement***
>
> Firstly, one needs to know not only the genera and species details of the organisms contained in the supplement, but also the strain details. Ideally, this should be detailed on the label, but if this is not clear, contact the manufacturer for further information. Secondly, the strains contained in the supplement will ideally display the desirable characteristics highlighted in Table 1. Thirdly, the right strain(s) with the desired action should be chosen for the clinical scenario at hand. Fourthly, there should be adequate amounts of viable organisms contained in the supplement at the time of consumption — for most strains this is currently considered to be $\geq 10^9$ colony-forming units of each organism per dose, but will vary depending on indication (see Dosage Range section below for more details).

CLINICAL USE

Restoring GIT microflora after antibiotic use

Antibiotic use frequently results in significant perturbations in the GIT microflora and gastrointestinal adverse events, such as diarrhoea (Rafii et al 2008). It was once believed that taking probiotics concurrently with antibiotics would be a waste of time and money as the antibiotic would be likely to destroy all the administered probiotic bacteria. However, research conducted over the past 20 years clearly shows that concurrent administration of specific probiotic strains alongside antibiotics is effective and significantly decreases the incidence of antibiotic-related side effects. Table 3 highlights the research examining the impact of probiotics on antibiotic-related gastrointestinal adverse events, primarily antibiotic-associated diarrhoea. As can be seen, the probiotic strains with the highest level of substantiating evidence are *L. rhamnosus* GG and *Saccharomyces cerevisiae* var. *boulardii* Biocodex, but a number of other strains have also demonstrated efficacy.

TABLE 3 IMPACT OF PROBIOTICS ON ANTIBIOTIC-RELATED GASTROINTESTINAL ADVERSE EVENTS (comments in italics)

Trial methodology	Strain(s) utilised	Results and comments
Meta-analysis 16 studies *n* = 3432 paediatric subjects	Various	In the per protocol analysis, the incidence of antibiotic-associated diarrhoea (AAD) in the probiotic group was 9% compared to 18% in the control group (2874 participants; relative risk [RR] 0.52; 95% confidence interval [CI] 0.38–0.72). An extreme-plausible intention to treat (ITT) analysis, where 60% of the drop-outs in the probiotic group was assumed to have AAD compared to only 20% of drop-outs in the control group, revealed no significant benefit to probiotic therapy (RR 0.81; 95% CI 0.63–1.04) (Johnston et al 2011). *The considerable bias against probiotic therapy built into the ITT analysis made the chance of a positive outcome very remote. Additionally, meta-analyses that combine the results of studies utilising different probiotic strains (such as this one) are actively discouraged as they are fundamentally flawed and fail to provide clinically relevant conclusions. Each strain is a unique therapeutic agent and should be evaluated as such. Meta-analyses such as this can only provide proof of concept data*
Meta-analysis 63 studies *n* = 11,811 subjects of all ages	Various	Probiotic administration was associated with a significant reduction in risk of AAD (RR = 0.58; 95% CI 0.50–0.68; $P < 0.001$) (Hempel et al 2012). *The same criticism of combining results on different probiotic strains is valid for this meta-analysis as well*
Meta-analysis two studies *n* = 307 paediatric subjects	*Lactobacillus rhamnosus* GG	70% reduced risk of developing AAD in children (95% CI 0.15–0.6; $P = 0.00003$) (Szajewska et al 2010). *This meta-anlaysis combines the data on a single probiotic strain, providing valuable clinically relevant information, demonstrating that this strain is effective in the prevention of AAD in paediatric populations being administered antibiotics*

TABLE 3 IMPACT OF PROBIOTICS ON ANTIBIOTIC-RELATED GASTROINTESTINAL ADVERSE EVENTS (comments in italics) *(continued)*		
Trial methodology	**Strain(s) utilised**	**Results and comments**
Meta-analysis five studies $n = 1076$ subjects of all ages	*Saccharomyces cerevisiae* var. *boulardii* Biocodex	Supplementation reduced the risk of AAD from 17.2% in controls to 6.7% (RR = 0.43; 95% CI 0.23–0.78) (Szajewska & Mrukowicz 2005)
R, DB, PC $n = 162$ adult subjects receiving antibiotic treatment for *Helicobacter pylori* infection	*Lactobacillus acidophilus* strains CUL-60 and CUL-21, *Bifidobacterium lactis* CUL-34 and *Bifidobacterium bifidum* CUL-20 (Lab4)	Coadministration of the probiotic combination with antibiotics prevented the increase in faecal *Candida albicans* populations immediately following antibiotic therapy ($P = 0.049$) (Plummer et al 2005)
R, DB, PC $n = 239$	*Lactobacillus plantarum* 299v	31% reduced risk of developing loose or watery stools (95% CI 0.52–0.92; $P = 0.012$); 49% reduced risk of experiencing nausea (95% CI 0.30–0.85; $P = 0.0097$) (Lonnermark et al 2010)
R, DB, PC $n = 40$ paediatric subjects	*Lactobacillus reuteri* MM53	Reduced incidence of a number of gastrointestinal symptoms relative to placebo in triple therapy-treated children — epigastric pain (15% vs 45%; $P < 0.04$), abdominal distension (0% vs 25%; $P < 0.04$), disorders of defecation (15% vs 45%; $P < 0.04$) and halitosis (5% vs 35%; $P < 0.04$) (Lionetti et al 2006)
R, DB, PC $n = 87$ subjects	*Lactobacillus rhamnosus* GG, *Lactobacillus acidophilus* LA5 and *Bifidobacterium lactis* Bb12	79% reduced risk of developing AAD ($P = 0.035$) (Wenus et al 2008)

R, randomised; DB, double-blind; PC, placebo-controlled.

P

Abdominal pain (functional)

A meta-analysis of trials evaluating LGG in the treatment of functional abdominal pain in children found LGG effective. LGG supplementation was associated with a significantly higher rate of treatment responders (defined as no pain or a decrease in pain intensity) in the overall population of children with abdominal pain-related functional gastrointestinal disorders (three trials: $n = 290$; relative risk [RR] 1.31, 95% confidence interval [CI] 1.08–1.59) and in the IBS subgroup (three randomised controlled trials; $n = 167$; RR 1.70, 95% CI 1.27–2.27, number needed to treat 4, 95% CI 3–8). There was also a significant decrease in the perception of pain intensity in children with functional abdominal pain (Horvath et al 2011).

Atopic eczema

The intestinal microflora plays a major protective role against the development of allergy because it reduces antigen transport through the intestinal mucosa and helps induce oral tolerance (Tanaka & Ishikawa 2004). Consequently, probiotics may have a protective role in the prevention and/or management of atopic dermatitis and eczema because of their proposed actions (Rosenfeldt et al 2004).

A number of clinical trials have investigated probiotic therapy to prevent atopic eczema development, and some have evaluated the efficacy of probiotic therapy in the treatment of atopic eczema.

Prevention of atopic eczema

The initial research detailing the efficacy of probiotics in the prevention of atopic eczema utilised the probiotic strain LGG (Kalliomaki et al 2001). Other studies assessing this same strain have since been published, with conflicting results (Boyle et al 2011, Kopp et al 2008). Table 4 provides details on these trials. As can be seen, the studies by Kalliomaki et al and Kopp et al had similar protocols, but contrasting results. The small differences in protocol are unlikely to explain the differences. The trial by Boyle et al only gave LGG to the mother from week 36 until delivery. Lack of apparent efficacy in this study might suggest that LGG needs to be given to the infant (either directly or via breast milk) for efficacy to be seen. More research is needed, however, to clearly define the role of LGG in the prevention of atopic eczema development.

A number of other probiotic strains have been evaluated for their effectiveness in the prevention of atopic eczema, with conflicting results. Pelucchi et al (2012) performed a meta-analysis of randomised controlled trials to investigate whether probiotic use during pregnancy and early life decreases the incidence of atopic eczema and IgE-associated atopic eczema in infants and young children. Eighteen publications based on 14 studies were included in the analysis. Meta-analysis demonstrated that probiotic use decreased the incidence of atopic dermatitis (RR = 0.79; 95% CI 0.71–0.88). The corresponding RR of IgE-associated atopic dermatitis was 0.80 (95% CI 0.66–0.96) (Pelucchi et al 2012). While the evidence on the whole supports the use of probiotics to decrease the incidence of atopic dermatitis in infancy and early childhood, some strains were not effective.

In a randomised, double-blind, placebo-controlled trial, Taylor et al (2007) administered *Lactobacillus acidophilus* strain LAVRI-A1 (3×10^9 colony-forming units [CFU]/day) to infants at high risk of allergic disease for the first 6 months of life. At both 6 and 12 months, the incidence of atopic dermatitis was similar in both the probiotic and the placebo group. The proportion of children with a positive skin prick test and atopic eczema was significantly higher in the probiotic group ($P = 0.045$) at 12 months, as was the rate of allergen sensitisation ($P = 0.030$). Hence, this strain was not effective in decreasing the incidence of atopic dermatitis development and may have actually increased allergen sensitisation, despite promising preliminary in vitro results (Taylor et al 2007).

Abrahamsson et al (2007) conducted a double-blind, randomised, placebo-controlled trial investigating the role of *Lactobacillus reuteri* strain ProGaia (MM53) in the prevention of atopic dermatitis development ($n = 232$). The mothers received *L. reuteri* ProGaia (1×10^8 CFU) daily from gestational week 36 until delivery. Their babies then continued with the same product from birth until 12 months of age. The incidence of eczema was found to be similar in both groups at 2 years of age. However, infants in the probiotic group did have less IgE-associated eczema

TABLE 4 ROLE OF *LACTOBACILLUS RHAMNOSUS* GG (LGG) IN THE PREVENTION OF ATOPIC ECZEMA

Trial design	Intervention details	Results
R, DB, PC *n* = 159 pregnant women with an atopic family history	1 × 10^{10} CFU/day LGG for 2–4 weeks before expected delivery. After delivery, breastfeeding mothers could take the capsules; otherwise infants received the agent directly for the following 6 months	There was a 49% reduced risk of eczema development at 2 years of age ($P = 0.008$), 43% reduced risk of eczema at 4 years of age ($P < 0.05$) and a 36% reduced risk at 7 years of age (Kalliomaki et al 2001, 2003, 2007)
R, DB, PC *n* = 105 pregnant women with an atopic family history	1 × 10^{10} CFU/day LGG for 4–6 weeks before expected delivery. After delivery, exclusively breastfeeding mothers took the LGG directly for the initial 3 months and it was administered directly to the infant for the following 3 months. Formula-fed infants received LGG directly for 6 months	The risk of atopic dermatitis in children on LGG was not decreased relative to placebo (relative risk [RR] = 0.96; confidence interval [CI] 0.38–2.33) (Kopp et al 2008)
R, DB, PC *n* = 250 pregnant women with an atopic family history	LGG 1.8 × 10^{10} CFU/day from 36 weeks' gestation until delivery only	Prenatal LGG treatment was not associated with reduced risk of eczema (34% probiotic, 39% placebo; RR 0.88; 95% CI 0.63–1.22) or immunoglobulin E-associated eczema (18% probiotic, 19% placebo; RR 0.94; 95% CI 0.53–1.68) (Boyle et al 2011)

R, randomised; DB, double-blind; PC, placebo-controlled; CFU, colony-forming unit.

(8 vs 20%; $P = 0.02$) and, in infants with allergic mothers, less skin prick test reactivity (14 vs 31%; $P = 0.02$) (Abrahamsson et al 2007).

Wickens et al (2008) performed a randomised, double-blind, placebo-controlled trial to assess the impact of two different probiotic strains on the development of atopic eczema. Pregnant women with an atopic family history were randomised to take *Lactobacillus rhamnosus* HN001, *Bifidobacterium animalis* subsp. *lactis* strain HN019 or placebo daily from 35 weeks' gestation until 6 months if breastfeeding, and their infants were randomised to receive the same treatment from birth to 2 years ($n = 474$). Infants in the *L. rhamnosus* HN001 group had a 49% reduced risk of eczema development at 2 years of age (95% CI 0.30–0.85; $P = 0.01$). On the other hand, there was no reduced risk of eczema development in infants receiving *Bifidobacterium animalis* subsp. *lactis* strain HN019 (Wickens et al 2008).

P

In another randomised, placebo-controlled, double-blind trial, the efficacy of *Lactobacillus paracasei* F-19 was evaluated. In this trial, the probiotic was administered to the infant (*n* = 179) directly at the time of weaning (mixed into food). Infants consumed the probiotic agent (1 × 10^8 CFU/day) from 4 to 13 months of age. Probiotic supplementation resulted in a significantly reduced cumulative incidence of eczema at 13 months of age (11 vs 22%; $P < 0.05$) and an improved Th1/Th2 ratio (West et al 2009).

In a further double-blind trial, women (*n* = 415) were randomised to receive either placebo or a probiotic milk (containing LGG, *Lactobacillus acidophilus* La5 and *Bifidobacterium lactis* Bb12) from 36 weeks' gestation to 3 months postnatally during breastfeeding. At 2 years old, the odds ratio (OR) for the cumulative incidence of atopic eczema was 0.51 in the probiotic group compared with the placebo (95% CI 0.30–0.87; *P* = 0.013). There were no significant effects on rates of asthma or atopic sensitisation (Dotterud et al 2010).

Treatment of atopic eczema

To determine whether probiotics are efficacious in treating atopic eczema, Michail et al (2008) performed a meta-analysis of randomised controlled trials. Eleven studies were located and data from 10 trials were available to pool and analyse (*n* = 678). There was an overall statistically significant difference favouring probiotics compared with placebo in reducing the Scoring of Atopic Dermatitis Severity Index score (mean change from baseline, −3.01; 95% CI −5.36 to −0.66; *P* = 0.01). Children with moderately severe disease appeared more likely to benefit. There was also a trend for greater improvement in IgE-sensitised patients (*P* = 0.07) (Michail et al 2008).

A randomised, double-blind study of 56 young children (aged 6–18 months) with moderate or severe atopic eczema found that treatment with *L. fermentum* VRI-003 PCC (1 × 10^9 twice daily) produced a significant reduction in the Severity Scoring of Atopic Dermatitis (SCORAD) index (Weston et al 2005). At week 16, 92% of children receiving probiotics had a SCORAD index that was significantly better than baseline compared with the placebo group (*n* = 17, 63%; *P* = 0.01). Another randomised double-blind study has found that supplementation of infant formula with viable, but not heat-inactivated, LGG may have benefits for the management of atopic eczema and cow's milk allergy, particularly in terms of acceleration of improvement (Kirjavainen et al 2003).

According to two other placebo-controlled studies, it appears that people with greater allergic responses may be better suited to treatment and experience superior effects. Rosenfeldt et al (2003) found that treatment with two *Lactobacillus* strains (lyophilised *L. rhamnosus* 19070-2 and *L. reuteri* DSM 122460) given in combination for 6 weeks to children aged 1–13 years with atopic dermatitis resulted in 56% experiencing improvement. Interestingly, the total SCORAD score did not change significantly. Allergic patients with a positive skin prick test response and increased IgE levels experienced a more pronounced response to treatment.

Similarly, a randomised, controlled trial by Sistek et al (2006) found that a combination of two probiotic strains (*Lactobacillus rhamnosus* HN001 and *Bifidobacterium lactis* HN019) given to children with established atopic eczema effectively reduced the SCORAD index among the food-sensitised children, but not in other children. Children in this study received 2 × 10^{10} CFU/g of probiotics or placebo daily as a powder mixed with food or water.

Gastrointestinal infections

Probiotics have a role in the management of various gastrointestinal infections, such as bacterial and viral-induced diarrhoea, *Helicobacter pylori*, traveller's diarrhoea (TD), recurrent *Clostridium difficile*-associated disease (CDAD) and pancreatitis.

Diarrhoea

Various probiotic strains have been subjected to clinical trials to evaluate their efficacy in diarrhoea of different origins.

Viral gastroenteritis — prevention

In a randomised, double-blind, placebo-controlled trial, infants admitted to a chronic medical hospital (average duration of stay 80 days) ingested formula that was supplemented with either placebo or a combination probiotic. The probiotic contained *Bifidobacterium lactis* Bb12 (1.9×10^8 CFU/g powdered formula) and the TH-4 strain of *Streptococcus thermophilus* (0.14×10^8 CFU/g powdered formula). Probiotic supplementation was found to significantly reduce diarrhoea incidence (7 vs 31%; $P = 0.035$) and rotavirus shedding (10 vs 39%; $P = 0.025$) (Saavedra et al 1994).

Another randomised, controlled trial found that the administration of LGG to hospitalised children reduced the risk of rotavirus gastroenteritis by 87% ($P = 0.02$) (Szajewska et al 2001).

Treatment

A meta-analysis of eight randomised controlled trials ($n = 988$) by Szajewska et al (2007) found that supplementation of LGG significantly reduced duration of rotavirus diarrhoea by 2.1 days in children ($P = 0.006$) and the risk of diarrhoea lasting >7 days was reduced by 75% ($P = 0.01$). The authors did caution, however, that the heterogeneity and methodological considerations of the studies limited the strength of the conclusions (Szajewska et al 2007).

In order to determine the dose-dependent effect of LGG on faecal rotavirus shedding, Fang et al (2009) conducted an open-label randomised study where 23 children with rotavirus gastroenteritis were treated for 3 days with a daily dose of LGG: 0 CFU/day (control group, $n = 6$); 2×10^8 CFU/day (low-dose group, $n = 9$); or 6×10^8 CFU/day (high-dose group, $n = 8$). The high-dose LGG group was the only group who experienced a significant reduction of rotavirus levels in stool samples (86% after 3 days).

A randomised, placebo-controlled trial comparing the efficacy of two different doses of *Lactobacillus reuteri* MM53 (1×10^{10} CFU/day or 1×10^7 CFU/day) with placebo in children with rotavirus-associated diarrhoea ($n = 66$) found that probiotic treatment reduced the duration of viral gastroenteritis-induced diarrhoea from 2.5 days in the placebo group to 1.9 days in the low-dose group and 1.5 days in the high-dose group ($P = 0.01$). By the second day of treatment watery diarrhoea persisted in 80% of the placebo, 70% of the low-dose group and 48% of the large-dose group ($P = 0.04$, large dosage vs. placebo) (Shornikova et al 1997).

Another double-blind, randomised, placebo-controlled study evaluated the efficacy of the multistrain probiotic preparation (VSL#3) in the treatment of rotavirus diarrhoea in children. Two hundred and thirty children were enrolled in the trial. By day 2, a lower mean stool frequency and improved stool consistency were noted in the VSL#3 group (both $P \leq 0.05$). On day 4 of treatment, 89% of VSL#3-treated children were recovered vs 40% of controls ($P < 0.001$) (Dubey et al 2008).

Bacterial gastroenteritis — traveller's diarrhoea

TD is the most common health problem in those visiting developing countries, affecting between 20% and 50% of tourists. Although it is usually short-lived and

P

self-limiting, TD represents a considerable socioeconomic burden for both the traveller and the host country. The most common enteropathogen is *Escherichia coli*, but a number of other microorganisms are also implicated (Ardley & Wright 2010). Recent research has highlighted the causative role of TD in the development of postinfectious IBS (Stermer et al 2006). Thus agents capable of preventing the development of TD are much needed.

Clinical trials with probiotics have thus far produced mixed results. In an attempt to clarify the role of probiotics in the prevention of TD, McFarland (2007) conducted a systematic review and meta-analysis on the area. Combining the data from 12 randomised, controlled trials indicated that probiotics significantly prevent the development of TD, with a pooled RR of 0.85 (95% CI 0.79–0.91; $P < 0.001$). While the data for probiotics as a whole were positive, a number of preparations were found to be ineffective: *Lactobacillus fermentum* VRI-003 (Katelaris & Salam 1995), Lactinex (unspecified strains of *Lactobacillus acidophilus* and *Lactobacillus helveticus* in combination) (de Dios Pozo-Olano et al 1978) and an unspecified strain of *Lactobacillus acidophilus* (Antibiophilus-Kapsein) (Kollaritsch et al 1989). Only strains with proven efficacy in TD should be utilised clinically (see below).

In a randomised, double-blind, placebo-controlled trial by Black et al (1989), the combination of *Lactobacillus acidophilus* La5 and *Bifidobacterium lactis* Bb12 was evaluated for the prevention of TD. Ninety-five Danish travellers touring Egypt took part in the trial and consumed either placebo or a probiotic preparation containing 1.8×10^{10} CFU/day of a combination of *Lactobacillus acidophilus* La5, *Bifidobacterium lactis* Bb12, *Lactobacillus delbrueckii* ssp. *bulgaricus* and *Streptococcus thermophilus* starting 2 days prior to travel. The first two strains constituted 90% of the mixture. The number of tourists developing diarrhoea was significantly reduced in the probiotic group — from 71% in controls to 43% ($P = 0.019$). This equated to a protection rate of 39.4% (Black et al 1989).

A large, randomised, placebo-controlled, double-blind study of the efficacy of LGG in preventing TD involved 820 people on holiday to Turkey to two destinations. The group was randomly assigned either LGG (2×10^9 CFU/day) or placebo in identical sachets. On the return flight, each participant completed a questionnaire indicating the incidence of diarrhoea and related symptoms during the trip. Of the original group, 756 (92%) subjects completed the study. The overall incidence of diarrhoea was 43.8% (331 cases), and the total incidence of diarrhoea in the LGG group was 41.0% compared with 46.5% in the placebo group, indicating an overall protection of 11.8%. Protection rates varied between two different destinations, with the maximum protection rate reported as 39.5% and no side effects reported (Oksanen et al 1990).

In another randomised, placebo-controlled trial investigating the efficacy of LGG (2×10^9 CFU/day) in the prophylaxis of TD, 245 subjects travelling from Finland to developing nations were enrolled. The risk of TD development for subjects taking LGG was reduced by 47% compared to the placebo-treated controls ($P = 0.05$) (Hilton et al 1997).

Utilising a randomised, placebo-controlled, double-blind trial design, Kollaritsch et al (1989) investigated the efficacy of two different doses of *Saccharomyces cerevisiae* var. *boulardii* strain Biocodex (250 mg/day and 500 mg/day) in the prevention of TD. Four hundred and six Austrian subjects travelling to tropical locales were enrolled. The rate of TD in the placebo group was 42.6%, versus 33.6% in the low-dose group and 31.8% in the high-dose group. This equates to a 21% reduction in incidence in the 250 mg/day group ($P < 0.007$) and 25% reduction with 500 mg/day ($P < 0.002$) compared to placebo (Kollaritsch et al 1989).

In another placebo-controlled double-blind study, two doses (250 and 1000 mg) of *Saccharomyces cerevisiae* var. *boulardii* strain Biocodex were administered prophylactically to 3000 Austrian travellers. A significant reduction in the incidence of diarrhoea was observed, with success depending directly on the rigorous use of the preparation. A tendency was noted for *S. cerevisiae* var. *boulardii* Biocodex to have a regional effect, which was particularly marked in North Africa and in Turkey. The effect was also dose-dependent, with participants taking the higher dose of probiotics experiencing the lowest incidence of TD (29%); little difference was observed between low-dose supplementation (34%) and placebo (39%). Treatment was considered very safe (Kollaritsch et al 1993).

Clostridium difficile-associated diarrhoea

Clostridium difficile is a common cause of diarrhoea associated with treatment with antimicrobial and/or antibiotic medication and can potentially progress to colitis, pseudomembranous colitis, toxic megacolon and death. In spite of antimicrobial therapy, recurrence is common, and increasingly, probiotic supplementation has been investigated as a potential treatment for CDAD.

A meta-analysis by McFarland (2006) assessed six blinded randomised controlled trials ($n = 354$ patients) that used a mixture of probiotics in the management of CDAD. The results showed that only *S. cerevisiae* var. *boulardii* supplementation resulted in a significant reduction in recurrence. These findings are in contrast to an earlier meta-analysis by Dendukuri et al (2005), where a role for probiotic use in CDAD was not supported in all the studies; the authors of this meta-analysis reported methodological flaws in some of the studies, although some benefit of probiotic therapy was seen in patient subgroups, particularly those characterised by severe CDAD and high use of vancomycin. Individual strains that have demonstrated efficacy in randomised, controlled trials for the prevention or treatment of CDAD include *S. cerevisiae* var. *boulardii* Biocodex (McFarland et al 1994, Surawicz et al 2000) and *Lactobacillus plantarum* 299v (Klarin et al 2008).

Vancomycin-resistant enterococci

Over the past 15–20 years, there has been a rapid increase in the prevalence of vancomycin-resistant enterococci (VRE). This has been associated with the widespread use of broad-spectrum antibiotics. VRE can be involved in the pathogenesis of persistent, hospital-acquired infections that often have poor outcomes. Additionally, they have the capacity to transfer their antibiotic resistance factors to other organisms. Non-antibiotic control measures of VRE are much needed. This randomised, double-blind, placebo-controlled trial was performed to assess the efficacy of LGG in the eradication of VRE. Twenty-seven VRE-positive hospital inpatients were randomly allocated to consume either a yoghurt containing LGG (100 g daily for 4 weeks) or an equivalent amount of pasteurised yoghurt. All subjects who received LGG yoghurt were cleared of VRE, compared to only 8% of controls ($P < 0.001$) (Manley et al 2007).

Pancreatitis

Probiotic therapy has been investigated in pancreatitis because of the increased risk of bacterial infections. Some animal studies have shown that the use of *L. plantarum* 299v (Mangiante et al 2001) and *S. cerevisiae* var. *boulardii* (Akyol et al 2003) reduced bacterial translocation. Human studies have investigated the use of single probiotic agents such as live *L. plantarum* 299v given to 22 patients compared with an inactivated form given to 23 patients; the probiotic-supplemented group had reduced rates of infection and abscess formation (Olah et al 2002).

P

However, these findings are in contrast to those of Besselink et al (2008), who used a novel preparation consisting of six different strains from six different species of lactic acid bacteria — *Lactobacillus acidophilus, L. casei, L. salivarius, Lactococcus lactis, Bifidobacterium bifidum* and *B. lactis* — in patients with severe acute pancreatitis. Use of this probiotic preparation was associated with significantly increased risk of bowel ischaemia (see section on Adverse Reactions, below). Thus not all probiotic preparations have a role for use as an adjunct treatment in pancreatitis.

Chemotherapy-induced diarrhoea

In an open-label trial, subjects ($n = 150$) undergoing 5-fluorouracil-based chemotherapy for colorectal cancer were randomly assigned to receive supplementation with LGG ($1–2 \times 10^{10}$ CFU/day). LGG supplementation was associated with a 41% reduced frequency of severe diarrhoea ($P = 0.027$), an 83% reduction in abdominal discomfort scores ($P = 0.025$) and 55% decreased frequency in bowel toxicity-induced dose reductions ($P = 0.0008$) compared to untreated controls (Osterlund et al 2007).

AIDS-related diarrhoea

In a small double-blind, placebo-controlled study, 24 women with AIDS/HIV, aged 18–44 years, who were not being treated with antiretrovirals and had moderate diarrhoea, were given either a yoghurt fermented with *Lactobacillus delbrueckii* ssp. *bulgaricus* and *Streptococcus thermophilus* (the typical yoghurt-making bacteria), supplemented with the probiotic strains *Lactobacillus rhamnosus* GR-1 and *L. reuteri* RC-14 or an unsupplemented yoghurt for 15 days. Women receiving the supplemented probiotic yoghurt experienced less diarrhoca, flatulence and nausea compared to those receiving the unsupplemented yoghurt. All probiotic-treated subjects were free of diarrhoea after 15 days' treatment vs 9% of controls. Additionally, there was an increase in CD4 counts observed in probiotic-treated subjects compared to a decrease in controls ($P < 0.02$) (Anukam et al 2008).

In an open-label trial, 17 HIV-positive patients with chronic diarrhoea were given *Saccharomyces cerevisiae* var. *boulardii* Biocodex strain (3 g/day) for 15 days. The mean number of stools per day decreased from 9.0 on enrolment to 2.1 on day 15. Patients gained a mean of 3.6 kg during the trial (McFarland & Bernasconi 1993, Saint-Marc et al 1991).

Trois et al (2008) investigated the effect of probiotics on the immune response in a randomised, double-blind, controlled trial of two groups of children (2–12 years) infected with HIV. The study of 77 children administered either a formula containing unspecified strains of *Bifidobacterium bifidum* and *Streptococcus thermophilus* — 2.5×10^{10} CFU/day (NAN2 probiotico Nestlé) — or a standard formula on a daily basis for 2 months. At the end of the study, there was an increase in CD4 cell count in the probiotic group (+118 cells/mm vs −42 cells/mm in controls; $P = 0.049$), suggesting that this probiotic combination has immunostimulatory properties.

Constipation

Constipation affects a significant proportion of the population. Probiotics have long been touted as useful for the treatment of constipation and recent randomised controlled trials have demonstrated efficacy for some probiotic strains.

In a randomised, controlled trial, Yang et al (2008) evaluated the effect of consuming a fermented milk containing *Bifidobacterium animalis* DN-173 010 (1.25×10^{10} CFU/day) on stool parameters in constipated women ($n = 135$). Compared to controls, stool frequency was significantly increased in the bifidobacteria group after 1 week (3.5 movements/week vs 2.5; $P < 0.01$) and after 2 weeks' consumption (4.17 vs 2.6; $P < 0.01$). Defecation condition and stool consistency also significantly improved after 1 and 2 weeks (all $P < 0.01$) of bifidobacteria consumption (Yang et al 2008).

Another randomised, double-blind, placebo-controlled trial compared the efficacy of placebo to a probiotic drink containing *Lactobacillus casei* Shirota (6.5×10^9 CFU/day) in constipated subjects ($n = 70$). After a 4-week treatment period, there was a significant decrease in the occurrence of moderate and severe constipation ($P < 0.001$) and in occurrence of hard stools ($P < 0.001$) in the probiotic group. There was also an increase in defecation frequency ($P = 0.004$) and improvement in stool consistency ($P < 0.001$). General wellbeing was also significantly improved in the probiotic group ($P = 0.008$) (Koebnick et al 2003).

Immune enhancement/infection prevention

The potential role of probiotics in the enhancement of immune function has been under investigation over the past few decades. The process started with in vitro and animal research, followed by studies evaluating the effects of probiotic administration on immune cell function in human subjects. More recently, well-conducted human trials with hard outcomes have been published.

In a systematic review, Vouloumanou et al (2009) assessed the data from randomised controlled trials (14 trials) that had investigated the role of probiotics for the prevention and treatment of respiratory tract infections (RTIs). Ten of the 14 trials did not find that the probiotic agents trialled reduced the incidence of RTIs compared to placebo; the remaining four trials found the incidence of RTIs to be significantly lower in probiotic-treated patients. A significant reduction in the severity of RTI symptoms associated with probiotic treatment was found in five of six randomised controlled trials that provided relevant data. In the remaining randomised controlled trial, no difference was noted. Three randomised controlled trials reported a significant decrease in duration of RTI symptoms associated with probiotic therapy, whereas nine did not (Vouloumanou et al 2009). The data suggest that some, but not all, probiotic preparations have the capacity to enhance immune function and decrease risk and duration of RTIs.

A number of probiotic strains have demonstrated the capacity to reduce the incidence of infections and/or shorten their duration. The results of these trials are detailed in Table 5.

Infantile colic

In a randomised, open-label trial, colicky breastfed infants ($n = 90$; aged 21–90 days) were supplemented with either simethicone (active control) or *Lactobacillus reuteri* MM53 (1×10^8 CFU/day) for 4 weeks. Significant reductions in daily crying time were noted by day 7 in the MM53 group compared to the simethicone group ($P = 0.005$). This improvement continued until day 28, when median crying time was reduced to 51 min/day in the MM53 group vs 145 min/day in controls ($P < 0.001$) On day 28, 95% of patients were responders in the probiotic group versus 7% in the simethicone group (Savino et al 2007).

Irritable bowel syndrome

Although the aetiology of IBS is still unknown, there is growing evidence that there is a persistent, mild inflammatory state with changes in mucosal function or structure and an associated imbalance of intestinal flora (Camilleri 2006). Dysbiosis has long been theorised to play a role in the pathophysiology of IBS and the first trial conducted investigating the efficacy of probiotics in IBS was

TABLE 5 PROBIOTICS IN THE PREVENTION OF INFECTIONS

Trial methodology	Strain(s) utilised	Results
R, DB, PC *n* = 201 infants 4–10 months old	*Bifidobacterium lactis* Bb12	Over a 3-month period, there was a reduction in fever episodes by 34% ($P < 0.001$), diarrhoea episodes by 58% ($P < 0.001$) and duration of diarrhoea episodes by 37% ($P < 0.001$) (Weizman et al 2005)
R, DB, PC *n* = 326 children 3–5 years of age	*Lactobacillus acidophilus* NCFM	Over a 6-month period, fever incidence was reduced by 53% ($P = 0.0085$) and coughing incidence by 41% ($P = 0.027$); use of antibiotics reduced by 68% ($P = 0.0002$); 32% reduction in days absent from child care ($P = 0.002$) (Leyer et al 2009)
R, DB, PC *n* = 326 children 3–5 years of age	*Lactobacillus acidophilus* NCFM and *Bifidobacterium lactis* Bi07	Over a 6-month period, fever incidence was reduced by 73% ($P = 0.0009$), coughing incidence by 62% ($P = 0.005$) and rhinorrhoea incidence by 59% ($P = 0.03$); use of antibiotics reduced by 84% ($P < 0.0001$); 28% reduction in days absent from child care ($P < 0.001$) (Leyer et al 2009)
R, DB, PC *n* = 215 infants aged 6–12 months	*Lactobacillus fermentum* CECT5716	Over a 6-month period, there was a 46% reduced incidence of gastrointestinal infections ($P = 0.032$), a 26% reduction in respiratory tract infections ($P = 0.022$) and a 30% reduction in the total number of infections ($P = 0.003$); the incidence of recurrent respiratory tract infections was reduced by 72% (Maldonado et al 2012)
R, DB, PC, CO *n* = 20 elite, male distance runners	*Lactobacillus fermentum* VRI-003	Over a 4-month winter period, distance runners taking the probiotic reported less than half the number of days of respiratory symptoms (30 vs 72; $P = 0.00006$) compared with placebo; illness severity was also decreased ($P = 0.06$) (Cox et al 2010).
R, DB, PC *n* = 201 infants 4–10 months old	*Lactobacillus reuteri* MM53	Over a 3-month period, fever episodes were reduced by 73% ($P < 0.001$), diarrhoea episodes by 94% ($P < 0.001$), duration of diarrhoea by 75% ($P < 0.001$) and child care absences by 67% ($P = 0.015$) in infants (Weizman et al 2005)

TABLE 5 PROBIOTICS IN THE PREVENTION OF INFECTIONS *(continued)*

Trial methodology	Strain(s) utilised	Results
R, DB, PC $n = 262$ healthy adults	*Lactobacillus reuteri* MM53	Over the 80-day trial period, there was a 58% reduction in number of subjects reporting sick days in the MM53 group compared to placebo ($P < 0.01$); amongst shift workers, 33% of those in the placebo group reported sick over the study period vs none in the MM53 group ($P < 0.005$) (Tubelius et al 2005)
R, DB, PC $n = 571$ children aged 1–6 years	*Lactobacillus rhamnosus* GG (LGG)	Over the 7-month winter period, there were 16% fewer days absent from day care in children in the LGG group ($P = 0.03$) and a 19% reduction in antibiotic use for respiratory tract infections ($P = 0.03$) (Hatakka et al 2001)
R, DB, PC $n = 281$ day-care-aged children	*Lactobacillus rhamnosus* GG	Over the 3-month intervention period, there was a 34% reduced risk of upper respiratory tract infections in toddlers in the LGG group, a 43% reduced risk of respiratory tract infections lasting longer than 3 days and significantly fewer number of days with respiratory tract symptoms (all $P < 0.001$). There was a trend for reduced number of days with gastrointestinal symptoms ($P = 0.06$) (Hojsak et al 2009)
R, DB, PC $n = 81$ infants < 2 months old	*Lactobacillus rhamnosus* GG and *Bifidobacterium lactis* Bb12	Over the 10-month period, there was a 56% reduced risk of otitis media in infants ($P = 0.014$), a 48% reduced risk of antibiotic prescription ($P = 0.015$) and a 49% reduced risk of recurrent respiratory tract infection ($P = 0.022$) (Rautava et al 2009)

R, randomised; DB, double-blind; PC, placebo-controlled; CO, crossover.

published in 1955 (Rafsky & Rafsky 1955). Many trials have been conducted since this time.

Moayyedi et al (2010) performed a systematic review and meta-analysis of randomised controlled trials that investigated the efficacy of probiotics in the treatment of IBS. Nineteen randomised controlled trials were included ($n = 1650$) in the review. Combining the data found probiotics to be significantly better than placebo in relieving IBS symptoms (relative risk of IBS not improving = 0.71; 95% CI 0.57–0.88) with a number needed to treat of four (95% CI 3–12.5). The authors concluded that probiotics appear to be efficacious in the treatment of IBS, but the magnitude of benefit and the most effective strains are uncertain (Moayyedi et al 2010).

A 2008 meta-analysis concluded that the use of probiotics can result in improved symptom relief in patients with IBS (McFarland & Dublin 2008).

Twenty randomised controlled clinical trials (n = 1404) were reviewed, and either single or multiple probiotics were used for varying time periods ranging from 2 to 24 weeks (median = 4 weeks). Probiotic use was associated with improvement in global IBS symptoms compared to placebo (pooled relative risk [RRpooled] 0.77, 95% CI 0.62–0.94). Probiotic use was also associated with less abdominal pain compared to placebo (RRpooled 0.78 [0.69–0.88], 95% CI 0.45–0.81). There were insufficient data, however, to draw conclusions about the most effective probiotic strains or the assessment of individual IBS symptoms.

Similarly, a systematic review and meta-analysis by Hoveyda et al (2009) reported that probiotic therapy for several weeks may result in modest improvement in the overall symptoms of IBS. A total of 14 randomised placebo-controlled trials of varying length (from 4 weeks to 6 months; although the majority lasted 8 weeks or less) were included in the analyses. The probiotic therapy varied in the strains utilised as well as the dose and strength; in addition, some studies used a single agent and others used combinations of multiple strains. It is important to note, however, that not all clinical studies have produced positive results. A large randomised, parallel-group, double-blind study by Drouault-Holowacz et al (2008) investigated the effects of four strains of lactic acid (LA) bacteria (1×10^{10} CFU *Bifidobacterium longum* LA 101 [29%], *Lactobacillus acidophilus* LA 102 [29%], *Lactococcus lactis* LA 103 [29%] and *Streptococcus thermophilus* LA 104 [13%]) on symptoms of IBS in 100 patients over a 4-week period. The probiotic combination was not significantly superior to the placebo in relieving symptoms of IBS, although symptomatic improvement was noted in some patient subgroups. Studies utilising LGG (in isolation) (O'Sullivan & O'Morain 2000), *Lactobacillus salivarius* UCC4331 (O'Mahony et al 2005a, 2005b) and *Lactobacillus acidophilus* NCFM (Newcomer et al 1983) also failed to demonstrate positive results. Probiotic preparations that have shown efficacy in the treatment of IBS are detailed in Table 6.

Inflammatory bowel disease

Probiotics are also being used as adjunctive therapy for Crohn's disease and ulcerative colitis (Goh & O'Morain 2003, Guslandi 2003a, 2003b, Kanauchi et al 2003, Karthik 2003, Marteau et al 2003, Rutgeerts 2003). Overall, present research indicates a limited role for probiotics in Crohn's disease; the results for ulcerative colitis are more promising, and there does seem to be a beneficial effect in pouchitis.

Crohn's disease

Only a limited number of studies have indicated a role for probiotics in the remission of Crohn's disease. In an open-label study, Guslandi et al (2000) compared *Saccharomyces cerevisiae* var. *boulardii* Biocodex plus mesalazine with mesalazine alone and found that adjunctive probiotic treatment resulted in fewer relapses (6% vs 38%; P = 0.04).

Supplementation with VSL#3 has also been evaluated. VSL#3 contains a high concentration of eight strains of lactic acid bacteria — *Bifidobacterium breve*, *B. longum*, *B. infantis*, *Lactobacillus acidophilus*, *L. plantarum*, *L. casei*, *L. bulgaricus* and *Streptococcus thermophilus*. A study of 40 patients randomised to 3 months of rifaximin followed by 9 months of VSL#3 or to 12 months of mesalazine also reported relapse prevention with probiotic therapy (Campieri et al 2000).

Other studies, including randomised, double-blind placebo-controlled trials, have suggested that LGG and *Lactobacillus johnsonii* La1 have no role to play in maintaining Crohn's disease in remission (Hedin et al 2007). Similarly, studies that have administered probiotics for the treatment of active Crohn's disease have also provided mixed results, mainly because of concurrent use of medications

TABLE 6 PROBIOTICS IN THE TREATMENT OF IRRITABLE BOWEL SYNDROME (IBS)		
Trial methodology	**Strain(s) utilised**	**Results**
R, DB, PC *n* = 34 female subjects with C-IBS	*Bifidobacterium animalis* strain DN-173010	After a 4-week treatment period, there was a significant reduction in abdominal distension ($P = 0.02$), an acceleration of gut transit time ($P = 0.049$) and a reduction in overall IBS symptom severity ($P = 0.032$). There were also reductions in abdominal pain/discomfort ($P = 0.044$), bloating ($P = 0.059$) and flatulence scores ($P = 0.092$) (Agrawal et al 2009)
R, DB, PC *n* = 362 female subjects with IBS	*Bifidobacterium infantis* 35624	After a 4-week treatment phase, there were significant reductions in abdominal pain/discomfort ($P = 0.023$), bloating/distension ($P = 0.046$), feeling of incomplete evacuation ($P < 0.04$), sense of straining at stool ($P < 0.02$), passage of gas ($P < 0.04$) and composite IBS symptom scores ($P = 0.013$) compared to controls. There was also a significant improvement in bowel habit satisfaction ($P < 0.02$) (Whorwell et al 2006)
R, DB, PC *n* = 52 subjects with IBS	*Lactobacillus acidophilus* strains CUL-60 and CUL-21, *Bifidobacterium lactis* CUL-34, and *Bifidobacterium bifidum* CUL-20 (Lab4)	After an 8-week treatment period, there were significant reductions in composite IBS symptom scores ($P = 0.0217$) and improvements in quality-of-life scores ($P = 0.0068$) compared to controls (Williams et al 2008)
R, DB, PC *n* = 48 subjects with IBS and bloating	VSL#3	After either a 4- or an 8-week treatment phase, there was a significant reduction in flatulence scores ($P = 0.011$). There were no significant changes in other IBS symptoms or bowel function, although colonic transit time was retarded in the VSL#3 group (Kim et al 2005)
R, DB, PC *n* = 214 subjects with IBS	*Lactobacillus plantarum* 299V	After a 4-week treatment phase, the frequency and severity of abdominal pain, bloating and feeling of incomplete evacuation scores were significantly reduced in the 299V group compared to controls (all $P < 0.05$). Stool frequency was significantly reduced in the 299V group ($P < 0.05$), and 78% of subjects in the 299V group scored the symptomatic effect as excellent or good vs 8% of controls ($P < 0.01$) (Ducrotte et al 2012)

R, randomised; DB, double-blind; PC, placebo-controlled; CO, crossover; C-IBS, constipation-predominant irritable bowel syndrome.

P

during the intervention period (e.g. prednisolone use or metronidazole) (Gupta et al 2000).

A Cochrane systematic review by Rolfe et al (2006) did not advocate a role for probiotics in Crohn's disease based on the available evidence, suggesting that, because all studies enrolled small numbers of patients, they may have lacked statistical power to show differences should they exist. Seven randomised controlled trials were identified that had utilised a variety of probiotics, such as LGG, *Escherichia coli* Nissle 1917 and *Saccharomyces cerevisiae* var. *boulardii*; most of the studies had a relatively small number of participants with different treatment protocols, probiotic strains and outcome measures, making it difficult for comparisons to be made.

Similar conclusions were reached in a recent systematic review of probiotics in Crohn's disease, where the authors stated there was no evidence from randomised controlled trials to support the use of probiotic therapy in Crohn's disease (Jonkers et al 2012).

Given the promising preliminary research on *Saccharomyces cerevisiae* var. *boulardii* Biocodex in Crohn's disease, the strain was evaluated using a more rigorous randomised, double-blind, placebo-controlled trial design. One hundred and sixty-five subjects with Crohn's disease that was currently in remission after treatment with steroids or salicylates were randomly allocated to receive either placebo or probiotic (1 g/day) for 12 months. Over the 12 months, the relapse rates were 47.5% in the probiotic group and 53.2% in the placebo group (a non-significant difference). The median time to relapse did not differ significantly between patients given probiotics (40.7 weeks) vs placebo (39.0 weeks). There were also no significant differences between groups in mean Crohn's disease activity index scores or erythrocyte sedimentation rates or in median levels of C-reactive protein. A post hoc analysis did reveal, however, that non-smokers given *S. cerevisiae* var. *boulardii* Biocodex were less likely to experience a relapse of Crohn's disease than non-smokers given placebo (OR 0.22, 95% CI 0.07–0.70; $P = 0.01$) (Bourreille et al 2013). The latter result requires confirmation in future research to ensure it was not a random finding, but in the meantime a trial of this probiotic strain would be warranted in non-smoking Crohn's disease patients.

Ulcerative colitis

A Cochrane review conducted in 2011 found four randomised controlled trials ($n = 587$) that evaluated probiotics for the maintenance of remission in ulcerative colitis. Combining the data from the three trials comparing probiotics to mesalazine found no significant difference in recurrence rates between the two treatments: 40.1% of subjects in the probiotics group and 34.1% in the mesalazine group relapsed over the treatment period. The final trial included a small placebo controlled trial ($n = 32$), and found no statistically significant difference in efficacy — 75% of probiotic patients relapsed at 1 year compared to 92% of placebo patients. The authors concluded that there is currently insufficient evidence to draw conclusions about the efficacy of probiotics for maintenance of remission in ulcerative colitis (Naidoo et al 2011).

A recent meta-analysis of randomised, controlled trials assessed the impact of probiotics on remission induction and maintenance in ulcerative colitis. Thirteen randomised controlled trials were included in the analysis. Seven reports evaluated remission rates ($n = 399$). When combined, the adjunct use of probiotics alongside standard care did not significantly alter remission rates. There was, however, marked heterogeneity in the results. Eight reports assessed the recurrence rate ($n = 709$). Compared to the placebo group, the use of probiotics was found to significantly reduce the ulcerative colitis recurrence rate (recurrence rate: 0.69,

95% CI 0.47–1.01; P = 0.05). Heterogeneity was again observed. The results suggest that using probiotics provides no additional benefit in inducing remission of ulcerative colitis, but probiotics auxiliary therapy is much better than non-probiotics therapy for maintenance of remission (Sang et al 2010). The significant heterogeneity observed in this study, which should have precluded the conduction of a meta-analysis, was most likely caused by the all-too-common error of combining research conducted on different probiotic strains or variations in study designs. Each strain must be viewed as a separate therapeutic agent.

Probiotic preparations that have shown efficacy in the treatment of ulcerative colitis are detailed in Tables 7 and 8.

Pouchitis

Probiotics have also been used in patients with relapsing or chronic pouchitis (Kailasapathy & Chin 2000). While studies have produced inconsistent results, overall there appears to be some evidence to support the therapeutic use of probiotics in postoperative pouchitis (Penner et al 2005) and the general view is that VSL#3 treatment can be effective in controlling this condition.

Studies by Gionchetti et al (2000, 2003) assessed the use of VSL#3 in both primary prevention of pouchitis and maintenance therapy for chronic relapsing pouchitis, demonstrating some success. In their randomised, controlled, double-blind study, 40 patients with relapsing pouchitis in remission received a 6 g daily dose of VSL#3 or a placebo for 9 months. Probiotic treatment resulted in a significantly reduced incidence of pouchitis (Gionchetti et al 2000), but when VSL#3 treatment was ceased, all patients relapsed 3 months later. In a subsequent randomised controlled study to investigate VSL#3 treatment for primary prophylaxis of pouchitis in 40 patients, Gionchetti et al (2003) reported that treatment with VSL#3 resulted in fewer relapses.

In another randomised, double-blind, controlled trial, Mimura et al (2004) also utilised VSL#3 in 36 patients with more severe recurrent pouchitis over a 1-year follow-up period and reported good results regarding maintenance of remission and improved quality of life in the patients.

A combination of probiotics also has been reported to result in beneficial effects; lactobacilli and bifidobacteria in fermented milk were administered to patients who had pouchitis after ulcerative colitis surgery, resulting in some resolution of disease activity (Laake et al 2005).

In contrast, in an uncontrolled study of 31 patients who were treated with antibiotics and were in remission, Shen et al (2005) found little benefit with VSL#3 administered for 8 months.

An open-label trial evaluated the efficacy of LGG in preventing pouchitis. Subjects with ulcerative colitis who had undergone an ileal pouch-anal anastomosis (n = 117) took part in the trial. LGG supplementation ($1–2 \times 10^{10}$ CFU/day) significantly delayed first onset of pouchitis compared to no-treatment controls (cumulative risk at 3 years: 7 vs 29%; P = 0.011) (Gosselink et al 2005).

Probiotics and diverticular disease

It has been suggested that altered bacterial flora is one of the causes of diverticular inflammation (White 2006). Consequently, some investigators have evaluated the role of probiotics in diverticular disease. In an open-label study, 15 patients with diverticular disease were treated with an antimicrobial and charcoal for the first symptomatic episode after enrolment and the second episode was treated with the same therapy, followed by *Escherichia coli* Nissle 1917 for 6 weeks. This second treatment resulted in a longer symptom-free duration of a mean of 14

TABLE 7 PROBIOTICS IN THE TREATMENT OF ULCERATIVE COLITIS (UC) — INDUCTION OF REMISSION

Trial methodology	Strain(s) utilised	Results
R, DB, C *n* = 116 patients with active UC	*Escherichia coli* Nissle 1917	Over a 12-month treatment period, *Escherichia coli* Nissle 1917 supplementation, in conjunction with standard inflammatory bowel disease therapy (corticosteroids), was equivalent to mesalazine in terms of remission rate ($P = 0.05$) and time to remission ($P = 0.009$). The duration of remission was also equivalent ($P = 0.017$) (Rembacken et al 1999)
R, DB, PC *n* = 90 patients with moderately active distal UC	*Escherichia coli* Nissle 1917	Intrarectal administration (via enema) of three different doses of *E. coli* Nissle 1917 (40, 20, or 10 mL) daily for 2 weeks did not significantly impact rates of remission in intention to treat analysis. There were a large number of protocol violations, however, and a per protocol analysis demonstrated a significant dose-dependent effect ($P = 0.0446$). Remission rates in the 40 mL group were 53%, 44% in the 20 mL group and 27% in the 10 mL group, compared to 18% in the placebo group (Matthes et al 2010)
R, DB, PC *n* = 147 subjects with mild to moderate active UC	VSL#3	At 6 weeks, 33% of VSL#3-treated subjects achieved >50% in the UC disease activity index versus 10% of controls ($P = 0.001$). At week 12, 43% of subjects in the VSL#3 group were in remission vs 16% of controls ($P < 0.001$) (Sood et al 2009)
R, DB, PC *n* = 29 children with active UC	VSL#3	In conjunction with standard UC therapy (steroids and mesalamine), remission was achieved in 93% of VSL#3-treated children vs 36% of controls ($P < 0.001$). Twenty-one per cent of VSL#3-treated subjects relapsed within 1 year versus 73% of controls ($P = 0.014$) (Miele et al 2009)
R, DB, PC *n* = 144 subjects with mild to moderate relapsing UC	VSL#3	In conjunction with standard UC therapy (stable doses of 5-aminosalicylic acid and/or immunosuppressants), the number of subjects experiencing a decrease in UC disease activity index scores of 50% or more was higher in the VSL#3 group than in the placebo group ($P = 0.031$). Rectal bleeding also improved significantly more in the VSL#3 group than controls ($P = 0.036$). Rates of remission were higher in the VSL#3 group, but not significantly so (43.6% vs 31.5%; $P = 0.132$) (Miele et al 2009)

R, randomised; DB, double-blind; PC, placebo-controlled.

TABLE 8 PROBIOTICS IN THE TREATMENT OF ULCERATIVE COLITIS (UC) — MAINTENANCE OF REMISSION

Trial methodology	Strain(s) utilised	Results
R, DB, C $n = 327$ UC patients in remission	*Escherichia coli* Nissle 1917	Over the 12-month trial period, *E. coli* Nissle 1917 treatment was found to be equally effective as mesalazine in preventing relapse (36.4% relapse vs 33.9%; $P = 0.003$) (Kruis et al 2004)
R, DB, C $n = 120$ UC patients in remission	*Escherichia coli* Nissle 1917	Over a 12-week period, relapse rates were 11.3% under mesalazine and 16.0% under *E. coli* Nissle 1917 (not significantly different). The mean relapse-free time was 103 ± 4 days for mesalazine and 106 ± 5 days for *E. coli* Nissle 1917 (not significantly different) (Kruis et al 1997)
R, OL $n = 187$ UC patients in remission	*Lactobacillus rhamnosus* GG	Subjects were randomised to receive either *Lactobacillus rhamnosus* GG (LGG) alone or in combination with mesalazine, or mesalazine alone. Over the 12-month trial period, there was no difference in relapse rates between the three groups. LGG supplementation was equally effective as mesalazine in maintaining clinical remission, but significantly more effective than mesalazine in prolonging the relapse-free time ($P < 0.05$) (Zocco et al 2006)
OL $n = 34$ UC patients in remission aged 11–18 years	*Escherichia coli* Nissle 1917	Over the 12-month treatment period, the relapse rate was 25% in probiotic-treated subjects vs 30% in the mesalazine group (Henker et al 2008)
OL $n = 20$ UC patients in remission	VSL#3	After 12 months, 15 of the 20 participants remained in remission, which compares favourably to rates of remission observed during long-term mesalazine therapy (Venturi et al 1999)

R, randomised; DB, double-blind; C, controlled; OL, open-label.

months compared to a mean of 2.4 months in the control group (Fric & Zavoral 2003).

Various studies have attempted to restore the altered microflora using probiotics, but most of these studies have been limited in their design and methods (Sheth & Floch 2009). However, results from these studies appear to be mostly positive, and randomised placebo-controlled studies are needed in order to make recommendations.

Alcohol-induced liver disease

In a prospective, randomised, clinical study, 66 men with advanced alcohol-induced liver disease received either *Bifidobacterium bifidum* (unspecified strain) and

Lactobacillus plantarum 8PA3 or standard therapy (no probiotics) for 5 days. At the end of the study, patients who had received the probiotic therapy had significantly increased numbers of both bifidobacteria (7.9 vs 6.81 log 10^9 CFU/g) and lactobacilli (4.2 vs 3.2 log 10^9 CFU/g) compared to the standard therapy group; likewise, the former group had a significant improvement in hepatic enzyme levels (Kirpich et al 2008).

Non-alcoholic fatty liver disease (NAFLD)

NAFLD comprises a spectrum of diseases ranging from simple steatosis to non-alcoholic steatohepatitis, fibrosis and cirrhosis. Probiotics have been proposed as a treatment option because of their modulating effect on the gut flora that could influence the gut-liver axis and there are now considerable data from animal models in support of this idea. A Cochrane systematic review conducted in 2007 found no human randomised controlled trials that evaluated probiotics in the treatment of NAFLD. The authors concluded that the lack of randomised controlled trials makes it impossible to support or refute the use of probiotics in NAFLD (Lirussi et al 2007).

In a randomised, double-blind, placebo-controlled trial, supplementation of obese children ($n = 20$; mean age 10.7 years) with persisting hypertransaminasaemia and ultrasonographic changes suggestive of NAFLD with LGG (1.2×10^{10} CFU/day) for 8 weeks resulted in a decrease in alanine aminotransferase concentration ($P = 0.03$) and in antipeptidoglycan-polysaccharide antibody levels ($P = 0.03$). Alanine aminotransferase levels normalised in 80% of LGG-treated subjects (Vajro et al 2011).

Hepatic encephalopathy

To date, there are only a few reports about the role of probiotics in hepatic encephalopathy; in addition to the conventional management with antibiotics and lactulose, probiotics may confer favourable changes in intestinal microflora in patients with hepatic encephalopathy.

A recent randomised, controlled, single tertiary centre study with open allocation by Bajaj et al (2008) investigated the effects of a probiotic yoghurt on minimal hepatic encephalopathy (MHE), a preclinical stage prior to full-blown hepatic encephalopathy. The probiotics *Streptococcus thermophilus*, *L. bulgaricus*, *L. acidophilus*, bifidobacteria and *L. casei* (unspecified strains) were administered in the form of a commercial yoghurt to a group of non-alcoholic MHE cirrhotic patients for 60 days; the study demonstrated a significant rate of MHE reversal (71% vs 0% in controls; $P = 0.003$).

Colon cancer

A number of factors may be involved in colon cancer risk, and it has been suggested that the colonic microbiota may be involved in the aetiology of colorectal cancer. A lower incidence of colon cancer has been associated with the consumption of lactobacilli or bifidobacteria. The exact mechanisms have not been fully elucidated (Fotiadis et al 2008), but may have to do with probiotic-induced reductions in colonic expression of β-glucuronidase, nitroreductase and azoreductase (Marotta et al 2003).

A randomised, controlled trial evaluated the efficacy of *Lactobacillus casei* Shirota in the prevention of colorectal cancer in patients ($n = 398$) who had had at least two colorectal tumours removed. Daily consumption of the probiotic over a 4-year period resulted in a significant reduction in the occurrence of colorectal tumours with moderate or severe atypia compared to the dietary instruction only group ($P < 0.05$) (Ishikawa et al 2005).

Clinical note — The hygiene hypothesis

The intestinal tract is the largest immune organ of the body. It produces more antibodies than any other part of the body and contains 80% of all antibody-producing cells. The intestinal mucosa functions as a barrier against infections, but it also provides communication between the different mucosal surfaces of the body (Ouwehand et al 2002).

At birth, the GIT is sterile. Normal gut flora develops gradually over time and is influenced by factors such as composition of the maternal gut microbiota, diet, degree of hygiene, use of antibiotics or other medications, the environment and possibly genetic aspects. Studies in germ-free mice have shown that, without these bacteria, the systemic immune system will not function normally (Vanderhoof & Young 2002).

In the absence of microbes, a mammal develops fewer Peyer's patches (part of the gut-associated lymphoid tissue) and less than 10% of the number of IgA-producing B cells compared with normal. However, on exposure to a normal microflora, previously germ-free animals develop their immune system very much like other animals. This indicates that the intestinal microflora is instrumental in the proper development of the immune system (Ouwehand et al 2002) and has led to the emergence of the 'hygiene theory of immune disorders'.

More specifically, the hygiene hypothesis suggests that improved hygienic conditions and vaccinations, which reduce early-life exposure to microbes, are associated with a heightened risk of allergic disease and other immune disorders. This is because reduced exposure may result in reduced stimulation of the immune system. As a result, lymphocytes that would normally differentiate to become Th1-type differentiate to Th2-type cells and produce inflammatory cytokines in the allergic response in much greater quantities. As such, very early stimulation of the immune system is important in dampening the Th2 dominance and reducing the development of IgE-mediated food reactions as well as other allergic reactions. In a closely observed cohort of 329 Finnish children, it was shown that the earlier an acute respiratory infection occurred, the greater the protective effect was against atopic eczema (Vanderhoof & Young 2003).

The obvious solution for increasing microbial exposure without increasing the health risk is the use of prebiotics and probiotics. Supplementation with probiotics has been shown to both reduce the risk and treat the symptoms of childhood eczema (see Atopic Eczema, above).

Modulating the intestinal microflora with probiotics and prebiotics may be an effective and safe therapy for the natural development of a balanced immune defence in infants and children. In adults and the elderly, prebiotics and probiotics may be used to improve the general functioning of the immune system.

High cholesterol

Some probiotics may have cholesterol-lowering effects due to several mechanisms, including enzymatic deconjugation of bile acids and metabolic utilisation of cholesterol (Brashears et al 1998, Liong & Shah 2005).

According to a meta-analysis of six studies of a probiotic dairy product containing *Enterococcus faecium*, treatment with the fermented yoghurt product produced a 4% decrease in total cholesterol and a 5% decrease in low-density lipoprotein cholesterol (Agerholm-Larsen et al 2000).

Since then, mixed findings have been reported regarding the use of encapsulated probiotics; a hypocholesterolaemic effect was not observed in some studies (Greany et al 2008, Hatakka et al 2008, Larsen et al 2006, Lewis & Burmeister 2005, Simons et al 2006), but Hlivak et al (2005) provided a daily dose of 10^9 CFU of probiotic bacteria and noted a hypocholesterolaemic effect. It is possible that lipid-lowering activity induced by probiotics is dependent on whether patients have high cholesterol levels (>6.0 mmol/L) (Agerback et al 1995, Bertolami et al 1999, Hlivak et al 2005, Xiao et al 2003) or lower to normal cholesterol levels (<5.4 mmol/L) (de Roos et al 1999, Greany et al 2004), although further randomised trials are required to confirm this observation. It is also possible that some probiotic strains have the capacity to lower serum cholesterol levels while others do not.

Most recently, two randomised, placebo-controlled studies failed to detect a significant lipid-lowering activity for different strains of probiotics. Greany et al (2008) conducted a randomised, single-blinded, placebo-controlled, parallel-arm study of 33 normocholesterolaemic women and 22 men aged 18–36 years. Subjects in the intervention group were treated for 3 months with probiotic capsules (three capsules daily) containing a total of 10^9 CFU *Lactobacillus acidophilus* strain DDS-1 and *Bifidobacterium longum* strain UABL-14 and 10–15 mg fructooligosaccharide. These probiotic strains had no effect on plasma lipid concentrations (Greany et al 2008).

Likewise, Hatakka et al (2008) conducted a double-blind, randomised, placebo-controlled, two-period crossover study to investigate the effects of taking on a daily basis two probiotic capsules containing viable *Lactobacillus rhamnosus* LC705 and *Propionibacterium freudenreichii* ssp. *shermanii* JS (2×10^{10} CFU of each strain) on serum cholesterol and triglyceride levels: the study of 38 mildly or moderately hypercholesterolaemic men aged 24–55 years found that probiotic treatment over 4 weeks did not have any effect on serum lipids.

Mastitis

Mastitis is an inflammatory condition of the breast that may, or may not, be associated with infection. It is a common reason for premature cessation of breastfeeding (Academy of Breastfeeding Medicine 2008). Recent research has found some probiotic strains to be of benefit in the treatment of mastitis and the prophylaxis of recurrent mastitis.

In a randomised, double-blind, placebo-controlled trial, 352 women with lactational mastitis were allocated into one of three groups: antibiotics, *Lactobacillus fermentum* CECT5716 or *L. salivarius* CECT (both at 1.0×10^9 CFU/day). After 3 weeks' treatment, both probiotic strains were found to be superior to antibiotics in decreasing levels of pathogenic bacteria in breast milk, increasing lactobacilli counts in breast milk and decreasing breast pain scores (all $P < 0.001$). They also significantly reduced the rate of recurrence compared to antibiotics: 10.5% in the *L. fermentum* CECT5716 group and 7.1% in the *L. salivarius* CECT5713 group versus 30.7% in the antibiotic group (both $P < 0.001$) (Arroyo et al 2010).

In another randomised, placebo-controlled trial, women (n = 20) with antibiotic-resistant mastitis were allocated to receive either placebo or a probiotic preparation (*Lactobacillus salivarius* CECT5713 and *L. gasseri* CECT5714; 2.0×10^{10} CFU/day) for 14 days. All mastitis signs were eliminated by day 14 in the probiotic group, whereas mastitis persisted in all women in the control group. There was also an ~100-fold decrease in milk staphylococcal counts in probiotic group (Jimenez et al 2008).

Postpartum obesity

Another novel area of research is using probiotics to prevent postpartum obesity. Ilmonen et al investigated the use of a probiotic combination product (containing LGG and *Bifidobacterium lactis* Bb12) in the prophylaxis of postpartum obesity. In the first trimester of pregnancy, 256 women were randomly assigned to receive no dietary counselling or nutritional counselling (low-fat and high-fibre diet) plus probiotics (LGG and Bb12; 2.0×10^{10} CFU/day) or counselling plus placebo. Interventions lasted until the end of exclusive breastfeeding for up to 6 months. At 6 months postpartum, the risk of central adiposity (defined as waist circumference 80 cm or more) was lowered in women in the diet/probiotics group compared with the control/placebo group (OR 0.30, 95% CI 0.11–0.85; $P = 0.023$ adjusted for baseline body mass index), while the diet/placebo group did not differ from the controls (OR 1.00, 95% CI 0.38–2.68; $P = 0.994$). The number needed to treat with diet/probiotics to prevent one woman from developing a waist circumference of 80 cm or more was four (Ilmonen et al 2011). At 12 months postpartum, central obesity occurred in 25% of diet/probiotic subjects versus 43% in the diet/placebo group. The proportion of body fat was also 3.5% lower in the diet/probiotic group ($P = 0.018$) (Laitinen et al 2009).

Urogenital infections

Probiotics are widely used in the treatment and prevention of urogenital infections. They can be administered both orally and locally, with several trials supporting their use. There are additional criteria needed for probiotic strains to be efficacious in urogenital applications. Strains must demonstrate the capacity to adhere to uroepithelial and vaginal cells, colonise the vagina, inhibit urogenital pathogen growth and/or attachment and ideally should produce hydrogen peroxide. Strains that will be administered orally must have sufficient tolerance to gastric acid and bile salts and the capacity to colonise the vagina after oral intake (Reid & Bruce 2001). Probiotic strains that do not exhibit these characteristics are unlikely to be therapeutic for urogenital applications.

The mechanisms by which some *Lactobacillus* strains reduce bacterial vaginosis, vaginal candidiasis and urinary tract infectionss appear to involve a combination of antiadhesion factors, byproducts such as hydrogen peroxide, bacteriocins and lactic acid, and destruction of urogenital pathogen biofilms, as well as immune modulation or modification of vaginal epithelial cell cytokine production (Kohler et al 2012, Korshunov et al 1999, McMillan et al 2011, Wagner & Johnson 2012).

Bacterial vaginosis

Bacterial vaginosis is the most prevalent vaginal infection worldwide and is characterised by an altered vaginal ecosystem — specifically depletion of the indigenous lactobacilli. Administration of exogenous lactobacilli strains has thus been an area of research interest (Martinez et al 2009a).

A Cochrane systematic review conducted in 2009 included four randomised controlled trials that examined probiotic agents in the treatment of bacterial vaginosis. Analysis suggested that probiotics were effective in enhancing microbiological cure rates, with the oral metronidazole/probiotic (*Lactobacillus rhamnosus* GR-1 and *L. reuteri* RC-14) regimen (OR 0.09; 95% CI 0.03–0.26) and the probiotic (unspecified strain of *Lactobacillus acidophilus*)/oestriol preparation (OR 0.02; 95% CI 0.00–0.47) showing effectiveness. The authors cautioned, however, that larger well-designed trials were needed before any firm conclusions could be made (Senok et al 2009). Research on specific strains that have demonstrated efficacy is highlighted below.

P

A randomised, controlled, open-label trial evaluated the efficacy of a probiotic combination (*Lactobacillus rhamnosus* GR-1 and *L. reuteri* RC-14; 2×10^9 CFU/day) in women with bacterial vaginosis. Women received either metronidazole gel or the probiotic preparation. Both preparations were applied intravaginally for 5 days. Application of probiotics resulted in a 90% cure rate by day 30. Follow-up at day 6, 15 and 30 showed cure of bacterial vaginosis in significantly more probiotic-treated subjects (16, 17 and 18/20, respectively) compared to metronidazole gel treatment (9, 9 and 11/20, respectively; $P = 0.016$ at day 6, $P = 0.002$ at day 15 and $P = 0.056$ at day 30) (Anukam et al 2006).

In a randomised, double-blind, placebo-controlled trial, 64 women diagnosed with bacterial vaginosis were randomly assigned to receive a single dose of tinidazole supplemented with either two placebo capsules or two capsules containing *Lactobacillus rhamnosus* GR-1 and *L. reuteri* RC-14 (2×10^9 CFU/day) taken orally every morning for the following 4 weeks. At the end of the trial, subjects in the probiotic group had a higher rate of bacterial vaginosis cure (88% vs 50%; $P = 0.001$). Vaginal flora normalised in 75% of probiotic-treated subjects compared to only 34% of controls ($P = 0.011$) (Martinez et al 2009a).

A more recent randomised, double-blind, placebo-controlled trial evaluated the efficacy of probiotics in isolation on bacterial vaginosis. Women diagnosed with bacterial vaginosis ($n = 544$) were randomly assigned to receive either oral placebo or probiotic therapy (*Lactobacillus rhamnosus* GR-1 and *L. reuteri* RC-14; $\sim 1 \times 10^9$ CFU/day) for 6 weeks. Restitution of a balanced vaginal ecosystem was reported in 27% of subjects in the placebo group compared to 62% in the probiotic group ($P < 0.001$). After an additional 6 weeks of follow-up, a normal vaginal ecosystem was still present in more than half (51%) of subjects in the probiotic group, but only in around one-fifth (21%) of subjects who were taking placebo ($P < 0.001$) (Vujic et al 2013).

A randomised, double-blind, placebo-controlled trial investigating the potential role of probiotics in the prevention and cure of bacterial vaginosis in women with HIV ($n = 65$) found 6 months' daily treatment with a probiotic preparation (*Lactobacillus rhamnosus* GR-1 and *Lactobacillus reuteri* RC-14; 2×10^9 CFU/day) to be ineffective in enhancing bacterial vaginosis cure rates in this population. Nor was there a difference in recurrence rates of bacterial vaginosis between the probiotics and the placebo groups. There was, however, a trend for a higher prevalence of normal vaginal flora in the probiotic group (53% normalised vs 25%; $P = 0.08$) (Hummelen et al 2010).

The strains to use in the prevention and treatment of bacterial vaginosis appear to be *Lactobacillus rhamnosus* GR-1 and *L. reuteri* RC-14.

Urinary tract infections

Grin et al (2013) performed this systematic review and meta-analysis to review the data on the potential effectiveness of lactobacilli in the prevention of recurrent urinary tract infections in women. Five randomised, controlled trials were included in the analysis. Combining the data from all the trials (294 patients) found no preventive effect of lactobacilli supplementation (RR = 0.85, 95% CI 0.58–1.25; $P = 0.41$). However, a sensitivity analysis was performed, excluding studies using ineffective strains and studies testing for safety only. Data from 127 patients in two trials were included. A statistically significant decrease in recurrent urinary tract infections was found in patients given lactobacilli, denoted by the pooled risk ratio of 0.51 (95% CI 0.26–0.99; $P = 0.05$) (Grin et al 2013).

A significant reduction in urinary tract infection recurrence rate was reported in a randomised, double-blind study involving 55 premenopausal women (Reid 2001). The study investigated the effectiveness of treatment for 1 year with a weekly suppository containing either 0.5 g *L. rhamnosus* GR-1 and *L. fermentum* B-54 or a *Lactobacillus* growth factor (skim milk). Treatment resulted in the urinary tract infection rate decreasing by 73% and 79%, respectively, with no adverse effects reported.

A recent, randomised, double-blind, non-inferiority trial compared the efficacy of 12 months of prophylaxis with antibiotics (trimethoprim-sulfamethoxazole; 480 mg/day) or oral probiotics (2×10^9 CFU/day of *Lactobacillus rhamnosus* GR-1 and *L. reuteri* RC-14) in the prevention of urinary tract infections in postmenopausal women with recurrent cystitis ($n = 252$). The number of symptomatic urinary tract infections over the 12-month treatment period was 2.9 in the antibiotic group and 3.3 in the lactobacilli group — a between-treatment difference of 0.4 episodes (95% CI −0.4 to 1.5) or 13.8%. In the year preceding the trial, the subjects experienced a mean of 6.9 urinary tract infections. The percentage of patients with at least one urinary tract infection at 12 months was 69.3% in the trimethoprim-sulfamethoxazole group and 79.1% in the lactobacilli group. The median times to first recurrence were 6 and 3 months, respectively. After 12 months of trimethoprim-sulfamethoxazole prophylaxis, all urinary *E. coli* isolates of asymptomatic women were resistant to trimethoprim-sulfamethoxazole and trimethoprim. Probiotic use, however, was not associated with increased antibiotic resistance. The authors stated that this lactobacilli combination may be an acceptable alternative for the prevention of urinary tract infections, especially in women who dislike taking antibiotics (Beerepoot et al 2012). While probiotic therapy appeared slightly less effective than antibiotic prophylaxis in postmenopausal women with recurrent urinary tract infections, their use does not damage the GIT ecosystem, nor create antibiotic-resistant organisms, and for these reasons, some have argued that this probiotic combination has a role to play in the prevention of recurrent urinary tract infections (Trautner & Gupta 2012).

The probiotic combination of *Lactobacillus rhamnosus* GR-1 and *L. reuteri* RC-14 appears to have the greatest evidence supporting its use in the prevention of urinary tract infections.

P

Vaginal candidiasis

Lactobacilli can impair the growth of *Candida albicans* via the production of lactic acid, which creates a low-pH environment, resulting in suppressed fungal growth. Cocultures of specific lactobacilli strains with *C. albicans* revealed that *C. albicans* cells lost metabolic activity and eventually died. Transcriptome analyses showed increased expression of stress-related genes and lower expression of genes involved in antifungal resistance (Kohler et al 2012).

A systematic review examining the role of lactobacilli probiotics in the treatment and prevention of vulvovaginal candidiasis (and other urogenital infections) was conducted by Abad and Safdar in 2009. Only four studies were found that evaluated lactobacilli supplementation in vulvovaginal candidiasis — two assessed preventive effects and two treatment effects. Only one prospective crossover trial found a significant benefit of probiotic therapy for the prevention of vulvovaginal candidiasis (RR 0.39; 95% CI 0.17–0.70). The authors concluded that there were insufficient data to make definitive conclusions at this point in time (Abad & Safdar 2009).

Some probiotic preparations have been shown to be ineffective in the treatment of vulvovaginal candidiasis — Lactobac (unspecified strains of *Lactobacillus rhamnosus* and *Bifidobacterium longum*) and Femilac (unspecified strains of *L. rhamnosus, L. delbrueckii* ssp. *bulgaricus, L. acidophilus* and *Streptococcus thermophilus*) (Pirotta et al 2004). Probiotic preparations that have shown efficacy in the treatment of vulvovaginal candidiasis are detailed in Table 9, although it should be highlighted that most of these trials were small in size.

TABLE 9 PROBIOTICS IN THE TREATMENT OF VULVOVAGINAL CANDIDIASIS (VC)

Trial methodology	Strain(s) utilised	Results
R, DB, PC *n* = 27 women with a history of recurrent VC	*Lactobacillus acidophilus* NAS as a vaginal suppository in isolation or with *L. acidophilus* NAS strain; *Bifidobacterium bifidum* Malyoth strain, and *Lactobacillus bulgaricus* LB-51 strain taken orally	In women who used the *L. acidophilus* NAS vaginal suppository, the incidence of recurrent VC was significantly reduced compared to controls (*P* = 0.005). Subjects who took both the suppository and the oral probiotic supplement also had a significant reduction in the number of infections compared to controls (*P* = 0.011). There was, however, no extra benefit seen from taking the oral probiotic preparation (Metts et al 2003)
R, DB, PC *n* = 55 women with VC	*Lactobacillus rhamnosus* GR-1 and *Lactobacillus reuteri* RC-14	After a single dose of fluconazole and 4 weeks' oral treatment with either probiotic or placebo, subjects in the probiotic group had reduced *Candida* colonisation (10% vs 39%; *P* = 0.014) and decreased vaginal discharge (10% vs 35%; *P* = 0.03) (Martinez et al 2009b)
R, PC, CO *n* = 33 women with a history of recurrent VC	*Lactobacillus acidophilus* LA5	The mean number of infections per 6 months decreased while in the probiotic phase compared to control phase of trial (0.38 vs 2.54; *P* = 0.001). The incidence of *Candida* colonisation also decreased during probiotic treatment (0.84 vs 3.23 per 6 months; *P* = 0.001) (Hilton et al 1992)
OL *n* = 28 women with a history of recurrent VC	*Lactobacillus rhamnosus* GG (LGG)	Twice-daily intravaginal application of LGG resulted in decreased symptoms of vulvovaginal candidiasis, as well as less erythema and discharge; 4/5 women who were positive for *Candida* at baseline had negative cultures at the end of 7 days (Hilton et al 1995)

R, randomised; DB, double-blind; PC, placebo-controlled; CO, crossover; OL, open-label.

OTHER USES

Probiotics may have many potentially important clinical applications, and current areas of active research include mostly animal studies investigating a range of diseases, including control or prevention of cancer (Fotiadis et al 2008) and prevention or treatment of graft-versus-host disease in transplant recipients (Gerbitz et al 2004).

DOSAGE RANGE

Probiotic doses are usually standardised in terms of the amount of living bacteria per unit of volume. Each living bacterium is referred to as a colony-forming unit or CFU.

The minimum concentration of probiotic bacteria needed to achieve therapeutic effects appears to be somewhat strain-dependent, in that, for some strains (e.g. *L. reuteri* MM53), 10^7 bacteria is a sufficient quantity to produce beneficial effects (Shornikova et al 1997), while for other strains, 10^9 viable bacteria is needed (e.g. *L. rhamnosus* GG) (Saxelin 1996). This situation, unfortunately, makes it hard to give firm dosage recommendations, as the minimum effective dosage appears to differ by strain. Thus it is best practice to ensure that supplements contain bacteria in concentrations $>10^9$ bacteria/dose, unless research has demonstrated that the specific strain contained in the supplement is effective in smaller amounts.

If a product contains multiple strains, then each strain should be present at levels of $\geq 10^9$ to ensure effectiveness. The viable bacteria are typically mixed in a suitable matrix, which may contain maltodextrin, cellulose, and small amounts of prebiotics, such as fructooligosaccharides and inulin.

Supplements are best taken with meals to enhance bacterial survival.

A serving of yoghurt containing fewer than 10^8 viable bacteria is unlikely to have any therapeutic activity beyond acting as a nutritional source.

ADVERSE REACTIONS

Probiotics are generally regarded as safe. However, probiotic therapy should be used with caution in the immunocompromised, as they may be at increased risk of adverse reactions. Infections, sepsis and meningitis have been reported in adult cases when administered lactobacilli (Land et al 2005, Mackay et al 1999, Rautio et al 1999). Cases of young children and infants have also been reported (Borriello et al 2003). Opportunistic pathogenicity is, however, considered low (Shanahan 2012).

There have been a number of cases of fungaemia reported in the literature from the oral administration of *Saccharomyces cerevisiae* var. *boulardii* (aka *S. boulardii*). These have occurred almost exclusively in immunocompromised or critically ill individuals, in particular those with intravascular catheters. Thus administration of strains of *S. cerevisiae* var. *boulardii* may best be limited to immunocompetent individuals — i.e. those with well-functioning immune systems (Enache-Angoulvant & Hennequin 2005, Lherm et al 2002, Riquelme et al 2003). Additionally, in hospitalised patients with a central venous catheter, supplementation with a strain of *S. cerevisiae* var. *boulardii* should be avoided to prevent inadvertent catheter contamination (Venugopalan et al 2010).

There is also concern in critically ill patients because impaired intestinal barrier function could result in infection as a result of bacterial translocation (Land et al 2005, Munoz et al 2005). Recently, there has been one report citing increased mortality in patients with severe acute pancreatitis who were administered a novel multispecies probiotic (Besselink et al 2008).

P

Practice points/Patient counselling

- Some probiotics may improve the long-term bowel flora; however, the benefits of probiotics extends well beyond this role.
- Studies have shown that probiotics are beneficial in the treatment of digestive disorders such as diarrhoea and some inflammatory bowel diseases and also other conditions, such as urogenital infections, antibiotic-induced and TD,

IBS, ulcerative colitis, food allergies, eczema and the prevention and treatment of paediatric atopic dermatitis.

- It is vital to note that, just because one strain of bacteria in a given species has a proven action or characteristic, it does not mean that another strain will too, even if they are closely related. Strains within the same species can have significantly different actions, properties and characteristics, as these are all essentially strain-specific qualities.
- Probiotics can be administered orally or intravaginally. They can also be taken as yoghurt or other cultured dairy products. It should be noted that only products containing actual probiotic strains will be beneficial. The so-called starter cultures (strains of *Lactobacillus delbrueckii* ssp. *bulgaricus* and *Streptococcus thermophilus*) have limited beneficial effects.
- For traveller's diarrhoea prevention, , it is recommended that the probiotic dose be started some days before travelling to ensure that the beneficial bacteria have colonised the gut; the dosage may vary depending on the probiotic strain.

SIGNIFICANT INTERACTIONS

Antibiotics

Concomitant administration of some strains of probiotics reduces gastrointestinal and genitourinary side effects according to clinical studies — combination can be safely used together and a beneficial interaction is likely.

CONTRAINDICATIONS AND PRECAUTIONS

Specific strains of probiotics are appropriate for different disorders. Probiotics are contraindicated in those people who are hypersensitive to any component of the probiotics-containing product. Strains of *Saccharomyces cerevisiae* var. *boulardii* may best be avoided in immunocompromised individuals

PREGNANCY USE

Likely to be safe in pregnancy; however, it is best practice to utilise strains that have demonstrated excellent safety profiles in clinical trials conducted on pregnant women.

PATIENTS' FAQs

What can probiotics do for me?
Studies have shown that probiotics are beneficial in the treatment of digestive disorders such as diarrhoea and some inflammatory bowel diseases and also other conditions not directly connected with the digestive tract, such as vaginal thrush and recurrent cystitis, antibiotic-induced and TD, IBS, food allergies and eczema.

When will they start to work?
Usually, probiotics can exert beneficial effects in digestive disorders within days, although continuous use for several weeks/months may produce long-term benefits and be necessary in the treatment of other disorders.

Are there any safety issues?

Generally, probiotics have a good safety profile; however, supplements should be used under supervision in the immunocompromised.

REFERENCES

Abad, C. L. & Safdar, N. 2009. The role of lactobacillus probiotics in the treatment or prevention of urogenital infections — a systematic review. J Chemother, 21, 243–52.

Abrahamsson, T. R., et al. 2007. Probiotics in prevention of IgE-associated eczema: a double-blind, randomized, placebo-controlled trial. J Allergy Clin Immunol, 119, 1174–1180.

Academy of Breastfeeding Medicine 2008. ABM clinical protocol #4: mastitis. Revision, May 2008. Breastfeed Med, 3, 177–80.

Agerback M, et al. Hypocholesterolemic effect of a new fermented milk product in healthy middle-aged men. Eur J Clin Nutr 49 (1995): 346–352.

Agerholm-Larsen L et al. The effect of a probiotic milk product on plasma cholesterol: A meta-analysis of short-term intervention studies. Eur J Clin Nutr 54.11 (2000): 856–860.

Agrawal, A., et al. 2009. Clinical trial: the effects of a fermented milk product containing *Bifidobacterium lactis* DN-173010 on abdominal distension and gastrointestinal transit in irritable bowel syndrome with constipation. Aliment Pharmacol Ther, 29, 104–14.

Ahmed, M., et al. 2007. Impact of consumption of different levels of *Bifidobacterium lactis* HN019 on the intestinal microflora of elderly human subjects. Journal of Nutrition, Health & Aging, 11, 26–31.

Ahrne, S. & Hagslatt, M. L. 2011. Effect of lactobacilli on paracellular permeability in the gut. Nutrients, 3, 104–17.

Ait-Belgnaoui, A., et al. 2006. *Lactobacillus farciminis* treatment suppresses stress induced visceral hypersensitivity: a possible action through interaction with epithelial cell cytoskeleton contraction. Gut, 55, 1090–4.

Akyol S et al. The effect of antibiotic and probiotic combination therapy on secondary pancreatic infections and oxidative stress parameters in experimental acute necrotizing pancreatitis. Pancreas 26.4 (2003): 363–367.

Anukam, K. C., et al. 2006. Clinical study comparing probiotic *Lactobacillus* GR-1 and RC-14 with metronidazole vaginal gel to treat symptomatic bacterial vaginosis. Microbes & Infection, 8, 2772–2776.

Anukam KC et al. Yogurt containing probiotic *Lactobacillus rhamnosus* GR-1 and *L. reuteri* RC-14 helps resolve moderate diarrhoea and increases CD4 count in HIV/AIDS patients. J Clin Gastroenterol 42.3 (2008): 239–243.

Ardley, C. & Wright, S. 2010. Travellers' diarrhoea. Medicine, 38, 26–29.

Arroyo, R., et al. 2010. Treatment of infectious mastitis during lactation: antibiotics versus oral administration of Lactobacilli isolated from breast milk. Clin Infect Dis, 50, 1551–8.

Arvola, T., et al. 1999. Prophylactic *Lactobacillus* GG reduces antibiotic-associated diarrhea in children with respiratory infections: a randomized study. Pediatrics, 104, 1–4.

Bajaj JS et al. Probiotic yogurt for the treatment of minimal hepatic encephalopathy. Am J Gastroenterol 103.7 (2008): 1707–1715.

Beerepoot, M. A., et al. 2012. Lactobacilli vs antibiotics to prevent urinary tract infections: a randomized, double-blind, noninferiority trial in postmenopausal women. Arch Intern Med, 172, 704–12.

Bengmark S. Ecological control of the gastrointestinal tract: the role of probiotic flora. Gut 42 (1998): 2–7.

Benno, Y., et al. 1996. Effects of *Lactobacillus* GG yoghurt on human intestinal microecology in Japanese subjects. Nutrition Today, 31, 9S–12S.

Bertolami MC, et al. Evaluation of the effects of a new fermented milk product (Gaio) on primary hypercholesterolemia. Eur J Clin Nutr 53 (1999): 97–101.

Besselink MG et al. Probiotic prophylaxis in predicted severe acute pancreatitis: a randomized, double-blind, placebo-controlled trial. Lancet 371 (2008): 651–659.

Black, F., et al. 1989. Prophylactic efficacy of Lactobacilli on travellers' diarrhea. Travel Med, 7, 333–335.

Borriello SP et al. Safety of probiotics that contain Lactobacilli or Bifidobacteria. Clin Infect Dis 36 (2003): 775–780.

Bougle, D., et al. 1999. Effect of propionibacteria supplementation on fecal bifidobacteria and segmental colonic transit time in healthy human subjects. Scand J Gastroenterol, 34, 144–8.

Bourreille, A., et al. 2013. *Saccharomyces boulardii* does not prevent relapse of Crohn's disease. Clinical Gastroenterology and Hepatology 11.8 982–987.

Boyle, R. J., et al. 2011. Lactobacillus GG treatment during pregnancy for the prevention of eczema: a randomized controlled trial. Allergy, 66, 509–516.

Brashears MM, et al. Bile salt deconjugation and cholesterol removal from media by *Lactobacillus casei*. J Dairy Sci 81 (1998): 2103–2110.

Buts, J. P., et al. 1986. Response of human and rat small intestinal mucosa to oral administration of *Saccharomyces boulardii*. Pediatr Res, 20, 192–6.

Buts, J. P., et al. 1994. *Saccharomyces boulardii* enhances rat intestinal enzyme expression by endoluminal release of polyamines. Pediatric Research, 36, 522–527.

Caballero-Franco, C., et al. 2007. The VSL#3 probiotic formula induces mucin gene expression and secretion in colonic epithelial cells. American Journal of Physiology — Gastrointestinal and Liver Physiology, 292, G315–G322.

Camilleri M. Probiotics and irritable bowel syndrome: rationale, putative mechanisms, and evidence of clinical efficacy. J Clin Gastroenterol 40.3 (2006): 264–269.

Campieri M et al. Combination of antibiotic and probiotic treatment is efficacious in prophylaxis of post-operative recurrence of Crohn's disease: A randomized controlled study vs mesalamine. Gastroenterology 118 (2000): G4179.

P

Castagliuolo, I., et al. 1999. *Saccharomyces boulardii* protease inhibits the effects of *Clostridium difficile* toxins A and B in human colonic mucosa. Infect Immun, 67, 302–7.

Cheigh, H. S., et al. 1994. Biochemical, microbiological, and nutritional aspects of kimchi (Korean fermented vegetable products). Critical Reviews in Food Science and Nutrition, 34, 175–203.

Corr, S. C., et al. 2009. Understanding the mechanisms by which probiotics inhibit gastrointestinal pathogens. Adv Food Nutr Res, 56, 1–15.

Cox, A. J., et al. Oral administration of the probiotic *Lactobacillus fermentum* VRI-003 and mucosal immunity in endurance athletes. Br J Sports Med, 14 (2010): 222–226.

D'Argenio, G. & Mazzacca, G. 1999. Short-chain fatty acid in the human colon. *In:* Zappia, V., et al. (eds.) Advances in Nutrition and Cancer, vol. 2. Springer US.

Dedicatoria RF, et al. The fermentation inoculation with lactic acid bacteria to increase the nutritive value of sauerkraut. Kalikasan 10 (1981): 214–2119.

De Dios Pozo-Olano, J., et al. 1978. Effect of a lactobacilli preparation on traveler's diarrhea. A randomized, double blind clinical trial. Gastroenterology, 74, 829–30.

Dendukuri N et al. Probiotic therapy for the prevention and treatment of *Clostridium difficile*-associated diarrhoea: a systematic review. CMAJ 173.2 (2005): 167–170.

de Roos NM, et al. Yoghurt enriched with *Lactobacillus acidophilus* does not lower blood lipids in healthy men and women with normal to borderline high serum cholesterol levels. Eur J Clin Nutr 53 (1999): 277–280.

Dotterud, C. K., et al. 2010. Probiotics in pregnant women to prevent allergic disease: a randomized, double-blind trial. Br J Dermatol, 163, 616–23.

Drouault-Holowacz S et al. A double blind randomized controlled trial of a probiotic combination in 100 patients with irritable bowel syndrome. Gastroenterol Clin Biol 32.2 (2008): 147–152.

Dubey, A. P., et al. 2008. Use of VSL#3 in the treatment of rotavirus diarrhea in children. J Clin Gastroenterol, 42, S126–S129.

Ducrotte, P., et al. 2012. Clinical trial: *Lactobacillus plantarum* 299v (DSM 9843) improves symptoms of irritable bowel syndrome. World J Gastroenterol, 18, 4012–8.

Enache-Angoulvant A, Hennequin C. Invasive *Saccharomyces* infection: a comprehensive review. Clin Infect Dis 41.11 (2005): 1559–1568.

Fang SB et al. Dose-dependent effect of *Lactobacillus* GG on quantitative reduction of faecal rotavirus shedding in children. J Trop Pediatr 55.5 (2009): 297–301.

FAO/WHO (Food and Agriculture Organization and World Health Organization). Expert consultation on evaluation of health and nutritional properties of probiotics in food including powder milk with live lactic acid bacteria. WHO: Geneva, 2001. Available online from www.who.int/foodsafety/publications/fs_management/en/probiotics.pdf (accessed September 2009).

Fotiadis CI et al. Role of probiotics, prebiotics and synbiotics in chemoprevention for colorectal cancer. World J Gastroenterol 14.42 (2008): 6453–6457.

Fric P, Zavoral M. The effect of non-pathogenic *Escherichia coli* in symptomatic uncomplicated diverticular disease of the colon. Eur J Gastroenterol Hepatol 15 (2003): 313–3115.

Fuller, R. & Gibson, G. R. 1997. Modification of the intestinal microflora using probiotics and prebiotics. Scandinavian Journal of Gastroenterology, 32(suppl 222), 28–31.

Garrote GL, et al. Chemical and microbiological characterisation of kefir grains. J Dairy Res 68 (2001): 639–652.

Gerbitz A, et al. Probiotic effects on experimental graft-versus-host disease: let them eat yogurt. Blood 103 (2004): 4365–4367.

Gibson GR, Roberfroid MB. Dietary modulation of the human colonic microbiota: introducing the concept of prebiotics. J Nutr 125.6 (1995): 1401–1412.

Gionchetti P, et al. Oral bacteriotherapy as maintenance treatment in patients with chronic pouchitis: a double-blind, placebo-controlled trial. Gastroenterology 119.2 (2000): 305–309.

Gionchetti P, et al. Prophylaxis of pouchitis onset with probiotic therapy: a double-blind, placebo-controlled trial. Gastroenterology 124.5 (2003): 1202–1209.

Goh J, O'Morain CA. Review article: nutrition and adult inflammatory bowel disease. Aliment Pharmacol Ther 17.3 (2003): 307–320.

Goldin, B. R. 1998. Health benefits of probiotics. British Journal of Nutrition, 80(suppl 2), S203–S207.

Gosselink, M. P., et al. 2005. Delay of the first onset of pouchitis by oral intake of the probiotic strain *Lactobacillus rhamnosus* GG. Diseases of the Colon & Rectum, 47, 876–884.

Greany KA et al. Probiotic consumption does not enhance the cholesterol-lowering effect of soy in postmenopausal women. J Nutr 134 (2004): 3277–3283.

Greany KA et al. Probiotic capsules do not lower plasma lipids in young women and men. Eur J Clin Nutr 62.2 (2008): 232–237.

Grin, P. M., et al. 2013. Lactobacillus for preventing recurrent urinary tract infections in women: meta-analysis. Can J Urol, 20, 6607–14.

Guarner, F., et al. 2011. Probiotics and prebiotics. World Gastroenterology Organisation Global Guideline 46.6 (2012); 468–481.

Guillot, C. C., et al. 1995. Effects of *Saccharomyces boulardii* in children with chronic diarrnea, especially cases due to giardiasis. Rev Mex de Puercultura y Pediatria, 2, 1–5.

Gupta P et al. Is lactobacillus GG helpful in children with Crohn's disease? Results of a preliminary, open-label study. J Pediatr Gastroenterol Nutr 31 (2000): 453–457.

Guslandi M. Of germs in inflammatory bowel disease and of how to fight them. J Gastroenterol Hepatol 18.1 (2003a): 115–16.

Guslandi M. Probiotics for chronic intestinal disorders. Am J Gastroenterol 98.3 (2003b): 520–1.

Guslandi M et al. *Saccharomyces boulardii* in maintenance treatment of Crohn's disease. Dig Dis Sci 45 (2000): 1462–1464.

Hasslof, P., et al. 2010. Growth inhibition of oral mutans streptococci and candida by commercial probiotic lactobacilli — an in vitro study. BMC Oral Health, 10, 18.

Hatakka, K., et al. 2001. Effect of long-term consumption of probiotic milk on infections in children attending day care centres: double-blind, randomised trial. British Medical Journal, 322, 1327.

Hatakka K et al. *Lactobacillus rhamnosus* LC705 together with *Propionibacterium freudenreichii* ssp *shermanii* JS administered in capsules is ineffective in lowering serum lipids. J Am Coll Nutr 27.4 (2008): 441–447.

Hawrelak, J. A. & Myers, S. P. 2004. Intestinal dysbiosis: A review of the literature. Alternative Medicine Review, 9, 180–197.

Hedin C, et al. Evidence for the use of probiotics and prebiotics in inflammatory bowel disease: a review of clinical trials. Proc Nutr Soc 66.3 (2007): 307–315.

Hempel, S., et al. 2012. Probiotics for the prevention and treatment of antibiotic-associated diarrhea: a systematic review and meta-analysis. JAMA, 307, 1959–69.

Henker, J., et al. 2008. Probiotic *Escherichia coli* Nissle 1917 (EcN) for successful remission maintenance of ulcerative colitis in children and adolescents: an open-label pilot study. Z Gastroenterol, 46, 874–875.

Hill MJ. Intestinal flora and endogenous vitamin synthesis. Eur J Cancer Prev 6 (1997): S43–S45.

Hilton E et al. Ingestion of yogurt containing *Lactobacillus acidophilus* as prophylaxis for candidal vaginitis. Ann Intern Med 116.5 (1992): 353–357.

Hilton, E., et al. 1995. Lactobacillus GG vaginal suppositories and vaginitis. Journal of Clinical Microbiology, 33, 1433.

Hilton, E., et al. 1997. Efficacy of Lactobacillus GG as a diarrheal preventive in travelers. Journal of Travel Medicine, 4, 41–43.

Hirayama K, Rafter J. The role of lactic acid bacteria in colon cancer prevention: mechanistic considerations. Antonie Van Leeuwenhoek 76.1–4 (1999): 391–394.

Hlivak P et al. One-year application of probiotic strain *Enterococcus faecium* M-74 decreases serum cholesterol levels. Bratisl Lek Listy 106 (2005): 67–72.

Hojsak, I., et al. 2009. Lactobacillus GG in the prevention of gastrointestinal and respiratory tract infections in children who attend day care centers: A randomized, double-blind, placebo-controlled trial. Clin Nutr, 125.5 (2010); 171–177.

Horvath, A., et al. 2011. Meta-analysis: *Lactobacillus rhamnosus* GG for abdominal pain-related functional gastrointestinal disorders in childhood. Aliment Pharmacol Ther, 33, 1302–10.

Hoveyda N et al. A systematic review and meta-analysis: probiotics in the treatment of irritable bowel syndrome. BMC Gastroenterol Feb 16.9 (2009): 15.

Hummelen, R., et al. 2010. *Lactobacillus rhamnosus* GR-1 and L. reuteri RC-14 to prevent or cure bacterial vaginosis among women with HIV. International Journal of Gynecology & Obstetrics, 111, 245–248.

Ilmonen, J., et al. 2011. Impact of dietary counselling and probiotic intervention on maternal anthropometric measurements during and after pregnancy: A randomized placebo-controlled trial. Clinical Nutrition, 30, 156–164.

Imaoka, A., et al. 2008. Anti-inflammatory activity of probiotic *Bifidobacterium*: enhancement of IL-10 production in peripheral blood mononuclear cells from ulcerative colitis patients and inhibition of IL-8 secretion in HT-29 cells. World J Gastroenterol, 14, 2511–6.

Ishikawa, H., et al. 2005. Randomized trial of dietary fiber and *Lactobacillus casei* administration for prevention of colorectal tumors. International Journal of Cancer, 116, 762–767.

Isolauri, E. 2012. Development of healthy gut microbiota early in life. Journal of Paediatrics and Child Health, 48, 1–6.

Jijon H et al. DNA from probiotic bacteria modulates murine and human epithelial and immune function. Gastroenterology 126 (2004): 1358–1373.

Jimenez, E., et al. 2008. Oral administration of *Lactobacillus* strains isolated from breast milk as an alternative for the treatment of infectious mastitis during lactation. Appl Environ Microbiol, 74, 4650–4655.

Johnson, A. C., et al. 2011. Effects of *Bifidobacterium infantis* 35624 on post-inflammatory visceral hypersensitivity in the rat. Dig Dis Sci, 56, 3179–86.

Johnston, B. C., et al. 2011. Probiotics for the prevention of pediatric antibiotic-associated diarrhea. Cochrane Database Syst Rev, CD004827.

Jonkers, D., et al. 2012. Probiotics in the management of inflammatory bowel disease: a systematic review of intervention studies in adult patients. Drugs, 72, 803–23.

Kailasapathy K, Chin J. Survival and therapeutic potential of probiotic organisms with reference to *Lactobacillus acidophilus* and *Bifidobacterium* spp. Immunol Cell Biol 78.1 (2000): 80–88.

Kajander K et al. Clinical trial: multispecies probiotic supplementation alleviates the symptoms of irritable bowel syndrome and stabilizes intestinal microbiota. Aliment Pharmacol Ther 27.1 (2008): 48–57.

Kalliomaki, M., et al. 2001. Probiotics in primary prevention of atopic disease: a randomised, placebo-controlled trial. Lancet, 357, 1076–1079.

Kalliomaki M et al. Probiotics and prevention of atopic disease: 4-year follow-up of a randomised placebo-controlled trial. Lancet 361.9372 (2003): 1869–1871.

Kalliomaki, M., et al. 2007. Probiotics during the first 7 years of life: A cumulative risk reduction of eczema in a randomized, placebo-controlled trial. J Allergy Clin Immunol, 119, 1019–1021.

Kanauchi O et al. Modification of intestinal flora in the treatment of inflammatory bowel disease. Curr Pharm Des 9.4 (2003): 333–346.

Karthik SV. Probiotics in inflammatory bowel disease. J R Soc Med 96.7 (2003): 370.

Katelaris, P. H. & Salam, I. 1995. Lactobacilli to prevent traveler's diarrhea. New England Journal of Medicine, 333, 1360–1361.

Kaur IP, et al. Probiotics: potential pharmaceutical applications. Eur J Pharm Sci 15.1 (2002): 1–9.

Kim, H. J., et al. 2005. A randomized controlled trial of a probiotic combination VSL#3 and placebo in irritable bowel syndrome with bloating. Neurogastroenterolgy and Motility, 17, 1–10.

Kirjavainen PV, et al. Probiotic bacteria in the management of atopic disease: underscoring the importance of viability. J Pediatr Gastroenterol Nutr 36.2 (2003): 223–227.

Kirpich IA et al. Probiotics restore bowel flora and improve liver enzymes in human alcohol-induced liver injury: a pilot study. Alcohol 42.8 (2008): 675–682.

Klarin, B., et al. 2008. *Lactobacillus plantarum* 299v reduces colonisation of *Clostridium difficile* in critically ill patients treated with antibiotics. Acta Anaesthesiol Scand, 52, 1096–1102.

Koebnick, C., et al. 2003. Probiotic beverage containing *Lactobacillus casei* Shirota improves gastrointestinal symptoms in patients with chronic constipation. Canadian Journal of Gastroenterology, 17, 655–659.

Kohler, G. A., et al. 2012. Probiotic interference of *Lactobacillus rhamnosus* GR-1 and *Lactobacillus reuteri* RC-14 with the opportunistic fungal pathogen *Candida albicans*. Infect Dis Obstet Gynecol, 2012, 636474.

Kollaritsch, H., et al. 1989. Prevention of traveller's diarrhea: comparison of different nonantibiotic preparations. Travel Med Int, 9–17.

Kollaritsch H et al. [Prevention of traveler's diarrhea with *Saccharomyces boulardii*: Results of a placebo controlled double-blind study.] Fortschr Med 111.9 (1993): 152–156.

Kontiokari, T., et al. 2001. Randomised trial of cranberry-lingonberry juice and *Lactobacillus* GG drink for the prevention of urinary tract infections in women. British Medical Journal, 322, 1571.

Kopp, M. V., et al. 2008. Randomized, double-blind, placebo-controlled trial of probiotics for primary prevention: no clinical effects of Lactobacillus GG supplementation. Pediatrics, 121, e850–e856.

Korshunov VM et al. The vaginal *Bifidobacterium* flora in women of reproductive age. Zh Mikrobiol Epidemiol Immunobiol 4 (1999): 74–78.

Kruis, W., et al. 1997. Double-blind comparison of an oral *Escherichia coli* preparation and mesalazine in maintaining remission of ulcerative colitis. Aliment Pharmacol Ther, 11, 853–8.

Kruis, W., et al. 2004. Maintaining remission of ulcerative colitis with the probiotic *Escherichia coli* Nissle 1917 is as effective as with standard mesalazine. Gut, 53, 1617–1623.

Laake KO et al. Outcome of four weeks' intervention with probiotics on symptoms and endoscopic appearance after surgical reconstruction with a J-configurated ileal-pouch-anal-anastomosis in ulcerative colitis. Scandinavian J Gastroenterol 40 (2005): 43–51.

Laitinen, K., et al. 2009. Dietary counselling and probiotic intervention initiated in early pregnancy modifies maternal adiposity over 12 months postpartum. Obesity Facts, 2 (suppl 2), 4.

Land MH et al. Lactobacillus sepsis associated with probiotic therapy. Pediatrics 115 (2005): 178–181.

Lankaputhra WE, Shah NP. Antimutagenic properties of probiotic bacteria and of organic acids. Mutat Res 397.2 (1998): 169–182.

Larsen CN et al. Dose-response study of probiotic bacteria *Bifidobacterium animalis* subsp *lactis* BB-12 and *Lactobacillus paracasei* subsp *paracasei* CRL-341 in healthy young adults. Eur J Clin Nutr 60 (2006): 1284–1293.

Lewis SJ, Burmeister S. A double-blind placebo-controlled study of the effects of *Lactobacillus acidophilus* on plasma lipids. Eur J Clin Nutr 59 (2005): 776–780.

Leyer, G. J., et al. 2009. Probiotic effects on cold and influenza-like symptom incidence and duration in children. Pediatrics, 124, e172–e179.

Lherm, T., et al. 2002. Seven cases of fungemia with *Saccharomyces boulardii* in critically ill patients. Intensive Care Medicine, 28, 797–801.

Ligaarden SC et al. A candidate probiotic with unfavourable effects in subjects with irritable bowel syndrome: a randomised controlled trial. BMC Gastroenterology 2010, 10:16

Link-Amster, H., et al. 1994. Modulation of a specific humoral immune response and changes in intestinal flora mediated through fermented milk intake. FEMS Immunology and Medical Microbiology, 10, 55–64.

Lionetti, E., et al. 2006. *Lactobacillus reuteri* therapy to reduce side-effects during anti-*Helicobacter pylori* treatment in children: a randomized placebo controlled trial. Aliment Pharmacol Ther, 24, 1461–1468.

Liong MT, Shah NP. Acid and bile tolerance and cholesterol removal ability of lactobacilli strains. J Dairy Sci 88 (2005): 55–66.

Lirussi, F., et al. 2007. Probiotics for non-alcoholic fatty liver disease and/or steatohepatitis. Cochrane Database Syst Rev, CD005165.

Lonnermark, E., et al. 2010. Intake of *Lactobacillus plantarum* reduces certain gastrointestinal symptoms during treatment with antibiotics. J Clin Gastroenterol, 44, 106–112.

Macfarlane, G. T. & Cummings, J. H. 1999. Probiotics and prebiotics: can regulating the activities of the intestinal bacteria benefit health. British Medical Journal, 318, 999–1003.

Mack, D. R., et al. 1999. Probiotics inhibit enteropathogenic E. coli adherence in vitro by inducing intestinal mucin gene expression. American Journal of Physiology, 276, G941–G950.

Mack, D. R., et al. 2003. Extracellular MUC3 mucin secretion follows adherence of *Lactobacillus* strains to intestinal epithelial cells in vitro. Gut, 52, 827–833.

Mackay AD et al. Lactobacillus endocarditis caused by a probiotics organism. Clin Microbiol Infect 5 (1999): 290–292.

Maldonado, J., et al. 2012. Human milk probiotic *Lactobacillus fermentum* CECT5716 reduces the incidence of gastrointestinal and upper respiratory tract infections in infants. J Pediatr Gastroenterol Nutr, 54, 55–61.

Mangiante G et al. *Lactobacillus plantarum* reduces infection of pancreatic necrosis in experimental acute pancreatitis. Dig Surg 18 (2001): 47–50.

Manley, K. J., et al. 2007. Probiotic treatment of vancomycin-resistant enterococci: a randomised controlled trial. MJA, 186, 454–457.

Marotta, F., et al. 2003. Chemopreventive effect of a probiotic preparation on the development of preneoplastic and neoplastic colonic lesions: an experimental study. Hepatogastroenterology, 50, 1914–8.

Marteau, P. 2011. Evidence of probiotic strain specificity makes extrapolation of results impossible from a strain to another, even from the same species. Annals of Gastroenterology & Hepatology, 2, 34–36.

Marteau, P., et al. 2002. *Bifidobacterium animalis* strain DN-173010 shortens the colonic transit time in healthy women: a double-blind, randomized, controlled study. Alimentary Pharmacology & Therapeutics, 16, 587–593.

Marteau P, et al. Manipulation of the bacterial flora in inflammatory bowel disease. Best Pract Res Clin Gastroenterol 17.1 (2003): 47–61.

Martinez, R. C., et al. 2009a. Improved cure of bacterial vaginosis with single dose of tinidazole (2 g), *Lactobacillus rhamnosus* GR-1, and *Lactobacillus reuteri* RC-14: a randomized, double-blind, placebo-controlled trial. Can J Microbiol, 55, 133–138.

Martinez, R. C., et al. 2009b. Improved treatment of vulvovaginal candidiasis with fluconazole plus probiotic *Lactobacillus rhamnosus* GR-1 and *Lactobacillus reuteri* RC-14. Lett Appl Microbiol, 48, 269–274.

Matamoros, S., et al. 2013. Development of intestinal microbiota in infants and its impact on health. Trends in Microbiology, 21, 167–173.

Matthes, H., et al. 2010. Clinical trial: probiotic treatment of acute distal ulcerative colitis with rectally administered *Escherichia coli* Nissle 1917 (EcN). BMC Complement Altern Med, 10, 13.

Mattila-Sandholm, T. & Salminen, S. 1998. Up-to-date on probiotics in Europe. Gastroenterology International, 11(suppl), 8–16.

McFarland LV. Meta-analysis of probiotics for the prevention of antibiotic associated diarrhoea and the treatment of *Clostridium difficile* disease. Am J Gastroenterol 101 (2006): 812–822.

McFarland LV. Meta-analysis of probiotics for the prevention of traveller's diarrhoea. Travel Med Infect Dis 5.2 (2007): 97–105.

McFarland, L. V. & Bernasconi, P. 1993. *Saccharomyces boulardii*'. A review of an innovative biotherapeutic agent. Microbial Ecology in Health and Disease, 6, 157–171.

McFarland LV, Dublin S. Meta-analysis of probiotics for the treatment of irritable bowel syndrome. World J Gastroenterol 14 (2008): 2650–2661.

McFarland, L. V., et al. 1994. A randomized placebo-controlled trial of *Saccharomyces boulardii* in combination with standard antibiotics for *Clostridium difficile* disease. JAMA: The Journal of the American Medical Association, 271, 1913–1918.

McKane, L. & Kandel, J. 1986. Microbiology: Essentials and Applications, New York, McGraw-Hill.

McKernan, D. P., et al. 2010. The probiotic *Bifidobacterium infantis* 35624 displays visceral antinociceptive effects in the rat. Neurogastroenterol Motil, 22, 1029–35, e268.

McMillan, A., et al. 2011. Disruption of urogenital biofilms by lactobacilli. Colloids and Surfaces B: Biointerfaces, 86, 58–64.

Meance, C. C., et al. 2001 A fermented milk with a Bifidobacterium probiotic strain DN-173010 shortened oro-fecal gut transit time in elderly. Microbial Ecology in Health and Disease, 13, 217–222.

Ménard, S., et al. 2004. Lactic acid bacteria secrete metabolites retaining anti-inflammatory properties after intestinal transport. Gut, 53, 821–828.

Metchnikoff, E. 1907. The Prolongation of Life: Optimistic Studies, London, William Heinemann.

Metts, J., et al. 2003. *Lactobacillus acidophilus*, strain NAS (H2O2 positive), in reduction of recurrent candidal vulvovaginitis. Journal of Applied Research, 3, 340–348.

Michail, S. K., et al. 2008. Efficacy of probiotics in the treatment of pediatric atopic dermatitis: a meta-analysis of randomized controlled trials. Annals of Allergy, Asthma & Immunology, 101, 508–516.

Miele, E., et al. 2009. Effect of a probiotic preparation (VSL#3) on induction and maintenance of remission in children with ulcerative colitis. Am J Gastroenterol, 104, 437–443.

Mimura T et al. Once daily high dose probiotic therapy (VSL#3) for maintaining remission in recurrent or refractory pouchitis. Gut 53.1 (2004): 108–114.

Moayyedi, P., et al. 2010. The efficacy of probiotics in the treatment of irritable bowel syndrome: a systematic review. Gut, 59, 325–32.

Mohan, R., et al. 2006. Effects of *Bifidobacterium lactis* Bb12 supplementation on intestinal microbiota of preterm infants: a double-blind, placebo-controlled, randomized study. J Clin Microbiol, 44, 4025–4031.

Munoz P et al. *Saccharomyces cerevisiae* fungemia: an emerging infectious disease. Clin Infect Dis 40 (2005): 1625–1634.

Naaber, P., et al. 2004. Inhibition of *Clostridium difficile* strains by intestinal *Lactobacillus* species. Journal of Medical Microbiology, 53, 551–554.

Naidoo, K., et al. 2011. Probiotics for maintenance of remission in ulcerative colitis. Cochrane Database Syst Rev, CD007443.

Newcomer, A. D., et al. 1983. Response of patients with irritable bowel syndrome and lactase deficiency using unfermented acidophilus milk. American Journal of Clinical Nutrition, 38, 257–263.

Ng, S. C., et al. 2009. Mechanisms of action of probiotics: Recent advances. Inflammatory Bowel Diseases, 15, 300–310.

Oksanen PJ et al. Prevention of travellers' diarrhoea by *Lactobacillus* GG. Ann Med 22.1 (1990): 53–56.

Olah A et al. Randomized clinical trial of specific lactobacillus and fibre supplement to early enteral nutrition in patients with acute pancreatitis. Br J Surg 89.9 (2002): 1103–1107.

O'Mahony L et al. A randomized, placebo-controlled, double-blind comparison of the probiotic bacteria lactobacillus and bifidobacterium in irritable bowel syndrome (IBS): symptom responses and relationship to cytokine profiles. Gastroenterology 128 (2005a): 541–551.

O'Mahony, L., et al. 2005b. Lactobacillus and *Bifidobacterium* in irritable bowel syndrome: symptom responses and relationship to cytokine profiles. Gastroenterology, 128, 541–551.

Osterlund, P., et al. 2007. Lactobacillus supplementation for diarrhoea related to chemotherapy of colorectal cancer: a randomised study. Br J Cancer, 97, 1028–1034.

O'Sullivan, M. A. & O'Morain, C. A. 2000. Bacterial supplementation in the irritable bowel syndrome: a randomised double-blind placebo-controlled crossover study. Digestive and Liver Disease, 32, 294–301.

Ouwehand A, et al. The role of the intestinal microflora for the development of the immune system in early childhood. Eur J Nutr 41.Suppl 1 (2002): 132–137.

Oyewole, O. B. 1997. Lactic fermented foods in Africa and their benefits. Food Control, 8, 289–297.

Pelucchi, C., et al. 2012. Probiotics supplementation during pregnancy or infancy for the prevention of atopic dermatitis: a meta-analysis. Epidemiology, 23, 402–14.
Penner R, et al. Probiotics and nutraceuticals: non-medicinal treatments of gastrointestinal diseases. Curr Opin Pharmacol 5.6 (2005): 596–603.
Pirotta, M., et al. 2004. Effect of lactobacillus in preventing post-antibiotic vulvovaginal candidiasis: a randomised controlled trial. BMJ, 329, 548.
Plummer, S. F., et al. 2005. Effects of probiotics on the composition of the intestinal microbiota following antibiotic therapy. Int J Antimicrob Agents, 26, 69–74.
Prioult, G., et al. 2003. Effect of probiotic bacteria on induction and maintenance of oral tolerance to β-lactoglobulin in gnotobiotic mice. Clinical and Diagnostic Laboratory Immunology, 10, 787–792.
Rachmilewitz D et al. Immunostimulatory DNA ameliorates experimental and spontaneous murine colitis. Gastroenterology 122 (2002): 1428–1441.
Rachmilewitz D et al. Toll-like receptor 9 signaling mediates the anti-inflammatory effects of probiotics in murine experimental colitis. Gastroenterology 126 (2004): 520–528.
Rafii, F., et al. 2008. Effects of treatment with antimicrobial agents on the human colonic microflora. Ther Clin Risk Manag, 4, 1343–58.
Rafsky, H. A. & Rafsky, J. C. 1955. Clinical and bacteriological studies of a new *Lactobacillus acidophilus* concentrate in functional gastrointestinal disturbances. American Journal of Gastroenterology, 24, 87–92.
Rajilic-Stojanovic, M., et al. 2007. Diversity of the human gastrointestinal tract microbiota revisited. Environ Microbiol, 9, 2125–36.
Rautava, S., et al. 2009. Specific probiotics in reducing the risk of acute infections in infancy — a randomised, double-blind, placebo-controlled study. Br J Nutr, 101, 1722–1726.
Rautio M et al. Liver abcess due to a *Lactobacillus rhamnosus* strain indistinguishable from a *L. rhamnosus* strain GG. Clin Infect Dis 28 (1999): 1159–1160.
Reid G. Probiotic agents to protect the urogenital tract against infection. Am J Clin Nutr 73 (Suppl) (2001): 437S–443S.
Reid, G. & Bruce, A. W. 2001. Selection of *Lactobacillus* strains for urogenital applications. Journal of Infectious Diseases, 183 (suppl 1), S77–S80.
Rembacken, B. J., et al. 1999. Non-pathogenic *Escherichia coli* versus mesalazine for the treatment of ulcerative colitis: a randomized trial. Lancet, 354, 635–639.
Riquelme, A. J., et al. 2003. *Saccharomyces cerevisiae* fungemia after *Saccharomyces boulardii* treatment in immunocompromised patients. Journal of Clinical Gastroenterology, 36, 41–43.
Rolfe VE et al. Probiotics for maintenance of remission in Crohn's disease. Cochrane Database Syst Rev 4 (2006): CD004826.
Rosenfeldt V et al. Effect of probiotic *Lactobacillus* strains in children with atopic dermatitis. J Allergy Clin Immunol 111.2 (2003): 389–395.
Rosenfeldt V et al. Effect of probiotics on gastrointestinal symptoms and small intestinal permeability in children with atopic dermatitis. J Pediatr 145.5 (2004): 612–6116.
Rousseaux C, et al. *Lactobacillus acidophilus* modulates intestinal pain and induces opioid and cannabinoid receptors. Nat Med 13 (2007): 35–37.
Rutgeerts P. Modern therapy for inflammatory bowel disease. Scand J Gastroenterol Suppl 237 (2003): 30–33.
Saavedra, J. M., et al. 1994. Feeding of *Bifidobacterium bifidum* and *Streptococcus thermophilus* to infants in hospital for prevention of diarrhoea and shedding of rotavirus. Lancet, 344, 1046–1049.
Saint Marc T, et al. Efficacy of *Saccharomyces boulardii* in the treatment of diarrhoea in AIDS. Ann Med Interne (Paris) 142 (1991): 64–5.
Salminen, S., et al. 2010. Interaction of probiotics and pathogens — benefits to human health? Current Opinion in Biotechnology, 21, 157–167.
Sang, L. X., et al. 2010. Remission induction and maintenance effect of probiotics on ulcerative colitis: a meta-analysis. World J Gastroenterol, 16, 1908–15.
Savino, F., et al. 2007. *Lactobacillus reuteri* (American type culture collection strain 55730) versus simethicone in the treatment of infantile colic: A prospective randomized study. Pediatrics, 119, e124–e130.
Schiffrin, E. J., et al. 1997. Immune modulation of blood leukocytes in humans by lactic acid bacteria: criteria for strain selection. American Journal of Clinical Nutrition, 66, 515S–520S.
Senok, A. C., et al. 2009. Probiotics for the treatment of bacterial vaginosis. Cochrane Database Syst Rev, CD006289.
Sgouras, D., et al. 2004. In vitro and in vivo inhibition of *Helicobacter pylori* by *Lactobacillus casei* strain Shirota. Applied and Environmental Microbiology, 70, 518–526.
Shanahan, F. 2012. A commentary on the safety of probiotics. Gastroenterology Clinics of North America, 41, 869–876.
Sheil B et al. Is the mucosal route of administration essential for probiotic function? Subcutaneous administration is associated with attenuation of murine colitis and arthritis. Gut 53 (2004): 694–700.
Shen B et al. Maintenance therapy with a probiotic in antibiotic-dependent pouchitis: experience in clinical practice. Aliment Pharmacol Ther 22.8 (2005): 721–728.
Sheth A, Floch M. Probiotics and diverticular disease. Nutr Clin Pract 24.1 (2009): 41–44.
Shornikova, A. V., et al. 1997. Bacteriotherapy with *Lactobacillus reuteri* in rotavirus gastroenteritis. Pediatr Infect Dis, 16, 1103–1107.
Simons LA, et al. Effect of *Lactobacillus fermentum* on serum lipids in subjects with elevated serum cholesterol. Nutr Metab Cardiovasc Dis 16 (2006): 531–535.
Sistek D et al. Is the effect of probiotics on atopic dermatitis confined to food sensitized children? Clin Exp Allergy 36.5 (2006): 629–633.
Sood, A., et al. 2009. The probiotic preparation, VSL#3 induces remission in patients with mild-to-moderately active ulcerative colitis. Clin Gastroenterol Hepatol, 7, 1202–1209.

Spinler, J. K., et al. 2008. Human-derived probiotic *Lactobacillus reuteri* demonstrate antimicrobial activities targeting diverse enteric bacterial pathogens. Anaerobe, 14, 166–171.

Stermer, E., et al. 2006. Is traveler's diarrhea a significant risk factor for the development of irritable bowel syndrome? A prospective study. Clin Infect Dis, 43, 898–901.

Sudo, N., et al. 1997. The requirement of intestinal bacterial flora for the development of an IgE production system fully susceptible to oral tolerance induction. The Journal of Immunology, 159, 1739–45.

Surawicz, C. M., et al. 2000. The search for a better treatment for recurrent *Clostridium difficile* disease: use of high-dose vancomycin combined with *Saccharomyces boulardii*. Clinical and Infectious Disease, 31, 1012–1017.

Szajewska, H. & Mrukowicz, J. 2005. Meta-analysis: non-pathogenic yeast *Saccharomyces boulardii* in the prevention of antibiotic-associated diarrhoea. Aliment Pharmacol Ther, 22, 365–72.

Szajewska, H., et al. 2001. Efficacy of *Lactobacillus* GG in prevention of nosocomial diarrhea in infants. J Pediatr, 138, 361–365.

Szajewska H et al. Meta-analysis: *Lactobacillus* GG for treating acute diarrhoea in children. J Aliment Pharmacol Ther 25.8 (2007): 871–881.

Szajewska, H., et al. 2010. Probiotics in the prevention of antibiotic-associated diarrhea in children: a meta-analysis of randomized controlled trials. J Pediatr, 149, 367–372.

Tanaka, K. & Ishikawa, H. 2004. Role of intestinal bacterial flora in oral tolerance induction. Histol Histopathol, 19, 907–14.

Taylor Al, et al. Probiotic supplementation for the first 6 months of life fails to reduce the risk of atopic dermatitis and increases the risk of allergen sensitization in high-risk children: A randomised controlled trial. J Allergy Clin Immunol 119 (2007): 184–191.

Tien, M.-T., et al. 2006. Anti-inflammatory effect of *Lactobacillus casei* on Shigella-infected human intestinal epithelial cells. The Journal of Immunology, 176, 1228–1237.

Trautner, B. W. & Gupta, K. 2012. The advantages of second best: comment on "Lactobacilli vs antibiotics to prevent urinary tract infections". Arch Intern Med, 172, 712–4.

Trois L, et al. Use of probiotics in HIV-infected children: a randomized double-blind controlled study. J Trop Pediatr 54.1 (2008): 19–24.

Tubelius, P., et al. 2005. Increasing work-place healthiness with the probiotic *Lactobacillus reuteri* : A randomised, double-blind placebo-controlled study. Environmental Health: A Global Access Science Source, 4, 25.

Vajro, P., et al. 2011. Effects of *Lactobacillus rhamnosus* strain GG in pediatric obesity-related liver disease. J Pediatr Gastroenterol Nutr, 52, 740–3.

Vandenplas Y et al. Probiotics in infectious diarrhoea in children: are they indicated? Eur J Pediatr 166.12 (2007): 1211–1218.

Vanderhoof JA, Young RJ. Probiotics in pediatrics. Pediatrics 109.5 (2002): 956–958.

Vanderhoof JA, Young RJ. Role of probiotics in the management of patients with food allergy. Ann Allergy Asthma Immunol 90.(6 Suppl 3) (2003): 99–103.

Venturi, A., et al. 1999. Impact on the composition of the faecal flora by a new probiotic preparation: preliminary data on maintenance treatment of patients with ulcerative colitis. Alimentary Pharmacology and Therapeutics, 13, 1103–1108.

Venugopalan, V., et al. 2010. Regulatory oversight and safety of probiotic use. Emerg Infect Dis, 16, 1661–5.

Vouloumanou, E. K., et al. 2009. Probiotics for the prevention of respiratory tract infections: a systematic review. International Journal of Antimicrobial Agents, 34, 197.e1–197.e10.

Vujic, G., et al. 2013. Efficacy of orally applied probiotic capsules for bacterial vaginosis and other vaginal infections: a double-blind, randomized, placebo-controlled study. Eur J Obstet Gynecol Reprod Biol, 168, 75–9.

Wagner, R. D. & Johnson, S. J. 2012. Probiotic lactobacillus and estrogen effects on vaginal epithelial gene expression responses to *Candida albicans*. J Biomed Sci, 19, 58.

Walker, W. A. 2008. Mechanisms of action of probiotics. Clinical Infectious Diseases, 46, S87–S91.

Waller, P. A., et al. 2011. Dose-response effect of *Bifidobacterium lactis* HN019 on whole gut transit time and functional gastrointestinal symptoms in adults. Scand J Gastroenterol, 46, 1057–64.

Weizman, Z., et al. 2005. Effect of a probiotic infant formula on infections in child care centers: comparison of two probiotic agents. Pediatrics, 115, 5–9.

Wenus, C., et al. 2008. Prevention of antibiotic-associated diarrhoea by a fermented probiotic milk drink. Eur J Clin Nutr, 62, 299–301.

West, C. E., et al. 2009. Probiotics during weaning reduce the incidence of eczema. Pediatr Allergy Immunol, 20, 430–437.

Weston S et al. Effects of probiotics on atopic dermatitis: a randomised controlled trial. Arch Dis Child 90.9 (2005): 892–897.

White JA. Probiotics and their use in diverticulitis. J Clin Gastroenterol 40 suppl 3 (2006): S160–S162.

Whorwell PJ et al. Efficacy of an encapsulated probiotic *Bifidobacterium infantis* 35624 in women with irritable bowel syndrome. Am J Gastroenterol 101 (2006): 326–333.

Wickens, K., et al. 2008. A differential effect of 2 probiotics in the prevention of eczema and atopy: A double-blind, randomized, placebo-controlled trial. J Allergy Clin Immunol, 122, 788–794.

Williams, E. A., et al. 2008. Clinical trial: a multistrain probiotic preparation significantly reduces symptoms of irritable bowel syndrome in a double-blind placebo-controlled study. Aliment Pharmacol Ther, 29, 97–103.

Xiao JZ et al. Effects of milk products fermented by *Bifidobacterium longum* on blood lipids in rats and healthy adult male volunteers. J Dairy Sci 86.7 (2003): 2452–2461.

Yang, Y. X., et al. 2008. Effect of a fermented milk containing *Bifidobacterium lactis* DN-173010 on Chinese constipated women. World J Gastroenterol, 14, 6237–43.

Zocco, M. A., et al. 2006. Efficacy of *Lactobacillus* GG in maintaining remission of ulcerative colitis. Aliment Pharmacol Ther, 23, 1567–1574.

S-Adenosyl-L-methionine (SAMe)

HISTORICAL NOTE SAMe was first discovered in Italy in 1952. About 20 years later, a stable salt was commercially manufactured and produced for injectable use. At first, it was investigated as a treatment for schizophrenia, for which it proved inappropriate; however, successful trials in depressed patients began in the 1970s and it was inadvertently found to improve symptoms of arthritis. Since then, numerous studies have been undertaken to examine the role of SAMe in treating depression, osteoarthritis and liver pathology. To date, more than 75 clinical trials have been conducted using SAMe as a therapeutic agent, involving over 23,000 people.

BACKGROUND AND RELEVANT PHARMACOKINETICS

SAMe is a naturally occurring molecule synthesised in the cytosol of every cell, with the liver being the major site of biosynthesis and degradation. SAMe is derived from two acids: methionine (an amino acid) and adenosine triphosphate (ATP: a nucleic acid). Up to half the daily methionine is converted to SAMe in the liver, where it is metabolised to *S*-adenosylhomocysteine (SAH) and then homocysteine. Being a central part of the one-carbon metabolism cycle, SAMe is intrinsically linked with the other methyl donors such as betaine (choline), folate and B_{12}. SAMe also plays a role in the synthesis of choline, which plays a critical role in cell membrane structural integrity, cholinergic neurotransmission, cell signalling and lipid metabolism (Imbard et al 2013). SAMe is the second most used cofactor in the cells after ATP, and is used by over 100 methyl transferases that act on DNA, RNA, proteins and for the synthesis of polyamides that stabilise DNA (Smith et al 2010).

SAMe naturally exists as diastereoisomers and it is presently unclear whether both the R and the S forms are biologically active in humans. Evidence from a rat model suggests that they are equipotent (Dunne et al 1998). Oral doses achieve peak plasma concentrations within 3–5 hours after ingestion of an enteric-coated tablet (400–1000 mg). Enteric coating of SAMe supplements is essential to ensure product stability and potency. Oral SAMe has low systemic bioavailability due to first-pass effects and rapid metabolism. In vitro research by Wagner et al (2009) found that SAMe absorption and the subsequent anti-inflammatory effects are enhanced by encapsulating SAMe in liposomes derived from cholesterol. The half-life is reported to be 100 minutes, and excretion occurs via both urine and faeces (Najm et al 2004).

MAIN ACTIONS

SAMe is involved in myriad biochemical processes and metabolic pathways, chiefly as a methyl donor, where it is important for transmethylation reactions, including the synthesis of creatine, acetylcholine, carnitine, melatonin, glutathione (GSH), phospholipids, proteins, adrenaline, amino acids L-cysteine and taurine and many small molecules, such as neurotransmitters, and for RNA and DNA methylation (Stabler et al 2009). SAMe is closely linked with the metabolism of folate, vitamin B_{12} and all sulfur-containing compounds.

This review only discusses those actions that have been confirmed clinically.

Antidepressant activity

SAMe supplementation produces a clinically significant antidepressant activity that has been demonstrated in numerous randomised controlled trials (RCTs).

The mode of antidepressant action is likely to involve several mechanisms. As a methyl donor, SAMe plays a role in the metabolism and synthesis of various central nervous system neurotransmitters that play an integral part in synaptic transmission and behaviour, such as noradrenaline, dopamine and serotonin (Bottiglieri 1996, 2013, Stanger et al 2009). SAMe improves tetrahydrobiopterin function, a cofactor required for the synthesis of monoamines (Felger & Lotrich 2013). Administration of oral SAMe (800 mg daily) for 2 weeks significantly increased concentrations of 5-hydroxyindoleacetic acid in cerebrospinal fluid, a marker for increased serotonin in the brain (Bottiglieri 2013). Supplementation with SAMe in depressed patients raises serotonin, dopamine and phosphatidylserine and improves neurotransmitter binding to receptor sites, resulting in increased activity (Pizzorno & Murray 2006). Evidence suggests that the dopaminergic activity is most prominent. One human study confirmed that 7 days of supplemental SAMe (400 mg/day) decreased the exaggerated plasma noradrenaline levels found in depressed patients (Sherer et al 1986).

SAMe is also involved in the formation of phosphatidylcholine, a major component of cell membranes and neurotransmission (Carney et al 1987). A recent review suggested that one mode of action in depression may be via the methylation of plasma phospholipids, altering the fluidity of the neuronal membrane and thereby modifying the response to monoamine neurotransmitters that traverse the membrane (Papakostas et al 2012). The results of studies on genetic, epigenetic and environmental components of neuropsychiatric conditions such as depression, schizophrenia, bipolar disorder and autism point to the importance of the folate-methionine transsulfuration hub as a novel target pathway for treatment development (Ozbek et al 2008).

Additionally, SAMe displays antioxidant, anti-inflammatory and neuroprotective activities which may all contribute to the antidepressant effect.

Anti-inflammatory

A substantial body of evidence has identified clinically significant anti-inflammatory activity for SAMe, with comparative trials showing it to be as effective as standard non-steroidal anti-inflammatory drugs (NSAIDs).

Although the mechanism of action remains unclear, it does not appear to be mediated by prostaglandins. SAMe stimulates the synthesis of proteoglycans by articular chondrocytes and exerts a chondroprotective effect, according to in vitro research and tests with experimental animals (Barcelo et al 1987, Clayton 2007, Harmand et al 1987). In vitro studies using cultured rabbit synovial cells has found that SAMe reduces tumour necrosis factor-alpha and fibronectin RNA expression (Gutierrez et al 1997). Clinical responses suggest a concomitant analgesic property. The mechanism for this was previously unknown; however Tsao et al (2012) noted that serotonin-induced pain hypersensitivity in mice is reduced by either SAMe pretreatment or by the combined administration of SAMe with selective antagonists for β_2- and β_3-adrenergic receptors, which have previously been shown to mediate pain signalling. This result highlights a potential analgesic mechanism.

S

Hepatoprotective and restorative effects

SAMe indirectly reduces oxidative stress in the liver by serving as a precursor for GSH. GSH is particularly important for reducing the toxic effects of free radical molecules generated by various substances, including alcohol and paracetamol.

The use of SAMe to prevent and reverse liver toxicity induced by paracetamol, cytokine, ethanol, carbon tetrachloride and ischaemia-reperfusion has been explored in animal models (Cederbaum 2010, Song et al 2004, Wallace et al 2002). An animal study confirmed that paracetamol reduces SAMe levels in liver tissue nuclei and mitochondria, and coadministration of SAMe prevented damage associated with paracetamol toxicity (Brown et al 2010). SAMe also acts as the main methylating agent in the liver. Research with people with alcoholic and non-alcoholic liver diseases confirms that SAMe supplementation significantly increases hepatic GSH levels (Vendemiale et al 1989). Additionally, in vitro and in vivo research has identified antifibrotic activity and enhanced production of interleukin-6, a key anti-inflammatory cytokine in the liver that assists regeneration and downregulation of tumour necrosis factor (Arteel et al 2003, Casini et al 1989, Song et al 2004). Furthermore, SAMe was found to minimise hepatic fibrogenesis by modulating nuclear factor-kappaB (NF-κB) signalling and inhibiting collagen processing (Thompson et al 2011).

Animal studies have shown that the availability of *S*-adenosylmethionine plays a critical role in the progression of liver regeneration via enhancement of GSH and polyamine synthesis (necessary for cell proliferation and differentiation), indicating that regulating hepatic transsulfuration reactions may be capable of modifying the recovery process after liver injury (Jung et al 2013).

Anticancer activity

Research using animal models demonstrates that SAMe is a natural growth regulator in hepatocytes and is antiapoptotic in healthy liver cells, but proapoptotic in hepatic carcinoma cells (Anstee & Day 2012, Lu & Mato 2005). SAMe has been shown to inhibit angiogenesis and endothelial cell proliferation in vitro and in vivo (Sahin et al 2011).

The folate-methionine transsulfuration hub has been found to be altered in cancer (Smith et al 2010). Aberrant DNA hypomethylation in the promoter regions of gene, which leads to inactivation of tumour suppressor and other cancer-related genes in cancer cells, has been shown to be one of the most well-defined epigenetic hallmarks in gastric cancer (Qu et al 2013) and epithelial ovarian cancer (Guerrero et al 2012). SAMe has been shown to ameliorate this hypomethylation in vitro and has also been shown to block mitogenic signalling in colon cancer cells in vitro (Chen et al 2007).

OTHER ACTIONS

Prolactin and thyroid-stimulating hormone (TSH) effects

A double-blind, placebo-controlled study involving 20 subjects with depression identified a significant reduction in prolactin concentrations following 14 days of SAMe treatment (Thomas et al 1987). The results of a study conducted in 1990, however, suggest that the effects on these hormones may be gender-specific, with women demonstrating an augmenting response of TSH and no effect on prolactin levels, whereas release of both TSH and prolactin was inhibited in male subjects (Fava et al 1990). If SAMe does exert dopaminergic effects, as presently suspected, then it should also be taken into consideration that dopamine naturally inhibits both TSH and prolactin secretion in humans.

Antioxidant

Previous in vitro experimental research suggested that SAMe acts as a direct antioxidant mainly by binding iron molecules in an inert form, thereby blocking iron-dependent interaction with molecular oxygen to generate reactive oxygen species (ROS), rather than by free radical scavenging (Caro & Cederbaum 2004). Recent in vitro research has shown that coadministration of SAMe and *Saccharomyces boulardii* (a probiotic yeast routinely used to prevent and treat gastrointestinal disorders) enhances the viability of *S. boulardii* in acidic environments, which may improve gastric survival in transit (possibly by preventing apoptosis via reduction of ROS) and the yeast's clinical efficacy (Cascio et al 2013).

CLINICAL USE

Although SAMe is administered as an oral supplement in Australia, it is also used in injectable dose forms in Europe. This is most likely to be because oral SAMe has poor bioavailability and is subject to significant first-pass effects. Manufacturers have been investigating different preparations to increase oral bioavailability, such as SAMe encapsulated in liposomes derived from cholesterol, which has demonstrated increased activity (Wagner et al 2009). This discussion will mainly focus on oral use.

Depression

Both oral and parenteral SAMe are effective treatments for major mood disorders according to a review of 45 RCTs involving depressed adults in Europe and the United States (Papakostas et al 2012). Papakostas et al (2012) and other authors' reviews have concluded that SAMe, at a dose of between 1200 and 1600 mg/day, is superior to placebo and as effective as standard tricyclic antidepressants (imipramine). It is also better tolerated in the treatment of depressive disorders, without any documented increased risk of suicide (Bressa 1994, Delle Chiaie et al 2002, De Vanna & Rigamonti 1992, Dhingra & Parle 2012, Qureshi et al 2013). There has been less research conducted with SAMe in combination with standard antidepressants, but what is available has been encouraging for partial responders to selective serotonin reuptake inhibitors (SSRIs) and serotonin noradrenaline reuptake inhibitors. Studies comparing SAMe to SSRIs found that SAMe has a faster onset of action (10 days) compared to SSRIs (21 days) and relatively few side effects, giving it an advantage (Mischoulon & Fava 2002).

SAMe alone or combined with other supplements has also been shown to alleviate depression associated with musculoskeletal disease, liver disease, Parkinson's disease and HIV/AIDS (Qureshi et al 2013).

Treatment-resistant depression

A number of early open-label studies found benefit of adjunctive treatment with SAMe in treatment-resistant depression, with remission rates ranging from 22% to 43% after treatment-resistant depression patients were augmented with SAMe (Alpert et al 2004, Rosenbaum et al 1990). A trial implementing 800–1600 mg/day SAMe as an adjunctive agent in 30 treatment-resistant patients over 6 weeks revealed a staggering 50% response rate, with 43% of the sample experiencing remission of symptoms (Alpert et al 2004).

More recently, a double-blind RCT of 73 patients with treatment-resistant major depressive disorder showed that coadministration of SAMe (800 mg twice daily) with SSRI treatment produced significantly higher response and remission rates compared to the addition of placebo, using the Hamilton Depression Rating and Clinical Global Impression scales. Furthermore, no serious adverse effects occurred during the trial (Papakostas et al 2010). A secondary analysis of this clinical trial by the same group also confirmed that the coadministration of SAMe improved the memory-related cognitive symptoms of major depressive disorder (Levkovitz et al 2012). Positive results such as these warrant further clinical investigation of SAMe in an adjunctive role in refractory depression, a view that was shared in recent reviews of treatment-resistant depression (Kupfer et al 2012, Shelton et al 2010).

Osteoarthritis

Treatment with SAMe (1200 mg/day) is effective in the management of osteoarthritis and equally as effective as standard treatments, including celecoxib, piroxicam, indomethacin, ibuprofen and naproxen, according to a 2011 meta-analysis of six RCTs (sample sizes 36–493 participants) (De Silva et al 2011). In all trials, SAMe was found to be equally as effective as the NSAID and more effective than placebo for pain and function. Drop-out rates were highest in the NSAID groups and lowest in the SAMe groups. Similar results were reported in a previous meta-analysis of 11 RCTs involving almost 1500 patients; it also concluded that SAMe was more effective than placebo and as effective as NSAIDs in reducing pain and improving functional limitation in patients with osteoarthritis of the knee. In addition, SAMe-treated patients were 58% less likely to experience adverse effects than those treated with NSAIDs (Soeken et al 2002). A 2009 Cochrane systematic review of the use of SAMe in osteoarthritis of the knee or hip (n = 656) was more conservative and acknowledged that the action of SAMe on both pain and function might be clinically significant; however larger trials are required for evidence to be definitive (Rutjes et al 2009).

The longest placebo-controlled study to date was conducted over 2 years and found that a loading dose of oral SAMe 600 mg/day taken over the first 2 weeks, followed by a maintenance dose of 400 mg, produced an improvement in symptoms within the first month and no serious adverse effects (Konig 1987).

Comparative studies

SAMe (1200 mg/day) was just as effective in reducing pain intensity as nabumetone (1000 mg/day) over a period of 8 weeks in a 2009 study of 134 Korean patients (Kim et al 2009). Other comparative studies in humans have found that oral SAMe (1200 mg) produces similar symptom-relieving effects as piroxicam (20 mg), ibuprofen (1200 mg), indomethacin (150 mg) or naproxen (750 mg) and celecoxib (200 mg/day) (Caruso & Pietrogrande 1987, Clayton 2007, Glorioso et al 1985, Maccagno et al 1987, Muller-Fassbender 1987, Vetter 1987).

In regard to celecoxib (200 mg/day), SAMe is as effective for symptom relief but has a slower onset of action according to a 16-week double-blind, crossover RCT of 61 individuals with osteoarthritis of the knee (Najm et al 2004). In this study, one month of treatment was required for full benefits to be observed.

Fibromyalgia

Four double-blind trials have investigated the effects of SAMe in fibromyalgia, with all reporting positive findings (Jacobsen et al 1991, Tavoni et al 1987, 1998, Volkmann et al 1997), such as reduced number of trigger points and areas of pain, improved mood and reduced fatigue (Sarac & Gur 2006). Two studies used injectable SAMe (200 mg daily).

The largest study involved 44 patients with primary fibromyalgia and found that, during week 5, the group receiving SAMe (800 mg/day) experienced improvements in clinical disease activity, pain, fatigue, morning stiffness and one measurement of mood. Although encouraging, not all parameters were improved beyond placebo, such as tender point score and isokinetic muscle strength (Jacobsen et al 1991).

These results should not be surprising, given that one-third of all fibromyalgia patients are reported to suffer from depression and a meta-analysis of the effectiveness of antidepressants (including SAMe) in fibromyalgia deemed them a successful treatment strategy (O'Malley et al 2000). It concluded that tricyclic antidepressants, SSRIs and SAMe all improved sleep, fatigue, pain and wellbeing, but not necessarily trigger points.

Schizophrenia

SAMe has been studied in the treatment of schizophrenia, largely based on biochemical considerations suggesting a possible benefit.

Meta-analyses have implicated polymorphisms in 5,10-methylenetetrahydrofolate reductase (MTHFR), encoding a critical enzyme in folate and homocysteine metabolism, in both schizophrenia and bipolar disorder (van Winkel et al 2010). These polymorphisms are functional and result in diminished enzyme activity, leading to lower folate and higher homocysteine levels, and both have been implicated in schizophrenia risk in two separate meta-analyses (Allen et al 2008, Shi et al 2008).

To date, only one small double-blind RCT has been conducted showing that SAMe (800 mg/day) taken for 8 weeks improved quality of life and reduced aggressive behaviour compared to placebo. The study included 18 people with long-term schizophrenia and also found female patients showed improvement of depressive symptoms and clinical improvement, but this did not correlate with serum SAMe levels. Additionally, two patients in the active group exhibited some exacerbation of irritability; however causality is difficult to determine (Strous et al 2009).

Parkinson's disease

High-dose SAMe (800–3600 mg/day) treatment was investigated in a pilot study involving 11 depressed patients with Parkinson's disease, all of whom had been previously treated with other antidepressant agents and had no significant benefit or intolerable side effects. After 10 weeks, 10 patients had at least a 50% improvement on the Hamilton Depression Scale, with only one patient showing no improvement. The mean score before treatment was 27.09 and was 9.55 after SAMe treatment (Di Rocco et al 2000).

Numerous studies have demonstrated that treatment with L-dopa in patients with Parkinson's disease induces high levels of homocysteine and depletes SAMe (Chao et al 2012, De Bonis et al 2010). When supplemented with SAMe, folate, vitamin B_{12} and vitamin B_6 homocysteine levels decrease in people with Parkinson's disease taking L-dopa (Lamberti et al 2005).

Further clinical trials in patients with Parkinson's are currently underway (Meissner et al 2011).

Liver cirrhosis

SAMe deficiency has been studied as a possible pathogenetic factor in several liver diseases, and its administration evaluated in the prevention and treatment of a variety of liver injuries, such as chronic hepatitis, pregnancy-induced liver injury, alcoholic hepatitis and paracetamol-induced liver damage (Vincenzi et al 2012). Depressed hepatic SAMe, especially together with a reduced SAM:SAH ratio, results in impaired transmethylation, producing increased fat deposition, apoptosis and accumulation of damaged proteins — all characteristic features of liver injury (Cave et al 2007, Kharbanda 2007). Primate studies have found that decreased hepatic SAMe concentrations and associated liver lesions, including mitochondrial injury, can be corrected with SAMe supplementation (Lieber et al 1990), with reduced markers of lipid peroxidation, histological evidence of liver injury and maintained mitochondrial GSH (Cave et al 2007).

Alcoholic liver disease

In alcoholic patients with advanced liver cirrhosis, hepatic SAMe concentration is greatly decreased through alcohol exposure, increasing the risk of nucleotide

S

imbalance, apoptosis and carcinogenesis (Cave et al 2007, Gao & Bataller 2011, Halsted 2013, Kharbanda 2007, Lieber 2002). While transient SAMe depletion is necessary for the liver to regenerate, chronic hepatic SAMe depletion may lead to malignant transformation as SAMe is a substrate for all DNA and histone methyltransferases, including those involved in activation of liver injury/repair genes (Halsted 2013, Lu & Mato 2005, 2008). A 2010 double-blind RCT of 13 participants with alcoholic liver disease asked to abstain from alcohol showed that both placebo and SAMe (1200 mg/day) for 24 weeks improved serum aspartate aminotransferase (AST), alanine aminotransferase (ALT) and bilirubin levels (due to abstinence from alcohol), but no significant improvements in steatosis, fibrosis or inflammation were noted in the SAMe group. These results may be due to the small sample size and likely underpowering of the study, relatively short treatment timeframe or high dropout rate (30%) due to resumption of alcoholism during the study (Medici et al 2011).

A small follow-up expansion of this study found similar non-significant results; however this study was severely limited due to all 12 participants suffering severe fibrosis and/or metaplasia, with very few functioning hepatocytes at baseline (Le et al 2013). Two previous European clinical studies suggested that a longer treatment period with oral 1200 mg SAMe may be effective in alcoholic liver disease, and in a 6-month Italian RCT of 17 patients with initially low hepatic GSH levels, oral SAMe (1200 mg/day) normalised levels (Vendemiale et al 1989). In a subsequent 2-year European multicentre trial of 123 patients with alcoholic liver disease, total mortality or liver transplant incidence was reduced from 30% in the placebo group to 16% in the SAMe group, but this was only noted after excluding the most severely ill patients from the analysis (Mato et al 1999).

A 2006 Cochrane review (updated in 2009) of SAMe in alcoholic liver disease analysed results from nine RCTs that included a heterogeneous sample of 434 patients (Rambaldi & Gluud 2006). The methodological quality was considered low; however, eight of the trials were placebo-controlled. As a result, the analysis was based mainly on one trial that found no significant effects of SAMe on all-cause mortality, liver-related mortality, liver transplantation or complications. The authors concluded that, based on such limited evidence, more long-term, high-quality randomised trials of SAMe for these patients are required before SAMe may be recommended for clinical practice. More recent reviews note that improved survival and reduction in liver transplants in patients receiving SAMe are important positive outcomes (Halsted 2013, Vazquez-Elizondo & Bosques-Padilla 2012).

Non-alcoholic fatty liver disease (NAFLD) or non-alcoholic steatohepatitis (NASH)

Human studies have demonstrated that patients with liver disease have an impaired ability to convert methionine to SAMe and decreased plasma and hepatic GSH levels (Cave et al 2007). SAMe has been shown to improve GSH in patients with liver disease after 6 months of oral therapy. Of particular interest is recent evidence from animal studies which suggest that SAMe depletion in the early stages of NASH may be a key point of disease progression into NAFLD (Lu & Mato 2008, Wortham et al 2008). Clinical trials have demonstrated benefit from SAMe therapy in various forms of liver disease, including alcoholic cirrhosis, intrahepatic cholestasis of pregnancy and chemotherapy-induced NASH (Vincenzi et al 2012). SAMe supplementation has also demonstrated attenuation of inflammation and liver injury in a nutritional deficiency model of steatohepatitis and clinical trials were carried out in NASH patients (Cave et al 2007). In lieu of more solid evidence to support SAMe as a therapeutic agent in NASH and NAFLD, the preferred current treatment is betaine, which by virtue corrects methylation by serving as a methyl donor and reduces SAMe depletion (Kharbanda 2007, Kwon 2009, Singal et al 2011).

Prevention of drug-induced liver toxicity

Paracetamol is the leading cause of drug-induced liver failure, hepatotoxicity, and is known to be one of the most frequent side effects associated with different chemotherapy regimens. A recent clinical trial of 78 patients noted that administration of 800 mg/day SAMe as adjunctive therapy was effective in reducing chemotherapy-induced liver toxicity from oxaliplatin plus bevacizumab in patients with metastatic colorectal cancer. AST, ALT, lactate dehydrogenase and total bilirubin were significantly reduced in the SAMe group compared to placebo, and SAMe supplementation significantly reduced chemotherapy course delay and dosage reductions due to liver toxicity (Vincenzi et al 2012). This study confirmed earlier research by the same group that determined SAMe supplementation reduces chemotherapy-induced liver toxicity; similarly, in that trial, SAMe supplementation was found to be associated with a significant lowering of AST and ALT values in 70% of the treated patients and also reduced chemotherapy delays or dose reductions due to transaminase elevation (Santini et al 2003).

OTHER USES

SAMe is used to reduce pain in migraine headache because analgesic activity was reported at a dose of 400–800 mg/day in a group of migraine sufferers (Gatto et al 1986). A case report of 5 paediatric cases of Lesch–Nyhan disease (a rare X-linked recessive neurogenetic disorder) showed significant improvement in self-injury and aggressive behaviour as well as a milder reduction of dystonia when SAMe was administered at a dose of 21–33 mg/kg/day (Chen et al 2013). It is also used in AIDS-related myelopathy and coronary artery disease, as these conditions have been associated with depleted SAMe levels. Supplementation has also been prescribed in cases of general fatigue, poor digestion and allergies.

Alzheimer's dementia (AD)

AD has a multifactorial aetiology that includes nutritional, genetic and environmental risk factors, none of which in isolation is sufficient to account for all cases of AD (Shea & Chan 2008). There is a growing body of evidence indicating that some SAMe-mediated reactions are compromised in AD and age-related neurodegeneration: SAMe is diminished and its metabolites SAH and homocysteine are increased, the accumulation of which also impairs SAMe reactions (Kennedy et al 2004). In patients with AD, decreased SAMe concentrations have been observed in cerebrospinal fluid along with increased concentrations of SAH in brain tissue (Bottiglieri 2013). Inhibited methylation reactions and hypomethylation of proteins that regulate levels of brain tissue phosphorylated-tau have also been noted in addition to hypomethylation of genes that affect the expression of β-amyloid protein (Bottiglieri 2013).

Interestingly, SAMe supplementation reduced amyloid production, increased spatial memory and reduced plaque spread in a 2012 in vivo study, suggesting a possible role in AD (Fuso et al 2012).

To date, no clinical trials have been published to investigate whether supplemental SAMe has benefits in AD, although the theoretical considerations make a good case for further investigation to be undertaken (Panza et al 2009).

Cholestasis of pregnancy

Cholestasis of pregnancy is characterised by elevated bilirubin and pruritus, and is associated with a high risk of a number of adverse perinatal outcomes, including preterm birth, meconium passage, fetal distress and fetal death (Anstee & Day 2012). A clinical trial of 78 pregnant volunteers with cholestasis showed that treatment with either SAMe or ursodeoxycholic acid (UDCA) effectively reduced pruritus; however the UDCA group showed greater improvement in bile acid secretion (Roncaglia et al 2004). However, a subsequent Cochrane review concluded that there was insufficient evidence to recommend either SAMe or UDCA for the treatment of cholestasis of pregnancy (Burrows et al 2010).

Hepatitis C management

An open-label pilot study of 29 patients with chronic hepatitis C who failed previous therapy with interferon-α and ribavirin were coadministered SAMe and betaine for 6–12 months, resulting in significant improvement of early virological response rates without significant additional adverse effects (Filipowicz et al 2010). SAMe was also found to improve early viral responses and interferon-stimulated gene induction in hepatitis C non-responders (Feld et al 2011). Larger trials are needed to confirm this combination as an effective adjunct treatment.

Cancer

There is a paucity of clinical trials exploring the role of SAMe supplementation in cancer; however, preclinical research and biochemical considerations provide a basis for its future investigation.

Hepatic cancer

Due to its role in the regulation of growth and apoptosis of hepatocytes, SAMe is being investigated as a possible preventive or treatment agent in hepatocellular carcinoma (Lu & Mato 2005, 2008), and has been administered in postradiofrequency ablation formulas to enhance recovery of hepatic tissue at an intravenous dose of 1000 mg for 2–3 days in conjunction with *Silybum marianum* (Feng et al 2012).

Colorectal cancer

There is considerable evidence that aberrant DNA methylation plays an integral role in oncogenesis, and genomic DNA hypomethylation has been reported in colorectal tumour tissue (Nagaraju & El-Rayes 2013). However few studies examine changes in intermediate methylation compounds: one study determined that folate concentration is diminished and SAMe and SAH is increased in neoplastic colonic mucosa when compared to healthy colon tissue (Alonzo-Aperte et al 2008). More studies are needed to confirm whether genomic DNA methylation measurements are functional biomarkers in colorectal cancer.

Breast and cervical cancer

A number of studies have explored the association between MTHFR C677T polymorphism and susceptibility to cervical and breast cancer and cervical intraepithelial neoplasia (Alshatwi 2010, Luo et al 2012). A recent meta-analysis confirmed that SAMe is known as an important DNA methylator, which may have a role in the prevention of pro-oncogene expression in cervical cancer; however, results remained controversial and further studies are needed (Luo et al 2012).

DOSAGE RANGE

Because SAMe is rapidly oxidised when exposed to air, the quality of the tablets is important in preserving potency. SAMe is better absorbed when taken at least 20 minutes before breakfast and 20 minutes before lunch. As an activating antidepressant, it can disturb sleep if taken after 4 pm (Bottiglieri 2013).

Based on clinical studies

- Depression: 1200–3200 mg/day in divided doses have been used in practice. Sometimes it is started as 200 mg twice daily, increased on day 2 to 400 mg twice daily and then increased again to 400 mg three times daily on day 10, until reaching a therapeutic dose of 400 mg four times daily by day 20.
- Osteoarthritis: 1200 mg/day in divided doses, taken as above, with a reduced dose of 400 mg/day used as a maintenance dose once a response occurs.
- Fibromyalgia: 600–800 mg/day in divided doses.
- Liver disease: 400–1200 mg/day in divided doses, although larger doses have been used.
- Parkinson's disease: 800–3600 mg/day in divided doses.
- Migraine: 400–800 mg/day in divided doses.
- Reducing aggression in schizophrenia: 800 mg/day (only under supervision).

ADVERSE REACTIONS

Orally, SAMe is generally well tolerated. Mild gastrointestinal discomfort (nausea) is the most common side effect reported in clinical studies, although anxiety, headache, urinary frequency, dizziness, nervousness, sweating and pruritus have also been reported (Ravindran & da Silva 2013). It has been reported that side effects are more likely with higher doses and may be minimised by consuming SAMe before food.

SIGNIFICANT INTERACTIONS

Controlled studies are not available; therefore, interactions are based on evidence of activity and are largely theoretical and speculative.

Tricyclic antidepressants and other serotonergic agents

Coadministration of SAMe with SSRIs has shown benefits in partial responders and may be a useful combination under professional supervision.

Hepatotoxic drugs

SAMe may reduce hepatic injury caused by agents such as paracetamol, alcohol and oestrogens — potentially beneficial interaction.

L-Dopa

SAMe methylates levodopa, which could theoretically reduce the effectiveness of levodopa given for Parkinson's disease; however, the effect has not been observed clinically — observe patients.

Thyroxine

Caution and monitoring may be warranted.

Betaine

In studies supplementing mice with betaine, significant increases in SAMe were observed with a threefold elevation of the activity of methionine adenosyltransferase — observe.

S

CONTRAINDICATIONS AND PRECAUTIONS

Previous case reports of agitation and mania in bipolar patients caution that SAMe should be avoided in people with bipolar disorder during the depressive phase (Andreescu et al 2008, Bogarapu et al 2008) and used with caution by people with schizophrenia or schizoaffective disorder (Guidotti et al 2007). However, separate research of coadministration of SAMe with SSRIs or venlafaxine reported no unmasking of hypomanic or manic symptoms (Alpert et al 2004, Papakostas et al 2010). Use under professional supervision to promote patient safety.

PREGNANCY USE

SAMe has been used intravenously in the last trimester of pregnancy with no adverse effects to mother or fetus. However, safety has not yet been conclusively established for either injectable or oral dose forms and possible effects on prolactin levels need to be considered.

PATIENTS' FAQs

What will this supplement do for me?
SAMe has anti-inflammatory, analgesic, antidepressant and protective effects on the liver. It effectively reduces pain and inflammation in osteoarthritis and elevates mood in depression. In fibromyalgia, SAMe reduces pain, fatigue and morning stiffness and may also reduce pain in migraine headache.
When will it start to work?
Beneficial effects are usually seen within 4–5 weeks for osteoarthritis, whereas antidepressant effects are experienced within 1 week. Benefits in fibromyalgia can take up to 6 weeks to establish.
Are there any safety issues?
SAMe should only be used under professional supervision by people with bipolar disorder, schizophrenia or schizoaffective disorder, Parkinson's disease or taking antidepressant medicines. Monitoring of homocysteine levels may be required with long-term supplementation.

Practice points/Patient counselling

- SAMe is involved in myriad biochemical reactions within the body. It is found within every cell and is a precursor for the synthesis of the antioxidant GSH and an important methyl donor.
- Clinically, it has significant anti-inflammatory, analgesic and antidepressant effects and is an effective treatment in depression and osteoarthritis.
- A 2011 meta-analysis concluded that SAMe is as effective as commonly used NSAIDs in reducing pain and improving functional limitation in patients with osteoarthritis without the adverse effects associated with NSAIDs. A recent study has found that it is as effective as celecoxib for providing symptom relief; however, SAMe has a slower onset of action.
- Clinical trials have also shown it to be a safe and effective treatment for depression — comparable with tricyclic antidepressant drugs, yet with a faster onset of action. SAMe also provides additional benefits when coadministered with SSRIs in treatment-resistant depression.

- It may also have benefits for patients with alcoholic liver disease and hepatitis C and for the prevention of drug-induced liver toxicity.
- SAMe may also be useful in fibromyalgia, and possibly migraine headache. Other uses include treatment of general fatigue, elevated homocysteine levels, allergies and poor digestion.

REFERENCES

Allen, NC et al. Systematic meta-analyses and field synopsis of genetic association studies in schizophrenia: the SzGene database. Nat. Genet. 40.7 (2008): 827–834.

Alonzo-Aperte E et al. Folate status and *S*-adenosylmethionine/*S*-adenosylhomocysteine ratio in colorectal adenocarcinoma in humans. Eur J Clin Nutr 62 (2008):295–298.

Alpert JE et al. *S*-adenosyl-L-methionine (SAMe) as an adjunct for resistant major depressive disorder: an open trial following partial or nonresponse to selective serotonin reuptake inhibitors or venlafaxine. J Clin Psychopharmacol 24.6 (2004): 661–664.

Alshatwi AA. Breast cancer risk, dietary intake, and methylenetetrahydrofolate reductase (MTHFR) single nucleotide polymorphisms. Food and Chem Toxicology 48 (2010):1881–1885.

Andreescu C, et al. Complementary and alternative medicine in the treatment of bipolar disorder — a review of the evidence. J Affect Disord 110.1–2 (2008): 16–26.

Anstee QM & Day CP. *S*-adenosylmethionine (SAMe) therapy in liver disease: A review of current evidence and clinical utility. J Hepatol 57 (2012): 1097–1109.

Arteel G et al. Advances in alcoholic liver disease. Best Pract Res Clin Gastroenterol 17 (2003): 625–647.

Barcelo HA et al. Effect of *S*-adenosylmethionine on experimental osteoarthritis in rabbits. Am J Med 83.5A (1987): 55–59.

Bogarapu S et al. Complementary medicines in pediatric bipolar disorder. Minerva Pediatr 60.1 (2008): 103–114.

Bottiglieri T. Folate, vitamin B_{12}, and neuropsychiatric disorders. Nutr Rev 54.12 (1996): 382–390.

Bottiglieri T. Folate, vitamin B_{12}, and *S*-adenosylmethionine. Psychiatric Clinics of North America (2013): 1–13.

Bressa GM. *S*-adenosyl-L-methionine (SAMe) as antidepressant: meta-analysis of clinical studies. Acta Neurol Scand Suppl 154 (1994): 7–14.

Brown JM et al. Temporal study of acetaminophen (APAP) and *S*-adenosyl-L-methionine (SAMe) effects on subcellular hepatic SAMe levels and methionine adenosyltransferase (MAT) expression and activity. Toxicol Appl Pharmacol. 247.1 (2010): 1–9.

Burrows RF et al. Interventions for treating cholestasis in pregnancy. Cochrane Database Sys Rev (2010).

Carney MW, et al. *S*-adenosylmethionine and affective disorder. Am J Med 83.5A (1987): 104–106.

Caro AA, Cederbaum AI. Antioxidant properties of *S*-adenosyl-methionine in Fe^{2+}-initiated oxidations. Free Radical Biol Med 36.10 (2004): 1303–1316.

Caruso I, Pietrogrande V. Italian double-blind multicenter study comparing *S*-adenosylmethionine, naproxen, and placebo in the treatment of degenerative joint disease. Am J Med 83.5A (1987): 66–71.

Cascio V et al. *S*-Adenosyl-L-Methionine protects the probiotic yeast, *Saccharomyces boulardii*, from acid-induced cell death. BMC Microbiology 13.35 (2013).

Casini A et al. *S*-adenosylmethionine inhibits collagen synthesis by human fibroblasts in vitro. Methods Find Exp Clin Pharmacol 11.5 (1989): 331–334.

Cave M et al. Nonalcoholic fatty liver disease: predisposing factors and the role of nutrition. J Nutr Biochem 18.3 (2007): 184–195.

Cederbaum AI. Hepatoprotective effects of *S*-adenosyl-L-methionine against alcohol- and cytochrome P450 2E1-induced liver injury. World J Gastroenterol 16.11(2010): 1366–1376.

Chao J et al Nutraceuticals and their preventive or potential therapeutic value in Parkinson's disease. Nutrition Reviews 70.7(2012):373–386.

Chen H et al Role of methionine adenosyltransferase 2A and *S*-adenosylmethionine in mitogen-induced growth of human colon cancer cells. Gastroenterology 133 (2007):207–218.

Chen BC et al. Treatment of Lesch–Nyhan disease with *S*-adenosylmethionine: Experience with five young Malaysians, including a girl. Brain & Development (2013) DOI: 10.1016/j.braindev.2013.08.013.

Clayton JJ. Nutraceuticals in the management of osteoarthritis. Orthopedics 30.8 (2007): 624–629.

Delle Chiaie R et al. Efficacy and tolerability of oral and intramuscular *S*-adenosyl-L-methionine 1,4-butanedisulfonate (SAMe) in the treatment of major depression: comparison with imipramine in 2 multicenter studies. Am J Cli Nutr. 76.5(2002): 1172S–1176S.

De Bonis ML et al. Impaired transmethylation potential in Parkinson's disease patients treated with L-dopa. Neuroscience Letters 468 (2010): 287–291.

De Silva V et al Evidence for the efficacy of complementary and alternative medicines in the management of osteoarthritis: a systematic review. Rheumatology 50 (2011):911–920.

De Vanna M, Rigamonti R. Oral *S*-adenosyl-L-methionine in depression. Curr Ther Res 52.3 (1992): 478–85.

Dhingra S, Parle M. Herbal remedies and nutritional supplements in the treatment of depression: a review. Bull Clinc Psychopharm 22.3 (2012): 286–92.

Di Rocco A et al. *S*-adenosyl-methionine improves depression in patients with Parkinson's disease in an open-label clinical trial. Mov Disord 15.6 (2000): 1225–1229.

Dunne JB et al. Evidence that *S*-adenosyl-L-methionine diastereoisomers may reduce ischaemia-reperfusion injury by interacting with purinoceptors in isolated rat liver. Br J Pharmacol 125 (1998): 225–233.

S

Fava M et al. Neuroendocrine effects of *S*-adenosyl-L-methionine: a novel putative antidepressant. J Psychiatr Res 24.2 (1990): 177–184.

Feld JJ, et al. *S*-adenosyl methionine improves early viral responses and interferon stimulated gene induction in hepatitis C nonresponders. Gastroenterology 140 (2011): 830–9.

Felger JC & Lotrich FE. Inflammatory cytokines in depression: neurobiological mechanisms and therapeutic implications. Neuroscience 246 (2013): 199–229.

Feng K et al A randomized controlled trial of radiofrequency ablation and surgical resection in the treatment of small hepatocellular carcinoma. J Hepatology 57 (2012): 794–802.

Filipowicz M et al. *S*-adenosyl-methionine and betaine improve early virological response in chronic hepatitis C patients with previous nonresponse. PLoS One 5.11 (2010): e15492.

Fuso A et al. *S*-adenosylmethionine reduces the progress of the Alzheimer-like features induced by B-vitamin deficiency in mice, Neurobiology of Aging 33 (2012):1482.e1–1482.e16.

Gao B, Bataller R. Alcoholic liver disease: pathogenesis and new therapeutic targets. Gastroenterology 141.5 (2011):1572–1585.

Gatto G et al. Analgesizing effect of a methyl donor (*S*-adenosylmethionine) in migraine: an open clinical trial. Int J Clin Pharmacol Res 6.1 (1986): 15–117.

Glorioso S et al. Double-blind multicentre study of the activity of *S*-adenosylmethionine in hip and knee osteoarthritis. Int J Clin Pharmacol Res 5.1 (1985): 39–49.

Guerrero K et al. A novel genome-based approach correlates TMPRSS3 overexpression in ovarian cancer with DNA hypomethylation. Gynecologic Oncology 125 (2012): 720–726.

Guidotti A et al. *S*-adenosyl methionine and DNA methyltransferase-1 mRNA overexpression in psychosis. Neuroreport 18.1 (2007): 57–60.

Gutierrez S et al. SAMe restores the changes in the proliferation and in the synthesis of fibronectin and proteoglycans induced by tumour necrosis factor alpha on cultured rabbit synovial cells. Br J Rheumatol 36 (1997): 27–31.

Halsted CH. B-vitamin dependent methionine metabolism and alcoholic liver disease. Clin Chem Lab Med 51.3(2013): 457–465.

Harmand MF et al. Effects of *S*-adenosylmethionine on human articular chondrocyte differentiation. An in vitro study. Am J Med 83.5A (1987): 48–54.

Imbard A et al. Plasma choline and betaine correlate with serum folate, plasma *S*-adenosyl-methionine and *S*-adenosyl-homocysteine in healthy volunteers. Clin Chem Lab Med 51.3 (2013): 683–692.

Jacobsen S, et al. Oral *S*-adenosylmethionine in primary fibromyalgia. Double-blind clinical evaluation. Scand J Rheumatol 20.4 (1991): 294–302.

Jung YS et al. Significance of alterations in the metabolomics of sulfur-containing amino acids during liver regeneration. Biochimie 95 (2013): 1605–1610.

Kennedy BP et al. Elevated *S*-adenosylhomocysteine in Alzheimer brain: influence on methyltransferases and cognitive function, J Neural Transm 111 (2004): 547–567.

Kharbanda KK. Role of transmethylation reactions in alcoholic liver disease. World J Gastroenterol 13.37 (2007): 4947–4954.

Kim J et al. Comparative clinical trial of *S*-adenosylmethionine versus nabumetone for the treatment of knee osteoarthritis: An 8-week, multicenter, randomized, double-blind, double-dummy, phase IV study in Korean patients. Clinical Therapeutics 31.12 (2009):2860–2872.

Konig BA. Long-term (two years) clinical trial with *S*-adenosylmethionine for the treatment of osteoarthritis. Am J Med 83.5A (1987): 89–94.

Kupfer D et al Major depressive disorder: new clinical, neurobiological, and treatment perspectives. Lancet 379 (2012): 1045–55.

Kwon DY. Impaired sulfur-amino acid metabolism and oxidative stress in nonalcoholic fatty liver are alleviated by betaine supplementation in rats. J Nutr (2009) 139(1):63–68.

Lamberti P et al. Hyperhomocysteinemia in L-dopa treated Parkinson's disease patients: effect of cobalamin and folate administration. Eur J Neurol. 12 (2005):365–368.

Le MD et al. Alcoholic liver disease patients treated with *S*-adenosyl-L-methionine: An in-depth look at liver morphologic data comparing pre and post treatment liver biopsies. Experimental and Molecular Pathology 95 (2013): 187–191.

Levkovitz Y et al Effects of *S*-adenosylmethionine augmentation of serotonin-reuptake inhibitor antidepressants on cognitive symptoms of major depressive disorder. Eur Psych 27 (2012): 518–521.

Lieber CS. *S*-Adenosyl-L-methionine and alcoholic liver disease in animal models: implications for early intervention in human beings. Alcohol 27.3 (2002): 173–177.

Lieber CS et al. *S*-adenosyl-L-methionine attenuates alcohol-induced liver injury in the baboon. Hepatology 11.2 (1990): 165–172.

Lu SC, Mato JM. Role of methionine adenosyltransferase and *S*-adenosylmethionine in alcohol-associated liver cancer. Alcohol 35.3 (2005): 227–234.

Lu SC, Mato JM. *S*-Adenosylmethionine in cell growth, apoptosis and liver cancer. J Gastroenterol Hepatol 23 (Suppl 1) (2008): S73–S77.

Luo YL et al Methylenetetrahydrofolate reductase C677T polymorphism and susceptibility to cervical cancer and cervical intraepithelial neoplasia: a meta-analysis. PLos One 7.9 (2012): e46272.

Maccagno A et al. Double-blind controlled clinical trial of oral *S*-adenosylmethionine versus piroxicam in knee osteoarthritis. Am J Med 83.5A (1987): 72–77.

Mato JM et al. *S*-adenosylmethionine in alcoholic liver cirrhosis: a randomized, placebo controlled, double-blinded, multicenter clinical trial. J Hepatol 30 (1999):1081–1089.

Medici V et al *S*-adenosyl-L-methionine treatment for alcoholic liver disease: A double-blinded, randomized, placebo-controlled trial. Alcohol Clin Exp Res 35.11 (2011): 1960–1965.

Meissner WG et al. Priorities in Parkinson's disease research. Nature Rev Drug Disc 10 (2011): 377–393.

Mischoulon D, Fava M. Role of *S*-adenosyl-L-methionine in the treatment of depression: a review of the evidence. Am J Clin Nutr 76.5 (2002): 1158S–61S.

Muller-Fassbender H. Double-blind clinical trial of *S*-adenosylmethionine versus ibuprofen in the treatment of osteoarthritis. Am J Med 83.5A (1987): 81–83.

Nagaraju GP, El-Rayes B. SPARC and DNA methylation: Possible diagnostic and therapeutic implications in gastrointestinal cancers. Cancer Letters 328 (2013):10–17.

Najm WI et al. *S*-adenosyl methionine (SAMe) versus celecoxib for the treatment of osteoarthritis symptoms: a double-blind cross-over trial. BMC Musculoskelet Disord 5 (2004): 6.

O'Malley PG et al. Treatment of fibromyalgia with antidepressants: a meta-analysis. J Gen Intern Med 15.9 (2000): 659–666.

Ozbek Z et al Effect of the methylenetetrahydrofolate reductase gene polymorphisms on homocysteine, folate and vitamin B_{12} in patients with bipolar disorder and relatives. Progress in Neuro-Psychopharmacology & Biological Psychiatry 32 (2008):1331–1337.

Panza F et al. Possible role of *S*-adenosylmethionine, *S*-adenosylhomocysteine, and polyunsaturated fatty acids in predementia syndromes and Alzheimer's disease. J Alz Dis 16 (2009): 467–470.

Papakostas GI et al. *S*-adenosyl methionine (SAMe) augmentation of serotonin reuptake inhibitors for antidepressant nonresponders with major depressive disorder: A double-blind, randomized clinical trial. Am J Psychiatry 167.8 (2010):942–948.

Papakostas GI et al. Folates and *S*-adenosylmethionine for major depressive disorder. Can J Psychiatry 57.7 (2012):406–413.

Pizzorno J, Murray M. Textbook of natural medicine, 3rd edn. St Louis: Elsevier, 2006.

Qu Y et al. Gene methylation in gastric cancer. Clinica Chimica Acta 424 (2013): 53–65.

Qureshi NA, Al-Bedah AM. Mood disorders and complementary and alternative medicine: a literature review. Neuropsych Dis Treat 9 (2013): 639–658.

Rambaldi A, Gluud C. *S*-adenosyl-L-methionine for alcoholic liver diseases. Cochrane Database Syst Rev 2 (2006): CD002235.pub2.

Ravindran AV, da Silva TL. Complementary and alternative therapies as add-on to pharmacotherapy for mood and anxiety disorders: A systematic review. J Affective Disorders 150 (2013): 707–719.

Roncaglia N et al. A randomized controlled trial of ursodeoxycholic acid and *S*-adenosyl-L-methionine in the treatment of gestational cholestasis. Br J Obstet Gynaecol 2 (2004): 17–21.

Rosenbaum JF et al. The antidepressant potential of oral *S*-adenosyl-L-methionine. Acta Psychiatr Scand 81.5 (1990): 432–6.

Rutjes AWS et al. *S*-adenosylmethionine for osteoarthritis of the knee or hip. CochraneDatabase of Systematic Reviews 4 (2009): CD007321.

Sahin M et al. Inhibition of angiogenesis by *S*-adenosylmethionine. Biochem Biophys Res Com 408 (2011): 145–148.

Santini D et al *S*-adenosylmethionine (AdoMet) supplementation for treatment chemotherapy-induced liver injury. Anticancer Res 23.6D (2003):5173–5179.

Sarac AJ, Gur A. Complementary and alternative medical therapies in fibromyalgia. Curr Pharm Des 12.1 (2006): 47–57.

Shea TB, Chan A. *S*-adenosyl methionine: a natural therapeutic agent effective against multiple hallmarks and risk factors associated with Alzheimer's disease. J Alz Dis 13 (2008): 67–70.

Sherer MA et al. Effects of *S*-adenosyl-methionine on plasma norepinephrine, blood pressure, and heart rate in healthy volunteers. Psychiatry Res 17.2 (1986): 111–1118.

Shelton RC et al Therapeutic options for treatment-resistant depression. CNS Drugs 24.2(2010): 131–161.

Shi J et al. Genetic associations with schizophrenia: meta-analyses of 12 candidate genes. Schizophr. Res. 104.1–3 (2008): 96–107.

Singal AK et al Antioxidants as therapeutic agents for liver disease. Liver Intl (2011):1432–48.

Smith CL et al Genomic and epigenomic instability, fragile sites, schizophrenia and autism. Current Genomics, 11 (2010): 447–469.

Soeken KL et al. Safety and efficacy of *S*-adenosylmethionine (SAMe) for osteoarthritis. J Fam Pract 51.5 (2002): 425–430.

Song Z et al. Modulation of endotoxin stimulated Interleukin 6 production in monocytes and Kupffer cells by *S*-adenosylmethionine (SAMe). Cytokine 28.6 (2004): 214–223.

Stabler SP et al. α-Lipoic acid induces elevated *S*-adenosylhomocysteine and depletes *S*-adenosylmethionine. Free Radical Biology & Medicine 47 (2009): 1147–1153.

Stanger O et al. Homocysteine, folate and B_{12} in neuropsychiatric diseases: review and treatment recommendations. Expert Rev. Neurother 9.9 (2009): 1393–1412.

Strous RD et al. Improvement of aggressive behavior and quality of life impairment following *S*-adenosyl-methionine (SAM-e) augmentation in schizophrenia. European Neuropsychopharmacology 19 (2009): 14–22.

Tavoni A et al. Evaluation of *S*-adenosylmethionine in primary fibromyalgia: a double-blind crossover study. Am J Med 83.5A (1987): 107–110.

Tavoni A, et al. Evaluation of *S*-adenosylmethionine in secondary fibromyalgia: a double-blind study. Clin Exp Rheumatol 16.1 (1998): 106–107.

Thomas CS et al. The influence of *S*-adenosylmethionine (SAM) on prolactin in depressed patients. Int Clin Psychopharmacol 2.2 (1987): 97–102.

Thompson KJ et al *S*-adenosyl-L-methionine inhibits collagen secretion in hepatic stellate cells via increased ubiquitination. Liver International (2011): 893–903.

Tsao D et al Serotonin-induced hypersensitivity via inhibition of catechol *o*-methyltransferase activity. Molecular Pain 8.25 (2012).

van Winkel R et al. MTHFR and risk of metabolic syndrome in patients with schizophrenia. Schizophrenia Research 121 (2010): 193–198.

Vazquez-Elizondo G, Bosques-Padilla FJ. Concise review: alcoholic hepatitis. Ann Gastro Hep 3.1(2012): 121–130.

Vendemiale G et al. Effects of oral *S*-adenosyl-L-methionine on hepatic glutathione in patients with liver disease. Scand J Gastroenterol 24.4 (1989): 407–415.

Vetter G. Double-blind comparative clinical trial with *S*-adenosylmethionine and indomethacin in the treatment of osteoarthritis. Am J Med 83.5A (1987): 78–80.

Vincenzi B et al The role of *S*-adenosylmethionine in preventing oxaliplatin-induced liver toxicity: a retrospective analysis in metastatic colorectal cancer patients treated with bevacizumab plus oxaliplatin-based regimen. Support Care Cancer 20 (2012):135–139.

Volkmann H et al. Double-blind, placebo-controlled cross-over study of intravenous *S*-adenosyl-L-methionine in patients with fibromyalgia. Scand J Rheumatol 26.3 (1997): 206–211.

Wagner EJ et al Liposome dependent delivery of *S*-adenosyl methionine to cells by liposomes: a potential treatment for liver disease. J Pharm Sc 98.2 (2009) 573–82.

Wallace KP et al. *S*-adenosyl-L-methionine (SAMe)for the treatment of acetaminophen toxicity in a dog. J Am Anim Hosp Assoc 38 (2002):246–254.

Wortham M et al. The transition from fatty liver to NASH associates with SAMe depletion in db/db mice fed a methionine choline-deficient diet. Dig Dis Sci 53.10 (2008): 2761–2774.

Schisandra

HISTORICAL NOTE Schisandra has an extensive history of use in traditional Chinese medicine (TCM). It has sour and warm qualities and is used to treat spleen and kidney 'deficiency', to restore Qi and also as a treatment for chronic cough, wheezing, diabetes, insomnia and palpitations.

OTHER NAMES

Chinese magnolia vine, gomishi, sheng-mai-san, wuweizi

BOTANICAL NAME/FAMILY

Schisandra chinensis (family Schisandraceae)

PLANT PART USED

Fruit

CHEMICAL COMPONENTS

Dibenzocyclooctene lignans (schisandrins A–C, deoxyshisandrin, γ-schisandrin, schizandrols, schisantherins, pregomisin, gomisins A–C, E–G, J, K and N), triterpenoids (schinchinenins A–H, schinchinenlactones A–C, henrischinins A–C, schicagenins A–C), essential oil, malic, tartaric, nigranoic and citric acids, resins, pectin, vitamins A, C and E, niacin, beta carotene, sterols, tannins and several minerals (MG Kim et al 2010, Shi et al 2011, Song et al 2013, Waiwut et al 2011, Wei et al 2013).

MAIN ACTIONS

Studies have been conducted with schisandra and a number of its constituents in isolation, such as schisandrin B and gomisin A. Currently, most evidence is derived from in vitro and animal studies, as it has not been significantly investigated in clinical studies. Many studies have also been conducted on schisandra in combination with other herbs. It is difficult to determine the individual efficacy of schisandra in these cases, and further studies of schisandra in isolation are required.

Antioxidant

In vitro and in vivo tests have identified antioxidant activity (Y Chen et al 2008, Chiu et al 2011, Kim et al 2009, S Ko et al 2008, Leong et al 2012, Liu et al 2009, Meng et al 2008, Ohsugi et al 1999, Smejkal et al 2010, Steele et al 2013, M Wang et al 2008, Yan et al 2009). Seven lignans isolated from schisandra have demonstrated stronger antioxidant activity than vitamin E at the same concentrations, with schisanhenol exhibiting the strongest effects (Lu & Liu 1992). The essential oil from *Schisandra* berries has also demonstrated antioxidant activity (X Chen et al 2012, Liu et al 2012a, Ma et al 2012).

Protective effects against ethanol-induced oxidative stress have been demonstrated by schisandra extract in vitro (Chen et al 2010) and schisandrin B in vivo (Lam et al 2010). While an in vitro study found that schisandra did not protect against oxidative stress-induced lymphocyte DNA damage (Szeto et al 2011), the herb has demonstrated a protective effect against heat stress (KJ Kim et al 2012) and silica-induced lung damage (Li et al 2009) in rats via antioxidant mechanisms. It appears that several constituents also have indirect antioxidant activity and can increase hepatic and myocardial glutathione levels (Yim & Ko 1999).

An extract of schisandra and the isolated constituent schisandrin B have both demonstrated the ability to significantly decrease alanine aminotransferase and increase glutathione levels in CCL4-damaged liver in vivo (Chiu et al 2002). Schisandrins B and C protected rats against solar irradiation-induced oxidative damage to epithelial tissue (Lam et al 2011). Schisandrin B also demonstrated genoprotective activity in mice with cisplatin-induced oxidative stress (Giridharan et al 2012), and long-term supplementation with schisandrin B enhanced mitochondrial antioxidant capacity and functionality in ageing mice, suggesting schisandrin B may have potential as an antiageing therapy (KM Ko et al 2008).

Deoxyschisandrin protected human intestinal epithelial cells against oxidative stress-induced apoptosis (Gu et al 2010). Schisandra polysaccharides have demonstrated analgesic activity in vivo, which may be due to its antioxidant capacity (Ye et al 2013).

Hepatoprotective activity

Decreases hepatotoxic damage

In vitro and in vivo studies have identified hepatoprotective effects with schisandra against carbon tetrachloride toxicity (Cai et al 2010, Chang et al 2009, Cheng et al 2013, Chiu et al 2007, Ip et al 1995, Mak & Ko 1997, Y Xie et al 2010, Yan et al 2009, Zhu et al 1999, 2000) and mercuric chloride toxicity (Stacchiotti et al 2009). Research with schisandrin B suggests that it is the main constituent responsible for these beneficial effects (Chiu et al 2007, Ip et al 1995, Mak et al 1996, Pan et al 2002). Further investigation reveals that schisandrin B increases the efficiency of the hepatic glutathione antioxidant system, thereby inhibiting carbon tetrachloride-induced lipid peroxidation; however, additional mechanisms appear likely (Ip et al 1995). More recently, the whole extract of schisandra fruit was shown to induce glutathione S-transferases in vitro (EH Choi et al 2008). Several lignans have been found to induce expression of phase II detoxification enzymes in vitro, a factor believed to be important in the prevention of liver cancer (SB Lee et al 2009).

Protection against paracetamol-induced liver damage has been demonstrated in two animal models using gomisin A (Kim et al 2008, Yamada et al 1993). In one study, gomisin A inhibited not only the elevation of serum aminotransferase activity and hepatic lipoperoxide content, but also the appearance of histological changes such as degeneration and necrosis of hepatocytes (Yamada et al 1993). In 2003, protection against paracetamol-induced liver damage and D-galactosamine-induced liver damage was confirmed for a fractionated extract of *S. chinensis* in an experimental model (Nakagiri et al 2003).

The hepatoprotective effects of gomisin N and γ-schizandrin have been analysed in interleukin-1β (IL-1β)-treated rat hepatocytes. Gomisin N and γ-schizandrin suppressed genetic expression of nitric oxide synthase (NOS), and decreased the transcription of IL1β and inflammatory chemokines (Takimoto et al 2013).

Gomisin A protected against D-galactosamine-induced hepatotoxicity in vivo (Kim et al 2008). The latter also protected against carbon tetrachloride-induced liver fibrosis in rats (HY Kim et al 2011).

Schisandrin B decreased hepatic total cholesterol and triglyceride levels in hypercholesterolaemic mice (Pan et al 2008) and protected mouse hepatocytes against hypoxia/reoxygenation-induced apoptosis (Chiu et al 2009).

An extract of schisandra lignans protected against restraint-induced liver damage in mice. The hepatoprotective effect was potentially mediated via antioxidant mechanisms (Pu et al 2012).

IN COMBINATION

Shengmai San (comprised of *S. chinensis, Panax ginseng,* and *Ophiopogon japonicus*) reduced hepatic lipids and lipid peroxidation in rats fed a high-cholesterol diet (Yao et al 2008). Another herbal combination preparation (*S. chinensis, Vitis vinifera* and *Taraxacum officinale*) protected against D-galactosamine-induced hepatotoxicity in vivo (JW Kang et al 2012).

Liver regeneration

Two animal studies have demonstrated that oral administration of gomisin A, a lignan isolated from *S. chinensis*, accelerates liver regeneration after partial hepatectomy and hastens recovery of liver function (Kubo et al 1992, Takeda et al 1987). The mechanism for these effects is not fully elucidated; however, gomisin A increases ornithine decarboxylase activity, which is important during the early stages of regeneration and suppresses fibrosis proliferation.

Anti-inflammatory

Schisandrin inhibits nitric oxide (NO) production, prostaglandin E_2 release, cyclooxygenase-2, inducible iNOS and nuclear factor-kappaB (NF-κB) in vitro (Guo et al 2008). In vitro and in vivo studies have identified anti-inflammatory activity for gomisin A, gomisin J, wuweizi C (Yasukawa et al 1992), schisandrin B (Checker et al 2012), schisandrin C, gomisin N (Oh et al 2010), α-iso-cubebene (Choi et al 2009), α-iso-cubebenol (YJ Lee et al 2010) and schisandrin derivatives (Blunder et al 2010). Several lignans from schisandra, including gomisin N and schisandrol A, have shown potent inhibition of nuclear factor of activated T cells (NFAT) in vitro (Lee et al 2003). Excessive activation of NFAT has a significant role to play in autoimmune disease, but further study is needed to assess schisandra's usefulness in immunopathological disease states.

Aqueous extracts of schisandra inhibited lipopolysaccharide-induced lung inflammation in mice (Bae et al 2012), and demonstrated potent effects in a mast cell line (Kang et al 2006). The extracts were found to inhibit tumour necrosis factor alpha (TNF-α), IL-6, IL-1 and granulocyte-macrophage colony-stimulating factor production (Park et al 2011). These effects may be due to schisandra inhibiting the degradation of IkappaB and therefore the translocation and activation of NF-κB. This may indicate a potential role for schisandra in the treatment of allergy. Similarly, another study found that schisandrin decreased scratching behaviour by inhibiting the IgE-antigen complex in vivo (Lee et al 2007).

IN COMBINATION

A herbal combination containing schisandra (Jianpi Huoxue) was found to inhibit the liver cytokine secretion pathway in rats (Peng et al 2008).

Immunomodulatory

Animal studies have found schisandra to possess immune-modulating activity (D Ma et al 2009). In mice, α-iso-cubebenol isolated from schisandra protected against induced sepsis by increasing the bactericidal activity of phagocytes, attenuating inflammatory cytokine production and inhibiting leucocyte apoptosis (SK Lee et al 2012). An in vitro follow-up study suggested the immunomodulatory activity of α-iso-cubebenol was due to stimulated neutrophil activity, including calcium increase, degranulation and chemotactic migration via interaction with chemokine receptor CXCR2 (Jung et al 2013). Alpha-iso-cubebene has demonstrated similar activity in vitro (Y Lee et al 2009).

Administration of schisandra polysaccharides to cyclophosphamide-induced immunosuppressed mice resulted in improved parameters of immune function, including increased phagocytic activity of peritoneal macrophages, increased serum haemolysin (Yang et al 2008), increased organ weight of the thymus and spleen and increased splenocyte proliferation (Y Chen et al 2012).

Antidiabetic

Schisandra exhibits multiple mechanisms of relevance in diabetes.

In vitro studies indicate that schisandra possesses antidiabetic activity (Gao et al 2009, Lau et al 2008, S Park et al 2009). Various lignans have been found to improve basal glucose uptake of hepatic cells (HepG2) in vitro. In particular, gomisin N demonstrated a greater effect than rosiglitazone, which has been used as an antidiabetic drug (J Zhang et al 2010).

Moreover, in vivo studies show that schisandra extracts reduce blood glucose levels, improve lipid metabolism, increase liver glycogen content and attenuate diabetes-induced weight loss and polydipsia in alloxan-induced diabetic mice (Gao et al 2009, Xv et al 2008, Zhao et al 2013a). Aqueous extracts of schisandra reduced postprandial blood glucose levels in rats via inhibition of α-glucosidase and α-amylase, enzymes responsible for absorption of monosaccharides in the small intestine (Jo et al 2011).

A fraction containing schizandrin, gomisin A and angeloylgomisin H increased glucose disposal rates and enhanced hepatic insulin sensitivity in type 2 diabetic rats (Kwon et al 2011).

IN COMBINATION

A TCM formula containing *S. chinensis, Coptis chinensis, Psidium guajava* and *Morus alba* significantly decreased non-fasting blood glucose in insulin-resistant mice (Wang & Chiang 2012).

Antiobesity

Treatment with schisandra resulted in decreased weight gain and adiposity in obese rats fed a high-fat diet. In vitro results suggest this effect may be mediated by inhibition of adipogenesis and adipocyte differentiation (HJ Park et al 2012).

IN COMBINATION

Gyeongshingangjeehwan (GGEx), a product containing *S. chinensis*, *Liriope platyphylla, Platycodon grandiflorum* and *Ephedra sinica*, promoted weight loss in one study of obese rats (Shin et al 2010) and decreased food intake, weight and abdominal fat gain, circulating triglycerides and hepatic lipid accumulation in another (Jeong et al 2008).

Antiallergic

Schisandra has demonstrated various antiallergic effects, including inhibition of eosinophil recruitment to lung epithelial cells in vitro (Oh et al 2009) and reduced severity of atopic dermatitis in vivo (Kang & Shin 2012). An aqueous extract of schisandra inhibited β-hexosaminidase release and expression of IL-4, IL-13 and TNF-α mRNA and protein in immunoglobulin E-antigen complex-stimulated rat basophilic leukaemia cells (mucosal mast cell-type cells) (Chung et al 2012). It appears that schisandra ameliorates the production of reactive oxygen species that drives allergic inflammation.

In in vitro studies, gomisin N inhibited the production of prostaglandin D_2, leukotriene C_4, β-hexosaminidase, IL-6 and cyclooxygenase-2 in bone marrow-derived mast cells (Chae et al 2011) and schizandrin has been found to inhibit the production of thymic stromal lymphopoietin (TSLP) in human mast cell lines. TSLP plays a key role in allergic diseases such as asthma and atopic dermatitis (Moon et al 2012). In vivo, schizandrin demonstrated significant antiasthmatic activity via inhibition of airway eosinophil accumulation, reduction of IL-4, IL-5, interferon-γ and TNF-α levels in bronchoalveolar lavage fluid, reduced oxidative stress, and inhibition of goblet cell hyperplasia and inflammatory cell infiltration in lung tissue (MY Lee et al 2010).

IN COMBINATION

Antiasthmatic activity was demonstrated by Xiao Qing Long Tang, a preparation of eight herbs, including *S. chinensis* (Wang et al 2012).

Nephroprotective

Schisandra significantly decreased the urine albumin excretion rate and urinary albumin/creatinine ratio, attenuated glomerulosclerosis and protected against podocyte loss in a mouse model of diabetic nephropathy (Zhang et al 2012).

In vitro pretreatment with schisandrin B protected against cyclosporin A-induced nephrotoxicity in mice and human proximal tubular epithelial cell line via antioxidant effects (Zhu et al 2012), and in vivo schisandrin B was also found to protect against mercuric chloride-induced (Stacchiotti et al 2011) and gentamicin-induced (Chiu et al 2008a) nephrotoxicity in rats.

Schizandrin significantly attenuated high-glucose-induced murine mesangial cell (MMC) damage by reducing the proliferation and protein synthesis of MMCs, reducing production of reactive oxygen species and inhibiting the activity of NADPH oxidase. These results suggest that it may be useful in the treatment of diabetic nephropathy (Jeong et al 2012).

Cardiovascular effects

Schisandrin B demonstrated protective effects against ischaemia–reperfusion-induced myocardial damage in animal models (Chiu et al 2008b, Yim & Ko 1999). The myocardial protection was associated with an enhancement in myocardial glutathione antioxidant status. Schisandrin B has also been found to inhibit signalling of transforming growth factor-β_1 (TGF-β_1) in vascular smooth-muscle cells (EJ Park et al 2012). TGF-β_1 is implicated in the pathogenesis of a number of vascular disease processes, including hypertension, atherosclerosis and restenosis. Schisandrin B stereoisomers protected rat cardiomyocytes against hypoxia/reoxygenation-induced apoptosis.

The whole extract, deoxyschizandrin, schisantherin A and gomisin A, has demonstrated vasorelaxant properties in isolated rat thoracic aorta, suggesting cardioprotective effects (JY Park et al 2007, J Park et al 2009a, Rhyu et al 2006, Seok et al 2011, X Yang et al 2011). An aqueous schisandra extract restored endothelial function in rats that underwent balloon-induced carotid artery injury. Similar to oestradiol therapy, it also reduced serum cholesterol levels and exhibited hypotensive effects in ovariectomised rats (EY Kim et al 2011).

Gomisin J (J Park et al 2012a) and gomisin A (J Park et al 2009b) have demonstrated vasorelaxant effects in vitro via increased activation of calcium-dependent endothelial NOS and subsequent production of endothelial NO. Administration of gomisin A to hypertensive mice ameliorated the increase in blood pressure and reactive oxygen species production, and decrease in aortic vascular NO and phosphorylated endothelial NOS induced by treatment with angiotensin II (J Park et al 2012b).

IN COMBINATION

A Cochrane review of nine randomised controlled trials assessed the use of Shengmai (a TCM combination of *Panax ginseng, Ophiopogon japonicus* and *S. chinensis*) in patients with heart failure. While issues of poor study design, small sample size and heterogeneity of particular outcomes were cited, there was some evidence to show that Shengmai may improve heart function in patients with heart failure (Chen et al 2012).

Antitumour

Extracts of schisandra and several isolated constituents have demonstrated anti-cancer activity against various cancer lines, including leukaemia, breast, liver, gastric, colon and lung in vitro (Gnabre et al 2010, Hwang et al 2011, Jie et al 2009, JH Kim et al 2010, JE Kim et al 2012, SJ Kim et al 2010, Lin et al 2008, 2011, Min et al 2008, Nishida et al 2009, C Park et al 2009, Waiwut et al 2012, Yim et al 2009, Yuezhen 2010, Zhao et al 2013b). Several schisandra lignans have been found to inhibit fatty acid synthase, a potential oncogenic enzyme (Na et al 2010). Gomisins J and N inhibited Wnt/β-catenin signalling in human colon carcinoma cells. The Wnt/β-catenin signalling pathway is involved in regulating cell growth and apoptosis, and has been implicated in the aetiology and progression of various forms of cancer (K Kang et al 2012).

Gomisin N was found to enhance apoptosis induced by TNF-α (Waiwut et al 2011) and TNF-related apoptosis-inducing ligand (TRAIL) (Inoue et al 2012) in vitro. A schisandra polysaccharide, WSLSCP, significantly inhibited the proliferation of lymphoma cells, increased secretion level of serum TNF-α, and improved survival rate of lymphoma-bearing mice. WSLSCP was also found to enhance phagocytic activity and NO and TNF-α secretion of macrophages in vitro (C Xu et al 2012). Another isolated schisandra polysaccharide (SCPP11) exhibited indirect cytotoxic activity against tumour cells in vitro, and significantly inhibited the growth of hepatic tumour cells (HepS) in vivo. SCPP11 also increased thymus indexes, serum IL-2 and TNF-α levels in vivo, and significantly enhanced NO production and phagocytosis in mouse macrophage-like cell lines in vitro (Zhao et al 2013b). These results suggest that schisandra's immunomodulatory activity may contribute to its antitumour effects.

Other constituents of the herb, such as deoxyschizandrin and γ-schizandrin, restored the cytotoxic action of the chemotherapy drug doxorubicin in multidrug-resistant human lung carcinoma cell lines. They also enhanced cellular accumulation of doxorubicin, and induced cell cycle arrest when combined with subtoxic doses of doxorubicin (Slaninova et al 2009).

Schisandra has been found to inhibit the proliferation of cancer cells in rodents with induced hepatocellular carcinoma (He et al 2010, Loo et al 2007). An extract of schisandra lignans inhibited hepatic metastases of mastocytoma tumour cells in mice (Tang et al 2011).

An isolated compound from schisandra (1-O-MFF) inhibited melanogenic processes in mouse melanoma cells (Oh et al 2010), and gomisin A has been found to inhibit skin cancer formation in mice (Yasukawa et al 2009).

IN COMBINATION

Shu Gan Liang Xue decoction, a TCM product that contains schisandra and is often used in menopause, inhibited the growth of human mammary epithelial carcinoma cell line, but did not display any oestrogenic activity (Zhang & Li 2009).

Neuroprotective

In vitro data suggest that certain lignans from schisandra (Kim et al 2004) are protective against L-glutamate-induced neurotoxicity in rat cortical cells. Schisandrin C has been shown to decrease the membrane action potential in glioma and neuronal cells lines (Y Choi et al 2008). Schisandrin has demonstrated neurogenic activity in rat hippocampal neurons (SH Yang et al 2011). and demonstrated the ability to reverse hyoscine-induced memory impairment in vivo by enhancing cholinergic function (Egashira et al 2008). Extracts of schisandra ameliorated the depressed hippocampal acetylcholinesterase activity and behavioural learning impairments seen in ovariectomised mice (X Xie et al 2010).

Schizandrin (N Zhang et al 2010) and schisandrin B (Zeng et al 2012) have been found to inhibit lipopolysaccharide-induced microglia activation and significantly ameliorate neuronal cell death in vitro and in vivo via inhibition of the microglial-mediated neurotoxic inflammatory response. Microglia activation is implicated in the pathophysiology of Alzheimer's and Parkinson's disease.

Extracts of schisandra (M Miao et al 2009, Y Miao et al 2009) and schisandrin B (N Chen et al 2008) have been shown to improve the outcome in cerebral ischaemia/reperfusion models in vivo. Schisandrin B protected against damage by enhancing the cerebral antioxidant status. Schisandrin B also exhibited significant neuroprotective effects in a rat model of transient focal cerebral ischaemia. Schisandrin B demonstrated inhibition of TNF-α and IL-1β, and decreased expression of matrix metalloproteinases-2 and -9, all of which are involved in microglial activation after ischaemic events (TH Lee et al 2012).

Schisandrin B appears to improve cognition and hepatic functions in mice treated with tacrine, the common Alzheimer's dementia medication (Pan et al 2002). Pretreatment with schisandrin B prevented scopolamine-induced oxidative stress and impairment of learning and memory in vivo. Schisandrin B was found to ameliorate the scopolamine-induced increase in acetylcholinesterase activity, and maintain normal acetylcholine levels (Giridharan et al 2011). Similarly, schisandrin was found to prevent dexamethasone-induced cognitive deficits in vitro and in vivo (X Xu et al 2012).

Schisandrins B and C reversed beta amyloid (Aβ) and homocysteine-induced neurotoxicity in vitro (Song et al 2011). Both deoxyschisandrin (Hu et al 2012) and ESP-806, a lignan-rich extract of schisandra (Jeong et al 2013), significantly ameliorated Aβ-induced memory impairment in mice. Deoxyschisandrin acted via antioxidative mechanisms, while ESP-806 attenuated the elevation of β-secretase activity, significantly inhibited hippocampal acetylcholinesterase activity and increased levels of reduced glutathione in the cortex and hippocampus. Deoxyschisandrin has also been found to inhibit the spontaneous and synchronous oscillations of intracellular Ca^{2+} in hippocampal neurons by depressing influx of extracellular calcium, and inhibiting spontaneous neurotransmitter release, suggesting deoxyschisandrin may be of benefit in regulating the excitability of neural networks (Fu et al 2008).

IN COMBINATION

A combined extract of *Schisandra chinensis, Angelica gigas* and *Saururus chinensis* is protective against L-glutamate-induced neurotoxicity in rat cortical cells (CJ Ma et al 2009). AdMax (Nulab, Florida), a product containing *Schisandra chinensis, Leuzea carthamoides, Rhodiola rosea* and *Eleutherococcus senticosus*, has been found to enhance expression of PANK2, which encodes the mitochondrial enzyme pantothenate kinase 2. Impaired PANK2 gene activity leads to pantothenate kinase-associated neurodegeneration (Antoshechkin et al 2008).

Gastrointestinal actions

Schisandra has demonstrated gastrointestinal antispasmodic activity in isolated rat colon (J Yang et al 2011a). Schisandra was also found to reverse visceral hypersensitivity in an irritable bowel syndrome rat model. The observed normalisation of elevated serotonin (5-HT) levels and a decline in the mRNA level of 5-HT receptors in the distal colon suggest the effect may be mediated via the colonic 5-HT pathway (Yang et al 2012). Extracts of schisandra inhibited acetylcholine- and 5-HT-induced contractions of guinea pig ileum, potentially via inhibition of both calcium ion influx and intracellular calcium ion mobilisation (J Yang et al 2011b).

Antibacterial

Schisandra has demonstrated bactericidal activity against *Staphylococcus epidermidis, S. aureus, Bacillus subtilis, Escherichia coli, Pseudomonas aeruginosa, Proteus vulgaris* (X Chen et al 2011, Wang 2008), *Bacillus anthracis, Shigella* (Wen-qiang 2009) and *Salmonella gallinarum* (Choi & Chang 2009).

OTHER ACTIONS

Lipid lowering

Schisandra may also help to reduce cholesterol, as it has been found to decrease triglycerides and low-density lipoprotein, and increase high-density lipoprotein cholesterol in vivo (Junshu & Anshan 2008). Schisandrin B (50–200 mg/kg) was coadministered with either a high-lipid diet or a cholesterol/bile salts mixture in vivo (Pan et al 2008). Hepatic total cholesterol and triglyceride levels were reduced by up to 50% and 52%, respectively, as compared to control animals. Similar results were found using an ethanol extract of schisandra (Pan 2011).

Improved erectile function

Corporeal smooth-muscle (CSM) relaxation is required for penile erection. Several schisandra lignans were found to induce CSM relaxation via inhibition of calcium ion influx (Han et al 2012). Schisandrol A, schisandrol B and an ethanol extract of schisandra were found to potentiate sildenafil citrate-induced relaxation of rabbit penile corpus cavernosum. Clinical studies are required to determine whether schisandra has a therapeutic role in patients with a poor response to sildenafil alone (HK Kim et al 2011).

IN COMBINATION

A combination of *Schisandra chinensis, Lycium chinense, Cornus officinalis, Rubus coreanus* and *Cuscuta chinensis* improved intracavernous pressure of corpus cavernosum in spontaneous hypertensive rats (Sohn et al 2008).

Anxiolytic and sedative

Schisandra has demonstrated sedative and hypnotic activity in mice, reducing sleep latency and prolonging sleep time (W Wang et al 2008a). Schisandra was found to decrease behavioural signs of anxiety in stressed mice, and ameliorated elevations in cerebral cortex noradrenaline, dopamine and 5-HT and plasma corticosterone levels (W Chen et al 2011). It is possible the anxiolytic effect is mediated by modulation of the hypothalamic-pituitary-adrenal axis activity.

Inhibits leukotriene formation

Various schisandra lignans decrease leukotriene production via inhibition of 5-lipoxygenase activity in vitro (Lim et al 2009). Gomisin A has been found to inhibit the biosynthesis of leukotrienes by preventing the release of arachidonic acid in vitro (Ohkura et al 1990).

Platelet-activating factor antagonist

Several lignans inhibit platelet-activating factor in vitro (Lee et al 1999). Pregomisin and gomisin N have demonstrated more potent inhibition of platelet-activating factor than aspirin (MG Kim et al 2010).

Enhanced exercise endurance

Schisandra (Cao et al 2009, W Wang et al 2008b) and ADAPT-232 (a standardised combination of *S. chinensis, Rhodiola rosea* and *Eleutherococcus senticosus*) (Panossian et al 2009) have been found to increase exercise endurance in mice.

Bone mineralisation

Lignans isolated from the fruit and seeds of schisandra may be able to protect against bone loss. An in vitro study using UMR 106 cells demonstrated that the lignans (extracted in 95% ethanol) stimulated the proliferation and activity of alkaline phosphatase in osteoblasts (Caichompoo et al 2009).

Cytochromes and P-glycoprotein

Schisandra extract and different isolated compounds have been tested for the effects of various cytochromes and P-glycoprotein in in vitro and animal model studies.

Cytochrome 3A4

In vitro evidence indicates that schisandrol A and gomisin A are inhibitors of CYP 3A4 (Wan et al 2010). Conflicting in vivo evidence has found schisandra to have both inhibitory and inducing effects on CYP 3A4 activity (Q Chen et al 2010, Iwata et al 2004, Li et al 2013, Su et al 2013, Wang et al 2011). In addition, schisandra has been found to increase the activation of the pregnane X receptor (PXR) signalling pathway. PXR is a transcription factor that, when activated, binds to the promoter region of CYP3A4 gene, resulting in increased CYP3A4 transcription (Yu et al 2011). The discrepancy between results from animal studies appears to be dependent on the duration of administration. Short-term treatment with schisandra (single dose) had an inhibitory effect on CYP 3A4, while longer-term treatment (6–14 consecutive days) resulted in induction of CYP 3A4 (Lai et al 2009, Yao et al 2011). Clinical studies are not available to clarify the effect of *S. chinensis* on CYP 3A4 in humans. One case study found that administration of deoxyschisandrin (22.5 mg after meals for 3 days) resulted in an increase of blood tacrolimus (a P-glycoprotein and CYP 3A4 substrate) concentration from 2.3 ng/mL to 17.7 ng/mL (Jiang et al 2010a). It was not clear whether the increased tacrolimus concentration was due to inhibition of P-glycoprotein, CYP 3A4, or a combination. Small-scale human studies have found that oral administration of *Schisandra sphenanthera* for 7–14 days resulted in increased area under the curve for tacrolimus (Jiang et al 2010b, Xin et al 2007) and midazolam (Xin et al 2009). Considering the two species share many of the same constituents (including deoxyschisandrin and schisandrin B), it is possible that *S. chinensis* may have the same effect.

It has been suggested that discrepancies between human and animal studies are due to lower mg/kg doses of schisandra in humans than animals, and the fact that gomisin C concentrations necessary for PXR activation in humans are twice those required for murine species (Gurley et al 2012). A 2012 review suggests that, based upon the human studies of *Schisandra sphenanthera*, *S. chinensis* is likely to have an inhibitory effect on CYP 3A4 in humans, and the potential for herb–drug interactions between schisandra extracts and drugs that are CYP 3A4 substrates is high (Gurley et al 2012).

P-glycoprotein

Various lignans from schisandra, including schisandrol A, gomisin A, schisandrin A and B and schisandrin B have demonstrated an inhibitory effect on P-glycoprotein in vitro (Fong et al 2007, Pan et al 2006, Qiangrong et al 2005, Wan et al 2006, Yoo et al 2007). Pretreatment with schisandrol B significantly increased the oral bioavailability of paclitaxel (a drug with notoriously poor oral bioavailability) in rodents, potentially via enhanced intestinal absorption due to inhibition of P-glycoprotein (Jin et al 2010). In vitro studies indicate that inhibition of P-glycoprotein by schisandra lignans can reverse multidrug resistance in cancer cells (Huang et al 2008); however clinical studies are required to confirm this.

In a small clinical trial ($n = 12$), pretreatment with schisandra extract (300 mg twice daily for 14 days) followed by a single dose of talinolol (100 mg) resulted in increased area under the curve and C_{max} of talinolol by 47% and 51% respectively, suggesting P-glycoprotein activity was inhibited (Fan et al 2009).

CLINICAL USE

While schisandra has not been extensively tested in clinical trials, it has been tested in numerous animal models and displays multiple mechanisms of action, thereby providing biological plausibility for some of its uses. It is often prescribed in combination with other herbal medicines, a factor which accounts for its investigation as part of multi-component treatments in some studies.

Liver damage, hepatoprotection

Traditionally, schisandra has been used to treat a variety of liver disorders. Hepatoprotective effects have been observed in test tube and animal studies; however, the clinical significance of these findings in humans remains unknown. Several encouraging clinical reports using an analogue of schisandrin C are available; however, it is not known whether these effects will be seen with *S. chinensis* (Akbar et al 1998). A pilot clinical study in 10 healthy subjects has evaluated the effects of schisandra and sesamin (a constituent of sesame oil) on blood fluidity due to the link between blood viscosity and liver dysfunction (Tsi & Tan 2008). The mixture was given for 1 week and blood fluidity was tested over 2 weeks, including 1 week postintervention. Blood passage time was reduced by 9.0% and 9.7% at 1 and 2 weeks, respectively, showing that the effect could be sustained for at least 1 week after cessation of treatment. The exact effects of schisandra in this formula are unknown.

Adaptogen

In TCM, schisandra is viewed as an adaptogen and prescribed with other herbs to increase resistance to physical and emotional stressors and to improve allostasis (see monograph on Siberian ginseng for further information about adaptogenic activity and allostasis).

IN COMBINATION

A randomised, double-blind, placebo-controlled pilot study assessed the effect of a single dose (270 mg) of ADAPT-232 (a standardised combination of *S. chinensis, Rhodiola rosea* and *Eleutherococcus senticosus*) on cognitive function in 40 healthy females aged 20–68 years. At 2 hours posttreatment, the treatment group demonstrated improvements in attention and increased speed and accuracy when performing stressful cognitive tasks compared to controls (Aslanyan et al 2010).

In a randomised, double-blind, placebo-controlled study, 30 subjects were assigned to three groups of 10: placebo group, *Rhodiola rosea* group (providing 144 mg SHR-5 extract twice daily) and ADAPT-232 group (140 mg of standardised combination twice daily) for 7 days. Experienced levels of fatigue significantly decreased in the *R. rosea* group but not in the ADAPT-232 group compared to placebo (Schutgens et al 2009).

Infection

Schisandra is also used in combination with other herbal medicines to treat infection. One double-blind, randomised, placebo-controlled pilot study found that a commercial product known as ImmunoGuard significantly reduced the duration, frequency and severity of attacks in patients with familial Mediterranean fever (Amaryan et al 2003). The dose regimen used was four tablets taken three times daily for 1 month. The ImmunoGuard product contains a fixed combination of *Andrographis paniculata* Nees., *Eleutherococcus senticosus* Maxim., *Schisandra chinensis* Bail. and *Glycyrrhiza glabra* L. special extracts, which are standardised for the content of andrographolide (4 mg/tablet), eleutheroside E, schisandrins and glycyrrhizin, respectively. Although these results are encouraging, it is not known to what extent schisandra contributed to the outcome.

A double-blind, placebo-controlled, randomised pilot study investigated the effects of another preparation known as Chisan (containing schisandra 51.0%, rhodiola 27.6% and Siberian ginseng 24.4%) on recovery time and quality-of-life scores in patients with acute non-specific pneumonia (Narimanian et al 2005). Sixty participants were randomised to receive the standard treatment of cephazoline, bromhexine and theophylline or the standard treatment plus the herbal mixture (20 mL twice a day standardised to contain schisandrin 0.177 mg/mL and gamma-schisandrin 0.105 mg/mL) for 10–15 days. Participants in the active group reported significant improvements in recovery time and quality-of-life scores. The requirement for antibiotics was on average 2 days shorter for those participants taking Chisan. All of these herbs have been celebrated for their adaptogenic effects and this may, at least in part, be responsible for the results. The individual effects of schisandra in this formula, however, are unknown.

OTHER USES

Traditionally, schisandra has been used to treat chronic cough and dyspnoea, diarrhoea, night sweats, irritability, palpitations and insomnia. Based on the herb's inhibitory effects on leukotriene biosynthesis and platelet-activating factor activity and anti-inflammatory effects, it is also used for asthmatic symptoms.

DOSAGE RANGE

As clinical research is lacking, the following dosages come from Australian manufacturers' recommendations.

- Dried fruit: 1.5–6 g/day.
- Liquid extract (1:2): 3.5–8.5 mL/day or 25–60 mL/week.

TOXICITY

Insufficient reliable information is available.

ADVERSE REACTIONS

Mild gastrointestinal discomfort

SIGNIFICANT INTERACTIONS

CYP3A4 substrates

Increased serum levels of drugs chiefly metabolised by CYP 3A4 are possible, based on current evidence. Practitioners are advised to carefully monitor patients who are already taking drugs that are CYP3A4 substrates to avoid inducing drug side effects caused by increased serum levels.

Schisandra should not be prescribed together with CYP3A4 substrates that have a narrow therapeutic index in order to avoid inducing drug toxicity.

P-glycoprotein substrates

Based on current evidence, it appears that P-glycoprotein inhibition is possible. As a result, serum levels of P-glycoprotein substrates could be increased. Practitioners are advised to carefully monitor patients who are already taking drugs that are P-glycoprotein substrates to avoid inducing drug side effects caused by increased serum levels.

Schisandra should not be prescribed together with P-glycoprotein substrates that have a narrow therapeutic index in order to avoid inducing drug toxicity.

Drugs metabolised by UGT1A3

Deoxyschizandrin and schisantherin A have demonstrated an inhibitory effect on UDP-glucuronosyltransferase 1A3 (UGT1A3) in vitro. This suggests a potential for herb–drug interactions between schisandra and drugs that mainly undergo UGT1A3-mediated metabolism; however the effect has not been confirmed clinically (Liu et al 2012b).

CONTRAINDICATIONS AND PRECAUTIONS

Insufficient reliable information is available.

PREGNANCY USE

Insufficient information is available to establish safety.

Practice points/Patient counselling

- *S. chinensis* is popular in TCM and is used to increase resistance to physical and emotional stressors and is regarded as an adaptogen.
- Traditionally, schisandra has been used to treat chronic cough and dyspnoea, diarrhoea, night sweats, irritability, palpitations and insomnia.
- It is commonly used as a liver tonic, and preliminary evidence has identified significant hepatoprotective effects.
- Schisandra exerts direct antioxidant activity and increases hepatic and myocardial glutathione levels, thereby increasing antioxidant systems within the heart and liver.
- Overall, little clinical evidence is available; therefore, much information is still speculative and based on in vitro and animal research and traditional use.

PATIENTS' FAQs

What will this herb do for me?

Schisandra is often prescribed to increase physical and emotional resilience and as a liver tonic. It has antioxidant activity, and early research suggests that it may have significant protective benefits for the liver.

When will it start to work?

This is uncertain due to insufficient research being available.

Are there any safety issues?

This is uncertain due to insufficient research being available.

REFERENCES

Akbar N et al. Effectiveness of the analogue of natural Schisandrin C (HpPro) in treatment of liver diseases: an experience in Indonesian patients. Chin Med J (Engl) 111.3 (1998): 248–251.

Amaryan G et al. Double-blind, placebo-controlled, randomized, pilot clinical trial of ImmunoGuard: a standardized fixed combination of *Andrographis paniculata* Nees, with *Eleutherococcus senticosus* Maxim, *Schizandra chinensis* Bail. and *Glycyrrhiza glabra* L. extracts in patients with familial Mediterranean fever. Phytomedicine 10.4 (2003): 271–285.

Antoshechkin A et al. Influence of the plant extract complex "AdMax" on global gene expression levels in cultured human fibroblasts. Journal of Dietary Supplements 5.3 (2008): 293–304.

Aslanyan G et al. Double-blind, placebo-controlled, randomised study of single dose effects of ADAPT-232 on cognitive functions. Phytomedicine 17.7 (2010): 494–9.

Bae H et al. Effects of *Schisandra chinensis* Baillon (Schizandraceae) on lipopolysaccharide induced lung inflammation in mice. Journal of Ethnopharmacology 142.1 (2012): 41–7.

Blunder M et al. Derivatives of schisandrin with increased inhibitory potential on prostaglandin E2 and leukotriene B4 formation in vitro. Bioorganic & Medicinal Chemistry 18.7 (2010): 2809–15.

Cai S et al. Protective effect of schisandrins extract on liver ultrastructure in rats with CCl_4 poisoning. Carcinogenesis, Teratogenesis & Mutagenesis 1.13 (2010).

Caichompoo W et al. Optimization of extraction and purification of active fractions from *Schisandra chinensis* (Turcz.) and its osteoblastic proliferation stimulating activity. Phytother Res 23.2 (2009). 289–292.

Cao S et al. Evaluation of anti-athletic fatigue activity of *Schizandra chinensis* aqueous extracts in mice. African Journal of Pharmacy and Pharmacology 3.11 (2009): 593–7.

Chae HS et al. Gomisin N has anti-allergic effect and inhibits inflammatory cytokine expression in mouse bone marrow-derived mast cells. Immunopharmacology and immunotoxicology 33.4 (2011): 709–13.

Chang C et al. Effect of schisandrin B and sesamin mixture on CCl4-induced hepatic oxidative stress in rats. Phytotherapy Research 23.2 (2009): 251–6.

Checker R et al. Schisandrin B exhibits anti-inflammatory activity through modulation of the redox-sensitive transcription factors Nrf2 and NF-ŒʃB. Free Radical Biology and Medicine 53.7 (2012): 1421–30.

Chen N, et al. Schisandrin B enhances cerebral mitochondrial antioxidant status and structural integrity, and protects against cerebral ischemia/reperfusion injury in rats. Biol Pharm Bull 31.7 (2008): 1387–1391.

Chen Y et al. Effects of Chinese herb medicine on performance, immune function and anti-oxidant capacity of broiler. Acta Ecologiae Animalis Domastici 4.16 (2008).

Chen ML et al. Biochemical mechanism of Wu-Zi-Yan-Zong-Wan, a traditional Chinese herbal formula, against alcohol-induced oxidative damage in CYP2E1 cDNA-transfected HepG2 (E47) cells. Journal Of Ethnopharmacology 128.1 (2010): 116–122.

Chen Q et al. Dual effects of extract of *Schisandra chinensis* Baill on rat hepatic CYP3A. Acta Pharmaceutica Sinica 45.9 (2010): 1194–8.

Chen W et al. Pharmacological studies on the anxiolytic effect of standardized schisandra lignans extract on restraint-stressed mice. Phytomedicine 18.13 (2011): 1144–7.

Chen X et al. Composition and biological activities of the essential oil from *Schisandra chinensis* obtained by solvent-free microwave extraction. LWT - Food Science and Technology 44.10 (2011): 2047–52.

Chen X et al. Chemical composition and antioxidant activity of the essential oil of *Schisandra chinensis* fruits. Natural Product Research 26.9 (2012): 842–9.

Chen Y et al. An immunostimulatory polysaccharide (SCP-IIa) from the fruit of *Schisandra chinensis* (Turcz.) Baill. International Journal of Biological Macromolecules. 50.3 (2012): 844–8.

Cheng N et al. Antioxidant and hepatoprotective effects of *Schisandra chinensis* pollen extract on CCl4-induced acute liver damage in mice. Food and Chemical Toxicology 55.0 (2013): 234–40.

Chiu PY et al. In vivo antioxidant action of a lignan-enriched extract of Schisandra fruit and an anthraquinone-containing extract of Polygonum root in comparison with schisandrin B and emodin. Planta Med 68.11 (2002): 951–956.

Chiu PY et al. Schisandrin B decreases the sensitivity of mitochondria to calcium ion-induced permeability transition and protects against carbon tetrachloride toxicity in mouse livers. Biol Pharm Bull 30.6 (2007): 1108–1112.

Chiu P et al. Schisandrin B enhances renal mitochondrial antioxidant status, functional and structural integrity, and protects against gentamicin-induced nephrotoxicity in rats. Biological & Pharmaceutical Bulletin 31.4 (2008a): 602–5.

Chiu P et al. Schisandrin B stereoisomers protect against hypoxia/reoxygenation-induced apoptosis and inhibit associated changes in Ca^{2+}-induced mitochondrial permeability transition and mitochondrial membrane potential in H9c2 cardiomyocytes. Life Sciences 82.21 (2008b): 1092–1101.

Chiu P et al. Schisandrin B stereoisomers protect against hypoxia/reoxygenation-induced apoptosis and associated changes in the Ca^{2+}-induced mitochondrial permeability transition and mitochondrial membrane potential in AML12 hepatocytes. Phytotherapy Research 23.11(2009): 1592–602.

Chiu P et al. Schisandrin B elicits a glutathione antioxidant response and protects against apoptosis via the redox-sensitive ERK/Nrf2 pathway in H9c2 cells. Molecular And Cellular Biochemistry 350.1–2 (2011): 237–50.

Choi I & Chang H. Antimicrobial activity of medicinal herbs against *Salmonella gallinarum* and Staphylococcus epidermidis. Korean Journal of Poultry Science 36.3 (2009): 231–8.

Choi EH et al. *Schisandra fructus* extract ameliorates doxorubicin-induced cytotoxicity in cardiomyocytes: altered gene expression for detoxification enzymes. Genes Nutr 2.4 (2008): 337–345.

Choi Y et al. Wuweizisu C from *Schisandra chinensis* decreases membrane potential in C6 glioma cells. Acta Pharmacologica Sinica 29.9 (2008): 1006–12.

Choi Y et al. Inhibition of endothelial cell adhesion by the new anti-inflammatory agent alpha-iso-cubebene. Vascular Pharmacology 51.4 (2009): 215–24.

Chung MJ et al. Suppressive effects of *Schizandra chinensis* Baillon water extract on allergy-related cytokine generation and degranulation in IgE-antigen complex-stimulated RBL-2H3 cells. Nutrition Research And Practice 6.2 (2012): 97–105.

Egashira N et al. Schizandrin reverses memory impairment in rats. Phytother Res 22.1 (2008): 49–52.

Fan L et al. Effect of *Schisandra chinensis* extract and Ginkgo biloba extract on the pharmacokinetics of talinolol in healthy volunteers. Xenobiotica; The Fate Of Foreign Compounds In Biological Systems 39.3 (2009): 249–54.

Fong WF et al. Schisandrol A from *Schisandra chinensis* reverses P-glycoprotein-mediated multidrug resistance by affecting Pgp-substrate complexes. Planta Med 73.3 (2007): 212–220.

Fu M et al. Deoxyschisandrin modulates synchronized Ca^{2+} oscillations and spontaneous synaptic transmission of cultured hippocampal neurons. Acta Pharmacologica Sinica 29.8 (2008): 891–8.

Gao X et al. Isolation, characterization and hypoglycemic activity of an acid polysaccharide isolated from *Schisandra chinensis* (Turcz.) Baill. Letters in Organic Chemistry 6.5 (2009): 428–33.

Giridharan VV et al. Prevention of scopolamine-induced memory deficits by schisandrin B, an antioxidant lignan from *Schisandra chinensis* in mice. Free Radical Research 45.8 (2011): 950–8.

Giridharan VV et al. Schisandrin B, attenuates cisplatin-induced oxidative stress, genotoxicity and neurotoxicity through modulating NF-κB pathway in mice. Free Radical Research 46.1 (2012): 50–60.

Gnabre J et al. Isolation of lignans from *Schisandra chinensis* with anti-proliferative activity in human colorectal carcinoma: Structure-activity relationships. Journal Of Chromatography. B, Analytical Technologies In The Biomedical And Life Sciences 878.28 (2010): 2693–700.

Gu BH et al. Deoxyschisandrin inhibits H2O2-induced apoptotic cell death in intestinal epithelial cells through nuclear factor-kappaB. International Journal Of Molecular Medicine 26.3 (2010): 401–6.

Guo LY et al. Anti-inflammatory effects of schisandrin isolated from the fruit of *Schisandra chinensis* Baill. Eur J Pharmacol 591.1–3 (2008): 293–299.

Gurley B, et al. Pharmacokinetic herb-drug interactions (part 2): drug interactions involving popular botanical dietary supplements and their clinical relevance. Planta Medica 78.13 (2012): 1490–514.

Han DH et al. Effects of *Schisandra chinensis* extract on the contractility of corpus cavernosal smooth muscle (CSM) and Ca^{2+} homeostasis in CSM cells. BJU International 109.9 (2012): 1404–13.

He Y, et al. The inhibit effect of *Fructus schizandrae* polysaccharide on the growth of tumor in mice with hepatocellular carcinoma and the primarily exploring on immunological mechanism. Information on Traditional Chinese Medicine 2.12. (2010).

Hu D et al. Deoxyschizandrin isolated from the fruits of *Schisandra chinensis* ameliorates AB1-42-induced memory impairment in mice. Planta Medica 78.12 (2012): 1332–6.

Huang M et al. Reversal of P-glycoprotein-mediated multidrug resistance of cancer cells by five schizandrins isolated from the Chinese herb *Fructus schizandrae*. Cancer chemotherapy and pharmacology 62.6 (2008): 1015–26.

Hwang D et al. A compound isolated from *Schisandra chinensis* induces apoptosis. Bioorganic & Medicinal Chemistry Letters 21.20 (2011): 6054–7.

Inoue H et al. Gomisin N enhances TRAIL-induced apoptosis via reactive oxygen species-mediated up-regulation of death receptors 4 and 5. International Journal Of Oncology 40.4 (2012): 1058–65.

Ip SP et al. Effect of schisandrin B on hepatic glutathione antioxidant system in mice: protection against carbon tetrachloride toxicity. Planta Med 61.5 (1995): 398–401.

Iwata H et al. Identification and characterization of potent CYP3A4 inhibitors in Schisandra fruit extract. Drug Metab Dispos 32.12 (2004): 1351–1358.

Jeong S et al. The Korean traditional medicine Gyeongshingangjeehwan inhibits obesity through the regulation of leptin and PPARα action in OLETF rats. Journal Of Ethnopharmacology 119.2 (2008): 245–51.

Jeong SI et al. Schizandrin prevents damage of murine mesangial cells via blocking NADPH oxidase-induced ROS signaling in high glucose. Food and Chemical Toxicology 50.3–4 (2012): 1045–53.

Jeong EJ et al. The effects of lignan-riched extract of *Schisandra chinensis* on amyloid-B-induced cognitive impairment and neurotoxicity in the cortex and hippocampus of mouse. Journal Of Ethnopharmacology 146.1 (2013): 347–54.

Jiang W, et al. The effect of deoxyschisandrin on blood tacrolimus levels: a case report. Immunopharmacology and immunotoxicology 32.1 (2010a): 177–8.

Jiang W et al. Effect of *Schisandra sphenanthera* extract on the concentration of tacrolimus in the blood of liver transplant patients. International Journal Of Clinical Pharmacology And Therapeutics 48.3 (2010b): 224.

Jie Y et al. Experimental study on isolation and purification of total lignans from *Schisandra chinensis* and the antitumor activity in vitro. China Pharmacist 12.18 (2009).

S

Jin J et al. Enhancement of oral bioavailability of paclitaxel after oral administration of Schisandrol B in rats. Biopharmaceutics & Drug Disposition 31.4 (2010): 264–8.

Jo SH et al. In vitro and in vivo anti-hyperglycemic effects of omija (*Schizandra chinensis*) fruit. International Journal of Molecular Sciences 12.2 (2011): 1359–70.

Jung YS et al. Role of CXCR2 on the immune modulating activity of Œ±-iso-cubebenol a natural compound isolated from the *Schisandra chinensis* fruit. Biochemical And Biophysical Research Communications 431.3 (2013): 433–6.

Junshu Y & Anshan S. Effect of *Schisandra chinensis* extract on blood biochemical index in broilers. Feed Industry 18.6 (2008).

Kang YH & Shin HM. Inhibitory effects of *Schizandra chinensis* extract on atopic dermatitis in NC/Nga mice. Immunopharmacology and immunotoxicology 34.2 (2012): 292–8.

Kang OH et al. Effects of the *Schisandra fructus* water extract on cytokine release from a human mast cell line. J Med Food 9.4 (2006): 480–486.

Kang JW et al. Protective effects of HV-P411 complex against D-galactosamine-induced hepatotoxicity in rats. The American Journal Of Chinese Medicine 40.3 (2012): 467–80.

Kang K et al. Dibenzocyclooctadiene lignans, gomisins J and N inhibit the Wnt/B-catenin signaling pathway in HCT116 cells. Biochemical And Biophysical Research Communications 428.2 (2012): 285–91.

Kim SR et al. Dibenzocyclooctadiene lignans from *Schisandra chinensis* protect primary cultures of rat cortical cells from glutamate-induced toxicity. J Neurosci Res 76.3 (2004): 397–405.

Kim S et al. Anti-apoptotic and hepatoprotective effects of gomisin A on fulminant hepatic failure induced by D-galactosamine and lipopolysaccharide in mice. Journal of pharmacological sciences 106.2 (2008): 225–33.

Kim SH, et al. Structural identification and antioxidant properties of major anthocyanin extracted from Omija (*Schizandra chinensis*) fruit. Journal of Food Science 74.2 (2009): C134–C140.

Kim JH et al. Apoptosis induction of human leukemia U937 cells by gomisin N, a dibenzocyclooctadiene lignan, isolated from *Schizandra chinensis* Baill. Food and Chemical Toxicology 48.3 (2010): 807–13.

Kim MG, et al. Anti-platelet aggregation activity of lignans isolated from *Schisandra chinensis* fruits. Journal of the Korean Society for Applied Biological Chemistry 53.6 (2010): 740–5.

Kim, SJ et al. Growth inhibition and cell cycle arrest in the G0/G1 by schizandrin, a dibenzocyclooctadiene lignan isolated from *Schisandra chinensis*, on T47D human breast cancer cells. Phytotherapy Research 24.2 (2010): 193–7.

Kim EY, et al. Cardioprotective effects of aqueous *Schizandra chinensis* fruit extract on ovariectomized and balloon-induced carotid artery injury rat models: Effects on serum lipid profiles and blood pressure. Journal Of Ethnopharmacology 134.3 (2011): 668–75.

Kim HK et al. The role of the lignan constituents in the effect of *Schisandra chinensis* fruit extract on penile erection. Phytotherapy Research 25.12 (2011): 1776–82.

Kim HY et al. Protective effect of HV-P411, an herbal mixture, on carbon tetrachloride-induced liver fibrosis. Food Chemistry 124.1 (2011): 248–53.

Kim JE et al. The a-iso-cubebenol compound isolated from *Schisandra chinensis* induces p53-independent pathway-mediated apoptosis in hepatocellular carcinoma cells. Oncology Reports 28.3 (2012): 1103–9.

Kim KJ et al. *Schisandra chinensis* prevents hepatic lipid peroxidation and oxidative stress in rats subjected to heat environmental stress. Phytotherapy Research 26.11 (2012): 1674–80.

Ko KM et al. Long-term schisandrin B treatment mitigates age-related impairments in mitochondrial antioxidant status and functional ability in various tissues, and improves the survival of aging C57BL/6J mice. Biofactors 34.4 (2008): 331–42.

Ko S et al. Comparison of anti-oxidant activities of seventy herbs that have been used in Korean traditional medicine. Nutrition Research And Practice 2.3 (2008): 143–51.

Kubo S et al. Effect of Gomisin A (TJN-101) on liver regeneration. Planta Med 58.6 (1992): 489–492.

Kwon DY et al. The lignan-rich fractions of Fructus Schisandrae improve insulin sensitivity via the PPAR-a pathways in in vitro and in vivo studies. Journal Of Ethnopharmacology 135.2 (2011): 455–62.

Lai L et al. Effects of short-term and long-term pretreatment of schisandra lignans on regulating hepatic and intestinal CYP3A in rats. Drug Metabolism and Disposition 37.12 (2009): 2399–407.

Lam PY et al. Schisandrin B co-treatment ameliorates the impairment on mitochondrial antioxidant status in various tissues of long-term ethanol treated rats. Fitoterapia 81.8 (2010): 1239–45.

Lam PY et al. Schisandrin B protects against solar irradiation-induced oxidative stress in rat skin tissue. Fitoterapia 82.3 (2011): 393–400.

Lau C et al. In vitro antidiabetic activities of five medicinal herbs used in Chinese medicinal formulae. Phytotherapy Research 22.10 (2008): 1383–8.

Lee IS et al. Structure-activity relationships of lignans from *Schisandra chinensis* as platelet activating factor antagonists. Biol Pharm Bull 22.3 (1999): 265–267.

Lee IS et al. Lignans with inhibitory activity against NFAT transcription from *Schisandra chinensis*. Planta Med 69.1 (2003): 63–64.

Lee B et al. Inhibitory effect of schizandrin on passive cutaneous anaphylaxis reaction and scratching behaviors in mice. Biol Pharm Bull 30.6 (2007): 1153–1156.

Lee SB et al. Induction of the phase II detoxification enzyme NQO1 in hepatocarcinoma cells by lignans from the fruit of *Schisandra chinensis* through nuclear accumulation of Nrf2. Planta Medica 75.12 (2009): 1314–8.

Lee Y et al. Identification of a novel compound that stimulates intracellular calcium increase and CXCL8 production in human neutrophils from *Schisandra chinensis*. Biochemical And Biophysical Research Communications 379.4 (2009): 928–32.

Lee MY et al. Anti-asthmatic effect of schizandrin on OVA-induced airway inflammation in a murine asthma model. International Immunopharmacology 10.1 (2010): 1374–9.

Lee YJ et al. Identification of a novel compound that inhibits iNOS and COX-2 expression in LPS-stimulated macrophages from *Schisandra chinensis*. Biochemical And Biophysical Research Communications 391.4 (2010): 1687–92.

Lee SK et al. a-Iso-cubebene, a natural compound isolated from *Schisandra chinensis* fruit, has therapeutic benefit against polymicrobial sepsis. Biochemical And Biophysical Research Communications 426.2 (2012): 226–31.

Lee TH, et al. Neuroprotective effects of Schisandrin B against transient focal cerebral ischemia in Sprague-Dawley rats. Food and Chemical Toxicology 50.12 (2012): 4239–45.

Leong PK et al. Cytochrome P450-catalysed reactive oxygen species production mediates the (-) schisandrin B-induced glutathione and heat shock responses in AML12 hepatocytes. Cell Biology International 36.3 (2012): 321–6.

Li SF et al. Protection of schisandrin B against silica-induced lung injury in rats. Chinese Journal of Comparative Medicine 5.7 (2009).

Li WL et al. In vivo effect of Schisandrin B on cytochrome P450 enzyme activity. Phytomedicine 20.8–9 (2013); 760–765.

Lim H et al. 5-Lipoxygenase-inhibitory constituents from *Schizandra fructus* and *Magnolia flos*. Phytotherapy Research 23.10 (2009): 1489–92.

Lin S, et al. Molecular mechanism of apoptosis induced by schizandrae-derived lignans in human leukemia HL-60 cells. Food Chem Toxicol 46.2 (2008): 590–597.

Lin RD et al. The immuno-regulatory effects of *Schisandra chinensis* and its constituents on human monocytic leukemia cells. Molecules 16.6 (2011): 4836–49.

Liu C, et al. Non-thermal extraction of effective ingredients from *Schisandra chinensis* Baill and the antioxidant activity of its extract. Natural Product Research 23.15 (2009): 1390–401.

Liu C et al. Chemical composition and antioxidant activity of essential oil from berries of *Schisandra chinensis* (Turcz.) Baill. Natural Product Research 26.23 (2012a): 2199–203.

Liu C et al. Strong inhibition of deoxyschizandrin and schisantherin A toward UDP-glucuronosyltransferase (UGT) 1A3 indicating UGT inhibition-based herb-drug interaction. Fitoterapia 83.8 (2012b): 1415–9.

Loo WT, et al. *Fructus schisandrae* (Wuweizi)-containing compound inhibits secretion of HBsAg and HBeAg in hepatocellular carcinoma cell line. Biomed Pharmacother 61.9 (2007): 606–610.

Lu H, Liu GT. Anti-oxidant activity of dibenzocyclooctene lignans isolated from Schisandraceae. Planta Med 58.4 (1992): 311–3113.

Ma CJ et al. ESP-102, a combined extract of *Angelica gigas, Saururus chinensis* and *Schizandra chinensis*, protects against glutamate-induced toxicity in primary cultures of rat cortical cells. Phytotherapy Research 23.11 (2009): 1587–91.

Ma D et al. Influence of an aqueous extract of *Ligustrum lucidum* and an ethanol extract of *Schisandra chinensis* on parameters of antioxidative metabolism and spleen lymphocyte proliferation of broilers. Archives Of Animal Nutrition 63.1 (2009): 66–74.

Ma C et al. Optimization of conditions of solvent-free microwave extraction and study on antioxidant capacity of essential oil from *Schisandra chinensis* (Turcz.) Baill. Food Chemistry 134.4 (2012): 2532–39.

Mak DH, Ko KM. Alterations in susceptibility to carbon tetrachloride toxicity and hepatic antioxidant/detoxification system in streptozotocin-induced short-term diabetic rats: effects of insulin and Schisandrin B treatment. Mol Cell Biochem 175.1–2 (1997): 225–232.

Mak DH et al. Effects of Schisandrin B and alpha-tocopherol on lipid peroxidation, in vitro and in vivo. Mol Cell Biochem 165.2 (1996): 161–165.

Meng X, et al. Study on extraction, purification and scavenging free radical of polysaccharide SCP-B II from *Schisandra chinensis*. Food Science 1.15 (2008).

Miao M, et al. Effect of *Schisandra chinensis* Baill distilled by ethanol on the ability of learning and memory in memory impairment mice model induced by repeated cerebral ischemia reperfusion. Chinese Journal of Modern Applied Pharmacy 5.4 (2009).

Miao Y et al. Effect of *Schisandra chinensis* Baill distilled by ethanol on energy metabolism in brain of repeated cerebral ischemia-reperfusion model mice. China Journal of Traditional Chinese Medicine and Pharmacy 9.37 (2009).

Min HY et al. Antiproliferative effects of dibenzocyclooctadiene lignans isolated from *Schisandra chinensis* in human cancer cells. Bioorg Med Chem Lett 18.2 (2008): 523–526.

Moon PD, et al. Effects of schizandrin on the expression of thymic stromal lymphopoietin in human mast cell line HMC-1. Life Sciences 91.11–12 (2012): 384–8.

Na M et al. Fatty acid synthase inhibitory activity of dibenzocyclooctadiene lignans isolated from *Schisandra chinensis*. Phytotherapy Research 24.2 (2010): S225–S8.

Nakagiri R, et al. Small scale rat hepatocyte primary culture with applications for screening hepatoprotective substances. Biosci Biotechnol Biochem 67.8 (2003): 1629–1635.

Narimanian M et al. Impact of Chisan (ADAPT-232) on the quality-of-life and its efficacy as an adjuvant in the treatment of acute non-specific pneumonia. Phytomedicine 12.10 (2005): 723–729.

Nishida H et al. Inhibition of ATR protein kinase activity by schisandrin B in DNA damage response. Nucleic acids research 37.17 (2009): 5678–89.

Oh B et al. Inhibitory effects of Schizandrae Fructus on eotaxin secretion in A549 human epithelial cells and eosinophil migration. Phytomedicine 16.9 (2009): 814–22.

Oh SY et al. Anti-inflammatory effects of gomisin N, gomisin J, and schisandrin C isolated from the fruit of *Schisandra chinensis*. Bioscience, Biotechnology and Biochemistry 74.2 (2010): 285–291.

Ohkura Y et al. Effect of gomisin A (TJN-101) on the arachidonic acid cascade in macrophages. Jpn J Pharmacol 52.2 (1990): 331–336.

Ohsugi M et al. Active-oxygen scavenging activity of traditional nourishing-tonic herbal medicines and active constituents of *Rhodiola sacra*. J Ethnopharmacol 67.1 (1999): 111–1119.

Pan S. Ethanol extract of Fructus Schisandrae decreases hepatic triglyceride level in mice fed with a high fat/cholesterol diet, with attention to acute toxicity. Evidence-Based Complementary and Alternative Medicine (2011); 2011: 729412.

Pan SY et al. Schisandrin B protects against tacrine- and bis(7)-tacrine-induced hepatotoxicity and enhances cognitive function in mice. Planta Med 68.3 (2002): 217–220.

Pan Q et al. Dibenzocyclooctadiene lignans: a class of novel inhibitors of P-glycoprotein. Cancer Chemother Pharmacol 58.1 (2006): 99–106.

Pan SY et al. Schisandrin B from *Schisandra chinensis* reduces hepatic lipid contents in hypercholesterolaemic mice. J Pharm Pharmacol 60.3 (2008): 399–403.

Panossian A et al. Adaptogens exert a stress-protective effect by modulation of expression of molecular chaperones. Phytomedicine 16.6–7 (2009): 617–22.

Park JY et al. Gomisin A from *Schisandra chinensis* induces endothelium-dependent and direct relaxation in rat thoracic aorta. Planta Med 73.15 (2007): 1537–1542.

Park C et al. Induction of G1 arrest and apoptosis by schisandrin C isolated from *Schizandra chinensis* Baill in human leukemia U937 cells. International Journal Of Molecular Medicine 24.4 (2009): 495–502.

Park J et al. The mechanism of vasorelaxation induced by *Schisandra chinensis* extract in rat thoracic aorta. Journal Of Ethnopharmacology 121.1 (2009a): 69–73.

Park J et al. Gomisin A induces Ca^{2+}-dependent activation of eNOS in human coronary artery endothelial cells. Journal Of Ethnopharmacology 125.2 (2009b): 291–6.

Park S et al. Huang-Lian-Jie-Du-Tang supplemented with *Schisandra chinensis* Baill. and *Polygonatum odoratum* Druce improved glucose tolerance by potentiating insulinotropic actions in islets in 90% pancreatectomized diabetic rats. Bioscience, Biotechnology, And Biochemistry 73.11 (2009): 2384–92.

Park SY et al. *Schisandra chinensis* a-iso-cubebenol induces heme oxygenase-1 expression through PI3K/Akt and Nrf2 signaling and has anti-inflammatory activity in *Porphyromonas gingivalis* lipopolysaccharide-stimulated macrophages. International Immunopharmacology 11.11 (2011): 1907–15.

Park EJ et al. Schisandrin B suppresses TGF-α signaling by inhibiting Smad2/3 and MAPK pathways. Biochemical Pharmacology 83.3 (2012): 378–84.

Park HJ et al. Anti-obesity effect of *Schisandra chinensis* in 3T3-L1 cells and high fat diet-induced obese rats. Food Chemistry 134.1 (2012): 227–34.

Park J et al. Gomisin J from *Schisandra chinensis* induces vascular relaxation via activation of endothelial nitric oxide synthase. Vascular Pharmacology 57.2–4 (2012a): 124–30.

Park J et al. Antihypertensive effect of gomisin A from *Schisandra chinensis* on angiotensin II-induced hypertension via preservation of nitric oxide bioavailability. Hypertension Research 35.9 (2012b): 928–34.

Peng JH et al. Effect of Jianpi Houxue decoction on inflammatory cytokine secretion pathway in rat liver with lipopolysaccharide challenge. World journal of gastroenterology 14.12 (2008): 1851.

Pu HJ et al. Correlation between antistress and hepatoprotective effects of schisandra lignans was related with its antioxidative actions in liver cells. Evidence-Based Complementary and Alternative Medicine (2012); 2012: 161062.

Qiangrong P et al. Schisandrin B: a novel inhibitor of P-glycoprotein. Biochem Biophys Res Commun 335.2 (2005): 406 411.

Rhyu MR et al. Aqueous extract of *Schizandra chinensis* fruit causes endothelium-dependent and -independent relaxation of isolated rat thoracic aorta. Phytomedicine 13.9–10 (2006): 651–657.

Schutgens F et al. The influence of adaptogens on ultraweak biophoton emission: a pilot-experiment. Phytotherapy Research 23.8 (2009): 1103–8.

Seok YM et al. Effects of gomisin A on vascular contraction in rat aortic rings. Naunyn-Schmiedeberg's Archives Of Pharmacology 383.1 (2011): 45–56.

Shi YM et al. Schicagenins A-C: three cagelike nortriterpenoids from leaves and stems of *Schisandra chinensis*. Organic Letters. 13.15 (2011): 3848–51.

Shin SS et al. The Korean traditional medicine Gyeongshingangjeehwan inhibits adipocyte hypertrophy and visceral adipose tissue accumulation by activating PPARα actions in rat white adipose tissues. Journal Of Ethnopharmacology 127.1 (2010): 47–54.

Slaninova I et al. Dibenzocyclooctadiene lignans overcome drug resistance in lung cancer cells — Study of structure-activity relationship. Toxicology in Vitro 23.6 (2009): 1047–54.

Smejkal K et al. Evaluation of the antiradical activity of *Schisandra chinensis* lignans using different experimental models. Molecules 15.3 (2010): 1223–31.

Sohn D et al. Elevation of intracavernous pressure and NO-cGMP activity by a new herbal formula in penile tissues of spontaneous hypertensive male rats. Journal of Ethnopharmacology 120.2 (2008): 176–80.

Song JX et al. Protective effects of dibenzocyclooctadiene lignans from *Schisandra chinensis* against beta-amyloid and homocysteine neurotoxicity in PC12 cells. Phytotherapy Research 25.3 (2011): 435–43.

Song, QY et al. Eleven new highly oxygenated triterpenoids from the leaves and stems of *Schisandra chinensis*. Organic & Biomolecular Chemistry 11.7 (2013): 1251–8.

Stacchiotti A et al. Schisandrin B stimulates a cytoprotective response in rat liver exposed to mercuric chloride. Food and Chemical Toxicology 4711 (2009): 2834–40.

Stacchiotti A et al. Different role of Schisandrin B on mercury-induced renal damage in vivo and in vitro. Toxicology 286.1–3 (2011): 48–57.

Steele M et al. Cytoprotective properties of traditional Chinese medicinal herbal extracts in hydrogen peroxide challenged human U373 astroglia cells. Neurochemistry International 62.5 (2013): 522–9.

Su T et al. Effects of unprocessed versus vinegar-processed *Schisandra chinensis* on the activity and mRNA expression of CYP1A2, CYP2E1 and CYP3A4 enzymes in rats. Journal Of Ethnopharmacology 146.1 (2013).

Szeto YT et al. In vitro antioxidation activity and genoprotective effect of selected Chinese medicinal herbs. American Journal of Chinese Medicine 39.4 (2011): 827–38.

Takeda S et al. Effects of TJN-101, a lignan compound isolated from Schisandra fruits, on liver fibrosis and on liver regeneration after partial hepatectomy in rats with chronic liver injury induced by CCl4. Nippon Yakurigaku Zasshi 90.1 (1987): 51–65.

Takimoto Y et al. Gomisin N in the herbal drug gomishi (*Schisandra chinensis*) suppresses inducible nitric oxide synthase gene via C/EBPβ and NF-kB in rat hepatocytes. Nitric Oxide 28.0 (2013): 47–56.

Tang SH et al. The protective effect of schisandra lignans on stress-evoked hepatic metastases of P815 tumor cells in restraint mice. Journal of Ethnopharmacology 134.1 (2011): 141–6.

Tsi D, Tan A. Evaluation on the combined effect of Sesamin and Schisandra extract on blood fluidity. Bioinformation 2.6 (2008): 249–252.

Waiwut P et al. Gomisin N enhances TNF-α-induced apoptosis via inhibition of the NF-κB and EGFR survival pathways. Molecular and Cellular Biochemistry 350.1–2 (2011): 169–75.

Waiwut P et al. Gomisin A enhances tumor necrosis factor-α-induced G1 cell cycle arrest via signal transducer and activator of transcription 1-mediated phosphorylation of retinoblastoma protein. Biological & Pharmaceutical Bulletin 35.11 (2012): 1997–2003.

Wan CK et al. Gomisin A alters substrate interaction and reverses P-glycoprotein-mediated multidrug resistance in HepG2-DR cells. Biochem Pharmacol 72.7 (2006): 824–837.

Wan C et al. Inhibition of cytochrome P450 3A4 activity by schisandrol A and gomisin A isolated from Fructus Schisandrae chinensis. Phytomedicine 17.8–9 (2010): 702–5.

Wang J. Study on the bacteriostatic and bactericidal activity of extract from *Schisandra chinensis*. Journal of Anhui Agricultural Sciences 16.83 (2008).

Wang HJ & Chiang BH. Anti-diabetic effect of a traditional Chinese medicine formula. Food & Function 3.11 (2012): 1161–9.

Wang M, et al. High throughput screening and antioxidant assay of dibenzo[a,c]cyclooctadiene lignans in modified-ultrasonic and supercritical fluid extracts of *Schisandra chinensis* Baill by liquid chromatography-mass spectrometry and a free radical-scavenging method. Journal of separation science 31.8 (2008): 1322–32.

Wang W et al. Sedative and hypnotic effects of each extract of Fructus Schisandrae in mice. Journal of Jiangsu University 2.9 (2008a).

Wang W et al. Effects of *Schisandra chinensis* Baill extract on anti-hypoxia and anti-fatigue in Mice. Journal of Inner Mongolia University for Nationalities 6.23 (2008b).

Wang B et al. Effects of *Schisandra chinensis* (Wuweizi) constituents on the activity of hepatic microsomal CYP450 isozymes in rats detected by using a cocktail probe substrates method. Acta pharmaceutica Sinica 46.8 (2011): 922.

Wang SD et al. Xiao-Qing-Long-Tang attenuates allergic airway inflammation and remodeling in repetitive *Dermatogoides pteronyssinus* challenged chronic asthmatic mice model. Journal of Ethnopharmacology 142.2 (2012): 531–8.

Wei B et al. Development of a UFLC-MS/MS method for simultaneous determination of six lignans of *Schisandra chinensis* (Turcz.) Baill. in rat plasma and its application to a comparative pharmacokinetic study in normal and insomnic rats. Journal of Pharmaceutical and Biomedical Analysis 77.0 (2013): 120–7.

Wen-qiang W. Study on in vitro antimicrobial effect of four Chinese herb medicines. Journal of Anhui Agricultural Sciences 6.83 (2009).

Xie X et al. Effects of Schisandra on behavioral learning and hippocampal AChE activity in ovariectomized mice. Journal of South China Normal University 3.24 (2010).

Xie Y et al. Integral pharmacokinetics of multiple lignan components in normal, CCl4-induced hepatic injury and hepatoprotective agents pretreated rats and correlations with hepatic injury biomarkers. Journal of Ethnopharmacology 131.2 (2010): 290–9.

Xin H et al. Effects of *Schisandra sphenanthera* extract on the pharmacokinetics of tacrolimus in healthy volunteers. British Journal of Clinical Pharmacology 64.4 (2007): 469–75.

Xin H et al. Effects of *Schisandra sphenanthera* extract on the pharmacokinetics of midazolam in healthy volunteers. British Journal of Clinical Pharmacology 67.5 (2009): 541–546.

Xu C et al. Inhibitory effect of *Schisandra chinensis* leaf polysaccharide against L5178Y lymphoma. Carbohydrate Polymers 88.1 (2012): 21–5.

Xu X, et al. Schizandrin prevents dexamethasone-induced cognitive deficits. Neurosci Bull. 2012 Oct;28(5):532–40

Xv G et al. Hypoglycemic effects of a water-soluble polysaccharide isolated from *Schisandra chinensis* (Turcz.) Baill in alloxan-induced diabetic mice. Journal of Biotechnology 136.0 (2008): S725.

Yamada S, et al. Preventive effect of gomisin A, a lignan component of shizandra fruits, on acetaminophen-induced hepatotoxicity in rats. Biochem Pharmacol 46.6 (1993): 1081–1085.

Yan F et al. Synergistic hepatoprotective effect of *Schisandrae* lignans with *Astragalus* polysaccharides on chronic liver injury in rats. Phytomedicine 16.9 (2009): 805–13.

Yang L et al. Study on immunological activity of coarse polysaccharides from ethanol-insoluble residue of Schisandra. Food Science 6.89 (2008).

Yang, J et al. Inhibitory effect of schisandrin on spontaneous contraction of isolated rat colon. Phytomedicine 18.11 (2011a): 998–1005.

Yang, J et al. Relaxant effects of *Schisandra chinensis* and its major lignans on agonists-induced contraction in guinea pig ileum. Phytomedicine 18.13 (2011b): 1153–60.

Yang SH et al. Schisandrin enhances dendrite outgrowth and synaptogenesis in primary cultured hippocampal neurons. Journal of the Science of Food and Agriculture 91.4 (2011): 694–702.

Yang X et al. Screening vasoconstriction inhibitors from traditional Chinese medicines using a vascular smooth muscle/cell membrane chromatography-offline-liquid chromatography-mass spectrometry. Journal of Separation Science 34.19 (2011): 2586–93.

Yang J et al. *Schisandra chinensis* reverses visceral hypersensitivity in a neonatal-maternal separated rat model. Phytomedicine: International Journal Of Phytotherapy And Phytopharmacology 19.5 (2012): 402–8.

Yao HT et al. Shengmai San reduces hepatic lipids and lipid peroxidation in rats fed on a high-cholesterol diet. Journal of Ethnopharmacology 116.1 (2008): 49–57.

Yao Q et al. Induction effects of the different processed Fructus schisandrae Chinensis on the hepatic microsomal cytochrome P450 in rats. West China Journal of Pharmaceutical Sciences 3.19 (2011).

Yasukawa K et al. Gomisin A inhibits tumor promotion by 12-*O*-tetradecanoylphorbol-13-acetate in two-stage carcinogenesis in mouse skin. Oncology 49.1 (1992): 68–71.

Yasukawa K et al. Gomisin A inhibits tumor promotion by 12-o-tetra-decanoylphorbol-13-acetate in two-stage carcinogenesis in mouse skin. Oncology 49.1 (2009): 68–71.
Ye C et al. Extraction optimization of polysaccharides of Schisandrae Fructus and evaluation of their analgesic activity. International Journal of Biological Macromolecules 57.1 (2013): 291–96.
Yim TK, Ko KM. Schisandrin B protects against myocardial ischemia-reperfusion injury by enhancing myocardial glutathione antioxidant status. Mol Cell Biochem 196.1–2 (1999): 151–156.
Yim SY et al. Gomisin N isolated from *Schisandra chinensis* significantly induces anti-proliferative and pro-apoptotic effects in hepatic carcinoma. Molecular Medicine Reports 2.5 (2009): 725–32.
Yoo HH et al. Effects of schisandra lignans on P-glycoprotein-mediated drug efflux in human intestinal Caco-2. Planta Med 73.5 (2007): 444–450.
Yu C et al. Identification of novel pregnane X receptor activators from traditional Chinese medicines. Journal of Ethnopharmacology 136.1 (2011): 137–43.
Yuezhen L. Effects of the different concentration Schisandrin B including multiplication and apoptosis in human gastric cancer cell line MGC-803. Journal of Mudanjiang Medical University 4.2 (2010).
Zeng KW et al. Schisandrin B exerts anti-neuroinflammatory activity by inhibiting the Toll-like receptor 4-dependent MyD88/IKK/NF-kB signaling pathway in lipopolysaccharide-induced microglia. European Journal of Pharmacology 692.1–3 (2012): 29–37.
Zhang Y & Li PP. Evaluation of estrogenic potential of Shu-Gan-Liang-Xue decoction by dual-luciferase reporter based bioluminescent measurements in vitro. Journal Of Ethnopharmacology 126.2 (2009): 345–9.
Zhang J, et al. Dibenzocyclooctadiene lignans from Fructus Schisandrae Chinensis improve glucose uptake in vitro. Natural Product Communications 5.2 (2010): 231–4.
Zhang N et al. Studies on chemical constituents of leaf of *Schisandra chinensis* and inhibitory effect of schizandrin on activation of microglia induced by LPS. Chinese Journal of Medicinal Chemistry 20.2 (2010): 110–5.
Zhang M et al. *Schisandra chinensis* fruit extract attenuates albuminuria and protects podocyte integrity in a mouse model of streptozotocin-induced diabetic nephropathy. Journal of Ethnopharmacology 141.1 (2012): 111–8.
Zhao T et al. Anti-diabetic effects of polysaccharides from ethanol-insoluble residue of *Schisandra chinensis* (Turcz.) Baill on alloxan-induced diabetic mice. Chemical Research in Chinese Universities 29.1 (2013a): 99–102.
Zhao T et al. Antitumor and immunomodulatory activity of a water-soluble low molecular weight polysaccharide from *Schisandra chinensis* (Turcz.) Baill. Food and Chemical Toxicology 55.0 (2013b): 609–16.
Zhu M et al. Evaluation of the protective effects of *Schisandra chinensis* on phase I drug metabolism using a CCl4 intoxication model. J Ethnopharmacol 67.1 (1999): 61–68.
Zhu M et al. Improvement of phase I drug metabolism with *Schisandra chinensis* against CCl4 hepatotoxicity in a rat model. Planta Med 66.6 (2000): 521–525.
Zhu S et al. Protective effect of schisandrin B against cyclosporine A-induced nephrotoxicity in vitro and in vivo. The American Journal of Chinese Medicine 40.3 (2012): 551–66.

Selenium

HISTORICAL NOTE During his travels in the 13th century, Marco Polo first reported what is thought to be selenium toxicity in grazing animals. He observed that certain grazing areas in China were associated with horses developing diseased hooves (Hendler & Rorvik 2001). It is now known that parts of China have the highest selenium soil concentrations in the world and diseased hooves were likely to be due to selenium toxicity. It was not until nearly 500 years later, in 1817, that selenium was actually discovered (Tinggi 2003), and the fact that it is essential in mammals was not discovered until 1957 (Navarro-Alarcon & Lopez-Martinez 2000). In 1979, the importance of selenium in human nutrition was further reinforced when Chinese researchers reported that selenium supplementation prevented the development of Keshan disease, a cardiomyopathy seen in children living in selenium-replete areas, and New Zealand workers reported a clinical response to selenium supplementation in a selenium-depleted patient (Shils et al 2006).

BACKGROUND AND RELEVANT PHARMACOKINETICS

Selenium is an essential trace element that enters the food chain through incorporation into plants from the soil. Selenium is mainly present in the form of selenite in acid soils, which is poorly assimilated by crops, whereas for alkaline soils it is in the form of selenate, which is more soluble and assimilated by crops. When taken in supplement form, animal and human trials demonstrate that bioavailability of organic forms of selenium (Se-methionine and Se-cysteine) is higher than that obtained for inorganic forms (selenite and selenate) (Navarro-Alarcon & Lopez-Martinez 2000).

The variation in selenium content of adult humans living in different parts of the world is testimony to the influence of the natural environment on the selenium content of soils, crops and human tissues. According to a WHO report, adults in New Zealand have approximately 3 mg selenium in their bodies and a daily intake of about 30 gm (100 gm/day is common) compared with 14 mg body content in some Americans and a daily intake around 100 g/day in North America. Intakes in Europe are in the range of 30 to 60 g/day.

Selenium is readily absorbed, especially in the duodenum and also in the caecum and colon. Vitamins A, E and C can modulate selenium absorption, and there is a complex relationship between selenium and vitamin E that has not been entirely elucidated for humans (Bates 2005). Selenium enters the body in two major forms: Se-methionine, which is derived from plants, and Se-cysteine, which is mainly derived from animal selenoproteins (Shils et al 2006). Metabolism is complex and occurs via several routes for the different selenoproteins. Se-methionine enters the methionine pool where it undergoes the same fate as methionine until catabolised. Once the selenium from Se-methionine is liberated by the trans-sulfuration pathway in the liver or kidney, it is able to be used by peripheral cells. Ingested selenite, selenate and selenocysteine are metabolised to selenide. Urinary excretion accounts for 50–60% of total excretion of selenium and homeostasis is achieved through regulation in the kidney. Volatile forms of selenium are exhaled when intake is very high and presents a significant route of excretion at this level.

CHEMICAL COMPONENTS

In human tissues, it is found as either L-selenomethionine or L-selenocysteine.

FOOD SOURCES

Most dietary selenium is in the form of selenomethionine which is virtually completely bioavailable. The amount of selenium in a food greatly depends on the amount of selenium in the soil where it was grown. As such, a single food plant can vary greatly in its selenium content. By contrast, animal and marine sources tend to have more consistent selenium content. In general, the most concentrated food sources are brewer's yeast, wheatgerm, meats, fish and seafood, Brazil nuts, garlic and organ meats.

DEFICIENCY SIGNS AND SYMPTOMS

Selenium deprivation reduces the activity of selenium-dependent enzymes and has widespread effects. Characteristic signs of selenium deficiency have not been described in humans, but very low selenium status is a factor in the aetiologies of a juvenile cardiomyopathy (Keshan disease) and a chondrodystrophy (Kashin-Beck disease) that occur in selenium-deficient regions of China.

Low selenium status has been associated with:

- loss of immunocompetence (Ongele et al 2002)
- increased risk of developing certain cancers (Clark et al 1998)
- reduced male fertility (Scott et al 1998, Xu et al 2003)
- poorer prognosis in HIV infection and AIDS (Baum et al 1997, Campa et al 1999)

- greater incidence of depression, anxiety, confusion and hostility (Rayman 2000)
- compromised thyroid hormone metabolism (particularly when iodine deficiency is also present) (Gartner et al 2002)
- asthma and atopy (Kadrabova et al 1996, Misso et al 1996, Omland et al 2002)
- rheumatoid arthritis (Zamamiri-Davis et al 2002)
- possibly, increased inflammatory processes (Zamamiri-Davis et al 2002)
- changes to drug-metabolising enzymes, including the cytochrome P450 system, with some activities increasing and others decreasing (Shils et al 2006).

Low selenium status may contribute to the aetiology of several diseases, while in others this state exacerbates disease progression, such as in HIV infection.

People at risk of marginal selenium deficiency include those living in areas of low environmental selenium, such as some regions of New Zealand, people receiving long-term total parenteral nutrition (TPN), low-protein diet associated with phenylketonuria and hyperphenylalaninaemia, alcoholics, and those with liver cirrhosis, hepatitis C virus infection, malabsorption syndromes, cystic fibrosis, coeliac disease and AIDS (Procházková et al 2013).

MAIN ACTIONS

Antioxidant

Selenium is an integral part of thioredoxin reductase and the glutathione peroxidases and therefore is intimately involved in the body's antioxidant systems. These enzymes are involved in controlling tissue levels of free radical molecules and maintain cell-mediated immunity.

Chemopreventative

Chemoprotective effects of selenium have been identified through RCTs and by experimental studies of selenium and known carcinogens in the development of specific cell lines. Several mechanisms have been postulated to explain the chemopreventive effect of selenium, including protection against oxidative damage, alterations to immune and metabolic systems, alterations to carcinogen metabolism, production of cytotoxic selenium metabolites, inhibition of protein synthesis, stabilisation of genetic material facilitating DNA repair by activation of p53, inhibition of nuclear factor-kappa B (NF-kappa B) and stimulation of apoptosis (Christensen et al 2007, Chun et al 2006, Clark et al 1996, El Bayoumy 2001, Schrauzer 2000, Seo et al 2002). One study demonstrated that combining vitamin E succinate and methylselenic acid produces a synergistic effect on cell growth suppression, primarily mediated by augmenting apoptosis (Zu & Ip 2003).

In humans, the chemopreventive effect is strongest for individuals with the lowest selenium status; however, it is still unclear whether low selenium status is implicated in the aetiology of cancer or whether it produces a state of increased susceptibility to the effects of carcinogens.

Immunomodulation

Confirmed in both animal studies and human trials, immunomodulation is in part due to improved activation and proliferation of B-lymphocytes and enhanced T-cell function (Gazdik et al 2002a, 2002b, Hawkes et al 2001, Kiremidjian-Schumacher & Roy 1998, Ongele et al 2002). A role for selenoprotein S in immune response has been proposed, with a study observing dose-dependent increased expression following influenza vaccine in selenium-supplemented adults

(Goldson et al 2011). Interestingly, selenium concentrations significantly decrease during stages of acute infection, suggesting increased use and/or excretion or decreased absorption during this period (Sammalkorpi et al 1988).

Thyroid hormone modulation

Selenium is required for normal thyroid hormone synthesis, activation and metabolism (Sher 2001). Three different selenium-dependent iodothyronine deiodinases (types I, II, and III) can both activate and inactivate thyroid hormone, making selenium an essential element for normal development, growth and metabolism through the regulation of thyroid hormones. However, it should be noted that selenium supplementation across a number of studies has been found to have no effect on thyroid hormone concentrations (Combs et al 2009, Hawkes et al 2008, Thomson et al 2011). In a randomised controlled trial of elderly UK residents ($n = 501$), supplementation with selenium (100–300 mcg/day) did not have any significant effects on thyroid function despite significant increases in plasma selenium concentration (Rayman et al 2008). A small, statistically significant increase in T_3 was observed in males; however, this did not correlate with a corresponding decrease in thyroid stimulating hormone, thus the clinical relevance on this increase in questionable (Combs et al 2009).

OTHER ACTIONS

Male fertility

Reduced selenium levels have been observed in infertile males, regardless of inflammatory status, which in turn has been associated with reduced percentage of normal sperm (Türk et al 2013). Selenium is required for testosterone synthesis, normal sperm maturation and sperm motility (Rayman & Rayman 2002). Two clinical studies have confirmed this association (Scott et al 1998, Vezina et al 1996) and identified selenium supplements as able to increase sperm motility. The effect of selenium in spermatogenesis may be due to several mechanisms, including the activity of the selenium-dependent enzyme phospholipid hydroperoxide glutathione peroxidase (GPX4) (Flohe 2007), altering oxidative stress-mediated apoptosis in germ cells (Kaushal & Bansal 2007a, 2007b), and the modulation of transcription factor NF-kappaB (Shalini & Bansal 2006, 2007a). Interestingly, animal studies suggest that detrimental effects on fertility are associated with either too little or excessive selenium intake (Shalini & Bansal 2007b, 2008).

Anti-inflammatory

Selenium deficiency produces a significantly increased COX-2 protein expression, as well as higher PGE_2 levels, according to one in vitro study (Zamamiri-Davis et al 2002). It has also been theorised that selenium may decrease leukotriene production (McCarty 1984). In vivo tests have identified anti-inflammatory activity in the lung with selenium, which is thought to relate to an increase in glutathione levels and immune parameters (Jeong et al 2002).

Reduces heavy metal toxicity

Selenium protects against toxicity of some heavy metals, such as cadmium, arsenic, lead, silver and mercury (Berry & Galle 1994, Bolkent et al 2008, Chuang et al 2007, El-Sharaky et al 2007, El-Shenawy & Hassan 2008, Li et al 2012, Lindh et al 1996, Navarro-Alarcon & Lopez-Martinez 2000, Yiin et al 1999a, 1999b, 2000, 2001). A physiological role for selenium in counteracting heavy metal poisoning has been proposed (Shils et al 2006). It appears that the form of selenium is important, as inorganic selenium has been shown to enhance the toxic effects of inorganic arsenic by increasing its retention in tissues and suppressing its metabolism in vitro (Styblo & Thomas 2001).

Antiatherogenic activity

Selenium supplementation reduces high-fat diet-induced atherosclerosis, according to an in vivo study (Kang et al 2001). In healthy subjects fed a test meal high in lipid hydroperoxides, selenium supplementation counteracted the postprandial synthesis of the atherogenic form of LDL (Natella et al 2007). By contrast, no association between toenail selenium and markers of subclinical atherosclerosis were found in a longitudinal study over an 18-year period (n = 3112) (Xun et al 2010).

According to studies with experimental models, beneficial effects on lipid metabolism are due to significant up-regulation of LDL receptor activity and mRNA expression (Dhingra & Bansal 2006a), and down-regulation of hypercholesterolaemia-induced changes in apolipoprotein B (apoB) and 3-hydroxy 3-methylglutaryl coenzyme A (HMG-CoA) reductase expression during experimental hypercholesterolaemia (Dhingra & Bansal 2006b).

Bone health

In healthy, euthyroid postmenopausal women, increased plasma selenium levels and selenoprotein P was associated with increased bone mineral density and reduced bone turnover (Hoeg et al 2012).

CLINICAL USE

Deficiency states: prevention and treatment

Traditionally, selenium supplementation has been used to treat deficiency or prevent deficiency in conditions such as malabsorption syndromes. In addition, the elderly are at increased risk of selenium deficiency. Poor levels are negatively associated with subjective indicators of quality of life (QOL) in older people, such as self-perceived health, chewing ability, physical activity (Gonzalez et al 2007), muscle strength (Beck et al 2007, Lauretani et al 2007) and cognitive function (Akbaraly et al 2007, Gao et al 2007). Supplementation in this population where deficiency has been demonstrated is warranted.

Cancer: prevention and possible adjunct to treatment

The first suggestion of a correlation between low selenium intake and increased cancer incidence arose in the 1970s, an observation which has been supported over time. However, it appears that selenium alone is not the only factor responsible for the protective effect. As such, it is not surprising that a recent Cochrane review determined that no reliable conclusions can be drawn regarding low selenium exposure and increased risk of cancer (Dennert et al 2011). The authors recommend that in many cases, results from available trials should be interpreted cautiously due to potential for confounding, bias and limited heterogeneity.

Chemoprevention

Collectively, evidence available from a range of human, animal and cell-based studies supports a protective role for selenium against the development of cancer; however, results are not always consistent. Further research is required to better determine characteristics of responders, optimal dosage and dose forms. Populations who live in low-selenium environments and have low selenium intakes tend to have higher cancer mortality rates. However, the results from epidemiological studies have been less consistent and show that the effect may be strongest in males.

Total cancer incidence and mortality

In a follow-up to the Linxian General Population Nutrition Intervention Trial, patients who received selenium in combination with vitamin E and beta-carotene had a lower overall mortality (HR 0.95, 95% CI 0.91–0.99) than placebo 10 years after the end of active intervention (Qiao et al 2009).

Several large-scale studies, including the Nutritional Prevention of Cancer (NPC) Trial and the Third National Health and Nutrition Examination Survey (NHANES III), have found that 200 mcg/day selenium is associated with reduced total cancer incidence and cancer mortality (Bleys et al 2008, Clark et al 1998, Reid et al 2008). Specifically, the NPC trial was a large multi-centre, double-blind randomised controlled trial (RCT) (*n* = 1312) of patients with a history of basal cell or squamous cell carcinoma which investigated the effects of 200 mcg/day selenium (as 500 mg brewer's yeast). Findings from this study suggest that while supplementation in this population did not alter future incidence of skin cancer, it significantly reduced total cancer mortality, total cancer incidence by 37% and the incidences of lung, colorectal and prostate cancers by 46%, 58% and 63%, respectively (Clark et al 1998). Further studies on this population suggest the protective effect of selenium may be restricted to people with low baseline plasma levels, and most pronounced for colorectal cancer and current smokers, whereas protective effects in prostate cancer were further restricted to lower baseline levels of prostate-specific antigen (PSA: ≤4 ng/mL) (Duffield-Lillico et al 2002, 2003, Reid et al 2002, 2006). Although 200 mcg/day selenium was associated with a lowered cancer incidence of 25%, this protective effect was not seen when a double dose was used (Reid et al 2008). At the 12-year follow-up of the NHANES III trial, both all-cause and cancer mortality were found to be reduced with increasing serum selenium levels up to <130 ng/mL, but a gradual increase in mortality was seen at higher levels exceeding 150 ng/mL (Bleys et al 2008).

Liver cancer

A trial involving 130,471 individuals living in a high-risk area for viral hepatitis and liver cancer (Quidong, China) found that table salt enriched with sodium selenite reduced the incidence of liver cancer by 35% during the 8-year follow-up period, whereas no changes were observed for the control groups (Yu et al 1997). Additionally, incidences of liver cancer began to rise after withdrawal of selenium supplementation. Patients with hepatocellular carcinoma had significantly lower serum selenium levels (along with iron, copper, and zinc) compared to those in the control group. The researchers speculated that lower levels of these minerals may act as biomarkers of the increased severity of viral hepatic damage (Lin et al 2006).

Prostate cancer

While much epidemiological and clinical data suggest that selenium may prevent prostate cancer, not all studies have shown a protective effect.

The Selenium and Vitamin E Cancer Prevention Trial (SELECT) (*n* = 35,533) determined that selenium (200 mcg/day) with or without concomitant vitamin E supplementation did not prevent prostate cancer among healthy men over age 50 (Se without vitamin E HR 1.09; Se with vitamin E HR 1.05) (Klein et al 2011). Secondary analyses corroborated these primary findings (Se without vitamin E HR 1.04; Se with vitamin E HR 1.05) (Lippman et al 2009). Similarly, among participants in the Prostate Cancer Prevention trial, secondary analysis found no association between selenium, either through dietary intake or supplementation, and risk of prostate cancer (Kristal et al 2010). A recent phase III randomised, double-blinded, placebo-controlled trial found that compared to placebo, selenium supplementation had no effect on incidence of prostate cancer in men (n = 699) who were at high risk of the disease (200 mcg/day HR 0.94; 400 mcg/day HR 0.90) (Algotar et al 2013).

Peters et al (2007) observed that there was no inverse association between prediagnostic serum selenium concentration and the risk of prostate cancer in a large cohort study with 724 cases and 879 matched controls. However, higher serum selenium levels may reduce prostate cancer risk in men who reported a high intake of vitamin E, in multivitamin users and in smokers (Peters et al 2007). Another prospective cohort study, the Vitamins And Lifestyle (VITAL) study, investigated the association of vitamin E and selenium supplementation with prostate cancer. No association was found between long-term selenium supplementation (average of 10 years) and prostate cancer risk, with an average intake of >50 microgram/day compared to non-users. Supplementation for longer than an average of 10 years, however, was associated with a statistically non-significant reduction in prostate cancer among older men (≥ 70 years) (Peters et al 2008).

Selenium supplementation has been found to have no significant effect on prostate cancer in a number of populations, men with localised non-metastatic prostate cancer not receiving active treatment (Stratton et al 2010), men with high-grade prostatic intraepithelial neoplasia (HGPIN) (Fleshner et al 2011, Marshall et al 2011). Subset analysis of the study by Marshall and colleagues (2011) found a non-significant reduced risk in men receiving selenium verses placebo in the lowest quartile of baseline plasma selenium, suggesting that future studies on this population alone may be of benefit.

By contrast, a large case-control study involved 33,737 males and identified an association between higher selenium status and a reduced risk of prostate cancer (Yoshizawa et al 1998). The study showed that men consuming the most dietary selenium (assessed indirectly by measuring toenail selenium levels) developed 65% fewer cases of advanced prostate cancer than those with the lowest intake.

Strong evidence for a protective effect of selenium against prostate cancer comes from the Nutritional Prevention of Cancer (NPC) trial, as described above, in which the incidence of prostate cancer was reduced in the selenium group by two-thirds as compared to placebo. Further follow-up has revealed that selenium supplementation continues to show a marked reduction on the incidence of prostate cancer with strongest effects seen in men with a PSA <4 ng/mL and those with the lowest serum selenium levels at study entry (Duffield-Lillico et al 2003). It is interesting to note that the NPC trial was conducted in an area with low soil selenium content, and this may in part explain the conflicting results in studies conducted in various countries around the world.

A meta-analysis of 20 epidemiological studies found an inverse association between selenium levels (assessed in studies by serum, plasma and toenail) and risk of prostate cancer (Brinkman et al 2006). This supports the findings of an earlier meta-analysis of 16 studies (Etminan et al 2005). Similarly, in a prospective, case-control study (n = 130), men with newly diagnosed prostate cancer had significantly lower serum selenium compared to healthy controls (66.3 microgram/L versus 77.5 microgram/L, respectively). An increase of 10 microgram/L in serum selenium concentration was associated with a significant decrease in risk of prostate cancer (Pourmand et al 2008).

Stomach and oesophageal cancers

A Cochrane review of five trials found that selenium appears to show significant beneficial effects against gastrointestinal cancer incidence (RR 0.59); however, four of these had a high risk of bias, therefore further RCTs are warranted (Bjelakovic et al 2008).

A large study of nearly 30,000 people demonstrated a protective effect for a combination of selenium, beta-carotene and vitamin E against the development of cancer of the gastric cardia and oesophagus (Mark et al 2000). Supplementation also reduced the cancer mortality rate compared with those not receiving supplementation. Protective effects on total cancer deaths developed slowly, appearing after 1 year of treatment, and the effect on stomach cancer appeared after 2 years. Gene–selenium interactions may influence an individual's susceptibility to oesophageal cancer. Individuals with polymorphisms in aldehyde dehydrogenase-2 Lys/Lys, X-ray repair cross-complementing 1399 Gln/Gln or Gln/Arg alleles, glutathione S-transferase isoenzyme Ile/Ile genotype or p53 (tumour suppressor gene) Pro/Pro genotype who consumed a low-selenium diet were at the greater risk of oesophageal squamous cell carcinoma, especially when combined with tobacco and alcohol intake (Cai et al 2006a, 2006b).

The protective role of selenium on gastric cancer risk may occur only in those with low baseline selenium. In a study where the levels of selenium were relatively high in both cases and controls, the lowest risk of gastric cancer was found in those with the lowest quartile of selenium level (assessed by toenail levels), whereas those with the highest risk were in the second highest quartile (Koriyama et al 2008).

Colorectal cancer

The incidence of colorectal adenomas, the precursor to most colorectal cancers, may be reduced by selenium. An inverse association between selenium and adenomas has been found in numerous studies, particularly among smokers and those with low baseline serum or plasma selenium (Clark et al 1993, Connelly-Frost et al 2006, Fernandez-Banares et al 2002, Jacobs et al 2004, Peters et al 2006, Reid et al 2006, Russo et al 1997). However, others have reported no association in risk (Early et al 2002, Wallace et al 2003). Compared to age-matched healthy controls, patients with colorectal cancer were found to have statistically lower serum selenium levels. Furthermore, a higher level of selenium was present in the cancerous tissue than in healthy tissue, though it is unclear whether this is the reason for the decreased selenium in the serum or whether the decreased serum levels occur prior to the development of colorectal cancer (Charalabopoulos et al 2006).

Premalignant skin lesions

Increased selenium status may reduce the incidence of arsenic-related premalignant skin lesions (Chen et al 2007, Huang et al 2008). This is consistent with several observational studies that found a protective association between plasma selenium level and the risk of non-melanoma skin cancer (Breslow et al 1995, Clark et al 1984, Karagas et al 1997). Long-term selenium supplementation may exert a protective effect against arsenic-induced premalignant skin lesions by reversing some of the changes in gene expression (Kibriya et al 2007).

Female reproductive

Selenium status measured by plasma levels and erythrocyte glutathione peroxidase activity was significantly lower in patients with cancer or benign neoplasia of the reproductive tract (uterus or ovary). Furthermore, examination of tissue margins of the tumours following surgery revealed significantly higher selenium concentrations compared to healthy tissue margins of healthy tissue. This suggests a protective role of selenium in the development of these reproductive tumours and a compensatory up-regulation of antioxidant defence systems in tumours due to persistent oxidative stress (Piekutowski et al 2007).

Oral cancer

Selenium levels are significantly associated with risk of oral squamous cell carcinoma, with lower levels found in patients compared to both healthy controls and those with precancerous lesions (oral submucous fibrosis and oral leucoplakia) (Khanna & Karjodkar 2006).

Lymphoma

In combination with chemotherapy, supplementation of selenium (as sodium selenite, 0.2 mg/kg/day) was found to have a synergistic effect, as observed through increased percentage of apoptotic lymphoma cells, reduced cervical and axillary lymphadenopathy, decreased splenic size and decreased bone marrow infiltration (Asfour et al 2009). This suggests that selenium may be a useful adjunct treatment in patients with non-Hodgkin's lymphoma; however, further studies are required with increased sample size and power to fully determine the effect of selenium supplementation.

Lung cancer

A randomised, double-blind, placebo-controlled, phase III trial, which looked at selenium supplementation in patients with resected stage I non-small-cell lung cancer found that while selenium (200 mcg/day for 48 months) was safe and well tolerated, it did not provide any significant benefit over placebo in the prevention of secondary primary tumours (Karp et al 2013).

Reducing radiotherapy-related adverse effects

In a multicentre, phase III clinical trial, selenium supplementation during radiotherapy for cerival and uterine cancers was found to be effective to reduce frequency and severity of radiotherapy-induced diarrhea in cervical and uterine cancers (Muecke et al 2010, 2013).

Reducing mortality from HIV infection

Selenium appears to be important in HIV infection, with plasma selenium a strong predictor of disease outcome in both adults and children (Baum & Shor-Posner 1998, Baum et al 1997, Campa et al 1999).

Low selenium status is common in HIV-positive patients and associated with a decline in Th (CD4) cell counts (Bates 2005). Low selenium is also associated with an increased incidence of mycobacterial diseases in HIV-1-seropositive drug users (Dworkin 1994, Dworkin et al 1986, 1989, Shor-Posner et al 2002).

In a double-blind, randomised, placebo-controlled trial, selenium supplementation (200 microgram/day) for 9 months suppressed the progression of HIV-1 viral burden and indirectly improved CD4 counts in adult HIV-infected men and women (Hurwitz et al 2007). One small intervention trial using low-dose selenium supplements (80 microgram/day with 25 mg vitamin E) over 2 months showed an improvement in general symptoms, but no alterations to immunological or haemotological parameters (Cirelli et al 1991).

In antiretroviral therapy-naïve adults, the combination of selenium with multivitamins over 24 months significantly reduced the risk of immune decline and morbidity association with HIV infection; however, neither selenium nor multivitamins alone resulted in any statistically significant changes (Baum et al 2013).

The protective role of selenium in HIV-infected pregnant women is less clear. A 2012 Cochrane review determined that while selenium may improve child survival and reduce maternal diarrhoeal morbidity, it did not delay maternal HIV progression or improve pregnancy outcomes (Siegfried et al 2012).

One study found that low plasma selenium status was associated with increased risk of intrapartum transmission of HIV, risk of fetal and child mortality and the risk of small-for-gestational age (Kupka et al 2005). Selenium supplementation (200 mcg/day) during pregnancy in an RCT was also associated with reduced diarrhoeal morbidity risk by 40% (RR 0.60, 95% CI 0.42–0.84) in HIV-infected women (Kupka et al 2009). By contrast, in a randomised, double-blind, placebo-controlled trial, 200 microgram/day of selenium during and after pregnancy did not improve HIV disease progression, fetal mortality, prematurity or small-for-gestational age birth. Supplementation may, however, improve child survival after 6 weeks (Kupka et al 2008).

Selenium and selenium-dependent glutathione peroxidase (GSH-Px) are important for antioxidant protection and reducing oxidative damage in HIV. Antioxidant defences are increased in selenium-replete HIV patients due to the increase in oxidative stress induced by the infection (Stephensen et al 2007). However, in those with poor selenium levels and subsequently reduced GSH-Px defences, the increased oxidative stress may increase HIV progression (Ogunro et al 2006).

Cardiovascular disease prevention

While a number of epidemiological studies have implicated a role for selenium in reducing cardiovascular disease mortality a recent Cochrane review of 12 RCTs (n = 19,715) found that of the data available, current evidence does not support the use of selenium for the primary prevention of cardiovascular disease (Rees et al 2013). A 2006 meta-analysis found that while analysis of RCTs had suggested there were no significant changes in coronary events following selenium supplementation, when analysing observational studies, 11 out of 14 cohort studies and 9 out of 11 case-control studies found an overall positive effect associated with selenium (Flores-Mateo et al 2006). These discrepancies may be due to observational studies, including selenium in combination with other vitamins/minerals, which may have confounded results.

No significant primary preventive effect was seen for selenium supplementation (200 microgram/day) and incidence of cardiovascular disease, myocardial infarction, stroke or all cardiovascular disease mortality in the NPC study (Stranges et al 2006). Lack of association was confirmed when analyses were further stratified by tertiles of baseline plasma selenium concentrations. Selenium has also been found to have no significant effect on endothelial function or pheripheral artery responsiveness in a randomised placebo-controlled trial of healthy men (Hawkes & Laslett 2009).

Many of the studies investigating selenium and cardiovascular disease have been conducted in European countries that have a lower selenium intake compared to countries such as the United States. It is possible that selenium is most effective at preventing cardiovascular disease in areas with intake levels less than those in the United States (Bleys et al 2008). The dose used in studies may also affect findings, with Bleys et al (2008) identifying that serum selenium levels below 120 ng/mL were associated with reduced cardiovascular and coronary heart disease mortality, while levels above this showed no statistically significant effect (Bleys et al 2008). It has been suggested that low selenium status may contribute to the development of hypertension. In a cross-sectional longitudinal study involving 710 Flemish subjects with an average baseline blood pressure of 130/77 mmHg, an inverse relationship was found between blood selenium and blood pressure in men at follow-up (median of 5.2 years). A 20-microgram/L higher baseline blood selenium concentration was associated with a 37% lower risk of developing high-normal BP or hypertension. No association was found in women (Nawrot et al 2007).

In non-Hodgkin's lymphoma patients receiving selenium supplementation as an adjunct to chemotherapy, supplementation prevented reductions in cardiac ejection fractions seen in patients who received chemotherapy alone, suggesting a possible cardioprotective effect (Asfour et al 2009).

Dyslipidaemia

Randomised, placebo-controlled, parallel-group study (*n* = 501) identified that selenium supplementation (100–300 mcg/day) had a beneficial effect on lipid profile in persons aged 60–74 years. Reductions at all doses were seen for total cholesterol and non-HDL cholesterol; however, improvement was seen at 300 mcg/day selenium only in HDL cholesterol (Rayman et al 2011).

Compared to premenopausal women, postmenopausal women had lower erythrocyte selenium levels, which were associated with significantly higher levels of total cholesterol, triglycerides and LDL cholesterol. This association remained after controlling for age, smoking status and body mass index (Karita et al 2008). Further studies with increased sample size and across a wider age range is recommended.

Diabetes

The relationship between selenium and diabetes is complex. It has been proposed that the association between selenium and cardiometabolic outcomes is U-shaped, with potential harm possible outside of the physiological range (Rayman & Stranges 2013, Zhou et al 2013). Inconsistent evidence available for selenium and its role in diabetes may be a result of differences in biomarker specificity, variability between trial subjects in baseline selenium status as well as inherent variations between population, age or racial groups (Rayman & Stranges 2013).

Selenium and selenoproteins appears to be involved in several key aspects of pancreatic beta-cell and islet function, increasing insulin content and secretion (Campbell et al 2008). Compared to healthy controls, diabetic patients have been found to have lower selenium levels (assessed by toenail levels) (Rajpathak et al 2005). Supplementation with selenium in diabetic patients has been found to reduce activation of NF-kappa B and levels of oxidative stress, and thus may help to prevent vascular complications (Faure et al 2004). Selenium has also been found to inhibit high glucose- and high insulin-induced expression of adhesion molecule via modulation of p38 pathway, and may therefore help to prevent the development of atherosclerosis in diabetics (Zheng et al 2008).

A randomised, double-blind, placebo-controlled trial (*n* = 84) determined that selenium supplementation (200 mcg/day) significantly lowered fasting serum insulin levels after 6 weeks, and, in combination with L-arginine (5 g/day), reduced the fasting nitric oxide concentration (Alizadeh et al 2012).

However, some evidence suggests that chronically high selenium levels in selenium-replete populations may increase the risk of developing diabetes. Results from the NHANES III found that those in the highest quintile of serum selenium had a statistically significant increased prevalence of diabetes compared with those in the first quintile (Bleys et al 2007). Similarly, secondary analysis of the NPC trial found that 200 microgram/day of selenium for an average of 7.7 years did not prevent diabetes and statistically significantly increased the risk of type 2 diabetes compared to the placebo group (Stranges et al 2007).

Selenium may play a protective role in gestational diabetes. A cross-sectional study involving 178 pregnant women (24–28 weeks of gestation) found a significant inverse correlation between selenium and blood glucose levels in patients with gestational diabetes mellitus or glucose intolerance having lower serum selenium levels compared to healthy controls (Kilinc et al 2008). This supports similar findings (Al-Saleh et al 2004, 2007, Bo et al 2005, Hawkes et al 2004, Molnar et al 2008, Tan et al 2001).

Adiposity

Associations between selenium and adiposity have been identified through a number of studies. A cross-sectional analysis of the National Diet and Nutrition Survey from the United Kingdom identified an inverse association between plasma selenium and waist circumference, and a positive association between red blood cell waist-to-hip ratio, although causality and underlying mechanisms were not investigated (Spina et al 2013).

Respiratory diseases

Asthma

Despite a number of observational studies suggesting that asthma, respiratory symptoms and ventilatory function may be associated with lowered circulatory selenium status and glutathione peroxidase activity (Devereux & Seaton 2005, Hasselmark et al 1990, Kadrabova et al 1996, Misso et al 1996, Omland et al 2002), a small number of intervention studies have been conducted, producing mixed results (Gazdik et al 2002a, 2002b, Hasselmark et al 1993).

Meta-analysis of data from a case-control study involving 569 asthmatic patients and 576 healthy controls in 14 European centres found no overall effect between plasma selenium levels and the risk of asthma (Burney et al 2008). These results are similar to those from a randomised, double-blind, placebo-controlled trial involving 197 asthmatic subjects given either a selenium supplement (high-selenium yeast preparation of 100 microgram) daily or placebo for 6 months. While the baseline plasma selenium levels increased by 48% in the treatment group, there was no significant difference between the groups with regard to either the primary outcome (asthma-related QOL score) or the secondary outcomes, including lung function, asthma symptom scores, peak flow and bronchodilator usage (Shaheen et al 2007).

A small randomised, double-blind study ($n = 24$) of patients with intrinsic asthma found that while 100 mcg sodium selenite daily for 14 weeks significantly increased serum selenium and platelet glutathione peroxidase activity, no significant improvements over baseline in any clinical parameters were observed (Hasselmark et al 1993). By contrast, a small pilot study of 17 asthmatics dependent on corticosteroid medication found that a dose of 200 microgram selenium daily taken over a 96-week period reduced both inhaled and systemic corticosteroid requirements. The same study observed selenium supplementation enhancing immunity (Gazdik et al 2002a, 2002b).

Selenium appears to have a protective role in reducing childhood wheezing. Low plasma selenium levels during early pregnancy and in the neonate have been found to increase the risk of early childhood wheezing, although this positive association was no longer found at the age of 5 (Devereux et al 2007). Similarly, in a study of 61 children aged 0.3–5 years with no atopic history, lower serum selenium levels were found in those with frequent wheezing compared with those in healthy controls, and selenium levels were significantly correlated with the number of wheezing episodes experienced in the previous year. This protective effect may be due to preventing the progression of respiratory infections, which subsequently contribute to the development of wheezing (Kocabas et al 2006).

UPPER RESPIRATORY TRACT INFECTION — IN COMBINATION

Echinacea purpurea in combination with selenium, zinc and ascorbic acid, but not *E. purpurea* alone, in chronic obstructive pulmonary disease patients with upper-respiratory tract infection significantly reduced severity and duration of infection compared to placebo. Further studies are warranted to determine the role of selenium within this multiple micronutrient supplementation (Isbaniah et al 2011).

Autoimmune thyroiditis

Selenium appears to play an important role in the health of thyroid gland function and the prevention of disease. In a study of differences in selenium levels between those with thyroid disease and those without, selenium levels were significantly decreased in those with both benign thyroid disease (subacute and silent thyroiditis) and malignant thyroid disease (follicular and papillary thyroid carcinoma) compared to healthy controls (Moncayo et al 2008). Similarly in a study of patients with Graves' disease, those with the highest serum selenium levels (>120 microgram/L) were more likely to be in disease remission (Wertenbruch et al 2007). Following 6 months selenium treatment (100 microgram twice daily), patients with mild Graves' orbitopathy were found to have a slowed disease progression and an increased quality of life compared to placebo in a randomised, controlled, clinical trial (Marcocci et al 2011). These data suggest selenium may be of benefit in those patients with Graves' disease.

Selenium supplementation may improve inflammatory activity in chronic autoimmune thyroiditis patients, as evidenced by a significant reduction in the concentration of thyroid peroxidase antibodies (TPO-Ab) to 63.8% in selenium-supplemented subjects versus 88% ($P = 0.95$) in placebo subjects (Gartner et al 2002). The randomised study of 70 females (mean age 47.5 years) compared 200 microgram sodium selenium daily orally for 90 days to placebo. A follow-up crossover study of 47 patients from the initial 70 was conducted for a further 6 months (Gartner & Gasnier 2003). The group that continued to take sodium selenite (200 microgram/day) experienced further significant decreases, whereas the group that ceased selenium use experienced a significant increase. The patients who received 200 microgram sodium selenite after placebo also experienced a significant decrease in levels of TPO-Ab.

A recent Cochrane review of four RCTs found that selenium supplementation in Hashimoto's thyroiditis determined that currently there was insufficient evidence to support use of selenium in this disorder (van Zuuren et al 2013). A total of 463 participants across four RCTs (279 selenium treated, 184 controls) were included in the meta-analysis, with duration of treatment ranging from 3 to 18 months. The Cochrane review concluded that there is a need for high-quality RCTs to properly evaluate the effects of selenium in this population, with three currently ongoing studies that may aid in clarifying current evidence.

In a prospective study of 80 patients with Hashimoto's thyroiditis receiving 200 microgram selenium (as selenomethionine) there was a significant 9.9% decrease in TPO-Ab levels after 6 months. In those patients who continued to take the selenium for another 6 months TPO-Ab levels decreased by another 8%, while those who ceased treatment experienced a 4.8% increase (Mazokopakis et al 2007).

Rheumatoid arthritis (RA)

Selenium supplements have been used in RA because of its antioxidant activity and the observation that some patients with RA have been reported with low selenium status (O'Dell et al 1991, Rosenstein & Caldwell 1999). One double-blind, placebo-controlled intervention study of 55 patients with moderate RA found that both placebo and selenium appeared to have significant effects on a number of symptoms; however, only selenium significantly improved arm movements and sense of wellbeing (Peretz et al 2001).

Lowered male fertility

Xu et al (2003) identified a significantly positive correlation between selenium levels and sperm density, sperm number, sperm motility and sperm viability in human volunteers. Similarly, Akinloye et al (2005) reported a significant inverse correlation between serum selenium level and sperm count and serum testosterone, and seminal plasma selenium with spermatozoa motility, viability and morphology (Akinloye et al 2005). Supplementation with selenium in selenium-replete subfertile men has been shown to improve sperm motility and the chance of successful conception in over half the treated patients (Scott et al 1998). When taken with vitamin E over 6 months, selenium produces a statistically significant increase in sperm motility, per cent live and per cent normal spermatozoa, with effects reversing after supplement cessation (Vezina et al 1996). Although results are encouraging, particularly for subfertile men with low selenium status, some studies have found no effect of selenium supplementation (Hawkes et al 2009, Iwanier & Zachara 1995).

General immune enhancement

Several intervention trials of either double-blind or open design have shown that selenium supplementation can enhance immune function and decrease the risk of developing certain infections in selenium-replete subjects, healthy adults and the elderly (Girodon et al 1999, Kiremidjian-Schumacher et al 1994, Roy et al 1994, Yu et al 1989).

The largest was a 3-year study of 20,847 people that showed substituting conventional table salt with table salt fortified with sodium selenite significantly reduced the incidence of viral hepatitis compared with controls provided with normal table salt (Yu et al 1989).

S

Critically ill patients

Selenoproteins play an important role in the immunomodulation of critically ill patients, and low levels of plasma selenium have been associated with increased markers of oxidative stress, risk of organ failure and higher mortality rates. Clinical trials of selenium supplementation in critically ill patients however have produced mixed results. A recent systematic review and meta-analysis found that selenium supplementation (≤500 microgram/day) may be associated with a beneficial effect on 28-day mortality in critically ill patients. However, it should be acknowledged that due to several factors relating to study quality, the authors state that further evaluation is required before routine adjuvant use of selenium is recommended in a clinical setting (Landucci et al 2014).

The long-term effect of selenium on mortality remains unclear. A 2011 RCT (n = 502) found selenium supplementation did not affect the risk of developing a new infection, 6-month mortality, length of stay, days of antibiotic use or modified sepsis-related organ failure assessment (Andrews et al 2011). One possible explanation suggested for negative findings is sodium selenite having a direct pro-oxidant action in these patients (Forceville 2007).

Daily infusion of 1600 microgram Se (as selenite) over 10 days was also found to significantly decrease incidence of hospital-acquired pneumonia, including early ventilator-associated pneumonia, in critically ill patients with SIRS (Manzanares et al 2011).

Mood elevation and reduced anxiety

Considering that low dietary intake of selenium has been linked with greater incidence of anxiety, depression and tiredness, several research groups have investigated whether higher dietary intake or selenium supplementation will elevate mood and/or reduce anxiety. Currently, results are equivocal; however, it appears that selenium-replete individuals are most likely to respond to supplementation, if a response is observed.

A randomised double-blind placebo-controlled trial of primigravida women (n = 166) found that 100 microgram/day selenium supplementation was associated with reduced symptoms of depression compared to those receiving placebo in the 8 weeks following delivery (Mokhber et al 2011).

Simiarly, an early double-blind, crossover study showed that short-term selenium supplementation (100 microgram/day for 5 weeks) significantly elevated mood and decreased anxiety, depression and tiredness, with effects most marked in people with low dietary intake (Benton & Cook 1991). A study of 30 selenium-replete men who were fed either a low (32.6 microgram/day) or a high (226.5 microgram/day) selenium diet for 15 weeks found that the mood of those with the higher selenium intake improved, whereas mood worsened with low intake (Finley & Penland 1998 as reported in Rayman 2005). Alternatively, another study involving 11 men of adequate selenium intake failed to show effects on mood when high (356 microgram/day) and low (13 microgram/day) selenium diets were followed for 99 days (Hawkes & Hornbostel 1996). Similarly, a large (n = 448) 2-year randomised study also failed to find evidence that additional selenium enhanced mood or any of its subscales, despite significant increases in plasma selenium levels (Rayman et al 2006). This study compared the effects of 100, 200 or 300 microgram/day of selenium to placebo for effects on mood and QOL. Selenium supplementation was given as high-selenium yeast, SelenoPrecise (Pharma Nord, Vejle, Denmark).

Reducing morbidity in preterm babies

Preterm infants are born with slightly lower selenium and glutathione peroxidase concentrations than full-term infants and have low hepatic stores of selenium. In very preterm infants, low selenium concentrations have been associated with an increased risk of chronic neonatal lung disease and retinopathy of prematurity (Darlow & Austin 2003). Although the full consequences of low selenium concentrations in this population are not fully known, observation from animal studies has found an association between selenium deficiency and increased susceptibility to oxidative lung injury. This has special significance for sick, very preterm infants as they are exposed to many possible sources of oxygen radical products, including high concentrations of inspired oxygen. A Cochrane review of three randomised studies that reported outcomes on 297 infants receiving selenium supplements and 290 control infants concluded that selenium supplementation in very preterm infants is associated with benefit in terms of a reduction in one or more episodes of late-onset sepsis, but is not associated with improved survival, a reduction in neonatal chronic lung disease or retinopathy of prematurity (Darlow & Austin 2003). It should be noted that most of the evidence derives from research conducted in New Zealand, a country with low soil and population selenium concentrations, and may not be readily translated to other populations. In one study, despite preterm infants having lower selenium levels compared to term infants, selenium levels did not correlate with chronic lung disease or septicaemia (Loui et al 2008).

OTHER USES

Used in combination with other antioxidants or administered intravenously, selenium has been used in pancreatitis and as adjunctive therapy in cancer patients.

Supplementation of selenium with coenzyme Q10 and vitamin E has been found to improve clinical conditions associated with severe psoriasis, including reduced oxidative stress markers in both plasma and lesional epidermis (Kharaeva et al 2009).

Oral sodium selenite (350 microgram/m^2 body surface area) was given daily for 4–6 weeks to 52 patients with extensive, persistent or progressive lymphoedema from radiation and resulted in the majority experiencing some reduction in oedema (Micke et al 2002). A further study (Micke et al 2003) of 48 patients found that sodium selenite supplementation had a positive effect on secondary lymphoedema caused by radiation therapy alone or by irradiation after surgery. The group consisted of 12 patients with oedema of the arm and 36 with oedema of the head and neck region. Increased dietary intake of selenium over 1 year was found to be positively correlated with capillary recruitment in skin of healthy men ($P = 0.038$), suggesting it may have a role in microvascular function and health (Buss et al 2013). In patients with leukaemia, undergoing allogenic haematopoietic stem cell transplantation, selenium treatment was found to reduce the incidence of oral mucositis, as well as the duration of objective oral mucositis compared to placebo (Jahangard Rafsanjani et al 2013).

Cancer treatment often induces toxicity associated with the oxidative damage to normal cells. A Cochrane review of selenium in the prevention of side effects associated with cancer treatment (Dennert & Horneber 2006) found only three trials that met inclusion criteria. One study found a lower incidence of recurrent erysipela infections of lymphoedematous upper limbs after breast cancer treatment in the selenium group, with a second study finding reduced facial swelling in selenium-treated patients in a 2-week period following surgical tumour resection. Preliminary results from another study suggest a lower incidence of diarrhoea in those receiving pelvic radiotherapy. On the whole, the authors concluded that there was still insufficient evidence to support selenium supplementation to reduce adverse effects of tumour-specific chemotherapy.

In an animal model, moderate selenium supplementation increased the total antioxidant activity leading to a lower generation of reactive oxygen metabolites, which helped to counteract the cardiotoxicity associated with the chemotherapeutic drug Adriamycin (Danesi et al 2006).

DOSAGE RANGE

The Therapeutic Goods Act altered the allowed amount of selenium in listed products to be raised to 150 microgram. Supplements containing selenium carry the following caution on their label: 'This product contains selenium which is toxic in high doses. A daily dose of 150 microgram for adults of selenium from dietary supplements should not be exceeded.'

Australian RDI

Children

- 1–3 years: 25 microgram
- 4–8 years: 30 microgram
- 9–13 years: 50 microgram

14–18 years

- Boys: 70 microgram
- Girls: 60 microgram

Adults

- Males >18 years: 70 microgram
- Females >18 years: 60 microgram
- Pregnancy: 65 microgram
- Lactation: 75 microgram

According to clinical studies

- Asthma: 100–200 microgram/day of sodium selenite.
- Cancer prophylaxis: 200 microgram/day selenium (supplied as 500 mg brewer's yeast).
- Infertility: 100 microgram/day.
- Mood disturbances: 100 microgram/day.
- Post myocardial infarction: selenium-rich yeast 100 microgram/day.
- Rheumatoid arthritis: 200 microgram/day.
- Autoimmune thyroiditis: 200 microgram/day sodium selenite.
- HIV-positive status: 80 microgram/day has been used but it is most likely that higher doses are required.

TOXICITY

Long-term ingestion of excessive levels of selenium (>1000 microgram/day) may produce fatigue, depression, arthritis, hair or fingernail loss, garlicky breath or body odour and gastrointestinal disorders or irritability (Fan & Kizer 1990). Chronic low-level overexposure has been associated with lethargy, dizziness, motor weakness and paraesthesia (Vinceti et al 2013).

ADVERSE REACTIONS

Nausea, vomiting, nail changes, irritability and fatigue have been reported.

The organic form of selenium found in high-selenium yeast is often preferred because it is less toxic.

The National Health and Medical Research Council of Australia states that selenium intake should not exceed 600 microgram/day.

SIGNIFICANT INTERACTIONS

Cisplatin

Selenium may reduce associated nephrotoxicity, myeloid suppression and weight loss, according to in vitro and in vivo tests (Camargo et al 2001, Ohkawa et al 1988) — potentially beneficial interaction.

Heavy metals (e.g. mercury, lead, arsenic, silver and cadmium)

Selenium reduces toxicity of heavy metals such as mercury, lead, arsenic, silver and cadmium by forming inert complexes — beneficial interaction.

Practice points/Patient counselling

- Selenium is a trace element that is essential for health.
- Low selenium states have been associated with a variety of conditions, such as cardiovascular disease, cancer, asthma, atopy, male subfertility, rheumatoid arthritis, depression and anxiety and compromised immune function.
- High-intensity sports training has been associated with a reduction in plasma selenium levels (Wang et al 2012).
- Studies have identified selenium deficiency in a significant number of people with the HIV infection and suggested a link between selenium levels and mortality rate.
- It is also involved in the detoxification of some heavy metals and xenobiotics.
- Selenium-enriched yeast is the safest way to supplement the diet, but other forms are also used.

CONTRAINDICATIONS AND PRECAUTIONS

Sensitivity to selenium.

PREGNANCY USE

Considered safe in usual dietary doses; safety at higher levels is unknown.

PATIENTS' FAQs

What will this supplement do for me?

Adequate selenium intake, and in some cases supplementation may reduce the risk of developing certain cancers and heart disease and help to improve a range of conditions such as rheumatoid arthritis, asthma, autoimmune thyroiditis, male subfertility, depression and anxiety.

When will it start to work?

If a protective effect is to occur with selenium against cancer or cardiovascular disease, the effect appears to develop slowly over several years' consistent intake.

Are there any safety issues?

High intakes of selenium above 1000 microgram/day have been associated with a number of adverse effects and should be avoided.

S

REFERENCES

Akbaraly TN et al. Plasma selenium over time and cognitive decline in the elderly. Epidemiology 18.1 (2007): 52–58.

Akinloye O et al. Selenium status of idiopathic infertile Nigerian males. Biol Trace Elem Res 104.1 (2005): 9–18.

Al-Saleh E et al. Maternal-fetal status of copper, iron, molybdenum, selenium and zinc in patients with gestational diabetes. J Matern Fetal Neonatal Med 16.1 (2004): 15–21.

Al-Saleh E et al. Maternal-foetal status of copper, iron, molybdenum, selenium and zinc in obese gestational diabetic pregnancies. Acta Diabetol 44.3 (2007): 106–113.

Algotar AM et al. Phase 3 clinical trial investigating the effect of selenium supplementation in men at high-risk for prostate cancer. Prostate 73.3 (2013): 328–335.

Alizadeh M et al. Effect of L-arginine and selenium added to a hypocaloric diet enriched with legumes on cardiovascular disease risk factors in women with central obesity: a randomized, double-blind, placebo-controlled trial. Ann Nutr Metab 60.2 (2012): 157–168.

Andrews PJ et al. Randomised trial of glutamine, selenium, or both, to supplement parenteral nutrition for critically ill patients. BMJ 342 (2011): d1542.

Asfour IA et al. High-dose sodium selenite can induce apoptosis of lymphoma cells in adult patients with non-Hodgkin's lymphoma. Biol Trace Elem Res 127.3 (2009): 200–210.

Bates CJ. Selenium. In: Benjamin C (ed), Encyclopedia of human nutrition., Oxford: Elsevier, 2005, pp. 118–125.
Baum MK, Shor-Posner G. Micronutrient status in relationship to mortality in HIV-1 disease. Nutr Rev 56.1 (1998): S135–S139.
Baum MK et al. Effect of micronutrient supplementation on disease progression in asymptomatic, antiretroviral-naive, HIV-infected adults in Botswana: a randomized clinical trial. JAMA 310.20 (2013): 2154–2163.
Baum MK et al. High risk of HIV-related mortality is associated with selenium deficiency. J Acquir Immune Defic Syndr Hum Retrovirol 15.5 (1997): 370–374.
Beck J et al. Low serum selenium concentrations are associated with poor grip strength among older women living in the community. Biofactors 29.1 (2007): 37–44.
Benton D, Cook R. The impact of selenium supplementation on mood. Biol Psychiatry 29.11 (1991): 1092–1098.
Berry JP, Galle P. Selenium-arsenic interaction in renal cells: role of lysosomes. Electron microprobe study. J Submicrosc Cytol Pathol 26.2 (1994): 203–210.
Bjelakovic G et al. Antioxidant supplements for preventing gastrointestinal cancers. Coch DB Syst Rev 2008 (2008): CD004183.
Bleys J, Navas-Acien A, Guallar E. Serum selenium and diabetes in U.S. adults. Diabetes Care 30.4 (2007): 829–834.
Bleys J et al. Serum selenium levels and all-cause, cancer, and cardiovascular mortality among US adults. Arch Intern Med 168.4 (2008): 404–410.
Bo S et al. Gestational hyperglycemia, zinc, selenium, and antioxidant vitamins. Nutrition 21.2 (2005): 186–191.
Bolkent S et al. Effects of vitamin E, vitamin C, and selenium on gastric fundus in cadmium toxicity in male rats. Int J Toxicol 27.2 (2008): 217–222.
Breslow RA et al. Serological precursors of cancer: malignant melanoma, basal and squamous cell skin cancer, and prediagnostic levels of retinol, beta-carotene, lycopene, alpha-tocopherol, and selenium. Cancer Epidemiol Biomarkers Prev 4.8 (1995): 837–842.
Brinkman M et al. Are men with low selenium levels at increased risk of prostate cancer? Eur J Cancer 42.15 (2006): 2463–2471.
Burney P et al. A case-control study of the relation between plasma selenium and asthma in European populations: a GAL2EN project. Allergy 63.7 (2008): 865–871.
Buss C et al. Long-term dietary intake of selenium, calcium, and dairy products is associated with improved capillary recruitment in healthy young men. Eur J Nutr 52.3 (2013): 1099–1105.
Cai L et al. Dietary selenium intake, aldehyde dehydrogenase-2 and X-ray repair cross-complementing 1 genetic polymorphisms, and the risk of esophageal squamous cell carcinoma. Cancer 106.11 (2006a): 2345–2354.
Cai L et al. Dietary selenium intake and genetic polymorphisms of the GSTP1 and p53 genes on the risk of esophageal squamous cell carcinoma. Cancer Epidemiol Biomarkers Prev 15.2 (2006b): 294–300.
Camargo SM et al. Oral administration of sodium selenite minimizes cisplatin toxicity on proximal tubules of rats. Biol Trace Elem Res 83.3 (2001): 251–262.
Campa A et al. Mortality risk in selenium-deficient HIV-positive children. J Acquir Immune Defic Syndr Hum Retrovirol 20.5 (1999): 508–513.
Campbell SC et al. Selenium stimulates pancreatic beta-cell gene expression and enhances islet function. FEBS Lett 582.15 (2008): 2333–2337.
Charalabopoulos K et al. Low selenium levels in serum and increased concentration in neoplastic tissues in patients with colorectal cancer: correlation with serum carcinoembryonic antigen. Scand J Gastroenterol 41.3 (2006): 359–360.
Chen Y et al. A prospective study of blood selenium levels and the risk of arsenic-related premalignant skin lesions. Cancer Epidemiol Biomarkers Prev 16.2 (2007): 207–213.
Christensen MJ et al. High selenium reduces NF-kappaB-regulated gene expression in uninduced human prostate cancer cells. Nutr Cancer 58.2 (2007): 197–204.
Chuang HY et al. A case-control study on the relationship of hearing function and blood concentrations of lead, manganese, arsenic, and selenium. Sci Total Environ 387.1–3 (2007): 79–85.
Chun JY et al. Mechanisms of selenium down-regulation of androgen receptor signaling in prostate cancer. Mol Cancer Ther 5.4 (2006): 913–918.
Cirelli A et al. Serum selenium concentration and disease progress in patients with HIV infection. Clin Biochem 24.2 (1991): 211–214.
Clark LC et al. Decreased incidence of prostate cancer with selenium supplementation: results of a double-blind cancer prevention trial. Br J Urol 81.5 (1998): 730–734.
Clark LC et al. Effects of selenium supplementation for cancer prevention in patients with carcinoma of the skin: a randomized controlled trial (Nutritional Prevention of Cancer Study Group). JAMA 276.24 (1996): 1957–1963.
Clark LC et al. Plasma selenium concentration predicts the prevalence of colorectal adenomatous polyps. Cancer Epidemiol Biomarkers Prev 2.1 (1993): 41–46.
Clark LC et al. Plasma selenium and skin neoplasms: a case-control study. Nutr Cancer 6.1 (1984): 13–21.
Combs GF Jr et al. Effects of selenomethionine supplementation on selenium status and thyroid hormone concentrations in healthy adults. Am J Clin Nutr 89.6 (2009): 1808–1814.
Connelly-Frost A et al. Selenium, apoptosis, and colorectal adenomas. Cancer Epidemiol Biomarkers Prev 15.3 (2006): 486–493.
Danesi F et al. Counteraction of adriamycin-induced oxidative damage in rat heart by selenium dietary supplementation. J Agric Food Chem 54.4 (2006): 1203–1208.
Darlow BA, Austin NC. Selenium supplementation to prevent short-term morbidity in preterm neonates. Cochrane Database Syst Rev 4 (2003): CD003312.
Dennert G et al. Selenium for preventing cancer. Coch DB Syst Rev 5 (2011): CD005195.
Dennert G, Horneber M. Selenium for alleviating the side effects of chemotherapy, radiotherapy and surgery in cancer patients. Cochrane Database Syst Rev 3 (2006): CD005037.

Devereux G et al. Early childhood wheezing symptoms in relation to plasma selenium in pregnant mothers and neonates. Clin Exp Allergy 37.7 (2007): 1000–1008.

Devereux G, Seaton A. Diet as a risk factor for atopy and asthma. J Allergy Clin Immunol 115.6 (2005): 1109–1117.

Dhingra S, Bansal MP. Hypercholesterolemia and LDL receptor mRNA expression: modulation by selenium supplementation. Biometals 19.5 (2006a): 493–501.

Dhingra S, Bansal MP. Modulation of hypercholesterolemia-induced alterations in apolipoprotein B and HMG-CoA reductase expression by selenium supplementation. Chem Biol Interact 161.1 (2006b): 49–56.

Duffield-Lillico AJ et al. Selenium supplementation, baseline plasma selenium status and incidence of prostate cancer: an analysis of the complete treatment period of the Nutritional Prevention of Cancer Trial. BJU Int 91.7 (2003): 608–612.

Duffield-Lillico AJ et al. Baseline characteristics and the effect of selenium supplementation on cancer incidence in a randomized clinical trial: a summary report of the Nutritional Prevention of Cancer Trial. Cancer Epidemiol Biomarkers Prev 11.7 (2002): 630–639.

Dworkin BM. Selenium deficiency in HIV infection and the acquired immunodeficiency syndrome (AIDS). Chem Biol Interact 91.2–3 (1994): 181–186.

Dworkin BM et al. Reduced cardiac selenium content in the acquired immunodeficiency syndrome. J Parenter Enteral Nutr 13.6 (1989): 644–647.

Dworkin BM et al. Selenium deficiency in the acquired immunodeficiency syndrome. J Parenter Enteral Nutr 10.4 (1986): 405–407.

Early DS et al. Selenoprotein levels in patients with colorectal adenomas and cancer. Am J Gastroenterol 97.3 (2002): 745–748.

El Bayoumy K. The protective role of selenium on genetic damage and on cancer. Mutat Res 475.1–2 (2001): 123–139.

El-Sharaky AS et al. Protective role of selenium against renal toxicity induced by cadmium in rats. Toxicology 235.3 (2007): 185–193.

El-Shenawy SM, Hassan NS. Comparative evaluation of the protective effect of selenium and garlic against liver and kidney damage induced by mercury chloride in the rats. Pharmacol Rep 60.2 (2008): 199–208.

Etminan M et al. Intake of selenium in the prevention of prostate cancer: a systematic review and meta-analysis. Cancer Causes Control 16.9 (2005): 1125–1131.

Fan AM, Kizer KW. Selenium: Nutritional, toxicologic, and clinical aspects. West J Med 153.2 (1990): 160–167.

Faure P et al. Selenium supplementation decreases nuclear factor-kappa B activity in peripheral blood mononuclear cells from type 2 diabetic patients. Eur J Clin Invest 34.7 (2004): 475–481.

Fernandez-Banares F et al. Serum selenium and risk of large size colorectal adenomas in a geographical area with a low selenium status. Am J Gastroenterol 97.8 (2002): 2103–2108.

Finley W, Penland JG. Adequacy or deprivation of dietary selenium in healthy men: clinical and psychological findings. J Trace Elem Exp Med 11 (1998): 1–27.

Fleshner NE et al. Progression from high-grade prostatic intraepithelial neoplasia to cancer: a randomized trial of combination vitamin-E, soy, and selenium. J Clin Oncol 29.17 (2011): 2386–2390.

Flohe L. Selenium in mammalian spermiogenesis. Biol Chem 388.10 (2007): 987–995.

Flores-Mateo G et al. Selenium and coronary heart disease: a meta-analysis. Am J Clin Nutr 84.4 (2006): 762–773.

Forceville X. Effects of high doses of selenium, as sodium selenite, in septic shock patients: a placebo-controlled, randomized, double-blind, multi-center phase II study–selenium and sepsis. J Trace Elem Med Biol 21 (Suppl 1) (2007): 62–65.

Gao S et al. Selenium level and cognitive function in rural elderly Chinese. Am J Epidemiol 165.8 (2007): 955–965.

Gartner R et al. Selenium supplementation in patients with autoimmune thyroiditis decreases thyroid peroxidase antibodies concentrations. J Clin Endocrinol Metab 87.4 (2002): 1687–1691.

Gartner R, Gasnier BC. Selenium in the treatment of autoimmune thyroiditis. Biofactors 19.3–4 (2003): 165–170.

Gazdik F et al. The influence of selenium supplementation on the immunity of corticoid-dependent asthmatics. Bratisl Lek Listy 103.1 (2002b): 17–21.

Gazdik F et al. Decreased consumption of corticosteroids after selenium supplementation in corticoid-dependent asthmatics. Bratisl Lek Listy 103.1 (2002a): 22–25.

Girodon F et al. Impact of trace elements and vitamin supplementation on immunity and infections in institutionalized elderly patients: a randomized controlled trial. MIN. VIT. AOX. geriatric network. Arch Intern Med 159.7 (1999): 748–754.

Goldson AJ et al. Effects of selenium supplementation on selenoprotein gene expression and response to influenza vaccine challenge: a randomised controlled trial. PLoS One 6.3 (2011): e14771.

Gonzalez S et al. Life-quality indicators in elderly people are influenced by selenium status. Aging Clin Exp Res 19.1 (2007): 10–15.

Hasselmark L et al. Lowered platelet glutathione peroxidase activity in patients with intrinsic asthma. Allergy 45.7 (1990): 523–527.

Hasselmark L et al. Selenium supplementation in intrinsic asthma. Allergy 48.1 (1993): 30–36.

Hawkes WC, Hornbostel L. Effects of dietary selenium on mood in healthy men living in a metabolic research unit. Biol Psychiatry 39.2 (1996): 121–128.

Hawkes WC, Laslett LJ. Selenium supplementation does not improve vascular responsiveness in healthy North American men. Am J Physiol Heart Circ Physiol 296.2 (2009): H256–262.

Hawkes WC et al. Selenium supplementation does not affect testicular selenium status or semen quality in North American men. J Androl 30.5 (2009): 525–533.

Hawkes WC et al. High-selenium yeast supplementation in free-living North American men: no effect on thyroid hormone metabolism or body composition. J Trace Elem Med Biol 22.2 (2008): 131–142.

Hawkes WC et al. Plasma selenium decrease during pregnancy is associated with glucose intolerance. Biol Trace Elem Res 100.1 (2004): 19–29.
Hawkes WC et al. The effects of dietary selenium on the immune system in healthy men. Biol Trace Elem Res 81.3 (2001): 189–213.
Hendler S, Rorvik D. PDR for nutritional supplements. Montvale NJ: Thomson Healthcare Publishers (2001).
Hoeg A et al. Bone turnover and bone mineral density are independently related to selenium status in healthy euthyroid postmenopausal women. J Clin Endocrinol Metab 97.11 (2012): 4061–4070.
Huang Z et al. Low selenium status affects arsenic metabolites in an arsenic exposed population with skin lesions. Clin Chim Acta 387.1–2 (2008): 139–144.
Hurwitz BE et al. Suppression of human immunodeficiency virus type 1 viral load with selenium supplementation: a randomized controlled trial. Arch Intern Med 167.2 (2007): 148–154.
Isbaniah F et al. Echinacea purpurea along with zinc, selenium and vitamin C to alleviate exacerbations of chronic obstructive pulmonary disease: results from a randomized controlled trial. J Clin Pharm Ther 36.5 (2011): 568–576.
Iwanier K, Zachara BA. Selenium supplementation enhances the element concentration in blood and seminal fluid but does not change the spermatozoal quality characteristics in subfertile men. J Androl 16.5 (1995): 441–447.
Jacobs ET et al. Selenium and colorectal adenoma: results of a pooled analysis. J Natl Cancer Inst 96.22 (2004): 1669–1675.
Jahangard-Rafsanjani Z et al. The efficacy of selenium in prevention of oral mucositis in patients undergoing hematopoietic SCT: a randomized clinical trial. Bone Marrow Transplant 48.6 (2013): 832–836.
Jeong DW et al. Protection of mice from allergen-induced asthma by selenite: prevention of eosinophil infiltration by inhibition of NF-kappa B activation. J Biol Chem 277.20 (2002): 17871–17876.
Kadrabova J et al. Selenium status is decreased in patients with intrinsic asthma. Biol Trace Elem Res 52.3 (1996): 241–248.
Kang BP, Mehta U, Bansal MP. Selenium supplementation protects from high fat diet-induced atherogenesis in rats: role of mitogen stimulated lymphocytes and macrophage NO production. Indian J Exp Biol 39.8 (2001): 793–797.
Karagas MR et al. Risk of squamous cell carcinoma of the skin in relation to plasma selenium, alpha-tocopherol, beta-carotene, and retinol: a nested case-control study. Cancer Epidemiol Biomarkers Prev 6.1 (1997): 25–29.
Karita K et al. Associations of blood selenium and serum lipid levels in Japanese premenopausal and postmenopausal women. Menopause 15.1 (2008): 119–124.
Karp DD et al. Randomized, double-blind, placebo-controlled, phase III chemoprevention trial of selenium supplementation in patients with resected stage I non-small-cell lung cancer: ECOG 5597. J Clin Oncol 31.33 (2013): 4179–4187.
Kaushal N, Bansal MP. Dietary selenium variation-induced oxidative stress modulates CDC2/cyclin B1 expression and apoptosis of germ cells in mice testis. J Nutr Biochem 18.8 (2007a): 553–564.
Kaushal N, Bansal MP. Inhibition of CDC2/Cyclin B1 in response to selenium-induced oxidative stress during spermatogenesis: potential role of Cdc25c and p21. Mol Cell Biochem 298.1–2 (2007b): 139–150.
Khanna SS, Karjodkar FR. Circulating immune complexes and trace elements (Copper, Iron and Selenium) as markers in oral precancer and cancer: a randomised, controlled clinical trial. Head Face Med 2 (2006): 33.
Kharaeva Z et al. Clinical and biochemical effects of coenzyme Q10, vitamin E, and selenium supplementation to psoriasis patients. Nutrition 25.3 (2009): 295–302.
Kibriya MG et al. Changes in gene expression profiles in response to selenium supplementation among individuals with arsenic-induced pre-malignant skin lesions. Toxicol Lett 169.2 (2007): 162–176.
Kilinc M et al. Evaluation of serum selenium levels in Turkish women with gestational diabetes mellitus, glucose intolerants, and normal controls. Biol Trace Elem Res 123.1–3 (2008): 35–40.
Kiremidjian-Schumacher L, Roy M. Selenium and immune function. Z Ernahrungswiss 37 (Suppl 1) (1998): 50–56.
Kiremidjian-Schumacher L et al. Supplementation with selenium and human immune cell functions. II: Effect on cytotoxic lymphocytes and natural killer cells. Biol Trace Elem Res 41.1–2 (1994): 115–127.
Klein EA et al. Vitamin E and the risk of prostate cancer: the Selenium and Vitamin E Cancer Prevention Trial (SELECT). JAMA 306.14 (2011): 1549–1556.
Kocabas CN et al. The relationship between serum selenium levels and frequent wheeze in children. Turk J Pediatr 48.4 (2006): 308–312.
Koriyama C et al. Toenail selenium levels and gastric cancer risk in Cali. Colombia. J Toxicol Sci 33.2 (2008): 227–235.
Kristal AR et al. Diet, supplement use, and prostate cancer risk: results from the prostate cancer prevention trial. Am J Epidemiol 172.5 (2010): 566–577.
Kupka R et al. Effect of Selenium Supplements on Hemoglobin Concentration and Morbidity among HIV-1–Infected Tanzanian Women. Clin Infect Dis 48.10 (2009): 1475–1478.
Kupka R et al. Randomized, double-blind, placebo-controlled trial of selenium supplements among HIV-infected pregnant women in Tanzania: effects on maternal and child outcomes. Am J Clin Nutr 87.6 (2008): 1802–1808.
Kupka R et al. Selenium status, pregnancy outcomes, and mother-to-child transmission of HIV-1. J Acquir Immune Defic Syndr 39.2 (2005): 203–210.
Landucci F et al. Selenium supplementation in critically ill patients: A systematic review and meta-analysis. J Crit Care 29.1 (2014): 150–156.
Lauretani F et al. Association of low plasma selenium concentrations with poor muscle strength in older community-dwelling adults: the InCHIANTI Study. Am J Clin Nutr 86.2 (2007): 347–352.
Li YF et al. Organic selenium supplementation increases mercury excretion and decreases oxidative damage in long-term mercury-exposed residents from Wanshan, China. Environ Sci Technol 46.20 (2012): 11313–11318.
Lin CC et al. Selenium, iron, copper, and zinc levels and copper-to-zinc ratios in serum of patients at different stages of viral hepatic diseases. Biol Trace Elem Res 109.1 (2006): 15–24.

Lindh U, Danersund A, Lindvall A. Selenium protection against toxicity from cadmium and mercury studied at the cellular level. Noisy-le-grand: Cell Mol Biol 42.1 (1996): 39–48.

Lippman SM et al. Effect of selenium and vitamin E on risk of prostate cancer and other cancers: the Selenium and Vitamin E Cancer Prevention Trial (SELECT). JAMA 301.1 (2009): 39–51.

Loui A et al. Selenium status in term and preterm infants during the first months of life. Eur J Clin Nutr 62.3 (2008): 349–355.

Manzanares W et al. High-dose selenium reduces ventilator-associated pneumonia and illness severity in critically ill patients with systemic inflammation. Intensive Care Med 37.7 (2011): 1120–1127.

Marcocci C et al. Selenium and the course of mild Graves' orbitopathy. N Engl J Med 364.20 (2011):1920–1931.

Mark SD et al. Prospective study of serum selenium levels and incident esophageal and gastric cancers. J Natl Cancer Inst 92.21 (2000): 1753–1763.

Marshall JR et al. Phase III trial of selenium to prevent prostate cancer in men with high-grade prostatic intraepithelial neoplasia: SWOG S9917. Cancer Prev Res (Phila) 4.11 (2011): 1761–1769.

Mazokopakis EE et al. Effects of 12 months treatment with L-selenomethionine on serum anti-TPO levels in patients with Hashimoto's thyroiditis. Thyroid 17.7 (2007): 609–612.

McCarty M. Can dietary selenium reduce leukotriene production? Med Hypotheses 13.1 (1984): 45–50.

Micke O et al. Selenium in the treatment of radiation-associated lymphedema. In: Prog Radio-Oncol VII Proc, 2002: 533–546.

Micke O et al. Selenium in the treatment of radiation-associated secondary lymphedema. Int J Radiat Oncol Biol Phys 56.1 (2003): 40–49.

Misso NL et al. Reduced platelet glutathione peroxidase activity and serum selenium concentration in atopic asthmatic patients. Clin Exp Allergy 26.7 (1996): 838–847.

Mokhber N et al. Effect of supplementation with selenium on postpartum depression: a randomized double-blind placebo-controlled trial. J Matern Fetal Neonatal Med 24.1 (2011): 104–108.

Molnar J et al. Serum selenium concentrations correlate significantly with inflammatory biomarker high-sensitive CRP levels in Hungarian gestational diabetic and healthy pregnant women at mid-pregnancy. Biol Trace Elem Res 121.1 (2008): 16–22.

Moncayo R et al. The role of selenium, vitamin C, and zinc in benign thyroid diseases and of selenium in malignant thyroid diseases: Low selenium levels are found in subacute and silent thyroiditis and in papillary and follicular carcinoma. BMC Endocr Disord 8 (2008): 2.

Muecke R et al. Impact of treatment planning target volumen (PTV) size on radiation induced diarrhoea following selenium supplementation in gynecologic radiation oncology — a subgroup analysis of a multicenter, phase III trial. Radiat Oncol 8 (2013): 72.

Muecke R et al. Multicenter, phase 3 trial comparing selenium supplementation with observation in gynecologic radiation oncology. Int J Radiat Oncol Biol Phys 78.3 (2010): 828–835.

Natella F et al. Selenium supplementation prevents the increase in atherogenic electronegative LDL (LDL minus) in the postprandial phase. Nutr Metab Cardiovasc Dis 17.9 (2007): 649–656.

Navarro-Alarcon M, Lopez-Martinez MC. Essentiality of selenium in the human body: relationship with different diseases. Sci Total Environ 249.1–3 (2000): 347–371.

Nawrot TS et al. Blood pressure and blood selenium: a cross-sectional and longitudinal population study. Eur Heart J 28.5 (2007): 628–633.

O'Dell JR et al. Serum selenium concentrations in rheumatoid arthritis. Ann Rheum Dis 50.6 (1991): 376–378.

Ogunro PS et al. Plasma selenium concentration and glutathione peroxidase activity in HIV-1/AIDS infected patients: a correlation with the disease progression. Niger Postgrad Med J 13.1 (2006): 1–5.

Ohkawa K et al. The effects of co-administration of selenium and cis-platin (CDDP) on CDDP-induced toxicity and antitumour activity. Br J Cancer 58.1 (1988): 38–41.

Omland O et al. Selenium serum and urine is associated to mild asthma and atopy: The SUS study. J Trace Elem Med Biol 16.2 (2002): 123–127.

Ongele EA et al. Effects of selenium deficiency in the development of trypanosomes and humoral immune responses in mice infected with Trypanosoma musculi. Parasitol Res 88.6 (2002): 540–545.

Peretz A, Siderova V, Neve J. Selenium supplementation in rheumatoid arthritis investigated in a double blind, placebo-controlled trial. Scand J Rheumatol 30.4 (2001): 208–212.

Peters U et al. Vitamin E and selenium supplementation and risk of prostate cancer in the Vitamins and lifestyle (VITAL) study cohort. Cancer Causes Control 19.1 (2008): 75–87.

Peters U et al. Serum selenium and risk of prostate cancer — a nested case-control study. Am J Clin Nutr 85.1 (2007): 209–217.

Peters U et al. High serum selenium and reduced risk of advanced colorectal adenoma in a colorectal cancer early detection program. Cancer Epidemiol Biomarkers Prev 15.2 (2006): 315–320.

Piekutowski K et al. The antioxidative role of selenium in pathogenesis of cancer of the female reproductive system. Neoplasma 54.5 (2007): 374–378.

Pourmand G et al. Serum selenium level and prostate cancer: a case-control study. Nutr Cancer 60.2 (2008): 171–176.

Procházková D et al. Controlled diet in phenylketonuria and hyperphenylalaninemia may cause serum selenium deficiency in adult patients: the Czech experience. Biol Trace Elem Res 154.2 (2013): 178–184.

Qiao Y-L et al. Total and Cancer Mortality After Supplementation With Vitamins and Minerals: Follow-up of the Linxian General Population Nutrition Intervention Trial. J Natl Cancer Inst 101.7 (2009): 507–518.

Rajpathak S et al. Toenail selenium and cardiovascular disease in men with diabetes. J Am Coll Nutr 24.4 (2005): 250–256.

Rayman MP. Selenium in cancer prevention: a review of the evidence and mechanism of action. Proc Nutr Soc 64.4 (2005): 527–542.

Rayman MP. The importance of selenium to human health. Lancet 356.9225 (2000): 233–241.

Rayman MP, Stranges S. Epidemiology of selenium and type 2 diabetes: Can we make sense of it? Free Radical Bio Med 65 (2013): 1557–1564.

Rayman MP et al. Effect of supplementation with high-selenium yeast on plasma lipids: a randomized trial. Ann Intern Med 154.10 (2011): 656–665.

Rayman MP et al. Randomized controlled trial of the effect of selenium supplementation on thyroid function in the elderly in the United Kingdom. Am J Clin Nutr 87.2 (2008): 370–378.

Rayman M et al. Impact of selenium on mood and quality of life: a randomized, controlled trial. Biol Psychiatry 59.2 (2006): 147–154.

Rayman MP, Rayman MP. The argument for increasing selenium intake. Proc Nutr Soc 61.2 (2002): 203–215.

Rees K et al. Selenium supplementation for the primary prevention of cardiovascular disease. Coch DB Syst Rev 1 (2013): CD009671.

Reid ME et al. Selenium supplementation and colorectal adenomas: an analysis of the nutritional prevention of cancer trial. Int J Cancer 118.7 (2006): 1777–1781.

Reid ME et al. Selenium supplementation and lung cancer incidence: an update of the nutritional prevention of cancer trial. Cancer Epidemiol Biomarkers Prev 11.11 (2002): 1285–1291.

Reid ME et al. The nutritional prevention of cancer: 400 mcg per day selenium treatment. Nutr Cancer 60.2 (2008): 155–163.

Rosenstein ED, Caldwell JR. Trace elements in the treatment of rheumatic conditions. Rheum Dis Clin North Am 25.4 (1999): 929–935: viii.

Roy M et al. Supplementation with selenium and human immune cell functions. I. Effect on lymphocyte proliferation and interleukin 2 receptor expression. Biol Trace Elem Res 41.1–2 (1994): 103–114.

Russo MW et al. Plasma selenium levels and the risk of colorectal adenomas. Nutr Cancer 28.2 (1997): 125–129.

Sammalkorpi K et al. Serum selenium in acute infections. Infection 16.4 (1988): 222–224.

Schrauzer GN. Anticarcinogenic effects of selenium. Cell Mol Life Sci 57.13–14 (2000): 1864–1873.

Scott R et al. The effect of oral selenium supplementation on human sperm motility. Br J Urol 82.1 (1998): 76–80.

Seo YR, Kelley MR, Smith ML. Selenomethionine regulation of p53 by a ref1-dependent redox mechanism. Proc Natl Acad Sci U S A 99.22 (2002): 14548–14553.

Shaheen SO et al. Randomised, double blind, placebo-controlled trial of selenium supplementation in adult asthma. Thorax 62.6 (2007): 483–490.

Shalini S, Bansal MP. Dietary selenium deficiency as well as excess supplementation induces multiple defects in mouse epididymal spermatozoa: understanding the role of selenium in male fertility. Int J Androl 31.4 (2008): 438–449.

Shalini S, Bansal MP. Alterations in selenium status influences reproductive potential of male mice by modulation of transcription factor NFkappaB. Biometals 20.1 (2007a): 49–59.

Shalini S, Bansal MP. Co-operative effect of glutathione depletion and selenium induced oxidative stress on API and NFkB expression in testicular cells in vitro: insights to regulation of spermatogenesis. Biol Res 40.3 (2007b): 307–17.

Shalini S, Bansal MP. Role of selenium in spermatogenesis: differential expression of cjun and cfos in tubular cells of mice testis. Mol Cell Biochem 292.1–2 (2006): 27–38.

Sher L. Role of thyroid hormones in the effects of selenium on mood, behavior, and cognitive function. Med Hypotheses 57.4 (2001): 480–483.

Shils M et al (eds). Modern nutrition in health and disease. Baltimore: Lippincott Williams and Wilkins, 2006. Available at: Clinicians health channel gateway.ut.ovid.com/gw1/ovidweb.cgi (accessed 13-06-06).

Shor-Posner G et al. Impact of selenium status on the pathogenesis of mycobacterial disease in HIV-1-infected drug users during the era of highly active antiretroviral therapy. J Acquir Immune Defic Syndr 29.2 (2002): 169–173.

Siegfried N et al. Micronutrient supplementation in pregnant women with HIV infection. Coch DB Syst Rev 2012 (2012): CD009755.

Spina A et al. Anthropometric indices and selenium status in British adults: The U.K. National Diet and Nutrition Survey. Free Radical Bio Med 65 (2013): 1315–1321.

Stephensen CB et al. Glutathione, glutathione peroxidase, and selenium status in HIV-positive and HIV-negative adolescents and young adults. Am J Clin Nutr 85.1 (2007): 173–181.

Stranges S et al. Effects of long-term selenium supplementation on the incidence of type 2 diabetes: a randomized trial. Ann Intern Med 147.4 (2007): 217–223.

Stranges S et al. Effects of selenium supplementation on cardiovascular disease incidence and mortality: secondary analyses in a randomized clinical trial. Am J Epidemiol 163.8 (2006): 694–699.

Stratton MS et al. Oral selenium supplementation has no effect on prostate specific antigen velocity in men undergoing active surveillance for localized prostate cancer. Cancer Prev Res (Phila) 3.8 (2010): 1035–1043.

Styblo M, Thomas DJ. Selenium modifies the metabolism and toxicity of arsenic in primary rat hepatocytes. Toxicol Appl Pharmacol 172.1 (2001): 52–61.

Tan M et al. Changes of serum selenium in pregnant women with gestational diabetes mellitus. Biol Trace Elem Res 83.3 (2001): 231–237.

Thomson CD et al. Minimal impact of excess iodate intake on thyroid hormones and selenium status in older New Zealanders. Eur J Endocrinol 165.5 (2011): 745–752.

Tinggi U. Essentiality and toxicity of selenium and its status in Australia: a review. Toxicol Lett 137.1–2 (2003): 103–110.

Türk S et al. Male infertility: Decreased levels of selenium, zinc and antioxidants. J Trace Elem Med Biol (2013) Corrected proof.

van Zuuren EJ et al. Selenium supplementation for Hashimoto's thyroiditis. Coch DB Syst Rev 6 (2013): CD010223.

Vezina D et al. Selenium-vitamin E supplementation in infertile men: Effects on semen parameters and micronutrient levels and distribution. Biol Trace Elem Res 53.1–3 (1996): 65–83.

Vinceti M et al. Selenium neurotoxicity in humans: Bridging laboratory and epidemiologic studies. Toxicol Letters (2013) Corrected proof.
Wallace K et al. Prediagnostic serum selenium concentration and the risk of recurrent colorectal adenoma: a nested case-control study. Cancer Epidemiol Biomarkers Prev 12.5 (2003): 464–467.
Wang L et al. Effects of high-intensity training and resumed training on macroelement and microelement of elite basketball athletes. Bio Trace Elem Res 149.2 (2012): 148–154.
Wertenbruch T et al. Serum selenium levels in patients with remission and relapse of Graves' disease. Med Chem 3.3 (2007): 281–284.
Xu DX et al. The associations among semen quality, oxidative DNA damage in human spermatozoa and concentrations of cadmium, lead and selenium in seminal plasma. Mutat Res 534.1–2 (2003): 155–163.
Xun P et al. Longitudinal association between toenail selenium levels and measures of subclinical atherosclerosis: the CARDIA trace element study. Atherosclerosis 210.2 (2010): 662–667.
Yiin SJ et al. Cadmium-induced liver, heart, and spleen lipid peroxidation in rats and protection by selenium. Biol Trace Elem Res 78.1–3 (2000): 219–230.
Yiin SJ et al. Cadmium induced lipid peroxidation in rat testes and protection by selenium. Biometals 12.4 (1999a): 353–359.
Yiin SJ et al. Cadmium-induced renal lipid peroxidation in rats and protection by selenium. J Toxicol Environ Health A 57.6 (1999b): 403–413.
Yiin SJ et al. Lipid peroxidation in rat adrenal glands after administration cadmium and role of essential metals. J Toxicol Environ Health A 62.1 (2001): 47–56.
Yoshizawa K et al. Study of prediagnostic selenium level in toenails and the risk of advanced prostate cancer. J Natl Cancer Inst 90.16 (1998): 1219–1224.
Yu SY et al. Chemoprevention trial of human hepatitis with selenium supplementation in China. Biol Trace Elem Res 20.1–2 (1989): 15–22.
Yu SY, Zhu YJ, Li WG. Protective role of selenium against hepatitis B virus and primary liver cancer in Qidong. Biol Trace Elem Res 56.1 (1997): 117–124.
Zamamiri-Davis F et al. Nuclear factor-kappaB mediates over-expression of cyclooxygenase-2 during activation of RAW 264.7 macrophages in selenium deficiency. Free Radic Biol Med 32.9 (2002): 890–897.
Zheng HT et al. Selenium inhibits high glucose- and high insulin-induced adhesion molecule expression in vascular endothelial cells. Arch Med Res 39.4 (2008): 373–379.
Zhou J et al. Selenium and diabetes—Evidence from animal studies. Free Radical Biol Med 65 (2013): 1548–1556.
Zu K, Ip C. Synergy between selenium and vitamin E in apoptosis induction is associated with activation of distinctive initiator caspases in human prostate cancer cells. Cancer Res 63.20 (2003): 6988–6995.

Ginseng — Siberian

HISTORICAL NOTE Siberian ginseng has been used for over 2000 years, according to Chinese medical records, where it is referred to as ci wu jia. It was used to prevent colds and flu and to increase vitality and energy. In modern times, it has been used by Russian cosmonauts to improve alertness and energy and to aid in adaptation to the stresses of life in space. It also has been used as an ergogenic aid by Russian athletes before international competitions (Mills & Bone 2000) and after the Chernobyl accident to counteract the effects of radiation (Chevallier 1996).

S

Clinical note — Allostasis

Allostasis is the body's adaptation to stress. Allostatic (adaptive) systems are critical to survival and enable us to respond to changes in our physical (such as asleep, awake, standing, sitting, eating, exercising and infection) and psychological states (such as anticipation, fear, isolation, worry and lack of control). The consumption of tobacco, alcohol and our dietary choices also induces allostatic responses (McEwan 1998). These systems are complex and have broad boundaries, in contrast to the body's homeostatic systems (e.g. blood pH and body temperature), which are maintained within a narrow range.

Most commonly, allostatic responses involve the sympathetic nervous system and the hypothalamic-pituitary-adrenal (HPA) axis. Upon activation (e.g. when a challenge is perceived), catecholamines are released from nerves and the adrenal medulla, corticotrophin is secreted from the pituitary and cortisol is released from the adrenal cortex. Once the threat has passed (e.g. the environment is more comfortable or infection is controlled), the system is inactivated and levels of cortisol and catecholamine secretion return to baseline.

Chronic exposure to stress can lead to allostatic load, a situation resulting from chronic overactivity or underactivity of allostatic systems. The situation is characterised by maladaptive responses whereby systems become inefficient or do not turn off appropriately. Currently, there is much interest in understanding the association between numerous diseases such as cardiovascular disease and overwhelming allostatic load.

One measure that is used to gauge an individual's allostatic response is the cortisol response to a variety of stressors. As such, cortisol is seen as the classical 'stress' hormone.

OTHER NAMES

Ci wu jia, devil's bush, devil's shrub, eleuthero, eleutherococcus, eleuthero root, gokahi, ogap'I, russisk rod, taigawurzel, touch-me-not, wu jia pi

BOTANICAL NAME/FAMILY

Eleutherococcus senticosus (synonym: *Acanthopanax senticosus*) (family Araliaceae)

PLANT PART USED

Root, rhizome

CHEMICAL COMPONENTS

Glycosides (eleutherosides A–M, including saponins, coumarins, lignans, phenylpropanoids, oleanolic acids, triterpenes, betulinic acid and vitamins), steroid glycoside (eleutheroside A), lignans (syringin, sesamin, chlorigenic acid), glycans (eleutherans A–G), triterpenoid saponins (friedelin), saponin (protoprimulagenin A), hydroxycoumarin (isofraxidin), phenolics, polysaccharides, lignans, coumarins and resin.

Nutrients include magnesium 723 mcg/g, aluminium 188 mcg/g and manganese 37 mcg/g and vitamins A and E (*Eleutherococcus senticosus* 2006, Meacham et al 2002, Nissen 2003, Panossian et al 1999, Skidmore-Roth 2001).

MAIN ACTIONS

Adaptogenic (modulates stress response)

Siberian ginseng appears to alter the levels of different neurotransmitters and hormones involved in the stress response, chiefly at the HPA axis. Various mechanisms have been proposed, including inhibition of catechol-*O*-methyltransferase, which inactivates catecholamines (Gaffney et al 2001a). As a result, catecholamine levels are not depleted and release of new catecholamines from nerve synapses is decreased (Panossian et al 1999). In theory, this may reduce the risk of the organism's adaptive responses becoming depleted and moving into the exhaustion phase of the stress response. In addition, eleutherosides have been shown to improve carbohydrate metabolism and energy provision and increase the synthesis of protein and nucleic acids, although the direct molecular targets responsible for this adaptive response remain unknown (Panossian et al 1999). Eleutherosides have also been reported to bind to receptor sites for progestin, oestrogen, mineralocorticoids and glucocorticoids in vitro and therefore may theoretically exert numerous pharmacological actions important for the body's stress response (Pearce et al 1982).

Owing to such actions, herbalists and naturopaths describe the herb's overall action as 'adaptogenic'. The term 'adaptogen' describes substances that increase the ability of an organism to adapt to environmental factors and to avoid damage from such factors (Panossian et al 1999). The term 'allostasis' (see Clinical note) has been adopted in the medical arena to describe 'the ability to achieve stability through change'.

Although the mechanism of action responsible is still unclear, several theories have been proposed to explain the effect of Siberian ginseng on allostatic systems, largely based on the pharmacological actions observed in test tube and animal studies. Depending on the stage of the stress response, Siberian ginseng can act in different ways to support the 'stress system'. Research suggests that there is a threshold of stress below which the herb increases the stress response and above which it decreases the stress response (Gaffney et al 2001b). Therefore, for example, if allostatic load is such that responses have become inadequate, then the resulting increase in hormone levels would theoretically induce a more efficient response. Alternatively, situations of chronic overactivity, also due to allostatic load, would respond to Siberian ginseng in a different way, with negative-feedback systems being triggered to inactivate the stress response (Gaffney et al 2001a).

The dosing regimen may also be significant. While multidose administration in chronic stress engages the HPA axis, balancing the switch-on and switch-off responses, single doses (~4 mL) in acute stress trigger a rapid response from the sympathoadrenal system, resulting in secretion of catecholamines, neuropeptides, adenosine triphosphate and nitric oxide (NO) (Panossian & Wagner 2005). Studies have demonstrated that maximal effects are achieved around 4 weeks but do not persist at the 8-week time point, which may help to explain the practice of giving Siberian ginseng for 6 weeks with a 2-week break before repeating.

Immunomodulation

Siberian ginseng appears to exert an immunomodulatory rather than just an immunosuppressive or stimulating action; however, evidence for the immune-enhancing effects of Siberian ginseng is contradictory. Clinical studies, in vitro and in vivo, have revealed stimulation of general non-specific resistance and an influence on T lymphocytes, natural killer (NK) cells and cytokines (Bohn et al 1987, Schmolz et al 2001), although other studies suggest that Siberian ginseng does not significantly stimulate the innate macrophage immune functions that influence cellular immune responses (Wang et al 2003). Alternatively, another in vitro study has demonstrated that activation of macrophages and NK cells does occur and may be responsible for inhibiting tumour metastasis both prophylactically and therapeutically (Yoon et al 2004).

The main constituents responsible appear to be lignans (sesamin, syringin) and polysaccharides, such as glycans, which demonstrate immunostimulant effects in vitro (Davydov & Krikorian 2000, Wagner et al 1984). Additionally, effects on the HPA axis will influence immune responses.

A liposoluble fraction from a crude extract of Siberian ginseng enhanced the forced swimming capacity of mice by decreasing muscle damage, effectively preventing the increase in blood urea nitrogen concentration and increasing fat utilisation (Huang et al 2010).

Antiviral

In vitro studies show a strong antiviral action, inhibiting the replication of ribonucleic acid-type viruses such as human rhinovirus, respiratory syncytial virus and influenza A virus (Glatthaar-Saalmuller et al 2001).

Anabolic activity

Syringin and other eleutherosides appear to improve carbohydrate metabolism and energy provision by increasing the formation of glucose-6-phosphate and activating glucogen transport (Panossian et al 1999), and Siberian ginseng extracts have been reported to improve the metabolism of lactic and pyruvic acids (Farnsworth et al 1985).

While initial animal studies showed promise for improving weight gain and increasing organ and muscle weight (Farnsworth et al 1985, Kaemmerer & Fink 1980), clinical studies confirming whether anabolic effects occur also in humans could not be located.

Anti-inflammatory

Excess production of NO is a characteristic of inflammation, and Siberian ginseng has been shown to significantly suppress NO production and inducible NO synthase (iNOS) gene expression in a dose-dependent manner (Lin et al 2008). The downregulation of iNOS expression may be the result of inhibition of intracellular peroxide production (Lin et al 2008) or through blocking c-Jun NH_2-terminal kinase (JNK) and Akt activation (Jung et al 2007). Cyanidin-3-*O*-(2″-xylosyl)-glucoside (C-3-*O*-(2″-xylosyl)-G), which was analysed as an active constituent from the fruit of Siberian ginseng, was shown to act by suppressing cyclooxygenase-2 expression and AP-1 and NF-κB transactivation and JNK, MAPKK3/6 and MEK/ERK1/2 phosphorylation (Jung et al 2013). *Acanthopanax senticosus* also exhibited significantly higher immunomodulatory activities against lymphocyte proliferation in vitro. It also demonstrated pronounced reductive power, strong hydroxyl radical-scavenging activity, moderate superoxide radicals and 2,2-diphenyl-1-picrylhydrazyl radical-scavenging activities. This however needs to be further explored for use in functional foods or medicine (Chen et al 2011).

Glycaemic control and insulin-sensitising effect

Animal studies have indicated a potential for hypoglycaemic effects when used intravenously. Syringin appears to enhance glucose utilisation (Niu et al 2008) and lower plasma glucose levels in animal experiments. The effect may be due to an increase in the release of acetylcholine from nerve terminals, stimulating muscarinic M_3 receptors in pancreatic cells to increase insulin release (Liu et al 2008). Syringin may also enhance the secretion of beta-endorphin from the adrenal medulla to stimulate peripheral micro-opioid receptors, resulting in a decrease of plasma glucose in insulin-depleted diabetic rats (Niu et al 2007).

Eleutherans A–G exert marked hypoglycaemic effects in normal and alloxan-induced hyperglycaemic mice (Hikino et al 1986), and eleutherosides show an insulin-like action in diabetic rats (Dardymov et al 1978). However, these effects have not been borne out in human studies (Farnsworth et al 1985). A glucose tolerance study in db/db mice orally administered *Acanthopanax senticosus* lowered plasma glucose levels more than the control group 30 minutes after sucrose loading, without affecting plasma insulin levels, and significantly inhibited α-glucosidase activity in the small-intestine mucosa (Watanabe et al 2010).

A small, double-blind, randomised, multiple, crossover study using 12 healthy participants actually showed an increase in postprandial plasma glucose at 90 and 120 minutes when 3 g Siberian ginseng was given orally 40 minutes before a

75-g oral glucose tolerance test (Sievenpiper et al 2004). More recently, oral administration of an aqueous extract of Siberian ginseng was shown to improve insulin sensitivity and delay the development of insulin resistance in rats (Liu et al 2005). As a result, further trials in people with impaired glucose tolerance and/or insulin resistance are warranted.

Hepatoprotective

Animal studies have demonstrated that an intravenous extract of Siberian ginseng decreased thioacetamide-induced liver toxicity when given before and after thioacetamide administration (Shen et al 1991). More recently, oral administration of aqueous extract and polysaccharide was found to attenuate fulminant hepatic failure induced by D-galactosamine/lipopolysaccharide in mice, reducing serum aspartate aminotransferase, alanine aminotransferase and tissue necrosis factor-alpha levels (Park et al 2004). The protective effect is thought to be due to the water-soluble polysaccharides. Coadministration of Siberian ginseng may also act to enhance the action of amtizole, improving the protective effect on hepatic antitoxic function and lipid metabolism (Kushnerova & Rakhmanin 2008). Diabetic rats treated with *Acanthopanax senticosus* plus metformin showed a more beneficial promotion for relieving the symptoms of diabetes and reversing liver and kidney damage to normal level than only metformin administration (Fu et al 2012).

Neuroprotective

Preliminary animal studies have suggested possible neuroprotective effects in transient middle cerebral artery occlusion in Sprague-Dawley rats. Infarct volume was reduced by 36.6% by inhibiting inflammation and microglial activation in brain ischaemia after intraperitoneal injection of a water extract of Siberian ginseng (Bu et al 2005). Similarly, intraperitoneal injection of Siberian ginseng was found to relieve damage to neurons following hippocampal ischaemia hypoxia and improve the learning and memory of rats with experimentally induced vascular dementia (Ge et al 2004). Siberian ginseng extract appears to protect against neuritic atrophy and cell death under amyloid beta treatment; the effect is thought to be due at least in part to eleutheroside B (Tohda et al 2008). The saponins present in Siberian ginseng have also been shown to protect against cortical neuron injury induced by anoxia/reoxygenation by inhibiting the release of NO and neuron apoptosis in vitro (Chen et al 2004).

Using a cerebral-ischaemic rat model, researchers demonstrated that an ethanolic extract of Siberian ginseng, given at the time of the ischaemic event and 90 minutes after, was protective against delayed neuronal cell death and also attenuated inflammatory markers, suggesting that some of the protective effect may be attributed to an anti-inflammatory effect (Lee et al 2012). In the Parkinson-induced mice model, oral administration of Siberian ginseng at low dose, 45 mg/kg, and high dose, 182 mg/kg, increased dopamine levels in the substantia nigra and enhanced coordination and motor function (Liu et al 2012). The researchers noted that more dopamine was present in the low-dose group (equivalent to 9 g/day for humans), suggesting that therapeutic effect is not necessarily a function of increasing dose.

In an in vitro depression model induced by stress hormone corticosterone, Siberian ginseng prolonged cell life and may account for the antidepressant effects reported in in vivo models (Wu et al 2013). And in sleep-deprived mice, treatment with eleutheroside E reduced the monoamines induced through sleep deprivation and restored their behaviour, suggesting that this component of Siberian ginseng could be valuable for the stress experienced from chronic sleeplessness (Huang et al 2011).

OTHER ACTIONS

Anticoagulant and antiplatelet effects

Animal studies have demonstrated prevention against thrombosis induced by immobilisation (Shakhmatov et al 2007), and the 3,4-dihydroxybenzoic acid constituent of Siberian ginseng has demonstrated antiplatelet activity in vivo (Yun-Choi et al 1987). A controlled trial using Siberian ginseng tincture for 20 days in 20 athletes detected a decrease in the blood coagulation potential and activity of the blood coagulation factors that are normally induced by intensive training of the athletes (Azizov 1997). Whether the effects also occur in non-athletes is unknown.

Antiallergic

In vitro studies demonstrate that Siberian ginseng has antiallergic properties in mast cell-mediated allergic reactions (Jeong et al 2001). The mechanism appears to involve inhibition of histamine, tumour necrosis factor-alpha and interleukin-6.

Antioxidant

Results using aqueous extracts of *Acanthopanax senticosus* indicated that it protects against oxidative stress which may be generated via the induction of Nrf2 and related antioxidant enzymes (Wang et al 2010). It was shown that *A. senticosus* orally administered to rats experienced significantly lower oxidative stress, as indicated by the expression of certain genes (Kim et al 2010).

Cardioprotective

Oral administration of Siberian ginseng (1 mL/kg) to rats for 8 days prevented stress-induced heart damage and chronic administration increased beta-endorphin levels and improved cardiac tolerance to D,L-isoproterenol and arrhythmia caused by adrenaline. The cardioprotective and antiarrhythmic effect may be related to an increase in endogenous opioid peptide levels (Maslov & Guzarova 2007). Benefits following a 45-minute coronary artery occlusion were not demonstrated in this study (Maslov & Guzarova 2007) but have been in studies using Siberian ginseng in a polypharmacy combination known as Tonizid (Lishmanov et al 2008).

Radioprotective

Animal studies have found that administration of Siberian ginseng prior to a lethal dose of radiation produced an 80% survival rate in mice (Miyanomae & Frindel 1988). Interestingly, α-difluoromethylornithine (DFMO), a chemotherapeutic drug which has a cytostatic effect, had a more pronounced effect than Siberian ginseng root tincture (SGRT) in radiation-induced carcinogenesis; however, in combination DFMO and SGRT increased survival rate and decreased frequency and multiplicity of malignant and benign tumours in irradiated rats (Bespalov et al 2013).

Vascular relaxant

In vitro studies have demonstrated vasorelaxant effects for Siberian ginseng. The effect is thought to be endothelium-dependent and mediated by NO and/or endothelium-derived hyperpolarising factor, depending on the size of the blood vessel. Other vasorelaxation pathways may also be involved (Kwan et al 2004).

CLINICAL USE

Due to its long history of use and myriad pharmacological actions, Siberian ginseng is used for many varied indications.

Stress

Siberian ginseng is widely used to treat individuals with nervous exhaustion or anxiety due to chronic exposure to stress or what is now termed 'allostatic load situations'. The biochemical effects on stress responses observed in experimental and human studies provide a theoretical basis for this indication (Abramova et al 1972, Gaffney et al 2001a).

One placebo-controlled study conducted over 6 weeks investigated the effects of an ethanolic extract of Siberian ginseng (8 mL/day, equivalent to 4 g/day dried root). In the study, active treatment resulted in increased cortisol levels, which may be consistent with animal research, suggesting a threshold of stress below which Siberian ginseng increases the stress response and above which it decreases the stress response (Gaffney et al 2001b). In a randomised, controlled study in 144 participants suffering from asthenia and reduced working capacity related to chronic stress, *Eleutherococcus senticosus* improved parameters over time and a significant difference was found in mental fatigue and restlessness, both in favour of *E. senticosus* versus 2-day professional stress management training (Schaffler et al 2013).

Fatigue

Siberian ginseng is used to improve physical and mental responses during convalescence or fatigue states. While traditional stimulants can produce a temporary increase in work capacity followed by a period of marked decrease, the initial increase in performance from adaptogens is followed by only a slight dip and performance remains above basal levels (Panossian et al 1999). The ability of Siberian ginseng to increase levels of noradrenaline, serotonin, adrenaline and cortisol provides a theoretical basis for its use in situations of fatigue. However, controlled studies are limited.

A randomised, double-blind, placebo-controlled trial of 300 mg/day (*E. senticosus* dry extract) for 8 weeks assessed health-related quality-of-life scores in 20 elderly people. Improvements were observed in social functioning after 4 weeks of therapy but did not persist to the 8-week time point. It would appear that improvements diminish with continued use (Cicero et al 2004), which may help to explain the practice of giving Siberian ginseng for 6 weeks with a 2-week break before repeating.

A randomised placebo-controlled trial evaluated the effectiveness of Siberian ginseng in chronic fatigue syndrome (CFS). No significant improvements were demonstrated overall; however, subgroup analysis showed improvements in fatigue severity and duration ($P < 0.05$) in CFS sufferers with less severe fatigue at 2-month follow-up (Hartz et al 2004). Further studies are required to determine whether Siberian ginseng may be a useful therapeutic option in cases of mild to moderate fatigue.

S

IN COMBINATION

A double-blind, placebo-controlled, randomised study of single-dose effects of a standardised fixed combination of *Rhodiola rosea, Schisandra chinensis* and *Eleutherococcus senticosus* extracts on mental performance, such as attention, speed and accuracy, in tired individuals performing stressful cognitive tasks showed that subjects gained improved attention and increased speed and accuracy during stressful cognitive tasks, in comparison to placebo (Aslanyan et al 2010).

Commission E approves the use of Siberian ginseng as a tonic in times of fatigue and debility, for declining capacity for work or concentration and during convalescence (Blumenthal et al 2000). In practice, it is often used in low doses in cases of fatigue due to chronic stress (Gaffney et al 2001a).

Cardioprotective

Due to its effects on vascular relaxation, stress response, anti-inflammatory and antioxidant activities, it is also believed to be a good tonic for the heart. Furthermore, a 2008 study shows that *Acanthopanax senticosus* significantly decreased serum low-density lipoprotein (LDL) (127.54 ± 29.79 mg/dL vs 110.33 ± 22.26 mg/dL) and the LDL/high-density lipoprotein ratio (2.40 ± 0.65 vs 2.11 ± 0.58) after supplementation in 40 postmenopausal women (Lee et al 2008).

Ergogenic aid

While initial animal studies showed promise for improving weight gain, increasing organ and muscle weight, improving the use of glycogen and metabolism of lactic and pyruvic acids (Farnsworth et al 1985, Wagner et al 1985), randomised controlled trials have produced inconsistent results in healthy individuals and athletes (Asano et al 1986, Dowling et al 1996, Eschbach et al 2000, Goulet & Dionne 2005, Kuo et al 2010, Mahady et al 2000). The evidence to date is inconsistent and further research is required to determine the potential role for Siberian ginseng in improving performance in sports.

In the mid-1980s, a Japanese controlled study conducted on six male athletes over 8 days showed that Siberian ginseng extract (2 mL twice daily) improved work capacity compared with a placebo (23.3 vs 7.5%) in male athletes, owing to increased oxygen uptake ($P < 0.01$). Time to exhaustion (stamina) also increased (16.3 vs 5.4%, $P < 0.005$) (Asano et al 1986). Other research however has failed to confirm these effects (Dowling et al 1996, Eschbach et al 2000).

A randomised, double-blind, crossover trial using a lower dose of 1200 mg/day Siberian ginseng for 7 days reported that treatment did not alter steady-state substrate use or 10-km cycling performance time (Eschbach et al 2000). Additionally, an 8-week, double-blind, placebo-controlled study involving 20 experienced distance runners failed to detect significant changes to heart rate, oxygen consumption, expired minute volume, respiratory exchange ratio, perceived exertion or serum lactate levels compared with placebo. Overall, both submaximal and maximal exercise performance were unchanged (Dowling et al 1996).

More recently, when recreationally trained males were treated for 8 weeks with *Eleutherococcus senticosus* supplementation there was marked enhancement in endurance time and elevated cardiovascular functions and this altered the metabolism of plasma free fatty acid and glucose after 8-week supplementation. This is the first well-controlled study that showed positive effects of Siberian ginseng on endurance exercise capacity in human clinical studies (Kuo et al 2010).

Siberian ginseng may however reduce blood coagulation factors induced by intensive training in athletes (Azizov 1997) and has been shown in combination with micronutrients to improve iron metabolism and immunological responsiveness in 39 high-grade unarmed self-defence sportsmen (Nasolodin et al 2006). Whether these effects also occur in other scenarios is yet to be established.

Siberian ginseng does not appear on the 2014 Prohibited List of the World Anti-doping Agency (WADA 2014).

Prevention of infection

Due to the herb's ability to directly and indirectly modulate immune responses, it is also used to increase resistance to infection. One double-blind study of 1000 Siberian factory workers supports this, reporting a 50% reduction in general illness and a 40% reduction in absenteeism over a 12-month period, following 30 days' administration of Siberian ginseng (Farnsworth et al 1985). More recently, a 6-month controlled trial in males and females with recurrent herpes infection found that Siberian ginseng (2 g/day) successfully reduced the frequency of infection by 50% (Williams 1995).

In practice, Siberian ginseng is generally used as a preventive medicine, as administration during acute infections is widely thought to increase the severity of the illness, although this has not been borne out in controlled studies using Siberian ginseng in combination with other herbs.

IN COMBINATION

A small randomised controlled trial demonstrated a significant reduction in the severity of familial Mediterranean fever in children using a combination of Siberian ginseng with licorice, andrographis and schisandra (Amaryan et al 2003), and a combination of Siberian ginseng with schisandra and rhodiola was found to expedite the recovery of patients with acute non-specific pneumonia (Narimanian et al 2005).

There is also clinical research conducted with an oral combination of Siberian ginseng and *Andrographis paniculata,* which is commonly known as Kan Jang, showing significant improvement of cold and flu symptoms (see Andrographis monograph for details).

Herpes simplex virus type 2 infection

Siberian ginseng (standardised to eleutheroside 0.3%) taken orally for 3 months reduced the severity, duration and frequency of genital herpes outbreaks; however more research is required before recommendations can be made about use (Ulbricht 2012).

Cancer therapy

A polypharmacy preparation known as AdMax, which contains *Eleutherococcus senticosus* in combination with *Leuzea carthamoides*, *Rhodiola rosea* and *Schizandra chinensis*, has been shown to boost suppressed immunity in patients with ovarian cancer who are subject to chemotherapy (Kormosh et al 2006). Which herb or combination of herbs is responsible for the effect is unclear.

OTHER USES

Given the herb's ability to increase levels of serotonin and noradrenaline in animal studies (Abramova et al 1972), a theoretical basis exists for the use of Siberian ginseng in depression.

In traditional Chinese medicine, Siberian ginseng is used to encourage the smooth flow of Qi and blood when obstructed, particularly in the elderly, and is viewed as a general tonic. It is therefore used for a myriad of indications, usually in combination with other herbal medicines. Numerous studies use Siberian ginseng in combination with other adaptogens, such as *Rhodiola rosea* and *Schisandra chinensis*, which may potentially act synergistically for improved effects.

S

> ***Clinical note — Case reports of Siberian ginseng need careful consideration***
>
> Some adverse reactions attributed to Siberian ginseng have subsequently been found to be due to poor product quality, herbal substitution and/or interference with test results. For example, initial reports linking maternal ginseng use to neonatal androgenisation are now suspected to be due to substitution with another herb, *Periploca sepium* (called Wu jia or silk vine), as American herb companies importing Siberian ginseng from China have been known to be supplied with two or three species of *Periploca* (Awang 1991). Additionally, rat studies have failed to detect significant androgenic action (Awang 1991, Waller et al 1992) for Siberian ginseng.

Another example is the purported interaction between digoxin and Siberian ginseng, which was based on a single case report of a 74-year-old man found to have elevated digoxin levels for many years (McRae 1996). It was subsequently purported that the herbal product may have been adulterated with digitalis. Additionally, Siberian ginseng contains glycosides with structural similarities to digoxin that may modestly interfere with digoxin fluorescence polarisation (FPIA), microparticle enzyme (MEIA) results, falsely elevating digoxin values with FPIA and falsely lowering digoxin values with MEIA (Dasgupta & Reyes 2005). It should be noted that measuring free digoxin does not eliminate these modest interferences in serum digoxin measurement by the Digoxin III assay (Dasgupta et al 2008).

DOSAGE RANGE

- 1–4 g/day dried root or equivalent preparations.
- Fluid extract (1 : 2): 2–8 mL/day (15–55 mL/week).
- Tincture (1 : 5): 10–15 mL/day.
- Acute dosing: 4 mL in a single dose before activity.

Extracts with standardised levels of eleutheroside E (syringin) (>0.5 mg/mL) are recommended. Russian and Korean sources appear to have higher levels of this constituent. So, variations in therapeutic activity may be predicted (Wagner et al 1982). As there can be a significant product variability in the level of eleutherosides between capsules and liquids, standardisation may be necessary for quality assurance (Harkey et al 2001).

In practice, Siberian ginseng is often given for 6 weeks with a break of at least 2 weeks before resuming treatment.

ADVERSE REACTIONS

Clinical trials of 6 months' duration have shown no side effects from treatment (Bohn et al 1987). High doses may cause slight drowsiness, irritability, anxiety, mastalgia, palpitations or tachycardia, although these side effects may be more relevant to *Panax ginseng*.

SIGNIFICANT INTERACTIONS

As controlled studies are not available, interactions are currently speculative and based on evidence of pharmacological activity and case reports. Studies have reported that normal doses of Siberian ginseng are unlikely to affect drugs metabolised by CYP2D6 or CYP3A4 (Donovan et al 2003).

Anticoagulants

An in vivo study demonstrated that an isolated constituent in Siberian ginseng has anticoagulant activity (Yun-Choi et al 1987), and a clinical trial found a reduction in blood coagulation induced by intensive training in athletes (Azizov 1997). Whether these effects also occur in non-athletes is unknown. Given that a study looking at the concomitant application of Kan Jang (Siberian ginseng in combination with andrographis) and warfarin did not produce significant effects on the pharmacokinetics or pharmacodynamics of the drug (Hovhannisyan et al 2006), a negative clinical effect is unlikely.

Chemotherapy

An increased tolerance for chemotherapy and improved immune function has been demonstrated in women with breast (Kupin 1984, Kupin & Polevaia 1986) and ovarian (Kormosh et al 2006) cancer undergoing chemotherapy treatment. Caution — as coadministration may theoretically reduce drug effects. However, beneficial interaction may be possible under medical supervision.

Diabetic medications

Claims that Siberian ginseng has hypoglycaemic effects are based on intravenous use in animal studies and not observed in humans, for whom oral intake may actually increase postprandial glycaemia (Sievenpiper et al 2004). Observe diabetic patients taking ginseng.

Influenza virus vaccine

Ginseng may reduce the risk of postvaccine reactions (Zykov & Protasova 1984), a possible beneficial interaction.

CONTRAINDICATIONS AND PRECAUTIONS

Some authors suggest that high-dose Siberian ginseng should be avoided by those with cardiovascular disease or hypertension (blood pressure > 80/90 mmHg) (Mahady et al 2000). Others merely suggest a caution, as reports are largely unsubstantiated (Holford & Cass 2001). As such, it is recommended that people with hypertension should be monitored.

Practice points/Patient counselling

- Siberian ginseng appears to alter the levels of different neurotransmitters and hormones involved in the stress response, chiefly at the HPA axis.
- It is widely used to treat individuals with nervous exhaustion or anxiety due to chronic exposure to stress or what are now termed 'allostatic load situations'. It is also recommended during convalescence or fatigue to improve mental and physical responses.
- Siberian ginseng may increase resistance to infection and has been shown to reduce frequency of genital herpes outbreaks with long-term use.
- The herb is popular among athletes in the belief that endurance, performance and power may improve with its use, but clinical studies have produced inconsistent results.
- It is not recommended for use in pregnancy, and people with hypertension should be monitored if using high doses.
- In a study of elderly people with hypertension, 8 weeks of Siberian ginseng use did not affect blood pressure control (Cicero et al 2004).
- Due to possible effects on glycaemic control (Sievenpiper et al 2004), care should be taken in people with diabetes until safety is established. Suspend use 1 week before major surgery.
- Traditional contraindications include hormonal changes, excess energy states, fever, acute infection, concurrent use of other stimulants and prolonged use.

PREGNANCY USE

Insufficient reliable information is available, but the herb is not traditionally used in pregnancy.

PATIENTS' FAQs

What will this herb do for me?

Siberian ginseng affects many chemicals involved in switching on and off the body's stress responses. As such, it is used to improve wellbeing during times of chronic stress and enhance physical performance and recovery from exercise. The scientific research has yet to fully investigate its use in this regard; however, experimental findings suggest that the neuroprotective, anti-inflammatory and antioxidant properties of the herb may be responsible.

It may also boost immune function and reduce the frequency of genital herpes outbreaks. Evidence for improved performance in athletes is inconsistent so its role remains unclear.

When will it start to work?

Effects on stress levels should develop within 6 weeks, whereas immune responses develop within 30 days.

Are there any safety issues?

It should not be used in pregnancy, and high doses should be used with care by those with hypertension.

REFERENCES

Abramova ZI et al. Lek Sredstva Dal'nego Vostoka 11 (1972): 106–8. In: Mills S, Bone K. Principles and practices of phytotherapy. London: Churchill Livingstone, 2000.

Amaryan G et al. Double-blind, placebo-controlled, randomized, pilot clinical trial of ImmunoGuard(R): a standardized fixed combination of *Andrographis paniculata* Nees, with *Eleutherococcus senticosus* Maxim, *Schizandra chinensis* Bail. and *Glycyrrhiza glabra* L. extracts in patients with Familial Mediterranean Fever. Phytomedicine 10.4 (2003): 271–85.

Asano K et al. Planta Med 3 (1986): 175–7. In: Mills S, Bone K. Principles and practices of phytotherapy. London: Churchill Livingstone, 2000.

Aslanyan G et al. Double-blind, placebo-controlled, randomised study of single dose effects of ADAPT-232 on cognitive functions. Phytomedicine (2010) 17(7):494–9

Awang DVC. Maternal use of ginseng and neonatal androgenization (so-called Siberian ginseng is probably *Periploca sepium*, or silk vine) [Letter]. JAMA 266.3 (1991): 363.

Azizov AP. Effects of eleutherococcus, elton, leuzea, and leveton on the blood coagulation system during training in athletes. Eksp Klin Farmakol 60.5 (1997): 58–60 [in Russian].

Bespalov V.G et al. Comparative effects of difluoromethylornithine and Siberian ginseng root tincture on radiation-induced carcinogenesis in rats and their lifespan. Advances in Gerontology, Jan 2013, Volume 3, Issue 1, pp 70–76

Blumenthal M, et al (eds). Herbal medicine expanded commission E monographs. Austin, TX: Integrative Medicine Communications, 2000.

Bohn B, et al. Flow-cytometric studies with *Eleutherococcus senticosus* extract as an immunomodulatory agent. Arzneimittelforschung 37.10 (1987): 1193–6.

Bu Y et al. Siberian ginseng reduces infarct volume in transient focal cerebral ischaemia in Sprague-Dawley rats. Phytother Res 19.2 (2005): 167–9.

Chen Y, et al. Protective effect of *Acanthopanax senticosus* saponins on anoxia/reoxygenation injury of neuron. Chin J Clin Rehab 8.31 (2004): 6964–5.

Chen R et al. Antioxidant and immunobiological activity of water-soluble polysaccharide fractions purified from *Acanthopanax senticosus*. Food Chemistry (2011) 127(2):34–440

Chevallier A. The encyclopedia of medicinal plants. London: Dorling Kindersley, 1996.

Cicero AF et al. Effects of Siberian ginseng (*Eleutherococcus senticosus* Maxim.) on elderly quality of life: a randomized clinical trial. Arch Gerontol Geriatr 38 (Suppl 1) (2004): 69–73.

Dardymov IV, et al. Rastit Resur 14.1 (1978): 86–9. In: Mills S, Bone K. Principles and practices of phytotherapy. London: Churchill Livingstone, 2000.

Dasgupta A, Reyes MA. Effect of Brazilian, Indian, Siberian, Asian, and North American ginseng on serum digoxin measurement by immunoassays and binding of digoxin-like immunoreactive components of ginseng with Fab fragment of antidigoxin antibody (Digibind). Am J Clin Pathol 124.2 (2005): 229–236.

Dasgupta A, et al. Effect of Asian ginseng, Siberian ginseng, and Indian ayurvedic medicine Ashwagandha on serum digoxin measurement by Digoxin III, a new digoxin immunoassay. J Clin Lab Anal 22.4 (2008): 295–301.

Davydov M, Krikorian AD. *Eleutherococcus senticosus* Maxim as an adaptogen: a closer look. J Ethnopharmacol 72.3 (2000): 345–93.

Donovan JL et al. Siberian ginseng (*Eleutheroccus senticosus*) effects on CYP2D6 and CYP3A4 activity in normal volunteers. Drug Metab Dispos 31.5 (2003): 519–22.

Dowling EA et al. Effect of *Eleutherococcus senticosus* on submaximal and maximal exercise performance. Med Sci Sports Exerc 28.4 (1996): 482–9.

Eleutherococcus senticosus. Altern Med Rev 11.2 (2006): 151–155.

Eschbach LF et al. The effect of Siberian ginseng (*Eleutherococcus senticosus*) on substrate utilization and performance. Int J Sport Nutr Exerc Metab 10.4 (2000): 444–51.

Farnsworth NR et al. Siberian ginseng (Eleutherococcus senticosus): current status as an adaptogen. In: Farnsworth NR (ed). Economic and medicinal plant research, vol. 1. London: Academic Press, 1985, p 178.

Fu J et al 2012. Anti-diabetic activities of *Acanthopanax senticosus* polysaccharide (ASP) in combination with metformin. Int J Biological Macromolecules, Vol 50, Issue 3, 1 April 2012, Pages 619–623.

Gaffney BT, et al. *Panax ginseng* and *Eleutherococcus senticosus* may exaggerate an already existing biphasic response to stress via inhibition of enzymes which limit the binding of stress hormones to their receptors. Med Hypotheses 56.5 (2001a): 567–72.

Gaffney BT, et al. The effects of *Eleutherococcus senticosus* and *Panax ginseng* on steroidal hormone indices of stress and lymphocyte subset numbers in endurance athletes. Life Sci 70.4 (2001b): 431–2.

Ge X et al. Effects of *Acanthopanax senticosus* saponins against vascular dementia in rats. Chin J Clin Rehab 8.34 (2004): 7734–35.

Glatthaar-Saalmuller B, et al. Antiviral activity of an extract derived from roots of *Eleutherococcus senticosus*. Antiviral Res 50 (2001): 223–8.

Goulet ED, Dionne IJ. Assessment of the effects of *Eleutherococcus senticosus* on endurance performance. Int J Sport Nutr Exerc Metab 15.1 (2005): 75–83.

Harkey MR et al. Variability in commercial ginseng products: an analysis of 25 preparations. Am J Clin Nutr 73.6 (2001): 1101–6.

Hartz AJ et al. Randomized controlled trial of Siberian ginseng for chronic fatigue. Psychol Med 34.1 (2004): 51–61.

Hikino H et al. Isolation and hypoglycemic activity of eleutherans A, B, C, D, E, F, and G: glycans of *Eleutherococcus senticosus* roots. J Nat Prod 49.2 (1986): 293–7.

Holford P, Cass H. Natural highs. Piatkus (2001): 90.

Hovhannisyan AS et al. The effect of Kan Jang extract on the pharmacokinetics and pharmacodynamics of warfarin in rats. Phytomedicine 13.5 (2006): 318–23.

Huang LZ et al. (2010) Antifatigue activity of the liposoluble fraction from *Acanthopanax senticosus*. Phytother. Res., 25: 940–943.

Huang LZ et al. The effect of Eleutheroside E on behavioral alterations in murine sleep deprivation stress model. Eur J Pharmacol (2011) 658(2–3):150–5

Jeong HJ et al. Inhibitory effects of mast cell-mediated allergic reactions by cell cultured Siberian Ginseng. Immunopharmacol Immunotoxicol 23.1 (2001): 107–17.

Jung CH et al. *Eleutherococcus senticosus* extract attenuates LPS-induced iNOS expression through the inhibition of Akt and JNK pathways in murine macrophage. J Ethnopharmacol 113.1 (2007): 183–7.

Jung SK et al. Cyanidin-3-*O*-(2″-xylosyl)-glucoside, an anthocyanin from Siberian ginseng (*Acanthopanax senticosus*) fruits, inhibits UVB-induced COX-2 expression and AP-1 transactivation. Food Science and Biotechnology, April 2013, Volume 22, Issue 2, pp 507–513

Kaemmerer K, Fink J. Prakt Tierarzt 61.9 (1980): 748, 750–2, 754, 759–60. In: Mills S, Bone K (eds). Principles and practices of phytotherapy. London: Churchill Livingstone, 2000: 538.

Kim KJ et al. The effects of *Acanthopanax senticosus* on global hepatic gene expression in rats subjected to heat environmental stress. Toxicol (2010) 278 (2):217–223

Kormosh N, et al. Effect of a combination of extract from several plants on cell-mediated and humoral immunity of patients with advanced ovarian cancer. Phytother Res 20.5 (2006): 424–5.

Kuo J et al. The effect of eight weeks of supplementation with *Eleutherococcus senticosus* on endurance capacity and metabolism in human. Chinese Journal of Physiology 53(2): 105–111, 2010.

Kupin VJ. Eleutherococcus and other biologically active modifiers in oncology. Medexport, Moscow, 1984: 21. In: Lininger SW et al (eds). A-Z guide to drug-herb-vitamin interactions. Healthnotes, 1999.

Kupin VI, Polevaia EB. Stimulation of the immunological reactivity of cancer patients by Eleutherococcus extract. Vopr Onkol 32.7 (1986): 21–6 [in Russian].

Kushnerova NF, Rakhmanin Iu A. [The impact of nitric oxide intoxication on hepatic metabolic reactions and the prevention of lesions.] Gig Sanit 1 (2008): 70–3.

Kwan CY et al. Vascular effects of Siberian ginseng (*Eleutherococcus senticosus*): endothelium-dependent NO- and EDHF-mediated relaxation depending on vessel size. Naunyn Schmiedebergs Arch Pharmacol 369.5 (2004): 473–80.

Lee YJ et al. The effects of A. senticosus supplementation on serum lipid profiles, biomarkers of oxidative stress, and lymphocyte DNA damage in postmenopausal women. Biochem and Biophysical Res Comm (2008) 375(1):Pages 44–48

Lee D et al. Neuroprotective effects of *Eleutherococcus senticosus* bark on transient global cerebral ischemia in rats. J Ethnopharmacol (2012) 139(1):Pages 6–11

Lin QY et al. Inhibition of inducible nitric oxide synthase by *Acanthopanax senticosus* extract in RAW264.7 macrophages. J Ethnopharmacol 118.2 (2008): 231–6.

Lishmanov IuB et al. [Cardioprotective, inotropic, and anti-arrhythmia properties of a complex adaptogen "Tonizid"]. Eksp Klin Farmakol 71.3 (2008): 15–22.

Liu T et al. Improvement of insulin resistance by *Acanthopanax senticosus* root in fructose-rich chow-fed rats. Clin Exp Pharmacol Physiol 32.8 (2005): 649–54.

Liu KY et al. Release of acetylcholine by syringin, an active principle of *Eleutherococcus senticosus*, to raise insulin secretion in Wistar rats. Neurosci Lett 434.2 (2008): 195–9.

Liu SM et al. Protective effect of extract of *Acanthopanax senticosus* harms on dopaminergic neurons in Parkinson's disease mice. Phytomedicine (2012) 19(7):631–638

Mahady GB et al. Ginsengs: a review of safety and efficacy. Nutr Clin Care 3.2 (2000): 90.

Maslov LN, Guzarova NV. [Cardioprotective and antiarrhythmic properties of preparations from *Leuzea carthamoides*, *Aralia mandshurica*, and *Eleutherococcus senticosus*]. Eksp Klin Farmakol 70.6 (2007): 48–54.

McEwan BS. Seminars in medicine of the Beth Israel Deaconess Medical Center: protective and damaging effects of stress mediators. N Engl J Med 338.3 (1998): 171–9.

McRae S. Elevated serum digoxin levels in a patient taking digoxin and Siberian ginseng. CMAJ 155.3 (1996): 293–5.

Meacham S et al. Nutritional assessments for cancer patients can be improved when mineral concentrations in dietary supplements are considered during medical nutrition therapy consultations. J Nutr 132.11 (2002): 3547S.

Mills S, Bone K. Siberian ginseng, principles and practice of phytotherapy. UK: Churchill Livingstone, 2000, pp 534–41.

Miyanomae T, Frindel E. Radioprotection of hemopoiesis conferred by *Acanthopanax senticosus* Harms (Shigoka) administered before or after irradiation. Exp Hematol 16.9 (1988): 801–6.

Narimanian M et al. Impact of Chisan® (ADAPT-232) on the quality-of-life and its efficacy as an adjuvant in the treatment of acute non-specific pneumonia. Phytomedicine 12.10 (2005): 723–9.

Nasolodin VV et al. [Prevention of iron deficiencies in high-qualification athletes.] Gig Sanit 2 (2006): 44–7.

Nissen D (ed). Mosby's drug consult, St Louis: Mosby, 2003, pp. 17.

Niu HS et al. Increase of beta-endorphin secretion by syringin, an active principle of *Eleutherococcus senticosus*, to produce antihyperglycemic action in type 1-like diabetic rats. Horm Metab Res 39.12 (2007): 894–8.

Niu HS et al. Hypoglycemic effect of syringin from *Eleutherococcus senticosus* in streptozotocin-induced diabetic rats. Planta Med 74.2 (2008): 109–13.

Panossian A, Wagner H. Stimulating effect of adaptogens: an overview with particular reference to their efficacy following single dose administration. Phytother Res 19.10 (2005): 819–38.

Panossian A, et al. Plant adaptogens. III. Earlier and aspects and concepts on their mode of action. Phytomedicine 6.4 (1999): 287–300.

Park EJ et al. Water-soluble polysaccharide from *Eleutherococcus senticosus* stems attenuates fulminant hepatic failure induced by D-galactosamine and lipopolysaccharide in mice. Basic Clin Pharmacol Toxicol 94.6 (2004): 298–304.

Pearce PT et al. Panax ginseng and *Eleutherococcus senticosus* extracts: in vitro studies on binding to steroid receptors. Endocrinol Jpn 29.5 (1982): 567–73.

Schaffler K et al. 2013. No benefit adding *Eleutherococcus senticosus* to stress management training in stress-related fatigue/weakness, impaired work or concentration, a randomized controlled study. Pharmacopsychiatry. E-pub ahead of print Apr 2013.

Schmolz MW, et al. The synthesis of Rantes, G-CSF, IL-4, IL-5, IL-6, IL-12 and IL-13 in human whole-blood cultures is modulated by an extract from *Eleutherococcus senticosus* L. roots. Phytother Res 15.3 (2001): 268–70.

Shakhmatov II et al. [Effect of eleutherococcus on hemostasis in immobilized rats]. Eksp Klin Farmakol 70.2 (2007): 45–7.

Shen ML et al. Immunopharmacological effects of polysaccharides from *Acanthopanax senticosus* on experimental animals. Int J Immunopharmacol 13.5 (1991): 549–54.

Sievenpiper JL et al. Decreasing, null and increasing effects of eight popular types of ginseng on acute postprandial glycemic indices in healthy humans: the role of ginsenosides. J Am Coll Nutr 23.3 (2004): 248–58.

Skidmore-Roth L. Mosby's handbook of herbs and natural supplements. St Louis: Mosby, 2001.

Tohda C et al. Inhibitory effects of *Eleutherococcus senticosus* extracts on amyloid beta(25-35)-induced neuritic atrophy and synaptic loss. J Pharmacol Sci 107.3 (2008): 329–39.

Ulbricht C. Herpes: An Integrative Approach. Alternative and Complementary Therapies. October 2012, 18(5): 269–276

WADA. The World Anti-Doping Code. The 2014 prohibited list: international standard. World Anti Doping Agency (2014).

Wagner H et al. Die DC-and HPLC-analyse der Eleutherococcus Droge DC-and HPLC-analysis of Eleutherococcus. Planta Med 44.4 (1982): 193–8.

Wagner H et al. Immunostimulant action of polysaccharides (heteroglycans) from higher plants: preliminary communication. Arzneimittelforschung 34.6 (1984): 659–61 [in German].

Wagner H et al. Economic and medicinal plant research. London: Academic Press, 1985, pp 155–215.

Waller DP et al. Lack of androgenicity of Siberian ginseng (Siberian ginseng fails to cause sex differentiation disorder in rats) [Letter]. JAMA 267.17 (1992): 232.

Wang H et al. Asian and Siberian ginseng as a potential modulator of immune function: an in vitro cytokine study using mouse macrophages. Clin Chim Acta 327.1–2 (2003): 123–8.

Wang X et al. The protective effects of *Acanthopanax senticosus* Harms aqueous extracts against oxidative stress: Role of Nrf2 and antioxidant enzymes. J Ethanopharmacol Volume 127, Issue 2, 3 February 2010, Pages 424–432

Watanabe K et al. Fundamental studies on the inhibitory action of *Acanthopanax senticosus* Harms on glucose absorption. J Ethnopharmacology, Vol 132, Issue 1, 28 October 2010, Pages 193–199

Williams M. Immunoprotection against herpes simplex type II infection by eleutherococcus root extract. Int J Alt Complement Med 13 (1995): 9–12.

Wu F et al. Protective effects of aqueous extract from *Acanthopanax senticosus* against corticosterone-induced neurotoxicity in PC12. J Ethnopharmacol (2013) 148(3):861–868

Yoon T et al. Anti-metastatic activity of *Acanthopanax senticosus* extract and its possible immunological mechanism of action. J Ethnopharmacol 93.2–3 (2004): 247–53.

Yun-Choi HS et al. Potential inhibitors of platelet aggregation from plant sources, III (Part 3). J Nat Prod 50.6 (1987): 1059–64.

Zykov MP, Protasova SF. Prospects of immunostimulating vaccination against influenza including the use of Eleutherococcus and other preparations of plants. In: New data on Eleutherococcus: proceedings of the second international symposium on Eleutherococcus. Moscow, 1984: 164–9.

Slippery elm

HISTORICAL NOTE The dried inner bark of the slippery elm tree was a popular remedy used by many Native American tribes, and subsequently taken up by European settlers. It was mixed with water and applied topically to treat wounds, bruises and skin irritations, and used internally for sore throat, coughs and gastrointestinal conditions. When mixed with milk, it was used as a nutritious gruel for children and convalescents. It also gained a reputation as an effective wound healer among soldiers during the American Civil War. From 1820 until 1960, it was listed in the US Pharmacopeia as a demulcent, emollient and antitussive (Ulbricht & Basch 2005). The name 'slippery elm' refers to the slippery consistency of the inner bark when it comes into contact with water.

COMMON NAME

Slippery elm

OTHER NAMES

American elm, Indian elm, moose elm, red elm, sweet elm, winged elm

BOTANICAL NAME/FAMILY

Ulmus fulvus or *Ulmus rubra* (family Ulmaceae)

According to current botanical nomenclature, it should now be referred to as *Ulmus rubra.*

PLANT PART USED

Dried inner bark

CHEMICAL COMPONENTS

The inner bark chiefly contains mucilage (various hexoses, pentoses, methylpentoses), glucose, polyuronides, tannins, galacturonic acid, L-rhamnose, D-galactose, starches, fat, phytosterols, sesquiterpenes, oxalate acid, flavonoids, salicyclic acid, capric acid, caprylic acid, decanoic acid and cholesterol (Beveridge et al 1969, Duke 2003, IM Gateway Database 2003, Newell et al 1996, Rousseau & Watts 2012). The bark provides 2740 kcal/kg. It contains a variety of nutritional factors, such as glucose, calcium, iron, vitamin C, thiamine, zinc, magnesium and potassium, providing support for its traditional use as a nutritious gruel.

Clinical note — Mucilages

Mucilages are hydrophilic structures, capable of trapping water, which causes them to swell in size and develop a gel-like consistency. The gels tend to have soothing properties and can be broken down by bowel flora when taken internally (Mills & Bone 2000). Mucilages are known to have beneficial effects on burns, wounds and ulcers when applied externally and on gastric inflammation, irritations and diarrhoea when taken internally.

S

MAIN ACTIONS

The pharmacological actions of slippery elm have not been significantly investigated in clinical studies. Therefore, information is generally based on what is known about key constituents found within the herb.

Soothes irritated and inflamed tissue

The large amount of mucilage found in slippery elm bark will coat the surface of mucous membranes or wounds and sores when it comes in contact with water, and form a gel-like layer. Mucilaginous medicinal plants, such as slippery elm, have beneficial effects on burns, wounds, ulcers, external and internal inflammations and irritations (Morton 1990). They provide a moist, protective barrier which can soothe and promote healing.

Nutritive demulcent

A number of constituents, such as starch, glucose, calcium, iron, vitamin C, thiamine, zinc, magnesium and potassium are present in slippery elm, making it a source of many nutritional factors (Duke 2003).

Antioxidant

In vitro studies show a free radical-scavenging activity that may relate to its anti-inflammatory action (Langmead et al 2002). Compounds with antioxidant activity are sometimes investigated for their tumoricidal activity; however an in vitro study found slippery elm to exhibit only weak tumoricidal properties (Mazzio & Soliman 2009).

CLINICAL USE

The therapeutic effectiveness of slippery elm has not been significantly investigated under clinical trial conditions, so evidence is derived from traditional, in vitro and animal studies.

Gastrointestinal conditions

Based on traditional evidence, slippery elm is taken internally to relieve the symptoms of gastritis, acid dyspepsia, gastric reflux, peptic ulcers, irritable bowel syndrome (IBS) and Crohn's disease.

It is widely accepted that, when orally ingested, the mucilage forms a physical barrier protecting the oesophageal and stomach walls from the damaging effects of stomach acid and possibly also exerting mild anti-inflammatory activity locally. Currently, clinical research is not available to determine the effectiveness of slippery elm in these conditions; however, anecdotally the treatment appears to be very successful and patients report rapid improvement in upper gastrointestinal symptoms.

Solid-dose tablets and capsules are used in the treatment of lower gastrointestinal conditions such as diarrhoea, where it is believed the fibre will slow down gastric transit time and act as a bulking agent. Although clinical studies are not available to determine its effectiveness, the high mucilaginous content and presence of tannins in the herb provide a theoretical basis for its use.

IN COMBINATION

A small, open pilot study investigated the use of a herbal formula containing slippery elm in the treatment of 31 patients with IBS, with promising results. Twenty-one patients with diarrhoea-predominant or alternating bowel habit IBS were given the herbal formula containing slippery elm (4.5 g), powdered bilberry fruit (10.0 g), agrimony (3.0 g) and cinnamon (1.5 g) twice daily for 3 weeks. Ten patients with constipation-predominant IBS were given a herbal formula containing slippery elm (7.0 g), lactulose (3.0 g), oat bran (2.0 g) and licorice root (1.5 g) twice daily for 3 weeks. The diarrhoea-predominant or alternating bowel habit IBS group reported no improvements in bowel habit, although they did report a significant improvement in a number of IBS symptoms, including straining, abdominal pain, bloating, flatulence and global IBS symptoms. There was a significant improvement in bowel habits in the constipation-predominant IBS group, with a 20% increase in bowel movement frequency and improvements in stool consistency, and IBS symptoms, including reductions in straining, abdominal pain, bloating and global IBS symptom severity (Hawrelak & Myers 2010). While some of these results are promising, the role of slippery elm in achieving the reported benefits is unclear. Further research is required to expand upon the findings of this pilot study.

Dermatitis and wounds

Slippery elm has also been used as a topical agent to soothe irritated and/or inflamed skin conditions, wounds and burns and to draw out boils and abscesses (Fisher & Painter 1996). When applied, it forms a protective gel-like layer, which is considered to have soothing properties.

Laryngeal 'soothing' effect

A single oral dose of 3 g of slippery elm taken in warm water as a tea had no 'soothing' effect according to a randomised, controlled, single-blind study of 24 volunteers without pharyngeal or laryngeal complaints (Rousseau & Watts 2012). A 'soothing' effect was defined as 'when the [tissue] surface feels as if it were coated with something, such as a layer of protective covering'. Further research should be conducted testing the preparation in people with current inflammation and discomfort.

OTHER USES

Traditionally, slippery elm is used to treat bronchitis, cystitis and intestinal parasites. Externally, it has been used to treat gout, inflamed joints and toothache (Fisher & Painter 1996).

DOSAGE RANGE

Owing to insufficient data available from clinical studies, doses have been derived from Australian manufacturers' recommendations.

S

Clinical note — Essiac tea

Slippery elm is one of the key ingredients in Essiac tea, which was reportedly developed by the Ojibwa tribe of Canada and named after an Ontario nurse (Rene Caisse) to whom the formula for the herbal tea was given by an Ojibwa healer in 1922 (Smith & Boon 1999). It is used to treat a variety of diverse conditions, such as allergies, hypertension and osteoporosis. The tea is made up of a mixture of four herbs, *Arctium lappa* (burdock root), *Rumex acetosella* (sheep sorrel), *Ulmus rubra* (slippery elm) and *Rheum officinale* (rhubarb) and is considered to possess antioxidant and, possibly, anticancer activities (Leonard et al 2006). As a result, it is used widely by North American cancer patients during chemo- and radiotherapies (Cheung et al 2005) for reduction in symptoms associated with cancer treatment and as a possible adjunctive treatment. In vitro tests with Essiac have identified anticancer activity, although its effects in vivo are controversial and evidence of efficacy is anecdotal (Leonard et al 2006). A recent study demonstrated that Essiac tea effectively scavenges several types of radicals and possesses DNA-protective effects (Leonard et al 2006). A retrospective cohort study of 510 women with breast cancer found that Essiac did not improve quality-of-life scores or mood (Zick et al 2006). Daily doses of Essiac range from 12 to 114 mL, with the average dose being 43.6 mL, corresponding to doses recommended on popular products. Duration of treatment ranged from 1 to 28 months, with the average being 11.1 months. The formula was well tolerated, with only two women reporting minor adverse events, while many women reported beneficial effects. In contrast, an in vitro study found Essiac tea stimulated the growth of human breast cancer cells via both oestrogen receptor-dependent and oestrogen receptor-independent mechanisms (Kulp et al 2006). Patients and health practitioners should consider these findings when making clinical decisions regarding treatment protocols.

Practice points/Patient counselling

- Slippery elm inner bark is a highly mucilaginous substance, which has been traditionally used as a topical application to soothe irritated and inflamed skin conditions and promote wound healing.
- It is used internally to soothe an irritated throat and is often combined with antiseptic herbs.
- Slippery elm is used to provide symptomatic relief in acid dyspepsia, gastrointestinal reflux and inflammatory bowel diseases, but has not been scientifically studied to any significant extent.
- Overall, slippery elm has not been significantly investigated in clinical studies, so most information is derived from traditional sources and the known activity or key constituents.

Gastrointestinal symptoms

- One to two capsules containing 150 mg of slippery elm before meals.
- Fluid extract (60%): 5 mL three times daily.
- Half a teaspoon of slippery elm bark powder is mixed with one cup of hot water and taken up to three times daily. For added flavouring, cinnamon or nutmeg can be added.

External use

- Mix the coarse powdered bark with enough boiling water to make a paste and use as a poultice (Hoffman 1983).

TOXICITY

Insufficient reliable information is available.

ADVERSE REACTIONS

Insufficient reliable information is available.

SIGNIFICANT INTERACTIONS

Controlled studies are unavailable, but interactions are theoretically possible with some medicines.

Since slippery elm forms an inert barrier over the gastrointestinal lining, it may theoretically alter the rate and/or extent of absorption of medicines with a narrow therapeutic range (e.g. barbiturates, digoxin, lithium, phenytoin, warfarin). The clinical significance of this is unclear. Separate doses by 2 hours.

CONTRAINDICATIONS AND PRECAUTIONS

Insufficient reliable information is available.

PREGNANCY USE

It is likely to be safe, but safety is still to be established.

PATIENTS' FAQs

What will this herb do for me?

The inner bark of slippery elm is highly mucilaginous, meaning that it forms a thick gel-like substance when combined with water. Traditionally, it has been used internally to relieve symptoms of dyspepsia and inflamed bowel conditions and topically to soothe irritated skin and promote wound healing.

When will it start to work?

Whether used internally for upper gastrointestinal symptoms (such as reflux and dyspepsia) or applied topically to irritated skin, it should theoretically provide quick symptomatic relief; however, research to confirm this is not available.

Are there any safety issues?

Although slippery elm has not been scientifically investigated, the US Food and Drug Administration has approved it as a safe demulcent substance.

REFERENCES

Beveridge RJ et al. Some structural features of the mucilage from the bark of *Ulmus fulvus*. Carbohydr Res 9 (1969): 429–439.

Cheung S, et al. Antioxidant and anti-inflammatory properties of ESSIAC and Flor essence. Oncol Rep 14 (2005): 1345–1350.

Duke JA. Dr Duke's phytochemical and ethnobotanical databases. Beltsville, MD: US Department of Agriculture–Agricultural Research Service–National Germplasm Resources Laboratory, Beltsville Agricultural Research Center, 2003. Available online: www.ars-grin.gov/duke (accessed March, 2008).

Fisher C, Painter G. Materia Medica for the southern hemisphere. Auckland: Fisher-Painter Publishers, 1996.

Hawrelak JA, Myers, SP. Effects of two natural medicine formulations on irritable bowel syndrome symptoms: a pilot study. The Journal of Alternative and Complementary Medicine 16.10 (2010):1065–71.

Hoffman D. The new holistic herbal. Dorset: Element Books, 1983.

IM Gateway Database. Slippery elm review. Available online: www.imgateway.com (accessed May 2003).

Kulp KS et al. Essiac and Flor-Essence herbal tonics stimulate the in vitro growth of human breast cancer cells. Breast cancer research and treatment 98.3 (2006): 249–59.

Langmead L et al. Antioxidant effects of herbal therapies used by patients with inflammatory bowel disease: an in vitro study. Aliment Pharmacol Ther 16.2 (2002): 197–205.

Leonard SS et al. Essiac tea: scavenging of reactive oxygen species and effects on DNA damage. J Ethnopharmacol 103.2 (2006): 288–296.

Mazzio EA, & Soliman KFA. In vitro screening for the tumoricidal properties of international medicinal herbs. Phytotherapy Research, 23.3 (2009): 385–98.

Mills S, Bone K. Principles and practice of phytotherapy. London: Churchill Livingstone, 2000.

Morton, JF. Mucilaginous plants and their uses in medicine. Journal of Ethnopharmacology 29.3 (1990): 245–66.

Newell CA, et al. Herbal medicines: a guide for health care professionals. London, UK: Pharmaceutical Press, 1996.

Rousseau B, Watts CR. Slippery elm, its biochemistry, and use as a complementary and alternative treatment for laryngeal irritation. Journal of Investigational Biochemistry, 1.1 (2012): 17–23.

Smith M, Boon HS. Counseling cancer patients about herbal medicine. Patient Educ Couns 38 (1999): 109–120.

Ulbricht CE, Basch EM. Natural standard herb and supplement reference. St Louis: Mosby, 2005.

Zick SM et al. Trial of Essiac to ascertain its effect in women with breast cancer (TEA-BC). J Altern Complement Med 12.10 (2006): 971–980.

St John's wort

HISTORICAL NOTE St John's wort (SJW) has been used medicinally since ancient Greek times when, it is believed, Dioscorides and Hippocrates used it to rid the body of evil spirits. Since the time of the Swiss physician Paracelsus (*c.* 1493–1541), it has been used to treat neuralgia, anxiety, neurosis and depression. Externally, it has also been used to treat wounds, bruises and shingles. The name 'St John's wort' is related to its yellow flowers, traditionally gathered for the feast of St John the Baptist, and the term 'wort' is the old English word for plant. SJW has enjoyed its greatest popularity in Europe and comprises 25% of all antidepressant prescriptions in Germany (Schrader 2000). In the past few decades, its popularity has grown in countries such as Australia and the United States.

OTHER NAMES

Amber, balsana, devil's scourge, goatweed, hardhay, hartheu, herb de millepertuis, hierba de San Juan, hypericum, iperico, johanniskraut, klamath weed, konradskraut, millepertuis, rosin rose, sonnenwendkraut, St Jan's kraut, tipton weed, witch's herb

BOTANICAL NAME/FAMILY

Hypericum perforatum (family Clusiaceae or Guttiferae)

PLANT PARTS USED

Aerial parts, flowering tops

CHEMICAL COMPONENTS

Naphthodianthrones (including hypericin and pseudohypericin). Flavonoids, mostly hyperoside, rutin, quercitrin, isoquercitrin, quercetin and kaempferol, phenolics, including hyperforin, procyanidins, essential oil, sterols (beta-sitosterol), vitamins C and A, xanthones and choline.

Clinical note — Pharmacologically important constituents

It has generally been considered that most of the pharmacological activities of SJW are attributable to hypericin and the flavonoid constituent, hyperforin. Besides contributing to the antidepressant activity, hypericin is the primary constituent responsible for the photosensitivity reactions reported with high intakes. Hyperforin is also a major contributor to the herb's antidepressant activity (Butterweck et al 2003a, Mennini & Gobbi 2004) and considered the main constituent responsible for inducing the cytochrome P-glycoprotein (P-gp) and thereby producing drug interactions. Besides this, it demonstrates many other pharmacological effects, such as antibacterial, anti-inflammatory and antineoplastic activities. Components previously considered void of activity have also been identified as important for pharmacological activity. For example, both procyanidin B2 and hyperoside increase the oral bioavailability of hypericin by 58% and 34%, respectively, and therefore, its clinical effects (Butterweck et al 2003b). A report published in June 2003 demonstrated that an extract devoid of both hyperforin and hypericin still exhibited antidepressant activity (Butterweck et al 2003a). Other constituents with antidepressant activity were identified and include hyperoside, isoquercitrin and miquelianin, and the 3-*O*-galactoside, 3-*O*-glucoside and 3-*O*-glucuronide of quercetin.

Manufactured products will vary in the concentrations and proportions of the different plant constituents present because these are influenced by the plant's place of origin, its harvest time and drying, extraction processes and storage conditions. Hyperforin, in particular, can be present in variable concentrations because it is unstable in light, air and most organic solvents (Mennini & Gobbi 2004). This is extremely important to remember when comparing studies, as variations in chemical composition could be responsible for differences in results. It also provides a rationale for lack of interchangeability between brands.

MAIN ACTIONS

SJW has demonstrated multiple mechanisms of action, due to the presence of multiple active constituents. Research has been undertaken to identify the key constituents responsible for each mechanism of action. Often, the resulting activity is due to a combination of phytochemicals and cannot be ascribed to a single chemical entity.

Antidepressant

Although SJW has been investigated extensively in scientific studies, there are still many questions about its pharmacology and mechanisms of action.

Collectively, the data show that SJW extract exerts significant pharmacological activity within several neurochemical systems believed to be implicated in the pathophysiology of depression. Recent investigations reveal that hyperforin and other constituents (e.g. adhyperforin, hypericins, flavanol glycosides) act synergistically through both pharmacodynamic and pharmacokinetic mechanisms to alleviate depression (Nahrstedt & Butterweck 2010). The synergistic antidepressive effects have been observed in vitro and in vivo (Fiebich et al 2011).

Inhibits synaptic reuptake of several neurotransmitters

Preclinical animal studies have found that SJW inhibits the synaptic reuptake system for serotonin, noradrenaline and dopamine (Nathan 1999, Wonnemann et al 2001). Studies using specific isolated constituents have demonstrated potent uptake inhibition of gamma-aminobutyric acid (GABA) and L-glutamate in vivo (Bilia et al 2002, Chatterjee et al 1998). These effects appear to be non-competitive, dose-dependent and mediated via sodium channels (Roz & Rehavi 2004).

Studies with hyperforin have shown that it does not interact directly with uptake transporters but instead acts by reducing the pH gradient across the synaptic vesicle membrane, resulting in diffusion of uncharged monoamines out of the vesicular compartment into the cytoplasm. The increase in cytoplasmic concentration decreases the transmembrane gradient of the neurotransmitters, causing an 'apparent' inhibition of synaptosomal uptake by hyperforin. Additionally, hyperforin elevates intracellular sodium concentration, thereby inhibiting gradient-driven neurotransmitter reuptake (Beerhues 2006). This is a novel mechanism of action, which differs from conventional antidepressant drugs.

Although hyperforin is the main constituent responsible for these effects, tests now show that a number of others are also involved (Gobbi et al 2001), such as adhyperforin, which has demonstrated a strong inhibitory effect on neurotransmitter uptake, and the oligomeric procyanidin fraction, which has demonstrated weak to moderate effects (Wonnemann et al 2001).

GABA receptor binding

SJW extracts have been shown to bind at GABA-A and -B receptors, to inhibit GABA reuptake, to evoke GABA release from synaptosomes and to exert an anxiolytic effect that is blocked by the benzodiazepine antagonist flumazenil (Perfumi et al 2002).

Upregulation of serotonin receptors

SJW significantly upregulates both 5-HT_{1A} and 5-HT_{2A} receptors and has a significant affinity for opiate sigma receptors, which may contribute to the antidepressant effect (Teufel-Mayer & Gleitz 1997).

Dopamine beta-hydroxylase inhibition

Studies on isolated constituents showed that hypericin and pseudohypericin can inhibit the enzyme dopamine beta-hydroxylase in vitro (Bilia et al 2002).

Inhibition of catechol-*O*-methyltransferase

This has been demonstrated in test tube studies (Thiede & Walper 1994).

Suppresses interleukin-6 (IL-6) synthesis

Various extracts from SJW produce a potent and dose-dependent inhibition of substance P-induced IL-6 synthesis (Fiebich et al 2001), which may also contribute to the herb's overall antidepressant effect.

Monoamine oxidase (MAO) inhibition

Inhibition of MAO by hypericin demonstrated in vitro was believed to be the primary mode of action; however, this has not been confirmed in several subsequent studies that have shown only weak inhibitory activity at doses in excess of usual therapeutic levels (Di Carlo et al 2001).

Anxiolytic

Several in vivo studies confirm the anxiolytic effects of SJW extract (Beijamini & Andreatini 2003, Jakovljevic et al 2000, Vandenbogaerde et al 2000). Activity at the GABA receptors and an increase in circulating GABA levels are likely to be involved. Whether the effect is clinically significant is unclear, as a recent systematic review concluded that there is insufficient evidence to conclude that SJW monotherapy is an effective anxiolytic treatment (Lakhan & Vieira 2010).

Cognitive effects

SJW extracts and hyperforin improve cognitive function in experimental models (Kiewert et al 2004); however, clinical studies have been less convincing (Siepmann et al 2002, Timoshanko et al 2001). In vivo studies with hyperforin have found that it induces the release of acetycholine from cholinergic terminals in the hippocampus and striatum, providing an explanation for the observed effects. Preventive administration of *Hypericum perforatum* (350 mg/kg orally) counteracted the working-memory impairments caused by repeated stress in male Wistar rats. The herb significantly improved hippocampus-dependent spatial working memory in comparison with control ($P < 0.01$) and alleviated some other negative effects of stress on cognitive functions (Trofimiuk & Braszko 2008). Interestingly, a small trial (n = 20) reported that smokers' cognitive function may benefit from taking

SJW (Remotiv, ZE117) while on nicotine replacement therapy (Nicabate CQ) (Camfield et al 2013).

Neuroprotective

A 2010 review of neurobiological effects of hyperforin and its potential role in Alzheimer's disease indicates that it has several mechanisms which are of relevance, including the ability to disassemble amyloid-beta aggregates in vitro, decrease of astrogliosis and microglia activation, as well as improving spatial memory in vivo (Griffith et al 2010). A recent in vivo study confirmed that mainly hyperforin and quercetin appear to be involved in the neuroprotective action of SJW standardised extracts (Gómez Del Rio et al 2013).

Anticonvulsant effects

A study in mice showed that SJW methanolic extract increased latency of seizure in the pretreated group (50 mg/kg) against seizure induced by picrotoxin. The higher dose of extract (200 mg/kg) significantly decreased the duration of seizure and death latency (Etemad et al 2011).

Effects on alcohol and food intake

Several reports indicate comorbidity between depression and ethanol abuse and that depressive disorders and ethanol abuse may be associated with similar changes in the activity of central neurotransmitters (Markou et al 1998). In vivo studies using SJW in animal models of alcoholism have found that it does not alter food and water intake, or the pharmacokinetics of alcohol, but a reduction in ethanol intake occurs (Panocka et al 2000).

In a model of binge eating (brought upon by stress and food restrictions), treatment with 250 and 500 mg/kg of SJW dry extract decreased the binge-eating episode (Micioni Di Bonaventura et al 2012).

Effects on morphine withdrawal syndrome

A study in morphine dependent rats suggests that SJW extract is capable of reducing the symptoms of opiate withdrawal. Its effectiveness may be equivalent to clonidine in reducing the opiate withdrawal syndrome (Feily & Abbasi 2009).

Anti-inflammatory and analgesic

SJW extract and several of its various isolated constituents have demonstrated effects on inflammation and pain pathways in different in vitro and animal models (Jakovljevic et al 2000, Raso et al 2002).

It potently inhibits binding to mu-, delta- and kappa-opioid receptors (Simmen et al 1998). In vivo tests also identify modulation of cyclooxygenase-2 (COX-2) expression for hypericum extract (Raso et al 2002). Studies with the isolated constituent hyperforin have shown that it potently inhibits COX-1 and 5-lipooxygenase in vitro (Albert et al 2002), and also demonstrates high effectiveness in vivo (Feisst et al 2009).

A more recent study found that hyperforin inhibits microsomal prostaglandin E_2 synthase-1 and suppresses prostaglandin E_2 formation in vivo (Koeberle et al 2011). Quercetin and other flavonoids contribute to the anti-inflammatory effect. Hyperoside (quercetin-3-*O*-galactoside) seems to exert its anti-inflammatory activity through the suppression of nuclear factor-κB activation, as detected in mouse peritoneal macrophages (Kim et al 2011).

A dried extract of SJW, as well as purified hyperforin and hypericin, induced a prolonged antinociception effect that persisted for 120 minutes after administration. The persistent thermal and chemical antinociception of SJW was mainly mediated by protein kinase C-inhibiting mechanisms (Galeotti et al 2010). Similarly, a single oral dose of a SJW dried extract (5 mg/kg orally) produced prolonged relief from pain hypersensitivity in vivo. Moreover, preventive SJW administration increased the latency to induction of hyperalgesia and reduced the duration of the painful symptomatology in a migraine model (Galeotti et al 2013a). Subsequently, hypericin was identified as a key component responsible for reversing nitric oxide-induced nociceptive hypersensitivity, whereas hyperforin and flavonoids were ineffective (Galeotti et al 2013b).

Anticancer effects

Hypericin, the photoactive compound of *Hypericum perforatum*, is probably the most powerful photosensitiser found in nature (Kacerovska et al 2008). It has minimal toxicity but exhibits potent photo-damaging effects in the presence of light (Olivo et al 2006). It is known to generate a high yield of singlet oxygen and other reactive oxygen species that are associated with photo-oxidative cellular damage (Karioti & Bilia 2010). The application of photodynamic therapy (PDT) with hypericin for the treatment of cancers such as recurrent mesothelioma and skin cancer has been validated in clinical trials. It may also have potential as a photodynamic agent in the treatment of nasopharyngeal cancer according to in vitro and in vivo models (Kacerovska et al 2008).

Hyperforin also exhibits antineoplastic potential based on the sum of its anticarcinogenic, antiproliferant, proapoptotic, anti-invasive and antimetastatic effects (Medina et al 2006). Hyperforin has been shown to effectively decrease the proliferation rates of a number of mammalian cancer cell lines, induce apoptosis of tumour cells and inhibit angiogenesis both in vitro and in vivo. For example, under hyperforin treatment in vivo, the growth of Kaposi's sarcoma — a highly angiogenic tumour — is strongly inhibited, with the resultant tumours reduced in size and vascularisation as compared with controls. Hyperforin inhibits neutrophil and monocyte chemotaxis in vitro and angiogenesis in vivo induced by angiogenic chemokines (CXCL8 or CCL2) (Lorusso et al 2009).

Besides hypericin and hyperforin, polyphenolic procyanidin B2 has also demonstrated an inhibitory effect on the growth of leukaemia cells, brain glioblastoma cells and normal human astrocytes in vitro (Hostanska et al 2003). Further, the inhibitory effects on leukaemic cell growth were synergistically strengthened when hypericin and hyperforin were tested together.

Antiretroviral, antifungal and antibacterial

Alcoholic SJW extracts (methanolic/ethanolic) have more pronounced antibacterial activity than aqueous extracts (Saddiqe et al 2010). The key antibacterial compound isolated to date from SJW is hyperforin, which has a higher antibacterial activity against Gram-positive than Gram-negative bacteria. More recently, a study found that an SJW extract was effective at inhibiting five non-pathogenic *Mycobacterium* isolates and *Bacillus subtilis*, but not *Escherichia coli*. Hyperforin isolated from this extract was more effective than hypericin or pseudohypericin (Mortensen et al 2012). This supports an earlier paper which identified hyperforin as a key constituent demonstrating antibacterial activities (Medina et al 2006).

Hyperforin exhibits effective antibacterial activity against methicillin-resistant *Staphylococcus aureus* and other Gram-positive bacteria, but no growth-inhibitory effect on Gram-negative bacteria or *Candida albicans* (Schempp et al 1999).

In a recent animal study SJW reduced the lung index and viral titre of mice infected with influenza A virus, decreasing mortality and prolonging the mean survival time (Xiuying et al 2012).

Although in vitro and studies in animal models have identified antiretroviral activity for hypericin and pseudohypericin (Meruelo et al 1988), two clinical trials could not confirm these effects, even when larger doses of hypericin were administered (Gulick et al 1999, Jacobson et al 2001).

The mechanism involved is not known; however, it is suspected to involve direct inactivation of the virus or prevention of virus shedding, budding or assembly at the cell membrane (Meruelo et al 1988). The presence of light is an important requirement for antiretroviral activity to be demonstrated, as the effect appears to be photoactivated (Hudson et al 1993, Miskovsky 2002).

Cardiovascular effects

New in vivo research revealed that SJW significantly lowered total cholesterol and low-density lipoprotein (LDL) cholesterol when tested in healthy rats. It significantly inhibited weight gain in high-fat-fed rats, and in fructose-fed rats, SJW normalised the dyslipidaemia induced by fructose feeding and improved the insulin sensitivity (Husain et al 2011a). The same authors showed that SJW significantly reduced elevated blood glucose levels in diabetic rats and exerted a significant anxiolytic effect in this test group (Husain et al 2011b). A significant decrease in blood glucose levels was also observed after 1 week's administrations of SJW extract (125 and 250 mg/kg) to streptozotocin-diabetic rats. It also improved their dysregulated metabolic parameters (Can et al 2011).

Hypolipidaemic activity and antiatherosclerotic effects were also seen in another study utilising hypercholesterolaemic rabbits being treated with hydroalcoholic SJW extract (150 mg/kg). The effect appeared to be stronger than that of lovastatin (10 mg/kg) (Asgary et al 2012).

Previously, SJW extracts were identified as inhibitors of adipogenesis of 3T3-L1 cells and shown to inhibit insulin-sensitive glucose uptake in mature fat cells. The same authors subsequently found that SJW extract limits the differentiation of pre-adipocytes and significantly induces insulin resistance in mature fat cells. These effects were not mediated by hyperforin and hypericin (Richard et al 2012)

Gastrointestinal effects

SJW exhibits antispasmodic activity, according to research conducted with an experimental animal model (Jakovljevic et al 2000), most likely mediated via GABA activity. Among the chemical constituents of SJW extract tested, hyperforin and, to a lesser extent, the flavonoids kaempferol and quercetrin inhibited acetylcholine-induced contractions in an animal model (Capasso et al 2008). SJW has a direct inhibitory effect on smooth muscle and could also possibly modulate gastric neurotransmission. A more recent in vivo irritable bowel syndrome study showed that SJW extract diminished the recruitment of inflammatory cells and tumour necrosis factor-α following restraint stress not in a dose-dependent manner and inhibited small-bowel and colonic transit acceleration like loperamide, but had minimal effect on gastric emptying (Mozaffari et al 2011).

S

OTHER ACTIONS

No clinically significant effect on platelet aggregation has been identified (Beckert et al 2007).

Induction of CYP3A4 activity in the intestinal wall

Human studies have identified CYP3A4 and 2C19 induction effects for standard SJW extracts (e.g. LI 160), but no effects on CYP1A2, CYP2C9 or CYP2D6 (Durr et al 2000, Gurley et al 2008a, Jiang et al 2004, Wang et al 2001, 2004a). Human studies have failed to identify significant CYP3A4, 2D6, 2C9, 1A2 or 2C19 induction for low-hyperforin SJW extracts, such as ZE 117, using the appropriate probe drugs (Arold et al 2005, Madabushi et al 2006, Mueller et al 2004).

Hyperforin is a potent ligand for the pregnane X receptor, an orphan nuclear receptor that regulates expression of the CYP3A4 mono-oxygenase (Moore et al 2000). Although it is considered the chief constituent responsible for the pharmacokinetic interactions reported, there are other, less potent constituents in SJW, which also modulate cytochrome enzymes (Obach 2000).

Results from an open-label clinical study suggest that the effects of standard SJW (LI 160) on CYP3A4 enzymes may be biphasic, where the initial dose leads to a minor inhibition, followed by significant induction during long-term use (Rengelshausen et al 2005). Clinical studies indicate that CYP3A activity returns progressively to the basal level approximately 1 week after cessation of SJW administration (Imai et al 2008).

Increases levels of intestinal P-glycoprotein

SJW extract produced a 3.8-fold increase of intestinal P-gp expression in vivo (Durr et al 2000). Hyperforin has been identified as the key constituent responsible for P-gp induction effects (Tian et al 2005), although in vitro tests suggest other less potent constituents also exist, such as quercetin, hypericin, biapigenin and kaempferol (Patel et al 2004, Weber et al 2004).

Once again, low-hyperforin SJW extracts do not appear to significantly induce P-gp (Arold et al 2005, Madabushi et al 2006, Mueller et al 2004).

In vitro and in vivo tests further indicate that P-gp effects caused by standard SJW (LI 160) are biphasic, with an initial inhibitory effect followed by induction after longer exposure (Rengelshausen et al 2005, Wang et al 2004a).

Decreases levels of P-glycoprotein at blood–brain barrier

Newer research shows that SJW extract and the constituents hyperforin, hypericin and quercetin decreased P-gp transport activity at the blood–brain barrier in a dose- and time-dependent manner. SJW extract and hyperforin directly inhibited P-gp activity, whereas hypericin and quercetin modulated transporter function through a mechanism involving protein kinase C (Ott et al 2010).

CLINICAL USE

SJW is one of the most clinically tested herbal medicines available. As a result, we have an understanding of the key mechanisms of action, clinical effects, safety issues and also how it compares to standard pharmaceutical treatments. Its strong evidence base provides a good rationale for every clinician to consider its use where appropriate. Various SJW extracts have been tested in clinical trials. Some trials conducted with SJW used a 0.3% hypericin water and alcohol extract, known as LI 160. Most newer studies use different preparations, such as WS 5573 (standardised to hyperforin) or ZE 117 (a low-hyperforin concentration preparation).

Depression

Overall, SJW preparations are mainly used for mood disorders in modern-day practice, although it demonstrates benefits for other indications. There is now strong evidence from several meta-analyses to conclude that SJW extract is an effective treatment in mild, moderate and major depressive disorder with efficacy comparable to tricyclic and selective serotonin reuptake inhibitor (SSRI) antidepressant drugs (Cipriani et al 2012, Linde et al 2005a, 2009, Nahas & Sheikh 2011, Sarris & Kavanagh 2009). Additionally, SJW is well tolerated and associated with fewer side effects than pharmaceutical antidepressants. There is also evidence indicating that it reduces relapse.

> ***Clinical note — The Hamilton Depression Scale (HDS)***
> The HDS is an observer-rated scale that focuses mainly on somatic symptoms of depression. Although the original version included 21 items, a similar version using 17 items is more commonly used in clinical trials. Most studies using the HDS report the number of 'treatment responders' (patients achieving a score less than 10 and/or less than 50% of the baseline score) (Linde et al 2005a).

Mild to moderate depression

SJW has shown efficacy as a successful treatment for mild to moderate depression in numerous double-blind, placebo-controlled trials, confirmed by several meta-analyses and systematic reviews. Moreover, the clinical guidelines for the management of major depressive disorder in adults published by the Canadian Network for Mood and Anxiety Treatments (CANMAT) conclude that level 1 evidence supports SJW in mild to moderate depressive disorder (Ravindran et al 2009).

A 2005 Cochrane review analysed data from 37 double-blind, randomised studies (n = 4925) that used monopreparations of SJW over a treatment period of at least 4 weeks (Linde et al 2005a). It concluded that SJW extracts were superior to placebo for improving symptoms and SJW produced effects similar to synthetic antidepressants (tricyclic antidepressants [TCAs] and SSRIs) in adults with mild to moderate depression. The same conclusion was found in a later systematic review (Sarris & Kavanagh 2009).

Kasper et al (2008a) reanalysed data from a subset of patients (n = 217) suffering from an acute episode of mild depression from controlled trials testing SJW extract WS 5570 from the 2005 Cochrane review. The analysis shows that SJW extract WS 5570 has a meaningful beneficial effect during acute treatment of patients suffering from mild depression and leads to a substantial increase in the probability of remission. The studies tested three different doses — 600, 900 or 1200 mg/day — or placebo for 6 weeks. Patients receiving active treatment with WS 5570 experienced decreases in the HDS total score by an average of 10.8 (600 mg/day), 9.6 (900 mg/day), and 10.7 (1200 mg/day) points between the pretreatment baseline value and the end of acute treatment, compared to 6.8 points in the placebo group. All differences were significant. The rates of responders were 73%, 64%, 71% and 37% for WS 5570 600 mg/day, 900 mg/day and 1200 mg/day and placebo, respectively.

Since then, a long-term, open, multicentre study testing 500 mg/day of SJW ZE117 extract over 52 weeks found that the herbal treatment produced a significant reduction in depression scores (HDS) and was associated with a lower side effect rate than for standard antidepressants, thereby confirming earlier results (Brattström 2009).

Melzer et al (2010) conducted a different type of trial in an attempt to see whether using SJW in a real practice setting, where patients were taking multiple medications and required individualised dosing, would still be effective in the treatment of depression. This open-label, German study (n = 1778, from 304 centres) utilised Helarium-425 capsules from Bionorica, Neumarkt, Germany, at different doses, individualised for the patient. The mean daily dose was 822.5 ± 205.4 mg dry ethanolic *Hypericum* extract at admission (range 425–1700 mg) and 754.4 ± 231.1 mg at the last visit. The most commonly prescribed dosage schedules were an intake twice or three times daily. Used in this way by outpatients, SJW treatment was effective as an antidepressant in the management of depression in daily practice and lower age and shorter duration of the disorder were associated with significantly better outcomes (Melzer et al 2010). The herbal drug was well tolerated, and no new or serious adverse drug reactions were identified. More specifically, the SJW treatment was an extract with 255–285 mg dry ethanolic extract per coated tablet, standardised to hypericin 0.3% and a hyperforin content of 2–3%, or Helarium-425 with 425 mg dry ethanolic extract per capsule (DER 3.5–6 : 1) or Helarium-425, which is standardised to hypericin 0.1–0.3% and has a hyperforin content of maximum 6%, flavonoid/rutoside minimum 6% in the extract.

Major depression

Although a 2005 Cochrane review stated that SJW shows only minimal benefits over placebo in major depression (Linde et al 2005a), an updated 2009 Cochrane systematic review has concluded that SJW extracts: (1) are superior to placebo in patients with major depression; (2) are similarly effective as standard antidepressants (SSRIs and TCAs); and (3) have fewer side effects than standard antidepressants (Linde et al 2009). A total of 29 randomised controlled trials (RCTs) were evaluated ($n = 5489$), including 18 comparisons with placebo and 17 comparisons with synthetic standard antidepressants. The standard antidepressants used as active comparators were fluoxetine (six trials, dosage 20–40 mg), sertraline (four trials, 50–100 mg), imipramine (three trials, dosage 100–150 mg), citalopram (one trial, 20 mg), paroxetine (one trial, 20–40 mg), maprotiline (one trial, 75 mg) and amitriptyline (one trial, 75 mg). Most trials used a dose range 500–1200 mg/day of SJW.

More recently, another double-blind, placebo-controlled, randomised study was conducted which involved 100 patients with moderate severity of major depression and vegetative features of atypical depression (Mannel et al 2010). The SJW extract LI 160 (600 mg/day) given over 8 weeks was significantly superior to placebo for producing an antidepressant effect (HDS) and also improved hypersomnolence. In addition, the secondary outcome variables were significantly improved by SJW treatment. These were the depression subscore of the Patient Health Questionnaire, the Clinical Global Impression (CGI), a patient's satisfaction scale and the Hamilton Anxiety Scale.

This result is clinically important as the effects of standard antidepressants over placebo are modest and, although SSRIs are better tolerated than older antidepressant drugs (such as monoamine oxidase inhibitors), side effects are still common.

Comparative studies

SJW vs SSRIs

SJW is as effective as the newer generation of antidepressants but with fewer adverse events and better tolerability. The most recent Cochrane review found no significant differences between SJW and SSRIs in the proportion of people responding (12 RCTs) and active treatment with SJW resulted in significantly fewer drop-outs due to side effects compared with SSRIs (11 RCTs, 1769 people). There were no significant differences between groups in the reporting of adverse effects, although the result was of borderline significance (nine RCTs, 1641 people; $P = 0.048$) (Cipriani et al 2011, Linde et al 2009). Similarly, a meta-analysis of SJW trials (13 controlled trials) in major depressive disorder found that SJW does not differ from SSRIs according to efficacy and adverse events. Once again, there were fewer drop-outs due to adverse events in the SJW group (Rahimi et al 2009).

A comparative analysis by Kasper et al (2010b) between paroxetine and SJW extract WS 5570 revealed a 10–38-fold higher adverse events rate for the synthetic comparator.

Citalopram

A double-blind study (n = 388) found SJW extract (900 mg daily of extract STW3-VI) to be as effective as citalopram (20 mg daily) in moderate depression (Gastpar et al 2006). Both antidepressants were significantly more effective than placebo. Significantly more adverse events were documented in the citalopram group (53.2%) than for SJW (17.2%) or placebo (30%). In contrast, a subsequent three-arm RCT (n = 81) found that neither SJW (810 mg/day, extract not further described) nor citalopram (20 mg/day) showed a statistically significant effect over placebo in the treatment of minor depression over a 12-week period. The authors state that both treatments were associated with a significant number of adverse effects during the treatment. However, the prevalence of adverse effects reported in the placebo arm was higher (91.3%) than in the SJW (84.6%) arm, confirming Gastpar's study (Rapaport et al 2011).

Sertraline

To study the long-term efficacy of SJW, a cohort of 124 participant 'responders' continued treatment after week 8, until week 26. They were randomly assigned SJW (900–1500 mg), sertraline (50–100 mg) or matching placebo during this extension phase. At week 26, the outcome was equivocal; although both SJW and sertraline were still therapeutically effective, a pronounced 'placebo effect' impeded calling a significant result at week 26 (Sarris et al 2012a).

SJW vs TCAs

The most recent Cochrane review found no significant differences between SJW and TCAs in the proportion of people responding (five RCTs in total, of which three RCTs used imipramine, one RCT used amitriptyline and one RCT used maprotiline). Additionally, significantly fewer participants withdrew for any reason or due to side effects with SJW treatment compared to older antidepressants (three RCTs, imipramine; one RCT, amitriptyline; one RCT, maprotiline) and significantly fewer reported any adverse effects (Cipriani et al 2011, Linde et al 2009). Importantly, SJW is not associated with orthostatic hypotension, a common adverse effect associated with TCAs and related drugs, the older MAO inhibitors and serotonin-noradrenaline reuptake inhibitors (SNRIs) (Darowski et al 2009).

SJW vs SSRI and SNRI and others (mirtazapine)

A Cochrane review analysing citalopram vs other antidepressants for depression found that SJW was equally effective as citalopram, mirtazapine or venlafaxine. They also found that citalopram was associated with a higher rate of patients experiencing side effects than SJW (odds ratio 1.69, 95% confidence interval 1.01–2.83; one trial, 258 participants). It was shown that citalopram was associated with a higher rate of patients experiencing gastrointestinal problems or vertigo (Cipriani et al 2012).

Clinical note — Which extracts are effective?

Since the constituents of SJW extract differ between the individual manufacturers, the efficacy cannot be extrapolated from one extract to another. Three RCTs have favourably compared low-hyperforin extracts (ZE 117) to fluoxetine or imipramine, suggesting that the absence of hyperforin does not hinder the antidepressant effect (Friede et al 2001, Schrader 2000, Woelk 2000). In a subsequent review of trials included in the clinical studies above, WS 5572, LI 160, WS 5570 and ZE 117 SJW extracts have all shown significantly greater efficacy than placebo and similar efficacy and better tolerability than standard antidepressant drugs (Kasper et al 2010a).

Clinical note — Is SJW cost-effective?

A recent study reports on using the Markov model to estimate the health and economic impacts of SJW versus antidepressants. Outcomes were treatment costs, quality-adjusted life years and net monetary benefits. SJW was shown to be a cost-effective alternative to generic antidepressants (Solomon et al 2011, 2013).

Similarly, a report commissioned by the National Institute of Complementary Medicine in Australia and undertaken by Access Economics concluded that, based on analyses of RCTs for SJW, it was found to be cost-effective and produced a cost saving compared to standard antidepressants for patients with mild to moderate depression (Access Economics 2010). More specifically, with treated mild and moderate depression estimated to affect 339,752 Australians in 2009, there could be around $50 million per annum in potential savings from switching to SJW from standard antidepressants.

In the sensitivity analysis, SJW dominated standard antidepressants for mild to moderate depression because it is cheaper than standard antidepressants and fewer patients withdraw from SJW than from standard antidepressants. Even if the unit cost of SJW was the same as that of standard antidepressants, SJW would remain dominant due to the lower changeover rates compared to standard antidepressants.

Paediatric use

Results from a postmarketing surveillance study of 101 children under 12 years with mild to moderate depression have suggested that SJW may be an effective and well-tolerated treatment in this population (Hubner & Kirste 2001). The number of doctors rating effectiveness of treatment with SJW as 'good' or 'excellent' was 72% after 2 weeks, 97% after 4 weeks and 100% after 6 weeks and ratings by parents were similar. Although encouraging, it is difficult to interpret the clinical significance of the results, as there was no placebo group and the final evaluation included only 76% of the initial sample. A subsequent study by Findling and colleagues (2003) evaluated the use of SJW in 33 children aged 6–16 years in an open-label design for 8 weeks, also finding good results. The initial dose was 150 mg three times daily and could be titrated up to 300 mg three times daily. Using the Children's Depression Rating Scale, 76% of the patients clinically improved and 93% continued therapy at the end of the study.

An 8-week open pilot study was conducted with SJW (300 mg three times daily) in 26 adolescents with major depressive disorder (Simeon et al 2005). The subjects were aged 12–17 years (mean 14.8 years). Only 11 patients completed the study; 9 (82%) of them showed significant clinical improvement based on CGI change scores. Of the 15 patients (58%) who did not complete the study, 8 patients were non-compliant and 7 patients were discontinued because of persisting or worsening depression. The interpretation of these results is difficult due to a large drop-out rate.

Preventing relapse of depression

A double-blind, placebo-controlled, multicentre trial conducted by Kasper et al (2008b) evaluated the efficacy and safety of hypericum extract WS 5570 in preventing relapse during 6 months' continuation treatment and 12 months' long-term maintenance treatment after recovery from an episode of recurrent depression.

After 6 weeks of single-blind treatment with 3 × 300 mg/day WS 5570, patients with score ≤2 on item 'Improvement' of the CGI scale and an HDS total score decrease ≥50% versus baseline were randomised to 3 × 300 mg/day WS 5570 or placebo for 26 weeks. This provided a total of 426 patients in the next study phase. Treatment with WS 5570 showed more favourable HDS and Beck Depression Inventory time courses and greater overall improvement (CGI) than controls. In long-term maintenance treatment, a pronounced prophylactic effect of WS 5570 was observed in patients with an early onset of depression as well as in those with a high degree of chronicity. Adverse event rates under WS 5570 were comparable to placebo.

A reanalysis of data obtained from a total of 154 patients responders, in a multicentre RCT after 6 weeks of treatment for an episode of moderate depression with either 20 mg citalopram or 900 mg SJW extract STW 3-VI, showed that SJW extract STW 3-VI is more efficient in lowering the relapse and recurrence rates of responders, when compared to citalopram and placebo. In addition, duration of response was increased in the group treated with SJW extract STW 3-VI (Singer et al 2011).

Postnatal depression

A 2009 systematic review found no clinically important results about the effects of SJW in postnatal depression (Craig & Howard 2009).

> ***Clinical note — Relative safety of SJW compared with pharmaceutical antidepressants***
>
> Much has been made of the known or suspected risks associated with the use of SJW, with far too little discussion focusing on the decisive question of its relative safety compared with pharmaceutical antidepressants. It has been estimated that approximately 1 in 30,000 people using SJW will experience an adverse reaction, including those attributed to drug interactions (Schulz 2006). An overview of 16 postmarketing surveillance studies involving different SJW preparations and 34,804 patients found that side effect incidence varied from 0 to 2.8% in short-term studies (4–6 weeks) and 3.4–5.7% in long-term studies (52 weeks) (Linde & Knuppel 2005). Gastrointestinal symptoms, sensitivity to light and other skin conditions and agitation were the most commonly reported side effects and were generally described as mild. The review found that serious side effects or interactions were not reported by any study. Taking this into account, the incidence of side effects to SJW is approximately 10-fold lower than for conventional antidepressants (SSRIs) (Schulz 2006). The most common adverse event among spontaneous reports is photosensitivity, which is estimated to occur in 1 in 300,000 treated cases. This can occur with a dose of 5–10 mg/day hypericin, which is 2–4-fold higher than the recommended dose. SJW has no significant effect on blood pressure or heart rate (Siepmann et al 2002), making it a safer choice than TCAs in patients with cardiovascular disease. It also lacks anticholinergic activity, so side effects such as dry mouth, urinary retention and blurred vision do not occur. In addition, the common side effects reported for SSRIs, such as anorexia, insomnia, sexual dysfunction, excessive sweating and visual disturbance, have not been reported for SJW. Similarly to all standard antidepressants, SJW can interact with other medicines and needs to be judiciously prescribed.

Obsessive-compulsive disorder (OCD)

Treatment with a fixed dose of 450 mg of SJW containing 0.3% hypericin twice daily over 12 weeks improved the condition in 5 of 12 patients, according to an open study (Taylor & Kobak 2000). Two recent systematic reviews, however, concluded that controlled studies suggest that SJW is ineffective in treating OCD (Camfield et al 2011, Sarris et al 2012b).

Autism

SJW was only modestly effective in the short-term treatment of irritability in some patients with autistic disorder in an open pilot study of three male participants (Niederhofer 2009).

Seasonal affective disorder (SAD)

Wheatley (1999) found that people with mild to moderate SAD experienced significant improvements with anxiety, loss of libido and insomnia after 8 weeks' treatment with SJW. The test group receiving SJW extract (Kira 300 mg) three times daily plus light therapy experienced superior sleep compared with the group receiving SJW as stand-alone treatment.

Polyneuropathy

Although SJW is sometimes used for nerve pain, a randomised, double-blind, crossover study of 54 patients identified a trend towards lower total pain score with SJW treatment, although none of the individual pain ratings was significantly changed (Sindrup et al 2001). The dose of SJW used provided 2.7 mg/day total hypericin and was taken over 5 weeks.

Menopause: psychological and psychosomatic symptoms

A 2013 meta-analysis has concluded that *Hypericum perforatum* L. extracts and its combination with other herbs were significantly superior to placebo in the treatment of menopause (Liua et al 2013). Importantly, SJW treatment had fewer side effects than the placebo arms of the studies analysed.

It appears that its effects are seen after at least 8 weeks of treatment, according to a placebo-controlled study showing SJW was an effective treatment for the vasomotor symptoms of perimenopausal or postmenopausal women ($n = 100$) (Abdali et al 2010). Other symptoms may also respond, as was seen in another study using SJW (160 mg effervescent tablet, Goldaru, three times a day), which significantly decreased psychomental changes, sleep disorders and vasomotor symptoms in 30 menopausal women throughout the third and the sixth week of the study (Fahami et al 2010). An early study not only confirmed that menopausal symptoms reduced or disappeared completely in the majority of women (76.4% by patient evaluation and 79.2% by doctor evaluation) but sexual wellbeing also improved in 80% of cases (Grube et al 1999). The study used 900 mg hypericum (Kira 300 mg three times daily) in the 12-week study.

A review of the evaluations given by women assessed in the VITamins And Lifestyle (VITAL) cohort ($n = 35{,}016$), of whom $n = 880$ had invasive breast cancer, found no risks associated with taking SJW for menopausal symptoms (Brasky et al 2010).

IN COMBINATION

SJW and black cohosh

A fixed combination of isopropanolic black cohosh (Remifemin; standardised to 1 mg triterpene glycosides) and ethanolic SJW (standardised to 0.25 mg total hypericin) was tested in 301 women with menopausal symptoms with pronounced psychological symptoms (Uebelhack et al 2006). The double-blind, randomised study found that 16 weeks of herbal treatment produced a significant 50% reduction in the Menopause Rating Scale score compared to 20% with placebo and a significant 42% reduction in the HDS score compared to only 13% in the placebo group.

A second study testing the effectiveness of combined SJW and black cohosh found that combination therapy was superior to stand-alone black cohosh therapy for the treatment of climacteric mood symptoms in general practice (Briese et al 2007). This was a prospective, controlled, open-label observational study which involved 6141 women attending 1287 outpatient gynaecologists in Germany.

A 2012 review similarly concluded that the combination of black cohosh and SJW showed an improvement of climacteric complaints in comparison to placebo, whereas most of the studies that compared black cohosh monotherapy with placebo did not show significant effects (Laakmann et al 2012).

SJW and chaste tree

The herbal combination of SJW and *Vitex agnus-castus* (chaste tree) was not found to be superior to placebo for the treatment of menopausal symptoms in an RCT with 93 women (van Die et al 2009a).

Perimenopause

Symptomatic perimenopausal women aged 40–65 years who experience hot flushes (three or more per day) may experience significant improvements to menopause-specific quality of life using SJW extract (900 mg t.i.d.) according to a double-blind, placebo-controlled study (Al-Akoum et al 2009). After 3 months of treatment, herbal treatment was significantly better than placebo for menopause-specific quality of life and also provided significant improvements for self-reported sleep problems. No significant effects were seen at 6 weeks, indicating that the effects have slow onset.

IN COMBINATION

SJW and chaste tree

It has been suggested that some of the symptoms typically attributed to menopause may be more related to premenstrual syndrome (PMS) than menopause, as perimenopausal women appear to be more prone to PMS-like symptoms, or at least to tolerate them less well. An RCT ($n = 14$, late perimenopausal women) conducted over 16 weeks found that the herbal combination was superior to placebo for total PMS-like scores ($P = 0.02$), PMS-depression ($P = 0.006$), and PMS-craving clusters ($P = 0.027$) and produced a significant reduction in anxiety ($P = 0.003$) and flushes ($P = 0.002$) (van Die et al 2009b).

S

Premenstrual syndrome

An early open study in patients with PMS found that a low dose of 300 mg SJW daily produced significant reductions in all outcome measures. The degree of improvement in overall PMS scores between baseline and the end of the trial was 51%, with over two-thirds experiencing at least a 50% decrease in symptom severity (Stevinson & Ernst 2000). Similarly, a 2009 systematic review concluded that SJW shows some benefit in PMS (Whelan et al 2009).

In a subsequent study Canning et al (2010) reported that SJW was more effective than placebo in the treatment of PMS. By measuring levels of serum sex hormones and inflammatory cytokines, they also excluded inflammatory or hormone regulation as a possible mechanism of action. Another subsequent RCT ($n = 170$ women with PMS for at least 6 months) showed that those receiving SJW (tablets, standardised to 680 mg of hypericin per day) had significantly lower

PMS scores compared with baseline and placebo. The biggest improvements in score occurred for crying (71%) and depression (52%) (Ghazanfarpour et al 2011).

Attention-deficit hyperactive disorder (ADHD)

A double-blind RCT found that SJW (300 mg three times daily of *H. perforatum* standardised to 0.3% hypericin) was ineffective for the symptomatic treatment of ADHD in children (Weber et al 2008). The study involved 54 children aged 6–17 years who met *Diagnostic and Statistical Manual of Mental Disorders* (Fourth Edition) criteria for ADHD by structured interview and was conducted over 8 weeks. Two subsequent reviews have also concluded that SJW is ineffective in ADHD (Rucklidge et al 2009, Sarris et al 2011).

Nervous agitation in children

IN COMBINATION

A multicentre, prospective observational study with 115 children aged between 6 and 12 years tested a herbal combination of SJW, valerian root and passionflower root dry extract for 4 weeks. According to the parents, a distinct improvement was observed in children who had attention problems, showed social withdrawal and/or were anxious/depressive. Based on the doctors' assessment, 82–94% of the affected children responded as they showed no or just mild symptoms at the end of the treatment period, an observation based on evaluated symptoms such as depression, school/examination anxieties, further anxieties, sleeping problems and different physical problems. Therapeutic success was not influenced by additional medication or therapies and treatment was well tolerated (Trompetter et al 2013).

Smoking cessation

Preliminary evidence from experimental models suggested that SJW may be of use in reducing nicotine withdrawal signs, although more recent research indicates no effect on abstinence rates. In the study, SJW significantly and dose-dependently reduced the total nicotine abstinence score (Catania et al 2003). In contrast, a placebo-controlled blinded RCT (n = 143) which tested 900 mg SJW or placebo tablets taken 2 weeks prior and 2 weeks after the quit day did not find that SJW increased absolute quit rates or affected withdrawal symptoms (Parsons et al 2009). Similarly, a placebo-controlled blinded RCT (n = 118) which tested 300 mg SJW, 600 mg SJW or placebo tablets three times daily also did not find that SJW increased smoking abstinence rates (Sood et al 2010).

Herpes infection

Based on its antiviral activity, SJW is also used clinically in the treatment of herpesvirus infections. One study of unknown design found that oral extract LI 160 (over a period of 3 months) reduced the frequency and severity of episodes of recurrent herpes labialis and herpes genitalis (Mannel et al 2000).

Topical use

SJW extract is used in a variety of skin conditions based on effects such as increased skin hydration, reduced the transepidermal water loss and promoted keratinocyte differentiation. For further information on the underlying mechanisms of these effects, please refer to Casetti et al (2011).

Atopic dermatitis

A cream containing SJW extract (standardised to 1.5% hyperforin) was shown to reduce the intensity of eczematous lesions when used twice daily in a prospective, double-blind study (Schempp et al 2003). Beneficial effects were already observed at the first visit, which was on day 7. A review evaluating plants for their effects in skin diseases also concluded that SJW appears promising for atopic dermatitis (Reuter et al 2010).

Treatment of acute and contused injuries

No controlled studies are available, but anti-inflammatory, analgesic and bactericidal activities provide a theoretical basis for its use.

Commission E approves the topical use of oily SJW preparations for this indication (Blumenthal et al 2000).

Herpes simplex 1 and 2

IN COMBINATION

A single-use, topical formulation containing copper sulfate pentahydrate and SJW (Dynamiclear) was compared to topical 5% aciclovir cream in an RCT (n = 149) for the treatment of herpes simplex virus type 1 and 2 lesions in adult patients. The SJW formulation was well tolerated and more effective in reducing burning, stinging, pain, erythema and vesiculation (Clewell et al 2012).

Myalgia

Although no controlled studies are available, anti-inflammatory and analgesic activities provide a theoretical basis for its use in this condition.

Commission E approves the topical use of oily SJW preparations for this indication (Blumenthal et al 2000).

First-degree burns

Although no controlled studies are available, anti-inflammatory, analgesic and bactericidal activities provide a theoretical basis for its use in this condition.

Commission E approves the topical use of oily SJW preparations for this indication (Blumenthal et al 2000).

Plaque-type psoriasis

SJW ointment applied twice daily for 4 weeks may be effective in reducing psoriasis area severity index scores in mild plaque-type psoriasis (Najafizadeh et al 2012).

Ultraviolet (UV)-protective effects

SJW cream significantly reduced UVB-induced erythema as opposed to the vehicle when tested on 20 volunteers in a randomised, double-blind, vehicle-controlled study (Meinke et al 2012).

Caesarean section

A placebo-controlled study of 144 volunteers supports the use of SJW ointment (applied three times daily for 16 days) following caesarean section to promote wound healing, improve scar formation and reduce pain and pruritus (Samadi et al 2010).

Diabetic foot

IN COMBINATION

A case report exists describing the successful use of an extract of SJW and neem oil (*Azadirachta indica*) for foot wounds with exposed bone in a patient with bilateral advanced diabetic ulcers (Labichella 2013).

Venous ulcers

IN COMBINATION

The therapeutic effects of the ointment Herbadermal (extracts of garlic, SJW and calendula) was tested over a 7-week period in 25 patients with ulceration of the lower leg (no longer than 2 months or recurrent ulceration during the last 6 months). The percentage of epithelialisation was 99.1% without significant effects on the microbial flora (Kundaković et al 2012).

Scalp wounds

IN COMBINATION

A retrospective, non-controlled analysis suggests that a mixture of SJW oil and neem oil (*Azadirachta indica*) is a therapy that is very simple to use, safe and potentially effective for the treatment of scalp wounds with exposed bone (Läuchli et al 2012).

Photodynamic therapy

A prospective study aimed at investigating the efficacy of PDT with topical application of an extract of *H. perforatum* in actinic keratosis, basal cell carcinoma (BCC) and morbus Bowen (carcinoma in situ) was conducted with 34 patients (8 with actinic keratoses, 21 with BCC and 5 with Bowen's disease) (Kacerovska et al 2008). Hypericum extract was applied on the skin lesions under occlusion and followed by irradiation with 75 J/cm^2 of red light 2 hours later. The treatment was performed weekly for 6 weeks on average. The percentage of complete clinical response was 50% for actinic keratoses, 28% in patients with superficial BCC and 40% in patients with Bowen's disease. There was only a partial remission seen in patients with nodular BCCs. A complete disappearance of tumour cells was found in the histological preparation of 11% of patients with superficial BCCs and 80% in the patients with Bowen's disease. Unfortunately, the combined treatment was poorly tolerated, as all patients complained of burning and painful sensations during irradiation.

Clinical note — PDT for tumour cells

PDT involves the administration of a photosensitiser, which is taken up and stored within tumour cells, followed by light irradiation with a specific wavelength, giving rise to irreversible tissue destruction (Kacerovska et al 2008). It is aimed at destroying tumour cells without damaging the surrounding normal tissues (Agostinis et al 2002). This combination approach results in the production of cytotoxic oxygen singlets within the tumour that cause irreversible cellular damage and tumour destruction.

OTHER USES

In practice, SJW is also used to treat fibrositis, nervous exhaustion, sciatica and gastrointestinal conditions, such as oesophagitis and peptic ulcers. Traditionally, SJW has been used for wound healing, as a diuretic, for melancholy, as pain relief, treatment for snake bites, for bedwetting in children, and in malaria and psychosis.

DOSAGE RANGE

- Dried herb: 2–5 g/day.
- Liquid extract (1:2): 3–6 mL/day.
- Tincture (1:5): 7.5–15 mL/day.
- Standardised extract containing 1.0–2.7 mg total hypericin daily.

- It is advised that patients using SJW long-term should have their doses reduced slowly when discontinuing its use.

External use

- Oily macerate: Macerate flowering tops in olive oil for several weeks and stir often, then drain through a gauze. Store in a dark bottle out of direct light. Apply oil directly to the affected area. To promote extraction of flavonoids, store in a sunny area for 6 weeks (oil will turn red).

According to clinical studies

Doses are for dried herb or equivalent.

- Mild to moderate depression: adult — doses ranging from 350 to 1800 mg/day have been used; children (aged 6–12 years) — 200–400 mg/day in divided doses.
- Major depression: 500 mg–1800 mg/day in divided doses.
- OCD: 450 mg twice daily of an extract containing 0.3% hypericin.
- Menopausal symptoms: 900 mg/day in divided doses.
- PMS: 300 mg/day (standardised to 900 mcg hypericin).
- SAD: 900 mg/day in divided doses.

Several pharmaceutical-grade preparations of SJW are commercially available, typically extracted from dried aerial parts. LI 160, produced by Lichtwer Pharma, Berlin, Germany, is standardised to contain 0.3% hypericin derivatives and 1–4% hyperforin. It is normally sold as 300 mg capsules. Similarly, the STEI 300 extract, produced by Steiner Arzneimittel of Berlin, Germany, contains 0.2–0.3% hypericin and pseudohypericin and 2–3% hyperforin. Capsules contain 350 mg of extract.

The extracts WS 5570, WS 5572 and WS 5573 are produced by Dr Willmar Schwabe Pharmaceuticals, Karlsruhe, Germany. In contrast to the previously mentioned extracts WS 5570 and WS 5572 contain a higher hyperforin amount (5–6%), whereas WS 5573 contains only low hyperforin levels (0.5%). WS 5570 is an 80% ethanolic extract of SJW with a plant-to-extract ratio of between 3 : 1 and 3 : 1–7 : 1. Tablets contain 300 or 600 mg of extract. The product WS 5572 has similar hyperforin and hypericin profiles to WS 5570, but has a plant-to-extract ratio of between 2.5 : 1 and 5 : 1.

In contrast, the hyperforin content of Ze 117 is only 0.2%, much lower than that of other products. Ze 117 is produced by Zeller, Switzerland. It is a 50% ethanolic extract with a herb-to-extract ratio of 4 : 1–7 : 1. The dosage of Ze 117 is 500 mg/day.

Helarium-425, produced by Bionorica, Neumarkt, Germany, contains 425 mg SJW 60% ethanolic extract with a plant-to-extract ratio of 3.5–6 : 1 (Kienow et al 2011).

S

Clinical note — Mechanisms responsible for reported interactions

Based on the herb's pharmacology, there are several mechanisms by which it may interact with drugs. Considering that SJW has significant serotonin reuptake inhibitor activity and significantly upregulates both 5-HT_{1A} and 5-HT_{2A} receptors, concomitant use of drugs that elevate serotonin levels, such as TCAs or SSRIs, may result in additive or synergistic effects and increase the risk of serotonergic syndrome. As the constituent hyperforin has a significant and selective induction effect on CYP3A4 and 2C19 activity (Durr et al 2000, Wang et al 2001) and induces the drug transporter P-gp, a number of pharmacokinetic interactions are possible with those drugs that are substrates for CYP3A4 or 2C19 and/or rely on P-gp transport. Refer to Chapter 8 for further information on interactions with herbs and natural supplements.

ADVERSE REACTIONS

It has been estimated that approximately 1 in 30,000 people using SJW will experience an adverse reaction, including those attributed to drug interactions (Schulz 2006). The incidence of side effects to SJW is approximately 10-fold lower than for conventional antidepressants (SSRIs). According to an overview of 16 postmarketing surveillance studies, gastrointestinal symptoms, sensitivity to light and other skin conditions and agitation were the most commonly reported side effects and were generally described as mild (Linde & Knuppel 2005). Recent reviews confirm earlier studies stating that adverse effects from SJW are infrequent and minor (Posadzki et al 2013).

Photosensitivity (unlikely at therapeutic doses)

The most common adverse event among spontaneous reports is photosensitivity, which is estimated to occur in 1 in 300,000 treated cases. This can occur with a dose of 5–10 mg/day hypericin, which is 2–4-fold higher than the recommended dose. Commission E has noted the possibility of photosensitivity reactions, particularly in fair-skinned people.

SIGNIFICANT INTERACTIONS

SJW is one of the few herbal medicines that has been subjected to controlled studies in order to determine the significance of its interaction with numerous drugs, which are mainly due to CYP450 enzyme induction and the induction of P-gp (Colalto 2010), and therefore mainly pharmacokinetic in nature (Tsai et al 2012). Although this can be reassuring, the clinical significance of many interactions is still unpredictable because of the variable chemical composition of products (Steinhoff 2012).

Hyperforin is a key mediator of SJW's antidepressive action and mainly responsible for the herb's drug interaction potential. It is a high-affinity ligand for human pregnane X receptor, an orphan nuclear receptor selectively expressed in the liver and intestine that mediates the induction of XME and efflux transporter gene transcription, resulting in decreased oral bioavailability, enhanced systemic clearance and reduced drug efficacy for many drugs.

Most SJW extracts are currently standardised to contain 3% hyperforin, yet several clinical studies have demonstrated that SJW extracts containing less than 1% hyperforin (e.g. ZE 117 extract) are both effective and less likely to produce clinically relevant pharmacokinetic herb-drug interactions (Arold et al 2005, Mai et al 2004, Mueller et al 2009).

Please also note that the enzyme induction may be unmasked after the withdrawal of a combination of SJW (a potent CYP3A inducer with a potent CYP3A inhibitor, e.g. ritonavir) leading to substantial drops in drug exposure of CYP3A substrates (e.g. midazolam). This may require substantial dose adjustments, particularly of orally administered drugs (Hafner et al 2010).

Alprazolam

Decreases serum levels of alprazolam via CYP induction. Monitor for signs of reduced drug effectiveness and adjust the dose if necessary or avoid.

Amitriptyline

Although SJW decreases serum levels of amitriptyline via CYP induction in vivo (Johne et al 2002), theoretically it could also induce increases in serotonin availability, which has an opposite effect; the clinical outcome of these two interacting mechanisms is unknown — monitor for signs of changed drug effectiveness and adjust the dose if necessary or avoid concurrent use.

Antidepressants (SSRIs and SNRIs)

Increased risk of serotonin syndrome possible; however, increased antidepressant activity is also possible with appropriate doses — avoid concurrent use unless under medical supervision, so that doses may be altered appropriately.

Anticonvulsants

Phenobarbitone, phenytoin: SJW may increase drug metabolism, resulting in reduced drug efficacy — avoid concurrent use unless under medical supervision, so that doses may be altered appropriately.

Antineoplastic drugs

Irinotecan imatinib mesylate: plasma levels decreased (He et al 2010, Mathijssen et al 2002). Reduction of toxicity — the combination might be of benefit (Rahimi & Abdollahi 2012).

Atorvastatin

SJW reduces the efficacy of atorvastatin, so lipid-lowering effects are compromised, according to a clinical study which tested a product called Movina (containing 300 mg of *Hypericum perforatum*), taken as one tablet twice daily (Andren et al 2007).

Bupropion

SJW decreased, to a statistically significant extent, the plasma concentrations of bupropion, probably by increasing the clearance of bupropion — avoid (Lei et al 2010).

Cisplatin

Cisplatin-induced histological abnormality of the kidney was blocked by pretreatment with SJW in vivo (Shibayama et al 2007). Total and free cisplatin concentration in serum was not influenced by SJW treatment, suggesting that this may be a beneficial interaction under professional supervision.

Clopidogrel

SJW might represent a valid option to increase the antiplatelet effect of clopidogrel in non-responders and/or hyporesponders. For example, SJW increased platelet inhibition by enhancement of CYP3A4 metabolic activity for clopidogrel in hyporesponsive volunteers (Lau et al 2011), and a recent study showed that residual platelet reactivity improved with SJW during the first month post percutaneous coronary intervention (Trana et al 2013).

Cyclosporin

Decreases plasma levels of cyclosporin significantly within 3 days of concomitant use via CYP induction (Bauer et al 2003) — avoid concurrent use.

A pharmacokinetic study with kidney graft recipients suggests that the effect is not significant when low-hyperforin products are used (Madabushi et al 2006).

Digoxin

Decreases serum digoxin levels significantly within 10 days of concomitant use (Johne et al 1999), chiefly due to induction of the P-gp. The interaction between digoxin and SJW in humans has been confirmed more recently by Gurley et al (2008) and is clinically significant — monitor patient for signs of reduced drug effectiveness and adjust the dose if necessary or avoid concurrent use.

Fexofenadine

In rats, SJW (1 g/kg) enhanced the elimination of fexofenadine, an antihistamine and P-gp substrate, into the bile when given once daily for 14 days (Turkanovic et al 2009).

Finasteride

SJW treatment for 2 weeks induced the metabolism of finasteride and caused a reduced plasma exposure of the drug (Lundahl et al 2009). A case report reported on an increased prostate-specific antigen value for a man who had started SJW 900 mg/day 10 weeks prior to the test and who was previously well controlled on finasteride (Lochner & Kirch 2011).

Gliclazide

Treatment with SJW significantly increases the apparent clearance of gliclazide, which is independent of CYP2C9 genotype, according to a crossover clinical study (Xu et al 2008). People with diabetes receiving this combination should be closely monitored to evaluate possible signs of reduced efficacy.

HIV non-nucleoside transcriptase inhibitors

Decreases serum levels — avoid concurrent use.
  Etravirine — potential effect (Kakuda et al 2011)
  Rilpivirine (Sharma & Saravolatz 2013).

HIV protease inhibitors

Decreases serum levels — avoid concurrent use.

Indinavir

Oral administration of either 150 or 300 mg/day SJW for 15 days significantly reduced indinavir plasma levels in rats. This interaction was attributable to the induction of indinavir metabolism by SJW (Ho et al 2009).

Ketamine

SJW greatly decreased the exposure to oral S-ketamine in healthy volunteers. Although this decrease was not associated with significant changes in the analgesic or behavioural effects of ketamine in the present study, usual doses of S-ketamine may need adjustment if used concomitantly with SJW (Peltoniemi et al 2012) — use with caution.

Methadone

Decreases serum levels via CYP induction — avoid concurrent use (Eich-Hochli et al 2003).

Methotrexate

Coadministration of 300 and 150 mg/kg of SJW significantly increased the systemic exposure and toxicity of methotrexate (Yang et al 2012).

Midazolam

Decreases serum levels of midazolam via CYP induction — monitor for signs of reduced drug effectiveness and adjust the dose if necessary or avoid.

Nifedipine

SJW was shown to induce nifedipine metabolism in vivo (Wang et al 2007) — monitor for signs of reduced drug effectiveness and adjust the dose if necessary or avoid.

Non-steroidal anti-inflammatory drugs (etoricoxib)

Decreases serum levels of the drug via CYP induction in vivo — avoid co-administration (Radwan et al 2012).

Omeprazole

Decreases serum levels via CYP induction (Wang et al 2004b) — monitor for signs of reduced drug effectiveness and adjust the dose if necessary or avoid.

Oral contraceptives

Breakthrough bleeding has been reported, which can indicate decreased effectiveness of oral contraceptives. In 2003, a controlled study confirmed that standard doses of SJW cause an induction of ethinyl oestradiol–norethindrone metabolism, consistent with increased CYP3A activity (Hall et al 2003) — use this combination with caution.

In 2002, a pharmacokinetic study found no significant interaction between low-hyperforin SJW and low-dose oral contraceptives (Madabushi et al 2006). This has been confirmed in a further clinical study using an SJW extract (Ze 117) with low hyperforin content on the pharmacokinetics of ethinyl oestradiol and 3-ketodesogestrel (Will-Shahab et al 2009) — low-hyperforin extracts appear to be safe.

OXYCODONE

SJW greatly reduced the plasma concentrations of oral oxycodone — avoid (Nieminen et al 2010).

Pegylated interferon-alpha (peginterferon-α)

The combination of peginterferon-α and SJW (taken for 6 weeks during 8 weeks' drug treatment) resulted in severe acute hepatitis in a 61-year-old woman. After 6 months of prednisone treatment, the liver function tests returned to baseline levels — avoid combination (Piccolo et al 2009).

Psoralen plus UVA therapy

High-dose hypericin may increase sensitivity to UV radiation — caution is advised.

Simvastatin

Decreases serum levels of simvastatin via CYP induction (Sugimoto et al 2001) — monitor for signs of reduced drug effectiveness and adjust the dose if necessary (no interaction is expected with pravastatin).

Tacrolimus

Decreases serum levels of tacrolimus via CYP induction (Mai et al 2003) — avoid this combination.

Verapamil

Decreases serum levels of verapamil via CYP induction — monitor for signs of reduced drug effectiveness and adjust the dose if necessary.

Warfarin

Metabolism of warfarin is chiefly by CYP2C9, and a minor metabolic pathway is CYP3A4, so theoretically it may interact with SJW. A clinical study found no change to international normalised ratio (INR) or platelet aggregation (Jiang et al

2004), but there are case reports suggesting that SJW may lower the INR. Caution is advised — monitor INR.

Zolpidem

Repeated administration of SJW decreases the plasma concentration of zolpidem, probably by enhancing CYP3A4 activity (Hojo et al 2011) — avoid.

CONTRAINDICATIONS AND PRECAUTIONS

People with fair skin undergoing UV treatment or with conditions which would be adversely affected by high UV exposure should use high doses of SJW with caution.

A case study reported on the occurrence of radiation-induced optic neuropathy, which may have been the result of radiosensitisation by temozolomide, which could have been strengthened by the hypericin the patient was also taking (Schreiber et al 2010).

People with cancer and undergoing treatment

Hypericum extract, by inducing both CYP3A4 and P-gp, can reduce the plasma concentrations of different antineoplastic agents such as imatinib, irinotecan and docetaxel, thus reducing the clinical efficacy of these drugs. Although these interactions are often predictable, the concomitant use of hypericum extract should be avoided in cancer patients taking interacting medications (Caraci et al 2011).

PREGNANCY AND LACTATION USE

A systematic review of the literature for evidence on the use, safety and pharmacology of SJW focusing on issues pertaining to pregnancy found there is in vitro evidence from animal studies that SJW during pregnancy does not affect cognitive development nor cause long-term behavioural defects, but may lower offspring birth weight (Dugoua et al 2006). A prospective study investigated 54 SJW-exposed pregnancies and 108 pregnancies in the two comparator groups (the second group was taking other pharmacological therapy for depression and a third group of healthy women was not exposed to any known teratogens). The rates of major malformations were similar across the three groups, and were not different from the 3–5% risk expected in the general population. The live birth and prematurity rates were also not different among the three groups (Moretti et al 2009).

A recent study comparing the effects of 7.5 mg/kg fluoxetine and 100 mg/kg SJW showed that maternal exposure to fluoxetine but not SJW could interfere with reproductive parameters in adult male rats (Vieira et al 2013). However, encouragingly, safe doses in pregnant women have not yet been determined. In practice, SJW is not recommended in pregnancy.

SJW appears to be relatively safe in lactation (Dugoua et al 2006, Howland 2010). A systematic review, which reported the results of observational studies, found weak evidence that SJW use during lactation did not affect maternal milk production or infant weight. However, in a few cases, it may cause infant colic, drowsiness or lethargy (Linde et al 2005b). A more recent review identified three studies in which SJW was used by breastfeeding mothers (one case report, one open-label and one cohort study). No adverse effects were reported for mothers and infants for any of these studies (Budzynska et al 2012).

PATIENTS' FAQS

What will this herb do for me?

SJW is an effective treatment for mild, moderate and severe depression and it reduces the risk of relapse. Its antidepressant effects are similar to pharmaceutical antidepressant drugs; however, it is better tolerated with fewer side effects. It may also be useful for PMS symptoms, in SAD and OCD and for menopausal and premenopausal women with psychological and psychosomatic symptoms. The oily preparations are also used topically to treat burns, injuries, allergic dermatitis and muscle pain.

When will it start to work?

It often starts to exert beneficial effects in depression within 2–4 weeks of continuous use; however, maximal effects in other conditions may take longer.

Are there any safety issues?

SJW is well tolerated and has far fewer side effects than pharmaceutical antidepressant drugs, but it can interact with a number of different medications. Patients with clinically diagnosed depression should be under the care of a healthcare professional.

Practice points/Patient counselling

- SJW contains numerous constituents with pharmacological activity, including antidepressant, analgesic, anti-inflammatory, antispasmodic, anxiolytic, antineoplastic, antiviral and bactericidal activities.
- The efficacy of SJW in the treatment of mild-to-moderate major depressive disorders is well established through numerous clinical studies. The most commonly studied extract is LI 160, although others have also been tested (e.g. WS 5573 [standardised to hyperforin], ZE 117 [a low-concentration hyperforin preparation], WS 550 and STW3-V1). Clinical effects are comparable to TCAs and SSRIs; it also reduces the incidence of depression relapse.
- With regard to safety, SJW is better tolerated than standard antidepressants (SSRIs and TCAs); however, it still needs to be prescribed judiciously to avoid interactions. Patients with clinically-diagnosed depression should be under the care of a healthcare professional.
- Low-hyperforin-containing SJW extracts do not have the same interaction potential as standard SJW extracts and may present a safer option for some individuals.
- Preliminary human studies have suggested a possible role in PMS, SAD, OCD and in menopausal and premenopausal women with psychological and psychosomatic symptoms.
- Oily preparations have been used topically to treat burns, acute and contused injuries, atopic dermatitis and myalgia.

S

REFERENCES

Abdali K, et al. Effect of St John's wort on severity, frequency, and duration of hot flashes in premenopausal, perimenopausal and postmenopausal women: a randomized, double-blind, placebo-controlled study. Menopause. 2010 Mar;17(2):326–31.

Agostinis P et al. Hypericin in cancer treatment: more light on the way. Int J Biochem Cell Biol 34.3 (2002): 221–241.

Al-Akoum M et al. Effects of *Hypericum perforatum* (St. John's wort) on hot flashes and quality of life in perimenopausal women: a randomized pilot trial. Menopause 16.2 (2009): 307–14.

Albert D et al. Hyperforin is a dual inhibitor of cyclooxygenase-1 and 5-lipoxygenase. Biochem Pharmacol 64.12 (2002): 1767–1775.

Andren L, et al. Interaction between a commercially available St. John's wort product (Movina) and atorvastatin in patients with hypercholesterolemia. Eur J Clin Pharmacol 63.10 (2007): 913–9116.

Arold G et al. No relevant interaction with alprazolam, caffeine, tolbutamide, and digoxin by treatment with a low-hyperforin St John's wort extract. Planta Med 71.4 (2005): 331–337.

Asgary S, et al. Effect of hydroalcoholic extract of *Hypericum perforatum* on selected traditional and novel biochemical factors of cardiovascular diseases and atherosclerotic lesions in hypercholesterolemic rabbits: A comparison between the extract and lovastatin. J Pharm Bioallied Sci. 2012 Jul;4(3):212–8.

Bauer S et al. Alterations in cyclosporin A pharmacokinetics and metabolism during treatment with St John's wort in renal transplant patients. Br J Clin Pharmacol 55.2 (2003): 203–211.

Beckert BW et al. The effect of herbal medicines on platelet function: an in vivo experiment and review of the literature. Plast Reconstr Surg 120.7 (2007): 2044–2050.

Beerhues L. Hyperforin. Phytochemistry 2006; 67: 2201–2207.

Beijamini V, Andreatini R. Effects of *Hypericum perforatum* and paroxetine on rat performance in the elevated T-maze. Pharmacol Res 48.2 (2003): 199–207.

Bilia AR, et al. St John's wort and depression: efficacy, safety and tolerability: an update. Life Sci 70.26 (2002): 3077–3096.

Blumenthal M, et al (eds), Herbal medicine: expanded Commission E monographs. Austin, TX: Integrative Medicine Communications, 2000.

Brasky TM, et al. Specialty supplements and breast cancer risk in the VITamins And Lifestyle (VITAL) Cohort. Cancer Epidemiol Biomarkers Prev. 2010 Jul;19(7):1696–708.

Brattström A Long-term effects of St. John's wort (*Hypericum perforatum*) treatment: a 1-year safety study in mild to moderate depression. Phytomedicine 2009;16(4):277–83.

Briese V et al. Black cohosh with or without St. John's wort for symptom-specific climacteric treatment — results of a large-scale, controlled, observational study. Maturitas 57.4 (2007): 405–414.

Budzynska K, et al. Systematic review of breastfeeding and herbs. Breastfeed Med. 2012;7(6):489–503.

Butterweck V et al. Step by step removal of hyperforin and hypericin: activity profile of different *Hypericum* preparations in behavioral models. Life Sci 73.5 (2003a): 627–39.

Butterweck V et al. Plasma levels of hypericin in presence of procyanidin B2 and hyperoside: a pharmacokinetic study in rats. Planta Med 69.3 (2003b): 189–92.

Camfield DA, et al. Nutraceuticals in the treatment of obsessive compulsive disorder (OCD): a review of mechanistic and clinical evidence. Prog Neuropsychopharmacol Biol Psychiatry. 2011 Jun 1;35(4): 887–95.

Camfield DA, et al. The Neurocognitive Effects of *Hypericum perforatum* Special Extract (Ze 117) during Smoking Cessation. Phytother Res. (2013): 27: 1605–1613..

Can ÖD, et al. Effects of treatment with St. John's Wort on blood glucose levels and pain perceptions of streptozotocin-diabetic rats. Fitoterapia. 2011 Jun;82(4):576–84.

Canning S, et al. The efficacy of *Hypericum perforatum* (St John's wort) for the treatment of premenstrual syndrome: a randomized, double-blind, placebo-controlled trial. CNS Drugs. 2010 Mar;24(3):207–25.

Capasso R et al. Inhibitory effect of the herbal antidepressant St. John's wort (*Hypericum perforatum*) on rat gastric motility. Naunyn Schmiedebergs Arch Pharmacol 376.6 (2008): 407–

Caraci, F., et al. 2011. Metabolic drug interactions between antidepressants and anticancer drugs: focus on selective serotonin reuptake inhibitors and hypericum extract. Curr.Drug Metab, 12, (6) 570–577.

Casetti F, et al. Dermocosmetics for dry skin: a new role for botanical extracts. Skin Pharmacol Physiol. 2011;24(6):289–93.

Catania MA et al. *Hypericum perforatum* attenuates nicotine withdrawal signs in mice. Psychopharmacology (Berl) 169.2 (2003): 186–189.

Chatterjee SS et al. Hyperforin as a possible antidepressant component of hypericum extracts. Life Sci 63.6 (1998): 499–510.

Cipriani A, et al., Depression in adults: drug and physical treatments. Clin Evid (Online). (2011) 2011: 1003.

Cipriani A, et al. Citalopram versus other anti-depressive agents for depression. Cochrane Database Syst Rev. (2012) 7: CD006534.

Clewell A, et al. Efficacy and tolerability assessment of a topical formulation containing copper sulfate and *Hypericum perforatum* on patients with herpes skin lesions: a comparative, randomized controlled trial. J Drugs Dermatol. 2012 Feb;11(2):209–15.

Colalto C Herbal interactions on absorption of drugs: Mechanisms of action and clinical risk assessment. Pharmacol Res. 2010 Sep;62(3):207–27.

Craig M, Howard L. Postnatal depression. Clin Evid (Online). 2009 Jan 26;2009. pii: 1407.

Darowski A, et al. Antidepressants and falls in the elderly. Drugs Aging. 2009;26(5):381–94.

Di Carlo G et al. St John's wort: Prozac from the plant kingdom. Trends Pharmacol Sci 22.6 (2001): 292–297.

Dugoua JJ et al. Safety and efficacy of St. John's wort (hypericum) during pregnancy and lactation. Can J Clin Pharmacol 13.3 (2006): e268–e276.

Durr D et al. St John's Wort induces intestinal P-glycoprotein/MDR1 and intestinal and hepatic CYP3A4. Clin Pharmacol Ther 68.6 (2000): 598–604.

Eich-Hochli D et al. Methadone maintenance treatment and St John's Wort: a case report. Pharmacopsychiatry 36.1 (2003): 35–37.

Etemad L, et al. Investigation of *Hypericum perforatum* extract on convulsion induced by picrotoxin in mice. Pak J Pharm Sci. 2011 Apr;24(2):233–6.

Fahami F, et al. A comparative study on the effects of *Hypericum perforatum* and passion flower on the menopausal symptoms of women referring to Isfahan city health care centers. Iran J Nurs Midwifery Res. 2010 Fall;15(4):202–7.

Feily A, Abbasi N. The inhibitory effect of *Hypericum perforatum* extract on morphine withdrawal syndrome in rat and comparison with clonidine. Phytother Res. 2009 Nov;23(11):1549–52.

Feisst C, et al. Hyperforin is a novel type of 5-lipoxygenase inhibitor with high efficacy in vivo. Cell Mol Life Sci. 2009 Aug;66(16):2759–71.

Fiebich B, et al. Inhibition of substance P-induced cytokine synthesis by St John's wort extracts. Pharmacopsychiatry 34 (Suppl 1) (2001): S26–S28.

Fiebich BL, et al. Pharmacological studies in an herbal drug combination of St. John's Wort (*Hypericum perforatum*) and passion flower (*Passiflora incarnata*): in vitro and in vivo evidence of synergy between *Hypericum* and *Passiflora* in antidepressant pharmacological models. Fitoterapia. 2011 Apr;82(3):474–80.

Findling R, et al. An open-label study of St. John's wort in juvenile depression. J Am Acad Child Adolesc Psychiatry 2003;42:908–14.

Friede M, et al. Differential therapy of mild to moderate depressive episodes (ICD-10 F 32.0; F 32.1) with St John's wort. Pharmacopsychiatry 34 (Suppl 1) (2001): S38–S41.

Galeotti N, Ghelardini C. St. John's wort relieves pain in an animal model of migraine. Eur J Pain. 2013a Mar;17(3):369–81.

Galeotti N, Ghelardini C. Reversal of NO-induced nociceptive hypersensitivity by St. John's wort and hypericin: NF-κB, CREB and STAT1 as molecular targets. Psychopharmacology (Berl). 2013b May;227(1):149–63.

Galeotti N, et al A prolonged protein kinase C-mediated, opioid-related antinociceptive effect of St John's Wort in mice. J Pain. 2010 Feb;11(2):149–59.

Gastpar M, et al. Comparative efficacy and safety of a once-daily dosage of hypericum extract STW3-VI and citalopram in patients with moderate depression: a double-blind, randomised, multicentre, placebo-controlled study. Pharmacopsychiatry 39.2 (2006): 66–75.

Ghazanfarpour M, et al. *Hypericum perforatum* for the treatment of premenstrual syndrome. Int J Gynaecol Obstet. 2011 Apr;113(1):84–5.

Griffith TN, et al. Neurobiological effects of Hyperforin and its potential in Alzheimer's disease therapy. Curr Med Chem. 2010;17(5):391–406.

Gobbi M et al. In vitro binding studies with two *Hypericum perforatum* extracts (hyperforin, hypericin and biapigenin) on 5-HT6, 5-HT7, GABA(A)/benzodiazepine, sigma, NPY-Y1/Y2 receptors and dopamine transporters. Pharmacopsychiatry 34 (Suppl 1) (2001): S45–S48.

Gómez Del Rio MA, et al. Neuroprotective properties of standardized extracts of *Hypericum perforatum* on rotenone model of Parkinson's disease. CNS Neurol Disord Drug Targets. (2013) 12: 665–679.

Grube B, et al. St John's Wort extract: efficacy for menopausal symptoms of psychological origin. Adv Ther 16.4 (1999): 177–186.

Gulick RM et al. Phase I studies of hypericin, the active compound in St John's Wort, as an antiretroviral agent in HIV-infected adults AIDS Clinical Trials Group Protocols 150 and 258. Ann Intern Med 130.6 (1999): 510–5114.

Gurley BJ et al. Clinical assessment of CYP2D6-mediated herb-drug interactions in humans: effects of milk thistle, black cohosh, goldenseal, kava kava, St. John's wort, and Echinacea. Mol Nutr Food Res 52.7 (2008a): 755–63.

Gurley BJ et al. Gauging the clinical significance of P-glycoprotein-mediated herb-drug interactions: comparative effects of St. John's wort, Echinacea, clarithromycin, and rifampin on digoxin pharmacokinetics. Mol Nutr Food Res 52.7 (2008b): 772–9.

Hafner V, et al. Effect of simultaneous induction and inhibition of CYP3A by St John's Wort and ritonavir on CYP3A activity. Clin Pharmacol Ther. 2010 Feb;87(2):191–6.

Hall SD et al. The interaction between St John's wort and an oral contraceptive. Clin Pharmacol Ther 74.6 (2003): 525–535.

Ho YF, et al. Effects of St. John's wort extract on indinavir pharmacokinetics in rats: differentiation of intestinal and hepatic impacts. Life Sci. 2009 Aug 12;85(7–8):296–302.

Hojo Y, et al. Drug interaction between St John's wort and zolpidem in healthy subjects. J Clin Pharm Ther. 2011 Dec;36(6):711–5.

Hostanska K et al. Hyperforin a constituent of St John's wort (*Hypericum perforatum* L) extract induces apoptosis by triggering activation of caspases and with hypericin synergistically exerts cytotoxicity towards human malignant cell lines. Eur J Pharm Biopharm 56.1 (2003): 121–132.

Howland RH. Update on St. John's Wort J Psychosoc Nurs Ment Health Serv. 2010 Nov;48(11):20–4.

Hubner WD, Kirste T. Experience with St John's Wort (*Hypericum perforatum*) in children under 12 years with symptoms of depression and psychovegetative disturbances. Phytother Res 15.4 (2001): 367–370.

Hudson JB, et al. The importance of light in the anti-HIV effect of hypericin. Antiviral Res 20.2 (1993): 173–178.

Husain GM, et al. Hypolipidemic and antiobesity-like activity of standardised extract of *Hypericum perforatum* L. in rats. ISRN Pharmacol. 2011a;2011:505247.

Husain GM, et al. Beneficial effect of *Hypericum perforatum* on depression and anxiety in a type 2 diabetic rat model. Acta Pol Pharm. 2011b;68(6):913–8.

Imai H et al. The recovery time-course of CYP3A after induction by St John's wort administration. Br J Clin Pharmacol 65.5 (2008): 701–707.

Jacobson JM et al. Pharmacokinetics, safety, and antiviral effects of hypericin, a derivative of St John's wort plant, in patients with chronic hepatitis C virus infection. Antimicrob Agents Chemother 45.2 (2001): 517–524.

Jakovljevic V et al. Pharmacodynamic study of *Hypericum perforatum* L. Phytomedicine 7.6 (2000): 449–453.

Jiang X et al. Effect of St John's wort and ginseng on the pharmacokinetics and pharmacodynamics of warfarin in healthy subjects. Br J Clin Pharmacol 57.5 (2004): 592–599.

Johne A et al. Pharmacokinetic interaction of digoxin with an herbal extract from St John's wort (*Hypericum perforatum*). Clin Pharmacol Ther 66.4 (1999): 338–345.

Johne A et al. Decreased plasma levels of amitriptyline and its metabolites on comedication with an extract from St John's wort (*Hypericum perforatum*). J Clin Psychopharmacol 22.1 (2002): 46–54.

Kacerovska D et al. Photodynamic therapy of nonmelanoma skin cancer with topical *Hypericum perforatum* extract — a pilot study. Photochem Photobiol 84.3 (2008): 779–785.

Kakuda TN, et al. Pharmacokinetic interactions between etravirine and non-antiretroviral drugs. Clin Pharmacokinet. 2011 Jan;50(1):25–39.

Karioti A, Bilia AR Hypericins as potential leads for new therapeutics. Int J Mol Sci. 2010 Feb 4;11(2):562–94.

Kasper S et al. Efficacy of St. John's wort extract WS 5570 in acute treatment of mild depression: a reanalysis of data from controlled clinical trials. Eur Arch Psychiatry Clin Neurosci 258.1 (2008a): 59–63.

Kasper S et al. Continuation and long-term maintenance treatment with *Hypericum* extract WS 5570 after recovery from an acute episode of moderate depression — a double-blind, randomized, placebo controlled long-term trial. Eur Neuropsychopharmacol 18.11 (2008b): 803–13.

Kasper, S., et al 2010a. Efficacy and tolerability of *Hypericum* extract for the treatment of mild to moderate depression. Eur. Neuropsychopharmacol. 20, 747–765.

Kasper, S., et al 2010b. Better tolerability of St. John's wort extract WS 5570 compared to treatment with SSRIs: a reanalysis of data from controlled clinical trials in acute major depression. Int. Clin. Psychopharmacol. 25, 204–213.

Kiewert C et al. Stimulation of hippocampal acetylcholine release by hyperforin, a constituent of St John's Wort. Neurosci Lett 364.3 (2004): 195–198.

Kim SJ, et al Anti-inflammatory activity of hyperoside through the suppression of nuclear factor-κB activation in mouse peritoneal macrophages. Am J Chin Med. 2011;39(1):171–81.

Koeberle A, et al. Hyperforin, an Anti-Inflammatory Constituent from St. John's Wort, Inhibits Microsomal Prostaglandin E(2) Synthase-1 and Suppresses Prostaglandin E(2) Formation in vivo. Front Pharmacol. 2011 Feb 18;2:7.

Kundaković T, et al. Treatment of venous ulcers with the herbal-based ointment Herbadermal®: a prospective non-randomized pilot study. Forsch Komplementmed. 2012;19(1):26–30.

Laakmann E, et al. Efficacy of *Cimicifuga racemosa, Hypericum perforatum* and *Agnus castus* in the treatment of climacteric complaints: a systematic review. Gynecol Endocrinol. 2012 Sep;28(9):703–9.

Labichella ML The use of an extract of *Hypericum perforatum* and *Azadirachta indica* in advanced diabetic foot: an unexpected outcome. BMJ Case Rep. (2013) 2013: pii:bcr2012007299..

Lakhan SE, Vieira KF. Nutritional and herbal supplements for anxiety and anxiety-related disorders: systematic review. Nutr J. 2010 Oct 7;9:42.

Lau WC, et al. The effect of St John's Wort on the pharmacodynamic response of clopidogrel in hyporesponsive volunteers and patients: increased platelet inhibition by enhancement of CYP3A4 metabolic activity. J Cardiovasc Pharmacol. 2011 Jan;57(1):86–93.

Läuchli S, et al. Post-surgical scalp wounds with exposed bone treated with a plant-derived wound therapeutic. J Wound Care. 2012 May;21(5):228, 230, 232–3.

Lei HP, et al. Effect of St. John's wort supplementation on the pharmacokinetics of bupropion in healthy male Chinese volunteers. Xenobiotica. 2010 Apr;40(4):275–81.

Linde K, Knuppel L. Large-scale observational studies of hypericum extracts in patients with depressive disorders: a systematic review. Phytomedicine 12.1–2 (2005): 148–157.

Linde K et al. St John's wort for depression. Cochrane Database Syst Rev 2 (2005a): CD000448.

Linde K, et al. St John's wort for depression: meta-analysis of randomised controlled trials. Br J Psychiatry 2005b;186:99–107.

Linde K, et al St John's wort for major depression. Cochrane Database Syst Rev 2009;(4):CD000448.

Liua, Y.R., et al 2013. *Hypericum perforatum* L. preparations for menopause: a meta-analysis of efficacy and safety. Climacteric Dec 27 (epub ahead of print).

Lochner S, Kirch W Does St. John's wort interact with finasteride? Dtsch Med Wochenschr. 2011 Aug;136(34–35):1746.

Lorusso G, et al Mechanisms of Hyperforin as an anti-angiogenic angioprevention agent. Eur J Cancer. 2009 May;45(8):1474–84.

Lundahl A, et al. The effect of St. John's wort on the pharmacokinetics, metabolism and biliary excretion of finasteride and its metabolites in healthy men. Eur J Pharm Sci. 2009 Mar 2;36(4–5):433–43.

Madabushi R et al. Hyperforin in St John's wort drug interactions. Eur J Clin Pharmacol 62.3 (2006): 225–233.

Mai I et al. Impact of St John's wort treatment on the pharmacokinetics of tacrolimus and mycophenolic acid in renal transplant patients. Nephrol Dial Transplant 18.4 (2003): 819–822.

Mai I, et al. Hyperforin content determines the magnitude of the St John's wort cyclosporine drug interaction. Clin Pharmacol Ther 2004; 76: 330–340 383.

Mannel M, et al. Oral hypericum extract LI 160 is an effective treatment of recurrent herpes genitalis and herpes labialis: 3rd International Congress on Phytomedicine. Phytomedicine 7 (II) (2000).

Mannel M, et al. St. John's wort extract LI160 for the treatment of depression with atypical features — a double-blind, randomized, and placebo-controlled trial. J Psychiatr Res. 2010 Sep;44(12):760–7.

Markou A, et al. Neurobiological similarities in depression and drug dependence: a self-medication hypothesis. Neuropsychopharmacology 18.3 (1998): 135–174.

Mathijssen RH et al. Effects of St John's wort on irinotecan metabolism. J Natl Cancer Inst 94.16 (2002): 1247–1249.

Medina MA et al. Hyperforin: more than an antidepressant bioactive compound?. Life Sci 79.2 (2006): 105–111.

Meinke MC, et al. In vivo photoprotective and anti-inflammatory effect of hyperforin is associated with high antioxidant activity in vitro and ex vivo. Eur J Pharm Biopharm. 2012 Jun;81(2):346–50.

Melzer J, et al. A hypericum extract in the treatment of depressive symptoms in outpatients: an open study. Forsch Komplementmed. 2010 Mar;17(1):7–14.

Mennini T, Gobbi M. The antidepressant mechanism of *Hypericum perforatum*. Life Sci 75.9 (2004): 1021–1027.

Meruelo D, et al. Therapeutic agents with dramatic antiretroviral activity and little toxicity at effective doses: aromatic polycyclic diones hypericin and pseudohypericin. Proc Natl Acad Sci U S A 85.14 (1988): 5230–5234.

Micioni Di Bonaventura MV, et al. Effect of *Hypericum perforatum* Extract in an Experimental Model of Binge Eating in Female Rats. J Obes. 2012;2012:956137.

Miskovsky P. Hypericin: a new antiviral and antitumor photosensitizer: mechanism of action and interaction with biological macromolecules. Curr Drug Targets 3.1 (2002): 55–84.

Moore LB et al. St John's wort induces hepatic drug metabolism through activation of the pregnane X receptor. Proc Natl Acad Sci U S A 97.13 (2000): 7500–7502.

Moretti ME, et al Evaluating the safety of St. John's Wort in human pregnancy. Reprod Toxicol. 2009 Jul;28(1):96–9.

Mortensen T, et al. Investigating the effectiveness of St John's wort herb as an antimicrobial agent against mycobacteria. Phytother Res. 2012 Sep;26(9):1327–33.

Mozaffari S, et al. Effects of *Hypericum perforatum* extract on rat irritable bowel syndrome. Pharmacogn Mag. 2011 Jul;7(27):213–23.

Mueller SC et al. Effect of St John's wort dose and preparations on the pharmacokinetics of digoxin. Clin Pharmacol Ther 75.6 (2004): 546–557.

Mueller SC et al. No clinically relevant CYP3A induction after St. John's wort with low hyperforin content in healthy volunteers. Eur J Clin Pharmacol 65.1 (2009): 81–87.

Nahas R, Sheikh O. Complementary and alternative medicine for the treatment of major depressive disorder. Can Fam Physician. 2011 Jun;57(6):659–63.

Nahrstedt A, Butterweck V. Lessons learned from herbal medicinal products: the example of St John's wort. J Nat Prod 2010; 73: 1015–1021.

Najafizadeh P, et al. The evaluation of the clinical effect of topical St Johns wort (*Hypericum perforatum* L.) in plaque type psoriasis vulgaris: a pilot study. Australas J Dermatol. 2012 May;53(2):131–5.

Nathan P. The experimental and clinical pharmacology of St John's Wort (*Hypericum perforatum* L). Mol Psychiatry 4.4 (1999): 333–338.

Niederhofer H. St John's Wort treating patients with autistic disorder. Phytother Res. 2009 Nov;23(11): 1521–3.

Nieminen TH, et al. St John's wort greatly reduces the concentrations of oral oxycodone. Eur J Pain. 2010 Sep;14(8):854–9.

Obach RS. Inhibition of human cytochrome P450 enzymes by constituents of St John's Wort, an herbal preparation used in the treatment of depression. J Pharmacol Exp Ther 294.1 (2000): 88–95.

Olivo M, et al. Hypericin lights up the way for the potential treatment of nasopharyngeal cancer by photodynamic therapy. Curr Clin Pharmacol 1.3 (2006): 217–222.

Ott M, et al. St. John's Wort constituents modulate P-glycoprotein transport activity at the blood-brain barrier. Pharm Res. 2010 May;27(5):811–22.

Panocka I et al. Effects of *Hypericum perforatum* extract on ethanol intake, and on behavioral despair: a search for the neurochemical systems involved. Pharmacol Biochem Behav 66.1 (2000): 105–111.

Parsons A, et al. A proof of concept randomised placebo controlled factorial trial to examine the efficacy of St John's wort for smoking cessation and chromium to prevent weight gain on smoking cessation. Drug Alcohol Depend. 2009 Jun 1;102(1–3):116–120.

Patel J et al. In vitro interaction of the HIV protease inhibitor ritonavir with herbal constituents: changes in P-gp and CYP3A4 activity. Am J Ther 11.4 (2004): 262–277.

Peltoniemi MA, et al St John's wort greatly decreases the plasma concentrations of oral S-ketamine. Fundam Clin Pharmacol. 2012 Dec;26(6):743–50.

Perfumi M et al. Blockade of gamma-aminobutyric acid receptors does not modify the inhibition of ethanol intake induced by *Hypericum perforatum* in rats. Alcohol Alcohol 37.6 (2002): 540–546.

Piccolo P, et al. Severe drug induced acute hepatitis associated with use of St John's wort (*Hypericum perforatum*) during treatment with pegylated interferon α. BMJ Case Rep. 2009;2009.

Posadzki P, et al. Adverse effects of herbal medicines: an overview of systematic reviews. Clin Med. 2013 Feb;13(1):7–12.

Radwan MA, et al Pharmacokinetics and cardiovascular effect of etoricoxib in the absence or presence of St. John's Wort in rats. Arzneimittelforschung. 2012 Jul;62(7):313–8.

Rahimi R, Abdollahi M. An update on the ability of St. John's wort to affect the metabolism of other drugs. Expert Opin Drug Metab Toxicol. 2012 Jun;8(6):691–708.

Rahimi R, et al. Efficacy and tolerability of *Hypericum perforatum* in major depressive disorder in comparison with selective serotonin reuptake inhibitors: a meta-analysis. Prog Neuropsychopharmacol Biol Psychiatry 33.1 (2009): 118–127.

Rapaport MH, et al. The treatment of minor depression with St. John's Wort or citalopram: Failure to show benefit over placebo. Journal of Psychiatric Research 2011;45(7):931–41.

Raso GM et al. In-vivo and in-vitro anti-inflammatory effect of Echinacea purpurea and *Hypericum perforatum*. J Pharm Pharmacol 54.10 (2002): 1379–1383.

Ravindran AV, et al Canadian Network for Mood and Anxiety Treatments (CANMAT) Clinical guidelines for the management of major depressive disorder in adults. V. Complementary and alternative medicine treatments. J Affect Disord. 2009 Oct;117 Suppl 1:S54–64.

Rengelshausen J et al. Opposite effects of short-term and long-term St John's wort intake on voriconazole pharmacokinetics. Clin Pharmacol Ther 78.1 (2005): 25–33.

Reuter J, et al. Botanicals in dermatology: an evidence-based review. Am J Clin Dermatol. 2010;11(4):247–67.

Richard AJ, et al. St. John's Wort inhibits insulin signaling in murine and human adipocytes Biochim Biophys Acta. 2012 Apr;1822(4):557–63.

Roz N, Rehavi M. Hyperforin depletes synaptic vesicles content and induces compartmental redistribution of nerve ending monoamines. Life Sci 75.23 (2004): 2841–2850.

Rucklidge JJ, et al. Nutrient supplementation approaches in the treatment of ADHD. Expert Rev Neurother. 2009 Apr;9(4):461–76.

Saddiqe Z, et al. A review of the antibacterial activity of *Hypericum perforatum* L. J Ethnopharmacol. 2010 Oct 5;131(3):511–21.

Samadi S, et al The effect of *Hypericum perforatum* on the wound healing and scar of cesarean. J Altern Complement Med. 2010 Jan;16(1):113–7.

Sarris J, Kavanagh DJ. Kava and St John's wort: current evidence for use in mood and anxiety disorders. J Altern Complement Med. 2009;15(8):827–836.

Sarris J, et al Complementary medicines (herbal and nutritional products) in the treatment of Attention Deficit Hyperactivity Disorder (ADHD): a systematic review of the evidence. Complement Ther Med. 2011a Aug;19(4):216–27.

Sarris J, et al. St John's wort (*Hypericum perforatum*) versus sertraline and placebo in major depressive disorder: continuation data from a 26-week RCT. Pharmacopsychiatry. 2012a Nov;45(7):275–8.

Sarris J, et al. Complementary medicine, self-help, and lifestyle interventions for obsessive compulsive disorder (OCD) and the OCD spectrum: a systematic review. J Affect Disord. 2012b May;138(3):213–21.

Schempp CM et al. Antibacterial activity of hyperforin from St John's wort against multiresistant *Staphylococcus aureus* and Gram-positive bacteria. Lancet 353.9170 (1999): 2129.

Schempp CM et al. Topical treatment of atopic dermatitis with St John's wort cream: a randomized, placebo controlled, double-blind half-side comparison. Phytomedicine 10 Suppl 4 (2003): 31–7.

Schrader E. Equivalence of St John's wort extract (Ze 117) and fluoxetine: a randomized, controlled study in mild-moderate depression. Int Clin Psychopharmacol 15.2 (2000): 61–68.

Schreiber S, et al Bilateral posterior RION after concomitant radiochemotherapy with temozolomide in a patient with glioblastoma multiforme: a case report. BMC Cancer. 2010 Oct 1;10:520.

Schulz V. Safety of St. John's Wort extract compared to synthetic antidepressants. Phytomedicine 13.3 (2006): 199–204.

Sharma M, Saravolatz LD. Rilpivirine: a new non-nucleoside reverse transcriptase inhibitor. J Antimicrob Chemother. 2013 Feb;68(2):250–6.

Shibayama Y et al. Effect of pre-treatment with St John's Wort on nephrotoxicity of cisplatin in rats. Life Sci 81.2 (2007): 103–108.

Siepmann M et al. The effects of St John's wort extract on heart rate variability, cognitive function and quantitative EEG: a comparison with amitriptyline and placebo in healthy men. Br J Clin Pharmacol 54.3 (2002): 277–282.

Simeon J et al. Open-label pilot study of St John's wort in adolescent depression. J Child Adolesc Psychopharmacol 15.2 (2005): 293–301.

Simmen U et al. *Hypericum perforatum* inhibits the binding of mu- and kappa-opioid receptor expressed with the Semliki Forest virus system. Pharm Acta Helv 73.1 (1998): 53–56.

Sindrup SH et al. St John's wort has no effect on pain in polyneuropathy. Pain 9.3 (2001): 361–365.

Singer A, et al. Duration of response after treatment of mild to moderate depression with Hypericum extract STW 3-VI, citalopram and placebo: a reanalysis of data from a controlled clinical trial. Phytomedicine. 2011 Jun 15;18(8–9):739–42.

Solomon D, et al. Potential of St John's Wort for the treatment of depression: the economic perspective. Aust N Z J Psychiatry. 2011 Feb;45(2):123–30.

Solomon D, et al Economic evaluation of St. John's wort (*Hypericum perforatum*) for the treatment of mild to moderate depression. J Affect Disord. 2013 Jun;148(2–3):228–34.

Sood A, et al. A randomized clinical trial of St. John's wort for smoking cessation. J Altern Complement Med. 2010 Jul;16(7):761–7.

Steinhoff B., Current perspectives on herb-drug interactions in the European regulatory landscape. Planta Med. 2012 Sep;78(13):1416–20.

Stevinson C, Ernst E. A pilot study of *Hypericum perforatum* for the treatment of premenstrual syndrome. Br J Obstet Gynaecol 107.7 (2000): 870–876.

Sugimoto K et al. Different effects of St John's wort on the pharmacokinetics of simvastatin and pravastatin. Clin Pharmacol Ther 70.6 (2001): 518–524.

Taylor LH, Kobak KA. An open-label trial of St John's Wort (*Hypericum perforatum*) in obsessive-compulsive disorder. J Clin Psychiatry 61.8 (2000): 575–578.

Teufel-Mayer R, Gleitz J. Effects of long-term administration of hypericum extracts on the affinity and density of the central serotonergic 5-HT1A and 5-HT2A receptors. Pharmacopsychiatry 30 (Suppl 2) (1997): 113–1116.

Thiede HM, Walper A. Inhibition of MAO and COMT by hypericum extracts and hypericin. J Geriatr Psychiatry Neurol 7 (Suppl 1) (1994): S54–S56.

Tian R et al. Functional induction and de-induction of P-glycoprotein by St John's wort and its ingredients in a human colon adenocarcinoma cell line. Drug Metab Dispos 33.4 (2005): 547–554.

Timoshanko A et al. A preliminary investigation on the acute pharmacodynamic effects of hypericum on cognitive and psychomotor performance. Behav Pharmacol 12.8 (2001): 635–640.

Trana C, et al. St. John's Wort in patients non-responders to clopidogrel undergoing percutaneous coronary intervention: a single-center randomized open-label trial (St. John's Trial). J Cardiovasc Transl Res. 2013 Jun;6(3):411–4.

Trofimiuk E, Braszko JJ. Alleviation by *Hypericum perforatum* of the stress-induced impairment of spatial working memory in rats. Naunyn Schmiedebergs Arch Pharmacol 376.6 (2008): 463–471.

Trompetter I, et al. Herbal triplet in treatment of nervous agitation in children. Wien Med Wochenschr. 2013 Feb;163(3–4):52–7.

Tsai HH, et al. Evaluation of documented drug interactions and contraindications associated with herbs and dietary supplements: a systematic literature review. Int J Clin Pract. 2012 Nov;66(11):1056–78.

Turkanovic J, et al. Effect of St John's wort on the disposition of fexofenadine in the isolated perfused rat liver. J Pharm Pharmacol. 2009 Aug;61(8):1037–42.

Uebelhack R et al. Black cohosh and St. John's wort for climacteric complaints: a randomized trial. Obstet Gynecol 107.2 (2006): 247–255.

Vandenbogaerde A et al. Evidence that total extract of *Hypericum perforatum* affects exploratory behavior and exerts anxiolytic effects in rats. Pharmacol Biochem Behav 65.4 (2000): 627–633.

van Die MD, et al *Hypericum perforatum* with Vitex agnus-castus in menopausal symptoms: a randomized, controlled trial. Menopause. 2009a Jan-Feb;16(1):156–63.

van Die MD, et al. Effects of a combination of *Hypericum perforatum* and Vitex agnus-castus on PMS-like symptoms in late-perimenopausal women: findings from a subpopulation analysis. J Altern Complement Med. 2009b Sep;15(9):1045–8.

Vieira ML, et al Could maternal exposure to the antidepressants fluoxetine and St. John's Wort induce long-term reproductive effects on male rats? Reprod Toxicol. 2013 Jan;35:102–7.

Wang EJ, et al. Quantitative characterization of direct P-glycoprotein inhibition by St John's wort constituents hypericin and hyperforin. J Pharm Pharmacol 56.1 (2004a): 123–8.

Wang LS et al. St John's wort induces both cytochrome P450 3A4-catalyzed sulfoxidation and 2C19-dependent hydroxylation of omeprazole. Clin Pharmacol Ther 75.3 (2004b): 191–7.

Wang XD et al. Rapid and simultaneous determination of nifedipine and dehydronifedipine in human plasma by liquid chromatography-tandem mass spectrometry: application to a clinical herb-drug interaction study. J Chromatogr B Analyt Technol Biomed Life Sci 852.1–2 (2007): 534–544.

Wang Z et al. The effects of St John's wort (*Hypericum perforatum*) on human cytochrome P450 activity. Clin Pharmacol Ther 70.4 (2001): 317–326.

Weber CC et al. Modulation of P-glycoprotein function by St John's wort extract and its major constituents. Pharmacopsychiatry 37.6 (2004): 292–298.

Weber W et al. *Hypericum perforatum* (St John's wort) for attention-deficit/hyperactivity disorder in children and adolescents: a randomized controlled trial. JAMA 299.22 (2008): 2633–2641.

Wheatley D. Hypericum in seasonal affective disorder (SAD). Curr Med Res Opin 15.1 (1999): 33–37.

Whelan AM, et al Herbs, vitamins and minerals in the treatment of premenstrual syndrome: a systematic review. Can J Clin Pharmacol. 2009 Fall;16(3):e407–29.

Will-Shahab L et al. St John's wort extract (Ze 117) does not alter the pharmacokinetics of a low-dose oral contraceptive. Eur J Clin Pharmacol 65.3 (2009): 287–294.

Woelk H. Comparison of St John's wort and imipramine for treating depression: randomised controlled trial. BMJ 321.7260 (2000): 536–539.

Wonnemann M et al. Evaluation of synaptosomal uptake inhibition of most relevant constituents of St John's wort. Pharmacopsychiatry 34 (Suppl 1) (2001): S148–S151.

Xiuying P, et al. Therapeutic efficacy of *Hypericum perforatum* L. extract for mice infected with an influenza A virus. Can J Physiol Pharmacol. 2012 Feb;90(2):123–30.

Xu H et al. Effects of St John's wort and CYP2C9 genotype on the pharmacokinetics and pharmacodynamics of gliclazide. Br J Pharmacol 153.7 (2008): 1579–1586.

Yang SY, et al St. John's wort significantly increased the systemic exposure and toxicity of methotrexate in rats. Toxicol Appl Pharmacol. 2012 Aug 15;263(1):39–43.

St Mary's thistle

HISTORICAL NOTE St Mary's thistle has a long history of traditional use since ancient times. Over the centuries, it has been touted as a remedy for snakebite, melancholy, liver conditions and promoting lactation. The name 'milk thistle' derives from its characteristic spiked leaves with white veins which, according to legend, were believed to carry the milk of the Virgin Mary.

S

OTHER NAMES

Carduus marianus, cardo blanco, cardo de burro, chandon marie, holy thistle, lady's milk, lady's thistle, Mariendistel, Marian thistle, Mary thistle, milk thistle, silybum, true thistle.

BOTANICAL NAME/FAMILY

Silybum marianum (family [Compositae] Asteraceae)

PLANT PART USED

Ripe seed

CHEMICAL COMPONENTS

Often silymarin is referred to as the active constituent of seeds from St Mary's thistle, but in fact it is a complex of at least seven flavonolignans, one flavonoid taxifolin and a bioflavonoid quercetin. The principal component of silymarin is silybin (more commonly referred to as silibinin), which makes up more than 50% of silymarin and is regarded as one of the most biologically active constituents (Jacobs et al 2002). Silibinin is not a single compound either, but rather a mixture of two diastereoisomers, silybin A and silybin B (Kroll et al 2007). Other flavonolignans include isosilybin, silychristin and silydianin, all of which exist as diastereoisomers. A new flavonolignan, silyamandin, was discovered in St Mary's thistle preparations (MacKinnon et al 2007). St Mary's thistle seeds also contain a fixed oil comprising linoleic, oleic and palmitic acids, tocopherol and sterols, including cholesterol, campesterol, stigmasterol and sitosterol.

MAIN ACTIONS

Silymarin has confirmed antioxidant (Aghazadeh et al 2011, Gazák et al 2010, Morazzoni & Bombardelli 1995, Shaker et al 2010), antifibrotic (Hernandez-Gea & Friedman 2011, Trappoliere et al 2009, Tzeng et al 2013), anti-inflammatory (Aghazadeh et al 2011, El-Zayadi et al 2005, Morishima et al 2010, Polyak et al 2007), hepatoprotective (Ferenci et al 1989, Fraschini et al 2002, Lieber et al 2003), antihypercholesterolaemic (Krecman et al 1998), antihyperglycaemic (Velussi et al 1997), immunomodulatory (Polyak et al 2007) and antiviral (Ahmed-Belkacem et al 2010, Ferenci et al 2008, Neumann et al 2010, Polyak et al 2007) pharmacological actions in vitro, in vivo and in human studies.

Hepatoprotective

Hepatoprotection is defined as several non-mutually exclusive biological activities including antiviral, antioxidant, anti-inflammatory and immunomodulatory functions (Polyak et al 2013).

Silymarin and silibin exert some of these mechanisms and have hepatoprotective effects (Abenavoli et al 2010). In particular, *Silybum marianum* achieves many of its pharmacological actions via its antioxidant mechanisms.

Specifically, in regards to *Amanita phalloides* (death cap mushroom) poisoning cases, silibinin as Legalon SIL appears to exert its hepatoprotective effects by competitive inhibition of amatoxin binding and uptake by hepatocytes (Jacobs et al 2002) and by the reduction of enterohepatic recirculation through the modulation of bile flow. Adjunct to these mechanisms, silibinin reduces the oxidative stress, consequent to necrotic cell death caused by amatoxin poisoning with anti-inflammatory and antifibrotic downstream effects. Silibinin also reduces damage through inhibition of TNF-α and helps recovery through the stimulation of protein synthesis for repair in damaged liver cells (Mengs et al 2012).

It has therefore been postulated that *Silybum marianum* protects the liver by preventing the uptake of toxins and viruses through the stabilisation of cell membranes, reducing the oxidative stress caused by the metabolism of toxins and reducing hepatic inflammation, fibrosis and aiding hepatic repair and regeneration (Polyak et al 2010).

The mechanisms of membrane stability have been researched in detail. Silymarin and silibinin alter the structure of hepatocyte cell membranes by being incorporated into the hydrophobic–hydrophilic interface of the microsomal bilayer (Parasassi et al 1984). Silibinin interacts with the surface rather than deeper regions of the bilayer, and therefore does not change significantly the biophysical properties of the deeper membrane regions (Wesolowska et al 2007). Additionally, inhibition of cyclic adenosine monophosphate (AMP)-dependent phosphodiesterase by silibinin has been shown in vitro, which results in increased cAMP and stabilisation of lysosomal membranes (Koch et al 1985).

Toxin blockade

Protection of liver cells has been demonstrated against the following substances in vitro or in vivo:

- Carbon tetrachloride-induced liver cirrhosis (Chrungoo et al 1997, Mourelle et al 1989, Muriel & Mourelle 1990, Tsai et al 2008).
- Ethanol (Das & Vasudevan 2006).
- Paracetamol-induced liver peroxidation (Chrungoo et al 1997, Muriel et al 1992).
- Cyclosporin (von Schonfeld et al 1997).
- Phenothiazine (Palasciano et al 1994).
- Butyrophenone (Palasciano et al 1994).
- Erythromycin (Davila et al 1989).
- Amitriptyline and nortriptyline (Davila et al 1989).
- Oestradiol (Morazzoni & Bombardelli 1995).
- *Amanita phalloides* (Floersheim 1976, Vogel et al 1984).
- Tacrine (Galisteo et al 2000).
- Iron overload (Choi 2012, Masini et al 2000, Pietrangelo et al 1995).
- Benzo(a)pyrene-induced lung cancer (Kiruthiga et al 2007).

CHELATES IRON AND DECREASES IRON EXCESS

Silybum marianum interacts with iron in a number of ways. Excess iron increases oxidative stress and *Silybum marianum* exerts antioxidant activity thereby decreasing the pathological consequences of excessive oxidative stress. *Silybum marianum* acts indirectly to reduce iron-induced damage by protecting the mechanisms, such as the expression of hepcidin, that regulates iron uptake (Choi 2012) and directly chelating iron to reduce its absorption (Hutchinson et al 2010) and reactivity (Borsari et al 2001).

Antioxidant

In vivo research suggests the key mechanisms of action responsible for the antioxidant activity of silymarin are:

- direct activity via redox reactions;
- indirect activity by inhibiting the activity of free radical producing enzymes; and
- indirect activity achieved by upregulating endogenous, antioxidant enzyme systems such as Nrf2 (Son et al 2008) and glutathione (Kim et al 2012, Lu et al 2010a).

In vivo research involving rats with induced-steatohepatitis found that treatment with *Silybum marianum* decreased the oxidative stress marker malondialdehyde (MDA) by 45%, while glutathione (GSH) was increased by 65% and TNF-α lowered by 47% all relative to the control group (Aghazadeh et al 2011).

Anti-inflammatory

The anti-inflammatory activity of silymarin is due to several different mechanisms, such as antioxidant and membrane-stabilising effects, and inhibition of the production or release of inflammatory mediators, such as arachidonic acid metabolites. Inhibitory activity on lipo-oxygenase, cyclo-oxygenase (COX) and prostaglandin (PG) synthetase has been demonstrated in several in vitro assays and animal studies (Alarcon de la Lastra et al 1992, Dehmlow et al 1996, Fiebrich & Koch 1979, Rui et al 1990, Zhao et al 1999). Furthermore, silymarin inhibits NF-kappaB signalling and suppresses tumour necrosis factor (TNF)-alpha, nitric oxide synthase (iNOS) and interleukin (IL)-1 (Agarwal et al 2006, Kim et al 2012, Polyak et al 2007).

Antifibrotic

Silymarin and silibinin demonstrate antifibrotic activity in a variety of preclinical models via multiple mechanisms of action.

Silymarin reduces markers for collagen accumulation in the liver and exerts antifibrotic activity, according to an animal model of liver fibrosis (Boigk et al 1997). Oral silibinin (25–50 microM) dose-dependently inhibited the transforming growth factor beta (TGF-β)-induced de novo synthesis of pro-collagen I directly, by reducing platelet derived growth factor (PDGF)-induced cell proliferation, and indirectly, by de novo reduction of TGF-β-induced synthesis of collagen type 1 in human hepatic stellate cells (Trappoliere et al 2009). This finding was confirmed in thioacetamide-induced hepatic fibrosis, where silibinin down-regulated hepatic MMP-2, MMP-13, TIMP-1, TIMP-2, AP-1, KLF6, TGFβ1, αSMA and COL-α1 (Chen et al 2012).

A silibinin-phosphatidylcholine complex (silibinin 200 mg per kg) taken for five weeks caused an improvement in liver steatosis and inflammation and reduced the levels of plasma insulin and TNF-α. These effects were associated with a reduction in membrane lipid peroxidation, decreased free radical release and restoration of GSH levels (Haddad et al 2011).

Oral silymarin reduced steatohepatitis, raised nuclear translocation of nuclear factor erythroid 2-related factor 2 (Nrf2), and reduced tumour necrosis factor (TNF)-α mRNA expression in the liver in insulin-resistant rats, suggesting its antifibrotic effect is achieved through anti-inflammatory, antioxidant and hepatoprotective effects (Kim et al 2012).

Antitumour effects

A variety of mechanisms attributed to silymarin show it has promise in the prevention and/or treatment of several different cancers.

Oxidative stress (OS) in chronic disease accelerates inflammation, fibrosis and necrosis, through damage to proteins, DNA, lipids, sensitising redox-regulated necrotic and inflammatory cell signalling pathways, affecting gene expression (Finkel & Holbrook 2000) and causing mitochondrial dysfunction and pathology (Kung et al 2011, Pias & Aw 2002, Pias et al 2003, Polyak et al 2007). Therefore it has been suggested that by ameliorating OS and inflammation, silymarin could theoretically have a role in reducing disease progression and cancer incidence (Ting et al 2013).

In vivo and in vitro research with silibinin has identified an ability to reduce proliferation and angiogenesis, and to promote cell cycle arrest and apoptosis (Agarwal et al 2013, Deep & Agarwal 2010, Kauntz et al 2012b, Li et al 2010, Zeng et al 2011). Recent in vitro studies have shown that silibinin also possesses strong anti-invasive and anti-metastatic efficacy (Agarwal et al 2013, Deep & Agarwal 2010).

At this stage, most studies investigating mechanisms of action and effects in cancer have been conducted in vivo and in vitro, whereas human trials are limited (Li et al 2010). There have also been preclinical trials in humans to investigate suitable doses, treatment safety and improvements in bioavailability with phytosome-based preparations (Flaig et al 2010).

Silibinin has been shown to regulate multiple cellular proliferative pathways in cancer cells, including receptor tyrosine kinases, androgen receptor, STATs, NF-κB, cell cycle regulatory and apoptotic signalling pathways in vivo and in vitro (Li et al 2010). In prostate cancer, in mice, silymarin treatment down-regulates androgen receptor, epidermal growth factor receptor, and nuclear factor-κB mediated signalling and induces cell cycle arrest (Deep & Agarwal 2007). Kim et al (2009) showed in in vitro studies that silibinin can prevent the degradation of certain proteins in breast cancer. By studying the effects of silibinin on matrix metalloproteinases (MMPs), whose abnormal expression is associated with carcinoma and vascular endothelial growth factor (VEGF) which is expressed by malignant and non-malignant cells, they propose that this constituent is a possible candidate for the therapy of tumour metastasis and angiogenesis. The action responsible appears to be inhibition of 12-*O*-tetradecanoyl phorbol-13-acetate (TPA)-induced MMP and VEGF expression in breast cancer cells (Kim et al 2009).

In colon carcinogenesis, in rats, silibinin shifted the disturbed balance between cell renewal and cell death through potent proapoptotic, anti-inflammatory and multi-targeted effects at the molecular level. The study concluded that the effective reduction of pre-neoplastic lesions by silibinin supports its use as a natural agent for colon cancer chemoprevention (Kauntz et al 2012a).

Brain, neuroprotective activity

Silymarin has been shown to reduce sepsis-induced lung and brain injury, partially through its antioxidant effects, inhibition of neutrophil infiltration and regulation of inflammatory mediator release (Nencini et al 2007, Toklu et al 2008). Additionally, pretreatment with silymarin, but not silibinin, dose-dependently reduced cerebral ischaemic/reperfusion induced brain infarction by 16–40% and improved neurological deficits in rats through antioxidant and anti-inflammatory mechanisms (Hou et al 2010). Another study in rats pre-treated with silymarin found it slowed neuronal injury in focal cerebral ischaemia and enabled functional recovery close to the baseline. Similar to previous studies, the authors suggest that the neuroprotective potential of silymarin is mediated through its antioxidative and antiapoptotic properties (Raza et al 2011).

According to an in vitro study, silibinin may have potential as both a preventive and an active treatment for Alzheimer's disease as it reduced the formation of amyloid plaque and also protected cells from amyloid plaque-induced oxidative stress in a dose-dependent manner (Yin et al 2011).

Nephroprotective effect

In vitro experiments with kidney cells damaged by paracetamol, cisplatin or vincristin demonstrate that administration of silibinin before or after the chemical-induced injury can lessen or avoid the nephrotoxic effects (Sonnenbichler et al 1999). Animal studies have confirmed the nephroprotective effect for cisplatin-induced injury (Karimi et al 2005). In one study, the effects of cisplatin on glomerular and proximal tubular function as well as proximal tubular morphology were totally or partly ameliorated by silibinin (Gaedeke et al 1996). In an in vivo study, silymarin significantly decreased gentamicin-induced nephrotoxicity when used as a single agent and when used in combination with vitamin E in comparison to the placebo group. Serum creatinine concentrations, but not urea concentrations, were significantly lower (Varzi et al 2007).

Gastroprotective effect

St Mary's thistle extract produces a dose-dependent antiulcerogenic activity against indomethacin-induced ulcers, which can be histologically confirmed, according to research with test animals (Khayyal et al 2001). This is associated with reduced acid output, increased mucin secretion, increased PGE_2 release and decreased leukotriene release. Experiments with silymarin have found it to be effective in the prevention of gastric ulceration induced by cold-restraint stress in rats (Alarcon de la Lastra et al 1992) and postischaemic gastric mucosal injury (Alarcon de la Lastra et al 1995).

IN COMBINATION

A herbal formulation known as STW 5, containing extracts of milk thistle fruit and eight other herbs (bitter candy tuft, lemon balm leaf, chamomile flower, caraway fruit, peppermint leaf, licorice root, angelica root and greater celandine) produced antiulcerogenic activity against indomethacin-induced gastric ulcers in rats as well as antisecretory and cytoprotective activities (Khayyal et al 2001). In addition, it was shown that STW 5 lowered the gastric acidity as effectively as commercial antacid preparations (i.e. Rennie, Talcid, Maaloxan), prevented secondary hyperacidity more effectively and, additionally, inhibited serum gastrin levels in rats (Khayyal et al 2006).

Antidiabetic effect

In type 2 diabetes (T2DM) amyloid deposits contribute to the dysfunction of β-cells and the loss of β-cell mass in T2DM patients. In vitro silibinin reduces the formation of amyloid deposits and enhances the viability of pancreatic β cells (Cheng et al 2012).

In vivo research showed that silibinin exerts pronounced effects on liver carbohydrate metabolism. The metabolic pathways that contribute to glycaemia maintenance, i.e. gluconeogenesis in the fasted condition and glycogenolysis and glycolysis in the fed condition, were both reduced by silibinin corroborating the role of the liver in the antihyperglycaemic effect of silibinin (Colturato et al 2012).

Antiviral effect

Silybum marianum, particularly silymarin and intravenous silibinin, block hepatitis C virus (HCV) infection and proliferation in vitro by blocking viral fusion, viral entry, viral RNA and protein synthesis, and virus transmission (Ahmed-Belkacem et al 2010, Blaising & Pecheur 2013, McClure et al 2012, Morishima et al 2010, Polyak et al 2007, 2010, 2013, Wagoner et al 2010, 2011). This mechanism would also apply to other viruses such as vesicular stomatitis virus, reovirus, and the influenza virus (McClure et al 2012). Guedj et al (2012) confirmed in vivo that intravenous silibinin may block both viral infection and viral production/release dose-dependently.

Intravenous silibinin reduced HCV RNA in previous non-responders to pegylated interferon and ribavirin in a clinical study (Ferenci et al 2008) and prevented HCV RNA re-infection after liver transplantation (Beinhardt et al 2011, Marino et al 2013, Neumann et al 2010). Intravenous silibinin has also been found to inhibit HIV in human cell lines (McClure et al 2012), previously confirmed in a HCV/HIV co-infected patient (Payer et al 2010).

Mast-cell stabilisation

Silibinin has shown mast-cell stabilisation activity in vivo (Lecomte 1975), which was confirmed some years later and found to be dose-dependent (Fantozzi et al 1986).

Asthma

Allergic asthma is a chronic inflammatory disease regulated by coordination of T-helper2 (Th2) type cytokines and inflammatory signal molecules. Previously, silymarin has been shown to exert protective effects in the early phase of asthma, most likely due to its influence on histamine release (Breschi et al 2002). More recently, research with an animal model of asthma showed that pretreatment with silibinin prevented the development of airway hyperresponsiveness, significantly inhibited airway inflammatory cell recruitment and peribronchiolar inflammation and reduced the production of various cytokines in bronchoalveolar fluid (Choi et al 2012).

Cytochromes

Effects on Phase I CYP450

There has been extensive investigation into the effects of various St Mary's thistle preparations on various cytochromes. Human studies with standard St Mary's thistle preparations have identified no clinically significant effect on cytochromes CYP 1A2, 2D6, 3A4 whereas 2C9 appears most vulnerable to inhibition (Gurley et al 2012, Hackett et al 2013, Hermann & von Richter 2012). The lack of effect may be due to poor bioavailability (Goey et al 2013). If this is the case, then preparations with greater bioavailability still require testing to confirm that clinically significant drug interactions are absent. Additionally, the use of isolated silymarin and silibinin preparations could produce different results (Loguercio & Festi 2011).

Tests with an animal model suggest inhibition of CYP 1A1 however human studies have not confirmed the findings (Kiruthiga et al 2013).

Effects on phase II conjugation pathways

Phytochemicals such as silymarin can increase levels of Nrf2 either by stimulating its release or inhibiting its proteolytic breakdown. Activated Nrf2 translocates into the nucleus where it interacts with small MAF family proteins bound to the antioxidant response element (ARE), allowing transcription of target genes including those that regulate antioxidant and phase II enzymes (Kim et al 2012, Son et al 2008).

An in vitro study on cardiomyocytes with a product called Protandim (*Bacopa monniera, Silybum marianum, Withania somnifera, Camellia sinensis* and *Curcuma longa*) resulted in nuclear accumulation of Nrf2, upregulation of key endogenous phase II antioxidant enzymes, and Nrf2-dependent protection of cardiomyocytes from apoptosis after an oxidative stress (Reuland et al 2012).

P-glycoprotein

No clinically significant effects are seen for St Mary's thistle preparations and P-gp (Gurley et al 2006a, 2006b, Hermann & von Richter 2012), despite an earlier in vitro study which identified that silymarin inhibited P-glycoprotein (P-gp) ATPase activity in such a way as to suggest direct interaction with P-gp substrate binding (Zhang & Morris 2003).

OTHER ACTIONS

Cholesterol lowering

Cholesterol reduction has been demonstrated for silymarin in three studies of rats fed a highcholesterol diet (Krecman et al 1998, Shaker et al 2010, Sobolova et al 2006).

Although the mechanism of action is unknown, it has been suggested that inhibition of HMG-CoA reductase (Skottova & Krecman 1998a) and inhibition of cholesterol absorption from dietary sources (Sobolova et al 2006) are involved. Considering that the herb also contains phytosterols, these too may play a role in cholesterol reduction.

CLINICAL USE

In practice, St Marys thistle is commonly used for treating digestive disorders and any indication whereby improved liver function or liver protection may be a benefit. Milk thistle fruits have a positive European Scientific Cooperative on Phytotherapy (ESCOP) monograph for the following therapeutic indications: toxic liver damage; supportive treatment in patients with chronic inflammatory liver conditions and hepatic cirrhosis (ESCOP 2009).

Dyspepsia

St Mary's thistle is commonly used to treat dyspeptic complaints, such as loss of appetite, poor digestion and upper gastrointestinal discomfort. Animal studies have identified a dose-dependent increase in bile flow and bile salt secretion for silymarin, achieved by stimulating the synthesis of bile salts (Crocenzi et al 2000). Silymarin has been found to impact on bile salt synthesis, bile secretion, biotransformation of cholestatic compounds and changes in transported expression and activity (Crocenzi & Roma 2006).

Commission E approves the use of crude milk thistle preparations for dyspeptic complaints (Blumenthal et al 2000).

Toxic liver damage

Mushroom poisoning (*Amanita phalloides*)

One of the best-documented uses of milk thistle is in the treatment of poisoning by the mushroom *Amanita phalloides*. Nausea, vomiting, abdominal cramps and severe diarrhoea usually occur 8–12 hours after ingestion, with extensive hepatic necrosis occurring 1–2 days later. A mortality rate of 20–30% has been observed but can be as high as 50% in children under 10 years of age (Floersheim et al 1982).

Since intervention studies would be unethical, a review of case reports and studied mechanisms of action are used as evidence to support its use.

A review of 154 cases of *Amanita phalloides* poisoning in Germany (1983–1992) showed a mortality rate of 15.2% in non-silibinin treated cases ($n = 38$) compared to 8.3% in patients treated with silibinin ($n = 116$) (Saller et al 2008). A more recent review of nearly 1500 documented cases concluded that the overall mortality in patients treated with Legalon SIL is less than 10% in comparison to more than 20% when using penicillin or a combination of silibinin and penicillin. Mengs et al (2012) recommend a daily dose of 20 mg silibinin/kg via continuous infusion over 24 hours, following a single loading dose of 5 mg silibinin/kg and to start treatment as soon as possible.

At the Poison Information Centre, Vienna, Austria; if silibinin is administered within 48 hours of poisoning, only mild to moderate liver injury is observed ($n = 18$) (Hruby et al 1983). After 48 hours, if left untreated, severe liver damage, coagulation disorders and coma are likely to occur. Hruby administered four divided doses of silibinin intravenously, each dose consisting of 20–50 mg/kg body weight/day; the dose varied depending on the severity of intoxication (Hruby et al 1983).

Silymarin protects against the *Amanita phalloides* toxins, α-amanita and phalloidin, by inhibiting the toxins binding to cell receptors by competitive inhibition of hepatocyte-specific OATP2 transporters; their uptake and interaction with cell components; binding with nuclear receptors and inhibiting protein synthesis and cell repair (Ferenci et al 1989, Hackett et al 2013). As silymarin reduces the uptake of toxins into cells, the earlier it is administered after exposure, the better the protective effects (Hruby et al 1983, Mengs et al 2012).

Clinical note — Hepatic fibrosis

Hepatic fibrosis is a pathological wound-healing process that occurs when the liver is injured chronically, such as in chronic alcohol abuse. The oxidative metabolite of ethanol, acetaldehyde, often in conjunction with viral or metabolic liver disease, is implicated as the major cause for liver fibrogenesis, which ultimately leads to cirrhosis (Schuppan et al 1995). Antifibrotic and antiviral interventions, which interrupt the continuous process of wound healing in the liver, are being investigated as strategies to prevent or reverse liver cirrhosis (Poynard et al 2009).

Environmental toxins and drugs

In animals, milk thistle reduces acute liver injury caused by paracetamol (Ali et al 2001, Muriel et al 1992), carbon tetrachloride (Favari & Perez-Alvarez 1997, Letteron et al 1990), radiation (Hakova & Misurova 1996, Kropacova et al 1998), iron overload (Masini et al 2000, Pietrangelo et al 1995), phenylhydrazine (Valenzuela & Guerra 1985) and D-galactosamine (Tyutyulkova et al 1981, 1983).

One randomised, double-blind study involving 222 patients showed that silymarin improves the tolerability of tacrine without altering the drug's cognitive effects (Allain et al 1999). Two other clinical trials have documented the effectiveness of silymarin in improving or preventing hepatotoxicity from chronic administration of phenothiazines or butyrophenone.

Supportive treatment in chronic liver diseases

Milk thistle fruits have a positive European Scientific Cooperative on Phytotherapy (ESCOP) monograph for supportive treatment in patients with chronic inflammatory liver conditions and hepatic cirrhosis (ESCOP 2009).

Numerous clinical trials have been conducted with St Mary's thistle preparations in various chronic liver diseases. The most studied treatments are Legalon (Madaus Corporation, Cologne, Germany) and silipide (Inverni Della Beffa Research and Development Laboratories, Milan, Italy), designed to improve oral absorption of silymarin.

A 1998 clinical review of St Mary's thistle concluded that it may be effective in improving the clinical courses of both acute and chronic viral, drug-induced, toxin-induced and alcoholic hepatitis (Flora et al 1998). A systematic review of efficacy for St Mary's thistle in chronic liver diseases stated that data are still too limited to detect a substantial benefit on mortality or recommend the herb in liver disease (Jacobs et al 2002).

Twelve clinical studies were located in which researchers have attempted to clarify the role of St Mary's thistle in the treatment of various liver diseases (Angulo et al 2000, Benda et al 1980, Buzzelli et al 1993, Ferenci et al 1989, Loguercio et al 2007, Lucena et al 2002, Magliulo et al 1978, Par et al 2000, Pares et al 1998, Salmi & Sarna 1982, Trinchet et al 1989, Velussi et al 1997). Much of the research focuses on the different forms of hepatitis and alcoholic liver cirrhosis with doses ranging from 100 to 300 mg three times daily, usually given in a standardised extract of 70–80% silymarin. Overall, results have been mixed, with nine trials showing generally positive results and three negative, suggesting that milk thistle is effective in only some forms of liver disease.

Alcoholic liver disease

A 2005 Cochrane review of 13 randomised clinical trials and a 2007 Cochrane review of 18 randomised clinical trials assessed milk thistle in 915 and 1088

S

patients, respectively, looking at its effect in alcoholic and/or hepatitis B or C virus liver diseases (Rambaldi et al 2005, 2007). The authors stated in both reviews that the methodological quality of the trials was low and that milk thistle versus placebo or no intervention had no significant effect on complications of liver disease or liver histology, and that milk thistle was not associated with a significantly increased risk of adverse events.

In comparison to the 2005 review, which concluded that liver-related mortality was significantly reduced by milk thistle in patients with alcoholic liver disease, the 2007 review found that liver-related mortality was significantly reduced by milk thistle in all trials, but not in high-quality trials (Rambaldi et al 2005, 2007).

A review of 36 papers concluded that silymarin may have a role in the treatment of liver cirrhosis, especially alcoholic cirrhosis. In five trials of patients with liver cirrhosis (n = 602), a significant but small (7%) reduction of liver-related mortality (not corrected for study duration) was attained with silymarin (Saller et al 2001). These findings were confirmed in a recent meta-analysis by the same author (Saller et al 2008).

Acute viral hepatitis

Several studies have investigated the use of milk thistle in this disease, reporting beneficial effects on serological outcomes (Bode et al 1977, Magliulo et al 1978, Tkacz & Dworniak 1983). However, these early studies were not clearly blinded.

More recently, a randomised, double-blind, placebo-controlled clinical trial involving 105 subjects with acute hepatitis (hepatitis A, B, C and E) patients tested a commercial St Mary's thistle product (Legalon 140 mg three times daily) taken for four weeks. The silymarin group had faster resolution of symptoms related to biliary retention, dark urine ($P = 0.013$), jaundice ($P = 0.02$) and scleral icterus ($P = 0.043$). However, the primary outcome measure of normalisation of bilirubin and hepatic enzymes did not differ between the herbal and placebo groups (El-Kamary et al 2009).

Hepatitis C infection

A 2003 systematic review of medicinal herbs for HCV infection concluded that compared with placebo, none of the herbs showed effects on HCV RNA or liver enzymes, except for the constituent silybin, which showed a significant reduction of serum aspartate aminotransferase (AST) and gamma-glutamyltranspeptidase levels in one trial (Liu et al 2003).

In a 4-week randomised, controlled clinical trial (n = 34) using 160 mg of milk thistle three times a day, AST, alanine aminotransferase (ALT) and viral load values decreased from baseline levels after 4 weeks although the effect was not significant. In comparison, values for ALT and viral load showed a significant increase in the control group over the same period. When treatment and control groups were then compared, a significant difference was observed for ALT and AST, but not for viral load (Torres et al 2004). Similarly, a 2005 review concluded that silymarin decreases serum AST and ALT levels, but does not seem to affect viral load or liver histology (Mayer et al 2005).

A randomised, double-blind, placebo-controlled, crossover study (n = 24) where subjects received 12 weeks treatment with 600 or 1200 mg milk thistle daily, viral load, ALT levels and quality of life scores (short-form (SF)-36) were not significantly different to placebo (Gordon et al 2006).

As part of the hepatitis C Antiviral Long-Term Treatment Against Cirrhosis (HALT-C) trial (n = 1145 participants), involving people with advanced chronic hepatitis C, non-responders to prior antiviral therapy continued taking pegylated interferon treatment with the addition of oral silymarin therapy; however, no changes to ALT and viral load were observed with adjunctive herbal treatment. Silymarin therapy did significantly lower liver-related symptoms and improved QOL parameters such as fatigue, nausea, liver pain, anorexia, muscle and joint pain, as well as general health (Seeff et al 2008).

Non-responders to pegylated interferon and ribavirin were treated with increasing doses of intravenous (IV) silibinin (Legalon, SIL; Madaus) (Ferenci et al 2008). A dose-dependent reduction of HCV RNA was achieved. Patients were given 15 or 20 mg/kg/day IV silibinin for 14 days, and 280 mg oral silymarin three times per day combined with pegylated interferon and ribavirin therapy from day 8. At week 12, 50% (7/14) previous non-responders had undetectable HCV RNA (Ferenci et al 2008). Despite the small numbers and lack of a control group, this was the first time that silibinin (intravenously) had shown a direct anti-HCV activity in chronic hepatitis C patients (Ferenci et al 2008). It identifies a new pharmacological action for silibinin in humans and provides useful information about effective doses of intravenous silibinin and oral silymarin. It is of clinical significance, because adding pegylated interferon and ribavirin to intravenous silibinin showed greater efficacy than silibinin or pegylated interferon and ribavirin alone, suggesting a synergistic effect.

A review found no evidence for a beneficial effect of oral silymarin on the progression of viral hepatitis, especially hepatitis C (Saller et al 2008). Negative results were also obtained in a 2012 double-blind placebo-controlled trial testing oral Legalon (420 mg or 700 mg three times a day) in people with chronic hepatitis C (CHC). The study of 154 CHC patients found treatment with silymarin for 24 weeks produced no significant change in serum ALT levels during or after the trial, compared to placebo. Additionally, other markers of advanced liver disease such as serum bilirubin, albumin and platelet counts were the same (Fried et al 2012).

The recent use of intravenous silibinin prevented HCV RNA re-infection after orthotopic liver transplantation (Neumann et al 2010). Neumann and colleagues (2010) started silibinin infusions (1400 mg daily for 14 days) administered eight hours after orthotopic liver transplantation, when HCV RNA levels measured 182 IU/mL. Three days later HCV RNA became undetectable (<15 IU/mL) and remained so 168 days later (Neumann et al 2010).

IN COMBINATION

More recently, a randomised, double-blind, placebo-controlled trial of 118 chronic hepatitis C participants showed that treatment with silymarin (720 mg silybin per day) and 12 vitamin and phytochemical based antioxidants achieved a higher rate of ALT normalisation compared to placebo ($P = 0.02$) or silymarin ($P = 0.003$) at Week 24. There was also a significant improvement in overall mental wellbeing (mental component summary scale) in the active treatment group (Salmond et al 2010).

A review concluded that silymarin 'is reasonable' to be employed as an adjunct therapy for alcoholic and grade Child A liver cirrhosis (Saller et al 2008).

S

Non-alcoholic fatty liver disease (NAFLD)

A phase III, double-blind clinical trial assessing the effects of silybin plus phosphatidylcholine on patients with nonalcoholic fatty liver disease showed positive outcomes over the 12-month treatment program. Patients were given Realsil, which is comprised of 94 mg silymarin, 194 mg phosphatidylcholine and 89.28 mg vitamin E acetate 50%. The study showed that there was substantial normalisation in ALT, AST and glutamyl-transpeptidase levels over the trial period. Blood glucose was 31% lower in the treatment group compared to placebo suggesting positive improvements in insulin resistance. Liver histology improvement was also noted via ultrasound (lobular inflammation, ballooning and fibrosis). In all measurements the active treatment group outperformed controls. It is suspected that the herb's antioxidant activity is chiefly responsible for the beneficial effects observed (Loguercio et al 2012).

IN COMBINATION

In 2013, another study was published testing silymarin (twice daily) in NAFLD producing positive results. The open study involved 72 patients who were on a restricted diet for 3 months and a food supplement containing vitamin E, L-glutathione, L-cysteine, L-methionine and *Silybum marianum* (Epaclin 3.5 g) taken twice a day. This treatment regimen reduced the biochemical, inflammatory and ultrasonic indices of hepatic steatosis and some parameters indicative of early stage of atherosclerosis (Cacciapuoti et al 2013). In particular, Steato test significantly ($P < 0.001$) reduced from baseline (0.71 ± 0.07) to the end of treatment (0.40 ± 0.05), ALT serum levels ($P < 0.01$) fell from a mean level of 109.48 ± 4.4 to 75.12 ± 3.3 U/L and AST recorded at baseline (72.39 ± 8.4 U/L) also significantly reduced ($P < 0.05$) after silymarin and diet (48.65 ± 3.2 U/L) (Cacciapuoti et al 2013).

> ***Clinical note — What is NAFLD?***
> Non-alcoholic fatty liver disease is the most common silent liver disease worldwide. It is characterised by fat accumulation in the liver (steatosis) and alterations in liver biochemical tests in people who do not consume high amounts of alcohol. Importantly, there are no obvious symptoms of disease. It has been estimated that the prevalence of NAFLD in Western countries is 20–30%. Obesity, type 2 diabetes and hyperlipidaemia are often associated with NAFLD (Cacciapuoti et al 2013).

Diabetes

Silymarin has also been investigated in people with type 2 diabetes both with and without cirrhosis. Velussi et al (1997) investigated whether long-term treatment with silymarin is effective in reducing lipoperoxidation and insulin resistance in diabetic patients with cirrhosis. The 6-month open trial found that silymarin treatment had several benefits. After the first month's treatment, fasting glucose levels showed a progressive and significant decline that, interestingly, did not lead to an increase in the frequency of hypoglycaemic episodes. Other observations revealed decreased glucosuria and levels of glycosylated haemoglobin also decreased significantly, indicating an overall improvement in glucose control. The dose used was 600 mg/day silymarin.

A 4-month randomised, double-blind, placebo-controlled trial in 51 type 2 diabetes patients receiving silymarin (200 mg three times daily) as an adjunct treatment to their conventional therapy showed a significant decrease in HbA_{1C}, fasting blood glucose, total cholesterol, LDL and triglyceride levels compared with placebo as well as with values at the beginning of the study in each group (Huseini et al 2006). Another randomised, double-blind, placebo-controlled trial of 4 months' duration involving 59 subjects with type 2 diabetes compared treatment with 200 mg silymarin/day plus 10 mg glibenclamide to placebo plus glibenclamide vs glinenclamide alone. The silymarin group had significant reductions in both fasting and postprandial glucose levels, HbA_{1C} and BMI compared to the placebo (Hussain 2007). A meta-analysis found the pooled mean difference (in the above two studies) in HbA_{1C} and fasting glucose were −1.92% ($P = 0.008$)

and −38.05 mg/dL ($P < 0.009$) in silymarin plus conventional treatment vs placebo plus conventional treatment (Suksomboon et al 2011). This meta-analysis concluded that treatment with *Silybum marianum* may improve glycaemic control in T2DM and called for further high quality studies to better elucidate the effects of these herbs on glycaemic control (Suksomboon et al 2011).

OTHER USES

Traditionally, the seeds have been used to treat jaundice, hepatitis, haemorrhoids and psoriasis, as a tonic for nursing mothers, and as a general 'liver-cleansing' agent.

Haemochromatosis

St Mary's thistle may have benefits in this condition, based on its mechanisms of action. Hutchinson et al suggested that silybin could chelate iron in the neutral pH of the duodenum and reduce the absorption of iron postprandially which they demonstrated in a crossover study with 10 people with haemochromatosis. Consumption of 140 mg of silybin with a meal resulted in a reduction in the postprandial increase in serum iron (AUC ± SE) compared with water (silybin 1726.6 ± 346.8 vs water 2988.8 ± 167; $P < 0.05$) and tea (silybin 1726.6 ± 346.8 vs tea 2099.3 ± 223.3; $P < 0.05$) (Hutchinson et al 2010).

Hypercholesterolaemia

In clinical practice, it is not unusual to find treatment with St Mary's thistle at the higher end of the dose range results in cholesterol-lowering effects. Several in vivo studies confirm that St Mary's thistle increases LDL cholesterol clearance and raises HDL cholesterol levels; however, only one clinical trial is available to determine whether the effect is clinically significant (Krecman et al 1998, Skottova & Krecman 1998b, Somogyi et al 1989). An open trial involving 14 subjects with type 2 hyperlipidaemia found that treatment with silymarin (420 mg/day) slightly reduced total cholesterol and HDL cholesterol levels (Somogyi et al 1989).

Cancer prevention and treatment

In the past two decades, silybin has demonstrated remarkable anti-cancer as well as cancer chemopreventive efficacy in preclinical cell culture and animal models of several cancer models including skin, breast, lung, bladder (Zeng et al 2011), colon, prostate, lung and kidney carcinomas (Deep & Agarwal 2010, Niture et al 2014). Silybin has also been tested in human phase I–II pilot clinical trials, where it was reported to be well tolerated and showed plasma and target-tissue bioavailability, though limited (Agarwal et al 2013, Flaig et al 2007, 2010).

S

Topical application of silymarin provided significant protection against different stages of UVB-induced skin carcinogenesis in mouse skin tumourigenesis models (Ahmad et al 1998, Lahiri-Chatterjee et al 1999).

A randomised, double-blind, placebo-controlled study of 37 men, 2–3 months after radical prostatectomy were randomised to receive 570 mg of silymarin and 240 mcg selenium ($n = 19$) or placebo ($n = 18$) daily for 6 months. The combination of silymarin and selenium significantly reduced two markers of lipid metabolism associated with prostate cancer (PCa) progression, LDL and total cholesterol which suggests that silymarin and selenium may be effective in reducing PCa progression (Vidlar et al 2010).

Chemotherapy support

Whether silymarin is a useful treatment to prevent organ toxicity due to chemotherapy remains to be tested. Based on its anti-inflammatory, antioxidant and hepatoprotective mechanisms, it could prove useful (Comelli et al 2007, Greenlee et al 2007). In a case of hepatotoxicity during chemotherapy which did not resolve with supportive care, there was an immediate response to milk thistle at 280 mg twice daily (McBride et al 2012).

Besides lowering toxicity, silybin strongly sensitises human prostate carcinoma cells to doxorubicin, cisplatin, carboplatin, and mitoxantrone-induced growth inhibition and apoptotic death. Similar synergistic effects of silybin with doxorubicin and cisplatin have also been reported in various other cancer cell lines (Agarwal et al 2013, Greenlee et al 2007). Further research is warranted to determine its role in practice and identify any safety issues.

Obsessive compulsive disorder

In a pilot randomised, double-blind trial of 35 adults with obsessive compulsive disorder (OCD) designed to compare the efficacy of silymarin to fluoxetine, both interventions provided equal and highly significant reductions on Yale-Brown Scale for OCD (Y-BOCS) ($P = 0.0001$). Patients were randomly assigned to receive either capsules of the *Silybum marianum* (600 mg/day taken in 200 mg capsules 3 times a day) or fluoxetine (30 mg/day taken in 10 mg capsules three times a day). There was also no significant difference between the two groups in terms of observed side effects (Sayyah et al 2010). Camfield suggests this effect is achieved through silibinin's inhibition of monoamine oxidase activity (Mazzio et al 1998) which increases serotonin levels in the cortex (Osuchowski et al 2004) and was shown to ameliorate decreases in dopamine and serotonin in the prefrontal cortex and hippocampus associated with methamphetamine abuse (Camfield et al 2011, Lu et al 2010b).

> ***Clinical note — Cisplatin***
> Cisplatin is one of the most active cytotoxic agents in the treatment of testicular cancer, head and neck, gastrointestinal, cervical, lung and bladder cancer. However, its clinical use is associated with side effects, such as severe nausea, ototoxicity, neurotoxicity and nephrotoxicity (Giacomelli et al 2002).

Pharmacokinetics of silymarin

Silymarin has low solubility in water and has poor oral bioavailability, similar to other flavonolignans, and undergoes rapid excretion (Loguercio & Festi 2011). Following oral administration, silymarin undergoes phase I and phase II metabolism, especially phase II conjugation reactions, forming chiefly monoglucuronides detectable in human plasma and in urine two hours after ingestion (Calani et al 2012). It undergoes multiple conjugation reactions and is primarily excreted into bile and urine (Pradhan & Girish 2006, Venkataramanan et al 2006, Wen et al 2008, Wu et al 2009).

A pharmacokinetic dosing study identified that oral doses of between 140 mg and 560 mg of silymarin resulted in increases in plasma silibinin A and silibinin B only whereas a higher dose of 700 mg silymarin resulted in six silymarin flavonolignans being detected in the plasma (Hawke et al 2010).

Due to its poor water solubility, research has been undertaken to find methods of improving silymarin bioavailability. This includes creating different preparations of more soluble derivatives of silybin creating silymarin nanoparticles, using a semisolid dispersion system and phytosomes of phosphatidylcholine as emulsifying agents (Filburn et al 2007, Hsu et al 2012, Hussein et al 2012, Loguercio & Festi 2011).

Efforts to improve silymarin bioavailability are important to obtain better clinical outcomes. For example, poor bioavailability with oral silymarin is correlated with liver inflammation (Hawke et al 2010, Loguercio & Festi 2011, Schrieber et al 2008). This supports the results and comments from the HALT-C trial (Freedman et al 2011). Ferenci's study (Ferenci et al 1989) and *A. phalloides* poisoning (Hruby et al 1983) showed that early administration of more bioavailable silymarin has better hepatoprotective activity.

To overcome oral bioavailability issues, intravenous silibinin has also been investigated. This method of use has recently been applied to patients with chronic hepatitis C, successfully clearing hepatitis C virus (HCV) infection in some patients even in monotherapy (Esser-Nobis et al 2013) and has also been successfully used to treat amatoxin poisoning (Mengs et al 2012).

DOSAGE RANGE

Studies show that the dose; route of administration; treatment duration; patient's diagnosed condition and any comorbidities; the inflammatory stage in the disease process (Loguercio & Festi 2011) and the genotype of the virus in HCV (Huber et al 2005) all impact the efficacy of silymarin treatment in liver disease. In summary:

- To show benefits in hepatic necroinflammation: 450 mg/day silymarin for 12 months achieved ALT normalisation in 15% of the CHC patients in a randomised study (El-Zayadi et al 2005);
- To improve liver histology: 420 mg/day silymarin for 41 months (mean) is required in alcoholic cirrhosis (Child-Pugh A, 5–7) (Fehér et al 1989, Ferenci et al 1989);
- To elicit antioxidant effects: 600 mg/day silymarin for 12 months reduced malondialdehyde in diabetic cirrhotics (Velussi et al 1997); and
- To elicit direct anti-HCV activity: 1400 mg/day intravenous silibinin administered for 14 days is needed (Biermer et al 2010, Ferenci et al 2008, Neumann et al 2010).

In most clinical trials the effective daily doses of silymarin range from 420 to 600 mg (Saller et al 2008). To obtain a midpoint of 500 mg of silymarin from a 1 : 1 herbal extract, assuming 1 mL of herbal extract contains 25 mg of silymarin, then 20 mL/day of the *Silybum marianum* extract is required. This is a higher level than is normally recommended in clinical practice.

- Liquid extract (1 : 1): 4–9 mL/day (Mills & Bone 2000).
- Silybin-phytosome: 13 g daily (Flaig et al 2007).

S

TOXICITY

Extremely low

Hawke et al (2010) showed that oral doses up to 2100 mg oral silymarin were non-toxic. Toxicity studies in rats and mice have shown that silymarin, even at daily doses as high as 2500–5000 mg/kg, produced no adverse toxic effects (Madaus 1989). In a 12-month study in rats and dogs given up to 2500 mg/day, no signs of toxicity were seen. Milk thistle products with a standardised content of silymarin (70–80%) were found to be safe for up to 41 months of usage (Francine 2005). Safety was further confirmed after comprehensive in vitro studies concluded that interference or heptatotoxicity of the dry extract from *S. marianum* at the recommended maximum daily dose of four Hepar-Pasc tablets, equivalent to 210 mg silibinin, is unlikely, and is to be considered safe (Doehmer et al 2011).

ADVERSE REACTIONS

Milk thistle is considered safe and well-tolerated when taken within the recommended dose range (Post-White et al 2007). A review of studies involving more than 7000 participants identified three cases of serious adverse reactions (two anaphylaxis and one gastroenteritis symptoms) (Jacobs et al 2002). In one clinical trial, patients with colorectal adenocarcinoma who received silipide (silybin with phosphatidylcholine) at dosages of 360, 720 or 1440 mg daily for 7 days found the administration of silipide to be safe (Hoh et al 2006). Another clinical trial ($n = 13$) reported hyperbilirubinaemia in 9/13 patients and increased ALT in 1/13 patients using silybin-phytosome (Flaig et al 2007), whereas all other trials reported only rare adverse events (Gordon et al 2006, Rainone 2005, Torres et al 2004), mostly gastrointestinal symptoms, even for intravenously administered silymarin (Ferenci et al 2008). Reviews concluded that silymarin has an excellent safety profile (Dryden et al 2006, Rainone 2005, Sagar 2007).

Overall, adverse effect frequency was the same as for placebo and had a low frequency, ranging from 2% to 12% in controlled trials. In practice, loose bowels and gastrointestinal symptoms have been reported.

SIGNIFICANT INTERACTIONS

In vitro studies using a standardised dry extract from *Silybum marianum* (Hepar-Pasc) state that according to FDA regulations, drug–drug interactions are possible for CYP2C8 and CYP2C9 but not likely, and are remote for CYP2C19, CYP2D6, and CYP3A4 (Doehmer et al 2011, Kiruthiga et al 2013). Although in vitro and some animal studies (Kiruthiga et al 2013) show possible drug interactions with silymarin these are not replicated in clinical interactions (Hackett et al 2013). A prospective human study of standard milk thistle extracts (non-phytosome) concluded that on the basis of current clinical data, the drug interaction risk for milk thistle products is minimal (Gurley et al 2012).

Cisplatin

Preliminary research has shown this combination may reduce toxic effects, yet enhance antitumour activity — theoretically adjunctive use may be beneficial when used under professional supervision however further research is required to confirm benefits (Agarwal et al 2013, Greenlee et al 2007).

Doxorubicin

Silymarin reduces cardiotoxicity and possibly chemosensitises resistant cells to anthracyclines — theoretically adjunctive use may be beneficial when used under professional supervision (Agarwal et al 2013, Greenlee et al 2007).

Hepatotoxic substances

General hepatoprotective effects reported for silymarin — adjunctive use may be beneficial when used under professional supervision.

CONTRAINDICATIONS AND PRECAUTIONS

Contraindicated in people with known allergy to the Asteraceae (Compositae) family of plants. One case of exacerbation of haemochromatosis due to ingestion of milk thistle has been reported (Whittington 2007); however, the association between herbal intake and outcome reported is unlikely (Kidd 2008).

PREGNANCY USE

An in vivo study concluded that silibinin was safe when used by pre-eclamptic pregnant women (Giorgi et al 2012). A review of four studies found no evidence of adverse effects in mothers and their offspring for silymarin when used by pregnant women with intrahepatic cholestasis, alcoholic and non-alcoholic liver cirrhosis, chronic and acute viral hepatitis, drug-induced liver toxicity, fatty degeneration of the liver (Hess 2013).

PATIENTS' FAQs

What will this herb do for me?

St Mary's thistle may improve digestion, particularly of fatty foods, and afford protection against the toxic effects of a number of drugs and environmental poisons. It is also used as supportive treatment in chronic liver diseases and high-cholesterol states.

When will it start to work?

This varies, depending on the indication.

Are there any safety issues?

St Mary's thistle is considered a very safe and well-tolerated herb. The most common side effects relate to gastrointestinal symptoms such as loose bowels.

Practice points/Patient counselling

- St Mary's thistle has hepatoprotective activity and has been shown to reduce the hepatotoxic effects of a variety of environmental toxins and medicines, such as paracetamol, erythromycin, carbon tetrachloride and death cap mushrooms (*Amanita phalloides* poisoning).
- It has direct and indirect antioxidant activities, accelerates the regeneration of hepatocytes after liver damage, has significant gastroprotective and nephroprotective activities, anti-inflammatory and antihistamine activities, and anti-tumour effects according to in vitro and animal studies.
- Numerous clinical studies have investigated its effects in a variety of liver diseases, many producing promising results however it's still too early to suggest the herb is used as routine treatment in chronic liver diseases. An individualised approach is best.
- In clinical practice, it is used to treat dyspepsia, toxic liver damage, as supportive therapy in chronic liver diseases and hypercholesterolaemia.
- Preliminary evidence suggests a possible role as adjunctive therapy with cisplatin and as a skin cancer preventive agent when applied topically.
- Dose and route of administration of silymarin preparations are important considerations in management of liver disease.

S

REFERENCES

Abenavoli, L., et al. (2010) Milk thistle in liver diseases: past, present, future. Phytother Res, 24, 1423–32.

Agarwal, C., et al. (2013) Anti-cancer efficacy of silybin derivatives — a structure-activity relationship. PLoS One, 8, e60074.

Agarwal R et al. Anticancer potential of silymarin: from bench to bed side. Anticancer Res 26.6B (2006): 4457–4498.

Aghazadeh, S., et al. (2011) Anti-apoptotic and anti-inflammatory effects of *Silybum marianum* in treatment of experimental steatohepatitis. Exp Toxicol Pathol, 63, 569–74.

Ahmad N et al. Skin cancer chemopreventive effects of a flavonoid antioxidant silymarin are mediated via impairment of receptor tyrosine kinase signaling and perturbation in cell cycle progression. Biochem Biophys Res Commun 247.2 (1998): 294–301.

Ahmed-Belkacem, A., et al. (2010) Silibinin and related compounds are direct inhibitors of hepatitis C virus RNA-dependent RNA polymerase. Gastroenterology, 138, 1112–22.
Alarcon de la Lastra AC et al. Gastric anti-ulcer activity of silymarin, a lipoxygenase inhibitor, in rats. J Pharm Pharmacol 44.11 (1992): 929–931.
Alarcon de la Lastra AC et al. Gastroprotection induced by silymarin, the hepatoprotective principle of *Silybum marianum* in ischemia-reperfusion mucosal injury: role of neutrophils. Planta Med 61.2 (1995): 116–1119.
Ali BH, et al. Effect of the traditional medicinal plants *Rhazya stricta, Balanitis aegyptiaca* and *Haplophylum tuberculatum* on paracetamol-induced hepatotoxicity in mice. Phytother Res 15.7 (2001): 598–603.
Allain H et al. Aminotransferase levels and silymarin in de novo tacrine-treated patients with Alzheimer's disease. Dement Geriatr Cogn Disord 10.3 (1999): 181–185.
Angulo P et al. Silymarin in the treatment of patients with primary biliary cirrhosis with a suboptimal response to ursodeoxycholic acid. Hepatology 32.5 (2000): 897–900.
Beinhardt, S., et al. (2011) Silibinin monotherapy prevents graft infection after orthotopic liver transplantation in a patient with chronic hepatitis C. J Hepatol, 54, 591–2; author reply 592-3.
Benda L et al. The influence of therapy with silymarin on the survival rate of patients with liver cirrhosis (author's transl). Wien Klin Wochenschr 92.19 (1980): 678–683.
Biermer, M., et al. (2010) Silibinin as a rescue treatment for HCV-infected patients showing suboptimal virologic response to standard combination therapy. J Hepatol, 52, S16.
Blaising, J. & Pecheur, E. I. (2013) Lipids: a key for hepatitis C virus entry and a potential target for antiviral strategies. Biochimie, 95, 96–102.
Blumenthal M, et al. (eds). Herbal medicine: expanded commission E monographs. Austin, TX: Integrative Medicine Communications, 2000.
Bode JC, et al. [Silymarin for the treatment of acute viral hepatitis? Report of a controlled trial. (author's transl)] Med Klin 72.12 (1977): 513–5118.
Boigk G et al. Silymarin retards collagen accumulation in early and advanced biliary fibrosis secondary to complete bile duct obliteration in rats. Hepatology 26.3 (1997): 643–649.
Borsari M et al. Silybin, a new iron-chelating agent. J Inorg Biochem 85.2–3 (2001): 123–129.
Breschi MC et al. Protective effect of silymarin in antigen challenge- and histamine-induced bronchoconstriction in in vivo guinea-pigs. Eur J Pharmacol 437.1–2 (2002): 91–95.
Buzzelli G et al. A pilot study on the liver protective effect of silybin-phosphatidylcholine complex (IdB1016) in chronic active hepatitis. Int J Clin Pharmacol Ther Toxicol 31.9 (1993): 456–460.
Cacciapuoti, F., et al. 2013. Silymarin in non alcoholic fatty liver disease. World J Hepatol., 5, (3) 109–113.
Calani, L., et al. 2012. Absorption and metabolism of milk thistle flavanolignans in humans. Phytomedicine, 20, (1) 40–46.
Camfield, D. A., et al. (2011) Nutraceuticals in the treatment of obsessive compulsive disorder (OCD): a review of mechanistic and clinical evidence. Prog Neuropsychopharmacol Biol Psychiatry, 35, 887–95.
Chen, I. S., et al. (2012) Hepatoprotection of silymarin against thioacetamide-induced chronic liver fibrosis. J Sci Food Agric, 92, 1441–7.
Cheng, B., et al. (2012) Silibinin inhibits the toxic aggregation of human islet amyloid polypeptide. Biochem Biophys Res Commun, 419, 495–9.
Choi, J. (2012) Oxidative stress, endogenous antioxidants, alcohol, and hepatitis C: pathogenic interactions and therapeutic considerations. Free Radic Biol Med, 52, 1135–50.
Choi, Y.H., et al. 2012. Silibinin attenuates allergic airway inflammation in mice. Biochem.Biophys.Res.Commun., 427, (3) 450–455.
Chrungoo VJ, et al. Silymarin mediated differential modulation of toxicity induced by carbon tetrachloride, paracetamol and D-galactosamine in freshly isolated rat hepatocytes. Indian J Exp Biol 35.6 (1997): 611–6117.
Colturato, C. P., et al. (2012) Metabolic effects of silibinin in the rat liver. Chem Biol Interact, 195, 119–32.
Comelli MC et al. Toward the definition of the mechanism of action of silymarin: activities related to cellular protection from toxic damage induced by chemotherapy. Integr Cancer Ther 6.2 (2007): 120–129.
Crocenzi FA, Roma MG. Silymarin as a new hepatoprotective agent in experimental cholestasis: new possibilities for an ancient medication. Curr Med Chem 13.9 (2006): 1055–1074.
Crocenzi FA et al. Effect of silymarin on biliary bile salt secretion in the rat. Biochem Pharmacol 59.8 (2000): 1015–1022.
Das SK, Vasudevan DM. Protective effects of silymarin, a milk thistle (*Silybum marianum*) derivative on ethanol-induced oxidative stress in liver. Indian J Biochem Biophys 43.5 (2006): 306–311.
Davila JC, et al. Protective effect of flavonoids on drug-induced hepatotoxicity in vitro. Toxicology 57.3 (1989): 267–286.
Deep, G. & Agarwal, R. (2007) Chemopreventive efficacy of silymarin in skin and prostate cancer. Integr Cancer Ther, 6, 130–45.
Deep, G. & Agarwal, R. (2010) Antimetastatic efficacy of silibinin: molecular mechanisms and therapeutic potential against cancer. Cancer Metastasis Rev, 29, 447–63.
Dehmlow C, et al. Scavenging of reactive oxygen species and inhibition of arachidonic acid metabolism by silibinin in human cells. Life Sci 58.18 (1996): 1591–1600.
Doehmer, J., et al. (2011) Assessment of a dry extract from milk thistle (*Silybum marianum*) for interference with human liver cytochrome-P450 activities. Toxicol In Vitro, 25, 21–7.
Dryden GW, et al. Polyphenols and gastrointestinal diseases. Curr Opin Gastroenterol 22.2 (2006): 165–170.
El-Kamary, S. S., et al. (2009) A randomized controlled trial to assess the safety and efficacy of silymarin on symptoms, signs and biomarkers of acute hepatitis. Phytomedicine, 16, 391–400.
El-Zayadi, A. R., et al. (2005) Non-interferon-based therapy: an option for amelioration of necro-inflammation in hepatitis C patients who cannot afford interferon therapy. Liver Int, 25, 746–51.
ESCOP (2009) ESCOP Monographs :The Scientific Foundation for Herbal Medicinal Products Supplement 2009, Stuttgart, Thieme.

Esser-Nobis, K., et al. 2013. Analysis of hepatitis C virus resistance to silibinin in vitro and in vivo points to a novel mechanism involving nonstructural protein 4B. Hepatology, 57, (3) 953–963.

Fantozzi R et al. FMLP-activated neutrophils evoke histamine release from mast cells. Agents Actions 18.1–2 (1986): 155–158.

Favari L, Perez-Alvarez V. Comparative effects of colchicine and silymarin on CCl4-chronic liver damage in rats. Arch Med Res 28.1 (1997): 11–117.

Fehér J et al. Liver-protective action of silymarin therapy in chronic alcoholic liver diseases. Orv Hetil 130.51 (1989): 2723–2727.

Ferenci P et al. Randomized controlled trial of silymarin treatment in patients with cirrhosis of the liver. J Hepatol 9.1 (1989): 105–113.

Ferenci P et al. Silibinin is a potent antiviral agent in patients with chronic hepatitis C not responding to pegylated interferon/ribavirin therapy. Gastroenterology 135.5 (2008): 1561–1567.

Fiebrich F, Koch H. Silymarin, an inhibitor of lipoxygenase. Experientia 35.12 (1979): 1548–1560.

Filburn CR, et al. Bioavailability of a silybin-phosphatidylcholine complex in dogs. J Vet Pharmacol Ther 30.2 (2007): 132–138.

Finkel, T. & Holbrook, N. J. (2000) Oxidants, oxidative stress and the biology of ageing. Nature, 408, 239–47.

Flaig TW et al. A phase I and pharmacokinetic study of silybin-phytosome in prostate cancer patients. Invest New Drugs 25.2 (2007): 139–146.

Flaig, T. W., et al. (2010) A study of high-dose oral silybin-phytosome followed by prostatectomy in patients with localized prostate cancer. Prostate, 70, 848–55.

Floersheim GL. Antagonistic effects against single lethal doses of *Amanita phalloides*. Naunyn Schmiedebergs Arch Pharmacol 293.2 (1976): 171–174.

Floersheim GL et al. Clinical death-cap (*Amanita phalloides*) poisoning: prognostic factors and therapeutic measures. Analysis of 205 cases. Schweiz Med Wochenschr 112.34 (1982): 1164–1177.

Flora K et al. Milk thistle (*Silybum marianum*) for the therapy of liver disease. Am J Gastroenterol 93.2 (1998): 139–143.

Francine R. Milk thistle. Am Fam Physician 72 (2005): 1285.

Fraschini, F., et al. (2002) Pharmacology of Silymarin. Clin Drug Investig, 22, 51–65.

Freedman, N. D., et al. (2011) Silymarin use and liver disease progression in the Hepatitis C Antiviral Long-Term Treatment against Cirrhosis trial. Aliment Pharmacol Ther, 33, 127–137.

Fried, M. W., et al. (2012) Effect of silymarin (milk thistle) on liver disease in patients with chronic hepatitis C unsuccessfully treated with interferon therapy: a randomized controlled trial. JAMA, 308, 274–82.

Gaedeke J et al. Cisplatin nephrotoxicity and protection by silibinin. Nephrol Dial Transplant 11.1 (1996): 55–62.

Galisteo M et al. Hepatotoxicity of tacrine: occurrence of membrane fluidity alterations without involvement of lipid peroxidation. J Pharmacol Exp Ther 294.1 (2000): 160–167.

Gazák, R., et al. (2010) Antioxidant and antiviral activities of silybin fatty acid conjugates. Eur J Med Chem, 45, 1059–67.

Giacomelli S et al. Silybin and its bioavailable phospholipid complex (IdB 1016) potentiate in vitro and in vivo the activity of cisplatin. Life Sci 70.12 (2002): 1447–1459.

Giorgi, V. S., et al. (2012) Silibinin modulates the NF-kappab pathway and pro-inflammatory cytokine production by mononuclear cells from preeclamptic women. J Reprod Immunol, 95, 67–72.

Goey, A. K., et al. (2013) Relevance of in vitro and clinical data for predicting CYP3A4-mediated herb-drug interactions in cancer patients. Cancer Treat Rev.

Gordon A et al. Effects of *Silybum marianum* on serum hepatitis C virus RNA, alanine aminotransferase levels and well-being in patients with chronic hepatitis C. J Gastroenterol Hepatol 21.2 (2006): 275–280.

Greenlee H et al. Clinical applications of *Silybum marianum* in oncology. Integr Cancer Ther 6.2 (2007): 158–65.

Guedj, J., et al. (2012) Understanding silibinin's modes of action against HCV using viral kinetic modeling. J Hepatol, 56, 1019–24.

Gurley BJ et al. Effect of milk thistle (*Silybum marianum*) and black cohosh (*Cimicifuga racemosa*) supplementation on digoxin pharmacokinetics in humans. Drug Metab Dispos 34.1 (2006a): 69–74.

Gurley B et al. Assessing the clinical significance of botanical supplementation on human cytochrome P450 3A activity: comparison of a milk thistle and black cohosh product to rifampin and clarithromycin. J Clin Pharmacol 46.2 (2006b): 201–13.

Gurley, B. J., et al. (2012) Pharmacokinetic herb-drug interactions (part 2): drug interactions involving popular botanical dietary supplements and their clinical relevance. Planta Med, 78, 1490–514.

Hackett, E. S., et al. (2013) Milk thistle and its derivative compounds: a review of opportunities for treatment of liver disease. J Vet Intern Med, 27, 10–6.

Haddad, Y., et al. (2011) Antioxidant and hepatoprotective effects of silibinin in a rat model of nonalcoholic steatohepatitis. Evid Based Complement Alternat Med, 2011, nep164.

Hakova H, Misurova E. Therapeutical effect of silymarin on nucleic acids in the various organs of rats after radiation injury. Radiats Biol Radioecol 36.3 (1996): 365–370.

Hawke, R. L., et al. (2010) Silymarin ascending multiple oral dosing phase I study in noncirrhotic patients with chronic hepatitis C. J Clin Pharmacol, 50, 434–49.

Hermann, R. & von Richter, O. (2012) Clinical evidence of herbal drugs as perpetrators of pharmacokinetic drug interactions. Planta Med, 78, 1458–77.

Hernandez-Gea, V. & Friedman, S. L. (2011) Pathogenesis of liver fibrosis. Annu Rev Pathol, 6, 425–56.

Hess, H. M. (2013) 23 — Herbs and Alternative Remedies. Clinical Pharmacology During Pregnancy. Waltham MA, Academic Press.

Hoh C et al. Pilot study of oral silibinin, a putative chemopreventive agent, in colorectal cancer patients: silibinin levels in plasma, colorectum, and liver and their pharmacodynamic consequences. Clin Cancer Res 12.9 (2006): 2944–2950.

S

Hou, Y. C., et al. (2010) Preventive effect of silymarin in cerebral ischemia-reperfusion-induced brain injury in rats possibly through impairing NF-kappaB and STAT-1 activation. Phytomedicine, 17, 963–73.
Hruby, K., et al. (1983) Chemotherapy of *Amanita phalloides* poisoning with intravenous silibinin. Hum Toxicol, 2, 183–95.
Hsu, W.C., et al. 2012. Characteristics and antioxidant activities of silymarin nanoparticles. J Nanosci.Nanotechnol., 12, (3) 2022–2027.
Huber, R., et al. (2005) Oral silymarin for chronic hepatitis C — a retrospective analysis comparing three dose regimens. Eur J Med Res, 10, 68–70.
Huseini HF et al. The efficacy of *Silybum marianum* (L.) Gaertn. (silymarin) in the treatment of type II diabetes: a randomized, double-blind, placebo-controlled, clinical trial. Phytother Res 20.12 (2006): 1036–1039.
Hussain, S. A. (2007) Silymarin as an adjunct to glibenclamide therapy improves long-term and postprandial glycemic control and body mass index in type 2 diabetes. J Med Food, 10, 543–7.
Hussein A, El-Menshawe S, Afouna M (2012) Enhancement of the in vitro dissolution and in vivo oral bioavailability of silymarin from liquid-filled hard gelatin capsules of semisolid dispersion using Gelucire 44/14 as a carrier. Pharmazie 67, 209–214.
Hutchinson, C., et al. (2010) The iron-chelating potential of silybin in patients with hereditary haemochromatosis. Eur J Clin Nutr, 64, 1239–41.
Jacobs BP et al. Milk thistle for the treatment of liver disease: a systematic review and meta-analysis. Am J Med 113.6 (2002): 506–515.
Karimi G, et al. Cisplatin nephrotoxicity and protection by milk thistle extract in rats. Evid Based Complement Altern Med 2.3 (2005): 383–386.
Kauntz, H., et al. (2012a) Silibinin, a natural flavonoid, modulates the early expression of chemoprevention biomarkers in a preclinical model of colon carcinogenesis. Int J Oncol, 41, 849–54.
Kauntz, H., et al. (2012b) The flavonolignan silibinin potentiates TRAIL-induced apoptosis in human colon adenocarcinoma and in derived TRAIL-resistant metastatic cells. Apoptosis, 17, 797–809.
Khayyal MT et al. Antiulcerogenic effect of some gastrointestinally acting plant extracts and their combination. Arzneimittelforschung 51.7 (2001): 545–553.
Khayyal MT et al. Mechanisms involved in the gastro-protective effect of STW 5 (Iberogast) and its components against ulcers and rebound acidity. Phytomedicine 13 (Suppl 5) (2006): 56–66.
Kidd R. Exacerbation of hemochromatosis by ingestion of milk thistle. Can Fam Physician 54.2 (2008): 182; author reply 182–3.
Kim, M., et al. (2012) Silymarin suppresses hepatic stellate cell activation in a dietary rat model of non-alcoholic steatohepatitis: analysis of isolated hepatic stellate cells. Int J Mol Med, 30, 473–9.
Kim, S., et al. (2009) Silibinin prevents TPA-induced MMP-9 expression and VEGF secretion by inactivation of the Raf/MEK/ERK pathway in MCF-7 human breast cancer cells. Phytomedicine, 16, 573–80.
Kiruthiga PV et al. Protective effect of silymarin on erythrocyte haemolysate against benzo(a)pyrene and exogenous reactive oxygen species (H2O2) induced oxidative stress. Chemosphere 68.8 (2007): 1511–15118.
Kiruthiga, P. V., et al. (2013) Silymarin prevents benzo(a)pyrene-induced toxicity in Wistar rats by modulating xenobiotic-metabolizing enzymes. Toxicol Ind Health 0748233713475524.
Koch HP, et al. Silymarin: potent inhibitor of cyclic AMP phosphodiesterase. Methods Find Exp Clin Pharmacol 7.8 (1985): 409–413.
Krecman V et al. Silymarin inhibits the development of diet-induced hypercholesterolemia in rats. Planta Med 64.2 (1998): 138–142.
Kroll DJ, et al. Milk thistle nomenclature: why it matters in cancer research and pharmacokinetic studies. Integr Cancer Ther 6.2 (2007): 110–1119.
Kropacova K, et al. Protective and therapeutic effect of silymarin on the development of latent liver damage. Radiats Biol Radioecol 38.3 (1998): 411–4115.
Kung, G., et al. (2011) Programmed necrosis, not apoptosis, in the heart. Circ Res, 108, 1017–36.
Lahiri-Chatterjee M et al. A flavonoid antioxidant, silymarin, affords exceptionally high protection against tumor promotion in the SENCAR mouse skin tumorigenesis model. Cancer Res 59.3 (1999): 622–632.
Lecomte J. General pharmacologic properties of silybin and silymarin in the rat. Arch Int Pharmacodyn Ther 214.1 (1975): 165–176.
Letteron P et al. Mechanism for the protective effects of silymarin against carbon tetrachloride-induced lipid peroxidation and hepatotoxicity in mice: evidence that silymarin acts both as an inhibitor of metabolic activation and as a chain-breaking antioxidant. Biochem Pharmacol 39.12 (1990): 2027–2034.
Li, L., et al. (2010) Targeting silibinin in the antiproliferative pathway. Expert Opin Investig Drugs, 19, 243–55.
Lieber, C. S., et al. (2003) Silymarin retards the progression of alcohol-induced hepatic fibrosis in baboons. J Clin Gastroenterol, 37, 336–9.
Liu J et al. Medicinal herbs for hepatitis C virus infection: a Cochrane hepatobiliary systematic review of randomized trials. Am J Gastroenterol 98.3 (2003): 538–544.
Loguercio, C. & Festi, D. (2011) Silybin and the liver: from basic research to clinical practice. World J Gastroenterol, 17, 2288–301.
Loguercio C et al. The effect of a silybin-vitamin e-phospholipid complex on nonalcoholic fatty liver disease: a pilot study. Dig Dis Sci 52.9 (2007): 2387–2395.
Loguercio, C., et al (2012) Silybin combined with phosphatidylcholine and vitamin E in patients with nonalcoholic fatty liver disease: a randomized controlled trial. Free Radic Biol Med, 52, 1658–65.
Lu, J. M., et al. (2010a) Chemical and molecular mechanisms of antioxidants: experimental approaches and model systems. J Cell Mol Med, 14, 840–60.
Lu, P., et al. (2010b) Silibinin attenuates cognitive deficits and decreases of dopamine and serotonin induced by repeated methamphetamine treatment. Behav Brain Res, 207, 387–93.
Lucena MI et al. Effects of silymarin MZ-80 on oxidative stress in patients with alcoholic cirrhosis: results of a randomized, double-blind, placebo-controlled clinical study. Int J Clin Pharmacol Ther 40.1 (2002): 2–8.

MacKinnon SL et al. Silyamandin, a new flavonolignan isolated from milk thistle tinctures. Planta Med 73.11 (2007): 1214–12116.
Madaus. Legalon booklet. Cologne: Madaus, 1989, pp 3–42. (As cited in Combest WL. Milk thistle. US Pharmacist 23.9 (1998).)
Magliulo E, et al. Results of a double blind study on the effect of silymarin in the treatment of acute viral hepatitis, carried out at two medical centres (author's transl). Med Klin 73.28–29 (1978): 1060–1065.
Marino, Z., et al. (2013) Intravenous silibinin monotherapy shows significant antiviral activity in HCV-infected patients in the peri-transplantation period. J Hepatol, 58, 415–20.
Masini A et al. Iron-induced oxidant stress leads to irreversible mitochondrial dysfunctions and fibrosis in the liver of chronic iron-dosed gerbils: the effect of silybin. J Bioenerg Biomembr 32.2 (2000): 175–182.
Mayer KE, et al. Silymarin treatment of viral hepatitis: a systematic review. J Viral Hepat 12.6 (2005): 559–567.
Mazzio, E. A., et al. (1998) Food constituents attenuate monoamine oxidase activity and peroxide levels in C6 astrocyte cells. Planta Med, 64, 603–6.
McBride, A., et al. (2012) *Silybum marianum* (milk thistle) in the management and prevention of hepatotoxicity in a patient undergoing reinduction therapy for acute myelogenous leukemia. J Oncol Pharm Pract, 18, 360–5.
McClure, J., et al. (2012) Silibinin inhibits HIV-1 infection by reducing cellular activation and proliferation. PLoS One, 7, e41832.
Mengs, U., et al. (2012) Legalon(R) SIL: the antidote of choice in patients with acute hepatotoxicity from amatoxin poisoning. Curr Pharm Biotechnol, 13, 1964–70.
Mills S, Bone K. Principles and practice of phytotherapy. London: Churchill Livingstone, 2000.
Morazzoni P, Bombardelli E. *Silybum marianum* (*Carduus marianus*). Fitoterapia 66 (1995): 3–42.
Morishima, C., et al. (2010) Silymarin inhibits in vitro T-cell proliferation and cytokine production in hepatitis C virus infection. Gastroenterology, 138, 671–81, 681.e1–2.
Mourelle M et al. Prevention of CCL4-induced liver cirrhosis by silymarin. Fundam Clin Pharmacol 3.3 (1989): 183–191.
Muriel P, Mourelle M. Prevention by silymarin of membrane alterations in acute CCl4 liver damage. J Appl Toxicol 10.4 (1990): 275–279.
Muriel P et al. Silymarin protects against paracetamol-induced lipid peroxidation and liver damage. J Appl Toxicol 12.6 (1992): 439–442.
Nencini C, et al. Protective effect of silymarin on oxidative stress in rat brain. Phytomedicine 14.2–3 (2007): 129–135.
Neumann, U. P., et al. (2010) Successful prevention of hepatitis C virus (HCV) liver graft reinfection by silibinin mono-therapy. J Hepatol, 52, 951–2.
Niture, S. K., et al. (2014) Regulation of Nrf2-an update. Free Radic Biol Med 66: 36–44.
Osuchowski, M. F., et al. (2004) Alterations in regional brain neurotransmitters by silymarin, a natural antioxidant flavonoid mixture, in BALB/c mice. Pharm Biol 42, 384–9.
Palasciano G et al. The effect of silymarin on plasma levels of malondialdehyde in patients receiving long-term treatment with psychotropic drugs. Curr Ther Res 55 (1994): 537–545.
Par A et al. Oxidative stress and antioxidant defense in alcoholic liver disease and chronic hepatitis C. Orv Hetil 141.30 (2000): 1655–1659.
Parasassi T et al. Drug-membrane interactions: silymarin, silybin and microsomal membranes. Cell Biochem Funct 2.2 (1984): 85–88.
Pares A et al. Effects of silymarin in alcoholic patients with cirrhosis of the liver: results of a controlled, double-blind, randomized and multicenter trial. J Hepatol 28.4 (1998): 615–621.
Payer, B. A., et al. (2010) Successful HCV eradication and inhibition of HIV replication by intravenous silibinin in an HIV-HCV coinfected patient. J Clin Virol, 49, 131–3.
Pias, E. K. & Aw, T. Y. (2002) Early redox imbalance mediates hydroperoxide-induced apoptosis in mitotic competent undifferentiated PC-12 cells. Cell Death Differ, 9, 1007–16.
Pias, E. K., et al. (2003) Differential effects of superoxide dismutase isoform expression on hydroperoxide-induced apoptosis in PC-12 cells. J Biol Chem, 278, 13294–301.
Pietrangelo A et al. Antioxidant activity of silybin in vivo during long-term iron overload in rats. Gastroenterology 109.6 (1995): 1941–1949.
Polyak SJ et al. Inhibition of T-cell inflammatory cytokines, hepatocyte NF-kappaB signaling, and HCV infection by standardized Silymarin. Gastroenterology 132.5 (2007): 1925–1936.
Polyak, S. J., et al H. (2010) Identification of hepatoprotective flavonolignans from silymarin. Proc Natl Acad Sci U S A, 107, 5995–9.
Polyak, S. J., et al. (2013) Silymarin for HCV infection. Antivir Ther. 18: 141–147.
Post-White J, et al. Advances in the use of milk thistle (*Silybum marianum*). Integr Cancer Ther 6.2 (2007): 104–109.
Poynard, T., et al. (2009) Peginterferon alfa-2b and ribavirin: effective in patients with hepatitis C who failed interferon alfa/ribavirin therapy. Gastroenterology, 136, 1618–28.e2.
Pradhan SC, Girish C. Hepatoprotective herbal drug, silymarin from experimental pharmacology to clinical medicine. Indian J Med Res 124.5 (2006): 491.
Rainone F. Milk thistle. Am Fam Physician 72.7 (2005): 1285–1288.
Rambaldi A et al. Milk thistle for alcoholic and/or hepatitis B or C liver diseases–a systematic cochrane hepato-biliary group review with meta-analyses of randomized clinical trials. Am J Gastroenterol 100.11 (2005): 2583–2591.
Rambaldi A, et al. Milk thistle for alcoholic and/or hepatitis B or C virus liver diseases. Cochrane Database Syst Rev 4 (2007): CD003620.
Raza, S. S., et al. (2011) Silymarin protects neurons from oxidative stress associated damages in focal cerebral ischemia: a behavioral, biochemical and immunohistological study in Wistar rats. J Neurol Sci, 309, 45–54.

S

Reuland, D. J., et al. (2012) Upregulation of phase II enzymes through phytochemical activation of Nrf2 protects cardiomyocytes against oxidant stress. Free Radic Biol Med, 56C, 102–111.

Rui YC et al. Effects of silybin on production of oxygen free radical, lipoperoxide and leukotrienes in brain following ischemia and reperfusion. Zhongguo Yao Li Xue Bao 11.5 (1990): 418–421.

Sagar SM. Future directions for research on *Silybum marianum* for cancer patients. Integr Cancer Ther 6.2 (2007): 166–173.

Saller R, et al. The use of silymarin in the treatment of liver diseases. Drugs 61.14 (2001): 2035–2063.

Saller R et al. An updated systematic review with meta-analysis for the clinical evidence of silymarin. Forsch Komplementmed 15.1 (2008): 9–20.

Salmi HA, Sarna S. Effect of silymarin on chemical, functional, and morphological alterations of the liver. A double-blind controlled study. Scand J Gastroenterol 17.4 (1982): 517–521.

Salmond, S. J., et al. (2010) Hep573 study–a randomised double-blind placebo-controlled trial of silymarin alone or combined with antioxidants in chronic hepatitis C. Proceedings of Digestive Diseases Week, AASLD. New Orleans, LA, Gastroenterology.

Sayyah, M., et al. (2010) Comparison of *Silybum marianum* (L.) Gaertn. with fluoxetine in the treatment of Obsessive-Compulsive Disorder. Prog Neuropsychopharmacol Biol Psychiatry, 34, 362–5.

Schrieber SJ et al. The pharmacokinetics of silymarin is altered in patients with hepatitis C virus and nonalcoholic fatty liver disease and correlates with plasma caspase-3/7 activity. Drug Metab Dispos 36.9 (2008): 1909–1916.

Schuppan D et al. Alcohol and liver fibrosis: pathobiochemistry and treatment. Z Gastroenterol 33.9 (1995): 546–550.

Seeff LB et al. Herbal product use by persons enrolled in the hepatitis C Antiviral Long-Term Treatment Against Cirrhosis (HALT-C) Trial. Hepatology 47.2 (2008): 605–612.

Shaker, E., et al. (2010) Silymarin, the antioxidant component and *Silybum marianum* extracts prevent liver damage. Food Chem Toxicol, 48, 803–6.

Skottova N, Krecman V. Dietary silymarin improves removal of low density lipoproteins by the perfused rat liver. Acta Univ Palacki Olomuc Fac Med 141 (1998a): 39–40.

Skottova N, Krecman V. Silymarin as a potential hypocholesterolaemic drug. Physiol Res 47.1 (1998b): 1–7.

Sobolova L et al. Effect of silymarin and its polyphenolic fraction on cholesterol absorption in rats. Pharmacol Res 53.2 (2006): 104–112.

Somogyi A et al. Short term treatment of type II hyperlipoproteinaemia with silymarin. Acta Med Hung 46.4 (1989): 289–295.

Son, T. G., et al. (2008) Hormetic dietary phytochemicals. Neuromolecular Med, 10, 236–46.

Sonnenbichler J et al. Stimulatory effects of silibinin and silicristin from the milk thistle *Silybum marianum* on kidney cells. J Pharmacol Exp Ther 290.3 (1999): 1375–1383.

Suksomboon, N., et al. (2011) Meta-analysis of the effect of herbal supplement on glycemic control in type 2 diabetes. J Ethnopharmacol, 137, 1328–33.

Ting, H., et al. (2013) Molecular mechanisms of silibinin-mediated cancer chemoprevention with major emphasis on prostate cancer. AAPS J, 15, 707–16.

Tkacz B, Dworniak D. [Sylimarol in the treatment of acute viral hepatitis]. Wiad Lek 36.8 (1983): 613–6116.

Toklu HZ et al. Silymarin, the antioxidant component of *Silybum marianum*, prevents sepsis-induced acute lung and brain injury. J Surg Res 145.2 (2008): 214–222.

Torres M et al. Does *Silybum marianum* play a role in the treatment of chronic hepatitis C? P R Health Sci J 23 (2 Suppl) (2004): 69–74.

Trappoliere, M., et al. (2009) Silybin, a component of silymarin, exerts anti-inflammatory and anti-fibrogenic effects on human hepatic stellate cells. J Hepatol, 50, 1102–11.

Trinchet JC et al. Treatment of alcoholic hepatitis with silymarin: a double-blind comparative study in 116 patients. Gastroenterol Clin Biol 13.2 (1989): 120–124.

Tsai JH et al. Effects of silymarin on the resolution of liver fibrosis induced by carbon tetrachloride in rats. J Viral Hepat 15.7 (2008): 508–514.

Tyutyulkova N et al. Hepatoprotective effect of silymarin (Carsil) on liver of D-galactosamine treated rats: biochemical and morphological investigations. Methods Find Exp Clin Pharmacol 3.2 (1981): 71–77.

Tyutyulkova N et al. Effect of silymarin (Carsil) on the microsomal glycoprotein and protein biosynthesis in liver of rats with experimental galactosamine hepatitis. Methods Find Exp Clin Pharmacol 5.3 (1983): 181–184.

Tzeng, J. I., et al. (2013) Silymarin decreases connective tissue growth factor to improve liver fibrosis in rats treated with carbon tetrachloride. Phytother Res. 27: 1023–1028.

Valenzuela A, Guerra R. Protective effect of the flavonoid silybin dihemisuccinate on the toxicity of phenylhydrazine on rat liver. FEBS Lett 181.2 (1985): 291–294.

Varzi HN et al. Effect of silymarin and vitamin E on gentamicin-induced nephrotoxicity in dogs. J Vet Pharmacol Ther 30.5 (2007): 477–481.

Velussi M et al. Long-term (12 months) treatment with an anti-oxidant drug (silymarin) is effective on hyperinsulinemia, exogenous insulin need and malondialdehyde levels in cirrhotic diabetic patients. J Hepatol 26.4 (1997): 871–879.

Venkataramanan R, et al. In vitro and in vivo assessment of herb drug interactions. Life Sci 78.18 (2006): 2105–2115.

Vidlar, A., et al. (2010) The safety and efficacy of a silymarin and selenium combination in men after radical prostatectomy — a six month placebo-controlled double-blind clinical trial. Biomed Pap Med Fac Univ Palacky Olomouc Czech Repub, 154, 239–44.

Vogel G et al. Protection by silibinin against *Amanita phalloides* intoxication in beagles. Toxicol Appl Pharmacol 73.3 (1984): 355–362.

von Schonfeld J, et al. Silibinin, a plant extract with antioxidant and membrane stabilizing properties, protects exocrine pancreas from cyclosporin A toxicity. Cell Mol Life 53.11–12 (1997): 917–920.

Wagoner, J., et al. (2010) Multiple effects of silymarin on the hepatitis C virus lifecycle. Hepatology, 51, 1912–21.

Wagoner, J., et al. (2011) Differential in vitro effects of intravenous versus oral formulations of silibinin on the HCV life cycle and inflammation. PLoS One, 6, e16464.
Wen Z et al. Pharmacokinetics and metabolic profile of free, conjugated, and total silymarin flavonolignans in human plasma after oral administration of milk thistle extract. Drug Metab Dispos 36.1 (2008): 65–72.
Wesolowska O et al. Influence of silybin on biophysical properties of phospholipid bilayers. Acta Pharmacol Sin 28.2 (2007): 296–306.
Whittington C. Exacerbation of hemochromatosis by ingestion of milk thistle. Can Fam Physician 53.10 (2007): 1671–1673.
Wu JW, et al. Drug–drug interactions of silymarin on the perspective of pharmacokinetics. J Ethnopharmacol 121.2 (2009): 185–193.
Yin, F., et al. (2011) Silibinin: a novel inhibitor of Abeta aggregation. Neurochem Int, 58, 399–403.
Zeng, J., et al. (2011) Chemopreventive and chemotherapeutic effects of intravesical silibinin against bladder cancer by acting on mitochondria. Mol Cancer Ther, 10, 104–16.
Zhang S, Morris ME. Effect of the flavonoids biochanin A and silymarin on the P-glycoprotein-mediated transport of digoxin and vinblastine in human intestinal Caco-2 cells. Pharm Res 20.8 (2003): 1184–1191.
Zhao J et al. Significant inhibition by the flavonoid antioxidant silymarin against 12-O-tetradecanoylphorbol 13-acetate-caused modulation of antioxidant and inflammatory enzymes, and cyclooxygenase 2 and interleukin-1alpha expression in SENCAR mouse epidermis: implications in the prevention of stage I tumor promotion. Mol Carcinog 26.4 (1999): 321–333.

Turmeric

HISTORICAL NOTE Turmeric is a perennial herb, yielding a rhizome that produces a yellow powder that gives curry its characteristic yellow colour and is used to colour French mustard and the robes of Hindu priests. It has been used in Hindu religious ceremonies, and Hindus also apply a mixture of turmeric and sandalwood powder on their foreheads (Jagetia & Aggarwal 2007). Turmeric was probably first cultivated as a dye, and then as a condiment and cosmetic. It is often used as an inexpensive substitute for saffron in cooking and in the 13th century Marco Polo marvelled at its similarities to saffron. In Chinese medicine, turmeric was used in the treatment of inflammatory and digestive disorders and was also used in tooth powder or paste (Anonymous 2001). In Ayurvedic medicine, it was used to treat a wide variety of disorders, including rheumatism, skin conditions, inflammation, intestinal worms, hepatic disorders, biliousness, dyspepsia, diarrhoea, constipation and colic (Jagetia & Aggarwal 2007). In addition to its use in cardiovascular disease and gastrointestinal disorders, research has focused on turmeric's antioxidant, hepatoprotective, anti-inflammatory, anticarcinogenic and antimicrobial properties (Anonymous 2001). Curcumin was first discovered from the rhizomes of turmeric by Harvard College laboratory scientists Vogel and Pelletier and published in 1815 (Gupta et al 2013). Turmeric is believed to promote the flow of *qi* (Jagetia & Aggarwal 2007).

COMMON NAME

Turmeric

OTHER NAMES

Chiang-huang, curcuma, curcumae longae rhizoma, curcuma rhizome, e zhu, haldi, haridra, Indian saffron, jiang huang, jiang huang curcumae rhizoma, turmeric rhizome, turmeric root, yellow root, yu jin, zedoary

BOTANICAL NAME/FAMILY

Curcuma longa (family Zingiberaceae [ginger])

PLANT PART USED

Dried secondary rhizome (containing not less than 3% curcuminoids calculated as curcumin and not less than 3% volatile oil, calculated on dry-weight basis).

CHEMICAL COMPONENTS

Turmeric rhizome contains 5% phenolic curcuminoids (diarylheptanoids), which give turmeric the yellow colour. The most significant curcuminoid is curcumin (diferuloylmethane). It also contains up to 5% essential oil, including sesquiterpene (e.g. Zingiberene), sesquiterpene alcohols, sesquiterpene ketones, and monoterpenes.

Turmeric also contains immune-stimulating polysaccharides, including acid glucans known as ukonan A, B and C (Evans & Trease 2002).

MAIN ACTIONS

Most research has focused on a series of curcumin constituents found in turmeric. Many of the animal studies involve parenteral administration as oral turmeric or curcumin was considered less active because curcumin is poorly absorbed by the gastrointestinal tract and only trace amounts appear in the blood after oral intake (Ammon & Wahl 1991). Curcumin possesses anti-inflammatory, antioxidant, immunomodulatory, wound-healing, anti-proliferative and antimicrobial activities (Dulbecco & Savarino 2013). Curcumin may, however, have significant activity in the gastrointestinal tract, and systemic effects may take place as a consequence of local gastrointestinal effects or be associated with metabolites of the curcuminoids.

ANTIOXIDANT

Studies have shown that turmeric, as well as curcumin, has significant antioxidant activity (Ak & Gulcin 2008, Bengmark 2006, Menon & Sudheer 2007, Shalini & Srinivas 1987, Soudamini et al 1992). Turmeric not only exerts direct free radical scavenging activity, it also appears to enhance the antioxidant activity of endogenous antioxidants, such as glutathione peroxidase, catalase and quinine reductase. Curcumin has been shown to induce phase II detoxification enzymes (glutathione peroxidase, glutathione reductase, glucose-6-phosphate dehydrogenase and catalase) (Iqbal et al 2003). Additionally, its antioxidant effects are 10-fold more potent than ascorbic acid or resveratrol (Song et al 2001). In addition to curcumin, turmeric contains the antioxidants protocatechuic acid and ferulic acid, and exhibits significant protection to DNA against oxidative damage in vitro (Kumar et al 2006).

Turmeric's antioxidant activity may protect against damage produced by myocardial and cerebral ischaemia (Al-Omar et al 2006, Fiorillo et al 2008, Shukla et al 2008) and diabetes (Farhangkhoee et al 2006, Jain et al 2006, Kowluru & Kanwar 2007). Turmeric has been shown to restore myocardial antioxidant status, inhibit lipid peroxidation and protect against ischaemia–reperfusion-induced myocardial injuries in two animal studies (Fiorillo et al 2008, Mohanty et al 2004). The mechanism is likely to be due to curcumin's antioxidant and anti-inflammatory effects. Curcumin has also been found to prevent protein glycosylation and lipid peroxidation caused by high glucose levels in vitro (Jain et al 2006) and to improve diabetic nephropathy (Srinivasan 2005) and retinopathy (Kowluru & Kanwar 2007). Turmeric has also been shown to suppress cataract development and collagen cross-linking, promote wound healing, and lower blood lipids and glucose levels (Jain et al 2006, Panchatcharam et al 2006).

Anti-inflammatory

There have been a large number of studies examining the anti-inflammatory effects of curcumin. There is strong molecular evidence published for curcumin's potency to target multiple inflammatory diseases (Henrotin et al 2013). Turmeric is a dual inhibitor of the arachidonic acid cascade. Curcumin has been shown to exert anti-inflammatory effects via phospholipase, lipo-oxygenase, COX-2, leukotrienes, thromboxane, prostaglandins, nitric oxide (NO), collagenase, elastase, hyaluronidase, monocyte chemoattractant protein-1, IFN-inducible protein, TNF-α and IL-12 (Chainani-Wu 2003, Lantz et al 2005, Rao 2007). Due to its anti-inflammatory effects, curcumin has shown promise in many chronic disorders such as arthritis, allergies, arteriosclerosis, colitis, diabetes, respiratory disorders, hepatic injury, pancreatic disease, intestinal disorders, eye diseases, neurodegenerative diseases and various cancers (Aggarwal et al 2007, Bengmark 2006).

The anti-inflammatory effect of curcumin was tested in adjuvant-induced chronic inflammation rats, where it was found that curcumin significantly reduced C-reactive protein, TNF-α, IL-1 and NO, with no significant changes observed in PGE_2 and leukotriene B_4 levels or lymphocyte proliferation (Banerjee et al 2003). Curcumin has also been shown to inhibit inflammation in experimental pancreatitis via inhibition of NF-κB and activator protein-1 in two rat models (Gukovsky et al 2003).

NF-kappa-B inhibition

The many and varied effects of curcumin may be partly associated with the inhibition of the transcription factor, nuclear factor-kappa beta (NF-κB), and induction of heat shock proteins (HSP). NF-κB is a transcription factor pivotal in the regulation of inflammatory genes and is also closely associated with the heat shock response, which is a cellular defence mechanism that confers broad protection against various cytotoxic stimuli. Inhibition of NF-κB may reduce inflammation and protect cells against damage (Chang 2001) and curcumin has been found to attenuate experimental colitis in animal models through a mechanism correlated with the inhibition of NF-κB (Salh et al 2003). The clinical significance of this is unclear.

Gastrointestinal effects

Hepatoprotective

Extracts of both turmeric and curcumin have been found to prevent and improve carbon tetrachloride-induced liver injury, both in vivo and in vitro (Abu-Rizq et al 2008, Deshpande et al 1998, Fu et al 2008, Kang et al 2002, Wu et al 2008). Curcumin also protects against dimethylnitrosamine-induced liver injury (Farombi et al 2008), reverses aflatoxin-induced liver damage in experimental animals (Soni et al 1992) and effectively suppresses the hepatic microvascular inflammatory response to lipopolysaccharides in vivo (Lukita-Atmadja et al 2002). An ethanol-soluble fraction of turmeric was shown to contain three antioxidant compounds — curcumin, demethoxycurcumin and bisdemethoxycurcumin — which exert similar hepatoprotective activity to silybin and silychristin in vitro (Song et al 2001).

Several different mechanisms may contribute to turmeric's hepatoprotective activity. Curcumin has been shown to prevent lipoperoxidation of subcellular membranes in a dosage-dependent manner, due to an antioxidant mechanism (Quiles et al 1998) and turmeric may also protect the liver via inhibition of NF-κB (see above), which has been implicated in the pathogenesis of alcoholic liver disease. Curcumin also appears to chelate hepatic and serum iron in vivo

(Jiao et al 2006, 2009). Iron is pro-oxidant to the liver, which may be problematic during hepatic disease. Recent research also suggests that curcumin may be useful in preventing hepatic fibrosis caused by chronic liver disease (Fu et al 2008, O'Connell & Rushworth 2008). Curcumin also blocks endotoxin-mediated activation of NF-κB and suppresses the expression of cytokines, chemokines, COX-2 and iNOS in Kupffer cells (Nanji et al 2003).

Cholagogue and hypolipidaemic

The extracts of turmeric and curcumin have shown dose-dependent hypolipidaemic activity in vivo (Asai & Miyazawa 2001, Babu & Srinivasan 1997, Keshavarz 1976, Manjunatha & Srinivasan 2007a, 2007b, Ramirez-Tortosa et al 1999, Soudamini et al 1992). One in vivo study suggests that curcumin may stimulate the conversion of cholesterol into bile acids, and therefore increase the excretion of cholesterol (Srinivasan & Sambaiah 1991). A further study demonstrated that supplementation with turmeric reduces fatty streak development and oxidative stress (Quiles et al 2002). Curcumin also increases LDL receptor mRNA (Peschel et al 2007). Oral curcumin has also been shown to stimulate contraction of the gall bladder and promote the flow of bile in healthy subjects (Rasyid & Lelo 1999).

Antispasmodic

Curcuminoids exhibit smooth muscle relaxant activity possibly mediated through calcium channel blockade, although additional mechanisms cannot be ruled out (Gilani et al 2005). Curcuminoids produced antispasmodic effects on isolated guinea pig ileum and rat uterus by receptor-dependent and independent mechanisms (Itthipanichpong et al 2003).

Cancer

Curcumin has been studied for its wide-ranging effects on tumourigenesis, angiogenesis, apoptosis and signal transduction pathways (Gururaj et al 2002, Mohan et al 2000, Thaloor et al 1998). It is known to inhibit oncogenesis during both the promotion and the progression periods in a variety of cancers (Anto et al 1996, Kuttan et al 1985, Menon et al 1999, Ruby et al 1995). Curcumin was found to possess chemopreventive effects against cancers of the skin, stomach, colon, prostate, and breast, as well as oral cancer in mice.

Chemoprevention

Chemoprevention refers to reversing, suppressing or preventing the process of carcinogenesis. Carcinogenesis results from the accumulation of multiple sequential mutations and alterations in nuclear and cytoplasmic molecules, culminating in invasive neoplasms. These events have traditionally been separated into three phases: initiation, promotion and progression. Typically, initiation is rapid, whereas promotion and progression can take many years. Ultimately, chemoprevention aims at preventing the growth and survival of cells already committed to becoming malignant (Gescher et al 1998, 2001).

Curcumin has been found to inhibit the invasion, proliferation and metastasis of various cancers in vivo (Kunnumakkara et al 2008). Curcumin has been found to effectively block carcinogen-induced skin (Azuine & Bhide 1992), colon (Rao et al 1995a, 1995b, 1995c, 1999) and liver (Chuang et al 2000) carcinogenesis in animals. It has been suggested that the chemoprotective activity of curcumin occurs via changes in enzymes involved in both carcinogen bioactivation and oestrogen metabolism. This is supported by the findings that curcumin treatment produced changes in CYP1A, CYP3A and GST in mice (Valentine et al 2006) and alleviated the CCl_4-induced inactivation of CYPs 1A, 2B, 2C and 3A isozymes in rats, possibly through its antioxidant properties, without inducing hepatic CYP (Sugiyama et al 2006).

Oral curcumin inhibited chemically-induced skin carcinogenesis in mice (Huang et al 1992) and curcumin prevented radiation-induced mammary and pituitary tumours in rats (Inano & Onoda 2002). Curcumin and genistein (from soybeans) inhibited the growth of oestrogen-positive human breast MCF-7 cells induced individually or by a mixture of the pesticides endosulfane, dichlorodiphenyltrichloroethane (DDT) and chlordane, or 17-beta oestradiol (Verma et al 1997). Another study found that curcumin inhibited breast cancer metastases in immunodeficient animals (Bachmeier et al 2007). This may be due to the ability of curcumin to reduce NF-κB and therefore downregulate the two inflammatory cytokines CXCL1 and CXCL2 (Bachmeier et al 2008).

Apoptosis

Apoptosis (programmed cell death) plays a crucial role in regulating cell numbers by eliminating damaged or cancerous cells. Curcumin has been shown to induce apoptosis in many different cancer cell lines, including breast, leukaemia, lymphoma, melanoma, ovarian, colorectal, lung and pancreatic in vitro (Kim et al 2001, Kuo et al 1996, Li et al 2007, Lin et al 2007, Lev-Ari et al 2006, Marin et al 2007, Skommer et al 2006, 2007, Tian et al 2008). Curcumin has also increased apoptosis in breast and ovarian cancers in vivo (Bachmeier et al 2007, Lin et al 2007). Curcumin has been demonstrated to induce apoptosis in human basal cell carcinoma cells associated with the p53 signalling pathway, which controls intracellular redox status, levels of oxidation-damaged DNA and oxidative stress-induced apoptosis (Jee et al 1998). Curcumin has also been found to induce apoptosis in human mutant p53 melanoma cell lines and block the NF-κB cell survival pathway and suppress the apoptotic inhibitor known as XIAP. Because melanoma cells with mutant p53 are strongly resistant to conventional chemotherapy, curcumin may overcome the chemoresistance of these cells and provide potential new avenues for treatment (Bush et al 2001).

Curcumin has also been found to inhibit prostate cancer cell growth in mice (Dorai et al 2001) and decrease proliferation and induce apoptosis in androgen-dependent and androgen-independent prostate cancer cells in vitro. This was found to be mediated through modulation of apoptosis suppressor proteins and interference with growth factor receptor signalling pathways (Dorai et al 2000). However, in a further study with rats curcumin did not prevent prostate carcinogenesis (Imaida et al 2001).

Antiproliferative

Reduction in proliferation and/or increased apoptosis will lead to tumour regression; however, a more potent effect will be achieved if the two mechanisms occur simultaneously. Curcumin has been shown to do this. The inhibition of cell proliferation is partly related to inhibition of various kinases, such as protein kinase and phosphorylase kinase (Reddy & Aggarwal 1994), and inhibition of several oncogenes and transcription factors. For example, turmeric inhibited epidermal growth factor receptor (EGF-R) signalling via multiple mechanisms, including downregulation of the EGF-R protein, inhibition of intrinsic EGF-R tyrosine kinase activity and inhibition of ligand-induced activation of the EGF-R (Dorai et al 2000). These mechanisms may be particularly important in preventing prostate cancer cells from progressing to a hormone refractory state (Dorai et al 2000). Curcumin has also been found to suppress the growth of multiple breast cancer cell lines and deplete p185neu, the protein product of the HER2/neu proto-oncogene, which is thought to be important in human carcinogenesis (Hong et al 1999).

Antimetastatic

Curcumin demonstrated the ability to reduce lung metastases from melanoma cells in mice. The activity of curcumin is varied. In cell adhesion assays, curcumin-treated cells showed a dose-dependent reduction in their binding to four extracellular matrix proteins (binding to proteins is associated with the spreading of the cancer). Another study found that curcumin effectively suppressed COX-2, vascular endothelial growth factor and intercellular adhesion molecules, while enhancing the expression of antimetastatic proteins, tissue inhibitor metalloproteases-2, non-metastatic gene 23 and E-cadherin, a transmembrane protein that plays an important role in cell adhesion (Kuttan et al 2007). Curcumin-treated cells showed a marked reduction in the expression of integrin receptors (integrins functionally connect the cell interior with the extracellular matrix, another process necessary for metastases).

Chemotherapy

Curcumin enhanced the cytotoxicity of chemotherapeutic agents in prostate cancer cells in vitro by inducing the expression of certain androgen receptor and transcription factors and suppressing NF-κB activation (Hour et al 2002). Curcumin enhanced the antitumour effect of cisplatin against fibrosarcoma (Navis et al 1999), fluorouracil and oxaliplatin in colorectal cancer (Du et al 2006, Li et al 2007) and gemcitabine and paclitaxel in bladder cancer (Kamat et al 2007). Curcumin also attenuated multidrug resistance in a non-small cell lung cancer cell line (Andjelkovic et al 2008) and acted as a radiosensitiser for cervical cancer in vitro (Javvadi et al 2008).

Curcumin, however, was found to significantly inhibit cyclophosphamide-induced tumour regression in an in vivo model of human breast cancer. It is suspected that this occurred as a result of inhibition of free radical generation and blockade of JNK function. As such, curcumin intake should be limited in people undergoing treatment for breast cancer with cyclophosphamide until further investigation can clarify the significance of these findings (Somasundaram et al 2002).

Immunomodulation

Curcumin administration was found to significantly increase the total white blood cell count and circulating antibodies in mice. A significant increase in macrophage phagocytic activity was also observed in curcumin-treated animals (Antony et al 1999). However, curcumin has also been demonstrated to have some immunosuppressive activity. Curcumin inhibits PAR2- and PAR4-mediated human mast cell activation by blocking the ERK pathway (Baek et al 2003).

An in vivo study using a cardiac transplant model found that curcumin also significantly reduced expression of IL-2, IFN-gamma and granzyme B (a serine protease associated with the activity of killer T-lymphocytes and NK cells) and increased mean survival time. Curcumin was further shown to work synergistically with the antirejection drug cyclosporin (Chueh et al 2003).

Curcumin also modulates other interleukins and has been shown in vitro to be a potent inhibitor of the production of the pro-inflammatory cytokine IL-8, thereby reducing tumour growth and carcinoma cell viability. Curcumin not only inhibited IL-8 production but also inhibited signal transduction through IL-8 receptors (Hidaka et al 2002) and inhibited cell proliferation, cell-mediated cytotoxicity and cytokine production most likely by inhibiting NF-κB target genes (Gao et al 2004).

Cardiovascular effects

Antiplatelet

Curcumin has been shown to inhibit platelet aggregation in vivo (Chen et al 2007, R Srivastava et al 1985, 1986) and in vitro (Jantan et al 2008, KC Srivastava 1989, KC Srivastava et al 1995). The anticoagulant effect of curcumin is weaker than that of aspirin, which is four-fold more potent than curcumin in treatment of collagen- and noradrenaline-induced thrombosis. Curcumin 100 mg/kg and aspirin 25 mg/kg resulted in 60% protection from thrombosis (Srivastava et al 1985).

Anti-atherogenic

A hydro-ethanolic extract of turmeric was found to decrease LDL oxidation, lower the oxidation of erythrocyte and liver membranes, as well as have a vitamin E-sparing effect in rabbits fed a diet high in saturated fat and cholesterol (Mesa et al 2003, Ramirez-Tortosa et al 1999). The atheroscleroprotective potential of turmeric was further demonstrated by an animal study that found turmeric lowered blood pressure and reduced the atherogenic properties of cholesterol (Zahid Ashraf et al 2005). Curcumin also inhibits the proliferation and migration of vascular smooth muscle cells in vitro (Yang et al 2006).

Many in vivo studies have investigated the effects of dietary curcumin on blood cholesterol in diabetic animals (Babu & Srinivasan 1997, Manjunatha & Srinivasan 2007a, 2007b, Pari & Murugan 2007). The two Manjunatha and Srinivasan studies found that curcumin significantly lowered plasma cholesterol, but only lowered hepatic cholesterol in animals with normal baseline cholesterol. Additionally, hepatic alpha-tocopherol and glutathione levels and serum glutathione peroxidase and glutathione transferase were increased. Babu and Srinivasan (1997) also found a significant decrease in blood triglyceride and phospholipid levels. In a parallel study in which diabetic animals were maintained on a high cholesterol diet, curcumin lowered cholesterol and phospholipid and countered the elevated liver and renal cholesterol and triglyceride levels seen in the diabetic animals (Babu & Srinivasan 1997).

Wound healing

Wound healing is a highly ordered process, requiring complex and coordinated interactions involving peptide growth factors, of which transforming growth factor-beta (TGF-beta) is one of the most important. Nitric oxide is also an important factor in healing, and its production is regulated by iNOS. Topical application of curcumin accelerated wound healing in normal and diabetic rats. The wound healing is partly associated with the regulation of the growth factor TGF-beta-1 and iNOS (Mani et al 2002). Curcumin's wound-healing ability has been confirmed in several other animal studies (Sidhu et al 1998, Sidhu et al 1999). Wounds of animals treated with curcumin showed earlier re-epithelialisation, improved neovascularisation, increased migration of various cells, including dermal myofibroblasts, fibroblasts and macrophages into the wound bed, and a higher collagen content (Sidhu et al 1999). It appears to be effective when used orally or as a local application.

Curcumin has also demonstrated powerful inhibition against hydrogen peroxide damage in human keratinocytes and fibroblasts (Phan et al 2001) and pretreatment with curcumin significantly enhanced the rate of wound contraction, decreased mean wound-healing time, increased synthesis of collagen, hexosamine,

DNA and NO and improved fibroblast and vascular densities in full thickness wounds in mice exposed to whole-body gamma-radiation (Jagetia & Rajanikant 2004).

Antibacterial/Antimicrobial

Curcumin is a highly pleiotropic molecule that was first shown to exhibit antibacterial activity in 1949 (Gupta et al 2013). Turmeric is used as an antimicrobial for preserving food (Jayaprakasha et al 2005) and has been found to have antifungal activity, as well as inhibiting aspergillus growth and aflatoxin production in feeds (Gowda et al 2004).

Curcumin has also been found to have dose-dependent, antiprotozoan activity against *Giardia lamblia* with inhibition of parasite growth and adherent capacity, induction of morphological alterations and apoptosis-like changes in vitro (Perez-Arriaga et al 2006). Curcumin has also shown in vitro and in vivo activity against malaria, with inhibition of growth of chloroquine-resistant *Plasmodium falciparum* in vitro and enhancement of survival in mice infected with *P. berghei* (Reddy et al 2005).

OTHER ACTIONS

Curcumin's anti-inflammatory and antioxidant actions may be useful in preventing neurodegenerative diseases, such as Alzheimer's disease and Parkinson's disease, and curcumin has been found to target multiple pathogenic cascades in preclinical models (transgenic and amyloid infusion models) of Alzheimer's disease (Cole et al 2005, Calabrese et al 2006). Curcumin has also been found to dose-dependently inhibit neuroglial proliferation, with low doses being as effective as higher doses, given a longer period of treatment (Ambegaokar et al 2003). It may also enhance immune clearance of amyloidosis in the brain (Zhang et al 2006).

Theracurmin, a highly absorptive curcumin dispersed with colloidal nanoparticles, recently exhibited an inhibitory action against alcohol intoxication after drinking in humans. This was shown by the reduced acetaldehyde concentration of the blood (Sasaki et al 2011).

Curcumin (20 mg/kg body weight) treatment significantly inhibited chemical (ovalbumin)-induced airway constriction and airway hyperreactivity in an animal model of asthma (Ram et al 2003), thereby inidcating potential anti-asthma effects.

Curcumin inhibits P-glycoprotein in numerous in vitro studies (Anuchapreeda et al 2002, Limtrakul et al 2004, Nabekura et al 2005). The clinical significance of this observation has yet to be determined.

CLINICAL USE

In practice, turmeric and the various curcuminoids are used in many forms and administered via various routes. This review will focus mostly on those methods of use that are commonly used and preparations, such as oral dose forms and topical applications. Turmeric may be used as a single therapeutic agent or in combination with other herbal medicines or nutrients, such as the omega-3 polyunsaturated fatty acids. There is strong molecular evidence published for curcumin's potency to target multiple inflammatory diseases (Henrotin et al 2013).

Arthritis

Curcumin is one of the most promising natural ingredients in the treatment of arthritis. It exhibits several mechanisms of action which make it an excellent candidate. In vitro studies have shown that curcumin inhibits NF-κB activation and translocation induced by IL-1β and the consequent expression of NF-κB induced pro-inflammatory genes, COX-2 and VEGF (Henrotin et al 2013). In a randomised, controlled, double-blind study, curcumin 1200 mg/day was compared with phenylbutazone in subjects with rheumatoid arthritis (RA).

Rheumatoid arthritis

Curcumin was found to be effective in improving morning stiffness, walking time and joint swelling; however, the effects of phenylbutazone were stronger (Deodhar et al 1980). A more recent randomised study involving 45 patients with active RA found that treatment with curcumin (500 mg/day) was more effective than diclofenac sodium (50 mg/day) for reducing the Disease Activity Score (DAS) 28, together with tenderness and swelling, as measured by the American College of Rheumatology (ACR) criteria (Chandran & Goel 2012). In particular, the treatment was safe and well tolerated.

Osteoarthritis

A proprietary complex of curcumin with soy phosphatidylcholine (Meriva, Indena SpA), which corresponded to 200 mg curcumin daily, was shown to decrease the global WOMAC score by 58% ($P < 0.05$) at 3 months, increase walking distance and significantly reduce C-reactive protein levels in volunteers with osteoarthritis, thereby indicating a significant anti-inflammatory effect. In comparison, the control group only experienced very modest effects (Belcaro et al 2010b). To test the long-term effects of curcumin treatment, a follow-up study of 100 people with OA was conducted, which showed significant improvements to both the clinical and biochemical end points for Meriva (1 gm/day) compared to controls at 8 months (Belcaro et al 2010a). The WOMAC score was decreased by more than 50%, whereas treadmill-walking performance was increased almost threefold. From a biochemical perspective, serum inflammatory biomarkers such as IL-1β,IL-6, soluble CD40 ligand, soluble vascular cell adhesion molecule-1, and erythrocyte sedimentation rate were also significantly decreased in the treatment group. Of particular importance, there was a significant decrease in the requirement for NSAIDs and reduced gastrointestinal complications.

IN COMBINATION

Curcumin combined with boswellia, withania and zinc produced a significant drop in pain and disability in osteoarthritis (OA) of the knee in a randomised, double-blind, placebo-controlled crossover study of 42 patients (Kulkarni et al 1991); however, the contribution of curcumin to these results is unknown.

Cancer

Epidemiological data suggest that curcumin consumption reduces the rate of colorectal cancer (Hergenhahn et al 2002) and curcumin has wide-ranging chemopreventive activity in preclinical carcinogenic models (Plummer et al 2001), most notably for gastrointestinal cancers (Ireson et al 2001). In 1987 Kuttan et al treated 62 patients with external cancerous lesions with topical curcumin and found remarkable symptomatic relieving activity (Kuttan et al 1987). There was a reduction in smell, itching, lesion size and pain. Interestingly, the effect lasted for several months in most patients. Since then, curcumin, either alone or in combination with other agents, has demonstrated potential against colorectal cancer, pancreatic cancer, breast cancer, prostate cancer, multiple myeloma, lung cancer, oral cancer, and head and neck squamous cell carcinoma (HNSCC) (Gupta et al 2013).

Curcumin appears to be a well-tolerated adjunctive treatment option for patients with pancreatic cancer. Twenty-five participants took 8 g of curcumin daily. Despite significant inter-patient variations in blood curcumin levels, NF-κB, COX-2 and phosphorylated signal transducer and activator of transcription 3 were all downregulated in peripheral blood mononuclear cells (Dhillon et al 2008).

In a phase 1 study, curcumin taken orally for 3 months at a starting dose of 500 mg/day was found to produce histological improvement in cases of bladder cancer, oral leucoplakia, intestinal metaplasia of the stomach, cervical intraepithelial neoplasm and Bowen's disease (Cheng et al 2001).

An ethanol extract of turmeric, as well as an ointment of curcumin, was found to produce remarkable symptomatic relief in patients with external cancerous lesions (Kuttan et al 1987) and there are clinical reports to suggest that curcumin could be safe and effective in the treatment of idiopathic inflammatory orbital pseudotumours (Lal et al 2000).

Curcumin has a potential use in breast cancer as it has been found to inhibit the migratory activity of breast cancer cells, proliferative rate, adhesion, and invasion through down-regulating the expression of NF-κB p65 (Liu & Chen 2013). Cell proliferation assays have shown that curcumin exhibited anti-proliferative effects on MDA-MB-231 and BT-483 breast cancer cells in a time- and dose-dependent manner. Curcumin decreased matrix metalloproteinases-1 expression in MDA-MB231 and BT-483 breast cancer cells. Down-regulation of NF-κB inducing genes (NF-κB p65) was also observed (Liu et al 2009). Curcumin may provide a clinically useful tool for the suppression of vascular endothelial growth factor (VEGF) in tumour cells. It has been found that curcumin suppressed breast tumour angiogenesis by negating osteopontin or medroxyprogesterone acetate-induced VEGF expression. Curcumin was found to inhibit α6β4 signalling and functions by altering intracellular localisation of α6β4, and prevented its association with signalling receptors such as the epidermal growth factor receptor (EGFR) and Protein Kinase B (Akt). In addition, the combination of epigallocatechin gallate (EGCG) and curcumin is efficacious in both in vitro and in vivo models of ERα-breast cancer. In these processes, the regulation of VEGFR-1 may play a key role in the antitumour activities (Liu & Chen 2013). Poly (ADP-ribose) polymerase 1 (PARP-1) plays a significant role in cellular protection against radiation. Targeting PARP-1 may provide an effective way of maximising the therapeutic value of curcumin and antioxidants for cancer prevention (Liu & Chen 2013). More research needs to be conducted for the potential use of curcumin in breast cancer patients.

Cardiovascular disease

Effects of curcumin on risk factors for atherosclerosis were investigated in a 6-month randomised, double-blind, placebo-controlled clinical trial (Chuengsamarn et al 2014).

Hyperlipidaemia

Turmeric may be associated with a decrease in the risk of cardiovascular disease and an intake of 200 mg of a hydro-ethanolic extract of turmeric may decrease total blood lipid peroxides as well as HDL- and LDL-lipid peroxidation, in addition to normalising plasma fibrinogen levels and apolipoprotein B/apolipoprotein A ratio (Miquel et al 2002).

A placebo-controlled, randomised, double-blind study investigated the effects of curcumin on the serum lipids in 36 elderly men and women (Baum et al 2007). The participants were randomised to receive 4 g/day of curcumin, 1 g/day of curcumin or placebo for 6 months. Neither active product significantly altered triglyceride or cholesterol levels at 1 or at 6 months. It was noted that the curcumin concentration was greater after capsule administration of curcumin compared to that of powder administration.

In an open trial, 10 healthy volunteers received 500 mg/day of curcumin for 7 days. A significant decrease in the level of serum lipid peroxides (33%), increase in HDL cholesterol (29%) and a decrease in total serum cholesterol (11.63%) were noted. It also reduced serum lipid peroxides (Soni & Kuttan 1992). In a subsequent study, a 45-day intake (by healthy individuals 27–67 years of age) of a turmeric hydro-alcoholic extract at a daily dose equivalent to 20 mg of curcumin resulted in a significant decrease in serum lipid peroxides (Ramirez-Bosca et al 1995). A daily intake of turmeric equivalent to 20 mg of curcumin for 60 days also decreased peroxidation of both HDL and LDL in 30 healthy volunteers ranging in age from 40 to 90 years. The effect was quite striking in the persons with high baseline values of peroxidised compounds in these lipoproteins, although no apparent change took place in the persons having low baseline values (Ramirez et al 1997). Larger trials are needed to test the efficacy of turmeric in dyslipidaemia.

Diabetes

Turmeric has been used for the treatment of diabetes in Ayurvedic and traditional Chinese medicine (Zhang et al 2013). A systematic review suggests that curcumin could favourably affect most of the leading aspects of diabetes, such as insulin resistance, hyperglycaemia, hyperlipidaemia, and islet apoptosis and necrosis, as well as diabetes-related liver disorders, adipocyte dysfunction, neuropathy, nephropathy, and vascular diseases. Increased inflammation and levels of circulating ROS have been identified in the progression of diabetes. Potential mechanisms in the treatment of diabetes include antioxidant, anti-inflammatory (reduced IL-6, NF-κB, TNFα) and delayed islet ROS production. The authors conclude that studies need to be carried out in humans to confirm the potential of curcumin in limitation of diabetes and other associated disorders.

A 9-month randomised, double-blind, placebo-controlled trial in a prediabetic population showed that curcumin significantly lowered the number of prediabetic individuals who eventually developed type 2 diabetes (16.4% vs 0%) (Chuengsamarn et al 2012). HbA_{1C}, fasting plasma glucose (FPG), and oral glucose tolerance test (OGGT) measured at 2 hours were significantly lower in the curcumin-treated group when compared with the placebo group ($P < 0.01$) in all visits at 3, 6 and 9 months. The curcumin-treated group showed a lower level of homeostasis model assessment-insulin resistance (HOMA-IR) (3.22 vs. 4.04; $P < 0.001$). In addition, the curcumin treatment appeared to improve overall function of β-cells, with very minor adverse effects.

Dyspepsia/peptic ulcers

A randomised, controlled, double-blind, prospective, multicentre pilot study compared the effects of dried extracts of greater celandine and turmeric with placebo in 76 patients with colicky abdominal pain in the right upper quadrant due to biliary dyskinesia. Abdominal pain was reduced more quickly with active treatment; however, other symptoms such as fullness, nausea and vomiting did not respond (Niederau & Gopfert 1999). Another randomised, placebo-controlled, double-blind study that investigated the efficacy of turmeric for treatment of dyspepsia and flatulence in 116 adult patients with acidic dyspepsia, flatulent dyspepsia or atonic dyspepsia found that 87% of patients receiving turmeric responded compared to 53% receiving placebo (Thamlikitkul et al 1989).

In a study of 24 patients with duodenal or gastric ulcers varying between 0.5 and 1.5 cm in diameter, 300 mg of turmeric given five times daily, 30–60 minutes before meals, at 4 pm and at bedtime, successfully healed 48% of ulcers after 4 weeks and 76% after 12 weeks. Of 20 patients who had erosion gastritis and dyspepsia, the same treatment produced a satisfactory reduction in abdominal pain and discomfort after the first and second week (Prucksunand et al 2001). Turmeric has also been positively compared to a liquid antacid for the treatment of gastric ulcer in a controlled clinical trial (Kositchaiwat et al 1993).

Irritable bowel syndrome (IBS)

Turmeric extract shows promise in the symptomatic treatment of IBS, according to a partially blinded, randomised study by Bundy et al (2004). The study of 207 volunteers with diagnosed IBS complying with the Rome II criteria were randomly assigned to receive either 72 mg or 144 mg of turmeric a day or placebo for 8 weeks (Bundy et al 2004). The group receiving the lower dose (72 mg/day) experienced a significant 53% decrease in irritable bowel symptoms, whereas higher treatment (144 mg/day) resulted in a 60% decrease when compared to placebo ($P < 0.001$). Abdominal discomfort was also reduced by 22% and 25% of patients in the 72 mg and 144 mg groups, respectively ($P < 0.001$). Approximately two-thirds of the participants in the active groups reported overall symptom improvement and had better quality-of-life scores.

Inflammatory bowel disease

An open-label pilot study has produced preliminary data to suggest that curcumin may be effective in inflammatory bowel disease (Holt et al 2005). Five patients with Crohn's disease received 360 mg of curcumin three times a day for 1 month, followed by four times a day for another 2 months. The Crohn's disease activity index (CDAI), C-reactive protein (CRP) and erythrocyte sedimentation rate (ESR) fell significantly in four out of five patients. Five patients with ulcerative proctitis were also enrolled and received 550 mg of curcumin twice a day for 1 month, then three times a day for another month. Overall, stool quality was greatly improved and frequency was significantly reduced. Two patients were able to eliminate their concomitant medications altogether, while another two patients were able to reduce them. The CRP and ESR also returned to within normal limits by the cessation of the study.

A randomised, double-blind, multicentre trial of 89 patients examined the efficacy of curcumin as a maintenance therapy in ulcerative colitis (Hanai et al 2006). Patients in the active group received 1 g of curcumin, twice a day (e.g. 1 g after breakfast and 1 g after the evening meal) with sulfasalazine or mesalazine as compared to placebo plus sulfasalazine or mesalazine. At the end of the study period, 4.7% of patients in the curcumin group relapsed during treatment compared to 20.5% in the placebo group ($P = 0.040$). The clinical activity index ($P = 0.038$) and endoscopic index ($P = 0.0001$) were also significantly improved. This is a promising result that may have great clinical significance.

Ophthalmology

Studies demonstrate the potential therapeutic role and efficacy of curcumin in eye relapsing diseases, such as dry eye syndrome, allergic conjunctivitis, anterior uveitis, glaucoma, maculopathy, and ischaemic and diabetic retinopathy (Pescosolido et al 2013). Curcumin treatment has resulted in a partial, but significant, inhibition of neuronal and vascular damage during ischaemic or oxidative stress, angiogenesis, and inflammatory diseases. The mechanism by which curcumin induces its effects is yet to be fully elucidated. A number of studies have shown its relevance as a potent anti-inflammatory and immunomodulating agent. In addition, curcumin with its pleiotropic activities can modulate the expression and activation of many cellular regulatory proteins such as chemokines, interleukins, haematopoietic growth factors, and transcription factors, which in turn inhibit cellular inflammatory responses and protect cells (Pescosolido et al 2013).

Psoriasis

A phase 2, non-blind, open-label trial investigated the effect of curcuminoid C3 complex (500 mg, 3 capsules three times a day) in 12 patients with plaque psoriasis for 12 weeks followed by a 4-week observation period (Kurd et al 2008). Results were poor with the intention-to-treat analysis response rate only reaching 16.7%. Of the eight patients who completed the trial, two participants responded with good results (83% and 88% improvement in symptoms); however, this could be due to a placebo effect. Overall, the medication was well tolerated with only mild side effects being reported, due to either gastrointestinal upset or hot flushing.

Topical curcumin reduced the severity of active, untreated psoriasis as assessed by clinical, histological and immunohistochemical criteria in an observational study of 10 patients. Curcumin was also found to decrease phosphorylase kinase, which is involved in signalling pathways, including those involved with cell migration and proliferation (Heng et al 2000). Topical administration of curcumin also induced normal skin formation in the modified mouse tail test (Bosman 1994). The effects are thought to be due to immune-modulating, anti-inflammatory and cyclo-oxygenase inhibitory actions. The downregulation of pro-inflammatory cytokines supports the view that turmeric antioxidants may exert a favourable effect on psoriasis-linked inflammation. Moreover, because IL-6 and IL-8 are growth factors for keratinocytes, their inhibition by those antioxidants may reduce psoriasis-related keratinocyte hyperproliferation (Miquel et al 2002).

OTHER USES

Chronic anterior uveitis

An open study of 32 patients found that orally administered curcumin improved symptoms and reduced recurrences of chronic anterior uveitis (a condition often associated with other autoimmune disorders) with an efficacy comparable to corticosteroid therapy, yet without significant side effects (Lal et al 1999).

Oral submucous fibrosis

Turmeric extract 3 g, oil 600 mg and oleoresin 600 mg effectively relieved symptoms and reduced the number of micronuclei (a sign of damage to the DNA and chromosomal integrity) in circulating lymphocytes and oral mucosal cells in patients with oral submucous fibrosis, a debilitating disease of the oral cavity mainly caused by chewing betel nut or tobacco (Hastak et al 1997).

Reducing alcohol intoxication

Theracurmin exhibited an inhibitory action against alcohol intoxication after drinking in humans, as evidenced by the reduced acetaldehyde concentration of the blood (Sasaki et al 2011).

DOSAGE RANGE

Internal use

- Tablet formulas are available, singular or in combination with other anti-inflammatory/antioxidant herbs, where the curcuminoids are formulated with phosphatidylcholine (phospholipid) to increase the relative absorption.
- Powdered turmeric: 1.5–3 g/day in water or cooking.

- Liquid extract (1:1) in 45% ethanol: 5–15 mL/day.
- Powdered extract standardised to 95% curcumin: 100–300 mg/day. Higher doses used for arthritis.

Due to its low solubility, oral bioavailability (Henrotin et al 2013; Pescosolido et al 2013) and systemic bioavailability (Henrotin et al 2013), the biomedical potential of curcumin is not easily realised unless it is taken in a bioavailable form such as theracurmin or Meriva (Indena TM). Multiple approaches are needed to overcome this limited solubility and poor bioavailability of curcumin. Some of these approaches include the synthesis of curcuminoids and development of novel formulations of curcumin, such as emulsions, sustained released tablets (Pescosolido et al 2013), nanoparticles and liposomal encapsulation (Pescosolido et al 2013, Zhang et al 2013).

Theracurmin is a highly absorptive curcumin dispersed with colloidal nanoparticles. Healthy human volunteers were administered orally 30 mg of Theracurmin or curcumin powder. The area under the blood concentration-time curve of Theracurmin was 27-fold higher than that of curcumin powder (Sasaki et al 2011). Something to note is the difference in particle size of Theracurmin vs curcumin (mean particle size (D50% diameter) was 0.19 mcm and 22.75 mcm, respectively). Water dispersion studies observed homogenised very small particles in the Theracurmin sample, while the curcumin powder showed crystal aggregates with various sizes around several dozen micrometres (Sasaki et al 2011).

Dose-escalating studies have indicated the safety of curcumin at doses as high as 12 g/day over 3 months (Gupta et al 2013). Pharmacologically, curcumin does not show any dose-limiting toxicity when it is administered at doses of up to 8 g/day for three months (Pescosolido et al 2013).

External use

- Turmeric powder of standardised powdered extract applied as a paste or poultice — half a cup of turmeric combined with 1 teaspoon of carbonate of soda and then mixed with hot water to make a paste; spread on gauze and apply to affected area.

ADVERSE REACTIONS

The safety of dietary curcumin is demonstrated by the fact that it has been consumed for centuries at levels of up to 10 mg/day by people in certain countries (Ammon & Wahl 1991). Curcumin was non-toxic to humans in doses up to 8000 mg/day when taken by mouth for 3 months (Cheng et al 2001). Multiple other human trials have also found it to be safe with no alteration of liver or renal function tests (Chainani-Wu 2003, Prucksunand et al 2001, Ramirez-Bosca et al 1995, Ramirez et al 1997, Sharma et al 2001). Nausea and diarrhoea are possible effects of curcumins ranging from 0.45 to 3.6 g/day when taken for 1 to 4 months. This also caused an increase in serum alkaline phosphatase and lactate dehydrogenase contents in human participants (Sharma et al 2004).

Large doses of turmeric powder may cause gastrointestinal irritation in some persons (Shankar et al 1980), and very high dosages have been shown to reduce fertility in male rats (human equivalent doses would be 35 g turmeric/70 kg adult) (Bhagat & Purohit 2001). Normal therapeutic dosages of turmeric are not expected to affect fertility. Contact dermatitis has been reported (Hata et al 1997), as has a single case of anaphylaxis (Robinson 2003).

SIGNIFICANT INTERACTIONS

Controlled studies are not available, so interactions are based on evidence of activity and are largely theoretical and speculative.

Antiplatelet drugs

Turmeric has a theoretical interaction with antiplatelet drugs; antiplatelet properties have been demonstrated for curcumin, therefore it may produce an additive effect. The clinical significance of this interaction is unclear and likely to be dose-dependent.

Anticoagulants

Theoretically, high-dose turmeric preparations may increase the risk of bleeding when used together with anticoagulant drugs — caution is advised.

Cyclophosphamide

Animal studies suggest that curcumin may reduce drug efficacy — avoid.

CONTRAINDICATIONS AND PRECAUTIONS

Turmeric is contraindicated in bile duct obstruction (Blumenthal et al 2000) and high doses are probably best avoided in males and females wanting to conceive.

Curcumin is also contraindicated in breast cancer patients treated with cyclophosphamide until the significance of an in vivo model of breast cancer, which found that curcumin reduced the tumour regression effects of chemotherapy, is clarified (Somasundaram et al 2002).

Due to antiplatelet activity and possible increased risk of bleeding, use of concentrated extracts should be suspended 1 week prior to major surgery; however, usual dietary intakes are likely to be safe.

PREGNANCY AND LACTATION USE

When used as a spice, this herb is most likely to be safe; however, the safety of therapeutic doses has not been established. Turmeric has been demonstrated not to be mutagenic in vitro (Nagabhushan & Bhide 1986) or to be teratogenic in mice (Garg 1974, Vijayalaxmi 1980). Constituents and/or metabolites of turmeric and curcumin were transferred to suckling pups, but no ill effect on the offspring was reported.

T

Practice points/Patient counselling

- In Ayurvedic medicine, turmeric is used to strengthen the overall energy of the body, relieve gas, dispel worms, improve digestion, regulate menstruation, dissolve gallstones, relieve arthritis and purify the blood (Blumenthal et al 2000).
- In Traditional Chinese medicine (TCM), turmeric is used for bruises, sores, ringworm, chest pain, toothache and jaundice. Turmeric was also recommended for abdominal pain, mass formation in the abdomen and amenorrhoea (Blumenthal et al 2000).
- Turmeric is commonly used in foods and is likely to be a safe and healthy addition to the diet.

- Turmeric has been shown to have antioxidant, anti-inflammatory and anti-atherosclerotic activities; however, further clinical evidence is needed before it can be recommended to treat specific conditions.
- Clinical evidence suggests that turmeric may provide benefit for people with dyspepsia, peptic ulcer, hyperlipidaemia and arthritis and there is emerging evidence to suggest that turmeric may help prevent a number of cancers as well as being useful as an adjuvant in cancer treatment.

PATIENTS' FAQs

What will this herb do for me?

In countries where people use turmeric extensively in cooking (generally in curries), the intake seems to be associated with a lower level of certain chronic conditions, possibly including cancer, gastrointestinal diseases and arthritis. There have been some encouraging studies supporting this. Curcumin has shown promising effects for symptomatic relief in numerous inflammatory conditions such as rheumatoid arthritis, osteoarthritis, inflammatory bowel disease, IBS, peptic ulcer, psoriasis and in various cancers, diabetes and eye conditions. Ideally, oral use of preparations where bioavailability has been improved is likely to give the best results.

When will it start to work?

In some studies, the effect began to be noticed after 2 weeks. However, as most of the conditions where turmeric may be beneficial are chronic in nature, treatment with turmeric should be considered long term.

Are there any safety issues?

Turmeric is considered very safe at normal dietary or therapeutic dosages with turmeric extracts. High doses are generally not recommended during pregnancy or for those wanting to conceive.

REFERENCES

Abu-Rizq HA et al. Cyto-protective and immunomodulating effect of Curcuma longa in Wistar rats subjected to carbon tetrachloride-induced oxidative stress. Inflammopharmacology 16.2 (2008): 87–95.

Aggarwal BB et al. Curcumin: the Indian solid gold. Adv Exp Med Biol 595 (2007): 1–75.

Ak T, Gulcin I. Antioxidant and radical scavenging properties of curcumin. Chem Biol Interact 174.1 (2008): 27–37.

Al-Omar FA et al. Immediate and delayed treatments with curcumin prevents forebrain ischemia-induced neuronal damage and oxidative insult in the rat hippocampus. Neurochem Res 31.5 (2006): 611–618.

Ambegaokar SS et al. Curcumin inhibits dose-dependently and time-dependently neuroglial cell proliferation and growth. Neuroendocrinol Lett 24.6 (2003): 469–473.

Ammon HP, Wahl MA. Pharmacology of Curcuma longa. Planta Med 57.1 (1991): 1–7.

Andjelkovic T et al. Synergistic effects of the purine analog sulfinosine and curcumin on the multidrug resistant human non-small cell lung carcinoma cell line (NCI-H460/R). Cancer Biol Ther 7.7 (2008): 1024–32.

Anonymous. Curcuma longa (turmeric) Monograph. Altern Med Rev 6 Suppl (2001): S62–6.

Anto RJ et al. Antimutagenic and anticarcinogenic activity of natural and synthetic curcuminoids. Mutat Res 370.2 (1996): 127–131.

Antony S et al. Immunomodulatory activity of curcumin. Immunol Invest 28.5–6 (1999): 291–303.

Anuchapreeda S et al. Modulation of P-glycoprotein expression and function by curcumin in multidrug-resistant human KB cells. Biochem Pharmacol 64.4 (2002): 573–582.

Asai A, Miyazawa T. Dietary curcuminoids prevent high-fat diet-induced lipid accumulation in rat liver and epididymal adipose tissue. J Nut 131.11 (2001): 2932–2935.

Azuine MA, Bhide SV. Chemopreventive effect of turmeric against stomach and skin tumors induced by chemical carcinogens in Swiss mice. Nutr Cancer 17.1 (1992): 77–83.

Babu PS, Srinivasan K. Hypolipidemic action of curcumin, the active principle of turmeric (Curcuma longa) in streptozotocin induced diabetic rats. Mol Cell Biochem 166.1–2 (1997): 169–175.

Bachmeier B et al. The chemopreventive polyphenol Curcumin prevents hematogenous breast cancer metastases in immunodeficient mice. Cell Physiol Biochem 19.1–4 (2007): 137–152.

Bachmeier BE et al. Curcumin downregulates the inflammatory cytokines CXCL1 and 2 in breast cancer cells via NFkappaB. Carcinogenesis 29.4 (2008): 779–789.

Baek OS et al. Curcumin inhibits protease-activated receptor-2 and -4-mediated mast cell activation. Clin Chim Acta 338.1–2 (2003): 135–141.
Banerjee M et al. Modulation of inflammatory mediators by ibuprofen and curcumin treatment during chronic inflammation in rat. Immunopharm Immunotoxicol 25.2 (2003): 213–224.
Baum L et al. Curcumin effects on blood lipid profile in a 6-month human study. Pharmacol Res 56.6 (2007): 509–514.
Belcaro G et al. Efficacy and safety of Meriva®, a curcumin-phosphatidylcholine complex, during extended administration in osteoarthritis patients. Altern Med Rev 15.4 (2010a): 337–344.
Belcaro G et al. Product-evaluation registry of Meriva®, a curcumin-phosphatidylcholine complex, for the complementary management of osteoarthritis. Panminerva Med 52.2 Suppl 1 (2010b): 55–62.
Bengmark S. Curcumin, an atoxic antioxidant and natural NFkappaB, cyclooxygenase-2, lipooxygenase, and inducible nitric oxide synthase inhibitor: a shield against acute and chronic diseases. JPEN J Parenter Enteral Nutr 30.1 (2006): 45–51.
Bhagat M, Purohit A. Antifertility effects of various extracts of Curcuma longa in male albino rats. Indian Drugs 38.2 (2001): 79–81.
Blumenthal M et al. (eds). Herbal medicine: expanded commission E monographs. Austin, TX: Integrative Medicine Communications, 2000.
Bosman B. Testing of lipoxygenase inhibitors, cyclooxygenase inhibitors, drugs with immunomodulating properties and some reference antipsoriatic drugs in the modified mouse tail test, an animal model of psoriasis. Skin Pharmacol 7.6 (1994): 324–334.
Bundy R et al. Turmeric extract may improve irritable bowel syndrome symptomology in otherwise healthy adults: a pilot study. J Altern Complement Med 10.6 (2004): 1015–1018.
Bush JA et al. Curcumin induces apoptosis in human melanoma cells through a Fas receptor/caspase-8 pathway independent of p53. Exp Cell Res 271.2 (2001): 305–314.
Calabrese V et al. Redox regulation of cellular stress response in neurodegenerative disorders. Ital J Biochem 55.3–4 (2006): 263–282.
Chainani-Wu N. Safety and anti-inflammatory activity of curcumin: a component of turmeric (Curcuma longa). J Altern Complement Med 9.1 (2003): 161–168.
Chandran B & Goel A. A randomized, pilot study to assess the efficacy and safety of curcumin in patients with active rheumatoid arthritis. Phytother Res 26.11 (2012): 1719–1725.
Chang DM. Curcumin: a heat shock response inducer and potential cytoprotector. Crit Care Med 29.11 (2001): 2231–2232.
Chen HW et al. Pretreatment of curcumin attenuates coagulopathy and renal injury in LPS-induced endotoxemia. J Endotoxin Res 13.1 (2007): 15–23.
Cheng AL et al. Phase I clinical trial of curcumin, a chemopreventive agent, in patients with high-risk or pre-malignant lesions. Anticancer Res 21.4B (2001): 2895–2900.
Chuang SE et al. Curcumin-containing diet inhibits diethylnitrosamine-induced murine hepatocarcinogenesis. Carcinogenesis 21.2 (2000): 331–335.
Chueh S-CJ et al. Curcumin enhances the immunosuppressive activity of cyclosporine in rat cardiac allografts and in mixed lymphocyte reactions. Transplant Proc 35.4 (2003): 1603–1605.
Chuengsamarn S et al. Curcumin extract for prevention of type 2 diabetes. Diabetes Care. 35.11 (2012): 2121–2127.
Chuengsamarn S et al. Reduction of atherogenic risk in patients with type 2 diabetes by curcuminoid extract: a randomized controlled trial. J Nutr Biochem. 25.2 (2014): 144–150.
Cole GM et al. Prevention of Alzheimer's disease: Omega-3 fatty acid and phenolic anti-oxidant interventions. Neurobiol Aging 26 Suppl 1 (2005): 133–136.
Deodhar SD et al. Preliminary study on antirheumatic activity of curcumin (diferuloyl methane). Indian J Med Res 71 (1980): 632–634.
Deshpande UR et al. Protective effect of turmeric (Curcuma longa L.) extract on carbon tetrachloride-induced liver damage in rats. Indian J Exp Biol 36.6 (1998): 573–577.
Dhillon N et al. Phase II trial of curcumin in patients with advanced pancreatic cancer. Clin Cancer Res 14.14 (2008): 4491–4499.
Dorai T et al. Therapeutic potential of curcumin in human prostate cancer. III. Curcumin inhibits tyrosine kinase activity of epidermal growth factor receptor and depletes the protein. Mol Urol 4.1 (2000): 1–6.
Dorai T et al. Therapeutic potential of curcumin in human prostate cancer. III. Curcumin inhibits proliferation, induces apoptosis, and inhibits angiogenesis of LNCaP prostate cancer cells in vivo. Prostate 47.4 (2001): 293–303.
Du B et al. Synergistic inhibitory effects of curcumin and 5-fluorouracil on the growth of the human colon cancer cell line HT-29. Chemotherapy 52.1 (2006): 23–28.
Dulbecco P, Savarino V. Therapeutic potential of curcumin in digestive diseases. World J Gastroenterol. 19.48 (2013): 9256–9270.
Evans W, Trease D. Pharmacognosy, 15th edn, Edinburgh: WS Saunders, 2002.
Farhangkhoee H et al. Differential effects of curcumin on vasoactive factors in the diabetic rat heart. Nutr Metab (Lond) 3 (2006): 27.
Farombi EO et al. Curcumin attenuates dimethylnitrosamine-induced liver injury in rats through Nrf2-mediated induction of heme oxygenase-1. Food Chem Toxicol 46.4 (2008): 1279–1287.
Fiorillo C et al. Curcumin protects cardiac cells against ischemia-reperfusion injury: effects on oxidative stress, NF-kappaB, and JNK pathways. Free Radic Biol Med 45.6 (2008): 839–846.
Fu Y et al. Curcumin protects the rat liver from CCl4-caused injury and fibrogenesis by attenuating oxidative stress and suppressing inflammation. Mol Pharmacol 73.2 (2008): 399–409.
Gao X et al. Immunomodulatory activity of curcumin: suppression of lymphocyte proliferation, development of cell-mediated cytotoxicity, and cytokine production in vitro. Biochem Pharmacol 68.1 (2004): 51–61.

Garg SK. Effect of Curcuma longa (rhizomes) on fertility in experimental animals. Planta Med 26.3 (1974): 225–227.

Gescher A et al. Cancer chemoprevention by dietary constituents: a tale of failure and promise. Lancet Oncol 2 (2001): 371–379.

Gescher A et al. Suppression of tumour development by substances derived from the diet: mechanisms and clinical implications. Br J Clin Pharmacol 45.1 (1998): 1–2.

Gilani AH et al. Pharmacological basis for the use of turmeric in gastrointestinal and respiratory disorders. Life Sci 76.26 (2005): 3089–3105.

Gowda NKS et al. Effect of some chemical and herbal compounds on growth of Aspergillus parasiticus and aflatoxin production. Animal Feed Sci Technol 116.3–4 (2004): 281–291.

Gukovsky I et al. Curcumin ameliorates ethanol and nonethanol experimental pancreatitis. Am J Physiol Gastrointest Liver Physiol 284.147–1 (2003): G85–95.

Gupta SC et al. Therapeutic roles of curcumin: lessons learned from clinical trials. AAPS J. 15.1 (2013): 195–218.

Gururaj A et al. Molecular mechanisms of anti-angiogenic effect of curcumin. Biochem Biophys Res Commun 297.4 (2002): 934–942.

Hanai H et al. Curcumin maintenance therapy for ulcerative colitis: randomized, multicenter, double-blind, placebo-controlled trial. Clin Gastroenterol Hepatol 4.12 (2006): 1502–1506.

Hastak K et al. Effect of turmeric oil and turmeric oleoresin on cytogenetic damage in patients suffering from oral submucous fibrosis. Cancer Lett 116.2 (1997): 265–269.

Hata M et al. Allergic contact dermatitis from curcumin (turmeric). Contact Dermatitis 36.2 (1997): 107–108.

Heng MCY et al. Drug-induced suppression of phosphorylase kinase activity correlates with resolution of psoriasis as assessed by clinical, histological and immunohistochemical parameters. Br J Dermatol 143.5 (2000): 937–949.

Henrotin Y et al. Curcumin: a new paradigm and therapeutic opportunity for the treatment of osteoarthritis: curcumin for osteoarthritis management. Springerplus. 2.1 (2013): 56.

Hergenhahn M et al. The chemopreventive compound curcumin is an efficient inhibitor of Epstein-Barr virus BZLF1 transcription in Raji DR-LUC cells. Mol Carcinogen 33.3 (2002): 137–145.

Hidaka H et al. Curcumin inhibits interleukin 8 production and enhances interleukin 8 receptor expression on the cell surface: impact on human pancreatic carcinoma cell growth by autocrine regulation. Cancer 95.6 (2002): 1206–1214.

Holt PR, Katz S, Kirshoff R. Curcumin therapy in inflammatory bowel disease: a pilot study. Dig Dis Sci 50.11 (2005): 2191–2193.

Hong RL, Spohn WH, Hung MC. Curcumin inhibits tyrosine kinase activity of p185neu and also depletes p185neu. Clin Cancer Res 5.7 (1999): 1884–1891.

Hour T-C et al. Curcumin enhances cytotoxicity of chemotherapeutic agents in prostate cancer cells by inducing p21WAF1/CIP1 and C/EBPbeta expressions and suppressing NF-kappaB activation. Prostate 51.3 (2002): 211–218.

Huang M-T et al. Inhibitory effects of curcumin on tumor initiation by benzo[a]pyrene and 7,12-dimethylbenz[a] anthracene. Carcinogenesis 13.11 (1992): 2183–2186.

Imaida K et al. Lack of chemopreventive effects of lycopene and curcumin on experimental rat prostate carcinogenesis. Carcinogenesis 22 (2001): 467–472.

Inano H, Onoda M. Radioprotective action of curcumin extracted from Curcuma longa LINN: inhibitory effect on formation of urinary 8-hydroxy-2'-deoxyguanosine, tumorigenesis, but not mortality, induced by gamma-ray irradiation. Int J Radiat Oncol Biol Phys 53 (2002): 735–743.

Iqbal M et al. Dietary supplementation of curcumin enhances antioxidant and phase II metabolizing enzymes in ddY male mice: possible role in protection against chemical carcinogenesis and toxicity. Pharmacol Toxicol 92.1 (2003): 33–38.

Ireson C et al. Characterization of metabolites of the chemopreventive agent curcumin in human and rat hepatocytes and in the rat in vivo, and evaluation of their ability to inhibit phorbol ester-induced prostaglandin E2 production. Cancer Res 61.3 (2001): 1058–1064.

Itthipanichpong C et al. Antispasmodic effects of curcuminoids on isolated guinea-pig ileum and rat uterus. J Med Assoc Thai 86 Suppl 2 (2003): S299–309.

Jagetia GC, Aggarwal BB. 'Spicing up' of the immune system by curcumin. J Clin Immunol 27.1 (2007): 19–35.

Jagetia GC, Rajanikant GK. Role of curcumin, a naturally occurring phenolic compound of turmeric, in accelerating the repair of excision wound, in mice whole-body exposed to various doses of [gamma]-radiation. J Surg Res 120.1 (2004): 127–138.

Jain SK, Rains J, Jones K. Effect of curcumin on protein glycosylation, lipid peroxidation, and oxygen radical generation in human red blood cells exposed to high glucose levels. Free Radic Biol Med 41.1 (2006): 92–96.

Jantan I et al. Inhibitory effect of compounds from Zingiberaceae species on human platelet aggregation. Phytomedicine 15.4 (2008): 306–309.

Javvadi P et al. The chemopreventive agent curcumin is a potent radiosensitizer of human cervical tumor cells via increased reactive oxygen species production and overactivation of the mitogen-activated protein kinase pathway. Mol Pharmacol 73.5 (2008): 1491–1501.

Jayaprakasha GK et al. Chemistry and biological activities of C. longa. Trends Food Sci Technol 16.12 (2005): 533–548.

Jee S-H et al. Curcumin induces a p53-dependent apoptosis in human basal cell carcinoma cells. J Invest Dermatol 111.4 (1998): 656–661.

Jiao Y et al. Iron chelation in the biological activity of curcumin. Free Radic Biol Med 40.7 (2006): 1152–1160.

Jiao Y et al. Curcumin, a cancer chemopreventive and chemotherapeutic agent, is a biologically active iron chelator. Blood 113.2 (2009): 462–469.

Kamat AM, Sethi G, Aggarwal BB. Curcumin potentiates the apoptotic effects of chemotherapeutic agents and cytokines through down-regulation of nuclear factor-kappaB and nuclear factor-kappaB-regulated gene products in IFN-alpha-sensitive and IFN-alpha-resistant human bladder cancer cells. Mol Cancer Ther 6.3 (2007): 1022–1030.

Kang H-C et al. Curcumin inhibits collagen synthesis and hepatic stellate cell activation in-vivo and in-vitro. J Pharm Pharmacol 54.1 (2002): 119–126.
Keshavarz K. The influence of turmeric and curcumin on cholesterol concentration of eggs and tissues. Poultry Sci 55.3 (1976): 1077–1083.
Kim MS, Kang HJ, Moon A. Inhibition of invasion and induction of apoptosis by curcumin in H-ras-transformed MCF10A human breast epithelial cells. Arch Pharm Res 24.4 (2001): 349–354.
Kositchaiwat C, Kositchaiwat S, Havanondha J. Curcuma longa Linn. in the treatment of gastric ulcer comparison to liquid antacid: a controlled clinical trial. J Med Assoc Thai 76.11 (1993): 601–605.
Kowluru RA, Kanwar M. Effects of curcumin on retinal oxidative stress and inflammation in diabetes. Nutr Metab (Lond) 4 (2007): 8.
Kulkarni RR et al. Treatment of osteoarthritis with a herbomineral formulation: a double-blind, placebo-controlled, cross-over study. J Ethnopharmacol 33.1–2 (1991): 91–95.
Kumar GS et al. Free and bound phenolic antioxidants in amla (Emblica officinalis) and turmeric (Curcuma longa). J Food Comp Anal 19.5 (2006): 446–452.
Kunnumakkara AB, Anand P, Aggarwal BB. Curcumin inhibits proliferation, invasion, angiogenesis and metastasis of different cancers through interaction with multiple cell signaling proteins. Cancer Lett 269.2 (2008): 199–225.
Kuo M-L, Huang T-S, Lin J- K. Curcumin, an antioxidant and anti-tumor promoter, induces apoptosis in human leukemia cells. Biochem Biophys Acta Mol Basis Dis 1317.2 (1996): 95–100.
Kurd SK et al. Oral curcumin in the treatment of moderate to severe psoriasis vulgaris: A prospective clinical trial. J Am Acad Dermatol 58.4 (2008): 625–631.
Kuttan G et al. Antitumor, anti-invasion, and antimetastatic effects of curcumin. Adv Exp Med Biol 595 (2007): 173–184.
Kuttan R et al. Potential anticancer activity of turmeric (Curcuma longa). Cancer Lett 29.2 (1985): 197–202.
Kuttan R et al. Turmeric and curcumin as topical agents in cancer therapy. Tumori 73.1 (1987): 29–31.
Lal B et al. Efficacy of curcumin in the management of chronic anterior uveitis. Phytother Res 13.4 (1999): 318–322.
Lal B et al. Role of curcumin in idiopathic inflammatory orbital pseudotumours. Phytother Res 14.6 (2000): 443–447.
Lantz RC et al. The effect of turmeric extracts on inflammatory mediator production. Phytomedicine 12.6–7 (2005): 445–452.
Lev-Ari S et al. Inhibition of pancreatic and lung adenocarcinoma cell survival by curcumin is associated with increased apoptosis, down-regulation of COX-2 and EGFR and inhibition of Erk1/2 activity. Anticancer Res 26.6B (2006): 4423–4430.
Li L et al. Liposomal curcumin with and without oxaliplatin: effects on cell growth, apoptosis, and angiogenesis in colorectal cancer. Mol Cancer Ther 6.4 (2007): 1276–1282.
Limtrakul P, Anuchapreeda S, Buddhasukh D. Modulation of human multidrug-resistance MDR-1 gene by natural curcuminoids. BMC Cancer 4 (2004): 13.
Lin YG et al. Curcumin inhibits tumor growth and angiogenesis in ovarian carcinoma by targeting the nuclear factor-kappaB pathway. Clin Cancer Res 13.11 (2007): 3423–3430.
Liu D, Chen Z. The effect of curcumin on breast cancer cells. J Breast Cancer. 16.2 (2013): 133–137.
Liu Q et al. Curcumin inhibits cell proliferation of MDA-MB-231 and BT-483 breast cancer cells mediated by down-regulation of NFkappaB, cyclinD and MMP-1 transcription. Phytomedicine. 16.10 (2009): 916–922.
Lukita-Atmadja W et al. Effect of curcuminoids as anti-inflammatory agents on the hepatic microvascular response to endotoxin. Shock 17.5 (2002): 399–403.
Mani H et al. Curcumin differentially regulates TGF-beta1, its receptors and nitric oxide synthase during impaired wound healing. Biofactors 16.1–2 (2002): 29–43.
Manjunatha H, Srinivasan K. Hypolipidemic and antioxidant effects of curcumin and capsaicin in high-fat-fed rats. Can J Physiol Pharmacol 85.6 (2007b): 588–596.
Manjunatha H, Srinivasan K. Hypolipidemic and antioxidant effects of dietary curcumin and capsaicin in induced hypercholesterolemic rats. Lipids 42.12 (2007a): 1133–1142.
Marin YE et al. Curcumin downregulates the constitutive activity of NF-kappaB and induces apoptosis in novel mouse melanoma cells. Melanoma Res 17.5 (2007): 274–283.
Menon LG, Kuttan R, Kuttan G. Anti-metastatic activity of curcumin and catechin. Cancer Lett 141.1–2 (1999): 159–165.
Menon VP, Sudheer AR. Antioxidant and anti-inflammatory properties of curcumin. Adv Exp Med Biol 595 (2007): 105–125.
Mesa MD et al. Oral administration of a turmeric extract inhibits erythrocyte and liver microsome membrane oxidation in rabbits fed with an atherogenic diet. Nutrition 19.9 (2003): 800–804.
Miquel J et al. The curcuma antioxidants: Pharmacological effects and prospects for future clinical use: a review. Arch Gerontol Geriatr 34.1 (2002): 37–46.
Mohan R et al. Curcuminoids inhibit the angiogenic response stimulated by fibroblast growth factor-2, including expression of matrix metalloproteinase gelatinase B. J Biol Chem 275.14 (2000): 10405–10412.
Mohanty I et al. Protective effects of Curcuma longa on ischemia-reperfusion induced myocardial injuries and their mechanisms. Life Sci 75.14 (2004): 1701–1711.
Nabekura T et al. Effects of dietary chemopreventive phytochemicals on P-glycoprotein function. Biochem Biophys Res Commun 327.3 (2005): 866–870.
Nagabhushan M, Bhide SV. Nonmutagenicity of curcumin and its antimutagenic action versus chili and capsaicin. Nutr Cancer 8.3 (1986): 201–210.

T

Nanji AA et al. Curcumin prevents alcohol-induced liver disease in rats by inhibiting the expression of NF-kappaB-dependent genes. Am J Physiol Gastrointest Liver Physiol 284.2 47–2 (2003): G321–327.

Navis I, Sriganth P, Premalatha B. Dietary curcumin with cisplatin administration modulates tumour marker indices in experimental fibrosarcoma. Pharmacol Res 39.3 (1999): 175–179.

Niederau C, Gopfert E. [The effect of chelidonium- and turmeric root extract on upper abdominal pain due to functional disorders of the biliary system: Results from a placebo-controlled double-blind study]. Med Klin 94.8 (1999): 425–430.

O'Connell MA, Rushworth SA. Curcumin: potential for hepatic fibrosis therapy? Br J Pharmacol 153.3 (2008): 403–405.

Panchatcharam M et al. Curcumin improves wound healing by modulating collagen and decreasing reactive oxygen species. Mol Cell Biochem 290.1–2 (2006): 87–96.

Pari L, Murugan P. Antihyperlipidemic effect of curcumin and tetrahydrocurcumin in experimental type 2 diabetic rats. Ren Fail 29.7 (2007): 881–889.

Perez-Arriaga L et al. Cytotoxic effect of curcumin on Giardia lamblia trophozoites. Acta Tropica 98.2 (2006): 152–161.

Peschel D, Koerting R, Nass N. Curcumin induces changes in expression of genes involved in cholesterol homeostasis. J Nutr Biochem 18.2 (2007): 113–119.

Pescosolido N. Curcumin: Therapeutical Potential in Ophthalmology. Planta Med. 2013 Dec 9. [Epub ahead of print].

Phan T-T et al. Protective effects of curcumin against oxidative damage on skin cells in vitro: Its implication for wound healing. J Trauma-Injury Infect Crit Care 51.5 (2001): 927–931.

Plummer SM et al. Clinical development of leukocyte cyclooxygenase 2 activity as a systemic biomarker for cancer chemopreventive agents. Cancer Epidemiol Biomarkers Prev 10.12 (2001): 1295–1299.

Prucksunand C et al. Phase II clinical trial on effect of the long turmeric (Curcuma longa Linn) on healing of peptic ulcer. Southeast Asian J Trop Med Public Health 32.1 (2001): 208–215.

Quiles JL et al. An ethanolic-aqueous extract of Curcuma longa decreases the susceptibility of liver microsomes and mitochondria to lipid peroxidation in atherosclerotic rabbits. Biofactors 8.1–2 (1998): 51–57.

Quiles JL et al. Curcuma longa extract supplementation reduces oxidative stress and attenuates aortic fatty streak development in rabbits. Arterioscler Thromb Vasc Biol 22.7 (2002): 1225–1231.

Ram A, Das M, Ghosh B. Curcumin attenuates allergen-induced airway hyperresponsiveness in sensitized guinea pigs. Biol Pharm Bull 26.7 (2003): 1021–1024.

Ramirez BA et al. Effects of the antioxidant turmeric on lipoprotein peroxides: Implications for the prevention of atherosclerosis. Age 20.3 (1997): 165–168.

Ramirez-Bosca A et al. Antioxidant Curcuma extracts decrease the blood lipid peroxide levels of human subjects. Age 18.4 (1995): 167–169.

Ramirez-Tortosa MC et al. Oral administration of a turmeric extract inhibits LDL oxidation and has hypocholesterolemic effects in rabbits with experimental atherosclerosis. Atherosclerosis 147.2 (1999): 371–378.

Rao CV et al. Chemoprevention of colon cancer by dietary curcumin. Ann NY Acad Sci 768 (1995b): 201–204.

Rao CV et al. Chemoprevention of colon carcinogenesis by dietary curcumin, a naturally occurring plant phenolic compound. Cancer Res 55.2 (1995c): 259–266.

Rao CV et al. Chemoprevention of colon carcinogenesis by phenylethyl-3-methylcaffeate. Cancer Res 55.11 (1995a): 2310–2315.

Rao CV et al. Chemoprevention of colonic aberrant crypt foci by an inducible nitric oxide synthase-selective inhibitor. Carcinogenesis 20.4 (1999): 641–644.

Rao CV. Regulation of COX and LOX by curcumin. Adv Exp Med Biol 595 (2007): 213–226.

Rasyid A, Lelo A. The effect of curcumin and placebo on human gall-bladder function: an ultrasound study. Aliment Pharmacol Ther 13.2 (1999): 245–249.

Reddy RC et al. Curcumin for malaria therapy. Biochem Biophys Res Commun 326.2 (2005): 472–474.

Reddy S, Aggarwal BB. Curcumin is a non-competitive and selective inhibitor of phosphorylase kinase. FEBS Lett 341.1 (1994): 19–22.

Robinson DM. Anaphylaxis to turmeric. J Allergy Clin 111.1 Suppl 2 (2003): S100.

Ruby AJ et al. Anti-tumour and antioxidant activity of natural curcuminoids. Cancer Lett 94.1 (1995): 79–83.

Salh B et al. Curcumin attenuates DNB-induced murine colitis. Am J Physiol Gastrointest Liver Physiol 285.1 (2003): G235–243.

Sasaki H et al. Innovative preparation of curcumin for improved oral bioavailability. Biol Pharm Bull. 34.5 (2011): 660–665.

Shalini VK, Srinivas L. Lipid peroxide induced DNA damage: protection by turmeric (Curcuma longa). Mol Cell Biochem 77.1 (1987): 3–10.

Sharma RA et al. Phase I clinical trial of oral curcumin: biomarkers of systemic activity and compliance. Clin Cancer Res 10.20 (2004): 6847–6854.

Shankar TN et al. Toxicity studies on turmeric (Curcuma longa): Acute toxicity studies in rats, guinea pigs and monkeys. Indian J Exp Biol 18.1 (1980): 73–75.

Sharma RA et al. Pharmacodynamic and pharmacokinetic study of oral Curcuma extract in patients with colorectal cancer. Clin Cancer Res 7.7 (2001): 1894–1900.

Shukla PK et al. Anti-ischemic effect of curcumin in rat brain. Neurochem Res 33.6 (2008): 1036–1043.

Sidhu GS et al. Curcumin enhances wound healing in streptozotocin induced diabetic rats and genetically diabetic mice. Wound Repair Regen 7.5 (1999): 362–374.

Sidhu GS et al. Enhancement of wound healing by curcumin in animals. Wound Repair Regen 6.2 (1998): 167–177.

Skommer J, Wlodkowic D, Pelkonen J. Cellular foundation of curcumin-induced apoptosis in follicular lymphoma cell lines. Exp Hematol 34.4 (2006): 463–474.

Skommer J, Wlodkowic D, Pelkonen J. Gene-expression profiling during curcumin-induced apoptosis reveals downregulation of CXCR4. Exp Hematol 35.1 (2007): 84–95.

Somasundaram S et al. Dietary curcumin inhibits chemotherapy-induced apoptosis in models of human breast cancer. Cancer Res 62.13 (2002): 3868–3875.

Song E-K et al. Diarylheptanoids with free radical scavenging and hepatoprotective activity in vitro from Curcuma longa. Planta Med 67.9 (2001): 876–877.

Soni KB, Kuttan R. Effect of oral curcumin administration on serum peroxides and cholesterol levels in human volunteers. Indian J Physiol Pharmacol 36.4 (1992): 273–275.

Soni KB, Rajan A, Kuttan R. Reversal of aflatoxin induced liver damage by turmeric and curcumin. Cancer Lett 66.2 (1992): 115–121.

Soudamini KK et al. Inhibition of lipid peroxidation and cholesterol levels in mice by curcumin. Indian J Physiol Pharmacol 36.4 (1992): 239–243.

Srinivasan K, Sambaiah K. The effect of spices on cholesterol 7 alpha-hydroxylase activity and on serum and hepatic cholesterol levels in the rat. Int J Vitamin Nutr Res 61.4 (1991): 364–369.

Srinivasan K. Spices as influencers of body metabolism: an overview of three decades of research. Food Res Int 38.1 (2005): 77–86.

Srivastava KC et al. Curcumin, a major component of food spice turmeric (Curcuma longa), inhibits aggregation and alters eicosanoid metabolism in human blood platelets. Prostaglandins Leukot Essent Fatty Acids 52.4 (1995): 223–227.

Srivastava KC. Extracts from two frequently consumed spices — cumin (Cuminum cyminum) and turmeric (Curcuma longa) — inhibit platelet aggregation and alter eicosanoid biosynthesis in human blood platelets. Prostaglandins Leukot Essent Fatty Acids 37.1 (1989): 57–64.

Srivastava R et al. Anti-thrombotic effect of curcumin. Thromb Res 40.3 (1985): 413–417.

Srivastava R et al. Effect of curcumin on platelet aggregation and vascular prostacyclin synthesis. Arzneimittel-Forschung 36.4 (1986): 715–717.

Sugiyama T et al. Selective protection of curcumin against carbon tetrachloride-induced inactivation of hepatic cytochrome P450 isozymes in rats. Life Sci 78.19 (2006): 2188–2193.

Thaloor D et al. Inhibition of angiogenic differentiation of human umbilical vein endothelial cells by curcumin. Cell Growth Differ 9.4 (1998): 305–312.

Thamlikitkul V et al. Randomized double blind study of Curcuma domestica Val for dyspepsia. J Med Assoc Thai 72.11 (1989): 613–620.

Tian B et al. Effects of curcumin on bladder cancer cells and development of urothelial tumors in a rat bladder carcinogenesis model. Cancer Lett 264.2 (2008): 299–308.

Valentine SP et al. Curcumin modulates drug metabolizing enzymes in the female Swiss Webster mouse. Life Sci 78.20 (2006): 2391–2398.

Verma SP, Salamone E, Goldin B. Curcumin and genistein, plant natural products, show synergistic inhibitory effects on the growth of human breast cancer MCF-7 cells induced by estrogenic pesticides. Biochem Biophys Res Commun 233.3 (1997): 692–696.

Vijayalaxmi. Genetic effects of turmeric and curcumin in mice and rats. Mutat Res 79.2 (1980): 125–132.

Wu SJ et al. Curcumin or saikosaponin a improves hepatic antioxidant capacity and protects against CCl4-induced liver injury in rats. J Med Food 11.2 (2008): 224–229.

Yang X et al. Curcumin inhibits platelet-derived growth factor-stimulated vascular smooth muscle cell function and injury-induced neointima formation. Arterioscler Thromb Vasc Biol 26.1 (2006): 85–90.

Zahid Ashraf M et al. Antiatherosclerotic effects of dietary supplementations of garlic and turmeric: Restoration of endothelial function in rats. Life Sci 77.8 (2005): 837–857.

Zhang DW et al. Curcumin and Diabetes: A Systematic Review. Evid Based Complement Alternat Med. (2013): 636053.

Zhang L et al. Curcuminoids enhance amyloid-beta uptake by macrophages of Alzheimer's disease patients. J Alzheimers Dis 10.1 (2006): 1–7.

Valerian

HISTORICAL NOTE The sedative effects of valerian have been recognised for over 2000 years, having been used by Hippocrates and Dioscorides in ancient Greece. Over the past 500 years, valerian has been widely used in Europe for nervousness or hysteria and also to treat dyspepsia and flatulence. Legend has it that the Pied Piper put valerian in his pockets to attract the rats out of Hannover. Valerian was widely used by the Eclectic physicians and listed in the United States Formulary until 1946.

COMMON NAME

Valerian and Mexican Valerian

OTHER NAMES

All-heal, amantilla, balderbrackenwurzel, baldrian, baldrianwurzel, fragrant valerian, heliotrope, herbe aux chats, katzenwurzel, phu germanicum, phu parvum, valeriana, wild valerian

BOTANICAL NAME/FAMILY

Valeriana officinalis, Valeriana edulis (family Valerianaceae)

PLANT PART USED

Rhizome

CHEMICAL COMPONENTS

Valtrates, didrovaltrates, isovaltrates, monoterpenes, sesquiterpenes, caffeic, gamma-amino butyric and chlorogenic acids, beta-sitosterol, methyl 2-pyrrolketone, choline, tannins, gum, alkaloids, a resin. Essential oils (0.5–2%) in the plant contain the compounds bornyl acetate and the sesquiterpene derivatives valerenic acid, valeranone and valerenal.

The chemical composition of valerian varies greatly depending on such factors as plant age and growing conditions. Processing and storage of the herb also affects its constituents, such as the iridoid esters, which are chemically unstable.

MAIN ACTIONS

Anxiolytic and hypnotic

Both in vivo and numerous clinical studies confirm sedative or hypnotic activity for valerian (Ammer & Melnizky 1999, Balderer & Borbely 1985, Della Loggia et al 1981, Donath et al 2000, Dorn 2000, Gerhard et al 1996, Gessner & Klasser 1984, Leathwood & Chauffard 1985, Leuschner et al 1993, Lindahl & Lindwall 1989, Schulz et al 1994, Wheatley 2001). Anxiolytic activity has been demonstrated, most recently seen with a valerian extract with high valerenic acid concentration (Felgentreff et al 2012). Antidepressant activity has been seen most recently with an ethanolic extract of valerian (Phytofin Valerian 368) in an experimental model (Hattesohl et al 2008).

Extensive pharmacological research has been conducted to identify the main active constituents responsible for these effects. It is apparent that multiple components are at work and several neurobiological mechanisms underlie these actions. Recent in vivo testing has identified that the chief component responsible for the anxiolytic activity of valerian is the valerenic acid content (Felgentreff et al 2012). In the study, two extracts of valerian were tested with different valerenic acid ratios. A stronger anxiolytic effect was seen in test animals for the higher concentration extract (12 : 1) compared to a lower ratio extract (1 : 1.5). Binding studies confirmed an affinity to GABAergic binding sites. In an in vitro cell culture model, valerenic acid and its derivatives, acetoxyvalerenic acid and hydroxyvalerenic acid, were shown to cross the blood–brain barrier (BBB) to a slower extent than the GABAA modulator diazepam. Valerenic acid was the slowest to permeate in the study, followed by hydroxyvalerenic acid and acetoxyvalerenic acid. The research suggested that these compounds do not cross into the CNS by passive diffusion and instead are transported over the BBB by an as yet unknown transport system (Neuhaus et al 2008).

In vitro tests so far have demonstrated that valerian stimulates the release of GABA, inhibits GABA reuptake and may modulate GABA activity at GABAA receptors (Ortiz et al 1999, Santos et al 1994). The sesquiterpenic acids (valerenic acid and acetoxyvalerenic acid) seem to be at least partly responsible for this effect. This was discovered when a valerian ethyl acetate extract containing high levels of valerenic acid exhibited strong enhancement of GABA receptor activation, whereas the removal of sesquiterpenic acids from the extract led to a loss of GABA enhancement (Trauner et al 2008).

An alternative explanation for the anxiolytic properties of valerian may be CNS depression via inhibition of glutamate receptors as suggested by in vitro and animal models (Del Valle-Mojica et al 2011a, 2011b, 2012). There is also evidence of agonist effects at the human A_1 adenosine receptor for the methanolic extract (Schumacher et al 2002).

Antispasmodic, vasorelaxant and anti-convulsant

Both in vitro and in vivo studies provide evidence of antispasmodic activity on smooth muscle using various models (Hazelhoff et al 1982, Occhiuto et al 2009, Estrada-Soto et al 2010, Rezvani et al 2010). Valerian extracts and valepotriates in aqueous and ethanolic extracts exhibited antispasmodic activity as demonstrated by decreasing uterine contractility in isolated human uterine muscle. The effect occurred in a concentration-dependent manner and is thought to be due to calcium-channel blocker activity (Occhiuto et al 2009). *Valeriana edulis* demonstrated a significant concentration-dependent vasorelaxant activity on isolated rat aorta which also appeared to be due to a calcium-channel blocker mechanism (Estrada-Soto et al 2010). Antiepileptic activity was observed for an aqueous extract of valerian (500 mg/kg) which reduced seizure activity in rats. The mechanism of action was thought to be activation of the adenosine system (Rezvani et al 2010).

OTHER ACTIONS

A pharmacokinetic study with healthy adults found that typical doses of valerian are unlikely to produce clinically significant effects on the CYP2D6 or CYP3A4 pathways of metabolism (Donovan et al 2004). These results were confirmed in another human pharmacokinetic study that found no evidence of valerian affecting CYP3A4/5, CYP1A2, CYP2E1 and CYP2D6 activity (Gurley et al 2005). There is some in vitro evidence that suggests valerian may increase glucuronidation via the UDP-glucuronosyltransferase (UGT) enzymes. However, this has not been confirmed in humans (Mohamed et al 2010, 2011).

CLINICAL USE

In practice, valerian is rarely used as a stand-alone treatment and is often combined with other sedatives or relaxant herbs, such as chamomile, passionflower, skullcap, lemon balm and hops.

Insomnia

Numerous randomised controlled trials (RCTs) have investigated the effects of different valerian preparations as a treatment for insomnia. Some studies have involved people with confirmed sleep disturbances and others involved healthy subjects with no sleep problems. Treatment time-frames varied from acute (1 dose) to longer term (over 1 month) and doses have varied considerably. Some studies use only subjective data such as self-reported sleep quality whereas others use objective measures such as polysomnographs. Additionally, some studies use herbal combinations which include valerian, whereas other use valerian alone as monotherapy. As a result, interpreting the evidence is difficult.

Overall, the research suggests that valerian improves the subjective quality of sleep and may reduce sleep latency, enabling people to fall asleep a little more quickly. It generally shows no significant effect among people without sleep disturbances. Some research also suggests that best results are obtained with continuous use after several days to weeks and in some studies, a herbal combination of valerian with lemon balm or hops is more effective than placebo.

Findings from a pharmacokinetic study indicate that valerian has a short period of activity as it demonstrated that valerenic acid (a pharmacologically active marker compound for valerian) was increased in serum within an hour of ingestion, reached maximal levels between 1 and 2 hours, then fell with a marked decrease within 4 hours and no detectable levels observed after 8 hours (Anderson et al 2005). This pharmacokinetic pattern is also consistent with the finding that valerian does not produce residual morning sedation.

A number of different valerian products have been studied in clinical trials (e.g. Baldosedron, Baldrien-Dispert, Euvegal, Harmonicum Much, Seda-Kneipp, Sedonium, Valdispert, Valverde and Valerina Nutt). The LI 156 valerian extract is one of the most studied.

One of the first major systematic reviews was conducted by Stevinson and Ernst (2000), who identified 19 studies involving valerian treatment that were published prior to May 1999. Of these, nine were chosen for inclusion because they were randomised, measured sleep parameters and tested single ingredient valerian products. Three studies considered the cumulative effects of long-term use of valerian, whereas six investigated the effects of single-dose treatment. Two of the three studies investigating repeated administration of valerian found that effects were established by 2 weeks. The most rigorous placebo-controlled study showed that valerian LI 156 (600 mg) produced improvement on nearly all measures between weeks 2 and 4 (Vorbach et al 1996 as reported by Stevinson & Ernst 2000). The 4-week study involved 121 volunteers and assessed clinical effectiveness using four validated rating scales. At the end of the study, valerian was rated better than placebo on the Clinical Global Impression Scale, and at study conclusion (day 28) 66% of patients rated valerian effective, compared to 26% with placebo. Of the six studies investigating acute effects, valerian produced positive results in three whereas in the other three it was no better than placebo.

Interpretation of study results is difficult because of varying research methodologies. For example, some studies used surveys whereas others used EEG readings; some were conducted at home and others in hospitals or sleep laboratories, and pre-bedtime variables (e.g. caffeine consumption) were not fully controlled. Additionally, some studies used healthy volunteers with no sleep disturbances with little scope to observe further improvements. Since then, several other studies have been published.

In 2007, a comprehensive systematic review conducted by Taibi et al identified 37 separate studies of which 29 were controlled trials which evaluated valerian for both efficacy and safety, and eight were open-label trials which evaluated for safety only (Taibi et al 2007). The search was not limited to English language publications, thereby identifying many additional studies published by European research groups, including 17 studies published in German. The review evaluated data from RCTs and trials of other designs that investigated ethanolic extracts of valerian, aqueous extracts of valerian and valerian herbal combination treatments in people with sleep disturbances and in those who were considered healthy.

Six randomised, double-blind studies of an ethanolic extract of valerian (mainly LI 156 Sedonium) at a dosage between 300 and 600 mg before bedtime were assessed (Taibi et al 2007). Two studies measured polysomnographic outcomes and four collected only subjective measures of sleep quality. Overall, the ethanolic extract was not found to significantly affect objective or subjective sleep outcomes compared to placebo, however it did improve subjective sleep quality ratings in a manner similar to benzodiazepines. If we assume benzodiazepines perform better than placebo, then this is a positive outcome.

Seven studies evaluated the effects of aqueous preparations of valerian (Valdispert, Dixa SA Switzerland) at doses ranging from 400 mg/night to 450 mg three times daily (Taibi et al 2007). Four studies involved healthy subjects, two were of elderly people with sleep disturbances and one study was of people with difficulties in sleep onset. Once again, methodologies were highly varied. Only one study excluded volunteers with medical conditions that could contribute to poor sleep. As may be expected with such variations, results were mixed. The two studies involving elderly volunteers produced contradictory results, whereas reduced subjective latency was demonstrated in people with sleep onset disturbances. Healthy volunteers appeared to gain no benefit from the treatment.

Five further studies used valerian extracts which were standardised to valepotriate content (Taibi et al 2007). Three of these studies used *V. edulis* (one used Harmonicum Much) as a source of valepotriates and one used *V. wallichii* (Valmane). The dose of valepotriates varied from 60 to 120 mg and one preparation of *V. officinalis* used a preparation standardised to 450 mg of valerenic acid (Mediherb, Queensland, Australia). While methodologies varied considerably, overall standardised extracts appeared to reduce sleep disturbances when compared to placebo. A dose of 100 mg valepotriates taken three times a day was found to significantly improve sleep quality ratings in people withdrawing from benzodiazepines when compared to placebo. Additionally, 60 to 120 mg valepotriates was similarly effective in people who had reported disturbed sleep.

Valerian herbal combinations

In the 2007 systematic review by Taibi et al, 10 studies evaluating valerian herbal combinations were reviewed. Four studies tested valerian–lemon balm and six studies tested valerian–hops in combination (Taibi et al 2007). The studies using valerian–lemon balm combinations were shown to reduce sleep latency and increase sleep quality in people suffering sleep disturbances, whereas no change was observed in healthy subjects. In contrast, studies with valerian–hops combinations found no significant improvements using polysomnographic equipment or subjective sleep outcomes (Taibi et al 2007). The hops–valerian treatments used were ZE 91019 (Alluna) or another product sHova (extraction unknown).

In 2007, a later randomised placebo controlled study was published that compared a valerian–hops combination (Ze 91019) to valerian monotherapy (Ze 911) (Koetter et al 2007). The herbal combination treatment contained the same amount of valerian (500 mg) as monotherapy, thereby allowing researchers to evaluate what contribution hops (120 mg) would make to the outcomes measured. Volunteers suffering from non-organic insomnia were given either treatment or placebo for 4 weeks. In contrast to previous studies cited by Taibi et al, the valerian–hops combination was significantly superior to placebo in reducing sleep latency, improving clinical global impression scores and increasing slow-wave sleep, while the single valerian extract failed to show benefits beyond placebo.

A 2008 randomised placebo-controlled double-blinded trial ($n = 42$) investigating a combined preparation of valerian and hops (Dormeasan) found that the time spent in deeper sleep was significantly higher for the active treatment group compared to the placebo group ($P < 0.01$) (Dimpfel et al 2008). The treatment was administered 15 minutes before an 8-hour EEG recording to a group of poor sleepers, as identified by a validated sleep questionnaire (Schlaffragebogen SF-B). An un-medicated first night was used as a reference and compared to a second night where volunteers received either treatment. The findings between the reference and medication night in regards to time spent in deeper sleep were also statistically significant ($P < 0.01$). This suggests that a single dose preparation may be effective in achieving deeper sleep. The dose used was 2 mL of a liquid extract (a 1 : 10 fresh-plant tincture of *Valeriana officinalis* radix equivalent to 460 mg plus a 1 : 12 fresh-plant tincture of *Humulus lupulus* strobilus equivalent to 460 mg in 61% ethanol).

Valerian monotherapy

A 2010 meta-analysis analysed results from 18 RCTs where valerian was used as monotherapy compared to placebo (Fernández-San-Martín et al 2010). Studies varied greatly in design with variations in sample size, population groups, diagnostic criteria, dosage and follow-up times. The outcome measures were improved sleep quality with a dichotomic variable, improved sleep quality identified through visual analogue scales and improved sleep latency (measured via polysomnography or self-reporting questionnaires). Analysis found that valerian did not demonstrate statistical significance in improving sleep latency, but did improve sleep quality when the outcome was measured as a dichotomous variable, but not using a visual analogue scale. This indicates that participants taking valerian subjectively perceived greater sleep quality however this was not confirmed with quantitative measurements. Adverse effects between valerian and placebo were comparable with the exception of diarrhoea. Diarrhoea was more frequent in patients taking Valerian (18%) compared with those taking a placebo (8%, $P = 0.02$).

Restless legs syndrome and insomnia

Whether valerian improves sleep quality and symptoms in people with restless legs syndrome (RLS) is unclear according to this triple-blind, placebo-controlled RCT (Cuellar et al 2009). Thirty-seven volunteers were treated for 8 weeks with either valerian capsules twice daily (800 mg dried *Valeriana officinalis radix* equivalent to 1.16 mg valerenic acid/day) or placebo. The primary aim was to assess sleep quality using the Pittsburgh Sleep Quality Index and sleepiness using the Epworth Sleepiness Scale. The secondary aim was to assess changes in RLS symptom severity using the International RLS Symptom Severity Scale. Although the treatment group displayed a greater improvement in the majority of RLS symptoms and sleep quality, the findings were not statistically significant.

POST-MENOPAUSAL WOMEN WITH INSOMNIA

A 2010 triple-blind, controlled trial involving 100 postmenopausal women aged 50 to 60 years experiencing insomnia found that more women treated with valerian capsules (Sedamin 530 mg concentrated valerian root extract per capsule) twice daily for 4 weeks experienced improved sleep quality (30%) compared to those taking placebo (4%; $P < 0.001$) (Taavoni et al 2011). The improvement in sleep quality was based on changes to the Pittsburgh Sleep Quality index, a self-rated questionnaire assessing subjective sleep quality, latency, duration, sleep disturbances, use of sleep medication and daytime dysfunction.

In contrast, a small ($n = 16$) randomised, double-blind, crossover, controlled trial of healthy women aged 55–80 years with insomnia, valerian capsules (300 mg of a concentrated *Valeriana officinalis* L. root extract Nature's Resource standardised to contain 0.8% valerenic acid /day) taken 30 minutes before bedtime for 2 weeks has no significant effect on sleep latency, sleep efficiency, wake after sleep onset or self-rated sleep quality (Taibi et al 2009). Interestingly, there was a significant increase (+17.7 ± 25.6 minutes, $P = 0.02$) in nocturnal wakefulness in the valerian group compared to placebo (+6.8 ± 26.4 minutes, NS) which the authors attributed to a paradoxical stimulating effect as cited in the traditional literature (Bone 2003). Side effects were minor and did not differ significantly between valerian and placebo. The study used results gathered over 9 nights in the laboratory using a self-reported morning sleep questionnaire and polysomnographic recordings and at home by daily self-reported sleep logs and actigraphy.

Comparisons with benzodiazepines

Three randomised studies have compared valerian monotherapy with benzodiazepine drugs. One double-blind trial found that subjects treated with either 600 mg valerian (ethanolic extract) or 10 mg oxazepam experienced significantly improved sleep, with no statistically significant differences detected between the treatments (Dorn 2000). Another study comparing the immediate sedative effects and residual effects of a valerian and hops preparation, a sole valerian preparation, flunitrazepam and placebo found that subjective perceptions of sleep quality were improved in all treatment groups; however, only flunitrazepam treatment impaired performance the morning after, as assessed both objectively and subjectively (Gerhard et al 1996). Furthermore, 50% of subjects receiving flunitrazepam reported mild side-effects compared with only 10% from the other groups.

A 2002 double-blind randomised trial compared the effects of valerian extract LI 156 (Sedonium) 600 mg/day to 10 mg oxazepam over 6 weeks in 202 patients with non-organic insomnia (Ziegler et al 2002). The multicentre trial took place at 24 study centres in Germany and found that valerian treatment was at least as efficacious as oxazepam, with both treatments improving sleep quality. Subjectively, 83% of patients receiving valerian rated it as 'very good' compared with 73% receiving oxazepam.

Children

The efficacy and tolerability of a valerian and lemon balm combination (Euvegal forte) was tested in a large, open, multicentre study of 918 children (aged under 12 years) with restlessness and nervous sleep disturbance (dyssomnia) (Muller & Klement 2006). Both investigators' and parents' ratings revealed a reduction in the severity of symptoms for most patients. The study reported that 81% of children with dyssomnia experienced an improvement and 70% of children with restlessness improved. Treatment was generally rated as good or very good and considered well tolerated. Each Euvegal forte tablet consisted of 160 mg valerian root dry extract (*Valeriana officinalis* L.) with a drug-extract ratio of 4–5 : 1 (extraction solvent ethanol 62% v/v) and 80 mg lemon balm leaf dry extract (*Melissa officinalis*) with a drug-extract ratio of 4–6 : 1 (extraction solvent ethanol 30% v/v). The standard dosage of Euvegal forte (4 tablets daily) was used by 75% of patients and chosen by the investigator.

Anxiety and psychological stress states

Less investigation has taken place to determine the role of valerian as a treatment for anxiety states.

A randomised study found that low-dose valerian (100 mg) reduced situational anxiety without causing sedation (Kohnen & Oswald 1988). Positive results were also obtained in a smaller open study of 24 patients suffering from stress-induced insomnia who found treatment (valerian 600 mg/day for 6 weeks) significantly reduced symptoms of stress and insomnia (Wheatley 2001). Another randomised trial compared the effects of a preparation of valepotriates (mean daily dose 81.3 mg) with diazepam (mean daily dose 6.5 mg) and placebo in 36 outpatients with GAD under double-blind conditions (Andreatini et al 2002). After 4 weeks' treatment, all groups had significant reductions in Hamilton anxiety (HAM-A) scale scores; however, only those receiving valepotriates or diazepam showed a significant reduction in the psychic factor of HAM-A.

Kava kava is a herbal medicine also used in the treatment of anxiety and found to be effective in clinical studies (Pittler & Ernst 2002). A study that compared the effects of kava kava to valerian and placebo in a standardised mental stress test found that both herbal treatments reduced systolic blood pressure, prevented a stress-induced rise in heart rate and decreased self-reported feelings of stress (Cropley et al 2002).

A 2006 Cochrane review concluded there is insufficient evidence to draw any conclusions about the efficacy or safety of valerian compared with placebo or diazepam for anxiety disorders (Miyasaka et al 2006). RCTs involving larger samples and comparing valerian with placebo or other interventions used to treat of anxiety disorders, such as antidepressants, are needed.

Obsessive-Compulsive Disorder (OCD)

High dose valerian treatment may have a role to play in OCD, according to a placebo-controlled RCT. Thirty-one adult outpatients who met the DSM-IV-TR criteria for OCD received valerian capsules (765 mg/day of concentrated dried valerian extract/day) or placebo for 8 weeks. Patients were assessed using the Yale-Brown Obsessive-Compulsive Scale (Y-BOCS) at weeks 2, 4, 6 and 8. Assessment at weeks 4, 6 and 8 found the treatment group displayed significantly lower scores compared to the placebo group ($P = 0.043$, $P = 0.07$, $P = 0.00$). In regards to frequency of side effects, no significant difference was found between the groups. However, there was a greater incidence of somnolence with valerian treatment compared to placebo ($P = 0.02$) (Pakseresht et al 2011).

Muscle spasm, cramping and dysmenorrhoea

Valerian preparations have long been used to treat a wide variety of gastrointestinal disorders associated with spasms such as diarrhoea, colic and irritable bowel syndrome. It has also been used to relieve cramping in dysmenorrhoea. Valerian is likely to exert some degree of antispasmodic activity based on its pharmacological actions.

Recently, a double-blind, randomised clinical trial involving 100 female students experiencing moderate to severe dysmenorrhoea found valerian treatment provided some significant benefits compared to placebo (Mirabi et al 2011). The study compared a valerian preparation (containing 255 mg of powdered valerian root per capsule) or placebo capsules which were taken 3 times daily for the first 3 days of each cycle and continued for two menstrual cycles. Pain severity was measured three times daily using a visual analogue scale (VAS) and a multidimensional verbal scoring system was used to assess the severity of associated symptoms (fatigue, lack of energy, nausea and vomiting, diarrhoea, headache, mood swings and syncope). Active treatment reduced pain severity from 7.45 out of 10 at baseline to 1.99 in the second cycle compared to the placebo group, where the change was from 7.06 to 4.41. The duration of pain in the intervention cycles was also shorter in the valerian group ($P = 0.01$). No statistically significant differences were seen in the severity of associated systemic symptoms, with the exception of syncope ($P = 0.006$).

OTHER USES

Fibromyalgia

One randomised study, which was investigator blinded, tested the effects of whirl baths with plain water or with water containing pine oil or valerian on pain, disturbed sleep and tender point count in 30 outpatients with generalised fibromyalgia. Valerian significantly improved wellbeing and sleep, together with decreasing tender point count, whereas baths with pine oil worsened pain and plain water baths reduced pain but had no effect on wellbeing and sleeplessness (Ammer & Melnizky 1999).

Benzodiazepine withdrawal

Although no clinical studies are available, the herb is also used in practice to reduce dependency on benzodiazepine drugs. Valerian is prescribed together with other herbal medicines and psychological counselling while the benzodiazepine dose is slowly reduced.

DOSAGE RANGE

- Infusion of dried root: 3–9 g/day.
- Liquid extract (1 : 2): 2–6 mL/day.
- Tincture (1 : 5): 5–15 mL/day.
- When used for insomnia, valerian should be taken approximately 1 hour prior to bedtime.

According to clinical studies

- Anxiety: 100 mg–600 mg/day of the dried root or valepotriates (mean daily dose 81.3 mg).
- Insomnia: doses above 600 mg/day of dried root taken 1 hour before bedtime. Ethanolic extract of valerian: 300–600 mg before bedtime. Aqueous preparations of valerian: 400 mg/night to 450 mg three times daily. Standardised extracts: 60–120 mg valepotriates or 450 mg of valerenic acid before bedtime.
- For benzodiazepine withdrawal: 100 mg valepotriates taken three times daily.
- Fibromyalgia: Bath — 20 mL liquid extract (ratio not specified) per 200 L of 36–37°C water, three times per week.

TOXICITY

A combined extract of *Valeriana officinalis, Passiflora incarnata* and *Crataegus oxyacantha* demonstrated no toxicity, genotoxicity or mutagenicity in rats, mice and dogs at high doses over 180 days (Tabach et al 2009). According to one case report, a dose of valerian taken at approximately 20-fold the recommended therapeutic dose appears to be benign (Willey et al 1995).

Hepatotoxicity

Two rare idiosyncratic reactions of valerian-associated hepatotoxicty have been reported. A 27-year-old woman displayed epigastric pain and fatigue for 2 weeks along with raised liver enzymes while taking a 300 mg capsule twice a day for the prior 3 months (Valerian Root, Mason Vitamins) (Cohen et al 2008). Another case report of hepatotoxicity in a 50-year-old woman was reported who had taken valerian tea for 3 weeks (5 cc extract of valerian root thrice weekly), along with consuming 10 tablets of vaimane (containing 125 mg dry valerian extract / tablet). The woman was asymptomatic, but routine blood tests revealed elevated liver enzymes and bilirubin along with inflammation on liver biopsy and a diagnosis of drug-induced hepatitis was made. Over 10 months her transaminase levels returned to normal. The patient did not undergo a rechallenge with valerian and the case report did not mention any preexisting health conditions, concomitant medications or state whether the valerian was tested to rule out adulteration, contamination or substitution (Vassiliadis et al 2009). It is not clear in either case whether the herbal treatment was tested for authenticity or contamination, making interpretation difficult.

ADVERSE REACTIONS

As with numerous pharmaceutical sedatives, next morning somnolence is a possible side-effect of therapy; however, evidence from two human studies suggests this is not associated with valerian use (Gerhard et al 1996, Kuhlmann et al 1999). Additionally, evidence from a pharmacokinetic study indicates this is highly unlikely.

Vivid dreams were reported in one study; however, this is considered rare by clinicians (Wheatley 2001).

Paradoxical stimulating effects have been observed in clinical practice and in one study of post-menopausal women; however, this also appears to be rare (Mills & Bone 2000).

Occasionally, headache and gastrointestinal symptoms have been reported (Ernst et al 2001).

Practice points/Patient counselling

- It appears scientific evidence supports the use of valerian as a treatment for insomnia; however, it appears that ongoing use may be more effective than single-dose use and effects on sleep progress over several weeks. It is often used together with other herbs for better effect, such as lemon balm and hops.
- It appears to be best suited to reducing sleep latency (i.e. time taken until falling asleep) and improves subjective assessments of sleep. Therefore valerian may be more effective for sleep onset insomnia than sleep maintenance insomnia.
- There is no evidence of next-day somnolence or significant adverse effects.
- Valerian may also relieve symptoms of stress and anxiety, with several studies observing effects similar to benzodiazepines; however, further research is required.
- Due to its pungent odour, solid-dose forms may be preferable.

SIGNIFICANT INTERACTIONS

Pharmaceutical sedatives / benzodiazepines

Theoretically, potentiation effects may occur at high doses; however, this has not been tested under clinical conditions — observe patients taking valerian concurrently with pharmaceutical sedatives. This interaction may be beneficial under professional supervision.

There is a case report of a 40-year-old male taking lorazepam (2 mg/24 hours) for 2 months without side effects and then self-medicating with valerian (*Valeriana officinalis*) and passionflower (*Passiflora incarnata*) infusion (dose unknown) for 2 nights. On the third night he took 3 tablets at 1-hour intervals before going to sleep (containing 300 mg of valerian and 380 mg of passionflower extract/tablet). This was repeated on the fourth night and strong handshaking, dizziness and palpitations were experienced, followed by a heavy drowsiness that made him fall asleep. These symptoms disappeared when the herbal treatment was discontinued. While this effect may be due to the herbal medicine increasing the inhibitory activity of benzodiazepines binding to the GABA receptors, until the preparation can be tested, causality remains unclear (Carrasco et al 2009).

Alcohol

RCTs have shown no potentiation effects with alcohol use (Ernst et al 2001).

Haloperidol

In a rat study, oxidative stress parameters in the liver were increased when haloperidol was taken in combination with valerian via a significant increase in lipid peroxidisation levels (enhanced oxidation of thiobarbituric acid reactive species and dichlorofluorescein reactive species, as well as an inhibition of hepatic d-ALA-D activity). The significance in humans is unknown — observe patients taking valerian concurrently with haloperidol (Dalla Corte et al 2008).

CONTRAINDICATIONS AND PRECAUTIONS

No known contraindications. Care should be taken when driving a car or operating heavy machinery when high doses are used.

PREGNANCY USE

No restrictions are known; however, safety has not been well established in pregnancy. No significant negative effects have been reported in toxicological tests with animals and none reported in clinical studies (Upton 1999). A combined extract of *Valeriana officinalis, Passiflora incarnata* and *Crataegus oxyacantha* in rats did not alter the oestrus cycle, did not affect fertility and did not induce teratogenesis in the offspring born from females treated during the entire pregnancy (Tabach et al 2009).

PATIENTS' FAQs

What will this herb do for me?
Valerian is classified as a mild, sedative herbal medicine. It can reduce the time it takes to fall asleep at night, improve the way people feel about their quality of sleep and may also relieve stress and anxiety during the day. When added to a bath, it may increase relaxation, wellbeing and reduce some forms of pain.
When will it start to work?
For some, valerian works within an hour of the first dose; however, research suggests it works best after several weeks of regular use for insomnia.
Are there any safety issues?
From the available evidence, next-day drowsiness is uncommon and physical addiction highly unlikely. Taking high doses during the day may increase drowsiness, so care is needed when driving a car or operating heavy machinery.

REFERENCES

Ammer K, Melnizky P. Medicinal baths for treatment of generalized fibromyalgia. Forsch Komplementarmed 6.2 (1999): 80–85.

Anderson G et al. Pharmacokinetics of valerenic acid after administration of valerian in healthy subjects. [abstract]. In: Pharmacokinetics of valerenic acid after administration of valerian in healthy subjects 19.9 (2005): 801–803.

Andreatini R et al. Effect of valepotriates (valerian extract) in generalized anxiety disorder: a randomized placebo-controlled pilot study. Phytother Res 16.7 (2002): 650–654.
Balderer G, Borbely AA. Effect of valerian on human sleep. Psychopharmacology (Berl) 87.4 (1985): 406–409.
Bone K. A clinical guide to blending liquid herbs: herbal formulations for the individual patient. St. Louis: Churchill Livingstone, 2003.
Carrasco MC et al. Interactions of Valeriana officinalis L. and Passiflora incarnata L. in a patient treated with lorazepam. Phytother Res 23.12 (2009):1795–1796.
Cohen DL, Del Toro Y. A case of valerian-associated hepatotoxicity. J Clin Gastroenterol 42.8 (2008): 961–962.
Cuellar NG, Ratcliffe SJ. Does valerian improve sleepiness and symptom severity in people with restless legs syndrome? Altern Ther Health Med. 15.2 (2009): 22–28.
Cropley M et al. Effect of kava and valerian on human physiological and psychological responses to mental stress assessed under laboratory conditions. Phytother Res 16.1 (2002): 23–27.
Del Valle-Mojica LM, Ortíz JG. Anxiolytic properties of Valeriana officinalis in the zebrafish: a possible role for metabotropic glutamate receptors. Planta Med 78.16(2012): 1719–1724.
Del Valle-Mojica LM et al. Selective Interactions of Valeriana officinalis Extracts and Valerenic Acid with [H] Glutamate Binding to Rat Synaptic Membranes. Evid Based Complement Alternat Med. (2011a): 403591.
Del Valle-Mojica LM et al. Aqueous and Ethanolic Valeriana officinalis Extracts Change the Binding of Ligands to Glutamate Receptors. Evid Based Complement Alternat Med. (2011b): 891819.
Dalla Corte CL et al. Potentially adverse interactions between haloperidol and valerian. Food Chem Toxicol 46.7 (2008): 2369–2375.
Della Loggia R et al. Evaluation of the activity on the mouse CNS of several plant extracts and a combination of them. Riv Neurol 51.5 (1981): 297–310.
Dimpfel W, Suter A. Sleep improving effects of a single dose administration of a valerian/hops fluid extract - a double blind, randomized, placebo-controlled sleep-EEG study in a parallel design using electrohypnograms. Eur J Med Res 13.5 (2008): 200–204.
Donath F et al. Critical evaluation of the effect of valerian extract on sleep structure and sleep quality. Pharmacopsychiatry 33.2 (2000): 47–53.
Donovan JL et al. Multiple night-time doses of valerian (Valeriana officinalis) had minimal effects on CYP3A4 activity and no effect on CYP2D6 activity in healthy volunteers. Drug Metab Dispos 32.12 (2004): 1333–1336.
Dorn M. Efficacy and tolerability of Baldrian versus oxazepam in non-organic and non-psychiatric insomniacs: a randomized, double-blind, clinical, comparative study. Forsch Komplementarmed Klass Naturheilkd 7.2 (2000): 79–84.
Ernst E et al. The desktop guide to complementary and alternative medicine: An evidence-based approach. St Louis: Mosby, 2001.
Estrada-Soto S et al. Vasorelaxant effect of Valeriana edulis ssp. procera (Valerianaceae) and its mode of action as calcium channel blocker. J Pharm Pharmacol 62.9 (2010):1167–1174.
Felgentreff F et al. Valerian extract characterized by high valerenic acid and low acetoxy valerenic acid contents demonstratesanxiolytic activity. Phytomedicine 19.13 (2012):1216–1222.
Fernández-San-Martín et al. Effectiveness of Valerian on insomnia: a meta-analysis of randomized placebo-controlled trials. Sleep Med 11.6 (2010): 505–511.
Gerhard U et al. Vigilance-decreasing effects of 2 plant-derived sedatives. Schweiz Rundsch Med Prax 85.15 (1996): 473–481.
Gessner B, Klasser M. Studies on the effect of Harmonicum Much on sleep using polygraphic EEG recordings. Z Elektroenzephalog Elektromyogr Verwandte Geb 15.1 (1984): 45–51.
Gurley BJ et al. In vivo effects of goldenseal, kava kava, black cohosh, and valerian on human cytochrome P450 1A2, 2D6, 2E1, 3A4/5 phenotypes. Clin Pharmacol Ther 77.5 (2005): 415–426.
Hattesohl M et al. Extracts of Valeriana officinalis L. s.l. show anxiolytic and antidepressant effects but neither sedative nor myorelaxant properties. Phytomedicine 15.1–2 (2008): 2–15.
Hazelhoff B, Malingre TM, Meijer DK. Antispasmodic effects of valeriana compounds: an in-vivo and in-vitro study on the guinea-pig ileum. Arch Int Pharmacodyn Ther 257.2 (1982): 274–287.
Koetter U et al. A randomized, double blind, placebo-controlled, prospective clinical study to demonstrate clinical efficacy of a fixed valerian hops extract combination (Ze 91019) in patients suffering from non-organic sleep disorder. Phytother Res 21.9 (2007): 847–851.
Kohnen R, Oswald WD. The effects of valerian, propranolol, and their combination on activation, performance, and mood of healthy volunteers under social stress conditions. Pharmacopsychiatry 21.6 (1988): 447–448.
Kuhlmann J et al. The influence of valerian treatment on reaction time, alertness and concentration in volunteers. Pharmacopsychiatry 32.6 (1999): 235–241.
Leathwood PD, Chauffard F. Aqueous extract of valerian reduces latency to fall asleep in man. Planta Med 2 (1985): 144–148.
Leuschner J et al. Characterisation of the central nervous depressant activity of a commercially available valerian root extract. Arzneimittelforschung 43.6 (1993): 638–641.
Lindahl O, Lindwall L. Double blind study of a valerian preparation. Pharmacol Biochem Behav 32.4 (1989): 1065–1066.
Mills S, Bone K. Principles and practice of phytotherapy. London: Churchill Livingstone, 2000.
Mirabi P et al. Effects of valerian on the severity and systemic manifestations of dysmenorrhea. Int J Gynaecol Obstet 115.3 (2011): 285–288.
Miyasaka LS et al. Valerian for anxiety disorders. Cochrane Database Syst Rev 4 (2006): CD004515.
Mohamed MF et al. Inhibitory effects of commonly used herbal extracts on UGT1A1 enzyme activity. Xenobiotica 40.10 (2010): 663–669.
Mohamed ME, Frye RF. Effects of herbal supplements on drug glucuronidation. Review of clinical, animal, and in vitro studies. Planta Med 77.4 (2011): 311–321.

Muller SF, Klement S. A combination of valerian and lemon balm is effective in the treatment of restlessness and dyssomnia in children. Phytomedicine 13.6 (2006): 383–387.
Neuhaus W et al. Transport of a GABAA receptor modulator and its derivatives from Valeriana officinalis L. s. l. across an in vitro cellculture model of the blood-brain barrier. Planta Med 74.11 (2008): 1338–1344.
Occhiuto F et al. Relaxing effects of Valeriana officinalis extracts on isolated human non-pregnant uterine muscle. J Pharm Pharmacol 61.2 (2009): 251–256.
Ortiz JG et al. Effects of Valeriana officinalis extracts on [3H]flunitrazepam binding, synaptosomal [3H]GABA uptake, and hippocampal [3H]GABA release. Neurochem Res 24.11 (1999): 1373–1378.
Pakseresht S et al. Extract of valerian root (Valeriana officinalis L.) vs. placebo in treatment of obsessive-compulsive disorder: a randomized double-blind study. J Complement Integr Med 8.1 (2011): Article 32.
Pittler MH, Ernst E. Kava extract for treating anxiety. Cochrane Database Syst Rev 2 (2002): CD003383.
Rezvani ME et al. Anticonvulsant effect of aqueous extract of Valeriana officinalis in amygdala-kindled rats: possible involvement of adenosine. J Ethnopharmacol 127.2 (2010): 313–318.
Santos MS et al. Synaptosomal GABA release as influenced by valerian root extract: involvement of the GABA carrier. Arch Int Pharmacodyn Ther 327.2 (1994): 220–231.
Schulz H et al. The effect of valerian extract on sleep polygraphy in poor sleepers: a pilot study. Pharmacopsychiatry 27.4 (1994): 147–151.
Schumacher B et al. Lignans isolated from valerian: identification and characterization of a new olivil derivative with partial agonistic activity at (A)1 adenosine receptors. J Nat Prod 65.10 (2002): 1479–1485.
Stevinson C, Ernst E. Valerian for insomnia: a systematic review of randomized clinical trials. Sleep Med 1.2 (2000): 91–99.
Taavoni S et al. Effect of valerian on sleep quality in postmenopausal women: a randomized placebo-controlled clinical trial. Menopause 18.9 (2011): 951–955.
Tabach R et al. Preclinical toxicological assessment of a phytotherapeutic product –CPV (based on dry extracts of *Crataegus oxyacantha L., Passiflora incarnata L.*, and *Valeriana officinalis L.*). Phytother Res 23.1 (2009): 33–40.
Taibi DM et al. A systematic review of valerian as a sleep aid: safe but not effective. Sleep Med Rev 11.3 (2007): 209–230.
Taibi DM et al. A randomized clinical trial of valerian fails to improve self-reported, polysomnographic, and actigraphic sleep in older women with insomnia. Sleep Med 10.3 (2009): 319–328.
Trauner G et al. Modulation of GABAA receptors by valerian extracts is related to the content of valerenic acid. Planta Med 74.1 (2008):19–24.
Upton R (eds). Valerian root, Santa Cruz: American Herbal Pharmacopoeia, 1999.
Vassiliadis T et al. Valeriana hepatotoxicity. Sleep Med 10.8 (2009): 935.
Wheatley D. Kava and valerian in the treatment of stress-induced insomnia. Phytother Res 15.6 (2001): 549–551.
Willey LB et al. Valerian overdose: a case report. Vet Hum Toxicol 37.4 (1995): 364–365.
Ziegler G et al. Efficacy and tolerability of valerian extract LI 156 compared with oxazepam in the treatment of non-organic insomnia: a randomized, double-blind, comparative clinical study. Eur J Med Res 7.11 (2002): 480–486.

Vitamin B_1

HISTORICAL NOTE The Chinese medical book *Neiching* describes beriberi in 2697 BC, but it was not known for a long time that vitamin B_1 deficiency was responsible. The neurological symptoms such as leg weakness characteristic of thiamin deficiency were also recorded in the 1890s in chicks fed a diet of polished rice. In 1912, thiamin was isolated from rice bran and in the mid-1930s the structure of vitamin B_1 was determined (Gropper & Smith 2013). Since it was found not to contain an amine group, the 'e' was dropped from its name (thiamine → thiamin).

BACKGROUND AND RELEVANT PHARMACOKINETICS

Vitamin B_1 is a water-soluble compound required by all tissues. It is also known as thiamin (previously thiamine), anti-beriberi factor, antineuritic factor and its active coenzyme form, thiamin diphosphate (TDP), also called thiamin pyrophosphate (TPP). Thiamin's phosphate ester functions as a coenzyme and its ability to shift between different degrees of phosphorylation makes it a key nutrient in energy pathways.

There are two sources of thiamin: dietary and bacterial, which is synthesised by normal intestinal microflora. Thiamin is absorbed, predominantly in the jejunum and ileum as free (unphosphorylated) thiamin, by a saturable rate-limiting transport mechanism and may be passive or active. Passive absorption occurs at high concentrations, while at physiological levels, two active thiamin transporters, ThTr1 and ThTr2, are utilised. The activity of these transporters is inhibited by alcohol. The absorption of thiamin in the gastrointestinal tract can also be impaired by the presence of naturally occurring antithiamin factors such as thiaminases, found in raw fish, and polyhydroxyphenols, found in coffee, tea, blueberries, red cabbage and Brussels sprouts (Groff & Gropper 2009). Interestingly, calcium and magnesium exacerbate the effect of the polyhydroxyphenols. Conversely, thiamin preservation in the gastrointestinal tract is enhanced by vitamin C and citric acid (Gropper & Smith 2013).

Thiamin is transported via the portal circulation, travelling in plasma either free, bound to albumin, or as thiamin monophosphate, to the liver, where it is phosphorylated to its TDP coenzyme form (80% total body thiamin), which is also its most active state. Magnesium is required as a cofactor for this conversion/ activation while alcohol has an inhibitory effect. Thiamin is taken up into brain by a blood–brain barrier transporter and via cerebrospinal fluid (CSF) (Fernstrom & Fenstrom 2013). Thiamin is excreted mainly by the kidneys. Thiamin is found in high concentrations in skeletal muscle, heart, liver, kidneys and brain and its half-life is approximately 15 days (Singleton & Martin 2001).

CHEMICAL COMPONENTS

Thiamin (vitamin B_1) is a water-soluble substance, composed of two heterocyclic moieties, substituted thiazole and pyrimidine rings joined by a methylene bridge (Rapala-Kozik 2011). It does not contain an amine group, as originally postulated.

FOOD SOURCES

Thiamin found in plant foods exists in its free form, while 95% of thiamin found in animal foods occurs primarily as TDP (Gropper & Smith 2013).

Brewer's yeast, lean meat and legumes are considered the richest sources of thiamin. Other sources include cereals, grains, pasta, wheat germ, soy milk, seeds and peanuts.

It is possible to lose up to 85% of the thiamin content in meat through cooking and canning, and up to 60% from cooking vegetables (Tanphaichitr 1999); cooking foods in water will further exacerbate the loss (Gropper & Smith 2013). There is also loss through refining of grains and polishing of rice (where the germ and bran have been removed, leaving only the endosperm). However, in Australia the fortification of wheat flour used for making bread with thiamin is mandatory to compensate for this loss (FSANZ 2012). Thiamin is not stable in alkaline environments; a pH of 8 or above destroys its activity (Gropper & Smith 2013).

DEFICIENCY SIGNS AND SYMPTOMS

The body only stores a small amount of thiamin and signs of deficiency tend to develop within 15–18 days of restricted intake.

Despite an expansive understanding of the role of thiamin at the cellular level, many aspects of the pathophysiological manifestations of thiamin deficiency remain unexplained (Gropper & Smith 2013). Beriberi (*beri* means weakness) is the classic deficiency state. General early or subclinical deficiency signs and symptoms include fatigue, weakness, rigidity (due to corresponding increase in lactic acid production), poor memory, sleep disturbances, chest wall pain, anorexia, abdominal discomfort and constipation. Other characteristic signs and symptoms include retarded growth, oedema, cardiomyopathy, bradycardia, heart failure and peripheral neuropathy (Combs 2012).

There are four forms of beriberi: dry, wet, acute and cerebral, otherwise known as Wernicke-Korsakoff syndrome. Dry beriberi is associated with muscle weakness and wasting, especially of the lower limbs, peripheral neurological changes and nerve conduction problems that may lead to symmetrical foot drop with calf tenderness (Gropper & Smith 2013). In addition to neurological changes, wet beriberi is associated with cardiovascular changes such as cardiomegaly and tachycardia. It is characterised by peripheral vasodilation, oedema due to sodium and water retention, increased cardiac output and myocardial failure, which can become fatal in severe cases. Acute beriberi occurs most commonly in infants and is associated with nausea and vomiting, convulsions, lactic acidosis, tachycardia and cardiomegaly; acute attacks may result in death if thiamin deficiency is not rapidly corrected.

Cerebral beriberi involves alterations to ocular and cognitive function secondary to bilateral symmetrical brain lesions in the paraventricular grey matter, producing ataxia, which can also be fatal. Ophthalmoplegia (paralyisis of the ocular muscles), nystagamus (involuntary, constant eyeball movement) and ataxia are the recognised triad of symptoms of Wernicke's encephalopathy. People with alcohol dependency are particularly at risk due to reduced consumption of food (thus thiamin intake), decreased absorption (Gropper & Smith 2013) and increased requirements due to decreased liver function (which impairs TDP formation).

Additionally, Wernicke–Korsakoff syndrome has been reported in several other conditions, such as hyperemesis gravidarum, hyperemesis due to gastroplasty (Kuhn et al 2012), acute psychosis after gastric bypass (Walker & Kepner 2012), gastric lap band (Becker et al 2012) and bariatric surgery (Lu'o'ng & Nguyen 2011, Sriram et al 2012), hyperthyroidism and inadequate parenteral nutrition (Bonucchi et al 2008, Gardian et al 1999, Ogershok et al 2002, Seehra et al 1996, Spruill & Kuller 2002, Tan & Ho 2001, Togay-Isikay et al 2001, Toth & Voll 2001). A 2007 case report of thrombocytopenia in a patient with Wernicke–Korsakoff syndrome, responsive to thiamin repletion, has introduced the possibility that this may constitute an unusual feature of the deficiency picture (Francini-Pesenti et al 2007).

While it is well recognised that the brain, heart and neuronal tissue are classically affected by thiamin deficiency, a recent in vivo study has found evidence of an endogenous self-preservation mechanism for brain and heart tissue that becomes established within 4 weeks of a thiamin-deficient diet (Klooster et al 2013). After this period, brain tissue transketolase activity remained constant and TDP (TPP) levels were significantly conserved in brain and heart tissue. The authors have suggested that other tissues could be suffering thiamin deficiency despite the absence of classical beriberi or Wernicke-Korsakoff syndrome (Lu'o'ng & Nguyen 2011, Sriram et al 2012). The length of time by which this self-preservation response can be effective during periods of low thiamin intake remains to be tested.

V

Clinical note — Thiamin deficiency is not uncommon in the elderly

Several observational studies have reported that thiamin deficiency is not uncommon in the elderly. A study of 118 elderly hospital patients identified a moderate deficiency incidence of 40% (Pepersack et al 1999). Similar results were obtained in another survey, where marginal thiamin deficiency had an incidence of 31% and frank deficiency of 17% in 36 non-demented elderly patients admitted to an acute geriatric unit. Delirium occurred in 32% of patients with normal thiamin status and 76% of thiamin-deficient patients ($P < 0.025$), although one or more other possible causes for delirium were present in all cases (O'Keeffe et al 1994). The importance of including thiamin deficiency in diagnostic work-ups of at-risk individuals is underscored by the high mortality rate in Wernicke–Korsakoff syndrome (10–20%), reported to be the direct result of underdiagnosis (Bonucchi et al 2008). Similarly, it is important to keep in mind that there is significant interindividual variability in both susceptibility to thiamin deficiency and its consequences (Al-Nasser et al 2006).

Preliminary research suggests that inadequate intake could also increase susceptibility to neurodegeneration, particularly in aged organisms (Nixon et al 2006, Pitkin & Savage 2004).

Clinical note — Thiamin food fortification in Australia and New Zealand
Australia New Zealand Food Standards Code, Standard 2.1.1 Amendment No. 111 2009 Cereals and Cereal Products, defines 'a number of products composed of cereals, qualifies the use of the term "bread", and requires the mandatory fortification of flour for bread making with thiamin in Australia' (Australian Government Comlaw 2009).

Primary deficiency

Primary deficiency is caused by inadequate dietary intake of thiamin, particularly in people subsisting mainly on highly polished rice (de Montmollin et al 2002) or unfortified refined grain products. Insufficient intake may also occur in anorexia. Historically, those receiving total parenteral nutrition (TPN) without adequate additional thiamin were at risk of a primary deficiency. Current TPN formulae include 3 mg thiamin (Merck Manual Professional 2009).

Secondary deficiency

Secondary deficiency is caused by an increased requirement, as in hyperthyroidism, pregnancy, lactation, fever, acute infection, increased carbohydrate intake, folate deficiency, malabsorption states, hyperemesis, prolonged diarrhoea, strenuous physical exertion, breastfeeding, adolescent growth and states of impaired utilisation such as severe liver disease, alcoholism, chronic haemodialysis, diabetes (types 1 and 2) and people taking loop diuretics long-term. Additionally, pyruvate dehydrogenase deficiency can result in deficiency (Beers & Berkow 2003, Thornalley et al 2007, Wardlaw et al 1997, Wahlqvist et al 2002). Alternatively, latent primary thiamin deficiencies produce overt clinical features when the patient is exposed to thiamin metabolism stressors, such as those listed above, e.g. pregnancy, surgery (Al-Nasser et al 2006).

MAIN ACTIONS

Coenzyme

Carbohydrate and branched-chain amino acid metabolism.

Thiamin serves as a cofactor for several enzymes involved in carbohydrate catabolism, including pyruvate dehydrogenase complex, where TDP/TPP converts pyruvate to acetyl CoA (Fattal-Valevski 2011), transketolase and alpha-ketoglutarate, and for the branched-chain alpha-keto acid dehydrogenase complex that is involved in amino acid catabolism (Singleton & Martin 2001). Some of these enzymes are also important in brain oxidative metabolism (Molina et al 2002).

Neurotransmitter biosynthesis

Thiamin is involved in the biosynthesis of a number of neurotransmitters, including acetylcholine and gamma-aminobutyric acid. As TTP, it may also be involved in nerve impulse transmission (Gropper & Smith 2013).

DNA

Thiamin is involved in the synthesis of DNA precursors, therefore its use is increased in people with tumours.

Neuropsychological actions and neurodegenerative diseases

Thiamin is taken up into brain by a blood–brain barrier transporter and via CSF (Fernstrom & Fenstrom 2013). It is involved in neurotransmitter biosynthesis and is required for neurotransmission, nerve conduction, blood CSF barrier functionality and muscle action.

In the form of TTP, it plays an essential role in the physiology of the nervous system as it concentrates in nerve and muscle cells and activates membrane ion channels. TTP represents the smallest percentage of thiamin forms in humans; however, its phosphorylation of key regulatory proteins and the activation of high-conductance anion channels in nerve cells demonstrate its vital role in nervous system physiology (Gangolf et al 2010, Rapala-Kozik 2011). Thiamin deficiency leads to impaired oxidative metabolism due to impaired thiamin-dependent enzyme activity, and subsequently results in a multitude of negative events in the brain, including oxidative stress, lactic acidosis, blood–brain barrier disruption, decreased glucose utilisation and inflammation (Jhala & Hazell 2011). The consequence of such impaired metabolism alters brain function and can result in structural damage, neurodegeneration and, ultimately, neuronal cell loss (Jhala & Hazell 2011, Rapala-Kozik 2011).

Severe thiamin deficiency in the nervous tissue of animals reduces TPP levels and causes loss of coordinated muscle control. Upon correcting thiamin levels these anomalies are reversed, suggesting no permanent neural damage or destruction (Fernstrom & Fenstrom 2013). However, evidence from animal studies suggests that impaired blood CSF barrier function, secondary to thiamin deficiency, allows passage of neuroactive substances into the brain, damaging the choroid plexus (Nixon et al 2006). In Wernicke-Korsakoff syndrome, selective damage of mammillary bodies, the thalamus and pons has been observed, and analysis at the cellular level shows microglial activation and astrocyte proliferation (Hazell 2009, Hazell et al 1998, Rapala-Kozik 2011, Wang & Hazell 2010). Furthermore, in Wernicke-Korsakoff syndrome, the activity of all TDP-dependent enzymes is reduced, which in turn leads to decreased glutamate, aspartate and gamma-aminobutyric acid production, mitochondrial disintegration, lactate accumulation, acidosis and ultimately neuronal cell loss (Rapala-Kozik 2011).

Energy production

The B vitamins collectively function as coenzymes particularly involved in mitochondrial energy production. TDP, specifically, is utilised as a cofactor in pyruvate dehydrogenase, alpha-ketoglutarate dehydrogenase and branched-chain alpha-keto acid dehydrogenase. Evidence suggests that impaired mitochondrial energy production and decreased antioxidant activity, secondary to thiamin deficiency, may be responsible for the neuronal damage associated with this deficiency.

Antioxidant

While thiamin does not have any direct free radical scavenging activity, it has been postulated that, in thiamin deficiency, the neuronal damage and cellular energy depletion may be due to oxidative stress; high nitric oxide synthase production and formation of peroxynitrites have been observed and may be responsible for the deactivation of ketoglutarate dehydrogenase (Gibson & Blass 2007, Huang et al 2010, Rapala-Kozik 2011).

Mood

In addition to thiamin's important roles in neurotransmitter production, neurotransmission and nerve conduction, a deficiency of thiamin impedes the brain's ability to utilise glucose for energy. Subsequent manifestations include a plethora of neuropsychological effects, including mental depression, anxiety, irritability, apathy, poor concentration, forgetfulness and dementia. An early study found that as little as 50 mg/day thiamin per day for 2 months improved thiamin status in deficient individuals and was associated with greater mental clarity (Benton et al 1997).

CLINICAL USE

Many of the clinical uses of thiamin supplements are conditions thought to arise from a marginal deficiency, but some indications are based on the concept of high-dose supplements acting as therapeutic agents. In practice, vitamin B_1 is usually recommended in combination with other B group vitamins.

Deficiency: treatment and prevention

Thiamin supplements are traditionally used to treat or prevent thiamin deficiency states in people at risk (see Secondary deficiency, above).

Hyperemesis

Although thiamin supplementation will not reduce the symptoms of hyperemesis, it may be necessary in cases of hyperemesis gravidarum and hyperemesis due to gastroplasty and gastric lap band surgery in order to avoid deficiency, which has been infrequently reported in these situations. Permanent multifocal neurological dysfunction has been reported in women, including adolescent women, within 3 months of undergoing gastroplasty and gastric lap band surgery and reporting hyperemesis (Becker et al 2012, Kuhn et al 2012, Towbin et al 2004, Walker & Kepner 2012). It may be precipitated in part by intravenous (IV) fluids containing dextrose, and is more commonly seen when the patient's liver transaminases are elevated, which may contribute to the encephalopathy (Becker et al 2012, Francini-Pesenti et al 2007, Gardian et al 1999, Kuhn et al 2012; Seehra et al 1996, Spruill & Kuller 2002, Tan & Ho 2001, Togay-Isikay et al 2001, Toth & Voll 2001, Welsh 2005).

Alcoholism

In alcoholism, a state of decreased intake, absorption, utilisation and increased requirement for thiamin occurs, necessitating increased intakes to avoid deficiency states (D'Amour et al 1991). In cases of Wernicke's encephalopathy, monitoring of thiamin status and prophylactic IV treatment will inhibit the progression to Korsakoff's psychosis (Thomson & Marshall 2005). Ongoing research has revealed that the cerebellar neurotoxicity associated with excess alcohol is more likely to be mediated predominantly by thiamin deficiency than by direct ethanol cytotoxicity, as previously believed (Mulholland et al 2005); however, there is growing evidence of a strong negative synergy between the two that extends well beyond the increased need for thiamin as a result of alcohol consumption (Nixon et al

2006). In the treatment of Wernicke's encephalopathy, two studies have found IV or intramuscular (IM) administration of 100–500 mg of thiamin over 30 minutes for 3 days necessary to sufficiently raise plasma thiamin levels, and improve thiamin uptake and transport across the blood–brain barrier (Francini-Pesenti et al 2009, Sechi & Serra 2007).

Total parenteral nutrition

Several case reports show that patients who have received TPN without proper replacement of thiamin are at risk of developing deficiency signs and Wernicke's encephalopathy (Francini-Pesenti et al 2007, Hahn et al 1998, van Noort et al 1987, Vortmeyer et al 1992, Zak et al 1991). Preliminary evidence suggests that current TPN formulations are not sufficient to ensure thiamin repletion in all patients (Francini-Pesenti et al 2009).

Hyperthyroidism

Although a somewhat rare sequela, a handful of case reports describe Wernicke–Korsakoff's syndrome in patients suffering thyrotoxicosis (Bonucchi et al 2008).

Surgical patients

Several case reports detailing Wernicke's encephalopathy in surgical patients highlight why this patient group should be considered 'high-risk' for thiamin deficiency: malnutrition, high stress levels, vomiting and ileus all increase thiamin requirements substantially (Al-Nasser et al 2006, Francini-Pesenti et al 2007). Several authors suggest that thiamin deficiency may be latent in the preoperative patient, with surgery or postoperative TPN precipitating clinical manifestation, and consequently recommend preoperative screening for thiamin status (Al-Nasser et al 2006).

Acute alcohol withdrawal

Several guidelines for the support of alcohol withdrawal recommend a dose of 100 mg thiamin administered IV or IM before routine administration of dextrose-containing solutions (Adinoff et al 1988, Erstad & Cotugno 1995).

Alzheimer's disease (AD)

Thiamin status has been investigated and found, amongst other nutrients, to have an inverse relationship with cognitive function in the elderly (Nourhashemi et al 2000). More specifically, AD has been associated with reduced plasma levels of thiamin, according to several clinical studies (Gold et al 1995, 1998, Molina et al 2002). One study analysing cerebral cortex samples from autopsied patients with AD found slight reductions in TDP levels compared with matched controls (Mastrogiacoma et al 1996). Others have demonstrated reduced activities of thiamin-dependent enzymes, together with a strong correlation between these reductions and the extent of the dementia pathology in autopsied brains (Gibson & Blass 2007). Proposed mechanisms for the relationship between thiamin and AD are varied, ranging from its role as an antioxidant and its critical contribution to the Krebs cycle to its involvement in the production of acetylcholine, disturbances of which have all been implicated in AD pathology (Bubber et al 2004, Butterfield et al 2002, Gibson & Blass 2007, Kruse et al 2004). Animal research points towards the shared features of thiamin deficiency and AD pathology in the brain, in particular, with increased oxidative stress and inflammation precipitating neuronal loss in specific brain areas and concomitant promotion of plaque formation (Karuppagounder et al 2009).

Investigation with high-dose thiamin supplementation in this population has produced mixed results (Blass et al 1988, Meador et al 1993, Mimori et al 1996).

One double-blind, placebo-controlled, crossover study showed that a dose of 3000 mg thiamin/day produced higher global cognitive ratings, as assessed by the Mini-Mental State Examination, compared with a niacinamide placebo. However, there were no changes to clinical state and behavioural ratings (Blass et al 1988). Another clinical study of unknown design found positive results with a dose ranging between 3 and 8 g/day of thiamin (Meador et al 1993), whereas a long-term study using high-dose supplementation produced negative results (Mimori et al 1996).

Although promising overall, a 2001 Cochrane review stated that it is still not possible to draw any conclusions about the effectiveness of thiamin supplementation in AD (Rodriguez-Martin et al 2001). In practice, it is often used as part of a broad-spectrum approach with other B group vitamins in age-related cognitive decline; however, further research is required to determine whether this method produces more consistent results, particularly as an adjunct to standard pharmaceutical treatments (Gibson & Blass 2007).

Diabetes

Given thiamin's essential role in the key carbohydrate metabolic enzymes transketolase, pyruvate dehydrogenase and alpha-ketoglutarate dehydrogenase and the glucose toxicity that occurs secondary to thiamin deficiency (Nixon et al 2006), there is growing interest in the therapeutic potential of this nutrient in diabetes. Preliminary research of thiamin status in diabetic patients reveals significantly high rates of deficiency (≈75% of type 1 and 2 diabetics), secondary to greatly increased renal losses (Thornalley et al 2007). It has been suggested that reduced thiamin availability may exacerbate diabetic metabolic dysfunction, particularly with respect to microvascular complications. This finding adds to the evidence produced earlier in test tube studies demonstrating that thiamin improves endothelial function, while protecting against insulin-mediated vascular smooth-muscle cell proliferation (Arora et al 2006).

In diabetes, benfotiamine, a synthetic derivative of thiamin (see section on Supplemental forms, below), induces key thiamin-dependent enzymes of the pentose shunt to reduce accumulation of toxic metabolites, including advanced glycation end products (Gibson et al 2013).

An investigation into high-dose thiamin (100 mg taken three times daily) over 3 months in a small sample of type 2 diabetes mellitus patients with microalbuminuria demonstrated reversal of early-stage nephropathy in the treatment group, without altering glycaemic control, dyslipidaemia or blood pressure (Rabbani et al 2009). Another study employing thiamin, this time in IV form, improved endothelium-dependent vasodilation in hyperglycaemic patients (both diabetic and non-diabetic); however, the mechanism of action remains unclear (Arora et al 2006).

Thiamin status in non-diabetic patients is typically assessed by the well-validated red blood cell transketolase activity test. However, an established limitation in this test is its inaccuracy in diabetic patients, complicating accurate assessment in this population (Thornalley et al 2007).

Clinical note — The link between glucose metabolism, Alzheimer's dementia and thiamin

A continuous supply of glucose is essential for normal brain function and a key feature and biomarker of progression of AD is reduced glucose metabolism (Gibson et al 2013). Changes in brain glucose metabolism occur decades before the development of symptoms (Reiman et al 2004). In a multicentre, longitudinal neuroimaging study (Alzheimer Disease Neuroimaging Initiative: ADNI) launched in 2004, in which 819 adult subjects, 55–90 years old, were investigated, it was found that brain glucose utilisation was the best predictor of developing and progressing from mild cognitive impairment to AD (Jack et al 2010).

Thiamin-dependent processes responsible for glucose metabolism are diminished in brains of AD patients at autopsy and have been correlated with worse outcomes on dementia rating scales (Gibson et al 2013). Furthermore, thiamin deficiency exacerbates plaque formation and impairs memory in animal studies, while benfotiamine diminishes plaques and reverses memory deficits. Despite the linkages between diminished glucose metabolism in the brain and AD, why glucose metabolism is diminished remains elusive.

Congestive heart failure (CHF)

A large trial published in 2006 confirmed that the incidence of thiamin deficiency is notable amongst CHF patients (Hanninen et al 2006). These results were echoed by a more recent review in which the majority of studies reflect a general trend of increased risk of thiamin deficiency amongst this patient group compared with individuals free from the condition (McKeag et al 2012). It is suspected that patients with existing heart failure are at increased risk of thiamin deficiency because of diuretic-induced depletion, advanced age, malnutrition and/or periods of hospitalisation. A cross-sectional study reported that approximately one-third of hospitalised patients with heart failure had tissue levels suggestive of thiamin deficiency (Keith et al 2009).

While a 2001 review concluded that there was insufficient evidence from large trials to confirm thiamin as a corrective treatment in CHF, a number of small interventional studies have assessed the effect of thiamin supplementation in patients with CHF, with promising results. In one pilot study of 6 patients treated with IV thiamin, such that their thiamin status returned to normal, there was increased left ventricular ejection fraction (LVEF) in 4 of 5 patients studied by electrocardiograph (Seligmann et al 1991). A randomised, placebo-controlled, double-blind study of 30 patients compared the effects of IV thiamin (200 mg/day) to placebo over 1 week followed by oral thiamin (200 mg/day) taken for 6 weeks. In the 27 patients completing the full 7-week intervention, LVEF rose by 22%. Other positive results have been reported from similar studies (Hanninen et al 2006). The current position of key researchers in this area is that, together with other micronutrients critical for myocardial energy production and control of oxidative stress (e.g. taurine), thiamin inadequacy is likely to exacerbate myocyte dysfunction and loss in this condition, making repletion an important therapeutic objective (Allard et al 2006).

IN COMBINATION

V

A Cochrane review of vitamin B complex for treating peripheral neuropathy, which included 13 studies (11 parallel RCTs and two quasi-randomised trials) involving 741 participants (488 treated with vitamin B alone) with alcoholic or diabetic neuropathy, concluded there are limited data and the evidence is insufficient to determine whether vitamin B complex is beneficial or harmful in these populations (Ang et al 2008).

One study using benfotiamine (see section on Supplemental forms, below), however, showed possible short-term benefit from 8-week treatment compared to placebo (Woelk et al 1998). Only 30 participants were treated with the oral benfotiamine in this study at a dosage of 320 mg/day during weeks 1–4 and 120 mg benfotiamine/day during weeks

5–8 (one capsule t.i.d.). Within the 8-week study period, benfotiamine led to a significant improvement of the threshold of vibration perception at the great toe, motor function and the overall symptom score. Marked improvement occurred in both pain and coordination (Woelk et al 1998). However, the strength of this evidence is weakened by the lack of other larger positive trials since this time.

Dysmenorrhoea

A Cochrane review of herbal and dietary therapies for primary and secondary dysmenorrhoea concluded that thiamin is an effective treatment when taken at 100 mg/day, although this conclusion is tempered slightly by its basis in only one large randomised controlled trial (Proctor & Murphy 2009). That trial was a randomised, double-blind, placebo-controlled, crossover design conducted over 5 months in 556 women and procured a positive improvement in >90% of the treatment cycle versus <1% in the placebo phase. The improvements observed during treatment appeared to have lasting effects, even after cessation of supplementation, for up to 3 months (Gokhale 1996). Due to the dramatic 'success' of this study, it has attracted scepticism regarding its methodology; certainly a question is why, with such positive results, an attempt to replicate the findings has not been undertaken since the mid-1990s (Fugh-Berman & Kronenberg 2003).

Epilepsy

A randomised, placebo-controlled trial involving 72 epileptic patients who had received long-term phenytoin treatment alone or in combination with phenobarbitone found that administration of thiamin (50 mg/day) over 6 months improved neuropsychological functions in both verbal and non-verbal IQ testing (Botez et al 1993). This study, interestingly, also found both folate supplementation (also typically depleted by the medication) and placebo ineffective. A 2009 Cochrane review investigating the role of B vitamins in controlling certain types of seizures found that thiamin supplementation improved neuropsychological functions related to psychomotor speed, visuospatial abilities, selective attention and verbal abstracting ability; however the sample was small and the authors concluded there is insufficient evidence that B vitamins improve seizure control or prevent harmful side effects of antiepileptic drugs in epileptic patients (Ranganathan & Ramaratnam 2009).

OTHER USES

Cataracts

A case-controlled study of 72 patients found that thiamin supplementation reduced the incidence of cortical, nuclear and mixed cataracts (Leske et al 1991).

Coma

A general approach to patients presenting to hospital with coma is to ensure adequate oxygenation, blood flow and treatment with hypertonic glucose and thiamin (Alguire 1990, Buylaert 2000).

Mortality in the elderly

In a recent study, higher intakes of vitamins B_1 and B_6 observed amongst Taiwanese elders were associated with increased survival rates by up to 10 years (Huang et al 2012). The Taiwanese Elderly Nutrition and Health Survey (1999–2000) interviewed 747 participants aged 65 years and over. Dietary and biochemical data were collected at baseline. Survivorship was determined until 31 December

2008. Controlled for confounders, and relative to the lowest tertile of vitamin B_1 or B_6 intakes, the hazard ratios (95% confidence interval) for tertile 3 were 0.74 (0.58–0.95) and 0.74 (0.57–0.97) (both $P < 0.05$). The authors concluded that deficiencies of vitamin B_1 and B_6 were found to be clearly predictive of mortality in elderly Taiwanese.

Polycystic ovarian syndrome

Insulin resistance is a key clinical feature in polycystic ovarian syndrome. Given the importance of thiamin in carbohydrate metabolism, it may suggest an important clinical role for thiamin in polycystic ovarian syndrome and improved insulin sensitivity (Hechtman 2011).

Tumour proliferation

In advanced cancer, thiamin deficiency, along with many other micronutrients, frequently occurs. However TPP is involved in ribose synthesis, required for cellular replication, and hence the concern about a proliferative role ensues. In a metabolic control analysis in vivo, a high stimulatory effect on tumour growth of 164% was found for thiamin doses at 25 times the recommended dietary allowance (RDA) compared to controls. However, in the same study when thiamin supplementation was 2500 times the RDA for mice, the opposite effect was observed and a 10% inhibition of tumour growth was recognised. This effect was heightened, resulting in a 36% decrease, when thiamin supplementation was administered from the 7th day prior to tumour inoculation (Comin-Anduix et al 2001). Human research is urgently needed in order to elucidate any potential benefits or risks for thiamin in cancer.

> ***Clinical note — No protection against insect bites***
>
> One claim that has been around for many years is that high oral doses of certain B vitamins could act as a deterrent to insects such as mosquitoes. Principally, the myth has centred on thiamin. A review of prophylaxis against insect bites found that neither topical application nor oral dosing of thiamin is an effective preventive strategy (Rudin 2005).

IN COMBINATION

The B group vitamins function as coenzymes in energy production and are a popular supplement taken by the public to lessen the impact of 'stress' and provide an energy boost. In one study, thiamin 10 mg/day significantly increased appetite, energy intake, body weight and general wellbeing and decreased fatigue, compared with placebo in a group of 80 randomly chosen women from a population with known marginal deficiency (Smidt et al 1991). Thiamin supplementation also tended to reduce daytime sleep time, improve sleep patterns and increase activity.

Fibromyalgia

Studies have detailed thiamin metabolism disorders in fibromyalgia patients (Eisinger et al 1994, Juhl 1998). Due to its importance in energy production, it is suggested that any subsequent deficiencies due to the metabolic alteration may negatively impact energy production, potentially exacerbating the fatigue already prevalent in fibromyalgia sufferers.

HIV

Several neuropathological reports have described brain lesions characteristic of Wernicke's encephalopathy in patients with AIDS. One study found a 23%

prevalence of thiamin deficiency in AIDS patients with no history of alcohol abuse (Butterworth et al 1991), which may correlate with symptoms of fatigue and lethargy related to HIV. Another study found a decreased progression to AIDS from HIV in patients replete in vitamins B and C (Tang et al 1993).

Neurogenic impotence

A dose of 25 mg thiamin taken orally resulted in normalisation of erection in a man with a history of chronic alcoholism and erectile dysfunction of 1 year's duration (Tjandra & Janknegt 1997). However, more recent evidence discussing the causes of neurogenic impotence suggests that thiamin deficiency is relatively rare (Finsterer 2005).

Maple syrup urine disease

Of four paediatric patients with maple syrup urine disease, three responded to thiamin therapy with a reduction in concentration of plasma and urinary branched-chain amino and keto acids (Fernhoff et al 1985).

IN COMBINATION

B vitamins were investigated for reducing sensitivity to painful stimuli in mice (Franca et al 2001), whereby thiamin and pyridoxine (50–200 mg/kg intraperitoneally [IP]) or riboflavin (3–100 mg/kg IP) induced an antinociceptive effect, not changed by naloxone (10 mg/kg IP), indicating that activity is not mediated by opiate pathways. The authors state that the B vitamins' antinociceptive effect may involve inhibition of the synthesis and/or action of inflammatory mediators. Furthermore, in an animal study the therapeutic effects of glucosamine hydrochloride and chondroitin sulfate as chondroprotection were enhanced by the addition of fursultiamine, a thiamin derivative, in the treatment of osteoarthritis (Kobayashi et al 2005).

Optic neuropathy

Several case reports suggest this condition can be caused by thiamin deficiency and successfully treated with supplementation. One case report of a man developing optic neuropathy as a result of receiving TPN without thiamin for 4 weeks found that supplementation with thiamin reversed the condition (Suzuki et al 1997). Two cases of symmetrical, bilateral optic neuropathy associated with thiamin deficiency were successfully treated with thiamin supplementation.

Fertility, preconception and health of the offspring

An animal study investigated the effects of thiamin deficiency in newly developing neuronal cells, reporting cellular membrane damage, apoptosis and irregular and ectopic cells (Ba 2008). The same paper postulates that thiamin repletion may stabilise neurons and prevent cellular death.

Another animal study by the same author investigated the impact of alcohol consumption and thiamin deficiency in the developing central nervous system (Ba 2011). Neurotoxicity caused by maternal thiamin deficiency during pre-, peri- and postnatal stages was compared with neurotoxicity caused by chronic maternal alcohol intake alone and finally compared with the combined effects. Neurodevelopmental abilities in the offspring were then measured. Both thiamin deficiency and ethanol exposure interfered with periods of intense cellular proliferation prenatally, and with cellular differentiation, synaptogenesis, axonogenesis and myelinogenesis during peri- and postnatal stages, producing neurofunctional alterations. Furthermore, perinatal effects of thiamin deficiency on primary cellular differentiation in the developing central nervous system were similar to those caused by alcohol exposure (Ba 2011).

Due to the imperative role of thiamin in female reproductive function, cellular differentiation and proliferation, and normal hormonal processes during gestation, a deficiency of thiamin during pregnancy may be implicated in an increased risk of miscarriage (Ba 2009). A limitation of this evidence is that the majority of investigations have been animal-based.

DOSAGE RANGE

- Prevention of deficiency (adult Australian recommended dietary intake [RDI]): 1.1–1.2 mg/day
- Treatment of marginal deficiency states: 5–30 mg/day
- Critical deficiency: 50–100 mg IV or IM for 7–14 days, after which oral doses are used (Tanphaichitr 1999)
- Therapeutic dose: generally 5–150 mg/day, atypical therapeutic doses >3 g daily
- CHF: when indicated, 100 mg twice daily IV for 1–2 weeks, then 200 mg/day orally
- Dysmenorrhoea: 100 mg/day orally
- Support of alcohol withdrawal: 100 mg given IV or IM
- Fatigue (when marginal deficiency likely): 10 mg/day
- Type 2 diabetes mellitus: 100 mg three times daily
- Wernicke's encephalopathy: 100–500 mg (IV or IM) over 30 minutes for 3 days
- Mental depression: 50 mg/day for 2 months
- Mood disorders: 10 mg/day with marginal deficiency.

Australian RDI

- Females >13 years: 1.1 mg/day.
- Males >13 years: 1.2 mg/day.

TOXICITY

Toxicity does not occur with oral thiamin as it is rapidly excreted by the kidneys (Tanphaichitr 1999), although there is some evidence that toxicity can occur with very large doses given parenterally (Jacobs & Wood 2003).

ADVERSE REACTIONS

Thiamin is well tolerated.

SUPPLEMENTAL FORMS

Thiamin hydrochloride is the most common form used in supplements, which consist of 89% thiamin and 11% HCl.

Benfotiamine is an *Allium*-derived, lipid-soluble derivative of thiamin that has better bioavailability than water-soluble salts. It is the preferred form in the treatment of alcoholic and diabetic neuropathies (Ang et al 2008, Stracke et al 1996) where supplementation with thiamin or benfotiamine in rat models revealed that equivalent doses of thiamin have a fivefold lower bioavailability than benfotiamine. Its higher cellular bioavailability is due to the thiazole ring that allows easier passage across cell membranes (Balakumar et al 2010).

Oral supplements are non-toxic, but should be used with caution in patients with cancer (Comin-Anduix et al 2001). (See Tumour proliferation section, above, and Cancer section, below.)

SIGNIFICANT INTERACTIONS

Antibiotics

Antibiotics can reduce the endogenous production of B group vitamins by gastrointestinal flora, theoretically resulting in lowered B vitamin levels. The clinical significance of this is unclear — increase intake of vitamin B_1-rich foods or consider supplementation.

Coffee, tea, blueberries, red cabbage and Brussels sprouts

Reduce the absorption of oral thiamin — separate doses by 2 hours (Groff & Gropper 2009).

Vitamin C and citric acid

May enhance oral bioavailability of thiamin (Gropper & Smith 2013).

Iron

Iron precipitates thiamin, thereby reducing its absorption — separate doses by 2 hours.

Loop diuretics

Chronic use may result in lowered levels of vitamin B_1 — increase intake of vitamin B_1-rich foods or consider long-term supplementation.

Other B vitamins

Thiamin deficiency commonly occurs in conjunction with poor B_2 and B_6 status (Jacobs & Wood 2003).

Sulfites

Concomitant intake may inactivate thiamin, which has been reported in TPN solutions (Bowman & Nguyen 1983).

Tannins

Tannins precipitate thiamin, thereby reducing its absorption — separate doses by 2 hours.

Horsetail (*Equisetum arvense*)

Theoretically, horsetail may destroy thiamin in the stomach due to the presence of a thiaminase-like compound found in the herb. Those who have a pre-existing thiamin deficiency or are at risk of thiamin deficiency may be advised to avoid concurrent use of horsetail (Shils et al 2005).

CONTRAINDICATIONS AND PRECAUTIONS

Cancer

There is some evidence of thiamin being associated with nucleic acid ribose synthesis of tumour cells in its biologically activated form (Boros 2000). In a metabolic control analysis in vivo in mice, a high stimulatory effect was observed with thiamin doses of 25 times the RDA on tumour growth of 164%, when compared to controls. However, in the same study, when thiamin supplementation was 2500 times the RDA for mice, the opposite effect was observed and a 10% inhibition of tumour growth was recognised (Comin-Anduix et al 2001).

As such, whether thiamin has any effect on tumour formation in humans remains unclear.

PREGNANCY USE

Safe during pregnancy and lactation.

Practice points/Patient counselling

- Thiamin is necessary for healthy functioning and is involved in carbohydrate and protein metabolism, the production of DNA and several neurotransmitters and nerve and muscle functions.
- Supplements are used to treat deficiency or prevent secondary deficiency in people at risk (e.g. alcoholism, malabsorption syndromes, hyperemesis, chronic diarrhoea, hyperthyroidism, pregnancy, lactation, fever, acute infection, folate deficiency, strenuous physical exertion, breastfeeding, adolescent growth, severe liver disease and chronic use of loop diuretics). There is a higher incidence of deficiency in people with CHF; however, it is not known whether correction of the deficiency will improve disease symptoms.
- High-dose thiamin supplements relieve symptoms of dysmenorrhoea, according to one large randomised controlled trial.
- Additionally, some early research has found an association between AD and low plasma thiamin levels, with supplementation producing some benefits; however, further investigation is still required.
- Some research has also suggested a potential use for thiamin in the improvement of vibration perception, motor function, pain and coordination associated with peripheral neuropathy. Further research is necessary.
- Oral supplements are non-toxic, but high doses should be used with caution in patients with cancer.

PATIENTS' FAQs

What will this vitamin do for me?

Thiamin is necessary for healthy functioning and is involved in carbohydrate and protein metabolism, the production of DNA and several brain chemicals and nerve and muscle functions. Supplements are taken to avoid deficiency states that can occur, for instance, in alcoholism, extreme vomiting, chronic diarrhoea or malabsorption syndromes. In high doses, it may relieve symptoms of painful menstruation and may be a useful adjunct in CHF.

When will it start to work?

Thiamin supplements can have dramatic effects on deficiency states within 24 hours. The response time for other conditions, such as dysmenorrhoea and CHF, also appears to be reasonably fast. Within two menstrual cycles, supplementation produced marked reductions in dysmenorrhoea, and CHF patients treated for only 7 weeks showed positive responses.

Are there any safety issues?

Taken orally, thiamin is considered non-toxic. People with cancer should consult with their doctor before taking high-dose thiamin supplements.

REFERENCES

Adinoff B et al. Acute ethanol poisoning and the ethanol withdrawal syndrome. Med Toxicol Adverse Drug Exp 3.3 (1988): 172–196.

Alguire PC. Rapid evaluation of comatose patients. Postgrad Med 87.6 (1990): 223–233: 8.

Allard ML, et al. The management of conditioned nutritional requirements in heart failure. Heart Fail Rev 11.1 (2006): 75–82.

Al-Nasser B, et al. Lower limb neuropathy after spinal anesthesia in a patient with latent thiamin deficiency. J Clin Anesth 18.8 (2006): 624–627.

Ang CD, et al. Vitamin B for treating peripheral neuropathy. Cochrane Database Syst Rev, 2008. CD004573.

Arora S et al. Thiamin (vitamin B_1) improves endothelium-dependent vasodilatation in the presence of hyperglycemia. Ann Vasc Surg 20.5 (2006): 75–82.

Australian Government ComLaw (2009) http://www.comlaw.gov.au/Details/F2009C00811. Viewed 20th April, 2013.

Ba A. Metabolic and structural role of thiamin in nervous tissue. Cell Mol Neurobiol 2008:28(7):943–53.

Ba A Alcohol and B_1 vitamin deficient-related stilbirths. J Maternal Foetal Neonatal Med, 2009;22(5):452–7.

Ba A Comparative effects of alcohol and thiamin deficiency on the developing central nervous system. Behavioural Brain Research 225 (2011) 235–242.

Balakumar, P., et al. The multifaceted therapeutic potential of benfotiamine. Pharmacological Research 61(2010)., 482–488.

Becker DA., et al. Dry beriberi and Wernicke's encephalopathy following gastric lap band surgery. Journal of Clinical Neuroscience 19 (2012) 1050–1052.

Beers MH, Berkow R (eds). The Merck manual of diagnosis and therapy, 17th edn. Whitehouse, NJ: Merck, 2003.

Benton D., et al. Thiamin supplementation mood and cognitive functioning. Psychopharmacology (1997) 129: 66–71.

Blass JP et al. Thiamin and Alzheimer's disease: a pilot study. Arch Neurol 45.8 (1988): 833–835.

Bonucchi J et al. Thyrtoxicosis associated Wernicke's encephalopathy. J Gen Intern Med 23.1 (2008): 106–109.

Boros LG. Population thiamin status and varying cancer rates between western. Asian and African countries. Anticancer Res 20.3B (2000): 2245–2248.

Botez MI et al. Thiamin and folate treatment of chronic epileptic patients: a controlled study with the Wechsler IQ scale. Epilepsy Res 16.2 (1993): 157–163.

Bowman BB, Nguyen P. Stability of thiamin in parenteral nutrition solutions. J Parenter Enteral Nutr 7.6 (1983): 567–568.

Bubber P, et al. Tricarboxylic acid cycle enzymes following thiamin deficiency. Neurochem Int 45.7 (2004): 1021–1028.

Butterfield DA et al. Nutritional approaches to combat oxidative stress in Alzheimer's disease. J Nutr Biochem 13.8 (2002): 444–461.

Butterworth RF et al. Thiamin deficiency and Wernicke's encephalopathy in AIDS. Metab Brain Dis 6.4 (1991): 207–212.

Buylaert WA. Coma induced by intoxication. Acta Neurol Belg 100.4 (2000): 221–224.

Combs GF Jr. The Vitamins (Fourth Edition). Chapter 10 — Thiamin. 2012, Pages 261–276. London: Elsevier

ComõÂn-Anduix BA, et al. The effect of thiamin supplementation on tumour proliferation A metabolic control analysis study. Eur. J. Biochem. 268, 4177–4182 (2001).

D'Amour ML, et al. Abnormalities of peripheral nerve conduction in relation to thiamin status in alcoholic patients. Can J Neurol Sci 18.2 (1991): 126–128.

de Montmollin D et al. Outbreak of beri-beri in a prison in West Africa. Trop Doct 32.4 (2002): 234–236.

Eisinger J., et al. Glycolysis abnormalities in fibromyalgia. J Am Coll Nutr 1994;24(2):144–8.

Erstad BL, Cotugno CL. Management of alcohol withdrawal. Am J Health Syst Pharm 52.7 (1995): 697–709.

Fattal-Valeski, A. Thiamin (vitamin B_1). Journal of Evidence-Based Complementary & Alternative Medicine 16 (1):12–20, 2011.

Fernhoff PM et al. Thiamin response in maple syrup urine disease. Pediatr Res 19.10 (1985): 1011–1016.

Fernstrom JD and Fenstrom MH Biology, metabolism, and nutritional requirements. In: Brain and Nervous System, 2013. Amsterdam: Elsevier.

Finsterer J. Mitochondrial neuropathy. Clin Neurol Neurosurg 107.3 (2005): 181–186.

Franca DS., et al. B vitamins induce an antinociceptive effect in the acetic acid and formaldehyde models of nociception in mice. European Journal of Pharmacology Volume 421, Issue 3, 15 June 2001, Pages 157–164.

Francini-Pesenti F et al. Wernicke's encephalopathy during parenteral nutrition. J Parenter Enteral Nutr 31.1 (2007): 69–71.

Francini-Pesenti F et al. Wernicke's syndrome during parenteral feeding: Not an unusual complication. Nutrition 2009a;25(2):142–146.

Francini-Pesenti F, et al. Wernicke's syndrome during parenteral feeding: not an unusual complication, Nutrition, 2009b; 25:142–46.

FSANZ Food Standards New Zealand and Australia (2012). http://www.foodstandards.gov.au/consumerinformation/fortification.cfm

Fugh-Berman A, Kronenberg F. Complementary and alternative medicine (CAM) in reproductive-age women: a review of randomized controlled trials. Reprod Toxicol 17.2 (2003): 137–152.

Gangolf, M., et al Thiamin triphosphate synthesis in rat brain occurs in mitochondira and is coupled to the respiratory chain. The Journal of Biological Chemistry, (2010), 285, 583–594.

Gardian G et al. Wernicke's encephalopathy induced by hyperemesis gravidarum. Acta Neurol Scand 99.3 (1999): 196–198.

Gibson GE, Blass JP. Thiamin-dependent processes and treatment strategies in neurodegeneration. Antioxid Redox Signal 9.10 (2007): 1605–1619.

Gibson GE, et al. Abnormal thiamin-dependent processes in Alzheimer's disease. Lessons from diabetes. Molecular and Cellular Neuroscience 55 (2013) 17–25.

Gokhale LB. Curative treatment of primary (spasmodic) dysmenorrhoea. Indian J Med Res 103 (1996): 227–231.

Gold M, et al. Plasma and red blood cell thiamin deficiency in patients with dementia of the Alzheimer's type. Arch Neurol 52.11 (1995): 1081–1086.

Gold M et al. Plasma thiamin deficiency associated with Alzheimer's disease but not Parkinson's disease. Metab Brain Dis 13.1 (1998): 43–53.

Groff, J., Gropper, S. Advanced nutrition and human metabolism, 5th edition. Belmont, CA: Wadsworth, Cengage Learning, 2009.

Gropper, S., Smith, J Advanced nutrition and human metabolism, 6th edition. Belmont CA: Wadsworth, Cengage Learning, 2013.

Hahn JS et al. Wernicke encephalopathy and beriberi during total parenteral nutrition attributable to multivitamin infusion shortage. Pediatrics 101.1 (1998): E10.

Hanninen SA et al. The prevalence of thiamin deficiency in hospitalized patients with congestive heart failure. J Am Coll Cardiol 47.2 (2006): 354–361.

Hazell, A. S. Astrocytes are a major target in thiamin deficiency and Wernicke's encephalopathy. Neurochemistry International (2009) 55, 129–135.

Hazell, A. S., et al. Mechanisms of neuronal cell death in Wernicke's encephalopathy. Metabolic Brain Disease (1998). 13, 97–122.

Hechtman, L. Clinical naturopathic medicine. Chatswood, NSW: Churchill Livingstone, Elsevier, 2011.

Huang, H. M., et al. (2010). Thiamin and oxidants interact to modify cellular calcium stores. Neurochemical Research 35, 2107–2116.

Huang, Y, et al. Prediction of all-cause mortality by B group vitamin status in the elderly. Clinical Nutrition 31 (2012) 191–198.

Jack Jr., C.R., et al 2010. Hypothetical model of dynamic biomarkers of the Alzheimer's pathological cascade. Lancet Neurol. 9, 119–128.

Jacobs P, Wood L. Hematology of malnutrition. II: Vitamin B_1. Disease-a-Month 49.11 (2003): 646–652.

Jhala SS & Hazell A S. Modeling neurodegenerative disease pathophysiology in thiamine deficiency: consequences of impaired oxidative metabolism. Neurochemistry International 58; 2011: 248–260.

Juhl JH. Fibromyalgia and the serotonin pathway. Altern Med Rev 1998;3(5):367–75.

Karuppagounder SS et al. Thiamin deficiency induces oxidative stress and exacerbates the plaque pathology in Alzheimer's mouse model. Neurol Aging 2009; 30: 1587–1600.

Keith ME., et al. B-Vitamin deficiency in hositalised patients with heart failure. Journal of American Dietetic Association, 2009; 109: 1406–1410.

Klooster, A., et al. Are brain and heart tissue prone to the development of thiamin deficiency? Alcohol (2013) 1–7.

Kobayashi T., et al. Fursultiamine, a vitamin B_1 derivative, enhances chondroprotective effects of glucosamine hydrochloride and chondroitin sulfate in rabbit experimental osteoarthritis. Inflamm Res 2005;54(6):249–55.

Kuhn AL., et al. Vitamin B_1 in the treatment of Wernicke's encephalopathy due to hyperemesis after gastroplasty. Journal of Clinical Neuroscience 19 (2012) 1303–1305.

Kruse M et al. Increased brain endothelial nitric oxide synthase expression in thiamin deficiency: relationship to selective vulnerability. Neurochem Int 45.1 (2004): 49–56.

Leske MC et al. The lens opacities case-control study: risk factors for cataract. Arch Ophthalmol 109.2 (1991): 244–251.

Lu'o'ng, K. V., & Nguyen, L. T. (2011). Role of thiamin in Alheimer's disease. American Journal of Alzheimer's Disease and Other Dementias, 26, 588e598.

Mastrogiacoma F et al. Brain thiamin, its phosphate esters, and its metabolizing enzymes in Alzheimer's disease. Ann Neurol 39.5 (1996): 585–591.

McKeag NA., et al. The role of micronutrients in heart failure. Journal of the Academy of Nutrition and Dietetics, 2012; 112: 870–886.

Meador K et al. Preliminary findings of high-dose thiamin in dementia of Alzheimer's type. J Geriatr Psychiatry Neurol 6.4 (1993): 222–229.

Mimori Y, et al. Thiamin therapy in Alzheimer's disease. Metab Brain Dis 11 (1996): 89–94.

Molina JA et al. Cerebrospinal fluid levels of thiamin in patients with Alzheimer's disease. J Neural Transm 109.7–8 (2002): 1035–1044.

Mulholland PJ et al. Thiamin deficiency in the pathogenesis of chronic ethanol-associated cerebellar damage in vitro. Neuroscience 135.4 (2005): 1129–1139.

Nixon PF et al. Choroid plexus dysfunction: the initial event in hyperglycemia. Ann Vasc Surg 20.5 (2006): 653–658.

Nourhashemi S et al. Alzheimer disease: protective factors. Am J Clin Nutr 71.2 (2000): 643–649s.

Ogershok PR et al. Wernicke encephalopathy in nonalcoholic patients. Am J Med Sci 323.2 (2002): 107–111.

O'Keeffe ST et al. Thiamin deficiency in hospitalized elderly patients. Gerontology 40.1 (1994): 18–24.

Pepersack T et al. Clin relevance of thiamin status amongst hospitalized elderly patients. Gerontology 45.2 (1999): 96–101.

Pitkin SR, Savage LM. Age-related vulnerability to diencephalic amnesia produced by thiamin deficiency: the role of time of insult. Behav Brain Res 148.1–2 (2004): 93–105.

Proctor M & Murphy PA. Herbal and dietary therapies for primary and secondary dysmenorrhoea. Cochrane Database Syst Rev 2001 (2009): CD002124.

Rabbani N et al. High dose thiamin therapy for patients with type 2 diabetes and microalbuminuria: a randomized, double-blind-placebo controlled pilot study. Diabetologia (2009): 52: 208–212.

Ranganathan LN., Ramaratnam S. Vitamins for epilepsy. Cochrane Database of Syst Rev (2009), Issue 2: CD004304.

Rapala-Kozik M. Vitamin B_1 (thiamin): a cofactor for enzymes involved in the main metabolic pathways and an environmental stress protectant. Advances in Botanical Research, Vol 58, 2011; 37–91.

Reiman, E.M., et al 2004. Functional brain abnormalities in young adults at genetic risk for late-onset Alzheimer's dementia. Proc. Natl. Acad. Sci. U. S. A. 101, 284–289.

Rodriguez-Martin JL, et al. Thiamin for Alzheimer's disease. Cochrane Database Syst Rev 2 (2001): CD001498.

Rudin W. Protection against insect bites. Ther Umsch 62.11 (2005): 713–7118.

Sechi G, Serra A. Wernicke's encephalopathy: new clinical setting and recent advances in diagnosis and management. Lancet Neurol, 2007; 6:442–55.

Seehra H et al. Wernicke's encephalopathy after vertical banded gastroplasty for morbid obesity. BMJ 312.7028 (1996): 434.

Seligmann H et al. Thiamin deficiency in patients with congestive heart failure receiving long-term furosemide therapy: a pilot study. Am J Med 91 (1991): 151–155.

Shils ME, et al. Modern nutrition in health and disease. 10th edn. Baltimore, MD: Lippincott Williams & Wilkins; 2005, 2146.

Singleton CK, Martin PR. Molecular mechanisms of thiamin utilization. Curr Mol Med 1.2 (2001): 197–207.

Smidt LJ et al. Influence of thiamin supplementation on the health and general well-being of an elderly Irish population with marginal thiamin deficiency. J Gerontol 46.1 (1991): M16–M22.

Spruill SC, Kuller JA. Hyperemesis gravidarum complicated by Wernicke's encephalopathy. Obstet Gynecol 99.5 (2002): 875–877.

Sriram, K., et al. (2012). Thiamin in nutrition therapy. Nutrition in Clinical Practice, 27, 41e50.

Stracke H, et al. A benfotiamine-vitamin B combination in treatments of diabetic polyneuropathy. Experimental and Clinical Endocrinology and Diabetes 1996;104(4):311–6.

Suzuki S et al. Optic neuropathy from thiamin deficiency. Intern Med 36.7 (1997): 532.

Tan JH, Ho KH. Wernicke's encephalopathy in patients with hyperemesis gravidarum. Singapore Med J 42.3 (2001): 124–125.

Tang AM., et al. Dietary micronutrient intake and risk of progression to acquired immunodeficiency syndrome (AIDS) in human immunodeficiency virus type-1 (HIV-1) infected homosexual men. Am J Epidemiol 1993;138:937–51.

Tanphaichitr V. Thiamin. In: Shils M (ed.), Modern nutrition in health and disease. Baltimore: Lippincott Williams & Wilkins, 1999.

The Merck Manual Professional, reviewed 2009. http://www.merckmanuals.com/professional/nutritional_disorders/nutritional_support/total_parenteral_nutrition_tpn.html#v883534. Viewed online 20th April, 2013.

Thomson AD, Marshall EJ. The natural history and pathophysiology of Wernicke's encephalopathy and Korsakoff's psychosis. Alcohol 41.2 (2005): 151–158.

Thornalley PJ et al. High prevalence of low plasma thiamin concentration in diabetes linked to a marker of vascular disease. Diabetologia 50.10 (2007): 2164–2170.

Tjandra BS, Janknegt RA. Neurogenic impotence and lower urinary tract symptoms due to vitamin B_1 deficiency in chronic alcoholism. J Urol 157.3 (1997): 954–955.

Togay-Isikay C, et al. Wernicke's encephalopathy due to hyperemesis gravidarum: an under-recognised condition. Aust NZ J Obstet Gynaecol 41.4 (2001): 453–456.

Toth C, Voll C. Wernicke's encephalopathy following gastroplasty for morbid obesity. Can J Neurol Sci 28.1 (2001): 89–92.

Towbin, A., et al. Beri beri after gastric bypass surgery in adolescence. J Pediatr 2004; 145:263–7.

van Noort BA et al. Optic neuropathy from thiamin deficiency in a patient with ulcerative colitis. Doc Ophthalmol 67.1–2 (1987): 45–51.

Vortmeyer AO, et al. Haemorrhagic thiamin deficient encephalopathy following prolonged parenteral nutrition. J Neurol Neurosurg Psychiatry 55.9 (1992): 826–829.

Wahlqvist M et al. Food and nutrition. Sydney: Allen & Unwin, 2002.

Walker J & Kepner A. Wernicke's encephalopathy presenting as acute psychosis after gastric bypass. The Journal of Emergency Medicine, Vol 43, No 5, pp. 811–814, 2012.

Wang, D. and Hazell, A. S. Microglial activation is a major contributor to neurologic dysfunction in thiamin deficiency. Biochemical and Biophysical Research Communications (2010). 402, 123–128.

Wardlaw G et al. Contemporary nutrition. 3rd edn. Brown and Benchmark, Dubuque, 1997.

Welsh A. Hyperemesis, gastrointestinal and liver disorders in pregnancy. Curr Obstet Gynaecol 15.2 (2005): 123–131.

Woelk H, et al. Benfotiamine in treatment of alcoholic polyneuropathy: an 8-week randomized controlled study (BAP I study). Alcohol and Alcoholism 1998;33(6):631–8.

Zak J III et al. Dry beriberi: unusual complication of prolonged parenteral nutrition. J Parenter Enteral Nutr 15.2 (1991): 200–201.

Vitamin B_{12}

BACKGROUND AND RELEVANT PHARMACOKINETICS

Vitamin B_{12} (cobalamin) is a water-soluble vitamin obtained mostly from animal protein products in the diet. In the stomach gastric acid is required to liberate protein-bound cobalamin, which is then immediately bound to R-binders (glycoproteins) that protect it from being denatured. When the contents of the stomach reach the duodenum, the R-binders are partially digested by pancreatic proteases, releasing them to bind to intrinsic factor (a glycoprotein), which is secreted by the parietal cells of the gastric mucosa. This complex is then absorbed in the terminal ileum and transported to cells, where it carries out its metabolic function, or to the liver, where it is stored until required (FAO/WHO 2002, Oh & Brown 2003). An alternative method of absorption, which is independent of intrinsic factor, also appears to exist and accounts for the absorption of approximately 1% of large oral doses (> 300 mcg) of B_{12} (Elia 1998). Absorption via intrinsic factor is limited to about 1.5–2.0 mcg/meal owing to limited receptor capacity (FAO/WHO 2002).

Clinical note — Nori: a source for vegetarians

While the majority of non-meat sources of vitamin B_{12} do not contain the biologically active form, it is possible to get B_{12} from some non-meat foods. In fact, improvements in B_{12} status have been observed following the ingestion of nori (seaweed). Nori is said to contain as much B_{12} as liver (Croft et al 2005), approximately 55–59 mcg/100 g dry weight. Five different biologically active vitamin B_{12} compounds have been identified in nori: cyanocobalamin, hydroxycobalamin, sulfitocobalamin, adenosylcobalamin and methylcobalamin (Takenaka et al 2001); the source of B_{12} appears to be bacteria (Croft et al 2005).

CHEMICAL COMPONENTS

Vitamin B_{12} is the largest of the B vitamins and is a complex structure containing a central cobalt atom. There are five forms of B_{12}: cyanocobalamin (a synthetic form that has a cyanide attached to the cobalt), hydroxycobalamin (hydroxyl group attached to the cobalt; it is produced for parenteral administration), aquacobalamin (water group bound to the cobalt) and the coenzymatically active forms (methylcobalamin and 5-deoxyadenosylcobalamin), in which a methyl group or a 5-deoxyadenosyl group is bound to the cobalt atom (FAO/WHO 2002, Freeman et al 1999).

FOOD SOURCES

Vitamin B_{12} is found in lamb's liver, sardines, oysters, egg yolk, fish, beef, kidney, cheese and milk. Up to 10% is lost in cooking (Wahlqvist 2002). Fortified breakfast cereals are also available.

Vitamin B_{12} bioavailability significantly decreases with increasing intake as the intrinsic factor-mediated intestinal absorption system is estimated to be saturated at about 1.5–2.0 mcg/meal for healthy adults with normal gastrointestinal function. The bioavailability of vitamin B_{12} from different sources is variable: fish (42%), lamb (56–89%), chicken (61–66%) and eggs (<9%) (Watanabe 2007).

Plants do not contain B_{12} because they have no cobalamin-dependent enzymes (Croft et al 2005). Most microorganisms, including bacteria and algae, synthesise B_{12}, which then makes its way into the food chain (FAO/WHO 2002). Human intestinal bacteria also synthesise B_{12}, but this is not absorbed to any considerable extent (Wahlqvist 2002). Vegans living in situations with more stringent hygiene are therefore more likely to develop deficiencies.

DEFICIENCY SIGNS AND SYMPTOMS

Vitamin B_{12} deficiencies manifest primarily as haematological and neurological disturbances. The elderly are particularly at risk, with vitamin B_{12} deficiency estimated to affect 10–15% of individuals over the age of 60 years (Baik & Russell 1999).

- Haemotological: macrocytic (megaloblastic) anaemia, pancytopenia (leucopenia, thrombocytopenia); symptoms may include lethargy, dyspnoea, anorexia, weight loss and pallor (Wahlqvist 2002).
- Neurological disturbances: paraesthesias, ataxia, optic neuropathy (reversible), peripheral neuropathy and demyelination of the corticospinal tract and dorsal columns (subacute combined systems disease).
- Psychological disturbances: impaired memory, irritability, depression, personality change, dementia, delirium and psychosis (Lee 1999, Lindenbaum et al 1988). A case report of vitamin B_{12} deficiency presenting as obsessive compulsive disorder has been described (Sharma & Biswas 2012).
- Various gastrointestinal symptoms can also develop, such as loss of appetite, intermittent constipation and diarrhoea, glossitis and abdominal pain.
- Folic acid supplementation may mask an underlying B_{12} deficiency, leading to the progression of neurological symptoms.

Primary deficiency

People at risk are those living in India, Central and South America, and selected areas in Africa (Stabler & Allen 2004), strict vegetarians and vegans, breastfed infants of vegetarian mothers with low B_{12} stores, elderly patients with 'tea and toast diets' and chronic alcoholics. Vitamin B_{12} deficiency exists more commonly among vegans than vegetarians, with depletion or deficiency of vitamin B_{12} found to occur irrespective of demographic, place of residency, age or type of vegetarian diet (Pawlak et al 2013). Approximately 62% of pregnant vegetarians are B_{12}-deficient as are 25–86% of vegetarian children, 21–41% of vegetarian adolescents and 11–90% of elderly vegetarians.

As vitamin B_{12} is stored to a considerable extent, even after complete depletion of food-ingested cobalamin, clinically relevant deficiencies will usually only develop after 5–10 years (Schenk et al 1999). This time frame increases to an average of approximately 18 years in strict vegetarians when intrinsic factor secretion is intact (Babior 1996). In this case, some enterohepatic recycling of cobalamin should occur in the distal ileum (Howden 2000).

Secondary deficiency

Vitamin B_{12} deficiency is more likely to result from inadequate absorption, defects in vitamin B_{12} metabolism or gastrointestinal disorders than a lack of dietary intake.

- Pernicious anaemia: an autoimmune condition affecting gastric parietal cells that produce intrinsic factor; common cause of megaloblastic anaemia, especially in persons of European or African descent (Stabler & Allen 2004).
- Methylmalonic acidaemia: inherited defect in B_{12} metabolism.
- Congenital absence of transcobalamin II.
- Medications that reduce gastric acidity (e.g. H_2 blockers and proton pump inhibitors [PPIs]).
- Atrophic gastritis/gastric atrophy: probably due to a decrease in acid output and intrinsic factor production (Schenk et al 1999). Gastric atrophy is more common in the elderly.
- Intestinal resection of the part of the ileum where absorption takes place or gastric resection, which affects the parietal cells and in turn production of intrinsic factor.
- Achlorhydria (Termanini et al 1998).
- Pancreatic insufficiency: the cobalamin-R-protein complex is split by pancreatic enzymes in the duodenum (Festen 1991).

- Ileal dysfunction (Howden 2000): may affect absorption at this site.
- Crohn's disease, irritable bowel disease, coeliac disease: reduced absorption.
- Bacteria and parasites in the intestine may also compete for B_{12}.
- Radiotherapy for rectal cancer: causes a rapid and persistent decrease in B_{12} status, as reflected by reduced serum B_{12} combined with increased serum methylmalonic acid (MMA) (Gronlie Guren et al 2004).
- Nitrous oxide may induce or potentiate B_{12} deficiency myelopathy (Hathout & El-Saden 2011).

The elderly deserve a separate mention as a population at risk of deficiency because of both primary and secondary causes, such as poor dietary intake, failure to separate vitamin B_{12} from food protein, inadequate absorption, utilisation and storage, as well as drug–food interactions leading to malabsorption and metabolic inactivation (Bradford & Taylor 1999, Dharmarajan et al 2003). Subtle signs of deficiency may include lethargy, weight loss and dementia (Dharmarajan et al 2003).

Elevated B_{12} levels

Elevated levels of serum cobalamin may be a sign of a serious, even life-threatening, disease such as chronic myelogenous leukaemia, promyelocytic leukaemia, polycythaemia vera, hypereosinophilic syndrome, acute hepatitis, cirrhosis, hepatocellular carcinoma and metastatic liver disease. Elevated B_{12} levels, therefore, warrant a full diagnostic workup to assess the presence of disease (Ermens et al 2003).

Liver failure mortality

A prospective study of patients with acute-on-chronic liver failure ($n = 105$) found that elevated vitamin B_{12} levels on hospital admission were associated with increased severity of liver disease and 3-month mortality rate (Dou et al 2012).

Clinical note — Testing for vitamin B_{12} deficiency

Numerous studies have indicated that serum B_{12} levels are an inadequate guide to B_{12} status (Briddon 2003, Carmel 1988, Kapadia 2000, Karnaze & Carmel 1990, Termanini et al 1998). The use of this test has led to poorly defined reference intervals for serum B_{12} (Briddon 2003), potentially delaying the diagnosis and allowing the progression of B_{12} deficiency. Approximately 50% of patients with subclinical disease have normal serum B_{12} levels and older patients present with neurological and psychiatric symptoms without haematological findings. In addition, use of the oral contraceptive pill may affect test results (Bor 2004). As a result, this method of testing has lost favour as an adequate measure of B_{12} status. A combination of two tests appears to be more conclusive. Elevated levels of total homocysteine in serum and plasma reflect deficiencies of either folate or B_{12}. MMA is a more specific marker of cobalamin function, but renal insufficiency may affect the results of this test. Therefore, a combination of the two is probably the clearest indicator (Bjorke Monsen & Ueland 2003, FAO/WHO 2002, Kapadia 2000). Preliminary evidence also suggests that overnight fasting urinary MMA concentrations correlate strongly with serum MMA; however, further investigations are required to confirm the application of this test in various populations (Kwok et al 2004). While the use of such markers may improve the assessment of B_{12} deficiency, establishing the cause of deficiency should also be part of the diagnostic approach (Schneede & Ueland 2005).

MAIN ACTIONS

Important cofactor

Vitamin B_{12} is essential for the normal function of all cells. It affects cell growth and replication, the metabolism of carbohydrates, lipids and protein and is involved in fatty acid and nucleic acid synthesis. It is also involved in the production of red blood cells in bone marrow, and activates folacin coenzymes for red blood cell production.

Homocysteine reduction

Methylcobalamin aids in the conversion of homocysteine to methionine by the action of methionine synthase, transferring a methyl group from methylfolate (folic acid).

After conversion from homocysteine, methionine is then converted to *S*-adenosyl-L-methionine (SAMe), important for methylation reactions and protein synthesis. An increase in homocysteine levels and decrease in SAMe levels have been implicated in depression and may also contribute to the neurological symptoms seen in pernicious anaemia (IMG 2003).

Nervous system

Vitamin B_{12} is involved in the synthesis of protein structures in the myelin sheath and nerve cells. As methylation is required for the production of myelin basic protein, a reduction in B_{12} and SAMe will result in demyelination of peripheral nerves and the spinal column (subacute combined degeneration; FAO/WHO 2002).

Immune system

Vitamin B_{12} acts as an immunomodulator for cellular immunity (Tamura et al 1999).

Liver

Vitamin B_{12} deficiency results in decreased serine dehydratase (SDH) and tyrosine aminotransferase activities in rat livers (Ebara et al 2008). In dimethylnitrosamine-induced liver injury in mice, vitamin B_{12} decreased the blood levels of aspartate aminotransferase and alanine aminotransferase, suggesting a possible hepatoprotective effect (Isoda et al 2008).

Antioxidant capacity

Recent studies have identified that vitamin B_{12} and its cobalamin-based derivatives are powerful antioxidants at pharmacological concentrations (Birch et al 2009, Moreira et al 2011, Weinburg et al 2009).

CLINICAL USE

Vitamin B_{12} supplementation is administered using various routes, such as intravenous and oral doses. This review will focus on oral supplementation as this is the form generally used by the public and is available over the counter. It is sometimes used in combination with other B group vitamins, in particular B_6 and folate.

Deficiency: treatment and prevention

Traditionally, vitamin B_{12} supplementation has been used to treat deficiency or prevent it in conditions such as pernicious anaemia and atrophic gastritis, but special consideration should be given to the elderly, who are at high risk.

Pernicious anaemia

Pernicious anaemia is caused by a deficiency of intrinsic factor, leading to malabsorption of vitamin B_{12}. Signs and symptoms include pallor, glossitis, weakness and neurological symptoms, including paraesthesias of the hands and feet, decreased deep-tendon reflexes and loss of sensory perception and motor controls (neurological symptoms may be irreversible). In more progressed conditions confusion, memory loss, moodiness, psychosis and delusional behaviour may be present. Achlorhydria and gastric mucosal atrophy may also occur, further complicating the condition.

Uncomplicated pernicious anaemia is characterised by mild or moderate megaloblastic anaemia without leucopenia, thrombocytopenia or neurological symptoms. In more advanced cases urgent parenteral administration of vitamin B_{12} and folic acid (typically 100 mcg of cyanocobalamin and 1–5 mg of folic acid) is given intramuscularly, as well as blood transfusions.

Atrophic gastritis

Elderly patients with atrophic gastritis appear to have higher rates of vitamin B_{12} deficiency ($P < 0.01$) which responds to B_{12} supplementation (Lewerin et al 2008).

Infants

In infants, severe vitamin B_{12} deficiency can cause neurological symptoms, including irritability, failure to thrive, apathy, anorexia and developmental regression which responds well to supplementation (Dror & Allen 2008). A large cohort study (n = 2001) found that vitamin B_{12} levels at birth did not affect asthma or eczema-related outcomes between birth and age 6 (van der Valk et al 2013).

Elderly

Vitamin B_{12} deficiency is common in the elderly, with estimates as high as 43% (Wolters et al 2004). Poor vitamin B_{12} status has been associated with vascular disease, depression, impaired cognitive performance and dementia. Elderly patients (>60 years) should be monitored for evidence of B_{12} deficiency (a minimum threshold of 220–258 pmol/L [300–350 pg/mL] is desirable in the elderly) and general supplementation with vitamin B_{12} (> 50 mcg/day) should be considered (Wolters et al 2004). Significantly higher doses may be required to correct deficiency. A randomised, parallel-group, double-blind, dose-finding trial found that the lowest dose of oral cyanocobalamin required to normalise mild vitamin B_{12} deficiency in the elderly is 647–1032 mcg/day, more than 200-fold the recommended dietary allowance (Eussen et al 2005). Conversely another randomised controlled trial (RCT) reported that even low doses of B_{12} could improve the vitamin status in elderly people with food-bound vitamin B_{12} malabsorption. The dose required to increase mean serum vitamin B_{12} by 37 pmol/L was 5.9 mcg/day (95% confidence interval [CI] 0.9–12.1) (Blacher et al 2007). In another study of elderly people with malabsorption taking 1000 mcg/day of crystalline cyanocobalamin for 1 month, 85% of subjects normalised their serum cobalamin concentrations, and all subjects corrected their initial macrocytosis and had medullar regeneration with a mean increase in reticulocyte count (Andres et al 2006). While hearing loss has been associated with poor B_{12} status in the elderly, short-term supplementation has so far failed to show benefits (Park et al 2006).

Pemetrexed treatment

To reduce the incidence of adverse effects, pretreatment with folate and vitamin B_{12} is recommended prior to treatment with pemetrexed, an antifolate chemotherapeutic used in non-small-cell lung cancer (Molina & Adjei 2003). No significant difference in adverse effects was noted in a trial which compared duration of folate and vitamin B_{12} (5–14 days versus less than 4 days: Kim et al 2013).

Hyperhomocysteinaemia

Vitamin B_{12} alone may not be sufficient to normalise elevated homocysteine levels (Yajnik et al 2007). As a result, vitamin B_{12} is often recommended in combination with folic acid and vitamin B_6 in conditions for which homocysteine is implicated as a possible causative factor.

> ***Clinical note — Oral forms are effective***
>
> Vitamin B_{12} is often given parenterally as an intramuscular injection, based on the understanding that oral doses will not be efficacious in cases of malabsorption.
>
> There is now considerable evidence that oral vitamin B_{12} therapy is comparable in efficacy to parenteral therapy, even when intrinsic factor is not present or in other diseases affecting absorption (Andres et al 2005a, 2005b, Castelli et al 2011, Delpre et al 1999, Oh & Brown 2003, Roth & Orija 2004, Vidal-Alaball et al 2005, Wellmer et al 2006). A 2005 Cochrane review suggested that 2000 mcg/day of oral vitamin B_{12} or 1000 mcg initially daily then weekly and monthly may be as effective as intramuscular injections in obtaining short-term haematological and neurological responses in vitamin B_{12}-deficient patients (Vidal-Alaball et al 2005). As rare cases of anaphylaxis may occur with parenteral administration, oral therapy is also considered a safer option with improved cost and compliance (Bilwani et al 2005, Bolaman et al 2003). At doses of 500 mcg/day, correction of serum B_{12} levels is likely to occur within 1 week to 1 month, with correction of haematological abnormalities after at least 3 months (Andres et al 2005b).

Cardiovascular protection

In practice, the relative safety and affordability of combined vitamin B supplementation (B_{12}, folic acid and B_6) make it an attractive recommendation in people with familial hyperhomocysteinaemia. Whether lowering total homocysteine improves cardiovascular mortality and morbidity is questionable, as large-scale clinical trials and meta-analyses have failed to demonstrate any benefits for either B_{12} alone or in combination for reducing overall cardiovascular risk, despite showing a reduction in homocysteine levels (Albert et al 2008, Clarke et al 2007, Mann et al 2008, Marcus et al 2007, Ray et al 2007). Furthermore, a 2013 Cochrane systematic review concluded that there was insufficient evidence to support the use of homocysteine-lowering interventions, including vitamin B_{12}, to prevent cardiovascular events (Martí-Carvajal et al 2013).

Failure of combined B vitamin therapy to reverse inflammatory processes associated with atherogenesis may partly explain the negative results (Bleie et al 2007). The consistent findings of an association between elevated plasma total homocysteine levels and vascular risk is yet to be fully explained; however it is possible that the association is a consequence rather than a cause of disease (Toole et al 2004).

Cardiovascular disease

There is very limited evidence from cohort studies that vitamin B_{12} deficiency predisposes for cardiovascular disease or diabetes according to a systematic review

(Rafnsson et al 2011). As such, current data do not support the use of vitamin B_{12} supplementation to reduce the risk of either of these diseases. An intervention study, VITATOPS, was a randomised, double-blind, placebo-controlled trial (n = 8164), which also found that daily administration of B_{12} in combination with folic acid and vitamin B_6 did not reduce the incidence of major vascular events such as stroke or transient ischaemic attacks (TIAs) in elderly patients with a recent history of stroke or TIA (VITATOPS Trial Study Group 2010).

Renal transplant recipients

Although studies investigating the effects of vitamin B_{12} as a stand-alone treatment in this condition are not available, several clinical studies have produced conflicting evidence for the use of combination vitamin B treatment (vitamin B_{12}, folic acid and B_6).

An RCT involving 56 renal transplant patients found that vitamin supplementation with folic acid (5 mg/day), vitamin B_6 (50 mg/day) and vitamin B_{12} (400 mcg/day) for 6 months reduced the progression of atherosclerosis. Patients taking the vitamin combination experienced a significant decrease in homocysteine levels and carotid intima media thickness, which is reflective of early atherosclerosis (Marcucci et al 2003). In another trial, 36 stable renal transplant recipients with hyperhomocysteinaemia received a similar combination of 5 mg folic acid and 50 mg B_6, in addition to either 1000 mcg B_{12} or placebo per day for 6 months. Supplementation decreased blood homocysteine and improved endothelium-dependent and independent vasodilation responses (Xu et al 2008). Despite these preliminary findings, combined therapy using even higher doses (40 mg folic acid, 100 mg B_6 and 2 mg B_{12}) did not improve survival (448 vitamin group deaths vs 436 placebo group deaths) (hazard ratio 1.04; 95% CI 0.91–1.18) or reduce the incidence of vascular disease (myocardial infarct, stroke and amputations) in patients with advanced chronic kidney disease or end-stage renal disease (Jamison et al 2007).

Restenosis after percutaneous coronary intervention

An RCT found that vitamin B_{12} (cyanocobalamin, 400 mcg/day), folic acid (1 mg/day) and vitamin B_6 (pyridoxine hydrochloride, 10 mg/day) taken for 6 months significantly decreased the incidence of major adverse events, including restenosis after percutaneous coronary intervention (Schnyder et al 2002).

Neural tube defects

Vitamin B_{12} is required to cleave folate, without which folate is not effective, and postpartum analysis of serum B_{12} levels has shown an increased risk of neural tube defects in women with low B_{12} status (Groenen et al 2004, Ray & Blom 2003, Suarez et al 2003). Some authors have called for combined fortification of food with folic acid and vitamin B_{12} because there are concerns about masking B_{12} deficiency (Czernichow et al 2005).

V

Noise-induced hearing loss

Homocysteine levels are significantly higher in subjects with noise-induced hearing loss as compared to healthy controls (Gok et al 2004) and elevated plasma B_{12} levels appear to play a protective role (Quaranta et al 2004).

Recurrent abortion

There appears to be a correlation between low serum B_{12} levels, increased homocysteine levels and early or very early recurrent abortion in some women (Reznikoff-Etievant et al 2002, Zetterberg et al 2002). One small study of five women with a history of very early recurrent abortion found that vitamin B_{12} supplementation resulted in four normal pregnancies (Reznikoff-Etievant et al 2002). Further research is required to investigate possible benefits.

Osteoporosis — inconclusive

Elevated homocysteine levels have been suggested as a risk factor for osteoporosis (Herrmann et al 2005); however, this remains uncertain. A meta-analysis of six studies identified that vitamin B_{12} and homocysteine levels were significantly increased in postmenopausal osteoporotic women compared to controls (Zhang et al 2014), whereas a more recent meta-analysis found no association between homocysteine, folate or vitamin B_{12} with bone mineral density in women (van Wijngaarden et al 2013). A small intervention study of women over 65 years of age ($n = 31$) with elevated homocysteine levels found that treatment with the combination of vitamin B_{12} and folate had no significant effect on bone turnover or bone health (Keser et al 2013).

Depression

Elevation of homocysteine and low levels of vitamin B_{12} and folate are commonly seen in depression (Coppen & Bolander-Gouaille 2005). Observational studies have found as many as 30% of patients hospitalised for depression to be deficient in vitamin B_{12} (Hutto 1997). A cross-sectional study of 700 community-living, physically disabled women over the age of 65 years found that vitamin B_{12}-deficient women were twice as likely to be severely depressed as non-deficient women (Penninx et al 2000). Similarly, a recent Finnish study found that, in subjects aged 45–74 years, vitamin B_{12} level was associated with melancholic depressive symptoms, but not with non-melancholic depressive symptoms (Seppälä et al 2013).

A study of 225 hospitalised acutely ill older patients receiving 400 mL of an oral nutritional supplement (106 subjects) or placebo (119 subjects) daily for 6 weeks reported significant increases in plasma vitamin B_{12} concentrations and red cell folate, and a decrease in depression scores (Gariballa & Forster 2007). Whether the study cohort were B_{12}-deficient at baseline was not clear.

AIDS and HIV

Low vitamin B_{12} levels are often observed in patients infected with HIV type 1 (Remacha & Cadafalch 1999, Remacha et al 1993). One study identified deficiency in 10–35% of all patients seropositive for HIV, presumably as a result of decreased intake, intestinal malabsorption and/or abnormalities in plasma-binding proteins or antagonism by the drug azidothymidine. Importantly, as serum cobalamin levels declined, progression to AIDS increased and neurological symptoms worsened.

Adjuvant treatment in hepatitis C infection

The combination of vitamin B_{12} with standard treatment significantly improved viral response compared to standard treatment only in antiviral-naïve patients with chronic hepatitis C virus infection (Rocco et al 2013).

Cognitive impairment and dementia

More than 77 cross-sectional studies including more than 34,000 subjects have reported a significant association between low blood levels of folate and B_{12} (or high levels of homocysteine) and prevalent dementia. The association has been described for different types of cognitive impairment, including vascular dementia,

Alzheimer's disease and mild cognitive impairment; however, it is not clear whether low B_{12} was a cause or consequence of dementia (Vogel et al 2009). A positive association between serum homocysteine levels and incidence of dementia has also been described in a recent meta-analysis of eight cohort studies ($n = 8669$; odds ratio 1.50; 95% CI 1.13–2.00) (Wald et al 2011).

Despite this possible association, few interventional studies using B_{12} supplementation have been conducted. A systematic review reports on six RCTs utilising B_{12} supplementation for effects on cognitive function; however, the range of doses and administration forms together with cognitive status of volunteers and measures used make interpretation difficult (Vogel et al 2009). Overall, the review concludes that there is insufficient evidence to suggest vitamin B_{12} supplementation to improve cognitive decline or incidence of dementia but also states there are several confounding factors to consider. Unfortunately, few studies considered taking fasting B_{12} blood samples at baseline: the possibility of misclassification of study subjects as cognitive-impaired (or demented) or healthy and classing subjects with normal scores on cognitive tests as healthy even though they have Alzheimer's disease at the preclinical state are other confounding factors.

This is important to bear in mind when considering that, while some interventional studies are negative, there are also positive studies showing that supplementation with vitamin B_{12} significantly reversed impaired mental function in individuals with pre-existing low levels (Healton et al 1991, Miller 2003, Refsum & Smith 2003, Tripathi et al 2001, Weir & Scott 1999).

Interestingly, women in the highest quartile of plasma vitamin B_{12} levels during midlife scored significantly higher on cognitive function tests in later years and were cognitively equivalent to those 4 years younger (Kang & Grodstein 2005). Another study of 370 non-demented 75-year-olds found a twofold increased risk of developing Alzheimer's dementia in subjects with low serum levels of vitamin B_{12} and folate over a 3-year period (Wang et al 2001).

Diabetic neuropathy

According to a 2005 review of seven RCTs, vitamin B_{12} supplementation may improve pain and paraesthaesia in patients with diabetic neuropathy (Sun et al 2005). The studies cited, however, were generally of low quality and more research is required to confirm these results and determine whether positive effects are due to the correction of deficiency or to alteration of abnormal metabolism.

Sleep disorders

A preliminary study investigated the effects of randomly assigned methyl- and cyanocobalamin on circadian rhythms, wellbeing, alertness and concentration after 14 days in 20 healthy subjects (Mayer et al 1996). Methylcobalamin supplementation led to a significant decrease in daytime melatonin levels, improved sleep quality, shorter sleep cycles, increased feelings of alertness, better concentration and a feeling of waking up refreshed in the morning. It appeared that methylcobalamin was significantly more effective than cobalamin.

Tinnitus

A group of 113 army personnel (mean age 39 years) exposed to military noise was studied, of which 57 had chronic tinnitus and noise-induced hearing loss (Shemesh et al 1993). Of this subset, 47% also had vitamin B_{12} deficiency. Treatment with vitamin B_{12} supplementation produced some improvement in tinnitus and associated symptoms.

OTHER USES

Human trials have shown vitamin B_{12} levels to be low in people with recurrent aphthous stomatitis, suggesting a possible aetiological factor (Piskin et al 2002). An inhalation of vitamin B_{12} mixed solution has been shown to be effective for the treatment of acute radiation-induced mucosal injury (Chen & Shi 2006).

Prostate cancer risk — no association

A large-scale population-based study (n = 317,000) found no association with vitamin B_{12} levels and prostate cancer risk (de Vogel et al 2013).

Erythema nodosum

A case report exists of a 38-year-old female diagnosed with erythema nodosum and B_{12} deficiency whose symptoms resolved completely without recurrence following vitamin B_{12} therapy (Volkov et al 2005). Testing for deficiency may be advised in such cases.

Atopic dermatitis

A novel use for B_{12} in a topical cream for atopic dermatitis was tested in a prospective, randomised, placebo-controlled phase III multicentre trial involving 49 patients. Subjects applied the B_{12} cream twice daily to one side of the body and a placebo cream to the contralateral side, according to the randomisation scheme, for 8 weeks. The B_{12} cream was reported to significantly improve the extent and severity of atopic dermatitis and was considered safe and very well tolerated (Stucker et al 2004).

Multiple sclerosis

Multiple sclerosis (MS) and vitamin B_{12} deficiency share common inflammatory and neurodegenerative characteristics and low or decreased levels of vitamin B_{12} have been demonstrated in MS patients and may correlate with early onset (<18 years) (Miller et al 2005). Considering vitamin B_{12} is a cofactor, and myelin formation has important immunomodulatory and neurotrophic effects (Loder et al 2002, Miller et al 2005, Sandyk & Awerbuch 1993), a theoretical basis exists for its use in MS.

Amyotrophic lateral sclerosis (ALS)

Early evidence suggests a possible benefit for long-term ultra-high-dose methylcobalamin (administered intravascularly or intramuscularly) for sporadic or familial cases of ALS (motor neuron disease) (Izumi & Kaji 2007); however, large-scale clinical trials are required to assess the efficacy and safety of this treatment.

Schizophrenia

An improvement in the negative symptoms of schizophrenia was seen following daily vitamin B_{12} (400 mcg) and folic acid (2 mg) supplementation during a 16-week multicentre RCT (Roffman et al 2013). Treatment response was affected by genetic variation in folic acid absorption. The effect of vitamin B_{12} in the absence of folic acid was not investigated.

DOSAGE RANGE

Australian recommended daily intake

- Adult >13 years: 2.4 mcg/day.
- Pregnancy: 2.6 mcg/day.
- Lactation: 2.8 mcg/day.

- Requirements may be higher for elderly people with impaired digestion or absorption.
- Sublingual cyanocobalamin: 1000–2000 mcg/day taken 30 min before breakfast.
- Pernicious anaemia: generally, vitamin B_{12} 1000 mcg intramuscularly 2–4 times weekly is given until haematological abnormalities are corrected, and then it is given once monthly. Alternatively, oral B_{12} can be given in very large doses (0.5–2 mg/day). Correction of haematological abnormalities usually occurs within 6 weeks of treatment, but neural improvement may take up to 18 months.
- Homocysteine lowering: 0.5 mg/day (Dusitanond et al 2005).

Note: Sublingual cobalamin is the preferred oral form for many practitioners, with methylcobalamin also becoming available in some regions.

ADVERSE REACTIONS

Although adverse effects to parenteral cobalamin have been reported, oral supplements appear to be well tolerated (Branco-Ferreira et al 1997, Hillman 1996).

SIGNIFICANT INTERACTIONS

Carbamazepine

In studies with children, long-term carbamazepine use led to a decrease in vitamin B_{12} levels (Karabiber et al 2003) — observe for signs and symptoms of B_{12} deficiency. Increased intake may be required with long-term therapy.

Colchicine

The use of colchicine may reduce the absorption of orally administered vitamin B_{12} — monitoring of serum B_{12} concentration is recommended, particularly if there is a history of deficiency.

Gastric acid inhibitors: PPI and H_2 receptor antagonists

Gastric acid is required to liberate protein-bound cobalamin. Therefore, vitamin B_{12} concentration may be decreased when gastric acid is markedly suppressed for prolonged periods (Laine et al 2000, Schenk et al 1999, Termanini et al 1998). Studies have shown that omeprazole therapy acutely decreases cyanocobalamin absorption in a dose-dependent manner (Marcuard et al 1994, Saltzman et al 1994) and deficiency may occur with long-term use (Valuck & Ruscin 2004). Additionally, a large-scale 2013 case-control study found that use of PPIs or H_2 receptor antagonists for 2 years or more was associated with an increased risk of vitamin B_{12} deficiency (Lam et al 2013). It should be noted that vitamin B_{12} supplements do not suffer the same fate, as they are not bound to protein — observe for signs and symptoms of B_{12} deficiency; vitamin B_{12} supplements may be required with long-term therapy.

Hydrochlorothiazide

There are a number of medications that have the ability to increase homocysteine levels, such as hydrochlorothiazide (Westphal et al 2003), therefore concurrent use of vitamin B_{12} (with folic acid) may be a useful adjunct — potential beneficial interaction.

Lithium

Lithium administration may result in a decrease in serum B_{12} concentration; however, the clinical significance of these findings is not yet clear (Cervantes et al 1999). Beneficial interaction is possible.

Metformin

In patients with type 2 diabetes, metformin has been shown to reduce levels of vitamin B_{12} (and folate) and increase homocysteine (Sahin et al 2007). This effect was not demonstrated in women with polycystic ovary syndrome who were taking metformin and receiving vitamin B_{12} and folate substitution, a daily oral multivitamin tablet, and dietary and lifestyle advice (Carlsen et al 2007). Supplementation may be beneficial.

Oral contraceptive pill

Users of the oral contraceptive pill showed significantly lower concentrations of cobalamin than controls in a 2003 clinical study (Sutterlin et al 2003). However, it would appear that this may be due to an effect on B_{12}-binding proteins in serum affecting test results, because total homocysteine and MMA markers were unchanged and no symptoms of deficiency were present (Bor 2004) — observe for signs and symptoms of B_{12} deficiency and conduct testing if deficiency is suspected.

Phenobarbitone and phenytoin

One clinical study reports that combined long-term use of phenobarbitone and phenytoin resulted in significantly increased serum levels of vitamin B_{12} (Dastur & Dave 1987) — observe patients taking this combination.

Prednisolone

Decreased vitamin B_{12} levels have been reported in the cerebrospinal fluid and serum of MS patients following high-dose (1000 mg daily for 10 days) intravenous methylprednisolone (Frequin et al 1993). Given the suggested importance of B_{12} in MS sufferers, a beneficial interaction is possible.

Sodium valproate

Administration of sodium valproate has been shown to increase plasma vitamin B_{12} concentrations, with one study citing increases of over 50% of baseline (Gidal et al 2005).

Tetracycline antibiotics

B complexes containing B_{12} may significantly reduce the bioavailability of tetracycline hydrochloride (Omray 1981) — separate doses by at least 2 hours.

Practice points/Patient counselling

- Vitamin B_{12} (cobalamin) is a water-soluble vitamin obtained mostly from animal protein products in the diet.
- There is considerable evidence that oral vitamin B_{12} therapy is comparable in efficacy to parenteral therapy, even when intrinsic factor is not present or in other diseases affecting absorption.
- As numerous studies have indicated that serum B_{12} levels are an inadequate guide to B_{12} status, a combination of total homocysteine and MMA is probably the clearest indicator, although discrepancies can still occur.
- Vitamin B_{12} deficiencies manifest primarily as haematological and neurological disturbances and are estimated to affect 10–15% of individuals over the age of 60 years.

- Traditionally, supplementation is recommended to treat deficiency states or prevent them in people at risk, such as in pernicious anaemia or atrophic gastritis.
- When administered together with folic acid and vitamin B_6 (pyridoxine), vitamin B_{12} is used to reduce homocysteine levels. In this way, vitamin B_{12} is sometimes recommended in conditions where homocysteine is implicated as a possible causative factor.
- Some evidence has shown supplementation can be useful in HIV and AIDS, depression, tinnitus and cognitive impairment when low vitamin B_{12} levels are also present. Preliminary evidence also suggests a possible role for supplementation in diabetic retinopathy and sleep disturbances.
- There are several commonly prescribed pharmaceutical medicines that can reduce vitamin B_{12} absorption when used long-term.

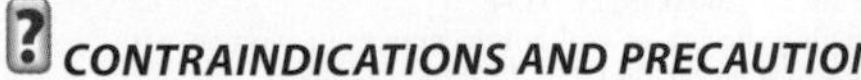

CONTRAINDICATIONS AND PRECAUTIONS

- Parenteral cyanocobalamin given for vitamin B_{12} deficiency caused by malabsorption should be given intramuscularly or by the deep subcutaneous route — never intravenously.
- Folic acid supplementation may mask a B_{12} deficiency.
- Treatment with cyanocobalamin should be avoided in cases of altered cobalamin metabolism or deficiency associated with chronic cyanide intoxication (Freeman et al 1999).

PREGNANCY USE

Vitamin B_{12} is considered safe in pregnancy.

Low-dose vitamin B_{12} (1–18 mcg/day) does not appear to impact on the circulating level of serum cobalamins or its binding proteins in lactating women (Morkbak et al 2007). If required, higher doses may need to be utilised.

PATIENTS' FAQs

What will this vitamin do for me?

Vitamin B_{12} is essential for healthy growth, development and health maintenance. It will reverse signs and symptoms of deficiency and can alleviate symptoms of tinnitus, poor memory, depression and HIV and AIDS when low vitamin B_{12} levels are also present. There is also some research suggesting some positive effects in diabetic retinopathy and sleep disturbances.

When will it start to work?

In cases of pernicious anaemia, the classical deficiency state, correction of blood abnormalities occurs within 6 weeks; however, correction of nervous system changes is slower and may take up to 18 months.

Are there any safety issues?

Vitamin B_{12} is considered a very safe nutrient.

REFERENCES

Albert CM et al. Effect of folic acid and B vitamins on risk of cardiovascular events and total mortality among women at high risk for cardiovascular disease: a randomized trial. JAMA 299.17 (2008): 2027–2036.

Andres E et al. Food-cobalamin malabsorption in elderly patients: Clinical manifestations and treatment. Am J Med 118.10 (2005a): 1154–1159.

Andres E et al. Usefulness of oral vitamin B_{12} therapy in vitamin B_{12} deficiency related to food-cobalamin malabsorption: Short and long-term outcome. Eur J Intern Med 16.3 (2005b): 218.

Andres E et al. Hematological response to short-term oral cyanocobalamin therapy for the treatment of cobalamin deficiencies in elderly patients. J Nutr Health Aging 10.1 (2006): 3–6.

Babior BM. Metabolic aspects of folic acid and cobalamin. In: Beutler E et al (eds). Williams haematology, 5th edn. New York: McGraw-Hill, 1996: 380–393.

Baik HW, Russell RM. Vitamin B_{12} deficiency in the elderly. Annu Rev Nutr 19 (1999): 357–377.

Bilwani F et al. Anaphylactic reaction after intramuscular injection of cyanocobalamin (vitamin B_{12}): a case report. J Pak Med Assoc 55.5 (2005): 217–2119.

Birch CS et al. A novel role for vitamin B12: Cobalamins are intracellular antioxidants in vitro. Free Radic Biol Med 47.2 (2009): 184–188.

Bjorke Monsen AL, Ueland PM. Homocysteine and methylmalonic acid in diagnosis and risk assessment from infancy to adolescence. Am J Clin Nutr 78.1 (2003): 7–21.

Blacher J et al. Very low oral doses of vitamin B_{12} increase serum concentrations in elderly subjects with food-bound vitamin B_{12} malabsorption. J Nutr 137.2 (2007): 373–378.

Bleie O et al. Homocysteine-lowering therapy does not affect inflammatory markers of atherosclerosis in patients with stable coronary artery disease. J Intern Med 262.2 (2007): 244–253.

Bolaman Z et al. Oral versus intramuscular cobalamin treatment in megaloblastic anemia: A single-center, prospective, randomized, open-label study. Clin Ther 25.12 (2003): 3124–3134.

Bor MV. Do we have any good reason to suggest restricting the use of oral contraceptives in women with pre-existing vitamin B_{12} deficiency? Eur J Obstet Gynecol Reprod Biol 115.2 (2004): 240–241.

Bradford GS, Taylor CT. Omeprazole and vitamin B_{12} deficiency. Ann Pharmacother 33.5 (1999): 641–643.

Branco-Ferreira M et al. Anaphylactic reaction to hydroxycobalamin. Allergy 52 (1997): 118–1119.

Briddon A. Homocysteine in the context of cobalamin metabolism and deficiency states. Amino Acids 24.1–2 (2003): 1–12.

Carlsen SM et al. Homocysteine levels are unaffected by metformin treatment in both nonpregnant and pregnant women with polycystic ovary syndrome. Acta Obstet Gynecol Scand 86.2 (2007): 145–150.

Carmel R. Pernicious anemia: The expected findings of very low serum cobalamin levels, anemia, and macrocytosis are often lacking. Arch Intern Med 148.8 (1988): 1712–1714.

Castelli MC et al. Comparing the efficacy and tolerability of a new daily oral vitamin B12 formulation and intermittent intramuscular vitamin B12 in normalizing low cobalamin levels: a randomized, open-label, parallel-group study. Clin Ther 33.3 (2011): 358–371.

Cervantes P et al. Vitamin B_{12} and folate levels and lithium administration in patients with affective disorders. Biol Psychiatry 45.2 (1999): 214–221.

Chen XL, Shi YS. [Effect of vitamin B_{12} mixed solution inhalation for acute radiation-induced mucosal injury.] Nan Fang Yi Ke Da Xue Xue Bao 26.4 (2006): 512–5114.

Clarke R et al. Effects of B-vitamins on plasma homocysteine concentrations and on risk of cardiovascular disease and dementia. Curr Opin Clin Nutr Metab Care 10.1 (v) (2007): 32–9.

Coppen A, Bolander-Gouaille C. Treatment of depression: time to consider folic acid and vitamin B_{12}. J Psychopharmacol 19.1 (2005): 59–65.

Croft MT et al. Algae acquire vitamin B_{12} through a symbiotic relationship with bacteria. Nature 438.7064 (2005): 90–93.

Czernichow S et al. Case for folic acid and vitamin B_{12} fortification in Europe. Semin Vasc Med 5.2 (2005): 156–162.

Dastur DK, Dave UP. Effect of prolonged anticonvulsant medication in epileptic patients: serum lipids, vitamins B_6, B_{12}, and folic acid, proteins, and fine structure of liver. Epilepsia 28.2 (1987): 147–159.

Delpre G et al. Sublingual therapy for cobalamin deficiency as an alternative to oral and parenteral cobalamin supplementation. Lancet 354.9180 (1999): 740.

de Vogel S et al. Serum folate and vitamin B12 concentrations in relation to prostate cancer risk — a Norwegian population-based nested case-control study of 3000 cases and 3000 controls within the JANUS cohort. Int J Epidemiol 42.1 (2013): 201–210.

Dharmarajan TS, et al. Vitamin B_{12} deficiency. Recognizing subtle symptoms in older adults. Geriatrics 58.3 (2003): 30–34, 37–8.

Dou JF et al. Serum vitamin B12 levels as indicators of disease severity and mortality of patients with acute-on-chronic liver failure. Clin Chim Acta 413.23–24 (2012): 1809–1812.

Dror DK, Allen LH. Effect of vitamin B_{12} deficiency on neurodevelopment in infants: current knowledge and possible mechanisms. Nutr Rev 66.5 (2008): 250–255.

Dusitanond P et al. Homocysteine-lowering treatment with folic acid, cobalamin, and pyridoxine does not reduce blood markers of inflammation, endothelial dysfunction, or hypercoagulability in patients with previous transient ischemic attack or stroke: a randomized substudy of the VITATOPS trial. Stroke 36.1 (2005): 144–146.

Ebara S et al. Vitamin B_{12} deficiency results in the abnormal regulation of serine dehydratase and tyrosine aminotransferase activities correlated with impairment of the adenylyl cyclase system in rat liver. Br J Nutr 99.3 (2008): 503–510.

Elia M. Oral or parenteral therapy for B_{12} deficiency. Lancet 352 (1998): 1721–1722.

Ermens AAM, et al. Significance of elevated cobalamin (vitamin B_{12}) levels in blood. Clin Biochem 36.8 (2003): 585–590.

Eussen SJ et al. Oral cyanocobalamin supplementation in older people with vitamin B_{12} deficiency: a dose-finding trial. Arch Intern Med 165.10 (2005): 1167–1172.

FAO/WHO (Food and Agriculture Organization/World Health Organization). Vitamin B_{12}: Report of a joint FAO/WHO expert consultation. Rome: WHO, 2002.

Festen HP. Intrinsic factor secretion and cobalamin absorption: Physiology and pathophysiology in the gastrointestinal tract. Scand J Gastroenterol Suppl 188 (1991): 1–7.

Freeman AG et al. Sublingual cobalamin for pernicious anaemia. Lancet 354.9195 (1999): 2080.

Frequin ST et al. Decreased vitamin B_{12} and folate levels in cerebrospinal fluid and serum of multiple sclerosis patients after high-dose intravenous methylprednisolone. J Neurol 240.5 (1993): 305–308.

Gariballa S, Forster S. Effects of dietary supplements on depressive symptoms in older patients: a randomised double-blind placebo-controlled trial. Clin Nutr 26.5 (2007): 545–551.

Gidal BE et al. Blood homocysteine, folate and vitamin B-12 concentrations in patients with epilepsy receiving lamotrigine or sodium valproate for initial monotherapy. Epilepsy Res 64.3 (2005): 161–166.

Gok U et al. Comparative analysis of serum homocysteine, folic acid and vitamin B_{12} levels in patients with noise-induced hearing loss. Auris Nasus Larynx 31.1 (2004): 19–22.

Groenen PMW et al. Marginal maternal vitamin B_{12} status increases the risk of offspring with spina bifida. Am J Obstet Gynecol 191.1 (2004): 11–17.

Gronlie Guren M et al. Biochemical signs of impaired cobalamin status during and after radiotherapy for rectal cancer. Int J Radiat Oncol Biol Phys 60.3 (2004): 807–813.

Hathout L and El-Saden S. Nitrous oxide-induced B_{12} deficiency myelopathy: Perspectives on the clinical biochemistry of vitamin B_{12}. J Neurol Sci 301.1–2 (2011): 1–8.

Healton EB et al. Neurologic aspects of cobalamin deficiency. Medicine (Baltimore) 70.4 (1991): 229–45.

Herrmann et al. Homocysteine: a newly recognized risk factor for osteoporosis. Clin Chem Lab Med 43.10 (2005): 1111–1117.

Hillman RS. Hematopoietic agents: growth factors, minerals, and vitamins. In: Hardman JG (eds). The pharmacological basis of therapeutics. New York: McGraw-Hill, 1996, pp 1311–40.

Howden C. Vitamin B_{12} levels during prolonged treatment with proton pump inhibitors. J Clin Gastroenterol 30.1 (2000): 29–33.

Hutto BR. Folate and cobalamin in psychiatric illness. Compr Psychiatry 38.6 (1997): 305–314.

IMG (Integrative Medicine Gateway). Unity Health 2001–06. Available at: www.imgateway.net (accessed 2003).

Isoda K et al. Hepatoprotective effect of vitamin B_{12} on dimethylnitrosamine-induced liver injury. Biol Pharm Bull 31.2 (2008): 309–311.

Izumi Y, Kaji R. [Clinical trials of ultra-high-dose methylcobalamin in ALS.] Brain Nerve 59.10 (2007): 1141–1147.

Jamison RL et al. Effect of homocysteine lowering on mortality and vascular disease in advanced chronic kidney disease and end-stage renal disease: a randomized controlled trial. JAMA 298.10 (2007): 1163–1170.

Kang JH, Grodstein F. Mid-life plasma folate and vitamin B_{12} levels and cognitive function in older women. Alzheimer Dementia 1.1 (Suppl 1) (2005): 28.

Kapadia C. Cobalamin [vitamin B_{12}] deficiency; Is it a problem for our aging population and is the problem compounded by drugs that inhibit gastric acid secretion? J Clin Gastroenterol 30.1 (2000): 4–6.

Karabiber H et al. Effects of valproate and carbamazepine on serum levels of homocysteine, vitamin B_{12}, and folic acid. Brain Dev 25.2 (2003): 113–1115.

Karnaze DS, Carmel R. Neurologic and evoked potential abnormalities in subtle cobalamin deficiency states, including deficiency without anemia and with normal absorption of free cobalamin. Arch Neurol 47.9 (1990): 1008–1012.

Keser I et al. Folic acid and vitamin B12 supplementation lowers plasma homocysteine but has no effect on serum bone turnover markers in elderly women: a randomized, double-blind, placebo-controlled trial. Nutr Res 33.3 (2013): 211–219.

Kim YS et al. The optimal duration of vitamin supplementation prior to the first dose of pemetrexed in patients with non-small-cell lung cancer. Lung Cancer 81.2 (2013): 231–235.

Kwok T et al. Use of fasting urinary methylmalonic acid to screen for metabolic vitamin B_{12} deficiency in older persons. Nutrition 20.9 (2004): 764–768.

Laine L et al. Review article: potential gastrointestinal effects of long-term acid suppression with proton pump inhibitors. Aliment Pharmacol Ther 14.6 (2000): 651–658.

Lam JR et al. Proton pump inhibitor and histamine 2 receptor antagonist use and vitamin B12 deficiency. JAMA 310.22 (2013): 2435–2442.

Lee GR. Pernicious anemia and other causes of vitamin B_{12} (cobalamin) deficiency. In: Lee GR et al (eds). Wintrobe's clinical hematology, 10th edn. Baltimore: Williams & Wilkins, 1999, pp 941–964.

Lewerin C et al. Serum biomarkers for atrophic gastritis and antibodies against *Helicobacter pylori* in the elderly: Implications for vitamin B_{12}, folic acid and iron status and response to oral vitamin therapy. Scand J Gastroenterol 43.9 (2008): 1050–1056.

Lindenbaum J et al. Neuropsychiatric disorders caused by cobalamin deficiency in the absence of anemia or macrocytosis. N Engl J Med 318 (1988): 1720–1728.

Loder C et al. Treatment of multiple sclerosis with lofepramine, L-phenylalanine and vitamin B(12): mechanism of action and clinical importance: roles of the locus coeruleus and central noradrenergic systems. Med Hypotheses 59.5 (2002): 594–602.

Mann JF et al. Homocysteine lowering with folic acid and B vitamins in people with chronic kidney disease–results of the renal Hope-2 study. Nephrol Dial Transplant 23.2 (2008): 645–653.

Marcuard SP et al. Omeprazole therapy causes malabsorption of cyanocobalamin (vitamin B_{12}). Ann Intern Med 120.3 (1994): 211–215.

Marcucci R et al. Vitamin supplementation reduces the progression of atherosclerosis in hyperhomocysteinemic renal-transplant recipients. Transplantation 75.9 (2003): 1551–1555.

Marcus J et al. Homocysteine lowering and cardiovascular disease risk: lost in translation. Can J Cardiol 23.9 (2007): 707–710.

Martí-Carvajal AJ et al. Homocysteine lowering interventions for preventing cardiovascular events. Cochrane Database Syst Rev (2013) CD006612.

Mayer G et al. Effects of vitamin B_{12} on performance and circadian rhythm in normal subjects. Neuropsychopharmacology 15.5 (1996): 456–464.

Miller AL. The methionine-homocysteine cycle and its effects on cognitive diseases. Altern Med Rev 8.1 (2003): 7–19.

Miller A et al. Vitamin B_{12}, demyelination, remyelination and repair in multiple sclerosis. J Neurol Sci 233.1–2 (2005): 93–97.

Molina JR and Adjei AA. The role of pemetrexed (Alimta, LY231514) in lung cancer therapy. Clin Lung Cancer 5.1 (2003): 21–27.

Moreira ES et al. Vitamin B_{12} protects against superoxide-induced cell injury in human aortic endothelial cells. Free Radic Biol Med 51.4 (2011): 876–883.

Morkbak AL et al. A longitudinal study of serum cobalamin and its binding proteins in lactating women. Eur J Clin Nutr 61.2 (2007): 184–189.

Oh RC, Brown DL. Vitamin B_{12} deficiency. Am Fam Physician 67.5 (2003): 979.

Omray A. Evaluation of pharmacokinetic parameters of tetracycline hydrochloride upon oral administration with vitamin C and B complex. Hindustan Antibiot Bull 23.VI (1981): 33–37.

Park S et al. Age-related hearing loss, methylmalonic acid, and vitamin B_{12} status in older adults. J Nutr Elder 25.3–4 (2006): 105–120.

Pawlak R et al. How prevalent is vitamin B(12) deficiency among vegetarians? Nutr Rev 71.2 (2013): 110–117.

Penninx BW et al. Vitamin B (12) deficiency and depression in physically disabled older women: epidemiologic evidence from the Women's Health and Aging Study. Am J Psychiatry 157.5 (2000): 715–721.

Piskin S et al. Serum iron, ferritin, folic acid, and vitamin B_{12} levels in recurrent aphthous stomatitis. J Eur Acad Dermatol Venereol 16.1 (2002): 66–67.

Quaranta A et al. The effects of 'supra-physiological' vitamin B_{12} administration on temporary threshold shift. Int J Audiol 43.3 (2004): 162–165.

Rafnsson SB et al. Is a low blood level of vitamin B12 a cardiovascular and diabetes risk factor? A systematic review of cohort studies. Eur J Nutr 50.2 (2011): 97–106.

Ray JG, Blom HJ. Vitamin B_{12} insufficiency and the risk of fetal neural tube defects. Q J Med 96.4 (2003): 289–295.

Ray JG et al. Homocysteine-lowering therapy and risk for venous thromboembolism: a randomized trial. Ann Intern Med 146.11 (2007). 761–767.

Refsum H, Smith AD. Low vitamin B-12 status in confirmed Alzheimer's disease as revealed by serum holotranscobalamin. J Neurol Neurosurg Psychiatry 74.7 (2003): 959–961.

Remacha AF, Cadafalch J. Cobalamin deficiency in patients infected with the human immunodeficiency virus. Semin Hematol 36.1 (1999): 75–87.

Remacha AF et al. Vitamin B_{12} transport proteins in patients with HIV-1 infection and AIDS. Haematologica 78.2 (1993): 84–88.

Reznikoff-Etievant MF et al. Low vitamin B(12) level as a risk factor for very early recurrent abortion. Eur J Obstet Gynecol Reprod Biol 104.2 (2002): 156–159.

Rocco A et al. Vitamin B12 supplementation improves rates of sustained viral response in patients chronically infected with hepatitis C virus. Gut 62.5 (2013): 766–773.

Roffman JL et al. Randomized multicenter investigation of folate plus vitamin B12 supplementation in schizophrenia. JAMA Psychiatry 70.5 (2013): 481–489.

Roth M, Orija I. Oral vitamin B_{12} therapy in vitamin B_{12} deficiency. Am J Med 116.5 (2004): 358.

Sahin M et al. Effects of metformin or rosiglitazone on serum concentrations of homocysteine, folate, and vitamin B_{12} in patients with type 2 diabetes mellitus. J Diabetes Complications 21.2 (2007): 118–123.

Saltzman JR et al. Effect of hypochlorhydria due to omeprazole treatment or atrophic gastritis on protein-bound vitamin B_{12} absorption. J Am Coll Nutr 13.6 (1994): 584–591.

Sandyk R, Awerbuch GI. Vitamin B_{12} and its relationship to age of onset of multiple sclerosis. Int J Neurosci 71.1–4 (1993): 93–99.

Schenk BE et al. Atrophic gastritis during long-term omeprazole therapy affects serum vitamin B_{12} levels. Aliment Pharmacol Ther 13.10 (1999): 1343–1346.

Schneede J, Ueland PM. Novel and established markers of cobalamin deficiency: complementary or exclusive diagnostic strategies. Semin Vasc Med 5.2 (2005): 140–155.

Schnyder G et al. Effect of homocysteine-lowering therapy with folic acid, vitamin B_{12}, and vitamin B_6 on clinical outcome after percutaneous coronary intervention: the Swiss Heart study: a randomized controlled trial. JAMA 288.8 (2002): 973–979.

Seppälä J et al. Association between vitamin b12 levels and melancholic depressive symptoms: a Finnish population-based study. BMC Psychiatry 13.1 (2013): 145.

Sharma V and Biswas D. Cobalamin deficiency presenting as obsessive compulsive disorder: case report. Gen Hosp Psychiatry 34.6 (2012): 578e7–578e8.

Shemesh Z et al. Vitamin B_{12} deficiency in patients with chronic tinnitus and noise-induced hearing loss. Am J Otolaryngol 14.2 (1993): 94–99.

Stabler SP, Allen RH. Vitamin B_{12} deficiency as a worldwide problem. Annu Rev Nutr 24 (2004): 299–326.

Stucker M et al. Topical vitamin B_{12}: a new therapeutic approach in atopic dermatitis-evaluation of efficacy and tolerability in a randomized placebo-controlled multicentre clinical trial. Br J Dermatol 150.5 (2004): 977–983.

Suarez L et al. Maternal serum B_{12} levels and risk for neural tube defects in a Texas-Mexico border population. Ann Epidemiol 13.2 (2003): 81–88.

Sun Y, et al. Effectiveness of vitamin B_{12} on diabetic neuropathy: systematic review of clinical controlled trials. Acta Neurol Taiwan 14.2 (2005): 48–54.
Sutterlin MW et al. Serum folate and Vitamin B_{12} levels in women using modern oral contraceptives (OC) containing 20 μg ethinyl estradiol. Eur J Obstet Gynecol Reprod Biol 107.1 (2003): 57–61.
Takenaka S et al. Feeding dried purple laver (nori) to vitamin B_{12}-deficient rats significantly improves vitamin B_{12} status. Br J Nutr 852 (2001): 699–70.
Tamura J et al. Immunomodulation by vitamin B_{12}: augmentation of CD8+ T lymphocytes and natural killer (NK) cell activity in vitamin B_{12}-deficient patients by methyl-B_{12} treatment. Clin Exp Immunol 116.1 (1999): 28–32.
Termanini B et al. Effect of long-term gastric acid suppressive therapy on serum vitamin B_{12} levels in patients with Zollinger-Ellison syndrome. Am J Med 104.5 (1998): 422–430.
Toole JF et al. Lowering homocysteine in patients with ischemic stroke to prevent recurrent stroke, myocardial infarction, and death: the Vitamin Intervention for Stroke Prevention (VISP) randomized controlled trial. JAMA 291.5 (2004): 565–575.
Tripathi M et al. Serum cobalamin levels in dementias. Neurol India 49.3 (2001): 284–286.
Valuck RJ, Ruscin JM. A case-control study on adverse effects: H2 blocker or proton pump inhibitor use and risk of vitamin B_{12} deficiency in older adults. J Clin Epidemiol 57.4 (2004): 422–428.
van der Valk et al. Neonatal folate, homocysteine, vitamin B12 levels and methylenetetrahydrofolate reductase variants in childhood asthma and eczema. Allergy 68.6 (2013): 788–795.
van Wijngaarden JP et al. Vitamin B12, folate, homocysteine, and bone health in adults and elderly people: a systematic review with meta-analyses. J Nutr Metab (2013) 2013: 486186.
Vidal-Alaball J et al. Oral vitamin B_{12} versus intramuscular vitamin B_{12} for vitamin B_{12} deficiency. Cochrane Database Syst Rev 3 (2005): CD004655.
VITATOPS Trial Study Group. B vitamins in patients with recent transient ischaemic attack or stroke in the VITAmins TO Prevent Stroke (VITATOPS) trial: a randomised, double-blind, parallel, placebo-controlled trial. Lancet Neurol 9.9 (2010): 855–865.
Vogel T et al. Homocysteine, vitamin B12, folate and cognitive functions: a systematic and critical review of the literature. Int J Clin Pract 63.7 (2009): 1061–1067.
Volkov I, et al. Successful treatment of chronic erythema nodosum with vitamin B_{12}. J Am Board Fam Pract 18.6 (2005): 567–569.
Wahlqvist ML (ed.). Food and nutrition, 2nd edn. Sydney: Allen & Unwin, 2002, p 260.
Wald DS et al. Serum homocysteine and dementia: Meta-analysis of eight cohort studies including 8669 participants. Alzheimers Dement 7.4 (2011): 412–417.
Wang HX et al. Vitamin B(12) and folate in relation to the development of Alzheimer's disease. Neurology 56.9 (2001): 1188–1194.
Watanabe F. Vitamin B_{12} sources and bioavailability. Exp Biol Med (Maywood) 232.10 (2007): 1266–1274.
Weinburg JB et al. Inhibition of nitric oxide synthase by cobalamins and cobinamides. Free Radic Biol Med 46.12 (2009): 1626–1632.
Weir GD, Scott MJ. Brain function in the elderly: role of vitamin B_{12} and folate. Br Med Bull 55.3 (1999): 669.14.
Wellmer J et al. [Oral treatment of vitamin B_{12} deficiency in subacute combined degeneration]. Nervenarzt 77.10 (2006): 1228–1231.
Westphal S et al. Antihypertensive treatment and homocysteine concentrations. Metabolism 52.3 (2003): 261–263.
Wolters M, et al. Cobalamin: a critical vitamin in the elderly. Prev Med 39.6 (2004): 1256–1266.
Xu T et al. Treatment of hyperhomocysteinemia and endothelial dysfunction in renal transplant recipients with B vitamins in the Chinese population. J Urol 179.3 (2008): 1190–1194.
Yajnik CS et al. Oral vitamin B_{12} supplementation reduces plasma total homocysteine concentration in women in India. Asia Pac J Clin Nutr 16.1 (2007): 103–109.
Zetterberg H et al. The transcobalamin codon 259 polymorphism influences the risk of human spontaneous abortion. Hum Reprod 17.12 (2002): 3033–3036.
Zhang H et al. Association of homocysteine, vitamin B12, and folate with bone mineral density in postmenopausal women: a meta-analysis. Arch Gynecol Obstet (2014) 289: 10039.

Vitamin B_2 — riboflavin

BACKGROUND AND RELEVANT PHARMACOKINETICS

Riboflavin was first discovered in 1917 and was originally referred to as vitamin G in the United States. Its name reflects both its structure and colour: *ribo* refers to the presence of a ribose-like side chain, and *flavus* is Latin for yellow (Gropper & Smith 2013). Structurally, it consists of a flavin isoalloxazine ring and a sugar alcohol side chain, ribitol.

Riboflavin is a water-soluble B group vitamin that is sensitive to light (including sunlight) and alkali conditions. It is resistant to heat, oxidation and acid; therefore most means of sterilisation, canning and cooking do not affect the riboflavin content of foods (Combs 2012).

Dietary B_2 occurs in three forms: flavin adenine dinucleotide (FAD), flavin mononucleotide (FMN) and riboflavin phosphate (see Food sources section, below). Prior to absorption these forms must all be freed to riboflavin, which requires specific gastrointestinal phosphatase enzymes for these conversions.

Riboflavin uptake occurs mainly in the proximal part of the small intestine and involves a specialised, saturable, energy-dependent, Na^+-independent carrier-mediated system, riboflavin transporter 2 (RFT2). Adaptive changes alter the number and/or activity of carriers, e.g. when large pharmacological doses of riboflavin are ingested, absorption occurs via simple diffusion. Approximately 95% of riboflavin from food is absorbed (Food and Nutrition Board 1998). There is evidence that bioavailability is optimal at 25 mg peak plasma levels, and doses in excess of this are poorly absorbed.

Absorption is enhanced by the presence of bile and the consumption of fresh foods and impeded by the presence of divalent metals (zinc, iron, copper and manganese), whereas alcohol has an inhibitory effect.

Once absorbed, much of the riboflavin is converted back into one of its active forms, as a component of two primary coenzymes, FAD (40%) and FMN (10%). Both of these belong to the class known as the flavin coenzymes (flavoenzymes, flavoproteins), which are active in redox reactions involving hydrogen transfer and consequently important for the body's energy production. The various forms are transported in blood by plasma proteins, including albumin, fibrinogen and immunoglobulins (Gropper & Smith 2013). Free riboflavin is the form that crosses most cell membranes and, in the case of the liver, calcium or calmodulin regulates riboflavin uptake. The liver, kidneys and heart contain the greatest concentrations of riboflavin.

FOOD SOURCES

There are two sources of riboflavin: dietary and bacterial; the latter, produced by normal gastrointestinal microflora, is dependent upon the type of diet consumed, with higher synthesis resulting from intake of vegetable-based diets than from meat-based diets (Said 2004).

Riboflavin is found in a wide variety of foods, especially those of animal origin. Milk and milk products such as cheese are thought to contribute the most dietary riboflavin, providing about one-half of total intake (Combs 2012, Gropper & Smith 2013). Other main food sources are organ meats, especially liver, eggs, legumes, yeast products (including Vegemite), almonds, wheatgerm, wild rice and mushrooms. It is also found to a lesser extent in fruits, vegetables and cereal grains. Refined grains are enriched with riboflavin due to its loss from the milling process that removes the bran and germ, resulting in a loss of about two-thirds of the riboflavin content (Gropper & Smith 2013). Maximum loss during cooking is 75% (Wahlqvist 2002).

Milk, eggs and enriched cereal grains contain either free or protein-bound riboflavin, while in most other foods it predominantly exists as its coenzyme derivatives or phosphorus-bound riboflavin.

DEFICIENCY SIGNS AND SYMPTOMS

Acute deficiency of riboflavin, known as ariboflavinosis, seldom occurs in isolation and is usually associated with a deficiency of other B group vitamins (Gropper & Smith 2013).

Primary deficiency

Primary deficiency is associated with inadequate dietary intake, such as vegetarianism and poor consumption of milk and other animal products (Combs 2012). Primary deficiency is reported to be more common in the elderly and adolescent girls.

Secondary deficiency

Secondary deficiencies can develop in chronic diarrhoea, liver disease, chronic alcoholism, alcohol and drug use, including use of the oral contraceptive pill, adrenal or thyroid hormone insufficiency, hyperthyroid, anorexia nervosa and postoperative situations in which total parenteral nutrition solutions lack riboflavin. In most cases, riboflavin deficiency is accompanied by other vitamin deficiencies, such as deficiencies of vitamin B_6, niacin and folic acid. Drugs that impair riboflavin absorption or utilisation by inhibiting the conversion of the vitamin to the active coenzymes include tricyclic antidepressants, chemotherapy drugs and psychotropic agents. There is also evidence suggesting an apparent increase in riboflavin requirements with increased physical exercise.

Signs and symptoms of deficiency

The body's 'storage capacity' is sufficient to provide riboflavin for 2–6 weeks when riboflavin is inadequate.

Initial symptoms of riboflavin deficiency are often non-specific and include weakness, fatigue, mouth pain, angular stomatitis, cheilosis and personality changes. In animals, general signs of anorexia, impaired growth and reduced efficiency of feed utilisation have occurred.

Clinical symptoms of deficiency appear after 3–4 months of inadequate intake. Because of the fundamental role of riboflavin in metabolism, deficiency manifestations initially occur in tissues with high and rapid cellular turnover, such as epithelial tissue and skin (Combs 2012). This will account for many of the early deficiency signs, including:

- Angular stomatitis, cold sores and cheilosis
- Glossitis (inflammation of the tongue), magenta tongue (Lo 1984)
- Red or bloody (hyperaemic) and swollen (oedematous) mouth or oral cavity
- Failure to grow in children
- Ocular and visual disturbances, with symptoms such as burning, itching, sensitivity to light and conjunctivitis
- Scaly and greasy dermatitis affecting the nasolabial folds, ears, eyelids, scrotum and labia majora (Lo 1984)
- Inflammatory skin conditions — desquamative dermatitis, seborrhoeic dermatitis
- Hair loss
- Poor wound healing
- Anaemia
- Peripheral nerve dysfunction (neuropathy).

V

MAIN ACTIONS

Riboflavin is involved in many different biological processes and is essential for maintaining health. The flavoproteins are central to carbohydrate, protein and lipid metabolism, are involved in adenosine triphosphate production, and are essential for immune function, tissue repair processes and general growth (required for the healthy growth of skin, nails and hair). Riboflavin extends the life of red blood cells and plays a key role in fatty acid oxidation and the metabolism of several other B vitamins. In particular, riboflavin activates vitamin B_6 and folate, which are essential cofactors in neurotransmitter formation and metabolism (Gropper & Smith 2013).

Coenzyme functions

Riboflavin exerts its functions as two flavin enzymes (flavoenzymes), FAD and FMN. These coenzymes are essential in carbohydrate, amino acid and lipid metabolism.

Flavoenzymes exhibit a range of redox potentials, acting as oxidising agents because of their ability to accept a pair of hydrogen atoms (Gropper & Smith 2013). Consequently, FMN and FAD function as coenzymes in cellular antioxidant protection and for a variety of oxidative enzyme systems (Combs 2012). Riboflavin increases intracellular levels of reduced glutathione (an essential antioxidant in itself) and maintains the glutathione redox cycle as part of the FAD-dependent enzyme glutathione reductase (Combs 2012). Other flavoproteins provide reducing equivalents to neutralise reactive oxygen species (free radicals).

CLINICAL USE

A number of clinical trials have been conducted in which patients presenting with different conditions have subsequently been found to have riboflavin deficiency. Treating the deficiency in some of these cases has been shown to improve the initial presenting condition.

Wound healing

Riboflavin deficiency lengthens the time to epithelialisation of wounds, slows the rate of wound contraction and reduces the tensile strength of incision wounds in vivo. Total collagen content is also significantly decreased, suggesting riboflavin deficiency will slow down wound-healing rate (Lakshmi et al 1989).

Migraine headaches: prophylaxis

Three clinical studies of varying design have found that treatment with high-dose riboflavin (400 mg) can reduce the frequency of migraines; however, one double-blind study that used it in combination with magnesium and feverfew failed to show any superior effects over low-dose riboflavin (25 mg) alone.

The first was an open pilot study testing the effects of 400 mg riboflavin over 3 months in 49 patients. The mean global improvement after therapy was 68.2% (Schoenen et al 1994). Based on these results, a second study with 55 subjects was conducted using a 3-month, randomised, placebo-controlled design, with similar positive findings (Schoenen et al 1998). Riboflavin treatment produced positive results, with 59% of the treatment group experiencing a reduction in migraine frequency of at least 50%. Using an intention-to-treat analysis, riboflavin was superior to placebo in reducing attack frequency ($P = 0.005$) and headache days ($P = 0.012$) and the number needed to treat for effectiveness was 2.3. More recently, a 2004 open-label study retested the same high dose of vitamin B_2 over 6 months, once again producing a significant reduction in headache frequency, from 4 days/month at baseline to 2 days/month after 3 and 6 months of treatment ($P < 0.05$). Use of abortive drugs reduced from 7 units/month to 4.5 units/month; however, the duration and intensity of each episode did not change significantly (Boehnke et al 2004).

Finally, a randomised, double-blind, controlled study using a combination of vitamin B_2 (400 mg), magnesium (300 mg) and feverfew (100 mg) failed to show benefits over riboflavin 25 mg alone, with both groups experiencing comparable significant reductions in number of migraines, migraine day and migraine index; however, in neither group was frequency successfully reduced by more than 50%, which was the primary outcome (Maizels et al 2004). Interestingly, the response obtained was greater than the placebo response reported in other migraine prophylaxis trials.

A Cochrane review intervention protocol (Exposito et al 2009) states there is no single theory or hypothesis that can explain all the phenomena that occur with migraines; therefore the manner in which riboflavin might prevent migraine headaches is also not clear (Bajwa & Sabahat 2008, as cited in Exposito et al 2009). Despite this, it is frequently suggested that where mitochondrial dysfunction and impaired metabolism are causal in migraine pathogenesis, riboflavin appears to be useful in its management (Maizels et al 2004, Markley 2012, Sandor 2005, Schoenen et al 1998). High-dose riboflavin assists in promoting cellular mitochondrial metabolism, thereby improving some headache symptomatology (Woolhouse 2005). These studies are important, as riboflavin displays high tolerance with a high index of safety and relatively few side effects.

Migraine prophylaxis in children

The first study to evaluate the efficacy of riboflavin for migraine prophylaxis in children was a randomised, double-blind study of 200 mg/day versus placebo in 48 children. No differences were found in primary efficacy measure (number of patients achieving a 50% or greater reduction in the number of migraine attacks per 4 weeks) nor secondary outcome measures (mean severity of migraine per day, mean duration of migraine, days with nausea or vomiting, analgesic use and adverse effects). The authors concluded that riboflavin is not an effective therapy for preventing migraine in children. A high placebo responder rate was also seen, with implications for other studies of paediatric migraine (MacLennan et al 2008). Similar negative findings were produced in another small study by Bruijn et al (2010); however, the authors did find a significant difference ($P = 0.04$) in the reduction of mean frequency of tension-type headaches in favour of riboflavin treatment.

A retrospective study of migraine prophylaxis in 41 paediatric and adolescent patients, who received higher riboflavin doses (200 or 400 mg/day for 3, 4 or 6 months), however, reported significantly decreased attack frequency and intensity ($P < 0.01$) during treatment. Additionally, during follow-up, 68.4% of cases had a 50% or greater reduction in frequency of attacks and 21% in intensity. The authors concluded riboflavin to be a well-tolerated, effective and low-cost prophylactic treatment in children and adolescents suffering from migraine (Condo et al 2009).

From these studies, it is perhaps evident that riboflavin has a positive prophylaxis effect in the reduction of attack frequency and intensity with higher doses (200–400 mg) combined with longer treatment times (more than 4 weeks). The effect of taking a daily riboflavin supplement from the adult studies was maximal after 3 months (Breen 2003). It would suggest further studies of longer duration are required.

V

> ***Clinical note — Causes of migraine***
>
> Numerous theories exist to explain the underlying pathology of migraine headache. One theory proposes a deficit of mitochondrial energy metabolism, as patients with migraine show decreased brain mitochondrial energy reserve between attacks. Interestingly, patients with mitochondrial encephalomyopathy, lactic acidosis and stroke-like episodes (MELAS) exhibit impaired mitochondrial energy metabolism, producing migraine-like headaches, which are in part ameliorated by prophylactic B_2 (Magis et al 2007).

Accordingly, riboflavin coenzyme Q10 and lipoic acid, as enhancers of mitochondrial energy efficiency, have been tested for prophylactic activity in migraine and appear to be promising agents (Magis et al 2007, Markley 2012, Schoenen et al 1994). Recent studies in experimental models add to our knowledge of the actions of riboflavin in migraine, with confirmation that it produces antinociception and anti-inflammatory effects. The analgesic activity observed is independent of opioid mechanisms (Granados-Soto et al 2004).

Comparative trial

A 4-month clinical trial comparing riboflavin supplementation (400 mg/day) with beta-adrenergic antagonists (metoprolol 200 mg/day and bisoprolol 10 mg/day) found that both treatments significantly decreased the frequency of migraine headache and improved the clinical symptoms of migraine headache (Sandor et al 2000). Analysis of their effects on cortical potentials showed that the two treatments achieve these results by working through different mechanisms.

Clinical note — Age-related cataract and antioxidants

Age-related cataract is an important public health problem, because approximately 50% of the 30–50 million cases of blindness worldwide result from leaving the condition untreated (Jacques 1999). The mechanisms that bring about a loss in transparency include oxidation, osmotic stress and chemical adduct formation (Bunce et al 1990). Besides traditional risk factors such as diabetes, nutrient deficiency is also being considered, particularly nutrients with antioxidant properties.

Age-related cataract prevention

Cataract was shown to be associated with riboflavin deficiency in animals in the 1930s and subsequently with deficiencies of amino acids, vitamins and some minerals (Wynn & Wynn 1996). This has been confirmed in human studies, in which lens opacities have been associated with lower levels of riboflavin, vitamins A, C and E, iron and protein status (Leske et al 1995, Mares-Perlman et al 1995).

Glutathione reductase is a key enzyme involved in lens protection. Riboflavin levels indirectly influence glutathione reductase activity, increasing the ability of the lens to deal with free radical formation (Head 2001). One study documented severe glutathione reductase deficiency in 23% of human lens epithelium specimens, possibly reflecting a dietary deficiency of riboflavin (Straatsma et al 1991). Another study found that a significant number of people with cataracts have inactive epithelial glutathione reductase (Horwitz et al 1987).

A large cross-sectional survey of 2873 volunteers aged 49–97 years detected a link between dietary vitamin supplement and a lower incidence of both nuclear and cortical cataract. Vitamin A, niacin, riboflavin, thiamine, folate and vitamin B_{12} all appeared to be protective, either in isolation or as constituents of multivitamin preparations (Kuzniarz et al 2001).

A sample of 408 women from the Nurses' Health Study aged 52–74 years at baseline participated in a 5-year study that assessed nutrient intake and the degree of nuclear density (opacification). Findings revealed that the geometric mean 5-year change in nuclear density was inversely associated with the intake of riboflavin (P = 0.03) and thiamin (P = 0.04), and most significantly with the duration of vitamin E supplement use (P = 0.006) (Jacques et al 2005).

The evidence currently suggests that higher intakes of riboflavin protect against the progression of age-related lens opacification.

Congestive heart failure

A recent review of micronutrients in heart failure summarised several observational studies investigating riboflavin status (McKeag et al 2012). While the authors state the results are inconclusive, one recent study they included produced significant findings. This study measured riboflavin and pyridoxine levels in 100 patients with heart failure (as defined by Framingham criteria). The percentage of individuals with evidence of riboflavin deficiency was 27% (erythrocyte glutathione reductase activity coefficient >1.2) and this was significantly higher in patients with heart failure compared with controls (27.0% vs 2.2%; P = 0.001) (Keith et al 2009). More research needs to be conducted in this area to determine if this could be a cause or consequence of the disease.

> ***Clinical note — Vitamin B_2 deficiency and protracted malaria recovery?***
> In a study of 35 of 64 children suffering malarial infection, riboflavin was assessed by measuring erythrocyte glutathione reductase activity (Das et al 1988). Interestingly, in the riboflavin-deficient group, the median parasite count was in fact lower than the non-deficient group; however, the correlation between activity coefficient and parasite count was significant (R = −0.49). Therefore the recovery process was slower in the deficient group, even though they had a relatively lower parasite count. The authors have thus inferred that riboflavin deficiency leads to inhibition of growth and multiplication of plasmodia. Its beneficial effects in malaria infection need further evaluation.

Anticarcinogenesis

Riboflavin deficiency may cause protein and DNA damage and prevent cellular differentiation in the G1 phase of cellular division, according to cell culture studies (Manthey et al 2006, as cited by Gropper & Smith 2013).

Riboflavin deficiency has been reported to enhance carcinogenesis (Combs 2012). In a rat study the formation of single-strand breaks in nuclear DNA was more pronounced on a riboflavin-deficient diet compared to that on a normal diet (Webster et al 1973). The introduction of riboflavin reversed this trend. The authors suggest that, as DNA damage and its altered repair may relate to carcinogenesis, modulation of these parameters by riboflavin suggests a potential chemopreventive role for this vitamin.

The proposed mechanism of action is that a decrease in riboflavin produces a reduction in antioxidant protection, increasing the activation of carcinogens and oxidative DNA damage. While clinical data relative to this possibility are few, recently an inverse relationship has been found between riboflavin status and cancer risk in three observational studies (de Vogel et al 2008 as cited by Combs 2012). The cancers were specifically oesophageal squamous cell cancer and colorectal cancer. More research is required in these areas.

V

Breast cancer

The majority of studies investigating the protective role of B vitamins in breast cancer have focused on folate, B_6 and B_{12}. Several case-controlled studies have reported protective associations (Chen et al 2005, Lajous et al 2006, Larsson et al 2007, Yang et al 2013), while cohort studies have shown inconsistent results (Cho et al 2007, Ericson et al 2007, Shrubsole et al 2011, Stevens et al 2010). Two of these studies also included an investigation of the role of riboflavin and found no risk reduction with B_2 (Shrubsole et al 2011, Yang et al 2013).

Breast cancer — adjunctive treatment to tamoxifen

Riboflavin's importance is recognised in a range of terminal disease states, most notably in breast cancer, where its cellular absorption is significantly enhanced (Bareford et al 2008). Based on its established antioxidant properties, its role in maintaining epithelial integrity, and its influence on prostaglandin synthesis and glutathione metabolism (Premkumar et al 2008a), vitamin B_2 (10 mg) has been tested in combination with coenzyme Q10 (100 mg) and niacin (50 mg) (known as CORN) together with tamoxifen in breast cancer patients. The results have consistently demonstrated augmenting actions — enhanced manganese superoxide dismutase expression, resulting in prevention of cancer cell proliferation (Premkumar et al 2008b), reduction of lipid peroxides (which are elevated in breast cancer and associated with tumour promotion) (Yuvaraj et al 2008), reduced tumour markers carcinoembryonic antigen (CEA) and CA15-3 and reduced serum cytokines (interleukin-1 [IL-1]-beta, IL-6, IL-8, tumour necrosis factor-alpha and vascular endothelial growth factor) (Premkumar et al 2008a). In addition to this, CORN supplementation reduced proangiogenic markers, with a corresponding increase in antiangiogenic markers. Given that the growth and metastasising capacity of any tumour (but particularly of breast tumours) are dependent upon angiogenesis, this could represent a means to improved prognoses (Premkumar et al 2008a). Finally, CORN supplementation was shown to moderate some of the negative side effects of tamoxifen treatment, with normalisation of lipid and lipoproteins following 90 days of treatment in postmenopausal breast cancer patients (Yuvaraj et al 2007).

Clinical note — Riboflavin carrier protein: a new marker to predict breast cancer

Interestingly, studies have shown that riboflavin carrier protein (RCP), an oestrogen-inducible protein that occupies a key position in riboflavin metabolism, is elevated in women with breast cancer. Oestrogen-inducible proteins such as RCP are upregulated and secreted into circulation in animal models and in women with neoplastic breast disease (Karande et al 2001). In a prospective blinded study, serum RCP levels were significantly elevated in women with breast cancer ($n = 52$) as compared with control subjects ($n = 50$; 6.06 ± 7.27 ng/mL vs 0.70 ± 0.19 ng/mL [mean ± SD], respectively; $P < 0.0001$). Furthermore, a serum RCP level of ≥1.0 ng/mL was highly predictive of the presence of breast cancer, detecting 88% of tumours in stages I–II and 100% of tumours in stages III–IV (Rao et al 1999). In another double-blind study, pre- and postmenopausal women with clinically diagnosed early and advanced breast cancer were compared with controls. This study also revealed that serum RCP levels in cycling breast cancer patients were three- to fourfold higher ($P < 0.01$) than in normal counterparts (Karande et al 2001). This difference in circulatory RCP levels is further magnified to nine- to 11-fold ($P < 0.005$) at the postmenopausal stage. Additionally, rising RCP levels are positively correlated with disease progression, as significantly higher RCP concentrations ($P < 0.005$) are encountered in patients with advanced (compared with early) metastasising breast cancer. A more recent study also noted elevated levels of RCP in breast cancer pathways, and the authors suggest it as a new marker to predict early-stage breast cancer (Shigemizu et al 2012). The current research is not suggesting any clear role, either preventive or causative, of riboflavin and breast cancer.

Role in folate and pyridoxine metabolism and the methylation pathologies

Effective one-carbon metabolism relies on nutrients beyond folate, B_6 and B_{12} — most notably B_2, which, although attracting significantly less research attention, is critical. Riboflavin, as FAD, is the cofactor for methylenetetrahydrofolate reductase (MTHFR), a key enzyme of the folate activation pathway, catalysing the interconversion of 5,10-methylene tetrahydrofolate and 5-methyltetrahydrofolate-converting folate into its active form (Bates 2013, Powers 2003, 2005, Sharp et al 2008). Consistent with this, there is emerging evidence of substantial interplay between folate and riboflavin in conditions previously associated principally with folate deficiency or ameliorated by folate treatment. For example, plasma levels of vitamin B_2 and homocysteine have been shown to correlate; that is, high homocysteine levels have in fact been found to be low in subjects with low riboflavin status (Combs 2012, de Vogel et al 2008, Ganji & Kafai 2004), especially in individuals with the MTHFR C677TT genotype (McNulty et al 2006).

Of several single-nucleotide polymorphisms affecting MTHFR, the best known are the C699T and A1298C variants. The first displays thermolability and lowered reductase activity exaggerated by the loss of FAD cofactor (Allen & Prentice 2013). Preliminary studies employing combinations of folate (400 mcg) and riboflavin (5 mg) have demonstrated improved efficacy over folate alone, for example in colorectal cancer (Powers 2005).

Additionally, high doses of folate alone have been reported to modestly but significantly reduce vitamin B_2 levels (Powers 2005). Taken together with the knowledge that riboflavin is central to pyridoxine metabolism (McCormick 2000), there is growing interest in the therapeutic potential of riboflavin in pathologies associated with poor methylation.

Fertility and pregnancy

Fetal and embyronic development require adequate riboflavin status (Karande et al 2001). In a 2010 study of mice, low dietary riboflavin status negatively affected embryonic growth and cardiac development (Chan et al 2010), with a greater incidence of delayed embryos and lower embryonic weights ($P < 0.05$, two-factor analysis of variance). The number of embryos with ventricular septal defects was significantly greater in the riboflavin-deficient mice ($P < 0.005$, Fisher's exact test).

Similarly, in humans, a case-controlled family study of 276 mothers of children with congenital heart defects has shown that mothers consuming a diet high in saturated fat and low riboflavin and niacin during the preconception period markedly increased the risk of congenital heart defects in the offspring (Smedts et al 2008). Thus, it has been extrapolated that ensuring adequate riboflavin status during preconception and pregnancy may prevent such complications.

A prospective cohort study of 1461 pregnancies found that low-birth-weight offspring are more common in women consuming diets low in vitamin C, riboflavin, pantothenic acid and sugars, even after adjustment for deprivation index, smoking, marital status and parity (Haggarty et al 2009).

Postpartum depression (PPD)

A prospective study of 865 Japanese women investigated the role of riboflavin consumption during pregnancy with risk of PPD (Miyake et al 2006). In this study, PPD was identified when subjects had an Edinburgh Postnatal Depression Scale score of ≥9 between 2 and 9 months postpartum. A total of 121 developed PPD and the results indicated that riboflavin adequacy reduced the risk of PPD (multivariate odds ratio 0.53, 95% confidence interval 0.29–0.95, $P_{trend} = 0.55$). The authors concluded that moderate consumption of riboflavin may be protective, e.g. 10–50 mg/day.

Pre-eclampsia

In a prospective study, 154 women at increased risk of pre-eclampsia were observed until delivery (Wacker et al 2000). Riboflavin deficiency was consistently found in 33.8%. The incidence of deficiency rose towards the end of the pregnancy, from 27.3% at 29–36 weeks' gestation compared with 53.3% at over 36 weeks. In the riboflavin-deficient group, mothers were 28.8% more likely to develop pre-eclampsia than in the riboflavin-adequate group (7.8%; $P < 0.001$, odds ratio 4.7). The authors concluded that riboflavin deficiency should be considered a possible risk factor for pre-eclampsia.

However, these results were not duplicated in a randomised, placebo-controlled, double-blind trial where a protective effect was not demonstrated in high-risk pregnant women supplemented with 15 mg of riboflavin (Neugebauer et al 2006). Such variability in results may be due to differences in study design and, in this study, the supplemental dose may be inadequate given that therapeutic levels of riboflavin ranges are 10–200 mg.

Sickle cell anaemia

Riboflavin supplementation (5 mg twice daily for 8 weeks) in patients with sickle cell anaemia resulted in improved haematological measurements compared with controls, suggesting that riboflavin enhances erythropoiesis (Ajayi et al 1993).

Rheumatoid arthritis

One study has suggested that patients with higher pain scores and active disease are at significantly greater risk of riboflavin deficiency than those with inactive disease (Mulherin et al 1996). In this study of 91 patients, pain score, articular index, C-reactive protein and erythrocyte sedimentation rate were all increased in those patients exhibiting riboflavin deficiency (all $P < 0.02$). It is unclear whether riboflavin deficiency influences pain threshold or is a result of the disease.

Osteoarthritis

B vitamins were investigated for reducing sensitivity to painful stimuli in mice (Franca et al 2001), whereby thiamin and pyridoxine (50–200 mg/kg, intraperitoneally [IP]) or riboflavin (3–100 mg/kg IP) induced an antinociceptive effect, not changed by naloxone (10 mg/kg IP). The authors state the B vitamins' antinociceptive effect may involve inhibition of the synthesis and/or action of inflammatory mediators. Furthermore, in an animal study the therapeutic effects of glucosamine hydrochloride and chondroitin sulfate as chondroprotective were enhanced by the addition of fursultiamine, a thiamine derivative, in the treatment of osteoarthritis (Kobayashi et al 2005).

OTHER USES

Riboflavin is also used to treat carpal tunnel syndrome and acne, although only case reports are available (Folkers et al 1984).

HIV/AIDS

A decreased progression of HIV to AIDS has been found in patients replete with vitamins B and C (Tang et al 1993).

DOSAGE RANGE

- Migraine prevention: 400 mg/day, taken for at least 3 months.
- Treating deficiency states: 10–20 mg/day until symptoms resolve or B_2 assays improve.
- Therapeutic levels: 10–200 mg/day.
- As an adjunct to tamoxifen in breast cancer treatment: 10 mg/day together with coenzyme Q10 100 mg/day and niacin 50 mg/day — based on preliminary evidence.
- Postpartum depression: 10–50 mg/day may be protective in at risk women.

Australian recommended dietary intake

<70 years

- Women: 1.1 mg/day.
- Men: 1.3 mg/day.

>70 years

- Women: 1.3 mg/day.
- Men: 1.6 mg/day.

Intake of vitamin B_2 causes a characteristic bright yellow-orange discolouration to urine.

TOXICITY

Riboflavin is considered an extremely safe supplement. Even at the high doses (e.g. 400 mg) used in some trials, no adverse effects are noted and riboflavin remains non-toxic.

ADVERSE REACTIONS

General side effects noted in trials using high doses were reasonably uncommon, but included diarrhoea and polyuria (Bianchi et al 2004). One case of anaphylaxis has been reported (Ou et al 2001).

SIGNIFICANT INTERACTIONS

Certain medicines can increase the body's requirements for riboflavin.

Antibiotics

Antibiotic drugs can reduce endogenous production of B group vitamins — increase intake of vitamin B_2.

Oral contraceptive pill

The oral contraceptive pill may increase demand for vitamin B_2 (Pelton et al 2000) — consider increasing intake with long-term use.

Tricyclic antidepressants

Reduce the absorption of riboflavin — may increase riboflavin requirements (Pelton et al 2000).

Amitryptyline

Increases the renal excretion of riboflavin (Bianchi et al 2004) — consider increased dietary intake with long-term use.

CONTRAINDICATIONS AND PRECAUTIONS

None known.

PREGNANCY USE

Considered safe.

> ***Practice points/Patient counselling***
>
> - Vitamin B_2 deficiency signs include poor wound healing, hair loss, greasy dermatitis, ocular disturbances, failure to grow in children, angular stomatitis, cold sores, cracked lips and magenta tongue.
> - Besides inadequate intake, deficiency can also result from chronic diarrhoea, liver disease and chronic alcoholism.
> - There is some evidence suggesting that high-dose supplements (400 mg daily) significantly reduce the frequency of migraine headaches.
> - Preliminary evidence suggests that regular supplementation with a multivitamin may also reduce the risk of developing cataracts.
> - Supplementation results in a characteristic yellow-orange discolouration of urine.

PATIENTS' FAQs

What will this vitamin do for me?

Vitamin B_2 is essential for health and is involved in many different biochemical processes in the body. Research has suggested that, when taken in high doses, it can significantly reduce the incidence of migraine headaches.

When will it start to work?

Deficiency is reversed rapidly with supplementation. If using riboflavin to prevent migraine headaches, 3–4 months' treatment is required to see significant effects.

Are there any safety issues?

The vitamin is considered a safe nutrient.

REFERENCES

Ajayi OA et al. Clinical trial of riboflavin in sickle cell disease. East Afr Med J 70.7 (1993): 418–421.

Allen L H & Prentice A. Encyclopedia of Human Nutrition (Third Edition) 2013. Amsterdam: Academic Press, Elsevier p. 162.

Bajwa ZH, Sabahat A. Pathophysiology, clinical manifestations, and diagnosis of migraine in adults. UpToDate 2008. Available at www.uptodate.com.

Bareford LM et al. Intracellular processing of riboflavin in human breast cancer cells. Mol Pharm 5.5 (2008): 839–848.

Bates CJ Encyclopedia of Human Nutrition. 3rd edn, Cambridge UK, 2013, pp. 158–165.

Bianchi A et al. Role of magnesium, coenzyme q10, riboflavin, and vitamin B_{12} in migraine prophylaxis. Vitamins Hormones 69 (2004): 297–312.

Boehnke C et al. High-dose riboflavin treatment is efficacious in migraine prophylaxis: an open study in a tertiary care centre. Eur J Neurol 11.7 (2004): 475–477.

Breen C. High dose riboflavin for prophylaxis of migraine. Can Fam Physician 2003;49:1291–3.

Bruijn J, et al. Medium-dose riboflavin as a prophylactic agent in children with migraine: A preliminary placebo-controlled, randomized, double-blind, cross-over trial. Cephalalgia December 2010 vol. 30 no. 12 1426–1434.

Bunce GE et al. Nutritional factors in cataract. Annu Rev Nutr 10 (1990): 233–254.

Chen J, et al. (2005) One-carbon metabolism, MTHFR polymorphisms, and risk of breast cancer. Cancer Res 65: 1606–1614.

Cho E, et al (2007) Nutrients involved in one-carbon metabolism and risk of breast cancer among premenopausal women. Cancer Epidemiology, Biomarkers & Prevention 16: 2787–2790.
Combs G. The Vitamins: Considering the Individual Vitamins. London: Elsevier 2012 pp 277–289.
Condo M, et al. Riboflavin prophylaxis in pediatric and adolescent migraine. J Headache Pain 2009 Oct;10(5):361–5.
Das BS, et al. Riboflavin deficiency and severity of malaria. Eur J Clin Nutr. 1988 Apr;42(4):277–83.
De Vogel S et al. Dietary folate, methionine, riboflavin, and vitamin B-6 and risk of sporadic colorectal cancer. J Nutr 138.12 (2008): 2372–2378.
Ericson U, et al (2007) High folate intake is associated with lower breast cancer incidence in postmenopausal women in the Malmo Diet and Cancer cohort [see comment]. Am J Clin Nutr 86: 434–443.
Exposito JA, et al. Riboflavin (vitamin B_2) for the prevention of migraine (Protocol). Cochrane Database of Systematic Reviews 2009, Issue 3. Art. No.: CD007889.
Folkers K et al. Enzymology of the response of the carpal tunnel syndrome to riboflavin and to combined riboflavin and pyridoxine. Proc Natl Acad Sci USA 81.22 (1984): 7076–7078.
Food and Nutrition Board. Dietary reference intakes for thiamin, riboflavin, niacin, vitamin B_6, folate, vitamin B_{12}, pantothenic acid, biotin and choline. Washington DC: National Academy Press, 1998 pp 87–122.
Franca DS., et al. B vitamins induce an antinociceptive effect in the acetic acid and formaldehyde models of nociception in mice. European Journal of Pharmacology Volume 421, Issue 3, 15 June 2001, Pages 157–164.
Granados-Soto V et al. Riboflavin reduces hyperalgesia and inflammation but not tactile allodynia in the rat. Eur J Pharmacol 492.1 (2004): 35–40.
Gropper, S., Smith, J Advanced Nutrition and Human Metabolism, 6th Edition. Belmont CA: Wadsworth, Cengage Learning, 2013.
Haggarty P, et al. Diet and deprivation in pregnancy. British Journal of Nutrition (2009), 102, 1487–1497.
Head KA. Natural therapies for ocular disorders, part two: cataracts and glaucoma. Altern Med Rev 6.2 (2001): 141–166.
Horwitz J et al. Glutathione reductase in human lens epithelium: FAD-induced in vitro activation. Curr Eye Res 6.10 (1987): 1249–1256.
Jacques PF. The potential preventive effects of vitamins for cataract and age-related macular degeneration. Int J Vitam Nutr Res 69.3 (1999): 198–205.
Jacques PF et al. Long-term nutrient intake and 5-year change in nuclear lens opacities. Arch Ophthalmol 123.4 (2005): 517–526.
Karande A A, et al. Riboflavin carrier protein: A serum and tissue marker for breast carcinoma. International Journal of Cancer 2001; 95:277–281.
Keith ME, et al. B-vitamin deficiency in hospitalized patients with heart failure. J Am Diet Assoc. 2009;109(8): 1406–1410.
Kuzniarz M et al. Use of vitamin supplements and cataract: the Blue Mountains Eye Study. Am J Ophthalmol 132.1 (2001): 19–26.
Lajous M, et al (2006) Folate, vitamin B_6, and vitamin B_{12} intake and the risk of breast cancer among Mexican women. Cancer Epidemiol Biomarkers Prev 15: 443–448.
Lakshmi R et al. Skin wound healing in riboflavin deficiency. Biochem Med Metab Biol 42.3 (1989): 185–191.
Larsson SC, et al (2007) Folate and risk of breast cancer: a meta-analysis. J Natl Cancer Inst 99: 64–76.
Leske MC et al. Biochemical factors in the lens opacities: Case-control study (The Lens Opacities Case-Control Study Group). Arch Ophthalmol 113.9 (1995): 1113–11119.
Lo CS. Riboflavin status of adolescents in southern China: Average intake of riboflavin and clinical findings. Med J Aust 141.10 (1984): 635–637.
MacLennan SC, et al. High-dose riboflavin for migraine prophylaxis in children: a double-blind, randomized, placebo-controlled trial. Child Neurol November 2008 vol. 23 no. 11 1300–1304.
Magis D et al. A randomized double-blind placebo-controlled trial of thioctic acid in migraine prophylaxis. Headache 47.1 (2007): 52–57.
Maizels M et al. A combination of riboflavin, magnesium, and feverfew for migraine prophylaxis: a randomized trial. Headache 44.9 (2004): 885–890.
Manthey K, et al. Riboflavin deficiency causes protein and DNA damage in HepG2 cells, triggering arrest in G1 phase of the cell cycle. J Nutr Biochem, 2006 17:250–256.
Mares-Perlman JA et al. Diet and nuclear lens opacities. Am J Epidemiol 141.4 (1995): 322–334.
Markley HG. CoEnzyme Q10 and riboflavin: the mitochondrial connection. Headache: The Journal of Head and Face Pain 2012 52(2):81–87.
McCormick DB. A trail of research on cofactors: an odyssey with friends. J Nutr 130 (2S Suppl) (2000): 323S–330S.
McKeag NA., et al. The role of micronutrients in heart failure. Journal of the Academy of Nutrition and Dietetics, 2012; 112: 870–886.
McNulty H et al. Riboflavin lowers homocysteine in individuals homozygous for the MTHFR 677C →T polymorphism. Circulation 113.1 (2006): 74–80.
Miyake Y, et al. Dietary folate and vitamins B_{12}, B_6, and B_2 intake and the risk of postpartum depression in Japan: The Osaka Maternal and Child Health Study. Journal of affective disorders 2006:96(1–2):133–138.
Mulherin DM et al. Glutathione reductase activity, riboflavin status, and disease activity in rheumatoid arthritis. Ann Rheum Dis 55.11 (1996): 837–840.
Neugebauer J, et al. Riboflavin supplementation and pre-eclampsia. International Journal of Gynecology & Obstetrics 2006;92(2):136–7.
Ou LS et al. Anaphylaxis to riboflavin (vitamin B_2). Ann Allergy Asthma Immunol 87.5 (2001): 430–433.
Pelton R et al. Drug-induced nutrient depletion handbook 1999–2000. Hudson, OH: Lexi-Comp, 2000.
Powers HJ. Riboflavin (vitamin B_2) and health. Am J Clin Nutr 77.6 (2003): 1352–1360.

Powers HJ. Interaction among folate, riboflavin, genotype, and cancer, with reference to colorectal and cervical cancer. J Nutr 135 (12 Suppl) (2005): 2960S–6S.
Premkumar VG et al. Anti-angiogenic potential of coenzyme Q10, riboflavin and niacin in breast cancer patients undergoing tamoxifen therapy. Vascul Pharmacol 48.4–6 (2008a): 191–201.
Premkumar VG et al. Co-enzyme Q10, riboflavin and niacin supplementation on alteration of DNA repair enzyme and DNA methylation in breast cancer patients undergoing tamoxifen therapy. Br J Nutr 100.6 (2008b): 1179–82.
Rao PN, et al. Elevation of serum riboflavin carrier protein in breast cancer. Cancer Epidemiol Biomarkers Prev. 1999 Nov;8(11):985–90.
Said HM. Recent advances in carrier-mediated intestinal absorption of water-soluble vitamins. Annu Rev Physiol 66 (2004): 419–446.
Sandor PS et al. Prophylactic treatment of migraine with beta-blockers and riboflavin: differential effects on the intensity dependence of auditory evoked cortical potentials. Headache 40.1 (2000): 30–35.
Schoenen J et al. High-dose riboflavin as a prophylactic treatment of migraine: results of an open pilot study. Cephalalgia 14.5 (1994): 328–329.
Schoenen J et al. Effectiveness of high-dose riboflavin in migraine prophylaxis. A randomized controlled trial. Neurology 50.2 (1998): 466–470.
Sharp L et al. Polymorphisms in the methylenetetrahydrofolate reductase (MTHFR) gene, intakes of folate and related B vitamins and colorectal cancer: a case-control study in a population with relatively low folate intake. Br J Nutr 99.2 (2008): 379–389.
Shigemizu D, et al. (2012) Using functional signatures to identify repositioned drugs for breast, myelogenous leukemia and prostate cancer. PLoS Comput Biol 8(2): e1002347.
Shrubsole MJ, et al. Dietary B vitamin and methionine intakes and breast cancer risk among Chinese women.Am J Epidemiol. 2011 May 15;173(10):1171–82.
Smedts HP, et al. Maternal intake of fat, riboflavin and nicotinamide and the risk of having offspring with congenital heart defects. Eur J Nutr 2008;47(7):357–365.
Stevens VL, et al (2010) Folate and other one-carbon metabolism-related nutrients and risk of postmenopausal breast cancer in the Cancer Prevention Study II Nutrition Cohort. Am J Clin Nutr 91: 1708–1715.
Straatsma BR et al. Lens capsule and epithelium in age-related cataract. Am J Ophthalmol 112.3 (1991): 283–296.
Tang AM., et al. Dietary micronutrient intake and risk of progression to acquired immunodeficiency syndrome (AIDS) in human immunodeficiency virus type-1 (HIV-1) infected homosexual men. Am J Epidemiol 1993;138:937–51.
Wacker J et al. Riboflavin deficiency and preeclampsia. Obstet Gynecol 96.1 (2000): 38–44.
Wahlqvist M (ed) Food and nutrition. Sydney: Allen & Unwin, 2002.
Webster, R. P., et al. (1973). Modulation of carcinogen-induced DNA damage and repair enzyme activity by dietary riboflavin. Cancer Res. 33, 1997.
Woolhouse M. Migraine and tension headaches: a complementary and alternative medicine approach. Australian Family Physician 2005;34:647–51.
Wynn M, Wynn A. Can improved diet contribute to the prevention of cataract? Nutr Health 11.2 (1996): 87–104.
Yang D, et al. Dietary intake of folate, B-vitamins and methionine and breast cancer risk among Hispanic and non-Hispanic white women. 2013 PLoS ONE 8(2): e54495.
Yuvaraj S et al. Ameliorating effect of coenzyme Q10, riboflavin and niacin in tamoxifen-treated postmenopausal breast cancer patients with special reference to lipids and lipoproteins. Clin Biochem 40.9–10 (2007): 623–628.
Yuvaraj S et al. Augmented antioxidant status in tamoxifen treated postmenopausal women with breast cancer on co-administration with coenzyme Q10, niacin and riboflavin. Cancer Chemother Pharmacol May 61.6 (2008): 933–941.

Vitamin B_5 — pantothenic acid

BACKGROUND AND RELEVANT PHARMACOKINETICS

The Greek word *pantos* means ‘everywhere’. As the name pantothenic acid implies, B_5 is widely distributed, present in nearly all plant and animal foods. Relatively unstable, it is sensitive to heat, freezing, canning and cooking and both acid and alkali, and considerable amounts are lost through the milling of cereal grains. The intestine is exposed to two sources of pantothenic acid: dietary and bacterial. Current research suggests that bacterial synthesis may be more dominant and important in ruminant species (Bates 1998).

Pantothenic acid is absorbed in the jejunum by passive diffusion at high concentrations, but at low concentrations it requires a sodium-dependent multivitamin transporter. Both biotin and lipoic acid share the multivitamin transporter. A study of placental tissue demonstrated that biotin uses the same transport mechanisms as pantothenic acid, which may indicate competition between these two nutrients in other tissues (Bates 1998).

Between 40% and 63% of pantothenic acid is bioavailable from the gastrointestinal tract, an amount that decreases to 10% when doses 10-fold greater than the recommended daily intake are taken (Gropper & Smith 2013). Rapid absorption seems to occur after oral doses, and increased tissue levels of coenzyme A (CoA) and other metabolites can occur within 6 hours. In leucocytes both CoA and pantothenic acid levels increase between 6 and 24 hours following oral ingestion (Kelly 2011).

In circulation, pantothenic acid is primarily found intracellularly in the red blood cells with a small amount in plasma. Organ uptake is via the same sodium-dependent multivitamin transporter and it is found as pantothenic acid, 4-phosphopantothenic acid and pantetheine in cells (Gropper & Smith 2013). The organ with the highest concentration of pantothenic acid is the liver, followed by the adrenal cortex, which reflects the large requirements of these tissues and is indicative of the biochemical role of the vitamin's coenzyme derivatives. There are contrasting opinions about whether a genuine storage capacity exists for this vitamin; however, if there is any at all, the consensus is that pantothenic acid is 'stored' in very limited amounts and in those tissues with the greatest requirements (Groff & Gropper 2009). Most pantothenic acid is used to synthesise or resynthesise CoA, which is found in high concentrations in the liver, adrenal gland, kidneys, brain and heart (Gropper & Smith 2013).

Following its absorption into cells, it can be converted to CoA or acyl carrier proteins (ACP), both of which are essential cofactors in fatty acid synthesis (Kelly 2011).

CHEMICAL COMPONENTS

Pantothenic acid is an amide and consists of β-alanine and pantoic acid joined by a peptide bond. In supplements, it is often found as calcium pantothenate.

FOOD SOURCES

The most concentrated sources are meats (especially liver), egg yolk, broad beans, legumes and potatoes, but it is also found in many other foods, such as whole grains, milk, peanuts, broccoli, avocado, mushroom and apricots. Royal jelly from bees also provides substantial amounts (Gropper & Smith 2013). Up to 50% can be lost through cooking (Wahlqvist 2002).

Approximately 85% occurs in food as a component of CoA, which is hydrolysed to pantothenic acid or pantethine during digestion.

DEFICIENCY SIGNS AND SYMPTOMS

Due to its widespread occurrence of pantothenate in foods, deficiencies are considered unlikely, and more often in conjunction with multiple nutrient deficiencies, as would occur in generalised malnutrition (Gropper & Smith 2013). Because pantothenic acid deficiency is so rare, most information regarding its signs and symptoms comes from experimental research in animals or cases of severe malnutrition. The deficiency picture appears to be generalised and species-specific (Bates 1998). Preliminary studies in humans using competitive analogues of pantothenic acid have produced the following symptoms:

- 'Burning feet syndrome': this affects the lower legs and is characterised by a sensation of heat (Gropper & Smith 2013, Kohlmeier 2003, Whitney 2011)

- Vomiting, fatigue, weakness, restlessness, dizziness, sleeplessness and irritability (Gropper & Smith 2013; Kohlmeier 2003)
- Neurological disturbances (Whitney et al 2011)
- Gastrointestinal disturbances, ulcers, abdominal distress (Hechtman 2012, Whitney et al 2011)
- Muscular weakness, burning cramps, paraesthesia (tingling sensation of toes and feet) (Hechtman 2012, Kohlmeier 2003)
- Loss of immune (antibody) function and increased susceptibility to infections (Kohlmeier 2003)
- Dermatitis, achromotrichia, alopecia (The Vitamins 2012)
- Adrenal hypofunction, with an inability to respond appropriately to stress. In late-stage deficiency, the adrenals atrophy and morphological damage occurs (Kelly 2011)
- Insensitivity to adrenocorticotrophic hormone
- Increased sensitivity to insulin.

Some conditions that have been associated with increased requirements are:

- Alcoholism (due to typically low intakes of vitamin B complex) (Gropper & Smith 2013)
- Diabetes mellitus (as a result of increased excretion) (Gropper & Smith 2013)
- Inflammatory bowel diseases (due to decreased vitamin absorption) (Gropper & Smith 2013).

MAIN ACTIONS

Pantothenic acid is involved in a myriad of important chemical reactions in the body as a result of its involvement in CoA and ACP.

Coenzyme function

CoA and the Krebs cycle

Numerous metabolic activities depend on adequate availability of pantothenate. Pantothenic acid is required for CoA synthesis and most pantothenate-dependent reactions use CoA as the universal donor and acceptor of acetyl and acyl groups (Kohlmeier 2003).

As part of CoA, pantothenate participates extensively in the metabolism of carbohydrate, lipids and protein (Gropper & Smith 2013). It plays a pivotal role in cellular respiration, the oxidation of fatty acids and acetylation of other molecules, so as to enable transportation. Together with thiamine, riboflavin and niacin, it is involved in the oxidative decarboxylation of pyruvate and alpha-ketoglutarate in the Krebs cycle and ultimately is important for energy storage and release (Gropper & Smith 2013).

Acyl carrier protein

Pantothenic acid functions in the body as a component of the acylation factors, CoA and 4'-phosphopantetheine (the prosthetic group for ACP) (Gropper & Smith 2013, Kohlmeier 2003). A few reactions use 4'-phosphopantetheine; most of these are related to lipid synthesis (Kohlmeier 2003).

Indirect antioxidant effects

New in vitro research supports an indirect antioxidant role for pantothenic acid through its ability to increase cellular adenosine triphosphate, which in turn creates increased levels of free glutathione and enhanced protection of cells against peroxidative damage (Slyshenkov et al 2004).

ADRENAL CORTEX FUNCTION AND NEUROTRANSMITTER SYNTHESIS

Pantothenic acid is essential in controlling stress and the ability to cope with stressful events, due to its involvement in the synthesis of the neurotransmitter acetylcholine. It plays an important role in adrenal function and, as CoA, is needed for proper adrenal cortex function and the synthesis of steroid hormones, namely cortisone. A consistent finding in animal studies conducted in the 1950s is that a deficiency of pantothenic acid initially causes adrenal hypertrophy, followed by progressive morphological and functional changes to the adrenal gland, resulting in adrenal hypofunction and an impaired stress response (Hurley & Morgan 1952, Kelly 2011).

Other functions

Pantothenate is required in the production of many secondary metabolites such as polyisoprenoid-containing compounds (e.g. ubiquinone, squalene and cholesterol), steroid hormones, vitamin D and bile acids, acetylated compounds such as *N*-acetylglucosamine, *N*-acetylserotonin, acetylcholine, and prostaglandins and prostaglandin-like compounds (Kelly 2011).

Pantothenic acid, thiamine, riboflavin and niacin participate in the oxidative decarboxylation of alpha-ketoglutarate to succinyl-CoA, an intermediate used with glycine to synthesise haem (Gropper & Smith 2013).

Lipid lowering

Pantethine, a metabolite of pantothenic acid, has been investigated in several clinical studies and found to exert significant lipid-lowering activity (Coronel et al 1991, Donati et al 1986, Gaddi et al 1984), with a 2005 study producing a 50% inhibition of fatty acid synthesis and an 80% inhibition of cholesterol synthesis (McRae 2005).

The mechanism of action relates to reduced insulin resistance and activation of lipolysis in serum and adipose tissue, according to in vivo research (Naruta & Buko 2001). Additionally, inhibition of HMG-CoA reductase, as well as more distal enzymes in the cholesterol synthetic pathway, is likely to be responsible (McCarty 2001).

As part of CoA, pantothenic acid is essential for the formation of acetyl CoA, an important substrate in the catabolism of fatty acids. Fat accumulation has been shown to increase with pantothenic acid deficiency, and refeeding pantothenic acid to rats originally fed a pantothenic acid-deficient diet decreased tissue fat (Shibata et al 2013).

Wound healing

Both oral and topical administration has been shown to accelerate closure of wounds and increase strength of scar tissue in vivo (Plesofsky 2002, Vaxman et al 1990). Both in vitro and in vivo studies reveal that topical dexpanthenol, the stable alcoholic analogue of pantothenic acid, induces activation of fibroblast proliferation, which contributes to accelerated re-epithelialisation in wound healing (Ebner et al 2002).

V

CLINICAL USE

Although pantothenic acid has been investigated in some studies, most investigation has occurred with several of its derivatives, chiefly an alcoholic analogue of pantothenic acid called dexpanthenol (Bepanthen; see below) and pantethine.

Deficiency states: prevention and treatment

Due to the widespread occurrence of pantothenate in foods, deficiencies are considered unlikely, and more often in conjunction with multiple nutrient deficiencies, as would occur in generalised malnutrition (Gropper & Smith 2013). Traditionally, pantothenic acid is recommended, together with other vitamin B complex nutrients, to treat generalised malnutrition or prevent deficiency in conditions such as alcoholism, diabetes mellitus and malabsorption syndromes (Gropper & Smith 2013). The interference from some prescription drugs (antimetabolites) may also interfere with pantothenate absorption and lead to deficiencies (Kohlmeier 2003).

Enhances wound healing

Pantothenic acid has been both used as an oral supplement and applied topically in a cream base to enhance wound healing; it has been shown to accelerate closure of wounds and increase strength of scar tissue in experimental animals (Plesofsky 2002, Vaxman et al 1990). Furthermore, fibroblast content of scar tissue has been shown to significantly increase following injections of pantothenate (20 mg/kg of body weight/24 hours) for 3 weeks (Aprahamian et al 1985). Skin dehydration and irritation have been found to be reduced with the use of dexapanthenol, a pantothente derivative (Biro et al 2003).

Although these results are encouraging, there has been little investigation in humans. One double-blind randomised controlled trial testing the effects of vitamin C (1000 mg) and pantothenic acid (200 mg) supplements over a 21-day period showed increased fibroblast proliferation but no significant alteration to wound healing during recovery from surgical tattoo removal (Vaxman et al 1995).

Topical use

In a randomised, double-blind trial in Mumbai, 207 women 30–60 years of age with epidermal hyperpigmentation were recruited and randomly assigned to apply a test or control facial lotion containing 4% niacinamide, 0.5% panthenol and 0.5% tocopheryl acetate to the face daily for 10 weeks (Jerajani et al 2010). Women who used the test lotion reportedly experienced significantly reduced hyperpigmentation, improved skin tone evenness, appearance of lightening of skin and positive effects on skin texture from as early as 6 weeks. Some evidence of a beneficial effect on barrier function was also observed. The authors state that these results concur with previous positive findings for topical niacinamide (Bissett 2002, Bissett et al 2005, Draelos et al 2005, Hakozaki et al 2002, Matts et al 2002) and panthenol (Biro et al 2003, Ebner et al 2002).

Bepanthen is a well-known dermatological preparation containing dexpanthenol, an alcoholic analogue of pantothenic acid. It has been investigated in numerous studies and found to act like a moisturiser, activate fibroblast proliferation, accelerate re-epithelialisation in wound healing, have anti-inflammatory activity against ultraviolet-induced erythema and reduce itch (Ebner et al 2002). Under double-blind study conditions, epidermal wounds treated with dexpanthenol emulsion showed a reduction in erythema, and more elastic and solid tissue regeneration. Another randomised, prospective, double-blind, placebo-controlled study published in 2003 investigated the efficacy of topical dexpanthenol as a protectant against skin irritation. The study involved 25 healthy volunteers who were treated with a topical preparation containing 5% dexpanthenol or a placebo and then exposed to sodium lauryl sulfate 2% twice daily over 26 days. Treatment with topical dexpanthenol provided protection against skin irritation, whereas a statistically significant deterioration was observed in the placebo group (Biro et al 2003).

Although Bepanthen is commonly used in radiotherapy departments to ameliorate acute radiotherapy skin reactions, a prospective study of 86 patients undergoing radiotherapy showed that topical use of Bepanthen did not improve skin reactions under these conditions (Lokkevik et al 1996). In an animal study by Dorr et al (2005), negative results were similarly obtained and it is not currently recommended for individuals undergoing radiotherapy.

Acne vulgaris

One hundred Chinese patients diagnosed with acne vulgaris (45 males and 55 females) were given oral pantothenic acid, 10 g a day in four divided doses, and a cream consisting of 20% by weight of pantothenic acid to apply to the affected areas four to six times a day. Within 1–2 days sebum production was noticeably reduced, frequency of new acne eruptions began to decline and existing lesions started to regress within 1–2 weeks. Patients who were categorised as suffering moderate-severity acne reported complete control of acne after 8 weeks with only occasional new eruptions, while in more severe cases complete control occurred after 6 months (Leung 1995b). The author notes that daily doses of 15–20 g/day of pantothenic acid did produce faster results in severe cases and a maintenance dose was 1–5 g/day of pantothenic acid.

Interestingly, it has been shown that dexpanthenol cream can help treat some mucocutaneous adverse reactions caused by isotretinoin, a chemotherapeutic drug used to treat acne (Romiti & Romiti 2002, as cited by Kelly 2011).

Nasal spray

A randomised controlled trial of 48 outpatients diagnosed with rhinitis sicca anterior found that dexpanthenol nasal spray is an effective symptomatic treatment for this condition (Kehrl & Sonnemann 1998). Two years later, another randomised controlled trial compared the effects of xylometazoline-dexpanthenol nasal spray versus xylometazoline nasal spray over a 2-week period in 61 patients with rhinitis after nasal surgery (Kehrl & Sonnemann 2000); it showed that the combination of xylometazoline-dexpanthenol nasal spray was significantly superior to the other treatment and well tolerated.

More recent studies support this emerging trend and point towards a reduction in ciliary and cytotoxic effects from nasal decongestants when 5% dexpanthenol is concurrently administered (Klocker et al 2003).

Elevated cholesterol and triglyceride levels

Several clinical studies confirm that pantethine, a metabolite of pantothenic acid, exerts significant lipid-lowering activity (Coronel et al 1991, Donati et al 1986, Gaddi et al 1984).

One double-blind study of 29 patients found that 300 mg of pantethine taken three times daily resulted in significant reductions to plasma total cholesterol, low-density lipoprotein (LDL) cholesterol and triglycerides, and an increase in high-density lipoprotein (HDL) cholesterol levels (Gaddi et al 1984).

A 2005 review analysed results from 28 clinical trials encompassing a pooled population of 646 hyperlipidaemic patients who were supplemented with a mean dose of 900 mg pantethine over an average trial length of 12.7 weeks (McRae 2005). The results of these studies suggest a response to pantethine that is time-dependent, with progressively greater reductions in LDL cholesterol and triacylglycerols between month 1 and 9. The most impressive results were observed at 9 months, with a reduction of total cholesterol by 20.5%, LDL cholesterol by 27.6% and triacylglycerols by 36.5% from baseline. Although minor increases were observed in HDL levels in the early stages of most trials, longer-term studies suggested that this is not sustained.

Of the trials studied, 22 were conducted in Italy and all were conducted between 1981 and 1991. The authors point out that no further clinical trials were published, and concluded that evidence to date has yielded positive and promising results, and further research is warranted.

Obesity and weight loss

An investigation of vitamin B_5 for weight loss was conducted with 100 Chinese volunteers (40 male) aged 15–55 years, following a strict calorie-controlled diet and supplemented with 2.5 g of pantothenic acid four times a day. The average weight loss was found to be 1.2 kg per week. Ketone bodies in urine were monitored regularly and were found to be absent in most circumstances and therefore did not explain the weight loss. While feelings of neither hunger nor weakness were reported, a sense of wellbeing was observed. To maintain the weight loss, the subjects required 1–3 g/day along with continual strict dietary advice. The author attributes the success to the role of CoA in carbohydrate, fat and protein metabolism, and its key role in the biosynthesis of many lipids and steroids (Leung 1995a). However, in the absence of a control group, the weight loss that occurred could be attributed to the calorie-controlled diet rather than the inclusion of pantothenic acid.

IN COMBINATION

Similarly, a double-blind, randomised, parallel-group, placebo-controlled study carried out on a product containing *Garcinia cambogia* extract with calcium pantothenate (standardised for the content of hydroxycitric acid and pantothenic acid) and extracts of *Matricaria chamomilla, Rosa damascena, Lavandula officinalis* and *Cananga odorata*, on body weight in overweight and obese volunteers during a 60-day treatment period found that the average reduction in body weight for the treatment group ($n = 30$) was 4.67% compared with 0.63% for placebo ($n = 28$; $P < 0.0001$). Weight losses of ≥3 kg were recorded for 23 subjects in the treatment group and only one in the placebo group (Toromanyan et al 2007).

Clinical note — Could pantothenic acid be an antiageing nutrient?

A contemporary theory of ageing implicates mitochondrial functional decline, or 'oxidative decay' of the mitochondria, as a major contributor. In light of this hypothesis, nutrients that possess a critical role in the mitochondria are being re-examined to determine their ability to prevent ageing in humans. The focus has been on pantothenic acid, biotin, lipoic acid, iron and zinc, because deficiencies of these micronutrients have been implicated in increased mitochondrial oxidation (Ames et al 2005, Atamna 2004). In addition, those with antioxidant capabilities are of particular interest, such as pantothenic acid, lipoic acid and zinc.

Because of the numerous nutrients implicated in mitochondrial health and disease, a broad-based multivitamin should be considered instead of a single-nutrient supplement for populations at increased risk of poor nutrition, such as the elderly, young, poor and obese (Ames et al 2005).

Life extension in animals supplemented with B_5 has been shown in several older studies (Gardner 1948a, 1948b, Pelton & Williams 1958). The first of these studies investigated the chemical components of royal jelly, a well-recognised antiageing supplement. Using *Drosophila melanogaster* (common fruit fly) as the testing medium, it was found that pantothenic acid was the primary antiageing factor (Gardner 1948a). In a follow-up study, the combination of biotin, pyridoxine and sodium yeast nucleate was shown to lengthen lifespan in *D. melanogaster,* and was further extended with pantothenic acid (Gardner 1948b). Furthermore, the mean lifespan for mice given 300 mcg/day supplementary calcium pantothenate was 653.1 days and that for the control mice was 549.8 days. The statistical difference between the two groups is $P = 0.05$ (t-test), 0.01 (U-test).

Clinical note — Could vitamin B_5 prevent neural tube defects?

Ongoing evidence from animal studies suggests that pantothenic acid may have a preventive role against neural tube defects independently of folic acid (Dawson et al 2006). Pharmaceuticals such as valproic acid that increase the risk of neural tube defect offspring have been shown also to reduce hepatic concentrations of CoA, an effect attenuated by coadministration of pantothenic acid. While the role of B_5 in neural tube closure remains unknown, it appears that it exerts actions both overlapping with and independent of folate.

OTHER USES

Pantothenic acid has been used for many other indications, but controlled studies to determine whether treatment is effective are lacking.

Stress

As vitamin B_5 is essential for adrenal cortex function and the synthesis of steroid hormones, it is often used together with other B vitamins during times of stress in order to improve the body's response and restore nutrient levels. In continual deficiency, a progressive morphological and functional degradation of the adrenal glands may occur, resulting in adrenal hypofunction, and an inability to respond to stress appropriately (Hurley & Morgan 1952, Kelly 2011, Melampy et al 1951). If pantothenic acid is supplied early enough after deficiency has been induced (i.e. before adrenal exhaustion occurs), the response to stress can be improved (Kelly 2011).

Interestingly, a large number of experiments from the 1950s (Dumm & Ralli 1953, Dumm et al 1955, Ershoff 1953, Hurley & Morgan 1952, Melampy et al 1951, Ralli & Dumm 1953) attempted to elicit the impact of pantothenic acid deficiency on adrenal function and stress response in animals; however, little research has been done since. One study in 2008 demonstrated that pantothenic acid enhanced the basal levels of corticosterone (and progesterone) in adrenal cells of male rats that had pantothenic acid (0.03%) added to their drinking water for 9 weeks. Increased sensitivity to stimulation with adrenocorticotrophic hormone and a slight non-significant increase in adrenal gland weight in the pantothenic acid group were also observed (Jaroenporn et al 2008).

Ulcerative colitis (UC)

In a pilot study of 3 patients, it was hypothesised that topically administered dexpanthenol may be beneficial in increasing tissue levels of CoA, improving fatty acid oxidation and ameliorating UC (Loftus et al 1997). It was proposed that a possible cause of UC is a block in the conversion of pantothenic acid to CoA, which reduces colonic CoA activity levels, inhibits short-chain fatty acid oxidation and contributes to distal UC. The patients received 4 weeks of dexpanthenol (1000 mg) enemas and the authors concluded that, despite increases in urinary pantothenic acid output, the treatment was ineffective (Loftus et al 1997). With such a minute sample size in this pilot study, further research is required to more appropriately ascertain its effectiveness. Interestingly, conditions of ulcers and colitis negatively impact the status and excretion rates of pantothenate (Bates 2013).

Coeliac disease

In 1972, a letter to the editor of the *British Medical Journal* suggested the use of pantothenic acid in patients with coeliac disease who respond only partially to a gluten-free diet as they may benefit from the administration of pantothenic acid (Monro 1972). Coeliac disease is a permanent enteropathy of the small bowel and may be characterised by ulceration and stricture formation, leading to narrowing and scarring. The author explains that pantothenic acid deficiency can produce atrophy of the small intestinal mucosa in animal species; in many species ulceration of the gastric and intestinal mucosa can occur, and this destruction may occur despite the sufferer consuming a gluten-free diet. Furthermore, Monro explains that 'pseudohypoadrenalism' and carbohydrate metabolism derangement with glucose intolerance are common features of both coeliac disease and pantothenic acid deficiency, suggesting a potential role in the management of these symptoms with pantothenic acid administration (Monro 1972).

Lupus erythematosus

The evidence for the use of pantothenic acid in persons with lupus erythematosus dates back to the 1950s. Kelly (2011) cites a study (Welsh 1954) that showed efficacy in lupus treatment using pantothenic acid (10–15 g/day) with 1500–3000 IU/day of vitamin E for 19 months.

One study administered doses of 10 g/day pantothenic acid, 2 g of vitamin C, 500 mg of B_1, 200 mg of B_6, 2 mg of B_{12} and two tablets of Super B and two tablets of multivitamins with minerals per day to females with systemic lupus erythematosus. After 4 weeks of treatment, there were varying degrees of improvement, particularly in fatigue. Later follow-up showed that the incidence of fever was decreased and no major flares were noted. In many cases, the original systemic lupus erythematosus medications could gradually be reduced (Leung 2004). More research needs to be conducted.

Ergogenic aid and athletic performance

Based on its role in carbohydrate metabolism as CoA, vitamin B_5 has been used to increase stamina and athletic performance.

Whether pantothenic acid supplementation improves overall exercise performance remains unclear. One study showed that blood lactate levels and oxygen consumption were decreased in endurance runners during prolonged exercise at 75% maximal oxygen uptake (VO_{2max}) (Litoff et al 1985). However, the time for highly trained distance runners to reach the point of exhaustion when taking 1 g/day of pantothenic acid for 2 weeks did not increase (Nice et al 1984).

In a randomised, double-blind, counterbalanced design study, cyclists ingesting either a placebo or a combination of 1 g of allithiamin (vitamin B_1 derivative) and 1.8 g of a 55%/45% pantethine/pantothenic acid compound for 7 days did not demonstrate any improvements in exercise metabolism or performance when completing a 2000-metre time trial (Webster 1998). Similarly, 1.5 g/day pantothenic acid and cysteine supplementation did not increase resting muscle CoA content, fuel selection or exercise performance in 8 males who cycled at 75% VO_{2max} until exhaustion (Wall et al 2012).

Reducing drug toxicity

Preliminary research in animal models shows that pantothenic acid reduces the toxicity effects of kanamycin and carbon tetrachloride and, when combined with carnitine, protects against valproate toxicity (Moiseenok et al 1984, Nagiel-Ostaszewski & Lau-Cam 1990, Thurston & Hauhart 1992).

Female alopecia — ineffective

According to a study of 46 women with symptoms of diffuse alopecia, calcium pantothenate (200 mg/day) over 4–5 months does not cause a significant improvement in this condition (Brzezinska-Wcislo 2001).

Testicular endocrinology, sperm motility and male fertility

In one study, the physiological roles of pantothenic acid on testicular endocrinology and sperm motility were investigated in 3-week-old male rats that were fed a B_5-free diet or a 0.0016% pantothenic acid diet (control) for 7 weeks. In the B_5-deficient group, sperm motility was significantly reduced, plasma concentrations of testosterone and corticosterone were significantly lower and testicular weight was significantly higher (Yamamoto et al 2009).

Female fertility

A prospective cohort study of 1461 pregnancies found that low-birth-weight offspring were more common in women consuming diets low in vitamin C, riboflavin, pantothenic acid and sugars, even after adjustment for deprivation index, smoking, marital status and parity (Haggarty et al 2009).

DOSAGE RANGE

Australian adequate intake

- Women: 4 mg/day (NHMRC nutrient reference values 2007).
- Men: 6 mg/day (NHMRC nutrient reference values 2007).
- Adults: 5 mg/day (Gropper & Smith 2013).
- Pregnancy: 5 mg/day (NHMRC nutrient reference values 2007) or 6 mg/day (Gropper & Smith 2013).
- Lactation: 6 mg/day (NHMRC nutrient reference values 2007) or 7 mg/day (Gropper & Smith 2013).
- Therapeutic dose: 20–500 mg/day.

According to clinical studies

- Wound healing: dexpanthenol cream 5% applied to affected areas up to two times daily (Biro et al 2003).
- Acne vulgaris: 15–20 g/day of pantothenic acid for 6 months for severe acne (Leung 1995b).
- Acne vulgaris: 1–5 g/day of pantothenic (Leung 1995b) acid maintenance dose.
- Lipid lowering: pantethine 300 mg three times daily (McRae 2005).

TOXICITY

No toxicity level known.

ADVERSE REACTIONS

Pantothenic acid is well tolerated, but contact dermatitis has been reported with topical dexpanthenol.

SIGNIFICANT INTERACTIONS

Antibiotics

Under in vitro conditions, experimental work from the 1950s suggests that pantothenic acid may interfere with the ability of some antibiotics (aureomycin, erythromycin and streptomycin) to inhibit the growth of certain microorganisms.

It has been speculated that these antibiotics might reduce endogenous production of vitamin B_5 by gastrointestinal flora or its downstream coenzymes (CoA or ACP); supplying pantothenic acid overcomes this enzyme inhibition (Watanabe et al 2010, as cited by Kelly 2011).

Oral contraceptive pill

Taking the oral contraceptive pill may increase the requirement for pantothenic acid. Increase vitamin B_5-rich foods or consider supplementation (Plesofsky 2002).

Isotretinoin

A single study reports that a 5% dexpanthenol cream can help treat mucocutaneous adverse reactions caused by using isotretinoin for acne (Romiti & Romiti 2002).

Acetylcholinesterase inhibitor drugs

A theoretical concern exists that pantothenic acid, since it is involved in the biosynthesis of acetylcholine, might increase the effects of acetylcholinesterase inhibitor drugs (Kelly 2011).

CONTRAINDICATIONS AND PRECAUTIONS

None known.

PREGNANCY USE

Considered safe when ingested at usual dietary doses.

PATIENTS' FAQs

What will this vitamin do for me?

Vitamin B_5 is essential for health and is used for many different conditions; for example, it is often used as part of a vitamin B complex supplement to aid the body during times of stress. In many of its uses research is not available to determine whether it is effective. Research generally supports its use in wound healing and in the form of pantethine to reduce cholesterol levels.

When will it start to work?

Pantethine reduces cholesterol levels within 2 months; however, optimal results are achieved with 9 months of supplementation. Xylometazoline-dexpanthenol nasal spray reduces symptoms of rhinitis within 2 weeks. It is not known how quickly the vitamin starts to work in most other conditions.

Are there any safety issues?

Pantothenic acid and pantethine are considered safe substances and are generally well tolerated.

Practice points/Patient counselling

- Deficiency is extremely rare, as pantothenic acid is widely distributed and present in nearly all plant and animal foods. Those at risk of reduced vitamin status are alcoholics, diabetics and people with malabsorption syndromes.
- Pantethine reduces total cholesterol levels significantly, according to controlled studies in both healthy and diabetic people.
- Dexpanthenol cream acts like a moisturiser, activates fibroblast proliferation, accelerates re-epithelialisation in wound healing, has anti-inflammatory activity against ultraviolet-induced erythema and reduces itch. When used in a nasal spray, it reduces symptoms of rhinitis.
- Vitamin B_5 supplements are commonly used together with other B vitamins during times of stress in order to improve the body's response and restore nutrient levels.
- Vitamin B_5 has also been used as adjunctive treatment for inflammatory conditions, such as dermatitis and asthma, as an ergogenic aid, to treat alopecia and to restore colour to greying hair, although no controlled studies are available to determine effectiveness in these conditions.

REFERENCES

Ames BN et al. Mineral and vitamin deficiencies can accelerate the mitochondrial decay of aging. Mol Aspects Med 26.4–5 (2005): 363–378.

Aprahamian M, et al. Effects of supplemental pantothenic acid on wound healing: experimental study in rabbit. Am J Clin Nutr 1985;41(3):578–89.

Atamna H. Heme, iron, and the mitochondrial decay of ageing. Age Res Rev 3.3 (2004): 303–318.

Bates CJ. Pantothenic acid. In: Physiology, dietary sources and requirements, Encyclopedia of human nutrition. St Louis: Elsevier, 1998, pp 1511–1515.

Bates CJ. Pantothenic acid. Encyclopedia of human nutrition. Elsevier, 2013 pp1–5.

Biro K et al. Efficacy of dexpanthenol in skin protection against irritation: a double-blind, placebo-controlled study. Contact Dermatitis 49.2 (2003): 80–84.

Bissett D. Topical niacinamide and barrier enhancement. Cutis 2002;70:8–12.

Bissett DL, et al. Niacinamide: A B vitamin that improves aging facial skin appearance. Dermatol Surg 2005;31:860–5.

Brzezinska-Wcislo L. Evaluation of vitamin B6 and calcium pantothenate effectiveness on hair growth from clinical and trichographic aspects for treatment of diffuse alopecia in women. Wiad Lek 54.1–2 (2001): 11–118.

Coronel F et al. Treatment of hyperlipemia in diabetic patients on dialysis with a physiological substance. Am J Nephrol 11.1 (1991): 32–36.

Dawson JE, et al. Folic acid and pantothenic acid protection against valproic acid-induced neural tube defects in CD-1 mice. Toxicol & App Pharmacol 211 (2006): 124–132.

Donati C et al. Pantethine improves the lipid abnormalities of chronic hemodialysis patients: results of a multicenter clinical trial. Clin Nephrol 25.2 (1986): 70–74.

Dorr W et al. Effects of dexpanthenol with or without Aloe vera extract on radiation-induced oral mucositis: preclinical studies. Int J Radiat Biol 81.3 (2005): 43–50.

Dumm ME, Ralli EP. Factors influencing the response of adrenalectomized rats to stress. Metabolism 1953;2:153–164.

Dumm ME, et al. Factors influencing adrenal weight and adrenal cholesterol in rats following stress. J Nutr 1955;56:517–531.

Draelos ZD, et al. Niacinamide-containing facial moisturizer improves skin barrier and benefits subjects with rosacea. Cutis 2005;76:135–41.

Ebner F et al. Topical use of dexpanthenol in skin disorders. Am J Clin Dermatol 3.6 (2002): 427–433.

Ershoff BF. Comparative effects of pantothenic acid deficiency and inanition on resistance to cold stress in the rat. J Nutr 1953;49:373–385.

Gaddi A et al. Controlled evaluation of pantethine, a natural hypolipidemic compound, in patients with different forms of hyperlipoproteinemia. Atherosclerosis 50.1 (1984): 73–83.

Gardner TS. The use of *Drosophila melanogaster* as a screening agent for longevity factors; pantothenic acid as a longevity factor in royal jelly. J Gerontol 1948a;3:1–8.

Gardner TS. The use of *Drosophila melanogaster* as a screening agent for longevity factors; the effects of biotin, pyridoxine, sodium yeast nucleate, and pantothenic acid on the life span of the fruit fly. J Gerontol 1948b;3:9–13.

Groff JL, Gropper SS. Advanced nutrition and human metabolism, 3rd edn. Belmont, CA: Wadsworth, 2009.

Gropper, S., Smith, J Advanced nutrition and human metabolism, 6th edition. Belmont CA: Wadsworth, Cengage Learning, 2013.

Haggarty P, et al. Diet and deprivation in pregnancy. British Journal of Nutrition (2009), 102, 1487–1497.

Hakozaki T, et al. The effect of niacinamide on reducing cutaneous pigmentation and suppression of melanosome transfer. Br J Dermatol 2002;147:20–31.

Hechtman, L. Clinical Naturopathic Medicine. Revised Edition. Churchill Livingstone, Elsevier, 2012.
Hurley LS, Morgan AF. Carbohydrate metabolism and adrenal cortical function in the pantothenic acid-defi- cient rat. J Biol Chem 1952;195:583–590.
Jaroenporn S, et al. Effects of pantothenic acid supplementation on adrenal steroid secretion from male rats. Biol Pharm Bull 2008;31:1205–1208.
Jerajani HR,et al. The effects of a daily facial lotion containing vitamins B3 and E and provitamin B5 on the facial skin of Indian women: A randomized, double-blind trial. Indian Journal of Dermatology, Venereolgy and Leprology 2010;76(1):20–26.
Kehrl W, Sonnemann U. Dexpanthenol nasal spray as an effective therapeutic principle for treatment of rhinitis sicca anterior. Laryngorhinootologie 77.9 (1998): 506–512.
Kehrl W, Sonnemann U. Improving wound healing after nose surgery by combined administration of xylometazoline and dexpanthenol. Laryngorhinootologie 79.3 (2000): 151–154.
Kelly, G S. Pantothenic acid. Alternative Medicine Review 2011;16(3):263–274.
Klocker N et al. The protective effect of dexpanthenol in nasal sprays. First results of cytotoxic and ciliary-toxic studies in vitro. Laryngorhinootologie 82.3 (2003): 177–182.
Kohlmeier, M. Nutrient Metabolism. Food science and technology. International series. London: Elsevier 2003.
Leung LH. Pantothenic acid as a weight-reducing agent: fasting without hunger, weakness and ketosis. Med Hypotheses 1995a;44:403–405.
Leung LH. Pantothenic acid deficiency as the pathogenesis of acne vulgaris, Med Hypotheses 1995b;44:490–492.
Leung LH. Systemic lupus erythematosus: a combined deficiency disease. Medical Hypotheses 62 (6) 2004, 922–924.
Litoff D, et al. Effects of pantothenic acid supplementation on human exercise. Med Sci Sports Exerc 1985;17:287.
Loftus EV Jr, et al. Dexpanthenol enemas in ulcerative colitis: a pilot study. Mayo Clin Proc 1997;72:616–620.
Lokkevik E et al. Skin treatment with bepanthen cream versus no cream during radiotherapy: a randomized controlled trial. Acta Oncol 35.8 (1996): 1021–1026.
Matts PJ, et al. A review of the range of effects of niacinamide in human skin. Int Fed Soc Cosmet Chem Mag 2002;5:285–90.
McCarty MF. Inhibition of acetyl-CoA carboxylase by cystamine may mediate the hypotriglyceridemic activity of pantethine. Med Hypotheses 56.3 (2001): 314–317.
McRae MP. Treatment of hyperlipoproteinemia with pantethine: A review and analysis of efficacy and tolerability. Nutr Res 25.4 (2005): 319–333.
Melampy RM, et al. Effect of pantothenic acid deficiency upon adrenal cortex, thymus, spleen, and circulating lymphocytes in mice. Proc Soc Exp Biol Med 1951;76:24–27.
Moiseenok AG et al. Antitoxic properties of pantothenic acid derivatives, precursors of coenzyme A biosynthesis, with regard to kanamycin. Antibiotiki 29.11 (1984): 851–855.
Monro J. Pantothenic acid and coeliac disease. Br Med J 1972; 4: 112–113.
Nagiel-Ostaszewski I, Lau-Cam CA. Protection by pantethine, pantothenic acid and cystamine against carbon tetrachloride-induced hepatotoxicity in the rat. Res Commun Chem Pathol Pharmacol 67.2 (1990): 289–292.
Naruta E, Buko V. Hypolipidemic effect of pantothenic acid derivatives in mice with hypothalamic obesity induced by aurothioglucose. Exp Toxicol Pathol 53.5 (2001): 393–398.
Nice C, et al. The effects of pantothenic acid on human exercise capacity. J Sports Med 1984;24:26–29.
Pelton RB, Williams RJ. Effect of pantothenic acid on the longevity of mice. Proc Soc Exp Biol Med 1958;99:632–633.
Plesofsky N. Pantothenic acid. Oregon: Linus Pauling Institute, 2002.
Ralli EP, Dumm ME. Relation of pantothenic acid to adrenal cortical function. Vitam Horm 1953;11:133–158.
Romiti R, Romiti N. Dexpanthenol cream significantly improves mucocutaneous side effects associated with isotretinoin therapy. Pediatr Dermatol 2002;19:368.
Shibata K, et al. Pantothenic acid refeeding diminishes the liver, perinephrical fats, and plasma fats accumulated by pantothenic acid deficiency and/or ethanol consumption. Nutrition 2013:1–6.
Slyshenkov VS et al. Pantothenic acid and pantothenol increase biosynthesis of glutathione by boosting cell energetics. FEBS Lett 569.1–3 (2004): 169–172.
Thurston JH, Hauhart RE. Amelioration of adverse effects of valproic acid on ketogenesis and liver coenzyme A metabolism by cotreatment with pantothenate and carnitine in developing mice: possible clinical significance. Pediatr Res 31.4 (1992): 419–423.
Toromanyan E, et al. Efficacy of Slim339 in reducing body weight of overweight and obese human subjects. Phytother Res 2007;21:1177–1181.
Vaxman F et al. Improvement in the healing of colonic anastomoses by vitamin B_5 and C supplements: Experimental study in the rabbit. Ann Chir 44.7 (1990): 512–520.
Vaxman F et al. Effect of pantothenic acid and ascorbic acid supplementation on human skin wound healing process. A double-blind, prospective and randomized trial. Eur Surg Res 27.3 (1995): 158–166.
Wahlqvist M (ed). Food and nutrition. Sydney: Allen & Unwin, 2002.
Wall B T, et al. Acute pantothenic acid and cysteine supplementation does not affect muscle coenzyme A content, fuel selection, or exercise performance in healthy humans. J Appl Physiol 2012; 112:272–278.
Watanabe T, et al. Dietary intake of seven B vitamins based on a total diet study in Japan. J Nutr Sci Vitaminol (Tokyo) 2010;56:279–286.
Webster MJ. Physiological and performance responses to supplementation with thiamin and pantothenic acid derivatives. Eur J Appl Physiol Occup Physiol 1998;77:486–491.
Welsh AL. Lupus erythematosus: treatment by combined use of massive amounts of pantothenic acid and vitamin E. AMA Arch Derm Syphilol 1954;70:181–198.
Yamamoto, T. et al. The effect of pantothenic acid on testicular function in male rats. Journal of Veterinary Medical Science 2009 71 No. 11 1427–1432.

Vitamin B_6

BACKGROUND AND RELEVANT PHARMACOKINETICS

Vitamin B_6 as pyridoxine was first isolated in 1938. Pyridoxal and pyridoxamine were later identified in the mid-1940s (Gropper & Smith 2013). In total, there are six different vitamin B_6 forms — pyridoxine, pyridoxal, pyridoxamine and their phosphorylated derivatives, pyridoxine phosphate (PNP), pyridoxal phosphate (PLP) and pyridoxamine phosphate (PMP), all of which are found in food. PLP is the active coenzyme important for amino acid metabolism.

For absorption, phosphorylated forms are hydroysed (dephosphorylated) to the free forms (pyridoxine, pyridoxal, pyridoxamine) by zinc-dependent alkaline phosphatase. (However, at high-ingested concentrations, the phosphorylated forms may be absorbed without dephosphorylation.)

Absorption of vitamin B_6 takes place in the jejunum by a passive, non-saturable process. The more acidic the environment, the greater is the absorption. Pyridoxine, pyridoxal and pyridoxamine are transported in the plasma and red blood cells to the liver, where they are metabolised predominantly to PLP. In all, 60–90% of vitamin B_6 found in systemic blood is in the form of PLP. Prior to cellular uptake, it must be enzymatically hydrolysed to free pyridoxal again, as extrahepatic tissues uptake only unphosphorylated forms (Gropper & Smith 2013). It is mainly stored in muscle tissue, and ultimately metabolised and excreted via the kidneys.

> ***Clinical note — Marginal B_6 deficiency***
>
> Although frank deficiency is rare, marginal deficiency appears to be common. One study found that 100% of 174 university students tested had some degree of vitamin B_6 deficiency (Shizukuishi et al 1981). A larger survey of 11,658 adults found that 71% of males and 90% of females did not meet the recommended daily intake (RDI) requirements for B_6 (Kant & Block 1990).

CHEMICAL COMPONENTS

Vitamin B_6 is a water-soluble vitamin and has six vitamer forms, of which pyridoxine hydrochloride is the main form, found in supplements and used to fortify foods, as it is particularly stable (Combs 2012). Pyridoxine is the alcohol form, pyridoxal the aldehyde form and pyridoxamine the amine form, each with a 5′-phosphate derivative (Gropper & Smith 2013).

FOOD SOURCES

All six forms of vitamin B_6 are found in food. Vitamin B_6 is widely distributed in animal and plant foods. Plant foods contain mainly pyridoxine, PNP and a conjugated pyridoxine glycoside, while animal products, such as sirloin steak, salmon and chicken, are the richest sources of pyridoxal, pyridoxamine, PLP and PMP (Gropper & Smith 2013). It occurs in the highest concentrations in meats (organ meats, beef, chicken, pork), salmon, wholegrain products, legumes, eggs, vegetables, some fruits (bananas) and nuts (Combs 2012, Gropper & Smith 2013). Per milligram, Vegemite is one of the richest sources.

On average, the bioavailability of vitamin B_6 from the most commonly consumed foods is between 61% and 92%. Prolonged heating, milling and refining grains and food storage contribute to substantial loss (Gropper & Smith 2013).

Up to 40% can be lost through cooking (Wahlqvist 1997); however, more recent sources suggest a variation of up to 70% (Combs 2012). Plant-derived foods lose very little vitamin B_6 from cooking, as they contain the most stable pyridoxine, whereas animal foods that contain mostly pyridoxal and pyridoxamine lose substantial amounts (Combs 2012).

DEFICIENCY SIGNS AND SYMPTOMS

Clinical signs and symptoms are non-specific because this vitamin is necessary for the proper functioning of over 60 enzymes (Pelton et al 2000, Wahlqvist 1997). Signs of deficiency can occur within 2–3 weeks of reduced intake, but may take up to 2½ months to develop (Gropper & Smith 2013). In adults with B_6 deficiency, chiefly dermatological, circulatory and neurological changes develop. In adults with chronic deficiency, a subacute or chronic neuropathy develops. In most cases, chronic deficiency is a result of the long-term use of vitamin B_6 antagonists such as isoniazid, hydralazine and penicillamine. Sensory symptoms appear first in the distal portion of the feet and then spread proximally to the knees and hands if medicine use continues (So & Simon 2012). In children, the central nervous system (CNS) is also affected. Signs and symptoms include:

- Seborrhoeic rash/dermatitis (similar to that seen in pellagra) on face, neck, shoulders and buttocks (Gropper & Smith 2013)
- Weakness, sleeplessness and fatigue
- Angular stomatitis and glossitis, and cheilosis (Combs 2012, Gropper & Smith 2013)
- Sideroblastic anaemia
- Hypochromic, microcytic anaemia due to impaired haem production (Gropper & Smith 2013)
- Impaired cell-mediated immunity and increased susceptibility to infection (Combs 2012)
- Renal calculi
- Elevated homocysteine levels (Lakshmi & Ramalakshmi 1998)
- Impaired niacin production from tryptophan (Combs 2012, Gropper & Smith 2013)
- Impaired glucose tolerance (Combs 2012)
- CNS effects such as irritability, confusion, lethargy, clinical depression, peripheral neuropathy, elevated seizure activity and convulsions (particularly in children) (Combs 2012, Gropper & Smith 2013), abnormal brain wave patterns and nerve conduction
- Birth defects such as cleft palate (associated with elevated homocysteine) (Weingaertner et al 2005).

Pyridoxine deficiency has also been associated with premature coronary artery disease and with impaired oxidative defence mechanisms (Miner et al 2001).

Primary deficiency

Primary deficiency is rare because this vitamin is widely available in many foods. Groups at risk of deficiency include breastfed babies born with low plasma B_6 levels, the elderly, those who consume large quantities of alcohol and individuals who are on dialysis due to abnormal vitamin loss (Groff & Gropper 2009).

Secondary deficiency

This may result from malabsorption syndromes, cancer, liver cirrhosis and alcoholism, hyperthyroidism, congestive heart failure or use of medicines that affect B_6 status or activity such as isoniazid, hydralazine, penicillamine, theophylline, monoamine oxidase inhibitors (Beers & Berkow 2003, Bratman & Kroll 2000, Wardlaw

1997), corticosteroids (promote vitamin B_6 loss), anticonvulsants (inhibit vitamin B_6 activity) and the oral contraceptive pill (Gropper & Smith 2013).

MAIN ACTIONS

Coenzyme

In the form of PLP, vitamin B_6 is associated with >100 enzymes and predominantly involved in amino acid metabolism (Gropper & Smith 2013). All except one amino acid, proline, rely on vitamin B_6 for their biosynthesis and catabolism (Combs 2012).

It is an important coenzyme in the biosynthesis of the neurotransmitters gamma-aminobutyric acid (GABA), dopamine and serotonin (Gerster 1996). It is also involved in protein metabolism, haemoglobin synthesis, gluconeogenesis, lipid metabolism, niacin formation, immune system processes, nucleic acid synthesis and hormone modulation (Bratman & Kroll 2000, Combs 2012, Wardlaw 1997).

Homocysteine

Homocysteine is formed from the essential amino acid methionine and about 50% is then remethylated to methionine via steps that require folic acid and vitamin B_{12}. Vitamin B_6 is required for another metabolic pathway and is a cofactor for cystathionine beta-synthase, which mediates the transformation of homocysteine to cystathionine (Wilcken & Wilcken 1998).

Serotonin, adrenaline and noradrenaline

Pyridoxine is required for the synthesis of many neurotransmitters, including serotonin, adrenaline and noradrenaline. It is a cofactor for the enzyme 5-hydroxytryptophan decarboxylase, which is involved in one of the steps that converts tryptophan to serotonin (Pelton et al 2000) and tyrosine carboxylase that converts tyrosine to dopamine, adrenaline and noradrenaline (Combs 2012). Deficiency states are therefore associated with alterations to mood and other psychological disturbances.

Niacin synthesis

Vitamin B_6 is a required cofactor for kynureninase and transaminases required for tryptophan conversion to niacin (Combs 2012).

Antioxidant

B_6 has been shown both in vitro and in vivo to display antioxidant activity (Anand 2005, Ji et al 2006, Kannan & Jain 2004, Matxain et al 2007).

Antitumour

In vitro and in vivo experiments have found evidence of some antitumour action on a number of cell lines, including breast and pituitary cells (Ren & Melmed 2006, Shimada et al 2005, 2006).

Reducing diabetic complications

According to Jain (2007), animal studies show that B_6 may reduce the incidence of several diabetic complications, such as retinopathy, nephropathy and dyslipidaemia. It is thought that advanced glycation end products (AGEs) contribute to the development of diabetic nephropathy and other diabetes complications, and, according to in vivo research, pyridoxamine (from the B_6 group of compounds) exerts antioxidant and anti-AGE action in the kidneys (Tanimoto et al 2007).

The anti-AGE action of PLP was confirmed in a diabetic rat model, where it prevented the progression of nephropathy (Nakamura et al 2007).

OTHER ACTIONS

Pyridoxine displayed a protective effect against neurotoxicity induced by glutamate in vivo, which may prove useful in hypoxic-ischaemic brain injury (Buyukokuroglu et al 2007). Another animal study indicated that neuroprotective activity preventing ischaemic damage may be due to a GABA-inhibitory effect (Hwang et al 2007).

Immune-stimulant actions, with an increase in T-helper and T-lymphocyte cells, were found in critically ill patients to whom B_6 was administered (Cheng et al 2006).

Myelin formation

PLP is required for the synthesis of sphingolipids for myelin sheath formation (Ang et al 2008).

Gene expression

In its non-coenzyme role, vitamin B_6 has been shown to affect gene expression by binding to DNA and modulating steroid hormones (including progesterone, androgens and oestrogens), binding to regulatory DNA regions (Oka 2001).

CLINICAL USE

Vitamin B_6 supplementation is used to treat a large variety of conditions and is mostly prescribed in combination with other B group vitamins.

Deficiency

It is traditionally used to treat vitamin B_6 deficiency.

Premenstrual syndrome (PMS)

Vitamin B_6 supplementation is used in doses beyond RDI levels for the treatment of PMS. A 1999 systematic review of nine clinical trials involving 940 patients with PMS supports this use, finding that doses up to 100 mg/day are likely to be of benefit in treating symptoms and PMS-related depression (Wyatt et al 1999). Another double-blind randomised controlled trial of 94 patients taking a dose of 40 mg B_6 twice a day found that active treatment significantly decreased PMS symptoms during the luteal phase. Benefits were most pronounced for mood and psychiatric symptoms (Kashanian et al 2008).

Comparative study

One randomised double-blind study compared the effects of pyridoxine (300 mg/day), alprazolam (0.75 mg/day), fluoxetine (10 mg/day) or propranolol (20 mg/day) in four groups of 30 women with severe PMS (Diegoli et al 1998). In this study, fluoxetine produced the best results (a mean reduction of 65.4% in symptoms), followed by propranolol (58.7%), alprazolam (55.6%), pyridoxine (45.3%) and placebo (39.4–46.1%). Symptoms responding well to pyridoxine were tachycardia, insomnia, acne and nausea (Diegoli et al 1998). Another comparative study of 60 women tested 100 mg of B_6 against bromocriptine and a placebo over 3 months. Both active treatments produced a significant reduction in symptoms compared to the control group; however, vitamin B_6 treatment was slightly more effective than bromocriptine and produced fewer side effects (Sharma et al 2007).

More recently, a systematic review investigated the role of herbs, vitamins and minerals advocated in the treatment of PMS and/or premenstrual dysphoric disorder (PMDD) to determine their efficacy in reducing the severity of PMS/PMDD symptoms (Whelan et al 2009). Data support the use of calcium for PMS, and suggest that chasteberry and vitamin B_6 may be effective (Whelan et al 2009).

Dysmenorrhoea

A Cochrane review of herbal and dietary therapies for primary and secondary dysmenorrhoea found one small trial with B_6 that showed it was more effective at reducing pain than both placebo (in this case ibuprofen) and a combination of magnesium and vitamin B_6 (Davis 1988) but, due to poor reporting of data, this was not included in the meta-analysis (Proctor & Murphy 2009).

Pregnancy

Vitamin B_6 has been associated with some benefits during pregnancy; however, more research is required to understand the role of B_6 supplementation in this population.

A 2006 Cochrane Review investigated the clinical effects of vitamin B_6 oral capsules or lozenges during pregnancy and/or labour to see whether there were any changes to Apgar score, birth weight, incidence of pre-eclampsia or preterm birth (Thaver et al 2006). Five trials (1646 women) were included. Vitamin B_6 as oral capsules or lozenges resulted in decreased risk of dental decay in pregnant women. A small trial showed reduced mean birth weights with vitamin B_6 supplementation, and no significant differences in the risk of eclampsia, pre-eclampsia or low Apgar scores at 1 minute between supplemented and non-supplemented groups. No differences were found in Apgar scores at 1 or 5 minutes, or breast milk production between controls and women receiving oral or intramuscular loading doses of pyridoxine at labour (Thaver et al 2006). The authors concluded there were not enough data to be able to make any useful assessments, and further research is required. Furthermore, three of the five studies were from the 1960s (Hillman et al 1962, 1963, Swartwout et al 1960); the other two were from the 1980s (Schuster et al 1984, Temesvari et al 1983). More updated information is required.

A more recent systematic review evaluated the risks and benefits of interventions with vitamins B_6, B_{12} and C during pregnancy on maternal, neonatal and child health and nutrition outcomes (Dror & Allen 2012). In this meta-analysis based on three small studies, vitamin B_6 supplementation had a significant positive effect on birth weight; however, there were no significant effects on other neonatal outcomes, including preterm birth, low birth weight and perinatal morbidity and mortality.

Homocysteine and recurrent miscarriages

A 2012 study assessed homocysteine levels and pregnancy outcomes in 50 cases of recurrent miscarriage. Active treatment consisted of B_{12} 1500 mcg, vitamin B_6 10 mg and folic acid 5 mg daily taken throughout the pregnancy (n = 25) or during the first trimester only (n = 25). Following treatment with the B group vitamins, homocysteine levels decreased by 37%. Miscarriage rate in patients with hyperhomocysteinaemia was 26.6% compared with 11.4% in patients with normal homocysteine. The authors concluded that hyperhomocysteinaemia was associated with a 2.5-fold increased risk of miscarriage (Agarwal et al 2012).

V

Morning sickness

A systematic review investigated the effectiveness and safety of a range of treatments for nausea and vomiting in early pregnancy and suggested there was low-quality evidence to support B_6 versus placebo for nausea but not vomiting

(Festin 2009). A Cochrane review in 2010 of 27 trials with 4042 women investigated the outcomes of vitamin B_6 supplementation, ginger and conventional drug therapy in reducing nausea and vomiting in early pregnancy (Matthews et al 2010). Two studies of 416 women compared vitamin B_6 with placebo (Sahakian et al 1991, Vutyavanich et al 1995) and showed that vitamin B_6 supplementation reduced nausea after 3 days. A well-designed, double-blind, randomised, controlled trial had similar results but over a 3-week period (Smith & Crowther 2005). It is unclear whether vomiting frequency also reduced, due to the heterogeneity of studies.

In the same review, the comparative effectiveness of ginger and vitamin B_6 for nausea and vomiting in early pregnancy found both interventions significantly reduced nausea and vomiting scores ($P < 0.05$, $P < 0.001$ respectively) (Chittumma et al 2007, Sripramote & Lekhyananda 2003). Two other studies (Ensiyeh & Sakineh 2009, Smith et al 2004) report improvements in vomiting frequency, nausea and retching (Matthews et al 2010). In an experimental study of 60 pregnant women experiencing nausea and/or vomiting (prior to the 12th week of gestation), 30 women were given 10 mg of vitamin B_6 and 30 were given 1.28 mg for 2 weeks to investigate the outcome on Pregnancy-Unique Quantification of Emesis and nausea (PUQE) score. Plasma B_6 concentration was significantly increased in both groups ($P < 0.05$), and the higher supplementation group had a greater decrease in PUQE score (Wibowo et al 2012), suggesting that the 10 mg dose of vitamin B_6 is effective in reducing both nausea and vomiting in early-stage pregnancy.

Another study (Bsat et al 2001) looked at the effectiveness of three different antiemetics (metoclopramide with vitamin B_6, prochlorperazine and promethazine). The authors report that approximately 65%, 38% and 40% of women in each group, respectively, responded that they felt better on the third day of treatment. The authors conclude that their results favour pyridoxine-metoclopromide over the other two regimens.

Based on current research, vitamin B_6 appears to be effective in reducing both nausea and vomiting in early stages of pregnancy in a number of individual clinical trials. Its effectiveness is equivalent to that of ginger and may occur within 3 days of starting supplementation. Furthermore, the combination of metoclopramide with vitamin B_6 appears to be more effective than other conventional treatment (prochlorperazine and promethazine), and this effect may also begin within 3 days of treatment. Although a number of the trials showed benefit of B_6 overall, the authors concluded there was limited evidence from trials to support the use of pharmacological agents, including vitamin B_6 (Matthews et al 2010).

Heart disease

A growing body of evidence in contemporary studies has suggested a subtle relationship between heart failure and micronutrient status (McKeag et al 2012). While the authors state the results are inconclusive, one recent study reviewed by them showed potentially significant results. This observational study measured riboflavin and pyridoxine levels in 100 patients (mean age 67.1 years, 58% males) with heart failure (as defined by Framingham criteria). It was found that the percentage of patients with evidence of pyridoxine deficiency was significantly higher in patients with heart failure (38.0% vs 19.0%; $P = 0.02$) (Keith et al 2009). Whether low B_6 is a causative factor or consequence of disease remains to be clarified.

Elevated homocysteine levels

In practice, the relative safety and affordability of combined vitamin B supplementation (B_{12}, folic acid and B_6) make it an attractive recommendation in people with familial hyperhomocysteinaemia. Whether lowering total homocysteine improves cardiovascular mortality and morbidity is questionable, as recent large-scale clinical trials and meta-analyses have failed to demonstrate any benefits for B group vitamins (including B_6) in reducing overall cardiovascular risk, despite showing a reduction in homocysteine levels (Albert et al 2008, Clarke et al 2007, CTSUESU 2006, den Heijer et al 2007, Mann et al 2008, Marcus et al 2007, Ray et al 2007). Negative results were obtained yet again in a 2013 Cochrane intervention review which evaluated the clinical effectiveness of homocysteine-lowering interventions (in the form of supplements of vitamin B_6, B_9 and B_{12}) at reducing the incidence of myocardial infarction, stroke or all-cause mortality as compared to placebo.

Twelve randomised controlled trials involving 47,429 participants both with and without pre-existing cardiovascular disease were included in the review, which concluded that the interventions did not significantly affect non-fatal or fatal myocardial infarction (pooled relative risk [RR] 1.02), stroke (pooled RR 0.91) or death by any cause (pooled RR 1.01) as compared with placebo (Martí-Carvajal et al 2013).

Failure of combined B vitamin therapy to reverse inflammatory processes associated with atherogenesis may partly explain the negative results (Bleie et al 2007). The consistent findings of an association between elevated plasma total homocysteine levels and vascular risk are yet to be fully explained; however, it is possible that the association is a consequence rather than a cause of disease (Toole et al 2004).

Venous thrombosis (VT)

A systematic review and meta-analysis investigated the association between B group vitamins and VT (Zhou et al 2012), given that a homocysteine-independent role for B group vitamins on VT development has been reported. In this review, significant standardised mean differences were obtained for plasma folic acid and vitamin B_{12}, suggesting that reduced levels of folic acid and vitamin B_{12} may be independent risk factors of VT. Moreover, a qualitative systematic review indicated that low level of vitamin B_6 was an independent risk factor of VT (Zhou et al 2012). Further prospective clinical studies are needed to provide additional evidence on the clinical benefits of B group vitamin supplementation for VT.

IN COMBINATION

In a 12-week, open-label, randomised, placebo-controlled trial, 85 hypertriglyceridaemic (triglycerides >150 mg/dL) males were randomised to one of five groups and given lysine (1 g/day), vitamin B_6 (50 mg/day), lysine (1 g/day) plus vitamin B_6 (50 mg/day), carnitine (1 g/day) or placebo for 12 weeks. Results showed that nutritional supplementation was associated with a significant reduction in total cholesterol by 10%. Additionally, plasma triglycerides were reduced by 36.6 mg/dL at 6 weeks compared with an increase of 18 mg/dL in the placebo group, although not statistically significant (Hlais et al 2012). The role of B_6 itself is unclear in achieving this result.

Reducing thromboembolism

A prospective cohort study of 757 patients experiencing first venous thromboembolism found that patients with lower plasma B_6 had a 1.8-fold higher risk of recurrence than those with higher levels of B_6 (Hron et al 2007). In contrast, no risk reduction was found in a secondary analysis of the HOPE-2 trial, which included over 5000 individuals with known cardiovascular disease or diabetes who were given a daily supplement of folic acid (2.5 mg), B_6 (50 mg) and B_{12} (1 mg) or a placebo for 5 years. In this analysis, vitamin therapy reduced homocysteine levels; however, it did not reduce the risk of venous thromboembolism, deep-vein thrombosis or pulmonary embolism (Ray et al 2007).

Improving outcomes after heart transplantation

Cardiac transplantation represents a potentially life-saving procedure for patients with end-stage cardiac disease. Short-term survival is improving because of improved immunosuppression, but long-term survival remains limited by an aggressive form of atherosclerosis known as transplant coronary artery disease (Miner et al 2001).

A randomised, double-blind placebo-controlled study showed that pyridoxine supplementation (100 mg/day) taken for 10 weeks improved endothelial function as assessed by flow-mediated dilatation in cardiac transplant recipients (Miner et al 2001). Interestingly, homocysteine levels remained unchanged with treatment, suggesting that other mechanisms are responsible.

IN COMBINATION

A randomised, double-blind, placebo-controlled study of 50 patients who were perceived to be at risk of cerebral ischaemia received B_6 (25 mg), folate (2.5 mg) and B_{12} (0.5 mg) or a placebo daily for a year. The study found that supplementation significantly reduced carotid intima-media thickness, which is a marker of atherosclerotic changes (Till et al 2005). In contrast, another small, double-blind, randomised and placebo-controlled trial of 30 individuals with a history of ischaemic stroke found that long-term treatment over 3.9 years with similar dosages of B_6 and B_{12} to the previous trial and slightly less folate (2 mg) produced no differences in carotid intima-media thickness and endothelial function (Potter et al 2007).

Cancer

A number of studies have investigated whether low B_6 may be associated with a higher prevalence of certain cancers and if higher levels have a chemopreventive effect. Some studies have focused on B_6 alone but often it is included as part of an investigation into the effects of folic acid, B_{12}, methionine and B_6 as a combination.

Theoretically, adequate B_6, B_{12}, folate and methionine might have a chemopreventive effect due to their roles in the one-carbon metabolism pathway, which is critical for DNA synthesis, methylation and repair (Harris et al 2012), and by reducing inflammation, cell proliferation and oxidative stress (Zhang et al 2013).

Ovarian cancer

The association between folate, methionine, vitamin B_6, vitamin B_{12} and alcohol among 1910 women with ovarian cancer and 1989 controls from a case-control study was conducted. An inverse association between dietary vitamin B_6 (covariate-adjusted odds ratio [OR] 0.76, 95% confidence interval [CI] 0.64–0.92; P_{trend} = 0.002) and methionine intake (covariate-adjusted OR 0.72, 95% CI 0.60–0.87; $P_{trend} < 0.001$) and ovarian cancer risk was found. The association with dietary vitamin B_6 was strongest for serous borderline (covariate-adjusted OR 0.49, 95% CI 0.32–0.77; P_{trend} = 0.001) and serous invasive (covariate-adjusted OR 0.74, 95% CI 0.58–0.94; P_{trend} = 0.012) subtypes. The authors concluded that methionine and especially vitamin B_6 may lower ovarian cancer risk (Harris et al 2012).

Breast cancer

The association of prediagnostic plasma concentrations of PLP with postmenopausal breast cancer risk was investigated in a case–control study of 706 cases and

706 controls. Women with higher plasma PLP concentrations had a 30% reduced risk of invasive breast cancer (CI 0.50–0.98) as compared with women with low PLP (P_{trend} = 0.02). The results suggest that higher circulating levels of vitamin B_6 are associated with a reduced risk of invasive postmenopausal breast cancer. The authors suggest a role for vitamin B_6 in the prevention of postmenopausal breast cancer, although further research is required (Lurie et al 2012).

The majority of studies investigating the protective role of B vitamins in breast cancer have focused on folate, B_6 and B_{12}. Several case-controlled studies have reported protective associations (Chen et al 2005, Larsson et al 2007, Lajous et al 2006, Yang et al 2013) while cohort studies have shown inconsistencies in results (Cho et al 2007, Ericson et al 2007, Shrubsole et al 2011, Stevens et al 2010). One investigated the association between dietary intakes of folate, B_2, B_6, B_{12} and methionine for breast cancer risk in Hispanic and non-Hispanic white women in the United States. Higher intakes of folate, B_{12} and methionine were associated with a lower risk of breast cancer; however there was no risk reduction with vitamin B_6 or B_2 (Yang et al 2013).

Other researchers, using the prospective cohort Shanghai Women's Health Study (1997–2008), including 718 Chinese breast cancer cases, investigated folate, B_6, B_{12}, niacin, riboflavin and methionine intakes and their association with breast carcinogenesis and again found no specific benefit from vitamin B_6 (Shrubsole et al 2011).

Bladder cancer

In an attempt to find a link between dietary components and incidence of bladder cancer, diet was assessed for 912 patients with bladder cancer and 873 controls by Garcia-Closas et al (2007). Individuals in the highest quintile for B_6 intake had a 40% reduced risk of bladder cancer compared with those in the lowest quintile.

Colorectal cancer

Current evidence suggests high dietary vitamin B_6 intake is associated with a reduced risk of colorectal cancer. One large longitudinal population study (n = 61; 433 women aged 40–76 years) used a food frequency questionnaire with a follow-up over 14.8 years and found that high dietary vitamin B_6 was associated with lower colorectal cancer risk, with protective effects most notably seen in women who drank alcohol (Larsson et al 2005). Similarly, a case-control study of 2028 people with colorectal cancer and 2722 controls confirmed a dose-dependent protective effect of B_6, with strongest protective effects observed for the highest intake and in people aged over 55 years (Theodoratou et al 2008). Another large population study of both men and women further confirmed that low dietary B_6 was associated with an increased risk in colorectal cancer, but the effect was specific for men and not for women. Protective effects were strongest in men with higher alcohol intake. These findings were from the large Japan Public Health Center-based Prospective Study, from which there were 526 cases of colorectal cancer (Ishihara et al 2007). A randomised controlled trial also found that high levels of plasma B_6 may be protective against colorectal adenomas (Figueiredo et al 2008).

A systematic review with meta-analysis of prospective studies assessed the association of vitamin B_6 intake or blood levels of PLP (the active form of vitamin B_6) with risk of colorectal cancer (Larsson et al 2010). Nine studies focused on vitamin B_6 intake and four studies on blood PLP levels. The pooled RRs of colorectal cancer for the highest vs lowest category of vitamin B_6 intake and blood PLP levels were 0.90 (95% CI 0.75–1.07) and 0.52 (95% CI 0.38–0.71), respectively. There was heterogeneity among studies of vitamin B_6 intake but not among studies of blood PLP levels. The risk of colorectal cancer decreased by 49% for every 100 pmol/mL increase in blood PLP levels (RR 0.51). Vitamin B_6 intake and blood PLP levels were inversely associated with the risk of colorectal cancer in this meta-analysis (Larsson et al 2010).

Another later study evaluated whether higher vitamin B_6 intake in the remote past is strongly associated with a lower risk of colorectal cancer than intake in the recent past. Vitamin B_6 intake was assessed every 4 years for up to 28 years using validated food frequency questionnaires from 86,440 women in the Nurses' Health Study and 44,410 men in the Health Professionals Follow-up Study. Total vitamin B_6 intake was significantly associated with an approximately 20–30% lower risk of colorectal cancer in age-adjusted results but these significant associations became attenuated and non-significant after adjustment for other colorectal cancer risk factors. Additionally, results did not differ by cancer subsite, source of vitamin B_6 (food or supplement) or intake of alcohol and folate (Zhang et al 2012).

Conversely, a randomised, double-blind, placebo-controlled trial of 5442 female health professionals at high risk for cardiovascular disease examined the effect of a combination pill of folic acid (2.5 mg), vitamin B_6 (50 mg) and vitamin B_{12} (1 mg) or placebo on the occurrence of colorectal adenoma. This study included 1470 participants who were followed up for as long as 9.2 years and underwent an endoscopy at any point during follow-up. The results indicated no statistically significant effect of the combination treatment on incidence of colorectal adenoma among this population. The risk of colorectal adenoma was similar among participants receiving treatment (24.3%, 180 of 741 participants) vs placebo (24.0%, 175 of 729 participants) (multivariable adjusted RR 1.00) (Song et al 2012).

Observational studies of dietary or dietary plus supplementary intake of vitamin B_6 and colorectal cancer risk have been inconsistent, with most studies reporting non-significant positive or inverse associations (Zhang et al 2013). However, a 30–50% reduction in colorectal cancer risk has been consistently reported in published studies where high circulating plasma levels of active vitamin B_6 (plasma POP) have been found. Zhang et al (2013) suggest that the discrepancy in the results may be due to dietary-based versus plasma-based studies, but why this is the case remains elusive. The age of vitamin B_6 repletion and the effect of repletion at different life stages, suboptimal levels, differing subtypes of colorectal cancer and genetic variants may also influence the results and explain such variations (Zhang et al 2013).

Lung cancer prognosis and vitamin B_6

The bioactive form of B_6, produced by pyridoxal kinase, has been found to exacerbate cisplatin- (cytotoxic agent used to treat non-small-cell lung cancer) mediated DNA damage and sensitise cancer cell lines to apoptosis, both in vitro and in vivo. Furthermore, low pyridoxal kinase activity, and thus low bioactive vitamin B_6, has been associated with poor disease outcome. The authors suggest pyridoxal kinase expression may be a marker for risk stratification in non-small-cell lung cancer patients (Galluzzi et al 2012).

Carpal tunnel syndrome (CTS)

It has been suspected that vitamin B_6 deficiency may play a role in the development of CTS, as several studies have found that patients with CTS and pyridoxine deficiency respond to supplementation (Ellis et al 1991). More recent evidence now casts doubt on the usefulness of B_6 supplementation in CTS. A 2002 review found no benefit with pyridoxine treatment in CTS (Gerritsen et al 2002). Similarly, a 2007 systematic review of treatments for CTS concluded that there was moderately strong evidence to suggest that B_6 was ineffective in the treatment of the condition (Piazzini et al 2007).

Autism

Overall, there is some research which suggests that supplementation with pyridoxine in combination with other nutrients, mainly magnesium, may improve some features of autism (Kuriyama et al 2002, Mousain-Bosc et al 2006, Pfeiffer et al 1995); however, larger trials with rigorous methodology are required before a more definitive conclusion can be made.

In 1997, a small, 10-week, double-blind, placebo-controlled trial found that an average dose of 638.9 mg pyridoxine and 216.3 mg magnesium oxide was ineffective in ameliorating autistic behaviours (Findling et al 1997). More recently, combination treatment with magnesium and B_6 was shown to improve symptoms such as social interaction, communication and general behaviour in autism (Mousain-Bosc et al 2006).

In a 2006 Cochrane systematic review, one study (Kuriyama et al 2002) concluded that pyridoxine was associated with improvement in verbal IQ scores; however it only included eight subjects and was a short-term study for 4 weeks. Overall, the review found that the quality and small sizes of the studies posed problems in evaluating the evidence that led to their conclusion that B_6-Mg therapy could not be recommended (Nye & Brice 2005). This review has been edited with no change to conclusions and republished in 2009. However, more current research needs to be conducted, including investigations on the clinical significance of the reduction in urinary dicarboxylic acid in autism.

Several studies have sought to explain how vitamin B_6 supplementation may provide benefits in this population.

Several studies have observed dietary deficiencies of vitamin B_2, vitamin B_6 and magnesium in autism (Kałuzna-Czaplinska et al 2009, Lakshmi Priya & Geetha 2011, Marlowe et al 1984, Xia et al 2010).

Increased homocysteine levels have been associated with autism (Kaluzna-Czaplinska et al 2013) as well as high levels of urinary dicarboxylic acids (an important marker of metabolism, energy production, intestinal dysbiosis and nutritional status in autistic children) (Kałuzna-Czaplinska et al 2011). Homocysteine levels can be lowered with a combination of vitamins B_6, B_{12} and folate; however it remains unclear whether this effect translates into a clinical benefit. Supplementation with magnesium (200 mg/day), pyridoxine (500 mg/day) and riboflavin (20 mg/day) for 3 months is able to reduce excretion of urinary dicarboxylic acid according to a study of 30 autistic children (Kałuzna-Czaplinska et al 2011). In this study, parents of the children being treated observed improvements in eye contact and the ability to concentrate, suggesting a possible clinical improvement.

Adams et al (2006) found that children with autism spectrum disorder had very high plasma levels of B_6 (without supplementation) compared to other children and suggested this may have occurred because of low activity of pyridoxal kinase to convert pyridoxine into PLP, which is the active cofactor for dozens of enzymatic reactions, including the formation of neurotransmitters. This may explain why high doses of B_6 seem necessary to produce benefits.

IN COMBINATION

A Cochrane review of vitamin B complex for treating peripheral neuropathy, which included 13 studies (11 parallel randomised controlled trials and two quasi-randomised trials) involving 741 participants (488 treated with vitamin B complex and 253 treated with placebo or another substance) with alcoholic or diabetic neuropathy, concluded there are only limited data, and the evidence is insufficient to determine whether vitamin B complex is beneficial or harmful (Ang et al 2008). Within this review, however, one trial suggested that 4-week treatment with high doses of oral vitamin B complex (thiamin 25 mg/daily and pyridoxine 50 mg/daily) was more efficacious than lower doses (1 mg each of thiamin and pyridoxine) in short-term reduction of pain, composite impairments, paraesthesiae and neuropathic symptoms (Abbas & Swai 1997). It is not clear if the results were due to the thiamin or pyridoxine or the combination. Given the age of this study, further investigations need to be conducted to attempt to elucidate similar findings.

Seizures

A study found that vitamin B_6-responsive seizures decrease or disappear following high-dose oral B_6 treatment (Ohtahara et al 2011). Vitamin B_6-responsive seizures or epilepsy are associated predominantly with West syndrome, but may also include Lennox-Gastaut syndrome, grand mal or partial motor seizures. In the study, 216 consecutive cases of West syndrome in children aged from 3 months to 5 years with both idiopathic and symptomatic seizures with organic brain lesions were administered high-dose B_6 and had an overall response rate of 13.9%. In responsive patients, long-term seizure and mental outcomes were noted. An increasing dose of 30 to 50–100 mg daily showed a slight clinical response, while doses of 100–400 mg/daily showed dramatic clinical improvements, with effects being noted within 1 week of treatment (Ohtahara et al 2011). In some cases the need for conventional antiepileptic medication was reduced.

This latter finding increases in significance and relevance in the clinical management of seizure control. A study found that 16/33 patients (48%) taking inducing antiepileptic drugs (AED) (phenytoin and carbamazepine) developed a vitamin B_6 deficiency compared with 9% in the control group. Of those that switched to non-inducing AED (levetiracetam, lamotrigine or topiramate), 21% were B_6-deficient (Mintzer et al 2012). The authors concluded that treatment with inducing AEDs commonly causes vitamin B_6 deficiency that is often severe.

Convulsions during a febrile episode

Two randomised trials have been conducted in children, producing conflicting results. One study of 65 children who had been admitted to hospital with febrile convulsions showed that a dose of 2–10 mg/kg PLP daily (orally or intravenously) produced a 100% success rate, whereas 43% in the control group experienced repeated convulsions (Kamiishi et al 1996). A second randomised trial found that a lower dose of 20 mg twice daily did not alter the incidence of febrile convulsions compared with placebo (McKiernan et al 1981).

Symptomatic treatment for stress

The term 'stress', as used by the public, is a subjective one and often described in different ways. One theoretical model that has been developed to predict psychological stress includes measures of life stressors, social support and coping style. Using this model, pyridoxine deficiency has been identified as a significant predictor of increased overall psychological stress during bereavement. More specifically, pyridoxine deficiency is significantly associated with increases in depression, fatigue and confused mood levels, but not with those of anxiety, anger or vigour (Baldewicz et al 1998).

One explanation is that pyridoxine is involved in neurotransmitter biosynthesis, such as GABA and serotonin, and therefore deficiency states that are associated with mood disturbances are improved with consequent supplementation (McCarty 2000).

Cognitive performance/Alzheimer's disease

Whether vitamin B_6 supplementation provides benefits in cognitive function and Alzheimer's disease (AD) remains to be clarified. It has gained some attention as a cheap and safe method of reducing homocysteine, which is implicated in the aetiology of AD and cognitive dysfunction; however, findings are equivocal.

One systematic review evaluated data from 16 studies that investigated the association between cognitive function in the elderly and B_6, folate and B_{12}. An association was found between folate and cognition in AD, but no association was found for vitamins B_6 or B_{12}. However, the authors suggested that heterogeneity in the methodology of the studies made interpretation problematic (Raman et al 2007).

A similar research group doing a systematic review of 14 trials found that most studies were small and of low quality. They found that three studies of B_6 and six trials of combined B vitamins revealed no effect, despite different dosages, on cognitive function. Only one of the trials found a significant improvement using B_6 to improve long-term memory. The review concluded that there was insufficient evidence to support a positive effect of B_6 on cognition. The reviewers suggested that larger, well-designed trials are needed to assess different groups of the population for any association between B_6 and cognitive function (Balk et al 2007).

A Cochrane systematic review on vitamin B_6 and cognition found no evidence for short-term benefit of vitamin B_6 in improving mood (depression, fatigue and tension symptoms) or cognitive functions (Malouf & Grimley Evans 2003). The review included two trials only (Bryan et al 2002, Deijen et al 1992) that used a double-blind, randomised, placebo-controlled design and involved 109 healthy older people. No trials of vitamin B_6 involving people with cognitive impairment or dementia were found, which may explain the negative results.

The development of cognitive impairment has been linked to elevated plasma homocysteine (Ford & Almeida 2012). A systematic review and meta-analysis of 19 randomised controlled trials was conducted to determine the effects of vitamins B_6, B_{12} and folic acid (commonly recognised homocysteine-lowering B vitamins) in individuals with and without cognitive impairment. It was found that these B vitamins, either alone or in combination, did not show an improvement in cognitive function for individuals with or without cognitive impairment. It remains to be established if prolonged treatment with B vitamins can reduce the risk of dementia in later life (Ford & Almeida 2012).

Homocysteine and Alzheimer's disease

According to one systematic review published in 2008, evidence is strong to suggest high homocysteine is a risk factor for AD and further randomised controlled trials are warranted to evaluate the association between B_6, folate, B_{12}, homocysteine levels and AD (Van Dam & Van Gool 2008).

Brain matter

Investigation of a healthy elderly population found a relationship between greater B_6 supplement intake and greater grey-matter volume (Erickson et al 2008). Another study with Alzheimer's patients found that low B_6 levels in patients were associated with white-matter lesions in the brain (Mulder et al 2005). The clinical significance of these findings remains to be clarified.

It has also been theorised that inflammation may be implicated in AD and dementia and that C-reactive protein, as a marker for systemic inflammation, may be a risk factor. A study of 85 individuals discovered that, where C-reactive protein was elevated, this was related to low B_6 levels and cerebral atrophy (Diaz-Arrastia et al 2006). This anti-inflammatory effect of B_6 may explain its possible role in neurodegenerative diseases; another interesting observation came from a study with older men, where levels of beta-amyloid levels were reduced with B_6, folate and B_{12} (Flicker et al 2008).

Schizophrenia

It has been suggested that high levels of homocysteine contribute to the pathogenesis of schizophrenia and the complex metabolic regulation of homocysteine that could be disrupted in schizophrenia (Petronijevic et al 2008).

To test whether supplementation could benefit this population, Levine et al (2006) conducted a randomised controlled trial of 42 schizophrenic patients with plasma homocysteine levels > 15 micromol/L. Treatment with oral folic acid, vitamin B_{12} and pyridoxine for 3 months reduced homocysteine and, more importantly, significantly improved clinical symptoms as measured by the Positive and Negative Syndrome Scale and neuropsychological tests overall, in particular the Wisconsin Card Sort (Levine et al 2006).

Tardive dyskinesia (TD)

TD is a significant clinical problem. Vitamin B_6 is a potent antioxidant and has a role in almost all of the possible mechanisms that are thought to be associated with the appearance of TD (Lerner et al 2007). To test whether supplementation would have any benefits, a 26-week, double-blind, placebo-controlled trial was conducted with 50 inpatients who had DSM-IV diagnoses of schizophrenia or schizoaffective disorder and TD. The randomised study found treatment with vitamin B_6 (1200 mg/day) significantly reduced symptoms of TD compared to a placebo.

Parkinson's disease (PD)

A higher dietary intake of vitamin B_6 was associated with a significantly decreased risk of PD, probably through mechanisms unrelated to homocysteine metabolism, according to findings from the Rotterdam Study — a prospective, population-based cohort study of people aged 55 years and older (de Lau et al 2006). The association between dietary intake of folate, vitamin B_{12} and vitamin B_6 and the risk of incident PD among 5289 participants was evaluated. After a mean follow-up of 9.7 years, the authors identified 72 participants with incident PD. Stratified analyses showed that this association was restricted to smokers. No association was observed for dietary folate and vitamin B_{12}.

Hyperhomocysteinaemia has been reported repeatedly in PD patients; the increase, however, seems mostly related to the methylated catabolism of L-dopa, the main pharmacological treatment of PD (Martignoni et al 2007).

OTHER USES

Vitamin B_6 supplements are effective for treating hereditary sideroblastic anaemia and refractory seizures in newborns, caused by pyridoxine withdrawal after delivery. Vitamin B_6 supplements have been used to prevent diabetic retinopathy and kidney stones, and to treat symptoms of vertigo, allergy to monosodium glutamate, asthma, photosensitivity and pervasive developmental disorders with hypersensitivity to sound. Women taking the oral contraceptive pill sometimes use supplemental B_6 to relieve mood disturbances and restore vitamin status. Whether supplementation has benefits in these circumstances remains unknown.

A small trial has shown some future potential clinical use in renal transplant patients with high homocysteine levels and endothelial dysfunction. A dose of folate (5 mg/day), B_6 (50 mg/day) and B_{12} (1000 mcg/day) was given to stable renal transplant patients for 6 months and homocysteine levels decreased and endothelial function was improved compared to the control patients (Xu et al 2008). Further trials are needed to confirm this finding.

Dream states

Many have suspected that pyridoxine supplements taken at night are able to influence dream states and sleep, causing disruption in some people. The results of a 2002 double-blind, placebo-controlled crossover study support this observation (Ebben et al 2002). Pyridoxine supplementation (250 mg) taken before bedtime was shown to significantly influence dream salience scores (a composite score containing measures for vividness, bizarreness, emotionality and colour), starting on the first night of treatment.

Leg cramps during pregnancy

A study of 84 pregnant women with leg cramps found that a combination of vitamin B_1 (100 mg/day) and B_6 (40 mg/day) improved symptoms 7.5-fold, and this was a better result than given by treatment with calcium carbonate (Sohrabvand et al 2006).

Irritable bowel syndrome (IBS)

In a cross-sectional study, IBS symptom score and dietary intake were assessed in 17 subjects with diagnosed IBS according to the Rome II criteria. The mean dietary intake was found to be 0.9 mg/day, below the recommended intake of 1.6 mg daily for men and 1.2 mg daily for women. The results indicated a high symptom score was associated with low vitamin B_6 intake ($P = 0.0002$) (Ligaarden & Farup 2011). This was a preliminary study, and the authors recognise the possibility of a type II error due to the small study group. However, this study may have clinical implications in the treatment and improvement of IBS symptoms with B_6 therapy, especially if given at therapeutic doses (minimum 5–25 mg to improve deficiency states). Further investigations need to be conducted to ascertain such possibilities.

Mortality in the elderly

A recent study identified that higher intakes of vitamins B_1 and B_6 observed among Taiwanese elders were associated with increased survival rates in this population by up to 10 years (Huang et al 2012). The Taiwanese Elderly Nutrition and Health Survey (1999–2000) provided data from 1747 participants 65 years and older. Dietary and biochemical data were collected at baseline and survivorship was determined until 31 December 2008. After controlling for confounders, a significant difference in mortality was found when comparing people in the lowest tertile to the highest tertile for both B_1 and B_6 dietary intakes (hazard ratios 0.74 and 0.74 respectively). The authors concluded that deficiencies of vitamin B_1 and B_6 were found to be clearly predictive of mortality in elderly Taiwanese.

DOSAGE RANGE

- Prevention of deficiency: Australian RDI for adults and children > 8 years: 1–1.7 mg/day.

- Treatment of deficiency: 5–25 mg/day.
- Morning sickness: 30–75 mg/day, sometimes taken as 25 mg three times daily. In clinical practice, monitored doses of 150 mg daily are often used.
- Symptoms of PMS: 100–500 mg/day.
- Elevated homocysteine levels: 100 mg/day (usually taken with B_{12} and folic acid).
- Leg cramps in pregnancy: vitamin B_1 100 mg/day and B_6 40 mg/day.
- Schizophrenic people with TD: vitamin B_6 (1200 mg/day).

TOXICITY

Symptoms of toxicity include paraesthesia, hyperaesthesia, bone pain, muscle weakness, numbness and fasciculation, most marked at the extremities (Dalton & Dalton 1987, Diegoli et al 1998). Some symptoms include unsteady gait, numbness of the hands and feet and impaired tendon reflexes. Excessive doses of vitamin B_6 cause degeneration of the dorsal root ganglia in the spinal cord, loss of myelination and degeneration of sensory fibres in the peripheral nerves.

The dose and time frame at which toxicity occurs vary significantly between individuals. Studies involving large population groups using 100–150 mg/day have shown minimal or no toxicity in 5–10-year studies, whereas studies of women self-medicating for PMS, taking 117 ± 92 mg for 2.9 ± 1.9 years, have reported increased incidence of peripheral neuropathy (Bernstein 1990, Dalton & Dalton 1987).

ADVERSE REACTIONS

Pyridoxine is considered non-toxic, although nausea and vomiting, headache, paraesthesia, sleepiness and low-serum folic acid levels have been reported.

Supplements taken at night may result in more vivid dreams and, for some individuals, disrupted sleep (Ebben et al 2002).

SIGNIFICANT INTERACTIONS

Amiodarone

Pyridoxine may increase the risk of drug-induced photosensitivity. Exercise caution with patients taking pyridoxine and amiodarone concurrently.

Antibiotics

Destruction of gastrointestinal flora can decrease endogenous production of vitamin B_6. Increase intake of vitamin B_6-rich foods or consider supplementation with long-term drug treatment.

Hydralazine

Hydralazine may induce B_6 deficiency according to a clinical study. Increased intake may be required with long-term drug therapy.

Isoniazid

Isoniazid increases vitamin B_6 requirements. Increase intake of vitamin B_6-rich foods or consider supplementation with long-term drug treatment.

L-dopa (without carbidopa)

In people with PD, L-dopa can cause hyperhomocysteinaemia, the extent of which is influenced by B vitamin status. To maintain normal plasma homocysteine concentrations, the B vitamin requirements are higher in L-dopa-treated patients than in those not on L-dopa therapy. B vitamin supplements may be warranted for PD patients on L-dopa therapy (Miller et al 2003).

Oral contraceptives

Oral contraceptives increase vitamin B_6 requirements. Increase intake of vitamin B_6-rich foods or consider supplementation with long-term drug treatment.

Penicillamine

This drug increases vitamin B_6 requirements. Increase intake of vitamin B_6-rich foods or consider supplementation.

Phenobarbitone, phenytoin

Vitamin B_6 supplements may lower plasma levels and efficacy of these drugs. Monitor for drug effectiveness, and exercise caution when these drugs are being taken concurrently.

Theophylline

May induce pyridoxine deficiency. Increased intake may be required with long-term drug therapy.

CONTRAINDICATIONS AND PRECAUTIONS

Monitor long-term use of high-dose pyridoxine supplements (>100 mg, although this level varies between individuals).

PREGNANCY USE

Pyridoxine supplements are commonly used during pregnancy to reduce symptoms of morning sickness, suggesting safety when used in appropriate doses.

Practice points/Patient counselling

- Vitamin B_6 is available in many foods; however, several surveys suggest that inadequate intakes are common.
- Deficiency can manifest with psychological symptoms of depression, irritability and confusion, and physical symptoms of lethargy, dermatitis, angular stomatitis, glossitis and impaired immunity.
- Overall, clinical research supports the use of vitamin B_6 supplements in relieving mild to moderate symptoms of PMS (particularly breast tenderness and mood disturbance), nausea in pregnancy and as a treatment for hyperhomocysteinaemia (usually with folate and B_{12}).
- Preliminary evidence suggests regular high dietary B_6 intake may have a protective effect in colorectal, breast, bladder and ovarian cancer risk, incidence of improvement of IBS symptomatology and possibly all-cause mortality.
- There is conflicting evidence as to whether vitamin B_6 supplements improve symptoms of CTS and autism (combined with magnesium), and whether they prevent febrile convulsions in children.
- Pyridoxine should not be used in high doses for the long term, as this can induce toxicity.

PATIENTS' FAQs

What will this vitamin do for me?

Vitamin B_6 is essential for the body's normal functioning. It has been used to treat many different conditions; however, scientific evidence generally supports its use in only a few conditions (e.g. morning sickness, mild to moderate PMS and elevated homocysteine levels).

When will it start to work?

This will depend on what is being treated. With regard to PMS symptoms, effects may take two to three menstrual cycles, whereas for morning sickness effects can be seen within 2–3 days.

Are there any safety issues?

High doses should not be taken for the long term, as this can cause toxicity.

REFERENCES

Abbas ZG, Swai ABM. Evaluation of the efficacy of thiamine and pyridoxine in the treatment of symptomatic diabetic peripheral neuropathy. East African Medical Journal 1997;74(12):803–8.

Adams JB et al. Abnormally high plasma levels of vitamin B_6 in children with autism not taking supplements compared to controls not taking supplements. J Altern Complement Med 12.1 (2006): 59–63.

Agarwal N, et al. Response of therapy with vitamin B_6, B_{12} and folic acid on homocystein level and pregnancy outcome in hyperhomocysteinaemia with unexplained recurrent abortions. International journal of Gynaecology and Obstetrics, 2012; 119(3):S759.

Albert CM et al. Effect of folic acid and B vitamins on risk of cardiovascular events and total mortality among women at high risk for cardiovascular disease: a randomized trial. JAMA 299.17 (2008): 2027–2036.

Anand SS. Protective effect of vitamin B_6 in chromium-induced oxidative stress in liver. J Appl Toxicol 25.5 (2005): 440–443.

Ang CD, et al. Vitamin B for treating peripheral neuropathy. Cochrane Database Syst Rev, 2008. CD004573.

Baldewicz T et al. Plasma pyridoxine deficiency is related to increased psychological distress in recently bereaved homosexual men. Psychosom Med 60.3 (1998): 297–308.

Balk EM et al. Vitamin B_6, B_{12}, and folic acid supplementation and cognitive function: a systematic review of randomized trials. Arch Intern Med 167.1 (2007): 21–30.

Beers MH, Berkow R (eds). The Merck manual of diagnosis and therapy, 17th edn. Whitehouse, NJ: Merck, 2003.

Bernstein AL. Vitamin B_6 in clinical neurology. Ann NY Acad Sci 585 (1990): 250–260.

Bleie O et al. Homocysteine-lowering therapy does not affect inflammatory markers of atherosclerosis in patients with stable coronary artery disease. J Intern Med 262.2 (2007): 141–272.

Bratman S, Kroll D. Natural health bible. Rocklin, CA: Prima Health, 2000.

Bryan J, et al. Short term folate vitamin B_{12} or vitamin B_6 supplementation slightly affects memory performance but not mood in women of various ages. Journal of Nutrition 2002;132(6):1345–56.

Bsat F, et al. Randomized study of three common outpatient treatments for nausea and vomiting of pregnancy [abstract]. American Journal of Obstetrics and Gynecology 2001;185(6 Suppl): S181.

Buyukokuroglu ME et al. Pyridoxine may protect the cerebellar granular cells against glutamate-induced toxicity. Int J Vitam Nutr Res 77.5 (2007): 336–340.

Chen J, et al. (2005) One-carbon metabolism, MTHFR polymorphisms, and risk of breast cancer. Cancer Res 65: 1606–1614.

Cheng CH et al. Vitamin B_6 supplementation increases immune responses in critically ill patients. Eur J Clin Nutr 60.10 (2006): 1207–1213.

Chittumma P, et al. Comparison of the effectiveness of ginger and vitamin B_6 for treatment of nausea and vomiting in early pregnancy: a randomized double-blind controlled trial. J Med Assoc Thai 90.1 (2007): 15–20.

Cho E, et al (2007) Nutrients involved in one-carbon metabolism and risk of breast cancer among premenopausal women. Cancer Epidemiology, Biomarkers & Prevention 16: 2787–2790.

Clarke R et al. Effects of B-vitamins on plasma homocysteine concentrations and on risk of cardiovascular disease and dementia. Curr Opin Clin Nutr Metab Care 10.1 (2007): 32–9.

Combs GF Jr. The Vitamins (Fourth Edition) Chapter 13 — Vitamin B_6. 2012, Pages 309–323. London: Elsevier

CTSUESU (Clinical Trial Service Unit and Epidemiological Studies Unit, Oxford, United Kingdom). Homocysteine-lowering trials for prevention of cardiovascular events: A review of the design and power of the large randomized trials. Am Heart J 151.2 (2006): 282–287.

Dalton K, Dalton MJ. Characteristics of pyridoxine overdose neuropathy syndrome. Acta Neurol Scand 76.1 (1987): 8–11.

Davis LS. Stress, vitamin B_6 and magnesium in women with and without dysmenorrhea: a comparison and intervention study [dissertation]. Austin (TX): University of Texas at Austin, December 1988.

Deijen JB, et al. Vitamin B_6 supplementation in elderly men effects on mood memory performance and mental effort. Psychopharmacology 1992;109(4):489–96.

De Lau LM et al. Dietary folate, vitamin B_{12}, and vitamin B_6 and the risk of Parkinson disease. Neurology 67.2 (2006): 315–3118.

Den Heijer MH et al. Homocysteine lowering by B vitamins and the secondary prevention of deep vein thrombosis and pulmonary embolism: A randomized, placebo-controlled, double-blind trial. Blood 109.1 (2007): 139–144.

Diaz-Arrastia R et al. P1-163: C-reactive protein in aging and Alzheimer's disease: Correlation with cerebral atrophy and low plasma vitamin B6. Alzheimers Dement 2.3, Supplement 1 (2006): S143.

Diegoli MS et al. A double-blind trial of four medications to treat severe premenstrual syndrome. Int J Gynaecol Obstet 62.1 (1998): 63–67.

Dror DK, Allen LH. Paediatric and Perinatal Epidemiology, 2012, 26 (Suppl. 1), 55–74.

Ebben M et al. Effects of pyridoxine on dreaming: a preliminary study. Percept Mot Skills 94.1 (2002): 135–140.

Ellis JM et al. A deficiency of vitamin B_6 is a plausible molecular basis of the retinopathy of patients with diabetes mellitus. Biochem Biophys Res Commun 179.1 (1991): 615–6119.

Ensiyeh J, Sakineh MAC. Comparing ginger and vitamin B_6 for the treatment of nausea and vomiting in pregnancy: a randomised controlled trial. Midwifery 2009;25(6):649–53.

Erickson KI et al. Greater intake of vitamins B_6 and B_{12} spares gray matter in healthy elderly: A voxel-based morphometry study. Brain Res 1199 (2008): 20–26.

Ericson U, et al (2007) High folate intake is associated with lower breast cancer incidence in postmenopausal women in the Malmo Diet and Cancer cohort [see comment]. Am J Clin Nutr 86: 434–443.

Festin, M Nausea and vomiting in early pregnancy. Clinical Evidence 2009;06:1405.

Figueiredo CJ et al. Vitamins B_2, B_6, and B_{12} and risk of new colorectal adenomas in a randomized trial of aspirin use and folic acid supplementation. Cancer Epidemiol Biomarkers Prev 17.8 (2008): 2136–2145.

Findling RL et al. High-dose pyridoxine and magnesium administration in children with autistic disorder: an absence of salutary effects in a double-blind, placebo-controlled study. J Autism Dev Disord 27.4 (1997): 467–478.

Flicker L et al. B-vitamins reduce plasma levels of beta amyloid. Neurobiol Aging 29.2 (2008): 303–305.

Ford AH, Almeida OP. Effect of homocysteine lowering treatment on cognitive function: a systematic review and meta-analysis of randomized controlled trials. J Alzheimers Dis. 2012;29(1):133–49.

Galluzzi L, et al. Prognostic impact of vitamin B_6 metabolism in lung cancer. Cell Reports 2012; 2:257–269.

Garcia-Closas R et al. Food, nutrient and heterocyclic amine intake and the risk of bladder cancer. Eur J Cancer 43.11 (2007): 1731–1740.

Gerritsen AA et al. Conservative treatment options for carpal tunnel syndrome: a systematic review of randomised controlled trials. J Neurol 249.3 (2002): 272–280.

Gerster H. The importance of vitamin B_6 for development of the infant: Human medical and animal experiment studies. Ernahrungswiss 35.4 (1996): 309–317.

Groff JL, Gropper SS. Advanced nutrition and human metabolism. Belmont, CA: Wadsworth, 2009.

Gropper, S., Smith, J Advanced nutrition and human metabolism, 6th edition. Belmont, CA: Wadsworth, Cengage Learning, 2013.

Harris, H. R., et al. (2012), Folate, vitamin B_6, vitamin B_{12}, methionine and alcohol intake in relation to ovarian cancer risk. Int. J. Cancer, 131: E518–E529.

Hillman RW, et al. The effects of pyridoxine supplements on the dental caries experience of pregnant women. American Journal of Clinical Nutrition 1962;10:512–5.

Hillman R, et al. Pyridoxine supplementation during pregnancy. Clinical and laboratory observations. American Journal of Clinical Nutrition 1963;12:427–30.

Hlais S, et al. Effect of lysine, vitamin B_6, and carnitine supplementation on the lipid profile of male patients with hypertriglyceridemia: a 12-week, open-label, randomized, placebo-controlled trial. Clinical Therapeutics, 2012; 34:8.

Hron G et al. Low vitamin B_6 levels and the risk of recurrent venous thromboembolism. Haematologica 92.9 (2007): 1250–1253.

Huang, Y, et al. Prediction of all-cause mortality by B group vitamin status in the elderly. Clinical Nutrition 31 (2012) 191–198.

Hwang IK et al. Time course of changes in pyridoxal 5'-phosphate (vitamin B_6 active form) and its neuroprotection in experimental ischemic damage. Exp Neurol 206.1 (2007): 114–125.

Ishihara J et al. Low intake of vitamin B-6 is associated with increased risk of colorectal cancer in Japanese men. J Nutr 137.7 (2007): 1808–1814.

Jain S. Vitamin B_6 supplementation and complications of diabetes. Metab 56.2 (2007): 168–1071.

Ji Y et al. Pyridoxine prevents dysfunction of endothelial cell nitric oxide production in response to low-density lipoprotein. Atherosclerosis 188.1 (2006): 84–94.

Kałużna-Czaplińska J, et al. Nutritional deficiencies in children an example of autistic children. Nowa Pediatria 2009;4:94–100.

Kałużna-Czaplińska J, et al. Vitamin supplementation reduces the level of homocysteine in the urine of autistic children. Nutr Research 31, 2011; 318–321.

Kaluzna-Czaplinska, J., et al. 2013. A focus on homocysteine in autism. Acta Biochim.Pol., 60, (2) 137–142.

Kamiishi A et al. A clinical study of the effectiveness of vitamin B_6 for the prevention of repeated convulsions during one febrile episode. Brain Dev 18 (1996): 471–478.

Kannan K, Jain SK. Effect of vitamin B_6 on oxygen radicals, mitochondrial membrane potential, and lipid peroxidation in H_2O_2-treated U937 monocytes. Free Radic Biol Med 36.4 (2004): 423–428.

Kant AK, Block G. Dietary vitamin B-6 intake and food sources in the US population: NHANES II, 1976–1980. Am J Clin Nutr 52.4 (1990): 707–716.

Kashanian M et al. The evaluation of the effectiveness of pyridoxine (vitamin B_6) for the treatment of premenstrual syndrome: A double blind randomized clinical trial. Eur Psychiatry 23 Supplement 2 (2008): S381.

Keith ME, et al. B-vitamin deficiency in hospitalized patients with heart failure. J Am Diet Assoc. 2009;109(8): 1406–1410.

Kuriyama S, et al. Pyridoxine treatment in a subgroup of children with pervasive developmental disorders. Developmental Medicine & Child Neurology, 2002; 44:283–286.

Lajous M, et al (2006) Folate, vitamin B(6), and vitamin B(12) intake and the risk of breast cancer among Mexican women. Cancer Epidemiol Biomarkers Prev 15: 443–448.

Lakshmi AV, Ramalakshmi BA. Effect of pyridoxine or riboflavin supplementation on plasma homocysteine levels in women with oral lesions. Natl Med J India 11.4 (1998); as cited by Court S. A controlled trial of pyridoxine supplementation in children with febrile convulsions. Clin Pediatr 20.3 (1981): 208–11.

Lakshmi Priya MD, Geetha A. Level of trace elements (copper, zinc, magnesium and selenium) and toxic elements (lead and mercury) in the hair and nail of children with autism. Biol Trace Elem Res 2011; 142: 142–158.

Larsson SC et al. Vitamin B_6 intake, alcohol consumption, and colorectal cancer: A longitudinal population-based cohort of women. Gastroenterology 128.7 (2005): 1830–1837.

Larsson SC, et al (2007) Folate and risk of breast cancer: a meta-analysis. J Natl Cancer Inst 99: 64–76.

Larsson SC, et al. Vitamin B_6 and risk of colorectal cancer: a meta-analysis of prospective studies. JAMA. 2010;303(11):1077–1083.

Lerner V et al. Vitamin B_6 treatment for tardive dyskinesia: a randomized, double-blind, placebo-controlled, crossover study. J Clin Psychiatry 68.11 (2007): 1648–1654.

Levine J et al. Homocysteine-reducing strategies improve symptoms in chronic schizophrenic patients with hyperhomocysteinemia. Biol Psychiatry 60.3 (2006): 265–269.

Ligaarden S C & Farup R G. Low intake of vitamin B_6 is associated with irritable bowel syndrome symptoms. Nutrition Research 31 (2011) 356–361.

Lurie, G, et al. Prediagnositic plasma pyridoxal 5-phosphate (Vitamin B_6) levels and invasive breast carcinoma risk: the multiethnic cohort. Cancer Epidemiol Biomarkers Prev 2012; 21(11); 1942–8.

Malouf R, Grimley Evans J. Vitamin B_6 for cognition. Cochrane Database of Systematic Reviews 2003, Issue 4. Art. No.: CD004393.

Mann JF et al. Homocysteine lowering with folic acid and B vitamins in people with chronic kidney disease — results of the renal Hope-2 study. Nephrol Dial Transplant 23.2 (2008): 645–53.

Marcus J et al. Homocysteine lowering and cardiovascular disease risk: lost in translation. Can J Cardiol 23.9 (2007): 707–10.

Marlowe M, et al. Decreased magnesium in the hair of autistic children. J Orthomol psychiatry 1984;13:117–22.

Martí-Carvajal AJ, et al. Homocysteine-lowering interventions for preventing cardiovascular events. Cochrane Database of Systematic Reviews 2013, Issue 1. Art. No.: CD006612.

Martignoni E et al. Homocysteine and Parkinson's disease: a dangerous liaison? J Neurol Sci 257.1–2 (2007): 31–37.

Matthews A, et al. Interventions for nausea and vomiting in early pregnancy. Cochrane Database of Systematic Reviews 2010, Issue 9. Art. No.: CD007575.

Matxain JM et al. Theoretical study of the reaction of vitamin B_6 with 1O2. Chemistry 13.16 (2007): 4636–4642.

McCarty MF. High-dose pyridoxine as an 'anti-stress' strategy. Med Hypotheses 54.5 (2000): 803–807.

McKeag NA., et al. The role of micronutrients in heart failure. Journal of the Academy of Nutrition and Dietetics, 2012; 1.12: 870–886.

McKiernan J et al. A controlled trial of pyridoxine supplementation in children with febrile convulsions. Clin Pediatr (Phila) 20.3 (1981): 208–211.

Miller JW et al. Effect of L-dopa on plasma homocysteine in PD patients: relationship to B-vitamin status. Neurology 60.7 (2003): 1125–1129.

Miner SE et al. Pyridoxine improves endothelial function in cardiac transplant recipients. J Heart Lung Transplant 20.9 (2001): 964–969.

Mintzer S, et al. B-Vitamin deficiency in patients treated with antiepileptic drugs. Epilepsy & Behavior 24 (2012) 341–344.

Mousain-Bosc M et al. Improvement of neurobehavioral disorders in children supplemented with magnesium-vitamin B_6. II. Pervasive developmental disorder-autism. Magnes Res 19.1 (2006): 53–62.

Mulder C et al. Low vitamin B_6 levels are associated with white matter lesions in Alzheimer's disease. J Am Geriatr Soc 53.6 (2005): 1073–1074.

Nakamura S et al. Pyridoxal phosphate prevents progression of diabetic nephropathy. Nephrol Dial Transplant 22.8 (2007): 2165–2174.

Nye C, Brice A. Combined vitamin B_6-magnesium treatment in autism spectrum disorder. Cochrane Database Syst Rev 4 (2005): CD003497.

Ohtahara S, et al. Vitamin B_6 treatment of intractable seizures. Brain & Development 33 (2011) 783–789.

Oka T. Modulation of gene expression by vitamin B_6. Nutr Res Rev. 2001; 14:257–65.

Pelton R et al. Drug-induced nutrient depletion handbook 1999–2000. Hudson, OH: Lexi-Comp, 2000.

Petronijevic ND et al. Plasma homocysteine levels in young male patients in the exacerbation and remission phase of schizophrenia. Prog Neuropsychopharmacol Biol Psychiatry 32.8 (2008): 1921–1926.

Pfeiffer SI et al. Efficacy of vitamin B_6 and magnesium in the treatment of autism: a methodology review and summary of outcomes. J Autism Dev Disord 25.5 (1995): 481–493.

Piazzini DB et al. A systematic review of conservative treatment of carpal tunnel syndrome. Clin Rehabil 21.4 (2007): 299–314.

Potter K et al. Long-term treatment with folic acid, vitamin B_6 and vitamin B_{12} does not improve vascular structure or function: A randomised double-blind placebo-controlled trial. Heart Lung Circ 16 Supplement 2 (2007): S168.

Proctor M & Murphy PA. Herbal and dietary therapies for primary and secondary dysmenorrhoea. Cochrane Database Syst Rev 2001 (2009): CD002124.

Raman G et al. Heterogeneity and lack of good quality studies limit association between folate, vitamins B-6 and B-12, and cognitive function. J Nutr 137.7 (2007): 1789–1794.

Ray JG et al. Homocysteine-lowering therapy and risk for venous thromboembolism: a randomized trial. Ann Intern Med 146.11 (2007): 761–767.

Ren SG, Melmed S. Pyridoxal phosphate inhibits pituitary cell proliferation and hormone secretion. Endocrinology 147.8 (2006): 3936–3942.

Sahakian V, et al. Vitamin B_6 is effective therapy for nausea and vomiting of pregnancy: a randomized, double-blind placebo-controlled study. Obstetrics & Gynecology 1991;78:33–6.

Schuster K, et al. Effect of maternal pyridoxine-HCl supplementation on the vitamin B-6 status of mother and infant and on pregnancy outcome. Journal of Nutrition 1984;114:977–88.

Sharma P et al. Role of bromocriptine and pyridoxine in premenstrual tension syndrome. Indian J Physiol Pharmacol 51.4 (2007): 368–374.

Shimada D et al. Effect of high dose of pyridoxine on mammary tumorigenesis. Nutr Cancer 53.2 (2005): 202–207.

Shimada D et al. Vitamin B_6 suppresses growth of the feline mammary tumor cell line FRM. Biosci Biotechnol Biochem 70.4 (2006): 1038–1040.

Shizukuishi S et al. Distribution of vitamin B_6 deficiency in university students. Tokyo: J Nutr Sci Vitaminol 27.3 (1981) 193–7.

Shrubsole MJ, et al. Dietary B vitamin and methionine intakes and breast cancer risk among Chinese women. Am J Epidemiol. 2011 May 15;173(10):1171–82.

Smith C, Crowther C. Ginger was as effective as vitamin B_6 in improving symptoms of nausea and vomiting in early pregnancy. Evidence-based Obstetrics & Gynecology 7.2 (2005): 60–61.

Smith C, et al. A randomized controlled trial of ginger to treat nausea and vomiting in pregnancy. Obstetrics & Gynecology 2004; 103(4):639–45.

So Y, Simon R. Chapter 57 Deficiency diseases of the nervous system. in Bradley's Neurology in Clinical Practice, 6th edn. Philadelphia, PA: Saunders, 2012.

Sohrabvand F et al. Vitamin B supplementation for leg cramps during pregnancy. Int J Gynaecol Obstet 95.1 (2006): 48–49.

Song, Y, et al. Effect of combined folic acid, vitamin B_6, and vitamin B_{12} on colorectal adenoma. JNCI J Natl Cancer Inst (2012) 104 (20): 1562–1575.

Sripramote M, Lekhyananda N. A randomized comparison of ginger and vitamin b6 in the treatment of nausea and vomiting in pregnancy. Journal of the Medical Association of Thailand 2003;86:846–53.

Stevens VL, et al (2010) Folate and other one-carbon metabolism-related nutrients and risk of postmenopausal breast cancer in the Cancer Prevention Study II Nutrition Cohort. Am J Clin Nutr 91: 1708–1715.

Swartwout JR, et al. Vitamin B_6, serum lipids and placental arteriolar lesions in human pregnancy. A preliminary report. American Journal of Clinical Nutrition 1960;8:434–44.

Tanimoto M et al. Effect of pyridoxamine (K-163), an inhibitor of advanced glycation end products, on type 2 diabetic nephropathy in KK-Ay/Ta mice. Metabolism 56.2 (2007): 160–167.

Temesvari P, et al. Effects of an antenatal load of pyridoxine (vitamin B_6) on the blood oxygen affinity and prolactin levels in newborn infants and their mothers. Acta Paediatrica Scandinavica 1983;72: 525–9.

Thaver D, et al. Pyridoxine (vitamin B_6) supplementation in pregnancy. Cochrane Database of Systematic Reviews 2006, Issue 2. Art. No.: CD000179.

Theodoratou E et al. Dietary vitamin B_6 intake and the risk of colorectal cancer. Cancer Epidemiol Biomarkers Prev 17.1 (2008): 171–182.

Till U et al. Decrease of carotid intima-media thickness in patients at risk to cerebral ischemia after supplementation with folic acid, vitamins B_6 and B_{12}. Atherosclerosis 181.1 (2005): 131–135.

Toole JF et al. Lowering homocysteine in patients with ischaemic stroke to prevent recurrent stroke, myocardial infarction and death. JAMA 291 (2004): 565–75.

Van Dam F, Van Gool WA. Hyperhomocysteinemia and Alzheimer's disease: A systematic review. Arch Gerontol Geriatr 48.3 (2008): 425–430.

Vutyavanich T, et al. Pyridoxine for nausea and vomiting of pregnancy: a randomized, double-blind, placebo-controlled trial. American Journal of Obstetrics and Gynecology 1995;173:881–4.

Wahlqvist M (ed). Food and nutrition. Sydney: Allen & Unwin, 1997.

Wardlaw G. Contemporary nutrition, 3rd edn. Madison, WI: Brown and Benchmark, 1997.

Weingaertner J et al. Initial findings on teratological and developmental relationships and differences between neural tube defects and facial clefting: First experimental results. J Cranio-Maxillofacial Surg 33.5 (2005): 297–300.

Whelan AM, et al. Herbs, vitamins and minerals in the treatment of premenstrual syndrome: a systematic review. Can J Clin Pharmacol. 2009 Fall;16(3):e407–29.

Wibowo N, et al. Vitamin B_6 supplementation in pregnant women with nausea and vomiting. International Journal of Gynecology and Obstetrics 116, 2012: 206–210.

Wilcken DE, Wilcken B. B vitamins and homocysteine in cardiovascular disease and aging. Ann NY Acad Sci 854 (1998): 361–370.

Wyatt KM et al. Efficacy of vitamin B-6 in the treatment of premenstrual syndrome: systematic review. BMJ 318.7195 (1999): 1375–1381.

Xia W, et al. A preliminary study on nutritional status and intake in Chinese children with autism. Eur J Pediatr 2010;169:1201–6.

Xu T et al. Treatment of hyperhomocysteinemia and endothelial dysfunction in renal transplant recipients with B vitamins in the Chinese population. J Urol 179.3 (2008): 1190–1194.

Yang D, et al. Dietary intake of folate, B-vitamins and methionine and breast cancer risk among Hispanic and Non-Hispanic white women. 2013 PLoS ONE 8(2): e54495.

Zhang X, et al. Prospective cohort studies of vitamin B_6 intake and colorectal cancer incidence: modification by time? Cancer Epidemiol Biomarkers Prev March 2012; 21; 560.

Zhang X-H, et al Vitamin B_6 and colorectal cancer: Current evidence and future directions. World J Gastroenterol 2013; 19(7): 1005–1010.

Zhou K, et al Association between B-group vitamins and venous thrombosis: systematic review and meta-analysis of epidemiological studies. Journal of Thrombosis and Thrombolysis 2012, Volume 34, Issue 4, pp 459–467.

Vitamin C

HISTORICAL NOTE Vitamin C deficiency has been known for many centuries as scurvy, a potentially fatal condition, dreaded by seamen in the 15th century, who were often forced to subsist for months on diets of dried beef and biscuits. It was also described by the European crusaders during their numerous sieges. In the mid-1700s Lind was the first doctor to conduct systematic clinical trials of potential cures for scurvy, identifying oranges and lemons as successful treatments (Bartholomew 2002). However, it was not until 1928 that vitamin C (then known as antiscorbutic factor) was isolated, leading to mass production in the mid-1930s.

Clinical note — Differences between major forms of vitamin C supplements

Here is a brief summary of the most common forms found in over-the-counter supplements.

- Ascorbic acid. The major dietary form of vitamin C.
- Mineral ascorbates (also known as non-acid vitamin C). These are buffered forms of vitamin C and believed to be less irritating to the stomach than ascorbic acid. Sodium ascorbate and calcium ascorbate are the most common forms. When mineral salts are taken, both the ascorbic acid and the mineral are absorbed. For example, sodium ascorbate generally provides 131 mg of sodium per 1000 mg of ascorbic acid, and calcium ascorbate provides 114 mg of calcium per 1000 mg of ascorbic acid.
- Vitamin C with bioflavonoids. Many bioflavonoids are antioxidant substances and are added to some vitamin C preparations in the belief that this increases the bioavailability or efficacy of vitamin C. Typically, the bioflavonoids are sourced from citrus fruits.
- Ascorbyl palmitate. A fat-soluble form of vitamin C formed by esterification with palmitic acid and most often used in topical creams.

BACKGROUND AND RELEVANT PHARMACOKINETICS

Vitamin C is an essential water-soluble nutrient for humans and required in the diet on a regular basis, as we are one of few species of animals that cannot synthesise it. This is because humans lack the enzyme L-gulonolactone oxidase, which is required for the conversion of glucose into vitamin C (Braunwald et al 2003).

The bioavailability of ascorbic acid is dependent on both intestinal absorption and renal excretion. Vitamin C, consumed either in the diet or as dietary supplements, is absorbed by the epithelial cells of the small intestine by the sodium vitamin C co-transporter 1 (SVCT1) and subsequently diffuses into the surrounding capillaries and then passes into the circulatory system (Li & Schellhorn 2007). Ultimately, the degree of absorption depends on the dose ingested and decreases as the dose increases. This is because, at low concentrations, most vitamin C is absorbed in the small intestine and reabsorbed from the renal tubule, but at high concentrations SVCT1 becomes saturated, which, combined with ascorbate-mediated SVCT1 downregulation, limits the amount of ascorbic acid absorbed from the intestine and reabsorbed from the kidney (Li & Schellhorn 2007). For this reason, oral vitamin C is best absorbed when it is ingested in small doses at regular intervals. Complete plasmatic saturation occurs at 1000 mg daily with a concentration of around 100 microM (Verrax & Buc Calderon 2008). Pectin and zinc are also able to impair oral absorption. These limitations are bypassed with the use of intravenously administered vitamin C, which can achieve much higher plasma levels than oral administration.

Following its absorption, ascorbic acid is ubiquitously distributed in the cells of the body. Within the body, the highest levels of ascorbic acid are found in the adrenal glands, the white blood cells, skeletal muscles and the brain, especially in the pituitary gland (Verrax & Buc Calderon 2008). Interestingly, the brain is the most difficult organ to deplete of ascorbate. As a polar compound with a relatively large molecular weight, vitamin C cannot readily cross the cell membrane by simple diffusion. The flux of vitamin C in and out of the cell is controlled by specific mechanisms, including facilitated diffusion and active transport, which are mediated by distinct classes of membrane proteins such as facilitative glucose transporters (GLUT) and SVCT respectively (Li & Schellhorn 2007). Once in cells, dehydroascorbic acid (the oxidised form of ascorbate) is rapidly reduced to ascorbate (Harrison & May 2009). Eventually it is metabolised in the liver, filtered by the kidneys and excreted in the urine. The biological half-life of vitamin C is 8–40 days (NHMRC 2006).

Clinical note — Deficiencies in smokers

It is well established that smokers have lowered vitamin C status than non-smokers and therefore have higher requirements for vitamin C. Vitamin C status is inversely related to cigarette use (Cross & Halliwell 1993). The depletion of plasma ascorbic acid associated with cigarette smoking was first described in the late 1930s. Reports have shown that low ascorbic acid concentrations in the plasma, leucocytes and urine of both male and female cigarette smokers are associated with increased numbers and activity of neutrophils, which suggests increased utilisation and lower intake, or reduced bioavailability, of vitamin C in smokers than in non-smokers (Northrop-Clewes & Thurnham 2007).

CHEMICAL COMPONENTS

Vitamin C exists as both its reduced form (L-ascorbic acid) and its oxidised form (L-dehydroascorbic acid). The two forms interchange in the body in a reversible equilibrium.

FOOD SOURCES

Vitamin C is found in many different fruits and vegetables. The most concentrated food sources are blackcurrants, sweet green and red peppers, hot red peppers, green chilli peppers, oranges and fresh orange juice, and strawberries. Other good sources are watermelon, papaya, citrus fruits, cantaloupe, mango, cabbage, cauliflower, broccoli and tomato juice. In practice, vegetables may be a more important source of vitamin C than fruits because they are often available for longer periods during the year.

The vitamin C content of food is strongly influenced by many factors, such as season, transportation, shelf-life, storage conditions and storage time, cooking techniques and chlorination of water (FAO/WHO 2002). Cutting or bruising food will reduce its vitamin C content; however, blanching or storing at low pH will preserve it.

Up to 100% of the vitamin C content of food can be destroyed during cooking and storing because the vitamin is sensitive to light, heat, oxygen and alkali

(Wahlqvist 2002). Additionally, using too much water during cooking can leach the vitamin from food and further reduce its vitamin C content.

DEFICIENCY SIGNS AND SYMPTOMS

In adults, scurvy remains latent for 3–6 months after reducing dietary intake to less than 10 mg/day (Beers & Berkow 2003). It manifests when the body pools fall below 300–400 mg (NHMRC 2006). Many of the features of frank vitamin C deficiency (scurvy) result from a defect in collagen synthesis.

Early symptoms are:

- weakness
- fatigue and listlessness
- muscular weakness
- petechial haemorrhages and ecchymoses (bruising)
- swollen gums
- poor wound healing and the breakdown of recently healed wounds
- poor appetite and weight loss
- emotional changes such as irritability and depression
- vague myalgias and arthralgias
- congested hair follicles.

Symptoms of more severe deficiency are:

- fever
- drying of the skin and mucous membranes
- susceptibility to infection
- bleeding gums and loosening of teeth
- oedema of the lower extremities
- anaemia
- joint swelling and tenderness, due to bleeding around or into the joint
- oliguria
- pain in the extremities
- haemorrhage
- convulsions
- shock
- eventually death if left untreated.

Although frank deficiency is uncommon in Western countries, marginal deficiency states are not uncommon.

Primary deficiency

This occurs if there is an inadequate dietary intake, which is often caused by a combination of poor cooking and eating habits. It occurs in areas of urban poverty, during famine and war, in young children fed exclusively on cow's milk for a prolonged period, in the institutionalised or isolated elderly, and in chronic alcoholics (Pimentel 2003, Richardson et al 2002). One Australian hospital identified that 73% of all new admissions had hypovitaminosis C and 30% had levels suggestive of scurvy (Richardson et al 2002).

Secondary deficiency

Factors that increase nutritional requirements include cigarette smoking, pregnancy, lactation, thyrotoxicosis, acute and chronic inflammatory diseases, major surgery and burns, infection and diabetes (Beers & Berkow 2003, FAO/WHO 2002, Hendler & Rorvik 2001, Wahlqvist 2002). Decreased vitamin C absorption in achlorhydria and increased excretion in chronic diarrhoea also increase the risk of deficiency, particularly when combined with poor dietary intake.

MAIN ACTIONS

Vitamin C is an electron donor (reducing agent or antioxidant), and this accounts for most of its biochemical and molecular functions. It is involved in many biochemical processes in the body, such as:

- energy release from fatty acids
- metabolism of cholesterol
- reduction of nitrosamine formation in the stomach
- formation of thyroid hormone
- carnitine biosynthesis
- modulation of iron and copper absorption
- corticosteroid biosynthesis
- protection of folic acid reductase, which converts folic acid to folinic acid
- collagen biosynthesis
- tyrosine biosynthesis and catabolism
- neurotransmitter biosynthesis.

The main actions of vitamin C are summarised below.

Antioxidant and pro-oxidant

At physiological concentrations, vitamin C is the most effective aqueous antioxidant in plasma, interstitial fluids and soluble phases of cells. As such, it is one of the most important water-soluble antioxidant substances in the body, acting as a potent free radical scavenger in the plasma, protecting cells against oxidative damage caused by reactive oxygen species (ROS). It scavenges free radical oxygen and nitrogen species such as superoxide, hydroxyl, peroxyl and nitroxide radicals and non-radical reactive species such as singlet oxygen, peroxynitrite and hypochlorite (FAO/WHO 2002, Hendler & Rorvik 2001). Besides having a direct antioxidant function, it also indirectly increases free radical scavenging by regenerating vitamin E (Vatassery 1987) and maintaining glutathione in reduced form. Much of the vitamin's physiological role stems from its very strong reducing power (high redox potential) and its ability to be regenerated using intracellular reductants such as glutathione, nicotinamide adenine dinucleotide and nicotinamide adenine dinucleotide phosphate (Chaudière & Ferrari-Iliou 1999).

In the presence of oxidised metal ions (e.g. Fe^{3+}, Cu^{2+}), high concentrations of ascorbic acid can have pro-oxidant functions at least in vitro, thereby promoting oxidative damage to DNA. The effect does not appear to be significant under normal physiological conditions in vivo; however, when used at higher pharmacological concentrations (0.3–20 mmol/L), ascorbic acid displays transition metal-independent pro-oxidant activity, which is more profound in cancer cells than healthy cells and causes cell death (Li & Schellhorn 2007).

Whether vitamin C functions as an antioxidant or pro-oxidant is determined by at least three factors: (1) the redox potential of the cellular environment; (2) the presence/absence of oxidised metal ions; and (3) the local concentrations of ascorbate (Li & Schellhorn 2007).

Maintenance of connective tissue

Vitamin C maintains the body's connective tissue and is essential for the formation of collagen, the major fibrous element of blood vessels, skin, tendon, cartilage and teeth (Morton et al 2001). If collagen is produced in the absence of vitamin C, it is unstable and cannot form the triple helix required for normal tissue structure. Vitamin C is involved in the biosynthesis of other substances important for connective tissue, such as elastin, proteoglycans, bone matrix, fibronectin and elastin-associated fibrillin (Hall & Greendale 1998).

These effects have been harnessed by the dermatological and cosmetic industries and are the rationale for producing topically applied products containing vitamin C.

Collagen stability

Vitamin C is necessary for the synthesis of collagen proteins, whereby it is involved in the hydroxylation of specific prolyl and lysyl residues of the unfolded procollagen chain. These reactions are catalysed by the enzymes prolyl 4-hydroxylase and prolyl 3-hydroxylase, which stabilise collagen molecules, and lysyl hydroxylase enzyme, responsible for collagen molecule cross-linking (Ochiai et al 2006, Traikovich 1999). In vivo and in vitro studies have explored topical vitamin C effects on melanogenesis and ageing.

Brain and nerve function

Ascorbate is involved in neurotransmitter synthesis. It is a cofactor required for the biosynthesis of noradrenaline from dopamine and hydroxylation of tryptophan to produce serotonin. It also acts as a modulator of glutaminergic, cholinergic and GABAergic transmission (Bornstein et al 2003, FAO/WHO 2002, Harrison & May 2009). Furthermore, it is involved in neural maturation and acts as a neuroprotective agent (Harrison & May 2009),

Immunostimulant

Ascorbic acid affects the immune system in several different ways and there is abundant evidence that the immune system is sensitive to circulating levels of vitamin C. Ascorbic acid modulates T-cell gene expression, specifically affecting genes involved with signalling, carbohydrate metabolism, apoptosis, transcription and immune function. It can also stimulate the production of interferons, the proteins that protect cells against viral attack and stimulate the synthesis of humoral thymus factor and antibodies of the immunoglobulin G (IgG) and IgM classes (Combs 2012).

Both in vivo and in vitro studies provide evidence of immunostimulant effects, generally at doses beyond recommended dietary intake (RDI) levels (Hendler & Rorvik 2001). In high doses, it is a potent immunomodulator and is preferentially cytotoxic to neoplastic cells. Vitamin C enhances the activity of natural killer cells in vivo and also both B- and T-cell activity (Drisko et al 2003).

Leucocytes maintain high levels of ascorbate which are correlated with their function. In fact, leucocyte ascorbate levels are 20–100 times higher than plasma levels. The uptake occurs via active transport which is temperature- and energy-dependent. Many infections and inflammatory diseases lower plasma and neutrophil ascorbate levels. Clinically, an association exists between recurrent infections and impaired neutrophil function. Adequate ascorbate nutrition improves several aspects of neutrophil activity, especially chemotaxis, proliferation and motility. Vitamin C can enhance neutrophil chemotaxis and motility, even in healthy individuals (Combs 2012, Muggli 1998).

In addition to these direct effects on the immune system, the antioxidant properties of vitamin C play a role. When neutrophils are activated during infection, they release free radicals. However, neutrophils are susceptible to free radical damage themselves. Protection against auto-oxidation is afforded by ascorbic acid together with other antioxidants and is essential during the mobilisation of host defences. Apart from its own effects, vitamin C helps immune function indirectly by protecting the antioxidant capacity of vitamin E, which is an immune-enhancing nutrient in its own right (Muggli 1998).

Antihistamine

Ascorbic acid is involved in histamine metabolism, acting with Cu^{2+} to inhibit its release and enhance its degradation (Combs 2012).

An inverse association has been identified between blood histamine levels and vitamin C status in humans (Johnston et al 1996). In that study, increasing vitamin C status with supplements (up to 250 mg/day) over 3 weeks was shown to decrease histamine levels. It is unclear whether single, high-dose supplementation also affects histamine levels, as two studies using 2 g doses have produced conflicting results (Bucca et al 1990, Johnston et al 1992).

Anticancer

In millimolar concentrations, vitamin C is selectively cytotoxic to many cancer cell lines and has in vivo anticancer activity when administered alone or together with other agents (Hoffer et al 2008). Importantly, pharmacological concentrations of ascorbic acid (0.3–20 mmol/L) are required to find evidence of cytotoxicity in vitro and in vivo, whereas physiological concentrations of ascorbic acid (0.1 mmol/L) do not have any effect on either tumour or normal cells (Li & Schellhorn 2007). The most reliable method of achieving these high doses is with intravenous (IV) administration of vitamin C and not via the oral route, which has limited absorption (Padayatty et al 2006). The effect is clearly dose-dependent and mediated via several mechanisms, such as immunomodulation, inhibition of cell division and growth, gene regulation and induction of apoptosis. One mechanism of cytotoxicity demonstrated in several models is the ability of ascorbate at pharmacological concentrations to exert pro-oxidant activity, generating hydrogen peroxide-dependent cytotoxicity towards a variety of cancer cells in vitro and in vivo without adversely affecting normal cells (Chen et al 2008, Tamayo & Richardson 2003).

Much investigation has been undertaken to understand how preferential cytotoxicity is achieved; however, the mechanisms are still largely unknown. For example, studies with radioactive-labelled vitamin C have found that tumour cells accumulate more vitamin C than healthy cells, whereas other studies have reported no differences in intracellular concentrations (Prasad et al 2002). There is also some preliminary evidence of synergistic cytotoxic effects and decreased drug toxicity with some pharmaceutical anticancer agents (Giri et al 1998).

One theory proposed to explain the preferential targeting of tumour cells relates to their overexpression of facilitative GLUTs (Gatenby & Gillies 2004) and dehydroascorbic acid, transported by GLUTs, accumulating within the tumour cells, which enables intracellular hydrogen peroxide levels to increase (Chen et al 2005, Verrax & Buc Calderon 2008, Zhang et al 2001). Other intrinsic properties of cancer cells may also be involved, such as reduced concentrations of antioxidant enzymes (e.g. catalase and superoxide dismutase) and increased intracellular transitional metal availability, both of which further augment free radical production (Li & Schellhorn 2007). Alternatively, it has been suggested that extracellular ascorbate is the source of this anticancer effect and is more important than intracellular vitamin C.

V

There are a number of factors that may be contributing to the inconsistent results obtained to date, such as the variable characteristics of the subjects studied, type of infecting virus, lack of control for dietary vitamin C intake and differences in measures of outcomes. Clearly, further investigation is required to clarify many issues surrounding the use of vitamin C supplements for upper respiratory tract infections (URTIs). In practice, naturopaths often recommend megadoses of vitamin C (taken frequently, in small amounts), which are well beyond the doses investigated so far, and often report good results. Although anecdotal, it is interesting to note that little research has investigated this method.

Modulation of gene expression

Many transcription factors, such as NF-κB, AP-1 or peroxisome proliferator-activated receptors, are redox-regulated, and moderate amounts of oxidative stress are known both to modulate gene expression and to signal transduction cascades by affecting kinases, phosphatases as well as Ca^{2+} signalling. L-ascorbic acid may modulate relatively unspecific gene expression by affecting the redox state of transcription factors and of enzymes involved in signal transduction (Table 1).

OTHER ACTIONS

High oral doses (4–12 g/day in divided doses) can acidify urine.

Ascorbic acid greatly enhances iron bioavailability from food. Within the body, ascorbic acid promotes the utilisation of haem iron, which appears to involve enhanced incorporation of iron into its intracellular storage form, ferritin. This effect involves facilitation of ferritin synthesis and enhanced ferritin stability (Combs 2012).

Vitamin C can also interact with other nutritional metals, reducing their toxicity, such as selenium, nickel, lead, vanadium and cadmium. This is achieved by interacting with them to create a reduced form which is poorly absorbed or more rapidly excreted (Combs 2012).

CLINICAL USE

Vitamin C is an important biological antioxidant and has been a popular nutritional supplement for decades. It is administered as intramuscular or IV injections and used topically and orally. This review will chiefly focus on oral and topical use, as these are the forms of vitamin C most commonly used by the public.

Deficiency: prevention and treatment

Traditionally, vitamin C supplements are used both to treat and to prevent deficiency. Treatment may include 250 mg vitamin C daily and encouragement to eat fresh fruits and vegetables on a regular basis (Kumar et al 2002), or 100 mg taken 3–5 times daily until 4000 mg has been reached (Braunwald et al 2003). Some deficiency symptoms start to respond within 24 hours, although most take from several weeks to months to resolve completely.

Iron-deficiency anaemia

Ascorbic acid is a potent enhancer of iron absorption. Vitamin C facilitates iron absorption by forming soluble complexes and may be used with an iron supplement and nutritious diet in the treatment of iron-deficiency anaemia. It is specifically helpful in increasing absorption of iron from plant-based foods. It is also recommended for women with menorrhagia in order to reduce the risk of iron deficiency.

Dermatological uses

Vitamin C is used as an oral supplement or topical application in a number of dermatological conditions.

Wound healing

Vitamin C is important for effective wound healing, as deficiency contributes to fragile granulation tissue and therefore impairs the wound-healing process (Russell 2001).

TABLE 1 KNOWN OR PUTATIVE GENES AND ENZYMATIC ACTIVITIES RESPONSIVE TO L-ASCORBIC ACID

Gene	Cellular process involved	Mechanism	Expression/ activity with L-ascorbic acid
h1-Calponin	VSMC phenotypic modulation	?	↑
h-Caldesmon	VSMC phenotypic modulation	?	↑
SM22α	VSMC phenotypic modulation	?	↑
α-SM actin	VSMC phenotypic modulation	?	↑
Collagen I	Matrix production	Transcription, mRNA stability	↑
Collagen III	Matrix production	Transcription, mRNA stability	↑
Elastin	Elasticity of arterial wall, VSMC phenotypic modulation	mRNA stability	↓
MMP2	Matrix degradation	?	↓
TIMP1	Inhibits matrix degradation	?	↑
Calponin 1	VSMC phenotypic modulation	?	↑
Myosin heavy chain-1	VSMC phenotypic modulation	?	↑
GATA4	Cardiac development	?	↑
Nkx2.5	Cardiac development	?	↑
ANF	Regulation of cardiac and vascular tone	?	↑
eNOS	Vascular homeostasis	Increased intracellular Ca^{2+}	↑
Prolyl hydroxylase	Stability and secretion of collagen	Cofactor	↑
ICAM-1	Cell adhesion	?	↓
Enzymes involved in carnitine synthesis	Fatty acid metabolism	Cofactor (epsilon-*N*-trimethyllysine hydroxylase and gamma-butyrobetaine hydroxylase)	↑

VSMC, vascular smooth-muscle cell.
Adapted from Villacorta et al (2007).

V

In vitro studies with skin graft samples have demonstrated that vitamin C extends cellular viability, promotes formation of an epidermal barrier and promotes engraftment (Boyce et al 2002). In this way, vitamin C is used to enhance wound healing before surgery has commenced.

Numerous case reports of surgical and dental patients generally suggest a use for vitamin C supplementation in doses beyond RDI as a means of enhancing the rate of wound healing (Ringsdorf & Cheraskin 1982). One early double-blind study found that vitamin C (500 mg twice daily) resulted in a significant mean reduction in pressure sore area of 84% after 1 month compared with 43% in the placebo group (Taylor et al 1974). The mean rates of healing were 2.47 cm^2 for vitamin C and 1.45 cm^2 for the placebo.

Photo-damaged skin

Two double-blind studies investigating the effects of topical preparations of vitamin C on photo-damaged skin have demonstrated good results after 3 months' use (Fitzpatrick & Rostan 2002, Humbert et al 2003). One study tested a topical application of 5% vitamin C in a cream base, whereas the other used a newly formulated vitamin C complex having 10% ascorbic acid (water-soluble) and 7% tetrahexyldecyl ascorbate (lipid-soluble) in an anhydrous polysilicone gel base.

Prevention of sunburn

One controlled study found oral vitamin C (2000 mg/day) in combination with vitamin E (1000 IU/day) had a protective effect against sunburn after 8 days' treatment in human subjects (Eberlein-Konig et al 1998). Similar results have been obtained for topical vitamin C preparations in several animal models (Darr et al 1992, 1996, JY Lin et al 2003) and a small human study (Keller & Fenske 1998). The latter found that application of an aqueous 10% L-ascorbic acid solution after ultraviolet B (UVB) radiation produced a significant reduction in the minimal erythema dose and a less intense erythematous response than controls.

As with many nutrients, studies associating dietary vitamin intake and disease risk are difficult to interpret. This is because it is difficult to separate the effects of the individual vitamin from the effects of other components in the diet. Where possible, an effort has been made to include information that will help in the interpretation of this type of data.

Hyperpigmentation

The beneficial effects of vitamin C on skin hyperpigmentation and ageing are mostly attributed to its antioxidant properties and key role in collagen production. The efficacy of vitamin C in hyperpigmentation disorders has been investigated in small studies, mostly as an adjunctive therapy. Hwang et al (2009) studied the efficacy of a formulation containing 25% L-ascorbic and a chemical penetration enhancer for the treatment of melasma. A 16-week open-label trial was conducted and 40 subjects were involved. The skin was assessed every month, and results showed significant decrease in pigmentation with the treatment. Espinal-Perez et al (2004) conducted a double-blind randomised trial comparing 5% L-ascorbic acid and 4% hydroquinone for melasma treatment. They concluded L-ascorbic acid to have beneficial effects on hyperpigmentation with minimal side effects, and therefore, to be a viable single or adjunctive long-term therapy for melasma (Espinal-Perez et al 2004). Results show that vitamin C has the ability to significantly improve abnormal skin pigmentation caused by chronic UV radiation exposure, including melasma.

Antiageing

Vitamin C antioxidant properties contribute to its antiageing effect as well, since ROS are known to interfere with fibroblasts and to destroy collagen and connective tissue structures. Vitamin C is a well-known potential antiageing agent due to its antioxidant effect and major role in collagen production (Humbert et al 2003, Park et al 2009, Taniguchi et al 2012, Traikovich 1999). A 3-month randomised double-blind vehicle-controlled study was conducted to determine the efficacy of topical vitamin C in photo-damaged skin. Clinical assessment showed significant improvement in many features, including fine wrinkles, tactile roughness, laxity and tone. Self-assessment questionnaire demonstrated that 84.2% of the subjects preferred the side treated with vitamin C. Photographic assessment showed vitamin C-treated skin to have 57.9% greater improvement compared to controls and optical profilometry analysis demonstrated improvement with active treatment up to 73.7% greater than control (Traikovich 1999).

Upper respiratory tract infections

Vitamin C is widely used both to prevent and to treat common URTIs, such as the common cold and influenza, largely based on its effects on the immune system, its ability to reduce histamine levels and the observations that the gastrointestinal absorption of vitamin C increases in the common cold (suggesting an increased demand for this nutrient) and that vitamin C concentrations in the plasma and leucocytes rapidly decline during infection (Wilson et al 1976, Wintergerst et al 2006). Although extremely popular, its usefulness in these conditions is widely debated.

A meta-analysis of 29 trials involving 11,306 participants was undertaken to assess the risk ratio (RR) of developing a cold while taking vitamin C regularly over the study period (Hemilä & Chalker 2013). To be eligible for inclusion, at least 200 mg daily of vitamin C was required and each study needed to have a placebo arm. The most promising results were obtained for children and athletes. Five trials involving a total of 598 marathon runners, skiers and soldiers on subarctic exercises yielded a pooled RR of 0.48, indicating that regular vitamin C supplementation significantly reduced the incidence of the common cold in this population. For the studies involving children, using a dose of 1–2 g/daily, vitamin C shortened the duration of colds by 18% and also reduced the severity of the cold infection. In regard to the general adult community (n = 10708), the pooled RR was 0.97, indicating similar effects to placebo and the duration was only slightly reduced, by 8% (3–12%), and in children by 14% (7–21%). Overall, the review concluded that routine vitamin C supplementation did not reduce the incidence of colds in the general population, yet vitamin C may be useful for people exposed to brief periods of severe physical exercise.

It has been suggested that the dose used may affect the magnitude of the benefit, there being on average greater benefit from ≥2 g/day compared to 1 g/day of vitamin C. In five studies with adults administered 1 g/day of vitamin C, the median decrease in cold duration was only 6%, whereas in two studies with children administered 2 g/day the median decrease was four times higher, 26% (Hemilä 1999).

Vitamin C taken in combination with zinc may be more successful, according to clinical trials. Both nutrients play a role in immune function and dietary intakes can be low. When the results of two double-blind, randomised, placebo-controlled trials utilising a combination of 1000 mg vitamin C plus 10 mg zinc in patients with the common cold are pooled together, the combination was significantly more efficient than placebo at reducing rhinorrhoea over 5 days of treatment.

Furthermore, symptom relief was quicker and the product was well tolerated (Maggini et al 2012).

Reduction in all-cause mortality

Several studies have identified an inverse association between plasma ascorbate levels, vitamin C intake and all-cause mortality. This means that low serum ascorbic acid levels are associated with higher all-cause mortality and in some studies, higher cardiovascular disease (CVD) mortality and cancer mortality.

In the Western Electric Company study, data on diet and other factors were obtained in 1958 and 1959 for a cohort of 1556 employed middle-aged men and an inverse association between vitamin C and mortality was identified (Pandey et al 1995). The next year, a prospective cohort study conducted with 725 older adults also identified an inverse relationship between vitamin C blood concentrations and total mortality during a 12-year follow-up (Sahyoun et al 1996). Similar results were obtained in the large European Prospective Investigation into Cancer and Nutrition (EPIC)-Norfolk study of 19,496 men and women aged 45–79 years (Khaw et al 2001). Plasma ascorbate concentration was inversely related to mortality from all causes, and from CVD and ischaemic heart disease in both men and women. Risk of mortality in the group with the highest intake was about half that of the low intake group and was independent of age, systolic blood pressure (SBP), serum cholesterol, cigarette smoking, diabetes or supplement use.

The Second National Health and Nutrition Examination Survey (NHANES II) mortality study further confirmed the inverse association between plasma ascorbate and risk of dying from all causes; however, this study identified a gender difference (Loria et al 2000). After adjustments for race, educational level, number of cigarettes smoked at baseline, serum total cholesterol, SBP, body mass index, diabetes status and alcohol consumption, men in the lowest serum ascorbate quartile (serum ascorbate concentrations <28.4 micromol/L) had a 57% higher risk of dying from any cause than did men in the highest quartile (>73.8 micromol/L). Additionally, men in the lowest serum ascorbate quartile had double the risk of dying from cancer than those in the highest quartile after adjustment for age. The dose corresponds to approximately 60 mg/day vitamin C. In contrast, among women no association was observed between quartiles of serum ascorbate concentration and total mortality or mortality from CVD or cancer.

As an extension to this, Simon et al (2001) identified that, amongst the 8453 Americans aged ≥ 30 years at baseline in the NHANES II, low serum ascorbic acid levels were marginally associated with an increased risk of fatal CVD and significantly associated with an increased risk for all-cause mortality (Simon et al 2001). Conversely, people with normal to high serum ascorbic acid levels had a marginally significant 21–25% decreased risk of fatal CVD (P for trend = 0.09) and a 25–29% decreased risk of all-cause mortality (P for trend < 0.001) compared to people with low level. Low serum ascorbic acid levels were also a risk factor for cancer death in men, but unexpectedly were associated with a decreased risk of cancer death in women. In other words, among men, normal to high serum ascorbic acid levels were associated with an approximately 30% decreased risk of cancer deaths, whereas such serum ascorbic acid levels were associated with an approximately twofold increased risk of cancer deaths among women.

A gender difference was also reported in the NHANES I Epidemiologic Follow-up Study (NHEFS) (Enstrom et al 1992). Vitamin C intakes >50 mg/day plus regular supplement use were associated with reduced mortality, compared with intakes <50 mg/day in men, but apparently not in women.

Prevention of cardiovascular disease

The association between vitamin C and CVD prevention is still unclear, although several themes are emerging as evidence accumulates.

In general, epidemiological studies show that low vitamin C intake is associated with higher CVD mortality and risk of heart failure and conversely higher levels are associated with lower risk, whereas interventional studies are less consistent (Carr & Frei 1999, Houston 2005, Khaw et al 2001, Knekt et al 2004, Kushi et al 1996, Lopes et al 1998, MRC/BHF 2002, Ness et al 1996, Nyyssonen et al 1997, Osganian et al 2003).

For example, subjects in NHANES I with the highest vitamin C intakes showed less cardiovascular death (standardised mortality ratio, 0.66; 95% confidence limits, 0.53–0.83) than subjects with lower estimated vitamin C intakes (Enstrom et al 1992). In the NHANES III survey of 8453 Americans, low serum ascorbic acid levels were marginally associated with an increased risk of fatal CVD (Simon et al 2001). A study by Toohey et al (1996) provides some rationale for the coronary heart disease (CHD)-preventive effects seen. In their trial, a significant inverse correlation was found between plasma ascorbic acid levels and both systolic ($P < 0.0001$) and diastolic blood pressure (DBP) ($P < 0.03$), and between plasma ascorbic acid and serum total cholesterol ($P < 0.03$), low-density lipoprotein (LDL)-cholesterol (LDL-C) ($P < 0.004$), and the ratio of LDL-cholesterol to high-density lipoprotein (HDL)-cholesterol (LDL-C : HDL-C) ($P < 0.004$). Serum HDL-cholesterol was positively related to plasma ascorbic acid ($P < 0.05$). When multiple regression analysis was applied, ascorbic acid was shown to be a significant independent contributor to the prediction of blood pressure and LDL-C concentration (Toohey et al 1996).

More recently, the European Prospective Investigation into Cancer and Nutrition study in Norfolk, United Kingdom, identified that the risk of heart failure decreased with increasing plasma vitamin C; the hazard ratios comparing each quartile with the lowest were 0.76 (95% confidence interval [CI] 0.65–0.88), 0.70 (95% CI 0.60–0.81) and 0.62 (95% CI 0.53–0.74) in age- and sex-adjusted analyses (*P* for trend < 0.0001) (Pfister et al 2011). This means that, for every 20 micromol/L increase in plasma vitamin C concentration, there was an accompanying 9% relative reduction in risk of heart failure after adjustment for age, sex, smoking, alcohol consumption, physical activity, occupational social class, educational level, SBP, diabetes, cholesterol concentration and body mass index, with similar result if adjusting for interim CHD. The study analysed results from 9187 healthy men and 11,112 women aged 39–79 years.

Possible mechanisms

Ascorbic acid is inversely related to several risk factors and indicators of atherosclerotic CVD, including hypertension and elevated concentrations of LDL, acute-phase proteins and haemostatic factors (Price et al 2001). More specifically, vitamin C inhibits oxidative modification of LDL cholesterol directly through free radical scavenging activity according to in vitro data, and indirectly by increasing glutathione and vitamin E concentrations within cell membranes. This has been demonstrated against the pro-oxidant combination of homocysteine and iron (Alul et al 2003) and may have implications for other diseases such as Alzheimer's dementia.

V

Other evidence suggests that other mechanisms are also likely to be involved. Vitamin C is linked to endothelial function and glucose metabolism. It improves endothelial dysfunction in smokers, renal transplant recipients, patients with CVD after a fatty meal, people with intermittent claudication diabetes and those with hypertension (Kaufmann et al 2000, Ling et al 2002, Silvestro et al 2002,

Solzbach et al 1997, Williams et al 2001), but not in healthy elderly people (Singh et al 2002). It is also required for collagen synthesis and metabolism, and has been shown to reduce arterial stiffness and platelet aggregation in healthy male volunteers, smokers and non-smokers, and diabetics (Schindler et al 2002, Wilkinson et al 1999). These effects are often observed with doses several times higher than current RDI levels. In vivo studies further indicate that vitamin C decreases carotid wall thickness, downregulates inducible nitric oxide (NO) synthase expression, normalises gene expression of antioxidant enzymes and inhibits plaque maturation (Kaliora et al 2006).

A 1997 review of epidemiological studies showed some inverse associations between SBP, DBP or both and vitamin C plasma concentration or intake (Ness et al 1997). Three more recent studies have supported this finding (Bates et al 1998, Block 2002, Block et al 2001). Four intervention studies investigated the effects of vitamin C supplementation, with three producing positive results (Duffy et al 1999, Fotherby et al 2000, Galley et al 1997, Ghosh et al 1994). The doses used were typically 250 mg twice daily for a period of 6–8 weeks, although effects have been reported after 4 weeks' treatment. The negative study by Ghosh et al showed a significant reduction in both SBP and DBP with ascorbic acid. This became non-significant when compared with the placebo responses, although the placebo and ascorbic acid groups were not evenly matched for baseline plasma ascorbate concentration.

Additionally, plasma ascorbate concentrations have been shown to be inversely correlated to pulse rate in one cross-sectional study involving 500 subjects (Bates et al 1998).

Nitrate tolerance

Preliminary studies seem to support the role of vitamin C in attenuating the development of nitrate tolerance. Three human studies have found that vitamin C administration prevents the development of nitrate tolerance (Bassenge et al 1998, Watanabe et al 1998a, 1998b). Although the mechanism responsible is not yet known, results from a double-blind study using an acute dose of 2 g have suggested that vitamin C is likely to protect NO from inactivation by oxygen free radicals (Wilkinson et al 1999), which could in part explain its observed effects.

Myocardial infarction (MI)

Two prospective studies in men have suggested that ascorbic acid deficiency and marginal deficiency predict subsequent MI, independently of classical risk factors. The first, a 5-year prospective population study of 1605 middle-aged Finnish men, free of coronary disease at baseline, found that a significantly higher percentage (13.2%) of the 91 men with baseline plasma vitamin C concentrations less than 11.4 micromol/L (2.0 mg/L) experienced MI, compared with men with higher plasma vitamin C levels (Nyyssonen et al 1997). These results are particularly impressive because low plasma ascorbate was the strongest risk factor of all the measured factors. The second, a 12-year follow-up study, revealed a significantly increased relative risk of ischaemic heart disease and stroke at initially low plasma levels of vitamin C (<22.7 micromol/L), independently of vitamin E and of the classical cardiovascular risk factors (Gey et al 1993).

In contrast, one smaller study involving 180 male patients with a first acute MI, but no recent angina, failed to detect an association between low plasma concentration of vitamin C and the risk of acute MI (Riemersma et al 2000). Similarly, analysis from the NHANES III survey, which involved 7658 men and women, found that among participants who reported no alcohol consumption, serum ascorbic acid concentrations were not independently associated with CVD prevalence (Simon & Hudes 1999). Among participants who consumed alcohol, serum ascorbic acid concentrations consistent with tissue saturation (1.0–3.0 mg/dL) were associated with a decreased prevalence of angina (multivariate odds ratio (OR) 0.48; 95% CI 0.23–1.03%; *P* for trend = 0.06), but were not significantly associated with MI or stroke prevalence.

Clinical studies involving vitamin C supplementation

Interventional studies with supplements have been performed; however, many use vitamin C in combination with other nutrients such as vitamin E, making it difficult to assess the contribution of vitamin C alone.

One review which analysed studies that only used supplemental vitamin C produced encouraging results. Knekt et al (2004) analysed results from nine prospective studies and a 10-year follow-up whereby 4647 major incident CHD events occurred in 293,172 subjects who were free of CHD at baseline (Knekt et al 2004). They found that people with higher supplemental vitamin C intake had a lower CHD incidence. Compared with subjects who did not take supplemental vitamin C, those who took >700 mg supplemental vitamin C daily had a relative risk of CHD incidence of 0.75 (0.60, 0.93; *P* for trend < 0.001). Interestingly, dietary intake of antioxidant vitamins was only weakly related to a reduced CHD risk after adjustment for potential non-dietary and dietary confounding factors and, compared with subjects in the lowest dietary intake quintiles for vitamins E and C, those in the highest intake quintiles had relative risks of CHD incidence of 0.84 (95% CI 0.71–1.00; *P* = 0.17) and 1.23 (95% CI 1.04–1.45; *P* = 0.07), respectively.

IN COMBINATION

The Women's Antioxidant Cardiovascular Study tested the effects of vitamin C (500 mg daily), vitamin E (600 IU every other day) and beta-carotene (50 mg every other day) on the combined outcome of MI, stroke, coronary revascularisation or CVD death among 8171 female health professionals at increased risk. Participants were 40 years of age or older, with a prior history of CVD or three or more CVD risk factors, and were followed for an average 9.4 years. The study's factorial design enabled a comparison to be made between individual test agents as well as combination therapy. Overall, there was no significant effect for the individual nutrients vitamin C, vitamin E or beta-carotene on the primary combined end point, or on the individual secondary outcomes of MI, stroke, coronary revascularisation or CVD death. A marginally significant reduction in the primary outcome with active vitamin E was observed among the prespecified subgroup of women with prior CVD (RR = 0.89, *P* = 0.04). With regard to combination therapy, people receiving both vitamins C and E experienced fewer strokes (*P* = 0.03), but there were no other significant findings (Cook et al 2007).

Effects on blood pressure

Although epidemiological evidence and prospective clinical trials point strongly to a role of vitamin C in reducing blood pressure in hypertensive and normotensive subjects, controlled studies have been inconsistent (Houston 2005). Interpretation of these results is difficult, as some studies lack a control group, have no baseline readings, use variable vitamin C doses and population characteristics, and do not report serum vitamin C or oxidative stress status. Overall, it appears that doses between 100 mg and 1000 mg of vitamin C daily are required for a reduction in blood pressure, with greater reduction in SBP than DBP and greater response in people with higher initial value.

There is a large body of evidence that ROS produced during myocardial ischaemia and reperfusion play a crucial role in myocardial damage and endothelial dysfunction. As a result, there has been some investigation to determine whether antioxidant supplementation (chiefly vitamins C and E) may improve the clinical outcome of patients with acute MI and limit the size of the infarct.

According to a large, randomised, double-blind, multicentre trial of 800 patients (mean age 62 years) with acute MI and receiving standard care, co-treatment with vitamin C (1000 mg/12 hours infusion) followed by 1200 mg/day orally and vitamin E (600 mg/day) for 30 days resulted in significantly less frequent incidence of reinfarction and other post-MI complications compared to a placebo (14% versus 19% respectively) (Jaxa-Chamiec et al 2005). Another randomised, double-blind, placebo-controlled study of 37 patients with acute MI investigated the effects of starting supplementation with vitamins C and E (600 mg/day each) on the first day of symptoms and continuing for a further 14 days (Bednarz et al 2003). Active treatment resulted in significantly lower exercise-induced QT-interval dispersion compared to a placebo, although baseline QT dispersion was similar in both groups. A prospective, randomised study of 61 patients further suggests that oral vitamin C administration (1 g/day) could be beneficial for patients at higher thrombotic risk post-MI, such as those with diabetes (Morel et al 2003).

Postmenopausal cardiovascular health

Across multiple large clinical trials, vitamin C supplementation, alone or in combination with vitamin E and betacarotene, appears to be ineffective at secondary prevention of CHD in pre- and postmenopausal women (Bjelakovic et al 2007, Cook et al 2007, Heart Protection Study Collaborative Group 2002, Waters et al 2002). However, observational studies evaluating vitamin C for primary prevention of CHD have found conflicting results in women (Gale et al 1995, Osganian et al 2003).

Cancer: prevention and treatment

One of the most important modifiable determinants of cancer risk is diet. Several research panels and committees have independently concluded that high fruit and vegetable intake decreases the risk of many types of cancer and, because vitamin C is present in large quantities in these foods, it is plausible that the reduction in cancer risk associated with the consumption of fruits and vegetables may be, at least in part, attributable to dietary vitamin C (Li & Schellhorn 2007).

Clinical note — Vitamin C for cancer: a historical perspective

More than three decades ago, the well-known team of Ewan Cameron and Linus Pauling started investigating the effects of high doses of continuous IV vitamin C and oral supplements in treating advanced, incurable cancer. The idea of using vitamin C was born out of the recognition that the outcome of every cancer is determined to a significant extent by the individual's inherent resistance, which in turn is influenced by the availability of certain nutritional factors such as ascorbic acid (Cameron 1982). They have published the results of several trials that have shown enhanced quality of life for some terminal patients and also improvements in objective markers. As a result, a protocol for the use of vitamin C in the treatment of cancer has been developed at the Vale of Leven Hospital, Scotland, the chief site of Cameron and Pauling's investigations (Cameron 1991). The protocol emphasises the importance of using an initial course of IV ascorbate, followed by a maintenance oral dose. Although their results are encouraging, they have been criticised because randomised double-blind principles were not adopted.

Prevention

Epidemiological evidence of a protective effect of dietary vitamin C for non-hormone-dependent cancers is strong (Block 1991a, 1991b). The majority of studies in which a dietary vitamin C intake was calculated have identified a statistically significant protective effect, with high intake conferring approximately a twofold protective effect compared with low intake. In general, most have shown that higher intakes of vitamin C are associated with decreased incidence of cancers of the mouth, throat and vocal cords, oesophagus and stomach, pancreas, colon, rectum, renal cell and lung (Cohen & Bhagavan 1995, FAO/WHO 2002, Jenab et al 2006, Negri et al 2000, You et al 2000). More recently, a case-control study of men in New York found that a higher intake of vitamin C was associated with reduced risk of prostate cancer (McCann et al 2005).

Two other large studies have identified inverse associations between dietary vitamin C and breast cancer risk (Michels et al 2001, Zhang et al 1999). More specifically, the Nurses' Health Study, which involved 83,234 women, detected a strong inverse association between total vitamin C from foods and breast cancer risk among premenopausal women with a positive family history of breast cancer (Zhang et al 1999). Those who consumed an average of 205 mg/day of vitamin C from foods had a 63% lower risk of breast cancer than those who consumed an average of 70 mg/day. A large Swedish population-based prospective study that comprised 59,036 women found that high dietary intakes of ascorbic acid (mean intake 110 mg/day) reduced the risk of breast cancer among women who were overweight and/or had a high intake of linoleic acid (Michels et al 2001).

More recently, a case–control study nested within the EPIC study identified an inverse risk of gastric cancer in the highest versus lowest quartile of plasma vitamin C (Jenab et al 2006). The inverse association was more pronounced in subjects consuming higher levels of red and processed meats, a factor that may increase endogenous *N*-nitroso compound production. It has been proposed that vitamin C protects against gastric cancer because it inhibits carcinogenic *N*-nitroso compound production in the stomach and acts as a free radical scavenger.

Overall, it appears that the protective effect is dose-dependent, with studies finding significant cancer risk reductions in people consuming at least 80–110 mg of vitamin C daily in the long term (Carr & Frei 1999).

Clinical studies

One of the first published studies by Cameron and Pauling (1974) was a phase I–II study in 50 patients with advanced, untreatable malignancies, in which both subjective and objective markers were evaluated. They observed that 27 patients failed to respond to treatment; however, three patients experienced stabilisation of disease, tumour regression occurred in five patients and tumour haemorrhage and necrosis occurred in four patients. Two years later, the same research team published a report that compared the survival rates of 100 terminal cancer patients given supplemental ascorbate as part of their routine management with 1000 patients who were not given the supplement, and observed the mean survival time to be more than 4.2 times longer for the ascorbate subjects (>210 days) than for the controls (50 days) (Cameron & Pauling 1976).

In subsequent years, two randomised, placebo-controlled studies investigating the effects of oral vitamin C supplementation (10 g/day) in terminal cancer patients failed to detect a significant difference in outcome (Creagan et al 1979, Moertel et al 1985). These two studies are often cited as evidence disproving the benefits of vitamin C in cancer treatment; however, the different routes of administration investigated in these studies is an important factor central to the discrepant results (Padayatty & Levine 2000). Maximal plasma vitamin C concentrations achievable by oral administration are limited by the kidney, which eliminates excess ascorbic acid through renal excretion, whereas IV injection bypasses the renal absorptive system, resulting in elevated plasma concentrations to high levels. As such, it has been argued that only IV administration of high-dose ascorbate can produce millimolar plasma concentrations that are toxic to many cancer cell lines.

Scientific interest in the interaction between ascorbic acid and cancer has been reawakened in recent years, with new evidence that in millimolar concentrations (only achievable after parenteral administration) vitamin C is selectively cytotoxic to many neoplastic cell lines, potentiates cytoxic agents and demonstrates anticancer activity alone and in combination with other agents in tumour-bearing rodents (Hoffer et al 2008). Simultaneously, theoretical interest has arisen in the potential of redox-active molecules like menadione, trolox and ascorbic acid to modify cancer biology, especially when administered with cytotoxic drugs.

Intravenous vitamin C

IV administration of vitamin C achieves much higher plasma and urine concentrations than oral dosing and has been proposed as the only viable means of achieving the high concentrations required to induce the antitumour effects exhibited by the vitamin (Padayatty et al 2004). Case studies suggest that this approach can improve patient wellbeing and, in some cases, reduce tumour size and improve survival (Padayatty et al 2006, Riordan et al 2005).

A safety study conducted in 2005 involved 24 late-stage terminal cancer patients who were administered continuous vitamin C infusions of 150–710 mg/kg/day for up to 8 weeks (Riordan et al 2005). This treatment regimen increased plasma ascorbate concentrations to a mean of 1.1 mmol/L and was considered relatively safe. The most common side effects reported were nausea, oedema and dry mouth or skin, and two 'possible' adverse events occurred. One was a patient with a history of renal calculi who developed a kidney stone after 13 days of treatment, and another was a patient who experienced hypokalaemia after 6 weeks. Interestingly, the majority of patients were vitamin C-deficient before treatment.

Clinical trials for phases I and II are currently being conducted using intravenously administered vitamin C in patients with solid tumours. The phase I study was primarily conducted to determine a recommended phase II dose, with secondary objectives to define any toxic effects, detect any preliminary antitumour effects and monitor for preservation of or improvement in quality of life. In the first phase I trial published in 2008, patients with advanced cancer or haematological malignancy were assigned to sequential cohorts infused with 0.4, 0.6, 0.9 and 1.5 g ascorbic acid/kg body weight three times weekly, delivered intravenously (Hoffer et al 2008). This protocol achieved plasma ascorbic acid concentrations of >10 microM for more than 4 hours, which is considered sufficient to induce cancer cell death according to in vitro research. In addition, all patients were provided with a daily multivitamin tablet (Centrum Select, Wyeth) and 400 IU D-alpha-tocopherol twice daily with meals, and, on non-infusion days, 500 mg ascorbic acid twice daily to obviate large shifts in plasma ascorbic acid concentrations. No unusual biochemical or haematological abnormalities were observed, and there were no changes in the social, emotional or functional parameters of quality of life in any cohort. Unlike in the previous case series by Cameron and Pauling (1974), in which acute tumour haemorrhage and necrosis were reported, these effects were not seen in this study (Hoffer et al 2008). Researchers concluded that the promise of ascorbic acid in the treatment of advanced cancer may lie in its combination with cytotoxic agents, where high concentrations might modify either toxicity or response. A phase I–II clinical trial is being planned that will combine IV ascorbic acid with chemotherapy as a first-line treatment in advanced-stage non-small-cell lung cancer, using the dose determined from this study.

Based on the available evidence of antitumour mechanisms and these case reports, further research into this approach is clearly warranted.

Adjunct to oncology treatments

Whether vitamin C improves or hinders responses to standard oncology treatment has been the focus of intense debate for many decades. There are in vitro studies showing that vitamin C can enhance the antitumour activity of cisplatin and doxorubicin (Abdel-Latif et al 2005, Kurbacher et al 1996, Reddy et al 2001, Sarna & Bhola 1993). In vivo evidence shows vitamin C enhances the effectiveness of 5-fluorouracil, doxorubicin, cyclophosphamide and vincristine (Lamson & Brignall 2000, Nagy et al 2003), whereas other studies find no change in drug effect. Although these results are promising, no large randomised studies are available to confirm their significance in humans.

Most recently, vitamin C inactivated the effects of bortezomib, a new proteasome inhibitor approved by the US Food and Drug Administration for the treatment of patients with relapsed multiple myeloma (Zou et al 2006). Interestingly, drug inactivation was not achieved through antioxidative mechanisms.

Evidence from experimental models suggests that vitamin C may also reduce drug toxicity in a dose-dependent manner (Giri et al 1998, Greggi Antunes et al 2000).

Breast cancer

There is limited evidence to support the use of vitamin C in the primary prevention of total cancer incidence, including breast cancer (Lin et al 2009, Moorman et al 2001, Poulter et al 1984). One of the largest studies in women found that vitamin C (500 mg daily) had no effect on the incidence of cancer after 9.4 years of follow-up (Lin et al 2009).

While vitamin C may not significantly reduce the risk of breast cancer, reduced risk of mortality was reported for vitamin C supplements taken after diagnosis, according to a recent meta-analysis of 10 prospective studies (Harris et al 2014). Harris et al (2014) found that postdiagnosis vitamin C supplement use was associated with a reduced risk of mortality. Dietary vitamin C intake was also statistically significantly associated with a reduced risk of total mortality and breast cancer-specific mortality. The studies involved 17,696 breast cancer cases and found the summary RR for postdiagnosis vitamin C supplement use was 0.81 for total mortality (95% CI 0.72–0.91) and 0.85 for breast cancer-specific mortality (95% CI 0.74–0.99). The summary RR for a 100 mg/day increase in dietary vitamin C intake was 0.73 for total mortality (95% CI 0.59–0.89) and 0.78 for breast cancer-specific mortality (95% CI 0.64–0.94) (Harris et al 2014).

Oral cancer

A recent systematic review showed that the pro-oxidant activity of pharmacological ascorbic acid is a part of its dose-dependent bimodal activity and is a result of the proposed Fenton mechanism. In vitro, animal and ex vivo studies of pharmacological ascorbic acid have yielded meritorious results proving vitamin C as an effective cytotoxic agent against oral neoplastic cells with potentially no harming effects on normal cells (Putchala et al 2013).

Clinical note — The debate continues ... to vitamin C or not?

One research group based at the University of Colorado has produced evidence that suggests that vitamin C and other antioxidant nutrients may not only protect healthy cells from damage, but also improve the antitumour effects of standard treatment (Gottlieb 1999). They are currently conducting further research to identify how cell selectivity occurs, but propose that cancer cells may have lost the normal homeostatic regulatory mechanism that stops excessive concentrations of antioxidants from entering the cell. As intracellular levels rise, a series of reactions occurs, resulting in growth inhibition and cell death. Another group at Memorial Sloan Kettering Cancer Center (Gottlieb 1999) argues that tumours already contain higher levels of ascorbic acid than normal cells and have identified a mechanism to explain this observation. As such, they advocate against the use of vitamin C when cytotoxic agents that rely on free radical production are being used.

Prevention of cataracts

Ascorbate has long been known to accumulate in tears and other biofluids, such as cerebrospinal fluid relative to plasma (Patterson & O'Rourke 1987), and lowered levels of vitamin C in the eye have been associated with increased oxidative stress in the human cornea (Shoham et al 2008). Ascorbic acid is thought to be a primary substrate in ocular protection because of its high concentration in the eye. Within the cell, vitamin C helps to protect membrane lipids from peroxidation by recycling vitamin E (May 1999). It is present at high concentrations in vitreous humour (Hanashima & Namiki 1999), cornea (Brubaker et al 2000) and tear film (Dreyer & Rose 1993).

Numerous observational and prospective clinical studies have been performed to examine the effect on cataracts of vitamin C alone or in combination with other antioxidants. Several epidemiological studies have identified an association between vitamin C and cataract incidence (Ferrigno et al 2005, Jacques & Chylack Jr 1991, Jacques et al 1988, Valero et al 2002); however, studies investigating whether supplementation is protective have produced mixed results (Chasan-Taber et al 1999, Chylack et al 2002, Hammond & Johnson 2002, Jacques et al 1997, 2001, Kuzniarz et al 2001, Seddon et al 1994, Taylor et al 2002).

Results from the Harvard Nurses' Health Study, Physicians' Health Study, the Beaver Dam Eye Study and the Australian Blue Mountains study suggest that if protective effects are to be seen, they are most likely when vitamin C is taken for a long period (5–10 years or more) and/or used as part of a multivitamin combination (Kuzniarz et al 2001, Mares-Perlman et al 2000, Seddon et al 1994, Taylor et al 2002).

It is suspected that vitamin C protects the lens of the eye from oxygen-related damage over time by both direct free radical scavenging activity and indirect activity. This is achieved primarily by protecting endogenous alpha-tocopherol (the major lipid-soluble antioxidant of retinal membranes) against oxidation induced by UV radiation and by regenerating it (Stoyanovsky et al 1995).

Diabetes

Vitamin C has several actions that provide a basis for its use in diabetes. It has been reported to lower erythrocyte sorbitol concentrations (important for preventing complications in type 1 diabetes), improve endothelial function (important for slowing atherosclerosis) and reduce blood pressure (Beckman et al 2001, Cunningham 1998). Plasma vitamin C levels seem to play a role in the modulation of insulin activity in aged healthy or diabetic subjects (Paolisso et al 1994) and are inversely related to glycosylated haemoglobin. Additionally, increased free radical production has been reported in patients with diabetes mellitus as a result of hyperglycaemia, which directly induces oxidative stress (Ceriello et al 1998).

Blood glucose

At this stage there are few studies that test the effects of supplemental vitamin C on plasma glucose levels directly. Although one early study demonstrated that an oral dose of 1500 mg vitamin C reduces plasma glucose levels in patients with type 2 diabetes (Sandhya & Das 1981), no further published studies confirm this result.

Endothelial function

The results of studies investigating the role of vitamin C on endothelial function in diabetes have attracted interest.

A double-blind, placebo-controlled study demonstrated that chronic oral vitamin C supplementation (500 mg/day) in type 2 diabetes significantly lowered arterial blood pressure and improved arterial stiffness compared with a placebo (Mullan et al 2002). After 1 month's treatment, SBP fell from 142.1 to 132.3 mmHg, mean pressure from 104.7 to 97.8 mmHg, DBP from 83.9 to 79.5 mmHg and peripheral pulse pressure from 58.2 to 52.7 mmHg, whereas placebo had no effect.

A randomised study of women with a history of gestational diabetes showed that ascorbic acid supplementation resulted in a significant improvement of endothelium-dependent flow-mediated dilatation, with no effect seen for a placebo (Lekakis et al 2000).

However, a randomised, double-blind, placebo-controlled study of vitamin C (800 mg/day for 4 weeks) concluded that high-dose oral vitamin C therapy resulted in incomplete replenishment of vitamin C levels and does not improve endothelial dysfunction and insulin resistance in type 2 diabetes (Chen et al 2006).

The mechanism of action appears to involve several steps, such as reduction in LDL oxidation, enhanced endothelial NO synthase activity and NO bioavailability and reduced insulin resistance, which can cause endothelium-dependent, NO-mediated vasodilation.

Eye health

Diabetes mellitus is associated with a number of ocular complications that can eventually lead to blindness. Vitamin C is found in high concentration in the eye and is thought to be important for protection against free radicals. This may have special significance for people with diabetes mellitus, as most studies have found that their circulating vitamin C levels are at least 30% lower than in people without the disease (Peponis et al 2002). Furthermore, a systematic review (Lee et al 2010) assessing five hospital-based, cross-sectional studies consistently reported that diabetic patients with retinopathy had lower vitamin C levels than those without retinopathy (Ali & Chakraborty 1989, Gupta & Chari 2005, Gurler et al 2000, Rema et al 1995, Sinclair et al 1992).

According to a 2008 Cochrane systematic review (Lopes de Jesus et al 2008) investigating the effectiveness of vitamin C in diabetic retinopathy, no research to date has adequately examined the treatment of diabetic retinopathy with vitamin C or superoxidase dismutase, so it remains unknown whether the intervention has a significant impact on the progress of this complication.

Because of its safety, cost-effectiveness and generally encouraging results, a strategy of adding 200–600 mg of vitamin C to a healthy diet is worth considering for individuals with diabetes type 1 or 2.

Clinical note — Do asthmatic lungs need more antioxidant protection?
In 1999, Kelly et al found that people with mild asthma have low levels of antioxidant nutrient vitamins E and C in their lung lining fluid, even though blood levels of these vitamins may be normal or increased. This observation, together with other factors, indicated that the asthmatic lung is exposed to greater oxidative stress in people with asthma than in non-asthmatics. The researchers suggested that the inflammatory cells in the lungs of asthmatic patients generate more free radical species than those in healthy people, adding to bronchoconstriction, increased mucus secretion and increased airways responsiveness. Given that oral supplementation in asthma has produced inconsistent results, chief researcher Frank Kelly suggests that future studies should focus on other administration forms, such as vitamin C inhalers (personal communication, Melbourne, 1998).

Pneumonia

Three prophylactic trials found a statistically significant (80% or greater) reduction in pneumonia incidence in the vitamin C group. These trials were assessed in a recent Cochrane review, which concluded that the prophylactic use of vitamin C to prevent pneumonia should be further investigated in populations who have a high incidence of pneumonia, especially if dietary vitamin C intake is low (Hemilä & Louhiala 2013).

Asthma

Vitamin C is the major antioxidant present in the extracellular fluid lining of the lung, where it protects against both endogenous free radicals (produced as a byproduct of inflammation) and environmental free radicals (such as ozone in air pollution). Theoretically, it may be of benefit in reducing symptoms of inflammatory airway conditions such as asthma, and may also be beneficial in reducing exercise-induced bronchoconstriction.

According to many epidemiological studies, dietary intake of vitamin C-rich foods or serum ascorbate is associated with improved lung function in both asthmatic and normal subjects (Devereux & Seaton 2005, Kelly 2005, McDermoth 2000). Oxygen metabolites can play a direct or indirect role in the modulation of airway inflammation. Many studies suggest that superoxide dismutase and free radical scavengers in the blood are significantly lower in asthma, and document a correlation between asthmatic severity and ROS products in asthmatic subjects (Shanmugasundaram 2001, Vural 2000). Not surprisingly, low blood concentrations of vitamin C have been found in mildly asthmatic subjects (Rahman 2006).

Despite a theoretical basis for its use in lung diseases such as asthma, its value in this disease is controversial. A 2001 Cochrane review of three studies concluded that current evidence is insufficient to recommend a specific role for vitamin C in the treatment of asthma and that a large-scale randomised controlled trial (RCT) is required to clarify its role (Kaur et al 2001). This was repeated in a Cochrane review published in 2004 that included new data from a study of 201 adults taking inhaled corticosteroids and came to a similar conclusion, stating that evidence is currently conflicting (Ram et al 2004).

A recent Cochrane review (Milan et al 2013) concluded that there is insufficient evidence to provide a robust assessment on the use of vitamin C in the management of asthma or exercise-induced bronchoconstriction. There was some indication that vitamin C was helpful in exercise-induced breathlessness in terms of lung function and symptoms; however, as these findings were provided only by small studies, more research is required before a conclusive recommendation can be made. Three human studies have produced positive results when vitamin C was used as pretreatment in doses ranging from 500 mg to 2000 mg (Cohen et al 1997, Miric & Haxhiu 1991, Schachter & Schlesinger 1982).

Asthma and atopy in children

A systematic review and meta-analysis (Nurmatov et al 2011) assessed 14 papers reviewing the association between vitamin C and asthma or atopic outcomes in children. While some of the studies showed some improvement in wheeze or allergy symptomatology overall, the body of evidence was judged to be methodologically weak and the possible effectiveness of vitamin C to prevent atopic outcomes remains unclear.

Bone mineral density (BMD)

Although the relationship between calcium, vitamin D and BMD is well known, other nutrients, such as vitamin C, are also critical for bone development, repair and maintenance (Ilich et al 2003). Epidemiological studies have demonstrated a positive association between BMD and intake of vitamin C (Hall & Greendale 1998, Leveille et al 1997). Low vitamin C intakes have been associated with a decline in BMD specifically at the femoral neck and total hip (Hall & Greendale 1998).

Data collected from 13,080 adults enrolled in NHANES III from 1988 to 1994 have identified an association between dietary and serum ascorbic acid, BMD and bone fracture (Simon & Hudes 2001). Dietary ascorbic acid intake was independently associated with BMD among premenopausal women and postmenopausal women without a history of smoking or oestrogen use. Additionally, fracture risk fell by 49% in postmenopausal women (with a history of smoking and oestrogen use) who had high serum vitamin C levels.

Vitamin C supplementation

Two controlled studies have investigated the effects of long-term vitamin C supplementation in postmenopausal women and found that it increases BMD (Hall & Greendale 1998, Morton et al 2001). Both studies identified a positive association with BMD in postmenopausal women with dietary calcium intakes of at least 500 mg or those taking calcium supplements. The effect was especially marked in those women taking calcium supplements and concurrent hormone replacement therapy.

The daily dose taken was generally in excess of the RDI and ranged from 100 mg to 5000 mg. More specifically, one study found that, for each 100 mg increment in dietary vitamin C intake, there was an associated increase of 0.017 g/cm^2 in BMD (femoral neck and total hip), and for those women with calcium intakes above 500 mg/day the increment increased to 0.019 g/cm^2 in BMD per 100 mg vitamin C.

An Australian study of 533 randomly selected women determined that vitamin C supplements may suppress bone resorption in non-smoking postmenopausal women (Pasco et al 2006).

In contrast to these results, no effect on BMD was observed for dietary or supplemental vitamin C in the Women's Health Initiative Observational Study and Clinical Trial, which involved 11,068 women aged 50–79 years (Wolf et al 2005). However, a significant beneficial interaction was observed between total vitamin C and hormone replacement therapy on total body, femoral neck, spine and total hip BMD.

Animal studies have detected an improved healing response in bone fractures with supplemental vitamin C, suggesting a further role in fracture healing (Yilmaz et al 2001).

Sports

Vitamin C supplementation is often used by athletes in order to improve recovery, restore immune responses, enhance wound healing and counteract oxidative stress and changes to adrenal hormones and inflammatory responses. It is often taken together with other antioxidant vitamins and minerals, such as vitamin E and zinc. One placebo-controlled study has shown that 20 mg of ascorbic acid twice daily over 14 days has some modest beneficial effects on recovery from unaccustomed exercise (Thompson et al 2001); however, no studies have reported improved performance for vitamin C supplementation.

Prevention of postendurance exercise infections

Athletes often use vitamin C supplements to prevent infections, as strenuous training and physiological stress appear to increase the body's need for vitamin C to a level above the usual RDI (Schwenk & Costley 2002). Additionally, the risk of infection after an intense aerobic training session or competition (such as a marathon) is increased (Jeurissen et al 2003).

A 2004 Cochrane review that analysed results from six trials involving a total of 642 marathon runners, skiers and soldiers on subarctic exercises found regular vitamin C supplementation significantly reduced the incidence of the common cold, supporting its use in this population (Douglas et al 2004).

Alterations to neurotransmitters and adrenal hormones

Several studies have been conducted with ultramarathon runners to investigate whether vitamin C supplementation, usually in doses of 1500 mg/day, is able to restore exercise-induced changes to neurotransmitters, adrenal hormones or inflammatory responses (Nieman et al 2000, Peters et al 2001a, 2001b). Overall, it appears that high-dose vitamin C supplements taken at least 7 days before racing do have some effect.

One study involving 45 ultramarathon runners found that doses of 1500 mg vitamin C taken for 7 days before the race, on the day of the race and for 2 days following the race significantly attenuated exercise-induced elevations in cortisol, adrenaline and interleukin-10 (IL-10) and IL-1 receptor antagonist levels compared with a placebo (Peters et al 2001a); however, the effect was transient.

Male infertility

A relationship between infertility and the generation of ROS has been established and extensively studied. Alterations in the testicular microenvironment and haemodynamics can increase production of ROS and/or decrease local antioxidant capacity, resulting in generation of excessive oxygen species. A large number of studies have elucidated the effects of increased oxygen species in the serum, semen and testicular tissues of patients.

Vitamin C (ascorbic acid), a major antioxidant found in extracellular fluid, is present in seminal fluid at a high concentration compared with that in blood plasma (364 versus 40 microM) and is present in detectable amounts in sperm (Patel & Sigman 2008). In infertile men, vitamin C has been found in reduced quantity in the seminal plasma (Lewis et al 1997). An association between oxidative stress and sperm DNA fragmentation has been identified and has led to studies looking for changes in semen DNA fragmentation as an outcome rather than just changes in semen parameters.

A review of the literature reveals that interventional studies have produced promising but inconsistent results and incomplete reporting of study outcomes. Sometimes changes to semen parameters are noted, but there is little or no information about successful pregnancies or characteristics of the study population, thereby hindering accurate interpretation of results. Clearly further research is required to better evaluate the effects of vitamin C in male fertility.

An RCT of 75 fertile, heavy smokers compared placebo to two different doses of vitamin C (200 mg and 1000 mg) and found that both supplemented groups experienced a significant improvement in sperm concentration, morphology and viability (Dawson et al 1992).

A randomised, placebo-controlled trial found that treatment with oral vitamin C and E of men with unexplained infertility associated with elevated sperm DNA fragmentation led to decreased DNA fragmentation without a change in semen parameters (Greco et al 2005b).

In an uncontrolled study of 38 men with an elevated percentage of fragmented spermatozoa (15%) and one prior failed intracytoplasmic sperm injection (ICSI) attempt, oral supplementation with vitamins E and C demonstrated a significant improvement in pregnancy rate (48.2% vs 6.9%) and implantation rate (19.6% vs 2.2%) when compared with their prior ICSI attempt (Greco et al 2005a).

A systematic review on the effect of oral antioxidants on male infertility evaluated results from 17 RCTs including a total of 1665 men, which differed in the populations studied and type, dosage and duration of antioxidants used. None of the studies assessed vitamin C as a single oral agent; however, when reviewing the effectiveness of vitamin C in conjunction with other antioxidants, the results were as follows. Sperm motility improved in two out of five studies (Omu et al 2008, Scott et al 1998), sperm concentration improved in one out of five studies (Galatioto et al 2008) and sperm DNA fragmentation index was reduced in two out of two studies (Greco et al 2005a, Omu et al 2008). However, sperm morphology did not improve in any of the five studies. Pregnancy rate after ICSI was significantly improved in the treatment group in one study ($P = 0.046$) (Tremellen et al 2007).

Pregnancy

A Cochrane systematic review evaluated results from five RCTs involving 766 women in which vitamin C supplementation was used (Rumbold & Crowther 2005). No difference was seen between women supplemented with vitamin C alone or in combination with other supplements compared with placebo for the risk of stillbirth, perinatal death, birth weight or intrauterine growth restriction. In regard to preterm birth, women supplemented with vitamin C were at increased risk compared to placebo. No difference was seen between women supplemented with vitamin C compared with placebo for the risk of neonatal death whereas a reduced incidence of pre-eclampsia was found with supplementation when using a fixed-effect model.

More recently, another three systematic reviews and meta-analyses concluded that combined vitamin C and E supplementation did not decrease the risk of pre-eclampsia and should not be offered to gravidas for the prevention of pre-eclampsia or other pregnancy-induced hypertensive disorders (Ahmet et al 2010, Conde-Agudelo et al 2011, Rossi & Mullin 2011).

Alzheimer's disease (AD)

A systematic review and meta-analysis reviewed eight RCTs, including a cohort of 223 people diagnosed with AD (da Silva et al 2013). Four studies showed statistically significantly lower plasma levels of vitamin C than in controls (unrelated to the classic malnourishment that is common in patients with AD). However, whether this means AD patients have increased oxidative stress and therefore increased antioxidant requirements which would benefit from vitamin C supplementation remains to be tested.

Periodontal disease

Nishida et al (2000) used data from the NHANES III study, which identified a statistically significant, albeit weak, association between decreased dietary vitamin C intake and increased risk of periodontal disease (OR 1.19). More recently, it was reported from the same NHANES III study that higher serum antioxidant levels were associated with lower ORs of severe periodontitis, with an OR of 0.53 for vitamin C (Chapple et al 2007). In a population of 413 non-institutionalised active older adults in Japan, a significant but weak association was found between serum vitamin C levels and clinical attachment loss (grade of severity of periodontal disease) (Amarasena et al 2005). Clinical attachment loss was 4% greater in subjects with lower serum vitamin C levels compared with subjects with higher serum vitamin C levels. The association was independent of other covariates, including smoking and random blood sugar levels. This result is in accordance with the findings from another study investigating the association of serum vitamin C levels with serology of periodontitis in a random subsample of Finnish and Russian men (Pussinen et al 2003).

Complex regional pain syndrome (CRPS)

A 2013 systematic review and meta-analysis assessed the use of high-dose vitamin C for CRPS (Shibuya et al 2013). Use of high-dose vitamin C has been recommended by the Evidence Based Guidelines for Type 1 CRPS for wrist fractures (oral administration of 500 mg of vitamin C per day for 50 days from the date of the injury) (Perez et al 2010). Quantitative synthesis showed a relative risk of 0.22 when daily vitamin C of at least 500 mg was initiated immediately after the extremity surgery or injury and continued for 45–50 days. A routine, daily administration of vitamin C may therefore be beneficial in foot and ankle surgery or injury to avoid CRPS.

Adjunct therapy for haemodialysis patients

Recent research highlights that vitamin C can potentiate the mobilisation of iron from inert tissue stores, and facilitates the incorporation of iron into protoporphyrin in haemodialysis patients being treated with epoetin. Eighteen published studies in the past decade have addressed this issue (Attallah et al 2006, Chan et al 2005, Deira et al 2003, Gastaldello et al 1995, Giancaspro et al 2000, Hörl 1999, Keven et al 2003, CL Lin et al 2003, Macdougall 1999, Mydlik et al 2003, Nguyen 2004, Sezer et al 2002, Taji et al 2004, Tarng & Huang 1998, Tarng et al 1999a, 1999b, 2004, Tovbin et al 2000).

Administration of IV vitamin C to haemodialysis patients with functional iron deficiency may promote better anaemia control and iron utilisation and has also been used successfully in patients with iron overload (Tarng & Huang 1998, Tarng et al 1999a, 1999b). Current recommendations for maintenance of haemodialysis patients advise supplementation with ascorbic acid 75–90 mg daily (Fouque et al 2007) during dialysis. In addition to the potential benefits of vitamin C for anaemia management, the importance of adequate vitamin C with regard to improving cardiovascular outcomes in haemodialysis patients is also the subject of research. A study by Deicher and colleagues of 138 haemodialysis patients examined baseline levels of plasma vitamin C and followed the cohort for occurrence of cardiovascular events (Deicher et al 2005). Results showed that low total vitamin C plasma concentrations (less than 32 micromol/L) were associated with an almost fourfold increased risk for fatal and major non-fatal cardiovascular events compared with haemodialysis patients who had higher plasma vitamin C levels (greater than 60 micromol/L).

OTHER USES

Vitamin C is used for numerous indications, although many have not been significantly studied, such as irritable bowel syndrome, osteoarthritis, menopausal hot flushes, cervical dysplasia, prevention of Alzheimer's dementia, allergies, treatment of lead toxicity and reducing delayed-onset muscle soreness.

Vitamin C supplements have also been used as part of antioxidant combination therapy in HIV. Preliminary research has shown that some antioxidant combinations reduce oxidative stress (Jaruga et al 2002), induce immunological and virological effects that might be of therapeutic value (Muller et al 2000) and produce a trend towards a reduction in viral load in HIV (Allard et al 1998).

For heroin withdrawal, high doses of oral ascorbic acid and vitamin E may ameliorate the withdrawal syndrome of heroin addicts after 4 weeks' treatment, according to one study (Evangelou et al 2000).

DOSAGE RANGE

Australian and New Zealand RDI

Infants

- 0–6 months: 25 mg.
- 7–12 months: 30 mg.

Children

- 1–8 years: 35 mg.
- 9–18 years: 40 mg.

Adults

- >19 years: 45 mg.

Pregnancy

- <19 years: 55 mg.
- >19 years: 60 mg.

Lactation

- <19 years: 80 mg.
- >19 years: 85 mg.

Deficiency

- 100 mg taken 3–5 times daily until 4000 mg has been administered, followed by a maintenance dose of 100 mg/day and encouragement to eat a diet with fresh fruit and vegetables.

V

- In cases of acute infection, complementary and alternative medicine practitioners frequently recommend vitamin C in doses of 1000 g (or more), to be taken in divided doses every few hours until loose bowels are experienced, otherwise known as 'bowel tolerance'. The rationale behind this dosage regimen is that body requirements during infection are dramatically increased, and not only does high-dose vitamin C meet these needs, but also maximum vitamin C absorption is attained when it is taken in divided doses rather than one large amount.

According to clinical studies

- Asthma: 500–2000 mg before exercise.
- Cancer: 10–100 g/day IV.
- CVD prevention: up to 1000 mg/day long-term.
- BMD: 750 mg/day long-term.
- Cataract protection: 500 mg/day long-term.
- Diabetes: 0.5–3 g/day long-term.
- Histamine-lowering effects: 250 mg to 2 g/day for several weeks.
- Respiratory infection: at least 2 g/day.
- Sunburn protection: oral vitamin C (2000 mg/day) in combination with vitamin E (1000 IU/day).
- Urinary acidification: 4–12 g taken in divided doses every 4 hours.

ADVERSE REACTIONS

Adverse effects of oral vitamin C include loose bowels and diarrhoea with high-dose supplements; however, the dose at which this occurs varies between individuals and also varies for each individual at different times.

Clinical note — Is the kidney stone risk overstated?

Most kidney stones consist of calcium oxalate, and higher urinary oxalate increases the risk of calcium oxalate nephrolithiasis (Taylor & Curhan 2007). Four mechanisms have been identified that account for increased oxalate excretion: increased dietary intake of oxalate, abnormally increased intestinal absorption of oxalic acid, a deficiency of oxalate-degrading bacteria (in particular *Oxalobacter formigenes*) and increased endogenous production of oxalate. Vitamins C and B_6 are both involved in the metabolic pathway of oxalate. While 40% of dietary vitamin C undergoes a non-enzymatic conversion to oxalate, vitamin B_6 has the opposite effect and metabolises oxalate (Gill & Rose 1985). Since vitamin C has been shown in some (but not all) studies to increase urinary oxalate, researchers speculated that it might have a detrimental role in increasing the risk of kidney stone formation.

Reports of a possible link between ascorbic acid and kidney stones started to appear in the literature in the 1980s (Griffith et al 1986, Power et al 1984). These findings have been challenged by several studies carried out in humans and in experimental animals since that time. In 1994, researchers discovered that vitamin C (in doses as high as 10 g/day) does not increase the amount of oxalate produced in the body in non-stone-forming people (Wandzilak et al 1994). Instead, urine tests used to detect oxalate levels were actually detecting oxalate formed by the conversion of ascorbate during the test procedure. As such, urine oxalate levels tested by this method do not genuinely represent in vivo oxalate when ascorbate is involved. Three studies that followed found no association between vitamin C intake and kidney stone risk. Two prospective studies of more than 85,000 women and 45,000 men found that doses ranging from less than 250 mg/day to more than 1500 mg/day taken over 6–14 years did not correlate with occurrence of kidney stones (Curhan et al 1996, 1999). The third was a controlled study measuring oxalate excretion and several other biochemical and physicochemical risk factors associated with calcium oxalate urolithiasis (Auer et al 1998, Curhan et al 1996, 1999).

Based on the available evidence, it appears unlikely that vitamin C supplements increase the risk of nephrolithiasis in the general population, particularly if they are used in the short to medium term.

SIGNIFICANT INTERACTIONS

Aluminium-based antacids

Vitamin C increases the amount of aluminium absorbed. Separate doses by at least 2 hours.

Aspirin

Aspirin may interfere with both absorption and cellular uptake mechanisms for vitamin C, thereby increasing vitamin C requirements (observed in animal and human studies). Increased vitamin C intake may be required with long-term therapy (Basu 1982).

Chitosan

According to a preliminary study in rats, taking vitamin C in combination with chitosan might provide additional benefit in lowering cholesterol. Potentially beneficial interaction.

Cisplatin

Vitamin C enhanced the antitumour activity of cisplatin in several in vitro tests (Abdel-Latif et al 2005, Reddy et al 2001, Sarna & Bhola 1993) and reduced drug toxicity in experimental models (Giri et al 1998, Greggi Antunes et al 2000). Potentially beneficial but difficult to assess.

Corticosteroids

Corticosteroids may increase the requirement for vitamin C based on in vitro and in vivo data (Chowdhury & Kapil 1984, Levine & Pollard 1983). Increased intake may be required with long-term drug therapy.

Clinical note — Does vitamin C interact with the oral contraceptive pill?

In 1981 a case was reported of a woman who had experienced heavy breakthrough bleeding as a result of stopping vitamin C supplementation while taking the oral contraceptive pill (Morris et al 1981). At the time, it was suspected that vitamin C in high doses increases the bioavailability of oestrogen and raises blood concentrations due to competition for sulfation (resulting in reduced drug metabolism) (Back & Orme 1990). Therefore, ceasing supplement use would have the opposite effect and potentially cause breakthrough bleeding, as reported in this case. Since then, further investigation has been conducted to evaluate whether this interaction is clinically significant. In 1993 a placebo-controlled study was conducted with 37 women and found that 1000 mg of vitamin C does not lead to an increased systemic bioavailability of ethinyl oestradiol, and therefore the purported interaction is unlikely to be of any clinical importance (Zamah et al 1993).

Cyanocobalamin

Vitamin C can reduce absorption of cyanocobalamin. Separate doses by at least 2 hours.

Cyclophosphamide

Vitamin C enhanced the therapeutic drug effect in vivo (Lamson & Brignall 2000). Potentially beneficial but difficult to assess.

Doxorubicin

Vitamin C enhanced the therapeutic drug effect and reduced drug toxicity in vivo (Lamson & Brignall 2000). Potentially beneficial but difficult to assess.

Etoposide

Vitamin C enhanced the antitumour activity of etoposide in vitro (Reddy et al 2001). Potentially beneficial but difficult to assess.

Fluorouracil

Vitamin C enhanced the antitumour activity of 5-fluorouracil in vitro and in vivo (Abdel-Latif et al 2005, Nagy et al 2003). Potentially beneficial but difficult to assess.

Iron

Vitamin C increases the absorption of iron. Potentially beneficial interaction.

L-Dopa

A case report of co-administration with vitamin C suggests this may reduce drug side effects (Sacks & Simpson 1975). Beneficial interaction.

Tamoxifen

Vitamin C enhanced the antitumour activity in vitro (Lamson & Brignall 2000). Potentially beneficial but difficult to assess.

Vincristine

Vitamin C enhanced the drug's effect in vivo (Lamson & Brignall 2000). Potentially beneficial but difficult to assess.

PS-341 (bortezomib, Velcade)

This is a proteasome inhibitor approved by the US Food and Drug Administration for the treatment of patients with relapsed multiple myeloma. Vitamin C inactivated drug activity in vitro (Zou et al 2006). Avoid until safety can be established.

CONTRAINDICATIONS AND PRECAUTIONS

In patients who are sensitive to iron overload, vitamin C supplementation may exacerbate iron toxicity by mobilising iron reserves. As such, vitamin C supplementation should be used with caution by people with erythrocyte glucose-6-phosphate dehydrogenase deficiency, haemochromatosis, thalassaemia major or sideroblastic anaemia.

Intravenous vitamin C

A dose-response study involving patients with solid tumours receiving high-dose IV vitamin C found virtually all the side effects that occurred were consistent with the side effects attending the rapid infusion of any high-osmolarity solution. The symptoms were preventable by encouraging patients to drink fluids before and during the infusion. Indeed, rather than provoking fluid overload, ascorbic acid acted like an osmotic diuretic which could induce volume depletion if patients did not compensate by increasing their voluntary fluid intake. Therefore, contraindications to the infusion of very-high-osmolarity ascorbic acid infusions are the same as for other osmotic diuretics: anuria, dehydration, severe pulmonary congestion or pulmonary oedema and a fixed low cardiac output (Hoffer et al 2008).

Laboratory tests

Supplemental vitamin C can affect the results of numerous laboratory tests and should be stopped prior to:

- carbamazepine
- lactate dehydrogenase
- serum aspartate transaminase
- serum bicarbonate
- serum cholesterol
- serum creatinine
- serum creatine kinase
- serum HbA_{1C}
- serum phosphate
- serum triglycerides
- serum urea nitrogen
- stool guiac
- theophylline
- urine 17-hydroxy corticosteroids
- urine 17-ketosteroids
- urine amphetamine
- urine and serum bilirubin
- urine and serum glucose
- urine and serum uric acid
- urine barbiturate
- urine beta-hydroxybutyrate
- urine iodide
- urine oxalate
- urine paracetamol
- urine protein.

V

Practice points/Patient counselling

- Vitamin C is an essential nutrient for humans, as we are one of the few animal species that cannot synthesise it endogenously.
- Although vitamin C is found widely in fruit and vegetables, up to 100% can be destroyed during cooking and storing, as it is sensitive to light, heat, oxygen and alkali.
- Although frank deficiency is uncommon in Western countries, marginal deficiency states are not uncommon, particularly in young children fed

exclusively on cow's milk for a prolonged period, the institutionalised or isolated elderly, chronic alcoholics, the urban poor and cigarette smokers.

- Vitamin C generally acts as an antioxidant and is involved in a myriad of biochemical processes in the body, such as neurotransmitter and hormone synthesis, maintenance of connective tissue, immune function and adrenal function.
- Many, but not all, studies have found a protective effect for dietary vitamin C intake on CVD and cancer incidence, emphasising the importance of adequate dietary intake of fresh fruit and vegetables.
- Oral vitamin C supplements have been investigated in many different conditions. Positive results have been obtained in some of these studies, such as for reducing incidence of the common cold in children, CHD prevention, prevention of several CVDs and BMD. Positive effects on mortality have been reported when vitamin C intake is increased after a diagnosis of breast cancer; however, use as a cancer treatment remains controversial. There are also possible benefits for bone density and cataract incidence and increasing intake after a diagnosis of breast cancer.
- Research shows that long-term supplements do not increase the risk of kidney stones and do not interact with oral contraceptives.

PREGNANCY USE

Vitamin C is safe in pregnancy; however, it is recommended to not exceed the therapeutic dose nor abruptly cease supplementation.

PATIENTS' FAQs

What will this vitamin do for me?

Vitamin C is necessary for health and wellbeing. Supplements have also been used for a variety of indications and in some cases shown to have benefits.

When will it start to work?

Studies have found that dietary or supplemental vitamin C may be required for at least 10 years before protection against heart disease or cancer incidence is detected. However, other benefits may be experienced more quickly, depending on the dose used and indication. Research also indicates that increasing vitamin C intake after a diagnosis of breast cancer may reduce mortality.

Are there any safety issues?

Vitamin C is considered very safe, although high doses may induce reversible loose bowels or diarrhoea. Supplements should be taken only under medical supervision by people with erythrocyte glucose-6-phosphate dehydrogenase deficiency, haemochromatosis, thalassaemia or sideroblastic anaemia.

REFERENCES

Abdel-Latif MM et al. Vitamin C enhances chemosensitization of esophageal cancer cells in vitro. J Chemother 17 (2005): 539–549.

Ahmet, B, et al Combined Vitamin C and E Supplementation for the Prevention of Preeclampsia: A Systematic Review and Meta-Analysis, Obstet Gynecol Surv, 2010 Oct 65(10):653–67.

Ali SM, Chakraborty SK. Role of plasma ascorbate in diabetic microangiopathy. Bangladesh Med Res Counc Bull 1989;15:47–59.

Allard JP et al. Effects of vitamin E and C supplementation on oxidative stress and viral load in HIV-infected subjects. AIDS 12.13 (1998): 1653–1659.

Alul RH et al. Vitamin C protects low-density lipoprotein from homocysteine-mediated oxidation. Free Radic Biol Med 34.7 (2003): 881–891.

Amarasena N, et al. Serum vitamin C–periodontal relationship in community-dwelling elderly Japanese. J Clin Periodontol 2005;32:93–7.
Attallah N et al. Effect of intravenous ascorbic acid in hemodialysis patients with EPOhyporesponsive anemia and hyperferritinemia. Am J Kidney Dis 47 (2006): 644–654.
Auer BL, et al. The effect of ascorbic acid ingestion on the biochemical and physicochemical risk factors associated with calcium oxalate kidney stone formation. Clin Chem Lab Med 36.3 (1998): 143–147.
Back DJ, Orme ML. Pharmacokinetic drug interactions with oral contraceptives. Clin Pharmacokinet 18.6 (1990): 472–484.
Bartholomew M. James Lind's treatise of the scurvy (1753). Postgrad Med J 78.925 (2002): 695–696.
Bassenge E et al. Dietary supplement with vitamin C prevents nitrate tolerance. J Clin Invest 102.1 (1998): 67–71.
Basu TK. Vitamin C–aspirin interactions. Int J Vitam Nutr Res Suppl 23 (1982): 83–90.
Bates CJ et al. Does vitamin C reduce blood pressure? Results of a large study of people aged 65 or older. J Hypertens 16.7 (1998): 925–932.
Beckman JA et al. Ascorbate restores endothelium-dependent vasodilation impaired by acute hyperglycemia in humans. Circulation 103.12 (2001): 1618–1623.
Bednarz B et al. Antioxidant vitamins decrease exercise-induced QT dispersion after myocardial infarction. Kardiol Pol 58 (2003): 375–379.
Beers MH, Berkow R (eds). The Merck manual of diagnosis and therapy, 17th edn. Whitehouse, NJ: Merck, 2003.
Bjelakovic G, et al. Mortality in randomized trials of antioxidant supplements for primary and secondary prevention. Systematic Review and Meta-Analysis. J Am Med Assoc 2007;297:842–57.
Block G. Epidemiologic evidence regarding vitamin C and cancer. Am J Clin Nutr 54.6 (Suppl) (1991a): 1310–14S.
Block G. Vitamin C and cancer prevention: the epidemiologic evidence. Am J Clin Nutr 53.1 (Suppl) (1991b): 270–82S.
Block G. Ascorbic acid, blood pressure, and the American diet. Ann NY Acad Sci 959 (2002): 180–187.
Block G et al. Ascorbic acid status and subsequent diastolic and systolic blood pressure. Hypertension 37.2 (2001): 261–267.
Bornstein SR et al. Impaired adrenal catecholamine system function in transgenic mice with deficiency of the ascorbic acid transporter (SVCT2). FASEB J 17 (2003): 1928–1930.
Boyce ST et al. Vitamin C regulates keratinocyte viability, epidermal barrier, and basement membrane in vitro, and reduces wound contraction after grafting of cultured skin substitutes. J Invest Dermatol 118.4 (2002): 565–572.
Braunwald E et al (ed). Harrison's principles of internal medicine. New York: McGraw Hill, 2003.
Brubaker RF et al. Ascorbic acid content of human corneal epithelium. Investig Ophthalmol Vis Sci 41 (2000): 1681–1683.
Bucca C et al. Effect of vitamin C on histamine bronchial responsiveness of patients with allergic rhinitis. Ann Allergy 65.4 (1990): 311–314.
Cameron E. Vitamin C and cancer: an overview. Int J Vitam Nutr Res Suppl 23 (1982): 115–127.
Cameron E. Protocol for the use of vitamin C in the treatment of cancer. Med Hypotheses 36.3 (1991): 190–194.
Cameron E, Pauling L. The orthomolecular treatment of cancer. I. The role of ascorbic acid in host resistance. Chem Biol Interact 9.4 (1974): 273–283.
Cameron E, Pauling L. Supplemental ascorbate in the supportive treatment of cancer: Prolongation of survival times in terminal human cancer. Proc Natl Acad Sci USA 73.10 (1976): 3685–3689.
Carr AC, Frei B. Toward a new recommended dietary allowance for vitamin C based on antioxidant and health effects in humans. Am J Clin Nutr 69.6 (1999): 1086–1107.
Ceriello A et al. Antioxidant defences are reduced during the oral glucose tolerance test in normal and non-insulin-dependent diabetic subjects. Eur J Clin Invest 28.4 (1998): 329–333.
Chan D, et al. Efficacy and safety of oral versus intravenous ascorbic acid for anemia in hemodialysis patients. Nephrology (Carlton) 10 (2005): 336–40.
Chapple IL, et al. The prevalence of inflammatory periodontitis is negatively associated with serum antioxidant concentrations. J Nutr 2007;137:657–64.
Chasan-Taber L et al. A prospective study of vitamin supplement intake and cataract extraction among U.S. women. Epidemiology 10.6 (1999): 679–684.
Chaudière J, Ferrari-Iliou R. Intracellular antioxidants: from chemical to biochemical mechanisms. Food Chem Toxicol 37 (1999): 949–962.
Chen Q et al. Pharmacologic ascorbic acid concentrations selectively kill cancer cells: action as a pro-drug to deliver hydrogen peroxide to tissues. Proc Natl Acad Sci USA 102 (2005): 13604–13609.
Chen H et al. High-dose oral vitamin C partially replenishes vitamin C levels in patients with type 2 diabetes and low vitamin C levels but does not improve endothelial dysfunction or insulin resistance. Am J Physiol Heart Circ Physiol 290.1 (2006): H137–H145.
Chen Q, et al. Pharmacologic doses of ascorbate act as a prooxidant and decrease growth of aggressive tumor xenografts in mice. Proc Natl Acad Sci USA 105 (2008): 11105–11109.
Chowdhury AR, Kapil N. Interaction of dexamethasone and DHEA on testicular ascorbic acid and cholesterol in prepubertal rat. Arch Andriol 12.1 (1984): 65–7; as cited in Pelton R et al. Drug-induced nutrient depletion handbook 1999–2000. Hudson, OH: Lexi-Comp, 2000.
Chylack LT Jr. et al. The Roche European American Cataract Trial (REACT): a randomized clinical trial to investigate the efficacy of an oral antioxidant micronutrient mixture to slow progression of age-related cataract. Ophthal Epidemiol 9.1 (2002): 49–80.
Cohen M, Bhagavan HN. Ascorbic acid and gastrointestinal cancer. J Am Coll Nutr 14.6 (1995): 565–578.

Cohen HA et al. Blocking effect of vitamin C in exercise-induced asthma. Arch Pediatr Adolesc Med 151.4 (1997): 367–370.
Combs Jr, G. F. 2012, "Chapter 9 — Vitamin C," In Combs GF (ed.) The Vitamins, Fourth Edition. San Diego: Academic Press, pp. 233–259.
Conde-Agudelo A, et al. Supplementation with vitamins C and E during pregnancy for the prevention of preeclampsia and other adverse maternal and perinatal outcomes: a systematic review and metaanalysis. Am J Obstet Gynecol 2011;204:503.e1–12.
Cook NR, et al. A randomized factorial trial of vitamins C and E and beta carotene in the secondary prevention of cardiovascular events in women: results from the Women's Antioxidant Cardiovascular Study. Arch Intern Med 2007;167:1610–8.
Creagan ET et al. Failure of high-dose vitamin C (ascorbic acid) therapy to benefit patients with advanced cancer: A controlled trial. N Engl J Med 301.13 (1979): 687–690.
Cross CE, Halliwell B. Nutrition and human disease: how much extra vitamin C might smokers need? Lancet 341 (1993): 1091.
Cunningham JJ. The glucose/insulin system and vitamin C: implications in insulin-dependent diabetes mellitus. J Am Coll Nutr 17.2 (1998): 105–108.
Curhan GC et al. A prospective study of the intake of vitamins C and B6, and the risk of kidney stones in men. J Urol 155.6 (1996): 1847–1851.
Curhan GC et al. Intake of vitamins B6 and C and the risk of kidney stones in women. J Am Soc Nephrol 10.4 (1999): 840–845.
Darr D et al. Topical vitamin C protects porcine skin from ultraviolet radiation-induced damage. Br J Dermatol 127.3 (1992): 247–253.
Darr D et al. Effectiveness of antioxidants (vitamin C and E) with and without sunscreens as topical photoprotectants. Acta Derm Venereol 76.4 (1996): 264–268.
da Silva, SL, et al Plasma nutrient status of patients with Alzheimer's disease: Systematic review and meta-analysis, Alzheimer's & Dementia, (2013)1–18.
Dawson EB et al. Effect of ascorbic acid supplementation on the sperm quality of smokers. Fertil Steril 58 (1992): 1034–1039.
Deicher, R.; et al. (2005) Low Total Vitamin C Plasma Level Is a Risk Factor for Cardiovascular Morbidity and Mortality in Hemodialysis Patients. J Am Soc Nephrol, Vol.16,No.6,pp. 1811–1818
Deira J et al. Comparative study of intravenous ascorbic acid versus low-dose desferrioxamine in patients on hemodialysis with hyperferritinemia. J Nephrol 16 (2003): 703–709.
Devereux G, Seaton A. Diet as a risk factor for atopy and asthma. J Allergy Clin Immunol 115 (2005): 1109–1117.
Douglas RM et al. Vitamin C for preventing and treating the common cold. Cochrane Database Syst Rev 2 (2004): CD000980.
Dreyer R, Rose RC. Lacrimal gland uptake and metabolism of ascorbic acid. Proc Soc Exp Biol Med 202 (1993): 212–2116.
Drisko JA et al. The use of antioxidant therapies during chemotherapy. Gynecol Oncol 88.3 (2003): 434–439.
Duffy SJ et al. Treatment of hypertension with ascorbic acid. Lancet 354.9195 (1999): 2048–2049.
Eberlein-Konig B et al. Protective effect against sunburn of combined systemic ascorbic acid (vitamin C) and d-alpha-tocopherol (vitamin E). J Am Acad Dermatol 38.1 (1998): 45–48.
Enstrom JE et al. Vitamin C intake and mortality among a sample of the United States population. Epidemiology 3 (1992): 194–202.
Espinal-Perez LE, et al. A double-blind randomized trial of 5% ascorbic acid vs. 4% hydroquinone in melasma. Int J Dermatol 2004;43:604e7.
Evangelou A et al. Ascorbic acid (vitamin C) effects on withdrawal syndrome of heroin abusers. In Vivo 14.2 (2000): 363–366.
FAO/WHO (Food and Agriculture Organization/World Health Organization). Report of a Joint FAO/WHO Expert Consultation, Bangkok, Thailand. FAO/WHO: Rome, 2002.
Ferrigno L et al. Associations between plasma levels of vitamins and cataract in the Italian–American Clinical Trial of Nutritional Supplements and Age-Related Cataract (CTNS): CTNS Report #2. Ophthal Epidemiol 12 (2005): 71–80.
Fitzpatrick RE, Rostan EF. Double-blind, half-face study comparing topical vitamin C and vehicle for rejuvenation of photodamage. Dermatol Surg 28.3 (2002): 231–236.
Fotherby MD et al. Effect of vitamin C on ambulatory blood pressure and plasma lipids in older persons. J Hypertens 18.4 (2000): 411–411.
Fouque, D.; et al. (2007) EBPG Guideline on Nutrition. Nephrol Dial Transplant, Vol.22, Suppl. 2,pp. ii45–ii87.
Galatioto, G.P., et al., 2008. May antioxidant therapy improve sperm parameters of men with persistent oligospermia after retrograde embolization for varicocele? World J. Urol. 26, 97–102.
Gale CR, et al. Vitamin C and risk of death from stroke and coronary heart disease in cohort of elderly people. Br Med J 1995;310:1563–6.
Galley HF et al. Combination oral antioxidant supplementation reduces blood pressure. Clin Sci (Lond) 92.4 (1997): 361–365.
Gastaldello K et al. Resistance to erythropoietin in iron-overloaded haemodialysis patients can be overcome by ascorbic acid administration. Nephrol Dial Transplant 10 (Suppl) (1995): 44–47.
Gatenby R, Gillies R. Why do cancers have high aerobic glycolysis? Nat Rev Cancer 4 (2004): 891–899.
Gey KF et al. Poor plasma status of carotene and vitamin C is associated with higher mortality from ischemic heart disease and stroke: Basel Prospective Study. Clin Invest 71.1 (1993): 3–6.
Ghosh SK et al. A double-blind, placebo-controlled parallel trial of vitamin C treatment in elderly patients with hypertension. Gerontology 40.5 (1994): 268–272.

Giancaspro V et al. Intravenous ascorbic acid in hemodialysis patients with functional iron deficiency (a clinical trial). J Nephrol 13 (2000): 444–449.
Gill HS, Rose GA. Idiopathic hypercalciuria. Urate and other ions in urine before and on various long term treatments. Urol Res 13.6 (1985): 271–275.
Giri A et al. Vitamin C mediated protection on cisplatin induced mutagenicity in mice. Mutat Res 421 (1998): 139–148.
Gottlieb N. Cancer treatment and vitamin C: the debate lingers. J Natl Cancer Inst 91 (1999): 2073–2075.
Greco E et al. Efficient treatment of infertility due to sperm DNA damage by ICSI with testicular spermatozoa. Hum Reprod 20 (2005a): 226–30.
Greco E et al. Reduction of the incidence of sperm DNA fragmentation by oral antioxidant treatment. J Androl 26 (2005b): 349–53.
Greggi Antunes LM et al. Protective effects of vitamin C against cisplatin-induced nephrotoxicity and lipid peroxidation in adult rats: a dose-dependent study. Pharmacol Res 41 (2000): 405–411.
Griffith HM et al. A case-control study of dietary intake of renal stone patients. I. Preliminary analysis. Urol Res 14.2 (1986): 67–74.
Gupta MM, Chari S. Lipid peroxidation and antioxidant status in patients with diabetic retinopathy. Indian J Physiol Pharmacol 2005;49:187–92.
Gurler B, et al. The role of oxidative stress in diabetic retinopathy. Eye 2000;14:730–5.
Hall SL, Greendale GA. The relation of dietary vitamin C intake to bone mineral density: results from the PEPI study. Calcif Tissue Int 63.3 (1998): 183–189.
Hammond BR Jr., Johnson MA. The Age-Related Eye Disease Study (AREDS). Nutr Rev 60 (2002): 283–288.
Hanashima C, Namiki H. Reduced viability of vascular endothelial cells by high concentration of ascorbic acid in vitreous humor. Cell Biol Int 23 (1999): 287–298.
Harris HR, et al . Vitamin C and survival among women with breast cancer: a meta-analysis. Eur J Cancer. 2014 May;50(7):1223–31
Harrison FE, May JM. Vitamin C function in the brain: vital role of the ascorbate transporter SVCT2. Free Rad Bio Med 46.6 (2009): 719–730.
Heart Protection Study Collaborative Group, MRC/BHF Heart Protection Study of antioxidant vitamin supplementation in 20536 high-risk individuals: a randomized placebo-controlled trials. Lancet 2002;360:23
Hemilä, H. Vitamin C supplementation and common cold symptoms: factors affecting the magnitude of the benefit. Medical hypotheses 52[2], 171–178. 1-2-1999.
Hemilä H, Chalker E. Vitamin C for preventing and treating the common cold. Cochrane Database of Systematic Reviews 2013, Issue 1. Art. No.: CD000980.
Hemilä H, Louhiala P. Vitamin C for preventing and treating pneumonia. Cochrane Database of Systematic Reviews 2013, Issue 8. Art. No.: CD005532.
Hendler SS, Rorvik D (eds). PDR for nutritional supplements. Montvale, NJ: Medical Economics, 2001.
Hoffer L et al. Phase I clinical trial of i.v. ascorbic acid in advanced malignancy. Ann Oncol 19.12 (2008): 2095.
Hörl WH. Is there a role for adjuvant therapy in patients being treated with epoetin? Nephrol Dial Transplant 14 (Suppl) (1999): 50–60.
Houston MC. Nutraceuticals, vitamins, antioxidants, and minerals in the prevention and treatment of hypertension. Prog Cardiovasc Dis 47 (2005): 396–449.
Humbert PG et al. Topical ascorbic acid on photoaged skin: Clinical, topographical and ultrastructural evaluation: double-blind study vs placebo. Exp Dermatol 12.3 (2003): 237–244.
Hwang SW, et al. Clinical efficacy of 25% L-ascorbic acid (C'ensil) in the treatment of melasma. J Cutan Med Surg 2009;13(2):74e 81.
Ilich JZ et al. Bone and nutrition in elderly women: protein, energy, and calcium as main determinants of bone mineral density. Eur J Clin Nutr 57.4 (2003): 554–565.
Jacques PF, Chylack LT Jr. Epidemiologic evidence of a role for the antioxidant vitamins and carotenoids in cataract prevention. Am J Clin Nutr 53 (1991): 352–355S.
Jacques PF et al. Nutritional status in persons with and without senile cataract: blood vitamin and mineral levels. Am J Clin Nutr 48 (1988): 152–158.
Jacques PF et al. Long-term vitamin C supplement use and prevalence of early age-related lens opacities. Am J Clin Nutr 66 (1997): 911–9116.
Jacques PF et al. Long-term nutrient intake and early age-related nuclear lens opacities. Arch Ophthalmol 119.7 (2001): 1009–1019.
Jaruga P et al. Supplementation with antioxidant vitamins prevents oxidative modification of DNA in lymphocytes of HIV-infected patients. Free Radic Biol Med 32.5 (2002): 414–420.
Jaxa-Chamiec T et al. Antioxidant effects of combined vitamins C and E in acute myocardial infarction: The randomized, double-blind, placebo controlled, multicenter pilot Myocardial Infarction and VITamins (MIVIT) trial. Kardiol Pol 62 (2005): 344–350.
Jenab M et al. Plasma and dietary vitamin C levels and risk of gastric cancer in the European Prospective Investation into Cancer and Nutrition (EPIC-EURGAST). Carcinogenesis 27.11 (2006): 2250–2257.
Jeurissen A et al. [The effects of physical exercise on the immune system]. Ned Tijdschr Geneeskd 147.28 (2003): 1347–1351.
Johnston CS et al. Antihistamine effect of supplemental ascorbic acid and neutrophil chemotaxis. J Am Coll Nutr 11.2 (1992): 172–176.
Johnston CS et al. Vitamin C depletion is associated with alterations in blood histamine and plasma free carnitine in adults. J Am Coll Nutr 15.6 (1996): 586–591.
Kaliora AC et al. Dietary antioxidants in preventing atherogenesis. Atherosclerosis 187 (2006): 1–17.

Kaufmann PA et al. Coronary heart disease in smokers: vitamin C restores coronary microcirculatory function. Circulation 102.11 (2000): 1233–1238.

Kaur B et al. Vitamin C supplementation for asthma. Cochrane Database Syst Rev 4 (2001): CD000993.

Keller KL, Fenske NA. Uses of vitamins A, C, and E and related compounds in dermatology: A review. J Am Acad Dermatol 39 (1998): 611–625.

Kelly FJ. Vitamins and respiratory disease: antioxidant micronutrients in pulmonary health and disease. Proc Nutr Soc 64 (2005): 510–526.

Kelly FJ et al. Altered lung antioxidant status in patients with mild asthma. Lancet 354.9177 (1999): 482–483.

Keven K et al. Randomized, crossover study of the effect of vitamin C on EPO response in hemodialysis patients. Am J Kidney Dis 41 (2003): 1233–1239.

Khaw KT et al. Relation between plasma ascorbic acid and mortality in men and women in EPIC-Norfolk prospective study: a prospective population study. European Prospective Investigation into Cancer and Nutrition. Lancet 357.9257 (2001): 657–663.

Knekt P et al. Antioxidant vitamins and coronary heart disease risk: A pooled analysis of 9 cohorts. Am J Clin Nutr 80 (2004): 1508–1520.

Kumar P et al. Clinical medicine, 5th edn. London: WB Saunders, 2002.

Kurbacher CM et al. Ascorbic acid (vitamin C) improves the antineoplastic activity of doxorubicin, cisplatin, and paclitaxel in human breast carcinoma cells in vitro. Cancer Lett 103 (1996): 183–189.

Kushi LH et al. Dietary antioxidant vitamins and death from coronary heart disease in postmenopausal women. N Engl J Med 334 (1996): 1156–1162.

Kuzniarz M et al. Use of vitamin supplements and cataract: the Blue Mountains eye study. Am J Ophthalmol 132 (2001): 19–26.

Lamson DW, Brignall MS. Antioxidants and cancer therapy II: quick reference guide. Altern Med Rev 5 (2000): 152–163.

Lee, CTC, et al Micronutrients and Diabetic Retinopathy – A Systematic Review, Ophthalmology 2010;117: 71–78

Lekakis JP et al. Short-term oral ascorbic acid improves endothelium-dependent vasodilatation in women with a history of gestational diabetes mellitus. Diabetes Care 23.9 (2000): 1432–1434.

Leveille SG, et al. Dietary vitamin C and bone mineral density in postemenopausal women in Washington State, USA. J Epidemiol Commun Health 1997;51:479–85.

Levine MA, Pollard HB. Hydrocortisone inhibition of ascorbic acid transport by Chromaffin cells. FEBS Lett 158.1 (1983): 13408; as cited in Pelton R et al. Drug-induced nutrient depletion handbook 1999–2000. Hudson, OH: Lexi-Comp, 2000.

Lewis SE et al. Comparison of individual antioxidants of sperm and seminal plasma in fertile and infertile men. Fertil Steril 67 (1997): 142–147.

Li Y, Schellhorn HE. New Developments and Novel Therapeutic Perspectives for Vitamin C. J Nutr 137.10 (2007): 2171–2184.

Lin CL et al. Low dose intravenous ascorbic acid for erythropoietin-hyporesponsive anemia in diabetic hemodialysis patients with iron overload. Ren Fail 25 (2003): 445–453.

Lin JY et al. UV photoprotection by combination topical antioxidants vitamin C and vitamin E. J Am Acad Dermatol 48.6 (2003): 866–874.

Lin J, et al. Vitamins C and E and beta carotene supplementation and cancer risk: a randomized controlled trial. J Natl Cancer Inst 2009;101:14–23.

Ling L et al. Vitamin C preserves endothelial function in patients with coronary heart disease after a high-fat meal. Clin Cardiol 25.5 (2002): 219–224.

Lopes C et al. [Diet and risk of myocardial infarction: A case-control community-based study]. Acta Med Port 11.4 (1998): 311–3117.

Lopes de Jesus CC, et al. Vitamin C and superoxide dismutase (SOD) for diabetic retinopathy. Cochrane Database of Systematic Reviews 2008, Issue 1. Art. No.: CD006695.

Loria CM et al. Vitamin C status and mortality in US adults. Am J Clin Nutr 72 (2000): 139–145.

Macdougall IC. Metabolic adjuvants to erythropoietin therapy. Miner Electrolyte Metab 25 (1999): 357–364.

Maggini, S., et al. 2012. A combination of high-dose vitamin C plus zinc for the common cold. J Int.Med Res., 40, (1) 28–42.

Mares-Perlman JA et al. Vitamin supplement use and incident cataracts in a population-based study. Arch Ophthalmol 118.11 (2000): 1556–1563.

May JM. Is ascorbic acid an antioxidant for the plasma membrane? FASEB J 13 (1999): 995–1006.

McCann SE et al. Intakes of selected nutrients, foods, and phytochemicals and prostate cancer risk in western New York. Nutr Cancer 53 (2005): 33–41.

McDermoth JH. Antioxidant nutrients: current dietary recommendations and research update. J Am Pharm Assoc 40 (2000): 785–799.

Michels KB et al. Dietary antioxidant vitamins, retinol, and breast cancer incidence in a cohort of Swedish women. Int J Cancer 91.4 (2001): 563–567.

Milan SJ, et al. Vitamin C for asthma and exercise-induced bronchoconstriction. Cochrane Database of Systematic Reviews 2013, Issue 10. Art. No.: CD010391.

Miric M, Haxhiu MA. Effect of vitamin C on exercise-induced bronchoconstriction. Plucne Bolesti 43.1–2 (1991): 94–97.

Moertel CG et al. High-dose vitamin C versus placebo in the treatment of patients with advanced cancer who have had no prior chemotherapy: A randomized double-blind comparison. N Engl J Med 312.3 (1985): 137–141.

Moorman PG, et al. Vitamin supplement use and breast cancer in a North Carolina population. Publ Health Nutr 2001;4(3):821–7.

Morel O et al. Protective effects of vitamin C on endothelium damage and platelet activation during myocardial infarction in patients with sustained generation of circulating microparticles. J Thromb Haemost 1 (2003): 171–177.
Morris JC et al. Interaction of ethinyl estradiol with ascorbic acid in man. BMJ 283 (1981): 503. Cited online: www.micromedex.com.
Morton DJ et al. Vitamin C supplement use and bone mineral density in postmenopausal women. J Bone Miner Res 16.1 (2001): 135–140.
MRC/BHF. Heart protection study of antioxidant vitamin supplementation in 20,536 high-risk individuals: a randomised placebo-controlled trial. Lancet 360.9326 (2002): 23–33.
Mullan BA et al. Ascorbic acid reduces blood pressure and arterial stiffness in type 2 diabetes. Hypertension 40.6 (2002): 804–809.
Muggli, R. 1998, "Vitamin C and the Immune System," In: Delves PJ (ed.) Encyclopedia of Immunology, Second Edition. Oxford: Elsevier, pp. 2491–2494.
Muller F et al. Virological and immunological effects of antioxidant treatment in patients with HIV infection. Eur J Clin Invest 30.10 (2000): 905–914.
Mydlik M et al. Oral use of iron with vitamin C in hemodialyzed patients. J Ren Nutr 13 (2003): 47–51.
Nagy B et al. Chemosensitizing effect of vitamin C in combination with 5-fluorouracil in vitro. In Vivo 17 (2003): 289–292.
Negri E et al. Selected micronutrients and oral and pharyngeal cancer. Int J Cancer 86.1 (2000): 122–127.
Ness AR et al. Vitamin C and cardiovascular disease: a systematic review. J Cardiovasc Risk 3.6 (1996): 513–521.
Ness AR et al. Vitamin C and blood pressure: an overview. J Hum Hypertens 11.6 (1997): 343–350.
Nguyen TV. Oral ascorbic acid as adjuvant to epoetin alfa in hemodialysis patients with hyperferritinemia. Am J Health-Syst Ph 61 (2004): 2007–2008.
NHMRC (National Health & Medical Research Council). Nutrient reference values for Australia and New Zealand. Canberra: NHMRC, 2006.
Nieman DC et al. Influence of vitamin C supplementation on cytokine changes following an ultramarathon. J Interferon Cytokine Res 20.11 (2000): 1029–1035.
Nishida M, et al. Dietary vitamin C and the risk for periodontal disease. J Periodontol 2000;71:1215–23.
Northrop-Clewes CA, Thurnham DI. Monitoring micronutrients in cigarette smokers. Clin Chim Acta 377 (2007): 14–38.
Nurmatov, U, et al. Nutrients and foods for the primary prevention of asthma and allergy: Systematic review and meta-analysis, J Allergy Clin Immunol 2011;127:724–33.
Nyyssonen K et al. Vitamin C deficiency and risk of myocardial infarction: prospective population study of men from eastern Finland. BMJ 314.7081 (1997): 634–638.
Ochiai Y, et al. A new lipophilic pro-vitamin C, tetra-isopalmitoyl ascorbic acid (VC-IP), prevents UV-induced skin pigmentation through its anti-oxidative properties. J Dermatol Sci 2006;44:37e44.
Omu, A.E., et al., 2008. Indication of the mechanisms involved in improved sperm parameters by zinc therapy. Med. Princ. Pract. 17, 108–116.
Osganian SK et al. Vitamin C and risk of coronary heart disease in women. J Am Coll Cardiol 42.2 (2003): 246–252.
Padayatty SJ, Levine M. Reevaluation of ascorbate in cancer treatment: emerging evidence, open minds and serendipity. J Am Coll Nutr 19.4 (2000): 423–425.
Padayatty SJ et al. Vitamin C pharmacokinetics: implications for oral and intravenous use. Ann Intern Med 140 (2004): 533–537.
Padayatty SJ et al. Intravenously administered vitamin C as cancer therapy: three cases. CMAJ 174 (2006): 937–942.
Pandey DK et al. Dietary vitamin C and beta-carotene and risk of death in middle-aged men: The Western Electric Study. Am J Epidemiol 142 (1995): 1269–1278.
Paolisso G et al. Plasma vitamin C affects glucose homeostasis in healthy subjects and in non-insulin-dependent diabetics. Am J Physiol 266.2 Pt 1 (1994): E261–E268.
Park HJ, et al. Vitamin C attenuates ERK signaling to inhibit the regulation of collagen production by LL-37 in human dermal fibroblasts. Exp Dermatol 2009;19:e258e64
Pasco JA et al. Antioxidant vitamin supplements and markers of bone turnover in a community sample of nonsmoking women. J Womens Health 15 (2006): 295–300.
Patel SR, Sigman M. Antioxidant therapy in male infertility. Urol Clin N Am 35 (2008): 319–330.
Patterson CA, O'Rourke MC. Vitamin C levels in human tears. Arch Opthalmol 105 (1987): 376–377.
Peponis V et al. Protective role of oral antioxidant supplementation in ocular surface of diabetic patients. Br J Ophthalmol 86.12 (2002): 1369–1373.
Perez RS, et al. Evidence based guidelines for complex regional pain syndrome type 1. BMC Neurol 10:20, 2010.
Peters EM et al. Vitamin C supplementation attenuates the increases in circulating cortisol, adrenaline and anti-inflammatory polypeptides following ultramarathon running. Int J Sports Med 22.7 (2001a): 537–43.
Peters EM et al. Attenuation of increase in circulating cortisol and enhancement of the acute phase protein response in vitamin C-supplemented ultramarathoners. Int J Sports Med 22.2 (2001b): 120–126.
Pfister, R., et al. 2011. Plasma vitamin C predicts incident heart failure in men and women in European Prospective Investigation into Cancer and Nutrition-Norfolk prospective study. Am Heart J, 162, (2) 246–253.
Pimentel L. Scurvy: Historical review and current diagnostic approach. Am J Emerg Med 21.4 (2003): 328–332.
Poulter JM, et al. Ascorbic acid supplementation and five year survival rates in women with early breast cancer. Acta Vitaminol Enzymol 1984;6:175–82.
Power C et al. Diet and renal stones: a case-control study. Br J Urol 56.5 (1984): 456–459.
Prasad KN et al. Pros and cons of antioxidant use during radiation therapy. Cancer Treat Rev 28 (2002): 79–91.
Price KD et al. Hyperglycemia-induced ascorbic acid deficiency promotes endothelial dysfunction and the development of atherosclerosis. Atherosclerosis 158.1 (2001): 1–12.

Pussinen PJ, et al. Periodontitis is associated with a low concentration of vitamin C in plasma. Clin Diagn Lab Immunol 2003;10:897–902.

Putchala, MC, et al. Ascorbic acid and its pro-oxidant activity as a therapy for tumours of oral cavity – A systematic review, Arch Oral Bio 58(2013)563–574

Rahman I. Oxidant and antioxidant balance in the airways and airway diseases. Eur J Pharmacol 533 (2006): 222–239.

Ram FS et al. Vitamin C supplementation for asthma. Cochrane Database Syst Rev 3 (2004): CD000993.

Reddy VG et al. Vitamin C augments chemotherapeutic response of cervical carcinoma HeLa cells by stabilizing P53. Biochem Biophys Res Commun 282 (2001): 409–415.

Rema M, et al. Does oxidant stress play a role in diabetic retinopathy? Indian J Ophthalmol 1995;43: 17–21.

Richardson TI et al. Will an orange a day keep the doctor away? Postgrad Med J 78.919 (2002): 292–294.

Riemersma RA et al. Vitamin C and the risk of acute myocardial infarction. Am J Clin Nutr 71.5 (2000): 1181–1186.

Ringsdorf J, Cheraskin E. Vitamin C and human wound healing. Oral Surg Oral Med Oral Pathol 53 (1982): 231–236.

Riordan HD et al. A pilot clinical study of continuous intravenous ascorbate in terminal cancer patients. Puerto Rica Health Sci J 24 (2005): 269–276.

Rossi, AC, Mullin, PM, Prevention of pre-eclampsia with low-dose aspirin or vitamins C and E in women at high or low risk: a systematic review with meta-analysis, European Journal of Obstetrics & Gynecology and Reproductive Biology 158 (2011) 9–16.

Rumbold A, Crowther CA. Vitamin C supplementation in pregnancy. Cochrane Database of Systematic Reviews 2005, Issue 1. Art. No.: CD004072.

Russell L. The importance of patients' nutritional status in wound healing. Br J Nurs 10.6 (Suppl) (2001): S42–4, S49.

Sacks W, Simpson GM. Ascorbic acid in levodopa therapy (Letter). Lancet 1.7905 (1975): 527. Cited online at: www.micromedex.com.

Sahyoun NR et al. Carotenoids, vitamins C and E, and mortality in an elderly population. Am J Epidemiol 144 (1996): 501–511.

Sandhya P, Das UN. Vitamin C therapy for maturity onset diabetes mellitus: relevance to prostaglandin involvement. IRCS I Med Sci 9 (1981): 618.

Sarna S, Bhola RK. Chemo-immunotherapeutical studies on Dalton's lymphoma in mice using cisplatin and ascorbic acid: synergistic antitumor effect in vivo and in vitro. Arch Immunol Ther Exp (Warsz) 41 (1993): 327–333.

Schachter EN, Schlesinger A. The attenuation of exercise-induced bronchospasm by ascorbic acid. Ann Allergy 49.3 (1982): 146–151.

Schindler TH et al. [Effect of vitamin C on platelet aggregation in smokers and nonsmokers]. Med Klin 97.5 (2002): 263–269.

Schwenk TL, Costley CD. When food becomes a drug: nonanabolic nutritional supplement use in athletes. Am J Sports Med 30.6 (2002): 907–916.

Scott, R., et al., 1998. The effect of oral selenium supplementation on human sperm motility. Br. J. Urol. 82, 76–80.

Seddon JM et al. The use of vitamin supplements and the risk of cataract among US male physicians. Am J Public Health 84 (1994): 788–792.

Sezer S et al. Intravenous ascorbic acid administration for erythropoietin hyporesponsive anemia in iron loaded hemodialysis patients. Artif Organs 26 (2002): 366–370.

Shanmugasundaram KR. Excessive free radical generation in the blood of children suffering from asthma. Clin Chim Acta 305 (2001): 107–114.

Shibuya, N, et al. Efficacy and Safety of High-dose Vitamin C on Complex Regional Pain Syndrome in Extremity Trauma and Surgery-Systematic Review and Meta-Analysis, J Foot Ankl Surg, 52(2013)62–66.

Shoham A et al. Oxidative stress in diseases of the human cornea. Free Radical Biology and Medicine 45.8 (2008): 1047–1055.

Silvestro A et al. Vitamin C prevents endothelial dysfunction induced by acute exercise in patients with intermittent claudication. Atherosclerosis 165.2 (2002): 277–283.

Simon, J.A. & Hudes, E.S. 1999. Serum ascorbic acid and cardiovascular disease prevalence in U.S. adults: the Third National Health and Nutrition Examination Survey (NHANES III). Ann.Epidemiol., 9, (6) 358–365

Simon JA, Hudes ES. Relation of ascorbic acid to bone mineral density and self-reported fractures among US adults. Am J Epidemiol 154.5 (2001): 427–433.

Simon, J.A., et al. 2001. Relation of serum ascorbic acid to mortality among US adults. J Am Coll. Nutr., 20, (3) 255–263.

Sinclair AJ, et al. An investigation of the relationship between free radical activity and vitamin C metabolism in elderly diabetic subjects with retinopathy. Gerontology 1992;38:268 –74.

Singh N et al. Effects of a 'healthy' diet and of acute and long-term vitamin C on vascular function in healthy older subjects. Cardiovasc Res 56.1 (2002): 118–125.

Solzbach U et al. Vitamin C improves endothelial dysfunction of epicardial coronary arteries in hypertensive patients. Circulation 96.5 (1997): 1513–15119.

Stoyanovsky DA et al. Endogenous ascorbate regenerates vitamin E in the retina directly and in combination with exogenous dihydrolipoic acid. Curr Eye Res 14.3 (1995): 181–189.

Taji Y et al. Effects of intravenous ascorbic acid on erythropoiesis and quality of life in unselected hemodialysis patients. J Nephrol 17 (2004): 537–543.

Tamayo C, Richardson MA. Vitamin C as a cancer treatment: state of the science and recommendations for research. Altern Ther Health Med 9 (2003): 94–101.

Taniguchi M, et al. Anti-oxidative and antiaging activities of 2-O-a-glucopyranosil-L-ascorbic acid on human dermal fibroblasts. Eur J Pharmacol 2012;674:126e31.

Tarng DC, Huang TP. A parallel, comparative study of intravenous iron *versus* intravenous ascorbic acid for erythropoietin hyporesponsive anaemia in haemodialysis patients with iron overload. Nephrol Dial Transplant 13 (1998): 2867–2872.

Tarng DC, et al. Erythropoietin hyporesponsiveness: from iron deficiency to iron overload. Kidney Int 55 (Suppl) (1999a): S107–18.

Tarng DC et al. Intravenous ascorbic acid as an adjuvant therapy for recombinant erythropoietin in hemodialysis patients with hyperferritinemia. Kidney Int 55 (1999b): 2477–86.

Tarng DC, et al. Effect of intravenous ascorbic acid medication on serum levels of soluble transferrin receptor in hemodialysis patients. J Am Soc Nephrol 15 (2004): 2486–2493.

Taylor EN, Curhan GC. Oxalate intake and the risk for nephrolithiasis. J Am Soc Nephrol 18.7 (2007): 2198–2204.

Taylor TV et al. Ascorbic acid supplementation in the treatment of pressure-sores. Lancet 304 (1974): 544–546.

Taylor A et al. Long-term intake of vitamins and carotenoids and odds of early age-related cortical and posterior subcapsular lens opacities. Am J Clin Nutr 75.3 (2002): 540–549.

Thompson D et al. Prolonged vitamin C supplementation and recovery from demanding exercise. Int J Sport Nutr Exerc Metab 11.4 (2001): 466–481.

Toohey, L., et al. 1996. Plasma ascorbic acid concentrations are related to cardiovascular risk factors in African-Americans. J Nutr., 126, (1) 121–128.

Tovbin D et al. Effectiveness of erythropoiesis on supervised intradialytic oral iron and vitamin C therapy is correlated with Kt/V and patient weight. Clin Nephrol 53 (2000): 276–282.

Traikovich SS. Use of topical ascorbic acid and its effects on photodamaged skin topography. Arch Otolaryngol Head Neck Surg 1999;125:1091e8.

Tremellen, K., et al., 2007. A randomized control trial of an antioxidant (Menevit) on pregnancy outcome during IVF-ICSI treatment. Aust. NZ J. Obstet. Gynaecol. 47, 216–221.

Valero MP et al. Vitamin C is associated with reduced risk of cataract in a Mediterranean population. J Nutr 132.6 (2002): 1299–1306.

Vatassery GT. In vitro oxidation of alpha-tocopherol (vitamin E) in human platelets upon incubation with unsaturated fatty acids, diamide and superoxide. Biochim Biophys Acta 926.2 (1987): 160–169.

Verrax J, Buc Calderon B. The controversial place of vitamin C in cancer treatment, Biocehem Pharmacol 76 (2008): 1644–1652.

Villacorta L, et al. Regulatory role of vitamins E and C on the extracellular matrix components of the vascular system. Mol Asp Med 28 (2007): 507–537.

Vural H. Serum and red blood cell antioxidant status in patients with bronchial asthma. Can Respir J 7 (2000): 476–480.

Wahlqvist M (ed). Food and nutrition, 2nd edn. Sydney: Allen & Unwin, 2002.

Wandzilak TR et al. Effect of high dose vitamin C on urinary oxalate levels. J Urol 151.4 (1994): 834–837.

Watanabe H et al. Randomized, double-blind, placebo-controlled study of the preventive effect of supplemental oral vitamin C on attenuation of development of nitrate tolerance. J Am Coll Cardiol 31.6 (1998a): 1323–1329.

Watanabe H et al. Randomized, double-blind, placebo-controlled study of ascorbate on the preventive effect of nitrate tolerance in patients with congestive heart failure. Circulation 97.9 (1998b): 886–891.

Waters DD, et al. Effects of hormone replacement therapy and antioxidant vitamin supplements on coronary atherosclerosis in postmenopausal women: a randomized controlled trial. J Am Med Assoc 2002;288:2432–40.

Wilkinson IB et al. Oral vitamin C reduces arterial stiffness and platelet aggregation in humans. J Cardiovasc Pharmacol 34.5 (1999): 690–693.

Williams MJ et al. Vitamin C improves endothelial dysfunction in renal allograft recipients. Nephrol Dial Transplant 16.6 (2001): 1251–1255.

Wilson CW et al. The metabolism of supplementary vitamin C during the common cold. J Clin Pharmacol 16.1 (1976): 19–29.

Wintergerst ES et al. Immune-enhancing role of vitamin C and zinc and effect on clinical conditions. Ann Nutr Metab 50 (2006): 85–94.

Wolf RL et al. Lack of a relation between vitamin and mineral antioxidants and bone mineral density: results from the Women's Health Initiative. Am J Clin Nutr 82 (2005): 581–588.

Yilmaz C et al. The contribution of vitamin C to healing of experimental fractures. Arch Orthop Trauma Surg 121.7 (2001): 426–428.

You WC et al. Gastric dysplasia and gastric cancer: *Helicobacter pylori*, serum vitamin C, and other risk factors. J Natl Cancer Inst 92.19 (2000): 1607–1612.

Zamah NM et al. Absence of an effect of high vitamin C dosage on the systemic availability of ethinyl estradiol in women using a combination oral contraceptive. Contraception 48.4 (1993): 377–391.

Zhang S et al. Dietary carotenoids and vitamins A, C, and E and risk of breast cancer. J Natl Cancer Inst 91.6 (1999): 547–556.

Zhang W et al. Synergistic cytotoxic action of vitamin C and vitamin K3. Anticancer Res 21 (2001): 3439–3444.

Zou W et al. Vitamin C inactivates the proteasome inhibitor PS-341 in human cancer cells. Clin Cancer Res 12 (2006): 273–280.

Vitamin D

HISTORICAL NOTE Vitamin D was identified as a nutrient in the early 1900s, when it was first realised that cod liver oil had an antirachitic effect in infants.

Is vitamin D really a vitamin?

Many characteristics of the vitamin D molecules vary substantially from the orthodox definition of a vitamin (Dusso et al 2005, NHMRC 2006, Vieth 2006) in that they:

- are not essential in the diet of all individuals, given adequate sun exposure (Dusso et al 2005, Holick 2008, Nowson & Margerison 2001, Nowson et al 2012)
- are structurally steroid derivatives (Gropper et al 2009, Valdivielso et al 2009)
- are inherently biologically inactive and require hydroxylation to produce the active form (Holick 2005, Kemmis et al 2006, Prietl et al 2013)
- produce 1,25(OH)$_2$D, which is a steroidal hormone (Dusso et al 2005)
- require vitamin D receptors (VDR) on cell surfaces, a member of the steroid receptor superfamily, to convey most, if not all, of their actions (Dusso et al 2005, Holick 2004, Hossein-nezhad & Holick 2013).

These discoveries and others have precipitated a revolution in vitamin D research over the last two decades (Dusso et al 2005, Holick 2004, 2005, Nowson et al 2012).

BACKGROUND AND RELEVANT PHARMACOKINETICS

The name 'vitamin D' actually refers to several related fat-soluble vitamin variants, all of which are sterol (cholesterol-like) substances. It is a pleiotropic steroid hormone, with its role being in the regulation of calcium and phosphorus levels (Zittermann et al 2014), involvement in vascular biology (Valdivielso et al 2009), bone mineralisation (Nowson et al 2012) and immunomodulation (Clancy et al 2013, Prietl et al 2013). Research over the last two decades has suggested that vitamin D has a role in autoimmune disease, cardiovascular disease, certain cancers, cognitive decline, depression, pregnancy complications, allergy, frailty and potential fetal epigenetics and brain development (Abrams et al 2013, Eyles et al 2013, Hossein-nezhad & Holick 2013, Liu et al 2013).

Cholecalciferol (D$_3$) is the form found in animal products and fish oils, whereas ergocalciferol (D$_2$) is the major synthetic form of provitamin D typically found in supplements and fortified foods; however, other forms also exist. These ingested forms have 50–80% bioavailability and enter the lymphatic circulation from the small intestine following emulsification by bile salts, and promote the absorption of calcium and phosphate from the gut (Nowson et al 2012).

Vitamin D (D$_3$) is also produced in the body through the conversion of a cholesterol-based precursor, 7-dehydrocholesterol, which is produced in the sebaceous glands of the skin. Exposure to sunlight (ultraviolet B [UVB]) converts this precursor into cholecalciferol over a 2–3-day period. Prolonged exposure to UVB can inactivate some of the newly formed vitamin D and its precursors, so that eventually a state of equilibrium is reached between vitamin D synthesis and catabolism. Therefore, short periods of sun exposure are considered more efficacious than long periods (Working Group 2005, 2012). Some vitamin D is stored in adipose tissue and can be mobilised during periods when exposure to sunlight is reduced or shortages develop (Nowson & Margerison 2002, Nowson et al 2012). This has implications for obesity research. Vitamin D and its metabolites are primarily excreted through bile, and the degraded active form is removed via the kidney. Losses are believed to be minor, owing to both reabsorption of vitamin D derivatives via the enterohepatic recirculation and limited filtration at the kidneys (Kohlmeier 2003). Parathyroid hormone (PTH), calcium, phosphorus and magnesium are involved in the regulation of vitamin D metabolism.

Traditionally associated with bone health, the identification of VDRs on a large and diverse number of cells has precipitated significant reconsideration of this nutrient (Dusso et al 2005, Holick 2004, 2006). VDRs are present in most tissues and cells in the body, including the brain, vascular smooth muscle, prostate, breast and macrophages (Hossein-nezhad & Holick 2013, Nowson et al 2012), and we now understand that vitamin D possesses two distinct action pathways dependent upon the site of bioactivation (Dusso et al 2005, Holick 2006). Renal hydroxylation of 25(OH)D produces 1,25$(OH)_2$D, primarily responsible for its traditional endocrine actions. In this two-step process, high-capacity cytochromes in the liver convert initially to D's major circulating form, 25-hydroxycholecalciferol (inactive) — 25(OH)D, and then further hydroxylation in the proximal tubular epithelial cells of the kidneys, to the biological active form: 1,25-dihydroxycholecalciferol — 1,25$(OH)_2$D, also known as calcitriol. This conversion is performed by CYP27B1 (25OH-1α-hydroxylase) (Clancy et al 2013, Nowson et al 2012). By contribution to regulation of extracellular calcium and phosphate homeostasis and through interaction with PTH, mineralisation of the skeleton is promoted, and regulation of muscle function (Angeline et al 2013). Importantly, as stated (Hossein-nezhad & Holick 2013, Nowson et al 2012), almost every nucleated cell expresses the VDR, and additionally, many extrarenal tissues have the capacity to make 1,25$(OH)_2$D. This is suggestive that vitamin D not only operates by the classical endocrine pathways, but through autocrine and paracrine pathways as well, implying that there are local synthesis and actions. This extrarenal bioactivation, by immune, prostate, breast, colon, beta and skin cells, however, results in non-genomic responses, characterised as autocrine rather than endocrine effects (Dusso et al 2005, Holick 2006, Kemmis et al 2006, Valdivielso et al 2009). Production of 1,25$(OH)_2$D at these sites does not fall under the same tight regulatory control as renal 1-alpha-hydroxylase (Dusso et al 2005, Kemmis et al 2006). This means that increasing concentrations of 25(OH)D provide a substrate for extrarenal bioactivation, with the rate of conversion mainly reliant upon local factors such as cytokines, which act to protect the internal cells from microbial invaders (Clancy et al 2013, Holick 2005, Lips 2006). Monocyte-macrophages contain CYP27B1, which enables intracellular production of active vitamin D, promoting an intracrine effect, which, by contrast to renal conversion, is not regulated by Ca^{2+} levels (Clancy et al 2013). It is instead driven by immune components such as chemokines like interferon-gamma (IFN-gamma) and Toll-like receptors (TLRs), which gives vitamin D the ability to act independently on the immune system. Its destruction by catabolic enzyme 24-hydroxylase (CYP24A1) is also initiated by its activation to the active form, but not in macrophages, which results in a prolonged signalling of vitamin D, which may provide insight into the potential mechanism of action in fighting intracellular organisms such as tuberculosis (Clancy et al 2013).

CHEMICAL COMPONENTS

Cholecalciferol (D_3) is considered to be the most important dietary form and is identical to the form produced in the body. Ergocalciferol (D_2) is produced by fungi and yeasts and is rare in the diet, but a common supplemental/fortificant form (Nowson & Margerison 2002, Nowson et al 2012). Some authors suggest that D_2 should not be classified as a nutrient, given that it has no natural place in human biology (Trang et al 1998, Vieth 2006) and, while both D_2 and D_3 were previously considered to be equipotent as supplements (FAO/WHO 2002, Nowson & Margerison 2002, Prietl et al 2013, Wahlqvist 2002), recent exploration of this issue points to marked discrepancies in favour of D_3. D_2 also comes under the names 1-alpha-OHD_2, calcifediol, calciferol, dihydrotachysterol, ergocalciferolum and ergosterol; D_3 may be referred to as 1-alpha-OHD_3, alfacalcidiol, calcitriol or rocaltrol (Micromedex 2003).

Quantification of any of the vitamin D forms is expressed in either international units (IU) or micrograms. The conversion is: 1 mcg = 40 IU.

Are all vitamin D forms alike?

Coincident with the recognition of 25(OH)D as the key marker of individual vitamin D status, the ability of cholecalciferol (D_3) and ergocalciferol (D_2) to increase serum levels of this marker has been compared (Trang et al 1998). Results from these studies reveal a 70% greater increase in serum 25(OH)D in response to cholecalciferol (D_3). Hypothesised reasons for this difference are based upon the distinct metabolic handling of the two different forms. D_3 demonstrates higher affinity for D-binding protein, making it less likely to be excreted in bile (Armas et al 2004, Dusso et al 2005, Hossein-nezhad & Holick 2013); D_3 produces more potent metabolites and is converted into 25(OH)D up to five times faster than D_2 (FSANZ 2007, Houghton & Vieth 2006, Trang et al 1998). The results of another study showed that serum 25(OH)D increases in response to D_2 supplementation were not sustained, and in fact fell below baseline values over 14 days, while the serum levels of those supplemented with D_3 continued to rise throughout the same period (Armas et al 2004). In addition to these concerns, the stability and purity of D_2 preparations are questionable (Houghton & Vieth 2006). This is confirmed by a recent systematic review reporting on 144 cohorts from 94 independent studies from 1990 to 2012. The review found that, in all four cohorts where D_2 was the supplement used, a decline in circulating 25(OH)D was observed. Further, in three of the four cohorts where D_2 and D_3 were reported separately, while an overall decline in 25(OH)D was noted, it is of interest that circulating 25(OH)D_2 increased significantly, but seemingly at the expense of 25(OH)D_3, which showed a marked decline (Zittermann et al 2014).

These findings have major ramifications for the interpretation of vitamin D research and the clinical implementation of such protocols. Every piece of vitamin D research must now be considered in the light of the supplemental form used. Clinically D_3's improved potency translates to significantly lower dose requirements, in the vicinity of 2.5–10 times less (FSANZ 2007, Houghton & Vieth 2006), compared with a D_2-based product (Glendenning 2002). Zittermann et al's (2014) review calculated that D_3 supplementation, compared with D_2, corresponded to an average increase of 20.19 nmol/L in circulating 25(OH)D. The review also found that concomitant calcium supplementation incurred a significant decrease in circulating 25(OH)D levels by an average of 6.34 nmol/L. Body weight, age and baseline circulating levels of 25(OH)D also impacted on circulating levels of 25(OH)D, with 54% of variability in levels being explained by these factors. Body weight was the main factor contributing more than one-third of the variance; however all these variables should be considered when reviewing or implementing the evidence, or planning new trials. The Working Group (2012) also discusses the concern of the effect of obesity on dosage regimens. Vitamin D enters adipose tissue and may not be readily available unless there is fat breakdown, which may result in lower circulating vitamin D following oral supplementation.

FOOD SOURCES

Small amounts are found in fatty fish, such as herring, salmon, tuna and sardines, beef and liver, butter, eggs and fortified foods such as margarine and milk (Gropper et al 2009). Cod liver oil is also a good source. Notably, meat products also contain some 25(OH)D, which is five times more active than D_3 (Nowson & Margerison 2001); however, the vitamin D content of all animal products is dependent upon the individual animal's vitamin D status and the use of fortified feed (Mattila et al 2004). There is therefore concern that, as a consequence of modern agricultural and aquacultural practices, vitamin D content is in decline, as demonstrated by a study which revealed a 75% decrease in the vitamin D content of farmed compared to wild salmon (Lu et al 2007). Naturally occurring D_2 is found only in mushrooms.

Current vitamin D fortification practices in Australia provide very little supplementation of D_3 in mandatory fortification (including edible oil spreads and table margarine) and voluntary fortification (modified and skim milks, powdered milk, yoghurt, cheese, butter, legume- and cereal-based analogue beverages) (FSANZ 2011, Nowson & Margerison 2001). There is one specially supplemented milk product in Australia that provides 200 IU per 250 mL serving. However dietary fortifications are not mandated as they are in other countries such as the United States and Canada, and remain an inadequate source of supplementation (Working Group 2012). Australian diet studies reveal that fortified margarine and edible oil spreads make the largest single contribution to vitamin D consumption (28–53%) (NHMRC 2006, Nowson & Margerison 2001). An Australian study found that average dietary consumption of vitamin D was 1.2 mcg/day and that only 7.9% of this sample took vitamin D supplements (van der Mei et al 2007).

DEFICIENCY SIGNS AND SYMPTOMS

Although the traditional understanding of hypovitaminosis D revolves around its critical role in calcium metabolism, the extensive presence of VDR throughout the body is providing the impetus for further research into actions, deficiency states and therapeutic applications (Gropper et al 2009). Its role in vascular biology and cardiovascular health in particular has been a focus of clinical studies in recent years. Some clinical studies have linked low levels of vitamin D metabolites with higher incidence of congestive heart failure and increases in mortality (Valdivielso et al 2009). Several studies have looked into the relationship between chronic kidney disease and vitamin D status (Palmer et al 2007). However, in the expert opinion piece by Valdivielso et al (2009), the importance of vitamin D research in relation to vascular effects has been highlighted. The authors state that a causal relationship has been established in several basic science experiments between vitamin D and cardiovascular diseases (atherosclerosis, hypertension, arterial dysfunction, left ventricular hypertrophy). Equally, nephrology research has shown a great deal of interest due to the low levels of calcidiol and calcitriol seen in patients with chronic kidney disease, and with a higher mortality rate. With targeted trials to evaluate therapeutic levels of vitamin D to control secondary hyperparathyroidism, and cardiovascular disease, which is the major cause of death, vitamin D status is an important marker for these two patient populations (Valdivielso et al 2009). These authors, however, caution against the routine use of vitamin D supplementation in healthy humans where no deficit exists, with the idea of a U-shaped curve of benefit in metabolite levels for individuals.

Primary deficiency

Unlike many other vitamins, vitamin D is not only ingested through the diet but also produced and stored in the body. As such, endogenous production, which is reliant on adequate exposure to sunlight, will greatly influence whether deficiency states develop. It has been estimated that exposing the skin to UVB radiation produces approximately 90% of the vitamin D_3 (cholecalciferol) that is bioavailable in the body. Currently, the National Health and Medical Research Council (NHMRC) reports that it is almost impossible to get sufficient vitamin D from dietary sources alone, stressing the importance of UVB exposure (NHMRC 2006, Working Group 2012).

Deficiency more prevalent than once thought

Inadequate vitamin D among Australians is now recognised as a substantial concern, given the significant percentage demonstrating a combination of poor dietary intake and inadequate sun exposure, according to the 2012 position statement released by the Working Group of the Australian and New Zealand Bone and Mineral Society, Endocrine Society of Australia and Osteoporosis Australia. This working group cites epidemiological data that estimate 31% of adults in Australia have inadequate vitamin D status, which they define as <50 nmol/L, and up to 50% of women during winter and spring (Nowson et al 2012).

Ongoing epidemiological research in Australia supports this view and has identified the wider community at risk of mild deficiency, with the results of numerous studies supporting this proposition. Using a cut-off of ≤50 nmol/L for serum 25(OH)D, vitamin D insufficiency has been found to affect >40% of healthy adults in Queensland (Kimlin et al 2007, van der Mei et al 2007), >65% Tasmanians (van der Mei et al 2007) and up to 74% of general medical inpatients (Chatfield et al 2007) — including 54% of the last group, who were taking vitamin D supplements. A study of maternal and neonatal levels in Sydney revealed that 15% of mothers (at 23–32 weeks' gestation) and 11% of neonates met the criteria for overt vitamin D deficiency (≤25 nmol/L) (Bowyer et al 2009). These rates increase dramatically if the reference range for optimal serum 25(OH)D is raised, as has been proposed in the scientific literature (Dawson-Hughes et al 2005, Vieth et al 2001, 2004). One group of researchers reanalysed population data based on the proposed cut-off of ≤80 nmol/L (Dawson-Hughes et al 2005, Heaney 2006, Holick 2005) and found that 70% of their sample of healthy Australians would, using this definition, be below optimal (van der Mei et al 2007).

More recently, in 2014, a cohort of community-dwelling elective cardiothoracic surgical patients attending the Alfred Hospital in Melbourne, Australia, was found to have a high prevalence of suboptimal vitamin D (Braun et al 2014). When fasting serum samples were taken on the day of surgery, 92.5% of patients had vitamin D levels <75 nmol/L, 67.5% had levels <60 nmol/L, 52.5% had levels between 30 and 59 nmol/L and 15% had levels <30 nmol/L (Braun et al 2014). The implications for surgical outcomes, healing and future cardiovascular events remain to be investigated.

Factors associated with lower 25(OH)D levels in Australia include:

- seasonal effects, with winter–early spring demonstrating peak incidence (Bowyer et al 2009, Chatfield et al 2007, Kimlin et al 2007, McGillivray et al 2007, van der Mei et al 2007)
- increasing latitude (Angeline et al 2013, Nowson et al 2012, van der Mei et al 2007)
- increasing skin pigmentation (Kimlin et al 2007, Nowson et al 2012), with one study calculating an odds ratio (OR) of 2.7 for dark skin (Bowyer et al 2009)

- non-Australian birthplace: OR 2.2 (Erbas et al 2008)
- hospitalisation, and institutionalisation and age (Bruyere et al 2009).

The institutionalised elderly are of particular concern, as their exposure to sunlight is often restricted and they have an estimated twofold reduction in capacity of the skin to produce D_3 (Wilson et al 1991), compromised final conversion in the kidneys, reduced tissue response and further reductions to calcium absorption independently of these pathways (Bouillon et al 1997, FAO/WHO 2002). The increasing risk with age is clearly demonstrated by the results of a Tasmanian study, which revealed that, although only 8% of 8-year-olds were considered vitamin D-deficient, deficiency escalated with increasing age to peak at 85% for people aged 60 years (RACGP 2003).

At the other end of the age spectrum, a 2-year surveillance of infants presenting with vitamin D deficiency-related problems at the Monash Medical Centre in Clayton, Victoria, found that the 13 infants admitted to hospital all had migrant parents and were predominantly or exclusively breastfed (Pillow et al 1995). This is a dangerous combination, with dark-skinned migrants at a significantly greater risk of deficiency (Bowyer et al 2009, Erbas et al 2008), particularly women who are veiled (OR 21.7) (Bowyer et al 2009, Grover & Morley 2001, Nowson & Margerison 2002, Wigg et al 2006), and breast milk is recognised as a poor source of vitamin D (Andiran et al 2002). Australian research demonstrates that recently immigrated infants or first-generation offspring of immigrant parents, especially Indian, Middle Eastern, African and Polynesian, are a key at-risk group: 40% of infants aged 4–12 months were found to be deficient (Nozza & Rodda 2001, Robinson et al 2006) and 87% of sampled East African children (0–17 years) living in Melbourne recorded serum 25(OH)D levels ≤50 nmol/L (McGillivray et al 2007).

Other populations at risk include obese individuals (Arunabh et al 2003, Blum et al 2008, Harris & Dawson-Hughes 2007, Hossein-nezhad & Holick 2013), psychiatric patients (Berk et al 2007), individuals with an intellectual disability (estimated deficiency prevalence 50–60%) (Vanlint et al 2008) and those observing requirements of modest clothing (Zittermann et al 2014).

Clinical note — The vitamin D dilemma

Between 80% and 100% of our vitamin D needs can be met through adequate sun exposure, with dietary intake only required to meet the shortfall (Nowson & Margerison 2001, 2002, Nowson et al 2012, Samanek et al 2006). Quantifying this shortfall, however, is complex and individualistic, as multiple variables influence the rate of endogenous production, such as age, weight, season, latitude, time of day, part of body exposed to sunlight and use of sunscreen. Researchers estimate that full-body sun exposure in Australia, sufficient to induce mild erythema (minimal erythemal dose), is equivalent to consuming 15,000 IU orally, and that exposure of around 15% of the body surface (arms and hands or equivalent) for a third of a minimal erythemal dose, near the middle of the day, will produce about 1000 IU (25 mcg) (Working Group 2005, 2012). Hence, we have the dilemma: while the majority of public health messages continue to promote sun protection, there is growing media coverage of the negatives associated with this and advocacy for exposure to UVB in order to prevent vitamin D deficiency (Scully et al 2008). The successful Slip Slop Slap campaign in Australia, which encourages covering up and reduced sun exposure, appears at odds with the vitamin D message and may have put many Australians at risk of poor vitamin D status. Australian research concurs with this, indicating that the public health message battle is currently being won by 'sun protection', with only 15% of surveyed Australians agreeing with the statement that 'sun protection may result in not having enough vitamin D' (Janda et al 2007).

Clearly, revision of the current public health messages regarding both vitamin D and safe sunlight exposure has been required for some time. In response, work has been undertaken to develop a message of compromise (Nowson & Margerison 2002, Working Group 2005, 2012), and the development of a vitamin D index, similar to a UV index, has been proposed (van der Mei et al 2007). Evidence from a study by Samanek et al (2006) supports the concept that safe sun exposure can yield vitamin D adequacy. Their research concluded that from October to March only 10–15 minutes of unprotected exposure to 15% of the body outside of the hours of 10 a.m. to 3 p.m. was sufficient; however, during other seasons, up to 1 hour of exposure was required. In addition to this, the authors themselves acknowledge that calculations were based on existing serum values, which have been widely contested by other researchers (Gomez et al 2003). In view of some of these concerns, the new NHMRC vitamin guidelines released in 2006 are now recommending an increased adequate intake of vitamin D, particularly for adults aged over 50 years. The guidelines also suggest varying lengths of time for sun exposure for different skin types in order to achieve adequate levels. Whether these initiatives are sufficient to prevent deficiency in the community remains to be seen. The Working Group (2012) recommendations range from 5 minutes exposure in Townsville, 7 minutes in Sydney, to 9 minutes in Hobart over the summer, and 16 min to 29 min for the rest of the year. They state that those with darker skin are likely to require exposure three to six times longer than suggested values, and those at risk of deficiency include very fair-skinned people who avoid exposure, those who may have clothing that blocks exposure, as well as those with chronic illness, or who are confined indoors.

Secondary deficiency

Malabsorption states such as coeliac disease, Crohn's disease, gastrectomy, intestinal resection, chronic cholestasis, cystic fibrosis and pancreatic disorders increase the risk of deficiency (Hendler & Rorvik 2001, Kumar & Clark 2002, Nowson et al 2012).

The use of certain anticonvulsants and chronic administration of glucocorticoids increase the risk of vitamin D deficiency. Several rare hereditary forms of rickets develop because the body cannot process (metabolise) vitamin D normally (Beers & Berkow 2003). Chronic liver disease will obstruct the first hydroxylation reaction, and end-stage kidney disease results in negligible conversion of 25(OH)D into 1,25(OH)D (Kumar & Clark 2002, Micromedex 2003). One large study also demonstrated that levels of serum 25(OH)D are inversely correlated with percentage of body fat and, as such, morbidly obese individuals have increased requirements (Arunabh et al 2003).

Signs and symptoms of deficiency

The previously determined serum concentrations of 25(OH)D believed to be indicative of deficiency (<20–25 nmol/L) are considered outdated (Gomez et al 2003). It is now apparent that much higher concentrations, deemed 'suboptimal' status, have deleterious effects (Dawson-Hughes et al 2005, Heaney

2006, Holick 2005, Nowson & Margerison 2002). Indications of deficiency include:

- alopecia with dilated hair follicles and dermal cysts (Dusso et al 2005)
- anaemia, decreased bone cellularity and extramedullary erythropoiesis (Brown et al 1999)
- cardiomegaly (Dusso et al 2005, Holick 2005, Valdivielso et al 2009)
- cardiovascular disease (atherosclerosis, hypertension, arterial dysfunction, left ventricular hypertrophy) (Valdivielso et al 2009)
- chronic kidney disease increased mortality from cardiovascular causes (Valdivielso et al 2009)
- chronic fatigue syndrome (deficiency may be misdiagnosed as this) (Holick 2004, Schinchuk & Holick 2007)
- chronic lower-back pain (Al Faraj & Al Mutairi 2003)
- excess PTH secretion and parathyroid hyperplasia
- fibromyalgia (it is estimated that 40–60% of patients diagnosed with this condition are actually suffering from vitamin D deficiency) (Holick 2004, 2005, Schinchuk & Holick 2007)
- hypertension (Dusso et al 2005, Forman et al 2007, Holick 2005)
- impaired glucose-mediated insulin secretion (Brown et al 1999)
- increased risk of fracture in the elderly (not limited to vitamin D's influence on bone mass)
- increased susceptibility to mycobacterial and viral infections (Dusso et al 2005)
- peripheral vascular disease with claudication (may be misdiagnosed or confounding factor) (Holick 2005)
- rickets and osteomalacia
- osteopenia and osteoporosis
- sarcopenia — skeletal muscle weakness and atrophy (Dusso et al 2005, Visser et al 2003)
- stunting.

Deficiency also significantly increases the risk of:

- autoimmunity, including multiple sclerosis (MS) (including increased severity of pre-existing cases) (Dusso et al 2005, Hall & Juckett 2013, Holick 2004), diabetes type 1 (Clancy et al 2013, Cooper et al 2011, Holick 2006) and inflammatory bowel disease (Hewison 2011, Holick 2004)
- cancer — breast, prostate, colon and skin cancers are among the 20 different cancer types demonstrating an inverse relationship with vitamin D levels (Holick 2004)
- heart failure in patients with cardiovascular disease (Holick 2005, Valdivielso et al 2009)
- non-insulin-dependent diabetes mellitus in high-risk populations — some studies (Pittas et al 2007), but not all (Reis et al 2007), show positive association
- pre-eclampsia — particularly if hypovitaminosis D is present at <22 weeks (Bodnar et al 2007, Hossein-nezhad & Holick 2013).

V

MAIN ACTIONS

Whereas vitamin D is considered a fat-soluble vitamin, its active metabolite $1,25(OH)_2D_3$ is considered to be more like a steroid hormone, because it can be produced by the body and moves through the systemic circulation to reach target tissues via receptors both at the cell membrane and at the nuclear receptor proteins. Vitamin D possesses two distinct action pathways dependent upon the site of bioactivation (Clancy et al 2013, Dusso et al 2005, Holick 2006). Renal hydroxylation of 25(OH)D produces 1,25$(OH)_2$D, primarily responsible for its traditional endocrine actions mentioned, as well as playing a role in intestinal detoxification and calcium absorption (Kutuzova & DeLuca 2007, Nowson et al 2012), healthy insulin secretion (Brown et al 1999, Dusso et al 2005, Mathieu & Badenhoop 2005) and blood pressure control, via inhibition of renin production and blunting cardiomyocyte hypertrophy (Dusso et al 2005, Holick 2005, Simpson et al 2007, Valdivielso et al 2009).

Extrarenal bioactivation, by immune, prostate, breast, colon, beta and skin cells, however, results in non-genomic responses characterised as autocrine rather than endocrine effects (Dusso et al 2005, Hewison 2011, Holick 2006, Kemmis et al 2006). These autocrine effects include controlling immune function (especially anti-inflammatory), cellular growth, maturation, differentiation and apoptosis (Dusso et al 2005, Hewison 2011, Holick 2005, Kemmis et al 2006, Lips 2006) as well as photoprotection (Dixon et al 2007), explaining vitamin D's role in immune function and cancer prevention.

Regulation of calcium and phosphorus levels

In conjunction with PTH, which is released under conditions of low calcium levels, vitamin D can stimulate calcium and phosphorus absorption in the intestines, reabsorption in the kidneys and release of calcium from the bones back into the blood. 1,25$(OH)_2D_3$ in turn is regulated by PTH, calcium, phosphorus and 1,25$(OH)_2D_3$ itself (Wahlqvist 2002). To achieve the maximal efficiency of vitamin D-induced intestinal calcium transport, the serum 25(OH)D concentrations must be at least 78 nmol/L (30 ng/mL). In deficiency, intestinal absorption of calcium can be halved in adults (Hossein-nezhad & Holick 2013, Holick 2004).

Modelling and remodelling of bone

Besides influencing bone by maintaining calcium and phosphorus homeostasis, vitamin D may also contribute to bone health in other ways.

One pathway involves binding of 1,25$(OH)_2D_3$ to DNA to promote transcription of specific mRNA, which codes for osteocalcin. Osteocalcin is then secreted by the osteoblasts, which bind calcium in new bone (Gropper et al 2009). Vitamin D also appears to play a role in oestrogen biosynthesis by increasing expression of the aromatase enzyme gene. It has demonstrated a synergistic effect in select tissues with the phyto-oestrogen genistein, with co-administration leading to a prolonged half-life of active vitamin D (Harkness & Bonny 2005, Swami et al 2005).

Cell differentiation, proliferation and growth

Some of the actions already described are the result of the vitamin's capacity to affect cell differentiation, proliferation and growth in many tissues (e.g. differentiation of stem cells into osteoclasts to facilitate bone resorption). Alternatively, 1,25$(OH)_2D_3$ can inhibit proliferation in many cells, including lymphocytes, keratinocytes, mammary, cardiac and both skeletal and smooth-muscle cells. This ability has led to its investigation as a treatment for proliferative disorders such as cancer (Brown et al 1999, Gropper et al 2009, Hossein-nezhad & Holick 2013, Kohlmeier 2003).

Reduction of PTH and regulation of growth of the parathyroid gland

Although PTH regulates the levels of 1,25$(OH)_2$D, its secretion is regulated by vitamin D, calcium and phosphorus. In deficiency, hypersecretion of this hormone can cause excessive growth of the parathyroid gland and secondary hyperparathyroidism (Brown et al 1999, Hewison 2011).

Immunomodulation

Increasing evidence for vitamin D's importance outside its classical role in bone metabolism is emerging. However the use of vitamin D to treat diseases has been used since Hippocrates first prescribed sunlight for tuberculosis (Clancy et al 2013). Vitamin D enhances the immune system's response to both bacterial and viral agents (Grant 2008c), primarily through promoting differentiation and activity of the macrophages, which means that immune responses can be tailored through the appropriate cell response (Brown et al 1999), but also through the induction of cathelicidin (Maalouf 2008). Vitamin D influences the cytokine production of immune cells, suppressing the release of interleukin-2 (IL-2), IFN-gamma and TNF-alpha, products of the Th1 line of cells, thereby reducing the propensity for a range of autoimmune conditions (Thien et al 2005). This reflects its propensity for inhibiting adaptive immunity while potentiating the innate response (Bikle 2008). There is speculation that, through this mechanism, vitamin D will promote a Th2 dominance and may predispose to the atopic diathesis. Supporting evidence comes from two studies that reveal supplementation with vitamin D in early life to be a potential precipitator of allergic disease (Hyppönen et al 2001); however, in other scenarios (e.g. autoimmunity) this effect would be considered to be therapeutic (Smolders et al 2008). In recent years, data have increasingly linked vitamin D deficiency with Th1 autoimmune disorders (Clancy et al 2013), such as MS, type 1 diabetes and Crohn's disease, suggesting a significant impact of vitamin D on immune function. Even increased susceptibility to infectious diseases, such as tuberculosis, is thought to have a link to low vitamin D levels (Hewison 2012). In a symposium paper from the Proceedings of the Nutrition Society, Hewison (2012) discusses that cells from the immune system are capable of converting the precursor 25-hydroxyvitamin D to the active 1,25-dihydroxyvitamin D, which stimulates a macrophage response to this active form in an antimicrobial fashion. Additionally, regulation of the maturation of antigen-presenting dendritic cells (DCs) occurs, from which vitamin D may control T-lymphocyte (T-cell) function. T cells, however, also have a direct response capacity to the active form of vitamin D in the activation of suppressor regulatory T cells. This suggests an immune adaptive response as well as innate immunity. Its influence on cytokine inflammatory markers, as mentioned above, may indicate a protective effect by reducing prolonged exposure to inflammation (Hewison 2012). Prietl et al (2013) also suggest that vitamin D-metabolising enzymes and VDRs, present in many cell types, are expressed extensively in immune cells, including antigen-presenting cells, T cells, B cells and monocytes, and purport that this not only modulates innate immune cells, but promotes a more tolerogenic immunological state.

OTHER ACTIONS

V

Our current understanding of the role of vitamin D appears to be only part of the picture. Ongoing discovery of previously unidentified receptors on tissues continues to broaden our understanding of its diverse effects. Recently, Nowson et al (2012), in the Working Group paper, state that almost every nucleated cell expresses the VDR, and that many extrarenal tissues have the capacity to make $1,25(OH)_2D$. This suggests evidence for not only classical endocrine operation, but also autocrine and paracrine pathways, which suggests vitamin D's role and importance in local synthesis and actions. This has major implications for vitamin D research and therapeutic value.

Haematopoietic tissues

VDRs have been identified on haematopoietic and lymphoid cells, suggesting the role of vitamin D in blood cell development and immune system function. The biologically active form of vitamin D, calcitriol, exerts an effect on erythropoiesis and bone cellularity. Calcitriol activates the VDRs, which appear to be the mediator of vitamin D's action, and may have a role in homing lymphoid cells to specific tissues. It has been found that VDRs are ubiquitous in human tissue, and that the gene for VDR, with its various polymorphisms (encoded on chromosome 12) and differences in transcription effects, is responsible for at least some of the variability among individuals, not only in vitamin D absorption and status, but in biologically diverse ways, such as adult height, bone mineral density and susceptibility to diseases such as tuberculosis (Hall & Juckett 2013).

Vitamin D has also been shown to inhibit clonal cell proliferation in some leukaemia lines and to promote leucocyte differentiation (Brown et al 1999). VDRs are expressed in various cells such as monocytes, thymocytes, activated B and T lymphocytes, as well as haematopoietic precursors in the haematopoietic system. The presence on activated lymphocytes suggests that there is an immune modulation role on differentiated cells. Changes in inflammatory cytokine profiles in VDR knockout mice suggest vitamin D's role in mediating inflammation (Hall & Juckett 2013). The expression of VDR on isolated DCs from lymphoid tissue further confirms the role of vitamin D in immunoregulation (Hewison 2012). DCs are critical in the adaptive immune response, in the establishment of immunological memory, and have the ability to induce a primary immune response in T lymphoctyes (Wieder 2003). Treatment with 1,25(OH)2D has been shown to suppress DC maturation, specifically in the myeloid DC, which is responsible for T-cell activation, and promote the more tolerogenic plasmacytoid DC (Hewison 2012).

Muscle function

Vitamin D maintains muscle strength and has an effect on skeletal muscle and smooth muscle, with proximal muscle weakness being a common feature of deficiency (Hossein-nezhad & Holick 2013). Early work performed in 1975 demonstrated a relationship between vitamin D and muscle function. Birge and Haddad found that phosphate regulation within the muscle cell promoted maintenance of muscle metabolism and function. In 2004, Holick suggested a link between fibromyalgia and vitamin D deficiency, with 40–60% of cases presenting with generalised muscle weakness and pain being estimated as undiagnosed hypovitaminosis. More recently, with VDR being identified on smooth-muscle cells, and with vitamin D's classic role in calcium and phosphate homeostasis, there are major implications for skeletal muscle function as well as smooth muscle in the respiratory, cardiovascular and reproductive systems. Cannell and colleagues (2009) describe the binding of $1,25(OH)_2D_3$ to the VDR, leading to gene transcription and increased cell protein synthesis and growth. Further, Bischoff-Ferrari et al (2004) show an age-related decline of VDR expression in muscle tissue, and abnormal development of muscle fibres and maturation have been demonstrated in VDR knockout mice (Minasyan et al 2009).

The cellular effect of vitamin D can be seen in a variety of cellular signalling cascades. Principal among them is the mitogen-activated protein kinase signalling pathway, which initiates muscle tissue cell genesis, proliferation and differentiation (Angeline et al 2013). Disruption of this pathway in deficient murine models and subsequent supplementation showed an increase in muscle mass through increased protein synthesis. Interestingly, however, exercise-induced muscle cell apoptosis was reduced in these animals (Cannell et al 2009, Ceglia 2009). Further clinical trials should be implemented to elucidate the implications of this effect.

The US Preventive Services Task Force report concluded that vitamin D supplementation is effective in preventing falls in community-dwelling adults over 65 years, but the evidence is less convincing about primary fracture prevention (Moyer 2013). With a demonstrated age-related decline in VDR expression (Bischoff-Ferrari et al 2004), and Minasyan et al's (2009) finding that their VDR knockout mice with abnormal muscle fibre development and maturation also showed poorer motor and balance function, the role of vitamin D in muscle health and strength may play at least a part in falls prevention and therefore fracture risk reduction in the elderly.

Vascular function

Local production of calcitriol acts as a regulator of certain cell functions. In both endothelial and vascular smooth muscle, the VDR activity suggests that vitamin D acts via an endocrine pathway as a regulator of vascular function. VDR is expressed in cells throughout the vascular system, including vascular smooth-muscle cells, endothelial cells and cardiomyocytes, which all produce CYP27B1 to convert into the active form calcitriol. Calcitriol has been shown to exhibit anti-inflammatory properties, through local control of cytokines, and also exhibit an inhibitory effect on vascular smooth-muscle cell proliferation, and help to regulate the renin-angiotensin system (Shapses & Manson 2011). Vitamin D has been found to exert a direct effect on the myocardium: $1,25(OH)_2D_3$ controls hypertrophy in cardiac monocytes and, together with 25(OH)D, improves the left ventricular function in patients with cardiomyopathies (Brown et al 1999). Cardiovascular pathology is the leading cause of death in patients with chronic kidney disease, and there is a relationship between cardiovascular health and vitamin D status. Metabolite levels are associated with a higher incidence of congestive heart failure and increases in mortality (Valdivielso et al 2009). Vitamin D deficiency has also been linked to an increased risk of developing incident hypertension (Forman et al 2007, Wang et al 2008). Observational studies have suggested considerable benefits from vitamin D dietary intake and supplementation; however, clinical trial evidence for hypertension and diabetes is inconsistent, and in subanalysis potentially suggests a benefit for those with the lowest levels of circulating vitamin D, and a potential detriment for normotensive individuals, or those with adequate circulating 25(OH)D levels, suggesting a U-shaped curve of benefit. While biological plausibility exists, the data have been less compelling in human subjects compared with animal models (Shapses & Manson 2011, Valdivielso et al 2009). Confounding factors such as obesity, age and exercise levels need to be considered in conducting robust large-scale randomised controlled trials (RCTs) with cardiovascular outcomes as the primary measure.

V

Pancreatic function

Vitamin D is essential for normal insulin secretion, as demonstrated in both animals and humans, and VDRs have been found in pancreatic beta cells, whose function improves following vitamin D repletion (Alemzadeh et al 2008, Mathieu & Badenhoop 2005, Palomer et al 2008). Enhanced insulin synthesis may be due to vitamin D's role in controlling intracellular calcium flux in islet cells which facilitates conversion of proinsulin to insulin, exocytosis of insulin and beta-cell glycolysis (Brown et al 1999, Palomer et al 2008). Vitamin D also modulates insulin receptor gene expression (Palomer et al 2008).

Brain function

Evidence over the past 10–15 years confirms that the steroid hormone vitamin D is essential for normal homeostasis and development of the brain (Eyles et al 2013). The data implicate 1,25$(OH)_2$D in the biosynthesis of neurotrophic factors, contribution to brain detoxification pathways with increased glutathione and reduced nitric oxide, neuroprotective effects, induction of glioma cell death and involvement in neurotransmitter synthesis, including acetylcholine and the catecholamines (Garcion et al 2002). The VDR and 1-alpha-hydroxylase activity has been demonstrated in specific brain regions (e.g. the hypothalamus), implying a potential role for vitamin D as a neuroactive hormone (Berk et al 2007, Eyles et al 2014, Obradovic et al 2006, Vieth et al 2004). There is also increasing evidence of vitamin D's modulation of several neurotransmitters, such as acetylcholine, catecholamines and serotonin (Jorde et al 2006, Obradovic et al 2006). Preliminary studies in rats have demonstrated an antiepileptic action (Kalueff & Tuohimaa 2005). Tentative links are being made between the aetiology/pathophysiology of Parkinson's disease and poor vitamin D status (Johnson 2001, Kim et al 2005). The extensive and interesting work of the Australian group of Eyles and colleagues has been presented in a series of papers, and has outlined the varied and far-reaching implications of vitamin D deficiency and absence in the developing fetal brain (Byrne et al 2005, Cui et al 2010, Eyles et al 2003, 2011, 2013, 2014, Harms et al 2011). Vitamin D affects an array of cellular functions, and the group has described in experimental mouse and rat models the effects of induced extreme deficiency, and developmental absence of vitamin D. These models show: a less differentiated brain; changes to neurotrophic factor expression; cytokine regulation; neurotransmitter synthesis; intracellular calcium signalling; antioxidant activity; greater number of proliferating cells (which elongates the shape of the developing brain); less apoptosis (further influencing distribution and shape of brain); expression of genes/proteins; structure and metabolism; and a reduction in factors associated with neuronal maturation (Eyles et al 2003, 2011, 2014). Additionally the group has demonstrated a persistent effect into adulthood of altered brain anatomy in structure and function (Eyles et al 2013), and neurochemistry (Eyles et al 2012) for fetuses exposed to deficiency or absence of vitamin D.

VDRs are shown to be nucleic in fetal life and readily apparent in the brain, although in lower amount than the more usual target organs of the gut and kidneys. However, in adulthood VDRs are demonstrated to be in the plasma membrane and more prominent in the gut and kidney, suggesting a change in function with maturation of the organs (Eyles et al 2014). Vitamin D deficiency has been linked to developmental psychiatric disorders, such as autism spectrum disorder, schizophrenia and Parkinson's disease, in observational and epidemiological studies (Eyles et al 2014). Correlations with greater risk associated with increasing latitude, seasonal variation as well as darker skin pigmentation in migrant groups have been well established for risk of schizophrenia (Cantor-Graae & Selten 2005, Davies et al 2003), depression (Byrne et al 2005), and are emerging for autism spectrum disorder (Cannell 2008, Grant & Soles 2009).

CLINICAL USE

Vitamin D is administered using various routes and can be prescribed as either a supplement or a drug, largely depending on dose and administration route. This review will focus on oral supplementation of D_2 or D_3 only and will not cover the variety of analogues that continue to be extensively studied. For many conditions that appear to require high doses, the race is on to develop and trial pharmaceutical analogues that retain, in particular, the antiproliferative nature of the vitamin, but are low-calcaemic in order to minimise the associated toxicity seen at such doses.

Deficiency states

Frank vitamin D deficiency in infancy or childhood produces rickets, which results from reduced sun exposure, deficient diet or metabolic or malabsorptive diseases. Vitamin D deficiency results in inadequate calcium and phosphorus levels for bone mineralisation (Beers & Berkow 2003). Diagnosis is confirmed with X-ray and serum assay of 25(OH)D. When occurring in adults, it is called osteomalacia, and its first presentation is often as chronic lower-back pain (Al Faraj & Al Mutairi 2003).

Defective vitamin D metabolism may be another cause, and consequently deficiency will not respond to standard oral treatment. In this situation, extremely high doses may be required, which should be monitored carefully for toxicity (Beers & Berkow 2003).

Pregnancy and lactation supplementation

Vitamin D's role in pregnancy is extremely complex, and points to its importance not only in establishing a pregnancy, but also in fetal and neonatal growth and development (Hossein-nezhad & Holick 2013). Vitamin D appears to be critical both to musculoskeletal and neurological growth and to the development of the infant. A recent Cochrane review, including six trials and reporting on a total of 1023 women, concluded that supplementation with vitamin D significantly improved women's vitamin D levels. The clinical significance of this finding and the potential use of vitamin D supplementation as a part of routine antenatal care are yet to be determined. (De-Regil et al 2012). The authors reported that data from three trials indicated that women who received vitamin D supplementation were slightly less likely to have a low-birth-weight (<2500 g) baby. However, no difference was apparent with regard to: pre-eclampsia; gestational diabetes; impaired glucose tolerance; caesarean section; gestational hypertension; or death in the mothers. For the newborns there was no difference in: preterm birth; stillbirth; neonatal death; neonatal admission to intensive care unit; low Apgar score; or neonatal infection (De-Regil et al 2012). In a study by Merewood and colleagues (2009), a strong association was found between vitamin D deficiency and increased risk of caesarean section. When all other factors were controlled for, having serum 25(OH)D <37.5 nmol/L increased the odds of having a caesarean delivery by 3.84. Women who had the highest serum 25(OH)D levels had the lowest risk of requiring a caesarean delivery. The authors hypothesise that, given that muscles contain VDRs, and that suboptimal muscle performance and weakness are associated with low serum 25(OH)D, this may be responsible for a potential failure to spontaneously begin labour or failure to progress in labour. Also, given the role of 25(OH)D in calcium regulation, this may also affect the action of smooth muscle required for efficient labour initiation and effective contractions (Merewood et al 2009).

An Australian study investigated the well-documented seasonal variation in birth weight to determine the parameters of anthropometric changes associated with this seasonal variation (McGrath et al 2005). Comparison of over 350,000 mean monthly birth weights of neonates at more than 37 weeks' gestation revealed that overall size, length, head size and skinfold thickness all display seasonal variation, but in particular greater limb length occurred with winter/spring births. Earlier animal studies imply that this may be a consequence of hypertrophy of the cartilage growth plates due to prenatal hypovitaminosis D (McGrath et al 2005).

Whether pregnant women require additional supplementation has been investigated in some studies. Trials involving more than 500 women conducted by Marya et al (1981, 1987), not included in the Cochrane Register review, have demonstrated statistically significant increased fetal birth weight, reduced prevalence of hypocalcaemia and hypophosphataemia, detected in both maternal and cord blood, and reduced blood pressure in non-toxaemic women. Additional evidence suggests a preventive role for a range of autoimmune conditions in the offspring when prenatal vitamin D levels are adequate (Holick 2004).

There is greater consensus regarding the need for vitamin D supplementation during lactation; breast milk is recognised as a poor source of this vitamin and infants are largely dependent on stored vitamin D acquired in utero (Andiran et al 2002, De-Regil et al 2012).

Children

The optimal regimen in relation to both route and dose of vitamin D for at-risk children remains controversial and is based on studies of limited size (Huh & Gordon 2008). The most common recommendation for infants is to supplement with D_2 or D_3 at 1000–2000 IU/day and up to 4000 IU/day in children older than 1 year. The US Institute of Medicine released a report in 2010 recommending dietary intakes of 400 IU/day for healthy infants and 600 IU for healthy children. The target circulating level of 25(OH)D was set at 50 nmol/L. This does not take into account the requirements for acutely or chronically unwell infants and children (Abrams et al 2013).

Treatment of deficiencies secondary to malabsorptive syndromes

Numerous studies have confirmed a high prevalence (25–75%) of hypovitaminosis D in patients with coeliac disease, Crohn's disease, small-bowel resection or cystic fibrosis. A positive correlation between low vitamin D status and clinical consequences, such as reduced bone mineral density and osteopenia, has been demonstrated in most studies. Interestingly, trials investigating the benefits of oral vitamin D supplements (400–800 IU/day) found limited success in patients. Owing to the theoretical advantage of supplementation in conditions associated with poor nutrient absorption, larger trials involving higher doses or different forms are expected to determine the most effective treatment (Abrams et al 2013, Buchman 1999, Congden et al 1981, Hanly et al 1985, Hoffmann & Zeitz 2000, Jahnsen et al 2002). A study of children with cystic fibrosis demonstrated 25(OH)D levels that were consistently >50 nmol/L with an average dose of 1405 IU/day.

Reducing all-cause mortality

Several large studies have identified an association between serum 25(OH)D concentrations and all-cause and cause-specific mortality, finding that, in particular, vitamin D deficiency (25(OH)D concentration <30 nmol/L) mortality was strongly associated with mortality from all causes, cardiovascular diseases, cancer and respiratory diseases (Schottker et al 2013, 2014). One German study investigated concentrations of 25(OH)D in 9578 people who were followed up over 9.5 years. For those people with vitamin D deficiency (<30 nmol/L) or insufficiency (30–50 nmol/L) was significantly increased (1.71 [1.43, 2.03] and 1.17 [1.02, 1.35], respectively) compared with that of subjects with sufficient 25(OH)D concentrations (>50 nmol/L). Vitamin D deficiency was also associated with increased cardiovascular mortality (1.39: 95% CI 1.02–1.89), cancer mortality (1.42: 95% CI 1.08–1.88) and respiratory disease mortality (2.50: 95% CI 1.12–5.56). The association of 25(OH)D concentrations with all-cause mortality proved to be a non-linear inverse association with risk that started to increase at 25(OH)D concentrations <75 nmol/L (Schottker et al 2013). Chowdery et al (2014) also concluded that evidence from observational studies indicates inverse associations of circulating 25-hydroxyvitamin D with risks of death due to cardiovascular disease, cancer and other causes. In particular, supplementation with vitamin D_3 significantly reduces overall mortality among older adults (Chowdhury et al 2014). The conclusion was based on study-specific relative risks from 73 cohort studies (849,412 participants) and 22 randomised controlled trials (vitamin D given alone versus placebo or no treatment; 30,716 participants). These were meta-analysed using random effects models and grouped by study and population characteristics.

The same group continued to explore the relationship in a larger study that involved a meta-analysis of individual participant data of eight prospective cohort studies from Europe and the United States. This involved data from 26,018 men and women aged 50–79 years. Comparing bottom versus top quintiles for vitamin D, a pooled risk ratio of 1.57 (95% CI 1.36–1.81) for all-cause mortality was observed. Risk ratios for cardiovascular mortality were similar in magnitude to that for all-cause mortality in subjects both with and without a history of cardiovascular disease at baseline. With respect to cancer mortality, an association was only observed among subjects with a history of cancer (risk ratio, 1.70: 1.00–2.88). Interestingly, no strong age, sex, season or country-specific differences were detected. The authors concluded that, despite levels of 25(OH)D strongly varying with country, sex and season, the association between 25(OH)D level and all-cause and cause-specific mortality was remarkably consistent (Schottker et al 2014).

Cancer prevention

In the 1930s it was reported that US navy personnel exposed to high-level UVB showed higher rates of skin cancer but lower rates of cancer malignancies (Giovannucci 2008, Grant 2008a). World Health Organization data from as early as 1955 have demonstrated latitudinal gradients in cancer mortality rates for breast, colon, lung, prostate, rectal and renal cancer (Grant 2008a); however, the hypothesis linking UVB, vitamin D and cancer was not formally proposed until 1980. Since this time, ongoing epidemiological evidence has demonstrated in both single and multiple-country studies that there is increasing cancer incidence or mortality with increasing distance from the equator (Garland et al 1999, Grant 2008a). Both advancing age and ethnicity have also been positively correlated with these cancers and this has been similarly explained in relation to reduced UVB exposure. Further epidemiological support comes from the inverse relationship between prospective serum 25(OH)D levels and cancer risk, season of cancer diagnosis and survival time and lower rates of cancer in high fish-consuming countries such as Iceland and Japan (Giovannucci 2008, Grant 2008a). In 2002 Grant identified 14 cancers for which there was strong evidence to support vitamin D sensitivity, including breast, colon, ovarian, prostate and rectal forms. Recently, Hossein-nazhad & Holick (2013) have outlined evidence to support the hypothesis of vitamin D's ability to regulate microRNA and its effect in several cancer cell lines, tissues and sera. They also suggest that local conversion of 25(OH)D in healthy cells in the colon, breast and prostate can help prevent malignancy. This prevention may occur due to 25(OH)D's capacity to induce cellular maturation, induce apoptosis and inhibit angiogenesis (Hewison 2011). Additionally, 25(OH) D may act to enhance the genes which control cellular proliferation and active detoxifying enzymes (Eyles et al 2013, Hossein-nazhad & Holick 2013).

Evidence from an interventional study of calcium (1400–1500 mg/day), alone or with vitamin D_3 (1100 IU/day), versus a placebo over 4 years supports a chemoprotective role for vitamin D (Lappe et al 2007). The study, involving

1179 women >55 years old, was primarily designed to assess reductions in fracture incidence, but upon further analysis also demonstrated significant risk reduction (relative risk [RR] 0.40) for all cancer incidence in the combined calcium and vitamin D group. When the analysis was restricted to those cancers diagnosed only after the first year of treatment, the RR became 0.23. While the group receiving calcium alone also demonstrated a reduced risk, the researchers speculate that this may not be robust and conclude that vitamin D is the key variable in reduced incidence of all cancer. Given the ability of vitamin D to inhibit abnormal proliferation, facilitate apoptosis, attenuate growth signals and reduce angiogenesis around tumours, its chemoprotective potential continues to be enthusiastically investigated through both in vitro studies and RCTss (Giovannucci 2008, Grant 2008a, Hossein-nazhad & Holick 2013). Risk reduction via protection against viral infections has also recently been hypothesised (Grant 2008b, Hewison 2012).

Improving cancer prognosis

According to a systematic review of 26 clinical studies, evidence now suggests that circulating 25-OHD levels may be associated with better prognosis in patients with breast and colorectal cancer (Toriola et al 2014).

Colorectal cancer and prevention of adenomatous polyps

Evidence of vitamin D's chemoprotective effect is strongest in relation to colorectal cancer (Giovannucci 2008) and comes from several different lines of investigation (Garland et al 1991, Giovannucci 2008, Grant & Garland 2004, Holt 2008, Holt et al 2002, Theodoratou et al 2008). A 2004 review of more than 20 epidemiological studies of vitamin D and colorectal cancer concluded that the overwhelming majority of studies have demonstrated an inverse relationship between dietary intake, serum 25(OH)D and incidence (Garland et al 2004). An estimate of daily requirements needed for prevention has been formulated using the data from the studies, suggesting that an oral intake of >1000 IU/day of vitamin D or serum 25(OH)D levels of >33 ng/mL (82 nmol/L) could reduce the risk of colorectal cancer by as much as 50%. Most intervention studies to date, however, have focused on calcium supplementation. Interestingly, some of these show that calcium's protective effect against recurrent adenomas is largely restricted to individuals with baseline serum 25(OH)D above the median (≈ 29 ng/mL). These data, together with later findings (Mizoue et al 2008), strongly point to a synergism between calcium and vitamin D for colorectal cancer and recurring adenoma risk reduction (Grau et al 2003, Holt 2008, Oh et al 2007, Theodoratou et al 2008).

An often-cited negative finding comes from the Women's Health Initiative (WHI), in which women supplemented with 1000 mg calcium and 400 IU vitamin D per day failed to demonstrate reduced cancer rates; however, several authors have published major criticisms of the study that include the inadequate dose of vitamin D administered and the time frame (Giovannucci 2008, Grant 2008a, Holt 2008). Reanalysis of the WHI findings has also elucidated oestrogen's critical modifying effect upon both nutrients, whereby higher oestrogen levels of both menstruating and postmenopausal women taking hormone replacement therapy negate calcium's otherwise protective effect (Ding et al 2008). Explanations for this phenomenon include competitive binding between vitamin D and oestrogen (Ding et al 2008, Oh et al 2007). Two recent meta-analyses reporting on more than 2000 participants each have shown a significant decrease in the risk of colorectal and rectal cancer in an inverse relationship with circulating levels of 25(OH)D (Chung et al 2011, Lee et al 2011). Stubbins et al (2012) show that the active form of vitamin D targets a β-catenin pathway by upregulating key tumour suppressor genes, which promote an epithelial phenotype. This is only possible when there is adequate VDR expression. This could provide useful targets for therapeutic administration.

Current evidence for a combined protective role of calcium, either dietary or supplemental, and vitamin D, particularly in men and postmenopausal women not taking hormone replacement therapy, is strong and further elucidation of the independent and combined effects of these nutrients will assist in the development of preventive protocols. Stubbins et al (2012) suggest that the recommended dietary intake should be increased to 2000 IU to target and increase serum 25(OH)D levels to above 30 ng/mL.

Prostate

Vitamin D's relationship to cancer is least clear with respect to prostate cancer, with inconsistent findings from numerous studies (Giovannucci 2008, Li et al 2007, Mucci & Spiegelman 2008). The belief that increased calcium, dairy consumption and vitamin D levels could increase risk has dominated, with epidemiological evidence from a number of substantial studies, including the Helsinki Heart Study, involving 19,000 men. This study showed that increased levels of circulating 1,25$(OH)_2D_3$ and low levels of 25(OH)D are inversely associated with prostate cancer, in both incidence and aggressiveness, and are associated with an earlier age of onset (Chen & Holick 2003, Mucci & Spiegelman 2008). However, evidence of the potentially protective effects of increased serum 25(OH)D and 1,25$(OH)_2D$ continue to emerge (Li et al 2007), while more comprehensive investigations of the relationship between dietary vitamin D intake and risk fail to show any effect (Huncharek et al 2008), largely due to globally poor intakes. Several explanations for these contrasting findings have been proposed, including that vitamin D status many years prior to diagnosis may be more predictive and relevant than levels just before or following diagnosis (Giovannucci 2008, Mucci & Speigelman 2008). In a recent review of ecological studies, there was strong evidence for a correlation with solar UVB irradiance and 15 types of neoplasms, and weaker, but significant, evidence of nine other types of cancer, including prostate (Grant 2012).

Experimental research with vitamin D has produced interesting results. Prostate cancer cells in vitro respond to vitamin D_3 with reduced proliferation, increased differentiation and apoptosis. More recently, reduced activity of the 1-alpha-hydroxylase enzyme in cancerous prostate cells when compared to healthy prostate tissue was discovered, resulting in a reduced ability to convert vitamin D to its active form. Therefore, prostates with cancer display partial resistance to the tumour-suppressing activity of 1,25$(OH)_2D_3$ (Ma et al 2004). Clinical trials using supplemental vitamin D at various stages of prostate cancer have yielded inconsistent results (Miller 1999).

Breast

Normal breast cells produce 1,25$(OH)_2D$, which in turn may contribute to healthy mammary function, inducing differentiation, inhibiting proliferation and modulating immune responses (Perez-Lopez 2008). VDRs in mammary tissue have also been shown to oppose oestrogen-driven proliferation of cells (Welsh et al 2003). In addition, there is growing epidemiological evidence to suggest an inverse association between vitamin D and breast cancer (Grant 2006, 2008c, 2012, Mohr et al 2008, Perez-Lopez 2008), with increasing UVB exposure reported to produce a RR of between 0.67 and 0.85 (Perez-Lopez 2008). One study that involved 179 breast cancer patients and 179 controls assessed vitamin D status of patients and polymorphisms of vitamin D, and identified an inverse relationship, possibly as high as sevenfold, between 25(OH)D levels and breast cancer risk (Lowe et al 2005). Interestingly, from a population-based case-control study in Ontario, there is evidence to suggest that sun exposure between the ages of 10 and 19 years is particularly protective against subsequent breast cancer diagnoses (Perez-Lopez 2008). This implies that vitamin D status may be especially important during breast development.

A more recent investigation of the effect of UVB exposure on breast cancer incidence in 107 countries also confirmed that increased UVB exposure is independently protective, with age-standardised incidence rates substantially higher at latitudes distant from the equator (Mohr et al 2008). The same study demonstrated that the protective effect was evident at serum levels above 22 ng/mL. Another study revealed that women with serum 25(OH)D ≥ 50 ng/mL halve their risk of breast cancer compared to those below this cut-off level (Perez-Lopez 2008).

A large meta-analysis of dietary studies initially failed to find a relationship between vitamin D intake and breast cancer risk. Restricting studies to only those with intakes > 400 IU/day, however, revealed a trend towards risk reduction with increasing vitamin D intake (RR 0.92) (Gissel et al 2008).

Autoimmune diseases

Autoimmune status is affected by multifactorial inputs: environmental contribution, as well as a genetic predisposition, and exposure to epidemiological risk factors are all key influencers of a person's immune state. Increasing prevalence of autoimmune disorders as well as geographical and seasonal variations have led to investigations of vitamin D insufficiency as a potential key factor. Autoimmune diseases such as type 1 diabetes mellitus (T1DM), MS, systemic lupus erythematosus (SLE), rheumatoid arthritis, Crohn's disease and other inflammatory bowel disease have been linked to significant epidemiological data which suggest associations with vitamin D (Hewison 2011, Prietl et al 2013). Treatment with calcitriol in animal models has shown to have preventive effects, or amelioration of disease (Bock et al 2012; Hewison 2011). Further, Bock et al (2012) present animal data from vitamin D-deficient or VDR knockout mice, showing increased inflammation and increased susceptibility to autoimmune disorders such as T1DM and Crohn's disease. Interestingly, they also demonstrate disturbed T-cell function, such as homing, and a lack of host protection from bacterial invasion and infection. Hall and Juckett (2013) elucidate the mechanism of action. Inflammatory cytokines, such as IL-2 and IFN-γ, stimulate a cellular immune response termed Th1, whereas IL-4, IL-6 and IL-10 drive a humoral immune response, termed Th2. Stimulation of VDR tends to favour the inflammatory mediating Th2 response by suppressing IFN-γ, which is implicated in innate and adaptive immunity, as well as autoimmune disease, when uncontrolled. Hewison (2011) also discusses regulation of cytokine synthesis and apoptosis of inflammatory cells with therapeutic administration of calcitriol in MS model mice.

Type 1 diabetes mellitus

Vitamin D deficiency has been linked to both types of diabetes mellitus, but the largest volume of evidence relates to an inverse association between prenatal and infant vitamin D levels and a child's overall risk of developing T1DM (Bailey et al 2007, Hyppönen et al 2001, 2010, Littorin et al 2006, Prietl et al 2013, Zipitis & Akobeng 2008). Incidence rates vary widely according to geographical location related to latitude. It is hypothesised that vitamin influences T1DM pathogenesis by reducing lymphocyte proliferation and cytokine production through immunomodulatory actions (Melamed & Kumar 2010). International epidemiological data confirm this marked geographical pattern of increasing incidence with increasing latitudes, together with significantly greater rates of diagnosis in autumn and winter (Svensson et al 2009, Zipitis & Akobeng 2008). In addition, assessment of T1DM patients reveals significantly lower 25(OH)D than age-matched controls. Given that the beta-cell destruction of T1DM frequently begins in infancy, with diagnosis typically occurring when 80% of cells have already been destroyed, much focus has been placed on the environmental and nutritional influences in early life as potential aetiological factors. Greer et al (2007) found in Australia that adolescents with newly diagnosed T1DM had a three times higher risk of having levels below 20 ng/mL than controls.

One birth cohort study published in the *Lancet* in 2001 involved the offspring of 12,055 pregnant Finnish women who gave birth in 1966. The families were assessed for vitamin D supplementation in the infant's first year of life and then the child was followed until 31 years of age to account for subsequent diagnoses of T1DM. It was shown that treatment of children with 2000 IU/day vitamin D from 1 year of age decreased the risk of developing the disease by 80% through the next 20 years; furthermore, children from the same cohort who were vitamin D-deficient at 1 year old had a fourfold increased risk of developing T1DM (Hyppönen et al 2001). Similar findings have been demonstrated in animal models, with pretreatment with $1,25(OH)_2D$ being effective in mitigating or preventing the onset of T1DM (Palomer et al 2008).

A case-control study conducted in Norway that involved 545 Norwegian children up to 15 years old with T1DM retrospectively assessed their cod liver oil and vitamin D use from birth to 12 months old. Children who had been given cod liver oil five times a week had a 26% lower incidence of the disease, whereas other forms of vitamin D appeared to bear no relationship (Stene & Joner 2003). Although this does not adequately assess vitamin D as a sole treatment agent and is not conclusive, it adds to the growing body of evidence implicating vitamin D in a preventive role against diabetes.

A meta-analysis of five studies of vitamin D supplementation in infancy, including the above two, concluded that supplementation during an infant's first year appears to be associated with a significant risk reduction for the development of T1DM later in life (OR 0.71) (Zipitis & Akobeng 2008). Current evidence points to the superiority of cod liver oil as a delivery form, but a lack of specific detail in many of the studies means that optimal dose, duration of supplementation and timing cannot currently be elucidated.

Research into the role of vitamin D metabolism genes demonstrates a consistent genetic predisposition to lower vitamin D metabolism and the risk of T1DM. Cooper and colleagues (2011) have shown consistent results indicating that circulating levels of calcitriol vary seasonally and are under the same genetic control as the normal population, but three key metabolism genes (CYP27B1, DHCR7 and CYP2R1) are much lower in those with T1DM. This indicates that there is a genetic role leading to vitamin D deficiency in T1DM, which has implications for the efficacy of supplementation and the dosages required in this population.

Seasonal variation suggests that the pathophysiology is multifactorial. Hewison (2011) indicates that low vitamin D status is linked to risk of developing T1DM, and that supplementation provides a protective effect. In knockout model mice, those under dietary restriction of vitamin D showed increased severity of disease. Further, genetic investigation reveals that polymorphic variations in genes for various aspects of vitamin D metabolisms and signalling affect diabetes susceptibility. In particular, the presence of specific VDR gene alleles is protective (Ramos-Lopez et al 2006), and variations in CYP27BI (conversion enzyme) impacts on susceptibility (Bailey et al 2007).

Type 2 diabetes mellitus (T2DM)

Epidemiological studies suggest that vitamin D deficiency places some populations (e.g. non-Hispanic blacks) at a higher risk of insulin resistance, impaired glucose homeostasis and metabolic syndrome (Palomer et al 2008). The mechanisms for this effect remain speculative, including suppression of PTH, reducing calcium influx and therefore limiting lipogenesis. Other theories relate to vitamin D's immunomodulatory actions. A range of elevated inflammatory markers has been identified to predate the onset of T2DM and many of these appear to be down-regulated by vitamin D, but direct evidence of this pathogenetic path is currently lacking (Palomer et al 2008, Shapses & Manson 2011). The relationship between diabetes and vitamin D, however, is likely to be a bidirectional one, with low levels of functioning insulin impairing bioactivation of vitamin D, and poor vitamin D status impeding correct insulin release and function.

Consistent evidence of an inverse relationship between serum 25(OH)D and adiposity highlights another domain of potential overlap and potential confounding between hypovitaminosis D and T2DM (Alemzadeh et al 2008, Palomer et al 2008). Consequently, vitamin D deficiency is common in T2DM patients (Sugden et al 2008). One study revealed that three-quarters of obese adolescents had levels <50 nmol/L, with a positive correlation between poor vitamin D status and glucose dysregulation (Alemzadeh et al 2008), while 49% of adult T2DM patients in another study demonstrated vitamin D deficiency (Sugden et al 2008). A meta-analysis concurs with these findings, while also adding calcium to the equation; it calculates an OR of 0.82 for incident T2DM among individuals with low vitamin D status, calcium or dairy intake (Pittas et al 2007).

Vitamin D supplementation in patients with mild T2DM and in non-diabetic patients with vitamin D deficiency can improve insulin secretion in response to oral glucose loads, but it is ineffective in patients with established or severe T2DM (Palomer et al 2008). In one clinical trial, 1332 IU/day oral vitamin D was administered for 1 month to 10 adult women with T2DM. Corresponding changes were observed in first-phase insulin secretion (34.3% increase) and serum 25(OH)D levels. Improvements observed in second-phase insulin secretion and insulin resistance were deemed non-significant (Borissova et al 2003). A more recent pilot study employed a single high dose of D_2 (100,000 IU) to vitamin D-deficient T2DM patients; this resulted in improved endothelial function, as evidenced by a highly significant reduction in systolic blood pressure. The proposed mechanisms for this effect are many and varied but remain hypothetical at this time (Sugden et al 2008). Intravenous administration of vitamin D to patients with gestational diabetes produces a transient reduction in both fasting glucose and insulin, suggesting improved insulin sensitivity rather than secretion (Palomer et al 2008).

It is important to note that single high-dose vitamin D actually increases blood glucose levels in patients with diabetes (Palomer et al 2008). While there is some biological plausibility for the role of vitamin D in the treatment of T2DM, and positive findings from observational studies, the results from clinical studies have been inconsistent, and insufficient to make recommendations (Maxwell & Wood 2011, Shapses & Manson 2011, Valdivielso et al 2009). There is some evidence to support a beneficial effect in people with very low levels of circulating 25(OH)D, but some evidence also points to a potential increase in risk at the highest levels, representing a U-shaped curve of effect (Shapses & Manson 2011). Pooled analysis shows inconsistent results; however results for insulin sensitivity seem to be more positive (Maxwell & Wood 2011, Shapses & Manson 2011). Well-designed large RCTs, with prespecified outcomes for T2DM, insulin resistance and cardiovascular outcomes, are required to establish whether vitamin D is effective for the treatment of these metabolic disorders.

Hypoparathyroidism

Vitamin D in combination with calcium has established benefits in the treatment of hypoparathyroidism, by promoting homeostasis of calcium, phosphorus, 25(OH)D and PTH levels (Hewison 2011, Mimouni et al 1986, Nowson et al 2012).

Secondary hyperparathyroidism

In a controlled study of 100 postmenopausal women with confirmed vitamin D deficiency (<18 nmol), supplementation with combination calcium and low-dose vitamin D showed more significant reductions in PTH levels over the 90-day trial period than supplementation with calcium alone (Deroisy et al 2002).

Hypophosphataemia

A combination of high-dose vitamin D and phosphorus results in improved phosphorus and calcium balance in these patients (Lyles et al 1982).

Osteoporosis and fracture prevention

One of the main functions of vitamin D is to maintain serum calcium and phosphorus levels in order to maintain healthy metabolic functions, transcription regulation and bone metabolism (Hossein-nezhad & Holick 2013). Both serum 25(OH)D and 1,25(OH)$_2$D levels are low in osteoporotic patients (Cranney et al 2008, Hunter et al 2000, Wilson et al 1991); however, conclusions regarding improvement of bone health with vitamin D supplementation alone have been mixed and largely hampered by methodological issues (e.g. accurate vitamin D assessment, accounting for and discriminating between different vitamin D sources, extricating effects of vitamin D from those of calcium) (Cranney et al 2008). A 2008 systematic review that included 17 RCTs of either D_2 or D_3 supplementation (300–2000 IU/day) in postmenopausal women or older men has found consistent evidence of a protective effect of D_3 at doses of ≥700 IU/day in combination with calcium (500–1200 mg/day) (Cranney et al 2008). Notably, however, vitamin D at these doses provided no additional benefits in black populations. A meta-analysis of 29 RCTs conducted in 63,897 individuals ≥50 years over an average of 3.5 years also concluded that calcium alone (≥1200 mg/day) or in combination with vitamin D (≥800 IU/day) reduced the risk of fracture by 12–24%, and reduced bone loss by 0.54% at the hip and 1.19% at the spine (Tang et al 2007). The greatest improvements were noted specifically in the elderly, institutionalised, underweight and calcium-deficient. In addition, an Australian trial that investigated the administration to 120 women aged 70–80 years of 1200 mg/day of calcium alone or in combination with 1000 IU vitamin D over 5 years yielded beneficial effects on bone mineral density and bone turnover markers for both treatment groups, with evidence of more sustained improvements in those also taking vitamin D (Zhu et al 2008). In a recent pooled analysis of the evidence, Bischoff-Ferrari et al (2012) state that doses of 20–50 mcg/day (800–2000 IU/day) have been demonstrated to prevent osteoporotic fractures in the elderly, and recommendations from the European Society for Clinical and Economic Aspects of Osteoporosis and Osteoarthritis state that up to 250 mcg (10,000 IU) daily is considered to be safe in this patient population (Rizzoli et al 2013).

Another study comparing the combined effects of calcium (500 mg/day) with either oral vitamin D_2 (700 IU/day) or calcitriol over 3 years demonstrated a protective effect of vitamin D_2 on the spine but not on the hip (Zofkova & Hill 2007).

Serum 25(OH)D levels in postmenopausal women are inversely associated with fracture risk, independent of number of falls, physical functionality, frailty and other associated risks (Cauley et al 2008). These data reveal that individuals with baseline serum levels <47.5 nmol/L have an increased risk of hip fracture rate over the next 7 years of 1.71 compared to those with values >70.7 nmol/L. Other studies of similar design concur with these results, while producing different cut-off values. Studies investigating vitamin D supplementation for fracture prevention in osteoporosis have produced some positive results. In the context of adequate or supplemented calcium, a 60% reduction in the incidence of peripheral fractures was observed by Cosman (700–800 IU/day), with a 40% reduction in hip fracture incidence specifically (Cosman 2005). A systematic review of 15 RCTs involving mostly D_3 supplementation (300–800 IU/day) found a non-significant reduction in fractures; however, methodological limitations, including the relatively low dose, could be a confounding issue (Cranney et al 2008).

One study has investigated the bone mineral density effects of co-supplementing silicon with calcium and vitamin D. In an RCT of 136 predominantly postmenopausal osteopenic women, 1000 mg calcium, 20 mcg vitamin D and 3 mg, 6 mg or 12 mg silicon in the form of orthosilicic acid was administered daily for 12 months to the treatment group. These subjects demonstrated significantly greater type I collagen, indicative of increased bone synthesis, compared to those receiving the placebo (Spector et al 2008). There was also a trend of decreasing resorption with increasing silicon dose.

The mechanisms behind vitamin D's bone actions are not limited to the suppression of PTH and improved calcium balance alone; evidence also exists of direct inhibition of bone resorption and reduced inflammatory markers. The active calcitriol interacts with its VDR in the small intestine to increase the efficiency of intestinal calcium and phosphorus absorption. It also interacts with VDR in osteoblasts to stimulate a receptor activator of the ligand of NF-κB, which works to produce immature preosteoclasts, stimulating them to become mature bone-resorbing osteoclasts, which then remove calcium and phosphorus from the bone to maintain blood calcium and phosphorus levels. In the kidneys, calcitriol stimulates calcium reabsorption from the glomerular filtrate (Hossein-nezhad & Holick 2013). There is also speculation regarding vitamin D's potentially positive effects on lean body mass, which would then convey an anabolic effect via increased mechanical load (Cauley et al 2008, Zofkova & Hill 2007).

Reducing falls in the elderly

The most recent recommendations from the Australian Working Group recognise vitamin D deficiency as an independent predictor of falls in older people, and have summarised the evidence for insufficient vitamin D and its association with impaired balance, increased muscle mass loss, lower-extremity muscle weakness, and impaired strength and physical function (Nowson et al 2012). Poor vitamin D status (e.g. low serum 25(OH)D, compromised VDR numbers or binding affinity, colder seasons) is independently associated with an increased risk of falling in the elderly, particularly in those aged 65–75 years (Prince et al 2008, Richy et al 2008, Snijder et al 2006) and in some studies with poorer physical performance generally (Brunner et al 2008). A 2004 review of double-blind RCTs of vitamin D in elderly populations concluded that vitamin D supplementation reduced the risk of falling by more than 20%. The results were significant only in women and appeared to be independent of calcium administration, type of vitamin D and duration of therapy (Bischoff-Ferrari et al 2006). More recent research has suggested an even greater effect, but the degree of risk reduction varies between studies. According to a double-blind randomised trial involving 64 institutionalised elderly women (age range 65–97 years; mean 25(OH)D levels 16.4 ng/mL), treatment with 1200 mg/day calcium plus 800 IU/day D_3 over 3 months reduced the rate of falls by 60% compared with calcium supplementation alone (Bischoff-Ferrari et al 2006). An Australian study of community-based women aged 70–90 years with baseline serum 25(OH)D < 24 ng/mL found that D_2 (1000 IU/day) in combination with 1000 mg calcium citrate over 1 year reduced falls by 19% (Prince et al 2008). An interesting finding was the marked seasonal variation in efficacy, with vitamin D's protective effect evident in winter/spring (months exhibiting increased risk of falls generally) but not in summer/autumn. This has been attributed to the decline in serum 25(OH)D during these months and has also been postulated as an explanation for the lack of effect seen in some larger long-term studies. The researchers also concluded that a serum level of <24 ng/mL is predictive of individuals who may benefit from vitamin D supplementation in this context.

In 2007 a pilot study of an osteopenic/osteoporotic elderly female population (≥65 years) investigated the possible additional clinical benefits of 3 months' exercise training and increased protein intake on top of year-long calcium and vitamin D supplementation (500–1000 mg/day and 400–800 IU/day, respectively) (Swanenburg et al 2007). Although the number of falls reduced dramatically in both groups, the group undertaking exercise training demonstrated greater and more sustained risk reduction (e.g. 100% at 6 months versus 40%). This multipronged approach appears promising and warrants further investigation. A systematic review funded by the US Office of Dietary Supplements of the National Institute of Health and the Agency for Healthcare Research and Quality included 14 RCTs of vitamin D for fall prevention and concluded that there was consistent evidence of benefit (OR 0.89) (Cranney et al 2008).

As a result of the accumulating evidence, routine vitamin D administration has been recommended for those institutionalised or housebound elderly who are already at risk of deficiency (Nowson et al 2012, Sambrook & Eisman 2002). The findings of an Australian study, however, suggest there are a significant number of community-dwelling elderly with sufficiently low vitamin D status who might also benefit from routine vitamin D (Prince et al 2008). One additional consideration is the best delivery form, with a comparative meta-analysis demonstrating superior results from vitamin D analogues, e.g. alfacalcidol and calcitriol, when compared to oral vitamin D (Richy et al 2008). These analogues, which override renal regulation of vitamin D bioactivation, may be particularly indicated in individuals who take high-dose glucocorticoids, exhibit impaired renal function or chronic inflammation, or who have T1DM.

In a recent systematic review on vitamin D supplementation on muscle strength, gait and balance in older adults, Muir and Montero-Odasso (2011) found that there was a significant improvement in postural sway, time to complete the timed up-and-go test for lower-extremity strength and balance with 800–1000 IU supplementation per day. They conclude that there were consistently demonstrated beneficial effects of vitamin D supplementation on strength and balance; however, gait was not affected.

In 2013, the American Geriatrics Society Workgroup on Vitamin D supplementation for Older Adults (American Workgroup) has recommended supplementation at 4000 IU/day to reduce the risk of falls and fractures for those with no underlying risk of hypercalcaemia. This larger dose recommendation is based on: the population's potential decreased adherence compared with trial participants, and increased requirement due to age and sun exposure likelihood.

Anticonvulsant-induced osteomalacia

Preliminary evidence has shown vitamin D to be an effective treatment for this condition; however, much emphasis has been placed on establishing the most superior form of D, D_2 or D_3, as they exhibit important metabolic differences in these patients (Hartwell et al 1989, Tjellesen et al 1985, 1986). More recent evidence suggests that the resultant bone disease in patients treated with anticonvulsant drugs mostly demonstrates bone remodelling rather than decreased mineralisation, some with significant turnover of bone, with manifest features of osteomalacia. Prophylactic vitamin D_3 supplementation of up to 2000 IU/day is recommended, and up to 2000–4000 IU/day in patients exhibiting osteopenic/osteoporotic disorders (Drezner 2004).

Hepatic and renal osteodystrophy

Both chronic liver disease and those conditions exhibiting end-stage renal disease result in compromised hydroxylation of vitamin D to produce its active metabolite. It has been reported that 50% of patients with chronic liver disease, especially those with primary or secondary biliary cirrhosis, present with associated osteodystrophy. This frequently leads to a vitamin D deficiency and manifests most commonly as metabolic bone disorders, hypocalcaemia and secondary hyperparathyroidism (Wills & Savory 1984). The resultant hypovitaminosis D can result in bone loss, cardiovascular disease, immune suppression and increased mortality in patients with end-stage kidney failure (Andress 2006). Consequently, correction of this deficiency has been one of many first-line treatments in these situations.

Although vitamin D_2 supplementation in combination with calcium, phosphorus and magnesium (where indicated) has shown some success in those patients with hepatic osteodystrophy (Compston et al 1979, Long & Wills 1978), recent trials and emerging research implicate other factors in the aetiology of these sequelae (Klein et al 2002, Suzuki et al 1998). As such, therapy with D_2 may need to be reviewed.

The treatment of renal osteodystrophy is reliant upon only the active forms or analogues of vitamin D, and natural supplementation is ineffective because of the inability to convert these precursors into 1,25-alpha-$(OH)_2D$ (Kim & Sprague 2002). In a recent Cochrane review of vitamin D for chronic kidney disease, it was found that, although the evidence was insufficiently powered to make clear recommendations, it did seem that vitamin D suppresses PTH in people with chronic kidney disease, but treatment was associated with clinically relevant serum elevations in both phosphorus and calcium. Observational data suggest improved survival rates in this population, but large RCTs are required to confirm these results.

Localised and systemic scleroderma

Although patients suffering from scleroderma do not show compromised D synthesis (Matsuoka et al 1991), vitamin D_3 has been investigated as a therapeutic agent to moderate the excessive proliferation and collagen production typically seen in this condition. An in vitro study assessing the action of vitamin D_3 on the behaviour of affected fibroblasts has confirmed a non-selective antiproliferative action (Boelsma et al 1995).

To date, clinical studies have produced mixed results. Clinical trials focusing on generalised scleroderma have involved small numbers and produced promising results, such as increased joint mobility, reduced induration and increased extensibility of the skin, with benefits lasting at least 1 year after discontinuation of treatment (Caca-Biljanovska et al 1999, Hulshof et al 1994). However, the largest RCT involving 27 patients (the majority of whom suffered a localised condition) found that treatment over 9 months with a similar dose of D_3 failed to produce any significant changes in any of the assessment criteria (Hulshof et al 2000). These results suggest that different therapies may be required for the two conditions; however, larger controlled studies are needed to confirm those positive results from the preliminary open trials. Pelago et al (2010) have criticised previous trials for dosage regimens being too low (40 IU/day) to demonstrate the potential benefits. Larger well-controlled randomised studies are required.

Prevention and treatment of infections and tuberculosis

The potential immune-enhancing effect of vitamin D was first described indirectly in 1849, when cod liver oil was attributed with being one of the most efficacious agents in the treatment of pulmonary tuberculosis (Maalouf 2008). However, the treatment of tuberculosis with sunlight was prescribed by Hippocrates. It is now understood that $1,25(OH)_2D$ is a potent suppressor for *Mycobacterium tuberculosis* proliferation in human monocytes (Hewison 2011). It was demonstrated under gene array analysis that macrophage expression of the converting enzyme CYP27B1 and the VDR was induced by the activation of TLR 2/1, which is a pathogen recognition receptor for Gram-positive bacteria and *M. tuberculosis* (Liu et al 2006). This antibacterial activity is, however, not restricted to macrophages and monocytes. Vitamin D-medicated induction by intracrine synthesis also induces the expression of the gene for cathelicidin (LL-37), which is an antimicrobial peptide that produces 1,25(OH)D only in primates (Hewison 2011, Reinholz et al 2012). The production or transcription of LL-37 is stimulated by the $1,25(OH)D_2$-VDR complex, and its bacterial killing response can be enhanced by simply increasing the precursor 25(OH) D. Studies conducted by Liu et al (2006) demonstrate this capacity, where the serum from vitamin D-deficient individuals produced lower levels of LL-37 following activation by TLR 2/1 compared with individuals who were vitamin D-sufficient.

Hewison (2011) describes the role of vitamin D, which has also been shown to promote increased levels of autophagy, and the formation of associated autophagosomes. These are known to be important for intracellular isolation of pathogens and their subsequent eradication by antibacterial proteins (Hewison 2011).

Remarkably, in spite of mounting evidence regarding the vast and potent immunomodulatory effects of vitamin D, the evidence supporting its use in the prevention and treatment of infections has not progressed substantially and the small number of in vivo studies conducted in this area possess marked methodological weaknesses. The most robust evidence to date comes from a small study of 67 patients with pulmonary tuberculosis, who received 10,000 IU/day in addition to standard antimycobacterial treatment and showed higher rates of sputum conversion and radiological improvement as a result. Several post hoc analyses of vitamin D supplementation studies using other primary outcomes (e.g. fracture) have revealed trends of decreasing infections, colds and flu for those individuals taking a minimum of 800 IU/day (Grant 2008b, Maalouf 2008). In a recent Australian study (D-Health), in a secondary analysis it was found that there was a 28% non-significant reduction in antibiotic use in the vitamin D group compared to the placebo group during the study period. When the data were stratified for age, there was a significant reduction in antibiotic use in the high-dose >70-year-old group, with an RR of 0.53. Dosages were high, at 60,000 IU/month (Tran et al 2014).

This is an area of potential growth and promise. Large clinical trials with primary antibacterial outcomes are required.

Depression

Patients with primary hyperparathyroidism, which secondarily impedes the bioactivation of vitamin D and raises serum calcium, frequently present with depressive disorders that normalise following successful PTH lowering (Hoogendijk et al 2008). Rodents deficient in VDR demonstrate mood abnormalities that include increased anxiety (Hoogendijk et al 2008, Jorde et al 2006, Obradovic et al 2006), and the presence of both VDR and 1-alpha-hydroxylase activity in specific brain regions (e.g. hypothalamus) implies a potential role for vitamin D as a neuroactive hormone (Berk et al 2007, Obradovic et al 2006, Vieth et al 2004). There is also increasing evidence of vitamin D's modulation of several neurotransmitters, such as acetylcholine, catecholamines and serotonin (Jorde et al 2006, Obradovic et al 2006). Yet in spite of such strong theoretical underpinning, concerted research into the links between vitamin D and mood has only recently begun in earnest.

Recent epidemiological data reveal a strong independent inverse relationship between serum 25(OH)D and both depression scores and cognitive impairment in elderly subjects (Hoogendijk et al 2008, Johnson et al 2008, Wilkins et al 2006), premenstrual syndrome, seasonal affective disorder, non-specific mood disorder and major depressive disorder in women (Murphy & Wagner 2008), depression and anxiety in fibromyalgia patients (Armstrong et al 2007), depression rating scores on the Beck Depression Inventory in overweight and obese patients (Jorde et al 2008) and significantly lower vitamin D levels in patients with uni- and bipolar depression compared with matched controls (Berk et al 2007).

Initial interventional studies of vitamin D supplementation produced mixed findings in depression, seasonal affective disorder and general wellbeing; however, notably low doses were used (400 IU/day over short durations and in small samples), which may partly explain this lack of effect in some studies (Berk et al 2007, Hoogendijk et al 2008, Lansdowne & Provost 1998). More recent study designs have attempted to account for such shortcomings and have produced more consistent results (Jorde et al 2008, Vieth et al 2004). In two studies, thyroid outpatients with low vitamin D status during summer received either 600 or 4000 IU/day over the following 6 months (a placebo treatment was deemed unethical, given confirmation of hypovitaminosis D of all subjects at baseline). When vitamin D status and wellbeing questionnaires were repeated the following winter, improvements in mood and self-reported health were noted, particularly in those patients taking 4000 IU/day and those with the lowest serum concentrations at baseline. Another study of 441 overweight and obese individuals, only some of whom had vitamin D deficiency, found that supplementation with either 40,000 IU/week or 20,000 IU per week in combination with 500 mg/day calcium over 1 year produced significant reductions in depression rating scores (Jorde et al 2008). The greatest effects were evident in those with higher depression scores at baseline and were independent of both body mass index and initial serum 25(OH)D values. Another study of elderly women supplemented with 800 IU/day and 1000 mg/day calcium, however, failed to produce improvements on mental health scores (Dumville et al 2006).

Vieth et al (2004) comment that previous studies have suggested gender-specific mood effects of vitamin D, with women being more susceptible to seasonally-dependent mood lability and more responsive to supplementation. They also identify many potential modulating influences upon vitamin D's mood effects, which future researchers must take into consideration in addition to baseline 25(OH)D: season, dose, duration, age and sex. More well-designed research is needed in this area to clarify the real therapeutic potential of vitamin D in depressed mood.

In a systematic review of the evidence to date, while high-quality trial data are still largely unavailable, the authors conclude that this is an association evident between vitamin D deficiency and depression. They examined a total of 31,424 participants in case-control, cross-sectional and cohort studies, and found lower vitamin D levels in depressed individuals compared with controls (standard mean difference = 0.60), and an increased OR of depression in the group with the lowest vitamin D levels versus the highest group in the cross-sectional studies of 1.31, or an increase of 31%, and an increase in the hazard ratio of lowest versus highest in the cohort studies (hazard ratio = 2.21). However, for establishing more robust causal relationship data, RCTs are needed (Anglin 2013).

Clinical note — A link between vitamin D and schizophrenia?

The epidemiological correlation between babies born in winter and spring and an increased prevalence of schizophrenia has been a long-established phenomenon and presented many riddles for researchers (Eyles et al 2013, Kendell & Adams 2002). The association has also been observed in cities where air pollution reduces UV irradiation, and, more recently, a 7–10-fold increased risk has been identified in second-generation dark-skinned migrants. These observations have led to the emergence of a neurodevelopmental theory of schizophrenia, which suggests that low prenatal vitamin D interferes with brain development by interacting with D-responsive/susceptible genes to create the currently recognised polygenic effects of schizophrenia (Mackay-Sim et al 2004).

A significant progression of this theory was made at the Queensland Centre for Schizophrenic Research, led by Professor John McGrath. The centre's work has taken the level of evidence beyond the early epidemiological findings, with research being conducted to assess the impact of vitamin D deficiency on animal brains and in vitro cultures. Research has also been conducted to measure third-trimester serum 25(OH)D levels in schizophrenic and schizoaffective mothers, while investigating the impact of vitamin D supplementation prior to 1 year of age in the infants and the subsequent risk reduction for the disease in later life (McGrath et al 2003, 2004a, 2004b). Subsequent investigations from the same group (Eyles et al 2013) have furthered the basic science evidence for the developmental basis of vitamin D deficiency and its association with schizophrenia. The evidence to date shows support for this hypothesis, with a consistent positive relationship appearing for males, and evidence pointing towards a stronger relationship in dark-skinned populations compared to fairer-skinned populations.

OTHER USES

Multiple sclerosis

There is strong evidence that vitamin D status is associated with risk of MS (Grant 2006, Kampman & Brustad 2008, Kragt et al 2009, Hewison 2011, Munger et al 2006, Niino et al 2008, Smolders et al 2008). A variety of observational studies illustrate a relationship between MS incidence and geographical location, with very low prevalence in the equatorial regions and increasing risk with increasing latitude in both hemispheres. Other demonstrated associations with MS incidence include the level of outdoor activity in adolescents and risk of onset later in life, while there is evidence of lower 25(OH)D levels in newly diagnosed patients when compared to controls and in relapsing patients compared to those in remission (Kampman & Brustad 2008, Niino et al 2008, Smolders et al 2008). Evidence is more mixed regarding VDR polymorphisms, month of birth and season of diagnosis.

In spite of these findings, strong evidence linking vitamin D to modulation of MS is currently lacking. A limited number of interventional studies using vitamin D also leave us without a firm conclusion. Some studies, including the Nurses' Health Study, point towards a protective effect in the years following regular supplement use, but the effects of vitamin D are difficult to extricate from other supplemented nutrients. In an open and uncontrolled study of 39 MS patients treated with 1000 IU/day for 6 months, changes in inflammatory markers were observed but clinical benefits were not investigated. The most promising study to date was conducted in 12 patients administered 1000 IU/day over 28 weeks, which reduced the number of gadolinium-enhancing lesions on the magnetic resonance imaging of one subject (Smolders et al 2008).

In the latest Cochrane review of vitamin D for the management of MS (Jagannath et al 2010), only one study was of sufficient quality to be included in the review. The results of this review suggest that there is some evidence of a beneficial effect of vitamin D supplementation, and a relative absence of any adverse events or risk of high serum calcium levels. A single trial assessed outcomes for 49 participants over a 52-week period. The study group (n = 25) were administered with escalating doses of vitamin D, and demonstrated a relative benefit in outcomes such as annualised relapse rate, suppression of T-cell proliferation and higher satisfaction scores. Hewison (2011) reviews evidence for the experimental autoimmune encephalomyelitis mouse model of MS, that shows an increased severity of disease under dietary restrictions of vitamin D, and a protective effect against symptoms when used therapeutically.

Crohn's disease and other inflammatory bowel disease

Crohn's disease is an autoimmune disease marked by an aberrant colonic immune response to enteric bacteria (Hewison 2012). Epidemiological evidence suggests that incidence of Crohn's disease and other inflammatory bowel diseases, in adult and paediatric patients, is related to levels of circulating vitamin D (Vagianos et al 2007). Research by Liu et al (2013) has identified that VDR expression on the intestinal epithelium is substantially reduced in patients with Crohn's disease or ulcerative colitis, and that in the knockout mouse model, gut epithelial VDR signalling has potent anticolitic activity that can be differentiated and is independent of non-epithelial immune VDR actions. Elevation of VDR expression by an approximate factor of 2 was protective against many experimental colitis models.

In another VDR gene knockout mouse study, aberrant gut migration of a specific cytotoxic T cell appears to be linked to an increased risk of inflammatory bowel disease (Yu et al 2008). In a study of vitamin D status in a paediatric population with inflammatory bowel disease, the prevalence of deficiency was reported to be 34.6%. Deficiency was more pronounced in children with darker skin, in winter months and in those not taking vitamin D supplementation (Pappa 2006). Hewison (2012) elucidates the aberrant or inadequate innate immune response of enteric microbiota as initiating an inflammatory adaptive immune response and its consequent damage. The effectiveness of vitamin D therapeutics may well function to both stimulate the innate immune response and suppress the inflammatory adaptive immune response.

Lupus (SLE)

There is growing evidence suggesting an aetiological role for vitamin D in SLE, as in MS and other autoimmune diseases. In addition to epidemiological studies showing low 25(OH)D in SLE patients compared to healthy controls, and inverse correlations between vitamin D status and disease severity, individuals with this condition are identified as being at high risk of vitamin D deficiency because of a range of factors (Cutolo & Otsa 2008, Kamen & Aranow 2008). These factors include increased photosensitivity, renal involvement impeding bioactivation and evidence of anti-D antibodies in select patient subsets. Data from animal and in vitro studies also point to vitamin D as an effective treatment, in particular reversing the characteristic immune abnormalities, while experimentally-induced deficiencies exacerbate clinical features. Additionally, given that SLE is a B-cell-related disorder, studies demonstrating the effect of 1,25(OH)D on VDR-expressing B cells indicate a suppression of proliferation and immunoglobulin production, and with the identification that B cells have a capacity to express CYP27B1 to activate conversion of vitamin D, this highlights the potential role of vitamin D in disorders such as SLE (Hewison 2012). Interventional studies in SLE patients are now required to confirm this indication.

Psoriasis

As a regulator of cellular growth and differentiation in various tissues, vitamin D has been investigated in psoriasis. The active form of vitamin D and its analogues have been found to suppress growth and stimulate the terminal differentiation of keratinocytes. Schauber et al (2011) have found that vitamin D may ameliorate the symptoms of psoriasis when treated with the antimicrobial peptide cathelicidin, whose production in the skin is stimulated by vitamin D.

Vaginal atrophy

Animal studies have revealed the presence of VDR in the cells lining the vagina (Yildirim et al 2004a). Given the established role of vitamin D in regulating growth and differentiation of tissues, especially those lining stratified squamous epithelium, a possible role for vitamin D in the prevention and treatment of vaginal atrophy associated with menopause is being considered (Yildirim et al 2004b). A number of studies involving co-administration with calcium have produced some positive results; however, a trial of calcium and D_3 (500 mg/day and 400 IU/day, respectively) used as a replacement for transdermal oestrogen replacement therapy in menopausal women over 1 year revealed an objective worsening of vaginal atrophy (Checa et al 2005). Dose, however, may be an issue.

DOSAGE RANGE

Acceptable daily intake (ADI)

The NHMRC vitamin guidelines released in 2006 make the following recommendations for ADI:

- Children and adults < 50 years: 200 IU/day.
- Adults 51–70 years: 400 IU/day.
- Adults over 70 years: 600 IU/day.

The ADI is based on the amount of vitamin D required to maintain serum 25(OH)D at a level of at least 27.5 nmol/L with minimal sun exposure. The level has been raised in the 51–70-year age group to account for the reduced capacity of the skin to produce vitamin D with ageing. The higher level recommended in the over-70-years group was made because this group tends to have less exposure to sunlight.

In a recent systematic review, recommendations were made on a 'per kg of body weight' dosage. The review found that up to 34.5% of variation in circulating 25(OH)D could be explained by body weight. The authors also found

V

that type of supplement (D_3 or D_2), age, concomitant calcium intake and baseline 25(OH)D could explain further variations in circulating levels (Zittermann et al 2014).

According to clinical studies

(D_3 supplemental form unless otherwise indicated.)

- Uncomplicated rickets: 1600 IU/day for the first month, gradually reducing the dose to 400 IU.
- Osteomalacia: 36,000 IU/day with calcium supplementation.
- Rickets and osteomalacia due to defective metabolism: 50,000–300,000 IU/day.
- Pregnancy supplementation: two large doses of 600,000 IU in the seventh and eighth months (Marya et al 1981).
- Reduction in fractures associated with osteoporosis: prevention of fractures has resulted from as little as 200 IU/day in combination with calcium, but the most effective dose is ≥800 IU/day in combination with ≥1200 mg/day calcium.
- Reduction in falls: 1000 IU/day in combination with 1000 mg/day calcium.
- Hyperparathyroidism: 2.5–6.25 mg/day.
- Hepatic osteodystrophy: 4000 IU/day.
- Anticonvulsant osteomalacia: 4000 IU D_2/day for 105 days, followed by 1000 IU/day.
- Systemic scleroderma: 0.75–1.25 mcg D_3/day for 6 months.

TOXICITY

Toxic ingestion of prescribed forms of vitamin D or excessive dietary consumption of either D_2 or D_3 has been reported in the vicinity of 50,000–100,000 IU/day or 10,000 IU/day taken routinely for several months. Obtaining such enormous amounts from unfortified foods is improbable. Traditionally the toxicity picture of vitamin D has been attributed to a secondary hypercalcaemia, which manifests as anorexia, nausea, vomiting, polyuria, muscle pain, unusual tiredness, dry mouth, persistent headache and secondary polydipsia. Over extended periods of time, this state of hypervitaminosis can result in metastatic calcification of soft tissues, including kidney, blood vessels, heart and lungs. Symptoms and signs at this later stage include cloudy urine, pruritus, drowsiness, weight loss, sensitivity to light, hypertension, arrhythmia, fever and abdominal pain. Toxic levels cannot be obtained from excessive sun exposure (FAO/WHO 2002, Gropper et al 2009). More recent research into vitamin D pharmacokinetics, however, points towards 25(OH)D's ability at high doses to displace $1,25(OH)_2D$ from VDR, therefore increasing free concentrations of the active form and subsequent gene transcription (Jones 2008).

ADVERSE REACTIONS

High doses of supplements may induce the following:

- arterial calcification
- arrhythmia
- gastrointestinal distress, including nausea, vomiting and constipation
- hypercalcaemia
- nephrotoxicity, manifesting as polyuria, polydipsia and nocturia.

SIGNIFICANT INTERACTIONS

Only those interactions relevant to the oral supplemental forms of vitamin D will be reviewed.

A number of pharmacokinetic and pharmacodynamic interactions are possible with vitamin D and a range of medicines and minerals.

Antituberculosis drugs

Drugs such as rifampicin and isoniazid have been reported to induce catabolism of vitamin D and in some cases manifest as reduced levels of metabolites. This may represent a concern in those patients already at risk of poor vitamin D status (Harkness & Bratman 2003).

Calcium channel blockers

Vitamin D supplementation may reduce the effectiveness of these drugs. Use with caution unless under medical supervision (Harkness & Bratman 2003).

Glucocorticoids

In high doses, these drugs directly inhibit vitamin D-mediated calcium uptake in the gastrointestinal tract and through unknown mechanisms may deplete levels of active vitamin D (Wilson et al 1991). During long-term therapy with either oral or inhaled corticosteroids, calcium and vitamin D supplementation should be considered.

Ketoconazole

This drug reduces the conversion of vitamin D to its active forms. Increased vitamin D intake may be required with long-term drug use.

Lipid-lowering drugs

Drugs such as cholestyramine and colestipol may compromise the absorption of all fat-soluble vitamins. To avoid the interaction, administer the supplement at least 1 hour prior to or 4–6 hours after ingestion of the drug (Harkness & Bratman 2003). Conversely, long-term use of statins is associated with increased 25(OH) D levels via an unknown mechanism (Aloia et al 2007).

Practice points/Patient counselling

- Vitamin D has a critical role in bone growth and development, but also has diverse roles throughout the body, including inhibiting abnormal proliferation of cells.
- Most vitamin D is endogenously produced through sun exposure and an activation process that involves both the liver and the kidneys; food sources represent a secondary and often unreliable source. Those groups in the community who have restricted sun exposure are at the greatest risk of a deficiency, including the elderly, newborns, institutionalised, adolescents and young children with marginal calcium intake during rapid growth periods, and those with dark skins.
- In the prevention of falls and prevention or treatment of osteoporosis, vitamin D supplements are most commonly given in combination with other nutrients, such as calcium.
- Other uses for vitamin D include: supplementation during pregnancy to increase fetal levels; correction of deficiencies that may result from medications or malabsorptive diseases such as coeliac disease, Crohn's disease and cystic fibrosis; as a protective agent against breast, prostate and colorectal cancer; and for a variety of metabolic bone disorders. Evidence suggests that higher circulating vitamin D levels may also be associated with better prognosis in patients with breast and colorectal cancer and vitamin D supplementation, reducing mortiality in the elderly.

Magnesium

Either an excess or inadequate level of magnesium can impact on vitamin D status. The final hydroxylation step to $1,25(OH)_2D_3$ is dependent upon magnesium and a deficiency would compromise this. However, high levels of magnesium, mimicking calcium, can suppress PTH secretion, also suppressing the activation phase (Groff & Gropper 2005). Therefore magnesium levels within the normal range will enhance activation of vitamin D to its active form.

Mineral oil

Mineral oil impairs absorption of all fat-soluble nutrients and may therefore deplete oral intake of vitamin D sources. Separate doses by at least 2 hours.

Oestrogens

Vitamin D works synergistically with oestrogens to prevent bone loss. Interaction is beneficial.

Orlistat

Although orlistat has been shown to reduce the absorption of some fat-soluble nutrients, its effect on vitamin D specifically remains unclear. Concurrent supplementation of a multivitamin with D is advised. Separate doses by a minimum of 4 hours either side of ingestion of orlistat (Harkness & Bratman 2003).

Phenytoin and valproate

The anticonvulsants induce catabolism of vitamin D through liver induction and prolonged use is associated with increased risk of developing rickets and osteomalacia.

CONTRAINDICATIONS AND PRECAUTIONS

- Hypersensitivity to vitamin D.
- Hypercalcaemia.
- Not to be taken in sarcoidosis or hyperparathyroidism without medical supervision.
- Possible interference with the action of calcium channel blockers.
- High doses require medical supervision in patients with arteriosclerosis and heart disease.
- High doses capable of inducing hypercalcaemia may precipitate arrhythmias in patients taking digitalis.

PREGNANCY USE

Vitamin D supplements as either D_2 or D_3 are exempt from pregnancy classification by the Therapeutic Goods Administration, which reflects their safety in pregnancy and lactation (Australian Drug Evaluation Committee 1999).

PATIENTS' FAQs

What will this vitamin do for me?

Vitamin D is essential for health and wellbeing. It plays a critical role in regulating calcium and phosphorus levels in the body, and is important for healthy bones and preventing abnormal cell changes, which may increase the risk of some cancers. Optimal levels of vitamin D appear to be associated with reduced mortality and supplementation for reducing mortality in the elderly.

When will it start to work?

This will depend on the condition being treated. In uncomplicated rickets, serum levels should begin to rise in 1–2 days, and after 3 weeks signs of calcium and phosphorus mineralisation appear on X-ray. For disease prevention, long-term adequate vitamin D status is recommended.

Are there any safety issues?

Vitamin D is considered a safe supplement when used in the recommended doses; however, it may interact with some medicines.

REFERENCES

Alemzadeh R et al. Hypovitaminosis D in obese children and adolescents: relationship with adiposity, insulin sensitivity, ethnicity, and season. Metabolism 57.2 (2008): 183–91.

Al Faraj S, Al Mutairi K. Vitamin D deficiency and chronic low back pain in Saudi Arabia. Spine 28.2 (2003): 177–9.

Aloia JF, et al. Statins and vitamin D. Am J Cardiol 100.8 (2007): 1329.

Andiran N, et al. Risk factors for vitamin D deficiency in breast-fed newborns and their mothers. Nutrition 18 (2002): 47–50.

Andress DL. Vitamin D in chronic kidney disease: A systemic role for selective vitamin D receptor activation. Kidney Int 69.1 (2006): 33–43.

Angeline M et al. The effects of vitamin D deficiency in athletes. Am J Sp Med 41 (2013): 461–464.

Anglin R. Vitamin D deficiency and depression in adults: systematic review and meta-analysis. Brit J Psych 202.2 (2013): 100–107.

Armas LA, et al. Vitamin D2 is much less effective than vitamin D3 in humans. J Clin Endocrinol Metab 89.11 (2004): 5387–91.

Armstrong DJ et al. Vitamin D deficiency is associated with anxiety and depression in fibromyalgia. Clin Rheumatol 26.4 (2007): 551–4.

Arunabh S et al. Body fat content and 25-hydroxyvitamin D levels in healthy women. J Clin Endocrinol Metab 88.1 (2003): 157–61.

Australian Drug Evaluation Committee. Prescribing medicines in pregnancy, 4th edn. Canberra: Therapeutic Goods Administration, 1999.

Bailey R et al. Association of the vitamin D metabolism gene CYP27B1 with type 1 diabetes. Diabetes 56 (2007): 2616–2621.

Beers MH, Berkow R (eds). The Merck manual of diagnosis and therapy, 17th edn. Whitehouse, NJ: Merck, 2003.

Berk M et al. Vitamin D deficiency may play a role in depression. Med Hypotheses 69.6 (2007): 1316–19.

Bikle DD. Vitamin D and the immune system: role in protection against bacterial infection. Curr Opin Nephrol Hypertens 17.4 (2008): 348–52.

Bischoff-Ferrari HA et al. Vitamin D receptor expression in human muscle tissue decreases with age. J Bone Miner Res 19.2 (2004): 265–69.

Bischoff-Ferrari HA et al. Is fall prevention by vitamin D mediated by a change in postural or dynamic balance? Osteoporos Int 17.5 (2006): 656–63.

Blum M, et al. Vitamin D(3) in fat tissue. Endocrine 33.1 (2008): 90–4.

Bodnar L et al. Maternal vitamin D deficiency increases the risk of pre-eclampsia. J Clin Endo Metab 92.9 (2007): 3517–22.

Boelsma E et al. Effects of calcitriol on fibroblasts derived from skin of scleroderma patients. Dermatology 191.3 (1995): 226–33.

Borissova AM et al. The effects of vitamin D3 on insulin secretion and peripheral insulin sensitivity in type 2 diabetic patients. Int J Clin Pract 57.4 (2003): 258–61.

Bouillon R et al. Ageing and calcium metabolism. Baillieres Clin Endocrinol Metab 11.2 (1997): 341–65.

Bowyer L, et al Vitamin D, PTH and calcium levels in pregnant women and their neonates. Clin Endocrinol (Oxf) 70.3 (2009): 372–7.

Braun, L.A., et al (2014) Prevalence of Vitamin D Deficiency Prior to Cardiothoracic Surgery. Heart, Lung and Circulation (0) available from: http://www.sciencedirect.com/science/article/pii/S1443950614001504

Brown A et al. Vitamin D. Am J Phys 277 (1999): F157–75.

Brunner RL et al. Calcium, vitamin D supplementation, and physical function in the Women's Health Initiative. J Am Diet Assoc 108.9 (2008): 1472–9.

Bruyere O et al. Highest prevalence of vitamin D inadequacy in institutionalized women compared with noninstitutionalized women: a case-control study. Women's Health (Lond Engl) 5.1 (2009): 49–54.

Buchman AL. Bones and Crohn's: problems and solutions. Inflamm Bowel Dis 5.3 (1999): 212–227.

Byrne J H et al. The impact of adult vitamin D deficiency on behavior and brain function in male Sprague-Dawley rats. Brain Rd Bull 65.2 (2005): 141–8.

Caca-Biljanovska NG et al. Treatment of generalized morphea with oral 1,25-dihydroxyvitamin D3. Adv Exp Med Biol 455 (1999): 299–304.

Cannell JJ. Autism and vitamin D. Med Hypotheses 70.4 (2008):750–9.

Cannell J et al. Athletic performance and vitamin D. Med Sci Sports Exerc. 41.5 (2009): 1102–1110.

Cantor-Graae E, Selten JP. Schizophrenia and migration: a meta-analysis and review. Am J Psychiatry 162.1 (2005):12–24.
Cauley JA et al. Serum 25-hydroxyvitamin D concentrations and risk for hip fractures. Ann Intern Med 149.4 (2008): 242–50.
Ceglia L. Vitamin D and its role in skeletal muscle. Curr Opin Clin Nutr Metab Care 12.6 (2009): 628–633.
Chatfield S et al. Vitamin D deficiency in general medical inpatients in summer and winter. Intern Med 37 (2007): 377–82.
Checa MA et al. A comparison of raloxifene and calcium plus vitamin D on vaginal atrophy after discontinuation of long-standing postmenopausal hormone therapy in osteoporotic women. A randomized, masked-evaluator, one-year, prospective study. Maturitas 52.1 (2005): 70–7.
Chen TC, Holick MF. Vitamin D prostate cancer prevention and treatment. Trends Endocrinol Metabol 14.9 (2003): 423–431.
Chowdhury R et al. Vitamin D and risk of cause specific death: systematic review and meta-analysis of observational cohort and randomised intervention studies. BMJ 348 (2014): g1903.
Chung M et al. Vitamin D with or without calcium supplementation for the prevention of cancer and fractures: an updated meta-analysis for the U.S. Preventive Services Task Forch. Arm Intern Med. 155.12 (2011): 827–838.
Clancy N et al. Vitamin D and neonatal immune function. J Matern Fetal Neoant Med 26.7 (2013): 639–646.
Compston JE et al. Treatment of osteomalacia associated with primary biliary cirrhosis with parenteral vitamin D2 or 25-hydroxyvitamin D3. Gut 20 (1979): 133–6.
Congden PJ et al. Vitamin status in treated patients with cystic fibrosis. Arch Dis Child 56.9 (1981): 708–14.
Cooper, J et al. Inherited Variation in Vitamin D Genes Is Associated With Predisposition to Autoimmune Disease Type 1 Diabetes. Diabet 60.5 (2011):1624–31.
Cosman F. The prevention and treatment of osteoporosis: a review. Med Gen Med 7.2 (2005): 73.
Cranney A et al. Summary of evidence-based review on vitamin D efficacy and safety in relation to bone health. Am J Clin Nutr 88.2 (2008): 513S–19S.
Cui X, et al. Maternal vitamin D deficiency alters the expression of genes involved in dopamine specification in the developing rat mesencephalon. Neurosci Lett 486.3 (2010): 220–3.
Cutolo M, Otsa K. Review: vitamin D, immunity and lupus. Lupus 17.1 (2008): 6–10.
Davies G, et al. A systematic review and meta-analysis of Northern Hemisphere season of birth studies in schizophrenia. Schizophr Bull 29.3 (2003):587–93.
Dawson-Hughes B et al. Estimates of optimal vitamin D status. Osteoporos Int 16.7 (2005): 713–16.
De-Regil LM et al. Vitamin D supplementation for women during pregnancy. Cochrane Datab Syst Rev. 2 (2012): DOI: 10.1002/14651858.
Deroisy R et al. Administration of a supplement containing both calcium and vitamin D is more effective than calcium alone to reduce secondary hyperparathyroidism in postmenopausal women with low 25(OH) vitamin D circulating levels. Aging Clin Exp Res 14.1 (2002): 13–17.
Ding EL et al. Interaction of estrogen therapy with calcium and vitamin D supplementation on colorectal cancer risk: reanalysis of Women's Health Initiative randomized trial. Int J Cancer 122.8 (2008): 1690–4.
Dixon K et al. In vivo relevance for photoprotection by the vitamin D rapid response pathway. J Steroid 103.3–5 (2007): 451–6.
Drezner MK. Treatment of anticonvulsant drug-induced bone disease. Epilep & Beh 5 (2004) S41–S4.
Dumville JC et al. Can vitamin D supplementation prevent winter-time blues? A randomised trial among older women. J Nutr Health Aging 10.2 (2006): 151–3.
Dusso A, et al. Vitamin D. Am J Physiol Renal Physiol 289 (2005): F8–28.
Erbas B, et al. Suburban clustering of vitamin D deficiency in Melbourne, Australia. Asia Pac J Clin Nutr 17.1 (2008): 63–7.
Eyles D et al. Vitamin D3 and brain development. Neuroscience 118 (2003): 641–653.
Eyles DW et al. Vitamin D in fetal brain development. Seminars in cell & devt boil 22 (2011): 629–636.
Eyles DW et al. Vitamin D, effects on brain development, adult brain function and the links between low levels of vitamin D and neurophychiatric disease. Front Neuroendocrin 34 (2013): 47–64.
Eyles DW et al. Intracellular distribution of the vitamin D receptor in the brain: comparison with classic target tissues and redistribution with development. Neurosci 268 (2014): 1–9.
FAO/WHO (Food and Agriculture Organization/World Health Organization). Report of a joint FAO/WHO expert consultation, Bangkok, Thailand. Rome: FAO/WHO, 2002.
Forman J et al. Plasma 25-hydroxyvitamin D levels and risk of incident hypertension. Hypertension 49.5 (2007): 1063–9.
FSANZ (Food Standards Australia New Zealand). Australia New Zealand Food Standards Code. Report no. 91. Canberra: FSANZ, 2007.
Garcion E et al. New clues about vitamin D functions in the nervous system. Trends Endocrinol Metab 13.3 (2002): 100–5.
Garland CF et al. Can colon cancer incidence and death rates be reduced with calcium and vitamin D? Am J Clin Nutr 54.1 (Suppl) (1991): 193–201S.
Garland CF et al. Calcium and vitamin D: Their potential roles in colon and breast cancer prevention. Ann NY Acad Sci 889 (1999): 107–19.
Garland CF et al. An epidemiologic basis for estimating optimal vitamin D3 intake for colon cancer prevention and a public health recommendation for greater vitamin D intake. AEP 15.8 (2004): 630.
Giovannucci E. Vitamin D status and cancer incidence and mortality. Adv Exp Med Biol 624 (2008): 31–42.
Gissel T et al. Intake of vitamin D and risk of breast cancer — a meta-analysis. J Steroid Biochem Mol Biol 111.3–5 (2008): 195–9.
Glendenning P. Vitamin D deficiency and multicultural Australia. Med J Aust 176.5 (2002): 242–3.
Gomez AC et al. Review of the concept of vitamin D 'sufficiency and insufficiency'. Nefrologia 23.2 (2003): 73–7.

Grant WB. Epidemiology of disease risks in relation to vitamin D insufficiency. Prog Biophys Mol Biol 92.1 (2006): 65–79.
Grant WB. Solar ultraviolet irradiance and cancer incidence and mortality. Adv Exp Med Biol 624 (2008a): 16–30.
Grant WB. Hypothesis — ultraviolet-B irradiance and vitamin D reduce the risk of viral infections and thus their sequelae, including autoimmune diseases and some cancers. Photochem Photobiol 84.2 (2008b): 356–65.
Grant WB. Differences in vitamin-D status may explain black–white differences in breast cancer survival rates. J Natl Med Assoc 100.9 (2008c): 1040.
Grant WB. Ecological studies of the UV-B-vitamin D-cancer hypothesis. Anitcancer Res 32.1 (2012): 223–236.
Grant WB, Garland CF. A critical review of studies on vitamin D in relation to colorectal cancer. Nutr Cancer 48.2 (2004): 115–23.
Grant WB, Soles CM. Epidemiologic evidence supporting the role of maternal vitamin D deficiency as a risk factor for the development of infantile autism. Dermatoendocrin 1.4 (2009):223–8.
Grau MV et al. Vitamin D, calcium supplementation, and colorectal adenomas: results of a randomized trial. J Natl Cancer Inst 95.23 (2003): 1765–71.
Greer RM, et al. Australian children and adolescents with Type 1 diabetes have low vitamin D levels. Med. J. Aust. 187.1 (2007): 59–60.
Groff JL, Gropper SS. Advanced nutrition and human metabolism. Belmont, CA: Wadsworth, 2005.
Gropper SS, et al. Advanced nutrition and human metabolism, 5th edition. Belmont, CA: Wadsworth, 2009.
Grover SR, Morley R. Vitamin D deficiency in veiled or dark-skinned pregnant women. Med J Aust 175 (2001): 251–2.
Hall A and Juckett M. The role of vitamin D in hematologic disease and stem cell transplantation. Nutr 5 (2013): 2206–2221.
Hanly JG et al. Hypovitaminosis D and response to supplementation in older patients with cystic fibrosis. Q J Med 56.219 (1985): 377–85.
Harkness LS, Bonny AE. Calcium and vitamin D status in adolescents: Key roles for bone, body weight, glucose tolerance and estrogen biosynthesis. J Pediatr Adolesc Gynecol 18 (2005): 305–11.
Harkness R, Bratman S. Mosby's handbook of drug–herb and drug–supplements interactions. St Louis: Mosby, 2003.
Harms L et al. Vitamin D and the brain. Best Prac & Res Clin Endocrin & Metab 25 (2011) 657–669
Harris SS, Dawson-Hughes B. Reduced sun exposure does not explain the inverse association of 25-hydroxyvitamin D with percent body fat in older adults. J Clin Endocrinol Metab 92.8 (2007): 3155–7.
Hartwell D et al. Metabolism of vitamin D2 and vitamin D3 in patients on anti-convulsant therapy. Acta Neurol Scand 79.6 (1989): 487–92.
Heaney R. Barriers to optimizing vitamin D3 intake for the elderly. J Nutr 136.4 (2006): 1123–5.
Hendler SS, Rorvik D (eds). PDR for nutritional supplements. Montvale, NJ: Medical Economics, 2001.
Hoffmann JC, Zeitz M. Treatment of Crohn's disease. Hepatogastroenterology 47.31 (2000): 90–100.
Holick MF. Vitamin D and health in the 21st century: bone and beyond: sunlight and vitamin D for bone health and prevention of autoimmune diseases, cancers, and cardiovascular disease. Am J Clin Nutr 80.6 (2004):1678–188S.
Holick M. The vitamin D epidemic and its health consequences. J Nutr 135 (2005): 2739S–48S.
Holick M. Vitamin D. In: Shils M (ed.), Modern nutrition in health and disease, 10th edn. Baltimore: Lippincott Williams & Wilkins, 2006, pp 376–95.
Holt PR. New insights into calcium, dairy and colon cancer. World J Gastroenterol 14.28 (2008): 4429–33.
Holt PR et al. Colonic epithelial cell proliferation decreases with increasing levels of serum 25-hydroxy vitamin D. Cancer Epidemiol Biomarkers Prev 11.1 (2002): 113–19.
Hoogendijk WJ et al. Depression is associated with decreased 25-hydroxyvitamin D and increased parathyroid hormone levels in older adults. Arch Gen Psychiatry 65.5 (2008): 508–12.
Hossein-Nezhad A, Holick MF. Vitamin D for health: A global perspective. Mayo Clinic Proc 88 (2013): 720–55.
Houghton LA, Vieth R. The case against ergocalciferol (vitamin D2) as a vitamin supplement. Am J Clin Nutr. 84.4 (2006): 694–7.
Huh SY, Gordon CM. Vitamin D deficiency in children and adolescents: epidemiology, impact and treatment. Rev Endocr Metab Disord 9.2 (2008): 161–70.
Hulshof MM et al. Oral calcitriol as a new therapeutic modality for generalized morphea. Arch Dermatol 130.10 (1994): 12990–3.
Hulshof MM et al. Double-blind, placebo-controlled study of oral calcitriol for the treatment of localized and systemic scleroderma. J Am Acad Dermatol 43.6 (2000): 1017–23.
Huncharek M, et al. Dairy products, dietary calcium and vitamin D intake as risk factors for prostate cancer: a meta-analysis of 26,769 cases from 45 observational studies. Nutr Cancer 60.4 (2008): 421–41.
Hunter D et al. A randomized controlled trial of vitamin D supplementation on preventing postmenopausal bone loss and modifying bone metabolism using identical twin pairs. J Bone Miner Res 15.11 (2000): 2276–83.
Hyppönen E et al. Vitamin D and increasing incidence of type 1 diabetes-evidence for an association? Diabet Obes Metab 12 (2010): 737–743.
Hyppönen E et al. Intake of vitamin D and risk of type 1 diabetes: a birth-cohort study. Lancet 358 (2001): 1500–3.
Jagannath V et al. Vitamin D for the management of multiple sclerosis. Cochrane Datab Syst Rev. 12 (2010): DOI:10.1002/14651858.
Jahnsen J et al. Vitamin D status, parathyroid hormone and bone mineral density in patients with inflammatory bowel disease. Scand J Gastroenterol 37.2 (2002): 192–9.
Janda M et al. Sun protection messages, vitamin D and skin cancer: out of the frying pan and into the fire? MJA 186.2 (2007): 52–3.
Johnson S. Micronutrient accumulation and depletion in schizophrenia, epilepsy, autism and Parkinson's disease? Med Hypotheses 56.5 (2001): 641–5.

V

Johnson MA et al. Age, race and season predict vitamin D status in African American and white octogenarians and centenarians. J Nutr Health Aging 12.10 (2008): 690–5.
Jones G. Pharmacokinetics of vitamin D toxicity. Am J Clin Nutr 88.2 (2008): 582S–6S.
Jorde R et al. Neuropsychological function in relation to serum parathyroid hormone and serum 25-hydroxyvitamin D levels. The Tromsø study. J Neurol 253.4 (2006): 464–70.
Jorde R et al. Effects of vitamin D supplementation on symptoms of depression in overweight and obese subjects: randomized double blind trial. J Intern Med 264.6 (2008): 599–609.
Kalueff AV, Tuohimaa P. Vitamin D: an antiepileptic neurosteroid hormone? Eur Neuropsychopharmacol 15 (Suppl 3) (2005): S618.
Kamen D, Aranow C. Vitamin D in systemic lupus erythematosus. Curr Opin Rheumatol 20.5 (2008): 532–7.
Kampman MT, Brustad M, Vitamin D: a candidate for the environmental effect in multiple sclerosis — observations from Norway. Neuroepidemiology 30.3 (2008): 140–6.
Kemmis C et al. Human mammary epithelial cells express CYP27B1 and are growth inhibited by 25-hydroxyvitamin D-3, the major circulating form of vitamin D-3. J Nutr 136 (2006): 887–92.
Kendell RE, Adams W. Exposure to sunlight, vitamin D and schizophrenia. Schizophrenia Res 54 (2002): 193–8.
Kim G, Sprague SM. Use of vitamin D analogs in chronic renal failure. Adv Renal Replace Ther 9.3 (2002): 175–83.
Kim JS et al. Association of vitamin D receptor gene polymorphism and Parkinson's disease in Koreans. J Korean Med Sci J 20.3 (2005): 495–8.
Kimlin M et al. Does a high UV environment ensure adequate vitamin D status? J Photochem Photobiol B 89.2–3 (2007): 139–47.
Klein GL et al. Hepatic dystrophy in chronic cholestasis: evidence for a multifactorial etiology. Pediatr Transplant 6.2 (2002): 136–40.
Kohlmeier M. Nutrient metabolism. London: Academic Press, 2003.
Kumar P, Clark M. Clinical medicine, 5th edn. London: WB Saunders, 2002.
Kutuzova G, DeLuca H. 1,25-dihydroxyvitamin D(3) regulates genes responsible for detoxification in intestine. Toxicol Appl Pharmacol 218 (2007): 37–44 (abstract).
Lansdowne AT, Provost SC. Vitamin D3 enhances mood in healthy subjects during winter. Psychopharmacology (Berl) 135.4 (1998): 319–23.
Lappe J et al. Vitamin D and calcium supplementation reduces cancer risk: results of a randomized trial. AJCN 85.6 (2007): 1586–91.
Lee JE et al. Circulating levels of vitamin D and colon and rectal cancer the Physicians' Health Study and a meta-analysis of prospective studies. Cancer Prev Res. 4.5 (2011): 735–743.
Li H et al. A prospective study of plasma vitamin D metabolites, vitamin D receptor polymorphisms, and prostate cancer. PLoS Med 4.3 (2007): e103.
Lips P. Vitamin D physiology. Prog Biophys Mol Biol 92.1 (2006): 4–8.
Littorin, B et al. Lower levels of plasma 25-hydroxyvitamin D among young adults at diagnosis of autoimmune type 1 diabetes compared with control subjects: Results from the nationwide Diabetes Incidence Study in Sweden (DISS). Diabetologia 49 (2006): 2847–2852.
Liu PT et al. Toll-like receptor triggering of a vitamin D-mediated human antimicrobial response. Science 311 (2006): 1770–1773.
Long RG, Wills MR. Hepatic osteodystrophy. Br J Hosp Med 20.3 (1978): 312–21.
Lowe C et al. Plasma 25-hydroxy vitamin D concentrations, vitamin D receptor genotype and breast cancer risk in a UK Caucasian population. Eur J Cancer 41 (2005): 1164–9.
Lu Z et al. An evaluation of the vitamin D3 content in fish: Is the vitamin D content adequate to satisfy the dietary requirement for vitamin D? J Steroid Biochem Mol Biol 103.3–5 (2007): 642–4.
Lyles KW et al. The efficacy of vitamin D2 and oral phosphorus therapy in X-linked hypophosphatemic rickets and osteomalacia. J Clin Endocrinol Metab 54 (1982): 307–15.
Ma JF et al. Mechanisms of decreased vitamin D 1 alpha hydrolase activity in prostate cancer cells. Mol Cell Endocrinol 221 (2004): 67–74.
Maalouf NM. The noncalciotropic actions of vitamin D: recent clinical developments. Curr Opin Nephrol Hypertens 17.4 (2008): 408–15.
Mackay-Sim A et al. Schizophrenia, vitamin D, and brain development. Int Rev Neurobiol 59 (2004): 351–80.
Marya RK et al. Effects of vitamin D supplementation in pregnancy. Gynecol Obstet Invest 12.3 (1981): 155–61.
Marya RK et al. Effect of calcium and vitamin D supplementation on toxaemia of pregnancy. Gynecol Obstet Invest 24.1 (1987): 38–42.
Mathieu C, Badenhoop K. Vitamin D and type 1 diabetes mellitus: state of the art. Trends Endocrinol Metab 16.6 (2005): 262–6.
Mattila P et al. Effect of vitamin D2- and D3-enriched diets on egg vitamin D content, production, and bird condition during an entire production period. Poult Sci 83.3 (2004): 433–40.
Matsuoka LY et al. Cutaneous vitamin D3 formation in progressive systemic sclerosis. J Rheumatol 18.8 (1991): 1196–8.
McGillivray G, et al. High prevalence of asymptomatic vitamin D and iron deficiency in East African immigrant children and adolescents living in a temperate climate. Arch Dis Child 92.12 (2007): 1088–93.
McGrath J et al. Low maternal vitamin D as a risk factor for schizophrenia: a pilot study using banked sera. Schizophrenia Res 63 (2003): 73–8.
McGrath JJ et al. Vitamin D3-implications for brain development. Steroid Biochem Mol Biol 89–90.1–5 (2004a): 557–60.
McGrath JJ et al. Vitamin D supplementation during the first year of life and risk of schizophrenia: a Finnish birth cohort study. Schizophrenia Res 67 (2004b): 237–45.
McGrath JJ et al. Seasonal fluctuations in birth weight and neonatal limb length: does prenatal vitamin D influence neonatal size and shape? Early Hum Dev 81 (2005): 609–18.

Melamed M & Kumar J. Low levels of 25-hydroxyvitamin D in the pediatric populations: prevalence and clinical outcomes. Pediatric Health 4.1 (2010): 89–97.

Merewood A, et al. Association between Vitamin D Deficiency and Primary Cesarean Section. J Clin Endorin Metab 94.3 (2009): 940–945.

Micromedex. Vitamin D. Thomson 2003. Available online at: www.micromedex.com.

Miller GJ. Vitamin D and prostate cancer: Biologic interactions and clinical potentials. Cancer Metastasis Rev 17 (1999): 353–60.

Mimouni F et al. Vitamin D2 therapy of pseudohypoparathyroidism. Clin Pediatr 25 (1986): 49–52.

Minasyan A et al Vestibular dysfunction in vitamin D receptor mutant mice. J Steroid Biochem Mol Biol 114.3–5 (2009): 161–166.

Mizoue T et al. Calcium, dairy foods, vitamin D, and colorectal cancer risk: the Fukuoka Colorectal Cancer Study. Cancer Epidemiol Biomarkers Prev 17.10 (2008): 2800–7.

Mohr SB et al. Relationship between low ultraviolet B irradiance and higher breast cancer risk in 107 countries. Breast J 14.3 (2008): 255–60.

Mucci LA, Spiegelman D. Vitamin D and prostate cancer risk — a less sunny outlook? J Natl Cancer Inst 100.11 (2008): 759–61.

Munger KL et al. Serum 25-hydroxyvitamin D levels and risk of multiple sclerosis. JAMA 296 (2006): 2832–2838.

Murphy PK, Wagner CL. Vitamin D and mood disorders among women: an integrative review. J Midwifery Women's Health 53.5 (2008): 440–6.

NHMRC (National Health & Medical Research Council). Nutrient reference values for Australia and New Zealand. Canberra, Australia Government of Health & Ageing, 2006.

Niino M et al. Therapeutic potential of vitamin D for multiple sclerosis. Curr Med Chem 15.5 (2008): 499–505.

Nowson C, Margerison C. Vitamin D status of Australians: impact of changes to mandatory fortification of margarine with vitamin D. Melbourne: Deakin University, 2001.

Nowson CA, Margerison C. Vitamin D intake and vitamin D status of Australians. Med J Aust 177.3 (2002): 149–52.

Nozza J, Rodda C. Vitamin D deficiency in mothers of infants with rickets. MJA 175 (2001): 253–5.

Obradovic D et al. Cross-talk of vitamin D and glucocorticoids in hippocampal cells. J Neurochem 96.2 (2006): 500–9.

Oh K et al. Calcium and vitamin D intakes in relation to risk of distal colorectal adenoma in women. Am J Epidemiol 165.10 (2007): 1178–86.

Palmer SC et al. Meta-analysis: vitamin D compounds in chronic kidney disease. Ann Intern Med 147 (2007): 840–53.

Palomer X et al. Role of vitamin D in the pathogenesis of type 2 diabetes mellitus. Diabetes Obes Metab 10.3 (2008): 185–97.

Pappa H. Vitamin D Status in Children and Young Adults With Inflammatory Bowel Disease. Pediatr 118.5 (2006): 1950–62.

Perez-Lopez FR. Sunlight, the vitamin D endocrine system, and their relationships with gynaecologic cancer. Maturitas 59.2 (2008): 101–13.

Pillow JJ et al. Vitamin D deficiency in infants and young children born to migrant parents. J Paediatr Child Health 31.3 (1995): 180–4.

Pittas A et al. The role of vitamin D and calcium in type 2 diabetes. A systematic review and meta-analysis. J Clin Endo Metab 92.6 (2007): 2017–29.

Prietl B et al. Vitamin D and immune function. Nutr 5 (2013): 2502–2521.

Prince RL et al. Effects of ergocalciferol added to calcium on the risk of falls in elderly high-risk women. Arch Intern Med 168.1 (2008): 103–8.

RACGP (Royal Australian College of General Practitioners). Proceedings of the RACGP Conference, Hobart, October 2003.

Ramos-Lopez E et al. Protection from type 1 diabetes by vitamin D receptory haploytpes. Ann N Y Acad Sci 1079 (2006): 327–334.

Reinholz, M, et al. Cathelicidin LL-37: An Antimicrobial Peptide with a Role in Inflammatory Skin Disease. Ann Dermatol. 24.2 (2012): 126–135.

Reis J et al. Vitamin D, parathyroid hormone levels, and the prevalence of metabolic syndrome in community-dwelling older adults. Diabetes Care 30.6 (2007): 1549–55.

Richy F, et al. Differential effects of D-hormone analogs and native vitamin D on the risk of falls: a comparative meta-analysis. Calcif Tissue Int 82.2 (2008): 102–7.

Robinson P et al. The re-emerging burden of rickets: a decade of experience in Sydney. Arch Dis Child 91 (2006): 564–8.

Samanek AJ et al. Estimates of beneficial and harmful sun exposure times during the year for major Australian population centres. Med J Aust 184.7 (2006): 338–41.

Sambrook PN, Eisman JA. Osteoporosis prevention and treatment. Med J Aust 172 (2002): 226–9.

Schauber J et al. Taming psoriasis with vitamin D. Sci Trans Med 3 (2011): 82ra38.

Schinchuk L, Holick M. Vitamin D and rehabilitation: improving functional outcomes. Nutr Clin Prac 22 (2007): 297–304.

Schottker, B., et al. 2013. Strong associations of 25-hydroxyvitamin D concentrations with all-cause, cardiovascular, cancer, and respiratory disease mortality in a large cohort study. Am J Clin Nutr., 97, (4) 782–793.

Schottker, B., et al. 2014. Vitamin D and mortality: meta-analysis of individual participant data from a large consortium of cohort studies from Europe and the United States. BMJ, 348, g3656.

Scully M, et al. Trends in news coverage about skin cancer prevention, 1993–2006: Increasingly mixed messages for the public. Aust N Z J Public Health 32.5 (2008): 461–6.

Simpson RU, et al. Characterization of heart size and blood pressure in the vitamin D receptor knockout mouse. J Steroid Biochem Mol Biol 103.3–5 (2007): 521–4.

Smolders J et al. Vitamin D as an immune modulator in multiple sclerosis, a review. J Neuroimmunol 194.1–2 (2008): 7–17.

Snijder MB et al. Vitamin D status in relation to one-year risk of recurrent falling in older men and women. J Clin Endocrinol Metab 91 (2006): 2980–5.

Spector TD et al. Choline-stabilized orthosilicic acid supplementation as an adjunct to calcium/vitamin D3 stimulates markers of bone formation in osteopenic females: a randomized, placebo-controlled trial. BMC Musculoskelet Disord 9 (2008): 85.

Stene LC, Joner G. Use of cod liver oil during first year of life is associated with a lower risk of childhood-onset type 1 diabetes: a large population-based, case-control study. Am J Clin Nutr 78.6 (2003): 1128–34.

Sugden JA et al. Vitamin D improves endothelial function in patients with Type 2 diabetes mellitus and low vitamin D levels. Diabet Med 25.3 (2008): 320–5.

Suzuki K et al. Hepatic osteodystrophy. Nippon Rinsho 56.6 (1998): 1604–8.

Svensson J et al. Danish Childhood Diabetes Registry. Long-term trends in the incidence of type 1 diabetes in Denmark: the seasonal variation changes over time. Pediatr Diabetes 2008 Nov 24 (Epub ahead of print). Available online at: http://www.ncbi.nlm.nih.gov/pubmed/19175901?ordinalpos=1&itool=EntrezSystem2.PEntrez.Pubmed.Pubmed_ResultsPanel.Pubmed_DefaultReportPanel.Pubmed_RVDocSum.

Swami S et al. Genistein potentiates the growth inhibitory effects of 1,25-dihydroxyvitamin D3 in DU145 prostate cancer cells: role for the direct inhibition of CYP24 enzyme activity. Mol Cell Endocrinol 241 (2005): 49–61.

Swanenburg J et al. Effects of exercise and nutrition on postural balance and risk of falling in elderly people with decreased bone mineral density: randomized controlled trial pilot study. Clin Rehabil 21.6 (2007): 523–34.

Tang BM et al. Use of calcium or calcium in combination with vitamin D supplementation to prevent fractures and bone loss in people aged 50 years and older: a meta-analysis. Lancet 370.9588 (2007): 657–66.

Theodoratou E et al. Modification of the inverse association between dietary vitamin D intake and colorectal cancer risk by a FokI variant supports a chemoprotective action of Vitamin D intake mediated through VDR binding. Int J Cancer 123.9 (2008): 2170–9.

Thien R et al. Interactions of 1 alpha,25-dihydroxyvitamin D3 with IL-12 and IL-4 on cytokine expression of human T lymphocytes. J Allergy Clin Immunol 116 (2005): 683–90.

Tjellesen L et al. Different actions of vitamin D2 and D3 on bone metabolism in patients treated with phenobarbitone/phenytoin. Calcif Tissues Int 37.3 (1985): 218–22.

Tjellesen L et al. Different metabolism of vitamin D2/D3 in epileptic patients treated with phenobarbitone/phenytoin. Bone 7.5 (1986): 337–42.

Toriola AT et al. Circulating 25-hydroxyvitamin D levels and prognosis among cancer patients: a systematic review. Cancer Epidemiol Biomarkers Prev 23.6 (2014): 917–933.

Tran B et al. Effect of vitamin D supplementation on antibiotic use: a randomized controlled trial. Amer J Clin Nutr 99.1 (2014): 156–61.

Trang HM et al. Evidence that vitamin D3 increases serum 25-hydroxyvitamin D more efficiently than does vitamin D2. Am J Clin Nutr 68.4 (1998): 854–8.

Vagianos, K et al. Nutrition assessment of patients with inflammatory bowel disease. J parenteral & ent nutr, 31.4 (2007): 311–319.

Valdivielso JM, et al. Vitamin D and the vasculature: can we teach an old drug new tricks? Expert Opin. Ther Targets 13.1 (2009): 29–38.

van der Mei IA et al. The high prevalence of vitamin D insufficiency across Australian populations is only partly explained by season and latitude. Environ Health Perspect 115.8 (2007): 1132–9.

Vanlint S, et al. Vitamin D and people with intellectual disability. Aust Fam Physician 37.5 (2008): 348–51.

Vieth R. Critique of the considerations for establishing the tolerable upper intake level for vitamin D. critical need for revision upwards. J Nutr 136 (2006): 1117–22.

Vieth R, et al. Efficacy and safety of vitamin D intake exceeding the lowest observed adverse effect level. AJCN 73 (2001): 288–94.

Vieth R et al. Randomized comparison of the effects of the vitamin D3 adequate intake versus 100 mcg (4000 IU) per day on biochemical responses and the wellbeing of patients. Nutr J 19.3 (2004): 8.

Visser M, et al. Low vitamin D and high parathyroid hormone levels as determinants of loss of muscle strength and muscle mass (sarcopenia): The Longitudinal Aging Study Amsterdam. J Clin Endo Metab 88.12 (2003): 5766–72.

Wahlqvist ML (ed). Food and nutrition, 2nd edn. Sydney: Allen & Unwin, 2002.

Wang TJ et al. Vitamin D deficiency and risk of cardiovascular disease. Circulation 117 (2008): 503–11.

Welsh JE et al. Vitamin D3 receptor as a target for breast cancer prevention. J Nutr 133 (2003): 2425–33S.

Wieder E. Dendritic Cells: A basic overview. Int Soc Cell Ther (2003).

Wigg A et al. A system for improving vitamin D nutrition in residential care. MJA 185.4 (2006): 195–8.

Wilkins CH et al. Vitamin D deficiency is associated with low mood and worse cognitive performance in older adults. Am J Geriatr Psychiatry 14.12 (2006): 1032–40.

Wills MR, Savory J. Vitamin D metabolism and chronic liver disease. Ann Clin Lab Sci 14.3 (1984): 189–97.

Wilson JD et al. Harrison's principles of internal medicine, 12th edn. New York: McGraw-Hill, 1991.

Working Group (of the Australian and New Zealand Bone and Mineral Society, Endocrine Society of Australia and Osteoporosis Australia). Vitamin D and adult bone health in Australia and New Zealand: a position statement. Med J Aust 182.6 (2005): 281–5.

Yildirim B et al. The effect of postmenopausal vitamin D treatment on vaginal atrophy. Maturitas 49 (2004a): 334–7.

Yildirim B et al. Immunohistochemical detection of 1,25-dihydroxyvitamin D receptor in rat epithelium. Fertil Steril 82.6 (2004b): 1602–8.

Yu S et al. Failure of T cell homing, reduced CD4/CD8αα intraepithelial lymphocytes and inflammation in the gut of vitamin D receptor KO mice. Proc Natl Acad Sci USA 105 (2008): 20834–20839.

Zhu K et al. Effects of calcium and vitamin D supplementation on hip bone mineral density and calcium-related analytes in elderly ambulatory Australian women: a five-year randomized controlled trial. J Clin Endocrinol Metab 93.3 (2008): 743–9.

Zipitis CS, Akobeng AK. Vitamin D supplementation in early childhood and risk of type 1 diabetes: a systematic review and meta-analysis. Arch Dis Child 93.6 (2008): 512–17.

Zittermann A et al. Vitamin D supplementation, body weight and human serum 25-hydroxyvitamin D response: a systematic review. Eur J Nutr 53 (2014): 367–374.

Zofkova I, Hill M. Long-term 1,25(OH)2 vitamin D therapy increases bone mineral density in osteopenic women. Comparison with the effect of plain vitamin D. Aging Clin Exp Res 19.6 (2007): 472–7.

Vitamin E

HISTORICAL NOTE Vitamin E was first discovered in 1922 at the University of California in Berkeley, when it was observed that rats required the nutrient in order to maintain their fertility (Evans 1925). In this way, vitamin E became known as the antisterility vitamin, which is reflected in its name, as *tokos* and *pherein* are the Greek words for 'offspring' and 'to bear or bring forth' (Saldeen & Saldeen 2005). Although considered an essential nutrient, it was not until the mid-1960s that deficiency states in humans were first identified (McDowell 2000). More specifically, deficiency was detected in children with fat malabsorption syndromes, and defects in genetic hepatic alpha-tocopherol transfer protein (Shils 1999, Traber et al 2006, Wahlqvist 2002). Most fat-soluble vitamins (A, D and K) have defined roles in human metabolism. However, vitamin E does not present an actual role; rather it is utilised in deficiency states, and is seen in malabsorptive and in genetic disorders. It is an antioxidant functioning via peroxyl radical-scavenging actions protecting membranous lipoproteins and polyunsaturated fats. Vitamin E depends on a complex network of other antioxidants and antioxidant enzymes to maintain efficacy and therefore rarely acts alone, as demonstrated by many journal papers (Blaner 2013, McDowell 2000, Saldeen & Saldeen 2005). Most of the research regarding vitamin E has been on alpha-tocopherols, with approximately 1% investigating tocotrienols (Wong 2012). This makes vitamin E as a single prescriptive supplement difficult to evaluate in human studies, rendering many studies equivocal (Blaner 2013, Traber et al 2006).

BACKGROUND AND RELEVANT PHARMACOKINETICS

Vitamin E is a collective term relating to all antioxidant activities of tocol and tocotrienol derivatives (Blaner 2013). Alpha-tocopherol is absorbed from the intestinal lumen and is dependent upon adequate fat digestion. After micellisation, it enters the lymphatic circulation and then the systemic circulation, where it is transported in chylomicrons. Breakdown of chylomicrons in the blood releases some vitamin E, which is then taken up by circulating lipoproteins such as low-density lipoprotein (LDL) and high-density lipoprotein (HDL). The remaining vitamin E is transported via chylomicron remnants to the liver. Here, the RRR alpha-tocopherol form is preferentially secreted back into the circulation in very-low-density lipoprotein (VLDL). It is suspected that hepatic alpha-tocopherol transfer protein is responsible for discriminating between the different types of tocopherol at this point (with the natural form preferentially taken up). Vitamin E is ultimately delivered to tissues when chylomicrons and VLDL are broken down by lipoprotein lipase. Vitamin E transported by LDL is also taken up by tissues via the LDL receptor. The bulk of vitamin E is stored in adipose tissue, although some storage also occurs in cell membranes, such as the plasma mitochondrial and microsomal membranes of the heart, muscles, testes, uterus, adrenal and pituitary glands, and blood (Borel 2013). Vitamin E molecules cannot be recycled. The inactive oxidated end product conjugates entering bile, and is mainly excreted in the faeces and urine, although the skin has also been implicated in its evacuation via sebaceous secretions (Shils 1999, Traber et al 2006). The efficiency of vitamin E absorption varies from 17% to roughly 79%, has an unknown saturation point, is enhanced by the presence of dietary lipids and is dependent upon adequate fat digestion, involving effective secretion of free fatty acids, monoglycerides and bile acids (Traber et al 2006).

CHEMICAL COMPONENTS

To date, there are eight identified naturally occurring compounds — 'tocochromanols' — collectively known as vitamin E 'vitamers', that display the biological activity of RRR-alpha-tocopherol, alpha-, beta-, gamma- and delta-tocopherol; and alpha-, beta-, gamma- and delta-tocotrienol. They all share the same chromanol structure and are divided into two classes: tocopherols (saturated side chain with 16 carbons) and tocotrienols (unsaturated side chain with 16 carbons). The various vitaminers cannot be interconverted by the body, and RRR-alpha-tocopherol is the most biologically active form meeting human requirements (Blaner 2013, Colombo 2010, Traber et al 2006). The human diet generally provides a mixture of compounds with vitamin E activity (Bender 2003). Natural vitamin E consists of four forms — alpha-, beta-, gamma- and delta-tocotrienol — and is labelled as 'D' forms. The synthetic forms are labelled 'dl' or 'all-*rac*' for clarification (Colombo 2010).

Relative strengths of the various forms of vitamin E

The relative strength of the different forms of vitamin E can be expressed as either alpha-tocopherol equivalents (alpha-TE) or international units (IU). One alpha-TE (IU) represents the activity of 1 mg RRR-alpha-tocopherol (D-alpha-tocopherol representing the highest biopotency), and the alpha-TE of natural forms of vitamin E can be calculated using mathematical calculations as follows. The number of milligrams of beta-tocopherol should be multiplied by 0.5, gamma-tocopherol by 0.1 and alpha-tocotrienol by 0.3, whereas any of the synthetic all-*rac*-alpha-tocopherols (DL-alpha-tocopherol) should be multiplied by 0.74 (FAO/WHO 2002).

More commonly, activity is described in terms of IU, where 1 mg of synthetic all-*rac*-alpha-tocopherol (DL-alpha-tocopherol) acetate is equivalent to 1 IU vitamin E. Relative to this, 1 mg of DL-alpha-tocopherol is equal to 1.1 IU, 1 mg of D-alpha-tocopherol acid succinate is equal to 1.21 IU and 1 mg of D-alpha-tocopherol acetate is equal to 1.36 IU (Table 1). The natural form of D-alpha-tocopherol has the highest biopotency, which is equal to at least 1.49 IU (Meydani & Hayes 2003).

FOOD SOURCES

Vitamin E is found in various forms in both animal and plant foods. The richest food sources of vitamin E are cold-pressed vegetable oils, with safflower oil being the highest source. Good alternative sources are wheatgerm oil, sunflower oil, and nuts and seeds, particularly almonds and sunflower seeds. Non-lipid sources include spinach, kale, sweet potatoes, yams, egg yolk, liver, soya beans, asparagus and dairy products such as butter and milk. Higher tocopherol sources are found

TABLE 1 EQUIVALENCE TABLE		
1 mg	DL-alpha tocopherol — synthetic	1 IU
1 mg	DL-alpha-tocopherol	1.1 IU
1 mg	D-alpha-tocopherol acid succinate	1.21 IU
1 mg	D-alpha-tocopherol acetate	1.36 IU
1 mg	D-alpha-tocopherol	1.49 IU

in olive oil, soya bean, corn and sunflower oils. Higher tocotrienol lipid sources include palm oil, coconut oil and cocoa butter, with non-lipid forms such as rice bran, legumes, and the bran and germ portions of cereal grains such as rice, barley and oats (Colombo 2010, NUTTAB 2010).

Similar to all fat-soluble vitamins, vitamin E is susceptible to oxidation and destruction during food preparation and storage, frying, processing, bleaching, milling and freezing. Therefore processed foods may not confer adequate intakes (Whitney et al 2011).

Fortified foods

Fortified foods contain esterified vitamin E (alpha-tocopherol acetate and succinate) prolonging the shelf-life and protecting its antioxidant property. It is suggested that the body efficiently hydrolyses and absorbs esters; however there is little supportive evidence (Leonard et al 2004).

Clinical note — Free radicals, antioxidant recycling and the antioxidant network

Oxygen-containing free radicals (such as the hydroxyl radical, superoxide anion radical, hydrogen peroxide, oxygen singlet and nitric oxide radical) are highly reactive species, capable of damaging biologically important molecules such as DNA, proteins, carbohydrates and lipids. Antioxidants can break the destructive cascade of reactions initiated by free radicals by converting them into harmless derivatives.

The term 'oxidative stress' refers to an imbalance of pro-oxidants over antioxidants. The term 'antioxidant capacity' is a measure of the sum of available endogenous and exogenous defence mechanisms that work synergistically to restore and maintain the oxidative balance. During the process of maintaining oxidative balance, antioxidants such as vitamin E become oxidised themselves. Other antioxidants, such as ubiquinone, ascorbate and glutathione, are then involved in recycling vitamin E back to its unoxidised state, allowing it to continue neutralising free radical molecules (Sen & Packer 2000). When these other antioxidants become oxidised in turn, they are also regenerated to their antioxidant forms by yet others, such as alpha-lipoic acid and cysteine. In this way, the recycling of various antioxidants occurs in an orchestrated manner. The interactions between antioxidant substances have been described as the 'antioxidant network', which comprises four parts that work together to provide a continuous defence against free radical damage (De Vita et al 2005). These are:

1. enzymes that destroy or detoxify common oxidants (e.g. catalase, glutathione peroxidase, which needs selenium)

2. antioxidant vitamins, notably vitamins E and C, and coenzyme Q10, which are continuously recycled, as discussed earlier
3. dietary antioxidants or phytochemicals (e.g. carotenoids, polyphenols and allyl sulfides).
4. proteins that sequester iron and copper so that free forms do not exist in the body.

The antioxidant network provides a basis for recommending combinations of foods and antioxidant nutrients to provide maximal benefits, rather than single entities in high doses.

DEFICIENCY SIGNS AND SYMPTOMS

Owing to the widespread availability of vitamin E in the food chain, it is generally accepted that primary vitamin E deficiency is rare; however, due to alpha-tocopherol transfer protein deficiency it does occur in genetic abnormalities, lipoprotein synthesis defects, fat malabsorpative syndromes and possibly with total parenteral nutrition. It may also manifest in low-birth-weight infants given infant formula or cow's milk with low vitamin E levels, diseases such as cystic fibrosis, Crohn's disease, cholestatic liver disease, pancreatitis and biliary obstruction. Due to the malabsorption of fats, people with conditions such as those listed may sometimes require water-soluble forms of vitamin E, e.g. tocopherol polyethylene glycol-1000 succinate (NIH 2013). Individuals limiting their dietary fat intake thereby reduce both vitamin E availability and absorption (Shils 1999, Traber et al 2006).

Ultimately, it is tissue uptake, local oxidative stress levels and polyunsaturated fat content that influence whether symptoms of deficiency develop.

Symptoms of deficiency tend to be vague and difficult to diagnose because of the nutrient's widespread actions, but the following signs and symptoms have been reported in humans (FAO/WHO 2002, Meydani & Hayes 2003, Traber et al 2006):

- haemolytic anaemia
- immunological abnormalities
- neurological disturbances (e.g. peripheral neuropathies and ataxia)
- platelet dysfunction
- leakage of muscle enzymes such as creatine kinase and pyruvate kinase into plasma
- increased levels of lipid peroxidation products in plasma.

Retinal degeneration

It is possible that there is an increased usage of vitamin E in intense physical training, in smokers and in polluted environments; however further research is needed (Dunford & Doyle 2012, Packer 2002).

MAIN ACTIONS

Vitamin E is an electron donor (reducing agent or antioxidant), and many of its biochemical and molecular functions can be accounted for by this function. It is involved in many biochemical processes in the body, but its most important biological function is that of an antioxidant and working within the antioxidant network. The actions of the electron donor activity relate to maintenance of membrane integrity in body tissue, providing protection from destructive reactive oxidation species, particularly during inflammation and tissue injury (Mittal et al 2014, Traber et al 2006).

Antioxidant

Vitamin E is considered to be one of the most important and potent lipid-soluble antioxidants, due to its oxidative inhibitory action, protecting cell membranes against lipid peroxidation. It prevents free radical damage to the polyunsaturated fatty acids (PUFAs) within the phospholipid layer of each cell membrane and oxidation of LDL. It has been estimated that, for every 1000–2000 molecules of phospholipid, one molecule of vitamin E is present for antioxidant defence (Rizvi et al 2014).

This is achieved by reacting with free radical molecules and forming a tocopheroxyl radical, which then leaves the cell membrane. Upon entering the aqueous environment outside the membrane, it reacts with vitamin C (or other hydrogen donors, such as glutathione) to become reduced and, therefore, regenerated (Vatassery 1987). In this way, vitamin E activity is influenced by what has been called the 'antioxidant network', which restores vitamin E to its unoxidised state, ready to act as an antioxidant many times over (see Clinical note for more information).

Taking a larger perspective, the collective antioxidant action at each cell membrane protects the body's tissues and organs from undue oxidative stress. Prolonged and/or excessive exposure to free radicals has been implicated in many conditions, such as cardiovascular disease (CVD), cancer initiation and promotion, degenerative diseases and ageing in general (FAO/WHO 2002, Rizvi et al 2014).

Regulates immunocompetence

Vitamin E increases humoral antibody production, resistance to bacterial infections, cell-mediated immunity, the T-lymphocyte response, tumour necrosis factor production and natural killer cell activity, thereby playing a role in immunocompetence. It also decreases prostaglandin E_2 production and therefore reduces its immunosuppressive effects and decreases levels of lipid peroxides that can adversely affect immune function. It is now considered an antiangiogenic vitamer due to the mediating effect on growth factor-alpha. Alpha, gamma and delta tocopherols have various actions in the inhibition of cancer, each having its own biochemical pathway in halting cancer growth (Meydani 1995, Rizvi et al 2014, Takahaski et al 2009).

OTHER ACTIONS

- Regulates vascular smooth-muscle cell proliferation
- Inhibits smooth-muscle cell proliferation by inhibiting protein kinase C activity
- Inhibits phospholipase A_2 activity, suppressing arachidonic acid metabolism
- Antiplatelet activity has been demonstrated in vitro, but in vivo tests have been inconsistent for D-alpha-tocopherol
- Modulates vascular function by regulating the enzymatic activities of endothelial nitric oxide synthase and NAD(P)H oxidase (Ulker et al 2003)
- Analgesic activity: most likely mediated via inhibitory effects on cyclooxygenase-2 and 5-lipoxygenase
- Promotes wound healing
- Exerts neuroprotective effects

- Gene regulation. Vitamin E modulates genes involved in cholesterol homeostasis, atherosclerosis, inflammatory pathways and cellular trafficking, including of synaptic vesicular transport and the synthesis pathways of neurotransmitters (Brigelius-Flohe 2009, Munteanu et al 2004).

More specifically, vitamin E regulates genes encoding proteins involved in apoptosis (CD95L, Bcl2-L1), cell cycle regulation (p27, cyclin D1, cyclin E), cell adhesion (E-selectin, L-selectin, intercellular adhesion molecule-1, vascular cell adhesion molecule-1, integrins), cell growth (connective tissue growth factor), extracellular matrix formation/degradation (collagen alpha-1(1), glycoprotein IIb, matrix metalloproteinase-1 [MMP-1, MMP-19), inflammation (interleukin-1β [IL-1β], IL-2, IL-4, transforming growth factor-beta), lipoprotein receptors (CD36, SR-BI, SR-AI/II, LDL receptor), transcriptional control (peroxisome proliferator-activated receptor-gamma), metabolism (CYP3A4, HMG-CoA reductase, gamma-glutamylcysteine synthetase), and other processes (leptin, a beta-secretase in neurons, tropomyosin), activation of the cellular retinoic acid-binding protein II (Brigelius-Flohe 2009).

Cell signalling

Under in vitro conditions efficiency of vitamin E is involved in the upregulation of Christmas factor, increasing blood coagulation and catalysing an increased conversion of testosterone to 5-alpha dihydrotestosterone, simultaneously upregulating enzymatic activity involved in the rate limitation of glutathione synthesis (Rimbach et al 2010).

Telomere length

In co-administration with vitamin C, vitamin E was associated with longer telomere production (in women), demonstrated by both foods containing the antioxidants and supplemental forms (Xu et al 2009).

CLINICAL USE

Although vitamin E supplementation is used to correct or prevent deficiency states, most uses are based on the concept of high-dose supplements acting as therapeutic agents to either prevent or treat various health conditions. The Scientific Committee of Food set a tolerable upper intake level for D-alpha tocopherol of 300 mg/day in adults. However, there are numerous clinical trials which have used higher doses and not shown any serious adverse effects. The Joint Expert Committee on Food additives suggests an acceptable daily intake at 0.15–2.0 mg/kg/day. These intakes are likely to have individual response differences dependent on uptake (Colombo 2010). In recent years, accumulating evidence has suggested that gamma tocopherol, mixed tocopherols and tocotrienols may have properties superior to alpha tocopherol and are being scientifically investigated.

Deficiency: prevention and treatment

Traditionally, vitamin E supplementation has been used to treat or prevent deficiency in conditions such as genetic abnormalities with alpha-tocopherol transfer protein, apolipoprotein B, or microsomal triglyceride transfer protein; and to treat fat malabsorption syndromes (e.g. chronic cholestasis, cystic fibrosis, short-bowel syndromes such as Crohn's disease, chronic steatorrhoea, coeliac disease, chronic pancreatitis and total parenteral nutrition) (Traber et al 2006).

Cardiovascular disease

Oxidative stress has been shown to play an integral role in the formation, progression and rupture of the atherosclerotic plaque via modification of proteins and DNA, alteration of gene expression, promotion of inflammation and endothelial dysfunction, enhancement of surface adhesion molecule expression, LDL oxidation, MMP production and consequently plaque rupture (Katsiki & Manes 2009). Vitamin E in the form of mixed tocopherols has an inhibitory effect on platelet aggregation and adhesion, and smooth-muscle cell proliferation has an anti-inflammatory effect on monocytes, improves endothelial function and decreases lipid peroxidation (Kaul et al 2001, Rizvi et al 2014). Based on these observations and evidence, largely from epidemiological studies, investigation of various antioxidant substances, in particular vitamin E, has been conducted to determine their role in primary and/or secondary prevention of CVD.

Vitamin E also modulates the expression of genes that are involved in atherosclerosis (e.g. scavenger receptors, integrins, selectins, cytokines, cyclins) (Munteanu et al 2004). Its ability to reduce oxidative stress, both directly and indirectly as part of the antioxidant network, is of particular importance as oxidation of LDL is a key process in atherogenesis, enhancing foam cell and early lesion formation (Terentis et al 2002).

In animal cell lines tocotrienols inhibit cholesterol synthesis, suppressing the key enzyme in sterologenic pathways 3-hydroxy-3-methylglutaryl CoA reductase enzyme. This has an effect of downregulating cholesterol biosynthesis in the liver. In humans, a study of tocotrienols combined with lovastatin (cholesterol-lowering medication) lowered cholesterol through different mechanisms. The outcome suggested that the combined therapy was effective, avoiding some of the detrimental effects of statin medication (Colombo 2010, McAnally et al 2007).

Based on these observations and evidence, largely from epidemiological studies, investigation of various antioxidant substances, in particular vitamin E, has been conducted to determine their role in primary and/or secondary prevention of CVD.

Epidemiological and clinical studies

Many epidemiological studies have observed an inverse association between cardiovascular disease (CVD) and dietary intake of vitamin E that contains mainly gamma tocopherol and alpha tocopherol; however, the results from intervention studies are more controversial. In humans, some clinical trials have reported a clear association between the reduction in the relative risk of CVD with high intake or supplementation of Vitamin E, whereas others have shown no association. The genetic background, type of vitamin E and dose used, baseline levels and dietary habits of test volunteers may have contributed to the different results and deserve further study. It was back in 1946 when a Canadian doctors first reported that vitamin E could protect against coronary heart disease; however, it was not until the results of two very large human studies were published nearly 50 years later that the greater scientific community and the public started to take note of vitamin E. In 1993, the prospective Nurses' Health Study and the Health Professionals' Follow-up study both reported that, compared to non-users, vitamin E supplementation at a dose of at least 100 IU for at least 2 years significantly reduced the risk of coronary disease by an estimated 40% (Rimm et al 1993, Stampfer et al 1993).

The prospective Nurses' Health Study followed 87,245 women aged 34–59 years without known coronary disease over 8 years and found that those women with the highest intake of vitamin E had the lowest relative risk of non-fatal myocardial infarction (MI) or death from coronary disease, compared to those with the lowest intake (Stampfer et al 1993). Interestingly, short-term use or dietary intake alone did not produce the same significant reduction. The Health Professionals' Follow-up study observed 39,910 men aged 40–75 years over 4 years and produced similar results, finding that long-term vitamin E (at least 100 IU/day) significantly reduced the relative risk of coronary disease compared to non-users (Rimm et al 1993).

Subsequently, a double-blind study conducted at Cambridge University, UK, and published in 1996 supported these results, but further suggested that higher doses could produce benefits more quickly and more dramatically (Stephens et al 1996). The placebo-controlled randomised study known as the Cambridge Heart Antioxidant Study (CHAOS) involved 2002 patients with angiographically proven coronary atherosclerosis, and compared the effects of two different strengths of alpha-tocopherol supplementation (400 IU and 800 IU) and a placebo over a median of 510 days. Treatment with either dose of vitamin E was seen to reduce the risk of cardiovascular death and non-fatal MI by over 75%, with effects established after 12 months.

In 1999, results from the large Gruppo Italiano per lo Studio della Sopravvivenza nell'Infarto miocardico (GISSI) trial were published, which were less convincing. However, the trial used synthetic vitamin E at a lower dose than the previously positive CHAOS study (Albert et al 1999, GISSI 1999). The trial, which involved 11,324 patients who had recently survived MI (<3 months), investigated the effects of three different treatment protocols compared to a placebo: 1 g omega-3 fatty acid/day, 300 IU synthetic vitamin E/day, fish oils plus vitamin E/day or a placebo. The four groups were observed for nearly 4 years for CVD morbidity and mortality. Results showed that the fish oil treatment groups had significantly decreased combined end points of death, non-fatal MI and stroke over this time, whereas the vitamin E treatment produced little effect. The trial has since been criticised because the form of vitamin E used was synthetic and the dose was relatively low compared to doses in other studies involving patients with pre-existing disease.

To date, 27 different randomised controlled trials (RCTs) in the peer-reviewed literature have evaluated the effects of vitamin E in people at risk of CVD or with clinically diagnosed CVD (Katsiki & Manes 2009). The larger studies — GISSI (1999), Women's Antioxidant Cardiovascular Study (WACS) and Alpha-Tocopherol Beta-Carotene (ATBC) cancer prevention study — have resulted in several published papers as researchers analyse effects in subgroups or results are re-evaluated using different models, with respect to the GISSI 2006 study, which tested the same daily intervention with slightly different patient characteristics (post-MI vs post-MI without congestive heart failure at baseline). Overall, eight RCTs have tested vitamin E as a sole treatment, five studies have studied vitamin E in combination with vitamin C supplementation, and 11 have used multiple vitamin combinations, which included vitamin E. Nine studies combined beta-carotene with vitamin E or in a multivitamin combination. The dose of vitamin E administered in the studies varies considerably, from 55 IU to 1,200 IU daily, and in at least nine studies, synthetic vitamin E was used. In general, studies using natural vitamin E tend to produce positive results, showing a benefit on cardiovascular outcomes, however, inconsistent results still remain. Additionally, RCTs conducted in people with established CVD were more likely to report a cardioprotective effect than primary prevention studies (Table 2). Most recently, new data has emerged that allows identification of a specific target population for vitamin E supplementation, namely patients with diabetes mellitus and the haptoglobin genotype 2-2 as being more likely to respond (Vardi et al 2013).

TABLE 2 SUMMARY OF POSITIVE FINDINGS FROM RANDOMISED STUDIES OF VITAMIN E IN PRIMARY OR SECONDARY CARDIOVASCULAR DISEASE (CVD) PREVENTION

Name of study	Prevention goal	Number of subjects	Characteristics	Daily intervention	Findings
CHAOS (Stephens et al 1996)	Secondary	2002	Coronary disease	Natural vitamin E (400 IU or 800 IU)	Vitamin E reduced risk of cardiovascular death and non-fatal MI by over 75%
SPACE (Boaz et al 2000)	Secondary	2198	End-stage renal disease — people on haemodialysis with pre-existing cardiovascular event	Natural vitamin E (800 IU)	Vitamin E caused a 50% reduction in cardiac events
CLAS (Azen et al 1996)	Secondary	146	Non-smoking 40–59-year-old men with previous coronary artery bypass graft surgery	Vitamin E (< or >100 IU) and vitamin C (< or >250 mg)	Higher vitamin E intake was associated with less carotid intima media thickness progression compared with low vitamin E users in people not treated with colestipol
DeMaio et al (1992)	Secondary	100	Restenosis	Dl tocopherol 1200 IU/day	35.5% reduction in restenosis versus 47.5% not statistically significant
ASAP (Salonen et al 2003)	Primary	520	Smoking/non-smoking men and postmenopausal women aged 45–69 years with elevated serum cholesterol	Twice daily either (136 IU) of D-alpha-tocopherol, 250 mg of slow-release vitamin C, a combination of these, or a placebo, for 3 years	The proportion of men with progression of carotid atherosclerosis was reduced by 74% with combination of vitamins E and C compared to the placebo; no significant effect was seen in women

Continued

V

TABLE 2 SUMMARY OF POSITIVE FINDINGS FROM RANDOMISED STUDIES OF VITAMIN E IN PRIMARY OR SECONDARY CARDIOVASCULAR DISEASE (CVD) PREVENTION *(continued)*

Name of study	Prevention goal	Number of subjects	Characteristics	Daily intervention	Findings
ASAP follow-up (Salonen et al 2003)	Primary	520	Smoking/non-smoking men and postmenopausal women aged 45–69 years with elevated serum cholesterol	Twice daily (136 IU) D-alpha-tocopherol, 250 mg of slow-release vitamin C, or a placebo, for 6 years	Effect was still significant after a further 3 years: combined vitamins E and C continued to slow down atherosclerotic progression in hypercholesterolaemic men
ATBC (Rapola et al 1996)	Primary: incidence of angina pectoris	29,134	Finnish male smokers aged 50–69 years with no history of MI	Synthetic vitamin E (55 IU), beta-carotene (20 mg), or both, or a placebo	Vitamin E was associated with a minor decrease in incidence of angina pectoris
ATBC (Virtamo et al 1998)	Primary and secondary	29,134	Finnish male smokers aged 50–69 years with no history of MI	Synthetic vitamin E (55 IU), beta-carotene (20 mg), or both, or a placebo	Vitamin E decreased incidence of primary major coronary events by 4%; no effect on incidence of non-fatal MI; vitamin E decreased incidence of fatal coronary heart disease by 8%
ATBC (subset) (Leppala et al 2000)	Primary: prevention of incident and fatal subarachnoid, intracerebral haemorrhage, cerebral infarction and stroke	29,134	Finnish male smokers aged 50–69 years with no history of MI	Synthetic vitamin E (55 IU), beta-carotene (20 mg), or both, or a placebo	Vitamin E prevented ischaemic stroke in high-risk hypertensive patients

St Francis (Arad et al 2005)	Primary	1005	Asymptomatic calcium scores >80th percentile	Atorvastatin 20 mg/day, vitamin C 1 g/day, vitamin E 1000 IU/day, aspirin 81 mg/day	Arteriosclerotic CVD event rate decreased 6.9% vs 9.9%
VEAPS (Hodis et al 2002)	Primary	353	LDL >3.37 mmol/L	DL-alpha-tocopherol 400 IU/day	Coronary carotid intimal thickness did not change, circulating LDL reduced
ATIC (Nanyakkara et al 2007)	Primary	93	Mild to moderate chronic kidney failure	Alpha-tocopherol, pravastatin and homocysteine-lowering therapy, consecutively introduced	Significant decrease in intima media thickness, endothelial dysfunction, albuminuria; no effect on renal output
IEISS (Singh et al 1996)	Secondary	125	Patients with suspected acute MI	Vitamin E (400 mg), vitamin A (50,000 IU), vitamin C (1000 mg), beta-carotene (25 mg)	Treatment reduced mean infarct size, angina pectoris and total arrhythmias; poor left ventricular function occurred less often with antioxidants; cardiac end points were significantly less in the antioxidant group (20.6% vs 30.6%, respectively)
Fang et al (2002)	Secondary	40	After cardiac transplantation	Twice-daily vitamin C (500 mg) plus vitamin E (400 IU)	Supplementation with vitamins C and E retarded early progression of transplant-associated coronary arteriosclerosis compared to the placebo

Continued

V

TABLE 2 SUMMARY OF POSITIVE FINDINGS FROM RANDOMISED STUDIES OF VITAMIN E IN PRIMARY OR SECONDARY CARDIOVASCULAR DISEASE (CVD) PREVENTION *(continued)*

Name of study	Prevention goal	Number of subjects	Characteristics	Daily intervention	Findings
WACS (Cook et al 2007)	Secondary	8171	Women with CVD or at least three risk factors	Vitamin C (500 mg/day), natural vitamin E (600 IU every other day) and beta-carotene (50 mg every other day)	Vitamin E significantly reduced incidence of stroke and produced a marginally significant reduction in the primary outcome (a combination of MI, stroke, coronary revascularisation or CVD death) in a prespecified subgroup of women with prior CVD
SPACE (Boaz et al 2000)	Secondary	196	-	DL-alpha-tocopherol 800 IU/day	Relative risk 0.46 in composite MI, ischaemic stroke, peripheral vascular disease and unstable angina

CHAOS, Secondary Prevention with Antioxidants of Cardiovascular disease in Endstage renal disease; MI, myocardial infarction; SPACE, Secondary Prevention with Antioxidants of Cardiovascular disease in Endstage renal disease; CLAS, Cholesterol Lowering Atherosclerosis Study; ASAP, Antioxidant Supplementation in Atherosclerosis Prevention; ATBC, Alpha-Tocopherol Beta-Carotene; VEAPS, Vitamin E Atherosclerosis Prevention Study; LDL, low-density lipoprotein; ATIC, Anti-oxidant Therapy in Chronic renal insufficiency; IEISS, Indian Experiment of Infarct Survival Study; WACS, Women's Antioxidant Cardiovascular Study; SPACE, Secondary Prevention with Antioxidants of Cardiovascular disease in Endstage renal disease.

TABLE 3 SUMMARY OF NEGATIVE FINDINGS FROM RANDOMISED STUDIES OF VITAMIN E IN PRIMARY OR SECONDARY CARDIOVASCULAR DISEASE (CVD) PREVENTION

Name of study	Prevention goal	Number of subjects	Characteristics	Daily intervention	Results
GISSI (Albert et al 1999)	Secondary	11,324	Post-MI	Synthetic vitamin E (300 mg/day), fish oils (1 g/day), combination of fish oil and vitamin E, or a placebo	There was no significant reduction in the combined end points of death, non-fatal MI and stroke
GISSI (Marchioli et al 2006)	Secondary	8415	Post-MI patients without CHF at baseline	Synthetic vitamin E (300 mg/day), fish oils (1 g/day), combination of fish oil and vitamin E, or a placebo	Vitamin E treatment was associated with a significant 50% increase of CHF in patients with left ventricular dysfunction (ejection fraction <50%)
HOPE (Yusuf et al 2000)	Primary and secondary	9541	2545 women and 6996 men 55 years of age or older who were at high risk of cardiovascular events because they had CVD or diabetes in addition to one other risk factor	Natural vitamin E (400 IU), and a placebo or angiotensin-converting-enzyme inhibitor (ramipril), or both	There was no significant effect on the primary outcome, which was a composite of MI, stroke and death from cardiovascular causes
MICRO-HOPE (Lonn et al 2005)	Secondary	3654	Middle-aged and elderly people with diabetes and CVD and/or additional coronary risk factor(s)	Vitamin E (400 IU) for an average of 4.5 years	Vitamin E had no effect on CV outcomes or nephropathy

Continued

V

TABLE 3 SUMMARY OF NEGATIVE FINDINGS FROM RANDOMISED STUDIES OF VITAMIN E IN PRIMARY OR SECONDARY CARDIOVASCULAR DISEASE (CVD) PREVENTION *(continued)*

Name of study	Prevention goal	Number of subjects	Characteristics	Daily intervention	Results
PPP (de Gaetano 2001)	Primary	4495	Those at risk of CVD: people with hypertension, hypercholesterolaemia, diabetes, obesity, family history of premature MI or the elderly	Vitamin E (300 mg)	There was no significant reduction in CV events
ATBC (subset) (Rapola et al 1997)	Secondary	1862	Finnish male smokers with previous MI	Synthetic vitamin E (55 IU), beta-carotene (20 mg), or both, or a placebo	Risk of fatal coronary heart disease increased in groups receiving either beta-carotene or vitamin E and beta-carotene. There was a non-significant trend of increased deaths in the vitamin E group
HPS (Parkinson Study Group 2002)	Secondary	20,536	High CVD risk: coronary disease, other occlusive arterial disease, or diabetes	Vitamin E (600 mg), vitamin C (250 mg), beta-carotene (20 mg)	There were no significant differences in all-cause mortality, or in deaths due to vascular or non-vascular causes; no significant reduction in incidence of non-fatal MI, coronary death, non-fatal or fatal stroke or coronary or non-coronary revascularisation

MVP (Tardif et al 1997)	Secondary: aimed to decrease incidence and severity of restenosis after angioplasty	317	Before and after coronary angioplasty	One month before angioplasty and for 6 months afterwards: multivitamins (30,000 IU beta-carotene, 500 mg vitamin C, and 700 IU vitamin E) twice daily and/or probucol, or a placebo 12 hours before angioplasty given an extra 1000 mg probucol, 2000 IU vitamin E, or both, or a placebo	Multivitamin ineffective at reducing the rate of restenosis
WAVE (Waters et al 2002)	Secondary	423	Postmenopausal women	Vitamin E 400 IU/day plus vitamin C 500 mg BID, HRT or placebo	Increased risk of death, MI and stroke
SUVIMAX (Zureik et al 2004)	Primary	1162	Healthy population	Vitamin C (120 mg), vitamin E (30 mg), beta-carotene (6 mg), selenium (100 mcg), and zinc (20 mg)	There was no beneficial effect on carotid atherosclerosis and arterial stiffness
PHS 11 (Sesso et al 2008)	Primary	14,641	Male >50 years old /94.9% were CVD-free at enrolment	Alpha-tocopherol 400 IU every other day, vitamin C or placebo	No effect on CV outcomes: associated with increased risk of haemorrhagic stroke

GISSI, Gruppo Italiano per lo Studio della Sopravvivenza nell'Infarto miocardico; MI, myocardial infarction; CHF, congestive heart failure; HOPE, Heart Outcomes Prevention Evaluation; PPP, Primary Prevention Project; ATBC, Alpha-Tocopherol Beta-Carotene; HPS, Heart Protection Study; MVP, Multivitamin Prevention; WAVE, Women's Angiographic Vitamin and Estrogen; HRT, hormone replacement therapy; PHS 11, Physician's Health Study 11.

V

Clinical note — Confusing results for vitamin E

To date, many in vitro, animal and epidemiological studies support the use of vitamin E in the prevention of CVD (Clarke & Armitage 2002). However, intervention studies are equivocal. Many factors could account for the lack of benefit on the primary end point in the majority of trials (Linus Pauling Institute 2008).

Dose selection

A closer look at the evidence shows that dose selection varies enormously, from levels just above the recommended dietary intake (RDI: 50 mg/day) to large doses of 2000 IU/day. Clinical research reveals that a daily dose of at least 400 IU is required for LDL to become less susceptible to oxidation (Brockes et al 2003, Miller et al 2005) and an effective threshold dose may be as high as 800 IU/day (Jialal & Devaraj 2005a, Traber et al 2006). However an RCT review suggests that a dose relationship with mortality exists with supplementation over 150 IU/day (Miller et al 2005). More recently, Colombo (2010) suggests a beneficial dose should reach 0.15–2.0 mg/kg body weight per day.

Biomarkers of oxidative stress

Just as the statin trials investigate subjects with high cholesterol levels rather than the general population, it can reasonably be assumed that antioxidant treatment is best suited to those people with increased oxidative stress rather than the general population, yet researchers consistently fail to consider this as a biochemical basis for patient inclusion (Meagher 2003). The levels of oxidised amino acids in urine and plasma can reflect those in tissues and identify people with high levels of oxidative stress; this may be one method of subject selection (Heinecke 2002). Brack et al (2013) suggest in both chronic and acute disease, such as CVD, amongst others, multiple abnormalities can be found, where a broad-spectrum approach to measuring numerous antioxidant profiles, including vitamin E status, is warranted (Niki 2014).

Type of supplement

In the specific case of vitamin E, the form of tocopherol used is crucial, as synthetic forms have less biological activity than RRR D-alpha-tocopherol. According to a 2002 FAO/WHO report, cross-country correlations between coronary heart disease mortality in men and the supply of vitamin E homologues across 24 European countries show a highly significant ($P < 0.001$) correlation for D-alpha-tocopherol, whereas all other forms of vitamin E do not achieve statistical significance.

In the last few years, it has further been proposed that the lack of efficacy of commercial tocopherol preparations in some clinical trials may be due to the absence of other natural tocopherols, primarily gamma- and delta-tocopherol. Preliminary studies provide some support for this view (Jialal & Devaraj 2005a, Saldeen & Saldeen 2005). Studies using different mixtures of alpha-, beta-, gamma- and delta-tocopherol have found that a mixture of gamma-, delta- and alpha-tocopherol with the ratio of 5:2:1 have a much better antioxidant effect than alpha-tocopherol alone. This mixture is similar to that found in nature. In human and animal studies, the mixed tocopherol preparation also had much more favourable effects on constitutive NO synthase and superoxide dismutase activity than alpha-tocopherol, and in a rat model was more effective in decreasing platelet aggregation and inhibiting thrombus formation. A mixed tocopherol preparation is also superior to alpha-tocopherol in terms of myocyte protection (Chen et al 2002). Similarly, Yoshida et al (2003) sustain a similar view. This view is not supported by Niki et al (2014) who remain steadfast in the view that alpha-tocopherol alone exerts antioxidant effects in vivo and in vitro. It is important to note that, in diets rich in mixed tocopherols such as Mediterranean diets, there is a lower incidence of heart disease; however this may be due to many other nutrient and lifestyle factors (Roehm 2009).

Plasma vitamin E levels

The measurement of plasma vitamin E levels in the supplemented groups has been inconsistent in studies, so it is uncertain whether levels significantly rose in response to treatment and subjects were compliant. For example, in the CHAOS, Antioxidant Supplementation in Atherosclerosis Prevention (ASAP), ASAP follow-up and Secondary Prevention with Antioxidants of Cardiovascular disease in Endstage renal disease (SPACE) studies, a significant increase in plasma antioxidant levels was reported and all studies found a benefit on the primary end point, whereas measurement of plasma levels has been inconsistent in the negative studies (Jialal & Devaraj 2005a).

Clearly, the optimal form/s, dosage regimen, duration of use and subpopulation best suited to primary and secondary preventive treatment still need to be clarified with future trials.

Identifying responders

New data is emerging to suggest that the specific target population for vitamin E supplementation appears to be patients with excessive oxidative stress, such as those undergoing haemodialysis and those with diabetes mellitus and the haptoglobin genotype 2-2 as likely responders (Vardi et al. 2013).

Restenosis

Restenosis is a major limitation to the long-term success of angioplasty. Therefore, measures that prevent or delay this occurrence are being investigated to extend the beneficial effects of the procedure.

While studies in experimental models have shown that vitamin E helps to stabilise atherosclerotic plaque after angioplasty and favours vascular remodelling (Orbe et al 2003), clinical trials to date have produced disappointing results.

An early double-blind study using oral synthetic vitamin E (1200 IU) for 4 months found that treatment did not significantly reduce the rate of restenosis after percutaneous transluminal coronary angioplasty, with restenosis defined as >50%. However, minor reductions were noted (treatment group 35.5% vs control group 47.5%) which did not reach statistical significance (DeMaio et al 1992, Vardi et al 2013).

V

In the Multivitamin Prevention (MVP) trial, Tardif et al (1997) aimed to decrease the incidence and severity of restenosis after coronary angioplasty (317 patients). The patients were randomly assigned one of four different treatments: (1) a combination of vitamins, including vitamin E (30,000 IU beta-carotene, 500 mg vitamin C and 700 IU vitamin E 2000 IU); (2) placebo; (3) probucol and MVP combination; or (4) probucol 500 mg. Treatment was given 1 month prior to surgery and 6 months postsurgery at a dose of twice daily, unless procedure-related complications were noted. Additionally all patients received an extra 1000 mg of probucol, and 2000 IU of vitamin E or placebo 12 hours prior to angioplasty. It was found that probucol treatment was the most effective in reducing restenosis (mean ± SD); there was a reduction in luminal diameter 6 months > angioplasty 0.12 ± 0.41 mm in the probucol group, 0.22 ± 0.46 mm in the combined treatment group, 0.33 ± 0.51 mm in the multivitamin alone group, and 0.38 ± 0.50 mm in the placebo group.

Angina pectoris

Low-dose vitamin E supplements (50 mg/day) produce a minor decrease in the incidence of angina pectoris in smokers without previous coronary heart disease, according to an RCT (Rapola et al 1996). A smaller study of 29 subjects with variant angina identified six patients who did not respond to calcium channel blockers and had lower plasma levels than normal, but who responded positively to supplementation with 300 mg/day vitamin E. Treatment resulted in a significantly reduced incidence of angina episodes (Miwa et al 1996). Several years later, the same research group identified a transcardiac reduction in plasma vitamin E concentrations concomitant with lipid peroxide formation, suggesting that oxidative stress and vitamin E depletion may be involved in the pathogenesis of coronary artery spasm (Kusama et al 2011, Miwa et al 1999).

Nitrate tolerance

Nitroglycerin (NTG) is utilised to prevent vasoconstriction in the acute treatment of angina, acute MI, pulmonary oedema and severe arterial hypertension. One limitation of treatment is that nitrate tolerance develops with continuous use of NTG over time (Klemenska & Bercsewicz 2009). Vitamin E supplements (200 mg three times daily) prevented nitrate tolerance when given concurrently with transdermal nitroglycerin (NTG 10 mg/24 hours) according to one randomised, placebo-controlled study in which 24 patients with ischaemic heart disease were compared with 24 healthy volunteers over a 6-day period (Watanabe et al 1997).

In animal studies of rats with angina pectoris, research indicates that continuous NTG infusion causes a time-dependent vitamin E depletion in plasma and tissue. Vitamin E dietary supplementation (0.5 g/kg) administered to the animals delayed the onset of, and extent of, tolerance, demonstrating vitamin E is beneficial in the prevention of nitrate tolerance (Minamiyama et al 2006). Yasue et al (2008) concur with animal study findings in that human trials demonstrate plasma vitamin E levels are low in coronary spasm disorders, with vasoconstriction causing oxygen free radical degradation. This suggests that vitamin E's antioxidant properties may be of use; however further trials are needed.

Hypertension

Vitamin E supplementation may reduce blood pressure and LDL oxidation and improve endothelial dysfunction in hypertension, according to clinical research.

An early double-blind, placebo-controlled study found that DL-alpha-tocopherol nicotinate (3000 mg) significantly reduced systolic blood pressure (SBP) from 151.0 to 139.2 mmHg within 4–6 weeks in hypertensive subjects; however, diastolic blood pressure (DBP) remained unchanged (Iino et al 1977). More recently, long-term vitamin E (200 IU/day) was shown to decrease SBP by 24% in mildly hypertensive patients compared with a 1.6% reduction with a placebo, according to a triple-blind placebo-controlled study conducted over 27 weeks (Boshtam et al 2002). The study involved 70 hypertensive patients (SBP 140–160 mmHg; DBP 90–100 mmHg) aged 20–60 years without other cardiovascular risk factors. Besides reducing SBP, DBP was reduced by 12.5% compared to 6.2% with a placebo.

Some studies have revealed that hypertensive patients have a higher susceptibility to LDL oxidation than normotensive subjects and, therefore, increased atherogenic potential. One study measured the effect of vitamin E (400 IU/day) on the resistance of LDL to oxidation in 47 volunteers (Brockes et al 2003). Comparisons made before and after 2 months' supplementation showed that vitamin E caused a significant increase in the lag time in normotensive and hypertensive patients, ultimately bringing hypertensive patients up to the same point as the healthy controls.

All-cause mortality (ACM)

There is substantial research indicating benefits for vitamin E supplementation in the treatment and prevention of various diseases, but regardless of these benefits, three meta-analyses have drawn the conclusion that vitamin E supplementation increases ACM (Bjelakovic et al 2007, 2013, Miller et al 2005). These findings have been unexpected and widely criticised, as they are based on the results of smaller studies of variable quality, often involving people with chronic disease and sometimes testing vitamin E as part of a multinutritional intervention and not as a stand-alone treatment. Based on recent reanalysis of the data by Berry et al (2009) and Gerss and Kopcke (2009), which are discussed below, the evidence is not convincing that vitamin E supplementation increases mortality.

In 2005, Miller et al published a meta-analysis of the dose–response relationship between vitamin E supplementation and total mortality using data from 19 RCTs consisting of a large study population (n = 135,967). A dose–response analysis showed a statistically significant relationship between vitamin E dosage and ACM. The authors suggested caution with doses of 400 IU/day or higher, while acknowledging that the high-dose studies (≥400 IU/day) analysed in the report were often small and performed in patients with chronic diseases.

This meta-analysis has several serious flaws and has been criticised on a number of accounts, inspiring over 40 letters to the journal's editor and hundreds of emails and telephone calls to the authors (Jialal & Devaraj 2005b). In summary, these responses centre on six major flaws. First, results from 12 clinical studies that reported fewer than 10 deaths each were excluded from the meta-analysis, which created the appearance of bias and would have given an artificial weight to studies in which more people died. Second, the meta-analysis included trials of different designs, treatment times, doses, combinations and end points. Pooling information together from such heterogeneous studies was considered inappropriate. Third, subjects in many studies had significant chronic diseases, such as Parkinson's disease (PD), end-stage renal disease, coronary artery disease, diabetes mellitus and Alzheimer's dementia (AD), which would have influenced their mortality risk. This also means that the results do not necessarily apply to healthy adults taking these supplements. Fourth, studies used different forms of vitamin E (natural and synthetic) and sometimes used vitamin E in combination with other nutrients; however, results of all these studies were pooled and not separated. Furthermore, subject adherence to the treatment protocol was considered in only one study (CHAOS). Lastly, the use of some statistical models has been questioned.

V

In 2007, Bjelakovic et al conducted a meta-analysis using data from 68 randomised trials involving 232,606 adults that compared beta-carotene, vitamin A, vitamin C (ascorbic acid), vitamin E and selenium, either singly or combined, to a placebo or to no intervention. When all trials of antioxidant supplements were pooled, there was no significant effect on mortality for vitamin E given singly in high (≥1000 IU) or low dose (<1000 IU). After exclusion of high-bias risk (studies with heterogeneity) and selenium trials, vitamin E given singly or combined with other antioxidants significantly increased mortality, with an estimate of increased mortality of about 5%. A closer look at the details of the study reveals that, of the 815 trials originally identified, 405 trials were excluded from the meta-analysis because mortality was zero (n = 40,000). Vitamin E was administered in doses ranging from 10 to 5000 IU daily, and populations studied were either healthy (primary prevention trials) or had a variety of established diseases such as cancer, CVD, renal disease, hepatitis, systemic lupus erythematosus, heart failure, cirrhosis, gastritis, MI or macular degeneration.

Gerss and Kopcke (2009) concur that the use of different methodological approaches yields contradictory results, with some statistical models finding an association and others not. They used the same data as that described in the Miller et al study (2005). The meta-analysis was augmented with 2495 additional participants receiving vitamin E doses from 136 to 5000 IU/day. Moreover in two of the originally included trials, the updated results of mortality at longer periods of follow-up were made available.

More specifically, hierarchical logistic regression analyses confirmed the former results, showing an increased mortality of patients receiving high-dose vitamin E, whereas application of a traditional methodological approach to meta-regression found that in certain trials increased mortality was not due to high-dose vitamin E, but could be explained by a higher proportion of male subjects in comparison to other trials (Gerss & Kopcke 2009). Overall, the causal relationship of vitamin E supplementation and increased ACM is questionable and, in particular, high-dose vitamin E supplementation cannot be regarded as 'proven' to increase mortality.

Similar findings were obtained by Berry et al (2009), who applied a Bayesian meta-analytical method to synthesise results from previous clinical trials of vitamin E. They used data from studies in the Miller et al (2005) meta-analysis, appended by 10 more recent studies, and concluded that vitamin E intake is unlikely to affect ACM, regardless of dose.

Re-evaluation of data from the original Framingham Heart Study has also failed to find an association between vitamin E supplementation and increased risk of ACM (Dietrich et al 2009). The Framingham Heart Study (n = 4270) began enrolling in 1948 to investigate the association between supplemental vitamin E and the 10-year incidence of CVD and ACM. Eleven per cent of people participating in the study used vitamin E supplements at baseline and the most commonly consumed dose was 300–500 IU/day. In all statistical models, age, diabetes and treatment for blood pressure were significant positive predictors of CVD and ACM, whereas no statistically significant associations were found between vitamin E supplement intake and CVD and ACM. In secondary analyses, the associations of vitamin E dose and duration of use with CVD and ACM were assessed. Once again, no statistically significant associations were observed in any of the analyses for CVD or ACM. The effects of potential confounders, such as use of aspirin, anticholesterol treatment and multivitamins, were minimised using multivariate models which did not change the results.

In a further attempt to suggest the effects of supplementation of beta-carotene, vitamin A, and vitamin E singly or in combination on increased ACM, Bjelakovic et al (2013) included 53 RCTs involving 241,883 participants. Meta-regression analysis revealed that doses of >15 mg of vitamin E increased mortality significantly. In rebuttal, Hemilä (2013: not peer-reviewed) states that the increase in ACM by 3% based on a pooling of studies does not correspond to an individual level analysis. The latest ATBC studies confirm the statement made by Hemilä casting doubt on the significance of the review by Bjelakovic et al (2013) (Kataja-Tuomola et al 2010, Lynch et al 2012).

Clinical note — LDL oxidation and vitamin E

Oxidative stress affects lipid metabolism by producing an oxidised LDL that has greater atherogenic potential than its original form. In the past, attention focused on investigating various antioxidants, such as vitamin E, for their ability to prevent LDL oxidation. In recent years, researchers have started to focus on identifying the biological oxidants responsible for initiating oxidation of LDL within the human arterial wall and on a better understanding of what makes oxidised LDL proatherogenic. In 2003, in vitro testing with LDL discovered that myeloperoxidase is a pathway that promotes LDL oxidation in the human artery wall, although others are also likely to exist. It is noteworthy that vitamin E failed to inhibit LDL oxidation by myeloperoxidase in vitro (Heinecke 2003), although it does reduce LDL oxidation in animals and humans when given in doses well above RDI (Brockes et al 2003). Oil palm vitamin E (tocopherols 70% and tocotrienols 30%) reduced atherogenesis in a recent animal model trial (Che Anishas et al 2014). In earlier studies the effect of palm oil vitamin E in humans suggests its use in lowering LDL and protecting HDL levels (Mukherjee & Mitra 2009). Supplemental forms of tocopherols are available from a palm oil source.

Clinical note — Neurodegenerative disease and oxidative stress

Neurodegenerative diseases are defined by the progressive loss of specific neuronal cell populations and are associated with protein aggregates. A growing body of evidence suggests that oxidative stress plays a key role in the pathophysiology of neurodegenerative disorders such as AD and PD. Reactive oxygen species are known to cause cell damage by way of three main mechanisms: lipid peroxidation, protein oxidation and DNA oxidation. Cells have developed several defence and repair mechanisms to deal with oxidative stress, and antioxidants such as vitamin E represent the first line of defence. In addition to its antioxidant properties, vitamin E can act as an anti-inflammatory agent, which may also be neuroprotective, and it regulates specific enzymes, thus changing the properties of membranes. The central nervous system is especially vulnerable to free radical damage because, compared to other tissues, it has a high oxygen consumption rate, abundant lipid content and a relative deficit in antioxidant systems. While it remains unclear whether oxidative stress is the primary initiating event associated with neurodegeneration or a secondary effect related to other pathological pathways, a growing body of evidence implicates it as being involved in the propagation of cellular injury (Ricciarelli et al 2007).

Parkinson's disease

Based on experimental and clinical data, it is well established that oxidative stress and lipid peroxidation are increased in the substantia nigra of people with PD and this may play an important role in the disease's aetiology. Vitamin E has therefore been the focus of research as a potential treatment. Using both in vitro and in vivo experimental model systems for PD, studies have demonstrated both vitamin E-mediated protection and lack of protection (Fariss & Zhang 2003). Similarly, inconsistent results have been obtained for vitamin E supplementation in the prevention and treatment of clinical PD. An open study using high doses of both tocopherol (3200 IU/day) and ascorbic acid (3000 mg/day) delayed the use of levodopa or dopamine agonists for 2 years in subjects with early PD (Fahn 1992). In contrast, the Deprenyl and Tocopherol Antioxidative Therapy of Parkinsonism (DATATOP) study found no effect on the progression of disability with a dose of alpha-tocopherol 2000 IU/day (Parkinson Study Group 1996). The same study found that vitamin E had no effect on mortality (Parkinson Study Group 1998). A meta-analysis six case-control, one cohort study and a cross-sectional study of several vitamins and the risk of PD found that vitamin E demonstrated a protective role seen in both high (less significant and warranting further trials) and moderate intakes, suggesting that vitamin E has a neuroprotective role attenuating risk (Mahyar et al 2005).

Alzheimer's dementia and cognitive decline

Alzheimer's disease occurs due to protein oxidation and lipid peroxidation. Beta amyloid proteins undergo oxidative stress via hydrogen peroxide, leading to neuronal death and decline into the disease. Vitamin E may block hydrogen peroxide production, slowing progression of cytotoxicity, resulting in reduced beta amyloid cell death (animal studies) (Rizvi et al 2014). The current standard of care for pharmacological management of the cognitive and functional disabilities of AD consists of a cholinesterase inhibitor and sometimes the addition of high-dose vitamin E (Bonner & Peskind 2002). The inclusion of vitamin E is largely based on a 1997 double-blind study that compared a large dose of synthetic vitamin E (1000 IU twice daily) with selegiline (5 mg twice daily) and placebo in a group of patients with moderately severe AD. The 2-year study found that vitamin E significantly slowed down the progression of the disease, delayed institutionalisation and increased survival rate (Sano et al 1997). In contrast to the positive 1997 study, a study involving 769 subjects with possible or probable AD using the same dose found no significant effects in patients with mild cognitive impairment and no change in the rate of progression to AD over a 3-year period (Petersen et al 2005).

Despite this, positive results were again achieved in a double-blind RCT which found that supplementation with alpha-tocopherol in mild to moderate AD was effective in slowing functional decline and decreasing caregiver burden (Dysken et al 2014). The study involved 613 patients with mild to moderate AD who received 2000 IU/day of alpha-tocopherol (n = 152), 20 mg/day memantine (n = 155), the combination (n = 154) or placebo (n = 152). Over a mean follow-up of 2.27 years, Alzheimer's Disease Co-operative Study — Activities of Daily Living (ADCS-ADL) inventory scores declined by 3.15 units (95% confidence interval [CI], 0.92–5.39; adjusted $P = 0.03$) less in the alpha-tocopherol group compared with the placebo group. In the memantine group, these scores declined 1.98 units less (95% CI, –0.24 to 4.20; adjusted $P = 0.40$) than the placebo group's decline. This change in the alpha-tocopherol group translates into a delay in clinical progression of 19% per year compared with placebo or a delay of approximately 6.2 months over the follow-up period.

Recent research suggests that in fact gamma-tocopherol may be more important than previously suspected in AD. A study by Morris et al (2014) found gamma-tocopherol concentrations were associated with lower amyloid load ($P = 0.002$) and lower neurofibrillary tangle severity ($P = 0.02$), whereas concentrations of alpha-tocopherol were not associated with AD neuropathology, except as modified by gamma-tocopherol. High alpha-tocopherol was associated with higher amyloid load when gamma-tocopherol levels were low and with lower amyloid levels when gamma-tocopherol levels were high (P for interaction = 0.03). Brain concentrations of gamma- and alpha-tocopherols may be associated with AD neuropathology in interrelated, complex ways (Morris et al 2014).

Prevention

Higher plasma vitamin E levels are associated with a significantly reduced risk of cognitive impairment and dementia in older adults. Protection is most consistently seen with vitamin E from food sources, but not always from vitamin E supplements (Cherubini et al 2005, Engelhart et al 2002, Morris et al 2005). Intervention studies using supplements have produced mixed results and focus on alpha-tocopherol only. The Cache County Study was a large study of 4740 people aged 65 years or older that found a combination of vitamins E (400 IU/day) and C (500 mg/day) taken for at least 3 years was associated with a reduced incidence of AD (Zandi et al 2004). No protective effects were seen when vitamin E or C was taken alone. In the Honolulu/Asia Aging Study, long-term use of vitamin E and C supplements was associated with an 88% reduction in the frequency of subsequent vascular dementia and appeared to improve cognitive function in later life; however, a protective effect against AD was not observed (Masaki et al 2000). A lack of association between dietary or supplemental vitamin E and risk of AD in elderly subjects was also found in the Washington Heights/Inwood Columbia Aging Project (WHICAP), which involved 980 older subjects (Luchsinger et al 2003). It must be noted that dietary intakes were assessed in this study with a limited food frequency questionnaire, which is likely to be less accurate than the more detailed surveys used in some other studies.

Immunity in the elderly

Immune cell function is influenced by the oxidant and antioxidant balance, so antioxidant supplements have been investigated clinically for their ability to enhance immune responses (Meydani et al 1998). Increased markers of T-cell-mediated immunity were enhanced with all doses of synthetic vitamin E tested, according to a randomised, double-blind study of 78 healthy elderly subjects. Doses used were 60, 200 and 800 mg/day for 4 months, with best overall responses obtained with the 200 mg dosage (Meydani et al 1997). Rizvi et al (2014) state that supplementation enhances immunity in the elderly, correlating higher plasma vitamin E levels with reduced number of infections over a 3-year period. Enhanced vaccine antibody response with no adverse side effects was also observed, with other authors stating that vitamin E improves resistance to respiratory infections in the aged (Rizvi et al 2014, Wu & Meydani 2008).

Common cold and respiratory disease

Low-dose vitamin E supplementation (50 mg/day) was found to reduce the incidence of the common cold by 28% in a subgroup of men enrolled in the ATBC cancer prevention study (Hemila et al 2006). Participants were older city-dwelling men (≥ 65 years) who smoked only 5–14 cigarettes/day. More recently, researchers re-evaluated the data and found that the effect of vitamin E diverged, depending on location of dwelling and smoking status. Among city-dwelling men considered to be low–moderate-level smokers (5–14 cigarettes/day), vitamin E significantly reduced common-cold risk, whereas among those smoking more and living away from cities, vitamin E increased common-cold risk. It appears that different modifying factors have an influence on whether vitamin E supplementation has beneficial or harmful effects. The ATBC study correlated vitamin E with a 14% higher incidence of pneumonia in smokers of five cigarettes a day aged 50–69 years over a 6-year period (Hemila & Kaprio 2008).

Haemodialysis (HD)

HD increases oxidative stress and triggers atherosclerosis and dialysis-related amyloidosis (Masatomi Sasaki 2006). Vitamin E supplementation may offer several benefits to patients on HD, who typically experience high levels of oxidative stress, as there is some evidence that supplementation reduces oxidative stress and LDL oxidability in this population (Badiou et al 2003, Diepeveen et al 2005, Galli et al 2001, Giray et al 2003). The SPACE study by Boaz et al (2000) found that high-dose vitamin E supplementation (natural vitamin E 800 IU/day) caused a 50% reduction in cardiac events. This is a highly significant outcome and worthy of further investigation.

HD patients also experience cramps, which appeared to respond to vitamin E supplementation according to a placebo-controlled, double-blind study of 60 subjects (Khajehdehi et al 2001). Treatment with a vitamin E dose of 400 mg/day for 8 weeks resulted in a 54% reduction in cramps, which increased to a 97% reduction when combined with vitamin C (250 mg/day). The benefits were not significantly associated with age, sex, aetiology of end-stage renal disease, serum electrolytes or HD duration, but showed a positive correlation ($P = 0.01$) with the type of therapy used.

According to one small study, vitamin E supplementation (500 mg/day) allowed for a reduction in erythropoietin dose (from 93 to 74 IU/kg/week) while maintaining stable haemoglobin concentrations (Cristol et al 1997).

Intradialytic hypotension is a condition plaguing diabetic HD patients where SBP may drop by up to 20% during treatment. In a small unrandomised trial of 62 diabetic HD patients, vitamin E-bonded polysulfone membrane dialysers were utilised to observe SBP. Two groups entered the trial. The groups were divided into those with very low SBP (28) requiring medication and those with low SBP (34) who were not medicated. Both groups demonstrated significantly improved SBP at 3 months (Koremoto 2012).

Premenstrual syndrome (PMS)

Treatment with D-alpha-tocopherol (400 IU/day) over three menstrual cycles significantly alleviated some affective and physical symptoms of PMS according to one randomised double-blind study (London et al 1987). Symptoms of anxiety, food craving and depression responded to active treatment, whereas effects on other measured parameters such as weight gain were not significant.

An earlier study of 75 women with benign breast disease found that D-alpha-tocopherol (150–600 IU/day) significantly decreased some symptoms of PMS compared with placebo; however, the study involved subjective patient evaluation, which may have influenced the findings (London et al 1983). Women who suffer from PMS do not statistically differ from other women in regard to biochemical deficiency. In a study of 62 women who presented with moderate to severe forms of PMS, cohorts were given either vitamin E 400 IU/day or placebo and both groups demonstrated significant benefits in physical and mental symptoms. Further observation and cross-over studies are obviously needed (Mandana et al 2013).

Dysmenorrhoea

According to two randomised placebo-controlled studies, taking 200 IU vitamin E twice daily or 500 IU daily, starting 2 days before menstruation and continuing for the first 3 days of bleeding, seems to reduce menstrual pain severity and duration and to decrease blood loss in teenage girls with primary dysmenorrhoea (Ziaei et al 2001, 2005). Beneficial effects can be seen after 2 months and reach maximal effect after 4 months.

Intermittent claudication

A Cochrane review of five placebo-controlled studies including a total of 265 volunteers (average age 57 years) concluded that, although further research is required to determine its effectiveness, vitamin E may have beneficial effects in intermittent claudication with no serious side effects (Kleijnen & Mackerras 2000). Treatment duration varied from 12 weeks to 18 months, and dosage regimens varied between the studies, which were considered generally small and of poor quality. A closer look at the evidence suggests that doses of at least 600 IU/day for a minimum of 12 weeks are required.

Since then a double-blind RCT testing vitamin E (400 IU/day) found no beneficial effects on perceived pain or treadmill-walking duration in people with claudication (Collins et al 2003).

A small study of 16 patients with stable claudication revealed that administration of vitamin E (200 mg/day) and vitamin C (500 mg/day) for 4 weeks reduces oxidative stress in this population, and therefore may also have an effect on the remote ischaemia-reperfusion damage (Wijnen et al 2001). Although mentioned as a possible supplement in the treatment of intermittent claudication, no further trials have been conducted (Brass 2013).

Cancer

Most of the epidemiological evidence suggests that vitamin E and other antioxidants decrease the incidence of certain cancers. Based on these observations, numerous prospective and intervention studies have been conducted in various populations. Very often, vitamin E is used in combination with other antioxidant nutrients, and sometimes the form of tocopherol administered is not stated, making it difficult to interpret study findings.

A review that systematically evaluated the scientific literature using guidelines developed by the US Preventative Services Task Force concluded that there is evidence to suggest that those individuals with higher serum vitamin E levels or who are receiving vitamin E supplementation have a decreased risk of some cancers, including lung, prostate, stomach and gastrointestinal carcinoma (Sung et al 2003). As can be expected, study design, differing treatment dose (nutritional levels or higher), form of vitamin used and population studied (general or high-risk) had an influence on outcomes. Since then, several new studies have been published that cast doubt on the cancer-protective effects of vitamin E for the general population. However, it seems likely that certain subpopulations (e.g. the poorly nourished) may benefit, and that lifestyle factors modify responses to supplementation (e.g. smoking). Research further suggests that differences in telomere length may be another factor affecting individuals' responses to vitamin E supplements (Shen et al 2009).

The role of vitamin E in cancer prevention remains controversial. The Cancer Institute of New Jersey states that gamma- and delta-tocopherols are preventive in prostate, lung, breast and colon cancer. Alpha-tocopherols had no effect. The Heart Outcomes Prevention Evaluation — The Ongoing Outcomes (HOPE-TOO) trial and the Women's Health Study found no significant reduction in risk with daily doses of 400–600 IU (Rizvi et al 2014).

All cancers

A large study of nearly 30,000 subjects was carried out in Linxian, China. It tested four combinations of vitamins and minerals (retinol and zinc; riboflavin and niacin; vitamin C and molybdenum; and beta-carotene, vitamin E and selenium) over a 5-year period in a population with a persistently low intake of several micronutrients (Blot et al 1995). Although no statistically significant effect on cancer incidence was achieved by any intervention, secondary analysis showed that the combination of selenium, beta-carotene and alpha-tocopherol was associated with a statistically significant lower total mortality rate, a 13% reduction (borderline significant) in total cancer mortality rate and a statistically significant lower mortality rate from stomach cancer (a major cancer in Linxian).

Results from the SUVIMAX study suggest that the protective effects of vitamin E may be gender-specific (Zureik et al 2004). In this trial, antioxidant supplementation (vitamin C 120 mg, vitamin E 30 mg, beta-carotene 6 mg, selenium 100 mcg and zinc 20 mg) was associated with a lower cancer incidence in men, but not in women. It is possible that men in the SUVIMAX trial benefited from supplementation due to their lower baseline levels of antioxidants.

More recently four large studies have found that vitamin E supplementation has no protective effect against cancer incidence. The Medical Research Council/British Heart Foundation study of 20,536 UK adults aged 40–80 years with coronary disease, other occlusive arterial disease or diabetes found that a daily antioxidant supplement containing 600 mg vitamin E, 250 mg vitamin C and 20 mg beta-carotene produced no significant reduction in the incidence of cancer or ACM (Parkinson Study Group 2002). The HOPE-TOO study, which used long-term natural vitamin E (400 IU/day) as a stand-alone supplement, failed to find a protective effect against cancer incidence or cancer deaths in people with pre-existing vascular disease or diabetes mellitus (Lonn et al 2005). Long-term use of natural vitamin E (600 IU) taken on alternate days provided no overall benefit for cancer incidence or total mortality in a large randomised study involving 39,876 healthy women of at least 45 years of age (Lee et al 2005).

Results from 7627 women free of cancer at bascline in the WACS found that long-term use (average 9.4 years) of vitamin C (500 mg/day), natural vitamin E (600 IU every other day) and beta-carotene (50 mg every other day) was not significantly associated with lowered incidence of total cancer or cancer mortality for any of the tested antioxidants (O'Donnell et al 2009).

When data were evaluated for effects on site-specific cancers, women receiving vitamin E supplements had a reduced risk (but not statistically significant) for colorectal cancer compared with the placebo group. This was largely due to a reduced risk of colon cancer. However, there was no statistically significant association of vitamin E supplementation with rectal or other cancers. Further subgroup analysis revealed that women in the vitamin E supplement group who currently smoked or had smoked in the past had lower rates of cancer death than those who never smoked. The *Cancer Prevention Research Journal* suggests that, at a nutritional level, all forms of vitamin E are protective against cancer. However supplementation has not been proven to reduce cancer incidence and supplementation did not alter cancer progression or prevention (Chung 2012). However in the Selenium and vitamin E Cancer Prevention Trial (SELECT 2008 and 2011 update) for prevention of prostate cancer, statistical significance was reached with a 17% relative increase in prostate cancer compared to placebo, whereas the selenium alone or E and selenium supplementation were not statistically significant (National Cancer Institute (NIH) 2014).

Urinary tract cancer

Analysis of data from the ATBC cancer prevention study, which tested synthetic vitamin E (50 mg/day) and beta-carotene (20 mg/day) in male Finnish smokers aged 50–69 years (n = 29,133), found neither supplement affected the incidence of urothelial cancer or of renal cell cancer (Virtamo et al 2000). Jacobs et al (2002) assessed the US Cancer Prevention Study II, where vitamin C and E supplements were trialled, to determine reduced risk in bladder cancer. In the

E group regular supplementation use ≥10 years demonstrated a reduced risk of bladder cancer mortality whereas shorter-duration supplementation did not prove beneficial. In a large epidemiological study plasma alpha-tocopherol and gamma-tocopherol with vitamin A were assessed. Researchers from Texas University suggest that gamma-tocopherol is not protective in isolation (Hernandez et al 2004). In the groups where plasma levels of all three nutrients were higher there was a reduction in the risk associated with bladder cancer, leading to the conclusion that there is a potentially protective effect in combination treatment (Liang et al 2008).

Respiratory tract cancers

Smoking and alcohol consumption are the major risk factors for upper aerodigestive tract cancers, and observational studies indicate a protective role for fruits, vegetables and antioxidant nutrients (Wright et al 2007). Analysis of data from the ATBC cancer prevention study testing long-term supplementation with synthetic vitamin E (50 mg/day) and beta-carotene (20 mg/day) in male Finnish smokers aged 50–69 years (*n* = 29,133) found no effect of either agent on the overall incidence of any upper aerodigestive tract cancer nor any effect on mortality from these neoplasms. In animal models oesophageal squamous cell carcinoma was visibly reduced by supplementation of selenium and vitamin E (80 IU/kg) in diet; this has yet to be proven in human trials (Yang et al 2012).

Breast cancer

Mixed results have been obtained for vitamin E in the primary prevention of breast cancer, although a 2003 study has detected a modest protective effect against recurrence of breast cancer and disease-related mortality in postmenopausal women previously diagnosed with the disease (Fleischauer et al 2003). Protective effects were established after 3 years' use, according to the study.

In a single study Chamras et al (2005) found a dose-responsive inhibition of cell proliferation in oestrogen receptor-positive cells. This trial is hopeful as the cell proliferation was reduced by 69–84%; vitamin E altered the expression of oestrogen receptor cells. This suggests that vitamin E may inhibit oestrogen receptor-positive cell growth and alter cellular response to oestrogen.

Ovarian cancer

Vitamin E supplements were protective against the incidence of ovarian cancer whereas consumption of antioxidants from diet was unrelated to risk according to another study (Fleischauer et al 2001). In analyses combining antioxidant intake from diet and supplements, vitamins C (>363 mg/day) and E (>75 mg/day) were associated with significant protective effects. In a human case-controlled study in Korean ovarian cancer patients, women with the highest tertile group for both alpha-tocopherol and gamma-tocopheral plasma levels presented >72% overall reduced risk compared to the lowest tertile group (Jeong et al 2009).

Colorectal cancer

Colorectal cancers are highly prevalent, with Australian levels reaching >12,000 diagnosed per year (ABS 2005). Studies investigating the association between vitamin E and incidence of colorectal cancer have produced inconsistent results. Prospective studies have shown that high serum levels of vitamin E are protective; however, only one of three intervention studies has produced positive results (Stone & Papas 1997). These results are difficult to interpret, as the studies have been criticised for not adequately distinguishing between cancer incidence and adenoma recurrence.

In the WACS (n = 7627), women receiving natural vitamin E (600 IU every other day) had a reduced risk (but not statistically significant) of colorectal cancer compared with the placebo group. This was largely because of a reduced risk of colon cancer; however, there was no statistically significant association of vitamin E supplementation with rectal or other cancers (O'Donnell et al 2009). The ATBC study also detected a somewhat lower incidence of colorectal cancer in the alpha-tocopherol arm compared with the no alpha-tocopherol arm, but this was not statistically significant (Virtamo et al 2000).

The World Cancer Research Fund (2011) suggests that vitamin E does not present with significant evidence of reduced incidence or prevalence of colorectal cancer. In a recent systematic review, although there was a concession that observational studies suggest vitamin E may be protective, experimental studies have had inconsistent results. From four studies Arain and Qadeer (2010) state that vitamin E as a primary prevention of colorectal cancer does not reduce incidence. In another review of dietary supplements where two trials regarding vitamin E were assessed, the conclusion remains steadfast (Posadzki et al 2013).

Prostate cancer

The ATBC cancer prevention study provided information about the incidence of prostate cancer with long-term use of synthetic alpha-tocopherol (50 mg), beta-carotene (20 mg), both agents or a placebo daily for 5–8 years (Albanes et al 2000). One of the most striking outcomes was a 32% decrease in the incidence of prostate cancer for volunteers receiving vitamin E (n = 14,564) compared to those not receiving it (n = 14,569) and a 41% reduction in mortality among men using vitamin E. Neither agent had any effect on the time interval between diagnosis and death (Heinonen et al 1998). The preventive effect of vitamin E on prostate cancer incidence was observed to be long-term according to later analysis of postintervention effects (Virtamo et al 2003).

One study has identified a decrease in serum androgen concentrations associated with long-term alpha-tocopherol supplementation, suggesting this may be one of the factors contributing to the observed reduction in incidence and mortality of prostate cancer (Hartman et al 2001). In contrast, SELECT (National Cancer Institute (NIH) 2014) determined that, in combination with selenium, there was an increased risk of prostate cancer with vitamin E. More specifically, there were 17% more prostate cancer cases diagnosed in the group of men assigned to take 400 IU of vitamin E (and no selenium) daily compared to the men taking two placebos (no vitamin E and no selenium), after an average of 7 years — 5.5 of the years on supplements followed by 1.5 years not taking supplements. Importantly, the vast majority of all of the cancers that were screened were very early-stage disease, and the rate of advanced or aggressive cancers in the vitamin E group was no higher than in the placebo group. Several theories have been proposed to explain the differences in results, such as a U-shaped response curve, where very low or very high blood levels of a nutrient are harmful but more moderate levels are beneficial. In other words, while the ATBC dose may have been preventive, the SELECT dose may have been too large to have a prevention benefit (http://www.cancer.gov/newscenter/qa/2008/selectqa).

Pancreatic cancer

Higher alpha-tocopherol concentrations may play a protective role in pancreatic carcinogenesis in male smokers, according to the ATBC cancer prevention study, which found that men with the highest serum tocopherol levels had a lower pancreatic cancer risk (highest compared with lowest quintile) (Stolzenberg-Solomon et al 2009). Polyunsaturated fat, a putative pro-oxidant nutrient, modified the association such that the inverse alpha-tocopherol association was most pronounced in subjects with a high polyunsaturated fat intake. Gong et al (2010) suggest that a positive association was noted in high intakes of monounsaturated palmitoleic and oleic fatty acids and polyunsaturated linolenic acid with vitamin C. In the study of a large population-based case-control study in San Francisco, it was found that vitamin C and vitamin E together or alone may reduce the risk of pancreatic cancer.

Adjunct with cisplatin

Bove et al (2001) made the observation that the neurotoxic presentation associated with cisplatin use was similar to that of vitamin E deficiency. They hypothesised that cumulative cisplatin use could induce vitamin E deficiency if patients' levels were not sufficiently high throughout treatment. To test the theory they started by measuring vitamin E in the plasma of five patients who developed severe neurotoxicity after cisplatin treatment and in another group of five patients before and after two or four cycles of cisplatin treatment. This produced preliminary data that supported the theory that inadequate vitamin E due to cisplatin treatment could be responsible for the peripheral nerve damage induced by free radicals (Bove et al 2001). Following this, four clinical trials were conducted where it was concluded that the incidence of chemotherapy-induced peripheral neuropathy was significantly reduced with vitamin E supplementation (Wolf et al 2008). Oral vitamin E (300 mg/day), taken before cisplatin treatment and continued for 3 months after cessation of treatment, significantly reduced the incidence and severity of neurotoxicity according to a randomised study ($n = 47$), in which the incidence of neurotoxicity was significantly lower in the group receiving vitamin E (30.7%) compared to those receiving the placebo (85.7%; $P < 0.01$) (Pace et al 2003). Shortly afterwards, Argyriou et al (2005) conducted a randomised study of 31 patients with cancer treated with six courses of cumulative cisplatin, paclitaxel or their combination regimens. Only 25% of patients randomly assigned to receive oral vitamin E (600 mg/day) during chemotherapy and for 3 months after its cessation developed neurotoxicity, compared to 73% in the control group. A year later, in another randomised study, 30 patients scheduled to receive six courses of cumulative cisplatin-based regimens were randomly allocated to receive either vitamin E (600 mg/day) during chemotherapy and for 3 months after its cessation or no adjunctive therapy (controls). This study again found a significantly reduced incidence of neurotoxicity with vitamin E (21.4%) compared to controls (68.5%) ($P = 0.026$) (Argyriou et al 2006).

While no data were included on the long-term survival of the patients involved, studies undertaken have failed to show a detrimental effect from combining vitamin E with chemotherapy (Ladas et al 2004, Pace et al 2003).

Arthritis

High-dose vitamin E supplements may be effective in relieving pain in osteoarthritis (OA) and rheumatoid arthritis (RA), according to several double-blind studies, with some studies finding that the effects are as strong as with diclofenac. Vitamin E supplements have been studied in people with OA, RA, spondylitis ankylosis, spondylosis and psoriatic arthritis. Comparisons have been made to placebos and non-steroidal anti-inflammatory drugs (NSAIDs).

Osteoarthritis

According to an early crossover study (Machtey & Ouaknine 1978), 52% of OA patients experienced less pain when treated with vitamin E (600 mg/day) compared to a placebo. Several years later, a double-blind randomised study of 50 volunteers with OA confirmed these findings and showed that vitamin E (400 IU/day) was significantly superior to a placebo in relieving pain, increasing mobility and reducing analgesic requirements (Blankenhorn 1986). Symptoms of pain at rest, during movement or with applied pressure all responded to treatment with vitamin E.

Vitamin E supplementation (500 IU/day) did not alter the loss of cartilage volume in knee OA according to a 2-year, double-blind, randomised, placebo-controlled study of 138 patients (American College of Rheumatology clinical and radiographic criteria) (Wluka et al 2002). Additionally, symptoms did not improve. Vitamin E also failed to alleviate symptoms in a shorter, 6-month double-blind study using the same dose (Brand et al 2001) and symptoms of pain, stiffness and function did not change at the 1-, 3- or 6-month assessments.

Research has continued in recent years, so that by 2007 a systematic review by Canter et al (2007) identified a total of seven RCTs that tested vitamin E in OA: four trials compared the treatment with a placebo, two tested against diclofenac and one against vitamin A. Of these, two placebo-controlled trials demonstrated the effectiveness of vitamin E for pain. One trial was considered methodologically weak, but the second was more robust and indicated greater effectiveness both for the whole patient sample and for a subgroup with OA of the knee and hip. Haflah et al's (2009) findings suggest that a dose of 400 mg/day has a potential role in reducing the symptoms of OA of the knee and may be as effective as glucosamine. This is in contrast to two earlier studies that involved patients with OA of the knee and produced largely negative results. Two equivalence trials comparing vitamin E to diclofenac produced more positive outcomes and suggested similar effectiveness for the two treatments, with one study reporting a statistically significant superiority of vitamin E over diclofenac (Canter et al 2007). The authors of the review have claimed that variable methodological rigour does not yet allow a definitive conclusion to be made about the effectiveness of vitamin E in OA. Further trials are needed; however it appears that the supplement of palm vitamin E is safe to use.

Rheumatoid arthritis

According to several double-blind studies, a dose of 1200 mg/day vitamin E significantly reduces pain symptoms in people with RA, but not always morning stiffness.

A double-blind study of 42 RA patients who received vitamin E (600 mg twice a day) over 12 weeks showed that pain parameters were significantly decreased with active treatment compared to a placebo (Edmonds et al 1997). The same study also found no change in the Ritchie Articular Index, duration of morning stiffness, swollen joint count or laboratory parameters with vitamin E supplementation compared to a placebo. A further study using the same dose detected a significant inverse correlation between vitamin E levels and pain score, whereas morning stiffness and sedimentation rate were not affected (Scherak & Kolarz 1991).

Edmonds et al (1997) enrolled 42 patients with RA in a double-blind randomised study in which alpha-tocopherol (600 mg twice a day) was compared to a placebo for 12 weeks. While laboratory measures of inflammatory activity and oxidative modification were unchanged with active treatment, pain parameters were significantly decreased after vitamin E treatment when compared with the placebo, suggesting that vitamin E may exert a small but significant analgesic activity independently of a peripheral anti-inflammatory effect. More recently, a combination of standard treatment (intramuscular methotrexate, oral sulfasalazine and indomethacin suppository at night) and vitamin E (400 mg three times daily) was compared to standard treatment and a combination of antioxidants or to standard treatment alone (Helmy et al 2001). Standard treatment started to produce tangible improvements after 2 months, whereas additional treatment with either vitamin E or antioxidants improved symptoms more quickly (after 1 month). Karlson et al (2008) suggest in a primary prevention Women's Health Study of females >45 years (randomised, double-blind, controlled) that, while inflammatory laboratory measures were unchanged in the active treatment group, pain parameters demonstrated significantly decreased levels after vitamin E treatment at 600 IU on alternate days. Although no significant associations were found in the primary end point in the prevention of RA, there was a suggestion of an inverse association with vitamin E treatment and seropositive RA; however it did not reach statistical significance. As seropositive RA is the more severe phenotype, this deserves further study. The limitations of the study were numerous, as discussed by the authors; larger numbers are needed to detect the risk reductions in seropositive and negative RA and inflammatory polyarthritis, due to previous findings of other authors reporting 28–56% reduction in risk with vitamin E supplement use (Cerhan et al 2003). In a systematic review of natural alternatives to RA treatment, McFarlane et al (2010) also suggest that vitamin E alleviates pain with no reported changes in laboratory measures of inflammation.

Comparisons with pharmaceutical medication

After 3 weeks' treatment with either high-dose vitamin E (400 mg RRR-alpha-tocopherol acetate three times daily) or diclofenac sodium, a significant improvement in all assessed clinical parameters was observed in hospitalised patients with established chronic RA ($n = 85$), according to a randomised, double-blind parallel-group trial (Wittenborg et al 1998). Duration of morning stiffness, grip strength and the degree of pain, assessed by a 10-cm visual analogue scale, reduced significantly with vitamin E as well as with diclofenac. Both treatments were considered to be equally effective by patients and doctors.

Menopausal symptoms

According to a review published by the Mayo Clinic in the United States, behavioural changes in conjunction with vitamin E (800 IU/day) are a reasonable initial approach for menopausal women with mild symptoms that do not interfere with sleep or daily function (Shanafelt et al 2002). The recommendation is based on a double-blind, randomised, placebo-controlled, crossover clinical trial that found that vitamin E (800 IU/day) was more effective than a placebo in controlling hot flushes in breast cancer survivors. Benefits have been confirmed in another double-blind, placebo-controlled trial, which found that treatment with 400 IU vitamin E daily significantly reduced hot flush severity and daily frequency as reported by participants (Ziaei et al 2007).

Male infertility

V

Lipid-soluble antioxidants such as vitamin E have been studied for their effects in male reproductive physiology because the membranes of germ cells and spermatozoa are very sensitive to oxidation (Bhardwaj et al 2000, Bolle et al 2002).

According to three of four studies, oral vitamin E supplementation can effectively treat some forms of male infertility (Geva et al 1996, Kessopoulou et al 1995, Rolf et al 1999, Suleiman et al 1996). Doses varied from 200 to 800 mg/day.

Kessopoulou et al (1995) compared vitamin E (600 mg/day) to a placebo over 3 months in 30 healthy men with high levels of reactive oxygen species generation in semen and a normal female partner. The randomised, crossover study found that active treatment improved zona binding, thereby showing that vitamin E significantly improved the in vitro function of human spermatozoa. Geva et al (1996) studied men enrolled in an in vitro fertilisation program who previously had had low fertilisation rates, and treated them with oral vitamin E (200 mg/day) for 3 months. After the first month, fertilisation rates increased significantly, from 19% to 29%. The same year, Suleiman et al (1996) treated asthenospermic patients with oral vitamin E, which significantly decreased the malondialdehyde concentration in spermatozoa and improved sperm motility. Of the 52 treated males, 11 (21%) impregnated their spouses; nine of the spouses successfully continued to have normal-term deliveries, whereas two aborted in the first trimester. No pregnancies were reported in the spouses of the placebo-treated patients.

The negative study used high-dose oral vitamin C (1000 mg/day), and vitamin E (800 mg/day) was tested over 56 days in 31 men with asthenozoospermia (<50% motile spermatozoa) and normal or only moderately reduced sperm concentration (>7×10^6 spermatozoa/mL) (Rolf et al 1999). Most recent studies combine vitamin E (400 IU/day) with selenium (and/or vitamin C) and are positively correlated with increased fertility and oligoasthenozoopermia syndrome; however it is not known whether vitamin E alone would have been just as effective (Kobori et al 2014, Moslemi & Tavanbakhsh 2011).

Dermatological conditions

Vitamin E is used both as an oral supplement and as a topical preparation in a variety of dermatological conditions. It is a popular ingredient in many moisturising preparations used to: alleviate dry and cracked skin; assist in the repair of abrasions, burns, grazes and skin lesions; prevent stretch marks; and diminish scar tissue. Vitamin E oil is used as a stand-alone preparation or incorporated into a cream or ointment base for these purposes.

Sunburn protection

Topical application of 1% alpha-tocopherol provided significant protection against erythema and sunburn in an experimental model. When combined with 15% ascorbic acid, the protective effect was enhanced (Lin et al 2003). Further improvements were seen when ferulic acid was added to the alpha-tocopherol (1%) and ascorbic acid (15%) solution, as this substance improves chemical stability of the antioxidants and doubles the photoprotective effect (Lin et al 2005).

Once again, it appears that not all forms of vitamin E exert a significant protective effect (McVean & Liebler 1999). According to an in vivo study, a 5% dispersion of alpha-tocopherol, gamma-tocopherol or delta-tocopherol in a neutral cream vehicle produced a statistically significant inhibition of thymine dimer formation, whereas alpha-tocopherol acetate and alpha-tocopherol methyl ether had no effect. Further research revealed that gamma-tocopherol and delta-tocopherol were five- to 10-fold less potent than alpha-tocopherol (McVean & Liebler 1997).

A comparison between topical vitamins E and C has demonstrated that vitamin E affords better protection against ultraviolet B radiation, whereas vitamin C is superior against ultraviolet A radiation (Baumann & Spencer 1999).

Although most research has focused on topical use, oral administration of a combination of high-dose vitamins E and C increases the threshold to erythema. The first study to show that the systemic administration of vitamins E and C reduces the sunburn reaction in humans was a small, double-blind, placebo-controlled trial that used ascorbic acid (2 g/day) combined with D-alpha-tocopherol (1000 IU/

day) (Eberlein-Konig et al 1998). The effect was seen after 8 days. The next to show reduction of the sunburn reaction was a 50-day study of 40 volunteers (20–47 years old), which showed that supplemental vitamin E (2 g/day) and C (3 g/day) protected against sunburn and resulted in increased vitamin E levels in keratinocytes (Fuchs & Kern 1998). This was once again confirmed in a controlled study of 45 healthy volunteers (Mireles-Rocha et al 2002). The doses used were lower in this study: 1200 IU/day of D-alpha-tocopherol in combination with vitamin C (2 g/day).

Scar tissue

Although vitamin E is widely used to diminish the appearance of scars, a small double-blind study of 15 patients who had undergone skin cancer removal found that applying an emollient preparation known as Aquaphor with added vitamin E after surgery either had no effect or worsened the appearance of scars compared to Aquaphor alone (Baumann & Spencer 1999). A larger study of 80 people with hypertrophic scars and keloids found that treatment with vitamin E and silicone gel sheets was successful in scar treatment (Palmieri et al 1995). After 2 months, 95% of patients receiving vitamin E and gel sheet treatment had improved by 50%, whereas 75% had improved by 50% without vitamin E.

Type 1 diabetes

Although the Heart Outcomes Prevention Evaluation (HOPE) study involving 3654 people with diabetes failed to detect a preventive effect for long-term vitamin E (400 IU/day) on CVD outcomes or nephropathy (Jain et al 1996, Lonn et al 2002), it is known that both types of diabetes demonstrate increased free radicals. It could be rationalised that the antioxidant effect on lipid peroxidation would be of some use; however metabolic parameters do not appear to improve in type 1 patients after vitamin E supplementation. There are limited trials and cohorts are relatively small (Gupta et al 2011).

Type 2 diabetes

In type 2 diabetes there is a similar increased production of free radicals as displayed in type 1 diabetes. Plasma measures of vitamin E are found to be lower in a small group of 52, with 36.2% diabetics with low alpha-tocopherol <12 micromol/L, 32.7% with a low alpha-tocopherol. Larger epidemiological and longitudinal studies are needed to confirm the use of vitamin E supplementation in this group (Illison et al 2011).

Chronic hepatitis C

According to a 2004 systematic review, significant improvements in biochemical responses were seen for vitamin E compared to a placebo (Coon & Ernst 2004). The authors report on one placebo-controlled trial in which a statistically significant reduction in liver enzyme (alanine aminotransferase [ALT]) was observed during vitamin E treatment but reductions were not consistent for all patients and complete normalisation of ALT levels did not occur. In the Middle East, where hepatitis C genotype is prevalent, ribavirin when used with pegylated interferon induces anaemia. Supplemental vitamin E 1000 IU/day demonstrated a protective impact on neutrophils and platelet counts, ameliorating the effect of haemolysis associated with ribavirin administration (Assem 2011).

Asthma and atopy

Studies have consistently demonstrated beneficial associations between dietary vitamin E and ventilatory function, and a few have demonstrated beneficial associations with asthma and atopy (Devereux & Seaton 2005). However, benefits do not extend to vitamin E supplements, as a randomised study (n = 72) using natural vitamin E (500 mg/day) over 6 weeks found no clinical benefit in subjects with mild to moderate asthma (Pearson et al 2004).

Age-related macular degeneration (AMD)

According to a review of RCTs comparing antioxidant vitamin and/or mineral supplement to controls, there is no evidence that antioxidant (vitamin E or beta-carotene) supplementation prevents AMD. However, there is evidence that supplementation with antioxidants (beta-carotene 15 mg, vitamin C 500 mg and vitamin E 400 IU) and zinc (elemental 80 mg) daily slows down the progression to advanced AMD and visual acuity loss in people with signs of the disease (Evans 2008). People with AMD, or early signs of the disease, may experience some benefit from taking supplements as used in the Age-Related Eye Disease Study (AREDS) (Sackett & Schenning 2002). Christen et al (2012) conducted an 8-year trial in well-nourished doctors of 400 IU every other day and vitamin C 500 mg/day. There appeared to be no beneficial or harmful effect on the risk of incidence of AMD. The dose for vitamin E was much lower than in the AREDS, at 400 IU/daily. Although this represents the largest study of its kind, it is not unreasonable to conclude that the dose was not high enough to exert effect and that the men were already nutritionally replete and perhaps at less risk.

Neurogenerative disease

Vitamin E supplementation may slow the rate of motor decline early in the course of Huntington's disease, according to a randomised, double-blind, placebo-controlled study of high-dose D-alpha-tocopherol treatment (Peyser et al 1995). The study of 73 patients with Huntington's disease found that treatment with D-alpha-tocopherol had no effect on neurological and neuropsychiatric symptoms in the treatment group overall; however, post hoc analysis revealed a significant selective therapeutic effect on neurological symptoms for patients early in the course of the disorder.

It now seems that the role of vitamin E has been established as essential for neurological function. In a recent review vitamin E was validated in the treatment of disorders of the central nervous system, specifically the use of vitamin E in the prevention or cure of Huntington's disease, tardive dyskinesia, amyotrophic lateral sclerosis (motor neuron disease [MND]), PD and AD (the last discussed earlier). Many trials for the use of vitamin E in the nervous system have been too small or the dose of vitamin E has been too low. Imounan et al (2012) suggest that in many neuropathic disorders vitamin E is revealing an important role.

OTHER USES

Oral supplements have been used to prevent or treat many other conditions, such as exercise-induced tissue damage, some types of senile cataracts, epilepsy and fibromyalgia.

Vitamin E prophylaxis in premature babies significantly reduces the risk of stage 3+ retinopathy by 52%, according to a 1997 meta-analysis of six randomised studies (Raju et al 1997).

Infusions of vitamin E are being investigated as a means of preventing ischaemic reperfusion injury in liver and heart surgery (Bartels et al 2004, Jaxa-Chamiec et al 2005).

DOSAGE RANGE

The body's requirement for vitamin E changes according to the amount and type of fat eaten in the diet. For example, vitamin E requirements increase when there is a high intake of PUFAs (Wahlqvist 2002).

Many scientists believe it is difficult for an individual to consume more than 15 mg/day of alpha-tocopherol from food alone, without also increasing fat intake above recommended levels.

Recommendations for adults (Australian adequate intake)

Adequate intake is used when there is insufficient scientific evidence derived from approximations of intakes in groups or a group of possibly healthy people (NHMRC 2014). It is at best a guide, not a therapeutic dose, and will not suffice where frank deficiency is observed.

- Men > 18 years: 10 mg/day alpha-tocopherol.
- Women > 18 years: 7 mg/day alpha-tocopherol.
- Upper level of intake: 300 mg/day alpha-tocopherol.
- Deficiency treatment: 800–1200 mg/day.

According to clinical studies

Both natural and synthetic forms of vitamin E have been evaluated in clinical trials at different doses and durations, and sometimes in combination with other nutrients that also exhibit antioxidant properties. Unless stated, dosages are for natural vitamin E (alpha-tocopherol).

- Alzheimer's disease: 2000 IU/day synthetic alpha-tocopherol.
- Anaemia in HD: 500 mg/day.
- Angina pectoris: 50–300 mg/day.
- Antioxidant effects: 400 IU/day.
- Cancer, to reduce cisplatin-induced neurotoxicity: oral vitamin E (600 mg/day) during chemotherapy and for 3 months after its cessation.
- Cerebral infarction prevention: 50 mg/day synthetic vitamin E.
- Colorectal cancer prevention: 50 mg/day long-term.
- CVD: primary prevention: 100–260 IU/day long-term (benefits uncertain with supplementation).
- CVD: secondary prevention: 100–800 IU/day long-term (benefits most likely in people with low baseline vitamin E and higher oxidative stress, e.g. people on haemodialysis and diabetics).
- Carotid atherosclerosis, slowing progression: 136 IU twice daily and vitamin C 250 mg (slow-release) twice daily.
- Dementia prevention: 400 IU/day alpha-tocopherol plus vitamin C 500 mg/day.
- HD, associated cramps: 400 mg/day alpha-tocopherol plus vitamin C 250 mg/day.
- Hypertension: 200 IU/day long-term.
- Immune system support in the elderly: 200 mg/day.
- Intermittent claudication: 600–1600 IU/day.
- Ischaemic stroke prevention in high-risk hypertension: 50 mg/day.
- Male infertility: 200–800 mg/day.
- Menopausal symptoms: 800 IU/day.
- Nitrate tolerance prevention: 200 mg three times daily.
- OA: 1200 IU/day.
- Ovarian cancer: >75 mg/day.
- Premenstrual symptoms: 400–600 IU/day.
- Prostate cancer prevention: 50 mg/day (200 mg detrimental).
- Retinopathy of prematurity: 100 mg/kg/day.
- RA: 1200 IU/day.

- Sunburn protection: 1000 IU/day up to 2000 mg/day plus vitamin C 2000–3000 mg/day.

TOXICITY

Vitamin E is relatively non-toxic. It is not stored as readily in the body as other fat-soluble vitamins and up to 60–70% of a daily dose is excreted in the faeces. Doses as high as 3200 mg/day have been used for 12 years with few adverse effects (Fariss & Zhang 2003).

In April 2000, the Food and Nutrition Board of the Institute of Medicine in the United States set an upper tolerable limit of 1500 IU of RRR-alpha-tocopherol as the highest dose unlikely to result in haemorrhage in most adults.

ADVERSE REACTIONS

Adverse effects are dose-related and tend to occur only at very high supplemental doses (>1200 IU/day); they include diarrhoea, flatulence, nausea and heart palpitations. Doses above this level should be used only under professional supervision.

SIGNIFICANT INTERACTIONS

Considering vitamin E is a fat-soluble vitamin, any medication that reduces the absorption of fats in the diet will also reduce the absorption of vitamin E. These include cholestyramine, colestipol, isoniazid, mineral oil, orlistat and sucralfate.

Oral contraceptive pill

A very small cross-sectional study suggests the oral contraceptive pill significantly lowered coenzyme Q10, and alpha-tocopherol levels. Further studies are needed (Palan et al 2006).

HMG-CoA reductase inhibitors (statins)

The effect of statins on lowering blood lipid levels of vitamin E has been suggested as a risk factor in the development of statin-associated myopathy. Further studies are warranted (Galli et al 2010).

Chloroquine

According to in vitro research, vitamin E inhibits drug uptake in human cultured fibroblasts. The clinical significance of this observation is unknown. Observe patients taking this combination (Scuntaro et al 1996).

Chlorpromazine

According to in vitro research, vitamin E inhibits drug uptake in human cultured fibroblasts. The clinical significance of this observation is unknown — observe patients taking this combination (Scuntaro et al 1996).

Cisplatin

A review of four clinical trials testing the effects of the combination of vitamin E with cisplatin has shown that in all trials the incidence of chemotherapy-induced peripheral neuropathy was significantly reduced (Wolf et al 2008). Beneficial interaction, but should be used under professional supervision.

Warfarin

Contradictory results have been obtained in clinical studies that have investigated whether vitamin E affects platelet aggregation or coagulation. A dose of

1200 IU/day (800 mg of D-alpha-tocopherol) taken for 28 days had no effect on platelet aggregation or coagulation according to one clinical study (Morinobu et al 2002). Similarly, a second clinical study found that a lower dose of 600 mg (900 IU) of RRR-alpha-tocopherol taken daily for 12 weeks did not alter coagulation activity (Kitagawa & Mino 1989). In contrast, increased risk of gingival bleeding at doses of 50 mg/day was found by another study (Liede et al 1998).

Overall, it appears that people with reduced levels of vitamin K may be more susceptible to the effects of vitamin E, potentiating warfarin activity. Until further research can clarify whether the interaction is clinically significant for most people, it is recommended that prothrombin time ratio, or international normalised ratio, should be closely monitored upon the addition and withdrawal of treatment with high-dose vitamin E supplements.

Doxorubicin

One study found that oral DL-alpha-tocopherol acetate (1600 IU/day) prevented doxorubicin-induced alopecia (Wood 1985). The same dose of oral DL-alpha-tocopherol acetate failed to prevent alopecia after doxorubicin treatment following mastectomy for breast cancer (Martin-Jimenez et al 1986). It also failed to prevent alopecia in a second study of 20 patients with different types of solid tumours (Perez et al 1986). Possible beneficial interaction but difficult to assess.

Nitrates

Oral vitamin E prevented nitrate tolerance when given concurrently with transdermal nitroglycerin (10 mg/24 hours), according to one randomised placebo-controlled study (Watanabe et al 1997). Beneficial interaction possible.

NSAIDs and simple analgesics

Vitamin E may enhance the pain-modifying activity of drugs. Beneficial interaction possible; drug dosage may require modification.

Propranolol

According to in vitro research, vitamin E inhibits drug uptake in human cultured fibroblasts. The clinical significance of this observation is unknown. Observe patients taking this combination (Scuntaro et al 1996).

Practice points/Patient counselling

- Vitamin E is actually a generic term used to describe any chemical entity that displays the biological activity of RRR-alpha-tocopherol, the most abundant form found in nature. The 'natural' form is the most potent of all eight forms of vitamin E, although there is evidence that other tocopherols also exhibit significant beneficial effects.
- It is involved in myriad biochemical processes such as immunocompetence and neurological function, but its most important biological function is that of an antioxidant.
- Vitamin E is used for many different indications. There is evidence to suggest that supplementation may be useful in:
  - secondary CVD prevention, although effects are inconsistent
  - slowing down progression of AD, although effects are inconsistent
  - enhancing immune function in the elderly•preventing anaemia and treating cramps in patients on HD
  - reducing PMS, dysmenorrhoea and menopause symptoms

- reducing pain in OA and RA
- improving some forms of male infertility
- reducing risk of stage 3+ retinopathy in premature babies
- preventing ischaemic stroke in high-risk hypertensive patients
- reducing incidence of some cancers, although effects are inconsistent
- preventing sunburn (when used with vitamin C)
- slowing down carotid atherosclerosis (when used with vitamin C)
- reducing blood pressure
- reducing nitrate tolerance
- reducing cisplatin-induced neurotoxicity.

- Oral supplements have been used to prevent or treat many other conditions, such as exercise-induced tissue damage, some types of senile cataracts, epilepsy and fibromyalgia.
- It is a popular ingredient in many moisturising preparations used to: alleviate dry and cracked skin; assist in the repair of abrasions, burns, grazes and skin lesions; prevent stretch marks; and diminish scar tissue. Vitamin E oil is used as a stand-alone preparation or incorporated into a cream or ointment base for these purposes.
- People with impaired coagulation, inherited bleeding disorders, a history of haemorrhagic stroke or vitamin K deficiency, or who are at risk of pulmonary embolism or thrombophlebitis should use high-dose supplements under medical supervision.

CONTRAINDICATIONS AND PRECAUTIONS

Vitamin E is considered to be a safe substance.

People with impaired coagulation, inherited bleeding disorders, a history of haemorrhagic stroke, vitamin K deficiency or at risk of pulmonary embolism or thrombophlebitis should use high-dose supplements under medical supervision.

Although it was thought that people with hypertension wanting to take supplements should start with low doses, evidence does not support the concern that high-dose supplements will significantly elevate blood pressure. Suspend use of high doses (>1000 IU/day) 1 week before major surgery.

PREGNANCY USE

Vitamin E is considered to be safe in pregnancy.

PATIENTS' FAQs

What will this vitamin do for me?

Vitamin E is essential for health and wellbeing. It is involved in many important biological processes in the body and may prevent serious diseases such as heart disease and some cancers; however, people with these conditions should seek professional advice. It is also used to reduce symptoms in common conditions such as arthritis, PMS and menopause. Vitamin E supplements enhance immune function in the elderly and may slow the progression of AD. Oral supplements have been used to prevent or treat many other conditions, such as exercise-induced tissue damage, some types of senile cataracts, epilepsy and fibromyalgia.

When will it start to work?

This depends largely on the reason for taking the supplement. In the case of disease prevention, studies suggest that long-term use is necessary (i.e. 2–3 years or longer). When using vitamin E to reduce symptoms, effects have generally been seen within 3 months.

Are there any safety issues?

People with impaired coagulation, inherited bleeding disorders, a history of haemorrhagic stroke or vitamin K deficiency, or who are at risk of pulmonary embolism or thrombophlebitis should use high-dose supplements under medical supervision. Additionally, vitamin E can interact with some medicines, so professional advice is recommended when using high-dose supplements.

REFERENCES

ABS 2005 Mortality and Morbidity: Colorectal Cancer. [Online] http://www.abs.gov.au/AUSSTATS/abs@.nsf/94713ad445ff1425ca25682000192af2/89be997ee1e35bd6ca25703b0080ccbd!OpenDocument [Accessed 10th may 2014].

Albanes D et al. Effects of supplemental alpha-tocopherol and beta-carotene on colorectal cancer: results from a controlled trial (Finland). Cancer Causes Control 11.3 (2000): 197–205.

Albert CM et al. Moderate alcohol consumption and the risk of sudden cardiac death among US male physicians. Circulation 100.9 (1999): 944–950.

Arad YLA, et al 2005. Treatment of asymptomatic adults with elevated coronary calcium scores with atorvastin, vitamin C, and vitamin E: the St Francis Heart Study randomized clinical trial. J Am Coll Cardiol 46: 166–172.

Arain MA, Qadeer A, 2010. Systematic review on 'vitamin E and prevention of colorectal cancer'. Pak J Pharm Sci 23;2:125–30.

Argyriou AA, et al. 2005. Vitamin E for prophylaxis against chemotherapy induced neuropathy: a randomized controlled trial. Neurology 64:26–31.

Assem, YM, (2011) Impact of pentoxifylline and vitamin E on Ribavirin-induced haemolytic anaemia in chronic hepatitis C patients: an Egyptian survey. Int J Hepatol: 530949.

Azen SP et al. Effect of supplementary antioxidant vitamin intake on carotid arterial wall intima-media thickness in a controlled clinical trial of cholesterol lowering. Circulation 94.10 (1996): 2369–2372.

Badiou S et al. Vitamin E supplementation increases LDL resistance to ex vivo oxidation in hemodialysis patients. Int J Vitam Nutr Res 73.4 (2003): 290–296.

Bartels M et al. Pilot study on the effect of parenteral vitamin E on ischemia and reperfusion induced liver injury: A double blind, randomized, placebo-controlled trial. Clin Nutr 23.6 (2004): 1360–1370.

Baumann LS, Spencer J. The effects of topical vitamin E on the cosmetic appearance of scars. Dermatol Surg 25.4 (1999): 311–3115.

Bender DA, 2003. Nutritional biochemistry of vitamins. 2nd edn. University College of London. Cambridge University Press.

Berry D, et al. Bayesian model averaging in meta-analysis: Vitamin E supplementation and mortality. Clin Trials 6.1 (2009): 28–41.

Bhardwaj A et al. Status of vitamin E and reduced glutathione in semen of oligozoospermic and azoospermic patients. Asian J Androl 2.3 (2000): 225–228.

Bjelakovic G et al. Mortality in randomized trials of antioxidant supplements for primary and secondary prevention: Systematic review and meta-analysis. JAMA 297.8 (2007): 842–857.

Bjelakovic G, et al 2013. Meta-regression analyses, meta-analyses, and trial sequential analyses of the effects of supplementation with beta-carotene, vitamin A and vitamin E singly or in different combinations on all-cause mortality: do we have evidence for lack of harm? PLOS ONE 8:9 e74558

Blaner WS, 2013. Vitamin E: the enigmatic one! Journal of Lipid Research, 54:2293–2294.

Blankenhorn G. Clinical effectiveness of Spondyvit (vitamin E) in activated arthroses. A multicenter placebo-controlled double-blind study. Z Orthop Ihre Grenzgeb 124.3 (1986): 340–343.

Blot WJ et al. The Linxian trials: Mortality rates by vitamin-mineral intervention group. Am J Clin Nutr 62.6 (Suppl) (1995): 1424S–6S.

Boaz M et al. Secondary Prevention with Antioxidants of Cardiovascular disease in Endstage renal disease (SPACE): randomised placebo-controlled trial. Lancet 356.9237 (2000): 1213–1218.

Bolle P et al. The controversial efficacy of vitamin E for human male infertility. Contraception 65.4 (2002): 313–315.

Bonner LT, Peskind ER. Pharmacologic treatments of dementia. Med Clin North Am 86.3 (2002): 657–674.

Boshtam M et al. Vitamin E can reduce blood pressure in mild hypertensives. Int J Vitam Nutr Res 72.5 (2002): 309–314.

Bove L et al. A pilot study on the relation between cisplatin neuropathy and vitamin E. J Exp Clin Cancer Res 20.2 (2001): 277–280.

Brack m, et al 2013. Distinct profiles of systemic biomarkers of oxidative stress in chronic human pathologies: Cardiovascular, psychiatric, neurodegenerative, rheumatic, infectious, neoplasmic and endogrinological diseases. Advances in Bioscience and Biotechnology, 2013, 4, 331–339.

Brand C et al. Vitamin E is ineffective for symptomatic relief of knee osteoarthritis: A six month double blind, randomised, placebo controlled study. Ann Rheum Dis 60.10 (2001): 946–949.

Brass EP, 2013. Intermittent Claudication: New targets for drug development. Drugs 73:999–1014.
Brigelius-Flohe R. Vitamin E: the shrew waiting to be tamed. Free Radic Biol Med 46.5 (2009): 543–554.
Brockes C et al. Vitamin E prevents extensive lipid peroxidation in patients with hypertension. Br J Biomed Sci 60.1 (2003): 5–8.
Canter PH, et al The antioxidant vitamins A, C, E and selenium in the treatment of arthritis: a systematic review of randomized clinical trials. Rheumatology (Oxford) 46.8 (2007): 1223–33.
Cerhan JR, et al 2003. Antioxidant micronutrients and risk of rheumatoid arthritis in a cohort of older women. Am J Epidemiol. 157(4):345–54.
Chamras H, et al 2005. Novel interactions of vitamin E and estrogen in breast cancer. Nutr Cancer 52:1;43–48.
Che Anishas C, et al 2014. Oil palm phenolics and vitamin E reduce atherosclerosis in rabbits, Journal of Functional Foods, 7; 550: 1756–4646.
Chen H et al. Mixed tocopherol preparation is superior to alpha-tocopherol alone against hypoxia-reoxygenation injury. Biochem Biophys Res Commun 291.2 (2002): 349–353.
Cherubini A et al. Vitamin E levels, cognitive impairment and dementia in older persons: the InCHIANTI study. Neurobiol Aging 26.7 (2005): 987–994.
Christen WG, et al 2012. Vitamins E and C and medical record confirmed age related macular degeneration in a randomized trial of male physicians. Ophthalmology 119:8;1642–1649.
Clarke R, Armitage J. Antioxidant vitamins and risk of cardiovascular disease. Review of large-scale randomised trials. Cardiovasc Drugs Ther 16.5 (2002): 411–415.
Collins EG et al. Pole striding exercise and vitamin E for management of peripheral vascular disease. Med Sci Sports Exerc 35.3 (2003): 384–393.
Colombo ML, 2010. An update on vitamin E, tocopherol and tocotrienol perspectives. Molecules, 15: 2103–2113.
Cook NR et al. A randomized factorial trial of vitamins C and E and beta carotene in the secondary prevention of cardiovascular events in women: Results from the Women's Antioxidant Cardiovascular Study. Arch Intern Med 167.15 (2007): 1610–1618.
Coon JT, Ernst E. Complementary and alternative therapies in the treatment of chronic hepatitis C: A systematic review. J Hepatol 40.3 (2004): 491–500.
Cristol JP et al. Erythropoietin and oxidative stress in haemodialysis: Beneficial effects of vitamin E supplementation. Nephrol Dial Transplant 12.11 (1997): 2312–23117.
De Gaetano G. Low-dose aspirin and vitamin E in people at cardiovascular risk: A randomised trial in general practice: Collaborative Group of the Primary Prevention Project. Lancet 357.9250 (2001): 89–95.
DeMaio SJ et al. Vitamin E supplementation, plasma lipids and incidence of restenosis after percutaneous transluminal coronary angioplasty (PTCA). J Am Coll Nutr 11.1 (1992): 68–73.
Devereux G, Seaton A. Diet as a risk factor for atopy and asthma. J Allergy Clin Immunol 115.6 (2005): 1109–1117.
De Vita VT, et al (eds). Cancer: principles and practice in oncology, 7th edn. Philadelphia: Lippincott, Williams and Wilkins, 2005
Diepeveen SH et al. Effects of atorvastatin and vitamin E on lipoproteins and oxidative stress in dialysis patients: a randomised-controlled trial. J Intern Med 257.5 (2005): 438–445.
Dietrich M et al. Vitamin E supplement use and the incidence of cardiovascular disease and all-cause mortality in the Framingham Heart Study: Does the underlying health status play a role? Atherosclerosis 205.2 (2009): 549–553.
Dunford M, Doyle J, 2012. Nutrition for sport and exercise, 3rd edn. Cengage learning.
Dysken, M.W., et al 2014. Effect of vitamin E and memantine on functional decline in Alzheimer disease: the TEAM-AD VA cooperative randomized trial. JAMA, 311, (1) 33–44.
Eberlein-Konig B et al. Protective effect against sunburn of combined systemic ascorbic acid (vitamin C) and d-[alpha]-tocopherol (vitamin E). J Am Acad Dermatol 38.1 (1998): 45–48.
Edmonds SE et al. Putative analgesic activity of repeated oral doses of vitamin E in the treatment of rheumatoid arthritis: Results of a prospective placebo controlled double blind trial. Ann Rheum Dis 56.11 (1997): 649–655.
Engelhart MJ et al. Dietary intake of antioxidants and risk of Alzheimer disease. JAMA 287.24 (2002): 3223–3229.
Evans, H.M. Invariable occurrence of male sterility with dietaries lacking fat soluble vitamin E. Proc. Natl. Acad. Sci. U.S.A. 1925: 11,373.
Evans J. Antioxidant supplements to prevent or slow down the progression of AMD: a systematic review and meta-analysis. Eye 22.6 (2008): 751–760.
Fahn S. A pilot trial of high-dose alpha-tocopherol and ascorbate in early Parkinson's disease. Ann Neurol 32 (Suppl.) (1992): S128–S132.
Fang JC et al. Effect of vitamins C and E on progression of transplant-associated arteriosclerosis: A randomised trial. Lancet 359.9312 (2002): 1108–1113.
FAO/WHO (Food and Agriculture Organization/World Health Organization). Vitamin E. In: Report of a Joint FAO/WHO Expert Consultation, Bangkok, Thailand. Rome: FAO/WHO, 2002.
Fariss MW, Zhang JG. Vitamin E therapy in Parkinson's disease. Toxicology 189.1–2 (2003): 129–146.
Fleischauer AT et al. Dietary antioxidants, supplements, and risk of epithelial ovarian cancer. Nutr Cancer 40.2 (2001): 92–98.
Fleischauer AT et al. Antioxidant supplements and risk of breast cancer recurrence and breast cancer-related mortality among postmenopausal women. Nutr Cancer 46.1 (2003): 15–22.
Fuchs J, Kern H. Modulation of UV-light-induced skin inflammation by d-alpha-tocopherol and l-ascorbic acid: A clinical study using solar simulated radiation. Free Radic Biol Med 25.9 (1998): 1006–1012.
Galli F et al. Vitamin E, lipid profile, and peroxidation in hemodialysis patients. Kidney Int Suppl 78 (2001): S148–S154.
Galli, F., et al. 2010. Do statins cause myopathy by lowering vitamin E levels? Med Hypotheses. 74(4):707 709.
Gerss J, Kopcke W. The questionable association of vitamin E supplementation and mortality — inconsistent results of different meta-analytic approaches. Cell Mol Biol 55 Suppl (2009): OL1111–20.

Geva E et al. The effect of antioxidant treatment on human spermatozoa and fertilization rate in an in vitro fertilization program. Fertil Steril 66.3 (1996): 430–434.

Giray B et al. The effect of vitamin E supplementation on antioxidant enzyme activities and lipid peroxidation levels in hemodialysis patients. Clin Chim Acta 338.1–2 (2003): 91–98.

GISSI. Dietary supplementation with n-3 polyunsaturated fatty acids and vitamin E after myocardial infarction: results of the GISSI-Prevenzione trial (Gruppo Italiano per lo Studio della Sopravvivenza nell'Infarto miocardico). Lancet 354.9177 (1999): 447–455.

Gong, Z, et al 2010. Intake of fatty acids and antioxidants and pancreatic cancer in a large population-based case-control study in the San Francisco Bay area. Int J Cancer. 127(8):1893–1904

Gupta S, et al 2011. Vitamin E supplementation may ameliorate oxidative stress in type 1 diabetes mellitus patients. Clin. Lab,Vol.57, No.5–6, pp.379–386

Haflah HM, et al 2009. Effects of palm vitamin E on osteoarthritis. Saudi Med 30:11; 1432–1437

Hartman TJ et al. Effects of long-term alpha-tocopherol supplementation on serum hormones in older men. Prostate 46.1 (2001): 33–38.

Heinecke JW. Oxidized amino acids: culprits in human atherosclerosis and indicators of oxidative stress. Free Radic Biol Med 32.11 (2002): 1090–1101.

Heinecke JW. Oxidative stress: new approaches to diagnosis and prognosis in atherosclerosis. Am J Cardiol 91.3A (2003): 12–16A.

Heinonen OP et al. Prostate cancer and supplementation with alpha-tocopherol and beta-carotene: incidence and mortality in a controlled trial. J Natl Cancer Inst 90.6 (1998): 440–446.

Hemilä H, 2013. Vitamin E may significantly increase and decrease mortality in some population groups [Comment]. PloS One, vol 8, e74558.

Hemila H, Kaprio J, 2008. Vitamin E supplementation and pneumonia risk in males who initiated smoking at an early age: effect modification by body weight and dietary vitamin C. Nutr J 7:33.

Hemila H et al. The effect of vitamin E on common cold incidence is modified by age, smoking and residential neighborhood. J Am Coll Nutr 25.4 (2006): 332–339.

Hernandez, L. M., et al. 2004. 95th Annual Meeting of the American Association for Cancer Research. Orlando, Florida, USA. March 27–31.

Hodis HN et al. Alpha-tocopherol supplementation in healthy individuals reduces low-density lipoprotein oxidation but not atherosclerosis: The Vitamin E Atherosclerosis Prevention Study (VEAPS). Circulation 106.12 (2002): 1453–1459.

Iino K et al. A controlled, double-blind study of dl-alpha-tocopheryl nicotinate (Juvela-Nicotinate) for treatment of symptoms in hypertension and cerebral arteriosclerosis. Jpn Heart J 18.3 (1977): 277–286.

Illison, V. K, et al 2011. The Relationship between plasma alpha-tocopherol concentration and vitamin E intake in patients with type 2 diabetes mellitus. Int J Vitam Nutr Res. 81(1):12–20.

Imounan F, et al 2012. Vitamin E in ataxia and neurodegenerative diseases: A review. World Journal of Neuroscience, 2;217–222.

Institute of Medicine, 2000. Food and Nutrition Board. Dietary Reference Intakes: Vitamin C, Vitamin E, Selenium, and Carotenoids. Washington, DC: National Academy Press.

Jacobs, E J, et al. 2002. Vitamin C and vitamin E supplement use and bladder cancer mortality in a large cohort of US men and women. American Journal of Epidemiology. 156(11):1002–1010.

Jain SK et al. Effect of modest vitamin E supplementation on blood glycated hemoglobin and triglyceride levels and red cell indices in type I diabetic patients. J Am Coll Nutr 15.5 (1996): 458–461.

Jaxa-Chamiec T et al. Antioxidant effects of combined vitamins C and E in acute myocardial infarction: The randomized, double-blind, placebo-controlled, multicenter pilot Myocardial Infarction and VITamins (MIVIT) trial. Kardiol Pol 62.4 (2005): 344–350.

Jeong, N. H, et al., 2009. Plasma carotenoids, retinol and tocopherol levels and the risk of ovarian cancer. Acta Obstet Gynecol Scand. 88(4):457–462.

Jialal I, Devaraj S. Scientific evidence to support a vitamin E and heart disease health claim: research needs. J Nutr 135.2 (2005a): 348–53.

Jialal I, Devaraj S. High-dosage vitamin E supplementation and all-cause mortality. Ann Intern Med 143.2 (2005b): 155.

Karlson EW, et al 2008. Vitamin E in the Primary prevention of Rheumatoid Arthritis: The Women's Health Study. Arthritis Rhuem.59:11;1189–1595

Kataja-Tuomola MJ, et al 2010. Effects of alpha-tocopherol and beta carotene supplementation on macrovascular complications and total mortality from diabetes: Results of the ATBC Study. 42 ;3: 178–186.

Katsiki N, Manes C. Is there a role for supplemented antioxidants in the prevention of atherosclerosis? Clinical Nutrition 28.1 (2009): 3–9.

Kaul N et al. Alpha-tocopherol and atherosclerosis. Exp Biol Med 226.1 (2001): 5–12.

Kessopoulou E et al. A double-blind randomized placebo cross-over controlled trial using the antioxidant vitamin E to treat reactive oxygen species associated male infertility. Fertil Steril 64.4 (1995): 825–831.

Khajehdehi P et al. A randomized, double-blind, placebo-controlled trial of supplementary vitamins E, C and their combination for treatment of haemodialysis cramps. Nephrol Dial Transplant 16.7 (2001): 1448–1451.

Kitagawa M, Mino M. Effects of elevated d-alpha(RRR)-tocopherol dosage in man. J Nutr Sci Vitaminol (Tokyo) 35.2 (1989): 133–42.

Kleijnen J, Mackerras D. Vitamin E for intermittent claudication. Cochrane Database Syst Rev 2 (2000): CD000987.

Klemenska E, Beresewicz A, 2009. Bioactivation of organic nitrates and the mechanism of nitrate tolerance. Cardiology Journal 16;1: 11–19

Kobori Y, et al 2014. Antioxidant cosupplementation therapy with vitamin C, vitamin E, and coenzyme Q10 in patients with oligoasthenozoospermia. Arch Ital Urol Andol 86;1

Kusama Y, et al 2011. Review: Variant angina and coronary artery spasm: The clinical spectrum, pathophysiology and management. J Nippon Med Sch;78:1.
Lee IM et al. Vitamin E in the primary prevention of cardiovascular disease and cancer: The Women's Health Study: a randomized controlled trial. ACC Curr J Rev 14.10 (2005): 10–111.
Leonard, SW, et al 2004. Vitamin E bioavailability from fortified breakfast cereal is greater than that from encapsulated supplements. The American Journal of Clinical Nutrition, 79:1, 86–92.
Leppala JM et al. Vitamin E and beta carotene supplementation in high risk for stroke: a subgroup analysis of the Alpha-Tocopherol, Beta-Carotene Cancer Prevention Study. Arch Neurol 57.10 (2000): 1503–1509.
Liang, D, et al 2008. Plasma vitamins E and A and risk of bladder cancer: a case-control analysis. Cancer Causes Control. 19:98
Liede KE et al. Increased tendency towards gingival bleeding caused by joint effect of alpha-tocopherol supplementation and acetylsalicylic acid. Ann Med 30.6 (1998): 542–546.
Lin JY et al. UV photoprotection by combination topical antioxidants vitamin C and vitamin E. J Am Acad Dermatol 48.6 (2003): 866–874.
Lin FH et al. Ferulic acid stabilizes a solution of vitamins C and E and doubles its photoprotection of skin. J Invest Dermatol 125.4 (2005): 826–832.
Linus Pauling Institute. Research newsletter – Spring/Summer 2008: 'Fatally Flawed' clinical trials of vitamin E. Oregan State University. [Online] http://lpi.oregonstate.edu/ss08/itamin.html [Accessed 2nd May 2014].
London RS et al. Evaluation and treatment of breast symptoms in patients with the premenstrual syndrome. J Reprod Med 28.8 (1983): 503–508.
London RS et al. Efficacy of alpha-tocopherol in the treatment of the premenstrual syndrome. J Reprod Med 32.6 (1987): 400–404.
Lonn E et al. Effects of vitamin E on cardiovascular and microvascular outcomes in high-risk patients with diabetes: results of the HOPE study and MICRO-HOPE substudy. Diabetes Care 25.11 (2002): 1919–1927.
Lonn E et al. Effects of long-term vitamin E supplementation on cardiovascular events and cancer: a randomized controlled trial. JAMA 293.11 (2005): 1338–1347.
Luchsinger JA et al. Antioxidant vitamin intake and risk of Alzheimer disease. Arch Neurol 60.2 (2003): 203–208.
Lynch SM, et al 2012. Abstract 13: Teleomere length and pancreatic cancer in the alpha-topherol beta carotene cancer prevention (ATBC) study. Cancer Epidemiol Biomarkers Prev. 21; 13.
Machtey I, Ouaknine L. Tocopherol in osteoarthritis: a controlled pilot study. J Am Geriatr Soc 26.7 (1978): 328–330.
Mahyar E, et al 2005. Intake of vitamin E, vitamin C and carotenoids and the risk of Parkinson's disease: A meta-analysis. The Lancet Neurology 4.6:362–5
Mandana Z, et al 2013. Evaluation the effect of vitamin E on treatment of premenstrual syndrome: A clinical randomized trial. Research and Reviews: Journal of Medical and Health Sciences 2:4.
Marchioli R et al. Vitamin E increases the risk of developing heart failure after myocardial infarction: Results from the GISSI-Prevenzione trial. J Cardiovasc Med (Hagerstown) 7.5 (2006): 347–350.
Martin-Jimenez M et al. Failure of high-dose tocopherol to prevent alopecia induced by doxorubicin. N Engl J Med 315.14 (1986): 894–895.
Masaki KH et al. Association of vitamin E and C supplement use with cognitive function and dementia in elderly men. Neurology 54.6 (2000): 1265–1272.
Masatomi Sasaki MS 2006. Development of vitamin E modified polysulfone membrane dialyzers. J Artif Organs 9:50–60.
McAnally, J.A, et al 2007. Tocotrienols potentiate lovastatin- mediated growth suppression in vitro and in vivo. Exp. Biol. Med. 232: 523–531
McDowell LR. (2000) Vitamins in animal and human nutrition. 2nd edn. Ames: Iowa State University Press, p156.
McFarlane GJ et al., 2010. Evidence for the efficacy of complementary and alternative medicines in the management of rheumatoid arthritis: systematic review. Rheumatology 50:9;1672–1683.
McVean M, Liebler DC. Inhibition of UVB induced DNA photodamage in mouse epidermis by topically applied alpha-tocopherol. Carcinogenesis 18.8 (1997): 1617–1622.
McVean M, Liebler DC. Prevention of DNA photodamage by vitamin E compounds and sunscreens: roles of ultraviolet absorbance and cellular uptake. Mol Carcinog 24.3 (1999): 169–176.
Meagher EA. Treatment of atherosclerosis in the new millennium: is there a role for vitamin E? Prev Cardiol 6.2 (2003): 85–90.
Meydani M. Vitamin E. Lancet 345.8943 (1995): 170–175.
Meydani M, Hayes KC. (2003) Vitamin E. Available online at: http.jn.nutrition.org (accessed 02-06-03).
Meydani SN et al. Vitamin E supplementation and in vivo immune response in healthy elderly subjects. A randomized controlled trial. JAMA 277.17 (1997): 1380–1386.
Meydani SN et al. Antioxidant modulation of cytokines and their biologic function in the aged. Z Ernahrungswiss 37 (Suppl 1) (1998): 35–42.
Miller ER III et al. Meta-analysis: high-dosage vitamin E supplementation may increase all-cause mortality. Ann Intern Med 142.1 (2005): 37–46.
Minamiyama Y et al. Vitamin E deficiency accelerates nitrate tolerance via a decrease in cardiac P450 expression and increased oxidative stress. Free Radic Biol Med 40.5 (2006): 808–816.
Mireles-Rocha H et al. UVB photoprotection with antioxidants: Effects of oral therapy with d-alpha-tocopherol and ascorbic acid on the minimal erythema dose. Acta Derm Venereol 82.1 (2002): 21–24.
Mittal M, et al 2014. Reactive oxygen species in inflammation and tissue injury. Antioxid Redox. Signal. 20(7): 1126–1167.
Miwa K et al. Vitamin E deficiency in variant angina. Circulation 94.1 (1996): 14–118.
Miwa K et al. Consumption of vitamin E in coronary circulation in patients with variant angina. Cardiovasc Res 41.1 (1999): 291–298.

Morinobu T et al. The safety of high-dose vitamin E supplementation in healthy Japanese male adults. J Nutr Sci Vitaminol (Tokyo) 48.1 (2002): 6–9.

Morris MC et al. Relation of the tocopherol forms to incident Alzheimer disease and to cognitive change. Am J Clin Nutr 81.2 (2005): 508–514.

Morris, M.C., et al 2014. Brain tocopherols related to Alzheimer's disease neuropathology in humans. Alzheimers Dement. doi: 10.1016/j.jalz.2013.12.015.

Moslemi, M. K, Tavanbakhsh S, 2011. Selenium-vitamin E supplementation in infertile men: effects on semen parameters and pregnancy rate. Int J Gen Med. 4:99–104.

Mukherjee S, and Mitra A, 2009. Health effects of palm oil. J Human Ecol 26:3: 197–203

Munteanu A et al. Anti-atherosclerotic effects of vitamin E: myth or reality? J Cell Mol Med 8.1 (2004): 59–76.

Nanyakkara PW et al. Effect of a treatment strategy consisting of pravastatin, vitamin E, and homocysteine lowering on carotid intima-media thickness, endothelial function and renal function in patients with mild to moderate chronic kidney disease: results from the Anti-odixant Therapy in Chronic Renal Insufficiency (ATIC) study. Arch Intern Med 167: 1262–1270.

National Cancer Institute (NIH) 2014 Selenium and Vitamin E Cancer Prevention Trial (SELECT). http://www.cancer.gov/newscenter/qa/2008/selectqa

NHMRC Nutrient Reference Values for Australia and New Zealand. Vitamin E Background. http://www.nrv.gov.au/nutrients/vitamin-e [Accessed 1st May 2014].

NIH (2013): Office of Dietary Supplements [Online], Vitamin E: Fact Sheet for Health Professionals. http://ods.od.nih.gov/factsheets/VitaminE-HealthProfessional/.[Accessed 06 May 14].

NUTTAB. 2010. Database Online. [Online] Available at: http://www.foodstandards.gov.au/science/monitoringnutrients/nutrientables/nuttab/Pages/default.aspx. [Accessed 06 May 14].

O'Donnell ME et al. The effects of cilostazol on exercise-induced ischaemia-reperfusion injury in patients with peripheral arterial disease. Eur J Vasc Endovasc Surg 37.3 (2009): 326–335.

Orbe J et al. Antioxidant vitamins increase the collagen content and reduce MMP-1 in a porcine model of atherosclerosis: Implications for plaque stabilization. Atherosclerosis 167.1 (2003): 45–53.

Packer L (2002), Handbook of antioxidants. Marcel Dekker Inc [Online]. NY 1016 Available at: http://lpi.oregonstate.edu/infocenter/vitamins/vitaminE/. [Accessed 07 May 14].

Palan, P. R., et al. 2006. Effects of menstrual cycle and oral contraceptive use on serum levels of lipid-soluble antioxidants. Am J Obstet Gynecol. 194(5):35–38.

Palmieri B et al. Vitamin E added silicone gel sheets for treatment of hypertrophic scars and keloids. Int J Dermatol 34.7 (1995): 506–509.

Parkinson Study Group. Impact of deprenyl and tocopherol treatment on Parkinson's disease in DATATOP patients requiring levodopa: Parkinson Study Group. Ann Neurol 39.1 (1996): 37–45.

Parkinson Study Group. Mortality in DATATOP: A multicenter trial in early Parkinson's disease. Parkinson Study Group. Ann Neurol 43.3 (1998): 318–325.

Parkinson Study Group. MRC/BHF Heart Protection Study of antioxidant vitamin supplementation in 20,536 high-risk individuals: A randomised placebo-controlled trial. Lancet 360.9326 (2002): 23–33.

Pearson PJK et al. Vitamin E supplements in asthma: A parallel group randomised placebo controlled trial. Thorax 59.8 (2004): 652–656.

Perez JE et al. High-dose alpha-tocopherol as a preventive of doxorubicin-induced alopecia. Cancer Treat Rep 70.10 (1986): 1213–12114.

Petersen RC et al. Vitamin E and donepezil for the treatment of mild cognitive impairment. N Engl J Med 352.23 (2005): 2379–2388.

Posadzki P, et al 2013. Dietary supplements and prostate cancer: a systematic review of double-blind, placebo-controlled randomised clinical trials, Maturitas, 75;2: 125–130.

Raju TN et al. Vitamin E prophylaxis to reduce retinopathy of prematurity: a reappraisal of published trials. J Pediatr 131.6 (1997): 844–850.

Rapola JM et al. Effect of vitamin E and beta carotene on the incidence of angina pectoris: A randomized, double-blind, controlled trial. JAMA 275.9 (1996): 693–698.

Rapola JM et al. Randomised trial of alpha-tocopherol and beta-carotene supplements on incidence of major coronary events in men with previous myocardial infarction. Lancet 349.9067 (1997): 1715–1720.

Ricciarelli R et al. Vitamin E and neurodegenerative diseases. Mol Aspects Med 28.5–6 (2007): 591–606.

Rimbach G, et al 2010. Gene regulatory activity of a- tocopherol. Molecules 2010, 15, 1746–1761.

Rimm EB et al. Vitamin E consumption and the risk of coronary heart disease in men. N Engl J Med 328.20 (1993): 1450–1456.

Rizvi S, et al 2014. The Role of Vitamin E in Human Health and Some Diseases. Sultan Qaboos Univ Med J. 14(2): e157–e165.

Roehm E, 2009. The evidence based Mediterranean diet reduces coronary heart disease risk, and plant derived monounsaturated fats may reduce coronary heart disease risk. Am J Clin Nutr 90:3:697–698.

Rolf C et al. Antioxidant treatment of patients with asthenozoospermia or moderate oligoasthenozoospermia with high-dose vitamin C and vitamin E: A randomized, placebo-controlled, double-blind study. Hum Reprod 14.4 (1999): 1028–1033.

Sackett CS, Schenning S. The age-related eye disease study: the results of the clinical trial. Insight 27.1 (2002): 5–7.

Saldeen K, Saldeen T 2005. Importance of tocopherols beyond alpha tocopherol: evidence from animal and human studies. Nutrition Research. 2005: 25; 877–889.

Salonen RM et al. Six-year effect of combined vitamin C and E supplementation on atherosclerotic progression: the Antioxidant Supplementation in Atherosclerosis Prevention (ASAP) Study. Circulation 107.7 (2003): 947–953.

Sano M et al. A controlled trial of selegiline, alpha-tocopherol, or both as treatment for Alzheimer's disease: The Alzheimer's Disease Cooperative Study. N Engl J Med 336.17 (1997): 1216–1222.

Scherak O, Kolarz G. Vitamin E and rheumatoid arthritis. Arthritis Rheum 34.9 (1991): 1205–1206.

Scuntaro I et al. Inhibition by vitamin E of drug accumulation and of phospholipidosis induced by desipramine and other cationic amphiphilic drugs in human cultured cells. Br J Pharmacol 119.5 (1996): 829–834.

Sen C, Packer L. Thiol homeostasis and supplements in physical exercise. Am J Clin Nutr 72 (s) (2000): 653–69s.

Sesso HD, et al 2008. Vitamins E and C in the prevention of cardiovascular disease in men: the Physician's Health Study 11 randomized controlled trial. JAMA 300: 2123–2133.

Shanafelt TD et al. Pathophysiology and treatment of hot flashes. Mayo Clin Proc 77.11 (2002): 1207–1218.

Shen J et al. Telomere length, oxidative damage, antioxidants and breast cancer risk. Int J Cancer 124.7 (2009): 1637–1643.

Shils M (ed). Modern nutrition in health and disease, 9th edn. Baltimore: Lippincott Williams & Wilkins, 1999.

Singh RB et al. Usefulness of antioxidant vitamins in suspected acute myocardial infarction (the Indian experiment of infarct survival-3). Am J Cardiol 77.4 (1996): 232–236.

Stampfer MJ et al. Vitamin E consumption and the risk of coronary disease in women. N Engl J Med 328.20 (1993): 1444–1449.

Stephens NG et al. Randomised controlled trial of vitamin E in patients with coronary disease: Cambridge Heart Antioxidant Study (CHAOS). Lancet 347.9004 (1996): 781–786.

Stolzenberg-Solomon RZ et al. Vitamin E intake, alpha-tocopherol status, and pancreatic cancer in a cohort of male smokers. Am J Clin Nutr 89.2 (2009): 584–591.

Stone WL, Papas AM. Tocopherols and the etiology of colon cancer. J Natl Cancer Inst 89.14 (1997): 1006–1014.

Suleiman SA et al. Lipid peroxidation and human sperm motility: protective role of vitamin E. J Androl 17.5 (1996): 530–537.

Sung L et al. Vitamin E: the evidence for multiple roles in cancer. Nutr Cancer 46.1 (2003): 1–14.

Takahashi S, et al 2009. Suppression of prostate cancer in a transgenic rat model via gamma-tocopherol activation of caspase signaling. Prostate. 69(6):644–51.

Tardif JC et al. Probucol and multivitamins in the prevention of restenosis after coronary angioplasty. Multivitamins and Probucol Study Group. N Engl J Med 337.6 (1997): 365–372.

Terentis AC et al. Vitamin E oxidation in human atherosclerotic lesions. Circ Res 90.3 (2002): 333–339.

Traber, MG, et al 2006. Vitamin E: Nutrition in Health and Disease. 10th edn. Baltimore, MD: Lippincott Williams & Wilkins.

Ulker S et al. Vitamins reverse endothelial dysfunction through regulation of eNOS and NAD(P)H oxidase activities. Hypertension 41.3 (2003): 534–539.

Vardi M, et al 2013. Vitamin E in the prevention of cardiovascular disease: the importance of proper patient selection. Journal of lipid research 54: 2013.

Vatassery GT. In vitro oxidation of alpha-tocopherol (vitamin E) in human platelets upon incubation with unsaturated fatty acids, diamide and superoxide. Biochim Biophys Acta 926.2 (1987): 160–169.

Virtamo J et al. Effect of vitamin E and beta carotene on the incidence of primary nonfatal myocardial infarction and fatal coronary heart disease. Arch Intern Med 158.6 (1998): 668–675.

Virtamo J et al. Effects of supplemental alpha-tocopherol and beta-carotene on urinary tract cancer: Incidence and mortality in a controlled trial (Finland). Cancer Causes Control 11.10 (2000): 933–939.

Virtamo J et al. Incidence of cancer and mortality following alpha-tocopherol and beta-carotene supplementation: A postintervention follow-up. JAMA 290.4 (2003): 476–485.

Wahlqvist ML (ed). Food and nutrition, 2nd edn. Sydney: Allen & Unwin, 2002.

Watanabe H et al. Randomized, double-blind, placebo controlled study of supplemental vitamin E on attenuation of the development of nitrate tolerance. Circulation 96.8 (1997): 2545–2550.

Waters DD, et al. 2002. Effects of hormone replacement therapy and antioxidant vitamin supplements on coronary atherosclerosis in postmenopausal women: a randomized controlled trial. JAMA. 288: 2432–2440.

Whitney E, et al 2011. A Understanding of Nutrition Australia and New Zealand. 2nd ed. Australia: Cengage Learning.

Wijnen MH et al. Antioxidants reduce oxidative stress in claudicants. J Surg Res 96.2 (2001): 183–187.

Wittenborg A et al. Effectiveness of vitamin E in comparison with diclofenac sodium in treatment of patients with chronic polyarthritis. Z Rheumatol 57.4 (1998): 215–221.

Wluka AE et al. Supplementary vitamin E does not affect the loss of cartilage volume in knee osteoarthritis: a 2 year double blind randomized placebo controlled study. J Rheumatol 29.12 (2002): 2585–2591.

Wolf S et al. Chemotherapy-induced peripheral neuropathy: Prevention and treatment strategies. Eur J Cancer 44.11 (2008): 1507–1515.

Wood LA. Possible prevention of adriamycin-induced alopecia by tocopherol. N Engl J Med 312.16 (1985): 1060.

World Cancer Research Fund International 2011. Colorectal Cancer. [Online] http://www.wcrf.org/cancer_research/cup/colorectal_cancer.php [Accessed 8th May 2014]

Wright ME et al. Effects of alpha-tocopherol and beta-carotene supplementation on upper aerodigestive tract cancers in a large, randomized controlled trial. Cancer 109.5 (2007): 891–898.

Wu D, Meydani SN, 2008. Age-associated changes in immune and inflammatory responses: impact of vitamin E intervention. J Leukoc Biol. 84:4: 900–914.

Xu Q1, et al 2009. Multivitamin use and telomere length in women. Am J Clin Nutr. 89(6):1857–63.

Yang CS, et al 2012. Does vitamin E prevent or promote cancer. Cancer Prev Res 5:701.

Yang, H, et al 2012. Time selective chemoprevention of vitamin E and selenium on esophageal carcinogenesis in rats: the possible role of nuclear factor kappaB signaling pathway. Int J Cancer. 131;7:1517–1527.

Yasue H, et al. Coronary artery spasm-Clinical features, diagnosis, pathogenesis, and treatment. Journal of Cardiology 2008:51:1;2–7.

Yusuf S et al. Vitamin E supplementation and cardiovascular events in high-risk patients: The Heart Outcomes Prevention Evaluation Study Investigators. N Engl J Med 342.3 (2000): 154–160.

Zandi PP et al. Reduced risk of Alzheimer disease in users of antioxidant vitamin supplements: The Cache County Study. Arch Neurol 61.1 (2004): 82–88.

Ziaei S et al. A randomised placebo-controlled trial to determine the effect of vitamin E in treatment of primary dysmenorrhoea. BJOG 108.11 (2001): 1181–1183.

Ziaei S, et al. A randomised controlled trial of vitamin E in the treatment of primary dysmenorrhoea. BJOG 112.4 (2005): 466–469.

Ziaei S, et al. The effect of vitamin E on hot flashes in menopausal women. Gynecol Obstet Invest 64.4 (2007): 204–207.

Zureik M et al. Effects of long-term daily low-dose supplementation with antioxidant vitamins and minerals on structure and function of large arteries. Arterioscler Thromb Vasc Biol 24.8 (2004): 1485–1491.

Zinc

BACKGROUND AND RELEVANT PHARMACOKINETICS

Zinc was recognised as being essential for the growth of numerous plant and animal species by the 1960s. However, it was not until a fortuitous meeting in 1961, between the clinical scientist Prasad and a group of young Iranian men with severe growth retardation and hypogonadism, that zinc essentiality in humans was considered (Prasad 2013). A decade of controversy followed, ending with the discovery that zinc deficiency was central to the pathology of acrodermatitis enteropathica, a rare autosomal recessive trait that produces severe multisystem disease shortly after infants start weaning. In 1974 the National Research Council of the National Academy of Sciences finally declared zinc to be essential in human nutrition and established a recommended dietary allowance (RDA) (Prasad 2013). In human nutrition this is a relatively recent discovery and, as such, explains why zinc research is still in its infancy.

Zinc is an essential trace element known to play an important role in all human living cells. The human body contains approximately 2 g zinc in total, distributed across all body tissues and fluids, with 60% found in skeletal muscle and 30% in bone mass (Wahlqvist et al 2002). In spite of being a dietary trace element, it is one of the most abundant elements within cells and a complex homeostatic system maintains cellular zinc concentrations within a narrow range (King 2011). Its wide distribution and diverse roles have attracted the label of the 'ubiquitous nutrient' given by some authors (Hambidge 2000, King & Cousins 2006). Zinc belongs to the class of type II nutrients which are considered the cellular building blocks (Golden 1996, King & Cousins 2006) and therefore zinc, together with the other type II nutrients (essential amino acids, magnesium, potassium, phosphorus, protein and sulfur), is required for the synthesis of any new tissue. They are not stored by the body and are under tight physiological control.

Dietary intake of zinc by healthy adults is 6–15 mg/day; however, less than half of this is absorbed (Beers & Berkow 2003). Zinc absorption is influenced by many factors and adequate dietary intake does not guarantee adequate zinc status. The International Zinc Nutrition Consultative Group (IZiNCG) concludes that the two key dietary influences on zinc bioavailability are phytates and calcium. Foods with high phytate content significantly reduce zinc absorption due to the formation of strong and insoluble complexes (Lonnerdal 2000) and a phytate : zinc molar ratio ≥ 15, e.g. whole grains, seeds and nuts, is reported to render the zinc virtually unobtainable (IZiNCG 2004). In addition to this, calcium in large amounts constitutes the main antagonistic mineral interaction and therefore calcium-rich diets may also precipitate zinc deficiency. Soy protein has been shown to negatively impact zinc bioavailability, above and beyond its phytate content (Lim et al 2013). In contrast, the amount of animal protein in a meal positively correlates to zinc absorption and the amino acids histidine and methionine, and various organic acids present in foods, such as citric, malic and lactic acids, can also increase absorption. As such, zinc, similarly to iron, is best absorbed from animal food sources (King 2003). These combined factors may partly explain why vegetarians are at risk of low zinc status, a finding reported in a 2013 meta-analysis of 26 studies (Foster et al 2013).

Zinc absorption is a saturable process occurring in the small intestine principally via ZIP4, ZnT1 and, to a lesser extent, DMT1 (the shared divalent metal transporter) and CTR1 (primarily a copper transporter) (Espinoza et al 2012, King 2010, 2011); however, there is evidence of unregulated paracellular uptake with very high doses. Regulated zinc uptake is influenced by current dietary intake of the mineral, i.e. as the total amount of zinc ingested increases, the fractional uptake decreases. This adjustment to high intakes is particularly apparent when single doses >20 mg are administered (Tran et al 2004). Several papers report that zinc bioavailability from supplements is significantly better than from food; however, longer-term studies have revealed that this diminishes over a few days of consecutive dosing, due to compensatory downregulation of zinc transporters, and quickly becomes comparable with the fractional absorption seen with food (Hambidge et al 2010, King 2010, Tran et al 2004). Studies assessing bioavailability using disparate methods and sources have produced contrasting figures, from 46% to 74% (Tran et al 2004). A recent study evaluating average uptake from a standard Brazilian diet which controlled for phytate levels found that, while bioavailability varied from 11% to 47%, mean uptake was 30% (Ribeiro et al 2013).

Zinc homeostasis principally occurs in the gastrointestinal tract, whereby zinc uptake is balanced with endogenous zinc losses (Hambidge et al 2010, King 2010) which are estimated to total 0.5–3 mg/day. Other losses occur via urine and skin (0.5–0.7 mg) and semen (1 mg/ejaculate) (Lim et al 2013). When dietary zinc intake is insufficient, the body's homeostatic response is to minimise zinc losses and increase gastrointestinal absorption. As there is only a small zinc pool within the body, deficiency features develop quickly if dietary intake remains low. In growing children, deficiency signs and/or symptoms can develop within days, whereas for adults, this happens in a few weeks. Once zinc intake is increased, repletion can occur quickly, with rapid improvement of the clinical picture within days of supplementation (King 2011). Metallothionein (MT) is a cysteine-rich molecule found all over the body which can bind ≤7 zinc molecules, as well as other metals such as copper and cadmium. Gut and pancreatic MT concentrations respond readily to changes in dietary zinc; for example, high intakes induce MT synthesis and limit zinc absorption by binding zinc within the enterocyte and inhibiting basolateral transfer. Low dietary zinc produces a decline in pancreatic and renal MT, facilitating the decline in faecal and urinary zinc losses (King 2011).

Zinc is mainly an intracellular nutrient; little is found in the cytoplasm or found 'free' (loosely bound). This is likely due to its role in second-messenger systems, which means zinc levels need to be tightly regulated (primarily via MT) and largely sequestered inside organelles (Lazarczyk & Favre 2008).

Typically, only 5% of body zinc is found extracellularly (King 2011). Inflammatory processes and increased glucocorticoids can cause redistribution of zinc, leading to sequestration by the liver and adipocytes (Ferro et al 2011). Two recent studies investigating altered zinc homeostasis in obesity (Feitosa et al 2013, Ferro et al 2011) found evidence of lower erythrocyte zinc, while Feitosa et al demonstrated an inverse relationship specifically with tumour necrosis factor-alpha

(TNF-alpha), consistent with the hypothesis that chronic inflammation in obesity will negatively impact zinc homeostasis.

Lastly, zinc homeostasis is altered in the elderly due to both higher intracellular levels of MT and defective zinc influx transporters, ultimately producing less available free intracellular zinc (Mocchegiani et al 2011).

CHEMICAL COMPONENTS

Zinc sulfate and gluconate are the most common forms of zinc found in commercially produced supplements. There is growing research on other forms, such as zinc picolinate and methionine and carnosine complexes, the latter specifically for gastrointestinal complaints. There is currently a lack of human research comparing the bioavailability of these forms; however, animal studies suggest that zinc sulfate is approximately twice as bioavailable as zinc oxide (in dogs, horses and rabbits), while zinc methionine and zinc propionate also produced significant increases in plasma zinc (Andermann & Dietz 1982, Wedekind & Lowry 1998, Wedekind et al 1992, 1994, Wichert et al 2002).

FOOD SOURCES

Meat, liver, eggs and seafood (especially oysters and shellfish) are the best sources both quantitatively and qualitatively. While zinc is also found in nuts, legumes, whole grains and seeds, the high phytate content (stored phosphate) of these foods makes them an inferior source. Phytates can be reduced through fermentation or sprouting, which in turn would improve zinc bioavailability in these foods. Other dietary sources include miso, tofu, brewers' yeast, mushrooms and green beans. It has been reported that, while zinc is found as organic complexes in meats, it is presented as inorganic salts in plant foods (Lim et al 2013) and this may in part explain the superior bioavailability of zinc from animal products and seafood.

DEFICIENCY SIGNS AND SYMPTOMS

Severe deficiency is rarely seen in industrialised countries, but marginal deficiency and inadequate intakes are not uncommon. According to a large national survey conducted in the United States of over 29,000 people, only 55.6% had adequate zinc intakes (based on total intakes of >77% of the 1989 US recommended daily intake (RDI) levels). Young children aged 1–3 years, female adolescents and older people aged ≥71 years had the lowest percentage of 'adequate' zinc intake, and were identified at greatest risk of deficiency (Briefel et al 2000).

Due to its important role in growth and development, zinc deficiency is characterised by impaired growth (linear growth velocity, weight or body composition) (Hambidge 2000). This will produce overt presentations in those life stages and tissues, necessitating rapid replication and turnover for health (Hambidge 2000), e.g. embryos, early childhood, adolescence, immune cells, epidermal and gastrointestinal tissue (Hambidge 2000, IZiNCG 2004, King 2000, King & Cousins 2006, Mahomed et al 1993), but often indiscernible pictures outside of these.

The clinical picture of mild zinc deficiency is subtle, ambiguous, idiosyncratic (Golden 1996, Hambidge 2000) and notoriously difficult to diagnose (Golden 1996, Wood 2000). King (2011) reminds us that, being a type II nutrient, zinc deficiency evokes sophisticated conservation mechanisms to limit endogenous losses and a metabolic adaptation to reduce the high-demand pathways for zinc such as growth and immunity. Altogether this can rapidly produce non-specific signs of metabolic or clinical dysfunction, such as malaise and apathy. Another prominent zinc researcher says, 'the ubiquity and versatility of zinc in subcellular metabolism suggest that zinc deficiency may well result in a generalised impairment of many metabolic functions' (Hambidge 2000, p 1345S).

Signs and symptoms of deficiency

Most consistently reported

- Anorexia, impaired sense of taste and smell
- Slowed growth and development
- Delayed sexual maturation, hypogonadism, hypospermia and menstrual problems
- Dermatitis, particularly around the body's orifices, as seen in acrodermatitis enteropathica
- Alopecia
- Chronic and severe diarrhoea
- Immune system deficiencies and increased susceptibility to infection, including bacterial, viral and fungal
- Impaired wound healing due to decreased collagen synthesis
- Night blindness; swelling and clouding of the corneas
- Behavioural disturbances such as mental fatigue and depression (King 2003).

Less consistently reported

- Erectile dysfunction
- Anergy
- Glossitis
- Nail dystrophy
- Hypopigmented hair
- Photophobia
- Photic injury
- Swelling and clouding of the corneas
- Reduced serum testosterone in males
- Reduced alcohol clearance
- Hyperammonaemia
- Impaired protein synthesis.

Zinc deficiency in pregnancy is associated with the following (Bedwal & Bahuguna 1994, Prasad 1996):

- Increased maternal morbidity, pre-eclampsia and toxaemia
- Prolonged gestation
- Inefficient labour
- Atonic bleeding
- Increased risk of abortion and stillbirths
- Teratogenicity
- Low-birth-weight infants
- Diminished attention in the newborn and poorer motor function at 6 months (Higdon 2003).

PRIMARY DEFICIENCY (Table 1)

Primary deficiency occurs as a result of inadequate intake, with greatest risks seen in vegetarians and individuals consuming high-phytate diets. This is particularly the case in many developing countries, with the World Health Organization estimating that suboptimal zinc nutrition affected nearly half the world's population in 2002 (Mistry & Williams 2011).

In developed countries, phytate levels are greatest in 'healthy high-fibre diets' with greater intake of wholegrains and legumes and can provide in excess of 1000 mg phytic acid/day. Hambidge et al (2010) used a mathematical model to determine that the RDA would need to be doubled for such individuals. A study of 20 women with type 2 diabetes consuming a high-fibre diet (1194 ±

TABLE 1 COMMON FEATURES OF MILD, MODERATE AND SEVERE ZINC DEFICIENCIES (PRASAD 2013)		
Mild deficiency	**Moderate deficiency**	**Severe deficiency**
↓ Serum testosterone	Growth retardation	Growth retardation
Oligospermia	Male adolescent hypogonadism	Male adolescent hypogonadism
↓ Natural killer cell activity	Rough skin	Bullous pustular dermatitis, especially around orifices and extremities
↓ Interleukin-2 activity	↓ Appetite	Blepharitis, conjunctivitis
↓ T-helper cells	Mental lethargy	Photophobia
↓ Serum thymulin activity	Delayed wound healing	Alopecia
Hyperammonaemia	Cell-mediated immune dysfunction	Diarrhoea and changes to small intestinal villi
Hypogeusia (impaired taste)	Abnormal neurosensory changes	Weight loss
↓ Dark adaptation		Emotional disorders, e.g. irritability, emotional instability
↓ Lean body mass		↓ Healing of ulcers
		Death

824 mg/day) found that this was a risk factor for zinc deficiency (Foster et al 2013). Recently a systematic review and meta-analysis of 26 studies examining the zinc status of vegetarians concluded that both dietary zinc intake and serum zinc were significantly lower in this group, with particular at-risk sub-groups being females, vegans and those living in developing countries (Foster et al 2013). As zinc is a type II nutrient (see Clinical note — Measuring zinc status is difficult), which is essential for cellular growth, the life stages that are most at risk of deficiency include childhood, adolescence and pregnancy.

SECONDARY DEFICIENCY

Factors which interfere with zinc absorption (i.e. malabsorption), distribution (i.e. inflammation), retention (i.e. weight loss), excretion (e.g. antihypertensive drugs) or significantly increase requirements (i.e. specific infections or periods of growth) can all play a part in producing a secondary zinc deficiency, as per the following (Gehrig & Dinulos 2010):

- Acrodermatitis enteropathica, a rare autosomal recessive defect in zinc transporters that manifests rapidly as severe zinc deficiency in infants after weaning
- Anorexia nervosa
- Antihypertensive medication (in particular angiotensin-converting enzyme inhibitors, angiotensin II receptor blockers and thiazide diuretics) (Braun & Rosenfeldt 2013)
- Breastfeeding

- Chronic alcoholism
- Malabsorption syndromes, e.g. Crohn's and coeliac disease (CD), ulcerative colitis, cystic fibrosis
- Renal impairments and dialysis
- Extensive cutaneous burns
- Hepatic or pancreatic insufficiency
- HIV infection
- Intestinal bypass procedures — percentage zinc absorption decreases significantly from 32.3% to 13.6% at 6 months after gastric bypass, with partial correction at 18 months (Ruz et al 2011)
- Prematurity with low zinc storage
- Penicillamine or chlorothiazide therapy
- *Yersinia enterocolitica* infection (Gehrig & Dinulos 2010)
- Obesity and cardiometabolic syndrome — redistribution due to chronic inflammation (Feitosa et al 2013, Ferro et al 2011, Foster & Samman 2012).

Clinical note — Measuring zinc status is difficult

According to the scientific evidence, there is currently no means of assessing zinc status in humans (particularly with respect to the detection of marginal deficiency states) that has demonstrated absolute accuracy, and the identification of such a test has been flagged as an area requiring urgent research (Bales et al 1990, Hambidge 2000, IZiNCG 2004, Wood 2000). The assessment of zinc in orthodox medicine currently utilises serum or plasma assays (Gropper et al 2009, IZiNCG 2004, Wood 2000). Principally validated as a tool to assess zinc adequacy of populations (IZiNCG 2004, Wood 2000), serum/plasma zinc lacks the sensitivity to accurately ascertain the zinc status of the individual, with decreased values reflective of end-stage depletion only (Gordon et al 1982, Gropper et al 2009, Hambidge 2000, 2003, IZiNCG 2004, Wood 2000). Multiple established confounding variables include diurnal variation, concomitant infections and inflammation, acute stress and trauma, haemodilution of pregnancy, low serum albumin, high white blood cell counts and the concomitant use of hormones and steroids (King & Cousins 2006, Wood 2000). Each of these scenarios is susceptible to producing false negatives, underpinning concerns regarding the specificity of serum/plasma zinc assessment (Hambidge 2003, Hotz et al 2003). In addition to this, data from the National Health and Nutrition Examination Survey (NHANES II) revealed significant differences in the mean values of 'healthy individuals' dependent on age and sex alone (IZiNCG 2004). In spite of these documented limitations, this test remains the first-line assay in orthodox medicine.

A range of other biochemical indices have been used to assess zinc, including red (Kenney et al 1984, Prasad 1985) and white blood cells (Bunker et al 1987, Prasad 1985), platelets (Baer & King 1984), hair (Bunker et al 1987, Erten et al 1978, Hambidge 2003, McBean et al 1971, McKenzie 1979), nails (McKenzie 1979), saliva (Bales et al 1990, Freeland-Graves et al 1981, Greger & Sickles 1979), sweat (Baer & King 1984, Eaton et al 2004) and urinary concentrations (Hambidge 2003, McKenzie 1979, Prasad 1985). All represent static measures and, as such, lack the sensitivity required to account for zinc's dynamic and complex homeostasis (Gropper et al 2009). Many researchers believe that an accurate indicator of zinc nutriture will therefore also need to be dynamic, similar to using ferritin as a marker for iron status (Hambidge

2000, 2003, Wood 2000) and measurement of both serum and erythrocyte metallothienein seems a likely candidate (King 2011).

One area of functional zinc assessment extensively researched since the 1970s is taste acuity testing (Gibson 1990, Gibson et al 1989, Henkin et al 1975b). Hypogeusia is recognised as an early indicator of zinc deficiency (Buzina et al 1980, Gibson 1990, Henkin et al 1975a, Kosman & Henkin 1981, Tanaka 2002, Wright et al 1981) and is believed to be the result of compromised gustin activity, a carbonic anhydrase zinc metalloenzyme which facilitates differentiation, growth and turnover of taste buds (Gibson et al 1989, Henkin et al 1975b, 1977, Law et al 1987, Thatcher et al 1998). The zinc taste response test (also known as the Bryce-Smith taste test) is a popular measure among naturopathic practitioners. It relies on patients detecting a taste after oral administration of 5–10 mL of a zinc sulfate heptahydrate solution. Delayed taste perception or lack of taste recognition is interpreted as a zinc deficiency state. This method is not particularly accurate and is hampered by variations in patients' subjective sense of taste and the fact that agents other than zinc influence taste perception. Clinical studies with zinc taste tests have confirmed the inconsistency of the results (Birmingham et al 2005, Eaton et al 2004, Garg et al 1993, Mahomed et al 1993) and a literature review of the zinc taste test, that remains popular in Australia and some other countries, reached the same conclusions (Gruner & Arthur 2012).

MAIN ACTIONS

Cofactor in many biochemical reactions

In humans, zinc metalloenzymes outnumber all the other trace mineral-dependent enzymes combined, with between 70 and 200 present in humans (Gropper et al 2009), found across all six different enzyme classes (Hambidge 2000). Consequently, zinc is involved in myriad chemical reactions that are important for normal body functioning, such as carbohydrate metabolism, protein and DNA synthesis, protein digestion, bone metabolism and endogenous antioxidant systems (Merck 2009, Wahlqvist et al 2002, Wardlaw et al 1997).

At the cellular level, zinc's functions can be divided into three categories: catalytic, structural and regulatory (King 2003, 2011). In its catalytic capacity, zinc metalloenzymes are defined as those apometalloenzymes which are dependent upon the binding of zinc for their activity, such as alkaline phosphatase. Structural roles are evident in a range of proteins, enzymes, e.g. CuZn, superoxide dismutase (SOD) and biomembranes. Of particular note is the zinc finger motif, which allows zinc to be bound in a tetrahedral complex with two cysteines within the protein.

Zinc's contribution as an intra- and intercellular regulatory ion continues to emerge and includes its profound role in gene expression, whereby zinc binds to a metal-binding transcription factor and a metal response element in the promoter of the regulated gene to stimulate transcription (King 2011). Other regulatory roles include receptor-mediated signal transduction, neurotransmitter release from synaptic vesicles, packaging of insulin into pancreatic granules and subsequent release, antigen-dependent T-cell activation and insulin-like growth factor receptor binding (Hambidge 2000, King 2011, King & Cousins 2006).

Growth and development

Zinc is essential for the formation of biomembranes and zinc finger motifs found in DNA transcription factors (Semrad 1999) and, belonging to the type II nutrient class, is required for the building of all new tissues (King 2011). Additionally, several studies of children with growth retardation and zinc deficiency have confirmed that repletion leads to increased levels and activity of growth hormone and insulin-like growth factor and insulin-like growth factor-binding proteins (Prasad 2013).

Normal immune responses

Zinc is involved in many aspects of immunological function. It is essential for the normal development and function of cells, for mediating non-specific immunity such as neutrophils, monocytes and natural killer cells and for affecting the development of acquired immunity and T-lymphocyte function. Deficiency primarily impacts on T-lymphocyte function, reducing both peripheral numbers and thymic cells, compromising function of the T-helper and cytotoxic cells and reducing serum levels of thymulin and T-helper subset 1 cell cytokines, e.g. interleukin-2 and interferon-gamma. In addition, zinc depletion rapidly diminishes antibody and cell-mediated responses in both humans and animals, altogether leading to increased opportunistic infections and mortality rates (Fraker et al 2000, Prasad 2009, 2013).

Animal models have shown that suboptimal zinc intake over 30 days can lead to 30–80% loss in defence capacity and that this occurs significantly earlier than changes in serum or plasma values (Prasad 2013). Investigation using a human model has demonstrated that even mild deficiency in humans adversely affects T-cell functions (Prasad 1998). Conversely, high-dose zinc supplementation (20-fold RDI) can also produce immune dysfunction due to an induced copper deficiency.

A key area of research interest currently relates to zinc's influence on cytokine production. Zinc is regarded as a key anti-inflammatory nutrient due to its ability to both reduce the source of oxidative stress, reactive oxygen species (ROS), and control the body's inflammatory response by reducing nuclear factor-kappaB (NF-κB), TNF-alpha and interleukin-beta (Feitosa et al 2013, Overbeck et al 2008, Prasad 2009, 2013). It is important to note, however, the new evidence of negative zinc redistribution that occurs in chronic inflammation that would hamper this anti-inflammatory role (Feitosa et al 2013).

Gastrointestinal structure and function

Numerous animal studies demonstrate the deleterious effects of zinc deficiency on villi (atrophy, reduced height), crypt cells (reduced number and depth), mucosal cells (increased apoptosis), tissue integrity (increased ulceration, disruption of junctional complexes and cytoskeleton disorganisation in $CaCo_2$ cells) and immune response (increased inflammation) (Scrimgeour & Condlin 2009, Tran et al 2011). Secondary to this is clear evidence of impaired function, including reduced expression of the brush border disaccharidases. New animal research suggests that, in part, these actions require not just adequate zinc but healthy levels of MT. Importantly, zinc supplementation (in individuals with normal MT production) corrects these observed gastrointestinal tract anomalies (Tran et al 2011).

Neurological function

Central nervous system zinc is found predominantly in the brain, specifically the hippocampus, amygdala and cortex, where it possesses both catalytic (cofactors) and regulatory roles (Szewczyk et al 2008). While 95% of brain zinc is bound to metalloproteins, the remainder is found in presynaptic vesicles. Neurons that contain these are known as zinc-enriched neurons (ZEN) (Frederickson & Danscher 1990, Frederickson & Moncrieff 1994, Frederickson et al 2000, Szewczyk et al 2008). Cerebellar ZEN are primarily associated with gamma-aminobutyric acid (GABA) neurotransmission, whereas in the other regions they are found in glutamate-producing neurons. Zinc therefore has the ability to inhibit both GABA and glutaminergic receptors, making it a candidate for neuronal excitability modulation. It also potentially plays an important role in synaptic plasticity (Szewczyk et al 2008). Other general actions include the stabilisation of certain stored macromolecules in presynaptic vesicles, the inhibition of GSK3 phosphorylation, which leads to increased brain-derived neurotrophic factor (BDNF) levels, and its anti-inflammatory functions, which are all important for the health and function of the brain.

Specific neurotransmitter actions include potent dopamine transporter inhibition, which allows dopamine to stay and engage with receptors longer within the synapse. Zinc is now considered an important regulator of dopamine transporter function (Stockner et al 2013). There is also evidence of zinc modulating serotonin uptake in vitro (Szewczyk et al 2008).

Prostate health

The prostate contains the highest zinc concentration of any soft tissue in humans. The concentration of zinc found in the prostate differs between the four lobes and is tightly regulated according to their different functions. The peripheral lobes hold the highest concentration and this relates to their central role in secretion of prostatic fluid, which contains ≈500 mcg/mL of zinc compared with plasma, 1–2 mcg/mL. With ageing, the zinc content of both the prostate and its fluid declines, a factor which has been linked with declining fertility. Beyond acting as a reservoir for the high zinc needs of prostatic fluid, zinc also plays an important role in making citrate available, which is also found in large amounts in prostatic fluid and zinc is at unusually high levels within prostatic mitochondria (unknown reason). Lastly, zinc has an antimicrobial role within the fluid and the greater gland itself (Kelleher et al 2011).

Low prostatic zinc has been linked to prostate disease and, while there is evidence of some dysregulation of zinc within the gland in these individuals, dietary zinc deficiency alone has been associated with increased DNA damage in the prostate during oxidative stress. This becomes a vicious circle, in that the greater the oxidative stress, the greater the prostate's need for zinc (Kelleher et al 2011).

Fertility

Zinc is important for both male and female fertility. In adult males, the testis and prostate have the highest concentration of zinc of any organ in the body (Bedwal & Bahuguna 1994). In moderate to severe zinc deficiency male hypogonadism has been well-documented (Prasad 2013). Zinc in humans is necessary for the formation and maturation of spermatozoa, for ovulation and for fertilisation (Favier 1992). Studies generally have shown a positive correlation between seminal zinc levels and sperm counts and motility. As an antioxidant, zinc protects vulnerable sperm from excess ROS, heavy metals, fluoride, cigarette smoke and heat (Sankako et al 2012, Talevi et al 2013, Yamaguchi et al 2009). An in vivo model of acute dietary zinc deficiency revealed that a zinc-deficient diet for 3–5 days preovulation (preconception) dramatically disrupted oocyte chromatin methylation and preimplantation development (Tian & Diaz 2013). Zinc also has multiple actions on the metabolism of androgen hormones, oestrogen and progesterone, and these, together with the prostaglandins and nuclear receptors for steroids, are all zinc finger proteins.

Pregnancy and lactation

Zinc is recognised as being a key nutrient during embryogenesis, fetal growth and development (Donangelo & King 2012, Mistry & Williams 2011). Severe deficiency results in a range of devastating outcomes, including multiple fetal malformations, growth retardation or death, embryonic death and potentially life-threatening complications in both pregnancy and delivery (Chaffee & King 2012, Donangelo & King 2012). The consequences of mild to moderate deficiency are less clear, although most studies demonstrate reduced birth weights and some found increased prematurity, possibly secondary to maternal infection. There is also specific interest in zinc's antioxidant and anti-inflammatory roles in pregnancy and prevention of pre-eclampsia and fetal growth restriction, both of which have oxidative stress as an essential component (Chen et al 2012, Mistry & Williams 2011).

While it has been reported that zinc requirements in pregnancy would theoretically necessitate an 18–36% increase in dietary intake, most pregnant women do not increase zinc consumption (Donangelo & King 2012). This has led researchers to conclude that the primary means of meeting these higher zinc needs is via homeostatic adjustment; however, the exact mechanisms remain unclear and fail to completely compensate when zinc intake is significantly inadequate.

Similarly, zinc is essential for healthy mammary gland function, specifically the expansion and reduction of mammary tissue dependent upon stage of pregnancy and lactation, differentiation into secretory tissue, proliferation of the mammary epithelial cells which line the acini and transfer nutrients into milk, and milk secretion (Kelleher et al 2011). When milk zinc levels are compromised, this results in failure to thrive, diarrhoea, irritability and dermatitis in the infant (Kelleher et al 2011). Zinc losses in breast milk are significant, e.g. mean 1.35 mg/day, and if this was to be met by diet alone, a 50% increase in zinc intake would be required; however, limited evidence points to some adaptive mechanisms such as increased intestinal absorptive capacity, reduced faecal losses and increased renal conservation. The greatest contribution to maternal zinc during the postpartum period is speculated to be through resorption of trabecular bone. During 6 months of exclusive breastfeeding, 4–6% of maternal bone mass is lost, and this would contribute about 20% of the breast milk zinc during this period (Donangelo & King 2012).

Antioxidant

Zinc limits oxidant-induced damage in a number of indirect ways. It protects against vitamin E depletion, controls vitamin A release, contributes to the structure of the antioxidant enzyme extracellular SOD, restricts endogenous free radical production, maintains tissue concentrations of MT, is a possible scavenger of free radicals, antagonising both iron and copper levels, and stabilises membrane structure (DiSilvestro 2000, Rai et al 2013). It was observed to decrease lipid peroxidation and protect mononuclear cells from TNF-alpha-induced NF-kappa-B activation associated with oxidative stress (Prasad et al 2004).

Supporting glycaemic control

Zinc pancreatic concentrations are very high, negatively impacted by deficiency and, not surprisingly, zinc possesses multiple related roles, including the processing, storage, secretion and action of insulin in β cells. In fact, as insulin and zinc are co-stored within the dense core vesicles (DCVs), when insulin is exocytosed (released), a substantial amount of ionic zinc is also released into local circulation, with important autocrine and paracrine effects on nearby cells (Li 2013, O'Halloran et al 2013), including 'switching off' glucagon release from the pancreatic α cells (Kelleher et al 2011). The co-storage of zinc and insulin within β cells appears critical, such that polymorphisms that reduce expression of the zinc transporters expressed on these DCVs are associated with significantly reduced insulin secretion, increased HbA_{1C} and an increased risk of type 2 diabetes (Chimienti 2013). Zinc is also an essential cofactor for insulin degradation, peripheral insulin signalling and several key zinc finger transcription factors are required for β-cell development and insulin gene expression (Kelleher et al 2011, O'Halloran et al 2013). Furthermore, zinc is necessary for activity of several gluconeogenic enzymes, including phosphoenolpyruvate carboxykinase, making zinc central in glucose metabolism regulation (Kelleher et al 2011).

Interestingly, another zinc-dependent enzyme, called insulin-responsive aminopeptidase (IRAP), is colocalised with GLUT4 transporters on cell membranes, with both upregulating in response to insulin (Kelleher et al 2011). Although the exact action of IRAP is yet to be elucidated, its membrane expression in muscle cells and adipocytes is reduced in type 2 diabetes, just like the GLUT4s, suggesting a strong link between zinc signalling and insulin activity.

Suboptimal zinc status decreases insulin secretion from the pancreas while during severe deficiency hyperglycaemia and hyperinsulinaemia can manifest (Kelleher et al 2011) and zinc supplementation has been shown to ameliorate some physiological aspects of diabetes.

CLINICAL USE

Most of the clinical uses of zinc supplements are for conditions thought to arise from a marginal zinc deficiency, but some indications are based on the concept that high-dose zinc supplements act as a therapeutic agent above and beyond the point of repletion.

Deficiency

Traditionally, zinc supplementation has been used to treat or prevent deficiency in conditions such as acrodermatitis enteropathica, anorexia nervosa, malabsorption syndromes, conditions associated with chronic, severe diarrhoea, alcoholism and liver cirrhosis, diabetes, HIV and AIDS, recurrent infections, severe burns, after major surgery, Wilson's disease and sickle cell anaemia. Zinc supplements are also popular among athletes in order to counteract zinc losses that occur through perspiration. There are numerous supplementation and fortification schemes which include zinc in developing countries, where deficiency is most prevalent.

Common cold

Oral zinc supplements, lozenges, nasal sprays and gels have been investigated in the prevention and treatment of the common cold. It has been demonstrated that a transient increase in zinc concentrations in and around the nasal cavity prevents rhinovirus binding to cells and disrupts infection (Novick et al 1996) and/or modulates inflammatory cytokines and histamine release, as well as astringes the trigeminal nerve, to reduce cold symptoms (Kurugöl et al 2007, Science et al 2012). There is also evidence to suggest that zinc inhibits viral replication and speculation regarding zinc's ability to change the activities of different transcription factors and thus the expression patterns of cellular and viral genes (Lazarczyk & Favre 2008).

Zinc's administration via a lozenge form appears particularly important regarding its efficacy in upper respiratory tract infections (URTIs). A prolific researcher in this area explains this via the 'mouth-nose biologically closed electric circuit' (BCEC) (Eby & Halcomb 2006). The BCEC moves electrons from the nose into the mouth and, in response to the electron flow, moves positively charged metal ions, such as ionic zinc, from the mouth into the nose, where it then exerts its key virucidal actions via competing with rhinoviruses for attachment to the intracellular adhesion molecule-1 receptor in nasal epithelium (Singh & Das 2013). If correct, this underscores the importance of using 'free' or ionic forms of zinc in the lozenge, rather than tightly bound ones (see Oral supplements, below).

Acute treatment

Nasal preparations

At least three placebo-controlled studies indicate that intranasal preparations containing zinc have benefits in the treatment of the common cold; however safety issues regarding transient anosmia limit its use in practice.

Administration of a zinc sulfate (0.12%) nasal spray reduced the total symptom score significantly better than placebo, according to a double-blind randomised controlled trial involving 160 people. The same treatment had no effect on the duration of cold symptoms or mean time to resolution (Belongia et al 2001). Two other placebo-controlled trials showed that zinc in a nasal gel formulation significantly reduced cold duration compared with placebo when used within 24–48 hours of symptom onset (Hirt et al 2000, Mossad 2003). The active nasal gel spray contained 33 mmol/L zinc gluconate and was administered as one dose per nostril four times daily until symptoms resolved or for a maximum of 10 days. Symptoms that responded included nasal drainage, hoarseness and sore throat (Mossad 2003).

Despite these promising results, concerns have been raised regarding temporary anosmia secondary to use of the zinc gluconate nasal preparations (Duncan-Lewis et al 2011). Based on consumer reports, in 2009 the US Food and Drug Administration issued a warning against the use of zinc nasal preparations, which were subsequently removed from the US market. The safety of these preparations has been the subject of debate between industry and government

Anosmia has been reported in animal models following the application of nasal zinc chloride or sulfate preparations and a more recent study which nasally irrigated rats with zinc gluconate further confirmed temporary anosmia compared with placebo. While the sensory loss is only transient and the mechanism remains unclear, any sensory loss is worrying (Duncan-Lewis et al 2011, Hemila 2011).

Oral supplements

According to two meta-analyses, zinc lozenges (≥75 mg/day) significantly reduce symptom duration compared to placebo in the acute treatment of URTIs but not symptom severity (Science et al 2012, Singh & Das 2013). Ideally, lozenges should be taken every 2 hours and started as soon as symptoms arise, thereby reducing symptom duration by about 1.65 days in adults (95% confidence interval −2.50 to −0.81) (Science et al 2012). They should not be taken with any food or beverage which may limit zinc absorption or ionisation (see Background and relevant pharmacokinetics, above).

While the body of evidence is positive, some adult studies do not demonstrate benefits, which may be due to differences in study methodology and whether zinc in the test preparation is accompanied by other ingredients which affect its release and/or absorption, such as citrate, tartrate, sorbitol or glycine, which decrease the level of free zinc ion (Hemila 2011). Since zinc ionisation is considered an important step in the clinical effectiveness of zinc, this is of particular concern. Ideally, future researchers should pay careful attention to exact lozenge composition in order to minimise this confounding factor (Hemila 2011, Silk & LeFante 2005). It has also been suggested that zinc lozenges be allowed to completely dissolve in the mouth without chewing and that citrus fruits or juices be avoided 30 minutes before or after dissolving each lozenge to avoid negating the therapeutic effects of zinc (Silk & LeFante 2005).

An updated Cochrane review of 16 double-blind randomised controlled trials (n = 1357) investigating zinc administration ≥75 mg/day for acute treatment of URTIs concluded there was a significant mean reduction in symptom duration compared to placebo (P = 0.003) and a smaller proportion of symptomatic individuals after 7 days in treatment groups; however, there was no significant difference in the severity of cold symptoms (Singh & Das 2013). Due to the heterogeneity of the studies, the authors urge caution regarding their calculated average estimates. Another 2013 systematic review and meta-analysis tried to improve upon the Cochrane methodology, including 17 trials (n = 2121) of oral zinc administration within 3 days of URTI symptom onset. They too concluded that, although no significant difference in symptom severity was evident, there was a mean reduction in duration (mean difference [MD] −1.65 days, 95% confidence interval [CI] −2.50 to −0.81). A subgroup analysis revealed that the effect was only significant in adults (MD −2.63, 95% CI −3.69 to −1.58) and was restricted to studies using a zinc acetate form and when administered at higher doses, e.g. ≥75 mg/day. The authors speculate that the lack of significance in paediatric cohorts is due to lower doses, reduced frequency of administration and alternative forms used, e.g. syrups rather than lozenges. Their findings would suggest that the impact of zinc administration on reducing URTI duration has previously been underestimated in studies that fail to attend to these important details (Science et al 2012).

An earlier systematic review focused specifically on zinc lozenges in acute URTI treatment, with all but one study conducted in adults (Hemila 2011). This review demonstrates, and argues convincingly for the merit of, several differences in statistical analysis. Firstly, the authors make the point that URTI symptom duration is highly variable independent of any treatment, and, as such, is more logical to calculate via relative effect on duration, rather than an absolute, e.g. percentage rather than days. When calculated like this, the authors found the evidence strengthened for zinc lozenge efficacy. The review also presents an extended discussion of lozenge dose and form, most notably pointing out that there is a sevenfold difference in total daily zinc dose across the included studies. Subgroup analysis found no effect was evident in the five trials using <75 mg/day. In contrast, the majority of studies using >75 mg/day demonstrated positive effects. The review also found greater reductions in symptom duration with zinc acetate (mean −42%, 95% CI 35–48) compared with other forms (mean effect −20%, 95% CI 12–28). These findings were recently echoed by Science et al (2012).

Prevention of colds

There is relatively little research dedicated to determining whether long-term zinc supplementation reduces URTI incidence. A 2013 Cochrane review included only two studies investigating zinc as a prophylactic treatment (n = 394) and concluded there was very low-level evidence of efficacy; however, the studies differed in many key variables, e.g, dose, form, duration of administration and still collectively produced an incident rate ratio of 0.64 (P = 0.006) (Singh & Das

2013). Critics of this review suggest that bias has insufficiently been accounted for and therefore the effect of zinc has possibly been overstated (Peters et al 2012).

In children

A recent double-blind randomised controlled trial not included in the Cochrane review of 100 8–13-year-old children showed that administration of zinc *bis*-glycinate 15 mg once a day for 3 months was not sufficient to reduce the incidence of URTIs but did reduce symptom severity and duration associated with colds if an URTI developed, as compared to placebo (Rerksuppaphol & Rerksuppaphol 2013).

In the elderly

Both zinc deficiency, due to poor dietary intake and altered homeostasis, and impaired cell-mediated immunity are commonly reported in the elderly (>55 years) and have been used to explain the increased infection rates observed in this population. A double-blind randomised controlled trial involving 50 healthy elderly subjects found that the majority had a marginal zinc deficiency and 35% were below the cut-off for frank deficiency, as measured via plasma zinc at baseline (Prasad et al 2007). Participants taking zinc gluconate supplements (45 mg/day) for 12 months experienced a significant reduction in infection incidence compared to placebo (88% vs 29%), with protective effects evident against URTIs (12% vs 24%), the common cold (10% vs 40%) and influenza (0% vs 12%). Also of note, while no individual in the treatment group experienced more than one infection in the 12-month period, six individuals taking placebo had two infections, and three subjects had three or more infections during the same period. Inflammatory cytokines and markers of oxidative stress were also investigated in this study, confirming zinc's role as both an anti-inflammatory and antioxidant in the elderly. Prior studies using much smaller zinc doses (15–20 mg/day) in multivitamin and mineral combinations failed to demonstrate efficacy in this cohort (Avenell et al 2005, Girodon et al 1999, Hemila 2011).

There is ongoing research interest in the relationship between zinc status and senescence, with preliminary in vivo studies pointing to zinc dysregulation being a key factor in the increasing inflammation and reduced immunocompetence seen with ageing (Mocchegiani et al 2011, Wong et al 2013).

Pneumonia

Worldwide, pneumonia is the leading cause of paediatric morbidity and mortality and approximately 95% of the pneumonia-related deaths occur in developing countries where zinc deficiency is most prevalent (Shah et al 2012). Several studies have investigated both prevention and treatment of paediatric pneumonia using zinc supplementation, usually as an adjunct to standard treatment.

Prevention

Supplemental zinc (70 mg/day) significantly reduced the incidence of pneumonia (relative risk [RR] 0.83) compared to placebo and significantly reduced mortality ($P = 0.013$) in a randomised controlled trial of 1665 poor, urban children aged < 12 months. In addition, active treatment resulted in a 49% decrease in the incidence of severe pneumonia and reduced URTI by 8% and reactive airways disease (bronchiolitis) by 12% (Brooks et al 2005).

Serum zinc concentrations have been shown to negatively correlate with pneumonia incidence in a study of nursing-home residents, prompting researchers to consider zinc as a potential prophylactic in this population also; however, there are currently no randomised controlled trials (Overbeck et al 2008).

Active treatment

In terms of acute treatment, positive findings include the study by Brooks et al (2004) — a randomised controlled trial involving 270 children aged between 6 and 12 months, hospitalised with pneumonia, which found that those given 20 mg/day of zinc (as acetate) experienced significant reductions in recovery time from severe pneumonia. Overall hospital stay duration was also reduced when used with standard antimicrobial therapy (Brooks et al 2004). Results from a similarly designed study, however, failed to corroborate zinc as an effective treatment (Bose et al 2006).

It is possible that the lack of differentiation between bacterial and non-bacterial pneumonia in these studies is an important feature. Another study which investigated the efficacy of adjunctive zinc treatment (10 mg zinc sulfate administered twice daily) in paediatric patients (<2 years) hospitalised for severe pneumonia identified that zinc supplementation in bacterial pneumonia had detrimental effects which were not seen in non-bacterial cases (Coles et al 2007). Further research is not available to confirm these results.

A Cochrane review includes four trials of zinc given as an adjunct to standard antimicrobial therapy in children (*n* = 3267) aged 2–35 months suffering with severe and non-severe pneumonia (Haider et al 2011). The studies by Brooks et al (2004) and Bose et al (2006) were included along with two other moderately-sized trials. All four studies tested 20 mg elemental zinc per day, except that by Valentiner-Branth et al (2010), who administered only 10 mg/day for <12 months. Duration of treatment varied from as little as 5 days to >14 days (discharge). The reviewers concluded that there was no significant reduction in clinical recovery in the groups receiving adjunctive zinc; however, none of the studies identified whether the aetiology was bacterial or viral, which, according to the findings of Coles et al (2007), limits the meaningfulness of these conclusions.

A 2012 meta-analysis of seven studies (*n* = 1066), including many of the ones already discussed, concludes that zinc supplementation fails to produce significant reductions in recovery time from paediatric pneumonia. The authors acknowledge several limitations of the review, including lack of distinction between bacterial and viral aetiologies (Das et al 2012). They also suggest that future studies should consider higher doses given the absence of adverse reactions and standardise definitions, recovery parameters, timing and doses of zinc before drawing definitive conclusions.

Since these two reviews were published, two other key studies have been conducted which provide additional insight. A Ugandan study of 352 children aged 6–59 months (Srinivasan et al 2012) provides us with a well-thought-out methodology, clearly taking into account the findings of recent research in this area, such as that by Coles et al (2007). Zinc gluconate was administered (<12 months received 10 mg/day, >12 months 20 mg/day) to the treatment group for 7 days. Both placebo and treatment groups also received vitamin A, in line with World Health Organization recommendations. Baseline plasma zinc levels were lower than seen in other studies (e.g. 4.4 micromol/L [1.3–8.0]) and the researchers confirmed that 17.7% of the sample were HIV-positive (highly active antiretroviral treatment-naïve). Interestingly, while zinc failed to reduce recovery time, it significantly reduced mortality (18.8% in placebo versus 6.7%; RR 0.3). This protective effect seen across the treatment group on further analysis was found to be greatest amongst the HIV-positive children (11% in placebo vs 0%; RR 0.2). Additionally, children with either bacterial or viral pneumonia when treated with zinc demonstrated reduced mortality; the majority of cases (75.5%) had a viral cause. The number needed to treat in order to save one life was 13 and, poignantly, the authors comment that this comes at a meagre cost of US$4.

Another study of adjunctive zinc (20 mg/day sulfate; administered for a maximum of 14 days) in paediatric (2–24 months) pneumonia (n = 550) where baseline plasma zinc averaged ≈9 micromol/L found that, in spite of significant increases in plasma zinc levels in the treatment group (4.3 ± 5.6 micromol), there was no significant reduction in time to recovery overall (Wadhwa et al 2013). Further analysis revealed that children diagnosed with very severe pneumonia at baseline did exhibit increased recovery time with zinc supplementation and there was a non-significant trend of reduced treatment failure in this subgroup.

Age-related macular degeneration (ARMD)

Both dietary and supplemental zinc have been investigated in the prevention and/or delayed progression of ARMD. This is not surprising as evidence that lifetime oxidative stress plays an important role in the development of ARMD is now compelling (Hogg & Chakravarthy 2004). ARMD is thought to be the result of free radical damage to photoreceptors within the macula, and therefore it is suspected that inefficient macular antioxidant systems play a role in disease development. After ageing, smoking is the next significant risk factor and a direct association between risk and the number of cigarettes smoked has been reported (Coleman et al 2008, Wills et al 2008a). Smokers have four times greater retinal cadmium concentrations than non-smokers and the associated morphological changes are reasonably consistent with ARMD pathology (Wills et al 2008a).

A 2005 study found that high dietary intake of zinc, beta-carotene and vitamins C and E was associated with a 35% reduced risk in elderly persons (van Leeuwen et al 2005). Similarly, the Blue Mountains Eye Study, an Australian prospective population-based cohort study conducted over 10 years, demonstrated protective effects of lutein and zeaxanthin, but also found that those individuals consuming the highest zinc had an RR of 0.56 for any ARMD and 0.54 for early ARMD compared with all other participants (Tan et al 2008). An interesting study has revealed that increased lifetime exposure to blue light appears to amplify the risk of low dietary antioxidants and zinc (Fletcher et al 2008). Originally it was believed that zinc simply acts as an antioxidant in this condition, yet ongoing discussions of zinc's possible actions in the prevention of this aetiology has produced new hypotheses.

A comparison of zinc and copper concentrations within the retinal pigment epithelium and choroid complex of eye donor subjects previously suffering from ARMD and those without the condition has revealed a 23–24% reduction in these metals in afflicted subjects (Erie et al 2009). Furthermore, in vitro studies confirm that zinc and copper, as well as manganese (the latter being most potent), effectively prevent the intracellular concentration of cadmium in retinal tissues and hence modulate its toxicity (Satarug et al 2008, Wills et al 2008b). Taken together, the knowledge that zinc and copper supplementation, in combination with antioxidants, has delayed progression of ARMD points towards a critical role for metal homeostasis in retinal health.

A 2006 Cochrane review assessed the effects of antioxidant vitamin and/or mineral supplementation on the progression of ARMD and found that evidence of effectiveness is currently dominated by one large trial that showed modest benefit in people with moderate to severe signs of the disease (Evans 2002). The study the authors refer to is the Age-Related Eye Disease Study (AREDS 2001), which showed that high-dose vitamins C and E, beta-carotene and zinc supplementation delayed the progression from intermediate to advanced disease by 25% over 5 years. The 11-centre, double-blind, prospective study involved 3640 volunteers aged between 55 and 80 years who were randomly divided into four treatment groups, receiving either antioxidant supplements (500 mg vitamin C, 400 IU vitamin E, and 15 mg beta-carotene daily), zinc oxide and cupric oxide (80 mg elemental zinc, 2 mg elemental copper daily), antioxidants plus zinc, or placebo. This treatment effect appeared to persist following 5 additional years of follow-up after the clinical trial was stopped. The AREDS formulation became the standard of care for persons who are at high risk for ARMD (Chew 2013); however, the actual contribution of zinc to this result is unknown (see Lutein monograph for more information about ARMD).

A more recent randomised controlled trial tested supplementation with zinc monocysteine (25 mg elemental zinc twice daily) as a stand-alone treatment to 80 ARMD patients over 6 months (Newsome 2008). Those in the treatment group experienced improved visual acuity, contrast sensitivity and reduced macular light flash recovery time when compared with the placebo group, with some benefits evident 3 months into the treatment.

Overall, current evidence suggests that zinc supplementation, either alone or in combination with other antioxidants, may help to prevent ARMD in those at least at moderate risk and delay progression of this condition in those suffering the early stages. Additional evidence suggests that genetic factors may be important when determining who will best respond to this treatment. Retrospective analyses of the AREDS study demonstrated a strong interaction between those individuals whose progression of the condition was delayed by zinc supplementation and the presence of the complement factor H genotype (Klein et al 2008, Lee & Brantley 2008). Substantiation of these findings could assist in the improved targeting of ARMD nutritional therapies.

Herpes simplex virus (HSV) infection

Various topical zinc applications have been studied, producing encouraging results in reducing the incidence, severity and duration of symptoms in HSV infection.

In a study of 90 volunteers with diagnosed genital herpes, three different concentrations of liquid zinc sulfate (1%, 2% and 4%) were compared. The strongest concentration (4%) gave the lowest risk of recurrence over a 6-month test period compared to the others or a control group using only distilled water (Mahajan et al 2013). The treatments were applied with a cotton bud to genital herpetic lesions every 5 days for a month, then every 10 days for 2 months and finally every 15 days for 3 months. This protective effect has also been demonstrated in vivo for topical zinc acetate (0.5–1%) in a carrageenan-based gel applied locally for 7 days prior to vaginal or rectal exposure to the virus (Kenney et al 2013).

A double-blind randomised controlled trial of 46 people with facial and circumoral herpes infection showed that prompt application of a zinc oxide and glycine cream every 2 hours reduced recovery time from 6.5 to 5 days. The people using active treatment also experienced a reduction in the overall severity of signs and symptoms, particularly blistering, soreness, itching and tingling, compared to controls. The only side effects reported were a burning and itching sensation (Godfrey et al 2001). Previously, another double-blind randomised controlled trial showed that a zinc sulfate (1%) gel applied every few hours resulted in 50% of patients with HSV-1 becoming symptom-free by day 5 compared to only 35% in the placebo group (Kneist et al 1995). Another study of 200 volunteers with herpes simplex found that a lower dose of only 0.25% zinc sulfate solution, started within 24 hours of lesion appearance and applied 8–10 times daily, cleared lesions within 3–6 days (Finnerty 1986). Not surprisingly, a randomised controlled trial using a far lower dose of 0.05% or 0.025% zinc sulfate found no effects on frequency, duration or severity of herpes attacks, suggesting that stronger concentrations are required for effectiveness (Graham et al 1985).

According to an experimental study using zinc oxide, the attachment of HSV-2 to target cells is inhibited by the presence of zinc (Antoine et al 2012). In vitro studies also confirm that zinc can inhibit the replication of HSV; however, the concentration required is much higher than possible in a physiological context (Overbeck et al 2008).

Interestingly, new research suggests that people with recurrent HSV-1 have significantly lower salivary zinc levels compared to healthy controls and that levels are lowest in the acute phase compared to the convalescent phase (Khozeimeh et al 2012).

Diabetes mellitus (type 1 and 2)

Zinc is abundant in the pancreas due to extensive roles in both its endocrine and exocrine functions. During deficiency, this is one of the few tissues that demonstrates reduced concentrations (Islam & Loots 2007). Limited data derived from both epidemiological studies and animal models suggest that increased dietary zinc intake may be protective against the development of both types of diabetes (Bolkent et al 2009, Islam & Loots 2007, Sun et al 2009). It is suspected that zinc may have a protective role due to its antioxidant activity, both directly and indirectly, via MT induction (Islam & Loots 2007). Decreasing oxidative stress may protect beta cells from damage and therefore assist in maintaining normal insulin secretion.

Zinc supplementation is sometimes used to avoid deficiency, a state synonymous with both type 1 and type 2 diabetes due to a combination of increased losses and reduced uptake (Chimienti 2013, Cunningham et al 1994). While animal studies have demonstrated improved glucose management with zinc, the results from human studies are less consistent (Chimienti 2013). It remains unclear whether simply addressing zinc deficiency or using high-dose zinc to induce other effects will be beneficial in the clinical management of diabetes, its complications or its prevention, as evidence from both animal and human studies has produced varying results (Baydas et al 2002, Cunningham et al 1994, Farvid et al 2004, Gupta et al 1998, Niewoehner et al 1986, Roussel et al 2003, Tobia et al 1998).

Several intervention studies utilising oral zinc have produced positive results in populations with type 1 diabetes, with evidence of reduced HbA_{1C} amongst individuals in the treatment group (30 mg/day elemental zinc for 3 months) when compared to controls (Al-Maroof & Al-Sharbatti 2006), improved blood lipid profiles following 12 weeks of zinc treatment (100 mg/day zinc sulfate) in another study (Partida-Hernández et al 2006) and improved glycaemic control and diabetic neuropathy in 20 patients administered 660 mg/day zinc sulfate over 6 weeks (Hayee et al 2005). Interestingly, new research has identified a fourth autoantibody common to type 1 diabetes which is made against the zinc transporter unique to islet cells (ZnT8) and therefore impairs zinc accumulation within the DCVs, making altered zinc regulation a potential cause (Chimienti 2013, O'Halloran et al 2013). Incredibly, since the 1930s it was known that the pancreas of diabetics contained only half of the zinc found in healthy individuals (Chimienti 2013).

Zinc supplementation to address the secondary multisystem effects of type 1 diabetes has been investigated with regard to vascular changes in mice. In control genetic type 1 diabetes mice, significant increases in aortic oxidative damage, inflammation, fibrosis and thickness were observed; however, in mice receiving $ZnSO_4$ 5 mg/kg over 3 months these changes were completely prevented, reportedly due to upregulation of both MT and Nrf2 (Miao et al 2013). In vitro studies of human endothelial cells have produced similar findings.

With respect to type 2 diabetes, a prospective, double-blind, clinical interventional study of 56 obese women with normal glucose tolerance randomised subjects to treatment with zinc, 30 mg/day, or placebo for 4 weeks (Marreiro et al 2002). Zinc treatment decreased insulin resistance from 5.8 to 4.3 and insulin decreased from 28.8 to 21.2 mU/mL, but was unchanged in the placebo group. These results are particularly noteworthy because the women were not zinc-deficient, suggesting a therapeutic role for zinc. Another small study of metformin-resistant patients with type 2 diabetes administered zinc (zinc acetate 50 mg/day) in combination with melatonin (10 mg/day) ± metformin to two treatment groups and placebo to a third (Hussain et al 2006). This combined treatment proved effective in improving fasting and postprandial glucose levels and augmented the action of the hypoglycaemic drug.

Zinc deficiency has been established as an independent risk factor for fatal coronary heart disease events in a large cohort of patients with type 2 diabetes, with serum zinc values < 14.1 micromol/L associated with 20.8% patients with fatal events versus 12.8% ($P < 0.001$) (Sarmento et al 2013, Soinio et al 2007). Studies investigating zinc's potential for reducing these secondary deleterious effects are still emerging. One randomised double-blind crossover study of 50 patients with type 2 diabetes with microalbuminuria, administered 30 mg/day elemental zinc over 3 months, revealed a significant reduction in homocysteine levels (from 13.71 ± 3.84 micromol/L to 11.79 ± 3.06 micromol/L; $P < 0.05$), a cardiovascular inflammatory mediator, while improving folate and B_{12} status. Other proposed protective effects are via both general anti-inflammatory and antioxidant actions as well as via MT induction (Miao et al 2013).

Regarding diabetic retinopathy, hypothesised protective mechanisms include zinc's inhibition of vascular endothelial growth factor, involved in the initiation and progression of neovascularisation and vascular leakage in diabetic retinopathy; however, clinical studies are lacking to date (Miao et al 2013).

Further studies with larger sample sizes are required to validate zinc as an effective treatment in type 1 and 2 diabetes and elucidate the optimal dosing and administration regimen. There is currently a study under way in Sri Lanka investigating zinc supplementation in prediabetics which may also further our knowledge in this area (Ranasinghe et al 2013).

Clinical note — Zinc deficiency and diabetes

Diabetes affects zinc homeostasis in many ways and is associated with increased urinary loss, decreased absorption and decreased total body zinc (Chausmer 1998, Cunningham et al 1994). The role of zinc and zinc deficiency in diabetes and its complications or prevention is currently unclear. It has been suggested that deficiency may exacerbate destruction of islet cells in type 1 diabetes and may adversely affect the synthesis, storage and secretion of insulin, a process that requires zinc. Furthermore, evidence indicates that patients with type 1 diabetes have a higher concentration of free radicals than healthy controls; this is due to increased oxidant production and/or decreased efficiency of endogenous antioxidant systems (Davison et al 2002). It is suspected that deficiency of key micronutrients (i.e. zinc, copper, manganese and selenium), which are integral components of important antioxidant systems, may be partly responsible.

Wound healing

Zinc is an essential cofactor in both wound healing and immune function. Therefore, zinc deficiency retards both fibroplasia and epithelialisation, and results in delayed wound healing in spite of maintained skin stores of zinc, except in instances of severe concomitant protein restriction (Lansdown et al 2007). Zinc supplements are used to restore zinc status in cases of wound healing associated with malnutrition and deficiency. Additionally, zinc administered orally or topically to wounds can promote healing and reduce infection, according to one major review (Lansdown 1996).

Oral application

In 2001, a randomised study demonstrated that oral zinc sulfate significantly improved healing of cutaneous leishmaniasis (Sharquie et al 2001). Results showed that the cure rate for a dose of 2.5 mg/kg was 83.9%, for 5 mg/kg it was 93.1% and for 10 mg/kg it was 96.9%, whereas no lesions showed any sign of healing in the control group. The results of several studies suggest a specific role for oral zinc in surgical wound repair (Lansdown et al 2007). Zinc redistribution and sequestration in the liver occur following both surgical trauma and infection. The corresponding reduction in serum zinc may then impair the individual's healing capacity, as demonstrated in a study of 80 total hip replacement patients (mean age 66 years), in whom serum zinc levels were significantly related to rates of infection and dehiscence (Lansdown et al 2007). Similarly, an interventional study of pre- and postoperative zinc infusion (30 mg/day) in patients undergoing major vascular reconstructive surgery attenuated the anticipated decline in serum zinc and produced significantly fewer wound-healing complications than placebo.

Topical application

Theoretically, topical zinc treatment is most suited to human wound healing that necessitates epithelialisation, e.g. suction blister wound, superficial small incision and split-thickness skin graft donor sites. While clinical trials have demonstrated its efficacy in relation to treatment of leg ulcers, pressure ulcers, diabetic foot ulcers and burn wounds (Lansdown et al 2007), one study also demonstrated that *Staphylococcus aureus* was cultured significantly less frequently in zinc oxide-treated wounds, which points to the additional antiseptic action. Topical zinc oxide promotes cleansing and re-epithelialisation of ulcers and reduces the risk of infection and deterioration of ulcers compared with placebo, according to one double-blind trial of leg ulcer patients with low serum zinc levels (Agren 1990). Evidence from animal and in vitro research suggests that topically applied zinc solution is more effective when combined with iron than when used alone, and can effectively enhance healing in acute partial-thickness and second-degree burn wounds (Feiner et al 2003). The form of zinc used topically may be of marked importance, with some studies investigating high concentrations of zinc sulfate delaying healing and increasing dermal inflammatory cell infiltration (Lansdown et al 2007). Preparations such as zinc oxide may be more suitable than readily water-soluble forms, providing a sustained release of bioavailable zinc at non-cytotoxic levels. Interestingly, pharmacopoeias attribute various zinc forms with different qualities/actions, e.g. zinc sulfate is regarded as a local astringent and antiseptic, insoluble zinc oxide as a mild antiseptic, astringent and protective agent, particularly indicated in inflamed skin and wounds.

Arterial and venous leg ulcers

Chronic leg ulcer patients often exhibit abnormal zinc metabolism and depressed serum concentrations (Lansdown et al 2007). A 2000 Cochrane review assessed six placebo-controlled trials of zinc sulfate supplementation (≈220 mg administered three times daily) in arterial and venous leg ulcers and concluded that, overall, there is no evidence of a beneficial effect on the number of ulcers healed. However, there is some evidence that oral zinc might improve healing of venous ulcers in people with low serum zinc levels (Wilkinson & Hawke 2000).

Double-blind studies producing encouraging results have used oral zinc (600 mg/day) combined with topical treatment and compression bandages (Haeger & Lanner 1974, Hallbook & Lanner 1972).

Acne and other skin conditions

Over the past two to three decades, tetracyclines and macrolide antibiotics have been widely prescribed for the treatment of acne; however, resistance has been reported, especially to erythromycin and clindamycin, with cross-resistance being widespread among strains of *Propionibacterium acnes* and increasing (Iinuma et al 2011). As a result, non-antibiotic treatments such as topical/oral zinc preparations have been investigated as both alternatives and adjunctive therapy.

Overall, there is increasingly consistent clinical evidence of the efficacy of zinc (both oral and topical) for the treatment of acne, showing it can improve skin condition. However, definitive conclusions are hampered by some poor-quality studies. Some studies utilise zinc supplementation in combination with other nutrients, making it difficult to ascertain the role of zinc but providing clinical guidance nonetheless.

Surprisingly, it is only recently that epidemiological research has demonstrated lower plasma zinc in acne patients ($P < 0.001$) and that blood zinc (and vitamin E) correlates with acne severity (Ozuguz et al 2014). Dietary analysis was not performed in this study, which still leaves the question of whether the low zinc is the cause or consequence of acne.

Oral supplementation

Numerous studies have been conducted investigating the effects of zinc supplementation in acne vulgaris (Dreno et al 1989, 1992, 2001, Goransson et al 1978, Hillstrom et al 1977, Orris et al 1978, Verma et al 1980, Weimar et al 1978, Weismann et al 1977). Doses between 90 mg and 200 mg (30 mg elemental zinc) daily taken over 6–12 weeks have been associated with generally positive results, whereas larger doses tend to be poorly tolerated.

Two double-blind studies have compared the effects of oral zinc supplementation with two antibiotic medicines, minocycline or oxytetracycline, over 3 months (Cunliffe et al 1979, Dreno et al 1989). Zinc sulfate (135 mg) was as effective as oxytetracycline after 12 weeks' use, decreasing acne scores by 65% in one study, whereas the same dose was not as effective as minocycline (500 mg) in the second study. An open study involving 30 subjects with inflammatory acne found that a lower dose of oral zinc gluconate (30 mg) taken daily reduced the number of inflammatory lesions after 2 months, regardless of whether *P. acnes* was present (Dreno et al 2005).

Both oral and topical zinc have also been investigated as an adjunct to antibiotic therapy under laboratory conditions. When administered in combination with erythromycin, it inhibits erythromycin-resistant propionibacteria according to two in vitro studies (Dreno et al 2005, Oprica et al 2002).

IN COMBINATION

A more recent open-label observational study involving 48 subjects with moderate acne vulgaris, treated with a zinc antioxidant combination (equivalent to 15 mg elemental zinc, 60 mg vitamin C, 15 IU vitamin E and 0.13 mg chromium) administered over 12 weeks produced a 79% response rate. Although a large clinical improvement (80–100%) was reported, particularly with respect to reduced inflammatory features, the absence of a control group and blinding of the intervention detract from the positive findings (Sardana & Garg 2010). Similarly, another open-label trial with positive findings in acne patients adds little to our evidence base for zinc, given the intervention was a multivitamin mineral containing forms of zinc and other minerals with poor bioavailability, i.e. oxides (Shalita et al 2012).

Topical application

A number of studies have investigated the effects of a topical erythromycin–zinc acetate (≈1.2%) formulation (Bojar et al 1994, Feucht et al 1980, Habbema et al 1989, Morgan et al 1993, Pierard & Pierard-Franchimont 1993, Pierard-Franchimont et al 1995, Schachner et al 1990).

Statistically significant effects have been observed within the first 12 weeks of treatment for acne severity grades, and for papule, pustule and comedo counts, with the effect of the combination superior to preparations containing erythromycin alone (Habbema et al 1989, Schachner et al 1990). A systematic review of acne treatments also concluded that topical erythromycin–zinc appears to be more effective than the antibiotic alone for the treatment of both inflammatory and non-inflammatory lesions (Purdy & de Berker 2011).

A 2013 review of 29 studies investigating zinc and acne concluded that there is inconsistent or limited quality patient-centred evidence for either oral or topical treatment with zinc; however, the review was funded and partly written by Galderma, a manufacturer of non-zinc-based acne treatments, thereby requiring confirmation by other researchers (Brandt 2013).

Human studies have identified antibacterial activity against *Propionibacterium* spp. in short-term treatment, which is mostly attributed to zinc (Fluhr et al 1999) and sebosuppressive effects (Pierard & Pierard-Franchimont 1993). New in vitro research, building on prior successful studies using topical ascorbic acid derivatives, has found superior antimicrobial activity in zinc ascorbate compared with other ascorbates, e.g. 0.064% concentration compared with 5% (Iinuma et al 2011). The study also confirms an additive effect when combined with some topical antibiotics (i.e. erythromycin and clindamycin) and, perhaps more impressively, demonstrated that zinc ascorbate was effective as a stand-alone treatment in inhibiting the proliferation of antibiotic-resistant strains of *P. acnes* (minimum inhibitory concentration 640 mcg/mL). The same researchers have shown topical zinc ascorbate similarly possesses potent antimicrobial activity against *Staphylococcus aureus* and, to a lesser extent, *Escherichia coli*, Gram-negative bacteria that typically act in concert with *P. acnes* in acne vulgaris. Again this is seen at significantly lower concentrations than with other ascorbate derivatives and ascorbic acid alone (Iinuma & Tsuboi 2012). Both zinc and ascorbic acid's capacity to inhibit ROS production (SOD-like activity) is speculated as an important attribute in acne treatment, with previous research demonstrating that elevated ROS and impaired SOD are characteristic features in acne patients, leading to an excess inflammatory response.

Reduced male fertility

Zinc deficiency leads to several clinical signs, such as decreased spermatogenesis, altered sperm morphology and impaired male fertility and, given zinc's pivotal role in DNA transcription, this is not surprising. Furthermore, zinc finger proteins are critical to the genetic expression of steroid hormone receptors. Together with zinc's additional antiapoptotic and antioxidant actions, these effects make zinc a promising contributor to healthy sperm (Ebisch et al 2007). The relationship between zinc concentrations in seminal fluid and semen fertility, however, remains somewhat unclear.

When zinc deficiency is not present, a 2002 survey found no statistically significant relationship between zinc in seminal plasma or serum and semen quality or local antisperm antibody of the immunoglobulin G (IgG) or IgA class (Eggert-Kruse et al 2002). Furthermore, zinc levels did not influence sperm capacity to penetrate cervical mucus in vitro or in vivo, nor affect subsequent fertility. However, a study of Chinese men (aged 20–59 years) revealed that, when serum zinc concentration was low, the risk of asthenozoospermia increased and the Cu/Zn ratio was higher in those with progressive motility abnormalities (Yuyan et al 2008).

In contrast to this, a small number of both animal (Kumar et al 2006) and human supplementation studies (Ebisch et al 2006) have produced positive results. The latter study, involving 40 subfertile and 47 fertile men treated for 26 weeks with 66 mg/day zinc sulfate and 5 mg/day folic acid or placebo, produced a 74% increase in normal sperm count in the subfertile subjects; however, more studies with larger sample sizes and measurement of pregnancy outcomes are required to substantiate these preliminary findings. In spite of this relative paucity of randomised controlled trial evidence, a trend of treatment has begun. A recent review of antioxidant supplementation in the treatment of idiopathic oligoasthenoteratospermia observes that, while elevated ROS is undoubtedly damaging to spermatids and mature spermatozoa and is implicated in male infertility, antioxidant treatment including zinc, which has become widely accepted, is yet to be established as efficacious (Agarwal & Sekhon 2010).

Impotence

In men, zinc deficiency may lead to impaired testosterone synthesis, resulting in hypogonadism and impotency. One placebo-controlled study has investigated whether oral zinc supplementation improves erectile dysfunction. The study involved 20 uraemic haemodialysis patients and showed that 6 months' treatment with oral zinc acetate (25 mg elemental zinc) taken twice daily 1–2 hours before meals resulted in greater libido, improved potency and more frequent intercourse compared to placebo (Mahajan et al 1982). Active treatment also resulted in significant increases in plasma zinc, serum testosterone and sperm count and decreases in serum levels of luteinising hormone and follicle-stimulating hormone.

Attention-deficit hyperactivity disorder (ADHD)

Zinc deficiency has been implicated in the pathogenesis of ADHD from numerous perspectives. With a critical role in neurological development and evidence of impaired learning and depressed psychomotor retardation in deficiency states, zinc may constitute a direct aetiological cause (Black 2003, Fanjiang & Kleinman 2007). An interesting longitudinal paediatric study found that children with malnutrition (protein, zinc and iron deficiencies) at 3 years of age demonstrated higher externalisation behaviour problems at 8, 11 and 17 years, when compared to replete children (Liu & Raine 2006), with this trifecta of deficiencies, a particularly common combination in young children.

Hypotheses of indirect actions of zinc deficiency include negative behavioural effects mediated via impaired fatty acid metabolism, blockage of the dopamine transporter to increase synaptic concentrations and through the exacerbation of heavy-metal effects.

In 1990, Arnold et al observed that boys aged 6–12 years with ADHD and a higher baseline hair zinc level had better responses to amphetamine therapy than children with hair concentrations indicative of mild zinc deficiency. At the time, it was suggested that poor/non-responders to drug therapy and those presenting with suboptimal zinc status would require zinc supplementation instead of amphetamine treatment to address the condition. Since then, numerous controlled studies have identified that children with ADHD have lower zinc tissue levels (serum, red cells, hair, urine, nails) than normal children (Arnold & DiSilvestro 2005). It is not certain why this occurs, but it may result from not sitting for long enough to consume a balanced diet, picky eating, stimulant-related appetite suppression, malabsorption or biochemical changes. Recently it has been suggested that zinc may be a proxy of poor diet quality in this group (Ghanizadeh & Berk 2013). Zinc status has also been also shown to correlate with the amplitude and latency of select brain waves, suggesting that zinc may particularly influence information processing in ADHD children (Yorbik et al 2008).

Three early double-blind studies, all conducted in Middle Eastern populations, investigated whether oral zinc supplementation has a beneficial effect in ADHD, producing promising results. One randomised study involving 400 Turkish children with a mean age of 9.6 years found that treatment with 150 mg zinc sulfate (equivalent to 40 mg of elemental zinc) daily for 12 weeks resulted in significant reductions in hyperactive, impulsive and impaired socialisation features, but not in reducing attention deficiency symptoms, as assessed by the ADHD scale (Bilici et al 2004). A significant difference between zinc and placebo was evident by week 4 ($P = 0.01$). Older children with low zinc and free fatty acid levels and high body mass index responded best to treatment.

A second placebo-controlled trial used a combination of 55 mg zinc sulfate (equivalent to 15 mg elemental zinc) and methylphenidate (1 mg/kg) daily for 6 weeks in Iranian children aged 5–11 years and reported significant benefits with the combination (Akhondzadeh et al 2004). Zinc (15 mg/day elemental) or placebo was administered to 218 grade three students in a low-income district of Turkey over 10 weeks, resulting in a reduced prevalence of clinically significant ratings of attention deficit and hyperactivity in the treatment group (Uçkardeş et al 2009). As all of these early studies were conducted in Middle Eastern countries where zinc deficiency is particularly prevalent, researchers were keen to see results of studies conducted in other regions and the chance arose with an American three-phased pilot study published in 2011 (Arnold et al 2011).

Being a pilot study, the numbers are small ($n = 52$, with only 28 assigned to zinc); however, the methodology is regarded as substantially superior to prior studies, including more comprehensive zinc assessment both pre- and posttreatment. The first phase was essentially a single-blind 8-week trial of zinc (15 mg/day as glycinate) compared with placebo, while the second phase added in open-label amphetamine (dosage according to body weight), maintained over 2 weeks. The third phase, which lasted 3 weeks, allowed clinicians to closely monitor and accordingly titrate the dose of amphetamine with no change to the zinc or placebo from the first phase. The findings were that zinc supplementation was not effective either alone or as an adjunct to amphetamines in the management of ADHD; however, it did reduce the effective dose necessary of the stimulant medication. What is particularly interesting about this study, the negative findings of which are given a lot of weight in a recent review by Ghanizadeh & Berk (2013), is the low zinc dose used and the subsequent failure to raise serum zinc in the supplemented group. In fact, in the third phase the researchers doubled this dose in 8 subjects, which produced greater improvements both on serum levels and behaviour ratings, begging the question of whether the dose administered to the majority was inadequate.

Somewhat similarly, two longer-term studies (6 months) conducted in Mexico and Guatemala failed to find a positive effect from zinc supplementation. However, in both instances, zinc oxide (a poorly absorbed form) was used to provide only 10 mg elemental zinc per day and there were numerous other confounding variables, e.g. lead intoxication (Kordas et al 2005) and lack of diagnostic criteria and selection for ADHD children only (DiGirolamo et al 2010).

The aforementioned systematic review includes the American study by Arnold and two of the mid-Eastern trials, ultimately concluding that there is insufficient evidence of efficacy for zinc in the management of ADHD and recommending that future studies correct for methodological flaws of the past (Ghanizadeh & Berk 2013). Until there is research of a higher standard with consistent outcomes, the case for zinc in ADHD is promising but requires further investigation to determine optimal dosage, treatment regimens and what symptoms are most likely to respond.

Depression

Zinc deficiency has been investigated as a contributing factor to the development of depression. Zinc supplementation has also been investigated as a treatment in depression, most commonly as an adjunctive therapy taken with standard pharmaceutical agents, for which there is positive evidence.

Epidemiological evidence has revealed an inverse relationship between serum zinc and depression-rating scores in depressed patients (Nowak et al 2005, Siwek et al 2010), the elderly (Marcellini et al 2006) and postpartum women (Wojcik et al 2006). Inadequate dietary intake has also been correlated with increased depression rates, particularly amongst women, in an American food frequency study (Maserejian et al 2012). A meta-analysis of 17 epidemiological studies (n = 1643 depressed individuals and 804 controls) investigating zinc levels and depression adds further weight to this association (Swardfager et al 2013), with 16 studies demonstrating a relationship. While meta-analysis found the actual difference in plasma/serum zinc to be small — approximately −1.85 micromol/L lower in depressed compared with control individuals ($P < 0.00001$) — the effect size increased in individuals with more severe depression, inpatients and studies with more robust methodology. It is important to note that these lower levels were typically still within the established reference range. While associations do not prove causality, there is also an increasing body of evidence piecing together how zinc might convey such antidepressant effects.

Zinc supplementation produces antidepressant-like effects in animal tests and models such as the forced-swim test and can augment the action of orthodox antidepressants in these scenarios (Nowak et al 2005). Theories regarding zinc's aetiological role in depression traditionally centred on its inhibition of *N*-methyl-D-aspartate receptor function and regulation of both hippocampal and cortical glutaminergic circuits and, interestingly, suicide victims demonstrate a statistically significant 26% decrease in zinc's antagonistic potency in hippocampal tissue, suggestive of an aberrant interaction between this mineral and the receptor underlying the psychopathology (Nowak et al 2003). There is current interest in the increased inflammatory markers evident in depressed individuals, which would, through redistribution of zinc, potentially create a pseudodeficiency (Marcellini et al 2006, Nowak et al 2005) and, via zinc's roles in both immunity generally and antioxidant defence specifically, improve with supplementation (Swardfager et al 2013, Szewczyk et al 2011). Other theories regarding mechanisms include zinc's capacity to increase synaptic dopamine levels (Stockner et al 2013), its critical role in fatty acid metabolism (Swardfager et al 2013), increased neural plasticity, increased hippocampal BDNF RNA and inhibition of the GSK-3 enzyme (Szewczyk et al 2008).

In spite of growing interest in zinc's antidepressant potential, there have been limited published interventional studies to date. Twenty patients with unipolar depression had an improved response to antidepressant medication when it was taken with zinc aspartate supplements (equivalent to 25 mg elemental daily), according to a small, double-blind pilot study (Nowak et al 2003). Significantly greater reductions in Hamilton Depression Rating Scale scores were achieved with zinc treatment compared to placebo by the 6th week and maintained until the end of the 12-week study. The same research group published the results of a study very similar in design, using ≈140 mg imipramine and 25 mg supplemental zinc (n = 30), compared with imipramine and placebo in the control group (n = 30) over 12 weeks, also with positive findings (Siwek et al 2009), and in a follow-up publication were able to show that treatment-resistant subjects had lower serum zinc (−14%) when compared with those subjects responsive to treatment, as did those who had had depression for a longer duration. They also found that serum zinc increased in all responders whether supplemented or not, concurrent with remission and a negative correlation between serum zinc and ratings on the Montgomery-Asberg Depression Rating Scale at the study's conclusion in all subjects (Siwek et al 2010). Based on their findings, Siwek et al go as far as to say that changes in serum zinc can be viewed as a state marker of depression and remission. A 2012 review paper which includes the Nowak et al and Siwek et al studies, as well as two others, concludes that there is consistent evidence of zinc's efficacy as an adjunct to antidepressants but less certainty as a stand-alone treatment (Lai et al 2012).

Diarrhoea

An updated 2013 Cochrane review of oral zinc treatment for paediatric diarrhoea which analysed results from 18 randomised controlled trials (n = 6165) concluded that zinc supplementation consistently reduced the duration and volume of both acute and persistent diarrhoea within a few days (for example, by day 3 of the intervention: RR 0.69, 95% CI 0.59–0.81; 1073 children, two trials) (Lazzerini & Ronfani 2013). While zinc-treated children were significantly more likely to experience vomiting as an adverse reaction to the supplement, it was concluded that the benefits of the treatment outweighed this side effect.

Typically, the intervention consisted of 10 mg/day of zinc, as a sulfate, acetate or gluconate salt, administered in a single or divided dose over 2 weeks to children aged 1 month to 5 years presenting with acute or persistent diarrhoea or dysentery. It is important to note that all except three of these trials were conducted in countries considered to be at high risk of widespread zinc deficiency and in such instances, due to the high rates of malnourishment, the RDA for zinc for <5-year-olds jumps to 2–4 mg/kg compared with only 3–5 mg/day in developed countries. Interestingly, however, there was no effect from geographical location, background zinc deficiency, supplemental form or general nutritional status. This review found no benefit in children less than 6 months old and it remains unclear at this time whether morbidity rates were impacted in children of any age.

Coeliac disease

Untreated coeliac patients demonstrate increased turnover and losses of intestinal zinc, although the mechanisms behind this appear to be greater than malabsorption alone (Tran et al 2011). In fact, researchers claim that zinc deficiency is the earliest and most pronounced nutritional issue in untreated CD adults (Scrimgeour & Condlin 2009), and researchers investigating zinc status in children undergoing investigation for CD concluded that a low serum zinc should be a prompt in this cohort for small-bowel biopsy (Hogberg et al 2009). A study of zinc homeostasis in children with CD found a correlation between impaired disaccharide digestion, reduced fractional zinc absorption and reduced zinc status and suggested that treated CD patients with ongoing gastrointestinal derangement are key candidates for zinc deficiency (Tran et al 2011). Interestingly, zinc is a potent inhibitor of the tissue transglutaminase (tTG) type 2 enzyme, therefore in zinc deficiency this will lead to greater activation of tTG, ultimately increasing the inflammation and villi atrophy at the core of CD pathology (Scrimgeour & Condlin 2009, Stenberg et al 2008). Recent research adds to concerns of zinc deficiency in the CD population, in finding that a gluten-free diet provides inadequate zinc levels for most individuals, therefore making supplementation a necessity (Shepherd & Gibson 2013). To date there are no published studies investigating the benefits of zinc supplementation in CD.

Crohn's disease

Zinc is important in the maintenance of gastrointestinal barrier function. Research has revealed that patients with inflammatory bowel disease with low mucosal zinc levels typically accumulate neutrophils in epithelial crypts and the intestinal lumen, resulting in the formation of crypt abscesses, which constitute a serious complication of the disease (Scrimgeour & Condlin 2009). Although reduced zinc status has long been associated with chronic diarrhoea and Crohn's disease (Sturniolo et al 1980), the results from a small open study demonstrated that oral zinc sulfate (110 mg three times daily) resolved intestinal permeability problems in people with increased permeability and decreased relapse rates (Sturniolo et al 2001). Given animal and human evidence suggesting that the supplemental form, zinc carnosine, has particular injury/ulcer-preventing actions (Mahmood et al 2007, Watari et al 2013), some researchers speculate whether this may be especially indicated in patients with inflammatory bowel disease (Scrimgeour & Condlin 2009).

Anorexia nervosa

Evidence suggests zinc deficiency may be intimately involved with anorexia nervosa, if not as an initiating cause, then as an accelerating or 'sustaining' factor for abnormal eating behaviours that may deepen the pathology of the anorexia in relation to neurological, immunological and metabolic aberrations (McClain et al 1992, Saito et al 2007, Shay & Mangian 2000). Zinc status is compromised due to an inadequate zinc intake, with supplementation (50 mg elemental zinc/day) shown to decrease depression and anxiety, stop body weight loss and improve weight gain (Katz et al 1987, Safai-Kutti 1990). According to one randomised, double-blind, placebo-controlled trial, 100 mg of zinc gluconate (14 mg/day elemental) doubled the rate of subjects with anorexia nervosa increasing their body mass index compared to placebo (Birmingham et al 1994); however, two other studies in a similiar cohort administered 50 mg zinc/day failed to show any improvement over placebo in weight gain (Flament et al 2012). Results from a series of animal studies suggest that zinc may stimulate food intake in short-term zinc-deficient rats through the afferent vagus nerve, with subsequent effects on hypothalamic peptides, such as increased expression of neuropeptide Y and orexin (Suzuki et al 2011). Accordingly, some key researchers advocate for routine prescribing of zinc for a minimum of 2 months in all anorexia nervosa patients (Birmingham & Gritzner 2006), in spite of reviewers concluding there is inadequate evidence to support this practice (Flament et al 2012).

Recent research has highlighted significantly greater serum zinc in recovered individuals when compared with those who remain ill; however, this is speculated to be largely due to altered dietary intake (Zepf et al 2012a) and, although leptin levels also increase during remission, a small epidemiological study failed to find a correlation between these two phenomena (Zepf et al 2012b).

Improves taste perception

Dysfunctional taste perception, or dysgeusia, is a condition that can at the least affect quality of life and occasionally can become life-threatening. Research into the aetiology of taste impairment has revealed a long list of possible causes and contributing factors, including various pathologies and drugs (Brown & Toma 1986, Deems et al 1991, Ikeda et al 2005, Kettaneh et al 2005, Osaki et al 1996, Rareshide & Amedee 1989, Zverev 2004). The pioneer of research in zinc-related taste acuity, Henkin, concluded in 1976 that zinc could not explain all cases of taste impairment (Henkin et al 1976). A subsequent review concurred: 'depletion of zinc can lead to decreased taste acuity but decreased taste acuity is not necessarily associated with depletion of zinc' (Catalanotto 1978).

Impaired gustatory function in the elderly is also well established (Bales et al 1986, Bartoshuk 1989, Deems et al 1991, Greger 1977, Greger & Geissler 1978, Ikeda et al 2005, Kettaneh et al 2005, Sandstead et al 1982, Schiffman 1983), particularly in relation to salt perception (Bales et al 1986, Greger & Sickles 1979, Sandstead et al 1982). Although zinc status also characteristically declines with age (Bales et al 1986, Greger 1977, Greger & Geissler 1978, Sandstead et al 1982), many studies have failed to demonstrate a consistent correlation between the two phenomena. While this has been challenged by the findings of a study (Stewart-Knox et al 2005), previous large-scale studies of elderly patients presenting with hypogeusia or ageusia have indicated that zinc deficiency represents the sole cause in <40% of elderly patients (Deems et al 1991, Ikeda et al 2005). Other major causes of taste impairment in this age group include the effect of medications and systemic diseases (Deems et al 1991, Ikeda et al 2005, Schiffman 1983). Consequently, confirmation of zinc deficiency in patients with taste impairment is necessary in order to determine the suitability of zinc as a treatment.

Several interventional studies investigating zinc as a treatment for taste impairment have produced generally positive findings. Zinc supplementation of 140 mg of zinc gluconate (20 mg/day elemental) in 50 patients with idiopathic dysgeusia improved gustatory function when compared with placebo (Heckmann et al 2005). In another study of 109 patients with idiopathic taste impairment, including some with low serum zinc, subjects were randomly assigned to either placebo or one of three zinc treatment groups: 17 mg/day, 34 mg/day or 68 mg/day zinc carnosine for 12 weeks (Sakagami et al 2008). Only those patients receiving 68 mg/day demonstrated significantly improved gustatory sensitivity over placebo. Two studies focusing specifically on improving taste perception in the elderly (Ikeda et al 2008, Stewart-Knox et al 2008) have been successful, particularly in relation to increased salt sensitivity and in the former study achieved a 74% response rate for improved gustatory function generally. However, benefit was only evident at doses ≥30 mg/day elemental zinc presented either as a gluconate or as a carnosine complex (Aliani et al 2013).

In contrast, treatment with zinc sulfate (45 mg three times daily) concomitant with and 1 month following radiotherapy treatment in patients suffering from head and neck cancers did not prevent taste alterations typically associated with this treatment and previously speculatively linked with poor zinc status (Halyard et al 2007). A more recent double-blind randomised controlled trial investigating zinc supplementation (50 mg elemental per day as a sulfate) over 3 months in taste disorders of patients receiving chemotherapy (n = 58) also failed to demonstrate any beneficial effect over placebo (Lyckholm et al 2012). Limitations of this study include the informal assessment of taste and lack of baseline zinc assessment, with the researchers concluding that more studies are necessary. New areas of research are investigating relationships between zinc status and specific genetic polymorphisms that impact taste (Noh et al 2013).

Tinnitus

In addition to its many diverse neurological roles, zinc has specifically been shown to modulate synaptic function in the cochlear nucleus through its involvement with glutamate receptors (Coehlo et al 2007). Also required for production of Cu/Zn SOD, the most abundant antioxidant enzyme in this tissue, zinc has a critical role in its healthy function through control of oxidation and the large amounts of generated ROS. There is also evidence that a deficiency of Cu/Zn SOD potentiates ear hair cell degeneration secondary to excessive oxidative damage. Other recent theories regarding zinc's role include its role in the structure of carbonic anhydrase, which removes free radicals in the vascular stria of the cochlea, and its ability to alter the endocochlear potential, altering cochlear electrophysiology (Ferreira et al 2009). In 1987, a report was published suggesting a link between reduced zinc status and intermittent head noises in people suffering with tinnitus (Gersdorff et al 1987). This has been further investigated in several studies; however, the poorly defined patient groups and use of serum zinc as the means of measuring zinc status make interpretation of results difficult to assess (Coehlo et al 2007). Results from these studies, however, suggest a non-significant trend of lower serum zinc values for patients suffering this condition compared to healthy controls.

In 1991 Paaske et al reported the results of a double-blind randomised controlled trial of 48 patients with tinnitus that failed to find a significant effect on symptoms with sustained-release zinc sulfate tablets. Of note, only one subject had low serum zinc levels. A study of 111 subjects aged 20–59 years found that individuals with tinnitus who had normal hearing had significantly lower serum zinc levels than controls, whereas zinc levels were normal for those with accompanying hearing loss (Ochi et al 2003). In addition, a significant correlation between average hearing sensitivity and serum zinc level was observed. Yetiser et al (2002) investigated serum zinc levels and response to supplementation in 40 patients with severe tinnitus of various origins. Some relief in tinnitus symptoms was reported by 57.5% of all subjects who received 220 mg of zinc daily for 2 months; however, the effect was considered minor. When results were divided by age, a different finding emerged, as 82% of people over 50 years of age experienced an improvement on the tinnitus scale compared to only 48% of younger subjects. There was no correlation between severity of tinnitus and serum zinc levels. Zinc supplementation (50 mg/day) was further studied in a randomised, placebo-controlled trial involving 41 Turkish patients with tinnitus of no known cause. Active treatment for 2 months produced clinically favourable progress in 46.4% of subjects; however, this result was not statistically significant (Arda et al 2003).

A review of these studies concluded that, although hampered by methodological weaknesses, zinc treatment may be beneficial in some tinnitus sufferers and, while an optimal dose for zinc has yet to be elucidated, most successful designs have employed 50–66 mg/day of elemental zinc in divided doses (Coehlo et al 2007). A randomised double-blind placebo-controlled cross-over trial designed by Coehlo et al tried to address the limitations of previous studies (Coehlo et al 2013). In a total sample size of 94, individuals were administered zinc 50 mg/day or placebo for a duration of 4 months followed by a 1-month washout and then treatment with the other for the same period. Final analysis revealed that 5% of individuals found their tinnitus improved with zinc and 2% with placebo, the difference being not statistically significant. Subsequently these authors concluded that zinc is not an effective treatment in tinnitus.

Warts

Oral zinc sulfate (10 mg/kg) supplements administered in three divided doses per day (up to 600 mg/day) for 2 months completely cleared recalcitrant viral warts in 87% of patients, according to a single-blind, placebo-controlled trial of 80 volunteers with at least 15 viral warts that were resistant to other treatments (Al Gurairi et al 2002). Warts were completely cleared in 61% of patients after 1 month of treatment, whereas none of the patients receiving placebo reported a successful response and some developed new warts. In both placebo and treatment groups, the drop-out rates were high: 50% and 45%, respectively. Interestingly, patients in the treatment group with low serum zinc baseline levels (mean 62.4 mcg/100 mL) reportedly exhibited no signs or symptoms of deficiency and zinc serum levels failed to rise in the patients who remained resistant to zinc therapy. Treatment with high-dose zinc supplements was accompanied by nausea and in some cases vomiting and mild epigastric pain, although these symptoms were described as mild and transient. A similar intervention was employed in a 2011 open-label study of 31 individuals with non-genital recurring warts with the same dose of zinc sulfate administered over 2 months. While 58% of subjects had deficient serum zinc at baseline, 50% were classed as responders, with full resolution of the warts and no recurrences within a 6-month follow-up (Mun et al 2011).

Wilson's disease

Due to the fact that zinc blocks copper absorption and increases its elimination in people with Wilson's disease, zinc supplementation is a common treatment in this condition. Patients with diagnosed Wilson's disease have increased hepatic glutathione and reduced oxidation when supplemented with zinc sulfate (220 mg three times daily) for 3 months, compared with those using penicillamine (Farinati et al 2003).

OTHER USES

Reducing the risk of cancer

Epidemiological studies suggest that zinc deficiency may be associated with increased risk of cancer (Prasad & Kucuk 2002). Research into mechanisms behind zinc and cancer prevention are being actively pursued via both in vitro (Hong et al 2012) and in vivo research and a key topic of discussion centres around evidence of zinc dysregulation in both prostate and breast cancer (Alam & Kelleher 2012, Ho et al 2011). As yet, however, there are no clinical trials or clear clinical directives from this research.

HIV and AIDS

Given zinc deficiency most profoundly compromises T-cell function, interest in zinc treatment for HIV and AIDS has been ongoing. Low plasma zinc concentration occurs in HIV infection, especially with advancing illness (Wellinghausen et al 2000). The balance of evidence favours the view that a low plasma zinc level is a marker for disease progression (Siberry et al 2002). A series of small interventional studies have produced mixed results, some demonstrating improved immune markers and reduced opportunistic infections (Mocchegiani et al 1995,

Zazzo et al 1989), while others suggesting either no therapeutic effect or increased risk of progression from HIV to AIDS (Tang et al 1996). These contrasting findings have been speculatively attributed to differences in baseline zinc status amongst subjects. One author points out that antiretroviral treatment has been shown to counteract zinc deficiency and therefore administering zinc to individuals taking this medication may enhance the risk of zinc toxicity and its associated immune impairment (Overbeck et al 2008). A small pilot study (n = 31) looked specifically at zinc supplementation in the treatment of immune discordance (defined as complete viral suppression without a rise in $CD4^+$ counts, which is associated with increased morbidity and mortality) amongst HIV-positive patients (Asdamongkol et al 2013). While the results found that 39% of these individuals had deficient plasma zinc, this is not strikingly dissimilar from the incidence in the general HIV population. They also reported that zinc supplementation (15 mg/day as a chelate for 6 months) resulted in increases in $CD4^+$ counts; however, due to the small numbers and lack of control group, their findings are weakened.

In a well-designed larger randomised placebo-controlled study of 231 HIV-positive adults, the treatment group received 12 mg (females) or 15 mg (males) zinc daily for 18 months. In comparison to placebo, zinc treatment was found to reduce the rate of immunological failure, defined as any $CD4^+$ count <200 cells/mm^3 fourfold (RR = 0.24; P < 0.002) and also significantly reduced the occurrence of diarrhoea (OR = 0.4; P = 0.019) (Baum et al 2010).

A 2010 Cochrane review, which does not include the studies cited here, included just two trials in adults (n = 559) and two in children (n = 128) and concluded that zinc supplementation is yet to be established as a beneficial adjunct in HIV management, except in the instance of prevention of diarrhoea in children, where there is a significant decrease in those treated with zinc (P = 0.001) (Irlam et al 2013). One of the limitations, however, of this review is the disparate nature of the HIV populations (from pregnant women to those suffering protracted diarrhoea), as well as heterogeneous design.

Malaria

Duggan et al (2005) identified low plasma zinc levels in children with acute malaria, including a significant correlation between evidence of illness severity, C-reactive protein levels and zinc status; however, this may be an artifact of the acute-phase effects on zinc homeostasis, rather than indicative of genuine depletion (Overbeck et al 2008). Similarly, a recent cross-sectional survey of children in Laos revealed a surprising inverse relationship between serum zinc and anti-*Plasmodium falciparum* IgG antibodies (e.g. an increase of 1 mcg/dL in serum zinc equated with −0.453 in antibody titre, P = 0.003) in individuals with active malaria; however, low zinc secondary to inflammation is flagged as a possible confounding variable by the researchers (Akiyama et al 2013).

Zinc supplementation (10 mg elemental) randomly allocated to preschool children residing in a malaria-endemic region of Papua New Guinea for 6 days a week over 46 weeks reduced morbidity due to *P. falciparum* (Shankar et al 2000). Further studies have produced contradictory findings in relation to zinc's capacity to prevent malaria, while studies of treatment regimens that include zinc as an adjuvant to standard chemotherapy have found no benefit (Overbeck et al 2008). A 2011 review into zinc treatment and the prevention of both morbidity and mortality in <5 years old in developing countries included four studies wherein zinc supplementation was assessed for effect on malaria incidence and found the pooled data failed to reach statistical significance (RR = 0.92; P = 1.04) (Yakoob et al 2011). Similarly, with regard to malaria-related mortality, there was a 10% non-significant reduction in association with zinc supplementation (RR = 0.90; $P = 1.06$).

IN COMBINATION

Subsequent to this review a study designed to investigate whether zinc adds to the preventive effects of vitamin A supplementation in malaria morbidity in Ghana infants administered either a one-off dose of 100,000 IU (<12 months old)/200,000 IU (>12 months old) vitamin A alone ($n = 88$) or additional elemental zinc of 10 mg/day for 6 months ($n = 87$) (Owusu-Agyei et al 2013). Follow-up was also performed 6 months after the conclusion of the supplementation phase. Results show a further 27% reduction in uncomplicated malaria incidence in those infants administered zinc ($P = 0.03$), which equates to reducing incidence from 62.5% in the vitamin A group to 46% in the combined treatment group. The combined intervention, however, failed to have any statistically significant impact on the incidence of other key morbidities such as diarrhoea, pneumonia and severe malaria over vitamin A alone: the reason for this is unknown. It is perhaps noteworthy that the change in plasma zinc from baseline to end point did not reach statistical significance in the supplemented group.

Alzheimer's dementia

There is significant ongoing discussion about the role of zinc deficiency in Alzheimer's disease in the scientific literature. Epidemiological studies have produced some mixed results (da Silva et al 2013, Kyumcu et al 2013, Szewczyk 2013), which may well be the result of disparate methodologies for assessment.

Cognitive performance was temporarily improved after 3 months of zinc supplementation (zinc chelate 15 mg) taken twice daily by six subjects with Alzheimer's disease (Potocnik et al 1997). Although the initial improvement was not maintained in this small open study, a modest cognitive improvement on psychometric testing was observed at 12 months for the four patients evaluated. A double-blind study tested 150 mg of a new zinc formulation per day (unknown elemental zinc content) or placebo for 6 months given to 58 subjects, 29 with Alzheimer's disease and 29 age- and sex-matched controls (Brewer & Kaur 2013). Zinc supplementation was found to raise serum zinc and reduce free copper as anticipated, but cognitive effects were limited to a non-significant trend towards improvement. Post hoc analysis, however, of those subjects >70 years in the treatment group ($n = 14$) revealed a significant cognitive benefit on all three tests ($P = 0.067$). While the researchers report these to be 'exciting' results, they also concede that the small sample size and need for post hoc analysis mean that much larger and better-designed studies are necessary to confirm their findings.

DOSAGE RANGE

Australian RDI

Children

- 1–3 years: 3 mg/day
- 4–8 years: 4 mg/day
- 9–13 years: 6 mg/day
- Males 14–18 years: 13 mg/day
- Females 14–18 years: 7 mg/day.

Adults

- Males >18 years: 14 mg/day
- Females >18 years: 8 mg/day.

Pregnancy

- <19 years: 10 mg/day
- ≥19 years: 11 mg/day.

Deficiency

- 25–50 mg elemental zinc daily.

According to clinical studies

- Common cold — zinc acetate lozenges are the most effective (free of sorbitol, mannitol or citric acid).
- Adults: 9–24 mg elemental zinc dissolved in the mouth, without chewing, every 2 hours for acute treatment. Total daily dose should provide ≥75 mg of elemental zinc.
- School-aged children: zinc acetate lozenges four times daily for acute treatment.
- It is recommended that citrus fruits or juices be avoided 30 minutes before or after dissolving each lozenge to avoid negating the effects of zinc.
- Improved immune function in elderly — 45 mg/day elemental zinc as zinc gluconate.
- Common cold — nasal gel sprays are no longer recommended due to the high incidence of temporary anosmia associated with their use.
- Pneumonia — 70 mg/day prophylactically or 20 mg/day in children suffering acute infection — especially in non-bacterial cases.
- Malaria — 10 mg/day elemental zinc.
- ARMD — zinc oxide (equivalent to 80 mg elemental zinc), together with 500 mg vitamin C, 400 IU vitamin E, taken daily, or 50 mg/day of zinc as zinc monocysteine as stand-alone treatment.
- ADHD — 30–40 mg elemental zinc daily.
- Depression – 25 mg elemental zinc per day.
- Type 1 diabetes — 30 mg/day (type of zinc unknown).
- Type 2 diabetes — 50 mg/day zinc acetate.
- Wound healing — 2.5 mg/kg zinc sulfate daily: zinc oxide form preferable topically.
- Leg ulcers — 600 mg zinc sulfate daily.
- Male fertility — 60 mg/day of zinc sulfate and 5 mg/day as folic acid.
- Acne vulgaris — 90–200 mg (50 mg elemental) daily.
- Crohn's disease — 110 mg zinc sulfate taken three times daily. However, a zinc carnosine preparation may be more appropriate.
- Diarrhoea — 10–20 mg/day elemental zinc in children between 6 months and 5 years for 2 weeks. Note: this dose was used in populations with a high prevalence of zinc deficiency.
- Herpes infection — 4% zinc sulfate solution applied via a cotton bud every 5 days for a month, then every 10 days for 2 months and finally every 15 days for 3 months.
- Anorexia nervosa — 14–50 mg elemental zinc daily.
- Dysgeusia — 20 mg/day elemental zinc as zinc gluconate and 68 mg/day as zinc carnosine.
- Tinnitus — 50–200 mg daily of zinc (salt unknown). Unclear benefit.

- Warts — 10 mg/kg zinc sulfate taken orally in three divided doses (up to 600 mg/day) for 1–2 months.

TOXICITY

Signs of toxicity are nausea, vomiting, diarrhoea, fever and lethargy and have been observed after ingestion of 4–8 g zinc according to a 2002 World Health Organization report. Single doses of 225–450 mg of zinc usually induce vomiting (King 2003).

Doses of zinc ranging from 100 to 150 mg/day interfere with copper metabolism and cause hypocuprinaemia, red blood cell microcytosis and neutropenia if used long-term.

ADVERSE REACTIONS

Mild gastrointestinal distress has been reported at doses of 50–150 mg/day of supplemental zinc (King 2003). According to a randomised, double-blind study, zinc gluconate glycine lozenge (104 mg, equivalent to 13.3 mg ionic zinc) taken every 3–4 hours is well tolerated (Silk & Lefante 2005). Of the side effects that were reported, dry mouth and a burning sensation on the tongue were probably related to use, whereas symptoms of nausea, dizziness, lightheadedness and upset stomach were considered as possibly related.

SIGNIFICANT INTERACTIONS

Calcium

High levels of dietary calcium impair zinc absorption in animals, but it is uncertain whether this occurs in humans — separate doses by 2 hours.

Angiotensin-converting enzyme inhibitors, angiotensin II receptor blockers and thiazide diuretics

These drugs reduce zinc status, most likely due to increased urinary excretion of zinc (Braun and Rosenfeldt 2013). Increased zinc intake may be required with long-term drug treatment.

Coffee

Coffee reduces zinc absorption — separate intakes by 2 hours (Pecoud et al 1975).

Copper

High zinc intakes (100–150 mg/day) interfere with copper metabolism and can cause hypocuprinaemia with long-term use. Avoid using high-dose zinc supplements long-term, or increase intake of copper.

Folate

Folate intake may reduce zinc levels — observe patient for signs and symptoms of zinc deficiency with long-term folate supplementation.

Iron

Supplemental (38–65 mg/day elemental) iron decreases zinc absorption (King 2003) — separate doses by 2 hours.

Non-steroidal anti-inflammatory drugs

Zinc interacts with non-steroidal anti-inflammatory drugs by forming complexes with these drugs (Dendrinou-Samara et al 1998) — separate dose by 2 hours.

Tetracyclines and quinolones

Complex formation between zinc and tetracycline results in reduced absorption of both substances with potential reduction in efficacy — separate dose by 2 hours.

Thiazide and loop diuretics

These diuretics increase urinary zinc loss — monitor for signs and symptoms of zinc deficiency with long-term drug use. Increased zinc intake may be required with long-term therapy.

Methylphenidate

The efficacy of this drug is improved by supplementation with zinc sulfate (15 mg elemental zinc) for 6 weeks in children with ADHD. There is no change to side effects reported (Akhondzadeh et al 2004).

Vaccinations

Zinc acetate improved seroconversion of vibriocidal antibodies in children given a cholera vaccination (Albert et al 2003) in both faecal and serum titres (Karlsen et al 2003).

Radiotherapy

Radiotherapy reduces plasma zinc levels (Ertekin et al 2004). Supplementation may be required with intensive radiotherapy treatment.

Interferon-alpha/ribavirin

Interferon-alpha and ribavirin treatment for hepatitis C patients is not affected by zinc supplementation (Ko et al 2005).

Orlistat

Orlistat has no significant effect on zinc levels (Zhi et al 2003).

Tricyclic antidepressants and selective serotonin reuptake inhibitors (SSRIs)

Zinc supplementation (25 mg elemental zinc daily) improves the efficacy of antidepressants such as tricyclic antidepressants and SSRIs after 2 weeks of intervention (Nowak et al 2003) — beneficial interaction possible.

CONTRAINDICATIONS AND PRECAUTIONS

Amiloride reduces zinc excretion and can lead to zinc accumulation (Reyes et al 1983). Therefore, supplementation should be used with caution.

PREGNANCY USE

Zinc is safe in pregnancy and may improve fetal heart rate in zinc-deficient mothers (in conjunction with iron and folic acid) (Merialdi et al 2004).

Practice points/Patient counselling

- Zinc is involved in many chemical reactions that are important for normal body functioning and it is essential for health and wellbeing.
- Although zinc supplements are traditionally used to treat deficiency, they are also used to prevent deficiency in conditions associated with low zinc status or deficiency, such as acrodermatitis enteropathica, anorexia nervosa, malabsorption syndromes, conditions associated with chronic diarrhoea, alcoholism, liver cirrhosis, diabetes, HIV and AIDS, recurrent infections, severe burns, postsurgery and sickle cell anaemia.
- Zinc supplements are also popular among athletes in order to counteract zinc loss that occurs through perspiration.
- Zinc lozenges have been used to prevent and treat the symptoms of the common cold and oral supplements have been used to treat acne vulgaris, improve wound healing and chronic leg ulcers, resolve intestinal permeability problems and reduce recurrences in Crohn's disease, treat recalcitrant warts, reduce symptoms of tinnitus and improve ADHD.
- Topical applications of zinc have been used to treat acne vulgaris (in combination with erythromycin) and herpes simplex and to promote wound healing.
- Numerous interactions exist between other minerals, foods and medicines and zinc.

PATIENTS' FAQs

What will this supplement do for me?

Zinc is found in every cell of the body and is essential for health and wellbeing. Some studies have found that supplements are not only useful to treat and prevent deficiency, but may also be useful in conditions such as the common cold, poor wound healing and leg ulcers, diabetes, Crohn's disease, acne vulgaris, warts, ADHD and tinnitus. Topical preparations may be useful in acne vulgaris (with erythromycin), herpes infection and chronic wounds.

When will it start to work?

This depends on the indication (refer to monograph for more details).

Are there any safety issues?

Used in high doses, zinc can cause nausea, vomiting, gastrointestinal discomfort and, if used long-term, reduce copper levels. Zinc also interacts with a number of other minerals, foods and medicines.

REFERENCES

Agarwal, A., & Sekhon, L. H. (2010). The role of antioxidant therapy in the treatment of male infertility. Hum Fertil (Camb), 13(4), 217–225.

Age-Related Eye Disease Study. A randomized, placebo-controlled, clinical trial of high-dose supplementation with vitamins C and E, beta-carotene, and zinc for age-related macular degeneration and vision loss: AREDS report no. 8. Arch Ophthalmol 119.10 (2001): 1417–36.

Agren MS. Studies on zinc in wound healing. Acta Derm Venereol Suppl (Stockh) 154 (1990): 1–36.

Akhondzadeh S, et al. Zinc sulfate as an adjunct to methylphenidate for the treatment of attention deficit hyperactivity disorder in children: a double blind and randomized trial. BMC Psychiatry 4.1 (2004): 9.

Akiyama, T., et al. (2013). Association between serum zinc concentration and the *Plasmodium falciparum* antibody titer among rural villagers of Attapeu Province, Lao People's Democratic Republic. Acta Trop, 126(3), 193–197.

Alam, S., & Kelleher, S. L. (2012). Cellular mechanisms of zinc dysregulation: a perspective on zinc homeostasis as an etiological factor in the development and progression of breast cancer. Nutrients, 4(8), 875–903.

Albert MJ et al. Supplementation with zinc, but not vitamin A, improves seroconversion to vibriocidal antibody in children given an oral cholera vaccine. J Infect Dis 187.6 (2003): 909–13.

Al Gurairi FT, et al. Oral zinc sulphate in the treatment of recalcitrant viral warts: randomized placebo-controlled clinical trial. Br J Dermatol 146 (2002): 423–31.
Aliani, M., et al. (2013). Zinc deficiency and taste perception in the elderly. Crit Rev Food Sci Nutr, 53(3), 245–250.
Al-Maroof RA, Al-Sharbatti SS. Serum zinc levels in diabetic patients and effect of zinc supplementation on glycemic control of type 2 diabetics. Saudi Med J 27.3 (2006): 344–50.
Antoine, T.E., et al. 2012. Prophylactic, therapeutic and neutralizing effects of zinc oxide tetrapod structures against herpes simplex virus type-2 infection. Antiviral Res., 96, (3) 363–375.
Arda HN et al. The role of zinc in the treatment of tinnitus. Otol Neurotol 24 (2003): 86–9.
Arnold LE, DiSilvestro RA. Zinc in attention-deficit/hyperactivity disorder. J Child Adolesc Psychopharmacol 15 (2005): 619–27.
Arnold LE et al. Does hair zinc predict amphetamine improvement of ADD/hyperactivity? Int J Neurosci 50 (1990): 103–7.
Arnold, L. E., et al. (2011). Zinc for attention-deficit/hyperactivity disorder: placebo-controlled double-blind pilot trial alone and combined with amphetamine. J Child Adolesc Psychopharmacol, 21(1), 1–19.
Asdamongkol, N., et al. (2013). Low plasma zinc levels and immunological responses to zinc supplementation in HIV-infected patients with immunological discordance after antiretroviral therapy. Jpn J Infect Dis, 66(6), 469–474.
Baer MT, King JC. Tissue zinc levels and zinc excretion during experimental zinc depletion in young men. Am J Clin Nutr 39 (1984): 556–70.
Bales CW et al. The effect of age on plasma zinc uptake and taste acuity. Am J Clin Nutr 44 (1986): 664–9.
Bales CW et al. Zinc, magnesium, copper, and protein concentrations in human saliva: age- and sex-related differences. Am J Clin Nutr 51.3 (1990): 462–9.
Bartoshuk LM. Taste. Robust across the age span? Ann N Y Acad Sci 561 (1989): 65–75.
Baum, M.K., et al. 2010. Randomized, controlled clinical trial of zinc supplementation to prevent immunological failure in HIV-infected adults. Clin Infect.Dis., 50, (12) 1653–1660
Baydas B, et al. Effects of oral zinc and magnesium supplementation on serum thyroid hormone and lipid levels in experimentally induced diabetic rats. Biol Trace Elem Res 88.3 (2002): 247–53.
Bedwal RS, Bahuguna A. Zinc, copper and selenium in reproduction. Experientia 50.7 (1994): 626–40.
Beers MH, Berkow R (eds). The Merck manual of diagnosis and therapy, 17th edn. Whitehouse, NJ: Merck, 2003.
Belongia EA, et al. A randomized trial of zinc nasal spray for the treatment of upper respiratory illness in adults. Am J Med 111.2 (2001): 103–8.
Bilici M et al. Double-blind, placebo-controlled study of zinc sulfate in the treatment of attention deficit hyperactivity disorder. Prog Neuropsychopharmacol Biol Psychiatry 28 (2004): 181–90.
Birmingham CL, Gritzner S. How does zinc supplementation benefit anorexia nervosa? Eat Weight Disord 11.4 (2006): e109–11.
Birmingham CL, et al. Controlled trial of zinc supplementation in anorexia nervosa. Int J Eat Disord 15.3 (1994): 251–5.
Birmingham CL et al. Reliability of the AccuSens Taste Kit(c) in patients with eating disorders. Eat Weight Disord 10.2 (2005): e45–8.
Black MM. The evidence linking zinc deficiency with children's cognitive and motor functioning. J Nutr 133 (5 Suppl 1) (2003): 1473S–6S.
Bojar RA et al. Inhibition of erythromycin-resistant propionibacteria on the skin of acne patients by topical erythromycin with and without zinc. Br J Dermatol 130.3 (1994): 329–36.
Bolkent S et al. The influence of zinc supplementation on the pancreas of streptozotocin-diabetic rats. Dig Dis Sci. 2009; 54: 2583–2587.
Bose A et al. Efficacy of zinc in the treatment of severe pneumonia in hospitalized children <2 y old. Am J Clin Nutr 83.5 (2006): 1089–96.
Brandt, S. (2013). The clinical effects of zinc as a topical or oral agent on the clinical response and pathophysiologic mechanisms of acne: a systematic review of the literature. J Drugs Dermatol, 12(5), 542–545.
Braun, L.A. & Rosenfeldt, F. 2013. Pharmaco-nutrient interactions — a systematic review of zinc and antihypertensive therapy. Int.J Clin Pract., 67, (8) 717–725.
Briefel RR et al. Zinc intake of the U.S. population: findings from the third National Health and Nutrition Examination Survey, 1988–1994. J Nutr 130 (2000): 1367–73S.
Brooks WA et al. Zinc for severe pneumonia in very young children: double-blind placebo-controlled trial. Lancet 363.9422 (2004): 1683–8.
Brooks WA et al. Effect of weekly zinc supplements on incidence of pneumonia and diarrhoea in children younger than 2 years in an urban, low-income population in Bangladesh: randomized controlled trial. Lancet 366.9490 (2005): 999–1004.
Brown JE, Toma RB. Taste changes during pregnancy. Am J Clin Nutr 43.3 (1986): 414–8.
Bunker VW et al. Metabolic balance studies for zinc and copper in housebound elderly people and the relationship between zinc balance and leukocyte zinc concentrations. Am J Clin Nutr 46 (1987): 353–9.
Buzina R et al. Zinc nutrition and taste acuity in school children with impaired growth. Am J Clin Nutr 33.11 (1980): 2262–7
Catalanotto F. The trace metal zinc and taste. Am J Clin Nutr 31 (1978): 1098–103.
Chausmer AB. Zinc, insulin and diabetes. J Am Coll Nutr 17.2 (1998): 109–15.
Coehlo CB, et al. Hyperacusis, sound annoyance, and loudness hypersensitivity in children. Progress in Brain Research. Elsevier; 2007: 279–85.
Coehlo, C., et al. (2013). Zinc to treat tinnitus in the elderly: a randomized placebo controlled crossover trial. Otol Neurotol, 34(6), 1146–1154.
Coleman HR et al. Age-related macular degeneration. Lancet 372.9652 (2008): 1835–45.

Coles CL et al. Infectious etiology modifies the treatment effect of zinc in severe pneumonia. Am J Clin Nutr 86.2 (2007): 397–403.

Cunliffe WJ et al. A double-blind trial of a zinc sulphate/citrate complex and tetracycline in the treatment of acne vulgaris. Br J Dermatol 101.3 (1979): 321–5.

Cunningham JJ et al. Hyperzincuria in individuals with insulin-dependent diabetes mellitus: concurrent zinc status and the effect of high-dose zinc supplementation. Metabolism 43.12 (1994): 1558–62.

Davison GW et al. Exercise, free radicals, and lipid peroxidation in type 1 diabetes mellitus. Free Radic Biol Med 33.11 (2002): 1543–51.

Deems DA et al. Smell and taste disorders, a study of 750 patients from the University of Pennsylvania Smell and Taste Center. Arch Otolaryngol Head Neck Surg 117.5 (1991): 519–28.

Dendrinou-Samara C et al. Anti-inflammatory drugs interacting with Zn(II), Cd(II) and Pt(II) metal ions. J Inorg Biochem 71.3–4 (1998): 171–9.

DiGirolamo, A. M., et al. (2010). Randomized trial of the effect of zinc supplementation on the mental health of school-age children in Guatemala. Am J Clin Nutr, 92(5), 1241–1250.

DiSilvestro RA. Zinc in relation to diabetes and oxidative disease. J Nutr 130 (5S Suppl) (2000): 1509–11S.

Dreno B et al. Low doses of zinc gluconate for inflammatory acne. Acta Derm Venereol 69.6 (1989): 541–3.

Dreno B et al. Zinc salts effects on granulocyte zinc concentration and chemotaxis in acne patients. Acta Derm Venereol 72.4 (1992): 250–2.

Dreno B et al. Multicenter randomized comparative double-blind controlled clinical trial of the safety and efficacy of zinc gluconate versus minocycline hydrochloride in the treatment of inflammatory acne vulgaris. Dermatology 203.2 (2001): 135–40.

Dreno B et al. Effect of zinc gluconate on *Propionibacterium acnes* resistance to erythromycin in patients with inflammatory acne: in vitro and in vivo study. Eur J Dermatol 15 (2005): 152–5.

Duggan C et al. Plasma zinc concentrations are depressed during the acute phase response in children with falciparium malaria. J Nutr 135.4 (2005): 802.

Eaton K, et al. Diagnosing human zinc deficiency. A comparison between the Bryce-Smith test and sweat mineral analysis. J Nutr Environ Med 14.2 (2004): 83–7.

Ebisch IM et al. Does folic acid and zinc sulphate intervention affect endocrine parameters and sperm characteristics in men? Int J Androl 29.2 (2006): 339–45.

Ebisch IM et al. The importance of folate, zinc and antioxidants in the pathogenesis and prevention of subfertility. Hum Reprod Update 13.2 (2007): 163–74.

Eby GA, Halcomb WW. Ineffectiveness of zinc gluconate nasal spray and zinc orotate lozenges in common-cold treatment: a double-blind, placebo-controlled clinical trial. Alt Ther Health Med 12.1 (2006): 34–8.

Eggert-Kruse W et al. Are zinc levels in seminal plasma associated with seminal leukocytes and other determinants of semen quality? Fertil Steril 77.2 (2002): 260–9.

Erie JC et al. Reduced zinc and copper in the retinal pigment epithelium and choroid in age-related macular degeneration. Am J Ophthalmol 147.2 (2009): 276–282.e1.

Ertekin MV et al. The effects of oral zinc sulphate during radiotherapy on anti-oxidant enzyme activities in patients with head and neck cancer: a prospective, randomized, placebo-controlled study. Int J Clin Pract 58.7 (2004): 662–8.

Erten J et al. Hair zinc levels in healthy and malnourished children. Am J Clin Nutr 31 (1978): 1172–4.

Evans JR. Antioxidant vitamin and mineral supplements for age-related macular degeneration. Cochrane Database Syst Rev 2 (2002): CD000254.

Fanjiang G, Kleinman RE. Nutrition and performance in children. Curr Opin Clin Nutr Metab Care 10.3 (2007): 342–7.

Farinati F et al. Zinc treatment prevents lipid peroxidation and increases glutathione availability in Wilson's disease. J Lab Clin Med 141.6 (2003): 372–7.

Farvid MS et al. The impact of vitamin and/or mineral supplementation on lipid profiles in type 2 diabetes. Diabetes Res Clin Pract 65.1 (2004): 21–8.

Favier AE. The role of zinc in reproduction: Hormonal mechanisms. Biol Trace Elem Res 32 (1992): 363–82.

Feiner AM et al. Evaluation of the effects of a zinc/iron solution on the migration of fibroblasts in an in-vitro incisional wound healing model. Wounds 15.4 (2003): A23–34.

Ferreira, G. D., et al. (2009). Vestibular evaluation using videonystagmography of chronic zinc deficient patients due to short bowel syndrome. Braz J Otorhinolaryngol, 75(2), 290–294.

Feucht CL et al. Topical erythromycin with zinc in acne: a double-blind controlled study. J Am Acad Dermatol 3.5 (1980): 483–91.

Finnerty EF. Topical zinc in the treatment of herpes simplex. Cutis 37.2 (1986): 130–1.

Flament, M. F., et al. (2012). Evidence-based pharmacotherapy of eating disorders. Int J Neuropsychopharmacol, 15(2), 189–207.

Fletcher AE et al. Sunlight exposure, antioxidants, and age-related macular degeneration. Arch Ophthalmol 126.10 (2008): 1396–403.

Fluhr JW et al. In-vitro and in-vivo efficacy of zinc acetate against propionibacteria alone and in combination with erythromycin. Zentralbl Bakteriol 289.4 (1999): 445–56.

Foster, M., et al. 2013. Effect of vegetarian diets on zinc status: a systematic review and meta-analysis of studies in humans. J Sci. Food Agric., 93, (10) 2362–2371

Fraker PJ et al. The dynamic link between the integrity of the immune system and zinc status. J Nutr 130 (2000): 1399–406S.

Frederickson CJ, Danscher G. Zinc-containing neurons in hippocampus and related CNS structures. Prog Brain Res 83 (1990): 71–84.

Frederickson CJ, Moncrieff DW. Zinc-containing neurons. Biol Signals 3.3 (1994): 127–39.

Frederickson CJ et al. Importance of zinc in the central nervous system: the zinc-containing neuron. J Nutr 130 (5S Suppl) (2000): 1471S–83S.

Freeland-Graves J et al. Salivary zinc as an indicator of zinc status in women fed a low-zinc diet. Am J Clin Nutr 34 (1981): 312–21.

Garg HK, et al. Zinc taste test in pregnant women and its correlation with serum zinc level. Indian J Physiol Pharmacol 37.4 (1993): 318–22.

Gersdorff M et al. A clinical correlation between hypozincemia and tinnitus. Arch Otorhinolaryngol 244 (1987): 190–3.

Ghanizadeh, A., & Berk, M. (2013). Zinc for treating of children and adolescents with attention-deficit hyperactivity disorder: a systematic review of randomized controlled clinical trials. Eur J Clin Nutr, 67(1), 122–124.

Gibson R. Principles of nutritional assessment. New York: Oxford University; 1990.

Gibson RS et al. A growth-limiting, mild zinc deficiency syndrome in some southern Ontario boys with low height percentiles. Am J Clin Nutr 49 (1989): 1266–73.

Godfrey, H.R., et al. 2001. A randomized clinical trial on the treatment of oral herpes with topical zinc oxide/ glycine. Altern. Ther. Health Med, 7, (3) 49–56

Golden M. Severe malnutrition. In: Weatherall D, Ledingham J, Warrell D, editors. Oxford textbook of medicine. 3rd edn. Oxford, UK: Ford Medical Publications; 1996. Vol. 1 pp. 1278–85.

Goransson K, et al. Oral zinc in acne vulgaris: a clinical and methodological study. Acta Derm Venereol 58.5 (1978): 443–8.

Gordon P et al. Effect of acute zinc deprivation on plasma zinc and platelet aggregation in adult males. Am J Clin Nutr 35 (1982): 113–9.

Graham RM, et al. Low concentration zinc sulphate solution in the management of recurrent herpes simplex infection. Br J Dermatol 112.1 (1985): 123–4.

Greger J. Dietary intake and nutritional status in regard to zinc of institutionalized aged. J Gerontol 32.5 (1977): 549–53.

Greger JL, Geissler AH. Effect of zinc supplementation on taste acuity of the aged. Am J Clin Nutr 31.4 (1978): 633–7.

Greger JL, Sickles VS. Saliva zinc levels: potential indicators of zinc status. Am J Clin Nutr 32 (1979): 1859–66.

Gropper S, et al. Advanced nutrition and human metabolism. 5th edn. Belmont: Wadsworth Thomson Learning; 2009.

Gupta R et al. Oral zinc therapy in diabetic neuropathy. J Assoc Physicians India 46.11 (1998): 939–42.

Habbema L et al. A 4% erythromycin and zinc combination (Zineryt) versus 2% erythromycin (Eryderm) in acne vulgaris: a randomized, double-blind comparative study. Br J Dermatol 121.4 (1989): 497–502.

Haeger K, Lanner E. Oral zinc sulphate and ischaemic leg ulcers. Vasa 3.1 (1974): 77–81.

Hallbook T, Lanner E. Serum-zinc and healing of venous leg ulcers. Lancet 2.7781 (1972): 780–2.

Halyard MY et al. Does zinc sulfate prevent therapy-induced taste alterations in head and neck cancer patients? Results of phase III double-blind, placebo-controlled trial from the North Central Cancer Treatment Group (N01C4). Int J Radiat Oncol Biol Phys 67.5 (2007): 1318–22.

Hambidge M. Human zinc deficiency. J Nutr 130 (2000): 1344S–9S.

Hambidge C. Biomarkers of trace mineral intake and status. J Nutr 133. Suppl 3 (2003): 948S–55S.

Hayee MA, et al. Diabetic neuropathy and zinc therapy. Bangladesh Med Res Counc Bull 31.2 (2005): 62–7.

Heckmann SM et al. Zinc gluconate in the treatment of dysgeusia: a randomized clinical trial. J Dent Res 84.1 (2005): 35–8.

Henkin RI et al. A syndrome of acute zinc loss. Cerebellar dysfunction, mental changes, anorexia, and taste and smell dysfunction. Arch Neurol 32.11 (1975a): 745–51.

Henkin RI, et al. Estimation of zinc concentration of parotid saliva by flameless atomic absorption spectrophometry in normal subjects and in patients with idiopathic hypogeusia. J Lab Clin Med 86.1 (1975b): 175–80.

Henkin RI et al. A double blind study of the effects of zinc sulfate on taste and smell dysfunction. Am J Med Sci 272.3 (1976): 285–99.

Henkin RI et al. Fractionation of human parotid saliva proteins. J Biol Chem 253.20 (1977): 7556–65

Higdon J. An evidence-based approach to vitamins and minerals. New York: Thieme, 2003: 197–205.

Hillstrom L et al. Comparison of oral treatment with zinc sulphate and placebo in acne vulgaris. Br J Dermatol 97.6 (1977): 681–4.

Hirt M, et al. Zinc nasal gel for the treatment of common cold symptoms: a double-blind, placebo-controlled trial. Ear Nose Throat J 79.10 (2000): 778–80, 782.

Ho, E., et al. (2011). Dietary factors and epigenetic regulation for prostate cancer prevention. Adv Nutr, 2(6), 497–510.

Hogberg, L., et al. (2009). Serum zinc in small children with coeliac disease. Acta Paediatr, 98(2), 343–345.

Hogg, R. & Chakravarthy, U. 2004. AMD and micronutrient antioxidants. Curr.Eye Res., 29, (6) 387–401

Hong, S. H., et al. (2012). Induction of apoptosis of bladder cancer cells by zinc-citrate compound. Korean J Urol, 53(11), 800–806.

Hotz C et al. Assessment of the trace element status of individuals and populations: the example of zinc and copper. J Nutr 133 (2003): 1563S–8S.

Hussain SA et al. Effects of melatonin and zinc on glycemic control in type 2 diabetic patients poorly controlled with metformin. Saudi Med J 27.10 (2006): 1483–8.

Iinuma, K., & Tsuboi, I. (2012). Zinc ascorbate has superoxide dismutase-like activity and in vitro antimicrobial activity against *Staphylococcus aureus* and *Escherichia coli*. Clin Cosmet Investig Dermatol, 5, 135–140.

Iinuma, K., et al. (2011). Susceptibility of *Propionibacterium acnes* isolated from patients with acne vulgaris to zinc ascorbate and antibiotics. Clin Cosmet Investig Dermatol, 4, 161–165.

Ikeda M et al. Taste disorders: a survey of the examination methods and treatment used in Japan. Acta Otolaryngol 125 (2005): 1203–10.

Ikeda M et al. Causative factors of taste disorders in the elderly, and therapeutic effects of zinc. J Laryngol Otol 122.2 (2008): 155–60.

Irlam, J. H., et al. (2013). Micronutrient supplementation for children with HIV infection. Cochrane Database Syst Rev, 10, CD010666.
Islam MS, Loots du T. Diabetes, metallothionein, and zinc interactions: a review. Biofactors 29.4 (2007): 203–12.
IZiNCG. Assessment of the risk of zinc deficiency in populations and options for its control. Food Nutr Bull 25 (2004): S91–S204.
Karlsen TH et al. Intestinal and systemic immune responses to oral cholerz toxoid B subunit whole-cell vaccine administered during zinc supplementation. Infect Immun 71.7 (2003): 3909–13.
Katz RL et al. Zinc deficiency in anorexia nervosa. J Adolesc Health Care 8.5 (1987): 400–6.
Kenney MA et al. Erythrocyte and dietary zinc in adolescent females. Am J Clin Nutr 39 (1984): 446–51.
Kenney, J., et al. (2013). A modified zinc acetate gel, a potential nonantiretroviral microbicide, is safe and effective against simian-human immunodeficiency virus and herpes simplex virus 2 infection in vivo. Antimicrob Agents Chemother, 57(8), 4001–4009.
Kettaneh A et al. Clinical and biological features associated with taste loss in internal medicine patients. A cross-sectional study of 100 cases. Appetite 44.2 (2005): 163–9.
Khozeimeh, F., et al. (2012). Comparative analysis of salivary zinc level in recurrent herpes labialis. Dent Res J (Isfahan), 9(1), 19–23.
King JC. Determinants of maternal zinc status during pregnancy. Am J Clin Nutr 71 (5 Suppl) (2000): 1334S–43S.
King J. Zinc. Oregon: The Linus Pauling Institute, 2003.
King J, Cousins R. Zinc. In: Shils M, et al. editors. Modern nutrition in health and disease. 10th edn. Baltimore: Lippincott Williams & Wilkins; 2006. pp. 271–85.
Klein ML et al. CFH and LOC387715/ARMS2 genotypes and treatment with antioxidants and zinc for age-related macular degeneration. Ophthalmology 115.6 (2008): 1019–25
Kneist W, et al. Clinical double-blind trial of topical zinc sulfate for herpes labialis recidivans. Arzneimittelforschung 45.5 (1995): 624–6.
Ko W-S et al. The effect of zinc supplementation on the treatment of chronic hepatitis C patients with interferon and ribavirin. Clin Biochem 38 (2005): 614–20.
Kordas, K., et al. (2005). Iron and zinc supplementation does not improve parent or teacher ratings of behavior in first grade Mexican children exposed to lead. J Pediatr, 147(5), 632–639.
Kosman DJ, Henkin RI. Erythrocyte zinc in patients with taste and smell dysfunction. Am J Clin Nutr 34.1 (1981): 118–9.
Kumar N et al. Effect of different levels and sources of zinc supplementation on quantitative and qualitative semen attributes and serum testosterone level in crossbred cattle (*Bos indicus* x *Bos taurus*) bulls. Reprod Nutr Dev 46.6 (2006): 663–75.
Kurugöl Z, et al. Effect of zinc sulfate on common cold in children: randomized, double blind study. Pediatr Int 49.6 (2007): 842–7.
Lai, J., et al. (2012). The efficacy of zinc supplementation in depression: systematic review of randomised controlled trials. J Affect Disord, 136(1–2), e31–39.
Lansdown AB. Zinc in the healing wound. Lancet 347.9003 (1996): 706–7.
Lansdown AB et al. Zinc in wound healing: theoretical, experimental, and clinical aspects. Wound Repair Regen 15.1 (2007): 2–16.
Law JS et al. Human salivary gustin is a potent activator of calmodulin-dependent brain phosphodiesterase. Proc Natl Acad Sci U S A 84 (1987): 1674–8.
Lazzerini, M., & Ronfani, L. (2013). Oral zinc for treating diarrhoea in children. Cochrane Database Syst Rev, 1, CD005436.
Lee AY, Brantley MA. C and LOC387715/ARMS2 genotypes and antioxidants and zinc therapy for age-related macular degeneration. Pharmacogenomics 9.10 (2008): 1547–50.
Liu J, Raine A. The effect of childhood malnutrition on externalizing behavior. Curr Opin Pediatr 18.5 (2006): 565–70.
Lonnerdal B. Dietary factors influencing zinc absorption. J Nutr 130 (2000): 1378–83S.
Lyckholm, L., et al. (2012). A randomized, placebo controlled trial of oral zinc for chemotherapy-related taste and smell disorders. J Pain Palliat Care Pharmacother, 26(2), 111–114.
Mahajan SK et al. Effect of oral zinc therapy on gonadal function in hemodialysis patients: a double-blind study. Ann Intern Med 97 (1982): 357–61.
Mahajan, B. B., et al. (2013). Herpes genitalis — Topical zinc sulfate: An alternative therapeutic and modality. Indian J Sex Transm Dis, 34(1), 32–34.
Mahmood, A., et al. (2007). Zinc carnosine, a health food supplement that stabilises small bowel integrity and stimulates gut repair processes. Gut, 56(2), 168–175.
Mahomed K et al. Failure to taste zinc sulphate solution does not predict zinc deficiency in pregnancy. Eur J Obstet Gynecol Reprod Biol 48.3 (1993): 169–75.
Marcellini F et al. Zinc status, psychological and nutritional assessment in old people recruited in five European countries: Zincage study. Biogerontology 7.5–6 (2006): 339–45.
Marreiro DN et al. Abstracts 1644-P, 569-P. In: Proceedings of the American diabetes association annual meeting, June 16–17, 2002.
Maserejian, N. N., et al. (2012). Low dietary or supplemental zinc is associated with depression symptoms among women, but not men, in a population-based epidemiological survey. J Affect Disord, 136(3), 781–788.
McBean L et al. Correlation of zinc concentrations in human plasma and hair. Am J Clin Nutr 24 (1971): 506–9.
McClain CJ et al. Zinc status before and after zinc supplementation of eating disorder patients. J Am Coll Nutr 11.6 (1992): 694–700.
McKenzie JM. Content of zinc in serum, urine, hair, and toenails of New Zealand adults. Am J Clin Nutr 32 (1979): 570–9.
Merialdi M et al. Randomized controlled trial of prenatal zinc supplementation and the development of fetal heart rate. Am J Obstet Gynecol 190.4 (2004): 1106–12.

Mocchegiani E et al. Benefit of oral zinc supplementation as an adjunct to zidovudine (AZT) therapy against opportunistic infections in AIDS. Int J Immunopharmacol 17.9 (1995): 719–27
Morgan AJ et al. The effect of zinc in the form of erythromycin-zinc complex (Zineryt lotion) and zinc acetate on metallothionein expression and distribution in hamster skin. Br J Dermatol 129.5 (1993): 563–70.
Mossad SB. Effect of zincum gluconium nasal gel on the duration and symptom severity of the common cold in otherwise healthy adults. QJM 96.1 (2003): 35–43.
Mun, J. H., et al. (2011). Oral zinc sulfate treatment for viral warts: an open-label study. J Dermatol, 38(6), 541-545.
Newsome DA. A randomized, prospective, placebo-controlled clinical trial of a novel zinc-monocysteine compound in age-related macular degeneration. Curr Eye Res 33.7 (2008): 591–8.
Niewoehner CB et al. Role of zinc supplementation in type II diabetes mellitus. Am J Med 81.1 (1986): 63–8.
Noh, H., et al. (2013). Salty taste acuity is affected by the joint action of alphaENaC A663T gene polymorphism and available zinc intake in young women. Nutrients, 5(12), 4950–4963.
Novick SG et al. How does zinc modify the common cold? Clinical observations and implications regarding mechanisms of action. Med Hypotheses 46 (1996): 295–302.
Nowak G et al. Effect of zinc supplementation on antidepressant therapy in unipolar depression: a preliminary placebo-controlled study. Pol J Pharmacol 55.6 (2003): 1143–7.
Nowak G, et al. Zinc and depression. An update. Pharmacol Rep 57 (2005): 713–8.
Ochi K et al. Zinc deficiency and tinnitus. Auris Nasus Larynx 30 (Suppl) (2003): S25–8.
Oprica C, et al. Overview of treatments for acne. Dermatol Nurs 14 (2002): 242–6.
Orris L et al. Oral zinc therapy of acne. Absorption and clinical effect. Arch Dermatol 114.7 (1978): 1018–20.
Osaki T et al. Clinical and physiological investigations in patients with taste abnormality. J Oral Pathol Med 25.1 (1996): 38–43.
Overbeck S, et al. Modulating the immune response by oral zinc supplementation: a single approach for multiple diseases. Arch Immunol Ther Exp (Warsz) 56.1 (2008): 15–30.
Owusu-Agyei, S., et al. (2013). Impact of vitamin A with zinc supplementation on malaria morbidity in Ghana. Nutr J, 12, 131.
Ozuguz, P., et al. (2013). Evaluation of serum vitamins A and E and zinc levels according to the severity of acne vulgaris. Cutan Ocul Toxicol.
Paaske PB et al. Zinc in the management of tinnitus: Placebo-controlled trial. Ann Otol Rhinol Laryngol 100 (1991): 647–9.
Partida-Hernández G et al. Effect of zinc replacement on lipids and lipoproteins in type 2-diabetic patients. Biomed Pharmacother 60.4 (2006): 161–8.
Pecoud A, et al. Effect of foodstuffs on the absorption of zinc sulfate. Clin Pharmacol Ther 17.4 (1975): 469–74.
Pierard GE, Pierard-Franchimont C. Effect of a topical erythromycin-zinc formulation on sebum delivery. Evaluation by combined photometric-multi-step samplings with Sebutape. Clin Exp Dermatol 18.5 (1993): 410–3.
Pierard-Franchimont C et al. A double-blind controlled evaluation of the sebosuppressive activity of topical erythromycin-zinc complex. Eur J Clin Pharmacol 49.1–2 (1995): 57–60.
Potocnik FC et al. Zinc and platelet membrane microviscosity in Alzheimer's disease: the in vivo effect of zinc on platelet membranes and cognition. S Afr Med J 87.9 (1997): 1116–9.
Prasad A. Laboratory diagnosis of zinc deficiency. J Am Coll Nutr 4.6 (1985): 591–8.
Prasad AS. Zinc deficiency in women, infants and children. J Am Coll Nutr 15.2 (1996): 113–20.
Prasad AS. Zinc and immunity. Mol Cell Biochem 188.1–2 (1998): 63–9.
Prasad, A.S. 2013. Discovery of human zinc deficiency: its impact on human health and disease. Adv.Nutr., 4, (2) 176–190
Prasad AS, Kucuk O. Zinc in cancer prevention. Cancer Metastasis Rev 21.3–4 (2002): 291–5.
Prasad AS et al. Antioxidant effect of zinc in humans. Free Radic Biol Med 37.8 (2004): 1182–90.
Prasad AS et al. Zinc supplementation decreases incidence of infections in the elderly: effect of zinc on generation of cytokines and oxidative stress. Am J Clin Nutr 85.3 (2007): 837–44.
Purdy, S., & de Berker, D. (2011). Acne vulgaris. Clin Evid (Online), 2011.
Rareshide E, Amedee R. Disorders of taste. J La State Med Soc 141.9 (1989): 9–11.
Reyes AJ et al. Urinary zinc excretion, diuretics, zinc deficiency and some side-effects of diuretics. S Afr Med J 64.24 (1983): 936–41.
Roussel A-M et al. Antioxidant effects of zinc supplementation in Tunisians with type 2 diabetes mellitus. J Am Coll Nutr 22.4 (2003): 316–21.
Safai-Kutti S. Oral zinc supplementation in anorexia nervosa. Acta Psychiatr Scand Suppl 361 (1990): 14–17.
Saito H et al. Malnutrition induces dissociated changes in lymphocyte count and subset proportion in patients with anorexia nervosa. Int J Eat Disord 40.6 (2007): 575–9.
Sakagami M et al. A zinc-containing compound, Polaprezinc, is effective for patients with taste disorders: randomized, double-blind, placebo-controlled, multi-center study. Acta Otolaryngol 26 (2008): 1–6.
Sandstead HH et al. Zinc nutriture in the elderly in relation to taste acuity, immune response, and wound healing. Am J Clin Nutr 36 (5 Suppl) (1982): 1046–59.
Sardana, K., & Garg, V. K. (2010). An observational study of methionine-bound zinc with antioxidants for mild to moderate acne vulgaris. Dermatol Ther, 23(4), 411–418.
Satarug S et al. Prevention of cadmium accumulation in retinal pigment epithelium with manganese and zinc. Exp Eye Res 87.6 (2008): 587–93.
Schachner L et al. Topical erythromycin and zinc therapy for acne. J Am Acad Dermatol 22.2 (1990): 253–60.
Schiffman S. Mechanisms of disease (first of two parts). N Engl J Med 308.21 (1983): 1275–9.
Scrimgeour, A. G., & Condlin, M. L. (2009). Zinc and micronutrient combinations to combat gastrointestinal inflammation. Curr Opin Clin Nutr Metab Care, 12(6), 653–660.
Semrad CE. Zinc and intestinal function. Curr Gastroenterol Rep 1.5 (1999): 398–403.

Shalita, A. R., et al. (2012). Inflammatory acne management with a novel prescription dietary supplement. J Drugs Dermatol, 11(12), 1428–1433.
Shankar AH et al. The influence of zinc supplementation on morbidity due to *Plasmodium falciparum*: a randomized trial in preschool children in Papua New Guinea. Am J Trop Med Hyg 62.6 (2000): 663–9.
Sharquie KE et al. Oral zinc sulphate in the treatment of acute cutaneous leishmaniasis. Clin Exp Dermatol 26.1 (2001): 21–6.
Shay NF, Mangian HF. Neurobiology of zinc-influenced eating behavior. J Nutr 130 (5S Suppl) (2000): 1493–9S.
Shepherd, S. J., & Gibson, P. R. (2013). Nutritional inadequacies of the gluten-free diet in both recently-diagnosed and long-term patients with coeliac disease. J Hum Nutr Diet, 26(4), 349–358.
Siberry GK, et al. Zinc and human immunodeficiency virus infection. Nutr Res 22.4 (2002): 527–38.
Silk R, LeFante C. Safety of zinc gluconate glycine (Cold-Eeze) in a geriatric population: a randomized, placebo-controlled, double-blind trial. Am J Ther 12 (2005): 612–7.
Siwek, M., et al. (2009). Zinc supplementation augments efficacy of imipramine in treatment resistant patients: a double blind, placebo-controlled study. J Affect Disord, 118(1–3), 187–195.
Siwek, M., et al. (2010). Serum zinc level in depressed patients during zinc supplementation of imipramine treatment. J Affect Disord, 126(3), 447–452.
Stenberg, P., et al. (2008). Transglutaminase and the pathogenesis of coeliac disease. Eur J Intern Med, 19(2), 83–91.
Stewart-Knox B et al. Zinc status and taste acuity in older Europeans: the Zenith study. Eur J Clin Nutr 59 (Suppl 2) (2005): S31–6.
Stewart-Knox BJ et al. Taste acuity in response to zinc supplementation in older Europeans. Br J Nutr 99.1 (2008): 129–36.
Stockner, T., et al. (2013). Mutational analysis of the high-affinity zinc binding site validates a refined human dopamine transporter homology model. PLoS Comput Biol, 9(2), e1002909.
Sturniolo GC et al. Zinc absorption in Crohn's disease. Gut 21.5 (1980): 387–91.
Sturniolo GC et al. Zinc supplementation tightens leaky gut in Crohn's disease. Inflamm Bowel Dis 7.2 (2001): 94–8.
Sun Q et al. A prospective study of zinc intake and risk of type 2 diabetes in women. Diabetes Care. 2009; 32: 629–634.
Suzuki, H., et al. (2011). Zinc as an appetite stimulator — the possible role of zinc in the progression of diseases such as cachexia and sarcopenia. Recent Pat Food Nutr Agric, 3(3), 226–231.
Swardfager, W, et al. (2013). Potential roles of zinc in the pathophysiology and treatment of major depressive disorder. Neuroscience & Biobehavioral Reviews, 37(5), 911–929.
Szewczyk, B. (2013). Zinc homeostasis and neurodegenerative disorders. Front Aging Neurosci, 5, 33.
Szewczyk, B., et al. (2008). Antidepressant activity of zinc and magnesium in view of the current hypotheses of antidepressant action. Pharmacol Rep, 60(5), 588–589.
Szewczyk, B., et al. (2011). The role of zinc in neurodegenerative inflammatory pathways in depression. Prog Neuropsychopharmacol Biol Psychiatry, 35(3), 693–701.
Tan JS et al. Dietary antioxidants and the long-term incidence of age-related macular degeneration: the Blue Mountains Eye Study. Ophthalmology 115.2 (2008): 334–41.
Tanaka M. Secretory function of the salivary gland in patients with taste disorders or xerostomia: correlation with zinc deficiency. Acta Otolaryngol Suppl 546 (2002): 134–41.
Tang AM, et al. Effects of micronutrient intake on survival in human immunodeficiency virus type 1 infection. Am J Epidemiol 143.12 (1996): 1244–56.
Thatcher B et al. Gustin from human partod saliva is carbonic anhydrase VI. Biochem Biophys Res Commun 250 (1998): 635–41.
Tobia MH et al. The role of dietary zinc in modifying the onset and severity of spontaneous diabetes in the BB Wistar rat. Mol Genet Metab 63.3 (1998): 205–13.
Tran, C. D., et al. (2011). Zinc homeostasis and gut function in children with celiac disease. Am J Clin Nutr, 94(4), 1026–1032.
Uçkardeş Y et al. Effects of zinc supplementation on parent and teacher behaviour rating scores in low socioeconomic level Turkish primary school children. Acta Paediatr 2009; 98: 731–736.
van Leeuwen R et al. Dietary intake of antioxidants and risk of age-related macular degeneration. JAMA 294 (2005): 3101–7.
Verma KC, et al. Oral zinc sulphate therapy in acne vulgaris: a double-blind trial. Acta Derm Venereol 60.4 (1980): 337–40.
Wahlqvist M et al. Food and nutrition. 2nd edn. Sydney: Allen & Unwin, 2002.
Wardlaw GM et al. Contemporary nutrition: issues and insights. 3rd edn. Boston: McGraw-Hill, 1997.
Watari, I., et al. (2013). Effectiveness of polaprezinc for low-dose aspirin-induced small-bowel mucosal injuries as evaluated by capsule endoscopy: a pilot randomized controlled study. *BMC Gastroenterol*, 13, 108.
Weimar VM et al. Zinc sulfate in acne vulgaris. Arch Dermatol 114.12 (1978): 1776–8.
Weismann K, et al. Oral zinc sulphate therapy for acne vulgaris. Acta Derm Venereol 57.4 (1977): 357–60.
Wellinghausen N et al. Zinc serum level in human immunodeficiency virus-infected patients in relation to immunological status. Biol Trace Elem Res 73.2 (2000): 139–49.
Wilkinson EA, Hawke CI. Oral zinc for arterial and venous leg ulcers. Cochrane Database Syst Rev 2 (2000): CD001273.
Wills NK et al. Cadmium accumulation in the human retina: effects of age, gender, and cellular toxicity. Exp Eye Res 86.1 (2008a): 41–51.
Wills NK et al. Copper and zinc distribution in the human retina: relationship to cadmium accumulation, age, and gender. Exp Eye Res 87.2 (2008b): 80–8.
Wojcik J et al. Antepartum/postpartum depressive symptoms and serum zinc and magnesium levels. Pharmacol Rep 58 (2006): 571–6.

Wood RJ. Assessment of marginal zinc status in humans. J Nutr 130 (2000): 1350–4S.

World Health Organization. Zinc: report of a joint FAO/WHO expert consultation, Bangkok, Thailand: WHO, 2002.

Wright A et al. Experimental zinc depletion and altered taste perception for NaCl in young adult males. Am J Clin Nutr 34.5 (1981): 848–52.

Yakoob, M. Y., et al. (2011). Preventive zinc supplementation in developing countries: impact on mortality and morbidity due to diarrhea, pneumonia and malaria. BMC Public Health, 11 Suppl 3, S23.

Yetiser S, et al. The role of zinc in management of tinnitus. Auris Nasus Larynx 2002; 29(4):329–333.

Yorbik O et al. Potential effects of zinc on information processing in boys with attention deficit hyperactivity disorder. Prog Neuropsychopharmacol Biol Psychiatry 32.3 (2008): 662–7.

Yuyan L et al. Are serum zinc and copper levels related to semen quality? Fertil Steril 89.4 (2008): 1008–11.

Zazzo JF et al Effect of zinc on the immune status of zinc-depleted AIDS related complex patients. Clin Nutr 8.5 (1989): 259–61.

Zepf, F. D., et al. (2012a). Differences in zinc status and the leptin axis in anorexic and recovered adolescents and young adults: a pilot study. Food Nutr Res, 56. doi: 10.3402/fnr.v56i0.10941

Zepf, F. D., et al. (2012b). Differences in serum zn levels in acutely ill and recovered adolescents and young adults with anorexia nervosa — a pilot study. Eur Eat Disord Rev, 20(3), 203–210.

Zhi J, et al. The effect of short-term (21-day) orlistat treatment on the physiologic balance of six selected macrominerals and microminerals in obese adolescents. J Am Coll Nutr 22.5 (2003): 357–62.

Zverev YP. Effects of caloric deprivation and satiety on sensitivity of the gustatory system. BMC Neurosci 5 (2004): 5

INDEX

Page numbers followed by 'f' indicate figures, 't' indicate tables, and 'b' indicate boxes.

D

I